DATE DUE

FEB 1 6 2005	
FEB 2 3 2005	
MAR 0 2 2005	
MAR 2 3 2006	

BRODART, CO.   Cat. No. 23-221-003

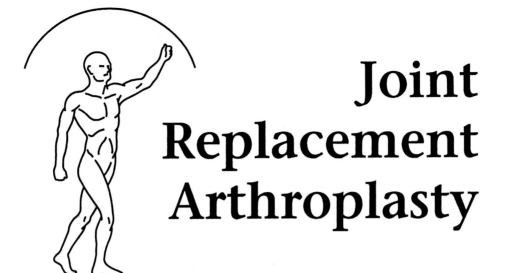

Joint
Replacement
Arthroplasty

Section Editors

Kai-Nan An, Ph.D.
Professor of Bioengineering and John Posy Krehbiel Professor
of Orthopedics, Mayo Medical School; Chair, Division of
Orthopedic Research; Consultant, Department of Orthopedic
Surgery, Mayo Clinic and Mayo Foundation, Rochester,
Minnesota
Section I: General Information

Robert H. Cofield, M.D.
Professor of Orthopedic Surgery, Mayo Medical School; Chair,
Department of Orthopedic Surgery; Consultant, Department
of Orthopedic Surgery, Mayo Clinic and Mayo Foundation,
Rochester, Minnesota
Section IV: The Shoulder

David G. Lewallen, M.D.
Professor of Orthopedic Surgery, Mayo Medical School;
Consultant, Department of Orthopedic Surgery; Chair,
Division of Adult Reconstruction Surgery, Mayo Clinic and
Mayo Foundation, Rochester, Minnesota
Section V: The Hip

William P. Cooney III, M.D.
Professor of Orthopedic Surgery, Mayo Medical School;
Vice Chairman and Consultant, Department of Orthopedic
Surgery, Mayo Clinic and Mayo Foundation, Rochester,
Minnesota
Section II: The Hand and Wrist

Harold B. Kitaoka, M.D.
Professor of Orthopedic Surgery, Section Head, Foot and
Ankle Surgery, Mayo Medical School: Consultant,
Department of Orthopedic Surgery, Mayo Clinic and Mayo
Foundation, Rochester, Minnesota
Section VII: The Foot and Ankle

Mark W. Pagnano, M.D.
Associate Professor of Orthopedic Surgery, Mayo Medical
School; Consultant, Department of Orthopedic Surgery, Mayo
Clinic and Mayo Foundation, Rochester, Minnesota
Section VI: The Knee

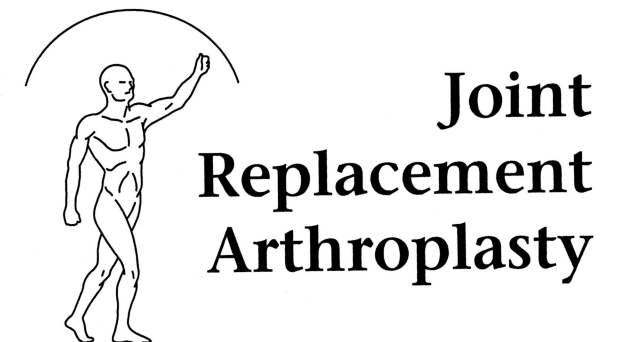

Joint
Replacement
Arthroplasty

Third Edition

Bernard F. Morrey, M.D.

Professor of Orthopedics
Mayo Medical School
Emeritus Chairman
Department of Orthopedics
Mayo Clinic and Mayo Foundation
Rochester, Minnesota

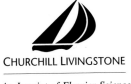

CHURCHILL LIVINGSTONE

An Imprint of Elsevier Science

CHURCHILL-LIVINGSTONE
An Imprint of Elsevier Science

The Curtis Center
Independence Square West
Philadelphia, PA 19106

Notice

Orthopaedics is an ever-changing field. Standard safety precautions must be followed, but as new
research and clinical experience broaden our knowledge, changes in treatment and drug therapy
become necessary or appropriate. Readers are advised to check the product information currently
provided by the manufacturer of each drug to be administered to verify the recommended dose,
the method and duration of administration, and contraindications. It is the responsibility of the
treating physician relying on experience and knowledge of the patient to determine dosages and
the best treatment for the patient. Neither the Publisher nor the editors assume any responsibility
for any injury and/or damage to persons or property.

The Publisher

First Edition 1991 © Mayo Foundation. Second Edition 1996 © Mayo Foundation

Library of Congress Cataloging-in-Publication Data

Joint replacement arthroplasty / [edited by] Bernard F. Morrey; section editors, Kai-Nan
An—[et al.]—3rd ed.
       p.; cm.
    Rev. ed. of: Reconstructive surgery of the joints. 1996.
    ISBN 0–443–06617–5
      1. Artificial joints. 2. Arthroplasty. I. Morrey, Bernard F., II. An, Kai-Nan. III. Reconstructive
surgery of the joints.
    [DNLM: 1. Arthroplasty, Replacement—methods. 2. Joint Prosthesis. WE 312 J7355 2003]
RD686 .J65 2003
617.4′720592—dc21   2002035195

Printed in the United States of America

Last digit is the print number   9   8   7   6   5   4   3   2   1

Dedication

The first edition of this book was appropriately dedicated to John Charnley and the second equally appropriately dedicated to the memory of Mark B. Coventry. As I considered who has had the greatest influence on my career and possibly that of the orthopedic community it became an easy choice to dedicate this third edition to my orthopedic partners at the Mayo Clinic. The insight, support, encouragement, and contributions which they provide, not only in the past, but on an ongoing basis, has been truly inspiring and has been the source of encouragement and confidence. This textbook series has evolved from one being principally focused on the Mayo Clinic approach and joint replacement arthroplasty to one of a more broad based literature but continuing with a strong emphasis of "how we do it at Mayo". In this context there can be no more appropriate dedication than that of my partners recognizing their unwavering dedication to patient care, to their passionate desire to document our experience and share it with the orthopedic community and their seemingly unending support of me and of this Department. Hence, I feel particularly fortunate to be able to consider this group not only my esteemed colleagues but also my treasured friends.

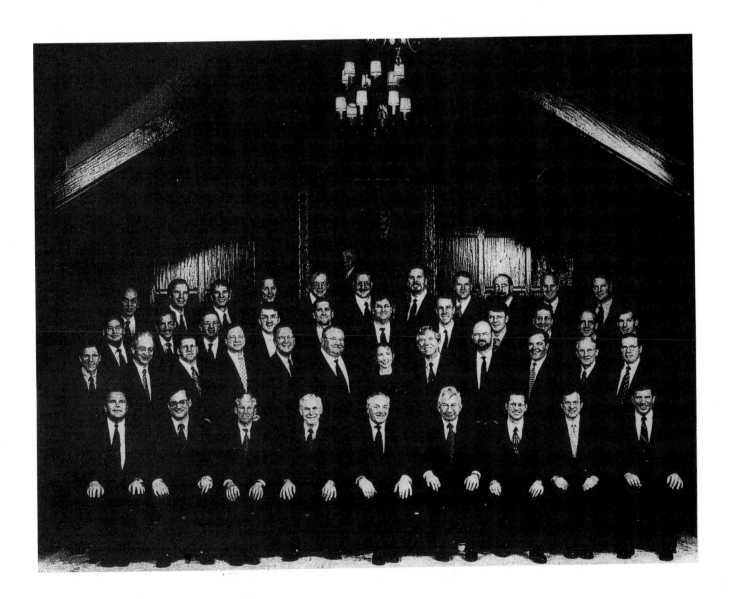

Contributors

R. A. Adams, M.A., R.P.A.
Assistant Professor and Program Director, Mayo School of Health Sciences; Associate, Department of Orthopedic Surgery, Mayo Clinic and Mayo Foundation, Rochester Minnesota
Results of Semiconstrained Replacement for Rheumatoid Arthritis

Abdul M. Ahmed, Ph.D.
Thomas Workman Professor of Mechanical Engineering, McGill University, Department of Mechanical Engineering, Montreal, Quebec, Canada
Polymethylmethacrylate

Alison Albrecht, M.D.
Assistant Professor of Anesthesiology, University of Illinois; Attending Anesthesiologist, Michael Reese Hospital, Chicago, Illinois
Anesthetic Considerations

Peter C. Amadio, M.D.
Professor of Orthopedic Surgery, Mayo Medical School; Consultant, Department of Health Science Research, Mayo Clinic; Consultant, Department of Orthopedic Surgery, Mayo Clinic and Mayo Foundation, Rochester, Minnesota
Outcome Studies, Measurement Tools, and Impairment Evaluation After Joint Replacement; Arthroplasty of the Proximal Interphalangeal Joint

Kai-Nan An, Ph.D.
Professor of Bioengineering and John Posy Krehbiel Professor of Orthopedics; Mayo Medical School; Chair, Division of Orthopedic Research; Consultant, Department of Orthopedic Surgery, Mayo Clinic and Mayo Foundation, Rochester, Minnesota
General Information; Practical Biomechanics; Relevant Biomechanics; Relevant Biomechanics

George C. Babis, M.D.
Assistant Professor of Orthopaedics; Ist Department of Orthopaedic Surgery, University of Athens, School of Medicine; "KAT" Hospital, Athens, Greece
The Young Patient: Indications and Results

Robert D. Beckenbaugh, M.D.
Professor of Orthopedic Surgery, Mayo Medical School; Consultant, Department of Orthopedic Surgery and Surgery of the Hand, Mayo Clinic and Mayo Foundation, Rochester, Minnesota
Arthroplasty of the Metacarpophalangeal Joint; Arthroplasty of the Wrist

Richard A. Berger, M.D., Ph.D.
Associate Professor of Orthopedic Surgery and Anatomy, Mayo Medical School; Consultant, Department of Orthopedic Surgery and Anatomy, Mayo Clinic and Mayo Foundation, Rochester, Minnesota
The Distal Radioulnar Joint

Daniel J. Berry, M.D.
Professor of Orthopedic Surgery, Mayo Medical School; Vice Chairman, Division of Adult Reconstruction; Consultant, Department of Orthopedic Surgery, Mayo Clinic and Mayo Foundation, Rochester, Minnesota
Cemented Femoral Components; Uncemented Femoral Components; The Young Patient: Indications and Results; Avascular Necrosis; Evaluation of the Painful Total Hip Arthroplasty; Acetabular Revision: Techniques and Results; Ectopic Bone; Periprosthetic Fractures Associated with Hip Arthroplasty

Allen T. Bishop, M.D.
Professor of Orthopedic Surgery, Mayo Medical School; Chair, Division of Hand Surgery, Department of Orthopedic Surgery; Section Head, Microsurgery, Division of Hand Surgery and Microvascular Surgery, Department of Orthopedic Surgery; Consultant, Department of Orthopedic Surgery, Division of Hand Surgery and Microvascular Surgery, Mayo Clinic and Mayo Foundation, Rochester, Minnesota
Anatomy and Surgical Approaches

Mark E. Bolander, M.D.
Professor of Orthopedic Surgery, Biochemistry, and Molecular Biology, Mayo Medical School; Consultant, Department of Orthopedic Surgery, Mayo Clinic and Mayo Foundation, Rochester, Minnesota
Individual Host Response to Foreign Materials

Miguel E. Cabanela, M.D.
Professor of Orthopedic Surgery, Mayo Medical School; Consultant, Department of Orthopedic Surgery, Mayo Clinic and Mayo Foundation, Rochester, Minnesota
Uncemented Femoral Components; Proximal Femoral Deformity; Femoral Revision Without Structural Augmentation

Donald C. Campbell II, M.D.
Assistant Professor, Retired, Mayo Graduate School of Medicine, Mayo Clinic and Mayo Foundation, Rochester, Minnesota
Prosthetic Intervention of the Great Toe

Richard J. Claridge, B.Sc., M.D.
Assistant Professor, Mayo Medical School; Consultant, Division of Foot and Ankle Surgery, Department of Orthopedic Surgery, Mayo Clinic and Mayo Foundation, Scottsdale, Arizona
Ankle Replacement Arthroplasty

Robert H. Cofield, M.D.
Professor of Orthopedic Surgery, Mayo Medical School; Chair, Department of Orthopedic Surgery; Consultant, Department of Orthopedic Surgery, Mayo Clinic and Mayo Foundation, Rochester, Minnesota
The Shoulder; Shoulder Arthroplasty: Anatomy and Surgical Approaches; Shoulder Arthroplasty for Arthritis; Shoulder Component Design and Fixation; Results of Shoulder Arthroplasty; Revision Shoulder Arthroplasty

William P. Cooney III, M.D.
Professor of Orthopedic Surgery, Mayo Medical School; Vice Chairman and Consultant, Department of Orthopedic Surgery, Mayo Clinic and Mayo Foundation, Rochester, Minnesota
The Hand and Wrist; Practical Biomechanics; Arthroplasty of the Metacarpophalangeal Joint; Arthroplasty of the Thumb Axis; The Distal Radioulnar Joint

Mark B. Coventry, M.D.*
Emeritus Professor of Orthopedic Surgery, Mayo Medical School; Emeritus Consultant, Department of Orthopedic Surgery, Mayo Clinic and Mayo Foundation, Rochester, Minnesota
The History of Joint Replacement Arthroplasty; Historical Perspective of Hip Arthroplasty

Diane L. Dahm, M.D.
Assistant Professor of Orthopedic Surgery, Mayo Medical School; Consultant, Department of Orthopedic Surgery, Mayo Clinic and Mayo Foundation, Rochester, Minnesota
Rehabilitation and Activities After Shoulder Arthroplasty

Gavan P. Duffy, M.D.
Assistant Professor of Orthopedic Surgery, Mayo Medical School; Consultant, Department of Orthopedic Surgery, Mayo Clinic and Mayo Foundation, Jacksonville, Florida
Cemented Femoral Components

Martin G. Ellman, D.P.M.
Instructor of Podiatric Medicine, Mayo Medical School; Consultant in Podiatric Medicine, Department of Orthopedic Surgery, Mayo Clinic and Mayo Foundation, Rochester, Minnesota
Anatomy and Surgical Approaches

Mark H. Ereth, M.D.
Associate Professor, Mayo Medical School; Consultant, Department of Anesthesiology, Mayo Clinic and Mayo Foundation, Rochester, Minnesota
Perioperative Mortality Associated with Hip and Knee Arthroplasty

Deborah A. Frassica, M.D.
Assistant Professor of Radiation Oncology; Residency Program Director, Department of Radiation Oncology; The Sidney Kimmel Comprehensive Cancer Center, Johns Hopkins University, Baltimore, Maryland
Ectopic Bone

Frank J. Frassica, M.D.
Robert A. Robinson Professor of Orthopaedic Surgery; Chair, Department of Orthopaedic Surgery; Professor of Oncology, The Sidney Kimmel Comprehensive Cancer Center, Johns Hopkins University, Baltimore, Maryland
Avascular Necrosis; Parkinson's Disease; Ectopic Bone

George J. Haidukewych, M.D.
Assistant Professor of Orthopedic Surgery, Mayo Medical School; Director, Orthopedic Trauma Service; Consultant, Department of Orthopedic Surgery, Mayo Clinic and Mayo Foundation, Rochester, Minnesota
Prosthetic Replacement for Intertrochanteric Fracture and Intertrochanteric Nonunion

Arlen D. Hanssen, M.D.
Professor of Orthopedic Surgery, Mayo Medical School; Consultant, Department of Orthopedic Surgery, Mayo Clinic and Mayo Foundation, Rochester, Minnesota
Prevention of Prosthetic Joint Infection; Anatomy and Surgical Approaches; Arthroplasty for Developmental Hip Dysplasia; Diagnosis and Treatment of the Infected Hip Arthroplasty; Posterior Cruciate-Substituting and-Sacrificing Total Knee Arthroplasty; Extensor Mechanism Problems Following Total Knee Arthroplasty; Management of the Infected Total Knee Arthroplasty

Steven J. Hattrup, M.D.
Assistant Professor of Orthopedic Surgery, Mayo Medical School; Consultant, Department of Orthopedic Surgery, Mayo Clinic Scottsdale, Scottsdale, Arizona
Shoulder Arthroplasty for Arthritis; Shoulder Arthroplasty for Osteonecrosis; Rotator Cuff Deficiency; Complications in Shoulder Arthroplasty

Guido Heers, M.D.
Department of Orthopedic Surgery, University of Regensburg, Germany
Arthroplasty for Acute Fractures of the Proximal Humerus

John A. Heit, M.D.
Professor of Medicine, Mayo Medical School; Director, Special Coagulation Laboratories; Consultant, Division of Cardiovascular Diseases; Consultant, Division of Hematology, Mayo Clinic and Mayo Foundation, Rochester, Minnesota
Venous Thromboembolism and Total Hip or Knee Replacement Surgery

---

*Deceased

Duane M. Ilstrup, M.S.
Associate Professor of Biostatistics, Mayo Medical School, Division of Biostatistics, Mayo Clinic and Mayo Foundation, Rochester, Minnesota
Statistical Considerations

Thomas R. Jenkyn, Ph.D.
Co-Director, Wolfe Orthopaedic Biomechanics Laboratory, Fowler-Kennedy Sport Medicine Clinic; Assistant Professor, School of Kinesiology, The University of Western Ontario, London, Ontario, Canada
Biomechanics

Kenton R. Kaufman, Ph.D., P. E.
Associate Professor of Bioengineering; Director, Motion Analysis Laboratory; Consultant, Department of Orthopedic Surgery, Mayo Clinic and Mayo Foundation, Rochester, Minnesota
Biomechanics of the Knee; Biomechanics and Design of Artificial Knee Joints

Todd A. Kile, M.D.
Assistant Professor of Orthopedic Surgery, Mayo Medical School; Chair, Division of Foot and Ankle Surgery, Department of Orthopedic Surgery, Mayo Clinic Scottsdale, Scottsdale, Arizona
Anatomy and Surgical Approaches

Harold B. Kitaoka, M.D.
Professor of Orthopedic Surgery, Section Head, Foot and Ankle Surgery, Mayo Medical School; Consultant, Department of Orthopedic Surgery, Mayo Clinic and Mayo Foundation, Rochester, Minnesota
The Foot and Ankle; Biomechanics; Ankle Replacement Arthroplasty; Complications of Replacement Arthroplasty of the Ankle

Jack E. Lemons, Ph.D.
Professor, Departments of Prostodontics and Materials, Division of Orthopedic Surgery, Depatment of Bioengineering, University of Alabama Schools of Dentistry and Medicine, Birmingham, Alabama
Metallic Alloys

Robert L. Lennon, D.O.
Supplimental Consultant, Mayo Foundation, Rochester, Minnesota
Anesthetic Considerations

David G. Lewallen, M.D.
Professor of Orthopedic Surgery, Mayo Medical School; Consultant, Department of Orthopedic Surgery; Chair, Division of Adult Reconstruction Surgery; Mayo Clinic and Mayo Foundation, Rochester, Minnesota
Perioperative Mortality Associated with Hip and Knee Arthroplasty; The Hip; Total Hip Arthroplasty After Acetabular Fracture; Acetabular Revision: Techniques and Results; Periprosthetic Fractures Associated with Hip Arthroplasty; Vascular Injuries Associated with Hip Arthroplasty

Stephen Li, Ph.D.
President, Medical Device Testing and Innovations, LLC, Sarasota, Florida
The History of Improved Ultra-High-Molecular-Weight Polyethylene: Past, Present, and Future

Ronald L. Linscheid, M.D.
Emeritus Professor of Orthopedic Surgery, Mayo Medical School; Emeritus Consultant, Department of Orthopedic Surgery; Consultant, Biomechanics Laboratory, Mayo Clinic and Mayo Foundation, Rochester, Minnesota
Arthroplasty of the Proximal Interphalangeal Joint; Arthroplasty of the Metacarpophalangeal Joint; Resurfacing Elbow Replacement Arthroplasty

Francisco Lopez-Gonzalez, M.D.
Assistant Professor of Orthopedic Surgery, University of Puerto Rico School of Medicine; Consultant, Department of Orthopedic Surgery, University District Hospital, San Juan, Puerto Rico
Arthroplasty for Acute Fractures of the Proximal Humerus

Zong-Ping Luo, Ph.D.
Associate Professor, Department of Orthopedic Surgery, Baylor College of Medicine, Houston, Texas
Biomechanics

Suzanne A. Maher, Ph.D.
Assistant Professor of Applied Biomechanics in Orthopaedic Surgery, Weill Cornell Medical College, Department of Surgery, Orthopedic Division; Assistant Scientist, Laboratory of Biomedical Mechanics and Materials, Hospital for Special Surgery, New York, New York
The Articulation

James T. McCarthy, M.D.
Professor of Medicine, Mayo Medical School; Division of Nephrology and Internal Medicine, Mayo Clinic and Mayo Foundation, Rochester, Minnesota
Care and Evaluation of the Patient with Renal Disease

S. Breanndan Moore, M.D.
Professor of Laboratory Medicine, Mayo Medical School; Chair, Division of Transfusion Medicine; Director, Histocompatibility Laboratory, Mayo Clinic and Mayo Foundation, Rochester, Minnesota
Blood and Blood Products

Bernard F. Morrey, M.D.
Professor of Orthopedics, Mayo Medical School; Emeritus Chairman, Department of Orthopedics, Mayo Clinic and Mayo Foundation, Rochester, Minnesota
Polymethylmethacrylate; Individual Host Response to Foreign Materials; The Elbow; Anatomy and Surgical Approaches; Relevant Biomechanics; Radial Head Prosthetic Replacement; Resurfacing Elbow Replacement Arthroplasty; Semiconstrained Total Elbow Replacement: Indications and Surgical Technique; Results of Semiconstrained Replacement for Rheumatoid Arthritis; Semiconstrained Elbow Replacement: Results in Traumatic Conditions; The Treatment of the Infected Total Elbow

Arthroplasty; Revision/Salvage Total Elbow Arthroplasty; Relevant Biomechanics; Historical Perspective of Hip Arthroplasty; Biomechanics; Cemented Acetabular Components; Uncemented Femoral Components; Conservative Replacement Designs: Metaphyseal Fixed Implants; The Young Patient: Indications and Results; Avascular Necrosis; Dislocation; Nerve Palsy After Total Hip Arthroplasty; Leg Length Inequality; Mobile-Bearing Knee; Managing Deformity: Total Knee Arthroplasty Techniques

Peter M. Murray, M.D.
Associate Professor of Orthopedic Surgery, Mayo Medical School; Senior Associate Consultant, Department of Orthopedic Surgery, Mayo Clinic and Mayo Foundation, Rochester, Minnesota
Arthroplasty of the Proximal Interphalangeal Joint

Thomas P. Nobrega, M.D.
Clinical Instructor, Mayo Medical School; Consultant, Department of Cardiovascular Disease, Mayo Clinic and Mayo Foundation, Rochester, Minnesota; Staff, Immanuel St. Joseph's Hospital, Department of Cardiology, Mankato, Minnesota
The Cardiac Patient

Shawn W. O'Driscoll, M.D., Ph.D.
Professor of Orthopedic Surgery, Mayo Medical School; Consultant, Department of Orthopedic Surgery, Mayo Clinic and Mayo Foundation, Rochester, Minnesota
Complications of Total Elbow Arthroplasty; Arthroscopy for Shoulder Arthritis and Applications to Shoulder Arthroplasty

Cedric J. Ortiguera, M.D.
Assistant Professor of Orthopedic Surgery, Mayo Medical School; Senior Associate Consultant, Department of Orthopedic Surgery, Mayo Clinic and Mayo Foundation, Jacksonville, Florida
Posterior Cruciate-Substituting and-Sacrificing Total Knee Arthroplasty

Douglas R. Osmon, M.D.
Associate Professor of Medicine, Mayo Medical School; Consultant, Division of Infectious Diseases, Department of Internal Medicine, Mayo Clinic and Mayo Foundation, Rochester, Minnesota
Prevention of Prosthetic Joint Infection; Diagnosis and Treatment of the Infected Hip Arthroplasty; Management of the Infected Total Knee Arthroplasty

Mark W. Pagnano, M.D.
Associate Professor of Orthopedic Surgery, Mayo Medical School; Consultant, Department of Orthopedic Surgery, Mayo Clinic and Mayo Foundation, Rochester, Minnesota
Arthroplasty for Developmental Hip Dysplasia; The Knee; Posterior Cruciate Ligament Retaining Total Knee Arthroplasty; Uncemented Total Knee Arthroplasty; Unicompartmental Knee Arthroplasty; Mobile-Bearing Knee; Revision Total Knee Arthroplasty: Techniques and Results

Panayiotis J. Papagelopoulos, M.D., D.Sc.
Assistant Professor and Consultant, Department of Orthopaedics, Athens University Medical School, Athens, Greece
Cemented Acetabular Components; Proximal Femoral Fracture and Femoral Neck Fracture; Uncemented Total Knee Arthroplasty

Javad Parvizi, M.D., F.R.C.S.
Assistant Professor of Orthopedic Surgery, Thomas Jefferson University Hospital, Rothman Institute, Philadelphia, Pennsylvania
Perioperative Mortality Associated with Hip and Knee Arthroplasty; Resurfacing Hip Arthroplasty; Hip Arthroplasty in Paget's Disease

Douglas J. Pritchard, M.D.
Professor of Orthopedics and Professor of Oncology, Department of Orthopedic Surgery, Mayo Medical School, Division of Orthopedic Oncology, Department of Orthopedic Surgery, Mayo Clinic and Mayo Foundation, Rochester, Minnesota
Neoplasms: Primary Pathologic Conditions

James A. Rand, M.D.
Professor of Orthopedic Surgery, Mayo Medical School; Consultant, Department of Orthopedic Surgery, Mayo Clinic Scottsdale, Scottsdale, Arizona
Posterior Cruciate Ligament Retaining Total Knee Anthroplasty; Uncemented Total Knee Arthroplasty; Unicompartmental Knee Arthroplasty; Revision Total Knee Arthroplasty: Techniques and Results; Management of the Infected Total Knee Arthroplasty

Michael G. Rock, M.D.
Professor of Orthopedic Surgery, Mayo Medical School; Consultant, Department of Orthopedic Surgery, Mayo Clinic and Mayo Foundation, Rochester, Minnesota
Oncogenesis and Foreign Materials; Neoplasms: Metastatic Disease

Jay H. Ryu, M.D.
Professor of Medicine, Mayo Medical School; Consultant, Division of Pulmonary and Critical Care Medicine and Internal Medicine, Mayo Clinic and Mayo Foundation, Rochester, Minnesota
Pulmonary Disease and Surgery

Joaquin Sanchez-Sotelo, M.D., Ph.D., FEBOT
Assistant Professor, University of Madrid; The Shoulder and Elbow Unit, Hospital La Paz, Universidad Autonoma de Madrid, Spain
Shoulder Arthroplasty for Arthritis; Shoulder Arthroplasty for Cuff-tear Arthropathy

Paula J. Santrach, M.D.
Assistant Professor of Laboratory Medicine, Mayo Medical School; Consultant, Division of Transfusion Medicine, Department of Laboratory Medicine and Pathology, Mayo Clinic and Mayo Foundation, Rochester, Minnesota
Blood and Blood Products

Thomas C. Shives, M.D.
Professor of Orthopedic Surgery, Mayo Medical School; Consultant, Department of Orthopedic Surgery, Mayo Clinic and Mayo Foundation, Rochester, Minnesota
Neoplasms: Primary Pathologic Conditions

Clarence Shub, M.D.
Professor, Division of Cardiology, Department of Internal Medicine, Mayo Medical School; Consultant, Division of Cardiology, Department of Internal Medicine, Mayo Clinic and Mayo Foundation, Rochester, Minnesota
The Cardiac Patient

Franklin H. Sim, M.D.
Professor of Orthopedic Surgery, Mayo Medical School; Chief, Division of Orthopedic Oncology; Consultant, Subsection of Orthopedic Oncology and Department of Orthopedic Surgery, Mayo Clinic and Mayo Foundation, Rochester, Minnesota
Proximal Femoral Fracture: Femoral Neck Fracture; Parkinson's Disease; Hip Arthroplasty in Paget's Disease

Jay Smith, M.D.
Associate Professor of Physical Medicine and Rehabilitation, Mayo Medical School; Consultant, Department of Physical Medicine and Rehabilitation, Mayo Clinic and Mayo Foundation, Rochester, Minnesota
Rehabilitation and Activities After Shoulder Arthroplasty

Mark J. Spangehl, M.D.
Assistant Professor of Orthopedic Surgery, Mayo Medical School; Senior Associate Consultant, Department of Orthopedic Surgery, Mayo Clinic and Mayo Foundation Scottsdale, Scottsdale, Arizona
Diagnosis and Treatment of the Infected Hip Arthroplasty; Extensor Mechanism Problems Following Total Knee Arthroplasty

John W. Sperling, M.D., M.S.
Assistant Professor of Orthopedic Surgery, Mayo Medical School; Senior Associate Consultant, Department of Orthopedic Surgery, Mayo Clinic and Mayo Foundation, Rochester, Minnesota
Shoulder Arthroplasty: Anatomy and Surgical Approaches; Results of Shoulder Arthroplasty; Revision Shoulder Arthroplasty

Scott P. Steinmann, M.D.
Assistant Professor of Orthopedic Surgery, Mayo Medical School; Consultant, Department of Orthopedic Surgery, Mayo Clinic and Mayo Foundation, Rochester, Minnesota
Shoulder Arthroplasty for Arthritis; Bone Deficiency in Total Shoulder Arthroplasty

Michael J. Stuart, M.D.
Professor of Orthopedic Surgery, Mayo Medical School Co-Director, Sports Medicine Center; Consultant, Department of Orthopedic Surgery, Mayo Clinic and Mayo Foundation, Rochester, Minnesota
Anatomy and Surgical Approaches; Posterior Cruciate-Substituting and-Sacrificing Total Knee Arthroplasty

Michael E. Torchia, M.D.
Associate Professor of Orthopedic Surgery, Mayo Medical School; Consultant, Department of Orthopedic Surgery, Mayo Clinic and Mayo Foundation, Rochester, Minnesota
Arthroplasty for Acute Fractures of the Proximal Humerus

Robert T. Trousdale, M.D.
Associate Professor of Orthopedic Surgery, Mayo Medical School Consultant, Department of Orthopedic Surgery, Mayo Clinic and Mayo Foundation, Rochester, Minnesota
Uncemented Acetabular Components; Resurfacing Hip Arthroplasty; Leg Length Inequality; Managing Deformity: Total Knee Arthroplasty Techniques

Norman S. Turner III, M.D.
Instructor of Orthopedic Surgery, Mayo Medical School; Associate Consultant, Department of Orthopedic Surgery, Mayo Clinic and Mayo Foundation, Rochester, Minnesota
Prosthetic Intervention of the Great Toe

Peter S. Walker, Ph.D.
Division of Biomedical Engineering, Royal National Orthopaedic Hospital Trust, Stanmore, Middlesex, United Kingdom
Biomechanics and Design of Artificial Knee Joints

Denise J. Wedel, M.D.
Professor, Department of of Anesthesiology, Mayo Medical School; Consultant, Department of Anesthesiology, Mayo Clinic and Mayo Foundation, Rochester, Minnesota
Anesthetic Considerations

Gordon G. Weller, D.P.M.
Instructor of Podiatric Medicine, Mayo Medical School; Consultant in Podiatric Medicine, Department of Orthopedic Surgery, Mayo Clinic and Mayo Foundation, Rochester, Minnesota
Anatomy and Surgical Approaches

James F. Wenz, M.D.
Assistant Professor of Orthopaedic Surgery; Chairman, Department of Orthopedic Surgery, Johns Hopkins Bayview Medical Center; Johns Hopkins University, Baltimore, Maryland
Parkinson's Disease

Timothy M. Wright, Ph.D.
Professor of Applied Biomechanics in Orthopaedic Surgery, Weill Medical College of Cornell University; Senior Scientist, Biomedical Mechanics and Materials, Hospital for Special Surgery, New York, New York
The Articulation

Ken Yamaguchi, M.D.
Associate Professor of Orthopaedics, Chief, Shoulder and Elbow Service, Department of Orthopaedic Surgery, Washington University School of Medicine, St. Louis, Missouri
The Treatment of the Infected Total Elbow Arthroplasty

Bruce R. Zimmerman, M.D.*
Associate Professor of Endocrinology, Mayo Medical School; Consultant, Division of Endocrinology, Department of Internal Medicine, Mayo Clinic and Mayo Foundation, Rochester, Minnesota
The Diabetic Patient

*Deceased

Foreword to the First Edition

The replacement of human joints was a sporadic event prior to the 1960s. At the time the groundwork was first laid with hip replacement, and in the following decade knee replacement procedures were developed. Since then every major (and minor) joint in the body has been intensely studied. Today, we have amassed almost 30 years of clinical experience and substantial research has been undertaken.

The Mayo Clinic has an orthopedic staff comprising all of the subspecialties of orthopedics. It is bolstered by researchers in physiology, biomechanics, statistics, and other significant areas. During this 30-year period, a vast amount of clinical and basic science data has been accumulated and documented. Our intention here is to share these data with the reader.

This book is unique because it is written almost entirely by current and former Mayo Clinic physicians. Although our own efforts are emphasized, the publications of others are included for completeness. In addition, the bibliographical references have been critically reviewed to ensure that they are current, specific, and immediately helpful; they are not, however, all inclusive.

This is a single-volume book. Considerable thought was given to the form of publication. We believed we could condense the important material we wished to present into one single, albeit large, volume. This would facilitate the use of this book as a reference. Virtually every joint is represented, except for the spine, for almost all joints in the body have been subject to some form of replacement.

The format of this book provides relatively short chapters oriented by topic. For example, "Dislocations" is a complete chapter, not one of several topics in a chapter about complications.

Strong emphasis is placed not only on the indications for joint replacement, but on two other major areas as well, namely, surgical techniques and results. We present the surgical techniques that are used primarily at the Mayo Clinic, granting, of course, that not all of us do the operation in exactly the same way. Where there is a choice of viable approaches, these are offered. The talent of one illustrator has been used throughout the book. The result is that the illustrations are of a uniform style. In effect, this book is also an atlas of surgical exposures for joint replacement arthroplasty.

The reporting of results can go on almost ad infinitum. We, however, stress the results obtained by us, and include the most current data possible. Of course, to give the reader the broadest range of information, results of others are included. But again, the stress is on what has been achieved at our institution. We have made a special effort to report our results according to the best methods of analysis, and have even included an entire chapter on how results should be analyzed and portrayed. This, too, is consistent and uniform throughout the book.

The structure of the book has been devised to make it well organized and easy for readers to find their way. Each section has its own outline and provides continuity within the chapters of that section. The same basic format is followed by each author.

Is a book of this nature, covering all types of joint arthroplasty, too vast and comprehensive? We have given much thought to this but truly believe that because of the similarities (acknowledging the very definite differences as well) among all types of joints in the body and our attempts to recreate these in an artificial fashion, putting all these ideas in one volume seems logical. We believe this book will serve the purpose for which it is intended, namely, a complete, contemporary, and ready reference for the orthopedist as he carries on with his attempts to alleviate the pain and suffering of patients with joint disease.

Mark. B. Coventry, M.D.
Emeritus Professor of Orthopedics
Mayo Medical School
Rochester, Minnesota

EDITOR'S NOTE:

Because this is a textbook largely focused on the Mayo Clinic's perception of the literature as well as our perception of indications and outcomes, it seems appropriate to maintain the foreword of our first edition written by the founder of our adult reconstruction section, Mark B. Coventry. As I read over the foreword which Dr. Coventry provided for the first edition I feel as though I can add little to this except to say that in keeping with the legacy which he provided to me and my partners, we have tried to be true to the goals and values that he exhibited in his life. Our hope is that the text is true to its promise as reflected in this foreword.

Preface

As was mentioned in the Preface of the second edition, the field of joint replacement arthroplasty continues to undergo almost meteoric change. In the second edition the focus was one of broadening the topic from joint replacement arthroplasty to joint reconstructive surgery. With the burgeoning interest, research and application focused specifically on joint replacement arthroplasty it seems appropriate to refocus this edition on joint replacement arthroplasty.

The overall approach to this volume, therefore, is a combination of the first and second editions. The intent is to have multiple relatively small chapters that are carefully focused on a specific topic. The goal is to be user friendly. The full spectrum of questions that arise referable to joint replacement as well as revision joint replacement are discussed. This edition also introduces new chapters on distal radio-ulnar joint replacement, uncoupled elbow replacement, resurfacing and other conservative hip procedures and mobile bearing knee replacement.

In this edition still greater emphasis has been placed on surgical technique as well as outcomes. It is hoped that the orthopedic surgeon who has the responsibility for a spectrum of patient pathology may find the answer to most of their questions referable to joint replacement in this text from the standpoint of indications, technique, and outcomes. Yet, controversial issues are also discussed and areas of uncertainty are clearly stated as such.

We feel very fortunate to have an opportunity to offer this text to the orthopedic community. This edition has been modified according to the feedback of friends and colleagues and it is hoped that this will be a useful resource for the orthopedic surgeon in training as well as the practicing orthopedic surgeon.

Acknowledgments

As mentioned in the dedication, I must acknowledge with great humility and gratitude the contributions of an exceptional group of individuals, my partners in the department of the Mayo Clinic. A text such as this is, of course, not possible without the dedication and contribution of a host of individuals. In this instance, this number includes virtually every member of our Orthopedic Department covering the full anatomic expression of joint replacement. So to my partners I wish to express my most sincere appreciation for their hard work in the sharing of their expertise in this volume, particularly Robert A. Rizza, M.D.

I wish to also acknowledge those individuals who have been an integral part of my professional life referring patients, asking questions, and participating in continuing medical education. It is also most appropriate to recognize the paramedical staff at Mayo who have been so supportive, not only in the execution of the surgical procedures but also in their personal inquisitiveness and for providing the data used in this volume. The surgical team at the Mayo Clinic deserves a specific note of recognition, particularly my scrub nurse, Denise Borowski, and our surgical coordinator, Donald Baltes. The ability to find the time for this project is due in great effort to my friend and colleague and the worlds best physician associate of 25 years, Bob Adams.

I should like to pay a special note of appreciation to Donna Riemersma who served as the typist and local project manager, as she interfaced with the publisher, the authors, and the artists. She has accomplished her responsibilities in an exemplary fashion in this edition just as she has in the first two. I would also like to recognize my secretary, Sherry Koperski, for her ongoing administrative support, particularly in the final stages of the project. A special note to Jim Postier, who not only served as the artist for the additional artwork but also helped to coordinate prior work as electronic communications. His dedication and time has been most appreciated.

Finally, as always and most appropriately, I wish to again recognize my wife, Carla, who has been my partner and associate for 36 years and without whose support and patience this textbook could not have come into existence. In the past I have recognized our children, Mike, Matt, Mark, and Maggie. Although they are now all grown and gone their support is no less felt. In this edition I wish to particularly thank Matthew who, as a professional medical illustrator, has served as an advisor and has assisted in some of the illustrations.

Contents

VI The Knee

MARK W. PAGNANO • SECTION EDITOR

VII The Foot and Ankle

HAROLD B. KITAOKA • SECTION EDITOR

I
General Information

KAI-NAN AN • SECTION EDITOR

1

The History of Joint Replacement Arthroplasty

• MARK B. COVENTRY

It is convenient to consider the development of joint reconstruction according to periods or phases. These correspond in general terms to the chronology of the development of joint reconstructive surgery. However, it may be more appropriate to consider this distinction as representing the evaluation of concepts rather than as being based on a strict chronology.

Phase 1 is the anthropologic documentation of joint disease that dates to prehistoric man. Over the millennia, little could be done for the painful joint other than rest and the use of a stick as a walking aid. Presumably, various oral analgesics and local antiphlogistines were used by the ancients. Heat and cold, tattooing, acupuncture, blistering with cantharides, wet and dry cupping, and cautery all continue to be used even today in some parts of the world. Nonsteroidal anti-inflammatories are the drugs now most commonly used.

Phase 2 was an attempt to alleviate pain by surgical means—specifically, joint débridement. Although surgical treatment was done occasionally before the advent of radiography, débridement in effect treated the radiographic image by removing spurs and loose bodies. Once the surgeon had inspected the exposed joint—usually the knee and, less commonly, the elbow and ankle—anything that looked abnormal, such as a torn meniscus and hypertrophic synovium, was also removed. This joint débridement was popularized by Magnuson.[19] It might be termed the "structural" approach to the degenerated joint. It has fallen into disrepute because it did not address the degenerative arthritis itself. Occasionally, joint arthrodesis also was done during this phase, often if and when the débridement procedure failed. During this period, resection of the joint was considered a viable alternative to joint arthrodesis. This was particularly effective at the hip and in circumstances involving septic arthritis.

Phase 3 of treatment is based on both physiologic and biomechanical aspects. Osteotomy about the hip to increase the weight-bearing area and, thus, remove focal overload commenced early with the work of Pauwels[24] and others[2] (Fig. 1–1). This was followed by correction of axial malalignment to treat unicompartmental joint disease of the knee.[9,16] Upper tibial valgus osteotomy changes the axial alignment and in a varus knee lessens the load on the cartilage and bone of the medial compartment.

The next phase in the treatment of joint afflictions, phase 4, is joint arthroplasty. Possibly the first attempt to replace the joint was that of Gluck in 1890. Using ivory, he reported experience with both hip and knee replacement.[13] Initially, this was done with fascia lata, chromicized pig bladder, or split-thickness skin. This was later followed by cup (mold) arthroplasty of the hip as practiced by Smith-Petersen. Then, the endoprosthesis, replacing the diseased head of the femur, was used. It was developed by A. T. Moore, Fred Thompson, and many others. Not until John Charnley and other pioneers developed metallic and plastic substances for joint replacement, however, did the present era of joint arthroplasty begin, and it has flourished since, being used for virtually all joints of the body. Replacement of the hip became a somewhat standard procedure in the 1960s.[5,6] Knee replacement was developed in the 1970s.[11,15] Subsequently, the elbow,[22] the ankle,[26,28] the wrist,[8] the finger joints,[27] the shoulder,[7,23] and the joints of the foot[17] were replaced.

Clinical interest in joint replacement flourished, and it became evident that more basic research into the materials used and forces acting on the joint was essential. Thus, refinement of the science of bioengineering to complement orthopedic surgery occurred simultaneously with the advent of joint replacement. Laboratory testing of forces about joints and of what could be expected of a replacement under certain situations of stress became essential. The materials of joint reconstruction came under intense scrutiny. Efforts were made to properly test each design in the laboratory before its incorporation into the human, a variance from practices during the early development of joint reconstruction. Now, we could be reasonably assured that the prostheses used would be of proper strength to resist fracture. Also, the stresses on and about the prostheses that could produce loosening in the host were evaluated in a laboratory environment by bunch testing or analytic simulation.

3

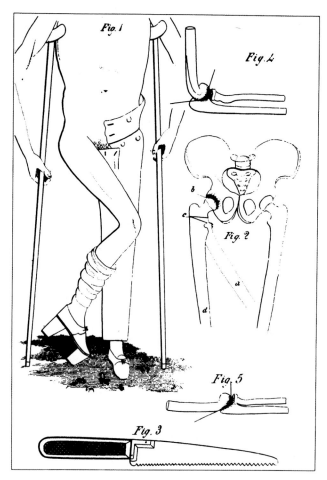

Figure 1–1. Early description of realignment of extremity for fixed deformity by John Barton. (From Barton JR: Osteotomy for ankylosis. N Am Med Surg J 3:274, 1827.)

Improvement in manufacturing technology has kept pace with improvement in our clinical and biomechanical knowledge. Controversy continues regarding the choice of metals (i.e., chrome-cobalt vs. titanium alloys). Specific tissue reactions to titanium alloy occur under certain circumstances.[1] Polyethylene fragments cause tissue reaction and synovial response, in turn producing bony lysis.[14] Ceramics have been intensely studied and utilized in Europe, and are being accepted in the United States as more experience is gained.[4,21]

SURVEILLANCE

The occasional clinical report of a few patients is of little value. Prospective studies of a sufficient number of patients must be carried out, evaluated according to current statistical modalities, and duly reported if our knowledge is to reach the stage where we can put in a specific prosthesis, with assurance that it will last a specified period of time under specific stresses. When the program of total hip replacement was started at the Mayo Clinic in March 1969, an elaborate protocol was established whereby, for a certain time period, all members of the Department of Orthopedics would do total hip arthroplasty by the same approach with the same prosthesis and the same follow-up protocol. A computerized data storage and retrieval system was established as a vital initial step in the development of this emerging clinical practice. In this way, we established a very large base of clinical experience, results could be evaluated, and we could thus determine if we were doing the right thing for our patients.

After this first study, certain variations were allowed with different prostheses and different approaches, all approved by our Joint Replacement Committee. These data have been accumulated, cataloged, and reported according to a follow-up protocol of 1, 5, 10, 15, and, now, 20 years.[3,10,18,25] It is by this critical analysis of indications, technique, and follow-up care that we are able to make a significant contribution, namely, the evaluation of a large number of patients, analyzed in different ways, according to a prospective protocol.

It must be evident that joint replacement is a multidisciplinary project. It is true that joint replacement originated with the orthopedic surgeon. However, it became evident almost immediately that the very close cooperation of experts in other fields was necessary in order to achieve the progress in joint replacement that we hoped for. John Charnley began this association with his studies of friction. The first collaborator was the bioengineer, and this person still is an absolutely essential member of the team. Then, the instrument (prosthesis) designer joined the effort, working closely with the surgeon and the engineer. The physiologic and pathologic effects of metal, polyethylene, and methyl methacrylate debris in joints remain the subjects of careful study. Biologic fixation has become a substitute for use of methyl methacrylate in certain patients and will bear careful scrutiny in the next few years, when its role will become better defined.[12] Finally, the statistician is a valuable part of this "team"; Chapter 24 is devoted to how statistical data should be gathered and evaluated, and these statistical methods are used through this work.

The Mayo Clinic is uniquely able to provide all these disciplines to study joint replacement. As we go to publication, almost 40,000 entries are recorded in the total joint registry. Our department members have designed hip, knee, shoulder, elbow, ankle, and finger joints. The accumulation of experience at the Mayo Clinic and the desire to share this experience are evident in the chapters that follow. The continued interaction of the practicing orthopedist with the basic laboratory scientist will give answers to the increasingly complex status of total joint replacement.

Phase 5 in the development of treatment for the arthritic joint is not surgical at all. It addresses the cartilage cell and its ability to differentiate or regenerate from a precursor cell and thus "heal" the arthritic joint.[20] A vast amount of experimental work continues in this area, including the use of cartilage allografts. In this era, the application of molecular biology to our discipline should allow us to effectively carry out this phase of our development. Is it possible that phase 5, the biologic phase, will witness a solution to the causes of joint arthritis?

Editor's Addendum

I believed that it was particularly appropriate to leave the foregoing statement intact in honor of Doctor Coventry's name and legacy (Fig. 1–2). The contributions of this man include the first total hip arthroplasty approved by the Food and Drug Administration in the United States in March 1969 (Fig. 1–3). The vision Coventry had and shared resulted in the present day Mayo Clinic Arthroplasty Database of more than 60,000 entries, dating from the first implant in 1969. This comprehensive resource includes data on more than 1000 elbow replacements, almost 2000 shoulder replacements, more than 30,000 knee replacements, and approximately 35,000 hip replacements (Table 1–1). It is of particular interest to note that the closing observations made by Coventry a decade ago are no less true today. The future of the management of joint afflictions rests in a biologic solution to the disease and a genomic answer to its development.

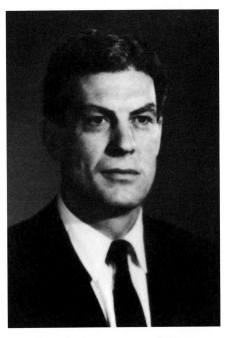

Figure 1–2. Dr. Coventry implanted the first FDA approved THA on March 10, 1969 at the Mayo Clinic, Rochester, Minnesota.

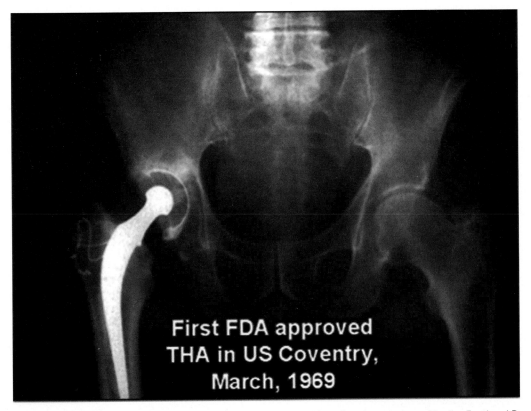

Figure 1–3. The immediate and 15 year follow-up of the first total hip arthroplasty approved by the Food and Drug Administration in the United States.

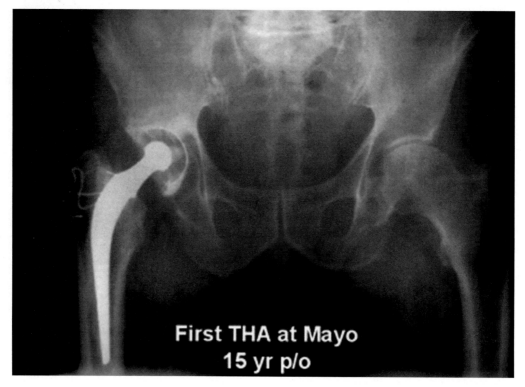

First THA at Mayo
15 yr p/o

Figure 1–3. *Continued.*

Table 1–1. JOINT REPLACEMENT: MAYO DATABASE (1969–2000)

Replacement	Primary	Revision	Total
Total hip arthroplasty	26480	8687	35167
Total knee arthroplasty	19223	3485	22708
Total shoulder arthroplasty	2590	365	2955
Total elbow arthroplasty	978	304	1282
Total	49271	12841	62112

References

1. Agins HJ, Alcock NW, Bansal M, et al: Metallic wear in failed titanium-alloy total hip replacements. J Bone Joint Surg 70A:347, 1988.
2. Barton JR: Osteotomy for ankylosis. N Am Med Surg J 3:274, 1827.
3. Beckenbaugh RD, Ilstrup DM: Total hip arthroplasty: A review of 333 cases with long follow-up. J Bone Joint Surg 60A:306, 1978.
4. Boutin P: L'Alumine et son utilization en chirurgie de la lauce (étude experimentale). Presse Med 79:639, 1971.
5. Charnley J: Anchorage of the femoral head prosthesis to the shaft of the femur. J Bone Joint Surg 42B:28, 1960.
6. Charnley J: Total hip replacement by low-friction arthroplasty. Clin Orthop 72:7, 1970.
7. Cofield RH: Total shoulder arthroplasty with the Neer prosthesis. J Bone Joint Surg 66A:899, 1984.
8. Cooney WP III, Beckenbaugh RD, Linscheid RL: Total wrist arthroplasty. Clin Orthop 187:121, 1984.
9. Coventry MB: Osteotomy of the upper portion of the tibia for degenerative arthritis of the knee. J Bone Joint Surg 47A:984, 1965.
10. Coventry MB, Beckenbaugh RD, Nolan DR, Ilstrup MS: 2,012 total hip arthroplasties: A study of postoperative course and early complications. J Bone Joint Surg 56A:273, 1974.
11. Coventry MB, Finerman GAM, Riley LH, et al: A new geometric knee for total knee arthroplasty. Clin Orthop 83:157, 1972.
12. Galante JO, Rostoker W, Lueck R, Ray RD: Sintered fiber metal composites as a basis for attachment of implants to bone. J Bone Joint Surg 53A:101, 1971.
13. Gluck T: As reported by LeVay M: History of Orthopedics. Park Ridge, NJ, Parthenon Press, 1990.
14. Goldring SR, Schiller AL, Roelke M, et al: The synovial-like membrane at the bone-cement interface in loose total hip replacements and its proposed role in bone lysis. J Bone Joint Surg 65A:575, 1983.
15. Gunston FH: Polycentric knee arthroplasty: Prosthetic simulation of normal knee movement. J Bone Joint Surg 53B:272, 1971.
16. Jackson JP, Waugh W: Tibial osteotomy for osteoarthritis of the knee. J Bone Joint Surg 43B:746, 1961.
17. Joplin RS: The digital nerve, vitallium stem arthroplasty and some thoughts about foot surgery in general. Clin Orthop 76:207, 1971.
18. Kavanagh BF, DeWitz M, Ilstrup D, et al: Charnley total hip arthroplasty with cement: 15 years results. J Bone Joint Surg 71A:1496, 1989.
19. Magnuson PB: Technic of débridement of the knee joint for arthritis. Surg Clin North Am 26:249, 1946.
20. Mankin HJ: The response of articular cartilage to mechanical injury. J Bone Joint Surg 64A:460, 1982.
21. Mittelmeier H, Harms GL: Derzeitiger Stand der zementfreien Verankerung von Kerasmik-Metall-Verbundprosthesen. Z Orthop 117:478, 1979.
22. Morrey BF, Bryan RS: Total joint replacement. In Morrey BF (ed): The Elbow and Its Disorders. Philadelphia, WB Saunders, 1985, p 546.
23. Neer CS II: Articular replacement for the humeral head. J Bone Joint Surg 37A:215, 1955.
24. Pauwels F: Biomechanics of the Locomotor Appparatus: Contributions on the Functional Anatomy of the Locomotor Apparatus. New York, Springer-Verlag, 1980.
25. Stauffer RN: Ten-year follow-up study of total hip replacement. J Bone Joint Surg 64A:983, 1982.
26. Stauffer RN, Segal NM: Total ankle arthroplasty; four years' experience. Clin Orthop 160:217, 1981.
27. Swanson AB: Flexible Implant Resection Arthroplasty in the Hands and Extremities. St. Louis, CV Mosby, 1973.
28. Waugh TR, Evanski PM, McMaster WC: Irvine ankle arthroplasty: Prosthetic design and surgical technique. Clin Orthop 114:180, 1976.

2
Polymethylmethacrylate

•ABDUL M. AHMED and BERNARD F. MORREY

In spite of the fact that bone cement has been used for more than 30 years, improvement of its mechanical properties and performance remains a topic of clinical and basic research. Because of the interdisciplinary nature of the investigations, the results are reported in such diverse publications as those dealing with orthopedic surgery, biomaterials, and bioengineering.

This chapter is intended to collect and summarize the various research findings in an integrated fashion. The first half of the chapter is concerned with investigations that are now substantially complete and their results, which have led to the development of the "contemporary" surgical procedures. The second half of the chapter, dealing chiefly with the problems of reduction of porosity in bone cement, discusses research areas that are still very active. The accumulating results within these areas, although having an impact on current surgical practice, have yet to allow a full resolution of the research objectives.

INITIAL USE OF BONE CEMENT

In the late 1950s, Dr. Dennis Smith, a dental materials scientist, introduced Sir John Charnley to the use of self-curing polymethylmethacrylate (PMMA) to anchor prostheses to bone. PMMA cures quickly without the addition of heat and has a modulus that falls between that of cancellous bone and cortical bone.

The introduction of bone cement, together with the use of ultra-high-molecular-weight polyethylene for the acetabular bearing material, led to the widespread acceptance of total hip replacement as a standard orthopedic procedure.*

COMPOSITION

There are approximately a dozen types of commercial bone cement. These fall into two broad categories: a "dough"-type cement, available since the 1950s, and a "low-viscosity" cement, developed in the early 1980s (to be used in conjunction with a "cement gun"), for better intrusion into cancellous bone. The exact clinical composition of each is proprietary information and is therefore unavailable. However, the general characteristics of bone cements are as follows.

Commercial bone cement is most commonly available in standard packages of 40 mg of polymer powder (PMMA) and 20 ml of liquid monomer (monomethacrylate). The cement powder consists mainly of preformed polymeric beads ranging from 30 to 150 μm in diameter (Fig. 2–1). The powder in some brands of cement may also contain a polystyrene copolymer, as in Simplex P (North Hill Plastics, London, England), or a methylacrylate polymer, as in Palacos R (FA Kulzer, Bad Homburg, West Germany). Two common additives in the powder are a radiopacifier, such as barium sulfate or zirconium dioxide, and a polymerization initiator, such as benzoyl peroxide.

The liquid monomer is prevented from spontaneously polymerizing by the presence of a small amount of stabilizer in the form of hydroquinone or a combination of hydroquinone and ascorbic acid.[57] Also present in the liquid monomer is N,N-dimethyl-p-toluidine (DMPT), which serves as an activator. When the liquid DMPT comes in contact with the benzoyl peroxide initiator in the polymer powder, benzoyl free radicals are generated.[57,66] The benzoyl free radicals then react with the monomer molecules to initiate polymerization. In some cement, when the liquid first comes in contact with the powder, the mixture has a granular texture akin to that of wet sand. This quickly turns into a liquid, and the process is commonly referred to as "wetting out." The dough-type cement remains in a low-viscosity state for only 1 to 2 minutes before becoming "doughy" and hardens at 8 to 14 minutes, depending on the brand of the cement and the environmental conditions. In contrast, the low-viscosity cement maintains a low-viscosity state for as long as 5 minutes and, after going through a brief doughy stage, hardens relatively rapidly in about 6 to 8 minutes.†

---

* The early success of bone cement fixation in hip arthroplasty initiated the development of similar procedures for other joint implants, particularly the knee.

† Some 25 years after the introduction of PMMA as a bone cement, Dr. Dennis Smith himself underwent bilateral total hip replacements with cemented femoral stems.[89]

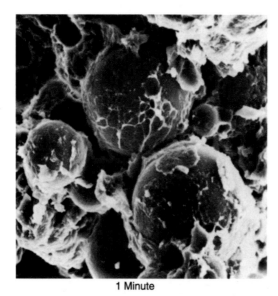
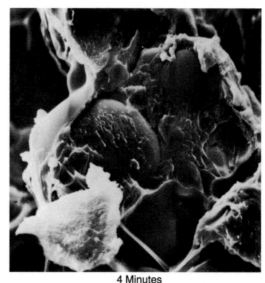

1 Minute   4 Minutes

Figure 2–1. Scanning electron micrograph of freshly mixed cement showing the polymer beads and the liquid monomer in the early stage of polymerization at 1 minute and 4 minutes after mixing (liquid nitrogen was used to terminate the reaction). (Courtesy of Dr. Klaus Draenert.)

Although hardening characteristics vary depending on the brand used, all are affected by environmental conditions in a similar manner. An increase of the ambient temperature causes the cement to harden earlier, roughly one minute per 1°C increase of the ambient temperature. The hardening time decreases by about 1 minute if the storage humidity is increased by about 50 percent. Therefore, it is possible in a warm, humid operating room for the bone cement to harden as much as 5 minutes earlier than anticipated.

The mechanical properties of bone cement are affected by the average value as well as by the distribution of molecular weight.[57,81] Therefore, it is theoretically possible to alter the mechanical properties of acrylic bone cement without changing the existing chemical composition by altering the degree of polymerization and thus the distribution and average molecular weight of the polymer.

LOOSENING

During revision surgery for loosening, it has been observed that either the cement was loose within the cavity or the cement mantle had fractured. The occurrence of loosening was found to be higher among younger, more active, and heavier patients,[11,69,88] suggesting that mechanical factors are important in the initiation and progression of loosening.

Mechanism of Loosening

The issue of loosening is complex. Mechanical failure of any one of several links—cement-bone interface, bulk cement, and cement-prosthesis interface—can precipitate loosening. It is noteworthy that the results of stress analysis show that fixation failure at either interface

leads to an increase in stress in the bulk cement (e.g., on the proximal-medial side in the case of a cemented femoral stem).[16,34,41]

The mechanical behavior of each of these three links has been the subject of intense investigation. In this chapter, results of studies on the two links representing the two interfaces are summarized in this section, and the results of completed and continuing investigations on the remaining link (i.e., bulk cement) are discussed in detail in the subsequent section.

Cement-Bone Interface

The increase in cement temperature because of exothermic polymerization at curing was believed to increase the adjacent bone temperature sufficiently to cause thermal necrosis of bone. However, the results of experimental and analytic studies[48,91] have largely discounted this possibility when the thickness of the cement layer is in the range used in surgery. However, one study has reported that the use of modern cementing techniques, including the method of cement mixing discussed earlier, increases the cement-bone interface temperature above the limit that might cause impaired bone regeneration in total hip replacement surgery.[92]

At this same time, considerable concern was focused on the possible toxicity of bone cement monomer,[75,77] but subsequent studies showed that chemical trauma is not as important as originally thought.[31,76] Bulk methyl methacrylate is essentially an immunologically inert implant material.[86] Histomorphologic and fractographic analyses of intact autopsy specimens confirmed that it is possible to have enduring close apposition of cement with trabecular bone in what appears to be "intimate osseointegration at the bone-cement interface."[68]

Apart from ensuring a clean bone surface, methods of improving cement intrusion into cancellous bone by the pressure injection of cement were also investigated as a mean of reducing loosening; these methods have now become part of the standard procedure in many operating theaters. With adequate penetration of cement into cancellous bone, the strength of the cement-bone interface is governed by the intrinsic strength of the cancellous bone, and it is now accepted that cement penetration into bone from 2 to 5 mm (4 mm optimal[ss]) is a desirable level for a secure interface. Newer formulations of decreased modulus have been shown to decrease PMMA bone cement interface shear and hence probably decrease the rate of loosening.[27]

Cement-Prosthesis Interface

Despite the apparent association of the cement-prosthesis interface failure with cement fracture (Fig. 2–2**A, B**), the importance of this interface was not widely recognized until the early 1980s. Migration of the femoral stem is possible only if there is a failure of the cement-prosthesis interface and a fracture in the cement mantle.[71,90] Also, results of studies using fractographic analysis on retrieved specimens suggest that debonding at the cement-prosthesis interface is the likely initiating mechanism for the loosening of cemented femoral stems in total hip replacements.[45,47,68] Although the prosthesis/cement interface behavior is quite design specific, in general, debonding at this interface greatly increases the risk of early mechanical failure of the cement mantle.[16,41,45,47]

Mechanical strength of the cement-prosthesis interface is known to depend on two mechanisms: mechanical interlock and specific adhesion.[80] Mechanical interlock is influenced by a number of variables, including the texture of the prosthetic surface, cement intrusion characteristics, and air entrapment at the interface.[37] One method of enhancing mechanical interlock is to consider a porous coating for the prosthesis,[95] but the clinical effectiveness of this design strategy is highly variable.

The second mechanism, specific adhesion, is the molecular interaction between the metal and the cement. The contribution of this mechanism to the strength of the interface is very much dependent on the surface characteristics of the metal and the state of the polymerizing cement. Enhancement of this mechanism may involve monomer pretreatment of the implant,[50] application of a bone cement layer on the implant before surgery,[7] and, finally, precoating of the implant with a thin layer of PMMA.[2,80] The latter approach toward improvement of

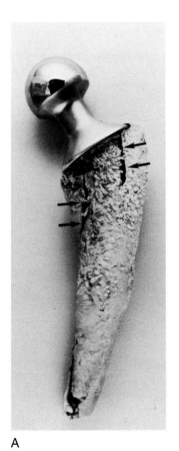
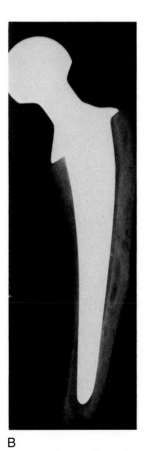
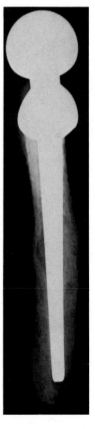

A   B

Figure 2–2. A, Fracture of cement mantle from a retrieved specimen at revision surgery. Longitudinal splits *(arrows)* start from the collar region and propagate distally, as described by Stauffer.[90] **B,** Radiograph of the same specimen. Note that the cracks are not visible either because of the shadow of the metal prosthesis *(anteroposterior view)* or because of the plane of projection relative to the plane of the fracture *(lateral view).* Typical appearance of a radiolucent zone in an area adjacent to the proximal lateral surface of the prosthesis, pathognomonic of cement mantle fracture. Note large amount of voids in cement mantle.

the strength of this interface has been studied in detail and been found to increase the interface fracture toughness and fatigue strength, an increase that remains effective even in a wet environment.[2,80] However, should this interface fail, the debris generation results in an aggressive osteolysis and early failure of the device (Fig. 2–3).[74]

MATERIAL PROPERTIES OF BONE CEMENT

Static Strength

The static strength of bone cement varies among brands and is known to be particularly sensitive to methods used in mixing and forming and to various environmental conditions.[51] Typical values of strength and modulus are shown in Table 2–1. Their percentages relative to that of cortical bone are also indicated. It is noted that the strength of bone cement in tension is only 30 to 50 percent of that in compression.[59,61,94]

Fatigue Strength

Testing of the fatigue strength of bone cement is displayed by plotting applied cyclic stress (S) versus number of cycles (N) to failure (the S-N curve) (Fig.

2–4A). The stress corresponding to failure at one cycle is the static strength of the material. With decreasing applied stress, the number of cycles to failure increases in a nonlinear manner. Acrylic bone cement is thought to be a material that has a stress level below which the material does not fail in fatigue. This stress level is called the *fatigue limit* or *endurance limit.* For many materials, the endurance limit is usually on the order of 20 to 30 percent of that of the static strength. The endurance limit of Simplex P has been estimated from less than 3 to greater than 12 MPa.[17,52] Because the fatigue life of bone cement influences the longevity of cemented fixation, factors affecting the fatigue life of this material should be discussed.

The fatigue life of a material can be prolonged in one of two ways.[48] As shown in Figure 2–4B, a modest decrease in applied stress can dramatically prolong the fatigue life of the material. Hence, good cementing technique and proper prosthesis design are important considerations. The second approach to increasing the fatigue life is to increase the static strength of the cement. As shown in Figure 2–4C, with only a modest increase in strength, the fatigue life is significantly prolonged.

As cautioned by Krause and Mathis[51] in their extensive review of the published literature on the fatigue properties of acrylic bone cements, the conclusions of

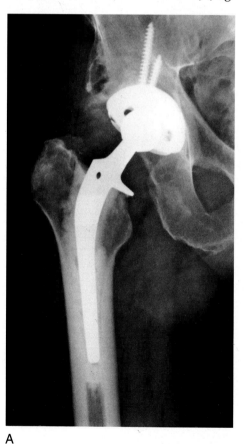
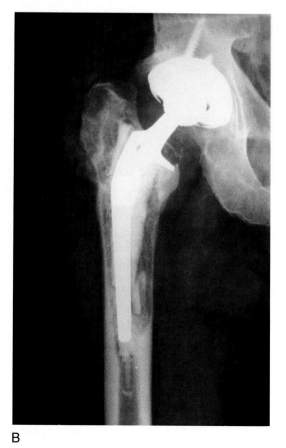

A

B

Figure 2–3. For reasons that are still unclear, the clinical application of precoat technology has not always been successful, and early and extensive osteolysis has occurred in some instances. This hip replacement reveals good cement technique (**A**), but massive osteolysis has occurred in just 3 years (**B**).

Table 2–1. STRENGTH AND MODULUS OF ELASTICITY OF POLYMETHYLMETHACRYLATE COMPARED WITH CORTICAL BONE

	MPa	% Cortical Bone
Tensile strength	32	25
Compressive strength	100	50
Modulus of elasticity	2700	15

the various investigators are valid only for a particular set of material parameters and experimental conditions under which specimens were tested. The internal porosity, batch-to-batch variation, presence of additives, and the fact that the polymerized cement is made of molecules of varying chain lengths all contribute to the scatter of the data.

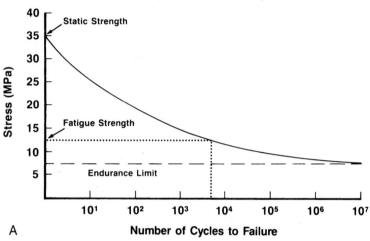

A

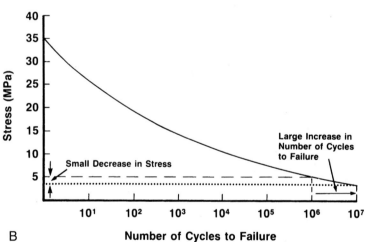

B

Figure 2–4. **A**, Schematic representation of a theoretical S-N curve for bone cement. **B**, Large increase in fatigue life with small decrease in the applied stress. **C**, Large increase in fatigue life with small increase in the strength of the bone cement.

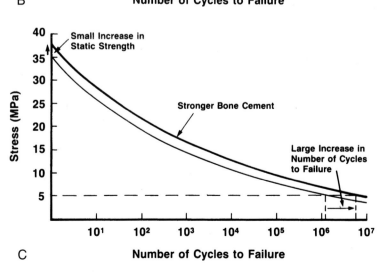

C

Effects of Additives

The inclusion of certain additives, such as radiopacifiers (e.g., barium sulfate) and antibiotics, may be desirable from a clinical point of view. However, such inclusions can potentially degrade the strength of bone cement. Barium sulfate is usually present in the amount of 10 percent of the weight of the bone cement powder. At this level, it appears that the decrease in shear strength of Simplex P is insignificant.[14] Furthermore, even the radiopaque additions have also been implicated as role players in osteolysis.[42]

The addition of up to 2 g of various types of antibiotic powder to a standard package of bone cement has been found to have no effect on the compressive and diametric tensile strength; however, when this amount is exceeded, a corresponding gradual decrease in these strengths has been observed.[55,56] Furthermore, antibiotic-impregnated cement, although having a strength similar to that of regular cement at the time of fabrication, has a dose-related decrease in compressive strength when exposed to a wet environment that becomes discernible at 6 months.[54] One antibiotic that does not cause a deterioration of mechanical strengths when added in large amounts (up to 3 g to a 40 g/20 ml pack of Simplex) is cefuzonam sodium, a third generation cephalosporin.[72] This is attributed to the relatively uniform spherical shape of this antibiotic and the possibility of the monomer's penetrating the antibiotic powder and thereby enhancing adhesion to the cement. When injectable liquid antibiotics that require a large volume of liquid are used, the static strength is significantly compromised.[55] The addition of up to 1 g of vancomycin or tobramycin to a 40 g/20 ml pack of air-mixed bone cement does not significantly alter the bending strength or the modulus. However, the improvement in bending strength for cement mixed under partial vacuum is negated by the addition of 1 g of the same antibiotic.[4] A possible explanation of these data is that porosity is a major determining factor for air-mixed bone cement. Partial vacuum mixing reduces porosity, thereby unmasking the weakening effect of the antibiotics on mechanical strength.

Only a few studies are available regarding the effect of additives on the fatigue life of bone cement. Barium sulfate decreases the fatigue life of Zimmer cement but does not appear to significantly affect Simplex P.[25] The addition of antibiotics has been reported not to affect the fatigue life of hand-mixed cements.[19,70] AKZ (Simplex P with 0.5 g of erythromycin and 0.24 g of colistin methane sulfonate) and Palacos R with 0.5 g of gentamycin are available bone cements that are commercially premixed with antibiotics. The fatigue strengths of these two cements were not significantly decreased by the presence of antibiotics, with or without centrifugation. Mixing of 1.2 g of tobramycin into a 40 g/20 ml pack of Simplex P bone cement also does not seem to affect the fatigue strength.

In summary, it appears that, when a reasonable amount of additive (such as 1 g of antibiotic powder to a 40 g/20 ml pack) is combined with bone cement, there is no significant decrease in mechanical strength. However, the weakening effect of the additives may become apparent when the porosity of the cement is eliminated. As discussed in detail later, porosity has a dominating effect in defining the mechanical strength of bone cement that, consequently, may overwhelm the effect of additives.

Effect of Storage

The data in the literature are unclear as to the effect of time on the static strength of bone cement in a wet environment. It is generally agreed that the modulus of elasticity and static strength increases during the first week[40,60] after curing. Holm called this the "after polymerization" effect and ascribed it to the increase in length of the molecular chains and possibly the polymerization of the residual monomer.[40] Other investigations have suggested that this increase in strength may go on for as long as a year.[54,60,83] Rostoker et al. reported that, although there is some decrease (9 percent) in flexural strength after 12 to 24 months of in vivo storage, the decrease is not statistically significant.[83] Jaffe et al. reported no significant change in static material properties of bone cement stored in bovine serum at 37°C for up to 2 years.[43] To date, there has been no report of a large amount of deterioration of static strength over time.

Regarding the effect of storage on fatigue strength of bone cement, the only available report indicates no significant deterioration of compressive fatigue behavior of Simplex-P and CMW bone cement in bovine serum at 37°C for up to 2 years.[43] However, compressive cyclic loading has little effect on the fatigue life of bone cement, which is defined primarily by the maximum cyclic tensile stress.[28] One study has further demonstrated that the method of mixing the cement is a more important variable influence on fatigue strength than the storage temperature.[62]

Porosity Reduction

Cement porosity is one of the most important variables dictating the mechanical behavior of PMMA. As early as 1975, Bayne et al. emphasized the importance of reducing porosity to improve the mechanical properties of the cement.[8] A subsequent series of investigations showed that reduction of porosity by centrifugation greatly prolongs the fatigue life of bone cement.[9,10,17,21,28,29] Concurrently, mixing under partial vacuum[3,53,63,64] and ultrasonic agitation has also been explored as an alternative method of porosity reduction,[85] but its efficacy has not yet been fully demonstrated.

Porosity is caused by the following:

1. Air entrapment during the mixing and transferring processes
2. Presence of air spaces between polymer beads
3. Void generation as a result of evaporation or boiling of monomer

4. Thermal expansion of existing bubbles
5. Presence of cavitation voids

Of these causes, the most common source of porosity, as well as the most easily controlled, is air entrapment during the mixing and transferring processes.

It is well known that vigorous mixing of cement by hand, under atmospheric conditions, increases the amount of air in the cement.[22,24,26,65] Because of the viscous nature of mixed bone cement, only large bubbles can easily migrate to the surface, leaving in the cement a substantial number of voids with a diameter of less than 1 cm.[46,97]

Greater porosity is noted in the proximal cement mantle.[12] In addition, porosity is preferentially concentrated at the cement-prosthesis interface of the cemented femoral stems of total hip replacements because of the rheologic behavior of bone cement during implant insertion.[44] This interfacial concentration of porosity cannot be reduced by prior centrifugation of the bone cement.

Porosity can be measured either as a percentage volume[8,97] or as a percentage cross-sectional area[46] occupied by voids. Both techniques result in values that range between 5 and 16 percent[8,26,46,97] for hand-mixed cement of regular viscosity.

When a stained section of hardened cement is examined, the voids can be classified into two categories, according to size. Voids that have a diameter of less than 500 μm, the detection of which is beyond the resolution of conventional radiography, can be referred to as *micropores*; voids whose diameters exceed this limit can be termed *macropores*. Regular hand-mixed, dough-type cement is characterized by a small number of macropores and a large number of micropores (Fig. 2–5). However, because of their size, macropores can account for up to half of the measured porosity. Because low-viscosity cements allow larger bubbles to escape, fewer macropores are present in such cements.

Mixing cement according to the manufacturer's instructions in an uncontrolled environment can produce a large variation of porosity in the cement.[24,65] The easiest method for minimizing the amount of air entrapped in the cement is gentle stirring for only the duration of time required to achieve complete mixing. The cement at this stage still has relatively low viscosity; if it is allowed to sit undisturbed, the larger air bubbles can rise to the surface. Simplex P cement prepared in this manner has approximately 5 percent porosity (i.e., at the lower limit of the reported range of porosity for hand-mixed cement). For Palacos R, 20 to 30 seconds of gentle kneading to rupture air bubbles after mixing is reported to reduce porosity.[24]

Porosity reduction can also be achieved by using centrifugation or mixing under partial vacuum. Centrifugation is achieved by pouring the chilled bone cement into sterile syringes immediately after mixing and spinning it at 3000 to 4000 rpm for a total time of 1 minute. For vacuum mixing, the chilled cement is placed in a sterile container and a partial vacuum is drawn. The cement is then mixed with a stirrer under vacuum.

Centrifugation has been found to be very effective in the removal of macropores but not micropores (see Fig. 2–5). The complexity, expense, and inconvenience of the process have lessened the popularity of this method.

Mixing cement under partial vacuum (ranging from 400 to 730 mm Hg below atmospheric pressure) has caused a significant reduction of porosity, from between 5 and 10 percent to 1 percent or less.[3,23,97] This reduction is the result of the elimination of most macropores and micropores (Figs. 2–5 and 2–6) and is effective for all types of cement considered. The partial vacuum level currently recommended is 550 mm Hg below atmospheric pressure.[97] This technique has become common practice since 1985, but the topic continues to be investigated. One study reports that vacuum mixing does not universally enhance mechanical characteristics, and the benefit may be cement specific.[30] Graham et al. further noted the fracture fatigue properties of vacuum mixing were not notable when done with non-ionized sterilized cement.[32]

The following sections discuss the effects of porosity reduction on the mechanical performance of bone cement.

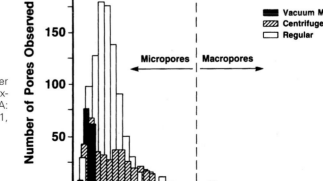

Figure 2–5. Pore-sized distribution of cement prepared under atmospheric condition, centrifugation, and partial vacuum mixing. (Adapted from Wixson RL, Lautenschlager EP, Novak MA: Vacuum mixing of acrylic bone cement. J Arthroplasty 2:141, 1987.)

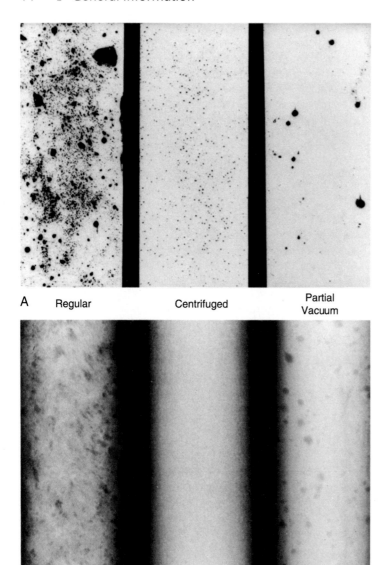

A   Regular   Centrifuged   Partial
                                        Vacuum

B

Figure 2–6. Comparison of stained section **A** and radiograph **B** of bone cement. Cement polymerized in a Miller cartridge was sectioned longitudinally and then stained with black shoe polish to visualize the voids. The same specimen was also radiographed to give an idea of how much porosity is present in the solid mass. Note that the porosity in these samples is exaggerated because of the high temperature resulting from the large mass of the polymerizing cement *(left)*. Micropores and macropores are present in large numbers in hand-mixed cement prepared under atmospheric pressure *(center)*. Centrifugation completely eliminates the macropores. Stained section shows the remaining micropores. These micropores are barely visible, even on the special high resolution radiographs *(right)*. Partial vacuum mixing eliminates many of the micropores as well as the macropores. Residual voids are still present. The residual porosity is most evident on the high-resolution radiographs.

Static Strength

In Table 2–2, the tensile strength of Simplex P, prepared by centrifugation or partial vacuum, is compared with that of the same cement mixed in the conventional manner, as reported by various investigators. The tensile strength is found to improve by 10 to 40 percent along with a reduction in standard deviation. The latter result points out that porosity contributes to the large scatter in the cement property data usually reported in the literature. Measurements under test conditions simulating some aspects of the femoral stem loading situation have confirmed that the static strength of bone cement is increased when porosity is reduced by centrifugation.[12,13]

Fatigue Strength

There is great variation in the fatigue strength of PMMA as documented in a study of 10 commercially available formulations.[36] The fact that porosity plays a major role in defining fatigue life in bone cement was identified in the early 1980s and is also a function of the specific formulation of the commercial product.[10,28,29] Centrifugation has also been used for the reduction of porosity and has confirmed a corresponding increase in fatigue life.[9] In addition, fatigue cracks initiate at internal pores, and there is a strong negative correlation between cross-sectional porosity and the cycles to failure.[44]

In a number of investigations using Simplex P cement, an improvement of two to nearly eight times the mean fatigue life was reported after centrifugation.[9,17,18,21] For partially vacuum-mixed cement, Wixson et al. reported a mean fatigue life seven times greater than that of conventionally mixed cement and generally greater than that of centrifuged cement.[97]

Some had argued that fatigue fracture was likely to be controlled more by the irregularities at the cement-bone interface than by internal pores. Therefore, porosity reduction in general, and centrifugation in particular,

Table 2–2. EFFECT OF POROSITY REDUCTION ON TENSILE STRENGTH (MPA) OF SIMPLEX P

Author (yr)[a]	Conventional	Centrifugation	↑[b]	Partial Vacuum	↑[b] (%)
Davies[17] (1987)	36.2 (10.1)[c]	44.7 (5.2)	23%		
Burke[9] (1984)	32.5 (10.5)	42.0 (5.5)	29%		
Noble[73] (1987)	37.4 (7.0)	43.5 (5.4)	16%	40.7 (7.2)	8
Wixson[97] (1987)	36.0 (5.0)	48.0 (3.0)	33%	52.0 (4.0)	44
Wixson[96] (1985)	44.8 (5.0)	58.5 (2.6)			31
Arroyo[3] (1986)	31.4 (5.1)	41.4 (4.3)			31

[a]The leading author of the referenced article and the year published.
[b]The percentage increase in tensile strength after porosity reduction.
[c]Figures in parentheses are standard deviations.

might not necessarily improve the survival of the cement mantle in the clinical situation. However, subsequent tests on specimens with surface irregularities, in the form of notches and trabecular bone interdigitations, showed that porosity reduction either by centrifugation or by partial vacuum mixing was still effective in prolonging the fatigue life of bone cement.[20,33]

Fracture Toughness

The effect of porosity reduction on fracture toughness is not immediately obvious. The elimination of stress concentration associated with the removal of pores might be negated by the removal of the beneficial effects of pores as crack terminators.

Rimnac et al. found that with compact tension specimens, porosity reduction by centrifugation did not lead to an improvement of fracture toughness.[81] In contrast, Lautenschlager et al., using thinner compact tension specimens (to avoid reintroduction of porosity via heat of polymerization), found that fracture toughness improved by 10 percent for centrifuged cement and by 20 percent for cement mixed under partial vacuum.[58] Nevertheless, the role of porosity reduction in fracture toughness of bone cement remains an active subject of continuing investigation. Additional efforts to enhance fracture toughness by means of a rubber toughening technique have been investigated. Unfortunately, as with other similar efforts, high residual monomer concentration seems to have limited the applicability of this approach.[79]

Shrinkage

The three generally recognized mechanisms in volume changes during the polymerization of bone cement are as follows[1,22,39]:

1. Polymerization shrinkage
2. Thermal expansion of entrapped gaseous bubbles
3. Thermal contraction of the hardened cement

Polymerization shrinkage occurs when the monomer molecules polymerize to form chains of PMMA. The resulting PMMA (density = 1.18 g/cm³), with a more compact molecular structure, occupies a smaller volume than methyl methacrylate monomer (density =

0.94 g/cm³).[22] During the polymerization process, an approximately 21 percent shrinkage in volume is accounted for by the monomer. In the standard bone cement mixture, the amount of monomer is approximately a third of the total weight; therefore, the theoretical maximal volume shrinkage resulting from polymerization alone is about 7 percent.

At the same time, during the temperature rise, the thermal expansion of the entrapped gaseous bubbles (and possibly some vaporization of the monomer when the temperature is sufficiently high) causes bulk volume expansion of the cement mass. The exothermic reaction during polymerization can result in a peak temperature of 60°C for a 3-mm-thick cement mass and of 107°C for a 10-mm-thick cement mass.[70] Therefore, experimental setups using a bulky mass of cement to measure volume changes would overestimate the contribution of thermal expansion of entrapped gaseous bubbles to volume changes.

After the cement has hardened and as it is cooling, the solid cement contracts. This component of the volume change is small, amounting to 4.5 μm for a 2-mm-thick cement layer that has cooled from 67°C to body temperature.[22]

To provide a better understanding of these complex volume changes, the curing process of the bone cement can be roughly divided into three phases (Fig. 2–7). During phase I, in the first few minutes after the completion of mixing, polymerization shrinkage is exhibited. In phase II, there is a rapid rise in temperature, but the cement is not yet fully hardened. Two rapid volumetric changes occur simultaneously: thermal expansion of the entrapped gaseous bubbles and accelerated polymerization shrinkage. In phase III, the cement is fully hardened and the polymerization is essentially completed. The cooling of the solid cement results in thermal contraction. A study has also documented the fact that cement characteristics and cement aging also alter the curing temperature characteristics[6] (Figs. 2–2 and 2–8).

The differences in volumetric changes between regular cement and low-porosity cement occur mostly during phase II of the curing process. For cement mixed in the regular fashion, the thermal expansion of the entrapped air partially compensates for the polymerization shrinkage. Therefore, as illustrated in Figure 2–7, the net shrinkage (V_0) of the low-porosity cement appears to be more than that of the regular cement (V_1).

Rimnac et al. found that centrifuged Simplex P cement contracts (4.3 percent) more than conventionally

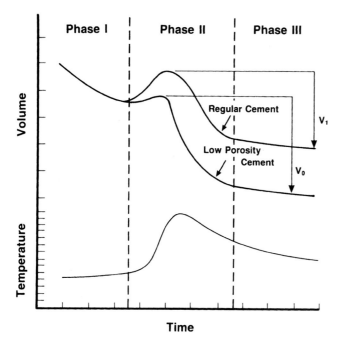

Figure 2–7. Schematic representation of volume change during polymerization of bone cement. During phase I, the volume change is mainly due to polymerization shrinkage. In phase II, there is simultaneous volume expansion as a result of thermal expansion of the gaseous bubbles and volume contraction as a result of polymerization. The volume change in phase III after solidification of the cement is due to thermal contraction as the cement cools.

mixed Simplex P cement (3.0 percent). However, later investigators, using a femoral stem model, found that there was no significant increase in diametric contraction of the cement mantle with porosity reduction with use of either centrifugation or partial vacuum mixing.[15,35] The combination of curing temperature and aging of the cement was also recently studied. These authors investigated the effect of temperature and aging on acrylic cement.[6]

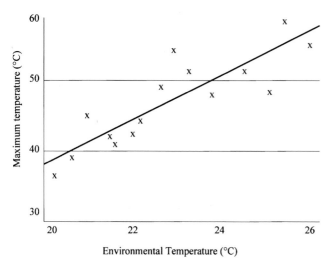

Figure 2–8. The relationship of environmental temperature and maximum temperature of the cured cement. (Modified from Baleani M, Cristofolini L, Toni A: Temperature and aging condition effects on the characterization of acrylic bone cement. J Eng Med 215:113, 2001.)

In conclusion, there is increased bulk volume shrinkage of cement when porosity is reduced. However, in cemented femoral stems, porosity reduction probably has no significant effect on diametric contraction of the cement mantle.

MODIFICATIONS OF BONE CEMENT

Alternate chemical formulations of PMMA aimed to reduce the modulus of cement are an area of intense interest. By decreasing the structural stiffness of the cement mantle (at least in the femoral hip replacement structure), the load transfer to the mantle becomes "smoother," resulting in decreased peak cement stresses.[41] One approach to the reduction of cement modulus is the incorporation of butylmethacrylate (a higher order methacrylate), either as the matrix[94] or the filler[67] component of the cement. Apart from reducing the modulus of the cement, such a formulation may also increase its ductility and toughness, thereby making it capable of absorbing more energy before failure. Although this formulation will reduce the interface shear stress, concern exists that a decreased modulus will also result in increased subsidence of the cemented femoral component.[98] Similarly, a two-solution acrylic formulation to enhance flexural strength is compromised in its clinical application by an increase in viscosity that may preclude adequate intrusion at the interface.[38]

Reinforcing agents such as carbon, glass, aramide, graphite, and titanium fibers have been added to bone cement in efforts to improve the tensile properties and fracture toughness.[78,82,84,87,93] However, such an approach for the improvement of cement properties has been hindered by the adverse effect of the reinforcing agents on the handling characteristics of the cement. In addition, the problems of nonuniform dispersion of the agents and of "filtration" of the agents by the cancellous bone at the bone-cement interface during pressurization remain unresolved.

References

1. Ahmed AM, Pak W, Burke DL, Miller J: Transient and residual stresses and displacements in self-curing bone cement. Part I: Characterization of relevant volumetric behaviour of bone cement. J Biomech Eng 104:21, 1982.
2. Ahmed AM, Raab S, Miller JE: Metal/cement interface strength in cemented stem fixation. J Orthop Res 2:105, 1984.
3. Arroyo NA: Physical and mechanical properties of vacuum mixed cement. In Transactions of the 12th Annual Meeting of the Society for Biomaterials. Minneapolis-St. Paul, 1986, p 187.
4. Askew MJ, Kufel MF, Fleissner PR Jr, et al: Effect of vacuum mixing on the mechanical properties of antibiotic-impregnated polymethylmethacrylate bone cement. J Biomed Mater Res 24:573, 1990.
5. Askew MJ, Steege JW, Lewis JL, et al: Effect of cement pressure and bone strength on polymethylmethacrylate fixation. J Orthop Res 1:412, 1984.
6. Baleani M, Cristofolini L, Toni A: Temperature and aging condition effects on the characterization of acrylic bone cement. J Eng Med 215:113, 2001.

7. Barb W, Park JB, Kenner GH, van Recum AF: Intramedullary fixation of artificial hip joint with bone cement precoated implants. J Biomed Mater Res 16:447, 1982.
8. Bayne SC, Lautenschlager EP, Compere CL, Wildes R: Degree of polymerization of acrylic bone cement. J Biomed Mater Res 9:27, 1975.
9. Burke DW, Gates EI, Harris WH: Centrifugation as a method of improving tensile and fatigue properties of acrylic bone cement. J Bone Joint Surg 66A:1265, 1984.
10. Carter DR, Gates EI, Harris WH: Strain-controlled fatigue of acrylic bone cement. J Biomed Mater Res 16:647, 1982.
11. Chandler HP, Reineck FT, Wixson RL, et al: Total hip replacement in patients younger than thirty years old. J Bone Joint Surg 63A:1426, 1981.
12. Chao EY, Chin HC, Stauffer RN: Roentgenographic and mechanical performance of centrifuged cement in a simulated total hip arthroplasty model. Clin Orthop 285:91, 1992.
13. Chin HC, Stauffer RN, Chao EY: The effect of centrifugation on the mechanical properties of cement: An in vitro total hip-arthroplasty model. J Bone Joint Surg 72A:363, 1990.
14. Combs SP, Greenwald AS: The effects of barium sulfate on the polymerization temperature and shear strength of surgical Simplex P. Clin Orthop 145:287, 1979.
15. Connelly TJ, Lautenschlager EP, Wixson RL: The role of porosity in the shrinkage of acrylic cement. In Transactions of the 13th Annual Meeting of the Society for Biomaterials, New York, 1987, p 114.
16. Crowninshield RD, Tolbert JR: Cement strain measurement surrounding loose and well-fixed femoral component stems. J Biomed Mater Res 17:819, 1983.
17. Davies JP, Burke DW, O'Connor DO, Harris WH: Comparison of the fatigue characteristics of centrifuged and uncentrifuged Simplex P bone cement. J Orthop Res 5:366, 1987.
18. Davies JP, O'Connor DO, Burke DW, Harris WH: Comparison of centrifugation and vacuum mixed Simplex P. Trans Orthop Res Soc 13:221, 1988.
19. Davies JP, O'Connor DO, Burke DW, Harris WH: Influence of antibiotic impregnation on the fatigue life of Simplex P and Palacos R acrylic bone cements, with and without centrifugation. J Biomed Mater Res 23:379, 1989.
20. Davies JP, O'Connor DO, Burke DW, et al: The effects of centrifugation on the fatigue life of bone cement in the presence of surface irregularities. Clin Orthop 229:156, 1988.
21. Davies JP, O'Connor DO, Greer JA, Harris WH: Comparison of the mechanical properties of Simplex P, Zimmer Regular, and LVC cements. J Biomed Mater Res 21:719, 1987.
22. Debrunner HU, Wettstein A, Hofer P: The polymerization of self-curing acrylic cements and problems due to the cement anchorage of joint prostheses. In Schaldach M, Holmann D (eds): Advances in Artificial Hip and Knee Joint Technology. Berlin, Springer-Verlag, 1976, p 294.
23. Demarest VA, Lautenschlager EP, Wixson RL: Vacuum mixing of acrylic cement. In Transactions of the 9th Annual Meeting of the Society for Biomaterials, Birmingham, AL, 1983, p 37.
24. Eyerer P, Jin R: Influence of mixing technique on some properties of PMMA bone cement. J Biomed Mater Res 20:1057, 1986.
25. Freitag TA, Cannon SL: Fracture characteristics of acrylic bone cements. II. Fatigue. J Biomed Mater Res 11:609, 1977.
26. Fumich RM, Gibbons DF: Rate of mixing and the strength of methylmethacrylate bone cements. Orthop Rev 8:41, 1979.
27. Funk MJ, Litsky AS: Effect of cement modulus on the shear properties of the bone-cement interface. Biomaterials 19:1561, 1998.
28. Gates EI, Carter DR, Harris WH: Tensile fatigue failure of acrylic bone cement. J Biomech Eng 105:393, 1983.
29. Gates EI, Carter DR, Harris WH: Comparative fatigue behaviour of different bone cements. Clin Orthop 189:294, 1984.
30. Geiger MH, Keating EM, Ritter MA, et al: The clinical significance of vacuum mixing bone cement. Clin Orthop 382:258, 2001.
31. Goodman SB, Fornasier VL, Kei J: The effect of bulk versus particulate polymethylmethacrylate on bone. Clin Orthop 232:255, 1988.
32. Graham J, Pruitt L, Ries M, Gundiah N: Fracture and fatigue properties of acrylic bone cement: The effects of mixing method, sterilization treatment, and molecular weight. J Arthroplasty 15:1028, 2000.
33. Hamati FI, Wixson RL, Novak MA, Lautenschlager EP: The effect of notching of Simplex P bone cement on the fatigue lives of regular versus vacuum-mixed specimens. Trans Orthop Res Soc 12:226, 1987.
34. Hampton SJ, Andriacchi TP, Galante JO: Three dimensional stress analysis of the femoral stem of a total hip prosthesis. J Biomech 13:443, 1979.
35. Hansen D, Jensen JS: Prechilling and vacuum mixing not suitable for all bone cements: Handling characteristics and exotherms of bone cements. J Arthroplasty 5:287, 1990.
36. Harper EJ, Bonfield W: Tensile characteristics of ten commercial acrylic bone cements. J Biomed Mat Res 53:605, 2000.
37. Harrigan TP, Davies JP, Burke DW, et al: On the presence or easy initiation of fracture in bone cement at the bone-cement interface in total hip arthroplasty. In Transactions of the 13th Annual Meeting of the Society for Biomaterials, New York, 1987, p 170.
38. Hasenwinkel JM, Lautenschlager EP, Wixson RL, Gilbert JL: A novel high-viscosity, two-solution acrylic bone cement: Effect of chemical composition on properties. J Biomed Mat Res 47:35, 1999.
39. Hass SS, Brauer GM, Dickson G: A characterization of polymethylmethacrylate bone cement. J Bone Joint Surg 57A:380, 1975.
40. Holm NJ: The modulus of elasticity and flexural strength of some acrylic bone cements. Acta Orthop Scand 48:436, 1977.
41. Huiskes R: Some fundamental aspects of human joint replacement. Acta Orthop Scand 185(Suppl):109, 1980.
42. Ingham E, Green TR, Stone MH, et al: Production of TNF-alpha and bone resorbing activity by macrophages in response to different types of bone cement particles. Biomat 21:1005, 2000.
43. Jaffe WI, Rose RM, Radin EL: On the stability of the mechanical properties of self-curing acrylic bone cement. J Bone Joint Surg 56A:1711, 1974.
44. James SP, Jasty M, Davies J, et al: A fractographic investigation of PMMA bone cement focusing on the relationship between porosity reduction and increased fatigue life. J Biomed Mater Res 26:651, 1992.
45. Jasty M, Burke D, Harris WH: Biomechanics of cemented and cementless prostheses. Chir Organi Mov 77:349, 1992.
46. Jasty M, Davies JP, O'Connor DO, et al: Porosity of various preparations of acrylic bone cements. Clin Orthop 259:122, 1990.
47. Jasty M, Maloney WJ, Bragdon CR, et al: The initiation of failure in cemented femoral components of hip arthroplasties. J Bone Joint Surg 73B:551, 1991.
48. Jefferiss CD, Lee AJC, Ling RSM: Thermal aspects of self-curing polymethylmethacrylate. J Bone Joint Surg 57B:511, 1975.
49. Johnston RC: The case for cemented hips. In The Hip: Proceedings of the 13th Open Scientific Meeting of the Hip Society. St. Louis, CV Mosby, 1987, p 351.
50. Keller JC, Lautenschlager EP, Mashall GW Jr, Meyer PR Jr: Factors affecting surgical alloy-bone cement interface adhesion. J Biomed Mater Res 14:639, 1980.
51. Krause W, Mathis RS: Fatigue properties of acrylic bone cements: Review of the literature. J Biomed Mater Res 22:37, 1988.
52. Krause W, Mathis RS, Grimes LW: Fatigue properties of acrylic bone cement: S-N, P-N, and P-S-N data. J Biomed Mater Res 22:221, 1988.
53. Kummer FJ: Improved mixing of bone cements. Trans Orthop Res Soc 10:238, 1985.
54. Lautenschlager EP, Black HR, Rapp GF: Effects of tobramycin antibiotic on the properties of Simplex P bone cement. In Transactions of the 9th Annual Meeting of the Society for Biomaterials, Birmingham, AL, 1983, p 32.
55. Lautenschlager EP, Jacobs JJ, Marshall GW, Meyer PR Jr: Mechanical properties of bone cements containing large doses of antibiotic powder. J Biomed Mater Res 10:929, 1976.
56. Lautenschlager EP, Marshall GW, Marks GW, et al: Mechanical strength of acrylic bone cements impregnated with antibiotics. J Biomed Mater Res 10:837, 1976.
57. Lautenschlager EP, Stupp SI, Keller JC: Structure and properties of acrylic bone cement. In Ducheyne P, Hastings GW (eds): Functional Behavior of Orthopaedic Biomaterials, vol II. Applications. Boca Raton, FL, CRC Press, 1984, p 88.
58. Lautenschlager EP, Wixson RL, Novak MA: Fatigue and fracture toughness of Simplex P. Trans Orthop Res Soc 11:118, 1986.
59. Lee AJC, Ling RSM, Vangala SS: The mechanical properties of bone cements. J Med Eng Tech May:137, 1977.

60. Lee AJC, Ling RSM, Vangala SS: Some clinically relevant variables affecting the mechanical behaviour of bone cement. Arch Orthop Trauma Surg 92:1, 1978.
61. Lee AJC, Ling RSM, Wrighton JD: Some properties of polymethylmethacrylate with reference to its use in orthopaedic surgery. Clin Orthop 95:281, 1973.
62. Lewis G: Effect of mixing method and storage temperature of cement constituents on the fatigue and porosity of acrylic bone cement. J Biomed Mat Res 48:143, 1999.
63. Lidgren L, Bodelind B, Moller J: Bone cement improved by vacuum mixing and chilling. Acta Orthop Scand 57:27, 1987.
64. Lidgren L, Drar H, Moller J: Strength of polymethylmethacrylate increased by vacuum mixing. Acta Orthop Scand 55:536, 1984.
65. Linden U: Porosity in manually mixed bone cement. Clin Orthop 231:110, 1988.
66. Linder L: The tissue response to bone cement. *In* Williams DF (ed): Biocompatibility of Orthopaedic Implants II. Boca Raton, FL, CRC Press, 1982, p 1.
67. Litsky AS, Rose RM, Rubin CT, Thrasher EL: A reduced-modulus acrylic bone cement: preliminary results. J Orthop Res 8:623, 1990.
68. Maloney WJ, Jasty M, Burke DW, et al: Biomechanical and histologic investigation of cemented total hip arthroplasties: A study of autopsy-retrieved femur after *in vivo* cycling. Clin Orthop 249:129, 1989.
69. McBeath AA, Foltz RN: Femoral components loosening after total hip arthroplasty. Clin Orthop 141:66, 1979.
70. Meyer PR, Lautenschlager EP, Moore BK: On the setting properties of acrylic bone cement. J Bone Joint Surg 55A:149, 1973.
71. Miller J, Burke DL, Staciewicz JW, et al: The pathophysiology of loosening of femoral components in total hip arthroplasty: A clinical and experimental study of cement fracture and loosening of the cement-bone interface. *In* The Hip: Proceedings of the 6th Open Scientific Meeting of the Hip Society. St. Louis, CV Mosby, 1978, p 84.
72. Morita M, Aritomi H: Bone cement not weakened by cefuzonam powder. Acta Orthop Scand 62:232, 1991.
73. Noble PC, Jay JL, Lindahl LJ, et al: Methods of enhancing acrylic bone cement. *In* Transactions of the 13th Annual Meeting of the Society for Biomaterials, New York, 1987, p 169.
74. Ohashi KL, Dauskardt RH: Effects of fatigue loading and PMMA precoating on the ahesion and subcritical debonding of prosthetic PMMA interfaces. J Biomed Mat Res 51:172, 2000.
75. Petty W: The effect of methylmethacrylate on chemotaxis of polymorphonuclear leukocytes. J Bone Joint Surg 60A:492, 1978.
76. Petty W: Methylmethacrylate concentrations in tissues adjacent to bone cement. J Biomed Mater Res 14:427, 1980.
77. Petty W, Caldwell JR: The effect of methylmethacrylate on complement activity. Clin Orthop 128:354, 1977.
78. Pillar RM, Blackwell R, Macnab I, Cameron HU: Carbon-fiber reinforced bone cement in orthopaedic surgery. J Biomed Mater Res 10:89, 1976.
79. Puckett AD, Roberts B, Bu L, Mays JW: Improved orthopaedic bone cement formulations based on rubber toughening. Crit Rev Biomed Eng 28:457, 2000.
80. Raab S, Ahmed AM, Provan JW: Thin film PMMA precoating for improved implant bone-cement fixation. J Biomed Mater Res 16:679, 1982.
81. Rimnac CL, Wright TM, McGill DL: The effect of centrifugation on the fracture properties of acrylic bone cements. J Bone Joint Surg 68A:281, 1986.
82. Robinson RP, Wright RP, Burstein AH: Mechanical properties of poly(methylmethacrylate) bone cements. J Biomed Mater Res 15:203, 1981.
83. Rostoker W, Lereim P, Galante JO: Effect of an in vivo environment on the strength of bone cement. J Biomed Mater Res 13:365, 1979.
84. Saha S, Subrata P: Improvement of mechanical properties of acrylic bone cement by fiber reinforcement. J Biomech 17:467, 1984.
85. Saha S, Warman ML: Improved compressive strength of bone cement by ultrasonic vibration. *In* Transactions of the 10th Annual Meeting of the Society for Biomaterials, Washington, DC, 1984, p 48.
86. Santavirta S, Konttinen YT, Bergroth V, Gronblad M: Lack of immune response to methyl methacrylate in lymphocyte cultures. Acta Orthop Scand 62:29, 1991.
87. Schnur DS, Lee D: Stiffness and inelastic deformation in acrylic-titanium composite implant materials under compression. J Biomed Mater Res 17:973, 1983.
88. Schurman DJ, Bloch DA, Segal MR, Tanner CM: Conventional cemented total hip arthroplasty: Assessment of clinical factors associated with revision for mechanical failure. Clin Orthop 240:173, 1989.
89. Smith D: Cementing the future [interview by P. Ralph Crawford]. J Can Dent Assoc 56:841, 1990.
90. Stauffer RN: Ten-year follow-up study of total hip replacement, with particular reference to roentgenographic loosening of the components. J Bone Joint Surg 64A:983, 1982.
91. Swenson LW, Schurman DJ: Finite element temperature analysis of a total hip replacement and measurement of PMMA curing temperatures. J Biomed Mater Res 15:83, 1982.
92. Toksvig-Larsen S, Franzen H, Ryd L: Cement interface temperature in hip arthroplasty. Acta Orthop Scand 62:102, 1991.
93. Topoleski LD, Ducheyne P, Cuckler JM: The fracture toughness of titanium-fiber-reinforced bone cement. J Biomed Mater Res 26:1599, 1992.
94. Weightman B, Freeman MAR, Revell PA, et al: The mechanical properties of cement and loosening of the femoral component of hip replacements. J Bone Joint Surg 69B:558, 1987.
95. Welsh RP, Pilliar RM, MacNab I: Surgical implants: The role of surface porosity in fixation to bone acrylic. J Bone Joint Surg 53A:963, 1971.
96. Wixson RL, Lautenschlager EP, Novak M: Vacuum mixing of methylmethacrylate bone cement. Trans Orthop Res Soc 10:327, 1985.
97. Wixson RL, Lautenschlager EP, Novak MA: Vacuum mixing of acrylic bone cement. J Arthroplasty 2:141, 1987.
98. Yetkinler DN, Litsky AS: Viscoelastic behaviour of acrylic bone cements. Biomaterials 19:1551–1559, 1998.

3

Metallic Alloys

•JACK E. LEMONS

GENERAL CHARACTERISTICS OF BIOMATERIALS

The synthetic-origin biomaterials currently used for the fabrication of orthopedic surgical implants may be broadly categorized into metals, ceramics, polymers, and composites of these substances. The use by number and weight is largest for metallic alloys based on the primary elements of iron (Fe), cobalt (Co), or titanium (Ti). Metals as single-element compositions, such as titanium or zirconium (Zr), do find applications; however, strength considerations of orthopedic devices are a significant limitation for most non-alloy structures. The ceramics and carbons include those that are based on aluminum or zirconium oxide (Al_2O_3 or ZrO_2), calcium aluminates and phosphates, glass and glass-ceramics, and carbon-silicon compounds. Polymers include polymethylmethacrylate (PMMA), ultra-high-molecular-weight polyethylene (UHMWPE), polytetrafluorethylene (PTFE), polyethylene-terephthalate (PET), polydimethylsiloxane (PDS or silicone), polyurethane, polypropylene, polysulfones (PSFs), and some copolymer systems.[29] Composites are sometimes used in which metals, ceramics, carbons, or polymers are bonded to one another to form new structures with specific properties that are different from the independent components. Since the early 1990s, a number of new and improved biomaterials have been developed with anisotropic properties that have been introduced through controlled compositions of metallic-based compounds and oxides (e.g., oxidized zirconium).[31] Also, a wide range of substances of biologic origin are being processed for use in musculoskeletal surgical reconstructions. This chapter emphasizes the metals and alloys and some specific properties related to the clinical use of these biomaterials.

The biomaterial components of devices have physical, mechanical, chemical, electrical, and biologic properties that depend directly on the material of constitution, the internal metallurgic conditions of the material, and the shape, form, and surface of the final device.[34] In broad categories, the ceramics are inert (biotolerant), hard, brittle nonconductors of heat and electricity, whereas carbons are also inert and brittle but are conductors of heat and electricity. After passivation to produce an oxide surface, the alloys are strong and ductile and are conductors of heat and electricity. In contrast, the polymers are softer, weaker, and more ductile, and, similar to ceramics, minimally conduct heat and electricity. The physical properties such as color, density, and conductivity characteristics of metallics are important when biodegradation phenomena, combinations of biomaterials for device construction, and clinical application near dermal surfaces are considered.

Implant designs are often determined on the basis of the biomaterial properties. For example, ceramics and carbons have limitations for hip device stems, intermedullary rods, plates, or screws because of their inherent lack of ductility. In contrast, the high hardness, inertness, and wear resistance of aluminum or zirconium oxides make them desirable candidates for articulating components such as total hip replacement femoral heads or acetabular cup liners. Polymers provide more resilient biomaterial properties and opportunities for use when lower density, flexibility, and compliance are critical considerations.

Design criteria are dependent on the basic elastic (modulus) and strength properties of synthetic substances for tissue replacement. For example, structural replacements for bone are most often made of metallic alloys or ceramics. In contrast, synthetic ligaments and tendons use polymers or fiber-reinforced, polymeric composites or biologics. These examples and applications have been based on more closely matching the material and the tissue properties of the regions being replaced. Elastic criteria for appropriate matching of relative implant and tissue properties are best interpreted by the modulus of elasticity.[9] This property is the slope of the mechanical stress-versus-strain relationship for each biomaterial or tissue. The modulus is a basic measurement of a substance's inherent elastic flexibility. Some confusion arises because of relative interpretations of moduli. Generally, this is because most clinicians consider elasticity as a measure of elastic strain or deformation before the beginning of permanent strain (called plastic deformation). In terms of bioengineering interpretations, high-magnitude elastic strains are directly correlated with lower elastic moduli biomaterials such as the polymerics. Conversely, higher elastic moduli materials, such as metallics and ceramics, have lower-magnitude elastic strain characteristics.

19

One reason for the extensive use of metallic alloys in orthopedic surgery is the availability of relatively strong and biotolerant materials over the past few years.[19,29] Before 1925, most available metallic systems had been evaluated, and the selection of the electrochemically noble elements (e.g., Au, Pt) was most common.[25,36] Alloys of iron and cobalt followed, with the introduction of titanium in 1951, and, since that time, most alloy systems have been based on iron, cobalt, or titanium.[33] In contrast to the noble metals, these alloys are used in an oxidized or passivated surface condition, which provides stability as related to corrosion. This has resulted in national (American Society for Testing Materials [ASTM] F4) and international (International Organization for Standardization [ISO]) material standards for most classes, metallurgic conditions, and surface finishes.[2,17] These specifications provide detailed requirements for nominal chemical analyses, mechanical properties, and surface conditions.[17,20] Limits with respect to consensus opinions on minimally acceptable property values are provided in these standards.

Because of the availability of specific property information and clinical experience, design criteria have evolved to optimize device longevity. New applications for devices are often simple changes of shape or surface conditions to better control the biomaterial-tissue interface. Some trends over the past few years have included porous surfaces on titanium and cobalt alloys for tissue ingrowth,[17,20] calcium-phosphate ceramic-like coatings to provide interfacial attachment with bone,[10] and surface compounds and/or oxides to enhance relative hardness (wear resistance) and smoothness for articulating surfaces.[10,34,35] These types of surfaces tend to alter the properties of the basic materials; therefore, basic design modifications of previously used devices are required. Interest in surface-altered biomaterials remains high, and considerable research and development efforts continue within the discipline.

METALS AND ALLOYS

Examples of orthopedic surgical implant components fabricated from metallic alloys are shown in Figures 3-1 through 3-4. Some total joint devices are shown in Figure 3-1, including femoral hip components fabricated from cast cobalt alloy (ASTM F 75). Fracture fixation plates from the same alloys are shown in Figure 3-2, and spinal implant systems made from iron alloy are shown in Figure 3-3. Surface modifications to include porosity for biologic ingrowth fixation are shown for cobalt and titanium alloys in Figure 3-4.

Spinal instrumentation devices are most often fabricated from iron-based surgical stainless steel because of its inherent strength, ductility, and toughness. However, this stainless steel should not be used for porous implants because of its susceptibility to crevice corrosion. Several iron-based alloys have been modified through the addition of elements to alter chemical constituents or residual strain to increase strength. These enhanced properties have been shown to have a positive influence on the alloys' biomechanical characteristics.[2]

The more commonly used metallic systems and selected properties are summarized in Table 3-1. The various metallic biomaterials exhibit significantly different magnitude moduli, strengths, and surface properties. It is useful to think of these property characteristics as a ratio to the similar measurements for compact bone. Comparative data and ratios are provided in Table 3-2.

It is noteworthy that all alloys have moduli of elasticity that are at least five times higher than those of compact bone. Also, strains (elongations) to fracture greatly exceed the limits of bone. These properties directly influence design criteria for prostheses.

The alloys of iron and cobalt have chromium oxide-based surfaces when prepared with a passivated (oxidized) surface condition.[23] The oxide is like a ceramic coating, although it is a very thin film and not visible under normal lighting. This ultrathin (nanometer) surface layer provides improved resistance to biodegradation. This resistance is most critical for the iron alloy systems, which are subject to crevice or pitting corrosion if the oxide surface layer is broken down in vivo.[11,12]

Titanium alloy forms a titanium oxide surface very rapidly in room-temperature air or normal physiologic fluids.[7] This oxide or passivation reaction makes the titanium systems (in general, the reactive group metals: Ti, Zr, hafnium [Hf], tungsten [W], and tantalum [Ta]) resistant to surface breakdown when they are used in a porous condition. The titanium-based systems have a lower modulus of elasticity compared with the iron or cobalt alloys. This basic material property is less by a factor of about two times and must be taken into account when designing load-bearing orthopedic devices. Design changes should include size or shape alterations to accommodate elastic property differences.

On a relative basis, the cast alloys of cobalt, iron, and titanium are weaker and have less ductility compared with the wrought alloy systems. This has resulted in some concern about mechanical stabilities for stemmed prostheses, especially when surface porosity is included in the design. Prosthesis designers must incorporate configuration restraints to minimize the possibilities of in vivo mechanical fracture characteristics.[20]

Electrochemical Properties

Another physical (and chemical/electrochemical) consideration in the selection and use of implant devices is the basic electrochemistry and property relationships of biodegradation phenomena. For metallic systems, these phenomena can be described by corrosion mechanisms, and a considerable body of literature has evolved in this general topic area.[2,5,6,27,34] One of the more useful characterizations of metallic materials is the galvanic series, which provides electrochemical comparisons in saline solutions. This series also permits theoretical predictions of galvanic coupling, or the relative corrosion behavior of two conductors that are electrically coupled within the host and therefore the same electrolyte environment. Examples are a cobalt-chromium-molybdenum

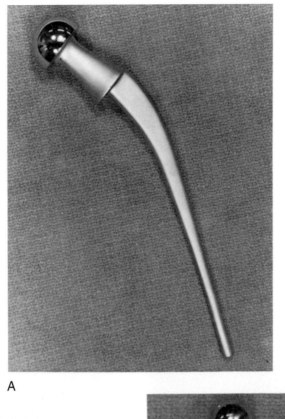

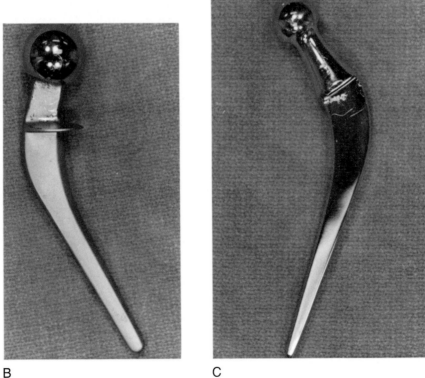

Figure 3–1. Examples of retrieved total hip replacements fabricated from (**A**) cobalt-, (**B**) titanium-, and (**C**) iron-based alloys.

(Co-Cr-Mo) femoral head on a titanium alloy (Ti-6Al-4V) stem for a total hip replacement or a stainless-steel wire wrapped onto a cobalt- or titanium-based alloy component. Galvanic coupling, with an associated enhancement of in vivo corrosion, is dependent on a number of environmental factors. The magnitude and rate of increased (or decreased) corrosion depends on the environment (e.g., fluid, soft tissue, or bone) and local transport phenomena; surface interactions such as wear (fretting or local oxide removal); relative surface area ratios of the components; galvanic potential differences; metallurgic conditions of the alloys; and localized

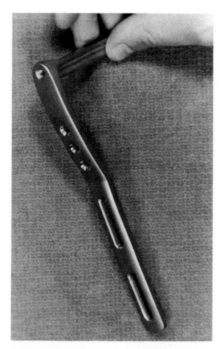

A

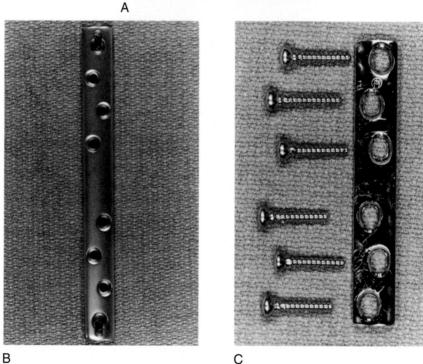

B   C

Figure 3–2. Examples of retrieved fracture fixation devices fabricated from (**A**) cobalt-, (**B**) titanium-, and (**C**) iron-based alloys. The surface damage is associated with clinical removal.

oxygen and ionic species concentrations and gradients.[11] Increases of in vivo corrosion are to be avoided because of biocompatibility considerations that emphasize the importance of this type of biomaterial-and-host information. A general rule is that surgical stainless steel should not be coupled with other alloys or carbon. In contrast, titanium, titanium alloys, and cobalt alloys have relatively similar electrochemical potentials.[13,21] Studies of the in vivo coupling of titanium- and cobalt-based alloys have not demonstrated significant increases

in the corrosion of either component.[22] Questions have been raised about adverse electrochemical phenomena for combination of cobalt and titanium alloys in the presence of fretting or assembly (modular design) debris. Most critically, the design, material, and manufacturing considerations must be optimized so that unanticipated biodegradation phenomena are not introduced as a result of environmental conditions that should not have existed for total joint replacement systems.

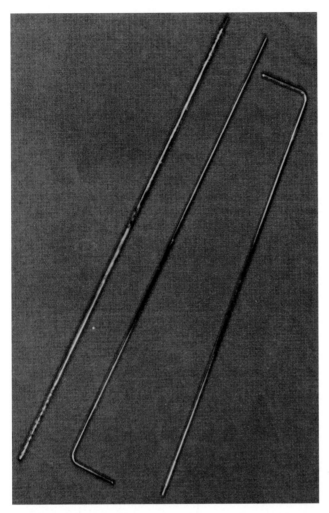

Figure 3–3. Examples of spinal instrumentation devices fabricated from iron-based alloys.

Potentiostatic and dynamic polarization data have provided detailed comparisons of solid and porous alloy implant systems (Table 3–3). Porous materials have higher surface areas, which can produce more in vivo corrosion. However, because most of the alloys are very corrosion resistant and have similar magnitude corrosion potentials (E_c), the corrosion currents (i_c) are within the same order of magnitude as the nonporous devices.[22]

Biomechanical Considerations

Correlations of biomaterial properties and in vivo outcomes have been major activities of the research and clinical communities. As a broad evaluation, materials have been selected with the highest possible strength, ductility and resistance to biodegradation and wear. However, these selections have also included the important considerations of availability, fabricability, and cost. Resistance-to-wear phenomena along articulating surfaces vary among biomaterial combinations. This resistance is dependent on the basic properties of the material, the surface finish (roughness) and chemistry, and the basic designs of the adjacent surfaces. Research, development, and application have shown UHMWPE to be relatively resistant to wear when articulating against smooth and polished alloy or ceramic surfaces under conditions of adhesive wear.[12,14,21,24,37] However, when debris is generated and in the presence of other particulates (e.g., PMMA bone cement), wear processes can be drastically altered. Polymeric components are quite susceptible to localized abrasion and "third-body" wear phenomena.[3,4] These same characteristics exist for the ceramics (i.e., if the abrasive particles are also ceramic particulate).[4,5,37] The wear characteristics of the highly

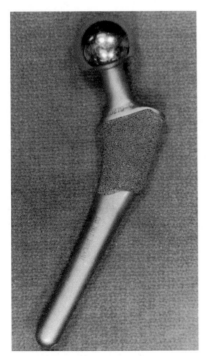

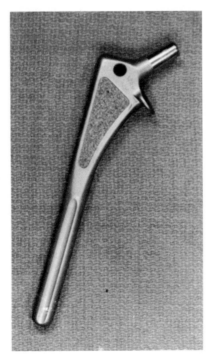

Figure 3–4. Examples of nonimplanted porous-surfaced total hip replacements fabricated from (**A**) cobalt- and (**B**) titanium-based alloys.

A

B

Table 3–1. METALLIC BIOMATERIALS COMMONLY USED FOR THE CONSTRUCTION OF ORTHOPEDIC SURGICAL IMPLANTS

Material	Nominal Composition (w/o)	Tensile Strength in MPa (ksi)	Modulus of Elasticity in GPa (psi × 10⁶)	Surface Condition
Cobalt alloys				
Cast	Co-27Cr-7Mo	655 (95)	235 (34)	Cr_xOy
Wrought	Co-26Cr-(Ni,Mo,W,Fe)	1172 (170)	235 (34)	Cr_xOy
Surgical stainless steel (316L)	Fe-18Cr-12Ni	480–1000 (70–145)	193 (28)	Cr_xOy
Titanium alloy	Ti-6Al-4V	860–896 (125–130)	117 (17)	Ti_xOy

Table 3–2. METALLIC BIOMATERIAL* AND TISSUE PROPERTIES

Material or Tissue	Modulus of Elasticity in GPa (psi × 10⁶)	Tensile Strength in MPa (ksi)	Elongation to Fracture (%)	Ratio (Material: Bone) Modulus	Ratio (Material: Bone) Strength	Fracture Elongation
Compact bone	21 (3)	138 (20)	1	1	1	1
Cobalt alloys	235 (34)	655–1172 (95–170)	>8	11	5–9	>8
Stainless steels	193 (28)	480–1000 (70–145)	>30	9 +	4–7	>30
Titanium alloy	117 (17)	860–896 (125–130)	>12	5 +	6–7	>12
Titanium	96 (14)	240–550 (25–70)	>15	5 +	1–4	>15

*Properties are provided from ASTM documents and represent minimum values for nominal composition.

Table 3–3. CORROSION DATA FROM POTENTIOSTATIC POLARIZATION

Material	Equilibrium Corrosion Potential and Rate From Potentiostatic Polorization E_c (mV)	Equilibrium Corrosion Potential and Rate From Potentiostatic Polorization i_c (μa/cm²)
Ti	−14	0.013
Solid		
Porous	−10	0.044
Ti-6Al-4V	−50	0.003
Solid		
Porous	−75	0.014
Co-Cr-Mo	−10	0.011
Solid		
Porous	−35	0.028
Fe-Cr-Ni (316L SS)	−49	0.008
Solid		

Data from previous studies of L. Lucas and R. Buchanan, University of Alabama at Birmingham.

cross-linked polyethylenes under conditions of third-body particulates continues to be an area of active laboratory research.[24,37]

Wear

Alloys demonstrate varying degrees of wear resistance. Most are susceptible to breakdown (fretting) if the localized contact stresses are excessive. However, cobalt alloys are more wear resistant than iron alloys, and both are more resistant than titanium alloys. Titanium alloys, if exposed to metallic contact and relative movement, undergo surface galling (roughening) and breakdown.[5,25–27] This phenomenon is characteristic for reactive-group metals and alloys and is related to the oxidation and environmental behavior of the metals involved. Titanium alloys, if used for articulating surfaces, require special surface modification treatments to minimize in vivo biodegradation associated with wear phenomena.[3] Surface treatments of titanium alloys have been shown to significantly reduce wear phenomena. In vivo breakdown associated with titanium is normally seen as a black zone within the tissues; cobalt alloys show green-blue; and iron alloys are noted as a dark brown coloration in the adjacent zones.

Biocompatibility

The principal alloying elements in Ti-6Al-4V and the more recently introduced beta-alloys have been evaluated with respect to in vivo biocompatibility.[5] Aluminum and vanadium ions in vivo have been associated with adverse tissue responses.[25,32,37] Thus, some manufacturers have initiated the introduction of alloys with other elements as principal constituents.[2,17] This is a most interesting situation in that corrosion potentials, currents, and device evaluations do not support significant clinical or tissue problems with the Ti-Al-V alloy. Comparisons of structure, property, and application relationships should provide greater insights into the long-term tissue responses to this alloy series.

Manufacturing quality control and assurance are aspects of device longevity. Industries fabricate implant devices with precision and accuracy standards that exceed most other industrial application requirements. Implant devices should have a "minimum defect" specification, and this is the desirable recommendation. National (ASTM F4) and international (ISO) consensus standards and recommended practices are available for most metallic materials used for orthopedic devices.[2,17] The ASTM F4 standards volume provides an excellent reference for biomaterials properties and standardized manufacturing practices. This publication also includes test methods, practices for biocompatibility testing, and arthroplasty-related documents on performance.

BIOLOGIC ASPECTS

Biodegradation from environmental exposure, articulating surface wear, or mechanical breakdown results in the entry of substances such as particulate and ionic forms into the in vivo milieu. Examples of situations in which breakdown products have demonstrated adverse sequelae are corrosion of metals; wear of metals, polymers, and ceramics; and mechanical fracture of alloys and polymers.[25,33–37]

The questions related to metallic ion release and tissue responses can be categorized into areas of local tissue reactions (toxicity), allergy or hypersensitivity, and carcinogenicity.[18,32] Well-known data document the fact that tissues have limited tolerance in relation to metallic product concentrations. Fortunately, the amount of product transferred from devices to local and systemic tissues has, for the most part, been within the tissue tolerance limits. This fact is demonstrated by a general evaluation of the numbers of metallic devices used over the past 50 years and the associated device longevity profiles. This limited tolerance may be related in part to the corrosion and ionization characteristics of metallic elements, especially particulate forms. The literature shows that hypersensitivity to metallic components should be considered in more detail.[6,20] A small but significant segment of the population reacts to nickel- or cobalt-based alloys. Because surgical stainless steel and cobalt alloys contain nickel, applications of these alloys in allergic patients should be carefully evaluated. Some reports exist on ion accumulations within organs and metallic debris at device or corrosion sites. Area-specific sarcomas have been reported at these locations, although the number of reports has been limited. This entire area has been of concern to all involved, and reporting of any available clinically relevant data is strongly recommended.[28]

A significant amount of information has been learned from device retrieval and analysis studies.[28] At this time, standard practices and protocols for these procedures are available.[2] Critical issues related to both materials and mechanics can often be resolved through multidisciplinary studies of retrieved components.[16] Interest in the direct bonding of bone to synthetic material surfaces (e.g., titanium, titanium alloy, calcium phosphate ceramics, A-W ceramics, or Bioglass) has expanded since the early 1990s, and many of the questions raised in this area may be answered only through retrieval and/or cadaveric analyses. Trends to provide surface coatings for tissue attachment produce as many potential disadvantages as advantages. Because of the complexities of device functions, human in vivo trials are required. Clearly, analysis of retrievals (if retrieved devices are available) represents one critical area of input toward future improvements. As a basis for comparison, synthetic substances that provide opportunities for bonding to bone are summarized in Table 3–4.[8] An example of a total hip replacement with a titanium alloy-to-bone interface region that demonstrated conditions of osteointegration is shown in Figure 3–5 (Voltz R: Personal communication).[28]

Dental root form and selected other dental implants have demonstrated direct bone-biomaterial interfaces for functional systems.[1] This process has been called *osteointegration*. These dental reconstructive devices have been fabricated from titanium and provide opportunities for staging the treatments so as to provide a protected time

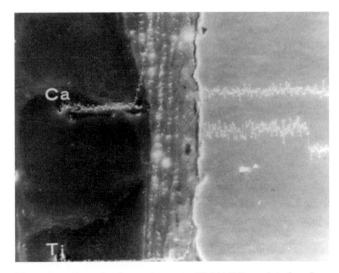

Figure 3–5. Example of osteointegrated Ti-6Al-4V bone interface from a retrieved total hip replacement. Scanning electron micrograph (SEM) trace for calcium (Ca) and titanium (Ti) are included on the SEM photograph.

Table 3–4. SELECTED BIOACTIVE COMPOUNDS PROPOSED FOR DIRECT BONDING OF LOAD-BEARING PROSTHESIS TO BONE

Material	Nominal Analysis	Modulus of Elasticity (GPa)	Tensile Strength (MPa)	Surface (Nominal)
Hydroxylapatite (HA)	99.99 +	80–120	40–300	$Ca_{10}(PO_4)_6(OH)_2$
Tricalcium phosphate (TCP)	99.99 +	90–120	40–120	$Ca_3(PO_4)_2$
Bioglass or ceravital	$Na_2O\text{-}CaO\text{-}P_2O_5\text{-}SiO_2$	40–140	20–350	$Ca\text{-}PO_4$ layer
AW ceramic	$(Al_2O_3)\text{-}M_9O\text{-}CaO\text{-}SiO_2\text{-}P_2O_5\text{-}CaF_2$	124	213	$Ca\text{-}PO_4$ layer
Ti and Ti-6Al-4V	99 + Ti	96	240–550	Ti_xO_y
	90 Ti-6Al-4V	117	860–896	Ti_xO_y

Data from Oonishi A, Sawai X (eds): Bioceramics, vol 1. Maryland Heights, MO, Ishiyaku EuroAmerica Inc., 1988.

for healing without applications of functional loads. This healing period without functional loading minimizes any micromotion during the bone adaptation and modeling phases. The first stage lasts normally at least 3 months. Between the years 2000 and 2002, the dental community has been evaluating the limits of "immediate loading," which is more similar to the orthopedic situation with respect to early biomechanical conditions. Surface analyses of dental systems have shown minimal soft tissue regions between the titanium (titanium oxide) and bone interfaces. This condition has been shown to exist over the long term for functional loading conditions.[30]

The direct transfer of mechanical load to the tissues through bonded interfaces could be a desirable feature for many orthopedic devices. Functional stimulation of bone could improve tissue maintenance, and, thereby, clinical longevity. Transfer of mechanical force through chemically (biochemically) bonded biomaterial-tissue interfaces could provide very significant advantages for orthopedic device designs and, one would hope, clinical longevity. Experience to date in the dental field indicates that there exist significant opportunities.[29,30]

FUTURE PERSPECTIVES

The past three decades have demonstrated multiple changes in synthetic biomaterials, device designs, surgical treatments, and clinical longevity. Continued improvements are anticipated.

In the 1960s, biomaterials were selected and designed to be more chemically inert (ceramics and carbons), and biocompatibility was evaluated by the presence or absence of foreign-body reactions. During the 1970s, interactions were emphasized, and the concept of "no mutual harm" was discussed in detail. Relative inertness was not judged to be so critically important.

During the 1980s, the emphasis shifted to controlling and directly influencing tissue response through the surface and bulk conditions of the synthetic biomaterial. In some situations, this was proposed through the use of mechanically and chemically anisotropic, fiber-reinforced components, whereas, in other cases, metallic alloys were coated with bioactive ceramics based on calcium phosphate or glass-ceramic systems. In both of these examples, proposals also included the addition of active biomolecules or synthetic compounds along the prosthesis-tissue interfaces. Since 1997, a number of new surface modifications, including metallic compounds and oxides, have been introduced. These continue to be areas of active research and development.

The various disciplines associated with biomaterials and biomechanics remain quite dynamic, and numerous changes in both orthopedic materials and designs for implant devices are expected before the year 2010.

References

1. Albrektsson T, Zarb G (eds): The Branemark Osseointegrated Implant. Chicago, Quintessence, 1989.
2. ASTM Annual Book of Standards: Medical Devices, vol 13.01. West Conshohocken, PA, ASTM Press, 2000.
3. Buchanan RA, Bacon RK, Williams JM, Beardsley GM: Ion implantation to improve the corrosive wear resistance of surgical Ti-6Al-4V. Trans Soc Biomater 6:106, 1983.
4. Buckhorn GH, Willert HG: Effects of plastic wear particles on tissue. In Williams DF (ed): Biocompatibility of Orthopaedic Implants. Boca Raton, FL, CRC Press, 1982, p 249.
5. Brown S, Lemons J (eds): Medical Applications of Titanium and Its Alloys [Am Soc for Testing and Mat]. West Conshohocken, PA, ASTM STP 1272, 1996.
6. Christel P, Meunier A, Dorlot JM, et al: Biomechanical compatibility and design of ceramic implants for orthopaedic surgery. In Ducheyne P, Lemons J (eds): Bioceramics: Material Characteristics Versus In Vivo Behavior. New York, New York Academy of Science, 1988, p 234.
7. Collings EW: The Physical Metallurgy of Titanium Alloys. Metals Park, OH, ASM Press, 1984.
8. Ducheyne P, Lemons JE (eds): Bioceramics: Material Characteristics Versus In Vivo Behavior. New York, New York Academy of Science, 1988, p 523.
9. Dumbleton JH, Black J: An Introduction to Orthopaedic Materials. Springfield, IL, Charles C Thomas, 1975.
10. Horowitz E, Parr J (eds): Characterization and Performance of Calcium Phosphate Coated Implants. Philadelphia, Am Soc for Testing and Mat, STP 1196, PA, 1994.
11. Fontana M, Greene ND: Corrosion Engineering. New York, McGraw-Hill, 1967.
12. Fraker A, Griffin C (eds): Corrosion and Degradation of Implant Materials. ASTM STP 859. Philadelphia, ASTM Press, 1985.
13. Griffin CD, Buchanan RA, Lemons JE: In vivo electrochemical corrosion of coupled surgical implant materials. J Biomed Mater Res 17:489, 1983.
14. Griffith M, Seidenstein MK, Williams D, Charnley J: Socket wear in Charnley low friction arthroplasty of the hip. Clin Orthop 37:137, 1978.
15. Gross UM: Biocompatibility: The interaction of biomaterials and host response. J Dent Educ 52:798, 1988.
16. Improving Medical Implant Performance Through Retrieval Information: Challenges and Opportunities, NIH Tech. Assess. Conf., Washington, DC, January, 2000.
17. ISO/TC Documents and Standards for Biomaterials, International Standards Organization, American National Standards Institute. New York, 1995.
18. Lang B, Morris H, Razzoog M: International Workshop: Biocompatibility, Toxicity and Hypersensitivity to Alloy Systems Used in Dentistry. Ann Arbor, University of Michigan Press, 1985.
19. Lemons JE: General characteristics and classifications of implant material. In Lin OCC, Chao EYS (eds): Perspectives in Biomaterials. Amsterdam, Elsevier, 1986, p 1.
20. Lemons JE (ed): Quantitative Characterization and Performance of Porous Implants for Hard Tissue Application. STP 953. Philadelphia, ASTM Press, 1987.
21. Lemons JE, Lucas LC: Properties of biomaterials. J Arthroplasty 1:143, 1986.
22. Lucas LC, Lemons JE, Lee J, Dale P: In vitro corrosion characteristics of Co-Cr-Mo/Ti-6Al-4V/Ti alloys. In Lemons JE (ed): Quantitative Characterization and Performance of Porous Alloys for Hard Tissue Applications. ASTM STP 953. Philadelphia, ASTM Press, 1987, p 124.
23. Mayor MB, Lemons JE: Medical device standards. ASTM Standardization News, 1986, p 40.
24. McKellop H, Hossenian A, Tuke M, et al: Superior wear of polymer hip prostheses. Trans Orthop Res Soc 10:322, 1985.
25. Mears DC: Materials and Orthopaedic Surgery. Baltimore, Williams & Wilkins, 1979.
26. Metallography, structures and phase diagrams, vol 8. In Metals Handbook. Metals Park, OH, ASM Press, 1973.
27. Nasser S, Campbell P, Amstutz HC: The unsuitability of titanium alloy as a bear surface in hip arthroplasty: A surface replacement model. Trans Soc Biomater 12:32, 1989.
28. Proceedings of the Symposium on Retrieval and Analysis of Surgical Implants and Biomaterials. Trans Soc Biomater 11:11, 1988.
29. Ratner B, Hoffman A, Schoen F, Lemons J (eds): Biomaterials Science. New York, Academic Press, 1996.
30. Rizzo T (ed): Proceedings of the NIDR Consensus Development Conference on Dental Implants. J Dent Educ 52:678, 1988.

31. Spector M, Ries M, Bourne R, Sauer W, et al: UHMWPE Wear Performance of Oxidized Zirconium Total Knee Femoral Components, Sci Exhibit No SE34, Am Acad Orthop Surg Annual Mtg. San Francisco, CA, 2001, pp 664–665.

32. Tharani R, Dorey F, Schmalzried T: The risk of cancer following total hip or knee arthroplasty. JBJS 83:774, 2001.

33. von Recum A (ed): Handbook of Biomaterials Evaluation. New York, Macmillan, 1986.

34. von Recum A (ed): Handbook of Biomaterials Evaluation, 2nd ed. Philadelphia, Taylor and Frances, 1999.

35. Willert H: From Alumina to Zirconia Hip Joint Heads: The Logical Evolution, Workshop 7 and Proceedings, Society for Biomaterials, Sixth World Congress, May, 2000, Kamuila, Hawaii, p 12.

36. Williams DF, Roaf R: Implants in Surgery. London, WB Saunders, 1973

37. Wright T, Goodman S: Implant Wear in Total Joint Replacement: Clinical and Biologic Issues, Material and Design Considerations. Rosemont, IL, Am Acad Orthop Surg, 2001.

4

The History of Improved Ultra-High-Molecular-Weight Polyethylene: Past, Present, and Future

Ultra-high-molecular-weight polyethylene molecular weight polyethylene (UHMWPE) has been the material of choice in total hip replacements since its first use by Sir John Charnley and Harry Craven in 1962. However, nearly since its introduction, there has been concern over the clinical consequences of wear debris.[30] This concern has led to the development and clinical use of several new, improved forms of UHMWPE. These attempts to improve the clinical performance of UHMWPE are reviewed here. The attempts include the use of carbon fiber reinforcement, changes in the method of sterilization, changes in the method of manufacturing, and, most recently, the use of higher doses of irradiation to increase the level of cross linking within the UHMWPE.

CHARNLEY'S ULTRA-HIGH-MOLECULAR-WEIGHT POLYETHYLENE MOLECULAR WEIGHT POLYETHYLENE

UHMWPE is a linear polymer of ethylene synthesized as a fine white powder in a variety of molecular weights, which typically range from 2 to 6 million. The average size of a powder particle is around 100 microns and may be as large as 500 microns. In the early 1990s, there were more than 10 different grades of UHMWPE available for use in orthopedic devices. These grades differed by their molecular weight, their location of manufacture, and the presence of calcium stearate. Today, there are only three grades available. The resins are 1020 and 1050 (2 and 6 million nominal molecular weight, respectively), supplied by Ticona (League City, TX), and 1900 (nominal molecular weight 4–6 million), supplied by Montel (Wilmington, DE). None of these three resins have calcium stearate added.

Montel 1900 is available only to a limited number of manufacturers who have agreed to limit the liability to Montel for use of the resin in medical devices. At this time, only Zimmer Orthopaedics (Warsaw, IN) and Biomet Orthopaedics (Warsaw, IN) continue to provide products made with 1900 resin.

The UHMWPE powder can be formed into an orthopedic device in one of three ways. The first is by directly molding the powder into the final device shape, with, typically, no machining of the articular surfaces. The second by first forming the powder into cylindrical bars by an extrusion process. The bars are then machined into their final form. The third method involves compression molding of the powder into large sheets. These sheets are typically 4 inches long by 8 inches wide (1.22 × 2.42 m) 1 to 12 (2.54–30.48 cm) inches thick. The effect of these different manufacturing methods and resin types on clinical performance is discussed in more detail in a later section.

CARBON-REINFORCED UHMWPE

In the 1970s, one of the first attempts to improve the performance of UHMWPE was the introduction of Poly II (Warsaw, IN), which was UHMWPE reinforced by carbon fibers. In laboratory evaluations, Poly II demonstrated lower wear, higher resistance to creep, and higher compressive strength than unreinforced UHMWPE. Poly II was used to make tibial inserts, patellas, and acetabular components. However, these carbon-reinforced materials were also found to have lower fatigue resistance compared with UHMWPE, and they suffered from manufacturing problems associated with incomplete molding.[32] Despite the better resistance to deformation, lower laboratory wear rates, and higher compressive and yield strengths, use of Poly II was

Table 4–1. EFFECT OF CRYSTALLINITY ON PHYSICAL PROPERTIES

Property	415GUR	Hylamer7 M	Hylamer7	Units
% Crystallinity	50	57	68	%
Density	0.934	0.946	0.955	g/cc
Melting point	135	147	149	C
Yield strength	23.3	26.5	28.6	MPa
Tensile strength	33.8	37.9	40.7	MPa
Elongation at break	339	369	334	%
Modulus	1.39	2.01	2.52	GPa
Creep	2.3	1.2	.9	%
Izod	950	1169	1196	J/m

discontinued approximately 7 years after its introduction to the marketplace.[31]

HYLAMER7 ORTHOPEDIC BEARING MATERIAL B ENHANCED POLYETHYLENE

In the early 1990s, Hylamer7 orthopedic bearing material was introduced as a new form of UHMWPE, which had significantly different physical properties from those of standard UHMWPE and which were achieved without the addition of any fillers or fibers. The property changes were effected by control of the morphology (crystalline structure) of the polymer, the result of exposing UHMWPE extruded bar to high pressures (>235MPa), high temperatures (>300E), and very slow cooling rates.[11] This process could alter the crystallinity of the UHMWPE from its normal range of 50 to 60 percent to values greater than 90 percent. As the crystallinity increased, the yield strength, resistance to deformation, and modulus increased as well. However, the modulus also generally increased at a faster rate than the other properties. The disproportionate increase in modulus compared with yield strength suggested that these materials might be at a disadvantage in designs that have high contact and subsurface shear stresses. The hip simulator determined wear rate of Hylamer7 was reported to be statistically equivalent to that of the 415GUR, from which it was made.[16]

Two commercial versions, Hylamer7 and Hylamer7 M (DuPont, Wilmington, DE), were introduced for use in acetabular cups and tibial inserts, respectively. These products were made by exposing extruded bars of 415GUR (Hoechst, League City, TX) to the process of high pressure and temperature and slow cooling rate described earlier. A comparison of the material properties as a function of crystallinity is provided in Table 4–1.

Does Hylamer Have High Wear?

The clinical performance of Hylamer7 has been mixed. The first reports of the Hylamer7 clinical performance were not favorable. Chmell and co-workers reported briefly on a retrospective examination of the results obtained from 143 of 193 cases treated by three surgeons.[2] At 34 months, five Hylamer7 liners (4.2%) were revised because of severe eccentric wear (>.36 mm/yr). Additionally, other devices in the series also exhibited high wear that was expected to result in revision surgery. The 4-year survivorship may be as low as 86 percent based on these projections. It should be noted that in this report, Hylamer7 cups were used with femoral stems and balls from seven different manufacturers.

In 1997, Livingston reported on 391 Hylamer7 liners that had been used in primary total hip replacements between January 1991 and December 1993.[14] Of these 391 cases, 191 were selected for examination based on the criteria of a 28-mm diameter and a femoral component made by either DePuy (Warsaw, IN) or Osteonics (Rutherford, NJ). Both cemented and cementless systems were used. These results were compared with those of 50 cases in which an Osteonics acetabular liner made of conventional UHMWPE was used in conjunction with an Osteonics femoral component. Table 4–2 summarizes the results in each of these four groups.

Table 4–2. COMPARISON OF RESULTS OF DIFFERENT PROSTHETIC GROUPS

Group	Stem Manufacturer	Femoral Head	Liner	Cement	No.	Age	Wear Rate (mm/yr)
1		CoCr		Yes	26	67	.13
				No	20	48	.29
1A	DePuy	Alumina	Hylamer	Yes	1	44	.33
				No	6	42	.33
2			Hylamer	Yes	114	67	.29
				No	24	44	.29
3	Osteonics	CoCr	Conventional	Yes	38	70	.12
				No	12	58	.12

CoCr = cobalt chromium.

The conclusion reached was that the average wear rate of all Hylamer liners in this study was greater than that of conventional UHMWPE, .27 versus .12 mm per year, respectively. However, on closer examination, there were many factors involved in addition to the type of UHMW-PE used in the acetabular liners. The patients could be divided into eight distinct groups based on combinations of cemented or cementless fixation, Hylamer7 or conventional UHMWPE, cobalt chromium (CoCr) or alumina femoral heads, and Depuy or Osteonics femoral heads. Table 4–2 presents a summary of the different prosthetic groups and wear rates reported. The patients who received Hylamer7 were also significantly younger than those who received conventional UHMWPE. These eight groups could be separated into two distinct wear rate regimes (<.13 mm/yr or >.29 mm/yr). The patients in the higher wear group could be categorized as young (<48 yr) and as having used either Hylamer7 liners or Hylamer7 rather than an Osteonics femoral head. The patients in the low wear groups were older than 58 years (with and without Hylamer7 liners). Although it is clear that Hylamer7 did not provide any clinical advantages over conventional UHMWPE, it is not possible to separate the effects of age, method of fixation, polyethylene type, or device manufacturer from these data. A more detailed discussion of the multifactorial nature of these results was provided by Schmalzreid.[24]

In contrast to the Livingston and Chmell reports described earlier, Sychertz reported that the clinical wear of Hylamer7 was less than that of conventional UHMWPE in a study that compared 80 Hylamer liners with 140 conventional UHMWPE liners.[28] In this study, all components were manufactured by Depuy (Warsaw, IN). In comparison with patients receiving conventional UHMWPE liners, patients receiving Hylamer liners were 10 years younger (54 vs. 64 years of age), were predominantly male (56% vs. 45%, respectively), and had a higher percentage of ceramic femoral heads (46% vs. 16%, respectively). Despite these differences, at average follow-up time of 3.6 years, the clinical wear rate of the Hylamer group was .15 mm per year versus .20 mm per year for the conventional group ($P < .10$). Some of this wear difference may have been due to differences in initial deformation between UHMWPE types because the difference in wear rates appeared to become smaller at longer implant times.

These data are in stark contrast to the early reports by Chmell and Livingston. The reason for the differences between the Livingston and Sychertz results is not clear. Nonetheless, it is clear that Hylamer did not appear to provide any greater clinical advantage than conventional UHMWPE. This experience should also serve as a reminder of the multifactorial nature of wear and of the fact that care must always be taken when the impact on clinical wear of any single variable, such as type of UHMWPE, is assessed.

Current View. Although there was no prospective clinical study, the reports discussed in the preceding paragraphs indicate that Hylamer did not appear to provide any long-term advantages over conventional UHMWPE. It is difficult to provide a true comparison of the clinical performance of Hylamer from the reported data, because covariables, such as patient age, femoral component manufacturers, or type of fixation prevent assessment of the effect of the material alone.

STERILIZATION METHODS

Since its commercial availability in the late 1960s, the dominant method for the sterilization of UHMWPE components has been gamma irradiation from a Co^{60} source. It has been known for some time that UHMWPE oxidizes after gamma sterilization and that physical properties may be adversely affected.[4,5,18,23] In the early 1990s, interest in oxidation was rekindled when factors that could influence the generation of particulate debris were sought out.[14–17] If the postirradiation aging is severe enough, the quality of a polyethylene component can be adversely effected, as evidenced by the presence of nonconsolidated particles, or the polyethylene can exhibit subsurface white bands on cross section.[10,13,15] In 1996, most manufacturers either modified the gamma sterilization process to minimize degradation or abandoned gamma sterilization in favor of nonirradiation methods such as ethylene oxide or gas plasma sterilization. It is important to note that these changes were made because of a desire to minimize degradation rather than wear.

It is now generally believed, in the vast majority of cases, that oxidation does not significantly or adversely influence clinical wear rate. This view is based on the reports described in the following paragraphs.

The rate of postirradiation aging of UHMWPE is very slow. It often takes more than 4 years of postirradiation aging for development of visible signs of degradation such as the formation of unconsolidated polyethylene particles or the presence of subsurface bands observed when components are sectioned for examination.[25] Because most devices are used less than 4 years after the time or sterilization, the on shelf oxidation is minimal.

There are no reports that can associate or correlate oxidation of UHMWPE with increased wear rate. In a report analyzing wear and oxidation levels of 100 retrieved Charnley acetabular cups, it was found that there was no correlation ($r^2 < .1$) between the oxidation state of the polyethylene and either radiographic or directly measured wear.

Hip simulation studies of acetabular cups with different postirradiation aging times up to 10 years showed that postirradiation did not affect the wear results.[26,29]

In three reports, the wear of gamma-irradiated (both in air and in inert atmosphere) inserts were shown to have thirty to forty-six percent lower hip simulator wear rates than inserts that were sterilized by ethylene oxide gas.[6,27] The reason for this result is that ethylene oxide gas causes neither degradation nor cross-linking of the polyethylene. These results demonstrate that the wear benefit of cross-linking is greater than any potential detriment of degradation.

Although oxidation does not appear to directly influence the wear rate of UHMWPE, it can be detrimental to the overall performance of either an acetabular cup or a tibial insert because oxidation does decrease the fracture toughness and fatigue resistance of the material (Fig. 4–1).

Current View. It is generally believed that gamma irradiation of UHMWPE is the preferred method of sterilization. Adverse effects of postirradiation aging are limited to decreased fracture and fatigue resistance and not to decreased wear. Postirradiation side effects can be minimized by irradiating components in a low oxygen environment (e.g., vacuum, nitrogen, Argon). The use of nonirradiation methods such as ethylene oxide gas provides products that do not oxidize because of irradiation and that have higher wear rates because of the lack of cross-linking.

EFFECT OF MANUFACTURING METHOD

As stated earlier, there are three methods of converting UHMWPE powder into an orthopedic bearing surface: machining of either (1) bar or (2) compression-molded sheet stock, or (3) direct molding of powder into the final form. The first report that the manufacturing method might play a role in clinical performance was made by Bankston et al., who compared the clinical wear rates of 162 TR28 (Zimmer, Warsaw, IN) total hip replacements with directly molded acetabular cups versus 74 Triad (Johnson and Johnson, St. Louis, MO) total hip replacements with machined acetabular liners. The average clinical wear rates were .05 mm per year for the TR28/ molded liners versus 12 mm per year for the Triad/ machined liners (*P* < .001).

Although the differences in wear are significant, there are too many cofactors (stem design, surgeon, etc.) to unequivocally attribute the lower wear of the TR28/molded group to the fact that the liners are directly molded. However, a hip simulator study published in 1996 compared the wear rates of directly molded cups made from 1900 resin with those of machined cups made from machined 4150 resin (HSS reference polyethylene).[1] All cups were gamma sterilized in air and articulated against a CoCr femoral head. Similar to the Bankston results, the molded 1900 cups had a 55 percent lower wear rate after 5 million cycles on the hip simulator (14 vs. 31 mg/million cycles).

Most recently, Ranawat et al. reported that the average linear head penetration rate for 235 directly molded, all polyethylene, cemented cups at a mean follow-up time of 6 years was .075 mm/year. This is 56 percent lower than the rate of .17 mm/year that he reported previously for the machined, uncemented, metal-backed cups of the same design.[21]

In addition to this apparent benefit of reduced wear, directly molded UHMWPE does not undergo postirradiation aging, even when the irradiation is done in the presence of oxygen. This has been shown for both retrieved and shelf-aged, directly molded tibial insert and acetabular liners after retrieval and shelf age times of more than 10 years.[7,8]

Current View. It appears that the manufacturing method can influence clinical wear. Directly molding acetabular cups with 1900 resin can provide wear rates 50 percent less than those of cups prepared by machining extruded non-1900 UHMWPE in both clinical and hip simulator environments.

THE LATEST IMPROVEMENTS: ELEVATED CROSS-LINKING

The most recent development in the effort to improve the wear performance of UHMWPE has been the use of high doses of irradiation to increase the levels of cross-linking. The concept was simply that if 24 to 40 kgrays could reduce the wear rate by 30 percent or more, a higher dose should provide more wear reduction. In the last three years, there have been more than 6 different new commercial products based on elevated cross-linking of UHMWPE. It should be noted that the use of elevated cross-linking to improve wear is not a new

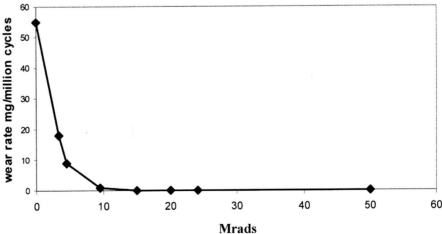

Figure 4–1. Wear rate of the ultrahigh molecular-weight polyethylene as a function of increasing dosage of gamma irradiation.

concept, and there are clinical reports of three examples of earlier cross-linking technology.

HISTORY OF HIGHLY CROSS-LINKED UHMWPE

Oonishi is credited with the first use of high-dose irradiation to reduce wear. It should be noted, however, that he used high-density polyethylene and not UHMWPE. Between 1971 and 1978, Oonishi implanted high-density polyethylene acetabular liners that had been irradiated at 100 Mrads.[19] The femoral components were made from COP alloy, which is stainless steel with 20 percent cobalt. The 100 Mrad dosage was determined via laboratory wear measurements of HDPE irradiated at many different doses. Several clinical series were conducted to compare the wear of unirradiated, highly irradiated, high-density polyethylene with the wear of stainless steel and ceramic femoral heads. It should be noted that cases in which the acetabular or femoral components were loosened or in which they migrated, metal-backed components and those not having well-defined radiographs were excluded from their evaluation. The results of the included cases are provided in Table 4–3.

The wear rate of highly cross-linked (100 Mrads) HDPE was less than that of unirradiated UHMWPE. However, the wear rate of highly cross-linked HDPE (.07 mm/yr) was not much lower than the .1 mm/year reported for UHMWPE irradiated at 2.5 to 4 Mrads. Further, the .07 mm/year rate is substantially higher than the 0 wear rate obtained from irradiating UHMWPE with doses greater than 20 Mrads. The .07 mm/year rate means that irradiating HDPE is either not the same as irradiating UHMWPE or that hip simulations underestimate the clinical wear for highly cross-linked UHMWPE.

In 1996, Wroblewski reported the clinical performance of XLP, which was UHWMPE which had been cross-linked with use of a silane coupling agent.[33] He implanted 19 XLP cups in 17 patients. He found that there was increased bedding in the period when the femoral head penetration into the liner was between .2 and .4 mm, which corresponded to an average head penetration rate of .29 mm/year. After 2 years, the average wear rate decreased to .022 mm/year. This was in contrast to the steady state (.07 mm/yr) of the metal against UHMWPE gamma sterilized between 2.5 and 4 Mrads.

The third example of an elevated cross-link cup was that of an acetabular cup that was exposed to 10 Mrad irradiation in the presence of acetylene gas. The acetylene gas was used to provide higher levels of cross-linking on the surface of the liner. Although more than 400 of these devices were implanted in the late 1970s and early 1980s, there is only complete clinical and radiographic follow-up of 61 cases. Of these 61 cases, 41 demonstrated no detectable wear, whereas the others demonstrated wear averaging .10 mm/year.

It is difficult to use these results for direct comparison with contemporary versions of elevated cross-linked products because of differences in starting material, femoral ball materials, and designs. These three examples suggest that clinical wear of elevated cross-linked cups may be higher than the nearly zero rate predicted by laboratory tests. It is also important to note that there are no long-term data in any of these cases to indicate that the types of elevated cross-linking technology used provided any overall clinical benefit.

CONTEMPORARY PRODUCTS

In the past few years, several manufacturers have introduced UHMWPE acetabular liners that have been irradiated above 4 Mrads with both electron beam and gamma irradiation. The wear rate of UHMWPE decreases with increasing gamma dosage, as seen in Figure 4–2. Note that there is little wear benefit in using gamma irradiation doses larger than 10 Mrads.

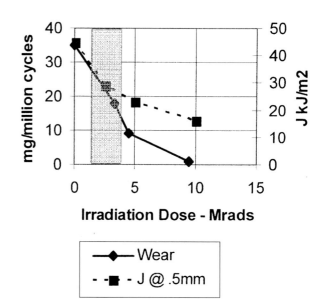

Figure 4–2. When considering decreased fracture toughness and enhanced wear, the optimum window of a gamma irradiation is between 2.5–4 Mrads.

Table 4–3. COMPARISON RESULTS

Stem	Femoral Ball	Polyethylene	No.	Wear Rate (mm/yr)
T28	T28	Nonirradiated UHMWPE	15	.25
SOM	SOM	100 Mrad HDPE	19	.076
SOM	Ceramic	Nonirradiated UHMWPE	71	.098
SOM	Ceramic	100 Mrad HDPE	9	.072

HDPE = high-density polyethylene; UHMWPE = ultra-high molecular-weight polyethylene.

References

1. Bennett AP, Wright TM, Li S: Global reference polyethylene: Characterization and comparison to commercial UHMWPE. Trans Orthop Res Soc 21:472, 1996.
2. Chmell MJ, Poss R, Thomas WH, Sledge CB: Early failure of Hylamer7 acetabular inserts due to eccentric wear. J Arthroplasty 11:351–353, 1996.
3. Dowd Sychertz CJ, Young Engh CA: Characterization of long term femoral head penetration rates: Association with and prediction of osteolysis. J Bone Joint Surg 82:1102–1107, 2000.
4. Eyerer P: Property changes of ultra high molecular weight polyethylene molecular weight polyethylene during Implantation. Trans Soc Biomater 8:184, 1985.
5. Eyerer P, Ke YC: Property changes of UHMW polyethylene hip endoprostheses during implantation. J Biomed Mater Res 21:275–291, 1987.
6. Furman BD, Lefebvre FK, Li S: Gamma irradiation does not adversely affect wear in total hip arthroplasty. Trans Soc Biomater 21:499, 1998.
7. Furman BD, Ritter MA, Li S: Effect of Polyethylene Type on Oxidation in Total Joint Replacement, [paper 479]. American Association of Orthopaedic Surgeons, 1997.
8. Furman BD, Ritter MA, Perone JB, et al: Effect of resin type and manufacturing method on UHMWPE oxidation and quality at long aging and implant times. Trans Orthop Res Soc 22:92, 1997.
9. Jahan MS, Wang C, Schwartz G, Davidson JA: Combined chemical and mechanical effects of free radicals in UHMWPE joints during implantation. J Biomed Mater Res 25:1005–1017, 1991.
10. Li S: The identification of defects in ultra high molecular weight polyethylene molecular weight polyethylene. Trans Orthop Res Soc 587, 1994.
11. Li S, Howard EG: Process for manufacturing ultra high molecular weight polyethylene molecular weight polyethylene shaped articles. U.S. Patent 5,037,928, issued August 6, 1991.
12. Li S, Nagy EV: Analysis of retrieved components via Fourier transform infrared spectroscopy. Trans Soc Biomater 13:274, 1990.
13. Li S, Saum K, Collier JP, Kazprzak D: Oxidation of UHMWPE over long time periods. Trans Soc Biomater 425, 1994.
14. Livingston BJ, Chmell MJ, Spector M, Poss R: Complications of total hip arthroplasty associated with the use of an acetabular component with a Hylamer7Liner. J Bone Joint Surg 79A:1529–1538, 1997.
15. Mayor MB, Wrona M, Collier JP, Jensen RE: The role of polyethylene quality in the failure of tibial knee components. Trans Orthop Res Soc 292, 1993.
16. McKellop HA, Liu B, Li S: Wear of acetabular cups of conventional and modification UHMWPE compared on hip joint simulator. Trans Orthop Res Soc 17:356, 1992.
17. Nagy EV, Li S: Fourier transform infrared spectroscopy techniques for the evaluation of polyethylene orthopaedic bearing surfaces. Trans Soc Biomater 13:109, 1990.
18. Nusbaum HJ, Rose RM: The effects of radiation sterilization on the properties of ultra high molecular weight polyethylene molecular weight polyethylene. J Biomed Mater Res 13:557–576, 1979.
19. Oonishi H, Takayama Y, Tsuh E: Improvement of polyethylene by irradiation in artificial Joints. Radiat Physics Chem 39:495–504, 1992.
20. Premnath V, Merrill E, Jasty M, Harris W: Melt irradiated UHMW-PE for total hip replacements: Synthesis and properties. Trans Orthop Res Soc 22:91, 1997.
21. Rasquinha VJ, Mohan V, Pardo LA, et al: Polyethylene Wear of Direct Compression Molded All Polyethylene Socket in Cemented Total Hip Arthroplasty. [poster PE334]. Sixty-eighth Annual Meeting, American Association of Orthopaedic Surgeons, 2001.
22. Rimnac CM, Wright TM, Klein RW, et al: Characterization of material properties of ultra high molecular weight polyethylene molecular weight polyethylene before and after implantation. Trans Soc Biomater Implant Retrieval Symp 15:16, 1992.
23. Roe RJ, Grood ES, Shastri R, et al: Effect of radiation sterilization and aging on ultra high molecular weight polyethylene molecular weight polyethylene before and after Implantation. J Biomed Mater Res 15:209–230, 1981.
24. Schmalzreid TP, Dorey FJ, McKellop HA: Commentary: Multifactorial nature of polyethylene wear in vivo. J Bone Joint Surg 80A:1234–1241, 1998.
25. Schroeder DW, Pozorski KM: Hip simulator testing of isostatically molded UHMWPE: Effect of EtO and gamma sterilization. Trans Orthop Res Soc 42:478, 1996.
26. Sommerich R, Flynn T, Schmidt MB, Zalenski E: The effects of sterilization on contact area and wear rate of UHMWPE. Trans Orthop Res Soc 42:486, 1996.
27. Sun DC, Schmidg G, Yau SS, et al: Correlations between oxidation, cross linking and wear performance of UHMWPE. Trans Orthop Res Soc 43:783, 1997.
28. Sycherts CJ, Shah N, Engh CA: Examination of wear in Duraloc acetabular components. J Arthroplasty 13:508–514, 1998.
29. Wang A. Polineni VK, Essner A, et al: Effect of shelf aging on the wear of ultra high molecular weight polyethylene molecular weight polyethylene acetabular cups: A 10 million cycle hip simulator study. Trans Orthop Res Soc 139, 1997.
30. Willert HG, Semlitsch M: Reactions of the articular capsule to wear products of artificial joint prostheses. J Biomed Mater Res 11:157–164, 1977.
31. Wright TM, Fukubayshi T, Burstein AH: The effect of carbon reinforcement on contact area, contact pressure and time-dependent deformation in polyethylene tibial components. J Biomed Mater Res 15:719–730, 1981.
32. Wright TM, Rimnac CM, Faris PM, Bansal M: Trans Orthop Res Soc 13:263, 1987.
33. Wroblewski BM: Prospective clinical and joint simulator studies of a new total hip arthroplasty using alumina ceramic heads and cross linked polyethylene cups. J Bone Joint Surg 78B:280–285, 1996.

5

The Articulation

•TIMOTHY M. WRIGHT and SUZANNE A. MAHER

THE NATURAL ARTICULATION

Restoration of function to diseased or damaged joints requires understanding of the dynamics, kinematics, mechanical properties, and shape of the opposing surfaces of a "normal" articulation. In a diarthroidal joint, cartilage surfaces roll and slide over one another, facilitated by the articular cartilage that covers the contacting surfaces and the synovial fluid that lubricates the joint. In the hip and shoulder, sliding predominates, whereas in the knee, both rolling and sliding occur simultaneously.[55]

The congruency of the joint surfaces contributes substantially to the kinematics of the joint. For example, the ball and socket configuration of the hip joint provides a stable, weight-bearing articulation but has only three degrees of freedom. The shoulder joint is another spheroidal joint, but because the humeral head is captured by much less of the glenoid than is the femoral head by the acetabulum, the joint is more susceptible to subluxation and dislocation. Thus, soft tissues forces (ligamentous constraints and muscle forces) play a significant role in stabilizing the joint. In even less conforming joints, soft tissue plays an even greater role. For example, in the knee, as the femur flexes on the tibia, its contact point on the tibia is displaced posteriorly; this action is controlled by the constraint provided by the posterior cruciate ligament, a motion allowed by the shapes of the joint surfaces.

A primary goal of joint arthroplasty is to provide normal function by selecting material combinations that provide a wear resistant, low-friction articulation in combination with surface profiles that are likened to the *natural joint*. However, depending on the degree to which the joint kinematics must be controlled to compensate for soft tissue insufficiency, the conformity, congruency, and constraint of the artificial joint are varied.

A BRIEF HISTORY OF ARTICULAR MATERIAL COMBINATIONS USED IN JOINT REPLACEMENTS

Significant advances in joint replacement over the past 100 years have led to outstanding clinical results, with reported survivorship of nearly 95 percent at 10 years for cemented hip replacements,[47] 87 percent at 12 years for total elbow prostheses,[72] 72 percent at 14 years for cemented total ankle replacements,[39] and 70 percent at 16 years for metacarpophalangeal joints.[15] The dominant long-term failure mechanism for joint replacements today, as was the case 100 years ago,[43] is implant loosening. The chronological order of events leading to implant loosening remains poorly understood (i.e., whether the loosening process is initiated by mechanical failure of the interfaces, by underlying bone, or by a biologic reaction to particulate wear debris).[50] However, it is now apparent that even the most well-fixed implant components are susceptible to failure in the face of submicron-sized wear particles and the periprosthetic osteolysis they induce. Although the wear problem has only recently gained overriding importance in improving the longevity of joint replacements, the history of joint replacement can be viewed as a quest to use materials that provide low friction with low wear rates (Fig. 5–1).

This chapter describes the concepts behind joint articular design and the choice of bearing material and considers how these concepts affect performance. The preclinical and clinical limitations of evaluating new joint articular materials and the future direction of joint evaluation are also addressed.

BASIC JOINT DESIGN CONSIDERATIONS

Designing the articulation of a joint replacement, as with any mechanical joint, requires consideration of both the shape (joint conformity and joint constraint) and the bearing materials used. Joint conformity describes how geometrically similar the two opposing joint surfaces are, whereas constraint describes the restriction in relative motion provided by the joint surfaces. For example, two perfectly flat surfaces are completely conforming (i.e., they both have an infinite radius of curvature), but they do not restrict relative motion (i.e., one surface could slide unconstrained in any direction on the other). However, two hemispheric surfaces could be made to be completely conforming (i.e., have the same radius of curvature), but the surfaces would be severely restricted in their relative motion (i.e., they would function as a three degree of freedom ball and socket).

Joint design is, for the most part, dictated by tradeoffs. In the knee joint, for example, the desire to control joint kinematics by choosing appropriate constraint must be counterbalanced against the desire to maintain sufficiently low bearing material stresses and implant fixation stresses by choosing appropriate conformity.

Of the material combinations that have been used in joint replacement, polyethylene—introduced to joint replacement in its high-density form by Sir John Charnley in the 1950s (see Fig. 5–1)—is arguably the only bearing material that has been universally accepted by the orthopedic community. Thus, joint design considerations are best discussed by focusing primarily on conventional articulations of metal on ultra-high-molecular-weight polyethylene (UHMWPE).

Tradeoffs in Knee Joint Design such as Wear Versus Function Versus Fixation

Knee joint design aims to recreate normal joint articulations by compensating for ligament insufficiency with joint conformity. Cruciate-preserving knee replacements are characterized by a low-conforming, low-constraint tibial tray, which offers little mechanical resistance to the action of the cruciate ligaments. Thus, joint stability is dependent on soft tissue tension rather than implant design. Taking low conformity to the extreme, a flat tibial component offers little resistance to translation of a curved femoral component; thus, tibial implant/bone interface shear stresses are minimized. However, because the contact area between the femoral prosthesis and the tray is at a minimum, polyethylene stresses in the tibial tray are at a maximum.

If the joint is made more toroidal or condylar because the tibial tray has been made more concave in order to better match the curved shape of the femoral component, polyethylene stresses are reduced (Fig. 5–2A), dramatically so if conformity in the medial/lateral direction is increased.[6] Lower polyethylene stresses reduce the tendency for the articular surfaces to pit or delaminate. However, the increased conformity increases resistance to femoral anteroposterior and medial-lateral sliding and internal and external rotation (see Fig. 5–2B) and causes transfer of increased shear forces to the implant interfaces. The tradeoff between the requirement for reduced polyethylene contact stresses and reduced fixation stresses is illustrated in Figure 5–2C and D.

Solutions to this tradeoff have stirred the controversy over the preservation or sacrifice and substitution of the posterior cruciate ligament (PCL). PCL substitution designs are advocated by those who believe that retaining the PCL does not help to maintain normal rollback kinematics[73] and that the unpredictable functionality of the retained PCL has a negative influence on the longevity of designs that rely on it for stability.[74] Many contemporary knee designs, even those that save the PCL, now employ articular surface design with increased joint conformity to compensate for the loss of stability. Designs that sacrifice the PCL usually compensate for its function by employing a cam and spine mechanism to ensure femoral rollback; these are the so-called posterior-stabilized designs.[34]

Reduced polyethylene stresses result from increased conformity (Fig. 5–2A), but implant fixation stresses are dependent on how much the joint kinematics induced by the articulation surfaces oppose the kinematics induced by surrounding soft tissue. Thus, fixation site

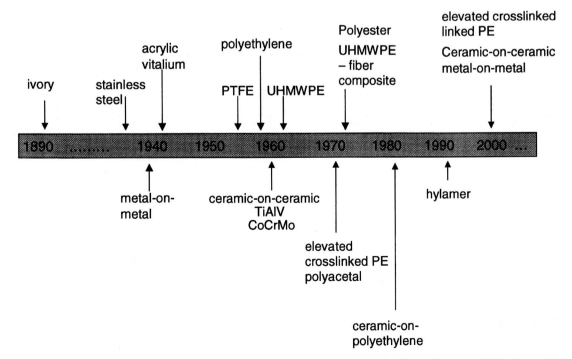

Figure 5–1. Bearing materials introduced over the past 100 years. (From Wright and Li, 2000; LeVay 1990; Wiles, 1958; Charnley, 1961.)

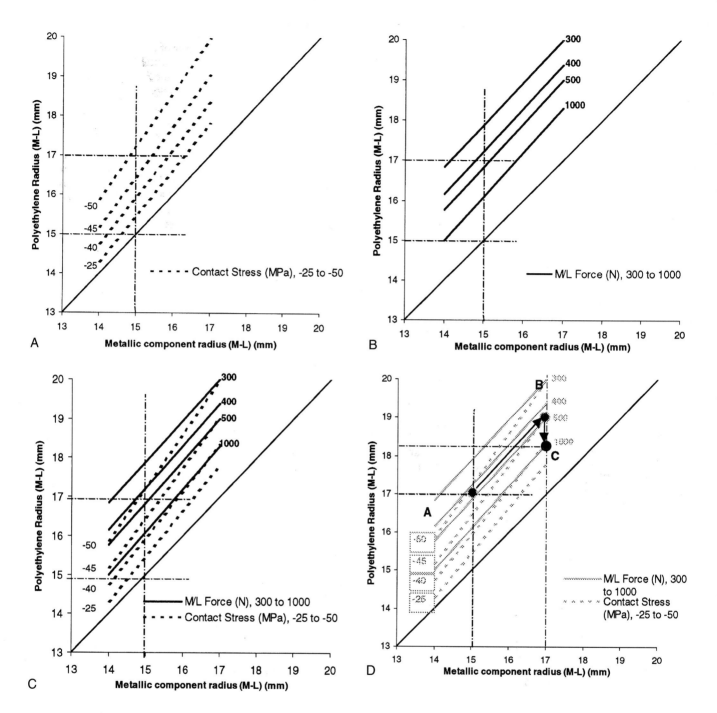

Figure 5–2. A, The effect of conformity between the metallic femoral component and the polyethylene tibial tray, on the poly-ethylene contact stresses, as generated from a finite element model (modified after Burnstein and Wright, 1994 from data produced by Don Bartel). Consider a perfectly conforming joint with metallic and polyethylene radii of 15 mm. This results in contact stresses of less than 25 MPa. If the radius of the polyethylene tibial tray is increased to 17 mm, the contact stress increases to about 50 MPa. Note: the applied load was 3000 N, and the polyethylene thickness was 7 mm. **B,** The effect of conformity between the metallic femoral component and the polyethylene tibial tray, on the M/L force – in other words, the force on the implant fixation site. Consider a perfectly conforming joint with metallic and polyethylene radii of 15 mm. This results in M/L forces in excess of 1000 N. If the radius of the polyethylene tibial tray is increased to 17 mm, the M/L forces decrease to about 500 N. **C,** The effect of conformity between the metallic femoral component and the polyethylene tibial tray, on the M/L force *and* on the contact stresses. **D,** The trade-offs associated with conformity between the metallic femoral component and the polyethylene tibial tray, on the M/L force *and* on the contact stresses. Consider a metallic component of 15 mm M-L radius, used with a tibial tray with 17 mm M-L radius: this results in M/L forces of 500 MPa and contact stresses of 50 N. To keep the M/L forces constant, but decrease the contact stresses, the polyethylene radius is increased from 17 mm to over 18 mm: this results in contact stresses of 45 N. If we are willing to sacrifice an increase in the forces at the implant fixation (M/L force) to 1000 N, we can further reduce the contact stresses to 40 N.

stresses are sensitive to surgical technique in relation to implant orientation.[60]

In an attempt to reduce implant fixation stresses, mobile-bearing designs combine high conformity (thereby lowering polyethylene stresses) with a second articulation between the back face of a tibial polyethylene insert and a metallic tray (reducing implant/bone interface stresses). Clinical results have shown little propensity for increased wear from the creation of a second articulation,[5] although laboratory tests indicate that the amount of wear is dependent on the allowable motions of the mobile bearings.[36] Clinical fluoroscopic studies have demonstrated that mobile bearing designs often have abnormal kinematics,[70] suggesting that current mobile bearing designs do not adequately account for the remaining soft tissue constraints.

Tradeoffs in Hip Joint Design: Wear Versus Stability Objectives

Total hip design aims to create a stable joint with a wide range of functional motion.[41] Maintaining the ball-and-socket geometry of the natural hip, few design choices remain to affect a metal on polyethylene articulation: femoral head size, clearance between the head and the acetabular component, and thickness of the acetabular component polyethylene. For example, wear of such a conforming articulation is dominated by abrasive and adhesive mechanisms that become more prevalent as contact pressure and sliding distance increase.[3] Femoral head size directly affects sliding distance; a 45-percent increase in head diameter (from 22 mm to 32 mm) causes a 45-percent increase in sliding distance for the same range of motion, with a concomitant increase in wear.[44] Thus, the increased stability afforded by a large head diameter is offset by the possibility of increased wear.

Similarly, the head-to-neck ratio can influence the articulation. As head-to-neck ratio increases, so too does the range of motion before impingement,[53] and hence stable range of motion. Impingement is a prevalent occurrence in hip arthroplasty, however, and can result in pitting and burnishing damage at the impingement site[26,81] as well as the potential for increased wear caused by increased stresses on the opposing wall of the acetabular component and by increased ingress of abrasive third-body particles.[63]

Replacement of Other Joints: Shoulder and Elbow

Designs for articulation of other joints, such as the shoulder and elbow, require consideration of the same types of tradeoffs as in the hip and knee. The goal remains to provide natural function while minimizing wear and maintaining fixation of the implant component to the surrounding bone. Pioneered by Neer in the 1950s, shoulder replacement has become an accepted treatment,[68] although more hemiarthroplasties (typically for treatment of complex fractures of the proximal humerus) are performed than total shoulder replacements. The articulation for a total shoulder joint must possess many of the features found in total knee replacement. The shoulder has a very large range of motion, and surrounding tissues provide more stability than bony geometry. The humeral head translates onto the glenoid by as much as 8 mm.[58]

To allow humeral head translation and to protect the implant/bone interface from loosening, unconstrained or minimally constrained shoulder joints are advocated. Indeed, unconstrained shoulder joints have historically had lower loosening rates than constrained joints.[66] However, as with knee implant design, the advantages of a minimally conforming, minimally constrained joint are at the expense of increased polyethylene stresses. Providing more joint constraint through the use of a polyethylene-on-metal articulation, which is much more conforming than the natural joint, leads to unacceptably high failure rates.[1]

The development of elbow prostheses has been likened to that of total knee joints.[27] Hinged designs were initially used; however, after high loosening rates at the cement/bone interface, total elbow replacement became dominated by partially constrained and semiconstrained ("sloppy" hinge) designs. Partially constrained, unlinked prostheses (e.g., the capitellocondylar prosthesis[61]) were designed to reproduce the anatomy of the ulna-humerus joint so that joint stability mainly relied on surrounding soft tissues. The competing objectives of low polyethylene stresses versus low interfacial stresses pose the same problem as encountered in total knee joints.

Hinged elbow designs, on the other hand, impart joint stability without relying on soft tissues. The articulation in a hinged joint is between a metallic axle and a polyethylene bushing. Sloppy hinge designs (e.g., the Coonrad-Morrey prosthesis[54]) seek to impart joint stability by striking a balance between soft tissue and the geometry of the articulation.[57] Sloppy hinge elbow designs may allow stable prosthesis/bone fixation; however, the large loads transferred to the hinge can result in increased bushing wear rates and increased likelihood of hinge dislocation; Madsen et al.,[47] for example, found significant bushing wear in clinically retrieved Pritchard-Walker sloppy hinge implants.

In summary, the wear performance record of total joint replacements suggests that although the wear problem can be minimized by attention to design, the need for appropriate kinematics limits the improvements that can be achieved. Effective designs therefore result in large contact stresses and long sliding distances, placing an extreme mechanical burden on the bearing materials.

BEHAVIOR OF CONVENTIONAL AND ALTERNATIVE ARTICULAR MATERIALS

For the purposes of the present discussion, the designation of *conventional* is restricted to variations of (UHMWPE) that articulate against metallic alloys (cobalt-chrome-molybdenum alloys, titanium-aluminum-vanadium alloys, or stainless steel). Polyethylene has undergone changes since it was first adopted for use in joint replacement in 1961. When it was introduced, polyethylene was a high-density material with molecular weight in the 500,000 range as opposed to today's UHMWPE, which has molecular weights exceeding four million. Because the newly introduced elevated cross-linked polyethylenes have the same basic chemistry, they are considered conventional as well.

All other material combinations are designated as *alternative* bearing materials. Alternative bearings have been advocated primarily for use in total hip replacement. Included in this usage are bearing combinations of ceramic (either alumina or zirconia) on polyethylene, ceramic on ceramic (alumina-on-alumina), and metal-on-metal (cobalt alloy-on-cobalt alloy). The respective advantages and disadvantages of both conventional and alternative bearings have been discussed in a number of excellent publications,[1,4,14,35,65,84,88] and are briefly summarized in Table 5–1.

Osteolysis: The Most Severe Local Effect Caused by Articulation

The significant bone resorption around implants noted on radiographs was initially attributed to a host reaction to bone cement (so-called *bone cement disease* attributed to the early work of Willert and colleagues). Later attention was focused on polyethylene wear as the culprit, but since the early 1990s, a considerable body of clinical and experimental evidence has been gathered to demonstrate that osteolysis can stem from a host reaction to wear debris from any origin, and hence the more correct terminology is *particle disease*.[28] The realization that particles generated from the articular surface could threaten implant stability has initiated widespread research into the host response to particles. Although many of the details remain unknown, the course of particle disease appears to begin with the attempt of macrophages to phagocytoze particulate debris. The cells in turn release various cytokines and other mediators of osteolysis.[24]

The macrophage response to particles is dictated to a large extent by the size, shape, and volume of particles present. The critical particle size to activate a macrophage response is believed to range from 0.2 μm to as large as 10 μm.[25,33] Because the wear mechanisms that occur in joint replacements depend on both design and bearing material, both factors affect particle size and, ultimately, the occurrence of osteolysis. For example, Shanbhag et al.[67] found that UHMWPE particles isolated from around failed knee joints (both cemented and uncemented) were predominantly spherical and ranged from 0.1 μm to 18 μm; 90 percent of the particles, however, were less than 3 μ in size, and 98 percent less than 10 μ. Shanbhag and colleagues also found that the distribution of particle sizes generated from failed knee replacements was skewed toward much larger particles than those isolated from around a comparative series of failed hip replacements (Fig. 5–3). Larger particles

Table 5–1. ADVANTAGES, DISADVANTAGES, AND UNKNOWNS ASSOCIATED WITH CONVENTIONAL AND ALTERNATIVE BEARING COMBINATIONS

Metal on Conventional Polyethylene		
Advantages	*Disadvantages*	*Unknowns*
History of clinical performance spanning 40 years	Potential for osteolysis	How can its wear characteristics be improved?
History of use in many design configurations	Aging characteristics	
History of use with many femoral head materials	Behavior after sterilization	

Metal on Elevated Cross-linked Polyethylene		
Advantages	*Disadvantages*	*Unknowns*
Low in vitro wear rates	Very short term follow-up	Clinical relevance of decreased fracture toughness
	Cost	Performance of new designs is unknown (e.g., performance of liner locking mechanisms)
		Impingement behavior

CERAMIC ON CERAMIC

Advantages	*Disadvantages*	*Unknowns*
Hydrophilic material	History of fracture, particularly of the femoral head	Influence of decreased fracture toughness on performance
Low friction articulation	Design sensitive	Design dependency
No ridges around scratches		Impingement and dislocation behavior
Suitable for young patients		Ease of clinical use
Less volume of particles generated: less osteolysis		

Metal on Metal		
Advantages	*Disadvantages*	*Unknowns*
Low wear rates in vitro	History of high loosening rates	Impingement behavior
Nanometer-sized particles: small risk for osteolytic response	Remote infiltration of wear particles	Systemic effect
	Scratch sensitive	

released from knees compared with hips support the dominance of pitting and delamination as damage modes on knee-bearing surfaces, as opposed to the adhesive and abrasive wear mechanisms that dominate in hip replacements. The tendency for a greater number of

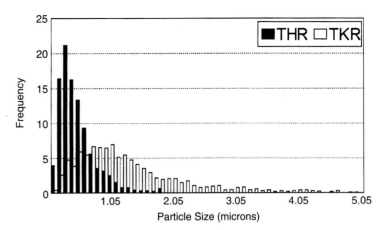

Figure 5–3. A schematic of the distribution of particle sizes found around failed total hip replacements and failed total knee replacements. (Adapted from data of Arun S. Shanbhag.)

large particles (too large for phagocytosis) to be present around knees may explain the lower incidence of osteolysis seen around knee implants.[51]

Other bearing materials generate submicron particles as well. Metallic particles of about 0.7 μm have been characterized by Maloney et al.[48] for titanium alloy and cobalt-chrome alloy articulations with UHMWPE. Lee et al.[42] characterized particles of 0.8 to 1.0 μ by 1.5 to 1.8 μ from titanium alloy cobalt chrome alloy, and stainless steel articulations with UHMWPE. Metal-on-metal articulations generate particles in the nanometer range,[17,23] which is thought to be below the threshold likely to elicit an osteolytic response.

Submicron-sized particles have been found from hip simulator studies of elevated cross-linked polyethylene acetabular cups.[21] However, the number of particles generated from in vitro simulations is significantly less than that found with conventional UHMWPE material.[19] Particles generated from ceramic-on-ceramic articulations have been found to range from 0.13 μm to 7.2 μm.[83] Despite initial suggestions that ceramic particles would be bioinert,[14] the biologic response to ceramic particles has been similar to that of other particles of comparable size[4] with the ability to elicit osteolysis.[83] However, the number of ceramic particles generated in a ceramic-on-ceramic hip joint is considerably less than the number of polyethylene particles generated in a conventional metal-on-UHMWPE joint,[9,56] possibly explaining the more benign biologic reaction compared with that observed with alumina-on-polyethylene and metal-on-polyethylene joints.[29] Despite the decreased biologic response, Sychertz et al.[71] found no difference in the radiographically measured wear performance of alumina over cobalt-chrome femoral heads when they were articulated with UHMWPE, emphasizing that a reduction in the biologic response to wear debris is only one of many factors that can influence implant longevity.

Systemic Effects

Debris generated from the articulation may also have systemic effects, particularly in young patients in whom joint replacements remain in place for long periods of time. Metallic bearing materials are the most worrisome

in this regard[35] because they can be transported as ionic species and because several of the metallic elements are present in forms that are detrimental biologically (e.g., vanadium and chromium). In a review of the systemic effect of orthopedic implants,[84] six reasons are given for why investigations into metal release from implants have taken on an increased level of urgency:

1. Identification of deposition of extensive metallic particulate debris in local and remote tissues
2. Reintroduction of metal-on-metal articulations
3. Observation of crevice corrosion processes in modular and multipart metallic joint replacement components (e.g., the amount of crevice corrosion in the modular femoral total hip replacement components was correlated with elevations in serum cobalt and urine chromium)[35]
4. Continued popularity of porous-coated cementless devices with high specific surface energies
5. Concern that metal degradation products could act directly as a stimulus to osteolysis by macrophage activation and indirectly by accelerating polyethylene debris generation
6. Realization that the serum transport of metallic degradation products is greater than has been previously appreciated (e.g., higher levels of chromium metal ions were found in the serum and urine of metal-on-metal hip replacement patients than were found in the serum and urine of patients with conventional bearing-material hip replacements).[30]

The toxicologic long-term consequences of elevated metallic ion levels are as yet unknown. It is difficult to attribute a particular systemic reaction to the presence of an implant; most events caused by systemic and remote toxicity can be expected to occur in a certain percentage of patients regardless of the presence of an implant.[84]

Modularity: Other Forms of Articulations

Implant modularity allows the following:

- Customization of generic implants for individual patients (e.g., choice of a modular head with a greater offset to increase stability in a patient with a total hip replacement)

- Use of alternative bearing materials that would not be suitable for implant fixation (e.g., a ceramic head for better wear press-fitted onto a porous-coated metallic stem for biologic fixation)
- More options should revision surgery be necessary (e.g., revising a worn UHMWPE liner in an otherwise well-fixed acetabular shell)
- Reduction in implant fixation stresses (e.g., mobile bearing knee replacements).

However, modularity can have disadvantages as well, depending on the bearing material used. The assembly of a ceramic liner into a metallic shell requires firm pressure to engage the taper lock, but with shock loading such pressure could generate critical flaws in the ceramic.[85] Similarly, care is required when metal-on-metal articulations are assembled; scratches on the bearing surfaces of either component can increase wear.

Modularity associated with conventional metal-on-UHMWPE total joint replacements can also be problematic. For example, polyethylene acetabular liners for total hip replacement are less sensitive to shock loading than ceramic liners, but failure can still occur if the locking mechanism between the liner and the shell fails, leading to liner dislodgment.[16] In fact, a potential shortcoming of elevated cross-linked polyethylenes is their decreased fracture toughness compared with conventional UHMWPE,[18] which causes concern for locking mechanisms that use polyethylene tabs or other features that rely on the material's resistance to fracture.

Modular metallic interfaces can add to the wear problem. Fretting—the micromotion that occurs between the interface under high loads—causes wear.[62] Corrosion and subsequent release of corrosion product also occur in the interface regions[38] and are accelerated by removal of the passive layer that protects the bulk material from the physiologic environment. Backside burnishing of UHMWPE components has been reported in acetabular components from total hip replacements and tibial components from fixed bearing total knee replacements.[22,31] The direct contribution of backside wear to clinical failures has not been well established, however. It remains to be seen whether the backside wear that may be associated with mobile bearing knees will significantly affect long-term performance (see section on tradeoffs in knee design).

Loosening and Loss of Stability

Although wear has been the primary reason for the introduction of new bearing materials in an effort to increase the longevity of joint replacements, alternative bearing material combinations may also influence implant longevity from another important standpoint: bone stress distribution. For example, acetabular loosening remains a serious clinical problem in hip arthroplasty. What role does increasing the stiffness of the acetabular liner (e.g., use of ceramic instead of UHMW-PE) play in changing load transfer from the component to the adjacent cancellous bone? Little work has been done in investigating such effects, although clinical evidence suggests that the problem could be important. In a retrospective analysis of the performance of 131 ceramic-on-ceramic total hip replacements, Sedel et al.[65] found survivorship (with failure measured as revision) of 93 percent at 12 years for patients younger than 40 years of age, whereas patients older than 40 years of age had a survivorship of only 83 percent at 12 years. Whether or not the counter-intuitive improved performance of ceramic-on-ceramic hip replacements in young patients could be associated with a more favorable bone stress distribution for bone/implant ingrowth and subsequent bone remodeling is unknown.

When the stability of an implant is compromised, the nature of the articulation dynamics alters. Load vectors change in magnitude and direction, and the location of contact forces deviates from the original path. In such situations, the ability of the implant components to continue to function depends in part on how the bearing materials perform. For conventional metal-on-UHMW-PE bearings, a bedding-in phase occurs that is caused by a combination of wear and of plastic deformation and creep of the polyethylene, with an increased rate of generation of wear debris immediately postoperatively in both hip[20] and knee joint replacements.[76] In the case of knee replacements, any change in the location of the contact area between the femoral and tibial component as a result of the bedding-in phase initiates new areas of contact. The potential for significant additional polyethylene wear debris generation is increased by the discontinuity between the initial worn area and the newly worn area.

Impingement Behavior

In a series of retrieved acetabular implants that were revised because of loosening, Yamaguchi et al.[81] found evidence of impingement in 40 percent of cases. Similarly, Shon et al.[82] found that 56 percent of retrieved acetabular liners showed evidence of impingement. Although repetitive cyclic impingement of the femoral neck on the rim of a UHMWPE liner may generate wear debris, the polyethylene deforms locally, thereby cushioning the impact. Alternative bearings using hard-on-hard articulations do not have this characteristic; thus, the impact forces at impingement are transferred more directly to the implant/bone interface. In the case of a metal-on-metal articulation, wear debris may result from the repetitive impingement of the neck on the liner.[30] Indeed, Iida et al.[32] reported a case of severe metallosis after only 1 year of implantation resulting from impingement of the femoral neck on the metallic shell (Fig. 5–4).

The concern for the brittle nature of ceramics has led to design modifications in ceramic-on-ceramic total hip replacements. The possibility of ceramic liner fracture resulting from repetitive neck/liner contact is a daunting prospect. To avoid fracture altogether, designs have been introduced in which the rim of the metallic

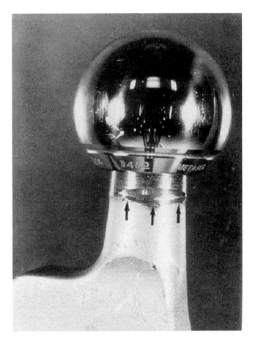

Figure 5–4. Retrieved femoral component showing a groove 11.7 mm long, 2.5 mm wide and 1.0 mm deep on the anteroinferior aspect of the neck caused by impingement of the neck on the metal acetabular shell. The patient exhibited severe metallosis. (From Iida H, Kaneda E, Takada H, et al: Metallosis due to impingement between the socket and the femoral neck in a metal-on-metal bearing total hip prosthesis. J Bone Joint Surg 81A:400–403, 1999, with permission.)

acetabular shell is elevated beyond the rim of the ceramic liner or in which a protective polyethylene layer is included to cushion impingement should it occur. Fortunately, few cases of ceramic liner fracture have been reported, and although retrieved Mittelmeier implants exhibited wear at the site of impingement, little evidence of fracture was found (Fig. 5–5). Metal-metal impingement has the potential to generate considerable additional wear debris. Again, the consequence of the reduced fracture toughness of elevated cross-linked UHMWPEs versus conventional polyethylene on impingement-type behavior is worrisome. Indeed, few hypotheses about alternative bearing material behavior under impingement-type load conditions compared with conventional materials have been tested, primarily because no accepted method exists for testing liners under impingement type loading.

Implant Surface Finish

Femoral head surface finish is typically described in orthopedic literature by quoting an R_a value (i.e., a *roughness average* value), which describes the distribution of peaks and valleys on a surface about a mean diameter. Falez et al.[87] measured the R_a of new femoral heads and found that ceramic heads had a more homogeneous and smooth surface compared with other materials (e.g., zircon [0.0152 μm] alumina heads [0.0129 μm], cobalt-chrome-molybdenum [0.0204 μm], cobalt-chrome with surface treatment with nitrogen ions

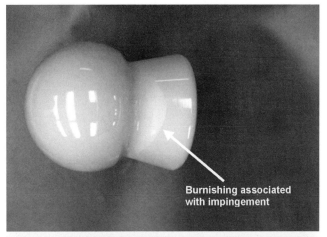

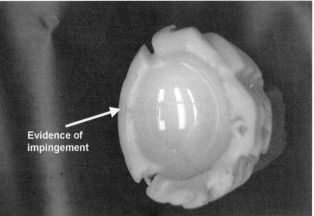

Figure 5–5. Retrieved ceramic component with evidence of impingement.

[0.0196 μm]). Minakawa et al.[52] measured the mean height of scratches (R_{pm}) on the damaged areas of retrieved femoral heads and also found smoother surfaces on ceramic heads ($R_{pm} = 0.023$ μm for alumina heads) compared with stainless steel heads ($R_{pm} = 0.400$ μm), titanium heads ($R_{pm} = 0.556$ μm) and cobalt-chrome heads ($R_{pm} = 0.446$ μm). They also found that the R_{pm} value was strongly correlated with wear volume as measured by in vitro wear tests. However, clinically, the association between femoral head roughness and wear generation appears less strong.[20]

SUMMARY

No material and design combinations for the articulations formed in total joint replacement have been proven superior. All have advantages and disadvantages (Table 5–1), and for now, the conventional articulation of metallic alloys on UHMWPE remains the clinical gold standard, having provided reasonable performance over implant lifetimes approaching thirty years. Renewed interest in alternative bearing combinations, such as metal-on-metal and ceramic-on-ceramic stem from the development of improved manufacturing processes[1,78] and quality assurance standards.[12]

Preclinical Limitations in Establishing Efficacy of "New" Articulations

Despite the efforts of regulatory agencies such as the Food and Drug Administration to establish safety and efficacy of medical devices before commercialization, failures in new technology introduced to the medical device marketplace remain too common an occurrence. New bearing materials, for example, have received approval from the Food and Drug Administration and been rapidly adopted by the market, but they have just as rapidly disappeared as premature failures were reported in the clinical literature. Two examples include Hylamer,[64] an enhanced form of UHMWPE intended to improve wear resistance of total hip replacements in acetabular components and Poly II, a carbon-reinforced UHMWPE[79] introduced into both hip and knee replacements with the same goal–better wear resistance than conventional UHMWPE.

The failure to predict the poor clinical performance of these materials before their introduction to the orthopedic community underscores shortcomings in the screening of bearing materials by means of preclinical evaluation. The usefulness of preclinical testing depends on how well the test simulates the clinical situation.[75] Ideally, preclinical testing should emphasize dominant failure modes and establish the performance of a new material (or design) in comparison with materials (or designs) known to have given satisfactory clinical performance.

Challenges to designing such tests include the following:

- Identifying dominant failure modes
- Knowing the magnitudes and directions of joint forces to simulate a worst-case scenario
- Understanding the temporal order of events that lead to implant failure
- Capturing the variability in implant performance found in vivo
- Combining biologic phenomena into mechanical testing
- Validating the test and the test conditions

Just learning about load magnitudes and directions is a formidable challenge. Few in vivo measurements of joint forces exist, and these were gathered primarily from studies of joint forces across the hip that used telemetrized implants.[7,40] No such data exist for knee replacements. Currently, consortium groups are in the process of combining clinically derived criteria with experimental and computational techniques, to find preclinical test methods that can test implant performance more effectively. An example of this process is demonstrated by a European Consortium project funded by the Standards, Measurement, and Testing program of the European Commission: contract SMT4–CT96–2076.[69] The consortium aims to use experimental and computational techniques to develop preclinical test cemented hip replacement implants.

Clinical Limitations in Establishing Efficacy of "New" Articulations

The current limitations in preclinical testing of new or alternative bearings direct more emphasis on post-market surveillance for establishing safety and efficacy. Unfortunately, adequate evaluation of joint replacements can require 5 to 10 years of follow-up. The problem is how to find the best way to introduce new technology without placing undue burdens on industry and, at the same time, to safeguard surgeons and their patients.

Few answers to this quandary currently exist. Radiostereometric analysis (RSA) has shown a strong correlation between implant migration 2 years postoperatively and subsequent premature failure resulting from loosening.[37] Experimentally, increased inducible migrations have been associated with increased loosening rates as measured clinically,[46] suggesting that such a technique might prove useful in preclinical testing of implant fixation. However, the true potential of RSA techniques lies in the ability to measure the wear rates of different bearing materials. This could pave the way for prospective randomized clinical trials in which all variables except the articulating surface material will be kept constant. The influence of an alternative bearing material on implant loosening rates could then be quantitatively assessed. This potential benefit has been discussed,[86] and initial studies on the applicability of RSA to this problem have been presented,[10] but, to date, RSA techniques have not been used extensively for this purpose.

Registry studies (e.g., the Swedish Hip Register[47]) have helped to identify and inform surgeons about implants with loosening rates that are higher than acceptable. The majority of implants fail because of loosening; however, the Swedish Hip Register does not identify the articular material associated with specific implant performance. Malchau et al.[47] recently reported that polyethylene wear accounted for only 0.5 percent of all hip revisions in Sweden. However, because exchange of an acetabular liner and/or femoral head component is not considered a revision, this percentage could be much higher. As these materials gain more popularity, the inclusion of alternative bearing materials as implant design variables should be an important consideration for registries.

Elevated cross-linked polyethylene materials have been introduced to the orthopedic market on the basis of the negligibly low wear rates found on in vitro simulator tests.[59] However, in contrast to the in vitro results, Martell et al.[49] found that volumetric wear rates of elevated cross-linked liners averaged 54 ± 70 mm^3/year 2 years postoperatively. The cause for the disparity between in vivo and in vitro results is unclear. However, for this alternative bearing material, as for others, widespread use on the basis of largely invalidated laboratory studies is risky. It is only through prospective randomized clinical studies that the true benefits of using alternative bearing materials can be assessed.

References

1. Amstutz HC, Grigoris P: Metal on metal bearings in hip arthroplasty. Clin Orthop S11–S34, 1996.
2. Amstutz HC, Thomas BJ, Kabo JM, et al: The Dana total shoulder arthroplasty. J Bone Joint Surg 70:1174–1182, 1988.
3. Archard JF: Contact and rubbing of flat surfaces. J Appl Phys 24:981–988, 1953.
4. Archibeck MJ, Jacobs JJ, Black J: Alternate bearing surfaces in total joint arthroplasty. Biologic Consideration. Clin Orthop 379:12–21, 2000.
5. Argenson J, O'Connor JJ: Polyethylene wear in meniscal knee replacement. A one to nine-year retrieval analysis of the oxford knee. J Bone Joint Surg 74B:228–232, 1992.
6. Bartel DL, Bicknell VL, Wright TM: The effect of conformity, thickness and material on stresses in ultra-high molecular weight components for total joint replacement. J Bone Joint Surg 68A:1041–1051, 1986.
7. Bergmann G, Graichen F, Rohlmann A: Hip joint forces in sheep. J Biomech 32:69–77, 1999.
8. Bizot P, Nizard R, Lerouge S, et al: Ceramic/ceramic total hip arthroplasty. J Orthop Sci 5:622–627, 2000.
9. Bohler M, Mochida Y, Bauer TW, et al: Wear debris from two different alumina-on-alumina total hip arthroplasties. J Bone Joint Surg 82B:901–909, 2000.
10. Bragdon CR, Yuan X, Perinchief R, et al: Precision and reproducibility of radiostereometric analysis (RSA) to determine polyethylene wear in a total hip replacement model. Trans Orthop Res Soc 2001, p 1005.
11. Burnstein AH, Wright TM: Fundamentals of Orthopaedic Biomechanics. Baltimore, Williams and Wilkins, 1994.
12. Cales B, Stefani Y: Risks and advantages in standardization of bores and cones for heads in modular hip prostheses. J Biomed Mater Res 43:62–68, 1998.
13. Charnley J: Arthroplasty of the hip. A new operation. Lancet 1:1129–1132, 1961.
14. Christel PS: Biocompatability of surgical-grade dense polycrystalline alumina. Clin Orthop 282:10–18, 1992.
15. Cook SD, Beckenbaugh RD, Redondo J, et al: Long-term follow-up of pyrolytic carbon metacarpophalangeal implants. J Bone Joint Surg 81A:635–648, 1999.
16. Della Valle AG, Ruzo PS, Li S, et al: Dislodgment of polyethylene liners in first and second-generation Harris-Galante acetabular components. J Bone Joint Surg 83A:553–559, 2001.
17. Doorn PF, Campbell PA, Worrall J, et al: Metal wear particle characterization from metal on metal total hip replacements: Transmission electron microscopy study of periprosthetic tissues and isolated particles. J Biomed Mater Res 24:103–111, 1998.
18. Duus LC, Walsh HA, Gillis AM, et al: A comparison of the fracture toughness of cross linked UHMWPE made from different resins, manufacturing methods and sterilization conditions. Trans Soc Biomat 384, 2000.
19. Edidin AA, Pruitt L, Jewett CW, et al: Plasticity-induced damage layer is a precursor to wear in radiation-cross-linked UHMWPE acetabular components for total hip replacement. J Arthroplasty 14:616–627, 1999.
20. Elfick AP, Smith SL, Unsworth A: Variation in the wear rate during the life of a total hip arthroplasty simulator and retrieval study. J Arthroplasty 15:901–908, 2000.
21. Endo MM, Barbour PS, Barton DC, et al: Comparative wear and wear debris under three different counterface conditions of crosslinked and non-crosslinked ultrahigh molecular weight polyethylene. J Biomed Mater Eng 11:23–35, 2001.
22. Engh GA, Koralewicz LM, Pereles TR: Clinical results of modular polyethylene insert exchange with retention of total knee arthroplasty components. J Bone Joint Surg 82A:516–523, 2000.
23. Firkins PJ, Tipper JL, Saadatzadeh MR: Quantitative analysis of wear and war debris form metal-on-metal hip prostheses tested in a physiological hip joint simulator. J Biomed Mater Eng 11:143–157, 2001.
24. Gelb H, Schumacher HR, Cuckler J, et al: In vivo inflammatory response to polymethylmethacrylate particulate debris: Effect of size, morphology, and surface area. J Orthop Res 12:83–92, 1994.
25. Green TR, Fisher J, Stone M, et al: Polyethylene particles of a 'critical size' are necessary for the induction of cytokines by macrophages in vitro. Biomaterials 19:2297–2302, 1998.
26. Hall RM, Siney P, Unsworth A, Wroblewski BM: Prevalence of impingement in explanted Charnley acetabular components. J Orthop Sci 3:204–208, 1998.
27. Hargreaves D, Emery R: Total elbow replacement in the treatment of rheumatoid disease. Clin Orthop 366:61–71, 1999.
28. Harris WH: Osteolysis and particle disease in hip replacement: A review. Acta Orthop Scand 65:113–123, 1994.
29. Henssge EJ, Bos I, Willman G: Al_2O_3 against Al_2O_3 combination in hip endoprostheses. Histological investigations with semiquantitative grading of revision and autopsy cases and abrasion measures. J Mater Sci 5:657–661, 1994.
30. Hodge WA, Harman MK, Banks SA, et al: Early clinical experience with a contemporary metal-on-metal total hip arthroplasty: A USA multicenter collaboration. Scientific exhibition, AAOS, 2001.
31. Huk OL, Bansal M, Betts F, et al: Polyethylene and metal debris generated by non-articulating surfaces of modular acetabular components. J Bone Joint Surg 76B:568–574, 1994.
32. Iida H, Kaneda E, Takada H, et al: Metallosis due to impingement between the socket and the femoral neck in a metal-on-metal bearing total hip prosthesis. J Bone Joint Surg 81A:400–403, 1999 .
33. Ingham E, Fisher J: Biological reactions to wear debris in total joint replacement. Proc Inst Mech Eng 214:21–37, 2000.
34. Insall JN, Lachiewicz PF, Burstein AH: The posterior stabilized condylar prosthesis: A modification of the total condylar design. Two to four-year clinical experience. J Bone Joint Surg 64A:1317–23, 1982.
35. Jacobs JJ, Urban RM, Gilbert JL, et al: Local and distant products from modularity. Clin Orthop 319:91–105, 1995.
36. Jones VC, Barton DC, Fitzpatrick DP, et al: An experimental model of tibial counterface polyethylene wear in mobile bearing knees: The influence of design and kinematics. J Biomed Mater Eng 9:189–96, 1999.
37. Karrholm J, Borssen B, Lowenhielm G, Snorrason F: Does early micromotion of femoral stem prostheses matter?—4–7 year stereoradiographic follow-up of 84 cemented prostheses. J Bone Joint Surg 76-B:912–916, 1994.
38. Kawalec JS, Brown SA, Payer JH, Merritt K: Mixed-metal fretting corrosion of Ti6Al4V and wrought cobalt alloy. J Biomed Mater Res 39:867–873, 1995.
39. Kofoed H, Sørensen TS: Ankle arthroplasty for rheumatoid arthritis and osteoarthritis. Prospective long-term study of cemented replacements. J Bone Joint Surg 80B:328–332, 1998.
40. Kotzar GM, Davy DT, Berilla J, Goldberg VM: Torsional loads in the early postoperative period following total hip replacement. J Orthop Res 13:945–955, 1995.
41. Krushell RK, Burke DW, Harris WH: Elevated-rim acetabular Components. Effect on range of motion and stability in total hip arthroplasty. J Arthroplasty 6(Suppl):S53–S58, 1991.
42. Lee JM, Salvati EA, Betts F, et al: Size of metallic and polyethylene debris particles in failed cemented total hip replacements. J Bone Joint Surg 74:380–384, 1992.
43. LeVay D: The History of Orthopaedics. An Account of the Study and Practice of Orthopaedics from the Earliest Times to the Modern Era. The Parthenon Publishing Group, Pearl River, NY, 1990.
44. Livermore J, Ilstrup D, Morrey B: Effect of femoral head size on wear of the polyethylene acetabular component. J Bone Joint Surg 72A:518–528, 1990.
45. Madsen F, Sojbjerg J, Sneppen O: Late complications with the Pritchard Mark 2 elbow prosthesis. J Shoulder Elbow Surg 3:17–23, 1994.
46. Maher SA, Prendergast PJ: Discriminating cemented femoral hip prostheses through migration and inducible displacement measurements [in press].
47. Malchau H, Herberts P, Söderman P, Odén A: Prognosis of total hip replacement. Update and validation of results form the Swedish National Hip Arthroplasty Registry 1979–1998. Scientific exhibition AAOS, 2000.
48. Maloney WJ, Smith RL, Schmalzried TP: Isolation and characterization of wear particles generated in patients who have had failure of a hip arthroplasty without cement. J Bone Joint Surg 77:1301–1310, 1995.

49. Martell J, Edidin A, Dumbleton J: Preclinical evaluation followed by randomized study of a crosslinked polyethylene for total hip arthroplasty at two year follow-up. Trans Orthop Res Soc 2001, p 1005.

50. McGee MA, Howie DW, Neale SD, et al: The role of polyethylene wear in joint replacement failure. Proc Inst Mech Engs 211:65–71, 1997.

51. Mikulak SA, Mahoney OM, dela Rosa MA, Schmalzried TP: Loosening and osteolysis with the press-fit condylar posterior-cruciate-substituting total knee replacement. J Bone Joint Surg 83A:398–403, 2001.

52. Minakawa H, Stone MH, Wroblewski BM, et al: Quantification of third-body damage and its effect on UHMWPE wear with different types of femoral head. J Bone Joint Surg 80B:894–899, 1998.

53. Morrey BF: Instability after total hip arthroplasty. Orthop Clin North Am 23:237–248, 1992.

54. Morrey BF, Adams RA, Bryan RS: Total replacement for post traumatic arthritis of the elbow. J Bone Joint Surg 73B:607–612, 1991.

55. Mow VC, Flatow EL, Foster RJ: Biomechanics. *In* Simon SS (ed): Orthopaedic Basic Science. American Academy of Orthopaedic Surgeons, 1994.

56. Nevelos JE, Prudhommeaux F, Hamadouche M, et al: Comparative analysis of two different types of alumina-alumina hip prosthesis retrieved for aseptic loosening. J Bone Joint Surg 83B:598–603, 2001.

57. O'Driscoll SW, An KN, Korinek S, Morrey BF: Kinematics of semi-constrained total elbow arthroplasty. J Bone Joint Surg 74B:297–299, 1992.

58. Poppen NK, Walker PS: Normal and abnormal motion of the shoulder. J Bone Joint Surg 58A:195, 1976.

59. Reis MD, Scott ML, Sauer WL: Relationship between the gravimetric wear and particle generation in hip simulators: Conventional versus crosslinked polyethylene, Scientific exhibit AAOS, 2001.

60. Rosenberg N, Henderson I: Medium term outcome of the LCS cementless posterior cruciate retaining knee replacements. Follow-up and survivorship study of 35 operated knees. Knee 8:123–128, 2001.

61. Ruth JT, Wilde AH: Capitellocondylar total elbow replacement. J Bone Joint Surg 74A:95–100, 1992.

62. Salvati EA, Lieberman JR, Huk OL, Evans BG: Complications of femoral and acetabular modularity. Clin Orthop Rel Res 319:85–93, 1995.

63. Scifert CF, Brown TD, Pedersen DR, et al: Development and physical validation of a finite element model of total hip dislocation. Comput Methods Biomech Biomed Eng 2:139–147, 1999.

64. Scott DL, Campbell PA, McClung CD, Schmalzried TP: Factors contributing to rapid wear and osteolysis in hips with modular acetabular bearings made of hylamer. J Arthroplasty 15:35–46, 2000.

65. Sedel L, Nizard RS, Kerboull L, Witvoet J: Alumina-alumina hip replacement in patients younger than 50 years old. Clin Orthop 298:175–183, 1994.

66. Severt R, Thomas BJ, Tsenter MJ, et al: The influence of conformity and constraint on translational forces and frictional torque in total shoulder arthroplasty. Clin Orthop 292:151–158, 1993.

67. Shanbhag AS, Bailey HO, Hwang DS, et al: Quantitative analysis of ultrahigh molecular weight polyethylene (UHMWPE) wear debris associated with total knee replacements. J Biomed Mater Res 53:100–110, 2000.

68. Skirving AP: Total shoulder arthroplasty—current problems and possible solutions. J Orthop Sci 4:42–53, 1999.

69. Standards, Measurement and Testing Programme of the European Commission Contract SMT4-CT96–2076: "Pre-clinical testing of cemented hip replacement implants: Pre-normative research for a European standard."

70. Stiehl JB, Dennis DA, Komistek RD, Keblish PA: In vivo kinematic analysis of a mobile bearing knee prosthesis. Clin Orthop 345:60–6, 1997.

71. Sychterz CJ, Engh CA, Young AM, et al: Comparisonof in vivo wear between polyethylene liners articulating with ceramic and cobalt chrome femoral heads. J Bone Joint Surg 82B:48–951, 2000.

72. Trail IA, Nuttall D, Stanley JK: Survivorship and radiological analysis of the standard Souter-Strathclyde total elbow arthroplasty. J Bone Joint Surg 81B:80–84, 1999.

73. Uvehammer J, Karrholm J, Brandsson S: In vivo kinematics of total knee arthroplasty. Concave versus posterior-stabilised tibial joint surface. J Bone Joint Surg 82B:499–505, 2000.

74. Wada M, Tatsuo H, Kawahara H, et al: In vivo kinematic analysis of total knee arthroplasty with four different polyethylene designs. Artif Organs 25:22–28, 2001.

75. Walker PS, Blunn GW, Perry JP, et al: Methodology for long-term wear testing of total knee replacements. Clin Orthop 372:290–301, 2000.

76. Walker PS, Sathasivam S: Design forms of total knee replacement. Proc Inst Mech Eng. Part H. 214:101–119, 2000.

77. Wiles P: The surgery of the osteo-arthritic hip. Br J Surg 45:488–497, 1958.

78. Willmann G: The evolution of ceramics in total hip replacement. Hip Int 4:193–203, 2000.

79. Wright TM, Astion DJ, Bansal M, et al: Failure of carbon fiber-reinforced polyethylene total knee components: Report of two cases. J Bone Joint Surg 70A:926–932, 1988.

80. Wright TM, Li S: Biomaterials. *In* Buckwalter JA, Einhorn TA, Simon SR (eds): Orthopaedic Basic Science, 2nd ed. Rosemont, IL, American Academy of Orthopaedic Surgeons, 2000.

81. Yamaguchi M, Akisue T, Bauer TW, Hashimoto Y: The spatial location of impingement in total hip arthroplasty. J Arthroplasty 15:305–313, 2000.

82. Shon WY, Wright TM, Baldini T, et al: Impingement in total hip arthroplasty: A study of retrieved acetabular components. Trans 47th ORS, 2001, p 1070.

83. Yoon TR, Rowe SM, Jung ST, et al: Osteolysis in association with a total hip arthroplasty with ceramic bearing surfaces. J Bone Joint Surg 80A:1459–1468, 1998.

84. Jacobs JJ, Goodman SB, Sumner DR, Hallab NJ: Biological Response to Orthopaedic Implants, Orthopaedic Basic Science, 2nd ed. American Academy of Orthopaedic Surgeons, 2000.

85. Hummer CD, Rothman RH, Hozack WJ: Catastrophic failure of modular zirconia-ceramic femoral head components after total hip arthroplasty. J Arthroplasty 10:848–850, 1995.

86. Linder L: Implant stability, histology, RSA and wear—more critical questions needed. A view point. Acta Orthop Scand 65:654–658, 1994.

87. Falez F, La Cava F, Panegrossi G: Femoral prosthetic heads and their significance in polyethylene wear. Int Orthop 24:126–129, 2000.

88. McKellop H, Shen FW, DiMaio W, Lancaster JG: Wear of gamma-crosslinked polyethylene acetabular cups against roughened femoral balls. Clin Orthop 369:73–82, 1999.

6

Individual Host Response to Foreign Materials

• BERNARD F. MORREY and MARK E. BOLANDER

Although poorly understood, the interaction of foreign body and host response is becoming a source of increasing interest. Clinical observation strongly suggests some variation in the manner and extent to which the host is influenced by and reacts to the presence of a foreign body. Pettersen observed that from 1966 to 1992, a total of 14,000 articles appeared in the literature regarding artificial implants; during the same period, 11,000 articles were written regarding allergic hypersensitivity and immunology.[12] However, only 45 articles appeared in the literature that addressed both topics. This has changed somewhat in the past few years.

Host response to a foreign stimulus takes one of several forms. The first category of adverse host response is an allergic hypersensitivity response to a material constituent of the implant. The second category of host response is a cell-mediated reaction to the materials of the implant. The third category is a toxic-type response to the implant, which is not mediated by the immune system. An example from the first category of host reaction is that of metal allergies. An example from the second category is that of macrophage responses to particulate debris. An example from the third category of adverse host response is the toxic effect of excess methyl methacrylate monomer on cells adjacent to the cement.

There is increasing awareness of the fact that the ultimate fate of a prosthetic joint replacement in some patients may be related to the individual host response characteristics to the implant itself or to wear particles. If the reaction to the device is dependent on individual host responses, potential treatment options may need to be based on this relationship as well.

HYPERSENSITIVE REACTION TO FOREIGN MATERIAL

Most orthopedic surgeons have had experience with clinical examples of what appear to be uncommon host responses to implants, which have led to loosening and failure of the devices (Fig. 6–1). In some, the loosening and failure may be explained as an atypical host response caused by a hypersensitivity reaction to foreign material (see Fig. 6–4).

Mechanisms

Exposure to an allergen that produces a hypersensitive state is the definition of an allergic response. The host may respond to an allergen by one of two cellular mechanisms. The first is by B-cell activation of the humeral immune system, and the second is by T-cell activation of cell-mediated immunity.

Several distinct clinical expressions of these allergic reactions have been described, and they are classified into four recognized types: type 1, anaphylactic reaction; type 2, cytotoxic hypersensitivity (transfusion reaction); type 3, complex-mediated hypersensitivity; and type 4, delayed hypersensitivity. Of these, only the latter two have clear orthopedic implications.[12]

Complex-Mediated Immune Response (Type 3)

The so-called type 3 reaction is characterized by activation of the complementary system in response to an antigen-antibody complex. Tissue-destructive enzymes are released as part of the cellular response to this complex. The cellular and histologic features typical of this response have been observed in 3 of 30 instances of atypical loosening of total hip arthroplasty reported by Langlais et al.[9] (as per Pettersen[12]). However, corroborative reports are limited, and it is believed that this type of immune response must represent a rare cause of implant failure. A report by Nakamura et al.[11] has provided strong evidence of the development of antibodies to red cells associated with metallosis.

Cell-Mediated Immunologic Response-Delayed Hypersensitivity (Type 4)

Best expressed clinically as contact dermatitis, this T-cell-mediated response is characterized by mononuclear

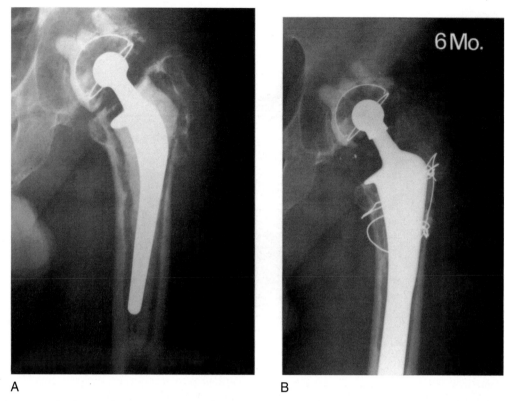

A   B

Figure 6–1. A 65-year-old man underwent a cemented hip replacement with adequate bone-cement interface. After 2 years, gross and progressive loosening occurred (**A**). This does not appear to be based on wear particles, nor does it have a mechanical explanation. Note that the acetabulum was intact at the time of revision (**B**).

cell infiltrates, including phagocytes and lymphocytes. Assays of the blood and urine reveal consistently increased concentrations of the metallic components of prostheses in these tissues, suggesting the possibility of developing toxicity or sensitivity to these agents.[1,4,5] Increased concentrations of virtually all of the metallic constituents of prosthetic devices have been reported, but vanadium concentration appears to be particularly high.[2]

Host response progresses to and is characterized by granuloma formation. Two distinct types of granulomatous bone have been recognized. In the first instance, granuloma formation follows what appears to be a common pathway of host response to particulate debris.[18] This reaction has no characteristics of B- or T-cell lymphocyte-mediated allergic reactions. The second type of granuloma reveals evidence of B- and T-cell lymphocytes, which are typically associated with hypersensitivity reaction. This form of reaction may be demonstrated by positive skin patch test results elicited by the constituent parts of the prostheses. Goldring further speculates that such responses may explain why some patients suffer pain from implants without an obvious source for the pain. He also speculates that such instances may eventually end in early loosening and revision.[18] In the experimental setting, particulate polymethylmethacrylate (PMMA) was demonstrated to incite a macrophage-initiated response that did not require the presence of lymphocytes.[8]

Clinical Implications

That the body may adversely react to foreign materials is well documented. Some materials, such as Teflon, elicit an intense reaction in virtually all patients. Other materials are well tolerated except in those patients who have a hypersensitivity to the agent. In this setting, the response can be so intense as to cause an obvious and deleterious result.

Other than specific case reports, only relatively small sample groups of patients have been studied with regard to constituent allergy. In a carefully controlled assessment of 66 patients, 15 percent developed a positive patch test reaction to one or more constituents of the prosthesis. Of the 10 control subjects who had positive test results, 1 (10 percent) developed aseptic loosening. In the control group, 5 percent had evidence of allergy to the elements tested before the prosthesis was inserted.[2] In a larger sample of 220 implants, 6 percent of the patients developed sensitivity to nickel, cobalt, or chromium. Fourteen percent of those with failed devices had positive patch test reactions to one or more of the metallic constituents. Although few studies report a frequency of implant sensitivity approaching the 28 percent reported by Bensen et al.,[1] it is likely that type 4 sensitivity develops in about 10 to 15 percent of patients. However, the implications referable to loosening are not clear.[2,4,5] In fact, sample groups of patients with known allergies to one or more components of the implant may exhibit no evidence of loosening or other expression of adverse host response.[3]

The issue is further clouded by the report of Rooker and Wilkinson, who observed that five of six patients with positive patch test results to nickel, chromium, or cobalt before implantation had negative test results after the procedure.[13] At this time, therefore, it may be reasonable to accept the fact that type 4 cell complex-mediated hypersensitivity does occur but is an infrequent, if not rare, cause of implant loosening (Fig. 6–2).

It is of interest to note that an allergic response to PMMA has also been documented in the four studies that specifically investigated this possibility.[2,4] One study was able to detect an allergic response to

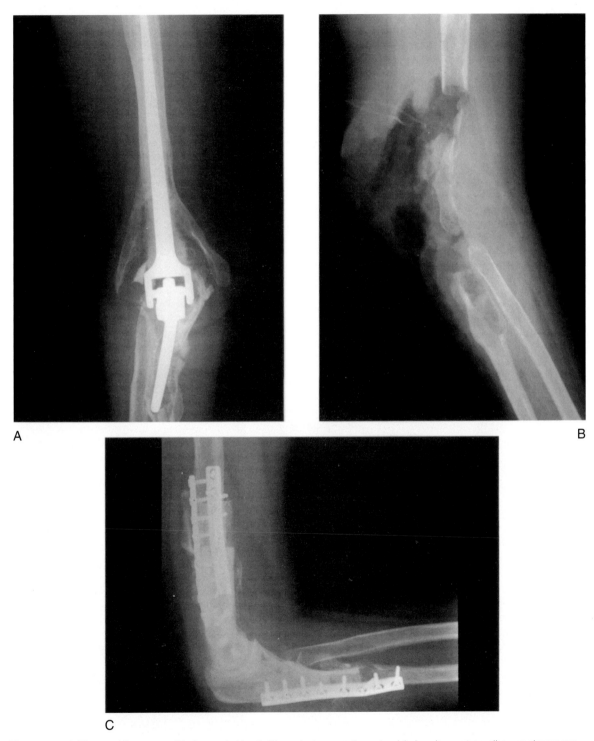

A

B

C

Figure 6–2. A 59-year-old woman with rheumatoid arthritis and a known allergy to nickel underwent an elbow replacement with a prosthesis comprised of nickel, cobalt, and chrome. **A**, After 4 years, both implants showed gross destruction. **B**, Extensive resection was required. **C**, Concern that this gross reaction may have been caused by the nickel allergy prompted an allograft replacement of the elbow.

N,N-dimethylparatoluidine (DMT), an accelerator used in bone cement. This response was directly correlated to early loosening.[7]

NONALLERGIC HOST RESPONSE TO PARTICULATE DEBRIS

Based on the foregoing discussion, there is little question that host sensitivity to the constituent materials of prosthetic joints does occur. There is considerable uncertainty as to the significance of this response, yet marked host response variation is seen after prosthetic replacement. Hence, it is reasonable to consider that clinically significant variability may be mediated as a nonallergic host response. Our understanding of the significance of particulate debris is continuing to develop, but observed clinical variations of implant integrity and survival prompt the question of whether this variation in intensity of response may be explained by factors of individual host response (Fig. 6–3). Radiographic observation of osteolysis is believed to be the most characteristic expression of the host response to particulate debris. This manifestation of bone resorption has, to date, been explained largely as a nonallergic granuloma formation that is dependent on the volume and rate of debris generation. However, the varied response to apparently similar radiographic expressions of wear is puzzling (Fig. 6–4). Because the mechanism by which particles induce osteolysis has not yet been fully explained, we should remain open to the prospect that individual response variation exists in a spectrum of particulate exposures.

Clinical Expression of Wear Debris Reaction

Most authorities believe that there is a "common final pathway" whereby a similar sequence of events occurs in reference to results in osteolysis regardless of what precise particle or biologic result mediates the reaction: PMMA, polyethylene, or metal.[15–17] It is generally accepted that the chief variables accounting for the specific response are the rate of generation of the debris and the size and shape of the particle.[10,14–17] Willert and his co-investigators have observed debris production, tissue reaction, host foreign body identification, and granuloma formation with osteolysis as a very consistent, reproducible process.[17] They believe that the response variation is due to mechanical factors, such as the amount and the size of the particles, rather than to individual host characteristics. This position is supported by Murray and Rushton,[10] who have shown that the variation in the amount of bone resorption is dependent on the particle type. Because phagocytosis of the particulate matter is mediated by prostaglandin E$_2$ production, these investigators concluded that all particles activate the macrophages in a similar fashion.[10] This line of reasoning supports the concept that the volume of particles released is the major factor initiating macrophage activation and hence bone resorption.

As noted earlier, an alternative argument was put forward by Goldring, who suggested two distinct types of granuloma reaction to foreign material, nonimmune and immune.[6] The immune granuloma is characterized by the identity of B- and T-cell lymphocytes, whereas the nonimmune granuloma is a volumetric response to nondigestable particles. Concern that response to wear

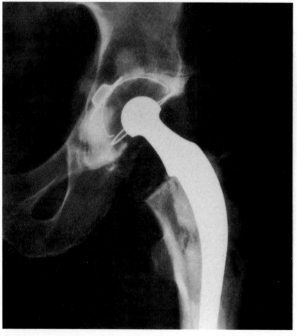
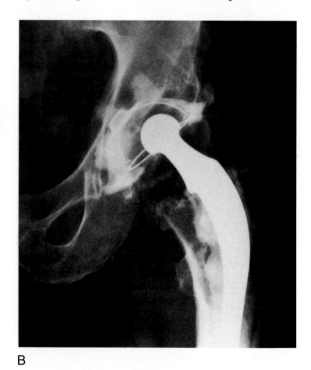

A   B

Figure 6–3. **A,** Cemented Charnley hip replacement 2 years after surgery. **B,** Significant acetabular wear revealed relatively little osteolysis at 15 years.

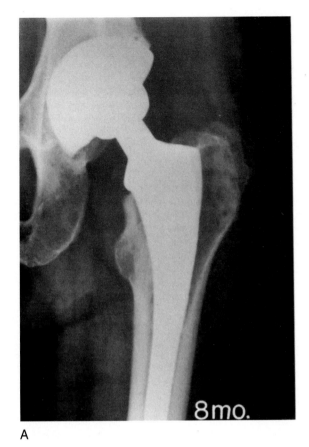
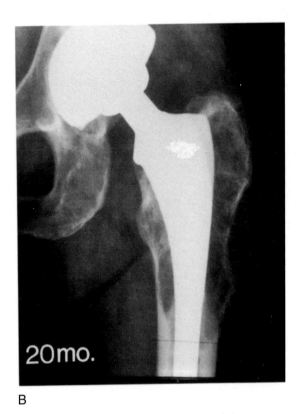

A   B

Figure 6–4. Patient with an uncemented titanium hip replacement after 8 months (**A**) shows the marked osteolytic response that replaced the entire proximal femur, with little radiographic evidence of wear after 20 months (**B**).

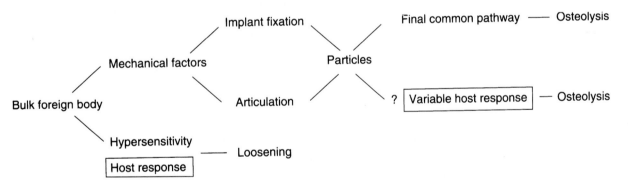

Figure 6–5. Potential sites of action of implant loosening influenced by host response variation.

debris may have individual host response features is supported by findings from our laboratory, which show regions of T-cell lymphocytes in the membrane of loose and reconstructed hip joints.[18]

The unanswered but central question is whether these granulomata form solely in response to the rate and size of debris particles, as most commonly suggested,[10,14,15] or whether nonallergenic individual host response occurs at the cellular level. The latter question is the topic of ongoing investigations. The issue may be summarized by the allergic versus nonallergic responses that were clinically observed to have occurred (Fig. 6–5). The issue of individual host response will benefit from

the exciting development in genetic research applied to the musculoskeletal system.

References

1. Bensen MKD, Goodwin PG, Bristoff J: Metal sensitivity in patients with joint replacement arthroplasties. Br Med J 4:374, 1975.
2. Cancilleri F, De Giorgis P, Verdoia C, et al: Allergy to components of total hip arthroplasty before and after surgery. Ital J Orthop Traumatol 18:407, 1992.
3. Carlsson A, Moller H: Implantation of orthopaedic devices in patients with metal allergy. Acta Derm Venereol 69:62, 1989.
4. Deutman R, Mulder TJ, Brian R, Nater JP: Metal sensitivity before and after total hip arthroplasty. J Bone Joint Surg 59A:862, 1977.

5. Elves MW, Wilson JN, Scale JT, Kemp HBS: Incidence of metal sensitivity in patients with total joint replacements. Br Med J 4:376, 1975.

6. Guyuron B, Lasa CI: Reaction to stainless steel wire following orthognathic surgery. Plast Reconstr Surg 89:540, 1992.

7. Haddad FS, Cobb AG, Bentley G, et al: Hypersensitivity in aseptic loosening of total hip replacements. The role of constituents of bone cement. J Bone Joint Surg 78B:546, 1996.

8. Jiranek W, Jasty M, Wang JT, et al: Tissue response to particulate polymethylmethacrylate in mice with various immune deficiencies. J Bone Joint Surg 77A:1650, 1995.

9. Langlais F, Postel M, Berry JP, et al: L'intolérance aux debris d'usure des prosthéses. Int Orthop 4:145, 1986.

10. Murray DW, Rushton N: Macrophages stimulate bone resorption when they phagocytise particles. J Bone Joint Surg 72B:988, 1990.

11. Nakamura S, Yasunaga Y, Ikuta Y, et al: Autoantibodies to red cells associated with metallosis—a case report. Acta Orthop Scand 68:495, 1997.

12. Pettersen AH: Allergy and hypersensitivity. *In* Morrey BF (ed): Biological Material and Mechanical Considerations of Joint Replacement. New York, Raven Press, 1993, p 353.

13. Rooker GD, Wilkinson JD: Metal sensitivity in patients undergoing hip replacement. J Bone Joint Surg 62B:502, 1980.

14. Wang JT, Goldring SR: The role of particulate orthopaedic implant materials in peri-implant osteolysis. *In* Morrey BF (ed): Biological Material and Mechanical Considerations of Joint Replacement. New York, Raven Press, 1993, p 119.

15. Willert HG, Bertram H, Buchhorn HG: Osteolysis in the alloarthroplasty of the hip: Role of bone and cement fragmentation. Clin Orthop Rel Res 258:108, 1990.

16. Willert HG, Buchhorn HG: Particle disease due to wear of ultrahigh molecular weight polyethylene. *In* Morrey BF (ed): Biological Material and Mechanical Considerations of Joint Replacement New York, Raven Press, 1993, p 87.

17. Willert HG, Buchhorn HG, Semlitsch M: Particle disease due to wear of metal alloys. *In* Morrey BF (ed): Biological Material and Mechanical Considerations of Joint Replacement. New York, Raven Press, 1993, p 425.

18. Witkiewicz H, Turner R, Rock M, et al: The local cellular response of components of total hip arthroplasty experiencing osteologies. *In* Morrey BF (ed): Biological Material and Mechanical Considerations of Joint Replacement. New York, Raven Press, 1993, p 129.

7

Oncogenesis and Foreign Materials

· MICHAEL G. ROCK

The introduction of implants to stabilize fractures and replace diseased joints has revolutionized orthopedic practice and afforded millions of patients levels of function that otherwise would not be achieved. Although the metal alloys that constitute these implants exhibit excellent resistance to corrosion, oxidation of these large components ultimately produces chlorides, oxides, and hydroxides in combination with particulate metal matter that is disseminated into the surrounding environment. Efforts to reduce the possibility of fatigue failure have included foraging, isostatic pressing, and ion implantation to produce a superior metal microstructure, thereby minimizing surface delamination. Additionally, modifications have been made to the plastic articulating segments to produce a much more consistent ultra-high-molecular-weight polyethylene. The perceived need to improve implant wear and design has been largely precipitated by the excessive soft tissue staining noted by orthopedic surgeons at the time of fixation removal or revision joint arthroplasty. The presence of particulate metal matter, polyethylene, and even fragments of polymethylmethacrylate in local tissue has been confirmed.[9,24,29] In spite of all of the modifications made in implant composition, implant fixation, and articulation, corrosion of these products persists.[1,6,17,43]

PHYSIOLOGIC RESPONSE TO DEBRIS

The body's response to the local presence of debris is dependent on the size and amount of the debris, as well as the rate of accumulation. The body attempts to neutralize these foreign particles by precipitating granulomatous foreign body reactions and/or removing them through local lymphatic channels. If the local accumulation of debris exceeds the body's ability to neutralize and/or transport it, the debris migrates from the site to remote areas, including the bone-cement or bone-implant surfaces, possibly contributing to if not initiating the phenomenon of loosening and osteolysis (Fig. 7–1).

Of equal or possibly even greater concern is the detection of metal ions, polyethylene, and even methylmethacrylate in areas remote from the implant, including serum, urine, and regional draining lymph nodes. Elevated serum levels of metal ions consistent with the composition of the implanted alloy have been confirmed in the experimental model[44] and in humans after total hip arthroplasty,[4] identifying serum levels of chromion, nickel, and titanium that are two- and three-fold higher than preoperative determinations. These figures are within the widely accepted normal range for these metallic ions in the human. Therefore, it is assumed that toxic levels of these foreign materials do not materialize. However, when the serum-to-urine concentration in patients subjected to conventional total hip arthroplasty is analyzed, it has become apparent that the urinary concentration of chromate in particular does not rise with the same magnitude as the serum level. This would suggest that the rise in serum values of metal ions, which occurs within the first several weeks postoperatively, exceeds the urinary ability to excrete them; therefore, it is entirely plausible that metal ions can accumulate in organs and tissues remote from implantation and that these concentrations, unlike those in the systemic circulation, could increase as a result of the unidirectional, intracellular ingestion of these particles.

Evidence for metallic debris accumulating in distant organs has been confirmed by Langkamer et al.[8,22] who identified widespread dissemination of particulate wear debris from hip prostheses to lymph nodes, liver, and spleen. They reported increases above normal levels in these organs of 30-fold for aluminum, chromium, and iron in the lymph node, and 10-fold in the spleen and liver. This was previously suggested by Steineman,[33] who calculated the potential release of metallic ions of 0.15 to 0.3 µg/cm²/day, which translates to between 11 and 22 mg/year in patients with total hip replacement. This incidentally coincides with the total body burden of such metallic ions in a 70-kg man. These findings suggest that concentrations of metal ions at remote sites may reach such proportions as to precipitate *altered cellular dynamics* in organs principally of the lymphoreticular system. It would only be logical to assume that local concentrations of such debris at the site of implantation would be even higher, although attempts at quantifying local concentrations have been fraught with inaccuracies, mostly resulting from sampling error and the inability to measure bioavailable or nonbioavailable metal species.

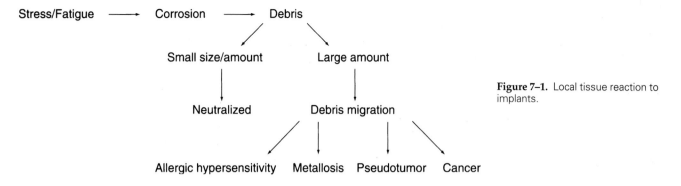

Figure 7–1. Local tissue reaction to implants.

What is potentially more disturbing is that these figures for serum concentrations and the identification of this debris in remote organs have come from patients who have been subjected to conventional cemented components. With the advent of uncemented porous-coated implants, particularly in younger patients, these figures would be expected to increase, creating the distinct possibility of toxic levels in the serum, tissues, and organs; these structures could respond with altered cellular dynamics and function.

CARCINOGENIC POTENTIAL OF METALS AND POLYMERS

Perhaps one of the greatest concerns with debris dissemination locally and within the systemic circulation is the possibility of inducing carcinogenesis (see Fig. 7–1). This is thought to be possible by one of two mechanisms:

1. A "solid-state" mechanism has been proposed, whereby a large foreign object implanted in vivo possibly stimulates mutagenesis of local cells, thereby creating tumor by its mere presence. Most large foreign objects, on implantation, initiate a very marked fibrous reaction. The cells within this fibrous reaction ultimately mutate and become cancer growths.
2. The other inescapable possibility is that either particulate metal matter or other sources of debris have an innate capacity to induce cancer.

Well-documented cases of carcinoma and sarcoma have developed in refinery workers who inhaled nickel and chromium and in miners who were exposed to iron, or even at local injection sites of iron dextran.[11] Aluminum has been linked to a high rate of lung and bladder cancer in exposed individuals, and titanium has been associated with experimental induction of lymphoreticular tumors and leukemia. Although the results have not been universally accepted, many animal experiments have shown a direct correlation between the initiation of sarcomas and the injection of particulate metal debris. This correlation appears to be related to the concentration, as well as the physical nature, of the metal implanted.[36] Metal ions, particularly cobalt, chromium, and nickel, are known to induce infidelity of DNA synthesis by causing the pairing of noncomplementary nucleotides and thereby creating a misinterpretation of the genetic code.

Further refinement to the animal model has been presented, in which a high incidence of malignant mesenchymal tumors arose around subcutaneously implanted biomaterials. Malignant tumors, such as malignant fibrous histiocytoma and pheomorphic sarcomas, were found in 25.8 percent of the implantation sites over a 6-month to 2-year period. What was unique about this study was the histologic confirmation of a spectrum of change within the capsule around the implanted biomaterials. This included changes from focal proliferative lesions through to preneoplastic proliferation, with ultimate evolution into incipient sarcoma. This study afforded the opportunity to witness defined stages in the development of mesenchymal malignancies as a by-product of implanted biomaterials.

Furthermore, it must be remembered that particulate metal matter may not be the only solid-form material that can be, and has been proved to be, carcinogenic in appropriate environments. In 1954, long before the first total hip arthroplasty was performed, Laskin[23] postulated the carcinogenic capabilities of polymethylmethacrylate after subcutaneous introduction of this material in mice. His conclusions suggested similar occurrences of tumor in humans who were being treated at that time with methyl methacrylate for dental deficiencies, and that this evolution of cancer may take up to 20 years of exposure given the proportional time of exposure before tumors were seen in the mice. A similar conclusion was reached by Carter and Rowe[7] regarding the use of polyethylene plastic before it was conventionally used in the management of arthritic joints. Regardless of form, whether powder or large solid segments, polyethylene plastic produced sarcomas in 25 and 35 percent of rats, respectively. Their conclusions also suggested a latent period of 20 years in humans before such an event could be expected to occur.

It is, therefore, noteworthy that investigators were forewarning the medical community of the carcinogenic effect of metals and polymers years before the development and introduction of joint replacement using these very same materials. In 1969, Sir John Charnley introduced total hip arthroplasty as an alternative in the management of arthritic hips. No other orthopedic procedure has been adopted with such enthusiasm. Thirty years later, we are still witnessing an incremental increase in the yearly utilization of this operation, attesting to its obvious success. According to some investigators, we may be coming into an era of increased tumor activity in the vicinity of, or possibly remote from, implantation sites of these orthopedic appliances.

CASE REPORTS OF OSTEOGENESIS NEAR OR AT ARTHROPLASTY SITES

In 1976, Harris et al.[16] were the first to describe an aggressive granulomatous lesion around a cemented femoral stem in a total hip replacement. This was a condition of localized tumor-like bone resorption that appeared radiographically as large lytic defects within the femur, approximating the cement mantle of the implant. Initially thought to be neoplastic, these lesions were surgically biopsied and found to be consistent with well-organized connective tissue containing numerous histiocytes, monocytes, and fibroblastic reactive zones. Immunohistologic evaluation revealed multinucleate giant cells and nonspecific esterase-positive monocyte macrophages. These findings suggest a foreign body-type reaction, and, with the subsequent isolation of polyethylene, methylmethacrylate, and metal debris, it was theorized that these constituents of the construct likely migrated down around the implant cement mantle in cemented prostheses and the implant-bone interface in ingrowth, noncircumferentially coated implants. Such a reaction suggests an excessive accumulation of debris at the site of articulation, which surpasses the body's ability to neutralize and/or transport the material, resulting in migration of debris to sites remote from the source. This rapid appearance of bone loss radiographically, which is often associated with a deteriorating clinical course, has been termed type II aseptic loosening.

In 1978, only 2 years after the introduction of pseudo-tumors of bone induced by the components of total hip arthroplasty, Arden and Bywaters[2] reported a case of a 56-year-old patient who developed a high-grade fibrosarcoma of soft tissue 2.5 years after receiving a metal-on-metal McKee-Farrar hip prosthesis. The tumor apparently did not have a direct association with the underlying bone or any components of the total hip arthroplasty. No formal analysis of the tumor for debris products was performed. This case drew attention to the possibility of tumors being initiated in the presence of large orthopedic appliances. It was not until 1984 that this concept became fashionable, in large part because of three articles that appeared simultaneously in the *Journal of Bone and Joint Surgery*, recounting two malignant fibrous histiocytomas and one osteosarcoma at the site of a total hip arthroplasty.[3,28,35]

This sudden and rather unexpected evolution prompted an editorial[15] in the same journal, addressing the issue of sarcoma and total hip arthroplasty and encouraging the orthopedic community worldwide to report such cases to a central registry to obtain more accurate figures on the incidence of such a problem. These tumors occurred 2, 4, and 5 years after hip replacement that was performed with various femoral and acetabular components, some with metal-on-metal articulations and others with metal on polyethylene. In two of these cases, the proximal femur was extensively involved with tumor that was in direct contact with the component. The remaining case was that of a soft tissue sarcoma not in direct approximation to the prosthesis. Two of these tumors were malignant fibrous histiocytomas, one of bone and one of soft tissue. The remaining tumor was an osteosarcoma. In this particular case, there was evidence of gray-brown pigmentation both intra- and extracellularly between the tumor and the femoral component. No formal metal analysis was performed. Three additional cases emerged before 1988 at 15 months, 4.5 years, and 2.0 years after implantation.[30,41,42]

In 1988, five cases were reported occurring 10 years[21,25] and 11 years[28,37,39] after implantation. The sarcomas included two osteosarcomas, two malignant fibrous histiocytomas, and one synovial sarcoma. Two of these were of soft tissue in a location with no direct association with the implant, yet in the case reported by Tait, there was evidence of nickel within tumor cells.[37] In the remaining three patients, all sarcomas had direct contact with either the cement or implant, with the tumor originating in bone.

In 1990, there were three additional reports in the literature, which included an osteosarcoma that developed at the site of a Charnley total hip arthroplasty 8 years[5] after implantation, a malignant fibrous histiocytoma that developed 15 years after a Charnley-Müller total hip arthroplasty,[38] and metastatic adenocarcinoma that developed at the site of a Freeman total knee arthroplasty 3 months after implantation.[20] In 1992, Jacobs et al.[18] presented a malignant fibrous histiocytoma that developed 0.5 year after implantation of a cementless AML total hip arthroplasty (Table 7–1). In that same journal volume, unpublished but submitted reports of five tumors that occurred around implants were brought to orthopedic attention.[14] These included two malignant fibrous histiocytomas around a Thompson and Müller total hip arthroplasty, an osteosarcoma around a Charnley total hip arthroplasty, a rhabdomyosarcoma of soft tissue in the vicinity of a Christiansen total hip arthroplasty, and a chondrosarcoma developing in a patient with Maffucci syndrome who had undergone a Charnley total hip arthroplasty. The intervals from implantation to tumor detection were 9, 3, 10, 9, and 1 years, respectively. More recently, a liposarcoma has been identified in the vicinity of a total joint prosthesis.[34] To this, we add two additional patients, neither of whom had their joint replacement done at the Mayo Clinic (Table 7–2). The first is that of a 79-year-old man who, 9 months previously, had received a total hip replacement with an uncemented Harris-Galante component; he was found to have a large malignant fibrous histiocytoma engulfing the proximal femur and extending to the implant. There was, however, no evidence of any particulate debris within the tumor cells removed. The second case was that of a 56-year-old man who developed a soft tissue osteosarcoma 14 months after a left total knee arthroplasty with conventional cemented

Table 7–1. PUBLISHED MALIGNANCIES ASSOCIATED WITH IMPLANTS

Author	Year	Implant	Time Interval (Years)	Tumor Type
Castleman	1965	Austin-Moore	1	Malignant fibrous histiocytoma
Rushford	1974	McKee-Farrar	0.5	Osteosarcoma
Arden & Bywaters	1978	McKee-Farrar	2.5	Fibrosarcoma
Bago-Granell	1984	Charnley-Müller	2	Malignant fibrous histiocytoma
Penman & Ring	1984	Ring	5	Osteosarcoma
Swann	1984	McKee-Farrar	4	Malignant fibrous histiocytoma
Weber	1986	Cemented TKA	4.5	Epithelioid sarcoma
Ryu	1987	Uncemented Vitallium	1.4	Malignant fibrous histiocytoma
Vives	1987	Charnley-Müller	2	Malignant fibrous histiocytoma
Van der List	1988	Charnley-Müller	11	Angiosarcoma
Lamovec	1988	Charnley-Müller	11	Synovial sarcoma
Lamovec	1988	Charnley-Müller	10	Osteosarcoma
Tait	1988	Charnley-Müller	11	Malignant fibrous histiocytoma
Martin	1988	Charnley-Müller	10	Osteosarcoma
Haag & Adler	1989	Weber-Huggier	10	Malignant fibrous histiocytoma
Brien	1990	Charnley	8	Osteosarcoma
Troop	1990	Charnley-Müller	15	Malignant fibrous histiocytoma
Kolstad & Högstorp	1990	Freeman TKA	0.25	Metastatic adenocarcinoma
Jacobs	1992	AML cementless	0.5	Malignant fibrous histiocytoma
Stephensen	1999	Titanium cemented	6	Liposarcoma

components. The tumor extended down to both the femoral and patellar components.

Thus, 27 tumors have been reported in direct contact or in close proximity to joint arthroplasty. The vast majority of these appeared with total hip arthroplasty (24), with a smaller number in conjunction with total knee arthroplasty (3). There have been no reported cases of malignant degeneration occurring in the vicinity of total shoulder and/or total elbow arthroplasty. Of the reported 27 cases, 7 tumors were of soft tissue origin, 19 were of primary bone pathology, and 1 was a metastatic gastric carcinoma. The histogenesis of the soft tissue tumors included two malignant fibrous histiocytomas, one synovial sarcoma, one soft tissue osteogenic sarcoma, one fibrosarcoma, one liposarcoma, and one rhabdomyosarcoma. The histogenesis of the primary bone tumors included 10 malignant fibrous histiocytomas, 6 osteosarcomas, 1 chondrosarcoma, 1 angiosarcoma, and 1 fibrosarcoma. Direct contact with the underlying tumor was noted in the 15 of 19 cases that provided sufficient information for such determinations to be made. In three of the cases, particulate metal matter was determined to be present in the tumor, including one case of a soft tissue sarcoma that appeared on image and exploration to be remote from the implant but had obvious evidence of nickel present within the tumor cells.

Many of these tumors have not had an appropriate latent interval between implantation and development to be seriously considered implant induced. Given that the interval to tumor induction from bone stimulation should be at least as long as the accepted 5-year interval from radiation therapy to sarcoma degeneration, 13 of the 27 patients would qualify, all of whom have had implants in total hip arthroplasties.

Apart from tumors developing at the site of prosthetic replacement, there have been 10 known malignant tumors that have developed at the site of previous internal fixation (Table 7–3). To date, there have been no malignancies noted around a titanium implant. The vast majority of malignancies both in the prosthetic and internal fixation groups have occurred in the vicinity of vitallium implants. This is not, however, to exonerate stainless steel, because tumors in the proximity of the implants made of this alloy have been reported in the animal literature as well as the human experience utilizing stainless steel as fixation devices for traumatology. It is interesting to note that, in 1976, veterinarians were encouraged within their own literature to report similar experiences of tumors around implants, 8 years before such concern was voiced regarding the application of these same metallic alloys in humans.

A review of the published literature on the subject indicates that the diagnosis of a tumor superimposed

Table 7–2. UNPUBLISHED MALIGNANCIES ASSOCIATED WITH IMPLANTS

Author	Year	Implant	Time Interval (Years)	Tumor Type
Harris	1992	Charnley	1	Chondrosarcoma
Surin	1992	Christiansen	9	Rhabdomyosarcoma
Lightowler	1992	Charnley	10	Osteosarcoma
Rees	1992	Thompson	3	Malignant fibrous histiocytoma
Nelson	1992	Müller	9	Malignant fibrous histiocytoma
Rock	1992	PCA ingrowth	8	Malignant fibrous histiocytoma
Rock	1992	PCA TKA	1.2	Osteosarcoma

Table 7-3. MALIGNANCY ASSOCIATED WITH INTERNAL FIXATION

Author	Year	Implant	Time Interval (Years)	Tumor Type
McDougall-McNally	1956	Stainless steel	30	Ewings
Delgado	1958	–	3	Undifferentiated
Dube-Fisher	1972	Stainless steel	36	Angiosarcoma
Tayton	1980	Vitallium	7.5	Ewings
McDonald	1981	Vitallium	17	Lymphoma
Dodion	1982	Vitallium	1.2	Lymphoma
Lee	1984	Vitallium	14	Malignant fibrous histiocytoma
Hughes	1987	Vitallium	29	Malignant fibrous histiocytoma
Ward	1990	Stainless steel	9	Osteosarcoma
Khurana	1991	Stainless steel	13	Malignant fibrous histiocytoma

on, or at least in proximity to, these replacements, carries with it a very dismal prognosis, suggesting an extremely aggressive course. Figures available suggest that the vast majority of patients succumb within the first year after diagnosis and many within several weeks to months from the time of tumor detection and management.

CRITICAL ANALYSIS AND ITS SIGNIFICANCE

As impressive as these cases may be, they must be put into perspective given the global use of internal fixation and prosthetic devices. Approximately 300,000 to 350,000 total hip joint replacements are performed worldwide on a yearly basis. It is assumed that approximately 5 million people will have had total hip arthroplasties performed by the end of 2002. To date, there have been 27 reports of malignant tumor arising in close proximity to these implants (24 total hip and 3 total knee arthroplasties). No direct contact was noted in 4 cases. If we assume a minimal latency of 5 years to suggest association between presence of implant and tumor, 13 of the 27 could have such an association. Therefore, the incidence of sarcomas in total joint replacement would be approximately 1 in 250,000. There are approximately 3000 new primary bone tumors and 5000 soft tissue sarcomas in the United States per year. This would give an incidence of approximately 1 in 100,000 for the general population to develop a primary bone sarcoma and 1 in 40,000 to develop a soft tissue sarcoma per year. These figures obviously are not stratified for age, given that many primary bone tumors develop in the second and third generations of life, yet it does afford the opportunity of putting this rather unusual event in perspective.

The prevalence of osteosarcoma among the osseous malignancies in this series is not entirely unexpected. Of the total number of cases of osteosarcoma, 15 to 20 percent occur in patients older than age 50 years. Most of these cases are superimposed on Paget's disease or occur in previously irradiated tissue, yet de novo cases of osteosarcoma do occur in this age group. Malignant fibrous histiocytoma of bone is somewhat less common. A review of the Mayo Clinic files reveals 71 cases, with more than half of these occurring in patients older than age 55. Malignant fibrous histiocytoma of soft tissue is the most common soft tissue sarcoma. It is not surprising, therefore, that two of six soft tissue tumors in the combined series are of this histogenesis. Thus, the distribution of sarcomas in the combined series could have been predicted from general population data given the age of the patients and the anatomic distribution.

There have been five separate reports that have critically analyzed the cancer risk after forms of arthroplasty.[10,12,13,26,27] The combined person-years of exposure after operation among these series was in excess of 500,000. The overall cancer incidence in the combined series did not appear to be any different from what was expected or anticipated in the general population. The cancer observed/expected ratio was especially low for the first 2 years after surgery, implying that patients undergoing these procedures are otherwise generally healthy. Although suggested in three series[10,13,40] a more recent extensive analysis of the Finnish cancer database would suggest no increased risk of hematopoietic cancers after 31,651 total hip arthroplasties had been performed. The latter study is particularly encouraging given that chronic stimulation of the immune system is likely to occur in this patient population owing to the predilection of particulate metal matter to accumulate in the reticulendothelial system.[8,22] This has been suggested by studies in animals subjected to metal implants, especially implants containing nickel; in these animals, there was an increase in malignancies of the lymphoproliferative system.[32] Because of the increased immune sensitivity, tumors of the breast, colon, rectum, and lung have shown a slight decrease relative to the general population as reported in several studies.[10,13]

One study suggests the possibility of metastasis as a cause of osteolysis and mechanical failure of implants precipitating revision surgery. In a series of 93 patients who underwent revision hip arthroplasty, 11.8 percent had a history of a previous malignancy. Two of these patients demonstrated obvious gross microscopic metastasis and was thought to have contributed to the mechanical failure of the original reconstruction. As such, when revision hip arthroplasty is considered, patients with a history of malignancy, particularly those who have a predilection to bone metastasis including thyroid, lung, breast, kidney and prostate, require additional preoperative assessment and appropriate biopsies at the time of revision arthroplasty to identify possible occult disease.[31]

SUMMARY

My interpretation of the literature suggests that implants commonly used for fixation and reconstruction may not be entirely inert. Accumulation of particulate debris occurs to some extent in all patients who have large metallic prosthetic devices. This includes the distinct possibility of systemic exposure to these foreign objects and as a by-product of a heightened immunologic sensitivity. In spite of these concerns and although theoretically possible, there is currently no convincing evidence to support the increased incidence of primary mesenchymal or lymphoproliferative malignancies as a by-product of biomaterials used for fixation and reconstruction in orthopedic practice. Furthermore, the International Agency for Research on evaluated carcinogenic risk to humans of surgical implants and other foreign bodies and concluded that orthopedic implants, including ceramics, were not classifiable as to their carcinogenicity to humans.[26]

References

1. Agins HJ, Allock NW, Bansal M, et al: Metallic wear in failed titanium alloy total hip replacements: A histological and quantitative analysis. J Bone Joint Surg 70A:347, 1988.
2. Arden GP, Bywaters EGL: Tissue reaction. In Arden GP, Ansel BM, (eds): Surgical Management of Juvenile Chronic Poly Arthritis. London, Academic Press, 1978, p 269.
3. Bago-Granell J, Aguirre-Canyadell M, Nardi J, et al: Malignant fibrous histiocytoma of bone at the site of a total hip arthroplasty: A case report. J Bone Joint Surg 66B:38, 1984.
4. Bartolozzi A, Black J: Chromium concentrations in serum blood clot and urine from patients following total hip arthroplasty. Biomaterials 6:2, 1985.
5. Brien WW, Salvati EA, Healey JH, et al: Osteogenic sarcoma arising in the area of a total hip replacement: A case report. J Bone Joint Surg 72A:1097, 1990.
6. Buchert BK, Vaughn BK, Mallory TH, et al: Excessive metal release due to loosening and spreading of sintered particles on porous coated hip prosthesis: Report of two cases. J Bone Joint Surg 68A:606, 1986.
7. Carter RL, Rowe FJC: Induction of sarcomas in rats by solid and fragmented polyethylene: Experimental observations and clinical implications. Br J Cancer 23:401, 1969.
8. Case CP, Langkamer BG, James C, et al: Widespread dissemination of metal debris from implants. J Bone Joint Surg 76B:701, 1994.
9. Coleman RF, Herrington J, Scales JT: Concentration of wear products in hair, blood, and urine after total hip arthroplasty. BMJ 1:527, 1973.
10. Coleman MP: Cancer risk from orthopedic prostheses. Ann Clin Lab Sci 26:139, 1996.
11. Doll R: Cancer of lung and the nose: nickel workers. Br J Indian Med 15:217, 1958.
12. Fryzek JP, Mellemkjaer L, McLaughlin JK, et al: Cancer risk among patients with finger and hand joint and temporomandibular joint prosthesis in Denmark. Int Cancer 81:723, 1999.
13. Gillespie WJ, Frampton CMA, Henderson RJ, et al: The incidence of cancer following total hip replacement. J Bone Joint Surg 70B:539, 1988.
14. Goodfellow J: Malignancy and joint replacement (editorial). J Bone Joint Surg 74A:645, 1992.
15. Hamblen DL, Carter RL: Sarcoma and joint replacement (editorial). J Bone Joint Surg 66B:625, 1984.
16. Harris WH, Schiller AL, Scholler JM, et al: Extensive localized bone resorption in the femur following total hip replacement. J Bone Joint Surg 58A:612, 1976.
17. Jacobs JJ, Skipor AK, Black J, et al: Release in excretion of metal in patients who have a total hip replacement component made of titanium base alloy. J Bone Joint Surg 73A:1475, 1991.
18. Jacobs JJ, Rosenbaum DH, Marshallhay R, et al: Early sarcomatous degeneration near a cementless hip replacement: A case report and review. J Bone Joint Surg 74B:740, 1992.
19. Kirkpatrick CJ, Alves A, Kohler H, et al: Biomaterial induced sarcoma. A novel model to study pre-neoplastic change. Am J Path 156:1455, 2000.
20. Kolstad K, Hogstrop H: Gastric carcinoma metastasis to a knee with a newly inserted prosthesis: A case report. Acta Orthop Scand 61:369, 1990.
21. Lamovec J, Zidar A, Cucek-Plenicar M, et al: Synovial sarcoma associated with total hip replacement: A case report. Addendum: Osteosarcoma associated with a Charnley-Mueller hip arthroplasty. J Bone Joint Surg 70A:1558, 1988.
22. Langkamer VG, Case CP, Heap P, et al: Systemic distribution of wear debris after hip replacement: A cause for concern? J Bone Joint Surg 74B:831, 1992.
23. Laskin DM: Experimental production in sarcomas by methylcrylate implant. Proc Soc Exp Biol Med 87:329, 1954.
24. Lux F, Zeisler R: Investigations of the corrosive deposition of components of metal implants and of the behavior of biologic trace elements in metallosis tissue by means of instrumental, multielement activation analysis. J Radiol Anal Chem 19:289, 1974.
25. Martin A, Bauer TW, Manley MT, et al: Osteosarcoma at the site of a total hip replacement. J Bone Joint Surg 70A:1561, 1988.
26. McGregor DB, Baan RA, Partensky C, et al: Evaluation of the carcinogenic risks to humans associated with surgical implants and other foreign bodies—a report of an IARC monographs program meeting, International Agency for Research on Cancer. Eur J Cancer 36:307, 2000.
27. Paavolainen P, Pukkala E, Eulkkinen P, Visuri T: Cancer incidence in Finnish hip replacement patients from 1980 to 1995: A nationwide cohort study involving 31,651 patients. J Arthroplasty 14:272, 1999.
28. Penman HG, Ring PA: Osteosarcoma in association with total hip replacement. J Bone Joint Surg 66B:632, 1984.
29. Rock MG, Hardie R: Analysis of local tissue response in 50 revision total hip arthroplasty patients. Presented at the Symposium on Retrieval and Analysis of Surgical Implants and Biomaterials, Snowbird, Utah, August 1988.
30. Ryu RKN, Bovill EG Jr, Skinner HB, Murray WR: Soft tissue sarcomas associated with aluminum oxide ceramic total hip arthroplasty: A case report. Clin Orthop 216:207, 1987.
31. Salai M, Zippel D, Perelman M, Chechik A: Revision hip arthroplasty in patients with a history of previous malignancy. J Surg Oncol 70:122, 1999.
32. Sinibaldi K: Tumors associated with metallic implants in animals. Clin Orthop 118:257, 1976.
33. Steineman SG: Corrosion of titanium and titanium alloys for surgical implant. In Lutergering G, Swicker U, Bunk W (eds): Titanium, Science, and Technology, vol 2. Berlin, Springer-Verlag, 1985, p 1373.
34. Stephensen SL, Schwarz Lausten G, Thomsen HS, Bjerregaard B: Liposarcoma in association with a total hip replacement. Int Orthop 23:187, 1999.
35. Swann M: Malignant soft tissue tumor at the site of a total hip replacement. J Bone Joint Surg 66B:269, 1984.
36. Swanson SAV, Freeman MAR, Heath JC: Laboratory tests on total joint replacement prosthesis. J Bone Joint Surg 55B:759, 1973.
37. Tait NP: Case reports, malignant fibrous histiocytoma occurring at the site of a previous total hip replacement. Br J Radiol 61:73, 1988.
38. Troop JK, Mallory TH, Fisher DA, Vaugh BK: Malignant fibrous histiocytoma after total hip arthroplasty: A case report. Clin Orthop 253:297, 1990.
39. Vanderlist JJJ: Malignant epithelioid hemangioendothelioma at the site of a hip prosthesis. Acta Orthop Scand 59:328, 1988.
40. Visuri T: Cancer risk after McKee-Farrar total hip replacement. Orthopedics 14:137, 1992.
41. Vives P, Sevestre H, Grodet H, et al: Histiocytome fibreux malin du fémur après prosthèses totale de hanche. Rev Chir Orthop 73:407, 1987.

42. Weber PC: Epithelioid sarcoma in association with total knee replacement. J Bone Joint Surg 68B:824, 1986.
43. Witt JD, Swann M: Methyl wear in tissue response and failed titanium alloy total hip replacements. J Bone Joint Surg 73B:559, 1991.
44. Woodman JL, Jacobs JJ, Gallante JO, Urbin RN: Methyl ion release from titanium based prosthetic segmental replacements of long bones in baboons: A long term study. J Orthop Res 1:421, 1984.

8

Transfusion Medicine and Orthopedic Surgery

BLOOD AND BLOOD PRODUCTS

• S. BREANNDAN MOORE and PAULA J. SANTRACH

BACKGROUND

The past two decades have brought changes in transfusion science so profound as to render today's practice almost unrecognizable to a modern Dr. Rip Van Winkle whose transfusion medicine experience antedated the mid-1980s. Unquestionably, the driving force for change has been the increased public awareness of the risks of transfusion. Patients fear, sometimes irrationally, acquired immunodeficiency syndrome (AIDS) and other transfusion-transmitted disease and clamor for a "zero-risk" blood supply. Physicians, although having a more sophisticated appreciation of potential risk, still tend to respond to their patients' fears as well as their own concerns about transfusion-transmitted disease.

These fears resulted in an extraordinary emphasis on the provision of autologous blood whenever possible and an equally intense effort to reevaluate transfusion practices with a goal of minimizing allogeneic exposures. Transfusion practices in general were changed, with much less blood being given per patient. Similarly, the widespread introduction of newer and more sensitive pathogen tests and the application of DNA amplification methods to blood-borne pathogen testing have led to an extraordinary level of safety of the current allogeneic blood supply. This in turn has led to a reexamination and revision of the previous emphasis on autologous transfusion (particularly preoperatively donated units).

RED BLOOD CELL TRANSFUSION BASICS

Obtaining a Transfusion History

Obtaining a transfusion history from a patient takes only a few minutes. One need only inquire about previous pregnancies, known transfusions, and events such as major surgery, which can involve transfusion unknown to the patient. If a patient is aware of a problem with a previous transfusion, it is usually an important signal. Often, there has been a significant, perhaps even life-threatening, reaction. Patients may possess cards or letters describing a transfusion problem because it is common, although not universal, practice for blood banks and hospitals to provide such documentation. Because the cause of a previous reaction may no longer be detectable by laboratory testing when information suggesting past transfusion problems is encountered, the hospital blood bank should be notified.

Typing, Screening, and Cross-matching for Red Blood Cell Transfusion

Typing a patient's blood before the administration of blood and blood products refers to the process of determining the ABO blood group and the Rh type (i.e., Rh positive or Rh negative). These are extremely important but simple tests once an appropriately collected and identified blood sample is available to the blood bank.

The *antibody screen* uses the patient's serum reacted with known reagent red cells in test tubes. The reagent red cells (two or three different donor red cells) are selected so that, between them, they contain nearly all of the important red cell antigens to which a patient might make an antibody; that is, the patient's serum is "screened" for red cell antibodies. A negative antibody screen provides more than 99.8 percent certainty that subsequent cross-matches will be compatible.[60] Determination of the ABO group and the Rh type together with antibody screening for red cell antibodies is known simply as a *"type and screen."*

The *cross-match* (compatibility testing) is similar to antibody screening in that the patient's serum is used in an attempt to detect antibodies in that serum. However, instead of being tested against reagent red cells, the patient's serum is reacted against red cells from the actual donor unit available for transfusion to the patient. That is, the cross-match is the in vitro correlate of the in vivo transfusion of the unit being tested. An antibody screen is always performed in conjunction with a cross-match, but a type and screen, by definition, does not include cross-matching.

Evidence of incompatibility can be elicited at two or three different points during the antibody screen or cross-match. The first of these occurs within 5 minutes of beginning the cross-match—the "first phase" or "immediate spin" part of the cross-match. The first phase of the cross-match provides a double check to ensure that the ABO group of the selected unit is compatible with that of the patient. In the absence of sufficient time to complete a full cross-match before transfusion, the completion of the first phase provides reassurance that the appropriate ABO selection—the most important element of most cross-matches—has been made for the patient.

The actual technical aspects of antibody screening and cross-matching require only approximately 30 to 45 minutes. However, obtaining a correctly identified sample, transporting that sample, testing, record keeping, labeling, and transportation of the blood product extend the approximate time for a complete cross-match to between 90 minutes and 4 hours, depending on the circumstances and the urgency of transfusion.

All of the activity associated with ABO and Rh typing, antibody screening, and cross-matching is directed at avoiding hemolytic transfusion reactions, which are potentially fatal. Antibodies directed at antigens in the ABO, Rh, Kell, Duffy, and Kidd blood group systems account for nearly all hemolytic reactions and associated deaths. The most important clinically significant antigens beyond the ABO system are the Rh system antigens D, C, c, E, e; the Kell system antigens K and k; the Duffy system antigens Fy^a and Fy^b; and Jk^a and Jk^b of the Kidd system. Although antibodies to many of the other 600+ red blood cell antigens identified to date are potentially hemolytic, they are seldom, if ever, encountered in a lifetime of orthopedic practice.

The cross-match is simply another test in the medical armamentarium, the usefulness of which depends on clinical considerations. Although life-threatening situations requiring transfusion are uncommon, delay in such situations while waiting for a cross-match can be a tragic mistake. Patients usually survive emergency transfusion of ABO-appropriate red cell units that are found incompatible on subsequent completion of the cross-match. Use of group O red blood cells avoids any possibility of a catastrophic ABO mismatch, and providing red cells as Rh-negative units avoids any possibility of Rh sensitization in women of childbearing age.

ABO Disasters

More than 60 percent of transfusion-related fatalities (not caused by transmitted viruses or bacteria) are caused by ABO blood group incompatibility.[54] Essentially, all ABO-related fatalities are the result of human error, and almost none are the result of mislabeling or mistyping of red cell units. These ABO disasters are nearly always the result of identification errors that are made either during the drawing of the patient's blood or during the administration of the blood. Physicians not only administer blood, but they also can be involved in drawing erroneous blood samples or in errors related to ordering (e.g., blood ordered for the wrong patient), which increase the likelihood of a mix-up during blood administration. The 131 deaths resulting from ABO incompatible transfusions reported to the Food and Drug Administration (FDA) during the years 1976 through 1985[54] represent but one death per approximately 1 million red blood cell transfusions— yet each was an avoidable tragedy. Physician insistence on meticulous identification procedures in the operating room and on the wards may avert such a catastrophic error.

TRANSFUSION PRACTICE IN THE NEW MILLENNIUM

Although the basic concepts of red blood cell transfusion discussed in the preceding paragraphs have been known for decades, much of transfusion medicine in the 2000s is new, representing recent innovations, application of new scientific knowledge, or alterations in practice in response to federal regulations and accrediting agency standards. Among the changes that are pertinent to orthopedic practice are (1) the development of relatively well-defined transfusion criteria and changes in the indications for transfusion of red blood cells and other blood products; (2) a greater awareness of the risks of transfusion coupled with a more reasonable perspective on those risks; (3) the necessity for documentation of transfusion practice, including the use of informed consent for transfusion; (4) a reappraisal of the role of autologous transfusion, the principal types of which are all applicable to orthopedic practice; (5) emphasis on appropriate transfusion practice, with cost-benefit analysis often becoming the key component of decision making; (6) a reevaluation of the use of "directed" donors; and (7) the increased complexity of tissue banking, including bone banking.

TRANSFUSION CRITERIA AND GUIDELINES FOR BLOOD COMPONENTS

Whole Blood

Whole blood from donors is now rarely used in an unmodified form. Instead, for maximum efficiency, the donated unit is divided into various fractions called components. Therefore, each donation can provide three components: red blood cells, platelets, and fresh frozen plasma (FFP) or cryoprecipitate. Autologous donations are sometimes maintained as whole blood. The remainder of this section discusses most of the available components.

Red Blood Cells and the "Transfusion Trigger"

Red blood cell transfusion is intended to provide oxygen-carrying capacity to maintain tissue oxygenation when intravascular volume and cardiac function are adequate for perfusion. Red blood cells (formerly called "packed cells") should be used only when time or underlying pathophysiology precludes other management of anemia (e.g., iron therapy or, when appropriate, erythropoietin). Red blood cells provided in the newer additive solutions (e.g., AS-1 or AS-3 red blood cells) are essentially a suspension of red cells in glucose and saline. A small volume of anticoagulant and approximately 30 to 50 ml of plasma are also present. Red blood cells should not be considered a source of plasma constituents. Today's typical red blood cell unit has a volume of 320 ± 50 ml and a hematocrit of 55 percent, and flows as readily as whole blood.

The red blood cell "transfusion trigger"—the point at which the risk of transfusion is thought to be balanced by the benefits—has clearly changed. A decade ago, a hemoglobin concentration below 10 g/dl (100 g/L) was frequently used as an indication for transfusion. When hemoglobin concentration is used as an indication for transfusion today, the level is more likely to be 7 or 8 g/dl.[48] Clinical signs and symptoms are more often taken into account than in the past, and current practice in many institutions requires or recommends documentation of the indications for red blood cell transfusion at hemoglobin levels above 7 to 8 g/dl (e.g., compromised cardiac, pulmonary, or cerebrovascular status). At the Mayo Clinic, the hemoglobin level was not found to influence the duration of hospitalization after hip replacement.[39]

The current bias is to avoid transfusion if at all possible, and, not surprisingly, concerns about undertransfusion are beginning to appear.[45,55] Enhanced ability to monitor tissue oxygenation will be a partial solution to transfusion dilemmas, but clinical judgment, based on knowledge of risks and benefits, will continue to be the ultimate determining factor in decisions about red blood cell transfusion for the foreseeable future.

Platelets

Platelets are intended for patients who are experiencing, or at significant risk of, hemorrhage as a result of thrombocytopenia or platelet dysfunction. In orthopedic patients, platelet transfusions have generally been limited to patients with preexisting platelet disorders and those with massive blood loss. Routine prophylactic transfusion of platelets has been shown not to be necessary in massive transfusion,[52] and, in general, platelets should be administered only in instances of small vessel (microvascular) bleeding in the presence of known or suspected platelet dysfunction or platelet counts less than 50×10^9/L (50,000/mm^3).[17] Dosage of platelets in most adults is from 4 to 6 units, depending on institutional practice, and each unit is expected to raise the platelet count by 5 to 10×10^9/L (5000 to 10,000/mm^3).

Fresh Frozen Plasma

FFP should be thought of as containing all the coagulation factors present in the same amount of normal plasma, except for factors associated with platelets. In orthopedics, FFP is used most often to correct coagulation factor deficiencies resulting from massive transfusion and for reversal of the coagulation defect associated with warfarin therapy in patients who require emergency procedures. Patients with congenital coagulation deficiencies for which safe factor concentrates are not available may require FFP before undergoing surgery.

Most authorities recommend transfusion of FFP in the situations previously discussed only if there is some documentation of a non–platelet-related coagulation defect, usually by a prothrombin time (PT) or activated partial thromboplastin time (APTT). Suggested "trigger" values are a PT greater than 1.5 times the midrange of normal (usually more than 18 seconds) and an APTT of 1.5 times the upper range of normal (more than 55 to 60 seconds).[15,57] FFP is often administered empirically, starting with a dose of two units (bags), with further therapy determined by coagulation studies performed after the initial infusion is completed.[17] In patients on warfarin-based anticoagulant therapy, an International normalized ratio (INR) of 1.4 or lower is usually considered adequate and does not require reversal before surgery.

Cryoprecipitate

Cryoprecipitate is a cold, insoluble fraction of FFP, and each bag contains approximately 80 to 100 units of factor VIII and 150 to 250 mg of fibrinogen in a volume of only 20 to 25 ml. Cryoprecipitate also contains factor XIII and von Willebrand's factor. Originally developed as a concentrated source of factor VIII to treat hemophilia, cryoprecipitate is now used almost exclusively as a concentrated source of fibrinogen for massively transfused patients and those with disseminated intravascular coagulation. (Although FFP contains fibrinogen, volume considerations limit its effectiveness in increasing fibrinogen levels in depleted patients. No FDA-approved commercial fibrinogen concentrate is available in the United States.)

Cryoprecipitate is often administered empirically as a source of fibrinogen in a dose of eight to ten bags (units) in adults. One rule of thumb is to administer 1 bag/5 kg of body weight.[17] If fibrinogen measurements are readily available, sufficient product to raise the patient's fibrinogen concentration above 100 mg/dl should be administered in the face of bleeding thought to be related to hypofibrinogenemia.[17]

Risks of Transfusion

Approximately 20 years ago, when it became clear that AIDS had contaminated the blood supply, there were several responses to this fact. The media began emphasizing the dangers of allogeneic transfusion relative to AIDS transmission to such an extent that the public began to think of transfusions as the primary source of the infection! In fact, more than 96 percent of cases of AIDS were not related to transfusions, even before there was a blood donor test for the virus! Nevertheless, this public anxiety—some justified, some hysterical—resulted in a major demand for the provision of autologous blood, especially for elective orthopedic and cardiac surgery. There was also significant congressional and legal activity, which resulted in a very laudatory reappraisal of both clinical transfusion practices and the actual safety of the blood supply. New federal regulations were introduced relative to donor screening interviews, pathogen testing, and other safety-related blood banking practices. Concomitantly, during the 1990s, basic science discoveries and developments led to identification, characterization, and tests for diagnosis of hepatitis C virus (HCV), as well as marked improvement in the sensitivity and specificity of several "generations" of the mandated pathogen testing of all donations. These changes have all resulted in significant improvements in the control of clinical transfusion practices and in the safety of the blood itself.

In early 2000, with strong encouragement from the FDA, testing of virtually all donations was begun by new and extremely sensitive nucleic acid amplification (NAT) tests for HCV and HIV. These tests detect the presence of the viral DNA or RNA itself and are designed to bypass the "biologic waiting period" needed for newly infected donors to develop antibodies, which are the target of the standard mandated generation of donor pathogen tests. In essence, by detecting DNA, the NAT method significantly reduces the so-called "window period" during which a donor may be infectious but has not yet produced the antibodies detectable by classical tests. Although this method has not yet been mandated by the FDA, virtually all blood collected (as of mid-2001) is actually NAT tested, and the mandate is expected soon.

With extensive data gathered from NAT results on over 10 million donations, figures projecting current residual risks from pathogens in the allogeneic blood supply have been presented at major national meetings.[20] Williams has calculated that the risk of HIV transmission was reduced 15.6-fold between 1995 and 2000! Similar dramatic improvements have occurred for HCV and, to lesser extent, for hepatitis B virus (HBV).

Because of the plethora of improvements in blood safety, evaluators of the latest NAT data have had to rely on conservative mathematical projections of residual risks because the yield from testing donors has been so low. For example, in one study, only 1 HIV (positive by NAT only) and 11 HCV (NAT only) positive results were found in 5.14 million donations from repeat donors. The figures for first-time donors were 11 positive results for HCV and none for HIV among 1.45 million donations.[20]

These data make it quite clear that (1) the residual risks are now extremely low, and (2) the DNA-based testing is going to become the new standard for donor testing. Based on the test data available in mid-2001, the approximate residual risks for transfusion transmission of HIV, HCV, and HBV are outlined in Table 8–1.

Each improvement in testing methods continues to incrementally increase blood safety, but it is important for patients to be aware that transfusions are not 100 percent safe and never will be. This fact must be kept in perspective, because nothing in life is completely safe. As discussed elsewhere in this chapter, even autologous blood is not without risk because it can be bacterially contaminated and, more importantly, can be transfused to the wrong recipient through clerical error.

When the risks of any procedure (including transfusions) are discussed, the patients need to be given realistic and balanced data and information. The risks of *not* being transfused must also be explained to them so that they can put the risks of being transfused into a reasonable perspective.

Documentation of Indications, Efficacy, and Consent for Transfusion

Awareness of the risks of transfusion has produced substantial alterations in transfusion practice. Informed patient consent for transfusion may be as necessary legally as is consent for other major procedures. This consent can be recorded on a document intended for this purpose, as recommended to hospitals by the American Association of Blood Banks, or, preferably, as a note in the medical record indicating that the risks and benefits have been discussed with and understood by either the patient or the patient's parent or guardian. Accrediting agencies, particularly the Joint Commission on Accreditation of Healthcare Organizations, insist on improved documentation of both the indication for and the results of transfusion episodes. The Joint Commission has charged the medical staff with this responsibility—usually fulfilled through the hospital transfusion committee.[38]

Table 8–1. APPROXIMATE RESIDUAL PATHOGEN RISKS PER UNIT

HBV	1:170,000
HCV	1:250,000—1:1.7 million
HIV	1:1.7 million—1:1.9 million

AUTOLOGOUS TRANSFUSION

Overview

Fear of AIDS and other adverse effects of allogeneic blood transfusion in the 1980s led to rapid growth in the use of autologous blood in orthopedic surgery. Provision of autologous blood is usually categorized into four main types: (1) preoperative collection, (2) immediate preoperative hemodilution, (3) perioperative blood salvage, and (4) perioperative component preparation. According to national surveys, preoperative autologous blood collections peaked in 1992 at an estimated 1.117 million units, which represented approximately 8 percent of all whole blood and red blood cell units collected in the United States.[62] However, subsequently, there has been a slow but steady decrease in this activity back to levels seen in the mid- to late 1980s.[30,61] In 1999, 367,000 units of autologous blood were transfused, a 12.6 percent decline from 1997.[58]

Numerous factors have influenced the use of autologous blood in surgical patients. Advantages related to the avoidance of allogeneic blood transfusion include decreased risks of transfusion-transmitted infection, alloimmunization, hemolytic and allergic transfusion reactions, and transfusion-associated graft-versus-host disease. Autologous blood transfusion can also lessen the pressure on the allogeneic blood supply to meet transfusion needs; currently, the incidence of blood shortages are increasing as the growth in transfusions outpaces the growth in availability of allogeneic blood donors.[58] Transfusion-related immunomodulation may also be reduced, although the clinical significance of this phenomenon is not ear.

On the other hand, the following issues have contributed to the decline in autologous activity:

1. Changes in costs and benefits: In preoperative autologous blood donation (PABD) programs, the number of units needed for surgery must be estimated. The need for a specific patient is often difficult to determine; needs may be overestimated and discard rates can be 50 percent or more.[53] When the expense of the discarded units is considered, the cost of autologous blood per unit transfused may be tremendous.[23] Decision analysis has suggested that the cost per quality adjusted life year (QALY) saved is high for PABD compared with other medical procedures. The cost of hip replacement surgery has been estimated between $235,000 and $373,000.[8,23] For postoperative autologous blood salvage programs in joint replacement surgery, the cost per QALY is calculated to be much higher, mostly related to the small number of red blood cells recovered and procedural costs that are incurred if even a small quantity of blood is salvaged.[36] The high cost-benefit ratio is made even worse by the continuing improvements in the safety of the allogeneic blood supply.

2. Questions regarding efficacy: The use of PABD has been shown to decrease the incidence of allogeneic transfusion in studies of selected patient populations.[27] However, it has also become clear that patients who donate blood typically have a lower preoperative hemoglobin level[14] and are much more likely to be transfused with any blood component.[3,27] The true benefit of PABD lies in its ability to stimulate erythropoiesis during the preoperative period. As a result, the patient can ultimately lose more red blood cells during surgery without having to receive an allogeneic transfusion. For patients who are unable to produce sufficient new red blood cells to replace those donated, PABD simply moves the "storage" of those red cells from the body to the refrigerator. This may also be true for patients with high predonation hemoglobin levels; donation may not induce much of an erythropoietic response.[49]

3. Recognition that autologous transfusion is not risk free: The use of autologous blood does not eliminate all of the risks associated with transfusion. Patients may be transfused with the blood from another patient because of errors made both inside and outside of the operating room.[44] Autologous blood transfusion may be associated with reaction rates similar to those seen with use of allogeneic blood.[22] Although 40 percent of these reactions were not related to transfusion, the remainder included febrile and allergic reactions, which may reflect cytokine generation during product storage. Other reported adverse effects of autologous blood transfusion involve bacterial contamination, hemolysis resulting from equipment malfunction, circulatory overload, and air embolism. These risks are particularly germane given the fact that the transfusion criteria for autologous blood appear to be less stringent in some institutions and that autologous blood may be infused simply "because it is available," regardless of the patient's clinical condition or hemoglobin level.

4. Recommendations against use for other patients: The FDA allows the transfusion of unused autologous blood into other patients as long as donors meet all the criteria for allogeneic donation. This practice has proved to be administratively challenging and is no longer recommended by either the American Association of Blood Banks[56] or the American Medical Association.[10]

5. Change in physician practices: Given all of the factors discussed, many physicians have been reassessing their practices regarding autologous blood. Some orthopedists have decided to no longer routinely recommend preoperative donation to all of their patients who are having joint replacement surgery. The current trend among these physicians is selective application of preoperative donation and perioperative blood salvage for patients most likely to benefit. Multiple studies have used patient-specific characteristics (e.g., the preoperative hemoglobin level and the type of surgical procedure) in algorithms to try to identify these patients more accurately.[16,19,33,37,41,46,49]

Selection of either one or a combination of the available perioperative autologous techniques may also be patient dependent.[4,7,32,35] These changes in physician practices are probably the major reasons for the decline in donations, because studies have shown that physician recommendations are the primary motivational factor for autologous donors.[21,42]

Preoperative Donation

Elective orthopedic procedures, particularly reconstructive joint surgery, lend themselves readily to the preoperative collection of autologous blood. Because most procedures are performed electively, can be delayed for several weeks to a month or more without harm to the patient, and are generally associated with significant and predictable blood loss, orthopedic surgery is an ideal area in which to perform preoperative collection for those patients who are most likely to benefit. Collection of up to three to four units of blood at weekly intervals may be accomplished within the month before surgery. Volume repletion after donation generally requires 48 to 72 hours and provides a practical limit to the interval between the last donation and surgery. The minimum hemoglobin level allowed for autologous donors is 11.0 mg/dL, and many patients benefit from the concurrent administration of oral iron therapy to optimize erythropoiesis.

Because of the changing nature of costs and benefits, physician groups and hospitals should strive to establish reasonable standards for autologous blood donation. Use of patient-specific approaches should be considered. Transfusion triggers for autologous units should be the same as allogeneic units owing to the risks described earlier. Although erythropoietin has been used in successful experimental trials to enable patients to donate more autologous units,[29,47,51] its use adds significantly to the cost of autologous blood, and clinical benefit may be realized only in patients who are initially anemic. More recent studies have focused on the use of erythropoietin alone as a means to stimulate erythropoiesis in patients with low initial hemoglobin concentrations, thereby avoiding the need for transfusion.[5,25,26]

Hemodilution

In immediate preoperative hemodilution (also known as acute normovolemic hemodilution or ANH), two to three units of autologous blood are collected in the operating room after the patient is anesthetized but before the onset of surgery. Crystalloid and/or colloid are administered to replace lost volume. Standard blood bags and anticoagulants are used, and the collected units are stored at room temperature in the operating room. The following rationales support the use of ANH: (1) the red cell content of each volume of blood lost after hemodilution is reduced; (2) patients with normal cardiac function can perfuse their tissues as adequately

with a hematocrit of 25 to 30 percent as with higher hematocrits; and (3) the procedure provides fresh autologous red cells, plasma, and platelets for administration after surgery. The use of ANH is attractive because of its low cost relative to other forms of autologous blood collection, but patients must be selected carefully to avoid adverse effects, and the procedure may delay the start of surgery. Widespread application of this technique has not occurred. Experimental trials suggest that the use of ANH can decrease the need for allogeneic transfusion.[12,28,31] However, application of perioperative transfusion protocols may achieve a similar effect.[12]

Intraoperative Salvage

Intraoperative blood salvage can be used effectively in orthopedic surgery; however, its use should be limited to procedures likely to cause significant blood loss, such as revision hip surgery as well as some spinal instrumentation cases. Primary reconstructive joint surgery is generally not associated with sufficient blood loss to justify the cost of intraoperative blood salvage.

In general, intraoperative collection of blood in orthopedic surgery is technically more difficult than in other types of surgery in which pooled shed blood in a body cavity is salvaged. Aspiration of blood with a large amount of air and at a high vacuum setting results in hemolysis and other damage to red cells. Accordingly, aspiration should be performed carefully at low vacuum. Effective filtering, hemoconcentration, and washing of the salvaged red blood cells are critical steps in the removal of free hemoglobin, tissue/bone debris, and other unwanted supernatant materials before reinfusion. Additional wash solution, micro aggregate filtering, and visible clearing of hemolysis in the waste line are often performed to ensure product quality.

Special efforts should also be made to avoid aspirating irrigation fluid and other crystalloids into the blood salvage system. In addition to the inefficient processing of salvaged blood that results from dilution, there are controversial reports of a condition characterized by coagulopathy and pulmonary dysfunction, the so-called "salvaged blood syndrome," which may be associated with such dilution.[13] Such irrigation solutions may also contain medications not intended for intravenous use, which may not be removed if washing is incomplete. Other relative contraindications to the use of blood salvage include malignancy, infection, and the use of collagen-based sealants, which heighten the risk of metastasis, sepsis, and thrombosis, respectively, after reinfusion.

Postoperative Salvage

On many occasions, collecting the drainage from a reconstructed joint postoperatively can yield the equivalent of a unit or more of red blood cells. After collection, the wound drainage can be directly reinfused through a filter or, alternatively, washed in a manner similar to that of most intraoperative blood salvage and then reinfused.

Postoperative wound drainage often contains elevated levels of the anaphylatoxic complement components C3a and C5a,[5,6] cytokines,[2] activated coagulation factors, fibrin split products,[9] methyl methacrylate,[34] fat, phospholipids, and lipolytic enzymes such as phopholipase A2,[40] in addition to markedly increased levels of free hemoglobin. Although most of the published reports indicate few clinical problems with the reinfusion of such unwashed salvaged blood, significant complications and reactions have occurred.[15,24,63] The consensus appears to be that patients can tolerate unwashed salvaged blood reinfusion in limited amounts (less than 1 liter) and within 6 hours of collection. When large amounts of drainage are expected, as in bilateral knee replacement surgery, washing with cell salvage instruments may be indicated.

Although the use of postoperative salvage was widespread in the early 1990s, its popularity has declined in the past few years. Both the efficacy and the cost-effectiveness of reinfusion of relatively small amounts of postoperatively salvaged blood have been questioned.

Perioperative Component Preparation

Devices are now available to prepare platelet-rich plasma and fibrin adhesive in the immediate preoperative period. Such products have been used topically in combination with bovine or human thrombin to promote wound hemostasis and healing, particularly in plastic surgery. Clinical trials of the use of these autologous platelet and plasma products in orthopedic surgery are lacking.

SUMMARY

Perioperative autologous blood collection and transfusion continue to have a role in the orthopedic surgery practice. In some circumstances, the patient's fear of transfusion drives the use of multiple autologous techniques in order to avoid allogeneic transfusion regardless of cost. However, for most practices, the experience gained since the mid-1980s has resulted in a more selective application that takes into account both the likelihood of significant blood loss and the individual patient's ability to tolerate and recover from such blood loss while still minimizing the use of allogeneic blood. Further changes in these practices are likely to occur depending on the status of the allogeneic blood supply, the clinical impact of transfusion-related immunomodulation, and the use of autologous component therapy.

Appropriateness and Cost-effectiveness Considerations

The issue of cost-effectiveness for any therapy should be determined by data on a number of factors. These include the statistical likelihood of defined adverse effects if the therapy in question is (or is not) used. The data should include realistic estimates of the costs of diagnosing these adverse reactions and devising therapy for them and must also take into account the demographics of the populations of patients in question. For instance, if the risks of disease transmission by allogeneic transfusion are significantly reduced by new donor screening and testing methods, the cost of avoiding any residual risk becomes significantly higher in the cost-effectiveness equation. Similarly, if the introduction of the "new" therapy (e.g., autologous transfusions) is associated with an increase in complexity of the operational systems required for its introduction (e.g., patient/donor evaluation, blood collection, testing, processing, storage and shipping), the potential for error (particularly clerical) is likely to be similarly increased. Thus, the new "safer" alternative may be attended by a considerable increase in the risk of the patient's actually receiving the wrong unit of blood! In fact, in some autologous (predeposited) donation systems, 1 in 16,000 units was reported to go to an unintended recipient.[43] This fact also has to be considered in the equation.

Although it may seem invidious to place a monetary value on life and health, common sense indicates that for health care expenditure to be evaluated before implementation, both costs and effectiveness must be determined so that a variety of competing programs can be reasonably compared. With growing pressures on health care providers to simultaneously reduce costs and increase the efficiency of health care delivery, the need to use a standardized method of determining cost-effectiveness assumes even greater importance. Such a system has been developed and utilized to establish a consensus figure for "acceptable" cost-effectiveness.[43] That figure in the 1990s was generally accepted to be $50,000. This means that an intervention would be considered to be cost-effective if the computed QALY was $50,000 or less for this particular intervention.

Based on the presumption that the rationale for preoperative autologous donation is avoidance of the risk of allogeneic pathogen transmission, the QALY figure for arthroplasty has been reported to be between $240,000 and $1,467,000 (clearly not cost-effective!), depending on whether the procedure was bilateral revision, unilateral hip, or unilateral knee surgery.[36] A major factor in this cost is the fact that, in general, 30 to 50 percent of predonated blood is never needed and is wasted because it cannot be used for other patients. This is because the majority of autologous donors (patients) would not be acceptable as allogeneic donors.

Although predonation programs are clearly not cost-effective any longer, intraoperative salvage of shed blood is a quite different consideration, largely because very little blood is wasted and because the procedure does not lead to preoperative anemia in the patient as preoperative donation often does.

In our practice, if we collect the equivalent of two units of red blood cells intraoperatively, the procedure is cost-effective. In assessing the question of cost-effectiveness of autologous donation, one must also be aware that the figures quoted earlier were developed before the new polymerase chain reaction (PCR)-based pathogen testing was introduced in 2000 for allogeneic donations. This advance in ensuring allogeneic blood safety would increase the QALY still higher and make autologous predonation even less cost-effective than was the case before 2000!

Blood from Directed Donors

Because of concerns about hepatitis and AIDS, patients may request that specific individuals donate blood for them. Such individuals are known as directed or designated donors. Usually, the patient cannot donate autologous blood and asks family members, friends, or even church or work groups to donate blood that is reserved for use exclusively by the patient. Such patients believe that they can select "safer" donors and thereby significantly reduce or eliminate the risk of transfusion-transmitted disease.

Overall, directed donors have not been shown to be a safer source of blood. Studies that examined disease markers for hepatitis and AIDS in directed donors compared with such markers in volunteer donors have demonstrated either similar or higher incidence of positive markers in the directed donors.[18,57] A higher prevalence of positive test results is seen when the directed donor group contains a significant proportion of "first-time" donors; comparable figures are seen with first-time volunteer donors. Therefore, the overall risk of transfusion-transmitted infectious disease is similar, and possibly higher, for blood products from directed and volunteer donors.

The use of blood from directed donors may, at least theoretically, decrease transfusion risks if the number of donors is limited. Such "minimal exposure transfusion" programs select only one or two individuals to provide for all of the anticipated blood needs of the patients.[11] In well-planned situations, one person may be able to provide multiple units of red blood cells and thus eliminate the need for blood from any other donors.

However, there are other theoretical and practical concerns regarding the use of directed donors. Such individuals may be under significant pressure to donate and thus may not be truthful regarding behavior that places them at risk for hepatitis or AIDS. Donor confidentiality may be difficult to maintain when blood is not usable because of abnormal test results or "high-risk" behavior or when disease transmission does occur. The increased handling and tracking of directed donor units to ensure their use by the intended patient can double the cost. The transfusion of blood from some related individuals can even have adverse effects, such as graft-versus-host disease.[50] It has also been shown that the complexities of autologous donation and processing are such that the risk of getting the wrong unit of blood is considerably higher for patients involved in autologous programs.

Clearly, the use of autologous blood is safest in terms of the transmission of infectious disease. The decision to use directed donors is best made on a case-by-case basis, taking into account the availability of a directed donor program, the patient's needs, and knowledge about the local blood supply.

Bone Banking

The availability of human banked bone over the past few years has added significant ammunition to the armamentarium of the orthopedist. In essence, one must treat the banking of bone in the same manner as the banking of blood! In fact, the FDA has recently moved to codify this approach in a comprehensive set of detailed regulations by which all tissue (including bone) banking will be regulated.

These regulations will parallel those developed to manage blood banking, will cover all aspects of bone banking, and are clearly designed to help ensure both the safety and efficacy of banked tissue. The regulations stipulate that all banked tissue must come from individuals tested and found negative for stipulated markers for HBV, HCV, HIV, human T-cell leukemia virus-I, and syphilis. The donors of such tissue must also not be in the designated high-risk groups for these diseases. In addition, the regulations spell out the details of how tissues must be acquired, tested, processed, and stored, and how the documentation of each of these steps must be formatted and kept. They even spell out the nature and content of the obligatory training that tissue bankers must undergo annually.

Clearly, tissue (bone) banking has changed from a loosely organized activity to a tightly regulated one. Orthopedic surgeons involved in bone banking would be well advised to peruse the FDA regulations and assess the personnel and equipment costs necessary to comply. In many cases, orthopedists who pioneered bone banking in their institutions are thankfully relinquishing their responsibility to those experienced in dealing with FDA regulation. We strongly encourage this approach.

SUMMARY

Since 1992, there have been profound changes in transfusion practices, with implications for all fields of medicine. Orthopedic surgeons and their patients stand to benefit more than most from an awareness of an appropriate application of new practices, knowledge, and standards. We hope both awareness and appropriate application are aided by this transfusion medicine perspective.

References

1. American Association of Blood Banks: 1983 Annual Report Arlington, VA,. American Association of Blood Banks, 1984.
2. Arnestad JP, Bengtsson A, Bengtson JP, et al: Release of cytokines, polymorphonuclear elastase and terminal C5b–9 complement complex by infusion of wound drainage blood. Acta Orthop Scand 66:334–338, 1995.

3. Audet A, Andrzejewski C, Popovsky M: Red blood cell transfusion practices in patients undergoing orthopedic surgery: A multi-institutional analysis. Transfus Pract Orthop Surg 21:851–858, 1998.

4. Ayers DC, Murray DG, Duerr DM: Blood salvage after total hip arthroplasty. J Bone Joint Surg 77:1347–1351, 1995.

5. Bengston J, Backman L, Stenqvist O, et al: Complement activation and reinfusion of wound drainage blood. Anesthesiology 73:376–380, 1990.

6. Bengtsson A, Lisander B: Anaphylatoxin and terminal complement complexes in red cell salvage. Acta Anaesthesiol Scand 34:339–341, 1990.

7. Billote D, Abdoue A, Wixson R: Comparison of acute normovolemic hemodilution and preoperative autologous blood donation in clinical practice. J Clin Anesth 12:31–35, 2000.

8. Birkmeyer JD, Goodnough LT, AuBuchon JP, et al: The cost-effectiveness of preoperative autologous blood donation for total hip and knee replacement. Transfusion 33:544–551, 1993.

9. Blaylock R, Carlson K, Morgan J, et al: In vitro analysis of shed blood from patients undergoing total knee replacement surgery. Am J Clin Pathol 101:365–369, 1994.

10. Blum L, Allen J, Genel M, Howe J: Crossover use of donated blood for autologous transfusion: Report of the Council on Scientific Affairs, American Medical Association. Transfusion 38:891–895, 1998.

11. Brecher ME, Taswell HF, Clare DE, et al: Minimal-exposure transfusion and the committed donor. Transfusion 30:599, 1990.

12. Bryson GL, Laupacis A, Wells GA: Does acute normovolemic hemodilution reduce perioperative allogeneic transfusion? A meta-analysis. Anesth Analg 86:9–15, 1998.

13. Bull B, Bull M: The salvaged blood syndrome: A sequel to mechanochemical activation of platelets and leukocytes? Blood Cells 16:5–23, 1990.

14. Churchill WH, McGurk S, Chapman RH, et al: The collaborative hospital transfusion study: Variations in use of autologous blood account for hospital differences in red cell use during primary hip and knee surgery. Transfusion 38:530–539, 1998.

15. Clements DH, Sculco TP, Burke SW, et al: Salvage and reinfusion of postoperative sanguineous wound drainage. J Bone Joint Surg 74A:646, 1992.

16. Cohen JA, Brecher ME: Preoperative autologous blood donation: Benefit or detriment? A mathematical analysis. Transfusion 35:640–44, 1995.

17. College of American Pathologists, Practice Guidelines Development Task Force: Practice parameter for the use of fresh-frozen plasma, cryoprecipitate, and platelets. JAMA 271:777, 1994.

18. Cordell RR, Yalon VA, Cigahn-Haskel C, et al: Experience with 11,916 designated donors. Transfusion 26:484, 1986.

19. Cushner FD, Scott WN: Evolution of blood transfusion management for a busy knee practice. Orthopedics 22:S145–S147, 1999.

20. Dodd RY, Aberle-Grasse JM, Stramel SL: The yield of nucleic acid testing (NAT) for HIV and HCV RNA in a population of US voluntary donors: Relationship to contemporary measures of incidence. Transfusion 40:(Suppl IS), 2000.

21. Domen RE, Ribicki LA, Hoeltge GA: An analysis of autologous blood donor motivational factors. Vox Sang 69:110–113, 1995.

22. Domen RE: Adverse reactions associated with autologous blood transfusion: Evaluation and incidence at a large academic hospital. Transfusion 38:296–300, 1998.

23. Etchason J, Petz L, Keeler E, et al: The cost effectiveness of preoperative autologous blood donations. N Engl J Med 332:719–724, 1995.

24. Faris P, Ritter M, Keating E, Valeri C: Unwashed filtered shed blood collected after knee and hip arthroplasties: A source of autologous red blood cells. J Bone Joint Surg [Am] 73:1169–1178, 1991.

25. Faris PM, Ritter MA, Abels RI, Group AES: The effects of recombinant human erythropoietin on perioperative transfusion requirements in patients having a major orthopaedic operation. J Bone Joint Surg 78A:62–72, 1996.

26. Feagen B, Wong C, Kirkley A, et al: Erythropoietin with iron supplmentation to prevent allogeneic blood transfusion in total hip joint arthroplasty—a randomized, controlled trial. Ann Intern Med 133:845–854, 2000.

27. Forgie MA, Wells P, Laupacis A, Fergusson D: Preoperative autologous donation decreases allogeneic transfusion but increases exposure to all red blood cell transfusion. Arch Intern Med 158:610–616, 1998.

28. Goodnough L, Monk T, Despotis G, Merkel K: A randomized trial of acute normovolemic hemodilution compared to preoperative autologous blood donation in total knee arthroplasty. Vox Sang 77:11–16, 1999.

29. Goodnough L, Price T, Friedman K, et al: A phase III trial of recombinant human erythropoietin therapy in nonanemic orthopedic patients subjected to aggressive removal of blood for autologous use: Dose, response, toxicity, and efficacy. Transfusion 34:66–71, 1994.

30. Goodnough LT, Brecher ME, Kanter MH, AuBuchon JP: Transfusion medicine: Blood transfusion. N Engl J Med 340:438–447, 1999.

31. Goodnough LT, Despotis GJ, Merkel K, Monk TG: A randomized trial comparing acute normovolemic hemodilution and preopertive autologous blood donation in total hip arthroplasty. Transfusion 40:1054–1057, 2000.

32. Grosvenor D, Goyal V, Goodman S: Efficacy of postoperative blood salvage following total hip arthroplasty in patients with and without deposited autologous units. J Bone Joint Surg 82A:951–954, 2000.

33. Hatzidakis A, Mendlick R, McKillip T, et al: Preoperative autologous donation for total joint arthroplasty. J Bone Joint Surg 82A:89–100, 2000.

34. Healy W, Wasilewski S, Pfeifer B, et al: Methylmethacrylate monomer and fat content in shed blood after total joint arthroplasty. Clin Orthop Res 286:15–17, 1993.

35. Huet C, Salmi L, Fergusson D, et al: A meta-analysis of the effectiveness of cell salvage to minimize perioperative allogeneic blood transfusion in cardiac and orthopedic surgery. Anesth Analg 89:861–869, 1999.

36. Jackson BR, Umlas J, AuBuchon JP: The cost-effectiveness of postoperative recovery of RBCs in preventing transfusion-associated virus transmission after joint arthroplasty. Transfusion 40:1063–1066, 2000.

37. Keating E, Meding J, Faris P, Ritter M: Predictors of transfusion risk in elective knee surgery. Clin Orthop 357:50–59, 1998.

38. Keeling MM, Schmidt-Clay P, Kotcamp WW, et al: Autotransfusion in the postoperative orthopedic patient. Clin Orthop 291:251, 1993.

39. Kim D, Brecher M, Estes T, Morrey BF: Relationship of hemoglobin level and duration of hospitalization after total hip arthroplasty: Implications for the transfusion target. Mayo Clin Proc 68:37, 1993.

40. Langton S, Sieunarine K, Lawrence-Brown M, et al: Lipolytic enzyme and phospholipid level changes in intraoperative salvaged blood. Transfusion Med 1:263–267, 1991.

41. Larocque B, Gilbert K, Brien WF: Prospective validation of a point score system for predicting blood transfusion following hip or knee replacement. Transfusion 38:932–937, 1998.

42. Lee SJ, Liljas B, Churchill WH, et al: Perceptions and preferences of autologous blood donors. Transfusion 38:757–763, 1998.

43. Linden JV: Errors in transfusion medicine. Arch Pathol Lab Med 123:563–565, 1999.

44. Linden JV: Autologous blood errors and incidents. Transfusion 34:28S, 1994.

45. Lundsgaard-Hansen P: Treatment of acute blood loss. Vox Sang 63:241, 1992.

46. Mercuriali F, Inghilleri G, Biffi E: Personalized approach to define transfusion support to surgical patients. Int J Artif Org 21:78–83, 1998.

47. Mercuriali F, Zanella A, Barosi G, et al: Use of erythropoietin to increase the volume of autologous blood donated by orthopedic patients. Transfusion 33:55–60, 1993.

48. National Institutes of Health Consensus Conference: Perioperative red blood cell transfusion. JAMA 260:2700, 1988.

49. Nuttall GA, Santrach PJ, Oliver WC, et al: Possible guidelines for preoperative autologous red blood cell donations for total hip arthroplasty patients based on the surgical blood order equation. Mayo Clin Proc 75:10–17, 2000.

50. Ohto H, Yasuda H, Noguchi M, Abe R: Risk of transfusion-associated graft-versus-host disease as a result of directed donations from relatives (letter). Transfusion 32:691, 1992.

51. Price TH, Goodnough LT, Vogler WR, et al: The effect of recombinant human erythropoietin on the efficacy of autologous blood donation in patients with low hematocrits: A multicenter, randomized, double-blind, controlled trial. Transfusion 36:29–36, 1996.

52. Reed RW II, Ciavarella D, Heimbach DM, et al: Prophylactic platelet administration during massive transfusion. Ann Surg 203:40, 1986.

53. Renner SW, Howanitz PJ, Bachner P: Preoperative autologous blood donation in 612 hospitals. Arch Pathol Lab Med 116:613–619, 1992.

54. Sazama K: Reports of 355 transfusion-associated deaths: 1976 through 1985. Transfusion 30:583, 1990.

55. Shibutani K, Frost EAM: Defining the low limit of hematocrit for surgical patients. Transfus Sci 14:335, 1993.

56. Standards for Blood Bank and Transfusion Services. Bethesda, MD, American Association of Blood Banks, 2000.

57. Starkey JM, MacPherson JL, Bolgiano DC, et al: Markers of transfusion-transmitted disease in different groups of blood donors. JAMA 262:3452, 1989.

58. Sullivan M: What is the State of the Nation's Blood Supply?: National Blood Data Resource Center, Bethesda, MD, 2001.

59. Vitale M, Stazzone E, Gelijns A, et al: The effectiveness of preoperative erythropoietin in averting allogeneic blood transfusion among children undergoing scoliosis surgery. Part B. J Pediatr Orthop 7:203–209, 1998.

60. Walker RH: What is a clinically significant antibody? In Polesky HF, Walker RH (eds): Safety in Transfusion Practices. Skokie, IL, College of American Pathologists, 1982, p 84.

61. Wallace EL, Churchill WH, Surgenor DM, et al: Collection and transfusion of blood and blood components in the United States, 1994. Transfusion 38:625–633, 1998.

62. Wallace EL, Churchill WH, Surgenor DM, et al: Collection and transfusion of blood and blood components in the United States, 1992. Transfusion 35:802–812, 1995.

63. Woda R, Tetzlaff J: Upper airway oedema following autologous blood transfusion from a wound drainage system. Can J Anaesth 39:290, 1992.

9A

The Cardiac Patient

•THOMAS P. NOBREGA and CLARENCE SHUB

The goal of the preoperative assessment of the cardiac patient is to minimize surgical morbidity and mortality. Risk stratification of a cardiac patient is fundamental to this goal and can often be accomplished using only the history, physical examination, electrocardiogram (ECG), and chest radiograph. Once risk stratification is accomplished, additional diagnostic testing, specialized monitoring, or even alteration of a planned surgical approach or its timing may be considered.

From the standpoint of perioperative risk, the three logical time frames to consider are the preoperative, the intraoperative, and the postoperative periods. The intraoperative responsibility for the patient with cardiac disease principally resides with the surgeon and the anesthesiologist. The pre- and postoperative periods may require the involvement of an internist or a cardiologist. Close communication between the physicians is essential. In general, patients with known, stable cardiac disease who are undergoing minor, low-risk procedures using local or regional anesthesia do not require the involvement of an internist or cardiologist. However, most patients with known cardiac disease who require general or spinal anesthesia for major orthopedic surgery should undergo preoperative cardiac evaluation. In selected cases, an internist or cardiologist should be involved in the postoperative care as well.

EVALUATION OF CARDIAC STATUS

Patients can be classified as high, intermediate, or low risk, based on clinical data acquired from the clinical assessment. Patients classified at intermediate risk may be further risk stratified using additional diagnostic tests. The risk stratification schemes developed by Goldman et al.[5] and Detsky et al.[4] found the following historical factors to be especially important: myocardial infarction (ever), unstable angina or myocardial infarction within the preceding 6 months, age older than 70 years, class III or IV angina, and recent or previous pulmonary edema. Physical examination variables associated with high risk included aortic stenosis, elevated jugular venous pressure, or a third systolic heart sound (S_3). Variables from the ECG associated with high risk included rhythm other than sinus or simple atrial premature contractions, or more than five premature ventricular contractions at any time before surgery. Patients with peripheral vascular disease represent a special high-risk group; the risk stratification schemes tend to underestimate risk in this group. Patients with diabetes mellitus also represent a special high-risk group, not only because they have a higher risk of underlying coronary artery disease but because they also have more frequent ischemia with no symptoms ("silent ischemia").

Coronary Artery Disease

The single most important factor with respect to cardiac risk of patients undergoing orthopedic surgery is coronary artery disease. Individuals with no prior clinical evidence of heart disease have a very low incidence of perioperative myocardial infarction. In patients with prior myocardial infarction, the risk is higher, particularly if the infarction occurs within the 6 months preceding surgery. This has prompted the recommendation to delay elective surgery for 6 months in such patients. However, in selected postinfarction patients who have been revascularized and have no significant ischemia on stress testing, the 6-month wait may not be necessary. Perioperative myocardial infarction, once it occurs, is associated with a high mortality.

Except for high-risk surgical procedures (Fig. 9A–1), most patients with mild, stable angina (class I or II) are at low risk for major cardiac events (perioperative myocardial infarction or death) and do not routinely require extensive preoperative cardiac testing (Fig. 9A–2).

Several authors have shown that the workload achieved on exercise stress testing is a significant predictor of perioperative cardiac events.[3] Orthopedic patients present special challenges because of their physical limitations. For example, a patient with severe osteoarthritis of the hips is usually so sedentary that functional limitation caused by angina pectoris, valve disease, or left ventricular dysfunction is not apparent. Although the use of wheelchairs and walkers may provide some clues to functional status, standard functional assessments are not applicable to many orthopedic patients. For some of these patients, pharmacologic stress testing may provide useful additional risk stratification.

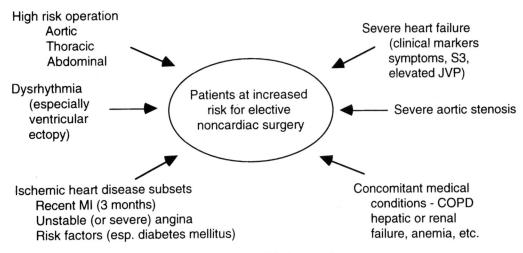

Figure 9A–1. Assessing risk of noncardiac surgery.

Valvular Heart Disease

Patients with severe aortic stenosis who are symptomatic should have aortic valve replacement before undergoing noncardiac surgery. However, there are groups of patients with significant aortic stenosis who either are not candidates for or refuse aortic valve replacement or who refuse to have the procedure done. O'Keefe et al.[8] have shown that in selected patients, with use of careful anesthetic techniques, it is possible to proceed with noncardiac surgery with a low risk of complications.

As a general rule, patients with symptomatic severe mitral stenosis should be considered as candidates for surgical correction or valvuloplasty. If, as in the case of the occasional patient, this is not feasible in occasional patients, medical therapy guided by intraoperative hemodynamic monitoring may be an alternative.

Regurgitant valvular lesions (mitral, aortic, and tricuspid regurgitation) are generally better tolerated than stenotic ones. Hence, patients with these lesions may be considered to be at lower risk as long as ventricular function is preserved.

Left Ventricular Dysfunction

Patients with a reduced ejection fraction should be maintained on their medications without interruption. Ideally, volume status should be optimized with the careful use of diuretics; heart failure, if present, should be treated before surgery. In patients with uncompensated congestive heart failure who require urgent surgery and have, preoperative and perioperative monitoring with a pulmonary artery catheter may be helpful.

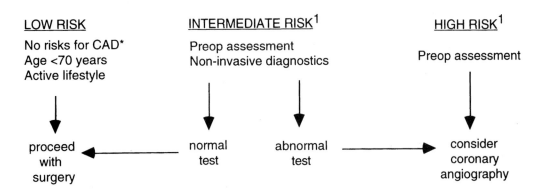

Figure 9A–2. Clinical approach to the cardiac patient.

Impact of Type and Urgency of Surgery

The overall risk of an orthopedic surgical procedure is determined by the urgency of the surgery as well as by the type of procedure. In general, orthopedic surgery is considered an intermediate risk procedure, particularly when compared with vascular, intrathoracic, or intraperitoneal surgery. However, patients undergoing procedures in which significant intravascular volume shifts take place and in patients requiring multiple transfusions, the risk level should be considered higher because there is greater potential for intravascular volume depletion or excess.

PREOPERATIVE CARE

Cardiac medications should be continued uninterrupted throughout the perioperative period. Although modifications in dose and route of administration may need to be considered, there is no reason to stop cardiac medications during the perioperative period (Table 9A–1). This is especially true for patients who are taking β-blockers, in whom β-blocker withdrawal may lead to a "rebound" phenomenon in which excessive increases in sympathetic discharge and heart rate may precipitate myocardial ischemia. Centrally acting α-blockers (e.g., clonidine) represent another class of drugs whose abrupt discontinuation may lead to severe rebound hypertension and provoke ischemia in a susceptible patient.

Perioperative myocardial ischemia is associated with an increased risk of morbidity and mortality. In a study of 52 consecutive patients undergoing elective hip arthroplasty by means of lumbar regional anesthesia, 31 percent of patients had episodes of myocardial ischemia perioperatively. Ninety-six percent of the ischemic events were clinically silent. No ischemic events were associated with heart rates of 50 beats per minute or less.[7]

Increasingly, evidence suggests there are many patients for whom perioperative β-blocker therapy should be considered. Perioperative β-blocker therapy was shown in a randomized trial to reduce short and long-term mortality in high-risk patients undergoing intermediate to high-risk procedures. The American College of Cardiology/American Heart Association guidelines support the use of perioperative β-blocker therapy (unless contraindicated) in patients with hypertension, coronary artery disease, or symptomatic arrhythmias.[1,6]

The perioperative risk of anticoagulant use poses special problems. The risk of a thrombotic event must be balanced against the risk of postoperative bleeding. Decisions regarding anticoagulation may be made jointly between the consulting cardiologist and the surgeon based on the specific procedure, the anticipated thromboembolic risk, anticipated blood loss, and like considerations. Patients taking anticoagulation therapy for chronic atrial fibrillation, depending on their embolic risk, can, in most cases, remain without anticoagulation for several days.

For patients with mechanical prosthetic valves, a variety of approaches may be taken. All anticoagulant therapy may be discontinued 1 to 3 days preoperatively and resumed approximately 2 days postoperatively; this has been associated with a 13 percent incidence of bleeding complications but no thrombotic events in one study.[9] An alternative approach involves using heparin anticoagulation until 6 hours preoperatively, and resuming heparin 12 to 24 hours postoperatively. The low molecular-weight heparins may expedite the transition back to warfarin in the postoperative period.

POSTOPERATIVE CARE

Most patients identified preoperatively as being at high risk should have an internist or cardiologist involved in their postoperative care. Decisions regarding the use of an intensive care unit or telemetry must be individualized and will depend to some extent on the intraoperative course. Intraoperative hypotension, significant tachycardia or bradycardia, ventricular ectopy, pulmonary edema, or the need for large volume replacement should all prompt the consideration of careful postoperative monitoring, possibly in an intensive care unit. Similarly, chest pain, pulmonary edema, or other cardiovascular complications in the postanesthesia recovery room should also prompt consideration of postoperative telemetry or intensive care unit placement.

Table 9A–1. CARDIAC MEDICATIONS

Medication Type	Use	Route of Administration	Comments
Nitrates	Antianginal	Oral, intravenous, topical	Continue pre- and perioperatively
Calcium channel blockers	Antianginal, antihypertensive, antiarrhythmic	Oral, intravenous	Continue pre- and perioperatively if possible
β-Blockers	Antianginal, antihypertensive, antiarrhythmic	Oral, intravenous	Potentially dangerous to discontinue pre- and perioperatively
Diuretics	Hypertension, congestive heart failure	Oral, intravenous	Assess for electrolyte disturbances
α-Blockers	Hypertension	Oral, intravenous (some α-blockers), topical	Centrally acting, dangerous to discontinue
Digoxin	Dysrhythmia, congestive heart failure	Oral, intravenous	Decreased dosage in renal failure

The key elements of postoperative care include minimizing triggers for ischemia, heart failure, or hemodynamic changes. Volume shifts, as fluid is mobilized, may occur as late as 48 to 72 hours postoperatively and can provoke cardiac ischemia or heart failure. It is particularly important that the surgeon recognize that excessive postoperative pain can also precipitate ischemia, and appropriate analgesia is especially important in high-risk patients.

SPECIAL CONSIDERATIONS

Subacute bacterial endocarditis prophylaxis should be given in patients with native or prosthetic valvular disease. These should be administered according to guidelines outlined by the American Heart Association.[13] As a general rule, asymptomatic conduction system disease noted on the preoperative ECG, such as bifascicular or even trifascicular block, does not warrant preoperative cardiac pacing. The patient with a permanent pacemaker generally requires consideration of antibiotic prophylaxis, and possibly pacemaker reprogramming after cautery is used in surgery.

References

1. ACC/AHA Task Force Report: Guidelines for perioperative cardiovascular evaluation for noncardiac surgery. JACC 27:910, 1996.
2. Ashton CM, Petersen NJ, Wray NP, et al: The incidence of perioperative myocardial infarction in men undergoing noncardiac surgery. Ann Intern Med 118:504, 1993.
3. Carliner NH, Fisher ML, Plotnick GD, et al: Routine preoperative exercise testing in patients undergoing major noncardiac surgery. Am J Cardiol 56:51, 1985.
4. Detsky AS, Abrams HB, McLauglin JR, et al: Predicting cardiac complications in patients undergoing non-cardiac surgery. J Gen Intern Med 1:211, 1986.
5. Goldman L, Caldera DL, Nussbaum SR, Southwick FS: Multifactorial index of cardiac risk in noncardiac surgical procedures. N Engl J Med 297:845, 1977.
6. Mangano DT, Layug EL, Wallace A, Tateo I: Effect of atenolol on mortality and cardiovascular morbidity after noncardiac surgery. Multicenter study of perioperative ischemia research group. N Engl J Med 335:1713, 1996.
7. Marsch SCU, Schaefer HG, Skarvan K, et al: Perioperative myocardial ischemia in patients undergoing elective hip arthroplasty during lumbar regional anesthesia. Anesthesiology 76:518, 1992.
8. O'Keefe JH, Shub C, Rettke SR: Risk of noncardiac surgical procedures in patients with aortic stenosis. Mayo Clin Proc 64:400, 1989.
9. Tinker JH, Tarhan S: Discontinuing anticoagulant therapy in surgical patients with cardiac valve prostheses: Observations in 180 operations. JAMA 239:738, 1978.

9B

Pulmonary Disease and Surgery

• JAY H. RYU

Postoperative pulmonary complications are commonly encountered in surgical patients. These include atelectasis, pneumonia, aspiration, pulmonary edema, respiratory failure, and pulmonary thromboembolism. In general, these problems are less frequent after orthopedic surgery than after thoracic or abdominal surgery, with the exception of pulmonary thromboembolism. In addition, fat embolism is usually associated with trauma and orthopedic procedures.

RESPIRATORY EFFECTS OF ANESTHESIA IN SURGERY

Several physiologic changes occur in the respiratory system with general anesthesia.[4] Virtually every anesthetic agent that is used in general anesthesia is a respiratory depressant. Effects include blunted ventilatory response to hypoxemia and hypercarbia, impaired respiratory muscle tone, and altered ventilatory pattern. Furthermore, mechanical ventilation is associated with ventilation-perfusion imbalance causing gas exchange abnormalities. Perioperative medications cause drying of secretions, decreased mucociliary clearance, and suppression of cough reflex, which impair defense mechanisms of the respiratory system. These effects extend into the postoperative period and pose risk, particularly in those patients with preexisting lung disease.

Avoidance of general anesthesia by using regional anesthesia generally lessens the likelihood of postoperative pulmonary complications. However, control of the airway with endotracheal tube and general anesthesia may facilitate management of certain patients who have excessive airway secretions and require frequent suctioning. Obviously, the anesthetic plan needs to be tailored to the individual patient's circumstances and the type of surgery to be performed (see Chapter 12).

RISK FACTORS FOR POSTOPERATIVE PULMONARY COMPLICATIONS

Preoperative assessment should include identification of risk factors for postoperative pulmonary complica-

tions to enable appropriate perioperative management. Risk factors are associated with patient-related factors, anesthesia, and the surgical procedure itself.[3]

Patient-related risk factors are sought by taking a comprehensive history and performing a careful examination. These factors include preexisting lung disease, current respiratory symptoms, general health status, smoking, obesity, and age.[3] Patients with suspected or known lung disorders should undergo a chest roentgenogram and pulmonary function testing to assess the degree of impairment. In many cases, a simple spirometry examination may suffice for assessment of pulmonary function. An arterial blood gas study may be needed to look for hypoxemia or hypercarbia in those patients with severe pulmonary dysfunction. However, it should be stated that the relationship between the severity of pulmonary dysfunction and the likelihood of postoperative pulmonary complications has not been firmly established for nonabdominal, nonthoracic surgery.[3] Severe pulmonary dysfunction, hypoxemia, or hypercarbia heightens concern regarding pulmonary complications, but these conditions may not be absolute contraindications for orthopedic surgery.

Duration of anesthesia, intraoperative events, and the nature of the surgical procedure also influence the postoperative course. Prolonged anesthesia and a complicated intraoperative period increase the chance of postoperative complications.

PERIOPERATIVE MANAGEMENT

Preoperative Considerations

Preoperative assessment allows identification of patients at risk and quantification of the predisposition to postoperative pulmonary complications. The intensity of perioperative management is determined based on this assessment. Measures to reduce the risk of pulmonary complications should begin with preoperative patient education.

Preoperative education should include cessation of smoking for smokers with or without known obstructive lung disease. For maximum benefit, smoking cessation should occur several weeks before surgery. If time allows, obese patients should undergo weight reduction. Patients with risk factors should be instructed in deep breathing exercises or incentive spirometry performed during every waking hour before and after surgery. Periodic coughing should be urged for those patients with excessive tracheobronchial secretions. Patients who have cough productive of discolored phlegm may benefit from a course of broad-spectrum antibiotics for several days before surgery. In patients with preexisting lung diseases, their usual pulmonary medications, such as bronchodilators and corticosteroids, should be continued perioperatively. Recent or current oral or parenteral corticosteroid usage requires consideration of possible adrenal suppression and increased corticosteroid dose perioperatively to mimic normal stress response. Use of corticosteroid inhalers in the usual dose range does not cause adrenal suppression, which may occur with high doses. Chest physiotherapy may help those patients with excessive respiratory secretions and those patients who are too weak or debilitated to raise their own secretions. An appropriate mode of deep venous thrombosis prophylaxis should be instituted before surgery (see Chapter 11). Lastly, pulmonary consultation should be considered for those patients with severe pulmonary dysfunction or recent deterioration in their pulmonary symptoms.

Intraoperative Considerations

Intraoperatively, vital functions require monitoring, which may include pulse oximetry, capnography, and arterial catheterization. Bronchodilators can be given via the inhalation route (Table 9B–1). Frequent suctioning controls secretions. Anesthesia time is reduced as is feasible, particularly for those patients at high risk for pulmonary complications.

Postoperative Considerations

Postoperatively, intensity of monitoring is tailored to the patient's risk for potential complications. In the early postoperative course, residual effects from anesthetics, muscle relaxants, and postoperative pain medications may produce detrimental effects on the respiratory function. In patients at high risk for pulmonary complications due to preexisting severe pulmonary disease or otherwise, one may choose to leave the endotracheal tube in place postoperatively until the patient is fully awake and strong enough to exhibit adequate ventilation and effective cough. Some patients may need postoperative mechanical ventilation and monitoring in the intensive care unit setting. Preoperative preventive measures undertaken to reduce pulmonary complications should be continued postoperatively. In addition, early mobilization and ambulation when the patient is able, along with adequate pain control, should be beneficial. Supplemental oxygen should be used when needed to maintain arterial oxygen saturation of at least 90 percent, with caution exercised for those patients with CO_2 retention. Humidification of inspired air may help those who have difficulty raising secretions. Expectorants and mucolytic agents are generally not helpful. Intermittent positive pressure breathing is not useful except for those patients with neuromuscular disease or restrictive chest wall defect in whom improved ventilatory capacity may be seen with its use.

Atelectasis. Atelectasis is the most commonly occurring pulmonary complication after surgical procedures. In many cases, the extent may be minimal and not require specific therapy. However, if the extent of atelectasis is significant enough to cause infiltrates and volume loss on the chest radiograph, along with fever, dyspnea, and hypoxemia, therapeutic maneuvers should be undertaken. In many cases, humidification, deep breathing, coughing, incentive spirometry, and chest physiotherapy may suffice to reverse atelectasis. Tracheal suctioning or continuous positive pressure mask may also help resolve atelectasis, particularly in those patients who are weak, debilitated, or uncooperative. In refractory cases, bronchoscopy can be employed to aid in clearing tracheobronchial secretions and mucous plugs.

Chronic Obstructive Pulmonary Disease. Patients with chronic obstructive pulmonary disease or asthma may have bronchospasm postoperatively. This usually responds to β-agonists given by metered dose inhaler or nebulizer (see Table 9B–1).[1] Severe cases may require oral or parenteral corticosteroids. Inhaled corticosteroids are not effective in the acute setting. Theophylline is less effective in bronchodilatation than β-agonists and has a limited role in treating acute bronchospasm. Wheezing can be caused by several processes other than

Table 9B–1. COMMONLY USED BRONCHODILATORS

Medication	Route	Usual Dose
β-agonist		
Albuterol	MDI[a]	2 puffs every 4–6 hr
	Nebulization	2.5 mg every 6 hr
Pirbuterol	MDI	2 puffs every 4–6 hr
Salmeterol (long-acting)	MDI	2 puffs every 12 hr
Anti-cholinergic		
Ipratropium	MDI	2 puffs every 6 hr
	Nebulization	500 mcg every 6–8 hr

[a]Metered dose inhaler.

bronchospasm; therefore, one should consider other entities such as pulmonary edema, pulmonary embolism, aspiration, pneumothorax, and drug or transfusion reaction. Wheezing may also be produced by upper airway difficulties such as laryngospasm, laryngeal edema, or upper airway injury owing to the presence of an endotracheal tube.

Aspiration. Aspiration is a potential complication, particularly for patients with depressed consciousness or impaired upper airway defense mechanisms. The effect may vary from minor lung infiltrates that are detected on the chest radiograph to severe hypoxemia with adult respiratory distress syndrome (ARDS). Prophylactic antibiotic usage is generally not helpful in this setting. Tracheal suctioning or bronchoscopy, if needed, may help clear large particulate matter from the airways. In the presence of extensive lung infiltrates and progressive hypoxemia, endotracheal intubation and mechanical ventilation is employed.

Pulmonary Embolism. Venous thromboembolism is a feared complication, particularly after knee and hip surgeries (and is discussed in detail in Chapter 11). The clinical picture usually includes dyspnea, chest pain, tachypnea, and tachycardia. When thromboembolism is suspected, intravenous heparin 5000 IU should be given (in the absence of absolute contraindications) before diagnostic studies are undertaken.[2] Diagnostic evaluation may include ventilation perfusion lung scan, computed tomography angiography, noninvasive evaluation of the lower extremity veins, or standard pulmonary angiography, depending on the clinical circumstances. In patients with contraindications to anticoagulation and confirmed venous thromboembolism, an inferior vena cava filter such as a Greenfield filter may be needed to prevent recurrence of pulmonary embolism. Thrombolytic therapy should be considered in those patients who have hemodynamic instability due to massive pulmonary embolism.[2]

Fat embolism. Fat embolism syndrome consists of respiratory insufficiency, cerebral disturbance, and, uncommonly, petechial rash. Therapy usually includes supportive measures such as supplemental oxygen and mechanical ventilation if needed. Although corticosteroids may have a role in prophylaxis, they do not appear to be efficacious in the treatment of fat embolism syndrome.

Pulmonary Edema. Pulmonary edema may occur postoperatively because of fluid overload, congestive heart failure, myocardial infarction, or ARDS. The latter, in turn, may be triggered by a variety of factors including aspiration, drug or transfusion reaction, sepsis, fat embolism, acute pancreatitis, and others. Dyspnea, tachypnea, tachycardia, crackles, diaphoresis, hypoxemia, and diffuse lung infiltrates develop. Pulmonary artery catheterization is frequently required to distinguish cardiogenic (hydrostatic) from noncardiogenic (permeability) pulmonary edema. Appropriate management is based on underlying causes and is usually carried out in an intensive care unit setting where mechanical ventilation with positive end-expiratory pressure may be needed.

Pulmonary Infections. Hospital acquired pneumonia is usually caused by gram-negative bacilli. *Staphylococcus aureus*, *Streptococcus pneumoniae*, anaerobes, and *Legionella* are less common causative agents. Choice of antibiotic for treatment of pneumonia may be based on sputum examination or empiric fashion. Aminoglycoside with an antipseudomonal penicillin or third-generation cephalosporin is commonly used.

References

1. Barnes PJ: Chronic obstructive pulmonary disease. N Engl J Med 343:269–80, 2000.
2. Hyers TM, Agnelli G, Hull RD, et al: Antithrombotic therapy for venous thromboembolic disease. Chest 114;561S–78S, 1998.
3. Smetana GW: Preoperative pulmonary evaluation. N Engl J Med 340:937–44, 1999.
4. Sykes LA, Bowe EA: Cardiorespiratory effects of anesthesia. Clin Chest Med 14:211–26, 1993.

9C

The Diabetic Patient

BRUCE R. ZIMMERMAN and BERNARD F. MORREY

It is estimated that, in the United States, 2.5 to 5 percent of the population has diabetes and an equal number of people have undiagnosed diabetes. Hence, the orthopedic surgeon performing joint reconstructive surgery is frequently faced with the coexistence of diabetes and its associated increased surgical and postoperative risks. Individuals with diabetes have more cardiovascular disease, renal impairment, and hypertension than people without diabetes. Poorly controlled diabetes increases the risk of postoperative wound infections.

PREOPERATIVE EVALUATION

Several aspects of the preoperative evaluation require more emphasis in the patient with diabetes.

With proper management of the blood glucose level, most studies find that the perioperative prognosis of patients with diabetes and no diabetic complications is similar to that in patients without diabetes.[3] In the patient with type 2 diabetes mellitus (previously called non—insulin-dependent diabetes mellitus), elective surgery should be delayed until control of the blood glucose level improves if the preoperative fasting blood glucose is greater than 200 mg/dl. Often institution of insulin treatment, even temporarily, is helpful. The preoperative evaluation should concentrate on identifying complications that might modify the surgical management. Clearly the major concern is cardiovascular disease, which is common in patients with diabetes. Clinical recognition of cardiovascular disease in people with diabetes is more difficult because the symptoms may be atypical and silent myocardial ischemia is common. How aggressively to test for coronary artery disease preoperatively depends on the extent and risk of the surgical procedure. Those patients with atherosclerosis obliterans have coronary artery disease. Cardiologic consultation is frequently helpful.

Cardiac arrest in patients with a severe cardiac autonomic neuropathy is an anesthesia risk that is not widely recognized in patients with diabetes. This possibility should be suspected in patients with extensive diabetic peripheral neuropathy or other forms of autonomic neuropathy, such as orthostatic hypotension, gastro-

paresis, or diabetic diarrhea. If the anesthesiologist is alert to this possibility, resuscitation is usually successful.[1]

The other complication that has a significant effect on surgical management is diabetic nephropathy. The earliest stage of nephropathy is identified by the presence of increased microalbuminuria. Proteinuria is found on the routine urinalysis test, and then the serum creatinine level becomes elevated when nephropathy progresses. At this stage, greater care is necessary in the management of fluids and the use of nephrotoxic medications. Nephropathy is frequently associated with hypertension and coronary artery disease, which further complicate the management of the patient.

Considerations During Anesthesia

During general anesthesia, hypoglycemia is difficult to recognize, and during regional anesthesia, medications may blunt the symptoms of hypoglycemia. Anesthesiologists rightly fear hypoglycemia, which sometimes incorrectly makes them reluctant to administer any insulin during surgery. The blood glucose level should be monitored at least hourly during surgery in patients with diabetes, particularly in patients receiving insulin, undergoing extensive procedures, or requiring large amounts of fluid replacement. Hyperglycemia should be treated with intravenous regular insulin, and hypoglycemia with intravenous dextrose. Serious problems intraoperatively should be rare with adequate blood glucose monitoring.

MANAGEMENT AFTER SURGERY

Unfortunately, there are no carefully done, randomized studies comparing the impact of several different approaches on perioperative morbidity and mortality. Several studies have demonstrated that intravenous insulin infusion protocols usually result in better blood glucose control, but it cannot be assumed that this result will translate into less morbidity or mortality for the patient.[2,4,5]

As a first step, it is important to recognize that the management approach is determined by the type of dia-

Table 9C–1. INTRAVENOUS (IV) INSULIN INFUSION ALGORITHM

Blood or Plasma Glucose (mg/dl)	Standard		Fluid Restricted	
	IV Infusion Rate (ml/hr)	Insulin Infusion Rate (Units/hr)	IV Infusion Rate (ml/hr)	Insulin Infusion Rate (Units/hr)
>400	16	8	8	8
351–400	12	6	6	6
301–350	8	4	4	4
250–300	6	3	3	3
200–249	5	2.5	2.5	2.5
150–199	4	2	2	2
120–149	3	1.5	1.5	1.5
100–119	2	1	1	1
<100	0	0	0	0

betes, present treatment of the diabetes, recent blood glucose control, and seriousness of the surgical procedure. Second, individualized blood glucose target ranges should be determined based on the medical condition and age of the patient. For most patients, target blood glucose values between 100 and 200 mg/dl are reasonable during the perioperative period. Third, if at all possible, patients with diabetes should be scheduled for surgery early in the day.

The details of management are rather involved and are best managed by those with expertise in this field. Examples of possible treatment protocols are shown in Table 9C-1.

STEROIDS

Corticosteroids are frequently given to orthopedic patients. They can cause a marked increase in the blood glucose level when given in large doses, and the blood glucose level should be monitored closely after their administration. Large-dose oral steroids cause an inordinate increase in the late afternoon blood glucose level and may require major adjustments in the insulin program. In these instances, the extra insulin may be given too late and in too small a dose. It is much better to give additional regular insulin at breakfast or noon to prevent the rise in the blood glucose level than to react to it after the fact late in the day.

CONCLUSION

Surgery in the patient with diabetes requires special care in preoperative evaluation and perioperative management. With proper care, diabetes alone is rarely a contraindication for surgery, and the presence of diabetes should result in no major increase in operative morbidity or mortality.

References

1. Ewing DJ, Campbell IW, Clarke BF: Assessment of cardiovascular effects in diabetic autonomic neuropathy and prognostic implications. Ann Intern Med 92:308, 1980.
2. Gavin LA: Management of diabetes mellitus during surgery. West J Med 151:525, 1989.
3. MacKenzie CR, Charlson ME: Assessment of perioperative risk in the patient with diabetes mellitus. Surg Gynecol Obstet 167:293, 1988.
4. Meyers EF, Alberts D, Gordon MO: Perioperative control of blood glucose in diabetic patients: A two-step protocol. Diabetes Care 9:40, 1986.
5. Schade DS: Surgery and diabetes. Med Clin North Am 72:1531, 1988.

9D

Care and Evaluation of the Patient with Renal Disease

• JAMES T. McCARTHY

I have elected to organize information for the surgeon in an outline form regarding the patient with renal disease. I hope this format may be effective in providing the surgeon a quick reference to information that may be needed in caring for arthroplasty patients with renal disease and assisting in their management.

Table 9D–1. PERIOPERATIVE CARE OF THE PATIENT WITH RENAL DISEASE*

General
    Maintain accurate record of intake and output
    Daily weight
    Check hemodialysis access daily for patency and infection
    Avoid venipuncture and intravenous lines in an extremity that has hemodialysis access
Nutrition
    Calories—30–35 kcal/kg/day
    Free fluids—800 ml/day + daily urine volume
    Protein—1.0 gm/kg/day (GFR 20–25 ml/min)
    —0.8 gm/kg/day (GFR 15–20 ml/min)
    —0.6 gm/kg/day (GFR < 15 ml/min; no dialysis)
    —1.2 gm/kg/day (dialysis)
    Sodium—60–90 mEq/day
    Potassium—60 mEq/day [urine volume < 400 ml/day]
    —80 mEq/day [urine volume > 400 ml/day]
    Phosphorus—800–1200 mg/day
Medications
    Advice for all medications
    Determine the GFR by measuring creatinine clearance or by estimating GFR with Cockcroft-Gault (or similar) formula*; dose
        adjustment is necessary for the renal patient.
Avoid (or use only with great caution)
    Potassium-containing intravenous fluids
    Magnesium-containing antacids or laxatives
    Potassium-sparing drugs (triamterene, spironolactone, amiloride, trimethoprim [rarely])
    Potassium supplements (standing order)
    Oral and parenteral nonsteroidal anti-inflammatory drugs (ketorolac)
    Meperidine (use great care in combining with morphine or propoxyphene)
    Angiotensin-converting enzyme inhibitors and angiotensin receptor blockers
    Iodinated intravenous radiographic contrast
    Low molecular weight (LMW) heparins (unpredictable effects on bleeding)
Dosage adjustment required (commonly encountered medications)
    Aminoglycoside antibiotics
    Vancomycin
    Codeine
    Digoxin
    H_2- blockers
    Labetalol
    Consult Pharmacy for all medications in renal failure
Other special medications
    Immunosuppressive medications (renal transplant patients)
    Erythropoeitin
    Calcitriol (or other vitamin D analogs)

Table continued on following page

Table 9D–1. PERIOPERATIVE CARE OF THE PATIENT WITH RENAL DISEASE* *Continued*

Oral multivitamins
Phosphate binders (calcium acetate, calcium carbonate, sevelamer)

*(GFR < 25 ml/min)
ClCr=Cockcroft-Gault estimate of creatinine clearance; GFR = glomerular filtration rate.

$$\frac{[140-\text{Age (yr)}] \times [\text{Weight (kg)}]}{[\text{Serum creatinine (mg/dl)}] \times 72}$$

Table 9D–2. PREOPERATIVE PREPARATION AND ASSESSMENT

Examination
   Volume status (lungs, heart, edema, blood pressure)
   Dialysis angioaccess (fistula, graft, or catheter)
   Signs of uremia (fetor, asterixis, pericardial rub, sensorium)
Laboratory and radiographic
   Chest radiograph (edema, effusions, cardiomegaly)
   Electrocardiogram (ischemia, rhythm, electrolyte effects)
   Blood tests (sodium, potassium, bicarbonate, creatinine, BUN, calcium, phosphorous, magnesium, albumin, AST, uric acid, hemoglobin, leukocytes, platelets)
Dialysis
   Should be done in the 24 hours just preceding surgery
Bleeding and transfusions
   Abnormal bleeding time (DDAVP, cryoprecipitate)
   Transfusions (may need leukocyte-poor or special blood if awaiting transplant)
Immediately preoperative and intraoperative
   Check potassium and check frequently (keep <6.0 mEq/l)
   Avoid large volumes of intravenous fluids
   Avoid potassium-containing fluids (e.g., lactated Ringer's solution)
   Carefully protect the hemodialysis angioaccess (fistula, graft, catheter)

AST = aspartate transaminase; BUN = blood urea nitrogen; DDAVP = l-deamino (8-D-arginine) vasopressin.

Table 9D–3. POSTOPERATIVE CARE AND ASSESSMENT

Examination
   Volume status (lungs, heart, edema, blood pressure)
   Dialysis angioaccess (fistula, graft, or catheter)
   Signs of uremia (fetor, asterixis, pericardial rub, sensorium)
Lab tests
   Daily (until stable) (sodium, potassium bicarbonate, creatinine, BUN, hemoglobin, leukocytes, platelets)
   Biweekly or weekly (albumin, calcium, phosphorous, magnesium, AST, uric acid)
Dialysis
   Avoid/minimize heparin
Special situations for renal patients
   Oligoanuria (bladder catheter usually not necessary)
   Treatment of hyperkalemia
   Arterial insufficiency (ulcers, delayed wound healing)
   Dialysis access infections
   Pulmonary edema
   Cognitive dysfunction from analgesics, sedatives, hypnotics
   Hepatitis B and C
   Preexisting hyperparathyroidism
   Persistent, resistant urinary tract infections

AST = aspartate transaminase; BUN = blood urea nitrogen.

10

Prevention of Prosthetic Joint Infection

• ARLEN D. HANSSEN and DOUGLAS R. OSMON

Although the efficacy of modern treatment methods has markedly improved, the cost and morbidity associated with treatment for established prosthetic joint infection (PJI) suggest that prevention rather than treatment is the best approach. The primary difficulty lies with establishing which methods of prevention are truly proven and determining which additional techniques are also reasonable despite the fact that they have not been proven in the clinical setting.

The development of infection requires introduction of bacteria into a wound of a given host. A classification that describes the mechanism by which the bacteria are presented to the wound environment includes surgical contamination, hematogenous spread, recurrent infection, and infection from direct inoculation or contiguous spread.[120] Although this classification clearly depicts the various mechanisms of bacterial delivery to the wound, the usefulness of this classification to prevent infection is limited. When deep periprosthetic infection occurs, the specific mechanism of bacterial delivery is often unknown and retrospective assignment as operative contamination or hematogenous infection is therefore arbitrary. Another classification characterizing three stages of periprosthetic infection based on the timing of the diagnosis of infection after surgery also has limited usefulness in the prevention or identification of the specific cause of infection and is better suited for guiding the treatment.[42]

Nonetheless, the question of whether infection after elective surgery is due to operating room contamination or to hematogenous seeding is often pondered. Usually, it is extremely difficult to prove the exact cause of the infection in an individual situation. Also, because bacterial contamination occurs in every operative wound, why do some patients develop infection whereas others do not? What can an individual surgeon do to minimize the incidence of deep infection?

The concept of an interdependent relationship among bacteria, wound, and host is most useful when considering the prevention of infection (Fig. 10–1). Establishment of infection is dependent on the inoculum size and virulence of the bacteria, the host's ability to eliminate those

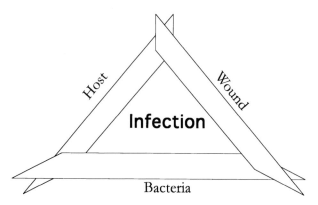

Figure 10–1. The interdependent relationship of bacteria, wound, and host in infection.

bacteria, and the status of the wound environment. Within this framework, there are multiple variables that contribute to the deposition of bacteria into the wound, numerous medical conditions or medications that may impair the patients' host defenses, and many vagaries of the wound environment that also potentiate the infectious process. Imbalance of any variable within this triad, such as the presence of a large prosthetic implant or an area of tissue necrosis, may facilitate the development of infection. Prevention of infection must address optimizing the wound environment, augmenting the host's ability to fight infection, and minimizing the number of bacteria dispensed into the wound. All three of these categories require vigilance in the preoperative, operative, and postoperative time periods (Table 10–1).

PREOPERATIVE PERIOD

Efforts focus on identifying patients with impaired *host* defenses, assessing operative sites that may provide a poor operative *wound* environment, and discovering remote sources of infection that increase the likelihood of *bacterial* inoculation into the wound. Variables such as remote sources of infection should be eliminated before surgery. Circumstances such as an impaired immune

Table 10–1. PREVENTION OF DEEP PERIPROSTHETIC INFECTION

	Preoperative Period	Operative Period	Postoperative Period
Host	Altered immune system Immunosuppressive medications Diabetes mellitus Rheumatoid arthritis Advanced age Malnutrition Anesthetic risk	Anesthetic agents Transfusions	Rheumatoid arthritis Altered immune system

Bacteria	Urinary tract infection
	Skin ulcers
	
	Poor dental hygiene
	Preoperative shaving
	
	Preoperative showers
	
	Prolonged hospitalization
		Instrument sterilization
		Operating room traffic
		
		Personnel ("dispersers")
		
		Face masks/hoods
		
		Exhaust suits
		Laminar airflow
		Ultraviolet light
		Prophylactic antibiotics
		Antibiotic-impregnated
		  PMMA
		Skin preparation
		Gloves
		Drapes/gowns
		Wound irrigants
		Sucker tips
		Splash basins
			Antibiotic prophylaxis
			Urinary tract
			  management
			Invasive procedures
			Remote sites of
			  infection
			Clean dental
			  procedures

Wound	Extensive scarring
	
	Prior surgery
	Prior infection
	Obesity
	Vascular disease
	Anatomic site
	Condition of skin
		Duration of procedure
		
		Surgical technique
		Sutures
		Implant selection
		Antibiotic impregnated
		  PMMA
		Bone graft
		Surgical drains
		Wound closure
			Postoperative
			  hematoma
			Wound drainage
			Skin necrosis
			Reoperation
			Loose prosthesis
			Particulate debris

PMMA, polymethylmethacrylate cement.

system or malnutrition can only be optimized, and conditions such as extensive scarring, which cannot be corrected, require careful preoperative planning.

Host

High-risk hosts include patients with immune systems altered by the presence of a congenitally defective defense mechanism, treatment with immunosuppressive medications,[103] systemic illnesses such as diabetes mellitus[38,42,83,88] malignancy,[15] rheumatoid arthritis,[42,111,144] advanced age,[40,44,93] and malnourishment.[33,44,51,64,125] Patients with a high anesthetic risk have an increased incidence of infection after total knee arthroplasty.[15,50] Acquired immunodeficiency syndrome as a risk factor for the development of infection after elective joint replacement is controversial and almost certainly depends on the degree of immunosuppression of the host caused by the human immunodeficiency virus infection.[63,112,139]

Laboratory assessment should be individualized. Appraisal of the patient's nutritional status may include evaluation of *anthropometric indicators* (arm muscle circumference, triceps skinfold thickness, percent weight loss, weight for height, and hand grip strength); *immunologic indicators* (total lymphocyte count and skin antigen testing); *biochemical indicators* (serum albumin, transferrin, and prealbumin levels, hematocrit and hemoglobin levels, total iron-binding capacity, and nitrogen balance).[33,51,64,125] Lymphocyte counts less than 1500 cells/mm and albumin levels less than 3.5 g/dl have been correlated with an increased incidence of wound complications in patients undergoing total hip and knee arthroplasty.[51] Serum transferrin levels, compared with lymphocyte counts and albumin levels, have been shown to be a more sensitive indicator of wound complications after total hip arthroplasty.[44] There is no current accepted standard for the definition of the malnourished patient, and additional study is required to evaluate the proper characterization of nutritional depletion in the assessment of the patient undergoing elective total joint arthroplasty.

Bacteria

Established infection at remote sites such as the oral cavity and the genitourinary and respiratory tracts, as well as skin lesions increase the risk of deep periprosthetic infection.[77,93] Preoperative assessment includes inspection for such infections. All sites of remote infection, including correction of poor dentition, should be treated before surgery. This type of preoperative care requires excellent communication between the internist, dentist, orthopedist, other health care providers, and the patient.

Preoperative shaving of the operative site has been associated with an increased risk of infection as a result of the rapid colonization of the small nicks induced by the razor.[86,123] Use of depilatory agents or avoidance of shaving until immediately before the operative procedure is more prudent. Preoperative showers with use of an antiseptic agent can reduce skin colonization; although the efficacy of these showers has not been demonstrated clinically, the practice does seem reasonable. A prolonged length of hospitalization before the surgical procedure has been associated with an increased incidence of infection. Whether this phenomenon is due to biased selection of a high-risk group of patients or to the colonization of those patients with nosocomial organisms is unknown.

Wound

A suboptimal wound environment is often present in patients with vascular disease, prior surgery, tissue affected by extensive scarring, and a history of prior infection at the operative site. Conditions such as psoriatic plaques adjacent to the operative site and obesity are potentially detrimental local wound factors, and the reported effect of these conditions has been conflicting.[16,42,84,117,129,130] Thin, atrophic skin should be noted for consideration of special wound care in the operating room and in the postoperative period. It is also known that certain anatomic sites, such as elbow and knee joints, are more vulnerable to occurrence of deep periprosthetic infection.[47,56,73,89,111,148]

THE OPERATING ROOM

Bacteria

In an effort to reduce bacterial contamination, the attention of the operating room team should remain focused on all aspects of the aseptic technique. Proper sterilization of instruments, operative site preparation, avoiding contact with objects outside the sterile field, and maintenance of fundamental aseptic protocols are essential practices for a successful outcome. Transport of the patient into the operating room should include disposal of ward bedding, restriction of traffic in and out of the operating room, and minimization of the number of personnel in the operating room.[93] An unoccupied operating room contains approximately one colony-forming unit of bacteria per cubic foot of air, and the addition of several operating room personnel increases the number of colony-forming units sixfold.[43] As a normal process from all individuals, incredible numbers of bacteria are shed every minute; however, a certain percentage of

individuals, known as dispersers, shed significantly more bacteria, and these individuals have been associated with an increased incidence of infection.[30,141] Furthermore, premenopausal women shed significantly fewer bacteria per minute than postmenopausal women or men.[30]

Conflicting evidence has been provided regarding the efficacy of face masks.[70,87,113,138] It has been shown that the use of face masks does not make any difference in the number of colony-forming units deposited on culture plates in an operating room or on the incidence of postoperative wound infection.[113,138] Conversely, an elegant study revealed that the method of mask use in combination with a surgical hood was an important factor in the reduction of airborne contamination.[70] Airborne contamination was most effectively reduced when the surgical mask was donned beneath an overlapping hood rather than applied over the hood, which allows dispersal of bacteria along the sides of the mask. This study also demonstrated that the use of a surgical hood and minimization of conversation does decrease airborne contamination in the operating room. If for no other reason, the use of masks and face shields seems advisable to protect the operating personnel from blood-borne contagions.

Clean Air

Reduction of airborne contamination by use of a ventilation system was mentioned in 1864, and yet implementation of this concept for the operating room did not occur until a century later.[23] Rather, the use of ultraviolet light to sterilize air particles carrying bacteria was initiated in 1936.[49] The absolute effectiveness of ultraviolet light in the clinical setting has not been determined because available studies are retrospective and compare infection rates with historical controls.[49,58,75] Because of the lack of conclusive clinical studies and concern about exposure of operating personnel, acceptance of the use of ultraviolet light has been tentative. Over the past few years, consideration of the cost-effectiveness of laminar airflow systems has provided a resurgence of interest in ultraviolet light, because it is considerably less expensive than laminar airflow system technology.[16,75]

Laminar airflow occurs when all air in a confined space is moved along parallel flow patterns at a uniform velocity with creation of a minimal number of eddies. Ultraclean air is provided to an operating room when laminar airflow is combined with high-efficiency particulate air filters that remove 99.8 percent of all particles larger than 0.3 μ. The standards of laminar airflow outlined for use in the aerospace industry were subsequently adapted to the operating room, and definitions of clean air have been meticulously detailed.[98]

Sir John Charnley's reports of a dramatic reduction in the incidence of postoperative infection with the clean air operating theater sparked considerable interest in the use of unidirectional airflow ventilation systems.[23,25] Charnley concluded that clean air was the most important factor but not the sole reason for the reduction in infection.[16,24] These observations created the perception, which continues to exist today, that the surgeon who is performing a total joint arthroplasty is obliged to ensure the use of a clean air ventilation system.[72]

The initial retrospective studies evaluating the efficacy of unidirectional airflow systems compared historical infection rates, and an excellent review details many of these studies.[96] A prospective randomized clinical trial initiated by the Medical Research Council to evaluate the effectiveness of ultraclean air during total hip and knee arthroplasties was published in 1982. This study, which detailed 6781 hip arthroplasties and 1274 knee arthroplasties performed at multiple centers between 1974 and 1979, demonstrated impressive results.[72] Infection occurred in 1.5 percent of the 4133 control patients and in only 0.6 percent of the ultraclean air group (*P*<.001). Although these results seemed to provide irrefutable evidence for the need of laminar airflow systems, the study design was flawed by lack of patient stratification, irregularities in the randomization process, and variable surgical technique and perioperative management; therefore, the use of prophylactic antibiotics was not controlled. In the patients receiving prophylactic antibiotics, the effect of ultraclean air technology was not significant.

Another large retrospective study of 2384 cementless total hip arthroplasties casts further doubt about the need for laminar airflow technology.[79] Between 1975 and 1978, when none of the patients received prophylactic antibiotics, infection occurred in 9 of 289 arthroplasties (3.11 percent) in the conventional operating room compared with 9 of 363 (2.47 percent) of the patients in the laminar airflow rooms. Because of the insignificant reduction of deep periprosthetic infection with the use of laminar airflow, the use of prophylactic antibiotics was initiated in 1979. With prophylactic antibiotics, infection occurred in 6 of 669 arthroplasties (0.89 percent) in the conventional operating room compared with 3 of 1063 (0.28 percent) of the patients in the laminar airflow rooms. This difference was not statistically significant. Finally, another large retrospective study of 3175 total hip and knee replacements, with and without a horizontal unidirectional filtered airflow system, demonstrated a paradoxical increase of infection after total knee arthroplasty performed in the laminar airflow rooms.[117] This increased rate of infection was attributed to positioning of the operating team between the patient and the airflow. This experience emphasizes the need for a diligent application of laminar airflow protocol and the detrimental effects associated with protocol breakdown.

MAYO CLINIC EXPERIENCE

In 1981, a randomized, blinded, prospective study was initiated at the Mayo Clinic to evaluate the effect of unidirectional airflow on the incidence of deep periprosthetic infection after total hip and knee arthroplasty. All procedures were performed at one hospital by the same group of surgeons in the same corridor of 10 operating rooms. All rooms were equipped with horizontal unidirectional filtered airflow systems, and randomization occurred by activation of the laminar airflow units determined by a randomization schedule. This method of randomization eliminated selection bias, such as use of prophylactic antibiotics, patient selection, and perioperative patient management, because the use of laminar airflow was blinded to the surgeons and the operating team.

Preliminary results of the first 7305 patients showed no statistically significant differences in the incidence of deep periprosthetic infection between the patients in rooms with activated laminar airflow and patients whose procedures were performed in the presence of conventional airflow.[41] The last patients were enrolled in this study in June 1993, and final follow-up data currently are being obtained for analysis of this study group, which includes 12,000 arthroplasties.

Antibiotics

Although once considered controversial, the use of prophylactic antibiotics is probably the single most effective method of reducing the incidence of postoperative wound infection.[1,2,48,54,59,94,99,102,145] Despite study design limitations in the available literature, all of these individuals and consensus panels support the routine use of systemic antimicrobial prophylaxis because the consequences of PJI are so severe.[45,59] The current controversies of prophylactic antibiotics include identification of the optimal antibiotic, the appropriate initiation and duration of antimicrobial prophylaxis, and whether or not systemic antimicrobial prophylaxis and ultraclean operating rooms used concurrently are additive in their ability to reduce the incidence of infection.

The optimal prophylactic antimicrobial agent should have (1) excellent in vitro activity against the common pathogens that cause surgical wound infection (i.e., staphylococci and streptococci), (2) maintain a relatively long serum half-life to provide coverage for the entire surgical procedure, provide good tissue penetration, and be relatively nontoxic and inexpensive. Heath and others reviewed the largest and most rigorous comparative clinical trials, but no single agent was shown to be superior.[1,20,32,39,48,105,110,126] We and others prefer cefazolin because it has been studied most extensively, has a long serum half-life, and is inexpensive compared with other agents. For patients who are known to have had a type I hypersensitivity reaction (e.g., immediate urticaria, bronchospasm, anaphylaxis) to penicillin, vancomycin is the preferred agent. The use of vancomycin in the penicillin-allergic patient can be decreased by focused perioperative allergy consultation and penicillin skin testing.[71]

Some have advocated the use of more broad-spectrum antimicrobials, including vancomycin, for perioperative prophylaxis because of an increasing frequency of nosocomial infections caused by organisms resistant to narrow-spectrum cephalosporins (see *www.aaos.org/wordhtml/papers/advistmt/vancomyc.htmaaos*).[1,39] Data are lacking regarding the efficacy or cost-effectiveness of this approach. Available data suggest that given a susceptible organism, β-lactams such as cefazolin have in vitro activity superior to that of vancomycin; moreover, vancomycin in the perioperative setting has toxic potential. For these reasons, we believe that decisions regarding this issue must be made on an individual basis after review of susceptibility patterns of organisms causing wound infection at any one institution and after consultation with the local infection control officer.[57,127]

Administration of prophylactic antimicrobial agents before the time of skin incision reduces the incidence of surgical wound infections.[21] A prospective clinical trial that enrolled 2847 patients undergoing a variety of clean and clean-contaminated surgical procedures (11 percent underwent joint replacement) demonstrated the lowest surgical wound infection rate with administration of prophylactic antimicrobial agents within a 2-hour period before the time of incision.[27] Currently, we recommend that systemic antimicrobial prophylaxis for prosthetic joint replacement be given within 30 minutes before the incision and 5 to 10 minutes before any tourniquet inflation.[1,9,21,48] For procedures with extensive blood loss or prolonged procedures exceeding the antimicrobial agent's half-life, an additional intraoperative dose is administered. In addition, we believe that because administering perioperative antimicrobial prophylaxis before the incision is of great importance in decreasing the risk of surgical wound infection, antimicrobial prophylaxis for revision surgery should not be withheld to obtain cultures with the exception of cases in which the index of suspicion of periprosthetic infection is high.[57]

The optimal duration of systemic antimicrobial prophylaxis is unknown.[61,80,110,147] Administration of the prophylactic agent for 24 to 48 hours appears as efficacious as administration for longer time periods. In a randomized clinical trial involving 2796 patients undergoing total hip arthroplasty, with a mean follow-up of 13 months, the incidence of superficial wound or deep prosthetic joint infection was comparable whether a single dose of cefuroxime or three doses of cefuroxime were given.[147] The power to detect meaningful statistical differences between patient groups in all of these studies is low, and it is therefore difficult to draw definitive conclusions. To reduce the possibility of additional antimicrobial toxicity, selection of resistant organisms, and additional expense, most authorities recommend a single preoperative dose or no more than two or three postoperative doses of a prophylactic antibiotic.[1,45,48,54,59,94,99,102] The estimated annual reduction in health care costs for 100,000 patients would be $7,700 million if prophylactic antibiotics were administered only once as an intraoperative dose rather than for 48 hours postoperatively.[93]

The use of antibiotic-impregnated bone cement for prophylaxis in primary total joint arthroplasty has also been shown to be effective in experimental models.[108] Although used extensively outside of the United States, its use for primary total joint arthroplasty remains controversial in North America because of the potential disadvantages of allergy, emergence of resistant organisms, and weakened bone cement.[22,66,76,81,137] It seems reasonable to add antibiotic to cement for patients at high risk, such as in the presence of prior infection; however, the proper role of antibiotic-impregnated cement for use as prophylaxis during primary total joint arthroplasty has not been clearly defined in randomized clinical trials, and we do not recommend its routine use in the absence of data from clinical trials.[57]

Surgical Preparation

Preparation of the patient's skin at the operative site should be performed with an antiseptic agent or the use of isopropyl alcohol; however, the optimal duration of the surgical preparation or the actual agent used has not been established.[46] A one-step, water-insoluble iodophor-in-alcohol solution is as effective in reducing skin bacterial counts as the traditional two-step, scrub-and-paint-skin preparation.[46] Although antiseptic agents effectively diminish the immediate bacterial count at the operative site, the presence of hair follicles prevents complete sterilization of the skin. Use of either an alcohol povidone-iodine or an alcohol chlorhexidine skin preparation, with or without a plastic skin drape preparation, allows the recolonization of the skin within 30 minutes, and these counts achieve normal bacterial levels by 3 hours.[65] In contrast, the use of a 95 percent isopropyl alcohol skin preparation followed by application of a slow-release iodophor-impregnated plastic drape effectively eliminated skin colonization for up to 3 hours.[65] At the end of long operative procedures, when the edges of the plastic drape are peeled away, it seems prudent to swab the exposed skin with a povidone-iodine solution to effectively reduce the bacterial colony count to zero for wound closure. Plastic adhesive drapes can harm thin and friable skin, and the use of a one-step, water-insoluble iodophor-in-alcohol solution without the drape (DuraPrep; 3M, St. Paul, MN) offers a satisfactory alternative to skin sterilization.

Similarly, surgical scrubbing of the operating room personnel's hands does not afford complete sterilization of the skin; it is the use of gloves that provides sterility. The use of double gloves is advisable because of the large number of perforations that occur during an orthopedic procedure. Double latex gloves have a significantly higher rate of inner glove puncture during orthopedic procedures than cloth outer gloves over inner latex gloves.[118] When double latex gloves are used, the number of punctures correlated directly with the duration of the operation, and all gloves were punctured in procedures lasting more than 180 minutes.[118] Routine changing of outer gloves during procedures lasting more than several hours may be advisable. During regloving, care must be taken to avoid contamination of the glove by the cuff of the surgical gown.

Surgical gowns and drapes should prevent the spread of bacteria that occurs because of airborne dispersion or direct contamination by capillary bleeding through the gown.[90,142] Some materials are significantly more effective than others; for example, Goretex (W.L. Gore and Associates, Flagstaff, AZ) prevents the dispersion of bacteria a thousand times more effectively than ordinary cotton gowns.[143] The operating team should try to avoid repetitive touching of the surgical gown with their gloves because bacteria do invariably progress to the surface of the gown.

Despite meticulous technique, operative sites are invariably contaminated with bacteria to some extent during the surgical procedure. Repetitive irrigation to maintain tissue viability, reduce bacterial colonization, and remove clot and tissue debris should be part of the disciplined approach to minimize the incidence of infection. Methods of wound decontamination include copious use of antibiotic irrigating solutions and employment of various techniques. Pulsatile lavage removes up to 99 percent of wound contaminants, but high-pressure lavage may damage tissue.[55] Concentrated antiseptic agents can damage tissue, and many of these agents are deactivated by plasma products present in the wound.[19,149] Chlorhexidine is not deactivated in the wound, and a 0.05 percent diluted solution applied with syringe lavage removes 99.8 percent of wound contaminants.[136] The use of antibiotic irrigating solutions has been shown to be effective in reducing bacterial contamination in experimental wounds.[14,108,116,119] Although the efficacy of antibiotic irrigating solutions has not been proven clinically to reduce the incidence of deep periprosthetic infection, their use seems reasonable. The potential for systemic aminoglycoside toxicity must be remembered when intraoperative transfusion retrieval systems are used concomitantly.

The Operating Environment

The sucker tip is a recognized source of surgical contamination.[52,82,132] Large volumes of air pass through the sucker, and airborne bacteria that collect on the sucker tip can be transferred to the wound. At the end of hip arthroplasty, 37 percent of sucker tips retained throughout the procedure were contaminated, compared with only 3 percent contamination when the sucker tip was exchanged before preparation of the femoral canal.[52] At an average time of 100 minutes, 55 percent of sucker tips were contaminated.[132] Frequent changing of sucker tips at 30-minute intervals, use of a clean "femoral sucker," and turning the suction system on only during use of suction helps to minimize this source of bacterial contamination.

Another source of contamination in the operating room is the splash basin.[8] In this study, at the end of the orthopedic procedure, 74 percent of splash basins were culture positive. The most common organism isolated was *Staphylococcus epidermidis*, the most common organism associated with deep periprosthetic infection, and 59 percent of the splash basins grew out multiple organisms. Contrary to usual practice patterns, instruments that have been placed into the splash basin should not be returned to the operative wound.

Wound

The large size of prosthetic joints and the extent of surgical dissection required to perform total joint arthro-

plasty create a fertile atmosphere for the evolution of infection. A prolonged operating time does influence the occurrence of deep periprosthetic infection.[42,44] Gentle handling of tissue to avoid the creation of devitalized and necrotic tissue undoubtedly contributes to the overall reduction of infection.

Incisions should be placed so as to avoid excessive tissue retraction and, if possible, preexisting scars should be excised. Use of existing scars to avoid postoperative skin necrosis is essential about the knee joint. Unnecessary dissection of subcutaneous tissue from the underlying fascia devitalizes the subcutaneous layer. Prolonged use of self-retaining retractors may induce large areas of devitalized tissue. Inappropriate tensioning or placement of sutures induces strangulation of tissue and facilitates the emergence of infection. Careful apposition of the epidermis is essential to allow early wound sealing, and a hasty wound closure with overlapped skin often precipitates prolonged postoperative wound drainage and provides a potential portal for the retrograde introduction of bacteria into the surgical wound.

The Foreign Body Effect

The increased susceptibility of the wound to infection in the presence of a foreign body is well known. Initial studies revealed that 2×10^2 staphylococci were required to create a suture abscess with a silk suture; however, 2 to 8×10^6 staphylococci were required to create a subcutaneous abscess in the absence of the suture.[37] The use of a monofilament synthetic suture is associated with a significantly lower infection rate than nonabsorbable sutures, nonsynthetic natural sutures such as catgut or silk, or braided absorbable synthetic sutures.[26,67,124]

The exact role of implant factors in the genesis of deep periprosthetic infection in the clinical setting is unknown. The physical and chemical characteristics of a biomaterial affect the efficiency of bacterial surface adhesion in such a way that coagulase-negative staphylococci exhibit preferential adhesion to polymers, whereas coagulase-positive staphylococci adhere more readily to metals.[53] The metabolic characteristics of bacteria adherent to a biomaterial appear to be altered and thereby to confer antibiotic resistance.[92] This effect appears to be independent of the presence of a glycocalyx, or slime covering, and is dependent on the biomaterial properties, because bacteria adherent to methyl methacrylate demonstrate a remarkably higher antibiotic resistance than bacteria adherent to metals.[53] The ability of bacteria to adhere to methyl methacrylate is inhibited by the presence of antibiotics within the bone cement.[100]

Methyl methacrylate impairs the chemotactic and phagocytic functions of human leukocytes.[107] In a canine model, the incidence of infection was significantly increased in the presence of various metal implants, but methyl methacrylate polymerized in vivo was associated with a higher incidence of infection than found with other types of biomaterials.[109] Based on these observations, it was postulated that a lower incidence of infection might occur with implants relying on tissue integration rather than the use of bone cement for prosthetic fixation. However, a large clinical series of 5000 primary total hip and total knee arthroplasties revealed no significant difference in the incidence of infection after cemented or uncemented hip or knee arthroplasty.[56] The use of metal-metal prostheses or structural bone graft are examples of other factors under the surgeon's discretion that appear to increase the incidence of infection.[111,121,145]

The ability of a tense hematoma to compromise the surrounding soft tissues and prevent antibiotic access has been demonstrated.[95] Careful suturing of tissue layers to eliminate dead space without inordinate tissue strangulation, attentive hemostasis (avoiding tissue destruction by excessive diathermy), and use of surgical drains are effective methods of minimizing a postoperative wound hematoma. Although some reports suggest that the routine use of surgical drains is not indicated for total hip and total knee arthroplasty, it should be emphasized that these studies include far too few numbers of patients to assess the effect of the drains on the incidence of infection.[10,115]

Host

Anesthetic agents have an immunosuppressive effect on the patient.[104] Regional anesthesia is used to avoid this phenomenon and also to potentially reduce the incidence of remote sites of infection such as the respiratory tract. Whether these uses have any effect on the incidence of deep periprosthetic infection is unknown. Transfusion of homologous blood products, as opposed to autologous blood products, has been associated with an increased incidence of postoperative infection, presumably caused by immunologic modulation of the recipient.[40,91] This information provides additional support for the use of autologous blood donation.

POSTOPERATIVE MANAGEMENT

Wound

Careful patient positioning and padding of bony prominences should be employed to prevent the development of skin ulcerations. A rapidly expanding hematoma should be evacuated in the operating room by formal débridement because the pressure from the hematoma devitalizes adjacent tissues and prevents the influx of antibiotic into the operative site.[95] Hematomas are commonly considered to be a significant factor in the development of infection.[43,47,93] Benign neglect of the superficial skin necrosis all too commonly progresses to deep periprosthetic wound infection. Superficial skin necrosis should be aggressively managed by formal débridement in the operating room and, if necessary, particularly about the knee joint, managed by local muscle transposition. Serious wound drainage may initially be managed by compressive dressings. Continued drainage may mandate the patient's return to the operating room for formal débridement, and the presence of this persistent drainage portends a higher risk of eventual deep infection.[15,135] Likewise, surgical intervention for a complication in the immediate postoperative period, such as hematoma evacuation or open reduction of a hip dislocation, carries a risk ratio of 4.4 for the eventual evolvement of infection.[135]

Bacteria

The questions that remain unanswered are what types of procedures or conditions provide a significant bacteremia, which prostheses are at risk for the development of infection when presented with these bacteremias, and what type of intervention(s) can be effectively applied to prevent this event.

The operative site is susceptible to hematogenous seeding because of the presence of inflammatory tissue changes and hematoma in the immediate postoperative period.[18] If possible, conditions or invasive procedures that may contribute to an episode of significant bacteremia should be avoided in the early postoperative period. Management of the urinary tract is an all too frequent problem in the arthroplasty patient, and there is no universal agreement on the proper postoperative protocol.[85,114,146] It seems reasonable to maintain antimicrobial coverage for manipulation of the genitourinary tract in the postoperative period. It has been suggested that the presence of peripheral Teflon catheters may be a distant focus of bacterial contamination to the operative site.[143]

Numerous authors have reported cases of PJI in the medical literature attributed to hematogenous seeding.[6,7,11,77,78,131] In the majority of cases, it has been difficult to document bacteremia preceding prosthesis infection, and more than 50 percent of these infections have been caused by *Staphylococcus aureus*, coagulase-negative staphylococci, and β-hemolytic streptococci, mainly considered to be from skin sources. Urinary tract, respiratory tract, and other remote infections have also been implicated as sources of hematogenous joint infection, and it seems prudent to aggressively diagnose and treat remote infections in patients with joint prostheses in order to prevent hematogenous seeding.[99] Patients with overt dental infection, such as dental abscesses, should receive appropriate empiric or culture-directed antibiotic treatment. Appropriate antimicrobial therapy, both empiric and directed, based on the clinical syndrome (dental abscess, pneumonia, UTI, etc.), the microbiology of the infection, and antibiotic allergies should be delivered as quickly as possible to avoid hematogenous infection.

Controversy stems from (1) the unsubstantiated belief that antimicrobial prophylaxis before invasive dental and medical procedures prevents infection, (2) the desire to avoid the complications of infection, (3) the high cost to eradicate infection, and (4) the concern about potential malpractice litigation if antimicrobial prophylaxis is not administered. Persons opposed to routine prophylaxis for these procedures cite the lack of formal epidemiologic data suggesting an association between invasive dental and medical procedures and deep periprosthetic infection, the risk of adverse reactions (1–0%),[74] including anaphylaxis and death due to administration of prophylactic antimicrobials, and concern about promoting antimicrobial resistance by the unnecessary use of antibiotics as reasons for their position. The risk of anaphylaxis or death from penicillin has been estimated to be 0.055 (range, 0.021 to 0.106) percent and 0.001 to 0.002 percent of treated patients, respectively.[74] The risk of anaphylaxis or death from cephalosporin prophylaxis is thought to be less of a risk than penicillin prophylaxis, but large studies are lacking.

The risk of PJI over the lifetime of the prosthesis is estimated in modern studies to be from 1 to 5 percent, depending on the type of prosthesis, number of revisions, host characteristics, and duration of follow-up in individual studies.[128] The overall rate (hazard) of PJI is highest in the first 6 months after prosthesis insertion and declines continuously thereafter. In the Mayo Clinic experience, the combined incidence rates of PJI during the first 2 years and years 2 through 10 postoperatively, are approximately 5.9 [95 percent CI: 5.3–6.5] and 2.3 [95 percent CI: 2.1–2.5] infections per 1000 joint-years, respectively.[128] The rate of total knee arthroplasty (TKA) infection is approximately twofold higher than the rate of total hip arthroplasty (THA) infection at any time period after implantation The cost of PJI is estimated to be three to four times the cost of a primary total joint arthroplasty and to exceed $50,000.[12,60,122]

It is true that dental and medical procedures, as well as routine daily activities such as tooth brushing and defecation, can cause transient bacteremia (Table 10–2).[34,35] The frequency of postprocedural bacteremia is highest for dental procedures, intermediate for genitourinary tract procedures, and lowest for gastrointesti-

nal procedures. However, there is a lack of data identifying invasive dental and medical procedures as risk factors for infective endocarditis or PJI derived from formal epidemiologic studies such as case control or cohort studies. In a large population-based case control study of 273 cases and matched controls, no association between dental treatment in the 3 months before the onset of infective endocarditis and development of infective endocarditis was found by Strom et al. (adjusted OR; 0.8 [95 percent CI: 0.4–1.5]).[133] Moreover, no association was seen with pulmonary, gastrointestinal, cardiac, or genitourinary procedures and the development of infective endocarditis.[134] The sample size was sufficient to detect associations with a twofold increase in risk for potential risk factors with a prevalence between 0.1 and 0.8. The American Heart Association routinely publishes recommendations regarding antimicrobial prophylaxis to prevent infective endocarditis in patients with high-risk cardiac lesions who are undergoing high-risk dental and medical procedures.[29]

No published controlled studies have assessed the association of PJI and invasive dental and medical procedures. The risk of hematogenous PJI due to infection located elsewhere (e.g., pneumonia, cellulitis) and due to invasive medical or dental procedures is estimated to be between 0.2 and 0.7 percent.[6,7,11,47,77,120] The majority (57 percent) of microorganisms isolated from suspected hematogenous PJI in a review of all published cases of hematogenous PJI before 1996 are *Staphylococcus aureus* or coagulase-negative staphylococci rather than oral flora such as viridans group streptococci or enteric flora that would be expected to be associated with dental, gastrointestinal, or genitourinary procedures.[31] Only 4 of 189 (2 percent) microorganisms isolated from suspected hematogenous infections of prosthetic joints were viridans group streptococci, microorganisms which constitute the majority of the facultative oral flora and are the most common blood

Table 10–2. FREQUENCY OF BACTEREMIA AFTER VARIOUS PROCEDURES

Procedure	Percent of Procedures followed by Bacteremia	Range (percent) N/A=Not available
Dental		
Tooth extraction	60	18–85
Peridontal surgery	88	60–90
Brushing teeth or irrigation	40	7–50
Gastrointestinal procedures		
EGD	4	0–8
Esophageal dilatation	45	N/A
ERCP	5	0–6
Barium enema	10	5–11
Colonoscopy	5	0–5
Flexible sigmoidoscopy	0	N/A
Rigid sigmoidoscopy	5	N/A
Proctoscopy		N/A
Genitourinary procedures		
Catheter insertion and removal	13	0–26
Prostatectomy (sterile urine)	12	11–13
Prostatectomy (infected urine)	60	58–82
Dilatation of strictures	28	19–86

Adapted from Durack DT: Prevention of infective endocarditis. *In* Mandell GL, Bennett JE, Dolin R (eds): Principles and Practice of Infectious Diseases, 5th ed. New York, Churchill Livingstone, 2000, pp 917–925; and Durack DT: Prevention of infective endocarditis. N Engl J Med 332:38, 1995.

culture isolate resulting from trauma to the gingiva. Sixteen percent were caused by normal gastrointestinal flora such as *B. fragilis*, *E. coli* or *E. faecalis*. Eighty one percent of 180 suspected hematogenous PJIs were thought to be due to infection at a remote site (e.g., cellulitis, urinary tract infection) rather than to an invasive medical or dental procedure. Only 17 (9 percent) and 4 (2.2 percent) of these infections were potentially attributed to a dental or gastrointestinal procedure, respectively. In 53 percent of these cases, an infection in the oral cavity preceded the dental procedure.

In two more studies published in 1997 and 1999, 9 (12.1 percent) of 74 late TKA infections between 1982 and 1993 and 3 (6 percent) of 52 late THA infections between 1982 and 1994 were attributed to dental procedure based on temporal association with a dental procedure.[68,140] These cases represented 0.2 percent of 3490 TKAs and 0.1 percent of 2973 THAs performed during the study period and are similar to the numbers reported in the 1996 review by Deacon et al.[31] Interestingly, all patients had had extensive dental procedures or prior oral infection and 7 (58 percent) had had either diabetes mellitus or rheumatoid arthritis. Nine (75 percent) of the 12 PJIs were due to usual oral flora and 2 (17 percent) were resistant to standard antibiotic prophylaxis regimens. One (8.3 percent) of the 12 patients received antimicrobial prophylaxis before the dental procedure.

A Consensus panel formed by the American Academy of Orthopedic Surgeons and the American Dental Association has recommended that routine antimicrobial prophylaxis before invasive dental procedures for all patients with a joint prosthesis is not necessary.[4] They did, however, recommend that prophylaxis be considered in high-risk patients undergoing high-risk dental procedures (Tables 10–3, 10–4, and 10–5). It is important to note that high-risk patients included those patients within 2 years of prosthesis implantation. A single dose

Table 10–3. PATIENTS AT POTENTIAL INCREASED RISK OF HEMATOGENOUS PROSTHETIC JOINT INFECTION

Risk Factor

Immunocomprimised/immunosuppressed patients
    Inflammatory arthropathies: rheumatoid arthritis and systemic lupus erythematosus
    Disease/drug/radiation induced immunosuppression
Other patients
    Insulin-dependent diabetes mellitus
    First two years following joint replacement
    Prior prosthetic joint infection
    Malnourishment
    Hemophilia

Adapted from Anonymous: Advisory statement. Antibiotic prophylaxis for dental patients with total joint replacements. American Dental Association; American Academy of Orthopaedic Surgeons. J Am Dent Assoc 1128:1004, 1997.

Table 10–4. DENTAL PROCEDURES AT INCREASED RISK OF TRANSIENT BACTEREMIA

Dental Procedure

Dental extraction
Periodontal procedures
Dental implants and reimplantation of avulsed teeth
Root canal or surgery only beyond the apex
Initial placement of orthodontic bands
Intraligamentary local anesthetic
Prophylactic cleaning where bleeding is anticipated

Adapted from Anonymous: Advisory statement. Antibiotic prophylaxis for dental patients with total joint replacements. American Dental Association; American Academy of Orthopaedic Surgeons. J Am Dent Assoc 1128:1004, 1997.

Table 10–5. SUGGESTED ANTIBIOTIC PROPHYLAXIS REGIMENS FOR HIGH-RISK PATIENTS WITH A JOINT PROSTHESIS UNDERGOING A HIGH RISK DENTAL PROCEDURE

Suggested Antibiotic Prophylaxis Regimens

Patients *not allergic* to penicillin:
Amoxicillin, cephalexin, or cephadrine 2 grams orally one hour prior to the procedure
Patients *not allergic* to penicillin and *unable* to take oral medication:
Ampicillin 2 grams or cefazolin 1 gram IM or IV one hour prior to the procedure
Patients *allergic* to penicillin:
Clindamycin 600 milligrams orally one hour prior to the procedure
Patients *allergic* to penicillin and *unable* to take oral medication:
Clindamycin 600 milligrams IV one hour prior to the procedure

Adapted from Anonymous: Advisory statement. Antibiotic prophylaxis for dental patients with total joint replacements. American Dental Association; American Academy of Orthopaedic Surgeons. J Am Dent Assoc 1128:1004, 1997.

within 60 minutes of the procedure was recommended to avoid the emergence of resistant organisms that can occur if prophylaxis is begun more than several hours before a dental procedure. The authors of this consensus statement say, "This statement provides guidelines to supplement practitioners in their clinical judgment regarding antibiotic prophylaxis for dental patients. It is not intended as the standard of care or as a substitute for clinical judgment . . . ." The statement goes on to postulate, "Practitioners must exercise their own clinical judgment in determining whether or not antibiotic prophylaxis is appropriate. Any perceived benefit of antibiotic prophylaxis must be weighed against the known risks of antibiotic toxicity, allergy, and selection of microbial resistance."

There are no data to provide a rational basis for any recommendation regarding antimicrobial prophylaxis for invasive gastrointestinal and genitourinary procedures. The American Society of Colon and Rectal Surgeons and the American Society for Gastrointestinal Endoscopy do not recommend antibiotic prophylaxis for their procedures.[5,101] If antimicrobial prophylaxis for the prevention of hematogenous prosthetic joint infection is recommended, the patient should be informed of the possibility of rare but life-threatening adverse reaction as well as the more common drug toxicities that may result. The antimicrobial agents that are chosen for prophylactic administration should be chosen on the basis of the in vitro susceptibilities of the flora at the site of the procedure.

Host

Many of the reports of hematogenous infection have detailed the importance of the host's ability to resist infection, and rheumatoid arthritis is frequently cited.[6,7,11,24,47,77,131] There are many other potential predisposing factors for the patient at risk for hematogenous infection. The presence of structural bone graft and use of metal-metal prostheses have been cited as additional risk factors.[11,111,121,144] These factors are more correctly considered as variables in the wound environment that impair the host's ability to clear the bacteria. Inflammation resulting from the presence of a loose prosthesis or synovitis induced by polyethylene or metallic debris are variables that may predispose the patient to hematogenous infection.[106] The identification of the various risk factors and the appropriate prophylaxis for these patients requires significant additional study.

References

1. Anonymous: ASHP therapeutic guidelines on antimicrobial prophylaxis in surgery. Am J Health-Syst Pharm 56:1839, 1999.
2. Anonymous: Antimicrobial prophylaxis in surgery. Med Lett Drugs Ther 41:75, 1999.
3. Anonymous: Recommendations for preventing the spread of vancomycin resistance. Recommendations of the Hospital Infection Control Practices Advisory Committee (HICPAC). MMWR—Morb Mortal Wkly Rep 44:1, 1995.
4. Anonymous: Advisory statement. Antibiotic prophylaxis for dental patients with total joint replacements. American Dental Association; American Academy of Orthopaedic Surgeons. J Am Dent Assoc 1128:1004, 1997.
5. Anonymous: Antibiotic prophylaxis for gastrointestinal endoscopy. Gastrointest Endosc 42:630, 1995.
6. Ahlberg A, Carlsson AS, Lindgren L: Hematogenous infection in total joint replacement. Clin Orthop 137:69, 1978.
7. Ainscow DAP, Denham RA: The risk of haematogenous infection in total joint replacements. J Bone Joint Surg 66B:580, 1984.
8. Baird RA, Nickel FR, Thrupp LD, et al: Splash basin contamination in orthopaedic surgery. Clin Orthop 187:129, 1984.
9. Bannister GC, Auchincloss JM, Johnson DP, Newman JH: The timing of tourniquet application in relation to prophylactic antibiotic administration. J Bone Joint Surg 70B:322, 1988.
10. Beer KJ, Lombardi AV Jr, Mallory TH, Vaughn BK: The efficacy of suction drains after routine total joint arthroplasty. J Bone Joint Surg 73A:584, 1991.
11. Bengtson S, Blomgren G, Knutson K, et al: Hematogenous infection after knee arthroplasty. Acta Orthop Scand 58:529,1987.
12. Bengtson S: Prosthetic osteomyelitis with special reference to the knee: risks, treatment and costs. Ann Med 25:523, 1993.
13. Bengtson S, Knutson K: The infected knee arthroplasty. A 6-year follow-up of 357 case patients. Acta Orthop Scand 62:301, 1991.
14. Benjamin JB, Volz RG: Efficacy of a topical antibiotic irrigant in decreasing or eliminating bacterial contamination in surgical wounds. Clin Orthop 184:114, 1984.
15. Berbari EF, Hanssen AD, Duffy MC, et al: Risk factors for prosthetic joint infection: A case control study. Clin Infect Dis 27:1247, 1998.
16. Berg M, Bergman BR, Hoborn J: Ultraviolet radiation compared to an ultra-clean air enclosure: Comparison of air bacteria counts in operating rooms. J Bone Joint Surg 73B:811, 1991.
17. Beyer CA, Hanssen AD, Lewallen DG, Pittelkow MR: Primary total knee arthroplasty in patients with psoriasis. J Bone Joint Surg 73B:258, 1991.
18. Blomgren G, Lindgren V: The susceptibility of total joint replacement to hematogenous infection in the early postoperative period. Clin Orthop 151:308, 1980.
19. Branemark PI, Ekholm R, Albrektsson B, et al: Tissue injury caused by wound disinfectants. J Bone Joint Surg 49A:48, 1967.
20. Bryan CS, Morgan SL, Caton RJ, Lunceford EM Jr: Cefazolin versus cefmandole for prophylaxis during total joint arthroplasty. Clin Orthop 228:117, 1988.
21. Burke JF: The effective period of preventative antibiotic action in experimental incisions and dermal lesions. Surgery 50:161, 1961.
22. Carlsson AS, Lidgren L, Lindberg L: Prophylactic antibiotics against early and late deep infections after total hip replacement. Acta Orthop Scand 48:405, 1977.
23. Charnley J: A clean-air operating enclosure. Br J Surg 51:195, 1964.
24. Charnley J: Postoperative infection after total hip replacement with special reference to air contamination in the operating room. Clin Orthop 87:167, 1972.
25. Charnley J, Eftekhar N: Postoperative infection in total prosthetic replacement arthroplasty of the hip joint with special reference to the bacterial content of the air in the operating room. Br J Surg 56:641, 1969.
26. Chu CC, Williams DF: Effects of physical configuration and chemical structure of suture material on bacterial adhesion: A possible link to wound infection. Am J Surg 147:197, 1984.
27. Classen DC, Evans RS, Pestotnik SL, et al: The timing of prophylactic administration of antibiotics and the risk of surgical wound infection. N Engl J Med 326:281, 1992.
28. Cruse PJE, Foord R: A five-year prospective study of 23,649 surgical wounds. Arch Surg 107:206, 1973.
29. Dajani AS, Taubert KA, Wison WR, et al: Prevention of bacterial endocarditis: Recommendations by the American Heart Association. JAMA 277:1794, 1997.
30. Davies RR, Noble WC: Dispersal of bacteria on desquamated skin. Lancet 2:1295, 1962.
31. Deacon JM, Pagliaro AJ, Zelicof SB, Horowitz HW: Prophylactic use of antibiotics for procedures after total joint replacement. J Bone Joint Surg Am 78:1755, 1996.
32. Debenedictis KJ, Rowan NM, Boyer BL: A double-blind study comparing cefonicid with cefazolin as prophylaxis in patients undergoing total hip or knee replacement. Rev Infect Dis 4(Suppl):901, 1984.
33. Dreblow DM, Anderson CF, Moxness K: Nutritional assessment of orthopaedic patients. Mayo Clin Proc 56:51, 1981.

34. Durack DT: Prevention of infective endocarditis. *In* Mandell GL, Bennett JE, Dolin R (eds): Principles and Practice of Infectious Diseases, 5th ed. New York, Churchill Livingstone, 2000, pp 917–925.

35. Durack DT: Prevention of infective endocarditis. N Engl J Med 332:38, 1995.

36. Edlich RF, Panek PH, Rodheaver GT, et al: Physical and chemical configuration in the development of surgical infection. Ann Surg 177:679, 1973.

37. Eleck SD, Conen PE: The virulence of *Staphylococcus pyogenes* for man: Study of the problems of wound infection. Br J Exp Pathol 38:573, 1957.

38. England SP, Stern SH, Install JN, Windsor RE: Total knee arthroplasty in diabetes mellitus. Clin Orthop 260:130, 1990.

39. Evard J, Doyan F, Acar JF, et al: Two-day cefamandole versus five-day cefazolin prophylaxis in 965 total hip replacements. Int Orthop 12:69, 1988.

40. Fernandez MC, Gottlieb M, Menitove JE: Blood transfusion and postoperative infection in orthopaedic surgery. Transfusion 32:318, 1992.

41. Fitzgerald RH Jr: Total hip arthroplasty sepsis: Prevention and diagnosis. Orthop Clin North Am 23:259, 1992.

42. Fitzgerald RH Jr, Nolan DR, Ilstrup DM, et al: Deep wound sepsis following total hip arthroplasty. J Bone Joint Surg 59A:847, 1977.

43. Fitzgerald RH Jr, Peterson LFA: Wound contamination and deep wound sepsis. *In* Eftekhar N (ed): Infection in Joint Replacement Surgery. St. Louis, CV Mosby, 1984.

44. Gherini S, Vaughn BK, Lombardi AV Jr, Mallory TH: Delayed wound healing and nutritional deficiencies after total hip arthroplasty. Clin Orthop 293:188, 1993.

45. Gillespie WJ: Infection in total joint replacement. Infect Dis Clin North Am 4:465, 1990.

46. Gilliam DL, Nelson CL: Comparison of a one-step iodophor skin preparation versus traditional preparation in total joint surgery. Clin Orthop 250:258, 1990.

47. Glynn MK, Sheehan JM: An analysis of the causes of deep infection after hip and knee arthroplasties. Clin Orthop 178:202, 1983.

48. Glenny AM, Song F: Antimicrobial prophylaxis in total hip replacement: A systematic review. Health Technol Assess 3:21, 1999.

49. Goldner JL, Allen BL: Ultraviolet light in orthopaedic operating rooms at Duke University: Thirty-five years' experience, 1937–1973. Clin Orthop 96:195, 1973.

50. Gordon SM, Culver DH, Simmons BP, Jarvis WR: Risk factors for wound infections after total knee arthroplasty. Am J Epidemiol 131:905, 1990.

51. Green KA, Wilde AH, Stulberg BN: Preoperative nutritional status of total joint patients: Relationship to postoperative wound complications. J Arthroplasty 6:321, 1991.

52. Greenough CG: An investigation into contamination of operative suction. J Bone Joint Surg 68B:151, 1986.

53. Gristina AG: Biomaterial-centered infection: Microbial adhesion versus tissue integration. Science 237:1588, 1987.

54. Gross PA, Barrett TL, Dellinger EP, et al: Quality standard for antimicrobial prophylaxis in surgical procedures. Clin Infect Dis 18:421, 1994.

55. Hamer ML, Robson MC, Krizek TJ, Southwick WO: Quantitative bacterial analysis of comparative wound irrigation. Ann Surg 181:189, 1975.

56. Hanssen AD, Fitzgerald RH Jr: Infection following primary cemented and uncemented total hip and knee arthroplasty. Presented at the 58th Annual Meeting of the AAOS, Anaheim, CA, March 9, 1991.

57. Hanssen AD, Osmon DR: The use of prophylactic antimicrobial agents during and after hip arthroplasty. Clin Orthop Dec:124, 1999.

58. Hart D: Sterilization of air in the operating room by bactericidal radiant energy: Results in over 800 operations. Arch Surg 37:956, 1938.

59. Heath AF: Antimicrobial prophylaxis for arthroplasty and total joint replacement: Discussion and review of published clinical trials. Pharmacotherapy 11:157, 1991.

60. Hebert CK, Williams RE, Levy RS, Barrack RL: Cost of treating an infected total knee replacement. Clin Orthop 331:140, 1996.

61. Heydemann JS, Nelson CL: Short-term preventative antibiotics. Clin Orthop 205:184, 1986.

62. Hill G, Flamant R, Muzas F, Evrard J: Prophylactic cefazolin versus placebo in total hip replacement. Lancet 1:795, 1981.

63. Hoekman P, Van De Perre P, Nelissen J, et al: Increased frequency of infection after open reduction of fractures in patients who are seropositive for human immunosufficiency virus. J Bone Joint Surg 73A:675, 1991.

64. Jensen JE, Jensen TG, Smith TK, et al: Nutrition in orthopaedic surgery. J Bone Joint Surg 64A:1263, 1982.

65. Johnston DH, Fairclough JA, Brown J, Hill RA: The rate of skin recolonization after surgical preparation: Four methods compared. Br J Surg 74:64, 1987.

66. Josefsson G, Gudmundsson G, Kolmert L, Wijkstriim S: Prophylaxis with systemic antibiotics versus gentamicin bone cement in total hip arthroplasty: A five-year survey of 1,688 hips. Clin Orthop 253:173, 1990.

67. Katz S, Izhar M, Mirelman D: Bacterial adherence to surgical sutures: A possible factor in suture induced infection. Ann Surg 194:35, 1981.

68. LaPorte DM, Waldman BJ, Mont MA, Hungerford DS: Infections associated with dental procedures in total hip arthroplasty. J Bone Joint Surg Br 81:56, 1999.

69. Laurence M: Ultra-clean air. J Bone Joint Surg 65B:375, 1983.

70. Letts RM, Doermer E: Conversation in the operating theater as a cause of airborne bacterial contamination. J Bone Joint Surg 65A:357, 1983.

71. Li JT, Markus PJ, Osmon DR, et al: Reduction of vancomycin use in orthopedic patients with a history of antibiotic allergy. Mayo Clin Proc 75:902, 2000.

72. Lidwell OM: Clean air at operation and subsequent sepsis in the joint. Clin Orthop 211:91, 1986.

73. Lidwell O, Lowburg E, Whyte W, et al: Effects of ultra-clean air in operating rooms on deep sepsis in the joint after total hip replacement: A randomized study. Br Med J 285:10, 1982.

74. Lin RV: A perspective on penicillin allergy. Arch Intern Med 152:930, 1992.

75. Lowell JD, Kundsin RB, Schwartz CM, Pozin D: Ultraviolet radiation and reduction of deep wound infection following hip and knee arthroplasty. Ann N Y Acad Sci 253:285, 1980.

76. Lynch M, Esser MP, Shelley P, Wroblewski BM: Deep infection in Charnley low-friction arthroplasty: Comparison of plain and gentamicin-loaded cement. J Bone Joint Surg 69B:355, 1987.

77. Maderazo EG, Judson S, Pasternak H: Late infections of total joint prostheses: A review and recommendations for prevention. Clin Orthop 229:131, 1988.

78. Maniloff G, Greenwald R, Laskin R, Singer C: Delayed postbacteremic prosthetic joint infection. Clin Orthop 223:194, 1987.

79. Marotte JH, Lord GA, Blanchard JP, et al: Infection rate in total hip arthroplasty as a function of air cleanliness and antibiotic prophylaxis: ten-year experience with 2,384 cement-less Lord Madreporic prostheses. J Arthroplasty 2:77, 1987.

80. Mauerhan DR, Nelson CL, Smith D, et al: Prophylaxis against infection in total joint arthroplasty: One day of cefuroxime compared with three days of cefazolin. J Bone Joint Surg 76A:39, 1994.

81. McQueen M, Littlejohn A, Hughes SPF: A comparison of systemic cefuroxime and cefuroxime loaded bone cement in the prevention of early infection after total joint replacement. Int Orthop 11:241, 1987.

82. Meals RA, Knoke L: The surgical suction tip: A contaminated instrument. J Bone Joint Surg 60A:409, 1978.

83. Menon TJ, Thjellesen D, Wroblewski BM: Chamley low-friction arthroplasty in diabetic patients. J Bone Joint Surg 65B:580, 1983.

84. Menon TJ, Wroblewski BM: Charnley low-friction arthroplasty in patients with psoriasis. Clin Orthop 175:127, 1983.

85. Michelson JD, Lotke PA, Steinberg ME: Urinary-bladder management after total joint-replacement surgery. N Engl J Med 319:320, 1988.

86. Mishriki SF, Law DJW, Jeffrey PJ: Factors affecting the incidence of postoperative wound infection. J Hosp Infect 16:223, 1990.

87. Mitchell NJ, Hunt S: Surgical face masks in modem operating rooms—a costly and unnecessary ritual? J Hosp Infect 18:239, 1991.

88. Moeckel B, Huo MH, Salvati EA, Pellicci PM: Total hip arthroplasty in patients with diabetes mellitus. J Arthroplasty 8:279, 1993.

89. Morrey BF, Bryan RS: Infection after total elbow arthroplasty. J Bone Joint Surg 65A:330, 1983.

90. Moylan JA, Fitzpatrick KT, Davenport KE: Reducing wound infections: Improved gown and drape barrier performance. Arch Surg 122:152, 1987.

91. Murphy P, Heal JM, Blumberg N: Infection or suspected infection after hip replacement surgery with autologous or homologous blood transfusions. Transfusion 31:212, 1991.

92. Naylor PT, Myrvik QN, Gristina A: Antibiotic resistance of bio-material-adherent coagulase-negative staphylococci. Clin Orthop 261:126, 1990.

93. Nelson CL: Prevention of sepsis. Clin Orthop 222:66, 1987.

94. Nelson CL: The prevention of infection in total joint replacement surgery. Rev Infect Dis 9:613, 1987.

95. Nelson CL, Bergfeld JA, Schwartz J, Kolczun M: Antibiotics in human hematoma and wound fluid. Clin Orthop 147:167, 1980.

96. Nelson JP: The operating room environment and its influence on deep wound infection. In The Hip: Proceedings of the Fifth Open Scientific Meeting of the Hip Society. St. Louis, CV Mosby, 1977, p 129.

97. Nelson JP, Fitzgerald RH Jr, Jaspers MT, Little JW: Prophylactic antimicrobial coverage in arthroplasty patients [editorial]. J Bone Joint Surg 72A:1, 1990.

98. Nelson JP, Glassburn AR, Talbott RD, McElhinney JP: Clean room operating rooms. Clin Orthop 96:179, 1973.

99. Norden CW: Antibiotic prophylaxis in orthopedic surgery. Rev Infect Dis 13:S842, 1991.

100. Oga M, Arizono T, Sugioka Y: Inhibition of bacterial adhesion by tobramycin-impregnated PMMA bone cement. Acta Orthop Scand 63:301, 1992.

101. Oliver G, Lowry A, Vernava A, et al: Practice parameters for antibiotic prophylaxis–supporting documentation. The Standards Task Force. The American Society of Colon and Rectal Surgeons. Dis Colon Rectum 43:1194, 2000.

102. Osmon DR: Antimicrobial prophylaxis in adults. Mayo Clin Proc 75:98, 2000.

103. Papagelopoulos PJ, Hay JE, Galanis E, Morrey BF: Infection around joint replacements in patients who have a renal or liver transplantation. J Bone Joint Surg Am 80:607, 1998.

104. Park SK, Brody JI, Wallace HA, et al: Immunosuppressive effect of surgery. Lancet 1:53, 1971.

105. Periti P, Jacchia E: Ceftriaxone as short term antimicrobial chemo-prophylaxis in orthopedic surgery: A 1-year multi-center follow-up. Eur Surg Res 21(Suppl 1):25, 1989.

106. Petrie RS, Hanssen AD, Osmon DR, Ilstrup DM: Metal-backed patellar failure of total knee arthroplasty: A potential risk factor for late infection. Am J Orthop 27:172, 1998.

107. Petty W: The effect of methylmethacrylate on bacterial phagocyt-osis and killing by human polymorphonuclear leukocytes. J Bone Joint Surg 60A:752, 1978.

108. Petty W, Spanier S, Schuster JG: Prevention of infection after total joint replacement: Experiments with a canine model. J Bone Joint Surg 70A:536, 1988.

109. Petty W, Spanier S, Schuster JG, Silverthorne C: The influence of skeletal implants on the incidence of infection. J Bone Joint Surg 67A:1235, 1985.

110. Pollard JP, Hughes SPF, Scott JE, et al: Antibiotic prophylaxis in total hip replacement. Br Med J 1:707, 1979.

111. Poss R, Thornhill TS, Ewald FC, et al: Factors influencing the inci-dence and outcome of infection following total joint arthroplasty. Clin Orthop 182:117, 1984.

112. Ragni MV, Crossett LS, Herndon JH: Postoperative infection fol-lowing orthopaedic surgery in human immunodeficiency virus-infected hemophiliacs with CD4 counts < or = 200/mm^3. J Arthroplasty 10:716, 1995.

113. Ritter MA, Eitzen H, French MLV, et al: The operating room envi-ronment as affected by people and the surgical mask. Clin Orthop 111:145, 1975.

114. Ritter MA, Faris PM, Keating EM: Urinary tract protocols follow-ing total joint arthroplasty. Orthopedics 12:1085, 1989.

115. Ritter MA, Keating EM, Faris PM: Closed wound drainage in total hip or knee replacement: A prospective, randomized study. J Bone Joint Surg 76A:35, 1994.

116. Rosenstein BD, Wilson FC, Funderburk CH: The use of bacitracin irrigation to prevent infection in postoperative wounds: An experimental study. J Bone Joint Surg 71A:427, 1989.

117. Salvati EA, Robinson RP, Zeno SM, et al: Infection rates after 3,175 total hip and total knee replacements with and without a horizontal unidirectional filtered air-flow system. J Bone Joint Surg 64A:525, 1982.

118. Sanders R, Fortin P, Ross E, Helfet D: Outer gloves in orthopaedic procedures: cloth compared with latex. J Bone Joint Surg 72A:914, 1990.

119. Scherr DD, Dodd TA: In vitro bacteriological evaluation of the effectiveness of antimicrobial irrigating solutions. J Bone Joint Surg 58A:119, 1976.

120. Schmalzried TP, Amstutz HC, Au MK, Dorey FJ: Etiology of deep sepsis in total hip arthroplasty: the significance of hematogenous and recurrent infection. Clin Orthop 280:200, 1992.

121. Schutzer SF, Harris WH: Deep wound infection after total hip replacement under contemporary aseptic conditions. J Bone Joint Surg 64A:724, 1988.

122. Sculco TP: The economic impact of infected joint arthroplasty. Orthopedics. 18:871, 1995.

123. Seroplan R, Reynolds BM: Wound infections after dipilatory versus razor shave. Am J Surg 121:251, 1971.

124. Sharp WV, Belden TA, King PH, Teague PC: Suture resistance to infection. Surgery 91:61, 1982.

125. Smith TK: Nutrition: Its relationship to orthopedic infections. Orthop Clin North Am 22:373, 1991.

126. Soave R, Hirsch JC, Salvati EA, et al: Comparison of ceforanide and cephalothin prophylaxis in patients undergoing total joint arthroplasty. Orthopedics 9:1657, 1986.

127. Southorn PA, Plevak DJ, Wright AJ, Wilson WR: Adverse effects of vancomycin administered in the perioperative period. Mayo Clin Proc 6:721, 1986.

128. Steckelberg JM, Osmon DR: Prosthetic Joint Infection. In Waldvogel FA, Bisno AL (eds): Infections Associated with Indwelling Medical Devices, 3rd ed. Washington, DC, ASM Press, 2000, pp 173–209.

129. Stern SH, Insall JN: Total knee arthroplasty in obese patients. J Bone Joint Surg 72A:1400, 1990.

130. Stern SH, Insall JN, Windsor RE, et al: Total knee arthroplasty in patients with psoriasis. Clin Orthop 248:108, 1989.

131. Stinchfield FE, Bigliani LU, Neu HC, et al: Late hematogenous infection of total joint replacement. J Bone Joint Surg 62A:1345, 1980.

132. Strange-Vognsen HH, Klareskov B: Bacteriologic contamination of suction tips during hip arthroplasty. Acta Orthop Scand 59:410, 1988.

133. Strom BL, Abrutyn E, Berlin JA, et al: Dental and cardiac risk factors for infective endocarditis. A population-based, case-con-trol study. Ann Intern Med 129:761, 1998.

134. Strom BL, Abrutyn E, Berlin JA, et al: Risk factors for infective endocarditis: Oral Hygiene and nondental exposures. Circulation 102:2842, 2000.

135. Surin VV, Sundholm K, Backman L: Infection after total hip replacement with special reference to a discharge from the wound. J Bone Joint Surg 65B:412, 1983.

136. Taylor GJS, Leeming JP, Bannister GC: Effect of antiseptics, ultraviolet light and lavage on airborne bacteria in a model wound. J Bone Joint Surg 75B:724, 1993.

137. Trippel SB: Antibiotic-impregnated cement in total joint arthro-plasty. J Bone Joint Surg 68A:1297, 1986.

138. Tunevall TG: Postoperative wound infections and surgical face masks: A controlled study. World J Surg 15:383, 1991.

139. Unger AS, Kessler CM, Lewis RJ: Total knee arthroplasty in human immunodeficiency virus-infected hemophiliacs. J Arthroplasty 10:448, 1995.

140. Waldman BJ, Mont MA, Hungerford DS: Total knee arthroplas-ty infections associated with dental procedures. Clin Orthop 343:164, 1997.

141. Walter CW, Kundsin RB: The airborne component of wound contamination and infection. Arch Surg 107:588, 1973.

142. Whyte W, Bailey PV, Hamblen DL, et al: Bacteriologically occlu-sive clothing system for use in the operating room. J Bone Joint Surg 65B:502, 1983.

143. Wilkins J, Patzakis MJ: Peripheral Teflon catheters. Clin Orthop 254:251, 1990.

144. Wilson MG, Kelly K, Thornhill TS: Infection as a complication of total knee-replacement arthroplasty: Risk factors and treatment in sixty-seven cases. J Bone Joint Surg 72A:87S, 1990.

144a. Wilson MG, Kelley K, Thomhill TS: Infection as a complicated deep sepsis in total hip arthroplasty: The significance of hematogenous and recurrent infection. Clin Orthop 280:200, 1992.

145. Wilson NI: A survey, in Scotland, of measures to prevent infection following orthopaedic surgery. J Hosp Infect 9:235, 1987.

146. Wroblewski BM, del Sel HJ: Urethral instrumentation and deep sepsis in total hip replacement. Clin Orthop 146:209,1980.

147. Wymenga A, van-Horn J, Theeuwes A, et al: Cefuroxime for prevention of postoperative coxitis: One versus three doses tested in a randomized multicenter study of 2,651 arthroplasties. Acta Orthop Scand 63:19, 1992.

148. Yamaguchi K, Adams RA, Morrey BF: Infection after total elbow arthroplasty. J Bone Joint Surg Am 80:481, 1998.

149. Zamaora JL, Price MF, Chuang P, Gentry LO: Inhibition of povidone-iodine's bacterial activity by common organic substances: An experimental study. Surgery 98:25, 1985.

11

Venous Thromboembolism and Total Hip or Knee Replacement Surgery

• JOHN A. HEIT

This chapter reviews venous thromboembolism (VTE) as it pertains to total hip replacement (THR) and total knee replacement (TKR) surgery. The natural history, pathogenesis, prevention, diagnosis, and treatment of VTE are reviewed from the perspective of the orthopedic surgeon. Because anticoagulant therapy is a frequent component of VTE management, the pharmacology and therapeutics of standard unfractionated heparin (UH), low-molecular weight heparin (LMWH), and vitamin-K antagonists (i.e., warfarin sodium) also are briefly reviewed. Finally, practical recommendations are given regarding the most cost-effective approach to all aspects of venous thromboembolic disease associated with joint replacement surgery.

The Natural History of Venous Thromboembolism

The key to the rational prevention and management of VTE is a basic understanding of its natural history. The vast majority of venous thromboses arise in the deep veins of the lower extremity or pelvis (DVT). Poorly adherent venous thrombi may detach and embolize to the lung (pulmonary embolism [PE]). Therefore, PE is a complication of DVT. Previously, only proximal DVT (popliteal or more proximal veins) were thought to embolize to the pulmonary arteries, whereas isolated calf vein thromboses were thought to embolize only after proximal propagation. This clearly is not the case. Isolated calf vein thromboses can embolize to the lung; however, symptoms of a PE are less frequent because these emboli are relatively small compared with emboli arising from the proximal deep veins.

DVT of the lower extremity typically becomes symptomatic when the thrombus progresses to completely occlude the vein lumen. Nonocclusive DVT may remain asymptomatic and yet produce symptomatic and even fatal PE. The pathophysiologic mechanism of fatal PE is hypotension resulting from the acute right ventricular failure that occurs with acutely elevated pulmonary artery pressure.[22] Although hypoxemia may be a prominent manifestation of PE, hypoxic patients seldom die in the absence of significant hypotension. Pulmonary emboli arising from isolated calf vein thrombosis usually are not large enough to occlude a sufficient portion of the pulmonary vasculature to cause acute pulmonary hypertension. However, in the patient with preexisting cardiac or pulmonary disease, cardiac or pulmonary functional reserve may be insufficient for the patient to tolerate even a small PE.

About 30 percent of patients with acute PE die within 7 days of onset[24]; most deaths occur within 30 minutes of the embolic event. For these patients, available time is insufficient for recognition, diagnosis, and initiation of therapy to alter the course of events. Therefore, prevention of VTE with appropriate prophylaxis is of paramount importance.

Incidence of Venous Thromboembolism after Total Hip or Knee Replacement

More than 200,000 patients per year in the United States suffer an incident episode of VTE.[53] Of these patients, approximately 25 percent have antecedent major surgery as at least one clinical risk factor for VTE.[27] Recent surgery increases the risk of VTE approximately 22-fold.[25] Clinical trials and cohort studies have provided a clearer picture of the natural history of acute VTE associated with major orthopedic surgery of the lower extremity and have also provided considerable information to guide decisions about prophylaxis.[18] Based on the results of venography performed on either control patients or patients randomized to receive placebo, the overall prevalence of asymptomatic DVT between 7 and 14 days after THR and TKR is about 50 percent to 60 percent (Table 11–1), with proximal DVT rates of about 25 percent and 15 percent to 20 percent, respectively. Although the operated leg is most commonly affected, the non-operated leg is also affected in about 20 percent of THR patients and between 8 percent and 14 percent of TKR patients. The incidence of asymptomatic PE is less certain. Intraoperative transesophageal echocardiography frequently shows "debris" transiting the right side of the heart, particularly during reaming of the bone. This debris, which includes both fat and thromboemboli,

Table 11–1. VENOUS THROMBOEMBOLISM PREVALENCE AFTER TOTAL HIP OR KNEE REPLACEMENT SURGERY

| Procedure | DVT* | | Pulmonary Embolism | |
	Total	Proximal	Total	Fatal
		%		
THR	45–57	23–36	0.7–30	0.1–0.4
TKR	40–84	9–20	1.8–7	0.2–0.7

*Total or proximal DVT prevalence among control or placebo groups in clinical trials using mandatory postoperative venography.
DVT = deep vein thrombosis; THR = total hip replacement; TKR = total knee replacement.
From Geerts WH, Heit JA, Clagett GP, et al: Prevention of Venous Thromboembolism. Sixth American College of Chest Physicians Consensus Conference on Antithrombotic Therapy. Chest 119:132S–175S, 2001.

often causes transient hypoxemia and pulmonary hypertension. However, serious clinical sequelae are uncommon. In studies that had a ventilation-perfusion lung scan performed routinely, about 7 percent to 11 percent of THR and TKR patients had a high probability scan within 7 to 14 days after surgery. New asymptomatic DVT and PE after hospital discharge are also common. Without postdischarge prophylaxis, 10 percent to 20 percent of patients develop an asymptomatic DVT within 4 to 5 weeks after hospital discharge, and about 6 percent develop an intermediate or high probability lung scan.

Compared with the incidence of asymptomatic VTE, the incidence of symptomatic, objectively documented DVT or PE after THR or TKR is far less common. For example, among a cohort of 1162 consecutive THR patients whose only prophylaxis was use of elastic stockings, the 6-month cumulative VTE incidence was 3.4 percent, with PE seen in 1.6 percent (0.3 percent fatal) and DVT diagnosed in an additional 1.9 percent.[60] Similarly, among TKR patients, the 3-month cumulative PE incidence was 1.5 percent (0.2 percent fatal).[37] Follow-up studies show that only between 1.3 percent and 3 percent of patients develop symptomatic VTE in the 3 months after hospital discharge despite an expected 25 percent to 40 percent prevalence of asymptomatic DVT at the time of hospital discharge.[6,26,39] These data suggest that most DVTs that develop despite prophylaxis resolve without causing symptoms. One cohort study of 213 elective THR or hip fracture patients with negative venography at hospital discharge reported no subsequent episodes of symptomatic VTE over the next 1 to 2 months.[1] Similarly, an overview of 2361 major orthopedic surgery patients with negative venography at hospital discharge found a 1.3 percent cumulative VTE incidence over the next 4 weeks.[49] Moreover, the proportion of patients developing venous stasis syndrome after major hip or knee surgery is low (4 percent to 6 percent)[17,21] and does not appear to be higher among patients with asymptomatic calf or proximal DVT than among patients with no DVT.[21]

Together, these data suggest the following hypothesis regarding the natural history of VTE after THR or TKR. Asymptomatic VTE (including proximal DVT and even PE) is common and, in the absence of prophylaxis, affects at least half of these patients. The majority of these thrombi resolve "spontaneously." For certain patients, however, the persistence of venous injury, prolonged immobility,[5,62] impaired natural anticoagu-

lant[42] or fibrinolytic system, or some as yet unidentified factor or factors allows a thrombus to propagate and become symptomatic because of either venous occlusion or embolization. A number of other clinical and hematologic risk factors for VTE have been identified (Table 11–2). The presence of one or more of these additional risk factors should prompt the use of adjunctive prophylaxis measures (i.e., an anticoagulant prophylaxis *plus* external pneumatic compression). For these patients, prophylaxis should be extended after hospital discharge for a total duration of 4 to 5 weeks from the date of surgery.[28] Similarly, higher intensity and prolonged prophylaxis should be considered for patients with chronic cardiopulmonary disease because these patients would least tolerate further impairment pulmonary or cardiac function by even small pulmonary emboli.

Pathogenesis of Deep Vein Thrombosis After Total Hip or Knee Replacement

The pathogenesis of venous thrombosis is poorly understood. Venous thrombosis may reflect an abnormality in the normal reparative response to venous endothelial injury. This hypothesis postulates a breakdown in the mechanisms that localize and confine a normal hemostatic plug (thrombus) to the site of vein injury. The unconstrained thrombus enlarges by continued clot accretion and eventually leads to vein occlusion, thrombus embolization, or both (e.g., a pathologic DVT).

Lower extremity joint replacement surgery may cause venous endothelial injury via several mechanisms. Direct venous trauma may occur through vein torsion at the time of hip or knee disarticulation. In addition, venous endothelium may be injured by the sustained external compression of the thigh cuff tourniquet used during TKR. Scanning electron microscopy studies have demonstrated venous "microtears" resulting from venodilation upstream from the point of venous occlusion. However, postoperative bilateral venography has demonstrated an 8 percent to 20 percent DVT incidence in the non-operated leg.[18] The cause of the venous endothelial injury that initiates these DVT is unclear; venodilatation associated with general anesthesia is one potential mechanism.[54] The lower DVT incidence associated with use of regional anesthesia or dihydroergotamine (both associated with less venodilatation) lends support to this hypothesis.[7,51]

Table 11–2. RISK FACTORS FOR VENOUS THROMBOEMBOLISM

Clinical Risk Factors	
Increasing age	Male gender
Obesity	White or African-American race
Surgery	Immobilization/paralysis
Trauma	Central venous catheter
Malignant neoplasm	Oral contraceptives
Prior venous thromboembolism	Estrogen replacement therapy

Hereditary (Familial or Primary) Thrombophilias	
Activated protein C (APC) resistance	Factor V R506Q (Leiden) mutation
Prothrombin 20210 G→A mutation	Hyperhomocysteinemia
Antithrombin III deficiency	Protein C deficiency
Protein S deficiency	Dysfibrinogenemia
Factor V HR2 haplotype	Factor XIII Val34Leu
Heparin cofactor II deficiency	Hypoplasminogenemia
Increased plasma factor II, VII, VIII, IX, and XI activity	
Tissue plasminogen activator (tPA) deficiency	
Increased plasminogen activator inhibitor (PAI-1) levels	

Acquired or Secondary Thrombophilia	
Nephrotic syndrome	Thrombotic thrombocytopenic purpura
Inflammatory bowel disease	Behçet's syndrome
Heparin-induced thrombocytopenia and thrombosis (HITT)	
Intravascular coagulation and fibrinolysis/disseminated intravascular coagulation	
Paroxysmal nocturnal hemoglobinuria (PNH)	
Lupus anticoagulant/anticardiolipin antibody	
Thromboangiitis obliterans (Buerger's disease)	
Systemic lupus erythematosis	

The events occurring after venous injury are less clear. Animal model data suggest that the earliest event after injury is platelet adhesion to adjacent venous endothelial cell junctions or exposed subendothelial basement membrane. Recruitment of additional platelets forms a local platelet thrombus. In addition, activation of the procoagulant system, possibly through exposure of vessel wall tissue factor or expression of tissue factor by adherent monocytes,[19] generates thrombin that cleaves fibrinogen to form fibrin and activates both platelets and factor XIII. Activated platelets secrete further procoagulant factors, vasoconstrictors, and platelet agonists that promote continued platelet aggregation and thrombus growth. An overlying fibrin network develops, which traps the red blood cells that give the thrombus its characteristic red appearance. Activated factor XIII cross-links fibrin and imparts further thrombus stability. However, the fact that thrombus initially has only a few venous wall adherence sites explains the propensity for detachment and embolization.

Forces opposing the initiation and growth of a venous thrombus include the fibrinolytic system and the natural anticoagulant system (protein C/thrombomodulin, protein S, antithrombin III).[15] In addition to vein injury, the plasma "acute phase" response to joint replacement surgery acts to inhibit both the fibrinolytic and natural anticoagulant systems. The acute phase response is mediated in part by lymphocytokines (IL-1, TNF-a)[11] and includes increases in procoagulant factor levels (fibrinogen, factor VIII, and von Willebrand factor)[3]; increased plasminogen activator inhibitor-1, which indirectly inhibits the fibrinolytic system; and decreased antithrombin III. Based on cell culture experiments, cytokine-induced expression of tissue-factor[3] and endocytosis of thrombomodulin on the cell surface may act in concert to increase thrombin levels. Expression of cell-surface receptors promotes the adhesion and emigration of leukocytes that contribute to local inflammation.[55] Taken together, these factors may promote both the continued growth and reduced clearance of thrombus at the site of local venous endothelial injury.

Venous Thromboembolism Prophylaxis

DVT prophylaxis has been divided into two categories: (1) primary prophylaxis with either anticoagulants or mechanical measures to reduce blood stasis and (2) secondary or "surveillance" prophylaxis. Theoretically, surveillance prophylaxis aims to detect the patient with an early, asymptomatic postoperative DVT by serially screening with a noninvasive diagnostic test (impedance plethysmography [IPG] or compression ultrasonography). Therapy would only be offered to those patients who develop a positive surveillance diagnostic test. If effective, this strategy would avoid exposure of anticoagulant-based prophylaxis and the associated bleeding risk to all patients. Unfortunately, none of the available noninvasive tests are sufficiently sensitive to detect asymptomatic postoperative DVT.[40,50] Consequently, surveillance prophylaxis remains theory at present.

General Prophylaxis Measures

Several nonpharmacologic prophylaxis methods have been applied to both THR and TKR and include *graduated* compression stockings, external pneumatic compression, and early ambulation. All are of proven benefit with DVT risk reductions of 25 to 60 percent (Table 11–3).[18] *Pneumatic plantar compression* using foot pumps may be moderately effective. However, because the published experience with the foot pump is small and the proximal DVT rates appear to be greater than with current anticoagulant prophylaxis, this modality is not recommended for primary prophylaxis. Compared with general anesthesia, *regional anesthesia* (spinal or epidural) may be associated with a significantly reduced incidence of postoperative DVT for THR surgery in the absence of other thromboprophylaxis interventions. However, the VTE prevalence after regional anesthesia remains substantial and warrants additional primary prophylaxis.

Inferior vena cava (IVC) filter placement has been suggested as a prophylaxis option for patients at extremely high risk for both postoperative VTE and bleeding. However, there are no randomized trials of prophylactic IVC filter insertion or of any studies that address the value of filters when added to recommended prophylaxis options. In DVT *treatment* studies, the incidence of subsequent PE was significantly reduced in the short term among patients receiving an IVC filter. However, mortality was not reduced in the filter group and filter patients had significantly more recurrent DVTs on follow-up.[10,64] Extrapolating these data to high-risk orthopedic surgery patients, prophylactic IVC filter placement may reduce the immediate risk of postoperative PE at the expense of an increased long-term risk for future DVT. Based on these issues, placement of an IVC filter as prophylaxis should be discouraged.

Total Hip Replacement

A number of anticoagulant-based prophylaxis regimens for THR surgery have been studied (Table 11–3).[18] Although meta-analyses have shown fixed *low dose* (mini-dose) *unfractionated heparin* (LDUH) or *aspirin* pro-

phylaxis to be more effective than no prophylaxis, both are less effective than other prophylaxis regimens in high-risk patients. Among 4088 hip and knee arthroplasty patients randomized to aspirin or placebo (with or without other prophylaxis measures), there was no benefit associated with aspirin use for either venous or arterial thromboembolic events.[48] Preoperative LDUH followed by postoperative heparin, dose adjusted to maintain the activated partial thromboplastin time at or just above the upper range of normal (*adjusted-dose heparin*), is safe and highly effective, and may be considered for patients at extremely high risk because of concomitant risk factors.[41] However, most surgeons consider adjusted-dose heparin prophylaxis to be impractical for routine use.

Adjusted-dose oral anticoagulation (e.g., warfarin sodium) is generally safe and effective prophylaxis and has been adopted by many orthopedic surgeons in North America (see Table 11–3).[18] Adjusted-dose warfarin has the potential advantage of allowing continued prophylaxis after hospital discharge. Oral anticoagulants should be administered at a dose sufficient to prolong the international normalized ratio (INR) to a target of 2.5 (range = 2.0 to 3.0). The initial oral anticoagulant dose should be administered either the evening before surgery or as soon after surgery as possible. However, even with early initiation of oral anticoagulants, the INR usually does not reach the target range until at least the third postoperative day.

LMWHs (low molecular weight heparins and heparinoids) have been studied extensively and are highly effective and generally safe as VTE prophylaxis after THR (see Table 11–3).[18] LMWH is more effective than LDUH, and is at least as effective or superior to adjusted-dose unfractionated heparin. Based on meta-analyses,[36,43] the pooled results of five randomized clinical trials,[16,23,32,33,57] and a large open-label trial,[6] LMWH is significantly more effective than warfarin in preventing asymptomatic and symptomatic in-hospital VTE.

Table 11–3. PREVENTION OF DEEP VEIN THROMBOSIS (DVT) AFTER TOTAL HIP REPLACEMENT*

Prophylaxis Regimen	Total DVT[†]		Proximal DVT[‡]	
	Prevalence (95% CI)	RRR	Prevalence (95% CI)	RRR
		%		
Placebo/control	54.2 (50–58)	—	26.6 (23–31)	—
Elastic stockings	41.7 (36–48)	23	25.5 (21–31)	4
Aspirin	40.2 (35–45)	26	11.4 (8–16)	57
Low-dose heparin	30.1 (27–33)	45	19.3 (17–22)	27
Warfarin	22.1 (20–24)	59	5.2 (4–6)	80
IPC	20.3 (17–24)	63	13.7 (11–17)	48
Lepirudin	16.3 (14–19)	70	4.1 (3–5)	85
LMWH	16.1 (15–17)	70	5.9 (5–7)	78
Danaparoid	15.6 (12–19)	71	4.1 (2–6)	85
Pentasaccharide	5.1 (4–6)	91	1.1 (0.5–1.6)	96
Adjusted-dose heparin	14.0 (10–19)	74	10.2 (7–14)	62

*Pooled DVT rates (total and proximal) determined by routine contrast venography from randomized trials.
[†]Patients with adequate venography.
[‡]The denominators for proximal DVT may be slightly different from those for total DVT because some studies did not report proximal DVT rates.
CI = confidence interval; IPC = intermittent pneumatic compression; LMWH = low molecular weight heparin; RRR = relative risk reduction.
From Geert WH, Heit JA, Clagett GP, et al: Prevention of Venous Thromboembolism. Sixth American College of Chest Physicians Consensus Conference on Antithrombotic Therapy. Chest 119:1325–1755, 2001.

However, the risk of surgical site bleeding and wound hematoma is slightly greater with LMWH. These conclusions are consistent with the more rapid onset of anticoagulant activity with LMWH compared with that of warfarin. The selection of LMWH or warfarin prophylaxis must be made at a specific hospital for an individual patient based on drug cost, convenience, availability of an infrastructure to provide safe oral anticoagulation, duration of planned prophylaxis, and potential bleeding and thrombosis risks. In a decision-analysis using Canadian health care costs, LMWH was preferred over adjusted-dose warfarin anticoagulation.[45] However, an analysis based on United States health care costs found adjusted-dose warfarin to be more cost-effective than LMWH.[34]

Three clinical trials have found subcutaneous *recombinant hirudin* (15 mg SC BID, initiated preoperatively) to be more effective than LDUH[12,13] or LMWH,[14] with no difference in bleeding. Although not approved for prophylaxis, recombinant hirudin (lepirudin, Refludan) is approved by the Food and Drug Administration (FDA) for therapy of heparin-induced thrombocytopenia (HIT). *Hirulog*, a synthetic peptide direct thrombin inhibitor that is based in part on hirudin structure, has been tested in one dose-ranging study as prophylaxis after major hip or knee surgery.[20] The highest Hirulog dose regimen tests (1.0 mg/kg SC [subcutaneously] q8h started after surgery) provided a 17 percent overall (2 percent proximal) venographic DVT rate. *Pentasaccharide* (fondaparinux), a synthetic indirect factor Xa inhibitor, has been tested in a dose-ranging study[59] and in two large phase III clinical trials[38,58] as prophylaxis after THR. In the European phase III trial,[38] pentasaccharide (2.5 mg qd started 6 hours after surgery, n=908) was clearly superior to enoxaparin sodium (40 mg qd, started 10 to 12 hours before surgery, n=919) (overall DVT rate: 4.1 percent vs. 9.2 percent, P<0.001; proximal DVT rate: 0.7 percent vs. 2.5 percent, P=0.002).[38] In the North American trial,[58] the same pentasaccharide dose regimen (n=787) provided similar efficacy and safety to enoxaparin sodium (30 mg SC b.i.d. started after surgery, n=797) (overall DVT rate: 6.1 percent vs. 8.3 percent, P=0.1; proximal DVT rate: 1.7 percent vs. 1.2 percent, P=NS).[58] For both trials, the rates of bleeding requiring re-operation and major bleeding with pentasaccharide were low (0.4 percent to 0.2 percent, and 3.7 to 1.6 percent) and did not differ significantly from rates with enoxaparin.

Total Knee Replacement

The overall DVT incidence rate after TKR is higher and the incidence of proximal DVT lower than after THR (Table 11–4). These DVTs, predominantly in the calf, are particularly recalcitrant to prophylaxis. Although major bleeding is not more common in TKR patients, the risk of hemarthrosis and its potential consequences is a major concern.

Several small studies suggest that *intermittent pneumatic compression IPC* is effective prophylaxis in TKR patients (see Table 11–4).[18] These devices are most effective when applied either intraoperatively or immediately postoperatively and should be worn continuously until the patient is fully ambulatory. Poor patient compliance, cost, and the inability to continue prophylaxis after hospital discharge limit the utility of IPC devices. IPC may be useful as an in-hospital adjunct to anticoagulant-based prophylaxis regimens. The *venous foot compression pump* has been shown to be effective in two small studies in TKR patients.[61,65] However, in two other trials, LMWH was considerably more effective than these devices.[4,44] *Continuous passive motion devices* have not been shown to reduce the DVT incidence in TKR patients compared with routine physiotherapy alone.

Low-dose unfractionated heparin (LDUH) and *aspirin* provide relatively small risk reductions for DVT and are not recommended after TKR (see Table 11–4). Based on postoperative venography, warfarin is only moderately effective, with total venographic DVT rates ranging

Table 11–4. PREVENTION OF DEEP VEIN THROMBOSIS (DVT) AFTER TOTAL KNEE REPLACEMENT*

Prophylaxis Regimen	Total DVT†		Proximal DVT‡	
	Prevalence (95% CI)	RRR	Prevalence (95% CI)	RRR
	%			
Placebo/control	64.3 (57–71)	—	15.3 (10–23)	—
Elastic stockings	60.7 (52–69)	6	16.6 (11–24)	—
Aspirin	56.0 (51–61)	13	8.9 (6–12)	42
Warfarin	46.8 (44–49)	27	10.0 (8–12)	35
LDH	43.2 (37–50)	33	11.4 (8–16)	25
VFP	40.7 (33–48)	37	2.3 (1–6)	85
LMWH	30.6 (29–33)	52	5.6 (5–7)	63
Pentasaccharide	12.5 (9–16)	81	2.4 (0.8–4)	84
IPC	28.2 (20–38)	56	7.3 (3–14)	52

*Pooled DVT rates (total and proximal) determined by routine contrast venography from randomized trials.
†Patients with adequate venography.
‡The denominators for proximal DVT may be slightly different from those for total DVT because some studies did not report proximal DVT rates.
CI = confidence interval; IPC = intermittent pneumatic compression; LMWH = low molecular weight heparin; RRR = relative risk reduction; VFP = ventricular filling pressure.
From Geerts WH, Heit JA, Clagett GP, et al: Prevention of Venous Thromboembolism. Sixth American College of Chest Physicians Consensus Conference on Antithrombotic Therapy. Chest 119:1325–1755, 2001.

from 36 percent to 55 percent and a pooled relative risk reduction of only 27 percent (see Table 11–4). However, in a clinical trial of 257 TKR patients receiving warfarin prophylaxis (target INR range = 1.8 to 2.5) for a mean duration of 10 days, the 3-month cumulative incidence of symptomatic VTE was only 0.8 percent.[50] Based on this study, adjusted-dose warfarin is as effective as prophylaxis after TKR.

LMWH has been studied extensively and is safe and effective prophylaxis after TKR surgery. The pooled overall DVT rates from the six randomized trials that directly compared oral anticoagulants with LMWH in TKR were 46.2 percent (505/1094) in the oral anticoagulant group and 31.5 percent (388/1231) in the LMWH group, whereas the proximal DVT rates were 10.2 percent and 6.7 percent, respectively. Based on the available data, LMWH is more effective than warfarin but probably causes more surgical site bleeding and wound hematomas, especially if LMWH is started within 24 hours after surgery. Similar to THR, the choice of LMWH or warfarin prophylaxis for TKR surgery should be tailored to the institution and the individual patient. In an analysis based on United States health care costs, adjusted-dose warfarin prophylaxis was slightly more cost-effective than LMWH.[34]

Pentasaccharide (2.5 mg qd started 6 hours after surgery) has been tested as prophylaxis after TKR in one large North American clinical trial.[2] The overall DVT rate was significantly reduced in the pentasaccharide group (*n*=361) compared that of enoxaparin sodium (30 mg SC b.i.d. started after surgery, *n*=363) (overall DVT rate: 12. percent vs. 27.8 percent, *P*<0.001); the proximal DVT rate was reduced by more than 50 percent in the pentasaccharide group, although this reduction did not reach statistical significance (proximal DVT: 2.4 percent vs. 5.4 percent, *P*=0.56). Bleeding leading to re-operation was uncommon for both pentasaccharide and enoxaparin (0.4 percent vs. 0.2 percent) and did not differ significantly between the two groups. However, the pentasaccharide group did have a higher major bleeding rate compared with the enoxaparin group (1.7% vs. 0%).

Other Prophylaxis Issues

COMPARISONS BETWEEN LOW-MOLECULAR WEIGHT HEPARINS

Currently, four LMW heparins (dalteparin, enoxaparin, nadroparin, tinzaparin) and one heparinoid (danaparoid) are available in the United States or Canada (Table 11–5). At the appropriate LMWH-specific dose and dosing schedule, all are safe and effective as prophylaxis after major orthopedic surgery. The few studies that directly compared two LMWHs showed no difference in efficacy and safety.[46,47] LMW heparins are effective and safe when administered at a fixed dose and without laboratory monitoring or dose adjustment.

PREOPERATIVE OR POSTOPERATIVE INITIATION OF LOW-MOLECULAR WEIGHT HEPARINS

In North America, the initial LMWH dose is generally administered 12 to 24 hours after surgery. However, in Europe, the first LMWH dose is usually administered the evening (10 to 12 hours) before surgery. A randomized

---

Table 11-5. VENOUS THROMBOEMBOLISM PROPHYLAXIS REGIMENS

Adjusted-dose Unfractionated Heparin

3500 U SC q8h and adjusted by ± 500 U per dose to maintain a mid-interval aPTT at high normal values

LMWH and Heparinoids*

Dalteparin sodium (Fragmin) 5000 U 8–12 h preoperatively and once daily starting 12–24 h postoperatively
Dalteparin sodium (Fragmin) 2500 U 4–6 h postoperatively; then 5000 U once daily (THR)
Danaparoid sodium (Orgaran) 750 U 1–4 h preoperatively and q12h postoperatively
Enoxaparin sodium (Lovenox) 30 mg q12h starting 12–24 h postoperatively
Enoxaparin sodium (Lovenox) 40 mg once daily starting 10–12 h preoperatively
Nadroparin 38 U/kg 12 h preoperatively, 12 h postoperatively, and once daily on postoperative days 1, 2, and 3; then increase to 57
  U/kg once daily
Tinzaparin sodium (Innohep) 75 U/kg once daily starting 12–24 h postoperatively
Tinzaparin sodium (Innohep) 4500 U 12 h preoperatively and once daily postoperatively

Pentasaceharide

2.5 mg once daily, started postoperatively

Warfarin Sodium

5–10 mg started the night before or the day of surgery; adjust the dose for a target INR 2.5 (range 2–3)

Lepirudin (Refludan)

15 mg SC b.i.d., started preoperatively and after placement of a regional anesthesia

Intermittent External Pneumatic Compression/Elastic Stockings

Start immediately before operation and continue until fully ambulatory

---

*Dosage expressed in anti-Xa units (for enoxaparin, 1 mg = 100 anti-Xa units).
SC = subcutaneously; THR = total hip replacement.
From Geert WH, Heit JA, Clagett GP, et al: Prevention of Venous Thromboembolism. Sixth American College of Chest Physicians Consensus Conference on Antithrombotic Therapy. Chest 119:1325–1755, 2001.

clinical trial found no difference in efficacy or safety when the first LMWH dose was administered either 2 hours before or 6 hours after surgery.[33] For patients at high risk for bleeding, the initial LMWH dose should be delayed until 12 to 24 hours after surgery. Regardless of the timing of the initial LMWH dose, the first postoperative dose should be delayed until hemostasis is assured (based on examination of the limb and drainage volumes).

ANTITHROMBOTIC DRUGS AND REGIONAL ANESTHESIA

Although paraspinal hematoma after neuraxial blockade (spinal or epidural anesthesia or epidural analgesia) is a rare complication of anticoagulant therapy or prophylaxis, the seriousness of the complication mandates cautious use of antithrombotic medication in patients who have neuraxial blockade. A 1997 FDA Public Health Advisory called attention to safety reports describing 43 United States patients who developed paraspinal hematoma after receiving the LMWH, enoxaparin, concurrently with spinal/epidural anesthesia. Many of these patients suffered neurologic impairment, including permanent paralysis, despite decompressive laminectomy. Factors suspected of predisposing patients to perispinal hematoma include the presence of an underlying hemostatic disorder, traumatic needle or catheter insertion, repeated insertion attempts or blood return, catheter insertion or removal in the presence of significant levels of anticoagulant, use of continuous epidural catheters, anticoagulant dosage, concurrent administration of medications known to increase bleeding, vertebral column abnormalities, older age, and female gender.[66] The problem has also been reported with LDUH, although with lower frequency.

Critical reviews of this problem provide guidelines for LMWH use in patients with spinal/epidural anesthetic interventions.[31] The following recommendations may improve the safety of neuraxial blockade in patients who have received or will receive anticoagulant prophylaxis: (1) regional anesthesia should generally be avoided in patients with a clinical bleeding disorder and in patients receiving drugs that may impair hemostasis (e.g., aspirin, other platelet inhibitors, or anticoagulants); (2) insertion of the spinal needle should be delayed until the anticoagulant effect of the medication is minimal (usually at least 8 to 12 hours after a prophylactic LMWH or heparin injection); (3) anticoagulant prophylaxis should be avoided or delayed if there is a hemorrhagic aspirate ("bloody tap") during the initial spinal needle placement; (4) removal of epidural catheters should be done when the anticoagulant effect is at a minimum (usually just before the next scheduled subcutaneous injection); and (5) anticoagulant prophylaxis should be delayed for at least 2 hours after spinal needle placement or catheter removal. All patients should be monitored carefully and frequently for the new onset of back pain and symptoms or signs of cord compression (e.g., progression of lower extremity numbness or weakness, or bowel or bladder dysfunc-

tion). For patients in whom spinal hematoma is suspected, diagnostic imaging and definitive surgical therapy must be performed as rapidly as possible to reduce the risk of permanent paresis.

DURATION OF THROMBOPROPHYLAXIS

The optimal duration of postoperative prophylaxis after hip and knee arthroplasty and hip fracture surgery remains uncertain. In previous trials, prophylaxis was continued for the duration of postoperative hospitalization and generally ranged from 7 to 14 days. Currently, the duration of hospitalization is often 5 days or less. However, the risk for DVT may persist for up to 2 months after total hip replacement surgery. Randomized clinical trials show that extended out-of-hospital LMWH prophylaxis for THR patients reduces the incidence of new asymptomatic DVT.[28] However, cohort studies found a very low incidence of new symptomatic VTE after hospital discharge. One double-blind, placebo-controlled trial found no significant difference in the combined symptomatic VTE and all-cause mortality rates among patients randomized to extended out-of-hospital LMWH prophylaxis or placebo.[26] Despite the low risk of symptomatic VTE seen in these follow-up studies, 45 percent to 80 percent of all symptomatic DVT and PE that are seen in hip and knee replacement patients occur after hospital discharge. The estimated median time from surgery to VTE was 17 days for THR patients and 7 days after TKR.[63] Although the optimal duration of prophylaxis after major orthopedic surgery has not yet been defined, prophylaxis with LWMH or warfarin should be continued for at least 7 to 10 days. Prolonged prophylaxis should be considered for patients with ongoing risk factors (e.g., continued immobilization, obesity) or a previous history of VTE. For these patients, subcutaneous LMWH (q.d. without laboratory monitoring or dose adjustment) is safe and effective for extended out-of-hospital prophylaxis. Based primarily on VTE treatment trials, adjusted-dose warfarin (target INR = 2.5, range = 2.0 to 3.0) probably is safe and effective for prolonged prophylaxis and an acceptable alternative to LMWH. However, LMWH is significantly more effective than warfarin as early (in hospital) prophylaxis after THR and TKR, and the risk of bleeding associated with extended out-of-hospital warfarin prophylaxis (INR 2.0–3.0) may be greater than with LMWH.

PREDISCHARGE SCREENING FOR DVT

Routine screening for asymptomatic DVT using duplex ultrasonography has not been shown to be useful. Only 3 of 1936 arthroplasty patients (0.15 percent) who received in-hospital LMWH prophylaxis and had predischarge ultrasonography, were found to have asymptomatic DVT.[39] In a trial that randomized hip and knee arthroplasty patients to predischarge duplex ultrasonography or a sham ultrasound procedure, the screening test detected DVT in 2.5 percent of patients, but this was not associated with any reduction in the rate of symptomatic VTE.[50]

Venous Thromboembolism Diagnosis

Because most postoperative DVTs are nonocclusive, the absence of symptoms does not preclude the presence of a postoperative DVT. On the other hand, the clinical symptoms and signs of both DVT (lower extremity pain and swelling) and PE (dyspnea, pleurisy, syncope, hemoptysis) are nonspecific and may be caused by several other diseases. Thus, objective diagnostic testing is required to confirm or refute the presence of a DVT or PE. All diagnostic tests for venous thromboembolism have strengths and limitations that depend on clinical factors specific to the individual patient. These factors are emphasized in the discussion of each individual diagnostic test.

Diagnostic Test Strategies for Deep Vein Thrombosis

VENOGRAPHY

Venography remains the gold standard for the diagnosis of deep vein thrombosis. Venography is the only reliable method for detecting isolated calf vein thrombosis. However, it is invasive, expensive, and associated with potential complications, including intravenous contrast allergy, delayed limb edema, contrast-induced nephropathy, and postvenography DVT. During a properly performed venogram, the injection of contrast should not be painful, especially if nonionic contrast is used. However, the recently operated hip or knee patient may experience discomfort caused by limb positioning necessary for proper film views. Poor contrast filling of the deep venous system resulting from either residuum from a prior DVT or extrinsic compression from hematoma may preclude interpretation and further impair venogram utility. Nevertheless, in the asymptomatic postoperative patient being screened for a DVT, only venography has sufficient sensitivity for adequate diagnosis. Furthermore, if in the surgeon's judgment it is important to detect an isolated calf vein thrombosis, a venogram should be performed.

IMPEDANCE PLETHYSMOGRAPHY

Impedance plethysmography (IPG) is a sensitive noninvasive method for the detection of *occlusive proximal* DVT. It is simple, portable, and inexpensive. However, IPG requires patient cooperation because the leg muscles must be completely relaxed and properly positioned. While the patient is supine, the leg is elevated approximately 30 degrees with slight external rotation at the hip and slight flexion at the knee. Because of its noninvasive nature, IPG testing is suitable for serial testing. However, the IPG test is inadequate for detecting asymptomatic DVT in postoperative patients because most of these thrombi are nonocclusive. Furthermore, it misses isolated calf vein thromboses in symptomatic patients. Compression duplex ultrasonography is more sensitive and has largely replaced IPG as the noninvasive diagnostic test of first choice.

COMPRESSION DUPLEX ULTRASONOGRAPHY

Real-time B-mode ultrasonography can image the veins of the upper leg from the common femoral to the popliteal level except for the femoral vein as it traverses the adductor canal. There are multiple deep veins in the calf that varies in anatomic location. Because it is impossible to be certain that all deep calf veins have been adequately visualized, a negative duplex ultrasound scan does not exclude the presence of an isolated deep calf vein thrombosis.

Under ultrasonographic visualization, the lumen of the normal vein can be obliterated by direct compression with the overlying ultrasound probe. In contrast, the vein lumen occupied by a DVT is "noncompressible." The finding of a noncompressible vein is very sensitive and specific for a DVT. Direct visualization of intraluminal thrombus is less reliable as a diagnostic criterion. Addition of pulsed gated Doppler to real-time B-mode ultrasonography (duplex ultrasonography) provides additional information regarding blood flow. The absence of venous flow provides indirect evidence of DVT but is unreliable for a definite diagnosis. Color-flow duplex ultrasonography adds little additional diagnostic information but does allow more rapid vein identification and shortens the examination time.

Compression duplex ultrasonography is safe, painless, and noninvasive but requires a skilled examiner. Patients must be prone for adequate examination of the popliteal system. Wound hematomas may distort proximal venous anatomy and complicate test interpretation. For the patient with clinical symptoms and signs of acute DVT, compression duplex ultrasonography is sensitive and specific for the detection of a proximal DVT. However, for the *asymptomatic* postoperative joint arthroplasty patient, compression duplex ultrasonography (including color-flow duplex ultrasonography) is inadequate for diagnosis.[9]

Diagnostic Test Strategies for Pulmonary Embolism

PULMONARY ANGIOGRAPHY

Pulmonary angiography remains the gold standard for the diagnosis of acute PE. A pulmonary angiogram is the procedure of choice for the postoperative patient with suspected acute PE and either an abnormal chest radiograph or an intermediate probability or indeterminate ventilation/perfusion lung scan. The complication rate (3 percent to 4 percent) and mortality rate (0.1 percent) associated with pulmonary angiography are quite low when the procedure is performed by an experienced examiner. However, pulmonary angiography is invasive, expensive, and may be associated with intravenous contrast allergy. Furthermore, many surgeons practice in locations where pulmonary angiography is unavailable.

VENTILATION/PERFUSION LUNG SCAN

In general, the ventilation/perfusion lung scan is the initial diagnostic test for the postoperative patient with suspected acute PE. However, lung scan accuracy may be limited by other common postoperative lung processes such as pulmonary atelectasis, pneumonia, or edema. An adequate quality chest radiograph must be reviewed before a lung scan is performed because the presence of an infiltrative lung process may prompt the surgeon to pursue alternative diagnostic tests (i.e., pulmonary angiography). Given the clinical setting of a suspected acute PE, a high-probability lung scan provides sufficient diagnostic certainty to warrant the initiation of anticoagulant therapy. Similarly, a normal lung scan virtually excludes PE and anticoagulant therapy can be withheld. Unfortunately, two thirds of all lung scans fall within the intermediate probability or indeterminate categories; thus, diagnostic certainty is insufficient to either commence or withhold anticoagulants. In this circumstance, additional diagnostic testing is warranted. Because most PEs originate in the deep veins of the leg, noninvasive diagnostic testing for DVT (e.g., compression duplex ultrasonography) is a reasonable diagnostic strategy because discovery of a DVT would prompt initiation of anticoagulant therapy. However, a negative ultrasound scan does not exclude a diagnosis of PE because the DVT could have completely embolized or the embolus could have originated from a pelvic vein or an isolated calf vein thrombosis that would be missed by the ultrasound. If the clinical suspicion of acute PE is high, these patients should undergo pulmonary angiography.

COMPUTED TOMOGRAPHY

High-resolution, high-speed, contrast-enhanced spiral (helical) or electron beam computed tomography (CT) is sensitive and specific for central or large PE[56] with less interobserver variability than the lung scan. Moreover, CT detects diseases other than PE.[8] Depending on the center, CT usually is less expensive than a ventilation/perfusion lung scan. Consequently, many centers now prefer CT as the diagnostic test of first choice for suspected acute PE. However, CT may miss emboli at the subsegmental artery size or smaller.[56] In addition, CT is associated with the risk of allergic reaction to intravenous contrast dye and requires a skilled interpreter. Additional testing is required for patients with a high clinical suspicion of PE in whom a CT scan is interpreted as negative. Such patients should undergo pulmonary angiography or testing for DVT.

Venous Thromboembolism Therapy

Standard Unfractionated Heparin

Standard unfractionated heparin (UH) is a sulfated glycosaminoglycan derived from either porcine intestinal mucosa or bovine lung. Heparin catalyzes antithrombin III inhibition of several procoagulant factors including thrombin.[29] UH binds to platelets, endothelial cells, and several non-anticoagulant-related plasma proteins. The anticoagulant effect of heparin becomes apparent only after these binding sites are occupied. Therefore, immediate heparin anticoagulation requires an intravenous

bolus dose. Many of these non-anticoagulant-related proteins are acute phase reactants (e.g., factor VIII). Thus, the plasma concentrations of these acute phase reactant proteins increase unpredictably during illness or after surgery. The differing plasma concentration among patients causes marked interindividual variability in the anticoagulant response (as measured by the activated partial thromboplastin time [aPTT]) such that aPTT monitoring and UH dose adjustment is required. The circulating plasma half-life of UH after intravenous administration is approximately 1 hour. The maximum anticoagulant effect of UH occurs approximately 3 hours after a subcutaneous injection, with a measurable effect lasting 12 hours.

The aim of anticoagulant therapy for VTE is to prevent further thrombus propagation and embolization. If there is no contraindication, immediate anticoagulant therapy should be given to the patient with a suspected acute DVT or PE.[35] The most common cause of recurrent VTE is failure to provide adequate early anticoagulant therapy. Successful UH anticoagulation may be delivered by either the intravenous or subcutaneous route at a total daily dose of approximately 30,000 to 40,000 U. The UH dose should be adjusted every 4 four hours initially until the aPTT is prolonged to between 1.5 and 2.5 times baseline. Failure to prolong the aPTT into the therapeutic range within the first 8 hours should prompt an additional 5000 U heparin IV bolus. The aPTT should be monitored at least daily as should the hemoglobin and platelet count. A relative platelet count decrease of 30 percent from baseline, or an absolute platelet count less than 100,000, raises the concern of heparin-induced thrombocytopenia (HIT). This potentially devastating complication of heparin therapy paradoxically causes widespread venous and arterial thrombosis. All heparin administration (including heparin "flush") must be discontinued whenever HIT is suspected.

Low Molecular Weight Heparin

Low molecular weight heparin (LMWH) is derived from chemical or enzymatic depolymerization of standard unfractionated heparin.[29] The lower molecular weight (e.g., 4000 to 6000 daltons) imparts several pharmacologic advantages to LMWH that avoid many of the problems associated with UH therapy. The main advantage is a marked reduction in LMWH binding to non–anticoagulant-related plasma proteins. Consequently, the LMWH anticoagulant response is unaffected by individual variation in acute phase reactant plasma protein levels. When dosed on a weight-adjusted basis, the LMWH anticoagulant response is very predictable and reproducible. LMWH is administered on a weight-adjusted basis and does not require laboratory monitoring or dose adjustment. Compared with UH, LMWH has a higher bioavailability after subcutaneous injection (90 percent vs. 30 percent) and longer plasma half-life (4 to 6 hours vs. 0.5 to 1 hour). The peak LMWH anticoagulant response occurs approximately 4 hours after SC injection, and there is no

Table 11–6. LOW MOLECULAR WEIGHT HEPARIN (LMWH) REGIMENS FOR VENOUS THROMBOEMBOLISM THERAPY

Low Molecular Weight Heparin	Regimen
Ardeparin sodium (Normiflo)	130 anti-X_a IU/kg SC 12 h (not FDA approved for venous thromboembolism therapy)
Dalteparin sodium (Fragmin)	200 anti-X_a IU/kg SC once daily (not FDA approved for venous thromboembolism therapy)
Enoxaparin sodium (Lovenox)	1 mg/kg SC 12 h (FDA approved for outpatient therapy of deep vein thrombosis)
	1 mg/kg SC 12 h, or 1.5 mg/kg SC once daily (FDA approved for inpatient therapy of deep vein thrombosis with or without pulmonary embolism)
Tinzaparin sodium (Innohep)	175 anti-X_a IU/kg SC once daily (FDA approved for inpatient therapy of deep vein thrombosis with or without pulmonary embolism)

FDA = Food and Drug Administration; SC = subcutaneously.

drug accumulation with repeated dosing over periods of up to 2 weeks. The LMWH anticoagulant effect can be partially reversed with protamine. Because LMWH is excreted primarily via the kidney, LMWH should be used with caution in patients with impaired renal function (e.g., serum creatinine > 2.0 mg/dl). For these patients, laboratory monitoring and dose adjustment to provide a peak LMWH level of 0.5 to 1.0 anti-Xa IU/L level may be appropriate. The incidence of HIT among patients receiving LMWH is lower than with UH. However, LMWH cannot be substituted for UH in patients with established HIT. These patients must be treated with either danaparoid sodium (Orgaran [a heparinoid]), recombinant hirudin ([lepirudin] Refludan), or argatroban.

The enhanced pharmacologic characteristics of LMWH make it an ideal choice for outpatient DVT therapy. Fixed-dose, unmonitored LMWH is effective and safe as outpatient therapy for acute DVT, and as inpatient therapy for acute PE.[28,35] Acute DVT patients with a high bleeding risk, active bleeding, or phlegmasia, should be hospitalized. In addition, DVT patients should receive adequate graduated compression stocking therapy (Table 11-6).

Oral Anticoagulants

Oral anticoagulants (i.e., warfarin sodium) inhibit the vitamin–K–dependent γ-carboxylation of procoagulant factors II (prothrombin), VII, IX, and X.[30] The delayed anticoagulant effect of warfarin is due to the relatively long plasma half-life of functional vitamin–K–dependent procoagulant factors formed before warfarin administration. For example, factor II has a normal circulating half-life for approximately 60 to 90 hours. Consequently, a 50 percent reduction in factor II activity requires approximately 4 to 5 days of warfarin therapy. A loading dose of warfarin has no effect on the plasma half-life of these factors and does not shorten the time required to reach therapeutic anticoagulation. On the other hand, the anticoagulant effects of warfarin can be reversed within hours by either oral or intravenous administration of vitamin K.[52] Consequently, factor replacement therapy in the form of cryoprecipitate or fresh frozen plasma (and the risk of blood-borne infection) is not warranted in the over-anticoagulated patient unless there is evidence of clinical bleeding.

Oral anticoagulant therapy is initiated when the diagnosis of VTE is confirmed. Heparin and warfarin should be given concurrently for at least 5 days, and until the International Normalized Ratio (INR) is within the therapeutic range (INR = 2.0 to 3.0) on two measurements performed at least 24 hours apart.[35] The INR adjusts for the inter-laboratory variability in prothrombin time assay methodology and standardizes the laboratory result. All laboratories should report both patient prothrombin time and INR levels. The patient should be started on the estimated daily maintenance dose; a loading dose should be avoided. The standard duration of oral anticoagulant therapy is 3 months. Patients with recurrent VTE or persistent risk factors for recurrent VTE (i.e., malignant neoplasm, serious neurologic disease with extremity paresis, antithrombin III deficiency, lupus anticoagulant/anticardiolipin antibody) should be considered for lifelong oral anticoagulant therapy.

Acknowledgments

Funded, in part, by grants from the National Institutes of Health (HL60279, HL66216) and the Centers for Disease Control and Prevention (3O0820), U.S. Public Health Service; the American Heart Association (99-50166N); and by Mayo Foundation.

References

1. Agnelli G, Ranucci V, Veschi F, et al: Clinical outcome of orthopaedic patients with negative lower limb venography at discharge. Thromb Haemost 74:1042–1044, 1995.
2. Bauer K: The PENTAMAKS Study: Comparison of the first synthetic factor Xa inhibitor with low molecular weight heparin for the prevention of venous thromboembolism after elective major knee surgery [abstract]. Blood 96:490a, 2000.
3. Bevilacqua MP, Pober JS, Majeau GR, et al: Recombinant tumor necrosis factor induces procoagulant activity in cultured human vascular endothelium: Characterization and comparison with the actions of interleukin 1. Proc Natl Acad Sci USA 83:4533–4537, 1986.
4. Blanchard J, Meuwly JY, Leyvraz PF, et al: Prevention of deep-vein thrombosis after total knee replacement. Randomised comparison between a low-molecular-weight heparin (nadroparin) and mechanical prophylaxis with a foot-pump system. J Bone Joint Surg Br 81:654–659, 1999.
5. Buehler KO, D'Lima DD Petersilge WJ, et al: Late deep venous thrombosis and delayed weightbearing after total hip arthroplasty. Clin Orthop 3:123–130, 1999.
6. Colwell CW Jr, Collis DK, Paulson R, et al: Comparison of enoxaparin and warfarin for the prevention of venous thromboembolic

disease after total hip arthroplasty. Evaluation during hospitalization and three months after discharge. J Bone Joint Surg Am 81:932–940, 1999.

7. Comerota AJ, Stewart GJ, White JV: Combined dihydroergotamine and heparin prophylaxis of postoperative deep vein thrombosis: Proposed mechanism of action. Am J Surg 150:39–44, 1985.

8. Cross JJ, Kemp PM, Walsh CG, et al: A randomized trial of spiral CT and ventilation perfusion scintigraphy for the diagnosis of pulmonary embolism. Clin Radiol 53:177–182, 1998.

9. Davidson BL, Elliott CG, Lensing AW: Low accuracy of color Doppler ultrasound in the detection of proximal leg vein thrombosis in asymptomatic high-risk patients. The RD Heparin Arthroplasty Group. Ann Intern Med 117:735–738, 1992.

10. Decousus H, Leizorovicz A, Parent F, et al: A clinical trial of vena caval filters in the prevention of pulmonary embolism in patients with proximal deep-vein thrombosis. Práevention du Risque d'Embolie Pulmonaire par Interruption Cave Study Group. N Engl J Med 338:409–415, 1998.

11. Dinarello CA, Mier JW: Lymphokines. N Engl J Med 317:940–945, 1987.

12. Eriksson BI, Ekman S, Kalebo P, et al: Prevention of deep-vein thrombosis after total hip replacement: Direct thrombin inhibition with recombinant hirudin, CGP 39393. Lancet 347:635–639, 1996.

13. Eriksson BI, Ekman S, Lindbratt S, et al: Prevention of thromboembolism with use of recombinant hirudin. Results of a double-blind, multicenter trial comparing the efficacy of desirudin (Revasc) with that of unfractionated heparin in patients having a total hip replacement. J Bone Joint Surg Am 79:326–333, 1997.

14. Eriksson BI, Wille-Jorgensen P, Kalebo P, et al: A comparison of recombinant hirudin with a low-molecular-weight heparin to prevent thromboembolic complications after total hip replacement. N Engl J Med 337:1329–1335, 1997.

15. Esmon CT: The regulation of natural anticoagulant pathways. Science 235:1348–1352, 1987.

16. Francis CW, Pellegrini VD Jr, Totterman S, et al: Prevention of deep-vein thrombosis after total hip arthroplasty. Comparison of warfarin and dalteparin. J Bone Joint Surg Am 79:1365–1372, 1997.

17. Francis CW, Ricotta JJ, Evarts CM, Marder VJ: Long- term clinical observations and venous functional abnormalities after asymptomatic venous thrombosis following total hip or knee arthroplasty. Clin Orthop 232:271–278, 1988.

18. Geerts WH, Heit JA, Clagett GP, et al: Prevention of Venous Thromboembolism. Sixth American College of Chest Physicians Consensus Conference on Antithrombotic Therapy. Chest 119:132S–175S, 2001.

19. Giesen PL, Rauch U, Bohrmann B, et al: Blood-borne tissue factor: Another view of thrombosis. Proc Natl Acad Sci USA 96:2311–2315, 1999.

20. Ginsberg JS, Nurmohamed MT, Gent M, et al: Use of Hirulog in the prevention of venous thrombosis after major hip or knee surgery. Circulation 90:2385–2389, 1994.

21. Ginsberg JS, Turkstra F, Buller HR, et al: Postthrombotic syndrome after hip or knee arthroplasty: A cross-sectional study. Arch Intern Med 160:669–672, 2000.

22. Grifoni S, Olivotto I, Cecchini P, et al: Short-term clinical outcome of patients with acute pulmonary embolism, normal blood pressure, and echocardiographic right ventricular dysfunction. Circulation 101:2817–2822, 2000.

23. Hamulyak K, Lensing AW, van der Meer J, et al: Subcutaneous low-molecular weight heparin or oral anticoagulants for the prevention of deep-vein thrombosis in elective hip and knee replacement? Fraxiparine Oral Anticoagulant Study Group. Thromb Haemost 74:1428–1431, 1995.

24. Heit JA, Silverstein MD, Mohr DN, et al: Predictors of survival after deep vein thrombosis and pulmonary embolism: A population-based, cohort study. Arch Intern Med 159:445–453, 1999.

25. Heit JA, Silverstein MD, Mohr DN, et al: Risk factors for deep vein thrombosis and pulmonary embolism: A population-based case-control study. Arch Intern Med 160:809–815, 2000.

26. Heit JA, Elliott CG, Trowbridge AA, et al: Ardeparin sodium for extended out-of-hospital prophylaxis against venous thromboembolism after total hip or knee replacement. A randomized, double-blind, placebo-controlled trial. Ann Intern Med 132:853–861, 2000.

27. Heit JA, O'Fallon WM, Petterson TM, et al: Relative impact of risk factors for deep vein thrombosis and pulmonary embolism: A population-based study [in press].

28. Heit JA: Low molecular weight heparin: The optimal duration of prophylaxis against postoperative venous thromboembolism after total hip or knee replacement. Thromb Res 101:163–173, 2001.

29. Hirsh J, Warkentin TE, Shaughnessy SG, et al: Heparin and low molecular weight heparin: Mechanisms of action, pharmacokinetics, dosing, monitoring, efficacy, and safety. Chest 119 (Suppl):64S–94S, 2001.

30. Hirsh J, Dalen JE, Anderson DR, et al: Oral anticoagulants; mechanism of action, clinical effectiveness, and optimal therapeutic range. Chest 119(Suppl):8S–21S, 2001.

31. Horlocker TT, Heit JA: Low molecular weight heparin: Biochemistry, pharmacology, perioperative prophylaxis regimens, and guidelines for regional anesthetic management. Anesth Analg 85:874–885, 1997.

32. Hull R, Raskob G, Pineo G, et al: A comparison of subcutaneous low-molecular-weight heparin with warfarin sodium for prophylaxis against deep-vein thrombosis after hip or knee implantation. N Engl J Med 329:1370–1376, 1993.

33. Hull RD, Pineo GF, Francis C, et al: Low-molecular-weight heparin prophylaxis using dalteparin in close proximity to surgery vs warfarin in hip arthroplasty patients: A double-blind, randomized comparison. The North American Fragmin Trial Investigators. Arch Intern Med 160:2199–2207, 2000.

34. Hull RD, Raskob GE, Pineo GF, et al: Subcutaneous low-molecular-weight heparin vs warfarin for prophylaxis of deep vein thrombosis after hip or knee implantation. An economic perspective. Arch Intern Med 157:298–303, 1997.

35. Hyers TN, Agnelli G, Hull RD, et al: Antithrombotic therapy for venous thromboembolic disease. Chest 119(Suppl):176S–193S, 2001.

36. Imperiale TF, Speroff T: A meta-analysis of methods to prevent venous thromboembolism following total hip replacement. JAMA 271:1780–1785, 1994.

37. Khaw FM, Moran CG, Pinder IM, Smith SR: The incidence of fatal pulmonary embolism after knee replacement with no prophylactic anticoagulation. J Bone Joint Surg Br 75:940–941, 1993.

38. Lassen MR: The EPHESUS Study: Comparison of the first synthetic factor Xa inhibitor with low molecular weight heparin for the prevention of venous thromboembolism after elective hip replacement surgery. Blood 96:490a, 2000.

39. Leclerc JR, Gent M, Hirsh J, et al: The incidence of symptomatic venous thromboembolism during and after prophylaxis with enoxaparin: A multi-institutional cohort study of patients who underwent hip or knee arthroplasty. Canadian Collaborative Group. Arch Intern Med 158:873–888, 1998.

40. Lensing AW, Doris CI, McGrath FP, et al: A comparison of compression ultrasound with color Doppler ultrasound for the diagnosis of symptomless postoperative deep vein thrombosis. Arch Intern Med 157:765–768, 1997.

41. Leyvraz PF, Richard J, Bachmann F, et al: Adjusted versus fixed-dose subcutaneous heparin in the prevention of deep-vein thrombosis after total hip replacement. N Engl J Med 309:954–958, 1983.

42. Lindahl TL, Lundahl TH, Nilsson L, Andersson CA: APC-resistance is a risk factor for postoperative thromboembolism in elective replacement of the hip or knee—a prospective study. Thromb Haemost 81:18–21, 1999.

43. Mohr DN, Silverstein MD, Murtaugh PA, Harrison JM: Prophylactic agents for venous thrombosis in elective hip surgery. Meta-analysis of studies using venographic assessment. Arch Intern Med 153:2221–2228, 1993.

44. Norgren L, Toksvig-Larsen S, Magyar G, et al: Prevention of deep vein thrombosis in knee arthroplasty. Preliminary results from a randomized controlled study of low molecular weight heparin vs foot pump compression. Int Angiol 17:93–96, 1998.

45. O'Brien BJ, Anderson DR, Goeree R: Cost-effectiveness of enoxaparin versus warfarin prophylaxis against deep-vein thrombosis after total hip replacement. CMAJ 150:1083–1090, 1994.

46. Planes A, Samama MM, Lensing AW, et al: Prevention of deep vein thrombosis after hip replacement—comparison between two low-molecular heparins, tinzaparin and enoxaparin. Thromb Haemost 81:22–25, 1999.

47. Planes A, Vochelle N, Fagola M, Bellaud M: Comparison of two low-molecular-weight heparins for the prevention of postoperative venous thromboembolism after elective hip surgery. Reviparin Study Group. Blood Coagul Fibrinolysis 9:499–505, 1998.

48. Pulmonary Embolism Prevention (PEP) Trial Collaborative Group: Prevention of pulmonary embolism and deep vein thrombosis with low dose aspirin: Pulmonary Embolism Prevention (PEP) trial. Lancet 355:1295–1302, 2000.

49. Ricotta S, Iorio A, Parise P, et al: Post discharge clinically overt venous thromboembolism in orthopaedic surgery patients with negative venography – an overview analysis. Thromb Haemost 76:887–892,1996.

50. Robinson KS, Anderson DR, Gross M, et al: Ultrasonographic screening before hospital discharge for deep venous thrombosis after arthroplasty: The post-arthroplasty screening study. A randomized, controlled trial. Ann Intern Med 127:439–445, 1997.

51. Sharrock NE, Go G, Mineo R, Harpel PC: The hemodynamic and fibrinolytic response to low dose epinephrine and phenylephrine infusions during total hip replacement under epidural anesthesia. Thromb Haemost 68:436–441, 1992.

52. Shields RC, McBane RD, Kuiper JD, et al: Efficacy and safety of intravenous phytonadione (Vitamin K_1) for correction of chronic oral anticoagulation. Mayo Clin Proc 76:260–266, 2001.

53. Silverstein MD, Heit JA, Mohr DN, et al: Trends in the incidence of deep vein thrombosis and pulmonary embolism: A 25-year population-based study. Arch Intern Med 158:585–593, 1998.

54. Stewart GJ, Lachman JW, Alburger PD, et al: Intraoperative venous dilation and subsequent development of deep vein thrombosis in patients undergoing total hip or knee replacement. Ultrasound Med Biol 16:133–40, 1990.

55. Stewart GJ: Neutrophils and deep venous thrombosis. Haemostasis 23(Suppl):127–140, 1993.

56. Teigen CL, Maus TP, Sheedy PF II, et al: Pulmonary embolism: Diagnosis with contrast-enhanced electron-beam CT and comparison with pulmonary angiography. Radiology 194:313–319, 1995.

57. The RD Heparin Arthroplasty Group: RD heparin compared with warfarin for prevention of venous thromboembolic disease following total hip of knee arthroplasty. J Bone Joint Surg Am 76A:1174–1185, 1994.

58. Turpie G: The Pentathlon 2000 Study: Comparison of the first synthetic factor Xa inhibitor with low molecular weight heparin in the prevention of venous thromboembolism after elective hip replacement surgery. Blood 96:491a, 2000.

59. Turpie AGG, Gallus AS, Hoek JA, for the Pentasaccharide Investigators: A synthetic pentasaccharide for the prevention of deep-vein thrombosis after total hip replacement. N Engl J Med 344:619–625, 2001.

60. Warwick D, Williams MH, Bannister GC: Death and thromboembolic disease after total hip replacement. A series of 1162 cases with no routine chemical prophylaxis. J Bone Joint Surg Br 77:6–10, 1995.

61. Westrich GH, Sculco TP: Prophylaxis against deep venous thrombosis after total knee arthroplasty. Pneumatic plantar compression and aspirin compared with aspirin alone. J Bone Joint Surg Am 78:826–834, 1996.

62. White RH, Gettner S, Newman JM, et al: Predictors of rehospitalization for symptomatic venous thromboembolism after total hip arthroplasty. N Engl J Med 343:1758–1764, 2000.

63. White RH, Romano PS, Zhou H, et al: Incidence and time course of thromboembolic outcomes following total hip or knee arthroplasty. Arch Intern Med 158:1525–1531, 1998.

64. White RH, Zhou H, Kim J, Romano PS: A population- based study of the effectiveness of inferior vena cava filter use among patients with venous thromboembolism. Arch Intern Med 160:2033–2041, 2000.

65. Wilson NV, Das SK, Kakkar VV, et al: Thromboembolic prophylaxis in total knee replacement. Evaluation of the A-V Impulse System. J Bone Joint Surg Br 74:50–52, 1992.

66. Wysowski DK, Talarico L, Bacsanyi J, Botstein P: Spinal and epidural hematoma and low-molecular-weight heparin. N Engl J Med 338:1774–1775, 1998.

12

Anesthetic Considerations

•ROBERT L. LENNON, DENISE J. WEDEL, and ALISON ALBRECHT

The practices of regional anesthesia and orthopedic surgery are closely linked. The site of surgery in orthopedic patients frequently makes them more suitable candidates for regional anesthetic techniques than other surgical patients. Although general anesthesia does have a role in orthopedic operative procedures, regional anesthetics offer tangible benefits. Care must be given to examine coexisting medical conditions that may influence anesthetic management. Additionally, the literature suggests that anesthetic management and preemptive analgesia may greatly influence perioperative morbidity and the quality of postoperative analgesia. With these considerations in mind, orthopedic anesthesia is discussed in relation to the particular influence of the surgical site on anesthetic management.

PREOPERATIVE ASSESSMENT

The anesthesiologist's preoperative assessment is crucial to the formation and execution of the anesthetic plan. During this assessment, the patient is evaluated for coexisting medical problems, previous anesthetic complications, potential airway difficulties, and considerations relating to intraoperative positioning. This evaluation, coupled with an appreciation of the surgical requirements, is used to formulate the anesthetic plan.

Elements of the History

As the general population ages, so do candidates for joint replacement surgery. Advancing age is often accompanied by changes in physiologic function that can progress to significant illness. Several of the more common medical conditions have been described in previous chapters. Therefore, the discussion here is limited to those medical illnesses with a significant bearing on anesthetic technique.

Hypertension

Hypertension is probably the most prevalent medical problem seen in patients undergoing joint replacement (see Chapter 9). Intraoperatively, hypertensive patients experience wider fluctuations in blood pressure than normotensive individuals. Noxious stimuli lead to exaggerated hypertensive responses. Conversely, once general or centroneuraxis anesthesia is induced, hypotension may occur, because hypertensive patients tend to be intravascularly depleted. Hypertensive patients should continue to take their antihypertensive medications perioperatively, particularly if they are using β- or α-blocking agents (see Chapter 9).

Coronary Artery Disease

Patients with coronary artery disease pose unique problems to the anesthesiologist (see Chapter 9). In the patient who has experienced a myocardial infarction, elective surgery should be delayed for 6 months to avoid significant cardiac morbidity and mortality.[11] Patients with unstable angina require a cardiac evaluation before undergoing elective surgery so that the extent of disease can be determined and appropriate interventions can be planned. Patients who are taking antianginal medications should continue these medications preoperatively. Intraoperatively, patients may require intravenous nitrates to improve coronary blood flow and β-blocking agents to control heart rate.

Rheumatoid Arthritis

Many patients undergoing joint replacement surgery have rheumatoid arthritis. These patients may have systemic manifestations of their disease, with pulmonary, cardiac, and musculoskeletal involvement. Particularly significant to the anesthesiologist are the involvement of the cervical spine, the temporomandibular joint, and the arytenoid cartilage of the larynx. Rheumatoid involvement of the cervical spine may result in limited neck range of motion, which interferes with airway management. Atlantoaxial instability, with subluxation of the odontoid process, can lead to spinal cord injury during neck extension. In this case, awake fiberoptic intubation may be the most appropriate method for securing the airway. Under direct visualization by means of a fiberoptic bronchoscope, the endotracheal tube can be placed with minimal movement of the patient's head and neck. Patients with rheumatoid arthritis often receive chronic steroid therapy. Patients who have taken steroids for more than 5 days in the preceding 12 months should receive steroid replacement perioperatively.[11] Guidelines for replacement therapy are presented in Table 12–1.[32]

Trauma

Management of orthopedic trauma involves unique considerations. It is assumed that trauma patients requiring emergency surgical intervention have full stomachs. Delayed gastric emptying secondary to the traumatic event and narcotic administration necessitate rapid-sequence induction or awake intubation if general anesthesia is indicated. Patients who have sustained cervical spine trauma require careful and controlled airway management to avoid further injury. In this situation, fiberoptic intubation while the patient is awake results in minimal cervical manipulation and allows for pre- and postintubation neurologic assessment. After the airway is established and cardiovascular stability ensured, surgery can proceed.

Anesthetic History

After the patient's medical history and current medical condition have been evaluated, the past anesthetic history of the patient and his or her family can be obtained. Facts gleaned from this review can have a significant impact on the anesthetic plan. A personal or family history of coagulation disorders associated with easy bruising or bleeding in the patient or the family may make regional anesthesia inadvisable. A history of porphyria dictates, to some extent, the anesthetic agents used. Some hereditary diseases, such as plasma cholinesterase disorders and malignant hyperthermia, may not even be diagnosed until the patient or a member of the family is anesthetized.

Physical Examination

After an adequate history is obtained, a focused physical examination is performed. The airway should be assessed for any limitation in mouth opening or neck extension, for adequacy of thyromental distance (measured from the lower border of the mandible to the thyroid notch), and for state of dentition. If difficulties are anticipated, the ability to control the airway must be assessed. The heart and lungs should be auscultated. In addition, the site of proposed injection for regional anesthesia should be examined for evidence of infection and anatomic abnormalities. At this time, the patient should also be evaluated for any potential positioning difficulties related to arthritic involvement of other joints or body habitus.

ANESTHETIC TECHNIQUE

After considering the history and physical examination, the duration and positioning requirements of surgery, and the surgeon's needs, an anesthetic plan is developed. Joint replacement surgery can be successfully completed under either regional or general anesthesia. The risks and benefits of each are discussed in the following sections.

General Anesthesia

General anesthesia provides the patient with amnesia, analgesia, hypnosis, and muscle relaxation. The agents used as general anesthetics result in reversible changes in neurologic function so that the patient does not respond to or recall intraoperative events. General anesthesia begins with induction, whereby the patient is rendered unconscious. This can be achieved by a variety of intravenous and inhalation anesthetic agents. Once the patient is unconscious, the airway must be protected. Manual ventilation, using a face mask or a laryngeal mask airway, can provide gas exchange during cases of short duration. For cases of longer duration, or when the patient may have retained gastric contents, the airway is secured with an endotracheal tube. This airway protection allows ventilation of the lungs, avoidance of aspiration of gastric contents, and, rarely, instillation of emergency resuscitative drugs. The anesthetic is maintained by inhalation agents, intravenous infusions, or a combination of both. When awakening is desired, the anesthetic agent is discontinued and the patient eliminates the agent by metabolism, excretion, or both.

Any patient who has an absolute contraindication to regional anesthesia is a candidate for general anesthesia.

Table 12–1. GUIDELINES FOR PERIOPERATIVE STEROID REPLACEMENT

Minor surgical procedures	1.5–2 times baseline steroid dose on day of surgery Normal dose on first postoperative day
Moderate surgical procedures	2 times baseline steroid dose on morning of surgery orally *or* 75 mg hydrocortisone IV intraoperatively and 50 mg hydrocortisone IV postoperatively Rapidly taper steroids to baseline dose over 48 h
Major surgical procedures	2 times baseline steroid dose orally or 50–100 mg hydrocortisone intraoperatively Postoperatively, 100 mg hydrocortisone q8h for 24 h Rapidly taper steroids over 24–72 h

IV = intravenously.
Modified from Chernow B, Alexander HR, Smallridge RC, et al: Hormonal responses to graded surgical stress. Arch Intern Med 147:1273, 1987.

In some cases, the patient may be reluctant to agree to regional anesthesia. If the patient's fears cannot be allayed, a general anesthetic is provided.

Regional Anesthesia

Orthopedic surgical procedures, because of their localized peripheral site, lend themselves to regional anesthetic techniques. A regional anesthetic provides the patient with surgical analgesia and muscle relaxation. Intravenous sedative can be used to provide mild sedation and amnesia during the operative procedure. Regional anesthetics include peripheral nerve blocks and central neuraxial blockade. The selection of the regional technique and the local anesthetic to be used depend on a variety of factors, including duration of surgery, desired length of postoperative analgesia, and indication for postoperative sympathectomy. Local anesthetics, if inadvertently injected intravascularly, can be associated with significant morbidity resulting from central nervous system and cardiovascular toxicity. Table 12–2 lists accepted dosing guidelines for the more commonly used local anesthetics. Regional anesthetics offer several advantages over general anesthetics, including improved postoperative analgesia, less respiratory and cardiac depression, improved perfusion via sympathetic block, reduced blood loss, and decreased risk of thromboembolism. Table 12–2 lists the pharmacologic and clinical characteristics of local anesthetics.[3]

It is clear that regional anesthesia offers more significant benefits than general anesthesia in patient groups who undergo orthopedic procedures. For patients who are to have arthroplastic procedures, it is important to explain these benefits and to encourage patients to choose regional anesthesia if appropriate.

Blood Loss

Historically, hypothermia and induced hypotension were used in an effort to control bleeding and reduce the use of blood products. Hypothermia was believed to decrease bleeding by inducing peripheral vasoconstriction. Prolonged hypothermia resulted in a coagulopathy related to platelet sequestration and inhibition of coagulation factors. Although it was believed that hypotension decreased intraoperative blood loss by decreasing tissue perfusion pressure, it did not provide more significant reductions in blood loss than normal surgical hemostasis. Consequently, the optimal method for controlling intraoperative blood loss is one that includes adequate surgical hemostasis and minimizes the duration of surgery.

Multiple studies have demonstrated significant reductions in intraoperative blood loss during total hip arthroplasty completed under central neuraxial blockade.[4] There is less blood loss during spinal and epidural anesthesia, than during general anesthesia. The reason for this reduced blood loss has been hypothesized but remains unproven. Central neuraxial blockade has been shown to decrease mean arterial pressure; in addition, blood flow redistributes to larger caliber vessels and venous pressure is reduced locally. It is likely that all these factors contribute to reduction of intraoperative blood loss. Decreased postoperative blood loss has not been as clearly demonstrated.

Deep Venous Thrombosis

Postoperative pulmonary thromboembolism (PTE) from deep venous thrombosis (DVT) is an important cause of morbidity and mortality in orthopedic surgical patients (see Chapter 11). Various authors have identified decreased incidence of DVT and PTE in patients whose surgery was conducted under centroneuraxial anesthesia. This benefit was identified in populations undergoing total hip arthroplasty, total knee arthroplasty, and hip fracture repair.[6] The explanation for this reduction in DVT and PTE has not been clearly elucidated, but it may be related to rheologic changes resulting in improved peripheral blood flow.

ANESTHETIC TECHNIQUES BY SURGICAL SITE

Distal Upper Extremity

Patients undergoing arthroplastic procedures of the elbow, hand, or wrist are usually positioned supine on the operating table. The patient should be comfortable, with care taken to ensure padding of bony prominences, particularly at the knee and elbow, where nerve damage is most common. Standard monitors (blood pressure cuff, electrocardiogram, pulse oximeter) and intravenous access are located conveniently for the anesthesiologist and the surgeon.

Regional anesthetic techniques pursuant to this location include brachial plexus block (axillary, supraclavicular, and infraclavicular approaches), wrist block, and Bier (intravenous regional) block.

Brachial Plexus Block

AXILLARY BLOCK

Axillary brachial plexus block involves anesthetizing the nerves of the brachial plexus as they emerge from the axilla. This block is well suited to procedures on the forearm and hand but may spare the elbow region and is not indicated for procedures on the shoulder. The majority of the brachial plexus is contained within a multicompartmental sheath at the level of the axilla. The notable exception is the musculocutaneous nerve, which often leaves the sheath before the level of the axilla. This nerve is anesthetized by injecting local anesthetic into the body of the coracobrachial muscle at the level of the axillary fold or by subcutaneous injection in a fanlike distribution lateral to the biceps tendon as the nerve traverses the antecubital fossa. To ensure adequate analgesia when a tourniquet is to be used, the intercostobrachial nerve (a branch of T2) must also be anesthetized separately. This nerve travels anterior to

Table 12–2. PHARMACOLOGIC AND CLINICAL CHARACTERISTICS OF LOCAL ANESTHETICS

Characteristics	Procaine (Novocaine)	Chloroprocaine (Nesacaine)	Lidocine (Xylocaine)	Prilocaine (Citanest)	Mepivacaine (Carbocaine)	Bupivacaine (Marcaine)	Tetracaome (Pontocaine)	Etodpcaome (Duracaine)
Physicochemical								
Potency ratio[a]	1	2	3	3	3	15	15	15
Toxicity ratio[a]	1	0.75	1.5	1.5	2.0	10	12	10
Anesthetic index (1)	1	3	3	2	1.5	1.5	1.25	1.5
pH of plain solution	5–6.5	2.7–4	6.5	4.5	4.5	4.5–6	4.5–6.5	4.5
pKa	8.9	8.7	7.9	7.7	7.6	8.1	8.6	7.7
Clinical								
Latency	Moderate	Fast	Fast	Fast	Fast	Moderate	Very slow	Fast
Penetrance	Moderate	Marked	Marked	Marked	Moderate	Moderate	Poor	Moderate
Duration	Short	Very short	Intermediate	Intermediate	Intermediate	Long	Long	Long
Duration ratio[a]	1	0.75	1.5–2	1.75–2	2–2.5	6–8	6–8	5–8
Concentration of Solution (%)								
Local infiltration	0.5	0.5	0.25–0.5	0.25–0.5	0.25–0.5	0.125–0.25	0.1–0.15	0.15–0.2
Regional IV	1	1	0.5	0.5	0.5	0.125–0.25	0.1–0.15	0.15–0.2
Small nerve sympathetic block	1	1	0.5	0.5	0.5	0.25	0.25	0.25
Block of nerve or plexus	2	2	1–1.5	1–2	1–1.5	0.375–0.5	0.15–0.3	0.5–1
Extradural block								
Analgesia	1.5	1.5	1	1	1	0.25–0.375	0.2–0.4	0.5–1
Motor block	3	3	2	2	2	0.5–0.75	0.3–0.5	1–1.5
Maximum single dose (mg/kg)	15	15	7	8	7	3	2.5	4

[a]Procaine used as standard of reference = 1; ratios vary according to techniques of regional anesthesia used. Anesthetic index = potency ratio/toxicity ratio.
From Bonica J, Loeser J, Chapman CR, et al: Regional analgesia and local anesthetics. In The Management of Pain, 2nd ed. Philadelphia, Williams & Wilkins, 1990.

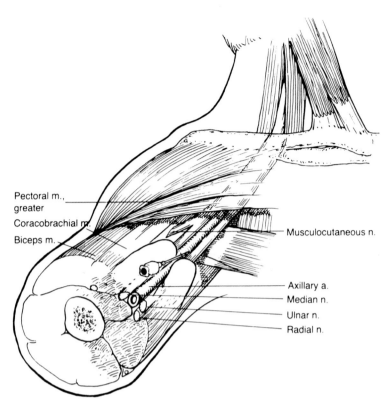

Pectoral m., greater

Coracobrachial m.

Biceps m.

Musculocutaneous n.

Axillary a.
Median n.
Ulnar n.
Radial n.

Figure 12–1. Axillary block. The arm is abducted at right angles to the body. Distal digital pressure is maintained during needle placement and injection of local anesthetic. (From Wedel DJ: Orthopedic Anesthesia. New York, Churchill Livingstone, 1993.)

the axillary sheath and is anesthetized by infiltrating local anesthetic over the pulsation of the axillary artery.

Complications of axillary blockade include intravascular injection, hematoma formation, persistent paresthesia, and infection. Frequent aspiration before injection reduces the risk of intravascular injection. The block should not be attempted if there is evidence of infection in the axilla. The axillary brachial plexus block has the advantage of being a reliable block that is safe and easy to perform (Fig. 12–1).[12]

SUPRACLAVICULAR BLOCK

The supraclavicular approach to the brachial plexus provides adequate analgesia for procedures on the elbow, forearm, and hand. With this technique, the trunks of the brachial plexus are approached at the level of the first rib. The classical method describes placing a needle superior to the midpoint of the clavicle and directing the tip caudally and slightly medially until a paresthesia is elicited or the first rib is contacted. The rib is usually encountered at a depth of 3 to 4 cm. This depth should not be exceeded, except in the obese patient, to avoid risk of pneumothorax. If the rib is encountered and no paresthesia has been obtained, the needle tip is walked along the rib anteriorly and posteriorly until a paresthesia is elicited. A nerve stimulator can also be used to identify the plexus. A second technique involves placing the needle at the intersection of the clavicle and the lateral insertion point of the sternocleidomastoid muscle. The needle tip is directed perpendicular to the skin or in a "plumb-bob" orientation, as demonstrated in Figure 12–2.[12] If a paresthesia is not

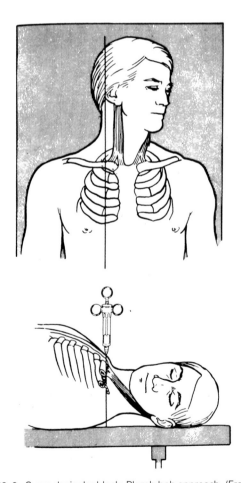

Figure 12–2. Supraclavicular block: Plumb-bob approach. (From Wedel DJ: Orthopedic Anesthesia. New York, Churchill Livingstone, 1993.)

elicited on the first pass, the needle tip is redirected slightly cephalad. This technique theoretically decreases the risk of pneumothorax and may be easier for some anesthesiologists to master.[12] To avoid intravascular injection, the needle should be aspirated to assess for the presence of blood before injection of the local anesthetic.

Pneumothorax occurs in 0.5 percent to 6 percent of patients, depending on the anesthesiologist's familiarity with the supraclavicular approach and the patient's anatomy. There may also be concurrent blockade of the recurrent laryngeal, phrenic, or cervical sympathetic nerves. When the supraclavicular approach is used, a lower dose of local anesthetic is required because of the compact structure of the brachial plexus at this level. Therefore, there is a reduced risk of side effects related to the local anesthetic.

INFRACLAVICULAR BLOCK

An alternative to the supraclavicular block for anesthesia of the elbow region is the infraclavicular approach to the brachial plexus. With this approach, the brachial plexus is anesthetized at a more proximal level than with the previously described axillary approach. This more proximal location affords a more reliable blockade of the axillary and musculocutaneous nerves. The approach to the brachial plexus is made at a point 2 cm below the midpoint of the clavicle, with the needle tip directed laterally and cephalad. The brachial plexus is identified by means of an insulated needle attached to a nerve stimulator. This device discharges low-amplitude electrical current, which, in the vicinity of a nerve, generates motor potentials that identify the nerve in proximity by characteristic muscle movement. The characteristic discharge of the brachial plexus is identified and maintained while the amplitude of current is

reduced, and the local anesthetic agent is instilled. Frequent aspiration is necessary to prevent inadvertent intravascular injection. There is a reduced risk of pneumothorax with this approach compared with the supraclavicular approach (Fig. 12–3).[8]

Wrist Block

The nerves that innervate the hand (i.e., median, radial, and ulnar) nerves can be anesthetized by the wrist block. The radial nerve is blocked by superficially infiltrating local anesthetic in a fanlike distribution at the base of the "anatomic snuffbox." The median nerve is blocked by injecting local anesthetic between the flexor carpi radialis and palmaris longus tendons at a point 2 cm proximal to the wrist crease. The ulnar nerve can be anesthetized by infiltration of local anesthetic on the radial side of the flexor carpi ulnaris tendon at the pisiform bone while the needle is directed medially (Fig. 12–4).[12] Because of the distal site of these blocks, a decreased amount of local anesthetic is needed, and there is a reduced risk of systemic toxicity with use of local anesthetic. The local anesthetic injected should not contain epinephrine because of the risk of impairing the peripheral circulation. A disadvantage of wrist blocks is that there is no provision for tourniquet analgesia.

Bier Block

The Bier block, or intravenous regional block, is highly useful for short surgical procedures on the upper extremity. A small-gauge intravenous catheter is inserted as distally as possible into the affected extremity. The patient's arm is then elevated and wrapped with an Esmarch bandage to exsanguinate the extremity. A

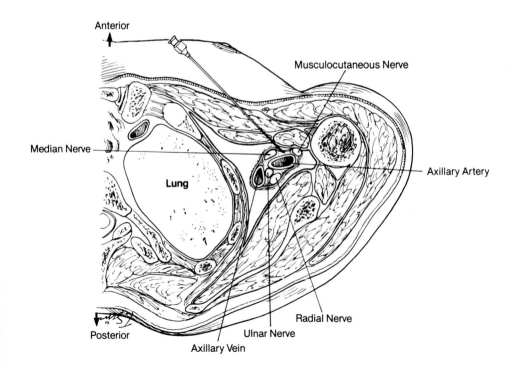

Figure 12–3. Infraclavicular approach to the brachial plexus, in transverse section of the axilla with its relations. The needle penetrates through the pectoralis major and minor before entering the brachial plexus sheath. Note the relationship of the neurovascular structures within the brachial plexus sheath. (From Raj PP, Pai V, Rawal N: Techniques of regional anesthesia in adults. *In* Raj PP [ed]: Clinical Practice of Regional Anesthesia. New York, Churchill Livingstone, 1991.)

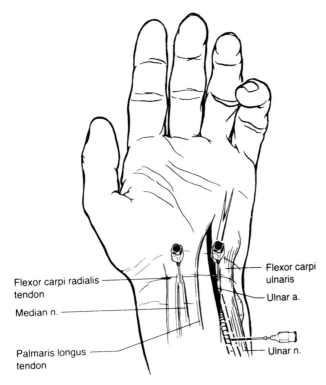

Figure 12–4. Anatomic landmarks for median and ulnar nerve block at the wrist are shown. (From Wedel DJ: Nerve blocks. *In* Miller RD [ed]: Anesthesia, 5th ed. New York, Churchill Livingstone, 1999.)

flated for at least 20 minutes after the injection. To decrease the potential for local anesthetic toxicity, the tourniquet may be deflated and inflated in 10-second cycles, resulting in delayed peak blood levels. It is imperative to have a reliable tourniquet for this procedure because premature tourniquet deflation may result in cardiovascular collapse caused by local anesthetic toxicity. The Bier block is highly useful for outpatient procedures because of the rapid onset and offset of anesthesia. However, because of the rapid offset time, provision for postoperative analgesia needs to be made shortly after the tourniquet is deflated.

Proximal Upper Extremity

In preparing the patient for shoulder surgery, specific concerns regarding positioning must be addressed. In many cases, the patient is positioned sitting upright in the "beach chair" position. This position allows anterior and posterior access to the shoulder joint and unobstructed rotation of the upper extremity. The patient is flexed at the hips and knees and placed in a slight Trendelenburg position that allows superior placement of the shoulder while elevation of the legs is maintained to improve venous return. After the table is positioned, the patient is moved laterally so that the shoulder to be repaired is free of the mattress. The hips and chest are secured to prevent further movement. The unoperated arm is positioned in the lap of the patient and secured. Padding is placed between the scapulae to elevate the shoulders. The head is then returned to a neutral position by elevation of the occiput. Next, the head is rotated away from the surgical site. Care must be taken to avoid excessive stretch on the brachial plexus during this maneuver. When the head is properly positioned, it is secured by straps at the chin and forehead to prevent lateral movement during surgery (Fig. 12–5).[13]

reliable double-cuff tourniquet is inflated to 100 mm Hg higher than the patient's systolic blood pressure. After cuff inflation, the Esmarch bandage is removed and local anesthetic is injected via the intravenous catheter. Half-percent lidocaine is the local anesthetic most commonly used because of its low risk of side effects. When surgery is complete, the tourniquet should not be de-

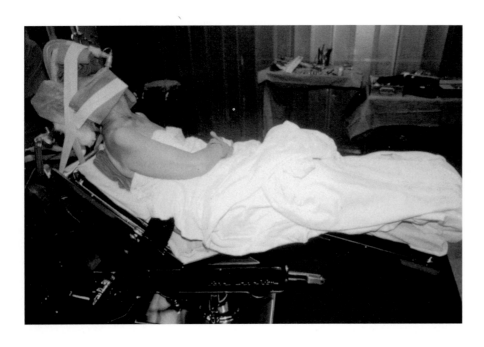

Figure 12–5. Lateral view of the upright shoulder position. (From Wedel DJ: Orthopedic Anesthesia. New York, Churchill Livingstone, 1993.)

Special Consideration: Venous Air Embolism

If the operative site is located 5 cm above the right atrium, there exists the theoretical possibility of entraining air into the systemic circulation via the surgical incision. When this occurs, the air may embolize to the pulmonary circulation, resulting in profound pulmonary vasoconstriction with ventilation-perfusion mismatch. If the volume of air entrained is significant, interstitial pulmonary edema and decreased cardiac output result from greatly elevated pulmonary vascular resistance and intracardiac outflow obstruction. Alternatively, air may paradoxically embolize to the cerebral or coronary circulation if a patent foramen ovale exists. Venous air embolism can be detected by mass spectrometry, precordial Doppler ultrasonography, and transesophageal echocardiography. On detection of an air embolism, attempts to prevent further air entrainment by flooding the surgical field and position change should be initiated to avoid cardiovascular collapse.

Interscalene Block

Surgical procedures on the shoulder can be completed under regional or general anesthesia. If general anesthesia is chosen, the interscalene brachial plexus block is useful for intraoperative and postoperative analgesia. If there is a high risk that brachial plexus injury may occur during the surgery (e.g., total shoulder arthroplasty), the block may be completed postoperatively after neurologic function has been assessed. The phrenic nerve is blocked on the ipsilateral side in 100 percent of patients receiving this block. For this reason, bilateral interscalene blocks are contraindicated, and this block is performed with caution in any patient with significant respiratory compromise. The block is performed with the patient positioned supine and with the head turned away from the side of the block. The interscalene groove is palpated at the level of the cricoid cartilage, which corresponds to the transverse process of C6. At this point, the needle is introduced perpendicular to the skin and directed caudad 45 degrees and slightly posterior. The brachial plexus is identified approximately 1 cm below the skin by elicitation of a paresthesia. If bone is encountered, the needle is walked anteriorly until the desired paresthesia is noted (Fig. 12–6).[12] Aspiration is done before injection because intravascular injection is a risk. Inadvertent injection into the vertebral artery can be catastrophic. This approach also carries a risk of anesthetizing the recurrent laryngeal nerve and the stellate ganglion and of injecting the epidural or subarachnoid space. Performance of the interscalene block is discouraged while patients are heavily sedated or under general anesthesia because there have been case reports of cervical spinal cord injury in four anesthetized patients after interscalene block.[13]

Hip

For patients undergoing hip surgery, the lateral decubitus position is often used to facilitate surgical exposure. Before positioning the patient, all necessary monitors should be in place. Appropriate intravenous access is obtained, and any other invasive monitoring devices indicated are placed with the patient supine. In transferring the patient from the supine to the lateral decubitus

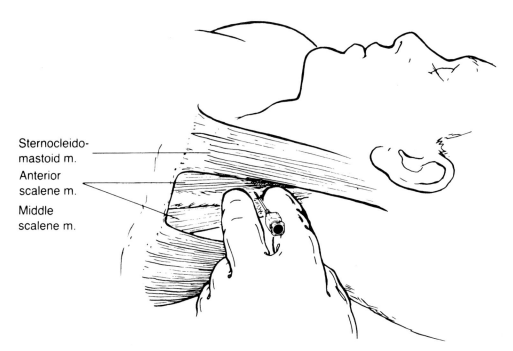

Sternocleido-mastoid m.

Anterior scalene m.

Middle scalene m.

Figure 12–6. Interscalene block. The fingers palpate the interscalene groove, and the needle is inserted with a caudad and slightly posterior angle. (From Wedel DJ: Nerve blocks. *In* Miller RD [ed]: Anesthesia, 5th ed. New York, Churchill Livingstone, 1999.)

position, care must be taken to maintain the head and shoulders in a neutral position. Ideally, one person is responsible for moving the legs, one the torso, one the shoulders, and one the head. The patient is supported in this position until secured with hip rests or other mechanical devices. The dependent arm is abducted and placed on a padded arm rest; a rolled towel is placed in the axilla to prevent compression of the brachial plexus and vascular structures. The upper arm is placed on a padded overarm board. With the patient properly positioned and padded, surgery may commence.

Regional anesthetic techniques are well suited to procedures involving the hip. Central neuraxial blockade, including spinal and epidural blockade, is commonly used. Addition of preservative-free narcotics to the local anesthetics used for these blocks provides excellent postoperative analgesia. Additionally, psoas compartment block can be used with a catheter for operative anesthesia or as a single shot for postoperative analgesia.

Central Neuraxial Block

Spinal anesthesia involves entering the subarachnoid space with a small-gauge needle and instilling small volumes of local anesthetics. The patient is blocked in the sitting position or in the lateral decubitus position. The lumbar spine is examined and an appropriate interspace is chosen below the level of the spinal cord. The skin site is prepared in a sterile fashion. After infiltration with local anesthetic, the spinal needle is introduced through the interspinous ligament until the characteristic change in resistance is noted as the needle tip passes through the ligamentum flavum and the dura. The stylet of the needle is removed to observe the flow of cerebrospinal fluid. The local anesthetic agent is then injected into the subarachnoid space. A dense sensory and motor block is established quickly. Adequate intravenous hydration before placement of the spinal block protects against a precipitous drop in blood pressure that can occur secondary to sympathetic blockade and peripheral vasodilatation. In any patient, there is a risk of postdural puncture headache, but this risk diminishes with increasing age and decreasing needle gauge. If the headache persists for 72 hours or is severe, postdural puncture headache can be effectively treated with placement of an epidural blood patch.

EPIDURAL ANESTHESIA

Epidural anesthesia involves introducing local anesthetic into the epidural space from where it then diffuses to the nerve roots and through the dura. At the nerve roots, the local anesthetic agents act to produce sensory and motor blockade. With the loss of resistance technique, an appropriate interspace is entered by a thin-walled 17- or 18-gauge needle that is advanced through the tissue planes until a characteristic increase in resistance is noted, representing penetration of the ligamentum flavum directly overlying the dura. At this point, the stylet is removed and a low-resistance glass syringe with a few milliliters of normal saline or air is attached

to the needle. The needle is advanced slowly, with constant pressure on the plunger of the syringe. While pressure is applied to the plunger of the syringe, a high resistance to the outflow of the saline or air is noted. Once the ligamentum flavum is passed, the resistance on the syringe is released, and the saline or air flows freely into the epidural space. With the needle tip located in the epidural space, the local anesthetic can be injected. Alternatively, a catheter can be inserted through the needle into the epidural space, allowing the anesthesiologist to provide prolonged surgical anesthesia and postoperative analgesia by redosing at intervals or maintaining a constant infusion.

Complications that may occur while epidural blockade is attempted include dural puncture, with increased risk of postdural puncture headache as a result of the large-gauge needle used. If a puncture of the dura is not identified, total spinal anesthesia with respiratory arrest may occur during subsequent administration of an epidural dose into the subarachnoid space. Intravascular injection can occur if the rich epidural venous plexus is entered with the needle tip or catheter. A test dose consisting of local anesthetic with epinephrine can identify intrathecal or intravascular injection before delivery of the full epidural dose.

Knee and Ankle

For knee arthroscopy or arthroplasty and ankle procedures, the supine position optimizes surgical conditions. Care must be taken to cushion the extremities and bony prominences. All standard monitoring devices are placed and intravenous access is obtained.

Regional anesthetic techniques that can be employed for surgical procedures on the knee include epidural and spinal anesthesia and various lower extremity blocks. Epidural and spinal anesthesia have been previously discussed in the section concerning hip surgery. Lower extremity blocks are increasingly being performed for a variety of operative procedures and for improving postoperative analgesia. To provide surgical anesthesia of the lower extremity using peripheral nerve blocks, each major nerve is blocked individually at separate locations. The exception to this is a block of the lumbar plexus that can anesthetize as many as three nerves at once. These blocks do offer the advantage of limiting symphathectomy to the extremity blocked. Also, if long-acting agents or indwelling catheters is used, significant postoperative analgesia can be provided. To provide complete surgical anesthesia for operative procedures on the knee, four nerves need to be blocked. These are the femoral, lateral femoral cutaneous, obturator, and sciatic nerves. Alternatively, general or central neuraxial anesthesia can be combined with psoas or femoral compartment block for analgesia.

Femoral Nerve Block

The femoral nerve innervates the anterior thigh muscles (quadriceps and sartorius) and provides sensation to the skin of the anterior thigh from the inguinal ligament to the knee and below the knee along the medial aspect of the lower leg to the big toe (saphenous nerve branch). The femoral nerve is blocked just below the level of the inguinal ligament lateral to the femoral artery. Location of the femoral nerve is confirmed by means of a nerve stimulator to elicit contraction of the quadriceps muscle identified by elevation of the patella, and local anesthetic is deposited at this site (Fig. 12–7).[12]

Lateral Femoral Cutaneous Nerve Block

The lateral femoral cutaneous nerve is divided into anterior and posterior branches after it emerges from the fascia lata. The anterior branch provides sensory innervation to the anterolateral thigh and down to the knee. The posterior branch supplies the skin of the lateral thigh from the hip to the midthigh. This nerve is included in the four-nerve block to provide relief of tourniquet pain. The lateral femoral cutaneous nerve can be anesthetized at a point 2 cm medial and 2 cm caudad to the anterior superior iliac spine. The needle introduced at this point is inserted to a depth between 1 and

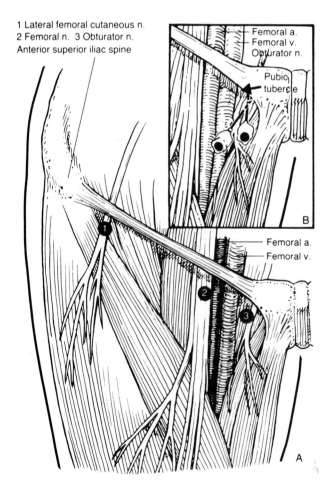

1 Lateral femoral cutaneous n.
2 Femoral n. 3 Obturator n.
Anterior superior iliac spine

Femoral a.
Femoral v.
Obturator n.

Pubic tubercle

Femoral a.
Femoral v.

B

A

Figure 12–7. A, Anatomic landmarks for the lateral femoral cutaneous, femoral, and obturator nerve blocks. **B,** Obturator nerve block. The needle is walked off the inferior pubic ramus in a lateral and caudad direction until it passes into the obturator canal. (From Wedel DJ: Nerve blocks. *In* Miller RD [ed]: Anesthesia, 5th ed. New York, Churchill Livingstone, 1999.)

3 cm or until the resistance of the fascia lata is passed. The local anesthetic solution is then infiltrated medially and laterally in a fanlike distribution both above and below the fascia.

Obturator Nerve Block

The obturator nerve bifurcates into anterior and posterior branches as it exits the obturator canal. The anterior segment provides an articular branch to the hip and innervates the anterior adductor muscles. There is a variable cutaneous branch to the lower medial thigh. The posterior segment innervates the deep adductor muscles with a variable articular branch to the knee. The obturator nerve is blocked as it emerges from the obturator canal. This block is accomplished by introducing the needle 1 to 2 cm laterally and 1 to 2 cm caudad to the pubic tubercle and advancing it 2 to 4 cm until the inferior pubic ramus is contacted. The needle tip is then walked laterally and caudad until it drops into the obturator canal. The local anesthetic is instilled after a negative aspiration is confirmed. All these peripheral blocks can be complicated by intravascular injection.

"3-in-1" Block

An alternative to these separate blocks is the 3-in-1 block. With this technique, the femoral nerve is approached in a manner similar to that previously described, with the needle directed cephalad. The needle tip passes under the inguinal ligament to introduce a moderate amount of local anesthetic into the sheath enveloping the lumbar plexus. The local anesthetic theoretically spreads in a cephalad direction to anesthetize the femoral, obturator, and lateral femoral cutaneous nerves. Complications are rare, but systemic local anesthetic toxicity can be associated with this approach because of the large volume of local anesthetic injected near major blood vessels. Evidence suggests that injection into the femoral nerve sheath does not reliably disperse injectate to the obturator nerve[9]; therefore, this block may be considered a "2-in-1" block. Additionally, a catheter may be placed during performance of this block for delivery of postoperative analgesia.

Psoas Compartment Block

The psoas compartment block is highly effective for postoperative analgesia after knee reconstructive surgery. Local anesthetic is deposited in proximity to the lumbar plexus in the psoas compartment, anterior to the transverse process of the L5 vertebra and posterior to the psoas muscle. The patient is placed in the lateral decubitus position, with the operative extremity uppermost. The line between the posterior superior iliac crests (Tuffier's line) is identified. The midpoint of this line corresponds to the L4 vertebra in most patients. A second line is identified 5 cm lateral and parallel to the vertebral column, and a point on this line 3 cm caudal to Tuffier's line is marked. At this site, a 22-gauge, 15-cm insulated needle is inserted and advanced until the transverse process of the L5 vertebra is contacted. The needle is then redirected cephalad until it passes the transverse process and enters the psoas compartment. The needle tip typically encounters the compartment at a depth of 12 cm plus or minus 2 cm and can be confirmed by use of a nerve stimulator to elicit a quadriceps twitch. At this time, a single injection of local anesthetic is given, or a continuous catheter is introduced. If anesthesia of the lower leg or posterior thigh is required, block of the sciatic nerve is also needed.

Sciatic Nerve Block

The sciatic nerve is the largest in the body, with a maximum width of 2 cm. It provides sensory innervation to the majority of the lower extremity, including the posterior thigh and the distal lower extremity, with the exception of a thin medial strip down to the great toe (an area innervated by the saphenous nerve). There are several techniques for blocking the sciatic nerve, including the classic approach of Labat (posterior), the anterior approach, and the lateral approach. With the classic approach of Labat, the patient is positioned laterally, with the leg to be blocked fully flexed and the ankle of the operative leg adjacent to the knee of the unoperated leg. The needle is introduced at the point indicated in Figure 12–8.[12] The needle is inserted until a paresthesia is noted or bone is contacted. If bone is contacted, the needle is walked medially and laterally until a paresthesia is noted. Alternatively, a nerve stimulator can be used to confirm proper needle placement. A moderate volume (25 to 30 ml) of local anesthetic is then injected.

The anterior approach involves blocking the sciatic nerve as it traverses below the lesser trochanter of the femur. A line is drawn from the anterior superior iliac spine to the pubic tubercle and divided in thirds. A second line is drawn parallel to this from the tuberosity of the greater trochanter. A perpendicular line dropped from the medial trisection point to the parallel line extending from the greater trochanter indicates the approximate position of the lesser trochanter (Fig. 12–9).[12] With this point noted, a needle is inserted and advanced approximately 5 cm until the lesser trochanter is encountered. The needle tip is then redirected medially until it walks off the lesser trochanter and is advanced about 5 cm until a paresthesia is elicited. After negative aspiration, the local anesthetic is injected.

Blocking the sciatic nerve leads to peripheral vasodilatation secondary to sympathetic blockade, which may be hemodynamically significant in compromised patients.

Ankle and Foot

For surgical procedures on the ankle and foot, the patient is positioned supine, with bony prominences padded as indicated. Standard monitoring devices are placed and intravenous access is obtained.

Regional anesthesia for ankle and foot surgery involves central neuraxial blockade, popliteal block, and peripheral nerve blocks at the ankle. Epidural and spinal anesthesia have been previously discussed in the section on the hip.

Popliteal Block

Popliteal block, or more accurately block of the sciatic nerve in the popliteal fossa, can be used intraoperatively

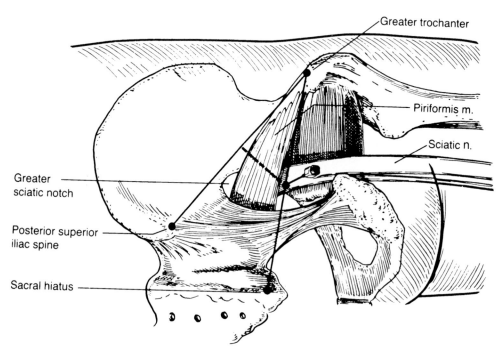

Figure 12–8. Anatomic landmarks for the posterior approach to the sciatic nerve block. (From Wedel DJ: Nerve blocks. *In* Miller RD [ed]: Anesthesia, 5th ed. New York, Churchill Livingstone, 1999.)

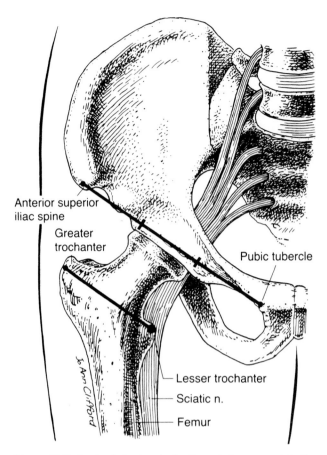

Figure 12–9. Anatomic landmarks for the anterior approach to the sciatic nerve block. (From Wedel DJ: Nerve blocks. *In* Miller RD [ed]: Anesthesia, 5th ed. New York, Churchill Livingstone, 1999.)

and is increasingly being used postoperatively. This block involves anesthetizing the sciatic nerve in the popliteal fossa, where it exists as the tibial and common peroneal nerves in the same sheath. The posterior approach can be performed with the patient in the prone, lateral, or supine (lithotomy) position. Needle insertion is performed 7 cm superior to the popliteal crease, at a point 1 cm lateral to a line that bisects the superior pole of the fossa. The needle is inserted at a 45-degree angle and advanced between 2.5 cm and 5 cm.

Alternatively, the popliteal block has more recently been described from a lateral[3] approach. This approach decreases the risk of intravascular injection because the vessels are positioned posterior and medial to the nerves and needle insertion site. With the patient in the supine position, the knee is extended and the foot flexed at 90 degrees. The needle is inserted at the point where a line extended from the upper pole of the patella intersects the groove between the biceps femoris tendon and the iliotibial tract. After skin puncture, the needle tip is directed 20 to 30 degrees posterior to the horizontal plane, with a slight caudad direction. Needle placement may be confirmed by use of a nerve stimulator. If anesthesia of the medial part of the ankle is required with any of these approaches to the popliteal fossa, a saphenous nerve block should also be performed.

Peripheral Nerve Blocks at the Ankle

The foot is innervated by the femoral nerve via the saphenous nerve and by the sciatic nerve via the posterior tibial, sural, and deep and superficial peroneal nerves (Figs. 12–10 and 12–11).[12] The posterior tibial nerve provides sensory innervation to the heel, sole, and plantar aspect of the toes and provides some motor innervation to the foot. This nerve is anesthetized by palpating the tibial artery at the level of the medial malleolus and inserting the needle posterior to this point. The needle is then directed toward the posterior aspect of the tibia and local anesthetic is instilled (see Fig. 12–10**B**).[12]

The sural nerve innervates the lateral aspect of the foot and little toe. This nerve can be anesthetized as it courses superficially between the lateral malleolus and the Achilles tendon. The needle is inserted lateral to the malleolus, and local anesthetic is infiltrated as the needle tip is advanced toward the Achilles tendon (see Fig. 12–10**C**).[12]

The deep peroneal nerve innervates the skin between the first and second toes and the short extensors of the toes. This nerve lies next to the anterior tibial artery between the tendons of the anterior tibial and hallucis longus muscles. Local anesthetic is infiltrated at this point. The superficial peroneal and saphenous nerves are anesthetized by infiltration of local anesthetic laterally and medially from the point where the deep peroneal nerve is anesthetized. The saphenous nerve innervates a strip along the medial aspect of the foot. The superficial peroneal nerve innervates the dorsum of the foot with the exception of the interdigital region of the first and second toes (see Fig. 12–11).[12] Secondary to

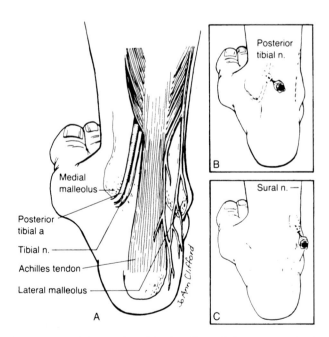

Figure 12–10. A, Innervation of the foot. **B** and **C,** Anatomic landmarks for the block of the posterior tibial (**B**) and sural (**C**) nerves. (From Wedel DJ: Nerve blocks. *In* Miller RD [ed]: Anesthesia, 5th ed. New York, Churchill Livingstone, 1999.)

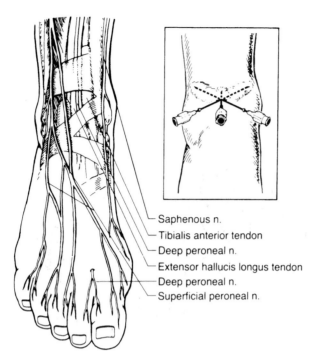

— Saphenous n.
— Tibialis anterior tendon
— Deep peroneal n.
— Extensor hallucis longus tendon
— Deep peroneal n.
— Superficial peroneal n.

Figure 12–11. Anatomic landmarks for the block of the deep peroneal, superficial peroneal, and saphenous nerves. (From Wedel DJ: Nerve blocks. *In* Miller RD [ed]: Anesthesia, 5th ed. New York, Churchill Livingstone, 1999.)

the peripheral site of these nerve blocks, epinephrine should not be included in the local anesthetic solution.

POSTOPERATIVE PAIN MANAGEMENT

Preemptive Analgesia

The anesthesiologist's role in patient care extends into the postoperative period with the provision of postoperative analgesia. Studies have suggested that preemptive analgesia may improve postoperative recovery and decrease morbidity. For this reason, intraoperative care emphasizes decreasing noxious stimuli by using either neural blockade or administration of adequate analgesics. Advances in techniques and equipment for performing continuous blocks are exciting. For this reason, regional anesthesia is gaining new importance as it relates to patient recovery and postoperative analgesia.

Patient-Controlled Analgesia

Patient-controlled analgesia (PCA) allows the patient to self-administer analgesics at the intervals required. The pump can be programmed and prevents the patient from receiving excessive amounts of pain medications. After an effective blood level of the analgesic is obtained, the patient can receive additional boluses as needed. Bolus doses are given on demand and followed by a predetermined lockout interval before the next

dose can be given. Patients are also limited to a maximal dose of medication per unit time, usually 4 hours. Patient satisfaction with PCA analgesia is higher than with standard analgesic administration. However, it must be remembered that PCA dosing is based on the assumption that patients have already attained adequate blood levels of analgesics and further dosing is used to maintain that therapeutic level. PCA technology can also be applied to continuous nerve blocks. Patients can self-administer local anesthetic and narcotic solutions via indwelling catheters by using PCA pumps. Outpatients can be discharged with spring-loaded syringes that continuously deliver analgesics without the need for a highly technical pump.

Continuous Central Neuraxial Analgesia

Epidural and spinal forms of anesthesia have been previously discussed in this chapter. Before the needle used to perform these blocks is withdrawn, a catheter can be inserted through the needle. The catheter can then be used for redosing intraoperatively and for postoperative analgesia. The use of an intrathecal catheter has not been shown to increase the risk of postdural puncture headache. Dilute local anesthetics, narcotics, or a combination of both may be used for postoperative pain management. Patients placed in passive range-of-motion devices postoperatively require more substantial levels of analgesia than do those who remain immobile. The synergistic effect of local anesthetics combined with narcotics may be beneficial in these patients. The density of the sensory block established by the local anesthetic must be monitored carefully. To avoid neurologic injury, patients must be able to distinguish excessive pressure at bony prominences. The use of dilute local anesthetics results in sympathectomy with vasodilatation and improved peripheral blood flow without excessive sensory blockade. As mentioned under the topic of PCA analgesia, central neuraxial analgesia can be provided in this manner.

Continuous Peripheral Nerve Analgesia

The principles of brachial plexus anesthesia have been previously discussed in this chapter. When the brachial plexus is blocked by use of the axillary and infraclavicular approaches, a catheter can be placed through the needle used to anesthetize the plexus. Because of the predictable location and compact size of the plexus, a catheter can be used to instill local anesthetics, providing postoperative analgesia and sympathectomy. Brachial plexus catheters have been used to augment peripheral blood flow, which promotes digit salvage and improves results of skin grafting. Dilute solutions of local anesthetic, such as 0.125 percent bupivicaine, can be used to provide sympathectomy and sensory blockade. Motor function remains intact, allowing physical therapy and early mobility. Additionally, catheters can be placed in proximity to individual nerves as the surgeon directly views them.

More recently described are continuous blocks of the lower extremity.[10] Although a convenient single location for catheter placement does not exist as in the upper extremity, continuous catheter techniques have been described for the lower extremity. Continuous psoas compartment, popliteal sciatic, and femoral nerve blocks are reliable and safe to perform; moreover, they provide excellent alternatives to standard postoperative analgesia. Catheters are inserted at these sites over the nerve stimulator needle. The catheters can then be used for prolonged analgesia postoperatively. The PCA technique can be used with these catheters to improve postoperative analgesia and level of patient satisfaction.

Intra-Articular Injections

Intra-articular local anesthetics can be used during arthroscopic procedures along with local infiltration to provide surgical anesthesia. These agents can be injected into the articular space before surgery or added to the irrigation solution. Longer-acting local anesthetic agents can provide postoperative pain relief, as can narcotic and nonsteroidal agents injected at the end of the procedure.

SPECIAL CONSIDERATIONS

Low Molecular Weight Heparin

With the advent of thromboembolism prophylaxis that uses low molecular weight heparin (LMWH) preparations, evidence of increased frequency of clinically significant epidural hematoma was noted in patients who received neuraxial anesthesia and analgesia. Therefore, guidelines have been established regarding the use of neuraxial blockade in patients who take these medications. Patients who have taken LMWH preoperatively must not receive a neuraxial anesthetic until 10 to 12 hours after they have taken their heparin dose. Patients who are to receive postoperative LMWH should receive their initial dose no earlier than 24 hours postoperatively. If an epidural catheter is provided for postoperative analgesia, it should be removed 2 hours before a dose is administered. If the catheter remains in place during LMWH administration, it should not be removed until 10 to 12 hours after a dose of LMWH. These guidelines were established to minimize the risk of neuraxial bleeding in patients receiving LMWH.

Malignant Hyperthermia

Malignant hyperthermia is a hypermetabolic disorder of skeletal muscle that is triggered by specific anesthetic agents. This syndrome is caused by a massive flux of calcium in skeletal muscle and is characterized by hyperthermia, muscle rigidity, and metabolic and respiratory acidosis. It is inherited as an autosomal dominant trait with variable penetration. Preoperative evaluation for a

family history of malignant hyperthermia can be helpful, but intraoperative monitoring for early signs of the syndrome (hypercarbia, tachycardia, and acidosis) is of the utmost importance. Triggering agents include the volatile anesthetic agents (halothane, isoflurane, enflurane, and desflurane) and the depolarizing muscle relaxant (succinylcholine). The patient who has been triggered into malignant hyperthermia must be cooled and the hypermetabolism must be regulated, but the integral component of therapy is administration of dantrolene sodium, 2 to 10 mg/kg. For the patient with a history of malignant hyperthermia, a regional technique or a nontriggering general anesthetic is used.

Methyl Methacrylate

Methyl methacrylate is an acrylic bone cement used during arthroplastic procedures. Insertion of this cement is associated with sudden onset of hypotension in some patients. This hypotension has been attributed to absorption of the volatile monomer of methyl methacrylate, embolization of air and bone marrow during reaming, lysis of blood cells and marrow induced by the exothermic reaction, and conversion of methyl methacrylate to methacrylic acid. Adequate hydration and maximization of the inspired oxygen concentration minimize the hypotension and hypoxemia that can follow cementing. Vigilance on the part of the anesthesiologist is of particular importance during this portion of the procedure.

Outpatient Anesthesia

Outpatient surgery represents a large and ever-increasing portion of orthopedic procedures. General and regional anesthetics are safe and effective for outpatient surgical procedures. Regional anesthetics are associated with shorter discharge times and excellent postoperative analgesia. Shorter-acting general anesthetic agents are being introduced, which have resulted in shortened discharge times after general anesthesia. In order to be discharged, patients must be able to care for themselves and not have excessive nausea, vomiting, or pain. Postoperative pain was found to be the most common reason for unplanned hospital admission in the postoperative orthopedic patient. Narcotics can exacerbate nausea and vomiting. This fact underscores the importance of controlling pain in the early postoperative period. To this end, regional anesthetic techniques, including continuous catheter administration of local anesthetics, are rapidly gaining popularity in the outpatient setting.

SUMMARY

Patients undergoing joint replacement require careful evaluation before surgery. Pre-existing medical conditions and their treatment can influence anesthetic management. Arthroplastic and arthroscopic procedures often lend themselves to regional anesthetic techniques. Postoperative pain control and pre-emptive analgesia can greatly influence the patient's postoperative course and are areas of active research and debate. Finally, as advances are made in anesthetic techniques and equipment, patient care, safety, and satisfaction will continue to improve.

References

1. Benumof JL: Permanent loss of cervical spinal cord function associated with interscalene block performed under general anesthesia. Anesthesiology 93:6, 2000.
2. Bonica J, Loeser J, Chapman CR, et al: Regional analgesia and local anesthesia. *In* The Management of Pain, 2nd ed. Philadelphia, Williams & Wilkins, 1990.
3. Bouaziz H, Narchi P, Zetlaoui P, et al: Lateral approach to the sciatic nerve at the popliteal fossa combined with saphenous nerve block. Tech Reg Anesth Pain Manage 3:19, 1999.
4. Brown DL, Bridenbaugh LD: Physics applied to regional anesthesia results in an improved supraclavicular block: The "plumb-bob" technique. Anesthesiology 69A:376, 1988.
5. Chernow B, Alexander HR, Smallridge RC, et al: Hormonal responses to graded surgical stress. Arch Intern Med 147:1273, 1987.
6. Keith I: Anesthesia and blood loss in total hip replacement. Anesthesia 32:444, 1997.
7. Modig J, Borg T, Earlstrom G, et al: Thromboembolism after total hip replacement: Role of general and epidural anesthesia. Anesth Analg 62:174, 1983.
8. Raj PP, Pai V, Rawal N: Techniques of regional anesthesia in adults. *In* Raj PP (ed): Clinical Practice of Regional Anesthesia. New York, Churchill Livingstone, 1991, p 271.
9. Ritter JW: Femoral nerve "sheath" for inguinal perivascular lumbar plexus block is not found in human cadavers. J Clin Anesth 7:470, 1995.
10. Singelyn FJE: Continuous femoral and popliteal sciatic nerve blockades. Tech Reg Anesth Pain Manage 2:90, 1988.
11. Tarhan S, Moffitt EA, Taylor WF, et al: Myocardial infarction after general anesthesia. JAMA 220:1451, 1972.
12. Wedel DJ: Nerve blocks. *In* Miller RD (ed): Anesthesia, 5th ed. New York, Churchill Livingstone, 1999.

13

Perioperative Mortality Associated with Hip and Knee Arthroplasty

• DAVID G. LEWALLEN, JAVAD PARVIZI, and MARK H. ERETH

Without question, the most devastating complication of total joint arthroplasty is death. The stress of a major operative procedure, blood loss, and anesthesia unavoidably subject patients to low-level risks of morbidity and mortality, but questions continue to be raised about the possible compounding effects of certain unique events observed at the time of arthroplasty.[16,17] In the early 1970s, reports of sudden intraoperative cardiovascular collapse and death associated with the cementation of hip implants were well known.[7,8,19,26,45,49] Potential etiologic factors include direct toxic effects of the methyl methacrylate monomer; peripheral vasodilatation, myocardial depression, activation of thrombosis and fibrinolysis in the lung; and embolism of air, fat, and the other intramedullary contents of bone.[51] The fat and marrow debris found within the pulmonary vasculature at autopsy in these early cases has been implicated in the initiation of the lethal physiologic response, but the fact that these same changes in the lungs are often seen after standard cardiopulmonary resuscitation also casts some doubt on this conclusion.[27] Subsequent investigations over the past two decades have centered around defining what occurs during placement of prosthetic implants for the average patient and understanding when, why, and in whom these physiologic changes are significant as causes of perioperative morbidity and mortality. Reports of fat embolism syndrome, neurologic compromise, and even sudden death associated with total knee arthroplasty have brought that procedure under scrutiny as well.[11,31,35]

HISTORICAL PERSPECTIVE

The initial case reports of sudden death during total hip arthroplasty did little to clarify the incidence or cause of this rare but catastrophic problem. However, numerous reports of the typically sudden dramatic temporal association of sudden death with the act of cementation of one of the hip components seemed to implicate this event. These early reports also made note of transient mild episodes of hypotension in one third or more of patients during surgery.[5,22] It is likely that these brief, benign hypotensive events represent one part of the spectrum of possible responses, which extends to cardiovascular collapse and, in some cases, death. These early reports also recognized the relationship between hip fracture prompting arthroplasty and the occurrence of fat embolism and sudden death.[8,19,49]

Duncan[13] reported mortality in 6 of 52 patients who had cemented endoprostheses inserted for subcapital fracture of the hip, a rate of 11.5 percent. Two additional patients recovered from severe bradycardia and hypotension that occurred within minutes of cementation of the femoral component. All those who died were elderly (between 70 and 86 years of age) and all had preoperative anesthesia risk assessed as grade III or IV by the American Society of Anesthesiologists. Because of this experience, we changed our implant selection to an uncemented bipolar device.

In a more recent prospective randomized study of patients with displaced subcapital fractures of the hip, which was designed to compare an uncemented endoprosthesis with a cemented bipolar device, the occurrence of two intraoperative deaths in the cemented group caused the investigators to abandon their protocol and revert to use of an uncemented endoprosthesis for all such patients.[29]

Patterson et al. reported seven patients who experienced cardiac arrest (four of whom died) as a result of arthroplasty with a cemented long-stemmed femoral component. Although the authors of this article concluded that use of a long-stemmed cemented device carried substantial risk, the fact not emphasized was that all seven patients had a fracture-related problem of some type involving the femur, two of which were associated with metastatic disease.[43]

Past reports of mortality related to total knee arthroplasty have been even more sporadic than those associated with THA and have largely been limited to isolated case reports.[31,35,37,52,54]

Incidence of Perioperative Mortality Associated with Hip Arthroplasty

One of the earliest efforts to obtain information on the incidence of mortality associated with hip arthroplasty was by Holiday et al., who undertook a review of the first 20 years of experience with hip arthroplasty at Mayo Clinic and reported on all instances of intraoperative death. A total of 19 deaths in 21,895 procedures occurred during surgery between 1969 and 1988. Those who died were predominantly female, elderly (mean age 82.6 years). Death resulted from sudden onslaught of hypotension and arrhythmia that at the time of insertion of a cemented component. Eighteen of the 19 deaths occurred in individuals with a history of prior cardiovascular disease, and 16 of the 19 patients underwent surgery for a fracture-related diagnosis. In fact, for patients undergoing arthroplasty for a fracture-related diagnosis in this review, the risk was nearly 1 percent (16 in 1690). This stands in marked contrast to the incidence seen in those undergoing elective arthroplasty for a non–fracture-related diagnosis with a risk of sudden death during surgery of only 0.015 percent (3 in 20,205) (P<.001). Those patients undergoing cemented arthroplasty for treatment of an intertrochanteric fracture had an intraoperative mortality rate of 3.3 percent (8 in 200) in this initial experience at that institution (P<.001).

From this initial review by Holiday et al., the profile of the patient most often affected by sudden intraoperative death was determined to be that of an elderly female with preexisting cardiovascular disease undergoing a cemented arthroplasty for treatment of a fracture-related problem.[24] In addition, based on the study by Patterson et al., the use of cemented long-stemmed femoral components was recognized as a potential risk factor when used in elderly arthroplasty patients, especially if associated with a pathologic process or hip fracture problem.[43]

Parvizi et al. have recently updated the 28-year Mayo experience and provided a longer-term, more comprehensive review from 1969 to 1997.[39] There was a total of 23 intraoperative deaths in 38,488 hip arthroplasties, an overall incidence of 0.06 percent. All deaths occurred during cemented primary arthroplasties. No intraoperative deaths occurred during any uncemented primary procedure or during any of the 8608 revision arthroplasties preformed over this time (P< .05). The incidence of intraoperative death during primary total hip arthroplasty is shown in Table 13–1. A significant fall in intraoperative mortality occurred over time during the years under study, with a 3.5-fold decrease from 0.087 percent between 1969 and 1988 to 0.024 percent between 1988 and 1997. This fall in mortality over time was related to improvements in medical management, improved anesthesia care, and methods to reduce the likelihood of venous embolization.

Thus, for the majority of patients, elective total hip surgery is not only effective but also extremely safe. Dearborn and Harris reported on 8 deaths out of 2736 patients (0.29 percent) occurring within 90 days of an elective hip arthroplasty.[9] More recently, Pedersen et al.

Table 13–1. MORTALITY AFTER 38,488 PRIMARY HIP REPLACEMENTS, MAYO EXPERIENCE, 1969–1997

	No. Deaths/Procedures	Percent
All Replacements	23/38,488	.06
Hemi	12/7,214	.17
Total	11/23,666	.05
Diagnosis		
Nonfracture	5/19,655	.03*
Fracture	18/10,245	.18
Neck	7/34,534	.2
Intertroch	11/706	1.6
Pathologic	3/70	4.3

*Statistically significant.

reported on another single surgeon's series that spanned 26 years, noting that by 90 days after surgery, there was an incidence of death of 0.98 percent in the 4967 hip arthroplasties performed.

Another review of 30-day mortality after hip arthroplasty at Mayo Clinic was undertaken to determine the patient and surgical factors that might increase the likelihood of death.[40] Thirty-day mortality data were compiled for 30,714 consecutive patients who underwent elective hip arthroplasty between 1969 and 1997. The patients who were undergoing arthroplasty for a fracture diagnosis were excluded. There were 90 deaths within 30 days of elective hip arthroplasty, yielding an overall mortality rate of 0.29 percent (90 in 30,714). Thirty-day mortality was significantly higher for patients with preexisting cardiovascular disease (P<0.0001), male patients (P<0.0001), and elderly patients (70 years of age or older) (P<0.0002). There was no difference in incidence of 30-day mortality for revision versus primary hip arthroplasty, cemented versus uncemented implants, or rheumatoid arthritis versus osteoarthritis. A significant decline in the incidence of 30-day mortality after elective hip arthroplasty was noted during the decade of the 1990s (P<0.0002), with a fall in overall mortality to 0.15 percent (23 in 14,989).

An additional analysis of the 28-year Mayo experience with 30-day perioperative mortality was compiled for those undergoing surgery for fracture.[41] Between 1969 and 1997, 7316 consecutive fracture patients undergoing hip arthroplasty were reviewed. The 30-day mortality incidence was 2.54 percent (186 in 7316). Mortality at 4.7 percent was significantly higher for patients who had received a cemented implant (143 in 3038) than for the 1 percent (43 in 4278) seen in those who had received an uncemented implant (P<0.0001). Thus, factors associated with increased incidence of mortality in this study were a cemented prosthesis, older age, diagnosis of intertrochanteric fracture, underlying malignancy, and history of prior cardiorespiratory disease.

Perioperative Mortality Associated with Total Knee Arthroplasty

Total knee arthroplasty is generally considered quite safe, with a very low perceived incidence of perioperative death resulting from the procedure. Previous reports of perioperative mortality associated with total knee arthroplasty are mainly in the form of case reports.[31,35,52,54] The precise incidence of perioperative mortality associated with total knee arthroplasty and risk factors associated with death are not clear. Fat embolization as a result of intramedullary instrumentation and pressurization has been implicated in hemodynamic instability, neurologic compromise, and sudden intraoperative death.[9,31,37] Changes in operative technique have been suggested, such as over-drilling of the femoral entry hole, suction of the medullary contents, use of fluted or cannulated rods within the canal, canal irrigation, slow insertion of intramedullary guides, and avoidance of intramedullary instrumentation in both femora and both tibial canals.[18,48,53]

The Mayo experience with 22,540 consecutive total knee arthroplasties from 1969 to 1997 was reviewed. The overall incidence of 30-day mortality was 0.2 percent (47 in 22,540)[42] (Table 13–2). All four of the patients who died subsequent to revision surgery received cemented long-stemmed implants. A history of prior cardiovascular pulmonary disease was present in 43 of 47 patients who died. Simultaneous bilateral total knee arthroplasty performed under the same anesthetic was associated with a significantly higher incidence of perioperative death ($P<0.002$). This study documented a significantly increased mortality after knee arthroplasty for patients 70 years of age or older, and for those with prior history of cardiovascular disease, primary versus revision knee surgery, use of a cemented prosthesis, and simultaneous bilateral knee arthroplasty.[42]

Potential Pathophysiologic Mechanisms for Increased Perioperative Mortality

Methyl Methacrylate Toxicity

Questions regarding the potential for direct toxic effects from the cement, especially the liquid monomer methyl methacrylate, were investigated in detail during the years soon after the introduction of total hip arthroplasty. Charnley,[5] in his classic text on acrylic cement, devotes a chapter to the systemic effects of monomers and notes that the evidence up to that time suggested low toxicity, with effects on the respiratory system rather than on the heart muscle and with requirements for large masses (1 lb or more) implanted in a liquid state in order to be lethal. Previous animal work by Charnley defined a lethal intravenous dose of 1.25 to 2.0 ml/kg in humans.[5] McLaughlin et al. performed a series of experiments on dogs, using a radiolabeled methacrylate monomer. Intravenous administration of monomer was also studied. Blood clearance by the lungs was noted to occur very rapidly, with decreased pulmonary function only when dosages of monomer were 35 times the amount liberated clinically during arthroplasty in humans.[33]

Modig et al., in a study of patients undergoing total hip arthroplasty, found that the release of tissue-thromboplastic products into the pulmonary circulation correlated with reduction of blood pressure and arterial oxygen saturation, which were measured after insertion of the femoral component. The pulmonary embolization of fat droplets and release of acrylic monomer measured in the blood seemed to be of little importance.[34]

Evidence suggests that cement is not a necessary prerequisite for these episodes. Studies have documented the embolic debris produced during reaming and intramedullary rodding of femoral and tibial fractures.[44] Any bone reaming, pressurization, or instrumentation can produce significant embolization of fat and marrow contents (Fig. 13–1). Sudden death has been reported during primary total knee arthroplasty after cementation of long-stemmed designs, both at the time of cementation and also after release of the tourniquet.[4,10,37] Fat embolization has also occurred during femoral reaming during revision total knee arthroplasty.[21] Significant reductions in oxygen saturation and end-tidal carbon dioxide tension have even been reported after insertion of the alignment rod into the femoral canal; these changes were eliminated by overdrilling the entry hole by 4.7 mm.[18,47]

Based on these and similar studies, attention has turned away from the direct effect of the monomer and cement. The focus is now on the materials released and embolized to the lungs as a result of preparation and pressurization of the bone and on the ensuing pulmonary response.

PULMONARY EMBOLIZATION OF MEDULLARY CONTENTS

Embolization of fat and other marrow elements during hip arthroplasty has been well documented. Several methods of investigation have been described, including examination of venous blood samples drawn proximal to the hip, histologic study of lung tissue from experimental animals, and use of an ultrasound probe placed over the femoral vein during surgery.[12,23,36]

Direct visualization of emboli as they pass through the chambers of the heart has been accomplished using transesophageal echocardiography[12,16] (Fig. 13–2). In a prospective study of 35 arthroplasty patients (19 cemented and 16 uncemented), venous embolization was observed as a result of surgery in all the patients studied but was significantly greater in the cemented patients. Increases in embolic material with reduction of the hip are likely caused by release of material "stored" within the compressed femoral vein while the leg was rotated into the dislocated position (Fig. 13–3).

Table 13–2. MORTALITY AFTER 22,540 PRIMARY KNEE REPLACEMENTS, MAYO EXPERIENCE, 1969–1999

	No. Deaths/Procedures	Percent
Overall	47/22,540	.2
Cemented	48/18,810	.2
Uncemented	0/3,730	0 (*P*<.001)
Primary	43/18,165	.24
Revision	4/4,375	.09 (*P*<.0003)

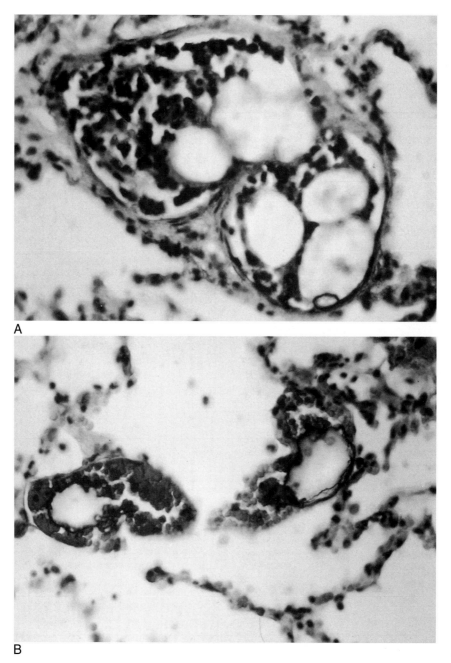

Figure 13–1. A, Histologic section from the lung of a patient who died during cementation of hip components showing marrow and fat in the pulmonary vasculature. **B**, Section of lung tissue showing apparent methyl methacrylate in pulmonary arteriole.

Although peak embolization was observed at the time of femoral stem insertion, significant amounts of echogenic material were also generated during acetabular preparation and cementation.[16] This is of some interest when considering the reports of two deaths during acetabular preparation from vascular collapse.[24]

One study has shown that similar echogenic material can be clinically viewed in humans at the time of tourniquet deflation during total knee arthroplasty.[38] Embolic material has also been demonstrated during femoral and tibial reaming before insertion of an intramedullary nail, and has been suggested as a possible cause of pulmonary insufficiency and a potential contributor to

the development of adult respiratory distress syndrome.[44] Venous embolization of intramedullary contents occurs when there is increased intramedullary pressure. Cemented total hip arthroplasty produces intramedullary pressures that can range as high as 575 mm Hg.[2,25,28]

Using a canine model, Orsini et al. compared a cemented femoral implant with an uncemented one and with a femoral implant inserted with bone wax. In a canine study, the number of fat emboli detected on histologic section of the lungs correlated with the pressures produced. Significant cardiorespiratory changes were observed in both the cemented and bone wax groups but not in the uncemented group. These changes

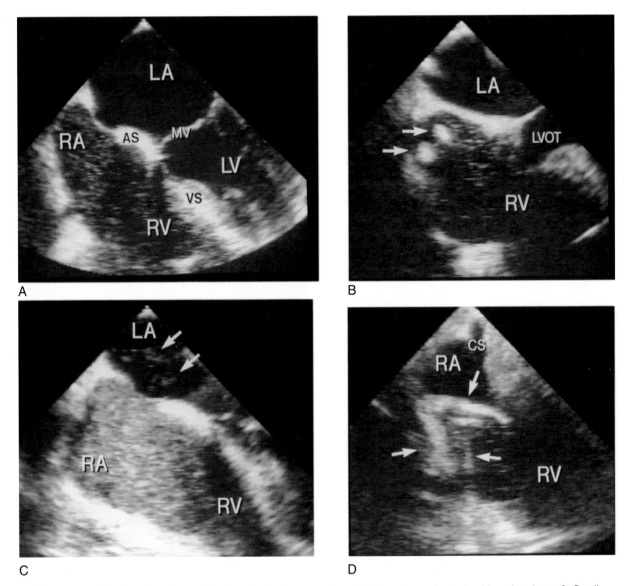

Figure 13–2. Four-chamber views of the heart using transesophageal echocardiography during hip arthroplasty. **A**, Small emboli in right atrium (RA) and right ventricle (RV). **B**, Small and medium-sized emboli in the right atrium (*arrows*). **C**, A large quantity of small emboli filling the entire right atrium with paradoxical emboli visible in the left atrium (LA) (*arrows*). **D**, Emboli over 10 mm in size (*arrows*). (From Ereth MH, WeberJG, Abel MD, et al: Cemented versus noncemented total hip arthroplasty: Embolism, hemodynamics, and intrapulmonary shunting. Mayo Clin Proc 67:1066, 1992.)

included decreased arterial oxygen tension, increased pulmonary arterial pressure, and increased intrapulmonary shunt fraction.[36]

It is apparent that embolization of echogenic material, which is probably a combination of fat, marrow elements, air, and bony debris, occurs to varying degrees during both cemented and uncemented (Fig. 13–4) hip arthroplasties. Factors that increase the amount of embolic material include higher pressures within the canal; use of cement, because this is a highly effective means of pressurizing the bone; and, possibly, poor cleaning of the medullary canal before implant or cement placement (Fig. 13–5). What is not clear is what is the key constituent or constituents responsible for causing severe hypotension and death. However, it seems unlikely that cement monomer plays any significant direct role. Information is accumulating regarding the

pulmonary activation of thrombosis, fibrinolysis, and release of inflammatory mediators such as the kallikrein, kininogen, and cytokine systems, but the exact cascade of events is still unclear.[16] What is especially perplexing is why the vast majority of patients tolerate this embolic insult without problems, whereas a few others are profoundly affected. A better understanding of the pathophysiology of this response in the future should assist physicians preventing or treating this problem.

PARADOXICAL EMBOLIZATION DURING HIP ARTHROPLASTY

Paradoxical embolization from the right side of the heart to the left-sided systemic circulation via a patent foramen ovale during hip arthroplasty[16,46] has been

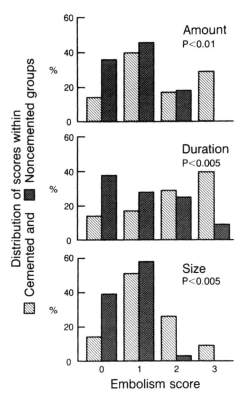

Figure 13–3. Distribution of embolism scores in the right atrium during the first minute after femoral stem insertion as determined by transesophageal echocardiographic analysis. (From Ereth MH, Weber JG, Abel MD, et al: Cemented versus noncemented total hip arthroplasty: Embolism, hemodynamics, and intrapulmonary shunting. Mayo Clin Proc 67:1066, 1992.)

hypothesized as potentially of clinical significance. Embolic debris can be seen flowing from the right atrium to the left atrium during hip arthroplasty when paradoxical embolization occurs (see Fig. 13–2C). A computed tomography (CT) scan can be of help in demonstrating areas of paradoxical cerebral embolization (Fig. 13–6). However, data suggest that both magnetic resonance imaging and single-photon emission CT scanning appear to be more sensitive than CT scan in detecting areas of hypoperfusion or infarction.[15]

A probe-patent foramen ovale is not uncommon and is present as an anatomic variant in 25 percent of patients examined at autopsy.[20] Hence, the potential for paradoxical embolization during surgery exists for an estimated 5 percent to 10 percent of the adult population.[1,6] There is likely to be a spectrum of neurologic dysfunction ranging from undetectable to profound produced by any paradoxical embolization that occurs relative to the amount, size, and ultimate localization of entrapped cerebral emboli.

Postoperative alteration of mental state may be more common than previously appreciated. Kilgus et al., in a review of total hip arthroplasty patients, hypothesized that the embolization of marrow contents produced during hip arthroplasty might produce significant neuropsychological brain dysfunction. Twenty-eight patients were monitored intraoperatively with transcranial Doppler scanning to detect bone embolization. Postoperatively, neuropsychological tests were repeated at 7 days and at 6 weeks. An alarming 71 percent of patients demonstrated intraoperative brain embolization by transcranial Doppler scan. Sixty-seven percent

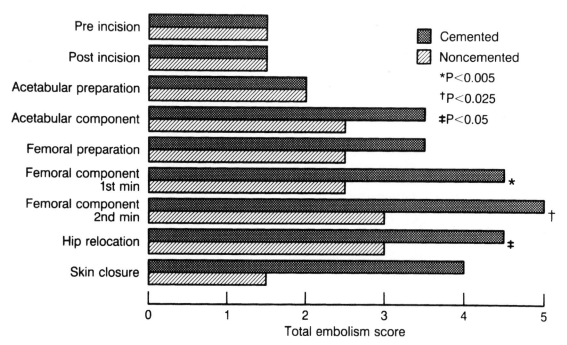

Figure 13–4. Comparison of the total embolism scores, derived from the sum of the median scores for amount, duration, and size of emboli passing through the right atrium, at indicated intervals during the operation. (From Ereth MH, Weber JG, Abel MD, et al: Cemented versus noncemented total hip arthroplasty: Embolism, hemodynamics, and intrapulmonary shunting. Mayo Clin Proc 67:1066, 1992.)

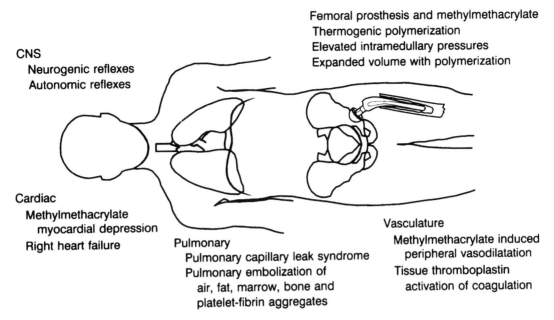

Femoral prosthesis and methylmethacrylate
Thermogenic polymerization
Elevated intramedullary pressures
Expanded volume with polymerization

CNS
Neurogenic reflexes
Autonomic reflexes

Cardiac
Methylmethacrylate
myocardial depression
Right heart failure

Pulmonary
Pulmonary capillary leak syndrome
Pulmonary embolization of
air, fat, marrow, bone and
platelet-fibrin aggregates

Vasculature
Methylmethacrylate induced
peripheral vasodilatation
Tissue thromboplastin
activation of coagulation

Figure 13–5. Some of the physiologic events associated with hip arthroplasty.

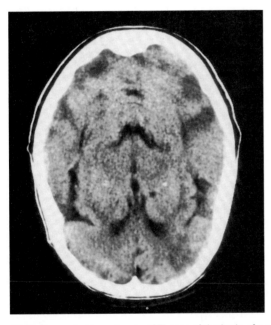

Figure 13–6. Computed tomography (CT) scan of the brain of a patient who experienced postoperative obtundation, coma, and, ultimately, death within days after cemented arthroplasty. A postoperative echocardiogram demonstrated a large right-to-left shunt at the atrial level. The head CT scan shows multiple dark cortical areas consistent with scattered fresh multifocal embolic infarcts, believed to be due to paradoxical embolization that occurred during component insertion.

of patients demonstrated a neuropsychological deficit. At 6 weeks after surgery, 29 percent of patients had a demonstrable neuropsychological dysfunction compared with their preoperative status. This study suggests that the embolic material from the medullary contents of bone during total joint arthroplasty is deliv-

ered, in a significant number of patients, to the cerebral circulation either by paradoxical embolization when a right-to-left shunt exists or through the pulmonary vasculature in other patients.[30]

PREVENTIVE MEASURES

Several options have been explored to reduce embolization during hip arthroplasty. Vent tubes within the femoral canal and drill holes near the tip of the stem have been suggested.[2,14] In a dog model, Sherman et al. showed that meticulous lavage of the distal femoral canal before insertion of a cemented rod was successful in eliminating the otherwise significant decreases in arterial oxygen saturation, increases in intrapulmonary shunt fraction, and elevations in pulmonary artery pressure otherwise seen in this model.[50] Byrick et al. showed a similar benefit from high-volume, high-pressure pulsatile lavage, which prevented pulmonary physiologic derangement; moreover, they documented a reduction in fat emboli in the lungs.[3] In a prospective double-blind study, retrograde filling of the canal with cement by means of a cement gun has been shown to reduce the amount of air embolized to the heart.[17]

Pulsatile lavage, the use of a cement gun, and distal plugging of the canal all were undisplaced at about the same time. Because canal plugging significantly increases the cement-induced bone pressurization,[32] the potential benefits of lavage and retrograde filling may be offset by the more efficient pressurization.

In elderly patients who have a history of significant cardiovascular or metastatic disease or fracture and who are considered to be at risk for cardiovascular collapse during arthroplasty, various methods for reducing embolization are worthy of consideration. Invasive cardiovascular monitoring may be of assistance in the management of these patients should embolic events produce significant cardiopulmonary compromise. For patients undergoing total knee arthroplasty, particularly those who are elderly or who have preexisting cardiovascular disease, avoidance of bilateral simultaneous procedures during the same anesthetic administration is recommended. Adequate hydration, fluid management, and careful monitoring are essential during the portions of the procedure (e.g., tourniquet release) known to be associated with increased release of embolic debris.

SUMMARY

Although a rare occurrence overall, sudden death during hip arthroplasty occurs in a characteristic fashion directly related to the preparation and pressurization of bone and the embolization of air, fat, and marrow contents that result. The patients most at risk are those who are elderly, those who have preexisting cardiovascular disease, and those whose surgery is being performed for fracture or metastatic disease. Cemented hip arthroplasty increases the risk of morbidity and mortality for these patients by virtue of the efficient pressurization of the intramedullary contents produced by femoral cementation, which is the point in the procedure at which embolization is greatest. Methods for reducing the amount of embolic material released should be considered in patients with identified risk factors. Communication between the orthopedist and the anesthesiologist regarding these issues is important before and during the management of these at-risk patients who are undergoing hip or knee arthroplasty. Improved understanding of the pathophysiology in the range of responses of different patients to the embolization that occurs during all arthroplasty procedures should improve the ability to anticipate, treat, and prevent this problem in the future.

Perioperative mortality rates for hip and knee arthroplasty are low, with the greatest risk of death occurring in elderly patients, in those with preexisting cardiovascular and hip disease, those undergoing emergent procedures for fracture, or those with oncologic diagnoses. Increased levels of surveillance and careful perioperative management by the entire medical team may help reduce the incidence of death in these higher-risk subgroups as well as help improve the overall safety profile of this already very safe and effective procedure.

References

1. Black S, Cucchiara RF, Nishimura RA, Michenfelder JD: Parameters affecting occurrence of paradoxical air embolism. Anesthesiology 71:235, 1989.
2. Breed AL: Experimental production of vascular hypotension and bone marrow and fat embolism with methylmethacrylate cement: Traumatic hypertension of bone. Clin Orthop 102:227, 1974.
3. Byrick RJ, Bell RS, Kay JC, et al: High-volume, high-pressure pulsatile lavage during cemented arthroplasty. J Bone Joint Surg 71A:1331, 1989.
4. Byrick RJ, Forbes D, Waddell JP: A monitored cardiovascular collapse during cemented total knee replacement. Anesthesiology 65:213, 1986.
5. Charnley J: Acrylic Cement in Orthopaedic Surgery. Edinburgh, Churchill Livingstone, 1970, p 72.
6. Cucchiara RF, Seward JB, Nishimura RA, et al: Identification of a patent foramen ovale during sitting position craniotomy by transesophageal echocardiography with positive airway pressure. Anesthesiology 71:235, 1985.
7. Cullen CA, Smith TC: The intraoperative hazard of acrylic bone cement: report of a case. Anesthesiology 35:547, 1971.
8 Dandy DJ: Fat embolism following prosthetic replacement of the femoral head. Injury 3:85, 1971.
9. Dearborn JT, Harris WH: Postoperative mortality after total hip arthroplasty. J Bone Joint Surg 80:1291, 1998.
10. DeBurge A: Guepar hinge prosthesis: Complication and results with two years follow-up. Clin Orthop 120:47, 1976.
11. Dorr LD, Merckel C, Mellman MF, Klein I: Fat emboli in bilateral total knee arthroplasty: Predictive factors for neurologic manifestations. Clin Orthop 248:112, 1989.
12. Drinker H, Panjabi M, Goel V: Acute cardiopulmonary toxicity of methacrylate pressurization in the dog femur. Orthop Trans 5:275, 1981.
13. Duncan JA: Intra-operative collapse or death related to the use of acrylic cement in hip surgery. Anaesthesia 44:149, 1989.
14. Engesaeter LB, Strand T, Raugstad TS, et al: Effects of a distal venting hole in the femur during total hip replacement. Arch Orthop Trauma Surg 103:328, 1984.
15. Erdem E, Namer IJ, Saribas O, et al: Cerebral fat embolism studied with MRI and SPECT. Neuroradiology 35:199, 1993.
16. Ereth MH, Weber JG, Abel MD, et al: Cemented versus noncemented total hip arthroplasty: Embolism, hemodynamics, and intrapulmonary shunting. Mayo Clin Proc 67:1066, 1992.
17. Evans RD, Palazzo MGA, Ackers WL: Air embolism during total hip replacement: Comparison of two surgical techniques. Br J Anaesth 62:243, 1989.
18. Fahmey NR, Chandler HP, Danychuk K, et al: Blood-gas and circulatory changes during total knee replacement: Role of the intramedullary alignment rod. J Bone Joint Surg 72A:19, 1990.
19. Gresham GA, Kuczynski A, Rosborough D: Fatal fat embolism following replacement arthroplasty for transcervical fractures of femur. BMJ 2:617, 1971.
20. Hagen PT, Scholz DG, Edwards WD: Incidence and size of patent foramen ovale during the first 10 decades of life: An autopsy study of 965 normal hearts. Mayo Clin Proc 59:17, 1984.
21. Hall TM, Calahan JJ: Fat embolism precipitated by reaming of the femoral canal during revision of a total knee arthroplasty: A case report. J Bone Joint Surg 76A:899, 1994.
22. Harris NH: Cardiac arrest and bone cement [letter]. BMJ 3:523, 1970.
23. Herndon JH, Bechtol CO, Crickenberger DP: Fat embolism during total hip replacement: A prospective study. J Bone Joint Surg 56A:1350, 1974.
24. Holiday AD Jr, Lewallen DG: Sudden death associated with hip arthroplasty. Presented at the 58th annual meeting of the American Academy of Orthopaedic Surgeons, Anaheim, CA, March 7–12, 1991.
25. Homsy CA, Tullos HS, Anderson MS, et al: Some physiological aspects of prosthesis stabilization with acrylic polymer. Clin Orthop 83:317, 1972.
26. Hyland J, Robins RHC: Cardiac arrest and bone cement [letter]. BMJ 4:176, 1970.
27. Jackson CT, Greendyke RM: Pulmonary and cerebral fat embolism after closed-chest cardiac massage. Surg Gynecol Obstet 120:25, 1965.
28. Kallos T, Enis JE, Golan F, Davis JH: Intramedullary pressure and pulmonary embolism of femoral medullary contents in dogs during insertion of bone cement and a prosthesis. J Bone Joint Surg 56A:1363, 1974.
29. Karpman RR, Lee TK, Moore BM: Austin-Moore versus bipolar hemiarthroplasty for displaced femoral neck fractures: A randomized prospective study. Presented at the 59th annual meeting of the American Academy of Orthopaedic Surgeons, Washington, DC, February 25, 1993.
30. Kilgus DJ, Colonna DM, Stump DA, et al: Total hip arthroplasty produces intraoperative brain embolization and neuropsychologic

dysfunction up to 6 weeks postoperatively. Proceedings of the 67th Annual meeting, AAOS, March 15–19, 2000, Orlando, FL, p 507.

31. Lachiewicz PF, Ranawat CS: Fat embolism syndrome following bilateral knee replacement with total condylar prosthesis. Report of two cases. Clin Orthop 160:106, 1981.

32. Markolf KL, Amstutz HC: In vitro measurement of bone acrylic interface pressure during femoral component insertion. Clin Orthop 121:60, 1976.

33. McLaughlin RE, DiFaxio CA, Hakala M, et al: Blood clearance and acute pulmonary toxicity of methylmethacrylate in dogs after simulated arthroplasty and intravenous injection. J Bone Joint Surg 55A:1621, 1973.

34. Modig J, Busch C, Olerud S, et al: Arterial hypotension and hypoxaemia during total hip replacement: The importance of thromboplastic products, fat embolism, and acrylic monomers. Acta Anaesth Scand 19:28, 1975.

35. Monto RR, Garcia J, Callaghan JJ: Fatal fat embolism following total condylar prosthesis: Report of two cases. Clin Orthop 160:106, 1981.

36. Orsini EC, Byrick RJ, Mullen BM, et al: Cardiopulmonary function and pulmonary microemboli during arthroplasty using cemented or non-cemented components: The role of intramedullary pressure. J Bone Joint Surg 69A:822, 1987.

37. Orsini EC, Richards RR, Mullen JMB: Fatal fat embolism during cemented total knee arthroplasty: A case report. Can J Surg 29:385, 1986.

38. Parmet JL, Berman AT, Horrow JC, et al: Thromboembolism coincident with tourniquet deflation during total knee arthroplasty. Lancet 341:1057, 1993.

39. Parvizi J, Holiday AD Jr, Lewallen DG, et al: Sudden death during hip arthroplasty. Clin Orthop 269:39, 1999.

40. Parvizi J, Johnson B, Rowland CR, et al: Thirty-day mortality following elective hip arthroplasty. J Bone Joint Surg 83A:Oct, 2001.

41. Parvizi J, Rowland CR, Ereth MH, Lewallen DG: Perioperative mortality following hip arthroplasty for fracture [unpublished data].

42. Parvizi J, Sullivan TA, Trousdale RT, Lewallen DG: Perioperative mortality associated with total knee arthroplasty. J Bone Joint Surg 83A:1157, 2001.

43. Patterson BM, Healy JH, Cornell CN, Sharrock NE: Cardiac arrest during hip arthroplasty with a cemented long-stem component. J Bone Joint Surg 73A:271, 1991.

44. Pell AC, Christie J, Keating JF, Sutherland GR: The detection of fat embolism by transesophageal echocardiography during reamed intramedullary nailing: a study of 24 patients with femoral and tibial fractures. J Bone Joint Surg 75B:921, 1993.

45. Phillips H, Cole PV, Lettin AWF: Cardiovascular effects of implanted acrylic bone cement. BMJ 3:460, 1971.

46. Propst JW, Siegel LC, Schnittger I, et al: Segmental wall motion abnormalities in patients undergoing total hip replacement: Correlations with intraoperative events. Anesth Analg 77:743, 1993.

47. Ries MD: Fat embolism associated with intramedullary alignment during total knee arthroplasty. Contemp Orthop 28:211, 1994.

48. Ries MD, Rauscher LA, Hoskins S, et al: Intramedullary pressure and pulmonary function during total knee arthroplasty. Clin Orthop 356:154, 1998.

49. Sevitt S: Fat embolism in patients with fractured hips. BMJ 2:257, 1972.

50. Sherman RMP, Byrick RJ, Kay JC, et al: The role of lavage in preventing hemodynamic and blood-gas changes during cemented arthroplasty. J Bone Joint Surg 65A:500, 1983.

51. Special Article: Acrylic cement and the cardiovascular system. Lancet 2:1002, 1974.

52. Stecker MS, Ries MD: Fatal pulmonary embolism during manipulation after total knee arthroplasty. A case report. J Bone Joint Surg 78A:111, 1996.

53. Stern SH, Sharrock N, Kahn R, Insall JN: Hematologic and circulatory changes associated with total knee arthroplasty instrumentation. Clin Orthop 143:211, 1979.

54. Weiss SJ, Cheung AT, Stecker MM, et al: Fatal paradoxical cerebral embolization during bilateral knee arthroplasty. Anesthesiology 84:721, 1996.

14

Outcome Studies, Measurement Tools, and Impairment Evaluation After Joint Replacement

• PETER C. AMADIO

MEASUREMENT OF OUTCOME AFTER JOINT REPLACEMENT

The assessment of clinical results after joint replacement has been the subject of many publications. Although the methods employed have varied, there are certain basic concepts that should be borne in mind whenever one attempts to assess results of a reconstructive procedure.

First is that results are multifactorial, and that combining dissimilar categories of outcome into a single score is a misguided attempt at simplicity that may obscure important factors.[16] Thus, for example, combining patient satisfaction or function with anatomic results eliminates any possibility of studying correlations between these factors. Rather than striving for simplicity, outcome assessment should aim to be accurate, reliable, and relevant. In addition, outcome assessment should be based on the premise that there are many different dimensions to outcomes. Although studies may appropriately focus on a limited subset of outcomes, it is important to remember that other dimensions exist and may well be relevant.

GENERAL CHARACTERISTICS OF OUTCOME ASSESSMENT

There are certain properties of all outcome assessment measures that must be borne in mind whenever one reviews a scientific study.[32] These properties are validity, reliability, responsiveness, and sensitivity (Fig. 14–1).

Validity is the relevance of the measure to the topic it purports to assess. Measurement of renal blood flow or visual acuity, for example, is not valid for assessment of outcome after hip arthroplasty. Validity can be assessed on its face by simply noting whether the measurement seems relevant (e.g., hip pain and hip surgery). Additional diligence is needed, though, to be sure that the measure is coherent. A valid scale is not affected by other, extraneous factors. A hip pain score should not, for example, be affected by headache pain. Walking

ability may be affected by pain but also by other factors such as weakness or balance. Ideally, any measure should be internally consistent as well. For questionnaires, statistical measures such as Cronbach's alpha or intraclass correlations may be used to show that individual items within a rating scale all tend to move in the same direction.

Validity is also assessed by determining whether the measure is affected by known correlates of the subject of interest; for example, a pain scale should reflect higher pain scores in patients with known painful conditions than in those without such conditions. A pain score may also be validated by showing that it correlates positively with the use of pain medications. Validity is clearly the most critical property of a measure; if a measure is invalid, it is of no use in studying the topic of interest. Fortunately, this property is usually easy to assess.

Reliability reflects the ability of a test to give identical results when administered repetitively, in circumstances when the factor of interest does not change. For tests in which an observer is involved, interobserver and intraobserver reliability should be noted. Many fracture rating systems, for example, have poor interobserver reliability; different observers reading the same films, even when given similar training, often come to dissimilar conclusions. In contrast, goniometry typically has fairly good interobserver reliability, on the order of plus or minus 5 to 10 degrees.[7] For questionnaires, test-retest reliability is measured. Reliability is also a critical property; measures that are not reliable cannot be compared across studies. Unfortunately, we often know little about the reliability even of commonly used measures, whether clinical or radiographic.

Responsiveness is the degree of change in a test after some intervention or lapse of time. Typically, responsiveness is measured in terms of effect size or standardized response mean (SRM); that is, the amount of change in terms of the standard deviation of the measure, or the standard deviation of the difference in measurements made before and after a test. Responsive measures affect sizes or SRMs of 1 or more. As with reliability, the responsiveness of a measure often is not

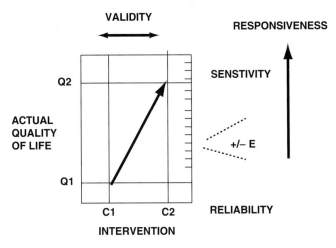

Figure 14–1. Essential properties of health status assessment. (Derived from Testa M, Simonson D: Assessment of quality-of-life outcomes. N Engl J Med 334:835–849, 1996.)

well defined. Without such data, it is difficult to know how many subjects to enroll in a study to obtain a clinically meaningful result. Davis et al.,[5] for example, reported on the results of different types of thumb arthroplasty. The results were inconclusive, in part because one of the measures used, range of motion, was not very responsive, and another, strength, was not very reliable.

Sensitivity is the fourth major property of a measure. Sensitivity is a reflection of how finely a measure can be divided. A goniometer calibrated in tenths of a degree is clearly more sensitive than one marked off in increments of 10 degrees, and, similarly, questionnaires with multiple questions are more sensitive than ones with fewer questions. Sensitivity, like validity, is a property that can be—but rarely is—assessed relatively quickly. Like responsiveness, sensitivity is an important factor in a measure's ability to identify differences between treatments or conditions.

OUTCOME DOMAINS

There are many different domains that are relevant to the assessment of outcome of joint replacement. Traditionally, orthopedic surgeons have used anatomic or physiologic measures, such as radiographic alignment, lucent lines, infection rates, and the like, as their primary outcome measures. Measures of patient function have often been rolled in to composite scores, such as the Harris Hip score, the Hospital of Special Surgery (HSS) score, the Knee Society Score, which make varying assumptions about the relative importance of pain, motion, and activity levels that often vary widely, based primarily on the judgment of the surgeons who designed the scales rather than on the responses of the patients with the conditions of interest. Such assessments may be discordant. One survey of patients with hip arthritis showed that symptoms interfering with sleep, hobbies, and sexual activity were very important; however, these are rarely surveyed in the traditional summary joint scores.[19]

Anatomy and Physiology

There are many valid and well-accepted anatomic and physiologic measures for the evaluation of joint replacement. For the most part, they are also reliable, but such measures may not be very responsive or sensitive, as meaningful chance may occur in only a small proportion of patients. Moreover, although these measures provide critical data about the mechanical status of the implant, they do not address the function of the patient. The assumption that a well-seated prosthesis means a satisfied patient has been shown to be unfounded in multiple studies. Clearly, these measures, although absolutely necessary, are not sufficient to provide a full understanding of the outcome of joint replacement.

Symptoms

Patients typically seek joint replacement not because of a concern about abnormal radiographic appearance but because of symptoms or functional complaints. Pain is the principal focus of these complaints, and, fortunately, there are many valid, reliable, and responsive measures to evaluate musculoskeletal pain. Pain severity can be measured quite reliably and with good sensitivity by a pain thermometer or a visual analogue scale. A variety of other questionnaire measures, such as the SF-36, Distress Alarm for the Severely Handicapped (DASH), and the American Academy of Orthopedic Surgeons (AAOS) Hip and Knee questionnaire, can detect patterns of joint pain frequency and its impact on daily activity. Such measures are a critical element in any clinical assessment of joint replacement outcome.

Function

According to the World Health Organization, physical function can be broken down into three basic conceptual areas. *Impairments* are physical or anatomic limitations of function, such as loss of a part, loss of motion, or loss of strength. These may or may not translate into *disabilities*, which are difficulties with specific tasks. Finally, disabilities may result in *handicaps*, or limitations on economic and social integration. Whether or not a disability results in a handicap depends not only on the disability but also on coping mechanisms, family and societal support, education, and a variety of other factors.[4] It should be clear that handicaps have the largest impact on an individual's life, and that the connection between impairments—typically measured by surgeons—and handicaps—which are most important to patients—is relatively obtuse.

Fortunately, there are many ways to measure disabilities and even handicaps, and these measures fulfill all four of the critical properties outlined earlier. Disability, or, to use its more positive counterpart, ability, can be assessed either by observation or by questionnaire. Observation takes one of two forms. One can actually observe patients over the course of a day or a week, and record what they can do, how easily they can do it, and so forth. Although theoretically possible, the cost of having a trained observer shadowing patients is clearly prohibitive, even without considering the problems of regulating interobserver variation or the effect that observation might have on performance, because it is well known that people behave differently when they are being observed. An option that retains the observer function but standardizes the evaluation so that it is less variable between patients involves the use of standardized simulations of various work tasks. Such measures as various step-up tests, manipulation rates, and the like can be reliable, sensitive, and even responsive but may not truly capture the activities that are most important to patients; therefore, these measures may lack some degree of validity.

In contrast to the two options just mentioned, there is questionnaire assessment. This method has considerable benefit because it can assess a variety of real-life activities simply by asking whether or not they have been or could be performed, and, if so, with what degree of inconvenience. Furthermore, the importance of these activities can also be assessed by direct questioning.[17,36] When self-administered, such tests have the double advantage of being inexpensive and unobtrusive. There is no necessity for interaction with an examiner who may possibly affect validity of the measurements. Although it is possible that the patient may not respond accurately, the responses can be validated by physical measures, if need be. Moreover, in practice, questionnaires are usually more reliable, sensitive, and responsive than other measures that require the use of an examiner. Such assessments make it clear that joint replacement is a highly successful procedure, which greatly improves function and overall quality of life in the vast majority of patients.[15,25]

Satisfaction

The ultimate measure of a therapy's worth lies not only in its biologic effect and its effect on activity but also on the sense of well being or satisfaction that the patient expresses. It seems clear that satisfaction is important not only in the final anatomic and functional results but also in the expectations that patients have preoperatively.[22,36] Cosmesis is also a relevant factor, especially in hand arthroplasty.[31] Again, an examiner tends only to confuse the matter, as patients are inclined to give more socially acceptable responses to an interviewer than they would to a self-completed questionnaire.

There is more than one kind of satisfaction. Satisfaction with the process of care is also of interest to payers as well as patients. Topics such as the politeness of the staff and attentiveness and communication skills of the surgeon are increasingly important elements of satisfaction.

Cost

The final dimension of outcome is cost. Without a financial analysis, one cannot assess the societal input that is needed to achieve whatever benefit the surgery provides.[10] Both direct (surgeon and hospital fees) and indirect (time lost from work by either patients or their caregivers) costs are relevant. A global assessment of the costs of joint replacement also takes into consideration lifetime expenses, including a discounted present value for the costs of possible revision surgery.

WHEN TO USE WHAT

It should be clear by this point that there are many ways to assess outcome after joint replacement, and, furthermore, there are no right or wrong methods. Instead, each method has specific strengths and weaknesses, and each addresses quite different aspects of the complex picture of results. Physical examination, laboratory, and radiographic assessment are critical for diagnosis and assessment of the mechanical status of the implant postoperatively. These data are clearly critical, but as discussed earlier, they are incomplete because they address the technical rather than the human aspect of total joint replacement outcomes. For the outcome from the perspective of the patient or of society, additional measures are needed. These include questionnaires and even financial analysis. But the question remains of when to use what.

Clearly, the answer depends in part on the aspect of outcomes that are of interest to the clinician or investigator, and in part also on the structure of the investigation. First, one must decide what to study. Technical outcomes are clearly important, but they do not need to be the focus of every investigation. A study designed to identify proper indications should include an analysis not only of procedures that might fail technically but also of those associated with the greatest perceived benefit to the patient in terms of functional improvement and satisfaction. Surveillance involves the use of simple, easy-to-use tools, such as short questionnaires; these lack detail, but large numbers of patients can be surveyed for major problems. Quality improvement studies need some process measures: Were the right tests done at the right time? What were the complications and what were the risk factors? Research projects require more detailed analyses and longer questionnaires.

The issue of longer questionnaires raises the problem of respondent burden. Longer questionnaires provide more detail but also take more time to complete. Questionnaires that are too long may not be completed by the patient because of fatigue; furthermore, longer questionnaires tend to have questions whose answers may be necessary for scoring but are irrelevant to the specific patient answering them. For example, a hypothetical mobility scale tests the full spectrum of mobility, from bedridden to full athletic ability. Such a scale requires many questions, a number of which would be irrelevant to individual subjects. If a patient has already expressed an inability to walk one block, there is little point in asking about the capability of walking a mile; similarly, if someone has stated a capability of running five miles, why ask about the ability of walking one mile? Fortunately, the new field of computer adaptive testing (CAT)[35] has come to the rescue. Using computer algorithms, one may first ask a question regarding maximum function; if that is answered affirmatively, there is no point in delving further into the lower regions of the scale. If that question is answered negatively, the algorithm may dictate a middle level question; based on that response, there may again be an intermediate question, until, after a series of perhaps four or five interrogations, the same quality data are obtained that would previously have required a scale of as many as 20 questions. The 20 questions are still there; they are just held in reserve and only asked to clarify the responses to a handful of key questions. Modified versions of the Short Form (SF)-36 and other questionnaires are under development and should give the investigator the best of both worlds—detail and brevity. Furthermore, by using a computer to ask the questions, the problem of data entry is eliminated. Finally, CAT technology allows crosswalks between different questionnaires with similar scales, so that, for example, one could compare a score of 50 on the DASH upper limb questionnaire with a score of 50 on the upper limb scale of the Short Musculoskeletal Functional Assessment (SMFA) questionnaire.

QUESTIONNAIRE ASSESSMENT OF TOTAL JOINT FUNCTION

At this point, it would be remiss not to identify at least a few commonly used and useful questionnaires for the assessment of outcome after joint replacement.

General Health and Quality of Life

For assessment of general health, quality of life, general pain, handicaps, and the like, there is little question but that the SF-36, a 36-item questionnaire that measures eight domains (physical function and role, emotional role, social function, mental health, bodily pain, vitality, and general health) is the current benchmark measure.[35] Although the SF-36 was designed for use in general medical patients, those who have had hip or knee replacement score remarkably well on this measure.[6,9,12–14,21,23,29] The improvement seen after joint replacement, as measured on the SF-36 in terms of improved health, physical function, and pain relief, exceeds that seen in patients after cardiac surgery. Shorter versions of this questionnaire (SF-20, SF-12, and SF-8) report only two summary scales: physical and mental well-being. Other questionnaires that can assess general health include the Sickness Impact Profile and the Nottingham Health Profile. Unfortunately, these questionnaires, which were designed to study function in medically ill patients, do not focus on occupational activities; thus, the upper limb is relatively underrepresented in each. More vigorous physical activity in general is also underrepresented, so healthy people tend to cluster at the ceiling of maximal function. Fortunately, other options are available, and these can provide more detailed assessment of musculoskeletal function.

Region and Joint-Specific Questionnaires

The assessment of musculoskeletal symptoms and function took a great step forward when the AAOS family of outcome questionnaires was developed between 1994 and 1996.[28] Designed to complement the SF-36, these questionnaires focus on musculoskeletal symptoms and function, both in everyday and work activities.[5] Unlike the SF-36 assessment, these questionnaires also attribute symptoms; instead of asking simply about pain, they ask about knee pain, hand pain, and so forth, depending on the questionnaire. Thus, using these instruments, one is able to sort out not only what the functional problem is, with a greater degree of precision (because many more musculoskeletal function questions are asked), but also where the problem is located, by using the attribution aspect of these questionnaires. In most cases, these tools have been designed to complement rather than replace the SF-36 assessment. There are currently 11 AAOS-endorsed questionnaires: DASH; Lower Limb; Sports Knee; Foot/Ankle; Hip/Knee; Pediatric (parent forms for infants and teens, and patient form for teens), and SMFA. Each has been validated, and normal data is also available for each (Table 14–1). The questionnaires are available, free of charge, at the AAOS web site (*www.aaos.org*), although a participation agreement must be signed to ensure that the questionnaires are not modified or commercialized without the consent of the AAOS. The normal data are also available through the AAOS.

Of course, there are also other tools that can be used to assess outcome after joint replacement. The Western Ontario/McMaster University osteoarthritis index is an excellent hip and knee function tool; like the SF-36 assessment, it is available in multiple language versions.[24,30] The Arthritis Impact Measurement Scale is designed to measure symptoms and functions as well as general well-being in patients with osteoarthritis or inflammatory arthritis.[18] There are also a host of joint-specific instruments.[2,20,34] These and many more (currently more than 800) questionnaires are available for review at a single web site, (*www.qlmed.org*), which also provides information regarding terms of use (most are free for scientific use but may have restrictions on commercialization).

OUTCOME REGISTRIES

Outcome data can be used for two main purposes: (1) to provide data for clinical trials, and (2) to provide data for ongoing, data-driven, evidence-based practice. The former purpose is, of course, important, particularly in comparing new with established technology, but the latter may have a greater impact on everyday practice. Built on the concepts of continuous quality improvement espoused by Deming and others,[27,33] evidence-based medicine invokes the quality improvement cycle (Fig. 14–2) to collect the evidence that then forms the basis of practice decisions. Critical to the proper functioning of such a process is the collection of accurate

Table 14–1. THE AAOS FAMILY OF OUTCOME QUESTIONNAIRES

Questionnaire	No. of questions	Normal values (median ± 25 percentile)	Domains
DASH*	30	4 (1, 13)	Upper limb symptoms, function; optional sport/work module
Sport knee	29	100 (91, 100)	Knee symptoms and function
Foot/ankle	30	99 (92, 100)	Foot/ankle symptoms and function
Hip/knee	12	96 (89, 100)	Joint specific symptoms and function
Lower limb	4	95 (86, 100)	Lower limb symptoms and function
Cervical spine	17	100 (87, 100)	Neck pain and neurologic symptoms
Lumbar spine	17	96 (80, 98)	Back pain and neurologic symptoms; optional scoliosis module
Pediatric/child (parent)	83	95 (89, 97)	Upper limb, lower limb, play, well-being
Pediatric/teen	83	99 (92, 100)	Upper limb, lower limb, play, well-being
Pediatric/teen Parent	83	98 (92, 100)	Upper limb, lower limb, play, well-being
SMFA†	40	4 (1, 16) (function index)	Emotion, ADL, function, arm/hand, mobility, bother

*DASH assessment codeveloped by AAOS and Institute for Work and Health, Toronto, Canada.
†SFMA assessment developed by University of Washington.
Note: DASH and SMFA are disability scales; 0 = best health and 100 = worst health. The others are ability scales; 0 = least ability and 100 = most ability.
AAOS = American Association of Orthopedic Surgeons; ADL = activities of daily living; DASH = disability of arm, shoulder, hand; SMFA = short-form musculoskeletal functional assessment.

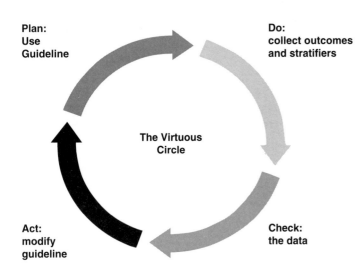

Figure 14–2. Evidence-based medicine.

and complete records on outcome and the factors affecting it. For this purpose, the total joint registry is an ideal tool.[1] A joint registry can be composed of the files of a single surgeon or those of an institution or of a national health system. The largest registry in the United States is probably that of the Mayo Clinic, which includes accurate follow-up until death or to the nearest 5-year follow-up point for more than 90 percent of all total joint replacements ever done at that institution.[3] Nearly 100,000 cases are on file, and the outcome data have served as the foundation for literally hundreds of publications. National registries in Sweden[11,26] and elsewhere[8] are similarly useful.

CONCLUSIONS

The assessment of the results of joint replacement is multifactorial. There is no one way to assess outcome that is correct in all circumstances. A sound foundation in the available tools, their proper use, and strategies to

implement the results into clinical practice are all essential elements of an outcome assessment program.

References

1. Amadio P, Naessens J, Rice R, et al: Effect of feedback on resource use and morbidity in hip and knee arthroplasty in an integrated group practice setting. Mayo Clin Proc 71:127–133, 1996.
2. Beaton DE, Richards RR: Measuring function of the shoulder. A cross-sectional comparison of five questionnaires. J Bone Joint Surg 78-A:882–890, 1996.
3. Berry DJ, Kessler M, Morrey BF: Maintaining a hip registry for 25 years. Mayo Clinic experience. Clin Orthop 344:61–68, 1997.
4. Bostrom C, Harms-Ringdahl K, Nordemar R: Relationships between measurements of impairment, disability, pain, and disease activity in rheumatoid arthritis in patients with shoulder problems. Scand J Rheum 24:352–359, 1995.
5. Davis AM, Beaton DE, Hudak P, et al: Measuring disability of the upper extremity: A rationale supporting the use of a regional outcome measure. J Hand Therapy 12:269–274, 1999.
6. Dunbar M, Robertsson O, Ryd L, Lidgren L: Appropriate questionnaires for knee arthroplasty: Results of a survey of 3600 patients from the Swedish Knee Arthroplasty Registry. J Bone Joint Surg 83B:339–344, 2001.

7. Garcia-Elias M, An K-Y, Amadio P, et al: Reliability of carpal angle determinations. J Hand Surg 14A:1017–1021, 1989.

8. Havelin LI: The Norwegian Joint Registry. Bull Hosp Joint Dis 58:139–147, 1999.

9. Hawker G, Wright J, Coyte P, et al: Health-related quality of life after knee replacement: Results of the knee replacement patient outcomes research team study. J Bone Joint Surg 80A:163–173, 1998.

10. Healy WL, Ayers ME, Iorio R, et al: Impact of a clinical pathway and implant standardization on total hip arthroplasty: A clinical and economic study of short-term patient outcome. J Arthroplasty 13:266–276, 1998.

11. Herberts P, Malchau H: How outcome studies have changed total hip arthroplasty practices in Sweden. Clin Orthop 344:44–60, 1997.

12. Hozack W, Rothman R, Albert T, et al: Relationship of total hip arthroplasty outcomes to other orthopaedic procedures. Clin Orthop 344:88–93, 1997.

13. Jones C, Voaklander D, Johnston D, Suarez-Almazor M: The effect of age on pain, function, and quality of life after total hip and knee arthroplasty. Arch Intern Med 161:454–460, 2001.

14. Katz JN, Phillips CB, Poss R, et al: The validity and reliability of a total hip arthroplasty outcome evaluation questionnaire. J Bone Joint Surg 77A:1528–1534, 1995.

15. Kay A, Davison B, Badley E, Wagstaff S: Hip arthroplasty: Patient satisfaction. Br J Rheum 22:243–249, 1983.

16. Konig A, Scheidler M, Rader C, Eulert J: The need for a dual rating system in total knee arthroplasty. Clin Orthop 345:161–167, 1997.

17. Kreibich DN, Vaz M, Bourne RB, et al: What is the best way of assessing outcome after total knee replacement? Clin Orthop 331:221–225, 1996.

18. Liang MH, Fossel AH, Larson MG: Comparisons of five health status instruments for orthopedic evaluation. Med Care 28:632–642, 1990.

19. Lieberman JR, Dorey F, Shekelle P, et al: Differences between patients' and physicians' evaluations of outcome after total hip arthroplasty. J Bone Joint Surg 78:835–838, 1996.

20. MacDermid JC, Richards RS, Donner A, et al: Responsiveness of the short form-36, disability of the arm, shoulder, and hand questionnaire, patient-rated wrist evaluation, and physical impairment measurements in evaluating recovery after a distal radius fracture. J Hand Surg 25:30–340, 2000.

21. Mancuso C, Salvati E, Sculco T, Williams-Russo P: Satisfaction with total hip arthroplasty: Overall versus expectation-Specific satisfaction. Arthritis Rheum 42:S267, 1999.

22. Mancuso CA, Salvati EA, Johanson NA, et al: Patients' expectations and satisfaction with total hip arthroplasty. J Arthroplasty 12:387–396, 1997.

23. Mangione C, Goldman L, Orav E, et al: Health-related quality of life after elective surgery: Measurement of longitudinal changes. J Gen Intern Med 12:686–697, 1997.

24. McGrory BJ, Harris WH: Can the Western Ontario and McMaster Unviersities (WOMAC) osteoarthritis index be used to evaluate different hip joints in the same patient? J Arthroplasty 11:841–844, 1996.

25. Rissanen P, Aro S, Slatis P, et al: Health and quality of life before and after hip or knee arthroplasty. J Arthroplasty 10:169–175, 1995.

26. Robertsson O, Scott G, Freeman MA: Ten-year survival of the cemented Freeman-Samuelson primary knee arthroplasty. Data from the Swedish Knee Arthroplasty Register and the Royal London Hospital. J Bone Joint Surg 82B:506–507, 2000.

27. Sahney V, Dutkewych J, Schramm W: Quality improvement process: The foundation for excellence in health care. J Soc Health Syst 1:17–29, 1989.

28. Simmons B, Swiontkowski M, Evans R, et al: Outcomes assessment in the information age: Available instruments, data collection, and utilization of data. Instructional Course Lectures 48, 1999.

29. Soderman P, Malchau H: Is the Harris Hip Score System useful to study the outcome of total hip replacement? Clin Orthop 1:189–197, 2001.

30. Soderman P, Malchau H: Validity and reliability of Swedish WOMAC osteoarthritis index: A self-administered disease-specific questionnaire (WOMAC) versus generic instruments (SF-36 and NHP). Acta Orthop Scand 71:39–46, 2000.

31. Synnott K, Mullett H, Faull H, Kelly EP: Outcome measures following metacarpophalangeal joint replacement. J Hand Surg 25B:601–603, 2000.

32. Testa M, Simonson D: Assessment of quality-of-life outcomes. N Engl J Med 334:835–840, 1996.

33. Townes C, Petit B, Young B: Implementing total quality management in an academic surgery setting: Lessons learned. Swiss Surg 1:15–23, 1995.

34. Turchin DC, Richards RR: Validity of observer-based aggregate scoring systems as descriptors of elbow pain, function, and disability. J Bone Joint Surg 80A:154–162, 1998.

35. Ware JE, Bjorner JB, Kosinski M: Practical implications of item response theory and computerized adaptive testing. A brief summary of ongoing studies of widely used headache impact scales. Med Care 38:II-73–II-82, 2000.

36. Wright JG, Young NL: The patient-specific index: Asking patients what they want. J Bone Joint Surg 79A:974–983, 1997.

15

Statistical Considerations

•DUANE M. ILSTRUP

The purpose of this chapter is to provide the reader with an overview of how clinical follow-up studies of total joint arthroplasty are conducted at the Mayo Clinic. The chapter is divided into parts that deal with (1) the history and importance of efforts to obtain up-to-date follow-up information about the current clinical status of Mayo patients; (2) the advantages and disadvantages of various study designs; retrospective, prospective, randomized, case-control, and population-based versus referral-based studies; (3) advantages and disadvantages of various methods of statistical analysis, including survivorship methodology; (4) new methods to correctly analyze multiple joints and multiple failures per patient; and (5) the relationship of study sample size to the ability to compare outcomes and to detect relationships between risk factors and clinical outcome.

SURVEILLANCE AND THE MAYO CLINIC TOTAL JOINT REGISTRY

In 1969, Mark Coventry of the Mayo Clinic performed the first total hip arthroplasty in the United States. Since that time, more than 64,000 total joints have been implanted at the Mayo Clinic, including 34,000 hip implants and 22,000 knee implants (Fig. 15–1).

It soon became clear that to be able to evaluate the success of this number of procedures, three areas of need had to be addressed: (1) standardized data recording, (2) data retrieval, and (3) a reliable follow-up system.

Data Recording

Clinical data on each patient had to be recorded in a standardized and concise fashion. The Mayo Clinic patient history is a unit record first designed at the turn of the 20th century. Clinical data are entered in both handwritten and online forms by Mayo physicians, whereas surgical data are entered by surgical recorders from dictation in the operating room area. Specific details about patient clinical status are retrievable to the extent that the individual physician enters them in the history, unless special forms are used. It was realized that the clinical information available would be inconsistent and poorly defined unless standardized data entry forms were designed for each type of total joint replacement. Thus, the first of many joint sheets, the Hip Sheet, was designed. Similar forms were designed for other joints. These sheets are kept in the patient history and are updated each time a patient returns for evaluation. This accomplishes two objectives. First, they facilitate the original purpose of obtaining consistent and well-defined patient data for subsequent analysis, and second, they provide the surgeon with a convenient tool during examination for easily evaluating changes in the patient's characteristics over time.

Retrieval

The potential existed for operations on thousands of patients with many different underlying operative diagnoses, many different preoperative risk factors, and many different types of prostheses. From this need, the idea of the Mayo Clinic Total Joint Registry (MCTJR) was born. Today's MCTJR is a computer data file of historical, surgical, follow-up, complication, and reoperation data. The history file contains the information that is most frequently used to identify specific patient groups for study. Patient listings can be printed, or magnetic files can be generated that form the skeletons of data files that the investigating surgeon can supplement by abstracting clinical data from the patient's history and total joint sheet. Clinical data are now also being entered into the MCTJR in a prospective fashion, and optical reading is being developed to facilitate the process.

Method of Follow-up

Today, because of reimbursement issues, not every patient returns for examinations at frequent and regular intervals, particularly at a national referral center such as the Mayo Clinic. If clinical evaluation studies contained data available only from the patient's history, these studies would contain incomplete and possibly biased information. Therefore, it is necessary to contact patients who have not returned to Mayo. The initial

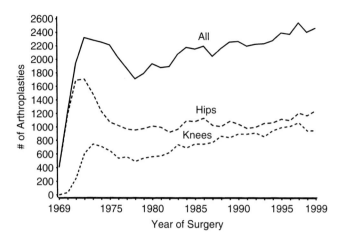

Figure 15–1. Number of arthroplasties at the Mayo Clinic by year.

attempt at patient follow-up is currently made by letter. If a patient does not respond, a second letter is sent. If this letter is not returned, an attempt is made to contact the patient or a relative by telephone. If no response is obtained, the patient's home physician may be contacted. Finally, if all these measures are unsuccessful, a request for a copy of the patient's death certificate is sent to the public health department of the patient's home state.

These follow-up attempts are made at various time intervals, depending on joint type. For example, follow-up contacts for hip replacements are made at 1, 2, 5, and 10 years. Some clinicians see their patients in person at these intervals. In addition to these time intervals, follow-up letters are sent whenever special studies are performed that require current patient data.

The follow-up letters are kept as a permanent part of the Mayo patient history, and information from them with respect to complications, reoperation, and clinical results is entered into the MCTJR. In all cases, an attempt is made to determine when a complication, reoperation, or death has occurred.

The importance of complete follow-up cannot be overemphasized. Patients who return for examination may be qualitatively different, either better or worse, than patients who choose not to return. In this manner, without follow-up letters, the results of clinical studies would be subject to bias. With frequent and current follow-up, the problems of bias may be overcome, and the results of clinical studies that use survivorship should be valid.[14] The validity of the questionnaire letter has been demonstrated in a prospective study by McGrory et al.[21] Ninety-seven percent of the patient responses were within one grade of the corresponding physician-recorded answers.

MEASURES OF SURGICAL SUCCESS

Implant survival and clinical function are the two main categories of surgical success. These are highly but imperfectly correlated variables. Pain, motion, ability to ambulate, limp, and use of walking aids are the chief components of clinical function. Pain is the chief reason patients seek the care of an orthopedic surgeon and therefore should be considered first when evaluating the efficacy of surgery. There are various composite measures of clinical function, called *joint scores*, which weigh the components of clinical function in a variety of ways in an effort to convert several variables into one summary measure. These scores are helpful when attempts are made to differentiate among large groups of patients but are not very useful on an individual patient basis, because, in the latter instance, the individual components of clinical function are more clinically relevant.

Implant survival or, conversely, implant failure may be, and has been, defined in several ways. The need for reoperation has been the most frequent definition. Roentgenographic loosening (also with various definitions) has also been used as a measure of implant failure. A composite definition of failure is needed, which combines the occurrence of either moderate or severe pain, reoperation, fracture, or roentgenographic loosening.[13]

There is increasingly heavy emphasis in the medical literature on the evaluation of patient "outcomes." Clinical, financial, functional, and psychosocial outcomes have been measured, as well as patient satisfaction.

SELECTION OF PATIENTS

Populations of patients chosen for study should represent the populations in which the prostheses will ultimately be used. If two prostheses are to be compared, it is essential that the study groups be as similar as possible on important prognostic factors.

STUDY DESIGNS

Retrospective Studies

In the past, the most frequently used study design was the retrospective or historical study. Although the value of such investigations has lessened, they do serve the purpose of providing long-term results that are essential for assessing the value of some procedures. When attempting to compare two prostheses, these studies are usually of the consecutive series type, in which all patients of a given type in a given time period are compared with all patients in another type in the same time period or, more typically, in a later time period. Another type of retrospective study is a matched or case-control study in which each patient with a given type of prosthesis is matched as closely as possible on several risk factors to one or more patients with another type of prosthesis. Both study designs, consecutive and matched, are subject to problems that usually preclude an unbiased estimation of which prosthesis is better. Although the matched study has fewer problems, these studies cannot separate the effects of the prosthesis from the impact of the surgeon when one surgeon preferentially uses one of the two prostheses and another surgeon preferentially uses the other. Even if each surgeon uses both prostheses, the choice of implants is usually made relative to which type the surgeon thinks will do better in that patient. This is called selection bias and is an inherent problem with historical studies.

Although it is difficult to compare treatment results in a historical study, such studies are still useful, if for no other reason than to provide the prospective patient with the experience of patients who have already had this procedure. It is only good medical practice to know what has happened to one's patients.

Prospective Nonrandomized Studies

If data are collected prospectively on two or more prosthetic designs, the evaluations will be made during the same time period and good data acquisition can be planned in advance. Patients in each group may still be qualitatively different because of surgeon selection bias.

Prospective Randomized Studies

If a patient is randomly assigned to the type of prostheses used, selection bias is eliminated. After a patient agrees to enter such a study, the prosthesis used is assigned by chance, not by the surgeon. Randomized studies that involve surgery are not easy to do. The surgeon must honestly admit to not really knowing which prosthetic design is better. Then the surgeon must convince the patient to participate willingly in the study.

Referral Bias and Population-Based Studies

The concept of referral bias has to do with the fact that patients who are referred to large medical centers may not be "typical" patients. They tend to be sicker patients and often have multiple medical conditions. It is problematic whether results of follow-up studies from a large medical center are applicable to patients seen on the front lines of orthopedic practice.

The Mayo Clinic has addressed the issue of referral bias[17,22] by comparing the results of patients referred to the Mayo Clinic from distant regions with the results of patients from Rochester, Minnesota, where almost all the care is provided by the Mayo Clinic. The Rochester population is a unique resource with which to do these studies because in few other communities can all patients with a given procedure be identified, followed, and evaluated.

STATISTICAL METHODS FOR SHORT-TERM ANALYSES

Unless one of two or more prosthetic designs being evaluated is a remarkably bad design, it is unlikely that there will be enough failures within the first years after surgery to reliably assess differences in failure rates. It is possible, however, to assess differences in clinical function, outcome measures, and patient satisfaction after only 1 or 2 years of surveillance. This may be particularly true when comparing cemented with uncemented prostheses, because patients with cemented prostheses tend to regain clinical function sooner than patients with uncemented designs. Methods are valid only when various assumptions about independence, underlying distributional form, equality of variance, and the like are met. Some statistical methods are more robust than others are when these assumptions are not met. It is recommended that the investigator consult with a professional statistician when questions arise about the appropriateness of alternative statistical methods, in particular when multivariate methods are employed.

If a variable is originally measured on a continuous scale, such as range of motion, or on an ordinal scale, such as pain (none, mild, moderate, severe), it is prudent to analyze the variable as originally measured, not in a categorized form. Investigators frequently categorize knee motion as less than 90 degrees or greater than or equal to 90 degrees rather than retaining the original measurement in degrees. In other studies, pain is categorized as none or mild versus moderate or severe rather than keeping the original ordinal scale. In both these instances, the investigators have made inefficient use of their data and may have sacrificed the ability to detect differences in clinical function. Continuous or ordinal variables should always be analyzed on their original scales before categorizing them.

The following statistical methods (Table 15–1) are appropriate when evaluating measurements that are made within a fixed time (e.g., 2 years after surgery).

Chi-square methods should be used for nominal variables such as the occurrence of superficial infection or dislocation.[8] For continuous variables, such as range of

Table 15–1. STATISTICAL METHODS BY NATURE OF VARIABLE AND STUDY DESIGN FOR FIXED TIME PERIODS

Study Design	Nominal	Continuous Gaussian	Continuous Non-Gaussian	Ordinal
Two-sample independent test	Chi-square	Two-sample t-test	Wilcoxon rank-sum test	Wilcoxon rank-sum
One-sample paired test	Sign test	Paired t-test	Wilcoxon signed-rank test	Wilcoxon signed-rank

motion or varus-valgus angulation, two-sample *tl*-tests for two prosthetic designs or one-way analysis of variance for more than two designs are appropriate when the underlying assumptions are met.[5,6] Wilcoxon rank-sum tests are appropriate for non-Gaussian (non-normal) continuous variables and for ordinal variables such as pain or distance walked.[11,24]

Multivariate methods should be used to adjust for differences in the distribution of risk factors that may influence the measure of outcome when comparing prosthetic designs. Multiple logistic regression may be used when comparing prosthetic designs on a discrete or ordinal outcome variable.[29] Multiple linear regression may be used to analyze continuous variables.[7]

All the methods mentioned assume that two or more independent groups of patients are being studied. If the same patient is being studied more than once (e.g., preoperatively versus postoperatively) or is being compared with himself (one side versus the contralateral side), or if patients are compared who have been matched on risk factors on a one-to-one basis, the above methods are inappropriate. In these instances, the paired *t*-test should be used when a continuous variable is analyzed, the sign test should be used when a nominal variable is analyzed, and the signed-rank test should be used a non-Gaussian continuous variable or an ordinal variable is analyzed.[4,9,10]

Finally, the data should always be graphed. Significance tests may help summarize the data, but one can seldom fully understand the information unless it is visualized. A Yogi Berra quote is very appropriate in this instance: "You can observe a lot just by watching."[2]

SURVIVORSHIP METHODS

Almost all adverse events in medicine, including orthopedics, are functions of time from some starting date. Because of this, it is important to know not only if but also when an event occurred. Berkson and Gage,[1] in 1950, advocated survival methods for cancer patients, and Dobbs,[12] in 1980, and Dorey and Amstutz,[13] in 1986, applied the use of survival methods to orthopedics.

If all patients arrived at the hospital for surgery on the same day, were observed for the same period, and the current status of their total joints was known, there would be no need for survival methods. However, all patients do not arrive for surgery on the same day and therefore have variable follow-up times relative to today's date. Some are "censored" because they are still being followed currently and their prostheses have not failed. Others are "lost to follow-up" on some date; that is, on that date they had not yet suffered a failure, and beyond that date their status is unknown.

Earlier methods of handling these problems were called actuarial methods because they were based on the life table methods that actuaries use.[1] In this method, survival time is lumped into time intervals, usually yearly intervals. Modern methods proposed by Kaplan and Meier[16] are now employed that use the actual time in days to failure.

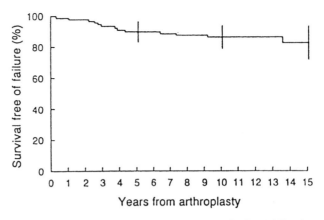

Figure 15–2. Typical Kaplan-Meier survivor curve for first MTP arthroplasty. The value of this type of data representation is that it considers all data and accommodates for differences in follow-up for each entry. (From Papagelopoulous PJ, Kitaoka HB, Ilstrup DM: Survivorship analysis of implant arthroplasty for the first metatarsophalangeal joint. Clin Orthop 302:164, 1994.)

The great advantage of survivorship methods is that they use *all* the available information and do not throw out data from patients because they have less than some minimum follow-up time. All patients contribute information to the survival curve until their joints fail or until their last day of follow-up. Figure 15–2 is an example of a survivorship curve from a study by Papagelopoulous et al.,[25] in which survivorship free of revision is plotted as a function of time from arthroplasty. A 95 percent confidence interval should always be included when survival curves are presented.

Another form of survival analysis that is most useful when attempting to demonstrate change in the probability of an event as a function of time is hazard function analysis.[18] The hazard function is sometimes known as the instantaneous rate of failure. It is a calculation of the conditional probability of the occurrence of an event at time = *t* given that the patient has not yet had the event before time = *t*. Figure 15–3 is an example of a hazard plot from a study by Morrey and Ilstrup of acetabular loosening versus femoral head size.[23]

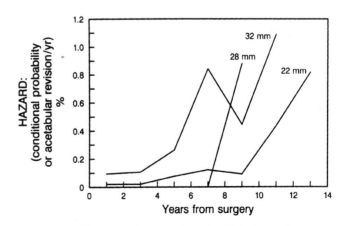

Figure 15–3. The hazard function relates the "risks" for a given event (i.e., revision) at a discrete time after surgery.

The most popular statistical method of comparing two or more survivorship curves is the log-rank test, which assumes that the survival curves continue to diverge proportionally from one another when plotted on a log scale.[26] When this is not the case, other Wilcoxon-type methods may be used that allow a better comparison of the curves.[19]

The Cox proportional hazards model, most often known simply as the Cox model, is the multivariate extension of the log-rank test.[3] Associations of survivorship with continuous variables, with several discrete variables, or with combinations of continuous and discrete variables may be estimated with this method. With real data, the assumptions of the Cox model are often not met, and experience and caution are necessary when this method is used. Most statisticians recommend that to develop a reliable multivariate model, there should be at least 10 events or failures for each risk factor evaluated in the model. For example, there should be at least 50 failures if 5 risk factors are evaluated in a Cox model.[15]

MULTIPLE JOINTS AND FAILURES PER PATIENT

Today, sophisticated statistical methods are available, which allow the clinical investigator to correctly analyze data when the patient may have more than one prosthesis (e.g., both right and left hips), or more than one event or failure (e.g., three occurrences of dislocation after total hip arthroplasty). These include Generalized Estimating Equations[20] and the extended Cox model,[28] with new methods being developed almost yearly. These methods to cannot be adequately described within the scope of this chapter. The reader should consult an experienced statistician when evaluating data of this nature.

SAMPLE SIZE

Several factors affect the number of patients needed to determine whether two prosthetic designs as study variables are statistically different. The nature of the end point directly affects the sample size. It usually takes far fewer patients to identify a difference in clinical function, such as hip score, than to identify a difference in implant failure, primarily because failure is much less common. It takes many patients to accrue enough failures for a difference to be detected.

The size of the difference that one would like to detect if, in fact, it should exist, also influences the sample size. Large differences are easier to detect than small differences. The smallest difference that would be clinically important is the ideal choice for most studies, but this can be a highly subjective and difficult concept on which to agree.

Another factor that affects sample size is how sure one wants to be of detecting the difference that may exist. This probability is typically set at 80 percent or 90 per-

cent and is called the *power* of the test. It is prudent to set the power of the test as high as economically possible.

Sample size is also affected by completeness of follow-up. The effective sample size is dramatically decreased and the power of the study is adversely affected when many patients are lost to follow-up early after surgery.

References

1. Berkson J, Gage RP: Calculation of survival rates for cancer. Proc Staff Meet Mayo Clin 25:270, 1950.
2. Berra Y: The Yogi Book. New York, Workman Publishing, 1998, p 95.
3. Cox DR: Regression models and life-table (with discussion). J R Stat Soc Serv B 34:187, 1972.
4. Dixon WJ, Massey FJ Jr: Introduction to Statistical Analysis, 3rd ed. New York, McGraw-Hill, 1969, p 98.
5. Dixon WJ, Massey FJ Jr: Introduction to Statistical Analysis, 3rd ed. New York, McGraw-Hill, 1969, p 116.
6. Dixon WJ, Massey FJ Jr: Introduction to Statistical Analysis, 3rd ed. New York, McGraw-Hill, 1969, p 150.
7. Dixon WJ, Massey FJ Jr: Introduction to Statistical Analysis, 3rd ed. New York, McGraw-Hill, 1969, p 212.
8. Dixon WJ, Massey FJ Jr: Introduction to Statistical Analysis, 3rd ed. New York, McGraw-Hill, 1969, p 237.
9. Dixon WJ, Massey FJ Jr: Introduction to Statistical Analysis, 3rd ed. New York, McGraw-Hill, 1969, p 335.
10. Dixon WJ, Massey FJ Jr: Introduction to Statistical Analysis, 3rd ed. New York, McGraw-Hill, 1969, p 341.
11. Dixon WJ, Massey FJ Jr: Introduction to Statistical Analysis, 3rd ed. New York, McGraw-Hill, 1969, p 344.
12. Dobbs HS: Survivorship of total hip replacement. J Bone Joint Surg 62B:168, 1980.
13. Dorey FJ, Amstutz HC: Survivorship analysis in the evaluation of joint replacement. J Arthroplasty 1:63, 1986.
14. Dorey FJ, Amstutz HC: Validity of survivorship analysis in total joint arthroplasty. Presented at the 56th Annual Meeting of the American Academy of Orthopaedic Surgeons, 1989.
15. Harrell FE, Lee KL, Califf RM, et al: Regression modeling strategies for improved prognostic prediction. Stat Med 3:143, 1984.
16. Kaplan EL, Meier P: Nonparametric estimation from incomplete observations. J Am Stat Assoc 53:457, 1958.
17. Lakhanpal S, Bunch T, Ilstrup D, Melton LJ III: Polymyositis-dermatomyositis and malignant lesions: Does an association exist? Mayo Clin Proc 61:645, 1986.
18. Lee ET: Statistical Methods for Survival Data Analysis. Belmont, CA, Lifetime Learning Publications, 1980, p 12.
19. Lee ET: Statistical Methods for Survival Data Analysis. Belmont, CA, Lifetime Learning Publications, 1980, p 131.
20. Liang KY, Zegar SL: Longitudinal data analysis using generalized linear models. Biometrika 73:13, 1986.
21. McGrory BJ, Morrey BF, Rand JA, Ilstrup DM: Correlation of patient questionnaire responses and physician history in grading clinical outcome following hip and knee arthroplasty: A prospective study of 201 joint arthroplasties. J Arthroplasty 11:47, 1996.
22. Melton LJ, Stauffer RN, Chao EYS, Ilstrup DM: Rate of total hip arthroplasty: A population based study. N Engl J Med 307:1242, 1982.
23. Morrey BF, Ilstrup DM: Size of the femoral head and acetabular revision in total hip replacement arthroplasty. J Bone Joint Surg 71A:50, 1989.
24. Moses LE, Emerson JD, Hosseini H: Analyzing data from ordered categories. N Engl J Med 311:442, 1984.
25. Papagelopoulous PJ, Kitaoka HB, Ilstrup DM: Survivorship analysis of implant arthroplasty for the first metatarsophalangeal joint. Clin Orthop 302:164, 1994.
26. Peto R, Peto J: Asymptotically efficient rank invariant procedure [with discussion]. J R Stat Soc Serv A 135:185, 1972.
27. Senghas RE: Statistics in the Journal of Bone and Joint Surgery: Suggestions for authors [editorial]. J Bone Joint Surg 74A:319, 1992.
28. Therneau TM, Grambsch PM: Modeling Survival Data: Extending the Cox model. New York, Springer-Verlag, 2000, p 169.

II

The Hand and Wrist

WILLIAM P. COONEY III • SECTION EDITOR

16
Anatomy and Surgical Approaches

• ALLEN T. BISHOP

GENERAL CONCEPTS

Arthroplasty of the wrist and hand requires a clear understanding of the functional and surgical anatomy of the hand in order to avoid injury to nerve and vascular structures, maintain tendon gliding, and preserve, as far as possible, the delicate balance of intrinsic and extrinsic forces. An ideal surgical incision should provide wide exposure of the involved joint, minimal risk of disabling scar and joint contracture, safe passage between cutaneous nerves, and the ability to be extended, if necessary.[12,16,22,29,32] Incisions should be placed along Langer's lines when possible (Fig. 16–1) and, in general, avoid crossing perpendicular to joint flexion creases.[6] Prolonged transverse incisions on the dorsum of the hand increase the risk of sensory neuropathy and may lead to edema and stiffness of digits. Exposure is generally more limited through a transverse approach, although the axis of the skin incision does not dictate the orientation of deeper dissection. Dorsally, subcutaneous veins are preserved as far as possible. Sharply angled incisions should be avoided on the dorsal side of the hand, where blood supply may be tenuous. Meticulous hemostasis during the initial dissection and before closure is imperative to avoid potentially serious complications of a hematoma. Placement of a subcutaneous drain is generally desirable, and a compressive bulky postoperative dressing is essential.

WRIST ARTHROPLASTY

Surgical Anatomy

The dorsal skin of the wrist and hand is loose and consists of fatty and fibrous layers which are embedded the cutaneous nerves and the majority of the venous and lymphatic vessels that drain the hand.[18] Typically, the cutaneous innervation of the dorsum of the hand is supplied by terminal branches of the superficial radial nerve and the dorsal sensory branch of the ulnar nerve (Fig. 16–2). However, considerable variability is the rule.[15,29] The lateral antebrachial cutaneous nerve may partially or completely overlap the terminal radial sensory fibers in 75 percent of specimens, as well as supply the radial aspect of the wrist and the base of the thumb palmar to the radial nerve.[24] The superficial radial nerve usually divides into five dorsal digital branches, supplying skin from the lateral thenar eminence to the fourth web space and the dorsum of the thumb, index, and middle fingers, as well as a portion of the ring finger. The dorsal sensory branch of the ulnar nerve passes from beneath the flexor carpi ulnaris to extend medially and dorsally onto the hand invested by superficial fascia. It then dividing into branches to the dorsal aspects of the middle, ring, and small fingers. The dorsal sensory branch is most vulnerable to trauma during a surgical exposure of the dorsal ulnocarpal area.

Dorsal Wrist Anatomy

Extensor Compartments

The extensor retinaculum (Fig. 16–3), 2 to 3 cm wide, is divided into six dorsal compartments by fibrous septa that attach to the periosteum of the underlying distal radius (Fig. 16–4). It originates on the radial side of the forearm from a bony attachment on the distal radius and from the transverse carpal ligament. Ulnarly, the retinaculum attaches to the triquetrum, pisiform, and transverse carpal ligament.

The first dorsal compartment, containing the abductor pollicis longus (APL) and the extensor pollicis brevis (EPB), frequently has an additional septum separating these two tendons. The EPB forms the radial-lateral boundary of the anatomic snuffbox.

The second compartment contains the radial wrist extensors, which are crossed superficially at the distal portion of the retinaculum by the tendon of the third compartment, the EPL. The EPL uses the radial (Lister) tubercle as a pulley, passing obliquely across the dorsum of the hand to the thumb to define the ulnar border of the snuffbox.

In the fourth compartment are found the extensor indicis proprius (EIP) and extensor digitorum communis tendons (EDC). Pressure from abnormal muscle bellies or ganglia in the fourth compartment may cause posterior interosseous nerve compresson.[14] The common extensor to the small finger is frequently absent or

141

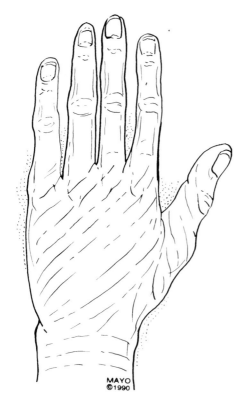

Figure 16–1. The distribution of Langer's lines on the dorsum of the hand.

very small.[28] The EIP lies deep to the EDC common extendor tendons at the wrist.

The fifth compartment contains the extensor digiti minimi, which usually consists of two or more slips. It is joined by the small finger communis tendon, if present, along the radial aspect of the small finger metacarpophalangeal (MCP) joint. Intertendinous connections, the junctura tendinum, occur most commonly between the ring finger extensor tendon and the adjoining middle and small finger extensor tendons.

The extensor carpi ulnaris (ECU) lies in the sixth dorsal compartment, within a groove on the distal aspect of the ulna. The extensor retinaculum here consists of two layers that constrain the ECU within the sixth extensor compartment. The extensor retinaculum proper is superficial, and the deeper portion (a subsheath) covers the compartment and is primarily responsible for maintaining stability of the ECU during wrist and forearm motion. The palmar floor of the sheath forms a portion of the triangular fibrocartilage complex.[26,27]

Capsule, Ligaments, and Neurovascular Structures

Deep to the extensor tendons and dorsal to the wrist capsule along the radial aspect of the fourth compartment lie the posterior interosseous nerve and artery. The nerve, which innervates the dorsal wrist capsule, ends in a ganglioform enlargement and may play a role in chronic wrist pain (Fig. 16–5).[7,9]

The dorsal wrist capsule contains capsular ligaments that are visible with retraction of the extensor tendons. These include the dorsal metacarpal and dorsal radiotriquetral ligaments. The dorsal carpal rete, formed from branches of the posterior terminal branch of the anterior interosseous artery, and the dorsal branches of the radial and ulnar arteries supply the dorsal aspect of the carpal bones (see Fig. 16–5).

Osseous Anatomy

The wrist consists of the eight carpal bones arranged in two rows, along with the five metacarpals and the forearm bones; these structures form the articulations of the wrist, together with the triangular fibrocartilage complex. They include the distal radioulnar, radiocarpal, midcarpal, and carpometacarpal joints. The distal radius has a palmar tilt of about 20 degrees and slopes ulnarward 15 to 30 degrees. A depression along its ulnar distal aspect, the sigmoid notch, forms the distal radioulnar joint, along with the head of the ulna. The carpal articular surface of the radius contains facets for articulation with the scaphoid and lunate, separated by a sagittally oriented ridge.

The distal radioulnar joint is separated from the radiocarpal joint by the articular disc (triangular fibrocartilage). The ulnar head is covered by articular cartilage over 270 degrees of its surface, including that distally beneath the triangular fibrocartilage. Stability of the distal radioulnar joint is provided by the triangular fibrocartilage complex as well as the geometry of the sigmoid notch, pronator quadratus, extensor retinaculum, and interosseous membrane. The distal radioulnar joint, in conjunction with the proximal radioulnar joint, enables forearm rotation (pronation-supination).

The triangular fibrocartilage complex, as described by Palmer and Werner, consists of the dorsal and volar radioulnar ligaments, ulnar collateral ligament, ulnocarpal meniscus homologue, volar ulnocarpal ligaments, articular disc, and ECU sheath (Fig. 16–6).[26] Strong palmar extrinsic ligaments link the carpal bones to the forearm. The dorsal and palmar portions lengthen and shorten with pronation and supination,[25] maintaining carpal stability and guiding carpal motion.

The midcarpal joint is bounded proximally by the interosseous ligaments of the proximal row and distally by the intercarpal interosseous ligaments. The trapeziotrapezoid interosseous ligament may be absent, allowing communication of the midcarpal and carpometacarpal joints. The carpometacarpal joints of the index, middle, ring, and small finger rays share a common joint capsule. Mobility is limited at the index and long carpometacarpal joints, but flexion and rotation of the ulnar digit rays up to 30 degrees can occur. This enables adjustment of the distal transverse arch to accommodate varied objects and tasks. Dorsal and volar carpometacarpal ligaments unite the distal row with the finger metacarpals of which the volar ligaments are the strongest.

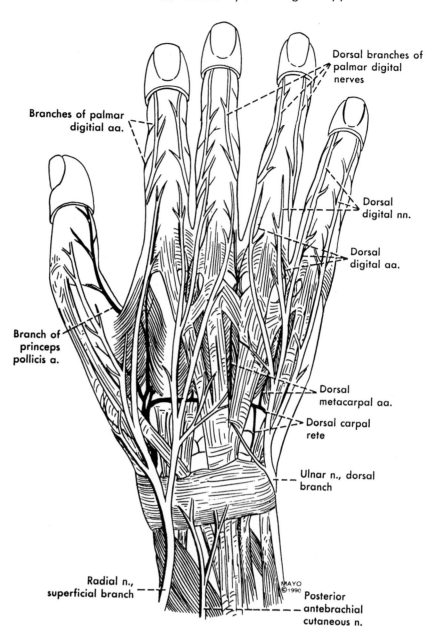

Branches of palmar digitial aa.

Dorsal branches of palmar digital nerves

Dorsal digital nn.

Dorsal digital aa.

Branch of princeps pollicis a.

Dorsal metacarpal aa.

Dorsal carpal rete

Ulnar n., dorsal branch

Radial n., superficial branch

Posterior antebrachial cutaneous n.

MAYO ©1990

Figure 16–2. The dorsum of the hand, demonstrating the distribution of cutaneous nerves.

Wrist Exposure

A dorsal approach to the wrist is used for soft tissue arthroplasty, total wrist arthroplasty, scaphoid excision and need carpal fusion, lunate excision and replacement, and proximal row carpectomy.[3,4,31] Surgical landmarks include Lister's tubercle, as well as the radial and ulnar styloid processes (Fig. 16–7). With the patient supine, a straight longitudinal incision is made over the mid-dorsum of the wrist. This is, in general, preferred to curvilinear incisions because of fewer skin problems. Narrow, acutely angled flaps should be avoided on the dorsum of the hand. The dissection is carried through the superficial fascia without undermining the skin or subcutaneous fatty layer to preserve dorsal skin blood supply and protect cutaneous nerves. The extensor retinaculum is thus exposed by elevation of medial and lateral skin flaps.

A variety of incisions to elevate the extensor retinaculum may be used, as shown in Figure 16-8, creating radial- and ulnar-based flaps of extensor retinaculum (see Fig. 16–8). Opening the third dorsal compartment is a utilitarian approach and is preferred for wrist replacement.[30] The wrist extensor tendons are retracted radially and the finger extensors ulnarly, and the posterior interosseous nerve is resected on the floor of the fourth compartment. Capsulotomy of the radiocarpal joint is then performed, reflecting the capsuloligamentous structures from the radius as an inverted T or a broad, distally based rectangular flap (Fig. 16–9). When the arthroplasty has been completed, the wound is closed in layers over a suction drain with capsular, retinacular, subcuticular, and cutaneous sutures placed after tourniquet release.

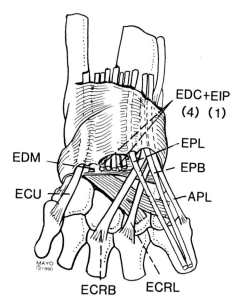

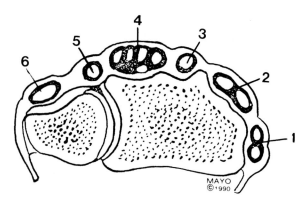

Figure 16–4. Cross-section of the distal forearm showing compartmentalization of the extensor tendons beneath the retinaculum.

Figure 16–3. The dorsum of the hand, demonstrating the extensor retinaculum and the extrinsic extensor tendons.

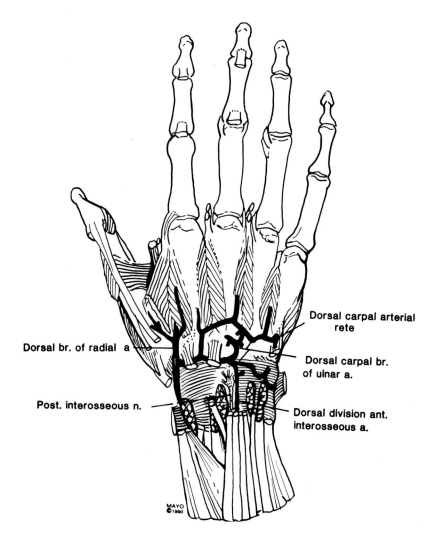

Figure 16–5. Dorsal wrist capsule, demonstrating the dorsal blood supply, posterior interosseous nerve, and dorsal wrist ligaments.

Dorsal carpal arterial rete

Dorsal br. of radial a

Dorsal carpal br. of ulnar a.

Post. interosseous n.

Dorsal division ant. interosseous a.

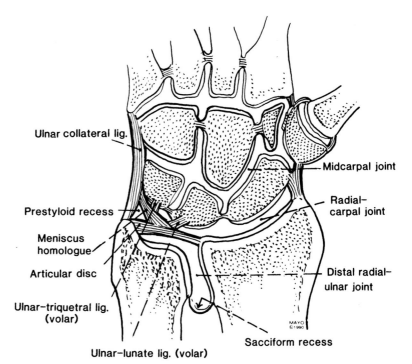

Figure 16–6. The triangular fibrocartilage complex.

ARTHROPLASTY IN THE HAND

Surgical Anatomy: Fingers

Each digit is normally composed of three phalanges and one metacarpal, and three joints (metacarpophalangeal, proximal interphalangeal, and distal interphalangeal). This chain of articulating segments is stabilized and controlled by a complex arrangement of intrinsic and extrinsic musculature as well as retinacular structures, allowing independent flexion and extension of the individual joints while preventing collapse of the intercalated middle segment.[19,20,23]

The MCP joints are multiaxial condyloid joints that permit flexion, extension, abduction and adduction, and slight axial rotation. Strong collateral ligaments maintain

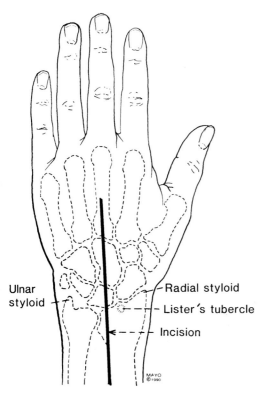

Figure 16–7. Dorsal wrist incision.

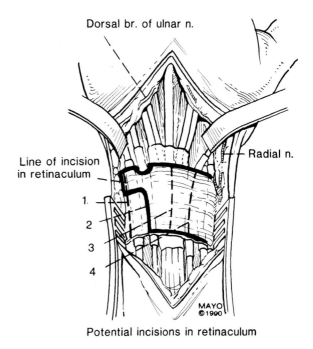

Figure 16–8. Commonly used retinacular incisions.

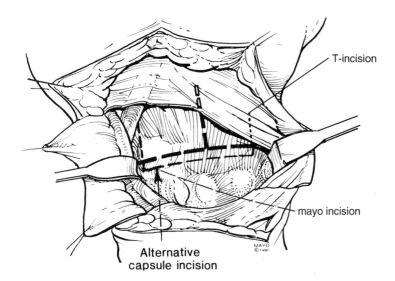

Figure 16–9. Dorsal wrist capsulotomy.

stability of the joint in flexion yet allow radial and ulnar deviation in extension.[2,19] The ligaments are oriented in a dorsal proximal-to-volar distal direction, originating in the lateral recesses of the metacarpal heads and attaching to the bases of the proximal phalanges (Fig. 16–10). Accessory collateral ligaments attach to the lateral margin of the stout volar plate, as does the deep transverse metacarpal ligament. The dorsal joint capsule, conversely, is thin and does not restrict motion. It is protected by the overlying extensor tendon and the sagittal band, which provide dorsal joint support and dynamic stability during grasp.

The collateral ligaments are tight in flexion but lax in extension, allowing some abduction and rotation. Motion at the MCP joint is a complex interaction between intrinsic and extrinsic flexors, all with a flexion moment, and the extrinsic extensors, which extend the joint via the extensor hood attachments to the joint capsule. The interphalangeal joints, in contrast, are ginglymoid (hinge) joints, without significant motion other than flexion-extension. The ligamentous constraints are identical in configuration to the MCP joint but, because of differences in the instantaneous center of rotation, are taut in all positions. The dorsal joint capsule is indistinguishable from the central slip of the extensor mechanism, with both inserting onto the proximal dorsal aspect of the middle phalanx. The volar plate of the proximal interphalangeal (PIP) joint has a strong distal attachment and a looser, meniscus-like arrangement

proximally, with a loose central attachment and strong lateral attachments.

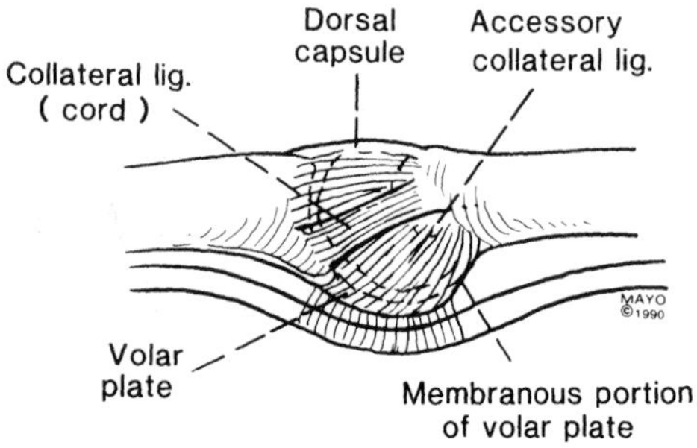

The extensor mechanism (Fig. 16–11) receives contributions from the dorsal and/or palmar interossei, the lumbricals, and the extrinsic extensor tendons (extensor digitorum communis and proprius tendons of the index and small fingers).[10,24] At the level of the MCP joint, it forms an expansion covering the metacarpal head. Sagittally directed fibers attach to the deep transverse intermetacarpal ligaments, constraining the extensor mechanism at the MCP joint and enabling MCP joint extension. More distally, the expanding extrinsic tendon fibers intermingle with the aponeurotic expansion of the interosseous and lumbrical tendons to form an elegantly balanced system that flexes the MCP joint and extends the PIP joint. Loose connections of the extrinsic tendons to the dorsal capsule are usually identifiable at the MCP joint. Over the proximal phalanx, the extensor mechanism narrows. Intertendinous laminae blend in a complex fashion, ultimately forming a central band that attaches to the base of the middle phalanx and two lateral bands that converge over the middle phalanx to form the terminal tendon at the distal interphalangeal (DIP) joint. The lateral bands are stabilized by the triangular ligament dorsally, preventing excessive lateral and palmar subluxation with flexion, and by the transverse retinacular ligament laterally, limiting excessive dorsal translation of the lateral bands with extension of the PIP joint.

The palmar digital arteries and nerves lie on either side of the fibro-osseous tunnel of the flexor tendons.[17] At the level of the PIP, the sheath has a thin annular pulley (A_3) and two associated cruciform pulleys (C_1 and C_2) (Fig. 16–12). Exposure of the PIP joint from a volar approach requires release of the A_3 pulley and retraction of the flexor tendons.

Surgical Anatomy: Thumb

A detailed study of articular "mismatch" failed to demonstrate this as an explanation of the high evidence

Collateral lig. (cord)   Dorsal capsule   Accessory collateral lig.

Volar plate   Membranous portion of volar plate

Figure 16–10. MCP joint, sagittal view.

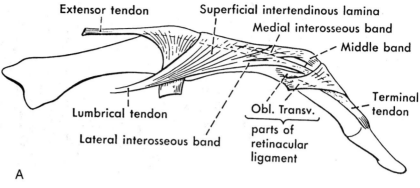

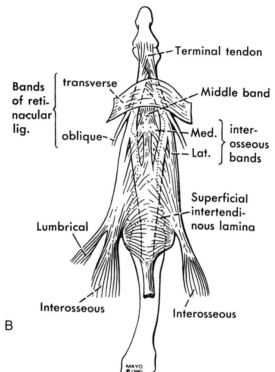

Figure 16–11. Dorsal (**A**) and lateral (**B**) views of the extensor mechanism.

of arthrosis of this joint.[1] The carpometacarpal (trapeziometacarpal) joint is a saddle-shaped or universal joint. The trapezium provides a saddle-shaped distal articular surface that fits congruently with the reciprocal surface of the first metacarpal base. A tubercle or rest provides attachment for the transverse carpal ligament, and a groove on the medial anterior surface accommodates the flexor carpi radialis. The carpometacarpal joint motion is controlled by the articular surfaces and capsular ligamentous constraints, including anterior and posterior oblique and intermetacarpal ligaments (Fig. 16–13).[13] The intermetacarpal ligaments provide the greatest constraint to radial and dorsal joint subluxation. The joint capsule is covered palmarly by the thenar musculature and dorsoradially by the tendons of the abductor pollicis brevis and the short and long thumb extensors.[11] The radial artery passes in proximity to the joint dorsally as it lies in the anatomic snuffbox (Fig. 16–14). Branches of the radial sensory, lateral antebrachial cutaneous, and palmar cutaneous branch of the median nerves provide cutaneous sensibility to the area.

The MCP joint of the thumb differs from those of the other digits. In many hands, its head is flattened and its arc of motion limited (average 75 degrees).[8] The metacarpal head articulates with the base of the proximal phalanx as well as the medial and lateral sesamoids (Fig. 16–15). The volar plate receives attachments from the transverse portion of the adductor pollicis tendon ulnarly and flexor pollicis brevis tendon radially. The proper collateral ligaments maintain stability in radial and ulnar deviation. Rotation is restricted by the accessory collateral ligaments. Dorsally, two extrinsic extensors cross the joint, receiving contributions from the adductor and abductor pollicis brevis to form the terminal extensor mechanism.

Metacarpophalangeal Joint Exposure

The MCP joints of the fingers may be approached either through individual longitudinal incisions centered over the metacarpal head or by a single transverse incision.

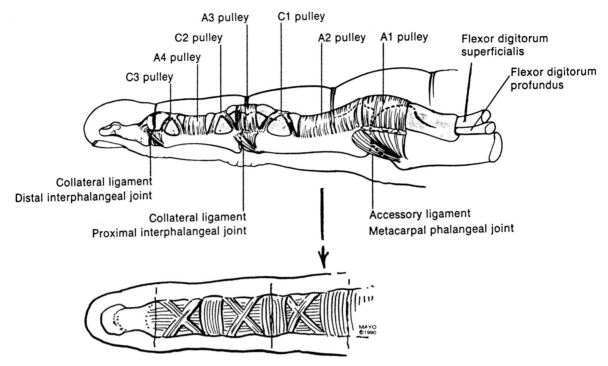

Figure 16–12. Relationship of the PIP joint to the flexor tendon sheath structures.

Occasionally, a pair of longitudinal incisions centered over the second and fourth intermetacarpal spaces may be considered (Fig. 16–16). If the latter two incisions are used, care must be taken not to injure the dorsal neurovascular structures in the intermetacarpal spaces. For procedures on multiple MCP joints, a transverse incision is generally preferred for MCP joint reconstruction;

individual longitudinal incisions provide more latitude when both MCP and PIP exposure is included. After the skin incisions are made, the underlying extensor mechanism is visualized and incised on the ulnar side of the extensor tendon (for the middle and ring fingers) or between the communis and proprius tendons (for the index and small fingers) (Fig. 16–17).

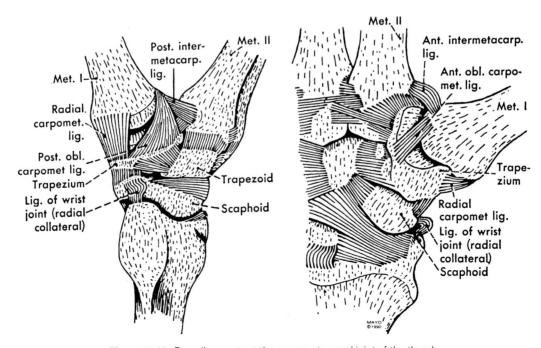

Figure 16–13. Deep ligaments at the carpometacarpal joint of the thumb.

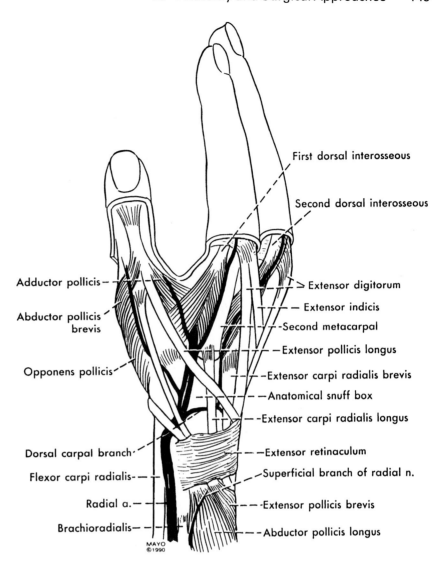

Figure 16–14. The anatomic snuffbox.

When significant ulnar drift deformity is present at the MCP joint, some surgeons prefer a radial incision through the extensor hood, partial ulnar release, centralization of the extensor tendon, and imbrication of a radial-based sagittal band flap to prevent recurrence of ulna extensor tendon displacement.[5] Careful division of the extensor mechanism preserves the dorsal joint capsule, which is then opened as a separate layer to allow exposure of the joint for arthroplasty. Release of the proper collateral ligaments from the metacarpal head origin is usually necessary for adequate exposure. With closure, they are reapproximated, often with proximal and dorsal advancement on the radial side to correct ulnar deviation and digit pronation.

Thumb Metacarpophalangeal Exposure

The thumb MCP joint is approached dorsally with a longitudinal or gently curvilinear incision (Fig. 16–18). The interval between the EPL and EPB is identified and opened, if necessary, detaching the EPB from its proximal phalanx insertion (Fig. 16–19). The joint is opened and synovectomy performed as needed before arthroplasty.[21]

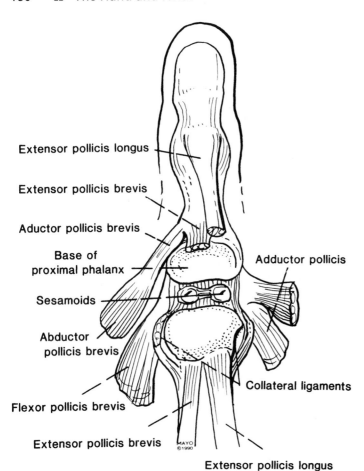

Extensor pollicis longus

Extensor pollicis brevis

Aductor pollicis brevis

Base of
proximal phalanx

Sesamoids

Abductor
pollicis brevis

Flexor pollicis brevis

Extensor pollicis brevis

Adductor pollicis

Collateral ligaments

Extensor pollicis longus

Figure 16–15. View of the volar surface, right thumb MCP joint.

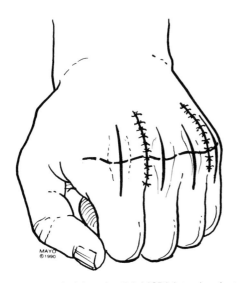

Figure 16–16. Incisions for digit MCP joint arthroplasty.

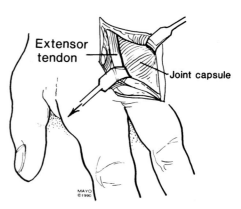

Extensor
tendon

Joint capsule

Figure 16–17. Incision of the extensor hood.

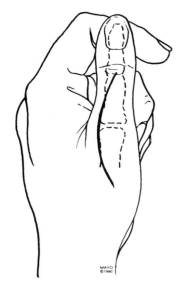

Figure 16–18. Exposure of the thumb MCP joint.

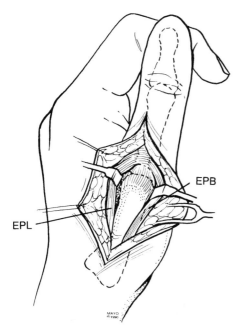

Figure 16–19. The interval between the EPL and EPB.

References

1. Athanasiou KA, Liu GT, Lavery LA, et al: Biomechanical topography of human articular cartilage in the first metatarsophalangeal joint. Clin Orthop 348:269, 1998.
2. Backhouse KM: The mechanics of normal digital control in the hand and an analysis of the ulnar drift of rheumatoid arthritis. J R Coll Surg Engl 43:154, 1968.
3. Beckenbaugh RD, Linscheid RL: Arthroplasty in the hand and wrist. In Green DP (ed): Operative Hand Surgery, 2nd ed. New York, Churchill Livingstone, 1988, p 167.
4. Birch R, Brooks D: The hand. In Dudly H, Carter DC (eds): Rob and Smith's Operative Surgery, 4th ed. St. Louis, CV Mosby, 1989.
5. Blatt G: Capsulodesis in reconstructive hand surgery. Hand Clin 3:81, 1987.
6. Bruner JM: Incisions for plastic and reconstructive (non-septive) surgery of the hand. Br J Plast Reconstr Surg 4:48, 1952.
7. Carr D, Davis P: Distal posterior interosseous syndrome. J Hand Surg 10A:873, 1985.
8. Coonrad RW, Goldman JL: A study of the pathological findings and treatment in soft tissue injury of the thumb metacarpophalangeal joint; with a clinical study of the normal range of motion findings of ligamentous structures in relation to function. J Bone Joint Surg 50A:439, 1968.
9. Dellon AL: Partial dorsal wrist denervation: Resection of the distal posterior interosseous nerve. J Hand Surg 10A:527, 1985.
10. Eyler DL, Markee JE: The anatomy and function of the intrinsic musculature of the fingers. J Bone Joint Surg 36A:1, 1954.
11. Fahrer M, Tubiana R: Palmaris longus: Anteductor of the thumb. Hand 8:287, 1976.
12. Fleeger EJ: Skin tumors. In Green DP (ed): Operative Hand Surgery, 2nd ed. New York, Churchill Livingstone, 1988, p 2323.
13. Haines RW: The mechanism of rotation of the first carpometacarpal joint. J Anat 78:44, 1944.
14. Hayashi H, Kojima T, Fukumoto K: The fourth-compartment syndrome: Its anatomical basis and clinical cases. Handchir Mikrochir Plast Chir 31:61, 1999.
15. Hollinshead WH: Anatomy for Surgeons: The Back and Limbs, vol III. Philadelphia, Harper & Row, 1982, p 226.
16. Hoppenfeld S, DeBoer P: Surgical exposures in orthopaedics: The anatomic approach. Philadelphia, JB Lippincott, 1984.
17. Kaplan EB: Embryological development of the tendinous apparatus of the fingers: Relationship to function. J Bone Joint Surg 32A:820, 1950.
18. Kuhlmann N, Meyer-Otetea G: Nerfs cutanées palmaires et voie d'abord de le face antérieure du poignet et de la paume. Ann Chir 30:859, 1976.
19. Landsmeer JMF: Anatomical and functional investigations of the articulations of the human fingers. Acta Anat (Basel) 25(Suppl):5, 1955.
20. Landsmeer JMF: The coordination of finger-joint motions. J Bone Joint Surg 45A:1654, 1963.
21. Lipscomb PR: Synovectomy of the distal two joints of the thumb and fingers in rheumatoid arthritis. J Bone Joint Surg 49A:1135, 1967.
22. Littler JW: Hand, wrist and forearm incisions. In Littler JW, Cramer LM, Smith JW (eds): Symposium on Reconstructive Hand Surgery. St. Louis, CV Mosby, 1974, p 89.
23. Long C, Brown ME: Electromyographic kinesiology of the hand: Muscles moving the long finger. J Bone Joint Surg 46A:1683, 1964.
24. Mackinnon SE, Dellon AL: The overlap pattern of the lateral antebrachial cutaneous nerve and superficial branch of the radial nerve. J Hand Surg 10A:522, 1985.
25. Nakamura T, Makita A: The proximal ligamentous component of the triangular fibrocartilage complex. J Hand Surg 25B:479, 2000.
26. Palmer AK, Werner FW: The triangular fibrocartilage complex of the wrist Banatomy and function. J Hand Surg 6:153, 1981.
27. Palmer AK, Werner FW: Biomechanics of the distal radioulnar joint. Clin Orthop 187:26, 1984.
28. Schenck RR: Variations of the extensor tendons of the fingers: Surgical significance. J Bone Joint Surg 46A:103, 1964.
29. Spinner M (ed): Kaplan's Functional and Surgical Anatomy of the Hand, 3rd ed. Philadelphia, JB Lippincott, 1984.
30. Swanson AB, Swanson GD: Flexible implant resection arthroplasty in the upper extremity. In Tubiana R (ed): The Hand, vol II. Philadelphia, WB Saunders, 1985, p 576.
31. Taleisnik J: The Wrist. New York, Churchill Livingstone, 1985.
32. Tubiana R: Surgical exposure and skin courage. In Tubiana R (ed): The Hand, vol II. Philadelphia, WB Saunders, 1985.

17

Practical Biomechanics

• KAI-NAN AN and WILLIAM P. COONEY III

Prosthetic joint replacement has been used for the treatment of hands impaired by rheumatoid arthritis, degenerative joint disease, and traumatic arthroses. However, the design and implementation of prosthetic replacements for the joints of the hand have been difficult because of the complexity of the anatomy and function of the human hand. Various criteria for the successful design of implants have been suggested by numerous investigators, including that the implant should restore the functional range of motion of the finger and thumb joints and provide sufficient functional strength with adequate joint stability. The long-term stability of the implant fixation and joint articulating surfaces is also important.

Based on biomechanical and functional analyses of the normal hand, information and improvements in implant design for the hand can be developed. In this chapter, several important biomechanical observations regarding the motion, force transmission, and joint constraints of the normal human hand are presented, and a comparison of a few finger joint implants currently available is discussed.

FUNCTIONAL ANATOMY

The human hand is a three-dimensional structure. From a biomechanical standpoint, the hand could be considered as a linkage system of intercalated bony segments balanced by muscle and tendon forces and joint constraints.

Skeletal Dimensions

The hand is relatively mobile and capable of conforming to the shape of objects to be manipulated. The mobility of the structure is possible through the unique arrangement and dimensions of its 27 bones. The ratios of the 19 metacarpal and phalangeal long bones closely follow a Fibonacci sequence.[11] Motion of the fingers from extension into flexion to the palm follows a "spiral nautilus" sequence similar to the reciprocal spiral coverage of a seashell or the tail of a lobster. Distances between the joint centers and joint articular surfaces of the five rays (Fig. 17–1A) provide the base-

line information of the longitudinal dimensions that must be restored by the joint replacement procedures. In the normal hand, the long shaft of the phalanges distal to the metacarpophalangeal (MCP) joints is more or less colinear. However, the longitudinal axis of the proximal phalanges is inclined ulnarly to the metacarpal axis[20] approximately 15 degrees for the index finger, 13 degrees for the middle finger, 0 degrees for the ring finger, and 7 degrees for the little finger (see Fig. 17–1B).

In terms of the cross-sectional geometry and dimensions of the long bones, however, there have been only a limited number of studies.[10,16]

The geometric shape of the joint articular surfaces is also important in the consideration of implant design. Sagittal contours of the metacarpal head and proximal phalanx grossly resemble the arc of a circle.[19] The radius of curvature of a circle fitted to the entire proximal phalangeal surface ranges from 11 to 13 mm, almost two times as large as that of the metacarpal head, which ranges from 6 to 7 mm (Fig. 17–2A). As a result, the local centers of curvature along the sagittal contour of the metacarpal heads are not fixed as a hinge joint but are rather polycentric to reflect the changing diameter and constraint of the proximal phalanx articulating on the metacarpal head. The locus of the center of curvature for the subchondral bony contour approximates the locus of the center for the acute curve of an ellipse. In contrast, the locus of the center of curvature for the articular cartilage contour approximates the locus of the obtuse curve of an ellipse (see Fig. 17–2B).

Physiologic and Mechanical Parameters of Hand Muscle

With contraction of the muscles, the joints of the hand move in a characteristic manner constrained by the interposing soft tissues and shape of the joint. Movement and balance of the hand are achieved by groups of extrinsic and intrinsic muscles. Biomechanically, there are several important parameters to describe the potential functions of each individual muscle (Tables 17–1 and 17–2).

The size and shape of the hand muscle can be described based on the fiber length, volume, and

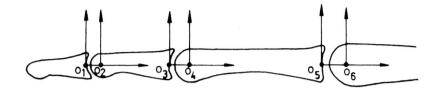

Distances Between Coordinate Systems
(mean and standard deviations)

	O_1O_2	O_2O_3	O_3O_4	O_4O_5	O_5O_6
Thumb	0.243 ± 0.035	1.0 ± 0	0.338 ± 0.042	1.424 ± 0.097	0.333 ± 0.047
Index	0.224 ± 0.034	1.0 ± 0	0.288 ± 0.036	1.919 ± 0.227	0.432 ± 0.058
Middle	0.184 ± 0.032	1.0 ± 0	0.233 ± 0.041	1.608 ± 0.087	0.365 ± 0.052
Ring	0.166 ± 0.031	1.0 ± 0	0.224 ± 0.041	1.576 ± 0.068	0.346 ± 0.030
Little	0.230 ± 0.042	1.0 ± 0	0.304 ± 0.046	1.797 ± 0.145	0.506 ± 0.082

A

Figure 17–1. A, Distances between the joint centers and joint articular surfaces of the five rays. **B,** Physiologic angles between the different skeletal structures of the hand. (**B,** From Tubiana R: The Hand. Philadelphia, WB Saunders, 1981.)

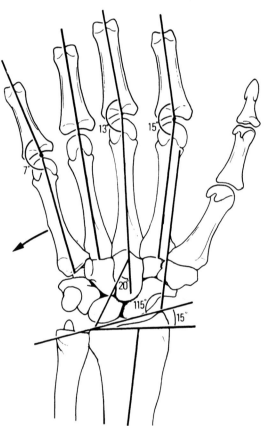

B

physiologic cross-sectional area (PCSA) of the muscle.[2,4] The length of the muscle fiber dictates the potential excursion of the muscle and associated tendon within a specific physiologic range. The PSCA is proportional to the potential tension (force) that could be generated by the muscle. Finally, the muscle volume represents the potential work that can be created by the muscle. For example, the first dorsal interosseous, a small intrinsic hand muscle, has a relatively small muscle volume and shorter mean fiber length but an equivalent PCSA compared with extrinsic muscles in the forearm, which have a large muscle volume and long mean fiber length. Any prosthetic design for finger or thumb joints must take into

consideration the potential forces that these muscle units transmit during pinch, prehensile grip, or power grip.

The efficiency of the muscles and tendons to move or balance a joint depends on the geometric relationship of the soft tissues spanning the joint. Biomechanically, these characteristics could be described by the orientation of the line of action and the moment arms of the tendons and muscles with reference to the joint coordinate systems. In general, the muscle functions three dimensionally at the joint. However, the extrinsic muscles of the hand pass adjacent to the finger and thumb joints, quite symmetrically dorsal and palmar to the shaft of the long bone. As a result, their functions are

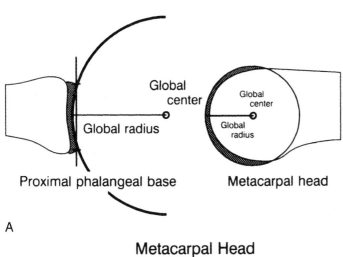

A

Metacarpal Head

B

Local center of bony contour

Local center of cartilage contour

Figure 17–2. A, Global centers of curvature of the MCP joint and proximal phalangeal[20] base were determined in each slice by use of the least-squares circle, fitted to the entire cartilage-covered area. The radius of curvature of the proximal phalangeal base is about twice as large as that of the metacarpal head. **B,** Loci of the local center of curvature for subchondral bony contour of the metacarpal head approximate the loci of the center for the acute curve of an ellipse. The loci of the local center of curvature for articular cartilage contour of the metacarpal head approximate the loci of the bony center of the obtuse curve of an ellipse.

Table 17–1. PHYSIOLOGIC AND MECHANICAL PARAMETERS OF THE INTRINSIC AND EXTRINSIC MUSCLES OF THE INDEX FINGER

| | | | | Moment Arm* | |
| | Muscle Volume (cm³) | Fiber Length (cm) | Muscle PCSA (cm²) | Flexion-Extension (cm) | Abduction-Adduction (cm) |
Muscle					
Dorsal interosseous	9.5	2.3	4.16	+0.37	−0.61
Volar interosseous	2.5	1.7	1.40	+0.66	+0.58
Lumbrical	1.7	4.7	0.36	+0.93	−0.48
Flexor profundus	27.6	6.7	4.10	+1.11	+0.11
Flexor sublimis	15.1	4.2	3.65	+1.19	+0.17
Extensor indicis	6.9	4.9	1.30	−0.9	+0.13
Extensor communis	6.5	6.1	1.1	−0.86	−0.02

*+ = flexion; − = extension; + = aduction; − = abduction; PCSA = physiologic cross-sectional area.

Table 17–2. PHYSIOLOGIC AND MECHANICAL PARAMETERS OF THE WRIST MUSCLES

| | | | | Moment Arm* | |
| | Muscle Volume (cm³) | Fiber Length (cm) | Muscle PCSA (cm²) | Flexion-Extension (cm) | Abduction-Adduction (cm) |
Muscle					
Flexor carpi radialis	11.6	5.5	2.0	+15	−8
Flexor carpi ulnaris	15.3	4.5	3.3	+16	+14
Extensor carpi radialis brevis	14.8	5.5	2.8	−12	−13
Extensor carpi radialis longus	15.1	8.5	2.0	−7	−19
Extensor carpi ulnaris	14.3	4.8	3.0	−6	+17

*+ = flexion; − = extension; + = ulnar deviation; − = radial deviation.

primarily flexion and extension and rarely abduction, adduction, or rotation. The intrinsic muscles, in comparison, approach the joints from the side and are responsible for most lateral movement, producing rotation and balancing the extrinsic flexor and extensor muscles. Restoration of the line of action and, ultimately, the ratio of the magnitude of the moment arm between flexion and extension or between abduction and adduction is of paramount importance. Otherwise, either normal hand function is not achieved or abnormal joint force is encountered, which is detrimental to the prosthetic implant.

MOTION

Global Range of Motion

Within the physiologic range of motion, the interphalangeal joints can be considered as hinge joints, providing flexion and extension motion. In the normal hand, each interphalangeal joint has between 60 (distal) and 110 (proximal) degrees of motion. The MCP joints are considered universal joints that provide not only flexion-extension motion (70 to 80 degrees) but also limited amounts of abduction-adduction motion (20 to 30 degrees) depending on the flexion-extension stance. There is greater abduction-adduction in MCP extension than in flexion as a result of the concentric shape of the MCP head, which tightens the collateral ligaments in flexion. The amount of abduction and adduction decreases with finger and thumb flexion. More precisely, the MCP joints of both the thumb and fingers as well as the carpometacarpal joint (CMC) of the thumb have the potential of three degrees of freedom in rotation. This particular point is further illustrated later in the section dealing with joint laxity and constraint.

Mathematically, the Eulerian angle concept has been adopted for description of the three-dimensional rotation of these two joints. The associated orientation angles of the index finger and thumb involved in pinch-and-grasp functions are shown in Table 17–3.[5,6] Again, for the ideal design of implants, these values should be considered.

Table 17–3. JOINT ORIENTATION ANGLES IN HAND FUNCTIONS (DEGREES)*

Function	Flexion-Extension	Radial-Ulnar	Pronation-Supination
Tip pinch			
Index MCP	+45.8	+11.6	−5.9
Thumb MCP	+10.1	−0.5	+16.1
Thumb CMC	+28.0	+18.0	+19.0
Grasp			
Index MCP	+65.2	+6.7	−15.6
Thumb MCP	+35.5	+1.0	+3.6
Thumb CMC	+25.0	+10.0	+20.0

*The normal range of motion of the thumb CMC joint has been found to be 53 plus or minus 11 degrees, 21 plus or minus 4 degrees, and 17 plus or minus 10 degrees in flexion-extension, abduction-adduction, and rotation, respectively.
+ = flexion; − = extension; + = radial deviation; − = ulnar deviation;
+ = pronation; − = supination; CMC = carpometacarpal; MCP = metacarpophalangeal.

Functionally, the wrist joint has been regarded as a universal joint with two degrees of freedom in flexion-extension and radial-ulnar deviation. The maximal wrist arc of motion is 130 degrees of combined flexion and extension and 40 degrees of combined radial and ulnar deviation.[14] However, for activities of daily living, it has been found that 40 degrees of extension, 40 degrees of flexion, and a combined 40-degree radioulnar deviation provide the minimal functional range of motion for normal populations.[15]

Articular Motion

An analysis of articulating motion of joints provides not only information about the mechanism of joint lubrication and wear but also specific kinematics regarding the locus of the center rotation of the joint during movement. Data regarding the joint center(s) of rotation are paramount for optimal implant design and maintenance of muscle balance in severely deformed hands. To date, there are only a few studies that have considered the center of rotation and tendon moment arms in the hand.

For the MCP joint of the finger, one of the more common finger joints that is replaced, the instantaneous center of rotation has been studied. Some suggest a fixed center of rotation,[7] whereas a majority[17,18,21] believe that a polycentric center of rotation exists. The other difference between these two concepts relates primarily to the experimental method used for analysis of center of rotation, wherein calculation analysis is prone to experimental error. Analytically, the instantaneous center of rotation of the MCP joint has been estimated.[13] Given the fact that the geometric shapes of the articular surfaces of the metacarpal head and proximal phalanx as well as the insertion location of the collateral ligaments significantly govern the articulating kinematics, the center of rotation does not appear to be fixed but rather moves as a function of the angle of flexion. The ratio of the moment arms for flexors and extensors caused by the shift of the center of rotation differs from that based on the fixed center of rotation. Rolling and sliding actions of articulating surfaces exist during the joint motion.

The articular kinematics of the trapeziometacarpal joint of the thumb has been studied.[9] The traces of the reference points on the head and base of the first metacarpal are monitored. The circumduction motion is accomplished by loading individual intrinsic and extrinsic muscles. The positions of the reference points of the head and base of the first metacarpal lie on the elliptical paths but move in opposite directions (Fig. 17–3). This pattern coincides with the characteristics of the reciprocal saddle joint surfaces and the locations of the axis of rotation. In flexion-extension motion, the axis of rotation is located within the trapezium, and the path of the head follows the same direction as the path of the base. Conversely, in abduction-adduction motion, the axis of rotation is located distal to the trapezium within the base of the first metacarpal, and the head and base move in opposite directions. This unique pattern of movement and its relationship to the ligamentous

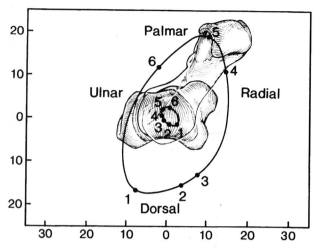

Figure 17–3. Under a loading condition of 500 g on each tendon, the positions of the base and head of the first metacarpal lay on the ellipsoid generated by circumduction (*left hand*). 1 = Extensor pollicis longus; 2 = extensor pollicis brevis; 3 = abductor pollicis longus; 4 = abductor pollicis brevis; 5 = flexor pollicis longus; 6 = adductor pollicis. (From Imaeda T, Niebur G, Cooney WP III, et al: Kinematics of the normal trapeziometacarpal joint. J Othop Res 12:197, 1994.)

constraint may predispose the joint to the early development and progression of osteoarthritis.

The wrist joint is composed of eight carpal bones and can be divided into two anatomic rows. The proximal carpal row consists of the scaphoid, lunate, triquetrum, and pisiform, and the distal row is composed of the trapezium, trapezoid, capitate, and hamate. The articular kinematics of carpal bones is complicated. In general, the tension of the wrist muscles applied to the base of the metacarpals generates motion starting at the distal carpal row. The relative intercarpal motion of the distal carpal row is slight. From full flexion to extension of the wrist, the average degrees of rotation at the hamate-capitate, capitate-trapezoid, and trapezoid-trapezium joints are between 6 and 12 degrees. The bones of the distal carpal row are considered as one functional unit. In wrist flexion, they all go into flexion and ulnar deviation. In wrist extension, the distal carpal row goes into extension and slight radial deviation. In radial deviation of the wrist, the distal carpal row goes into extension, supination, and radial deviation. In ulnar deviation of the wrist, they go into flexion, ulnar deviation, and pronation.

The bones of the proximal carpal row are less tightly bounded. In general, with wrist joint motion, the intercarpal motion could be in the range of 30 degrees on the radial side and 15 degrees on the ulnar side. In wrist flexion, the scaphoid, lunate, and triquetrum go into flexion and ulnar deviation, whereas during wrist extension they extend and radially deviate. Furthermore, the three proximal carpal bones move synergistically from a flexed position in wrist radial deviation to an extended position in wrist ulnar deviation. This flexion-extension adaptive mechanism, present in the normal wrist, allows a constant spatial congruency between the distal carpal row and the radius no matter what wrist position is adopted.[8]

FORCE

The magnitude and manner of force transmission through the joints probably are the most important pieces of information for implant design. Most of this information has been obtained through either two-dimensional or three-dimensional analytic estimation. Numerous technical difficulties are usually encountered in terms of analytic determinations of joint and muscle forces, which may affect some of the results. Nevertheless, the ranges of joint and muscle forces for the finger and thumb joints have been obtained.[1,5,6]

During tip-pinch function of 50 N of force at the tip of the index finger, for example, there are about 100, 250, and 200 N of compressive force generated at the distal interphalangeal, proximal interphalangeal (PIP), and MCP joints individually (Fig. 17–4). In addition, there are also 15, 50, and 100 N of shear force applied dorsally at the proximal ends of each phalanx of the three joints as well. A moderate amount of shear force in the radial direction at each of the joints is also encountered. Torsional forces may be even more significant. Consider the torque applied from the thumb against the index or long finger in pinch. Five kilograms of force working over 8 cm of finger length produces 40 kg-cm of torsional load. No wonder that fixed implants at the MCP joint failed by torsion, as noted by spiral fracture of polyethylene and torsional weakening of Silicone metacarpal implants, despite the effect of grommets or changes in the implant material. It should be recognized, therefore, that the magnitudes of the joint constraint forces passing through the hand joints are not trivial. In normal joints, these forces are balanced and resisted by the synergistic contribution of articular surfaces and surrounding capsuloligamentous structures. For an ideal implant design, either the implant should be strong enough to resist these constraint forces or the assistance of the

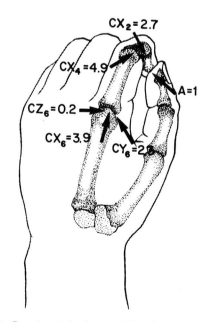

Figure 17–4. Resultant joint forces during tip-pinch function of one unit force. A = 1.

ligamentous contributions should be incorporated in the design consideration.

Moments at the wrist joint can be generated by the load applied on the hand or even on the tension of the hand extrinsic muscles. Balance of these moments by the wrist muscles creates significant amounts of compressive and shear forces at the joint. In general, with the wrist and forearm in neutral position, approximately 80 percent of the axial compressive force is transmitted through the distal radius and 20 percent through the distal ulna.[22] Wrist position affects the distribution of forces on the radius and ulna (Table 17–4). With ulna deviation or forearm pronation, there is an increase in the force transmission on the ulna. There is a corresponding decrease in the ulna force with radial deviation and forearm supination.

Dynamic forces in the tendon depend on the relative moment arms of the muscle at given joint positions. Joint replacement would disturb the nature of joint kinematics and thus the associated moment arms of the muscles. The tendon tension required to balance the wrist after joint replacement has been studied. In general, regarding both radial-ulnar deviation and flexion-extension motion, the wrist with an implant requires greater radial deviator forces and smaller or equivalent ulnar deviator forces than an intact wrist.[22]

STABILITY AND JOINT CONSTRAINT

Joint stability and constraint are provided by the joint articular surfaces, the joint capsule, the collateral ligaments, and active musculotendinous units. Primary joint stability is related to muscle and tendon response to sustained pinch and grasp forces.[3] In contrast, the ligaments and capsules appear to play the role of initial stabilizer against instantaneous joint load and provide a second line of defense in maintaining joint stability. Understanding the anatomic characteristics and function of the capsuloligamentous structure is important for proper implant design, especially for implants of the resurfacing or semiconstrained types. In fact, the ideal concept of implant design incorporates capsuloligamentous reconstruction after joint replacement. Because the load sharing is assumed by the active capsuloligamentous structure, there should be a reduction in the load and an elongated life of the "inert" implant material.

Table 17–4. PERCENT FORCE DISTRIBUTION IN THE INTACT WRIST

Position	Radius	Ulna
Neutral	81.6	18.4
Ulnar deviation	71.6	28.4
Radial deviation	87.2	12.8
Forearm pronation	63.0	37.0
Forearm supination	86.0	14.0

From Werner FW, An KN, Palmer AK, Chao EYS: Force analysis. In An KN, Berger RA, Cooney WP III (eds): Biomechanics of the Wrist Joint. New York, Springer-Verlag, 1991, p 77.

Soft Tissue Constraints

The collateral ligament stabilizers of all joints in the hand are important soft tissues. Depending on the orientation of the fibers, various portions of the collateral ligament play different roles in joint stability (Fig. 17–5A, B). By examination of a series of anatomic studies in which different areas of the collateral ligaments were sectioned, we found that each portion of the collateral ligament has its own characteristics in terms of lengthening and shortening throughout the range of joint motion. Each part of the ligament thus makes its own characteristic contribution to resist forces and moments under various loading and displacement conditions.

The locations of the bony insertion and the fiber orientations of the collateral ligaments around the finger and thumb joints have been extensively studied and reported in the literature.[12] This information is essential in designing nonconstrained finger joint prostheses. On the anteroposterior view, the insertions of the radial collateral ligament (RCL) are closer to the centerline of the metacarpal (x axis) than those of the ulnar collateral ligament (UCL) (see Fig. 17–5C, D). The dorsal fibers originating from the metacarpal head are more distal than those of the volar portion. Conversely, the insertion on the proximal phalanx is just the opposite.

With a clear understanding of these anatomic relationships, the preservation or reconstruction of collateral ligamentous attachments can be planned during joint replacement and the joint stability can be improved. The distance between the ligamentous insertions or the apparent ligament length changes with joint flexion angle can be analyzed. When the ligaments are taut, the ligament lengths that average 23 and 22 mm for the RCL and UCL, respectively, can be set during reconstructive procedures on the hand.

At the thumb trapeziometacarpal joint, ligament constraints are quite essential; loss of the anterior oblique ligament tautness appears to be the initiating factor in thumb trapeziometacarpal arthritis. Secondary ligament laxity of the intermetacarpal and posterior oblique follow, and thumb metacarpal subluxation during pinch is the result. Therefore, it is quite important that ligamentous contributions to joint constraint be studied. Linear or angular measurement of the resistive forces and moments when the joint is displaced is important. During supination and pronation rotation of the MCP joint, for example, we have found that the curve of the torque or moment versus the joint angle can be obtained and resembles the typical curve for soft tissue (Fig. 17–6). At the neutral position with minimal rotation, the joint is relatively compliant. Between 10 degrees of pronation and supination rotation, a minimal amount of torque is observed. This amount of rotation can be defined as the rotational laxity of the MCP joint. This is what was meant earlier when it was stated that, actively, the MCP joints have two degrees of freedom that are voluntarily controlled. Moreover, passively, this joint can be considered to have three degrees of rotational freedom or at least a certain amount of laxity in axial rotation.

The relative contributions of the RCL and UCL in resisting joint displacement have been further studied

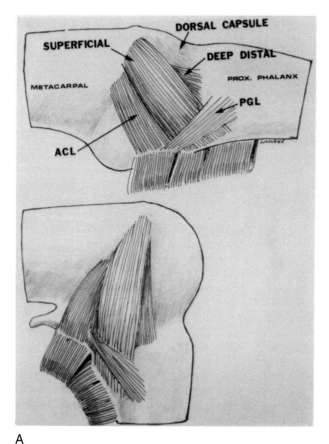

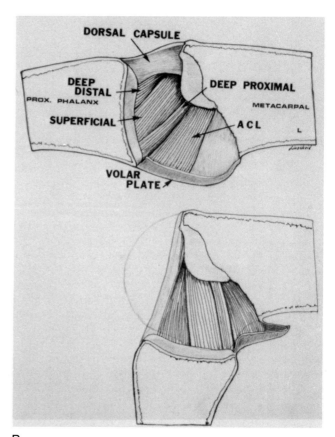

A

B

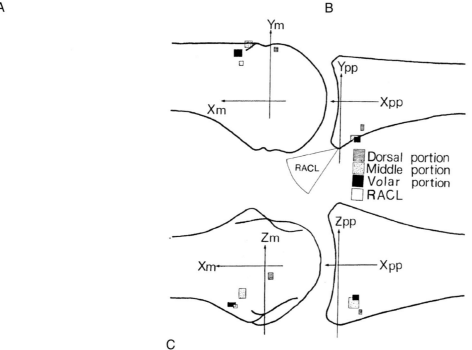

C

Figure 17–5. Morphologic findings of the ligamentous structure of the MCP joint. **A**, External view. Extended position (*top*) and flexed position (*bottom*). The collateral ligament appears to be separable into two components, the superficial and the deep. The deep distal component is hidden beneath the superficial portion of the collateral ligament when the joint is in extension but becomes increasingly taut and visible as the joint is flexed. **B**, Internal view. The specimen is reversed by rotating about the vertical axis to indicate the view from the interior of the joint. Extended position (*top*) and flexed position (*bottom*). The deep layer of the collateral ligament appears to be separable into two portions, the deep distal and the deep proximal. The deep proximal component shortens in flexion and lengthens in extension. These fibers bulge laterally during joint flexion. **C**, Location of origin and insertion of the RCL and radial accessory collateral ligament. Lateral view (*top*) and anteroposterior view (*bottom*). **D**, Location of origin and insertion of the UCL and ulnar accessory collateral ligament. Lateral view (*top*) and anteroposterior view (*bottom*). ACL = accessory collateral ligament; PGL = phalangioglenoidal ligament.

Illustration continued on opposite page

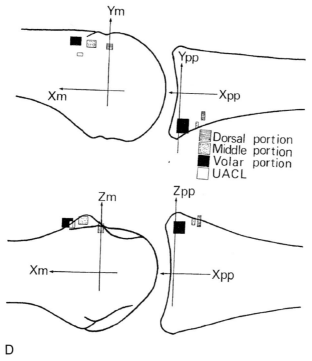

D

Figure 17–5. *Continued.*

by sequential sectioning or removal of the individual ligaments (see Fig. 17–6). The reduction of load caused by the removal of each ligamentous structure represents the contribution of that ligament. In general, the RCL contributes 70 percent in resisting pronation, 40 percent in palmar subluxation, and 90 percent in adduction. However, the UCL contributes about 60 percent in supination, 60 percent in palmar subluxation, and 90 percent in abduction. When the joint is distracted, the UCL contributes slightly more than the RCL.

Articulating Constraint

Depending on the shape and congruity of the joint articular surface, contributions to joint shear force have varied. For the MCP joint, the joint surfaces contribute primarily axial compressive force. The size and location of joint contact areas have been observed to change as a function of the joint flexion angle (Fig. 17–7). The radioulnar width of the contact area becomes narrow in the neutral position and expands in both the hyperextended and fully flexed

Figure 17–6. Load-displacement curves were obtained by measuring the restraining torques when the MCP joints were placed in supination and pronation. Curve *a* represents the torques with the entire capsule-ligament complex intact. Curves *b* and *c* represent the torques when the palmar and dorsal portions of the RCL were sectioned, respectively. Curves *d* and *e* represent the restraining torques when the palmar and dorsal portions of the UCL were sectioned, respectively. The difference in load between each curve for a given displacement indicates the contribution of that particular sectioned element. For example, the difference in load between curves *a* and *b* represents the contribution of the palmar portion of the RCL. N-m = newton-meter.

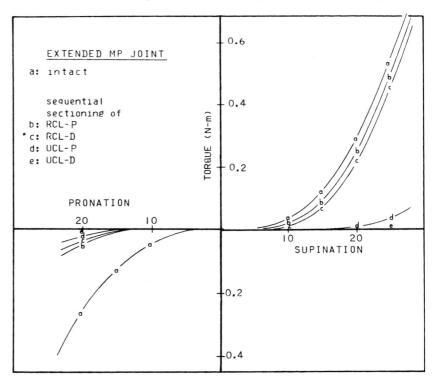

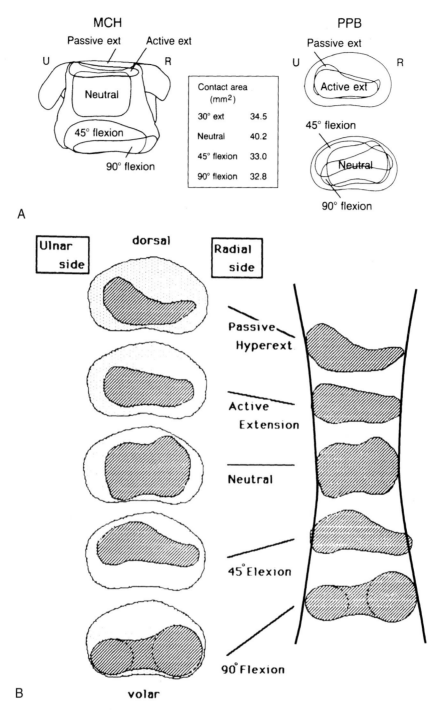

Figure 17–7. A, Contact area of the MCP joint in five joint positions. **B,** End-on view of the contact area on each of the proximal phalanx bases. The radioulnar width of the contact area becomes narrow in the neutral position and expands in both the hyperextended and fully flexed positions.

positions.[19] In the neutral position, the contact area is located in the center of the phalangeal base; this area is slightly larger on the ulnar than on the radial side.

The intrinsic stability of the resurfacing MCP joint depends on the joint surface curvature and the compressive force across the joint. Such constraint can be evaluated based on the stability ratio, which is defined as the maximal force required to cause subluxation of the joint in a given direction divided by the axially applied

compressive force. A study has been performed to compare the stability ratio of a resurfacing MCP implant with that of the anatomic joint (Fig. 17–8).

IMPLANT CONSIDERATIONS

Current joint implants for the PIP and MCP joints of the fingers and the MCP and CMC joints of the thumb

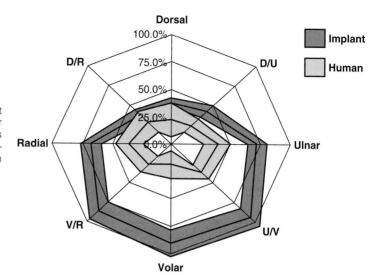

Figure 17–8. Average stability ratio of both human and implant MCPs at zero degrees of flexion. Shaded area represents plus or minus one standard deviation. The stability ratio is defined as the maximal force at subluxation/axial load. The directions represent movement of the proximal phalange base in the direction of motion.

are reviewed in subsequent chapters of this book. There are new resurfacing implant designs for the finger PIP and MCP joint and thumb MCP joint that show promise. These joints include ligament reconstruction as an essential component of the procedure so that the joint is not subjected to the high stresses mentioned earlier. We believe that it is important to insert anatomic-like joints that reproduce normal anatomy. Silastic joints serve as biologic spaces but do not function as true joint replacement prostheses. As a result of high torsion and shear forces, these implants fail through the stem-joint interface within 3 to 5 years. Hinge silicone or metal PIP joint implants also failed as a result of overfixation and no adaptation for soft tissue compliance. Within the thumb, constrained MCP joints have proved to be unsuccessful and have been all but abandoned with the exception of one. Within the finger PIP and MCP joints, our work continues to evaluate different prosthetic designs that combine important elements of soft tissue construction. We believe that it is important to consider not only the joint articular surface construct but also the soft tissue ligament and extensor tendon balance.

To date, there has been increased clinical or experimental studies on unconstrained finger joint prostheses, in comparison with constrained finger joints. Surface replacement finger joints with appropriate collateral ligament and capsule reconstruction appear superior to that of more constrained prostheses and to silicone prostheses. Our own anatomic and biomechanical studies as well as clinical experience shows advances in joint resurfacing prostheses.

Finally, in the hand there exists the different issue of implant fixation in bone. Silastic prostheses have no fixation, whereas mechanical implants have cement fixation. Neither method is fully suitable. Bone cement, in particular, may be contraindicated because it leads to the excessive heat of polymerization, bone necrosis, and eventual loosening. New techniques of fixation between intramedullary bone and the implants with pyrolytic carbon or tantalum

may offer promise. On the horizon are new methods of biologic fixation such as porous polyethylene or osseous integration, and these methods may prove to be fruitful. Testing of new fixation systems will be welcome to examine new implant and fixation designs.

References

1. An KN, Chao EY, Cooney WP, Linscheid RL: Forces in the normal and abnormal hand. J Orthop Res 3:202, 1985.
2. An KN, Hui FC, Morrey BF, et al: Muscles across the elbow joint: A biomechanical analysis. J Biomech 14:659, 1981.
3. Basmajian JV: Muscles Alive. Baltimore, Williams & Wilkins, 1962.
4. Brand PW, Beach RB, Thompson DE: Relative tension and potential excursion of muscles in the forearm and hand. J Hand Surg 6:209, 1981.
5. Chao EY, Opgrande JD, Axmear FE: Three-dimensional force analysis of finger joints in selected isometric hand functions. J Biomech 9:387, 1976.
6. Cooney WP III, Chao EY: Biomechanical analysis of static forces in the thumb during hand function. J Bone Joint Surg 59A:27, 1977.
7. Flatt AE: The Pathomechanics of Ulnar Drift : A Biomechanical and Clinical Study. Final Report, SRS Grant RD 2226M, 1971.
8. Garcia-Elias M, Horii E, Berger RA: Individual carpal bone motion. In An KN, Berger RA, Cooney WP III (eds): Biomechanics of the Wrist Joint. New York, Springer-Verlag, 1991, p 61.
9. Imaeda T, Niebur G, Cooney WP III, et al: Kinematics of the normal trapeziometacarpal joint. J Orthop Res 12:197, 1994.
10. Lazar GT, Schulter-Ellis FP: Intramedullary structure of human metacarpals. J Hand Surg 5:477, 1980.
11. Littler JW: On the adaptability of man's hand (with reference to the equiangular curve). Hand 5:187, 1973.
12. Minami A, An KN, Cooney WP III, et al: Ligament stability of the metacarpophalangeal joint: A biomechanical study. J Hand Surg 10A:255, 1985.
13. Pagowski S, Piekarski K: Biomechanics of the metacarpophalangeal joint. J Biomech 10:205, 1977.
14. Palmer AK, Werner FW, Murphy D, Glisson R: Functional wrist motion: Biomechanical study. J Hand Surg 10A:39, 1985.
15. Ryu J, Cooney WP III, Askew LJ, et al: Functional range of motion of the wrist joint. J Hand Surg 16A:409, 1991.
16. Schulter-Ellis FP, Lazar GT: Internal morphology of human phalanges. J Hand Surg 9A:490, 1984.
17. Schultz RJ: Metacarpophalangeal Joint Replacement. Memphis, Richards Manufacturing Co., 1975.

18. Swanson AB: Flexible Implant Resection Arthroplasty in the Hand and Extremities. St. Louis, CV Mosby, 1973.
19. Tamai K, Ryu J, An KN, et al: Three-dimensional geometric analysis of the metacarpophalangeal joint. J Hand Surg 13A:521, 1988.
20. Tubiana R: The Hand. Philadelphia, WB Saunders, 1981.
21. Walker PS, Erhman MJ: Laboratory evaluation of a metaplastic type of metacarpophalangeal joint prosthesis. Clin Orthop 112:349, 1975.
22. Werner FW, An KN, Palmer AK, Chao EYS: Force analysis. p 77. *In* An KN, Berger RA, Cooney WP III (eds): Biomechanics of the Wrist Joint. New York, Springer-Verlag, 1991.

18

Arthroplasty of the Proximal Interphalangeal Joint

• PETER C. AMADIO, PETER M. MURRAY, and RONALD L. LINSCHEID

The proximal interphalangeal (PIP) joint normally has the greatest arc of motion of any finger joint. Whether the fingers are positioned over a musical instrument, extended to enable grasp of large objects, or flexed in a variable cascade to hold an object of irregular shape, the PIP joint plays a critical role in hand function.

PATIENT EVALUATION

Examination of the impaired PIP joint should be performed in the context of a complete hand examination. Handedness, occupation, and avocations are important to decision making. For example, more PIP flexion is required in the hand that fingers the frets of a guitar than in the one that strums it. For a laborer who needs power grip, functional needs may best be served by a stable fused joint rather than by a mobile one that is likely to have less lateral stability and, possibly, less longevity. Specific patient needs may also suggest nonsurgical options, such as built-up tool handles to compensate for limited flexion. Many PIP joints afflicted with osteoarthritis are cosmetically undesirable but functionally adequate for the patient's needs. Furthermore, the motion that the patient desires or needs may be unachievable by current arthroplasty techniques. The average arc of motion after PIP arthroplasty is reported to be between 40 and 60 degrees in most series; if the arc of finger motion is already in this range, restoration of motion is probably an unreasonable goal. Arthroplasty may still be appropriate to redirect the arc of motion that is present (e.g., from hyperextension to flexion in cases of swan-neck deformity, or from flexion to extension in cases of flexion contracture), but a painless PIP joint that extends fully or nearly so and flexes to 60 degrees cannot, in general, be reliably helped by arthroplasty. Finally, as a prerequisite to PIP arthroplasty, bone stock must be sufficient to receive the stems of the implant; supple, full-thickness skin cover must be available; finger sensibility and circulation must be adequate; and tendons should be normal or able to be reconstructed.

Fingers work best in concert. An impaired digit must always be assessed in relation to its neighbors. A single fused PIP joint in an otherwise normal hand, unless it is the index joint as mentioned earlier, is likely to limit the function of its neighbors through the *quadriga* effect. The PIP joint must also be assessed in the context of its ray. The function level of a digit with combined PIP and metacarpophalangeal (MCP) arthroplasties may be less than that of one with arthroplasty of the MCP joint and PIP fusion. Function after PIP arthroplasty is also less likely to fare well in a digit with tendon imbalance (boutonnière or swan-neck deformity) than in one with simply contracture or joint surface incongruity.[27,28]

In examining the PIP joint, certain tests help distinguish features that may affect the result of arthroplasty. Collateral ligament instability is best tested in some flexion to relax the volar plate and accessory collateral ligaments.[15] Joint opening of more than 20 degrees suggests complete collateral ligament disruption. If arthroplasty is to be considered in such a joint, ligament reconstruction needs to be considered as well.

Both active and passive ranges of motion should be measured. A difference between the two suggests tendon insufficiency or adhesions that need to be addressed at the time of arthroplasty. Motion of the PIP joint may be limited by intrinsic tightness. A reduction in passive motion with the MCP joint in extension suggests intrinsic tightness, which again must be addressed at the time of arthroplasty, either by intrinsic release or by bone shortening. Distal interphalangeal (DIP) function and motion should also be assessed, because the PIP and DIP joints may have reciprocal deformities. Hyperextension of the DIP joint is common with central slip insufficiency, creating the typical boutonnière deformity. Hyperextension of the DIP joint may also occur after profundus tendon rupture, but the PIP deformity in such cases is not associated with extensor insufficiency. For this reason, active DIP flexion should be assessed. Similarly, the typical swan-neck deformity may be due either to proximal intrinsic tightness or to a distal extensor insufficiency (mallet deformity) with secondary overpull of the extensors at the PIP level. Active DIP extension should therefore be noted as well; improvement with PIP flexion suggests that the terminal tendon is intact.

Once the examination is completed, the surgeon can formulate a treatment plan. Even if the impairment is significant, the patient with a painless arc of 60 degrees of PIP motion in good position may be best advised to avoid surgery. A patient who has psoriatic or rheumatoid arthritis with poor bony stock at the PIP level and severe flexion contracture[2] or a patient with fixed swanneck deformity often regains little motion after arthroplasty. For such patients, arthrodesis may be the preferred treatment modality.

IMPLANT OPTIONS

If arthroplasty is elected, the list of implant options is short. Metallic hinge prostheses such as the Brannon and Flatt designs are no longer available, because of problems of bony erosion, subsidence, and wear fret-ting. Constrained metal and polyethylene hinge devices, which often were simply downscaled MCP prostheses, required excessive joint excision and had largely disappointing results. Another one-piece implant devised by Heipel for the PIP level was the Biomeric prosthesis composed of titanium stems cemented to a thin hinge of polyolefin with a proprietary industrial adhesive. This device had a built-in flexion range of approximately 30 degrees. Late results were disappointing as a result of failure of the material.[25]

The one early device that remains in common use is the Swanson implant. Swanson devised a flexible hinge of silicone rubber for MCP arthroplasty in the early 1960s and began using it at the PIP level in 1965 (Fig. 18–1).[27,28] This implant has the largest number of reported series and, although the results are far from normal, they are predictable, and salvage has proved easier than for most of its successors. Another silicone device from

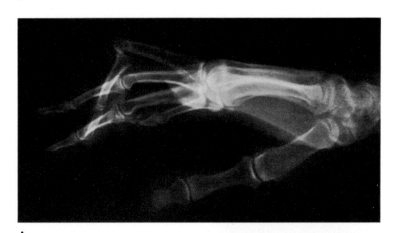

A

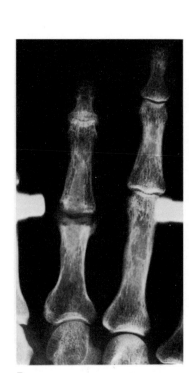

B

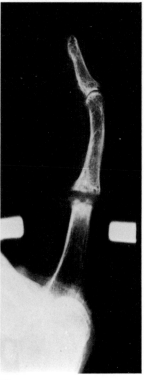

C

Figure 18–1. A, PIP flexion contracture resulting from psoriatic arthritis involving the right ring finger in a 49-year-old woman. **B**, One year after intra-articular bone shortening and PIP arthroplasty with Swanson implant, anteroposterior view shows satisfactory alignment. **C**, Lateral view also shows satisfactory positioning. PIP range of motion went from a 15-degree flexion contracture to 80 degrees of flexion.

the same era developed by Niebauer was laminated onto a Dacron template and covered with a Dacron mesh for the purpose of developing a fibrous fixation. The results were disappointing in the reported series.

In 1978, our own interest in PIP prosthesis shifted to a minimally constrained two-component surface replacement design that closely followed anatomic contours.[18] This device was designed to reduce the amount of joint excision to a minimum so as to preserve the stability provided by the collateral ligaments. The design provided additional lateral stability by retaining the chevron configuration of the articular surfaces and by allowing the palmar shift of the lateral bands during flexion.[21] Centering the components to provide optimal beam lengths for the tendons was achieved by aligning the proper size prosthesis with the dorsal aspect of the phalangeal cortices. Several minor modifications of stem and articular contour were made in the intervening years. Three different series of approaches—lateral, palmar and dorsal—were evaluated. The components were cemented with polymethylmethacrylate. The most recent modification has shot blasted, roughened stems, contoured so as to more closely match the endosteal surfaces. This modification allows the option of press fitting or cementing the components in place.

SURGICAL TECHNIQUE

Silicone Replacement Arthroplasty

The technique of PIP arthroplasty varies somewhat, depending on the etiology of the joint deformity and the type of prosthesis chosen. Swanson has carefully outlined his approach to PIP arthroplasty with use of a Silastic spacer.[27,28]

Surgery should be done under tourniquet hemostasis. The approach selected should provide an optimal chance to preserve the function of the central slip and diminish the chances for adversely affecting the function of the rest of the delicate extensor expansion. A dorsal, volar, or midaxial approach may be used in the finger, depending on the angular deformity of the finger. The dorsal approach is more commonly used. A curved dorsal incision keeps skin and tendon suture lines from overlapping (Fig. 18–2). As many dorsal veins as possible should be preserved. Swanson advises splitting of the extensor insertion to the dorsum of the middle phalanx and elevating the resulting halves of the extensor mechanism laterally to expose the joint. This of necessity releases the central slip insertion, and one may wish to carefully prepare suture holes in the dorsal cortex of the midphalanx for later repair of the insertion site (Fig. 18–3). If the joint is suppler, it may also be possible to split the extensor mechanism between the central slip and a lateral band, dislocating the head of the proximal phalanx through this interval.

In stiffer joints, an alternative is to remove the head of the proximal phalanx with a bur or rongeur before mobilizing the central slip. These central slip-preserving procedures may facilitate mobilization postoperatively.

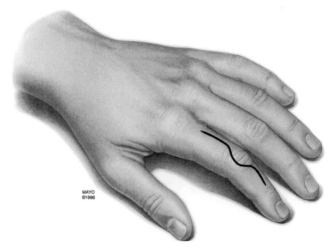

Figure 18–2. Dorsal skin incision. (By permission of Mayo Foundation for Medical Education and Research.)

Whatever method is chosen, the goal of this part of the operation is to remove the head of the proximal phalanx and flex the joint, which enables the base of the middle phalanx to be seen (Fig. 18–4**A**). Osteophytes and articular cartilage should be removed from the middle phalanx. If possible, the subchondral bone of the middle phalanx is preserved. In cases of flexion contracture, the volar plate can also be released. With severe contracture, more bone may need to be removed from both sides of the joint. If this requires collateral ligament release, it should be done proximally, and the ligaments should be released subperiosteally and preserved for later reattachment. The next step is to broach the intramedullary cavities of the two phalanges. This step may be

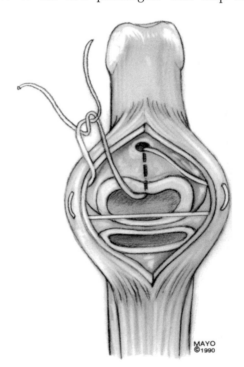

Figure 18–3. Dorsal mid-line tendon splitting incision. Reconstruction requires bringing the tendon slips together dorsally, and attaching them through a drill hole in the base of the middle phalanx.

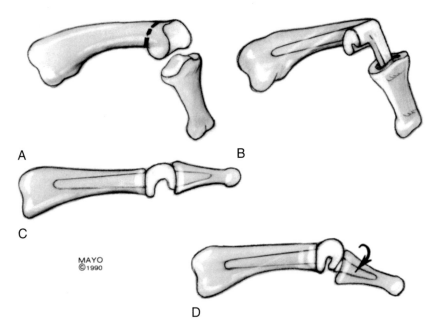

A

B

C

D

MAYO
©1990

Figure 18–4. **A,** Bone resection is primarily from the distal proximal phalanx. **B,** After implant insertion, the implant stem should be able to piston slightly within the medullary canals. **C,** Proper implant positioning permits gliding motion of middle phalanx into flexion. **D,** With inadequate bone resection or soft tissue release, the implant is too tight, and a hinging flexion occurs; however, this may limit flexion and result in early implant failure.

performed with use of either power or hand tools, depending on the consistency of the bone encountered. The resulting edges and interior surfaces should be carefully smoothed to diminish implant abrasion.

A trial implant reduction is done (see Fig. 18–4**B**). The implant should not be so wide as to bulge beyond the outer cortical margins of the phalanges. The dorsal cut edges of the phalanges should not impinge on the implant in extension (see Fig. 18–4**C**). Flexion should be a smooth, rolling motion, as in the normal digit. Hinging on the palmar edges of the phalanges (as opposed to hinging through the prosthetic hub) is undesirable and usually indicates that more bone needs to be resected (see Fig. 18–4**D**). If the implant does not seat against the bone ends but seems appropriate in width, an alternative to using a smaller implant is to shorten the stem tip. This can be done simply by removing the acral portion of the stem as desired with a scalpel blade. The piston-like behavior of the stem is a normal and desirable phenomenon of the Swanson Silastic implant; therefore, it is important that the stem be slightly shorter than the reamed intramedullary canal.

Once the implant size has been determined, the bones are prepared for tendon and ligament reattachment. A 0.5-mm Kirschner wire can be used to make drill holes at the reinsertion sites (usually at the dorsolateral aspect of the proximal phalanx for collateral ligaments and the dorsal base of the middle phalanx for the central slip). Fixation sutures are passed before implant insertion and tied after the implant is in place (Fig. 18–5). Passive range of motion should now be checked. At least 70 degrees of PIP flexion should be possible, with good lateral stability. It is our practice to deflate the tourniquet and achieve hemostasis before skin closure. If needed, small drains of silicone tubing may be inserted. A bulky, conforming dressing is used for 3 to 5 days, after which active motion may be started. A splint holds the finger extended at night for 3 to 6 weeks. To concentrate tendon force on the PIP joint, it is often helpful during exercises to block the MCP joint in extension. Dynamic

flexion assist can be added if necessary after 3 weeks, and strengthening may begin at 6 weeks. Swanson has a number of publications that specifically address the important issue of aftercare, to which the reader is referred for more details.[27,28]

A midaxial incision may be elected to provide access to an adherent flexor system or to obtain a better view of a deficient collateral ligament (Fig. 18–6). It may, however, be more difficult to see the extensor mechanism, and especially the opposite collateral ligament, through this approach. Thus, it may be less useful than a dorsal approach, and we use it rarely. The palmar approach may be useful when there is no static flexion deformity or when there are flexor tendon problems. A palmar zigzag incision is used, and the A3 pulley is released so

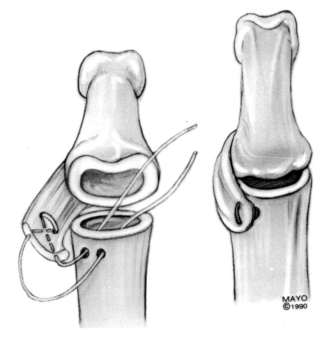

MAYO
©1990

Figure 18–5. Reattachment of the collateral ligament.

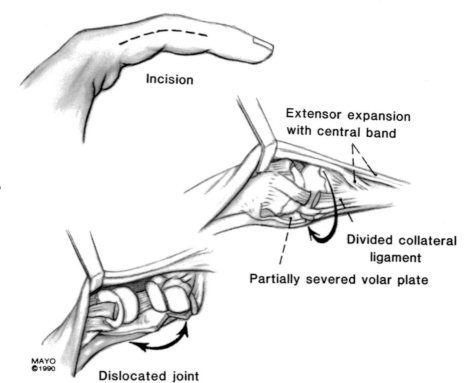

Incision

Extensor expansion
with central band

Divided collateral
ligament

Partially severed volar plate

Dislocated joint

Figure 18–6. Lateral approach to the PIP joint.

that the flexors may be pulled aside, exposing the volar plate (Fig. 18–7). After the volar plate is released, the joint is hyperextended to expose the joint surfaces. The advantage of this approach is that both the extensor mechanism and the collateral ligaments can be observed and protected. In a comparative study, Herren and Simmen[11] have shown, however, that this may be just a theoretical advantage. They followed 59 PIP arthroplasties in 38 patients for a minimum of 12 years. Thirty-eight implants were inserted through a palmar approach, and 21 dorsally. The patients were similar in terms of age, indication, and preoperative motion. Final arc of motion averaged 51 degrees in both groups. Lin et al. reported comparable results.[17] It has been our impression, however, that, although the final results are similar, the postoperative management is much simpler with the palmar approach. For cases in which osteoarthritis or traumatic arthritis is the indication and only a single digit is operated on, often the only rehabilitation needed is simple buddy taping of the operated digit to an adjacent sound digit. Complex splinting regimens and therapy programs can thus be avoided, at

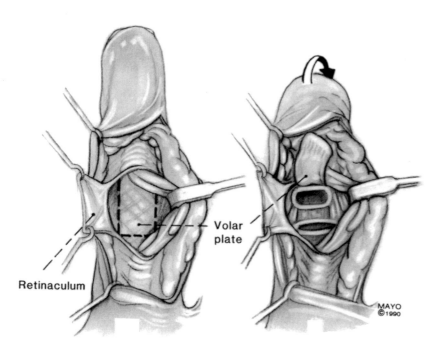

Retinaculum

Volar plate

Figure 18–7. Volar approach to the PIP joint.

least in this special (although not, in our experience, all that unusual) case.

Reconstruction for boutonnière deformity is similar to the procedure used for the dorsal approach described earlier, except that the extensor system must be rebalanced. This requires shortening of the central slip before reattachment and often lengthening of the terminal tendon to improve DIP flexion. Postoperatively, the boutonnière finger is splinted continuously in extension for 2 to 3 weeks, although DIP flexion exercises are started immediately. Nighttime extension splinting should continue for 3 months.

Correction of swan-neck deformity requires lengthening of the central slip, palmar relocation of the lateral bands, and, on occasion, palmar plate reattachment (Fig. 18–8). For cases of severe swan-neck deformity, arthrodesis may be a better option than arthroplasty.

Surface Replacement Arthroplasty

A similar dorsal midline incision, splitting the central slip in half, and reflecting the extensor mechanism subperiosteally from the middle phalanx may be used for surface replacement arthroplasty.[19] The method of Chamay preserves the central slip insertion by reflecting a triangular flap of the central slip distally for exposure of the joint and then repairing the extensor mechanism with fine sutures[4] (Fig. 18–9). We often use a modification of this approach with a longer rectangular flap of the central tendon. This places the primary retaining

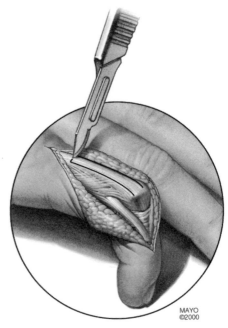

Figure 18–9. Distally based central slip incision. (By permission of Mayo Foundation for Medical Education and Research.)

sutures through a thicker, more robust area of the tendon proximally and allows a number of fine sutures to be placed along the parallel incisions in the extensor apparatus.[19] The sutures should be placed very close to either edge to avoid constricting the interval between the lateral bands and the central slip. Iselin and Pradet[13] have described a transverse incision in the extensor mechanism.

Only 2 to 3 mm of the middle phalangeal base and proximal phalangeal head are removed (Fig. 18–10). An oscillating saw is used to make the cuts as smooth as possible. It is important to preserve as much of the integrity of the collateral ligaments as possible. The intramedullary cavities are prepared with the broaches supplied with the prostheses to effect a close fit of the roughened stems with the endosteal surfaces (Fig. 18–11). This fit is important, particularly when the prosthesis is used in the noncemented mode. Alignment of the components in all three planes is important. The dorsal aspect of the components should align with the dorsal cortices of the phalanges to place the center of rotation in the optimal position. With the joint reduced,

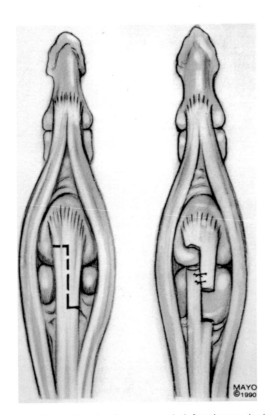

Figure 18–8. Reconstruction for swan-neck deformity require lengthening of the central slip.

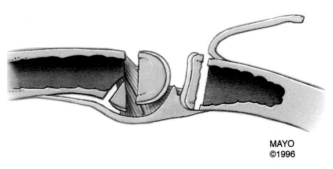

Figure 18–10. Extent of limited bone resection for surface replacement arthroplasty. (By permission of Mayo Foundation for Medical Education and Research.)

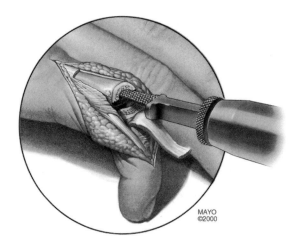

Figure 18–11. Preparation of intramedullary cavity with custom broaches. (By permission of Mayo Foundation for Medical Education and Research.)

the finger should passively extend to neutral and flex to 90 degrees with minimal resistance (Fig. 18–12). The position and alignment of the components should be checked under the image intensifier and adjusted as necessary.

If the trial components do not fit snugly into the intramedullary cavities, liquid polymethylmethacrylate is injected into the bone through a No. 12 intravenous catheter or through the tip of a 5-mm syringe (Fig. 18–13). The permanent components are seated in the cement, and the excess cement is carefully wiped away. The joint is held reduced in extension until the cement is set. Saline lavage helps to carry away the heat of polymerization. The central slip is repaired with an intraosseous nonabsorbable suture. If the modified Chamay procedure is used, two or three 4-0 or 5-0 sutures are placed in the thickened central tendon proximally. Multiple 5-0 or 6-0 sutures are placed close to the edges of the longitudinal cuts so as not to constrict the matrix of interlacing fibers connecting the lateral bands and the central slip.

Postoperatively, the finger is held extended at the PIP joint, but active DIP motion may be begun immediately. This motion tends to relax tension on the central tendon. If the tendon repair was secure at surgery, the PIP motion may begin in small increments after the second day. The finger is maintained in an extension outrigger splint to ensure that the joint is returned to neutral after each movement (Fig. 18–14). Flexion is increased progressively at a rate of 10 to 15 degrees per week, provided that active extension of the PIP joint is maintained.

RESULTS OF PROXIMAL INTERPHALANGEAL ARTHROPLASTY

In 1959, Brannon and Klein reported on a series of 14 patients who received metallic constrained prostheses; the majority of these patients experienced pain relief and a functional return of motion.[3] In 1961, Flatt introduced his modification of the metallic hinged prosthesis, which employed two proximal and distal prongs to prevent the rotational instability observed with the Brannon prosthesis. He reported encouraging short-term results in 57 implanted prostheses.[9] However, both he and Brannon recognized the potential for loosening and migration of this particular prosthesis, including the cortical erosions and subsequent penetrations typically observed with the Flatt device. In 1971, Niebauer and Landry reported their experience with the replacement of 13 PIP joints.[24] Their technique required a midlateral incision, with sacrifice of the collateral ligaments. Breakage of the prosthesis was not observed. Dryer and colleagues reported on the results of 93 PIP joint arthroplasties in patients with rheumatoid hands.[7] The average range of motion of patients with Flatt prostheses was 15 degrees, and that of patients with Niebauer prostheses was 19.5 degrees. Nearly 80 percent of the Flatt prostheses displayed cortical perforations. The average follow-up in this series was 6.2 years after implantation.

The results of PIP arthroplasty with the Swanson implant have been reported by many investigators. In 1985, Swanson reported his personal series of 424 implants observed for a minimum of 1 year.[27,28] Slightly more than two thirds of these fingers had more than 40 degrees of PIP motion at final follow-up, averaging between 38 and 60 degrees depending on the etiology of the contracture. Results were best in fingers with minimal deformity, and worst in those with rheumatoid swan-neck deformity and post-traumatic ankylosis. Five percent of the implants fractured and 11 percent

Figure 18–12. With the joint reduced and the trial implants in place, the finger should passively extend to neutral and extend to 90 degrees with minimal resistance. (By permission of Mayo Foundation for Medical Education and Research.)

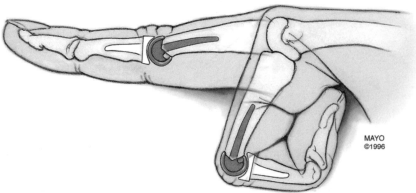

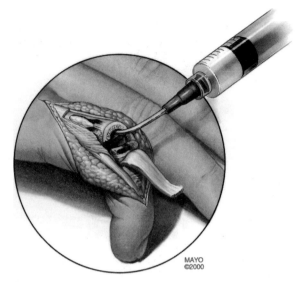

Figure 18–13. Liquid polymethylmethacrylate is injected into the bone through a small intravenous catheter. (By permission of Mayo Foundation for Medical Education and Research.)

required revision, usually including reimplantation. There were only three infections. Moore et al.[22] reported on 78 implants at a minimum of 2 years' follow-up; all of these procedures were done for osteoarthritis or post-traumatic arthritis. Although the revision rate was much higher (nearly 40 percent), salvage by reimplantation was still usually possible. Again, results were worst in the post-traumatic group. The fracture rate in this series was nearly 15 percent. In 1988, Ferencz and Millender[8] reported 11 patients with post-traumatic arthritis observed for a minimum of 18 months. In this series, there were no fractures or revisions and motion averaged 64 degrees. Iselin and Pradet,[13] in a series of 120 arthroplasties in fingers with post-traumatic contractures observed for at least 2 years, had satisfactory results in two thirds of cases. Belsky et al.[2] reported on a series of patients with psoriatic arthritis. Silastic arthroplasty was done in 11 fingers. The average range of motion was only 20 degrees. In one long-term study of patients with rheumatoid arthritis treated with PIP

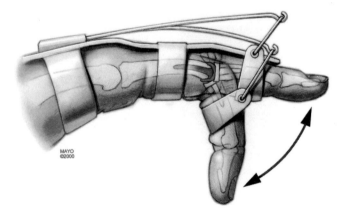

Figure 18–14. Extension outrigger splint allows early motion with protection of the extensor mechanism. (By permission of Mayo Foundation for Medical Education and Research.)

arthroplasty, the average range of motion at 3 years was 42 degrees, but at 10 years, it was only 26 degrees. Recurrent swan-neck deformity is a major problem, occurring in roughly one fourth of patients, as noted in several series.[7,16,27,28]

Pellegrini and Burton[25] retrospectively reviewed 43 PIP joint reconstructive procedures in 24 patients. Thirty-six procedures were performed in patients with erosive osteoarthritis, five in patients with psoriatic arthritis, and two in patients with post-traumatic arthrosis. Twenty-six Swanson arthroplasties were performed (24 in patients with erosive osteoarthritis, 1 in a patient with psoriatic arthritis, and 1 in a patient with post-traumatic arthritis), seven Biomeric designs were implanted (all erosive osteoarthritis patients), and arthrodesis was performed on 10 joints. At a mean follow-up of 3.4 years, all patients enjoyed excellent pain relief. The mean follow-up of the 26 Swanson implants was 3 years, 9 months. The mean active range of motion of the patients with Swanson PIP joint prostheses was 56 degrees (extension, minus 3.2 degrees; flexion, plus 59.2 degrees). Although no Swanson PIP implants in this particular study required revision, 27 percent displayed periprosthetic erosions at an average of 4 years after implantation. In this particular series, no Swanson implants were performed in index fingers. Five of the seven Biomeric arthroplasties in this same series required revision because of symptomatic failure of the synthetic elastomer hinge. At a mean follow-up of 2 years, the average range of motion of patients with the Biomeric implants was 66.4 degrees (extension, minus 12.2 degrees; flexion, plus 78.6 degrees). Five Biomeric implants in this series were performed in index fingers; all of these patients developed a static angular deformity. In the 10 patients who received a PIP joint arthrodesis, 9 obtained a solid union. Comparatively, the hands with PIP joint arthrodeses obtained key pinch strength superior to the hands with a PIP joint arthroplasty. Five of the 10 arthrodeses performed in this series were index PIP joints.

Stern and Ho[26] caution against the use of Swanson silicone implants in the index and middle PIP joints, especially in the young, active patient. They highlight the usual necessity of detaching the radial and ulnar collateral ligament origins from the proximal phalanx in order to resect the proximal phalangeal head through its neck. They contend that resultant stresses on the radial collateral ligament are significant in key pinch and may lead to ultimate implant failure. They recommend arthrodesis of the index and long PIP joints when these joints are destroyed, reserving arthroplasty for the ring and small PIP joints. Others, however, continue to advocate the use of Swanson hinged interposition implant arthroplasty for the painful, destroyed index and long finger PIP joints as long as these digits are well aligned and the collateral ligaments are in good condition.[18,19,22] Ashworth et al.[1] have emphasized the durability and lasting pain relief of the Swanson PIP joint hinged interposition arthroplasty despite limited range of motion and a significant fracture rate. This series followed 99 PIP joint arthroplasties in 45 patients for an average of

5.8 years. The average range of motion was 29 degrees, the fracture rate was 7 percent, and bone resorption occurred in 12 percent. Survivorship, however, was 91 percent at 2 years, 87 percent at 5 years, and 81 percent at 9 years, when revision surgery was used as an endpoint. Similar results have been reported by Hage et al. in follow-up of 16 PIP Swanson implants,[10] and by Iselin and Conti.[12] Mathoulin and Gilbert[20] have reported similar results in short-term follow-up with the Sutter silicone implant.

The reported experience with the silicone Dacron device designed by Niebauer is less extensive and less promising. That particular device is no longer available.[24] There is little follow-up information available on the Sutter thin-hinged silicone device manufactured by Avanta Orthopedics or the Neuflex device manufactured by DePuy. A report of an implant of alumina ceramic[6] had a short follow-up (12 to 31 months). Motion only averaged 30 degrees at the PIP level and no further information was available. Condamine has reported several series of the surface replacement prosthesis of his design. This has a unique method of stem fixation that uses a ribbed plastic bone insert into which the metal stem of the components is reduced. Preliminary results are promising.[5]

The unpublished Mayo Clinic experience with 106 Mayo Mark I and II implants, as well as 13 Steffee, 72 Biomeric, and 10 Buchholtz implants, suggests complication rates in the range of 50 percent at 2 to 10 years' follow-up (Fig. 18–15), more than double that in 125

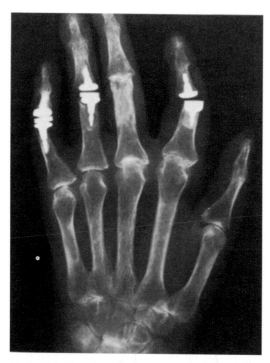

Figure 18–15. This 56-year-old woman with long-standing rheumatoid arthritis had biomeric implants. After 3 years, the index implant is broken and painful, the ring implant is lose and painful, and the little finger has only 20 degrees of motion. After these radiographs were taken, the index finger implant was removed and the index PIP joint was fused.

Swanson implants, for which our results parallel those reported in the literature.

Linscheid[18,19] developed a surface replacement arthroplasty (Mayo Mark II) for the PIP joint that allows preservation of the collateral ligaments. The components are anatomic designs of the head of the proximal phalanx and the base of the middle phalanx (Fig. 18–16). The proximal phalangeal component is a chromium-cobalt alloy with a stem designed to fit the internal contours of the medullary canal, which sacrifices only a minimal amount of bone. The middle phalangeal component has a titanium metal body and stem supporting a biconcave articular tray stamped from high-density polyethylene. Eighty-five surface replacement arthroplasties for the PIP joint have been implanted in 52 patients over a 19-year period (1980 to 1999). Forty-seven surface replacement arthroplasties have been implanted in patients with osteoarthrosis, 124 in patients with post-traumatic arthrosis, and 14 in patients with rheumatoid or psoriatic arthritis. Complete follow-up data are available for 74 of the 85 joints. Twenty-nine joints have been implanted in the long finger, 18 in the ring finger, 38 in the index finger, and 7 in the small finger. An additional 8 have been implanted in the IP joint of the thumb. At an average follow-up of 41.6 months, 58 of the patients had nonpainful joints, 5 had mild pain, and 12 had moderate pain. The average range of motion increased from 35.5 degrees preoperatively (extension, minus 13.0 degrees; flexion, plus 48.9 degrees) to 47.5 degrees (extension, minus 16.3 degrees; flexion, plus 63.8 degrees) postoperatively. Component failure has not been a problem. Frank loosening has occurred in two fingers in this series. The stability of the index PIP joint has been maintained with the use of this prosthesis. Complications have included boutonnière and swan-neck deformities and joint subluxation. The complication rate is currently approximately 20 percent, compared 10 percent in a concurrent (unpublished) series of Swanson implants at the same institution. Both implants are currently used at our institution (Fig. 18–17).

The digital joint operative arthroplasty implant is one of several new metalloplastic devices available in Europe.[5] Condamine et al. have reported similar performance characteristics (i.e., 50-degree arc of motion and good pain relief but some radiographic changes in short-term follow-up). In the publications describing its use, the authors state that they are pursuing improvements in implant design and surgical approach to improve their results.

Other reconstructive issues include conversion of PIP joint arthrodesis to arthroplasty as well as immediate PIP joint arthroplasty for severe intra-articular PIP joint fractures. Nagle et al.[23] reported on eight patients with immediate Swanson PIP joint hinged interposition arthroplasty for nonsalvageable fractures of the PIP joint. Their retrospective review shows an average range of motion of only 29 degrees at a follow-up of 26 months. Iselin et al.[14] report more encouraging results for conversion of PIP joint arthrodesis to the Swanson PIP joint hinged interposition arthroplasty. In this series, 12 patients with conversion of arthrodesis to a Swanson

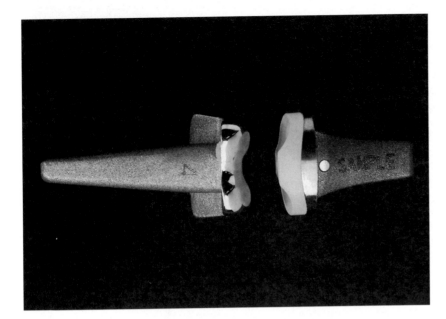

Figure 18–16. Metal and plastic surface replacement arthroplasty implants.

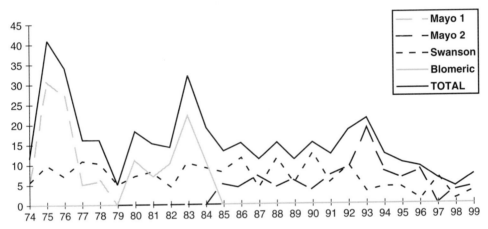

Figure 18–17. PIP arthroplasty at the Mayo Clinic, 1974–1999 (print of graph).

PIP joint interposition arthroplasty were reviewed at an average follow-up of 39 months. The criteria for conversion included the preservation of normal bony length and the presence of an articular fusion in "good position." Eleven of the 12 patients were satisfied, and there was a reported mean gain in active range of motion of 56.8 degrees.

COMPLICATIONS

Complications of silicone PIP arthroplasty include joint stiffness, lateral instability, implant fracture, implant deformation, progressive loss of motion, and infection. For the cemented surface replacement implants, loosening, subsidence, dislocation, tendinous adhesion, malalignment, and bone fracture have been noted. Ankylosis after arthroplasty generally functions as an arthrodesis and does not often require—or improve from—revision. Instability and infection generally are revised by arthrodesis. The Swanson implant is usually easily removed, but cemented implants are difficult to extract. Frequently, only a thin cortical shell remains around the device. Great care must be taken to preserve as much bone stock as possible. To preserve digit length after implant removal, arthrodesis may be accomplished with a block of bone graft shaped to resemble the removed implant. Fixation with Kirschner wires is usually adequate. Revision for implant fracture is not always necessary, particularly for the Silastic device (Fig. 18–18). Silicone synovitis, a problem with carpal bone implants, has not been reported at the PIP level. Lateral instability is the most common problem seen with implant fracture. The sudden onset of lateral instability several years after arthroplasty is a common mode of presentation. Usually, reimplantation can successfully salvage a fractured Swanson implant although we have successfully converted these to surface replacement arthroplasties as well. Attention to surgical detail is, however, as important as in primary arthroplasty; the bone surfaces must be reprepared and the ligaments restabilized. Fracture of other implants may be more difficult to salvage by reimplantation. Deficient bone stock in such cases may oblige performance of an arthrodesis.

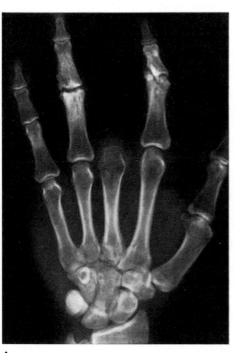
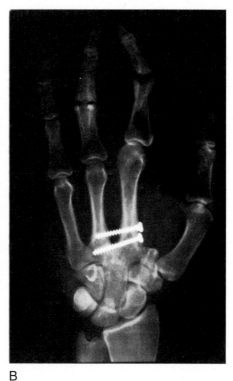

A   B

Figure 18–18. **A**, An industrial accident left this 22-year-old man with ankylosis of the PIP joints of the ring fingers, absent flexor tendon systems in both fingers, and amputation of the middle finger. **B**, After ray transportation, PIP arthroplasty, and two-stage flexor tendon reconstruction, function was improved, but after 5 years, a fracture of the ring implant and lateral instability of the index implant are noted. There is no pain and motion remains good, with full extension and 50 degrees of flexion of the index PIP joint and full extension and 55 degrees of flexion of the ring PIP joint. The patient continues to work as a clerk.

AUTHORS' PREFERENCE

Our current preference for PIP arthroplasty is dependent on the condition of the bones and soft tissue findings. Metalloplastic prostheses have shown the ability to function for longer than two decades, whereas silicone implants have been in constant use, with little design modification, for more than 35 years. There are certain circumstances in which the metalloplastic prosthesis seems to be the better choice. Lateral stability is significantly better with the metalloplastic prostheses than with silicone devices.[21] This is particularly an issue in the index finger, which experiences more lateral deviation forces than the ulnar digits. Bony fixation remains an issue, but the introduction of shot-blasted stems for both the proximal and distal stems provides the opportunity for either cemented or noncemented insertion. Careful preservation of central slip function through better surgical technique appears to be improving the results as well. There are instances in which the Swanson or other silicone implant seems to be a more prudent choice, such as the ulnar side of the hand, especially when there is a concern, on the part of either the surgeon or the patient, about the magnitude of any revision surgery. Although there is little literature on revision PIP arthroplasty, there is no question that a failed cemented metalloplastic prosthesis is more likely to result in a short, stiff finger than a failed silicone implant. Nevertheless, the silicone implant is far from an ideal solution to PIP joint replacement. The PIP joint remains a challenging problem for the arthroplasty surgeon.

References

1. Ashworth CR, Hansraj KK, Dukhram AO, et al: Swanson PIP arthroplasty in patients with rheumatoid arthritis. Clin Orthop 342:34, 1997.
2. Belsky MR, Feldon P, Millender LH: Hand involvement in psoriatic arthritis. J Hand Surg 7:203, 1982.
3. Brannon E, Klein G: Experiences with a finger joint prosthesis. J Bone Joint Surg 41A:87, 1959.
4. Chamay A: A distally based dorsal and triangular tendinous flap for direct access to the interphalangeal joint. Ann Chir Main 7:179, 1988.
5. Condamine JL, Fourquet M, Marucci L, Pichereau D: Primary metacarpophalangeal and proximal interphalangeal arthrosis. Indications and results of 27 DJOA arthroplasty. Ann Chir Main Memb Super 16:68, 1997.
6. Doi K, Kuwata N, Kawai S: Alumina ceramic finger implants: A preliminary biomaterial and clinical evaluation. J Hand Surg 9A:740, 1984.
7. Dryer RF, Blair WF, Shurr DG, Buckwalter JA: Proximal interphalangeal joint arthroplasty. Clin Orthop 185:187, 1985.
8. Ferencz CC, Millender LH: Long-term evaluation of silastic arthroplasty of the proximal interphalangeal joint for post-traumatic arthritis. 18th Annual Meeting of the American Association of Hand Surgeons, Toronto, Canada, 1988.
9. Flatt A, Ellison M: Restoration of rheumatoid finger joint function. J Bone Joint Surg 54A:1317, 1972.
10. Hage JJ, Yoe EPD, Zevering JP, deGroot PJM: Proximal interphalangeal silicone arthroplasty for posttraumatic arthritis. J Hand Surg 24A:73, 1999.

11. Herren DB, Simmen BR: Palmar approach in flexible implant arthroplasty of the PIP joint. Clin Orthop 371:131, 2000.
12. Iselin F, Conti E: Long-term results of proximal interphalangeal resection arthroplasty with a silicone implant. J Hand Surg 20A:S95, 1995.
13. Iselin F, Pradet G: Resection arthroplasty with Swanson's implant for posttraumatic stiffness of proximal interphalangeal joints. Bull Hosp Joint Dis Orthop Inst 44:233, 1984.
14. Iselin F, Pradet G, Gouet O: Conversion to arthroplasty from proximal interphalangeal joint arthrodesis. Ann Chir Main 7:115, 1988.
15. Kiefhaber TR, Stern PJ, Grood ES: Lateral stability of the PIP joint. J Hand Surg 11A:661, 1986.
16. Lane CS: The Dacron-silicone prosthesis for the interphalangeal joints of the hand (Niebauer design): Follow-up of 20 interphalangeal joint prostheses and introduction of a new "adaptable" prosthesis. Ann Chir 29:1011, 1975.
17. Lin H, Wyrick JD, Stern PJ: Proximal interphalangeal joint silicone replacement arthroplasty: Clinical results from an anterior approach. J Hand Surg 20A:123, 1995.
18. Linscheid RL, Dobyns JH, Beckenbaugh RD, Cooney WP III: Proximal interphalangeal joint arthroplasty with a total joint design. Mayo Clin Proc 54:227, 1979.
19. Linscheid RL, Murray P, Vidal MA, Beckenbaugh RD: Development of a surface replacement arthroplasty for the proximal interphalangeal joint. J Hand Surg 22A:286, 1997.
20. Mathoulin C, Gilbert A: Arthroplasty of the PIP joint using the Sutter implant. J Hand Surg 24:565, 1999.
21. Minamikawa Y, Imaeda T, Amadio PC, et al: Lateral stability of proximal interphalangeal joint replacement. J Hand Surg 19A:1050, 1994.
22. Moore MM, Powell RG, Strickland JW: Long-term evaluation of the performance of silicone rubber arthroplasty of the proximal interphalangeal joint. 41st Annual Meeting of the American Association of Hand Surgeons, New Orleans, LA, 1986.
23. Nagle DJ, Ekenstam FWA, Lister GD: Immediate Silastic arthroplasty for nonsalvageable intraarticular phalangeal fractures. Scand J Plast Reconstr Surg Hand Surg 23:47, 1989.
24. Niebauer J, Landry R: Dacron-silicone prosthesis for the metacarpophalangeal and interphalangeal joints. Hand 3:55, 1971.
25. Pellegrini VD Jr, Burton RI: Osteoarthritis of the proximal interphalangeal joint of the hand: Arthroplasty or fusion? J Hand Surg 15:194, 1990.
26. Stern PJ, Ho S: Osteoarthritis of the proximal interphalangeal joint. Hand Clin 3:405, 1987.
27. Swanson AB: Flexible implant arthroplasty of the proximal interphalangeal joint of the fingers. Ann Plast Surg 3:346, 1979.
28. Swanson AB, Maupin BK, Gajjar NV, Swanson G: Flexible implant arthroplasty in the proximal interphalangeal joint of the hand. Hand Surg 10A:796, 1985.

19

Arthroplasty of the Metacarpophalangeal Joint

•WILLIAM P. COONEY III, RONALD L. LINSCHEID, and ROBERT D. BECKENBAUGH

Arthroplasty of the metacarpophalangeal (MCP) joint is the most common procedure in the rheumatoid hand and has been advanced recently by improvement in joint arthroplasty. Combined with soft tissue reconstruction, physical therapy, and improved medical regimens for rheumatoid disease, MCP arthroplasty can improve motion, strength, and function of the rheumatoid hand.

The MCP joints of the four fingers continue to represent a distinct challenge with respect to soft tissue reconstruction and long-term success of joint replacements[4,7,9,19,29] (Fig. 19–1). The problems encountered have to do with (1) the difficulty in matching the positioning and function of four adjacent joints; (2) adjusting the position of an MCP replacement and soft tissue balance to provide normal motion of the interphalangeal (IP) joints; (3) adjusting the soft tissue balance to maintain alignment with the metacarpals throughout the flexion-extension arc; (4) preventing the subsidence and loosening problems inherent with all arthroplastic procedures; and (5) duplicating the kinematics of the normal joint to allow abduction and adduction in extension while permitting flexion along a more or less fixed plane as the dominant motion.[12,56]

MCP arthroplasty is indicated primarily in rheumatoid arthritis, in which there is progressive deformity and diminished function.[12,20,31,43,50] There are indications for MCP joint arthroplasty also in post-traumatic and degenerative arthritis[16]; however, these arthroses do not have the soft tissue reconstructive challenges of the rheumatoid hand. Long-term results, although limited in number, appear sustained for the nonrheumatoid arthritic conditions and suggest that earlier treatment of the rheumatoid hand might offer better function and longer sustained results as well.

ANATOMY AND FUNCTION

The MCP joint is a complex diarthrodial joint at the apex of the longitudinal arch of the hand.[2,39] The anatomic aspects are discussed in detail in Chapter 16. The MCP joint allows more than simple grasping motion because evolutionary refinements in the motor controls of the digits, particularly the extensor apparatus, have permitted reciprocal angulation to occur simultaneously between the MCP and IP joints. Along with the progressive development of the opposable thumb, this makes possible the dexterity that is the quintessential trait of our species.[39]

To accomplish the grasp and pinch functions necessary, the thumb must open widely to accommodate a wide range of spatially diverse objects. This action requires simultaneous MCP and IP extension with abduction at the carpometacarpal (CMC) joint. Grasp occurs with coordinated flexion at the three joints of the finger, which takes place sequentially at proximal interphalangeal (PIP), distal interphalangeal (DIP), and MCP joints. Prehensile grasp is functionally more important than power grasp (grip) in the rheumatoid hand.[8,26]

Pinch is a dynamic action in which manipulation of an object is possible by a rolling action between the opposed thumb and the digital pulps (Fig. 19–2). Key, tip, and palmar pinch are variations on the theme, with pulp to pulp pinch the more common need in the rheumatoid hand. Pinch requires a reciprocal angulation between the IP and MCP joints, whereby flexion occurs in one and extension in the other, followed by reversal.

A stable thumb (IP and MP joints) opposed to stable index and long fingers provides the most useful pinch. The force supplied by the thumb opposition must be resisted by the finger in a plane that is roughly perpendicular to the plane of flexion-extension. The collateral ligaments of the MP and IP joints, along with the intrinsic radial abductors of the index and long fingers, must provide the primary restraint to the thumb (Fig. 19–2). The ulnar fingers add additional lateral stability when partially flexed.[25,57,69,74] The role of these soft tissue constraints is an important consideration in determining arthroplasty versus joint fusion in an effort to obtain useful pinch.[33,36]

Finger flexion and extension is a complex action that must occur with synchrony and balance at all three finger joints. At the MCP joint, the reciprocal finger motion requires that the extensor hood passing dorsal to the MCP must slide over the MCP to its distal attachments

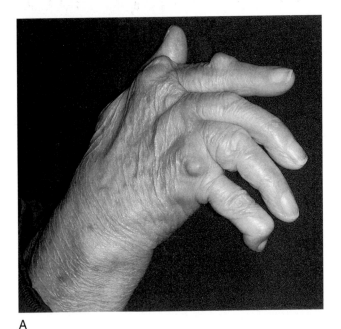

A

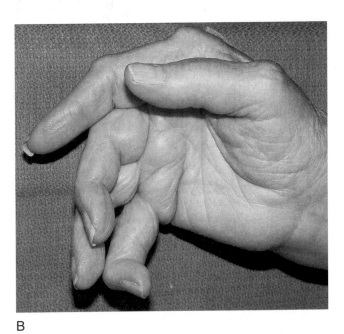

B

Figure 19–1. A, Rheumatoid hand deformity, dorsal view. Dislocation of index, long, ring, and little MCP joints with ulnar drift, multiple rheumatoid nodules, and ulnar displacement of extensor tendons. **B,** Rheumatoid hand, polar view. Limitation of finger extension with flexion deformity of long, ring, and little finger MCP joints.

on the middle and distal phalanges[37,39,74] (Fig. 19–3). Transverse laminae or sagittal bands descend around the MCP to insert at the conjoined palmar plate and base of the proximal phalanx. Extension of the MCP joint is achieved by means of a lifting action of the sagittal bands and transverse laminae at the base of the proximal phalanx, because there is no direct insertion of the extensor tendon at the base of the proximal phalanx.

These structures also act to prevent subluxation of the proximal phalanx by transferring partial extensor force to the proximal phalanx. The oblique tendons of the intrinsic muscles that originate volar to the MCP center of rotation exert moderate tension that increases flexion moment at the MCP joint while providing essential force for extension of the proximal and distal interphalangeal joints. The MCP flexion moment of the intrinsic muscles

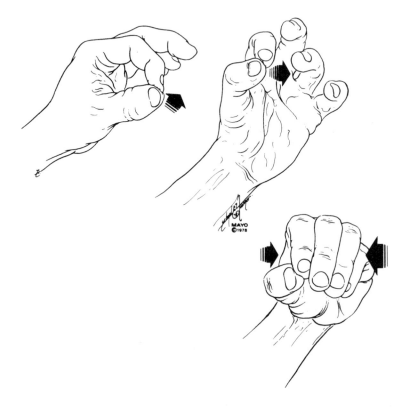

Figure 19–2. Apposition pinch of pulp of index finger and thumb induces torque at interphalangeal joints, which stresses radial collateral ligaments. During apposition pinch, support of adjacent ulnar fingers helps resistance of this torque. (From Linscheid RL, Dobyns JH, Beckenbaugh RD, Cooney WP: Proximal interphalangeal joint arthroplasty with a total joint design. Mayo Clin Proc 54:227, 1979, by permission of Mayo Foundation.)

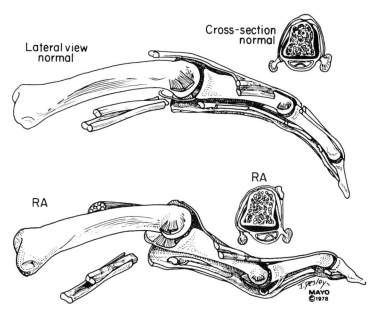

Figure 19–3. Sagittal representation of (**top**) normal alignment of metacarpals and phalanges obtained through ligamentous constraints about joints. Tendons are closely applied about the joint. Sagittal representation (**bottom**) of progressive deformity associated with rheumatoid arthritis, in which there is a volar subluxation at the MCP joint and lengthening of capsular ligaments through attenuation by synovitis. There is a secondary loss of cartilage height by erosion and, frequently, a secondary change in bony architecture, producing flattening of the metacarpal head and settling and erosion of the dorsal lip of the proximal phalanx. This deterioration causes proximal migration and volar subluxation of the proximal phalanx, often associated with synovitis in the flexor tendon sheath and volar distraction of the flexor tendons. These conditions provide a much larger flexion moment arm at the MCP joint. Ulnar drift of the finger is attributable to ulnar bowstringing of the flexor tendons and ulnar pull on the intermetacarpal ligament by the hypothenar musculature. On cross section, the volar plate is displaced volarly and ulnarly on the stretched collateral ligaments and radial sagittal band of the extensor apparatus. Such displacement tends to be associated with progressive myofascial contracture of the ulnar interosseous muscles and displacement of attachment of the radial interosseous muscles. (From Linscheid RL, Dobyns JH: Total joint arthroplasty: The hand. Mayo Clin Proc 54:516, 1979, by permission of Mayo Foundation.)

is a potentially recurring palmar force that needs to be addressed in the rheumatoid hand.[58] The root of the problem in designing functional arthroplasties is to overcome the flexion forces produced by the intrinsic muscles in combination with flexor superficialis and profundus tendon forces. For the reciprocal motion to work, the length-tension parameters of both the skeletal and soft tissue must not vary appreciably more than a millimeter or two in length, and regaining this balance is the key to effective correction of deformities of the hand.[25]

Once the finger soft tissues and joint systems are destabilized beyond a certain point, further deformity is progressive. This, unfortunately, happens frequently in rheumatoid arthritis, with a spectrum of deformity that can begin with radial deviation of the wrist and secondary ulnar deviation of the fingers at the MCP joint. Added to this is the intrinsic muscle tightness of flexing the MCP joint and producing swan-neck deformity or other variations of complex deformities at the PIP joint.[13,14,34,48,63,70]

Kinematic considerations of the MCP joint are also important for effective hand function. Contact on the metacarpal head occurs centrally in extension but shifts laterally during abduction-adduction. After some 60 degrees of flexion, the contact shifts laterally to either side of the proximal phalanx base, where it articulates with the bicondylar aspect of the metacarpal head.

Because this is also the position of maximal collateral ligament tautness, the MCP is at its most stable position with flexion greater than 60 degrees.[2,51]

On transverse section, the metacarpal heads are wedge shaped, and therefore, as the collateral ligaments pass around the metacarpal head in flexion, a greater portion of the ligament is rendered taut and has also passed proximal to the center of rotation.[34,47] This has a serious implication for the success of arthroplasty. Proximal displacement of the proximal phalanx is resisted by the vulnerable distal fibers of the collateral ligament.

The collateral ligaments possess the greatest strength in the constraint system of the MCP, accounting for virtually all the resistance to palmar displacement, distraction, and abduction-adduction.[52] Laxity of the collateral ligaments contributes to the ulnar deviation and volar subluxation so characteristic of the rheumatoid hand. For this reason, a reasonable effort at repair, advancement, or reconstruction of the collateral ligaments should be made to restore joint stability. Although the palmar plate accounts for some 20 percent of the resistance to dorsal subluxation and the dorsal capsule to 20 percent of excessive flexion, their respective roles are likely small in providing support to the MCP joint in the rheumatoid hand.[51]

Landsmeer[39] has shown the collateral ligaments to be most oblique to the joint on the radial aspect of each joint, but both ligaments become progressively more longitudinal in orientation from the index finger to the small finger. Each metacarpal head is also unique, with that of the ring finger having a symmetric contour in both the coronal and sagittal plane. The third metacarpal head is intermediate in appearance between those of the index and ring fingers, whereas the small finger metacarpal head is a less pronounced and smaller version of the index with the asymmetry reversed.[48,59] These anatomic variations are important if anatomic replacement of the metacarpophalangeal joint is considered.[1,9,27,40,41]

RHEUMATOID DEFORMITY

Rheumatoid arthritis produces profound changes in the MCP joints, which result progressively in palmar subluxation, ulnar transposition, and supination of the proximal phalanx (Fig. 19–1A, B). These deformities are due to ligament laxity associated primarily with rheumatoid synovitis and are secondary to internal forces of the intrinsic interosseous and extrinsic finger flexors that are displaced and act on this attenuated joint ligament system. This results in ulnar transposition of the flexor tendon complex and finger extensors at the MCP level and progressive swan-neck deformities at the PIP level.[23,33,59] The latter change appears to be effected primarily by subtle increases of tension in the components of the extensor tendon as they progress to the central slip and lateral bands as a result of the volar subluxation of the MCP. The lateral bands tighten over the dorsum of the PIP, increasing the tension in the central slip. It then becomes increasingly difficult to initiate PIP flexion as the first angular deflection of the flexing finger. The tension in the flexor profundus is transferred to the DIP. Flexion of the DIP in turn increases tension in the dorsally displaced lateral bands, which encourages PIP extension. This becomes the pattern of the swanneck or intrinsic plus deformity.[66,76] Acting in concert with the extensor imbalance, the restraining volar plate becomes attenuated by the joint synovitis and flexor tenosynovitis, diminishing the potential for flexion of the PIP joint.

The initial event at the MCP joint is capsular distention with secondary collateral ligament laxity and then displacement of the extensor tendon mechanism.[25,50] With joint distention, the natural tendency is for the more oblique radial collateral ligament to be stretched.[37] This in turn allows the proximal phalanx to supinate and sublux in a palmar and ulnar direction. The radial collateral ligament becomes increasingly stretched by the forces induced by the flexor profundi and superficialis as well as the intrinsic muscles, whose vector forces lie palmar to the center of rotation. These forces act through or in close proximity to the force nuclei at either side of the MCP joints, where the proximal tendon sheath pulley, sagittal bands, palmar plates, and transverse intermetacarpal ligaments coalesce. At the index and middle fingers, the flexors approach the plane of flexion of the fingers from an ulnar angle of 15 and 8 degrees, respectively. This further augments the ulnar deviation tendency.[33,48,59,60]

The palmar angulation of the fourth and fifth metacarpals during grasp in effect changes the trigonometric status of the relative position of the metacarpal heads. This has the effect of increasing the tension on the relatively inextensible intermetacarpal ligaments in such a way as to pull the palmar plate assemblage of the adjacent metacarpal ulnovolarly.[76]

Initially, the radial intrinsics and radial sagittal bands resist these forces, but the weakened underlying ligamentous structures fail to provide adequate static support. At some point, the ability to resist further deformity is exhausted and the ulnovolar capsular structures undergo permanent contracture. The ulnar aspect of the extensor hood also contracts and fixes the dorsal positioning of the ulnar lateral band. The ulnar intrinsic muscles become contracted and lose most of their excursion properties. Contour changes occur in the joint as a result of uneven wear and erosion of the cartilage as well as collapse of the subcortical trabecular structure. This is especially noted on the dorsal rim of the proximal phalanx and the distal convexity of the metacarpal head.[13,26,34,50,63,66,72,73]

Concomitant collapse deformities at the wrist may accelerate the changes in the fingers. The combination of ulnar translation, radial deviation, and intercarpal supination produced by attenuation of wrist soft tissues and deficient support of a diseased extensor carpi ulnaris increase the ulnar deviation forces at the MCP joints. These deforming forces must be corrected or neutralized if MCP joint reconstruction is to be successful. Loss of height of the carpus moves the strength of the extrinsic tendons to the left on the length-tension slope of the Blix curve, further weakening the support at the MCP joints afforded by the sagittal bands.[34,57]

TREATMENT

Conservative treatment is based primarily on the ability to decrease the inflammatory conditions in the affected joints with medications such as nonsteroidal antiinflammatory drugs. Medical treatments also include chemotherapeutic agents such as hydroxychloroquine (Plaquenil), cyclophosphamide (Cytoxin), sulfasalazine (Azulfedme), and methotrexate. The role of cox-2 inhibitors and the new tumor necrosis factor alpha neutralizers infliximab, leflunomide, and etanercept continue to be studied. There appears to be an increased role for chondroitin sulfate and glucosamine. Wrist and hand splints are recommended at night and intermittently during the day, and, significantly, after reconstructive surgery of the hand and wrist, as an important part of the rehabiliation after surgery. Intra-articular steroid injections at both the MCP and PIP joints have a place in diminishing inflammation, although their effect may be only temporary. Arthroscopic synovectomy is used in the wrist but, to date, not within the MCP joints. Physical therapy measures are also helpful in the context of overall support and prophylaxis but are beyond the scope of this chapter.

SURGICAL TREATMENT

Synovectomy and Other Soft Tissue Options

Synovectomy of the MCP joint combined with collateral ligament advancement and capsulorrhaphy with centralization of the extensor tendons are considered when the integrity of the joint surfaces has been maintained to a reasonable degree. If as much as 50 to 60 percent of the joint surface remains, the original joint should be retained. If there is more than 50 percent joint loss as well as extensive synovitis or significant volar subluxation that cannot be corrected without MCP joint replacement, a joint arthroplasty should be performed. As to synovectomy, the results have been satisfactory in many instances, although recurrent synovitis may lead to further destruction.[23,36,75] Arthroscopic synovectomy of the wrist and thumb CMC joints has been performed, but we are not aware of this technique having been applied to the finger MCP joint.

Smith-Peterson suggested resection arthroplasty of the MCP joint in 1940.[3,20,26] Fowler and Riordian described a technique that included a wedge-shaped metacarpal arthroplasty and a tenodesis of the extensor tendon to the base of the proximal phalanx.[26a] Vainio et al.[70,71,75] introduced the redundant extensor into the defect created by metacarpal head resection to produce a fibrous arthroplasty in conjunction with realignment of the MCP joint. Tupper introduced a variation in which the palmar plate was detached proximally and sutured to the osteotomized metacarpal neck dorsally, thereby reducing the subluxation and providing a fibrous interposition. These operative approaches are rarely used today except for salvage procedures such as performed after sepsis of a previous MCP arthroplasty.

Joint Replacement

A variety of prosthetic replacements have been designed for the MCP joint (Fig. 19–4), beginning with simple metallic hinged joint prostheses (Flatt)[26] and through a number of constrained ball-socket designed prostheses using metalloplastic designs.[8,61] In addition there have been several snap-fit constrained devices with a variety of bone fixation options, including metal pegs, titanium screws, and porous polyethylene grommets. Most of these prostheses have had very little in the way of clinical trials. All have relied on intramedullary fixation, usually augmented by ridging or fluting to stimulate fibrous fixation, bony ingrowth, or polymethylmethacrylate cementing.[1,8,27]

Virtually all these devices have encountered problems that have limited their usefulness such that few are currently marketable devices. Our past report on the Steffee MCP joint was presented in earlier editions of this book.[61] It represents a theoretical good concept for a constrained prosthetic design, but it had many problems, including implant subsidence and loosening, plastic deformation or fracture, stem angulatory erosion, dislocation, metal deformation or fracture, and malpositioning (Fig. 19–5). There is, in addition, with all of these internally constrained devices, a tendency for the center of rotation to displace dorsally on flexion and palmarly on extension.[40] The volar displacement decreases the moment arm for the extensor tendons and increases the moment arm for the flexor tendons, thereby altering the usual physiologic tendency of a joint to encourage the antagonist of the prevailing angulation. This imbalance produces a tendency for the joint to develop a contracture in the direction of most instability, usually flexion and ulnar deviation. This problem is enhanced by the difficulty in precisely positioning the center of rotation in these designs of fixed centers of rotation of

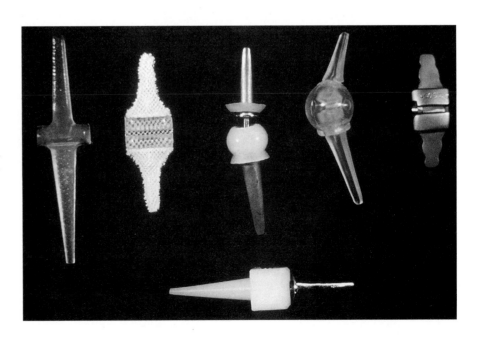

Figure 19–4. Metacarpophalangeal implants (**left to right**). At the bottom, Strickland constrained MCP joint. *Top,* Silicone implant from Swanson AB, silicone implant from Niebauer JJ, constrained implant from Steffee A.

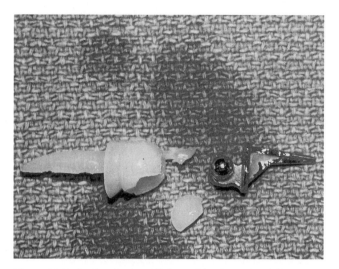

Figure 19–5. Steffee implant. Failure of implant related first to cold flow and then to plastic deformation and dislocation of implant.

the MCP joint. Today, there are no constrained MCP joints being applied in the reconstruction of the rheumatoid hand.

Silicone Joint Replacement

Silicone replacement of the MCP joint (Fig. 19–6) is the primary arthroplasty procedure used worldwide in rheumatoid hand reconstructive procedures.[3,11,19,21,28,30,31,35,38,47,56,60,64,68] This approach employs a one-piece viscoelastic device made of silicone alone or with reinforced materials (Dacron). The design of the prostheses varies by location and function of the silicone hinge. The Swanson device, which has a dorsal, based hinge with favors joint extension by its viscoelastic

properties but has a smaller moment arm for the extensor tendons.[64,65] The Avanta implant is a hinged silicone implant with a dorsal center of rotation[28] (Fig. 19–7) and assumes a fixed axis of motion of the MCP joint, which favors the flexor tendons. The Neuflex implant system is a silicone implant that has a more volar placed center of rotation with a 30-degree neutral angle.[72] It favors the extensor tendon moment arm and potentially provides 90 degrees of MCP joint flexion (Fig. 19–8). The main differences among implants relate to concepts in design such that the Swanson device involves a pistoning of the prosthesis within bone, seeking the best center of rotation, whereas the Avanta and Neuflex systems have a fixed hinge that attempts to simulate the true center of rotation. The mid-area of the Swanson design reportedly has a thicker hub to resist torsional and tensile stresses. It has a curved geometry to encourage movement through the hub. It is reportedly thick enough to resist compression but does not account for rotational stress about the MCP joint (Fig. 19–9).[65]

The problems that have affected viscoelastic (silicone) replacements of the MCP joint include delamination of the composite devices, cold flow deformation, subsidence, and late-developing capsular contractures (Fig. 19–10). These findings appear to be present in all three current types of silicone joint replacements. Fracture of the implants is not a uncommon occurrence, although it is argued that it does not affect joint function.[3,11,12,19,21,28,30,31,47,54,56,60,64] Modifications using titanium grommets with the Swanson design to shield the prosthesis from sharp bone surfaces have had limited success in reducing complications. The silicone implants provide a relative ease of insertion and thus allow time for soft tissue reconstruction, including recommended dorsal advancement or repair of the collateral ligaments.

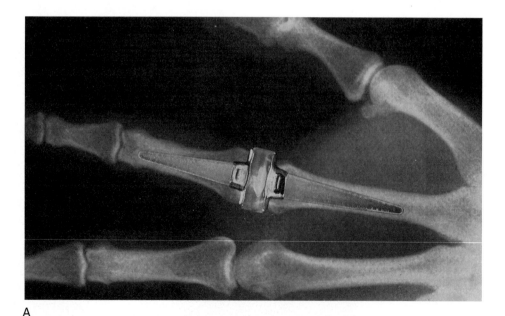

A

Figure 19–6. Silicone joint (Swanson design). **A,** Silicone MCP implant overlayed at the MCP joint with a grommet.
Illustration continued on opposite page

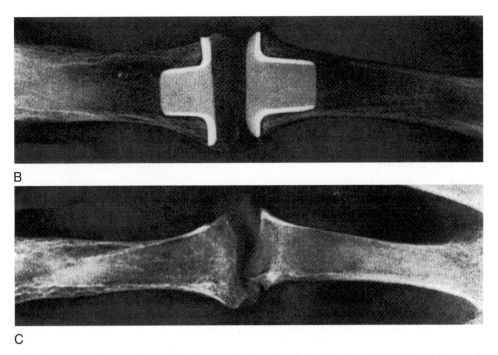

Figure 19–6. *Continued.* **B**, Silicone MCP implant with implant fracture and subsidence. **C**, Revision with new silicone implant 24 months later, with proximal and distal grommets.

Surface Replacements

Anatomic replacement of the finger MCP joint is now possible with two new designs that replace the surface of the MP joint—so-called re-surfacing joint replacements. The goal of these implants is to closely mimic the natural joint. One resurfacing design is made of pyrolytic carbon (Fig. 19–11), which has shown up to 8 years of long-term benefit.[5,17] The second design is metal on plastic resurfacing design that is quite anatomic in producing the change of curvature of the metacarpal head from extension to flexion (Fig. 19–12**A**, **B**). The unique

configuration or design of the MCP joint, however, requires careful soft tissue balance, including the repair or advancement of the collateral ligaments and recognition that each finger in the hand is different, thereby necessitating several sizes and right-left patterns. The complex curvature surface replacement design has been used in clinical trial and appears to have success in providing improved range of motion and strength compared with silicone implants (Fig. 19–13**A**–**D**). This design attempts to simulate the contours of the normal articulation while requiring minimal joint resection. This helps preserve the collateral and

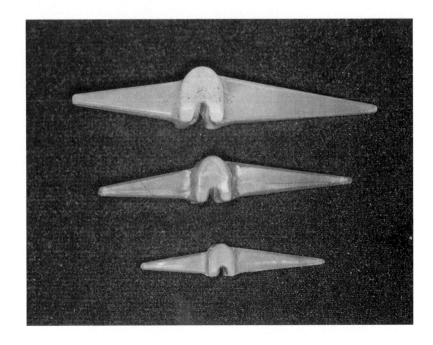

Figure 19–7. Sutter MCP implant. Thicker hinge component with a fixed axis of motion that forces the flexor tendons.

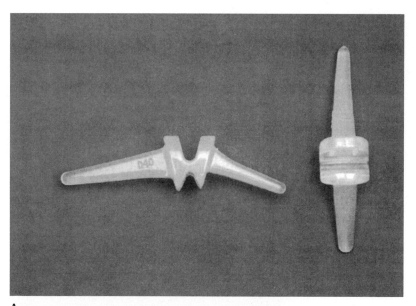

A

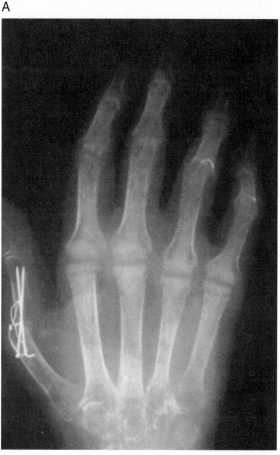

B

Figure 19–8. A, Neuflex implant system. Silicone construction with a 30-degree neutral angle and volar placement of center of rotation. **B**, Clinical case of MCP arthroplasty—Neuflex—showing excellent alignment of MCP joints.

accessory collateral ligaments. Contact areas change with flexion-extension to aid stability in flexion (Fig. 19–14). Computer-aided design and machining allow greater flexibility in manufacture of design and sizes for the various fingers.

Fixation of the pyrolytic carbon implant is by fibrous tissue ingrowth, whereas the resurfacing metal-plastic prosthesis requires bone cement (polymethylmethacrylate). Alternating methods of fixation for resurfacing implants are being studied, including titanium-backed implants for bone ingrowth.[29] Soft tissue reconstruction in rheumatoid arthritis will not be solved by any implant and will continue to require individual assessment and modification at the time of surgery.

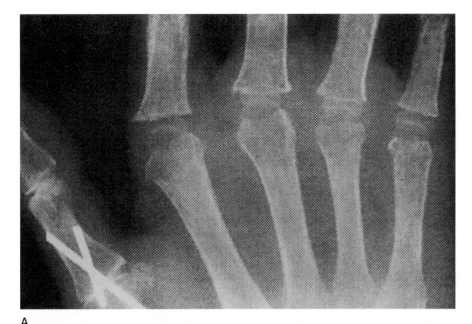

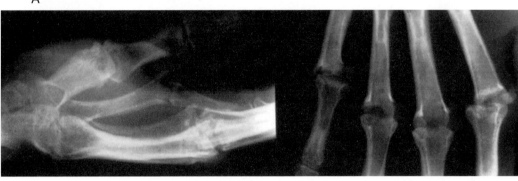

A

B

Figure 19–9. Silicone MCP joints. **A**, Status after implant insertion. Good alignment of implants and correction of ulnar drift. **B**, Anteroposterior and lateral radiograph of fractured silicone prostheses. Displacement of index finger and bone spur with fracture of the little finger. (From Beckenbaugh RD, Dobyns JH, Linscheid RL, Bryan RS: Review and analysis of silicone-rubber metacarpophalangeal implants. J Bone Joint Surg 58A:483, 1976.)

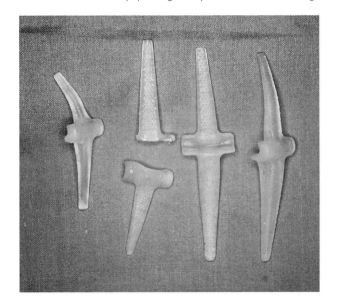

Figure 19–10. Failure of silicone implants (Swanson design). Cold flow deformity (**left**), spiral fracture (**center**), and intact, minimally deformed implants (**right**).

Correcting Deformity

Correction of soft tissue deformity and rebalancing the extensor mechanism are essential for success finger joint replacement. Various techniques for correcting the swan-neck and ulnar deviation deformities have been tried in combination with centralization of the extensor tendons. A simple resection of the triangular oblique fibers of the extensor hood just distal to the sagittal bands was seldom sufficient by itself (Littler technique).[44] Release of the ulnar intrinsics to overcome the static ulnarly deviating force was followed by crossed intrinsic transfers in which the ulnar wing tendon in continuity with the ulnar intrinsic muscle was transferred to the radial lateral band on the adjacent finger.[12] Transferring this restraint to the base of the proximal phalanx was judged more physiologic but difficult to achieve, so that attachment to the collateral ligament is more common in practice. The ulnar intrinsic is represented by a palmar interosseous on the index and ring finger but by a conjoined dorsal and palmar interosseous on the middle finger. The ulnar intrinsics of the little finger are also quite troublesome. Both the

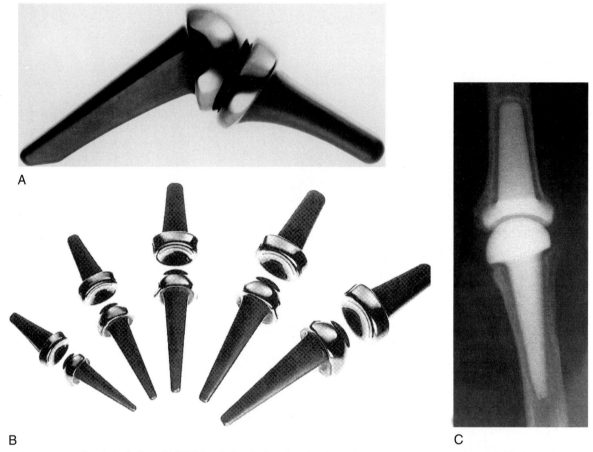

Figure 19–11. Pyrolytic design of MCP joint. **A**, Pyrolytic carbon implant with polished articular surfaces. **B**, Five sizes (small to large) of pyrolytic carbon implants for an MCP joint. **C**, Fine lucent line around carbon implant 3 years postoperatively represents appositional bone growth adjacent to the translucent pyrocarbon layer over radiopaque carbon substrate. (**B**, From Beckenbaugh RD: Preliminary experiences with a noncemented nonconstrained total joint arthroplasty for the metacarpophalangeal joint. Orthopedics 6:962–965, 1983.)

abductor digiti quinti and the volar interossei are diffi-cult to mobilize, and each of these muscles in the advanced deformity is usually devoid of useful contrac-tility.[21,35]

A swan-neck deformity that has persisted usually has an attenuated palmar plate at the PIP joint so that re-balancing of the soft tissues proximally is of little bene-fit. Cutting the ulnar half of the superficialis tendon in the distal palm allows decompression of the flexor sheath, often already compromised by tenosynovitis, and provides a convenient tendon for tenodesis of the PIP joint in slight flexion. This is effective if it is sutured into bone after being extracted from the tendon sheath or by looping through the A_2 pulley if good pulley sub-stance is present.[44,49]

SURGICAL INDICATION

The primary indication for MCP arthroplasty is relief of pain and improved appearance. The surgical procedure of arthroplasty of the MCP joints allows restoration of lost extension and correct longitudinal malalignment (ulnar drift) of the digits. These two goals are reasonable and reliable and have provided good initial short-term results. Recurrence of the disease process and persist-ence of deforming forces, however, may limit the long-term maintenance of the extensile and longitudinal stance. Pain relief is a reliably predictable result after replacement of the MCP joint and is the main indication for surgery in the majority of patients.[7,12,65]

The functional improvement after MCP joint arthro-plasties can be very difficult to assess and to measure objectively. In general, the hand is brought from a flexed and ulnar-deviated central arc of motion of approxi-mately 50 to 100 degrees to an extensile arc of motion of 10 to 50 degrees[10,19,32,47,70] (Fig. 19–14). If the distal joint motion is satisfactory preoperatively, this will result in excellent stability of the hand and a very functional grip. If the IP motion is not satisfactory preoperatively, how-ever, it will not improve postoperatively and the recon-structed hand will only be available to correct and establish a large grip.

The second major indication for MCP arthroplasty is correction of deformity and improved function. The major structural indication for reconstructive surgery of the MCP joints is found in the patient who has flexion/subluxation of the MCP joint with ulnar devia-tion and limited extension. This is a patient who is unable to open the hand to grasp larger items such as a bottle or a glass. Because the procedure may limit the total flexibility of the digits into the palm, it may be

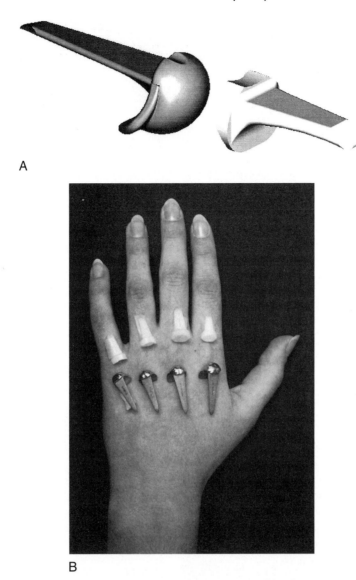

A

B

Figure 19–12. A, Resurfacing design metal-plastic MCP joint. Broad metacarpal head to provide cam-effect to heighten the collateral ligaments and flat dorsal surface of the proximal phalanx for the extensor tendon. **B,** Overlay of surface replacement (SR) implants at the MCP joints. Four sizes presented with metacarpal and proximal phalanx variations.

preferable to perform the surgery to open the hand on one side and leave the other hand in its uncorrected position for more of a tight, closed-fist grip. Others prefer to have both hands in a better position for prehensile grasp and pinch, and they are not concerned with power grip. A number of hand therapists suggest that a functional arc of motion is clearly preferred to one of tight fingers held into the palm of the hand.

The third indication for MCP arthroplasty is improvement of appearance (cosmesis). This is not uncommonly a serious complaint in a patient crippled with rheumatoid arthritis, especially when multiple joints are involved. Cosmesis is coupled with correction of deformity to improve function. Some patients have particular sensitivity to the appearance of their hands, particularly in public service occupational and vocational areas, and in these individuals this represents a very distinct and appropriate indication for surgical intervention.

SURGICAL TECHNIQUE: SILICONE IMPLANTS

Swanson[65,66] has demonstrated the technique using the silicone rubber devices of his design. He prefers to consider the device a spacer that encourages the development of fibrous capsule, which maintains the integrity of the joint against further deformation and directs the encapsulation to provide the correct plane of motion. The sliding action of the stems of the device within the intramedullary cavities is necessary to develop sufficient mobility of the dorsal capsule for adequate flexion. The interested reader is referred to Swanson's writings for further insight.[64] Many of the basic concepts of surgical incision, release of extensor expansion, collateral ligament advancement, and closure with rebalance of extensor expansion are included in these writings. They are incorporated into the surgical description that follows.

In the mid-1980s, under the direction of several hand surgeons, the Avanta Corporation (formerly Sutter) developed a new silicone-based MCP joint arthroplasty.[4,28,54] This particular device is a hinged silicone rubber implant with squared bases and stems to control implant position and interfaces. The operative procedure for the Avanta implant is identical to that of the Swanson implant, but it is noteworthy that the device appears to offer a slightly increased ease in rotational alignment within the intramedullary canals of the MCP joint. The hinge also represents a fixed center of rotation and it is not clear whether this implant pistons within the intramedulary canals as is proposed for the Swanson Silastic implant.

In the late 1990s a further refinement of the silicone design resulted in the Neuflex silicone implant.[72] The insertion principles for this implant are similar to those of the Swanson and Avanta silicone designs, with emphasis on correct level of resection of the metacarpal head and careful broaching of the intermedullary canal. The implant is designed to not piston within the intramedullary canals and to favor greater MCP flexion with a 30-degree prebent flexion starting position. It is believed to more closely reflect the center of rotation of the MCP joint.

However, a study of tendon excursion and moment arm comparison of three silicone implants versus the normal joint showed relatively little difference.

AUTHORS' PREFERENCE

Exposure

The MCP arthroplasty is performed through a transverse incision proximal to the web spaces of the fingers or through individual curved longitudinal incisions (Fig. 19–15A). The latter incision is preferred for single digits or if surgical correction at the PIP joint is anticipated. The extensor tendons and sagittal bands are exposed, with attention to the juncturae tendinae, transverse lamina, and position and location of the extensor tendons (Fig. 19–15B). If there is a small amount of ulnar displacement of the extensor tendons, the radial sagittal band is released adjacent to the extensor tendon and reflected from the underlying capsule. For the index and little fingers with two extensor tendons, the incision should split between the two tendons. If the amount of displacement of the extensor

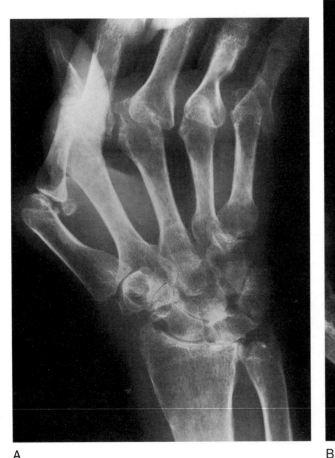

A

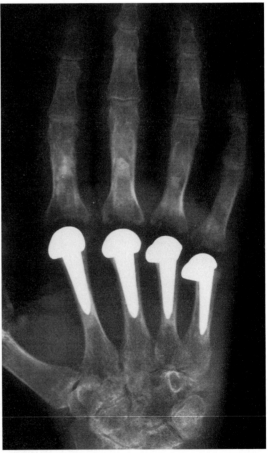

B

Figure 19–13. A, Rheumatoid hand deformity with dislocation-subluxation of the MCP joints of the index, long, ring, and little fingers with ulnar drift. **B,** Correction of the deformity with metal-plastic SR MCP joints. Fixation with methylmethacrylate. Centralization of the extensor tendon complex.

Illustration continued on opposite page

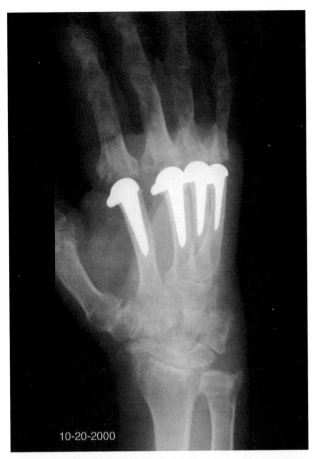

10-20-2000

C

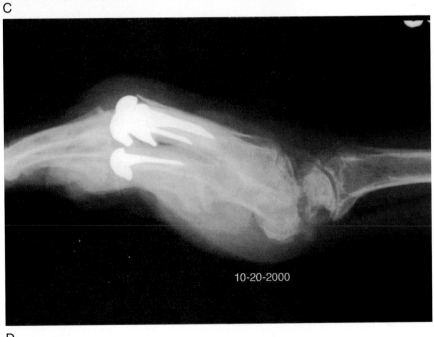

10-20-2000

D

Figure 19–13. *Continued.* **C**, Oblique views at 2 years of follow-up. Maintained MCP joint alignment. **D**, Lateral view at 2 years of follow-up.

tendon is significant (i.e., the tendon lies in the gutter between the metacarpal heads), the ulnar sagittal band and transverse lamina are released as well so that the tendon will be freed sufficiently for replacement over the dorsum of the metacarpal head during closure (Fig. 19–15**C**). The extensor expansion is freed from the joint capsule if possible and divided in the midline. A synovectomy of the joint is performed. The radial and

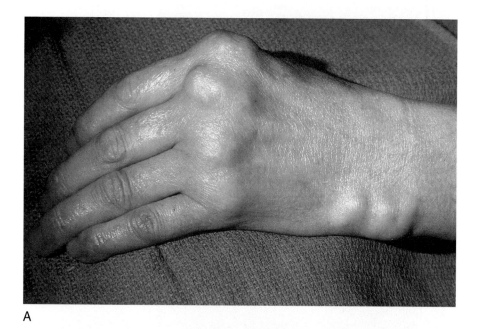

A

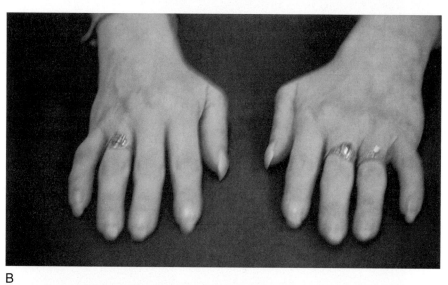

B

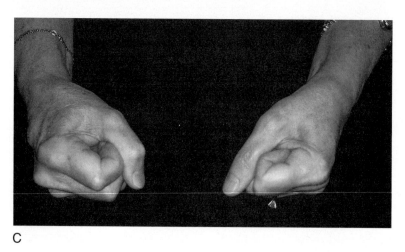

C

Figure 19–14. Rheumatoid hand resurfacing implants. **A**, Preoperative dorsal view. MCP joint synovitis and volar subluxation of MCP joints with ulnar drift. **B**, Dorsal view of both hands. Left hand at 1 year and right hand at 3 years of follow-up. **C**, MCP flexion with both hands.

Illustration continued on opposite page

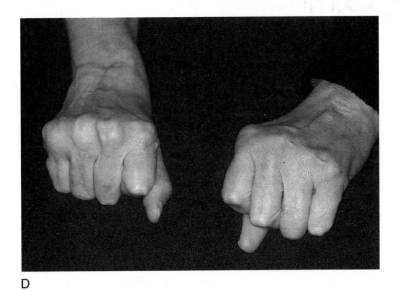

D

Figure 19–14. *Continued.* **D,** MCP flexion, axial view, in a different patient, showing the potential for joint replacement. Unoperated (**left**) and postoperative (**right**) MCP arthroplasty.

ulnar collateral ligaments are next carefully exposed and released from the metacarpal head. The metacarpal head is next resected with an oscillating saw. The size of the implant and degree of volar subluxation of the proximal phalanx determine the amount of metacarpal head resection (Fig. 19–15**D**). A minimum of 1 cm of space is needed between the metacarpal neck and the proximal phalanx for full MCP joint extension. If joint subluxation is not extreme, the collateral ligament attachments may be preserved; usually, they are separated free from the capsule and sagittal bands and protected for secondary repair at closure. After resection of the metacarpal head, additional synovectomy of the MCP joint is performed by sharp dissection and the use of fine ronguers, especially beneath the collateral ligaments and between the metacarpal neck and palmar plate.

Preparation

Soft Tissue Reconstruction and Closure

Soft tissue balancing is necessary using techniques such as crossed intrinsic transfers, release of the ulnar wing tendons, or radial collateral ligament reconstruction. With the prosthesis in place, the collateral ligaments are advanced on the metacarpal shaft. We recommend nonabsorbable sutures (3–0 mersilene) for reattachment of the collateral ligaments. The capsule is closed with fine absorbable sutures with a minimum of raw surface. The extensor tendon is then centralized over the underlying approximated sagittal bands, or the radial sagittal band is imbricated to the extensor if the ulnar sagittal band is sufficiently long. With the MCP joint in full extension, it is recommended that a vest-over-pants closure be made with use of a resorbable polyglygolic acid-based suture.

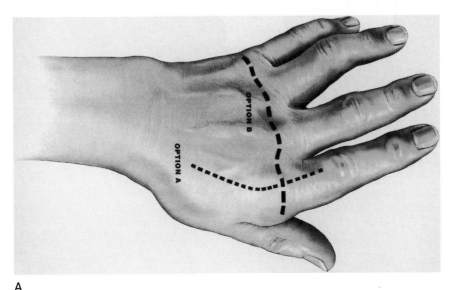

OPTION B

OPTION A

A

Figure 19–15. Surgical approach. **A,** Option A: longitudinal incision, single joint; option B: transverse incision, multiple joints.

Illustration continued on following page

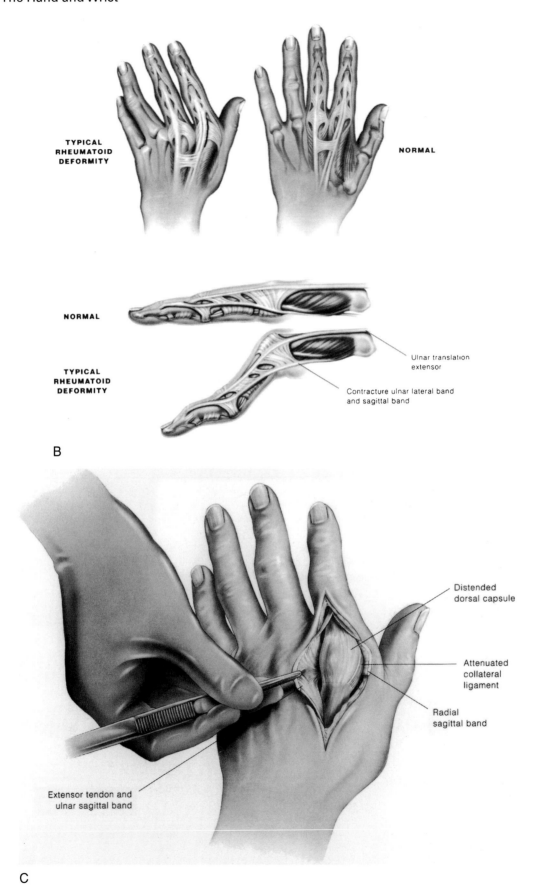

TYPICAL
RHEUMATOID
DEFORMITY

NORMAL

NORMAL

TYPICAL
RHEUMATOID
DEFORMITY

Ulnar translation
extensor

Contracture ulnar lateral band
and sagittal band

B

Distended
dorsal capsule

Attenuated
collateral
ligament

Radial
sagittal band

Extensor tendon and
ulnar sagittal band

C

Figure 19–15. *Continued.* **B**, Surgical anastomy—extensor hood. Surgical release is performed along the radial border of the extensor tendon at the MCP joint. Rheumatoid hand deformity (**left**), extensor tendon. Normal extensor tendon mechanism (**right**). **C**, Reflection of the extensor tendon mechanism and the ulnar sagittal band.

Illustration continued on opposite page

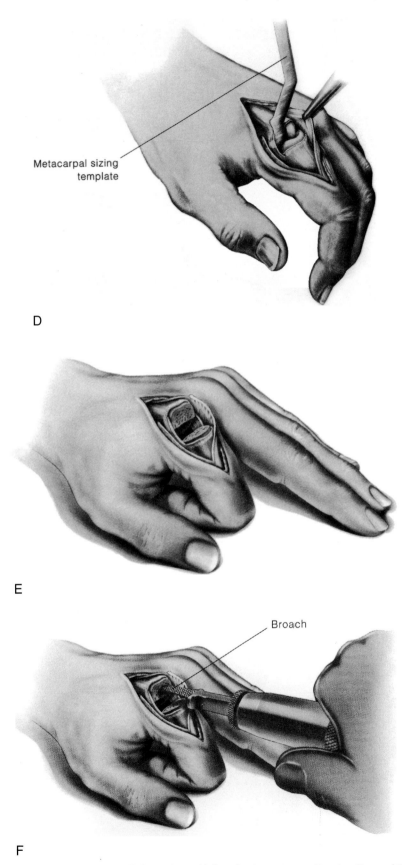

Metacarpal sizing
template

D

E

Broach

F

Figure 19–15. *Continued.* Surgical approach. **E**, Resection guidelines for the metacarpal head and base of the proximal phalanx. Increased metacarpal head resection will be needed to correct the volar subluxation of the MP joint. Limited resection of the proximal phalanx base will be required to preserve the volar plate and the collateral ligament origins. **F**, Broaching of the metacarpal canal to the size of the predetermined prosthesis.

Illustration continued on following page

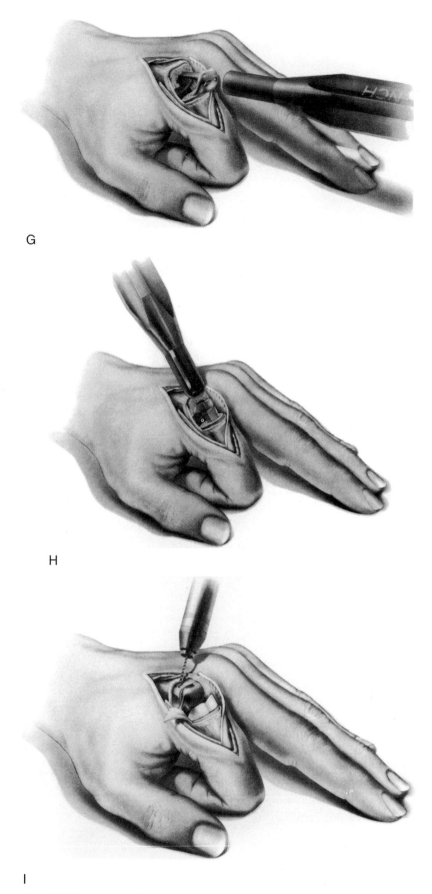

G

H

I

Figure 19–15. *Continued.* **G**, Trial prosthesis insertion into the metacarpal and proximal phalanx. **H**, Metacarpal and proximal phalanx. **I** and **J**, Drilling through the metacarpal head for suture (2–0 or 3–0 nonresorbable suture) for repair and advancement of the radial and ulnar collateral ligaments. Proximal phalanx and metacarpal prostheses are inserted.

Illustration continued on opposite page

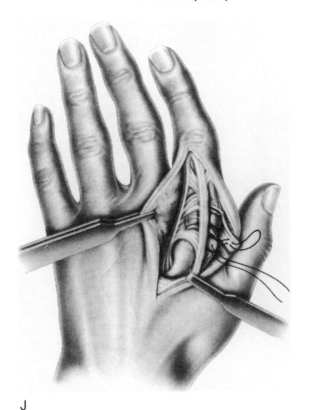

J

K

Radial collateral
ligament tightened

Figure 19–15. *Continued.* **J,** Drilling through the metacarpal head for suture (2–0 or 3–0 nonresorbable suture) for repair and advancement of the radial and ulnar collateral ligaments. Proximal phalanx and metacarpal prostheses are inserted. **K,** Collateral ligament repair tightened with MCP joint in full extension with the joint fully reduced and aligned.

Illustration continued on following page

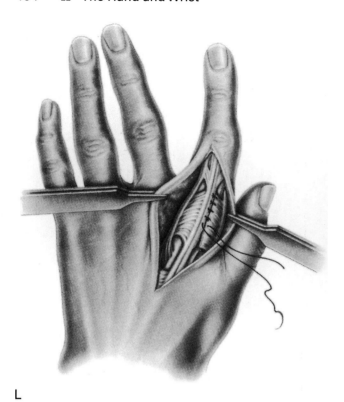

L

Figure 19–15. *Continued.* **L**, Extensor head centralized by radial repair or reefing of sagittal bands and extensor tendon pants-over-vest.

Resurfacing Arthroplasty: SR MCP Implant

The surgical approach for the resurfacing arthroplasty is similar to that used for the silicone arthroplasty up to the point of resection of the joint (see company brochures on surgical technique from Avanta Orthopedics, San Diego, CA). For the metal-plastic implant, trial prostheses guides are used to provide precise resection of the metacarpal head and base of the proximal phalanx. The resection of the metacarpal head must be proximal enough to allow full MCP extension. The base of the proximal phalanx resection must be minimal in order to preserve the origins of the volar plate and the proper collateral ligaments (Fig. 19–15**E**). There are specifically sized broaches for the metacarpal canal and the proximal phalanx canals; a separate series of broaches is provided for each (Fig. 19–15**F**). Trial implants are available to ensure proper depth, fit, and size of the prostheses. For the metal-plastic resurfacing implant, bone cement is currently used. We insert the metacarpal and proximal phalanx components at the same time and cement each finger in separately (Fig. 19–15**G, H**), beginning with the index and moving ulnarly. It is important to have exact anatomic alignment of the prosthesis so that with flexion the fingers do not overlap. After each finger joint is inserted, we proceed stepwise with collateral ligament advancement (Fig. 19–15**I, J**), capsule closure, and centralization of the extensor tendon (Fig. 19–15 **K, L**). It is best to place the collateral ligament suture into the metacarpal neck before inserting the bone cement and prosthesis, and then advance the collateral ligament with the MCP joint in full extension.

Resurfacing Arthroplasty: Pyrolytic Carbon

Pyrolytic carbon, a pure carbon material like graphite and diamond, has desirable features of both. Pyrolytic carbon in implants is made by super-heating a gas, such as methane CH_4, which splits off carbon molecules from hydrogen to form a pure carbon gas. A pyrocarbon joint is made of a super-strong graphite core that is passed through a chamber with the carbon gas.[24] The pyrolytic carbon surface is a .5-mm layer added on to the graphite subtrate core. It is polished to an extremely low friction surface for articulation and demonstrates high strength, fatigue resistance, and nearly wear-free characteristics in clinical and laboratory testing. It has an elastic modulus similar to that of cortical bone (as opposed to cement, metal, and ceramics) and has been shown to fix in medullary canals of bone through appositional bone growth; therefore, it does not require cement for bony fixation.[18] The procarbon MCP joint is a simple ball and socket design (see Fig. 19–11**A**).[6] It is available in five sizes (see Fig. 19–11**B**). Stems are designed in a physiologic shape complementing the normal medullary canal configuration. These stems have planar subarticular collars that allow precise press fitting into the metacarpal and proximal phalanx. The subarticular collar planes are angulated to allow preservation of the collateral ligament attachments and to enhance dorsal expansion to increase stability against subluxation. (The dorsal tip of the phalangeal component is extended proximally.)

The graphite substrate is impregnated with a small amount of tungsten to make it radiopaque. The pyrocarbon coating, however, does not have tungsten; therefore, as bone grows adjacent to the implant, a lucent line is seen, unlike other metal and ceramic prostheses and/or cemented devices. This lucent line is a good sign and signifies bony fixation, not loosening (Fig. 19–11**B**).

SURGICAL TECHNIQUE

The operation is performed through a normal dorsal transverse or longitudinal incision (Fig. 19–15**A**). In conditions without extensor tendon displacement, the extensor mechanism is split longitudinally over the joint. In subluxed extensor mechanisms, the hood is incised on the radial side of the central tendon (Fig. 19–15**B**). The extensor hood is separated from the capsule, if possible, and the capsule is incised longitudinally to expose the joint (Fig. 19–15**C**). Excess synovium is removed. The alignment awl is inserted into the head of the metacarpal and down the shaft (Fig. 19–16**A**). A saw guide is placed on the alignment guide and used to start a cut dorsally to the center of the guide at the proper (27.5 degrees) angle (Fig. 19–16**B**). The angle cut is completed by free hand after removal of the guide (Fig. 19–16**C**).

An identical sequence is then used to resect the base of the proximal phalanx at a 5-degree backward angulation (Fig. 19–16**D**).

The medullary canals are now impacted or reamed to the appropriate sized implant. In general, the largest size implant that fits the proximal phalanx is used as a sizing method. Implant sizes cannot be mismatched. The sized reamers are fit minimally below the actual implant size to allow implant impaction (Fig. 19–16E). After reaming is complete, the implant trials are tapped into place with the plastic impactors. The joint is reduced. After reduction, the goal is to achieve passive

mobility of the MCP through an arc of 0 to 90 degrees of flexion, without excessive tension. This may require release of the volar plate, but the joint resection is usually too small to allow inspection of the flexor tendons, as is possible in silicone arthroplasty. The intrinsics are tested; if tight, they are released. All ulnar structures are

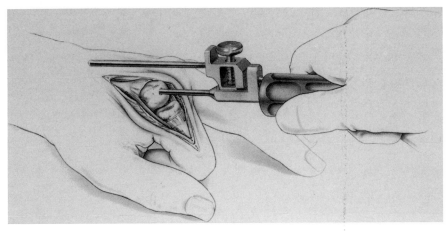

A

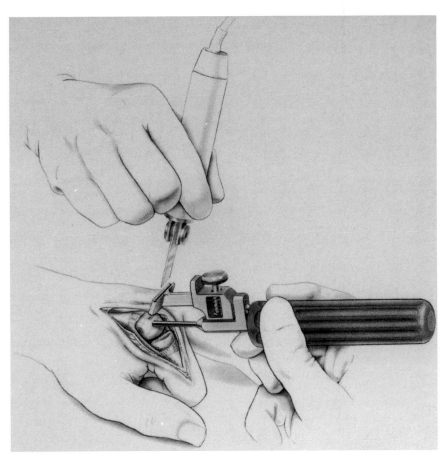

B

Figure 19–16. Pyrolytic carbon surgical technique. **A,** Awl is inserted down metacarpal and dorsal guide bar is inserted to orient alignment of the awl within the medullary canal of the metacarpal in a radio ulnar and anteroposterior plane. **B,** Dorsal guide bar is replaced by saw alignment guide, and the dorsal half of the metacarpal head is cut.

Illustration continued on following page

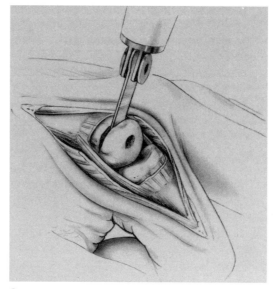

C

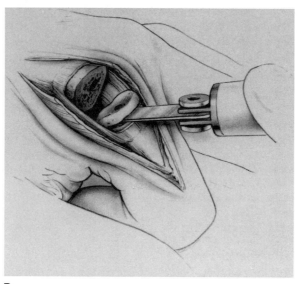

D

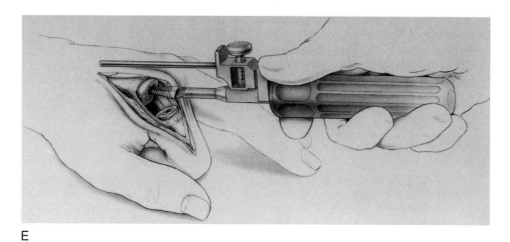

E

Figure 19–16. *Continued.* **C**, The second half of the cut is completed free hand with the plane of the dorsal saw being used for a guided cut. **D**, The proximal phalanx saw cut is also guided.

Illustration continued on opposite page

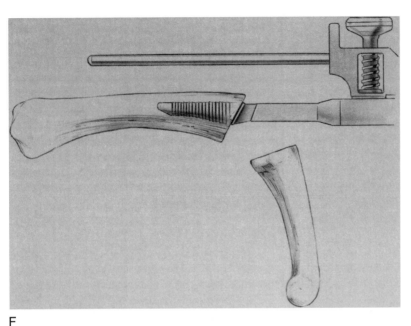
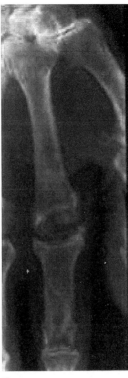

F   G

Figure 19–16. *Continued.* **E** and **F**, With use of the alignment guide rod on the broach of the medullary canals, the broach is press fit within the medullary canal. **G**, Ten-year follow-up of pyrocarbon MCP implant with a zero to 70-degree range of motion and biologic fixation. It is noteworthy that the original design had no tungsten in the substrate.

released, including the metacarpal origin of the collateral ligament, if necessary, to allow full passive extension and correction of any ulnar deviation.

The trials are removed, and the real implants are gently impacted in place. Dorsal palmar instability is tested and corrected with soft tissue reconstruction of the capsule, collateral ligament, or extensor tendon and hood, as required. The capsule, if present, is repaired snugly over the prosthesis. The radial collateral ligament may be repaired to the metacarpal, if necessary. The extensor mechanism is closed with radial imbrication of the hood to centralize it over the metacarpal joint. If the ulnar hood is too tight to allow imbrication radially, the ulnar hood can be cut free of the central tendon and repaired to the radial hood. The central tendon is then repaired to the radial hood and may be sutured into the base of the proximal phalanx to enhance stability, if necessary. The remainder of the wound is closed in the usual manner, and a bulky compression dressing is applied to maintain the digits in extension at the MCP and to ensure functional flexion at the IP joints. Check radiographs are taken to ensure proper position and articulation of the implants after the postoperative dressing is applied.

POSTOPERATIVE CARE

As the joints are intrinsically nonjoined, it is necessary for soft tissues to heal to create stability. In general, the hand is immobilized in full extension at the MCP joints for 3 to 4 weeks, with the IP joints free after 1 to 2 weeks. Early motion as performed after silicone arthroplasty should not be done in patients with rheumatoid arthritis with nonconstrained resurfacing prostheses, because motion of 80 degrees or more can be obtained and may lead to recurrent ulnar drift or instability. The exception is in patients with osteoarthritis or traumatic arthritis, in whom soft tissue stability is good, and motion may begin at 3 to 4 days.

After removal of the postoperative cast/splint at 3 to 4 weeks, a carefully supervised program of motion, protected by custom-made dynamic and static splints, is begun under the daily guidance of a therapist who is a specialist in hand therapy. The goals are to achieve 0 to 45 degrees of balanced motion by 3 months postoperatively in patients with rheumatoid arthritis. Dynamic splints to guide joint position by day are used for 3 months postoperatively, and static resting splints are recommended at night indefinitely.

PRINCIPLES AND GUIDELINES

In the use of pyrolytic carbon ball and socket implants, it is necessary to remember that successful joint replacement requires the capability of reconstructing a stable soft tissue envelope that allows bony fixation by appositional bone growth. The ideal indication, therefore, is in patients with osteoarthritis and post-traumatic arthritis. In rheumatoid patients with soft medullary and thin cortical bone, the implant should be used with caution. Although impaction bone grafting or cement may be considered, there is no long-term information on these newer techniques (of bone grafting). If there is severe deformity (> 60 degrees of extension lag and > 45 degrees ulnar deviation), soft tissue reconstruction may not be sufficient to provide stability, and conversion to silicone arthroplasty may be necessary at the time of primary surgery. In cases of complete MCP dislocation with more than 1 cm of proximal migration of the proximal phalanx, the implant should not be used. If there is a significant degree of intercarpal supination and radial deviation with ulnar translation, the wrist position should be corrected before implant surgery of the MCP.

The pyrolytic carbon MCP replacement offers the benefit of producing a fixed fulcrum, more normal "articulated" joint function. A limited number of pyrolytic carbon implants were used in rheumatoid and osteoarthritic patients on a custom basis in the 1980s. The results of this study have demonstrated that obtaining biologic fixation is viable and desirable. The potential for relief of pain, improvement in cosmesis, improvement in fixation, and long-term durability is excellent.[17] The greatest potential problem with the design is subluxation and/or recurrent ulnar deviation. With careful surgical technique and postoperative care, a stable, painfree, functional arthroplasty is achievable (Fig. 19–16**F**).

Adjunctive Procedures

When the PIP joints are markedly eroded, displaced, or have an uncorrectable swan-neck deformity, arthrodesis in functional flexion generally allows the MCPs to gain a better range of motion than is obtainable if the PIP joints are left alone. PIP fusion is generally set at 30 degrees for the index finger, progressing to 45 degrees at the little finger. Proximal interphalangeal arthroplasty may be performed in combination with fusion and soft tissue reconstruction of the MCP joint, but[41] replacing both the MCP and PIP joints is not advised.[42] Soft tissue rebalancing at PIP joint for both swan-neck and boutonnière deformity should always be performed after the MCP arthroplasties.

The thumb is an extremely important component of the crippled rheumatoid hand. The most common anomaly is the duckbill deformity with flexion and radial angulation of the MCP joint and hyperextension deformity of the IP joint.[53] This makes a dexterous tip pinch difficult to perform. Arthrodesis of the MCP joint in slight flexion provides release for the taut IP extensors, allowing the IP joint to regain flexion. An alternative is to fuse the IP joint and transfer the extensor pollicis longus (EPL) to act as an extensor of the MCP joint. Occasionally, arthroplasty of the MCP joint of the thumb[10] may be desirable, particularly with fusion of the thumb MCP joint. Finally, the base of the thumb, the metacarpotrapezial joint, may be unstable with dorsoradial subluxation and an adducted metacarpal with hyperextension of the thumb MCP. A fibrous arthroplasty (the Eaton-Littler or the Burton ligament reconstruction tendon interposition procedure) is indicated with resection of the trapezium, adductor release, and soft tissue stabilization of the TMC joint.

After Care: Silicone Implants

Small silicone rubber drains are left beneath the incisions. A bulky, compressive, absorptive dressing is applied with the MCP joints in full extension and radial deviation. The PIP joints should also be splinted in nearly full extension. The arm is elevated, and ice bags may be helpful in minimizing swelling. The dressing change and drain removal is performed within 4 days. For the silicone MCP joints, dynamic extension splints are applied, with the goal of MCP extension assist with radial deviation. The principle is actively assisted extension with active flexion of the MCP joints. We commonly use a volar gutter splint across the PIP joint so that all motion is directed at the MCP joint. After 5 to 7 days, active flexion may be commenced under supervision of a hand therapist. A static support splint is used at night, with MCP full extension and PIP in slight flexion. A progressive increase in motion is then used by the hand therapist, with a goal of maintaining nearly full extension and a gain of up to 50 degrees of MCP flexion. Flexion slings are added only after the fourth or fifth week if flexion is lagging. Controlled motion within the splints is continued for at least 6 weeks, and rest splinting is continued indefinitely.[46,55]

After Care: Resurfacing Implants

With the resurfacing MCP joints, soft tissue stability is of paramount importance; therefore, the postoperative program is one of rest for 3 to 4 weeks, then active assisted motion. Within 2 to 3 days after the surgical procedure, we cast the hand and wrist with the MCP joint in full extension and slight radial deviation. The wrist is in extension for 20 degrees and ulnar deviation is present. At 3 weeks (or 4 weeks if there was considerable soft tissue laxity of the MCP joints, so-called wet rheumatoid hand), the dynamic splinting is started (Fig. 19–17). The progress to active motion is dependent on MCP joint stability and the need for static splinting during the day as well as at night (Fig. 19–17**B**). Splinting is necessary to prevent MCP joint subluxation.

RESULTS

Silicone Implants

Results in patients with silicone rubber prostheses have now been reported by a number of investigators as well as by Swanson and associates.[19,28,30–32,47,65] These studies show excellent relief of pain and generally increased hand function. The cosmetic appearance of the hands improved considerably in most instances. Total active motion of the MCP joints has varied in different reports from 34 to 57 degrees, with an average of 45 degrees. Extension lags range from 7 to 27 degrees, with an average of 15 degrees. A slow deterioration of motion over time has been seen. Recurrence of ulnar drift and volar subluxation are the major concerns.[62]

The increase in grip and pinch strength is modest with silicone procedures, but patients report overall improved hand function, and the majority are pleased with the results of the procedure. Stabilization of the thumb MCP and IP joints also improves pinch and dexterity[55,75] and is a recommended associated procedure with MCP arthroplasty.

From a long-term perspective, silicone joints have demonstrated satisfactory results for longer than 8 to 10 years. From Kaplan Meier survival curve analysis, the

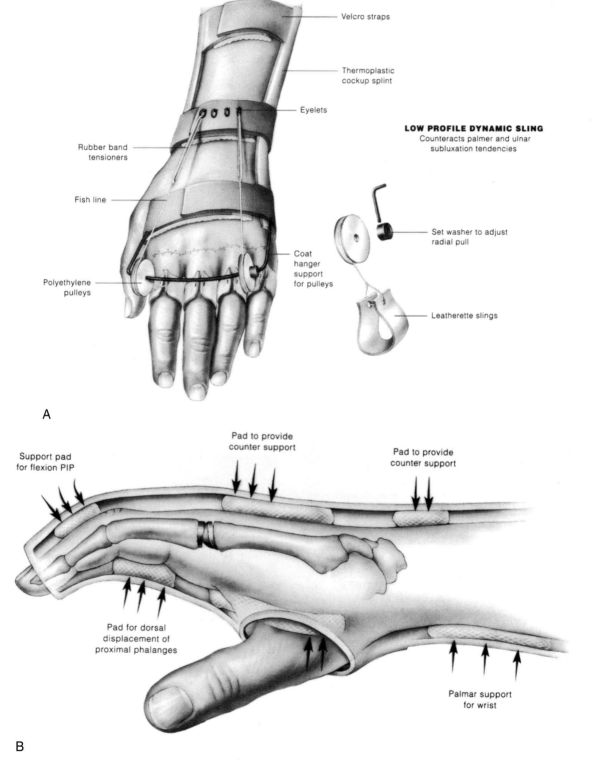

Figure 19–17. A, Low-profile dynamic splinting after MCP arthroplasty. The principle of extension and the radial deviation of the MCP joint are shown. **B**, Orthoplast splint with low profile MCP extension and prehensile pinch between the thumb and the index and long fingers.

Illustration continued on following page

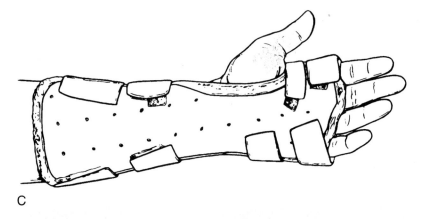

C

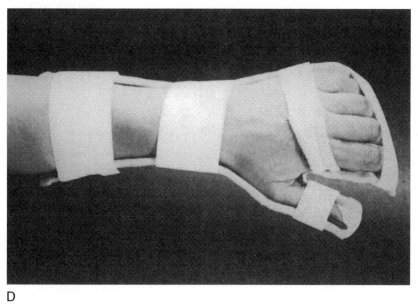

D

Figure 19–17. *Continued.* **C**, Static splinting across the MCP for day use; the PIP joints are free. **D**, Static night splinting holding the MCP joints in extension, the PIP joints in slight flexion, and the thumb in abduction.

rate of failure leading to revision surgery (reoperation representing the endpoint) extends to a 70 percent survival level up to 10 years and then begins to move downward with subsequent years. The results from the Neuflex implant show improved range of motion over other silicone implants, as reported in a reference publication by the design originators.[72] In 46 patients with 168 implants with a mean follow-up of 14 months, the authors reported good results with average motion of 12 to 73 degrees of flexion and no complications. Improvement in grip and pinch strength as well as functional activity changes, however, were not reported.

The major complication with silicone joint prostheses is fracture of the prostheses and recurrence of ulnar drift. The occurrence of silicone fracture has varied from 0 percent to as high as 26 percent.[3,4,7,12,20,22,25,41] Fracture was higher in the original silicone joints than in the later version. It has occurred with a result of both torsion and bending forces. However, the degree of fracture and recurrence of ulnar drift may not affect the long-term outcome. Several authorities question whether fracture matters at all. In one recent experience, for example, the

authors report, with a minimum 5-year follow-up, a high satisfaction rate. All patients denied pain and were pleased with the results,[38] despite the fact that by radiographic examination, 30% of implants had fractured. Fractures occur primarily in the hub of the prosthesis or at the juncture with the stems. Unfortunately, the use of metal grommets has not affected this complication. In addition, cold flow deformation of the silicone can be seen after prolonged use. Discoloration from apparent imbibition of lipids also is known. Subsidence from pressure of the prosthesis against the cut cortical surfaces has been reported as generally minimal but occasionally extensive. Slow narrowing of the width between the cortical surfaces of the base of the proximal phalanx and the metacarpal joint correspond to a gradual loss of mobility. Particulate synovial inflammation (silicone synovitis) is much less of a problem than with the carpal implants.

Our Experience with Silicone Implants

In 1976, Beckenbaugh et al.[5] reported the Mayo Clinic results with silicone implants, including a series of

Niebauer prostheses as well as Swanson prostheses. At that time, our results showed an average range of motion of 38 degrees of flexion and extension. The breakage rate was assessed at 38 percent for the Niebauer prosthesis and 26 percent for the Swanson prosthesis. An interesting observation was the frequent limitation of motion of the ulnar two fingers compared with the radial fingers. This may be explained in part by the necessity of releasing the intrinsic musculature to a greater degree on the ulnar fingers, especially the abductor digiti minimi. This release effectively removes the primary flexion force from the proximal phalanx.

A more recent review of silicone MCP joints included both Swanson and Sutter designs. We found a similar rate of implant deformation and fracture (30%) but continued reasonable function and a range of motion that averaged 40 degrees. Currently, silicone replacement athroplasty remains the standard in MCP joint replacement. Because it is not a true joint arthroplasty, it is difficult to call it the gold standard for MCP joint replacement. We consider silicone implants very useful in most advanced cases of rheumatoid arthritis and prefer to recommend them to patients for correction of ulnar deviation and flexion deformity, with a goal of motion of 10 to 15 degrees of lack of extension and up to 45 to 50 degrees of joint flexion. Silicone implants are recommended for all patients with resorptive arthropathy. Hence, we recommend silicone replacement of the MCP joint and fusion of the PIP joints. In our experience, there have not been any substantial differences in the results between the different types of silicone implants.

Resurfacing Implants

In the past 5 years, there have been improvements in the design and clinical use of resurfacing implants. Our first experience was with the pyrolytic carbon implant. In 1999, Cook et al.[17] reported an 8-year follow-up of 40 patients with good long-term results up to 10 years after surgery. This information provides encouragement to develop further improved designs of resurfacing MCP implants. Since 1994, we have had experience with a metal-plastic MCP joint replacement in selected patients with early rheumatoid or degenerative arthritis (Fig. 19–14A–D). The results to date with use of anatomically designed duplicates of joint articular surfaces are encouraging. Preliminary results of a Food and Drug Administration clinical trial in 20 patients with 60 implants, comparing resurfacing implants with silicone implants demonstrate increased range of motion of 60 degrees of total motion, with only 10 degrees lack of extension at 70 degrees of flexion. Similar results have been reported for pyrolytic carbon implants. Resurfacing implants have, for the most part, provided good relief of pain and little recurrence of ulnar drift. Grip and pinch strength are improved. There is not, however, long-term follow-up, and potential complications that may arise include recurrence of MCP flexion and ulnar drift, implant loosening, component failure, and subsidence. As mentioned earlier, a very different postoperative program of joint support is needed, and, in most cases,

the collateral ligaments must be reattached and protected until healing back to the metacarpal neck shaft has occurred. The Food and Drug Administration has given permission to use both the pyrolytic carbon implant and the resurfacing metal on plastic implants as approved devices for MCP arthroplasty in patients with degenerative, post-traumatic, and rheumatoid arthritis. We believe that use of these devices is warranted in the early to middle stages of rheumatoid disease, but, at this time, not in advanced rheumatoid disease of the MCP joints or the "wet" progressive rheumatoid.

SPECIAL CASES

Isolated rheumatoid arthritis, traumatic arthrosis, or degenerative joint disease may occasionally affect the performance of the adjacent fingers. These types of problems would seem to be ideal for a surface replacement prosthesis. Commercially available metal on plastic resurfacing implants and the pyrolytic carbon prostheses have been used in patients with these conditions. We have used these implants in cases of failed silicone arthroplasty, in which added stress by forceful use of the hands is anticipated or demonstrated by early fracture of the silicone implants. The resurfacing implants may have a special role in treatment of patients with localized degenerative arthritis whose soft tissue stability and collateral ligaments have not been compromised.

THE FUTURE

There may remain major impediments to the successful design of a long-lasting, clinically effective MCP arthroplasty, but improved designs are encouraging. Foremost is the problem of designing a joint replacement that can simulate the function of the normal joint. The new pyrolytic and metal on plastic implants appear to have attained this first goal. The second problem is overcoming the soft tissue contractures and reinforcing the attenuated tissues. This problem may require replacement of damaged ligaments with composite tissues and reinforcements for the extensor tendon mechanism. Bioengineering is on the way to meet these demands. The development of new rheumatoid medications will also slow the synovitic process and allow early effective joint replacements. Hand surgeons will need to work closely with rheumatologist to effect a treatment algorithm that best suits each individual patient with hands and wrist affected by rheumatoid arthritis

References

1. Adams BD, Blair WF, Shurr DG: Schultz metacarophalangeal arthroplasy. Long term followup. J Hand Surg 15A:641, 1990.
2. An KN, Chao EYS, Cooney WP, et al: Normative model of the hand for biomechanical analysis. J Biomechan 12:775, 1979.
3. Aptekar RG, Duff IF: Metacarpophalangeal joint surgery in rheumatoid arthritis. Clin Orthop 83:123, 1972.

4. Bass RL, Stern PJ, Nairus JG: High implant fracture with Sutter silicone metacarpophalangeal joint arthroplasties. J Hand Surg 64A:813, 1996.
5. Beckenbaugh RD: Preliminary experiences with a noncemented nonconstrained total joint arthroplasty for the metacarpophalangeal joint. Orthopedics 6:962, 1983.
6. Beckenbaugh RD: Pyrolytic carbon implants. In Simmen B, Allieu Y, Lluch A, Stanley J (eds): Hand Arthroplasties. London, Martin Dunitz, 1999.
7. Beckenbaugh RD, Daubers JH, Linscheid RL, Bryan RS: Review and analysis of silicone-rubber metacarpophalangeal implants. J Bone Joint Surg 58A:483, 1976.
8. Beckenbaugh RD, Linscheid RL: Arthroplasty in the hand and wrist. In Green DP (ed): Operative Hand Surgery, 3rd ed., vol. I. New York, Churchill Livingstone, 1993.
9. Beevers DJ, Seedholm BB: Metacarpophalangeal joint prosthesis. A review of the clinical results of past and current designs. J Hand Surg 20B:125, 1995.
10. Beckenbaugh RD, Steffee AD: Total joint arthroplasty of the MCP joint of the thumb. Orthopedics 4:298, 1981.
11. Bieber EJ, Weiland AJ, Volenec-Dowling S: Silicone rubber implant arthroplasty of the metacarpophalangeal joints for rheumatoid arthritis. J Bone Joint Surg 68A:206, 1986.
12. Blair WF, Shurr DG, Buckwalter JA: Metacarpophalangeal joint implant arthroplasty with a Silastic spacer. J Bone Joint Surg 66A:365, 1984.
13. Brewerton DA: Hand deformities in rheumatoid disease. Ann Rheum Dis 16:183, 1957.
14. Bunnell S: Surgery of the rheumatic hand. J Bone Joint Surg 37A:757, 1955.
15. Cao H: Mechanical performance of pyrolytic carbon in prosthetic heart valve applications. J Heart Valve Dis 5(Suppl 1):S32, 1996.
16. Conolly WB, Rath S: Silastic implant arthroplasty for post-traumatic stiffness of the finger joints. J Hand Surg 16:286, 1991.
17. Cook SD, Beckenbaugh RD, Redondo J, et al: Long term follow-up of pyrolytic carbon metacarpophalangeal implants. J Bone Joint Surg 81A:635, 1999.
18. Cook SD, Beckenabugh RD, Weinstein AM, Klawitter JJ: Pyrolite carbon implants in the metacarpophalangeal joint of baboons. Orthopedics 6:952, 1983.
19. Derkash RS, Niebauer IJ, Lane CS: Long-term follow-up of metacarpophalangeal arthroplasty with silicone Dacron prostheses. J Hand Surg 11A:553, 1986.
20. Dobyns JH, Linscheid RL: Rheumatoid hand repairs. Orthop Clin North Am 2:629, 1971.
21. el-Gammal TA, Blair WF: Motion after metacarpophalangeal joint reconstruction in rheumatoid disease. J Hand Surg 18A:504, 1993.
22. Ellison MR, Flatt AE, Kelly KJ: Ulnar drift of the fingers in rheumatoid disease. J Bone Joint Surg 53A:1061, 1971.
23. Ellison MR, Kelly KJ, Flatt AE: The results of surgical synovectomy of the digital joints in rheumatoid disease. J Bone Joint Surg 53A:1041, 1971.
24. Ely JL, Emken MR, Accuntius JA, et al: Pure pyrolytic carbon: Preparation and properties of a new material, On-X carbon for mechanical heart valve prostheses. J Heart Valve Dis 7:626, 1998.
25. Flatt AE: The Pathomechanics of Ulnar Drift. Final Report. Social and Rehabilitation Services, Grant No. RD 2226M, 1971.
26. Flatt AE: Care of the Rheumatoid Hand, 3rd ed. St. Louis, CW Mosby, 1974.
26a. Fowler SB: Arthroplasty of the metacarpophalangeal joint in rheumataid arthritis. J Bone Joint Surg 44:1037, 1962.
27. Gillespie TE, Flatt AE, Youm Y, Sprague BL: Biomechanical evaluation of metacarpophalangeal joint prosthesis designs. J Hand Surg 4:508, 1979.
28. Goldner JL: Metacarpal phalangeal arthroplasty with silicone Dacron prosthesis (Niebauer type): six and a half years' experience. J Hand Surg 2:200, 1977.
29. Houpt P: Cemented and non cemented biological fixation and osseointegration. Design and clinical behavior. In Simmen B, Allieu Y, Lluch A, Stanley J (eds): Hand Arthroplasties. London, Martin Dunitz, 1999.
30. Gschwend N, Zimmerman J: Analyse von 200 MCP-arthroplastiken. Handchirurgie 6:7, 1974.
31. Hagert CG: Metacarpophalangeal joint implants. II. Scand J Plast Reconstr Surg 9:158, 1978.

32. Hagert CG, Eiken O, Ohleson NM, et al: Metacarpophalangeal joint implants. I. Roentgenographic study on the Silastic finger joint implant, Swanson design. Scand J Plast Reconstr Surg 9:147, 1978.
33. Hakstian RW, Tubiana R: Ulnar deviation of the fingers: The role of joint structure and function. J Bone Joint Surg 49A:299, 1967.
34. Hastings DE, Evans JA: Rheumatoid wrist deformities and their relation to ulnar drift. J Bone Joint Surg 57A:930, 1975.
35. Hellum C, Vainio K: Arthroplasty of the metacarpophalangeal joints in rheumatoid arthritis with transposition of the interosseous muscles. Scand J Plast Reconstr Surg 2:139, 1968.
36. Henderson ED, Lipscomb PR: Surgical treatment of the rheumatoid hand. JAMA 175:431, 1961.
37. James DF, Clark IP, Colwill JC, Halsall AP: Forces in metacarpophalangeal joint due to elevated fluid pressure. Analysis, measurements and relevance to ulnar drift. J Biomech 15:73, 1982.
38. Kirschenbaum D, Schneider LH, Adams DC, Cody RP: Arthroplasty of the metacarpophalangeal joints with use of Silastic rubber implants in patients who have rheumatoid arthritis: Long-term results. J Bone Joint Surg 75A:3, 1993.
39. Landsmeer JMF: A report on the coordination of the interphalangeal joints of the human finger and its disturbances. Acta Morphol Neerl Scand 2:59, 1958.
40. Linscheid RL, Beckenbaugh RD, Dobyns JH, Cooney WP III: Metacarpal arthroplasty with Steffee prostheses. In Inglis AE (ed): Symposium on Total Joint Replacement of the Upper Extremity. American Academy of Orthopaedic Surgeons. St. Louis, CV Mosby, 1982, p 187.
41. Linscheid RL, Dobyns JH: Total joint arthroplasty: The hand. Mayo Clin Proc 54:516, 1979.
42. Linscheid RL, Dobyns JH, Beckenbaugh RD, Cooney WP: Proximal interphalangeal joint arthroplasty with a total joint design. Mayo Clin Proc 54:227, 1979.
43. Linschied RL: Metacarpophalangeal arthroplasties: Prosthetic design considerations. In Simmen B, Allieu Y, Lluch A, Stanley J (eds): Hand Arthroplasties. London, Martin Dunitz, 1999.
44. Littler JW, cited by Harris C Jr, Riordan DC: Intrinsic contracture in the hand and its surgical treatment. J Bone Joint Surg 36A:10, 1954.
45. Lundborg G, Branemark PI, Carlson I: Metacarpophalangeal joint arthroplasty based on the osseointegration concept. J Hand Surg 18B:693, 1993.
46. Madden JW, De Vore G, Arem AJ: A rational postoperative management program for metacarpophalangeal joint implant surgery. J Hand Surg 2:358, 1977.
47. Mannerfelt L, Anderson K: Silastic arthroplasty of the metacarpophalangeal joints in rheumatoid arthritis: Long term results. J Bone Joint Surg 57A:484, 1975.
48. McMaster M: The natural history of the rheumatoid metacarpophalangeal joint. J Bone Joint Surg 54B:687, 1972.
49. Milford L: The hand. In Edmonson AS, Crenshaw AH (eds): Campbell's Operative Orthopaedics, vol. I. St. Louis, Mosby, 1980, p 110.
50. Millender LH, Nalebuff EA, Feldon PG: Rheumatoid arthritis. In Green DP (ed): Operative Hand Surgery. New York, Churchill Livingstone, 1982, p 1161.
51. Minami A, An KN, Cooney WP, et al: Ligamentous structures of the metacarpophalangeal joint: A quantitative anatomic study. J Orthop Res 1:361, 1984.
52. Minami A, An KN, Cooney WP III, et al: Ligament stability of the metacarpophalangeal joint: A biomechanical study. J Hand Surg 10A:255, 1985.
53. Nalebuff EA: Diagnosis, classification and management of rheumatoid thumb deformities. Bull Hosp Joint Dis 29:119, 1968.
54. Niebauer JJ, Shaw JL, Doren WW: The silicone Dacron hinge prosthesis: Design, evaluation, and application [abstract]. J Bone Joint Surg 50A:634, 1968.
55. Opitz JL, Linscheid RL: Hand function after metacarpophalangeal joint replacement in rheumatoid arthritis. Arch Phys Med Rehabil 59:162, 1978.
56. Rothwell AG, Cragg KJ, Oneill LB: Hand function following silicone arthroplasty of the metacarpophalangeal joints in rheumatoid arthritis. J Hand Surg 22B:90, 1997.
57. Shapiro JS: A new factor in the etiology of ulnar drift. Clin Orthop 68:32, 1970.

58. Smith EM, Juvinall RC, Bender LF, Pearson TR: Role of the finger flexors in rheumatoid deformities of the metacarpophalangeal joints. Arthritis Rheum 7:467, 1964.
59. Smith RJ, Kaplan EB: Rheumatoid deformities at the metacarpophalangeal joints of the fingers. J Bone Joint Surg 49A:31, 1967.
60. Stanley JK, Evans RA: What are the long term followup results of silastic metacarpophalangeal and poximal interphalangeal joint replacements. Br J Rheumatol 31:839, 1992.
61. Steffee AD, Beckenbaugh RD, Linscheid RL, Dobyns JH: The development, technique, and early clinical results of total joint replacement for the metacarpophalangeal joint in the finger. Orthopaedics 4:175, 1981.
62. Stothard J, Thompson AE, Sherris D: Correction of ulnar drift during Silastic metacarpophalangeal joint arthroplasty. J Hand Surg 16B:61, 1991.
63. Straub L: Deformity in the hand affected by rheumatoid arthritis. Bull Hosp Joint Dis Orthop Inst 21:322, 1960.
64. Swanson AB: Flexible implant arthroplasty for arthritic finger joints. J Bone Joint Surg 54A:435, 1972.
65. Swanson AB, deGroot GA: Flexible implant resection arthroplasty: A method for reconstruction of small joints in the extremities. Instr Course Lect 27:27, 1978.
66. Swanson AB, deGroot GA, Hehl RW, et al: Pathogenesis of rheumatoid deformities in the hand. *In* Cruess RL, Mitchell N (eds): Surgery of Rheumatoid Arthritis. Philadelphia, JB Lippincott, 1971, p 143.
67. Swanson AB, Swanson G, DeHeer DH: Small joint implant arthroplasty: 3+ years of research and experience. *In* Simmon B, Allieu Y,

Lluch A, Stanley J (eds): Hand Arthroplasties. London, Martin Dunitz, 2000.
68. Vahvanen V, Viljakka T: Silicone rubber implant arthroplasty of the metacarpophalangeal joint in rheumatoid arthritis: A follow-up study of 32 patients. J Hand Surg 11A:333, 1986.
69. Vainio K, Oka M: Ulnar deviation of the fingers. Ann Rheum Dis 12:122, 1953.
70. Vainio K, Reimar I, Pulkki T: Results of arthroplasty of the metacarpophalangeal joints in rheumatoid arthritis. Reconstr Surg Traumatol 9:1, 1967.
71. Weilby A, Tupper AW: Resection arthroplasty of the metacarpophalangeal joint using interposition of the volar plate. Scand J Plast Reconstr Surg 11:239, 1977.
72. Weiss APC: Neuflex prosthesis. *In* Simmen B, Alleiu Y, Lluch A, Stanley J (eds): Hand Arthroplasties. London, Martin Dunitz, 1999.
73. Wilkes LL: Ulnar drift and metacarpophalangeal joint subluxation in the rheumatoid hand: Review of the pathogenesis. South Med J 70:965, 1977.
74. Wise KS: The anatomy of the metacarpophalangeal joints, with observations of the etiology of ulnar drift. J Bone Joint Surg 57B:485, 1975.
75. Wood VE, Ichtertz DR, Yahiku H: Soft tissue metacarpophalangeal reconstruction for treatment of rheumatoid hand deformity. J Hand Surg 14A:163, 1989.
76. Zancolli E: Structural and Dynamic Bases of Hand Surgery, 2nd ed. Philadelphia, JB Lippincott, 1979, p 325.

20

Arthroplasty of the Thumb Axis

•WILLIAM P. COONEY III

The joint most commonly affected with arthritis in the upper extremity is the trapeziometacarpal (TMC) joint.[12,21] The disease most commonly affects women in the fifth and sixth decades. Approximately one quarter of women older than age 40 are affected, and one fifth of those require surgical treatment.[11,18] The etiology of TMC arthritis includes osteoarthritis, post-traumatic arthritis, and rheumatoid arthritis.[5,15,27]

Disabling pain from osteoarthritis of this joint is a progressive problem that most commonly affects women after the age of 40. The pathophysiology is increasingly related primarily to laxity of ligaments (and capsule), with secondary displacement leading to altered joint contact.[16,55,56] As a consequence of ligament laxity (perhaps estrogen related), joint asymmetry and increased contact forces result. Trapezial tilt may be a contributing factor.[7,65] This combination of factors results in shear forces and compressive loads associated with repetitive use of the hand leading to wear and degeneration of the joint articular surfaces.[16,55] Approximately one out of every four women develops some element of degenerative arthritis of the TMC joint, and out of these, 20 percent require surgical treatment.[6,7]

Patients typically have pain and swelling around the base of the thumb. Antecedent trauma is rare. The pain is aggravated by activities requiring forceful key pinch, strong grasp, or a wringing motion. Patients also have difficulty with activities requiring even modest amounts of abduction, including opening a door or picking up a glass. The pain improves with rest. Night symptoms are rare. Positive physical findings include pain and swelling at the TMC joint. There may be crepitus of the joint combined with dorsal or volar joint tenderness. Opposition, radial, and palmar abduction are limited. There may be an adduction contracture of the first web combined with a metacarpophalangeal hyperextension deformity.

Patients who have a clinical picture of TMC arthritis should first undergo a period of conservative treatment. A combination of nonsteroidal anti-inflammatory medication, splinting, and steroid injections should be attempted. If the patient remains significantly symptomatic, surgical intervention is warranted. Multiple surgical procedures for treating TMC arthritis have been described. Alternatives include total joint arthroplasty

arthrodesis, osteotomy, and resection arthroplasty with and without ligament reconstructions. Goals of the surgery should be pain relief and a functional range of motion.[1,5,8,11,14,20,24,29,44,59,62,64]

Second in prevalence, we find rheumatoid arthritis, which is a multisystem disease that commonly involves both the hand and wrist.[27] The thumb TMC joint is second to the metacarpophalangeal (MCP) joints of the fingers and thumb in frequency of involvement.[15] In rheumatoid arthritis, loss of ligament support of this joint commonly leads to an adduction contracture of the first metacarpal, with dorsoradial subluxation of the joint and thumb MCP and carpometacarpal (CMC) instability.[26] Collapse of the thumb ray typically involves the interphalangeal (IP), MCP, and TMC joints in a variety of clinical presentations; distinguishing the different types of instability assists in the determination of treatment.

The presence of either osteoarthritis or rheumatoid arthritis can have a devastating effect on the function of the hand. When it results in the loss of support of the thumb TMC joint or, occasionally, the MCP joint, joint arthroplasty may be indicated. The purpose of this chapter is to describe the most common presentations of arthritis involving the thumb IP, MCP, and TMC joints with primary emphasis on the TMC joint, and to designate the specific indications for joint arthroplasty. In particular, I hope to present the rationale for total joint arthroplasty, excisional arthroplasty, and joint fusion in light of current clinical practice, biomechanical considerations and personal experience. The current status of Silastic interposition arthroplasty of the TMC joint and its relationships to the incidence of Silastic synovitis are also discussed.

THUMB BASAL JOINT ARTHRITIS

Indications for Treatment

The preferred treatment of patients with thumb basal joint arthritis is based on patient demographics, including age, sex, and occupation, as well as the extent of the disease. The patient involved in heavy, repetitive manual activities with fewer requirements for dexterity than strength may have more success with a fusion than with an arthroplasty. Younger patients as well may find a stronger, more stable thumb after arthrodesis.[14,40] Amadio and DeSilva, in 1990, however, demonstrated no statistically significant difference in pinch strength between arthrodesis and arthroplasty with a 2-year follow-up and suggested that arthroplasty in the younger patient may be appropriate.[5] They noted that results were poorer in those who perform heavy labor.

Classification is important in deciding on the treatment for patients with TMC arthritis. We utilize the Eaton radiographic classification[21,23,31] of carpometacarpal arthritis to classify all of our patients and help in the treatment plan (Fig. 20–1; Table 20–1). This classification has distinctive treatment application. In stage I or early stage II disease, there are surgical options of arthroscopic débridement, cheilotomy and capsulorrhaphy, metacarpal osteotomy, ligament reconstruction (Eaton-Littler technique), and tenotomy of accessory slips of the abductor pollicis longus (APL), and cheilectomy.[10,24,28,29,48,58,65] For more advanced arthritis (late stage II or stage III), resection of the trapezium with soft tissue interposition or joint arthroplasty or arthrodesis is preferred.[1,5,38,44,52,58] With pantrapezial involvement stage

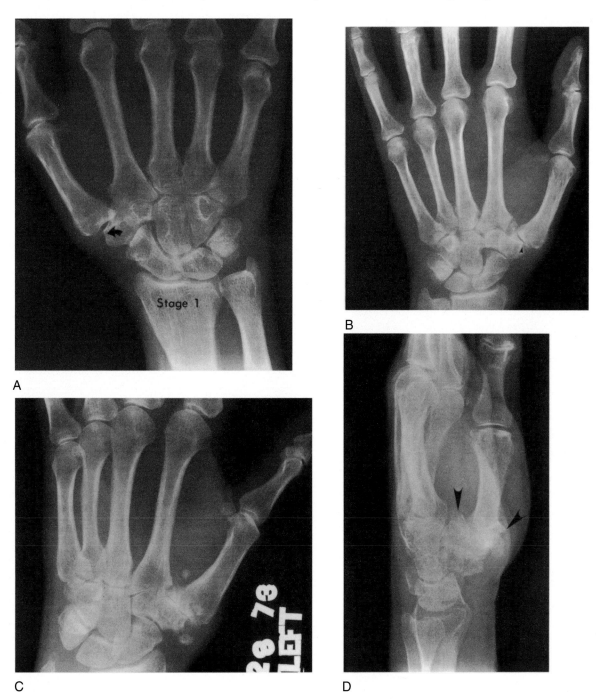

Figure 20–1. Eaton-Littler classification (radiographic) of TMC arthritis. **A**, Stage I: a slight joint space narrowing only (*arrow*). **B**, Stage II: joint narrowed; margina, osteophytes; mild joint subluxation (*arrowhead*). **C**, Stage III: joint space obliterated; heterotopic bone; joint subluxation. **D**, Stage IV: pantrapezial arthritis (*arrowheads*).

Table 20–1. RADIOGRAPHIC STAGES OF
TRAPEZIOMETACARPAL ARTHRITIS

Stage I	Normal articular contours
	Slight joint space narrowing (widening) if joint effusion is present
Stage II	Joint space narrowed; normal articular contours
	Marginal osteophytes (<2 mm)
	Subluxation up to one third of articular surface
Stage III	Joint space obliterated; loss of normal contours
	Marginal osteophytes (>2 mm)
	Subluxation greater than one third of articular surface
Stage IV	Pantrapezial involvement

IV, resection arthroplasty with ligamentous reconstruction or a suspensionplasty is required.

Clinical Anatomy and Biomechanics

The base of the thumb TMC joint is designated as a *saddle joint* (Fig. 20–2)[17,35] and is an exact mechanical equivalent of a universal joint with the one exception of a small degree of independent axial rotation.[56] The MCP joint is designated as a ball-and-socket joint and the IP joint as a hinge joint. The architectural design of the joint articular surfaces provides natural stability in positions of full opposition for pinch and power grasp. The joints are supported by quite strong collateral ligaments at the IP and MCP joints and by three palmar-ulnar ligaments (intermetacarpal, volar collateral, and anterior oblique) at the TMC joint. Bettinger et al. described 16 ligaments that support and stabilize the trapezium and trapeziometacarpal joint[7] (Fig. 20–3). The dorsoradial and deep anterior oblique ligaments play a substantial role in stabilizing the TMC joint. Other ligaments prevent cantilever bending forces on the trapezium.

In the closed-pack position of MacConnail, in which the thumb rotates into pronation and abduction or adduction and supination, the thumb is stable.[39,56] There is a small amount of obligatory rotation, the result of the geometry of the articular surfaces, which produces pronation during abduction and flexion and supination during extension and adduction at both the TMC and MCP joints.[17] A stable position is achieved when the thumb is in full abduction during flexion and extension for prehensile grasp, whereas a less stable position is present when the thumb is in adduction and supination for either a power grip, such as holding a hammer, or a lateral or key pinch.

Unstable positions of the thumb are present in the mid-rotation position of prehensile tip-to-tip pinch and palmar pinch, as well as when the thumb is opposed to the index and long fingers in a prehensile grasp. In these positions, substantial rotational torque is placed across the TMC and MCP joints, straining the support ligaments and stressing the articular cartilage of the joint.[16] In time, excessive stress leads to wear of the cartilage and degenerative arthritis, especially at the TMC joint.

Anatomic and biomechanical studies of the thumb have demonstrated the important ligaments needed to maintain a stable thumb at the TMC joint.[7,21,35,39] The dorsoradial, anterior obliques and first intermetacarpal ligaments are probably the most important ligaments because they support the base of the first metacarpal to the second metacarpal, resisting the shear forces of pinch and grasp (Fig. 20–3). The anterior oblique ligament and dorsoradial ligaments resist axial torsion and lateral shear forces. To effectively restore stability, ligament reconstruction of the thumb joints must replace these important structures.

To illustrate the sizable forces across the joints of the thumb, mechanical studies have demonstrated that

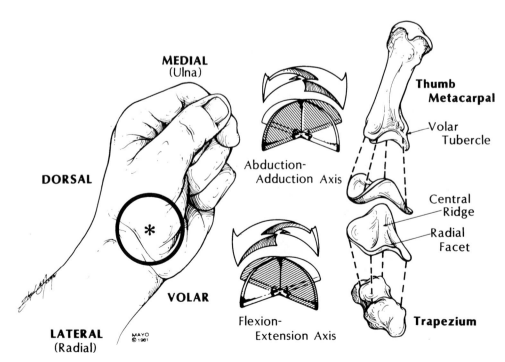

Figure 20–2. Anatomy of the TMC joint. There are two principal axes of motion: Abduction-adduction and flexion-extension. The anatomy of the joint is the mechanical equivalent of a universal joint. (From Cooney WP, Lucca MJ, Chao EYS, Linscheid RL: The kinesiology of the thumb trapeziometacarpal joint. J Bone Joint Surg 63A:1371, 1981. By permission of Mayo Foundation.)

MEDIAL
(Ulna)

DORSAL

LATERAL
(Radial)

VOLAR

Abduction-Adduction Axis

Flexion-Extension Axis

Thumb Metacarpal

Volar Tubercle

Central Ridge

Radial Facet

Trapezium

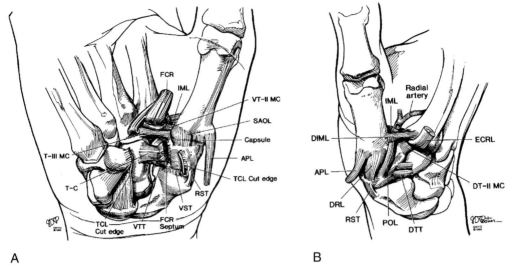

A   B

Figure 20–3. A, The volar ligaments that stabilize the trapezium and the TMC joint. **B,** The dorsal ligaments that stabilize the trapezium and TMC joint. T-C, trapeziocapitate; TCL, transverse carpal ligament; FCR, flexor carpi radialis; VST, volar scapho-trapezial; RST, radial scaphotrapezial; APL, abductor pollicis longus; SAOL, superficial anterior oblique; IML, intermetacarpal; DIML, dorsal intermetacarpal; POL, posterior oblique; ECRL, extensor carpi radialis longus. (From Bettinger PC, Smutz WB, Linschied RL, et al: Material properties of the trapezial and trapeziometacarpal ligaments. J Hand Surg 25A:1085, 2000. Copyright with the Mayo Clinic, 1995.)

compressive load and shear force at the thumb joints can be magnified significantly during pinch and grasp. The contracting intrinsic and extrinsic muscle forces that balance the prehensile forces applied during pinch and grasp can multiply the applied pinch or grasp load by a factor of 4 at the IP joint, by a factor of 6 at the MCP joint, and by a factor of 13 at the TMC joint (Fig. 20–4).[16] In addition, dorsal as well as lateral subluxing force or shear force occurs during pinch. There is a substantial torque moment along the central axis of the thumb that increases the tendency of the thumb to sublux or displace into an unstable position. With firm pinch, subluxating force at TMC joint can be estimated to be six times that of the applied load (Fig. 20–4). We have observed that 5 kg of pinch force results in compressive loads of 60 kg, lateral shear of 6 kg, and torsional moment of 8 kg/cm. During pathologic conditions, the applied force is substantially magnified and concentrated on the radial side of the trapezium.

Radiographically, there is attenuation of the intermetacarpal and anterior oblique ligaments with secondary calcification, as well as osteophytes adjacent to the anterior and posterior oblique ligaments of the thumb metacarpal. The result of these joint forces produces lateral (radial) and dorsal subluxation of the thumb metacarpal. Clinically, one can demonstrate the instability of the joint by examining the thumb during the act of key pinch or tip pinch. The thumb force required either to hold or to reduce the base of the trapezium gives one a sense of the instability that is involved.

Thumb Kinematics

Motion of the IP joint is a simple hinge action, whereas both the MCP and TMC joints can rotate on any of three planes. Thumb positioning is usually a composite motion

at one or more joints that is clinically observed along variable axes of rotation. At the base of the thumb, the thumb metacarpal is oriented in position away from the other metacarpals (45 degrees from the plane of the finger metacarpals) and has its own axis of flexion-extension and abduction-adduction.[17] From biomechanical studies, we have determined that the thumb TMC joint has approximately 40 degrees of flexion-extension, 52 degrees of abduction-adduction, and 17 degrees of axial rotation. The MCP joint has 45 to 60 degrees of flexion, 20 degrees of abduction-adduction in each direction, and 25 degrees of rotation. Most of the thumb motions described previously are combinations of components of flexion-extension, abduction-adduction, or rotation rather than one action alone. Conjunctive rotation,[39] for example, employs full range of motion and contributes to prehensile functions by placing the hand in opposition (abduction-flexion) and retroposition (adduction-extension) during pinch and grasp. Preserving a full complement of motion in the thumb joints is essential to the prehensile function of the hand.

OSTEOARTHRITIS OF THE THUMB TRAPEZIOMETACARPAL JOINT

Clinical Classification

The degree of osteoarthritis that affects the thumb TMC joint has been analyzed by both clinical and anatomic studies, and a radiologic classification has been prepared by Eaton and co-workers.[23,31] Clinical staging is based on joint stability and radiographic appearance (Fig. 20–1). The first clinical stage of degenerative arthritis (stage I) involves the TMC joint alone without evidence of joint instability (Fig. 20–1**B**). There is usually

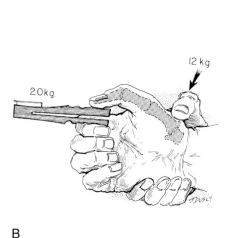

A

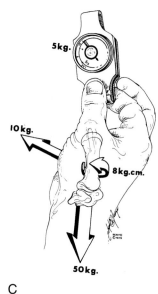

B   C

Figure 20–4. A, Muscle forces that resect from applied pinch of 1 kg of force. Intrinsic and extrinsic muscles carry equal force. FPL, flexor pollicis longus; OPP-FB, opponens and flexor pollicis brevis; APB, abductor pollicis brevis; APL, abductor pollicis longus. **B,** With a lateral tip pinch of 2 kg, the joint torsion and shear force produce 12 kg of subluxing force, which can be estimated by the palpating thumb. **C,** Forces across the thumb TMC joint associated with firm pinch (5 kg). Note joint compression force (50 kg), shear force (10 kg), and torque (8 kg/cm).

pain on direct palpation of the joint, increased discomfort on axial rotation (the longitudinal grind test), and decreased pinch strength. Radiographs of the thumb are completely normal. The next clinical stage (stage II) involves loss of the joint articular cartilage associated with lateral or dorsal subluxation of the TMC joint (Fig. 20–1**B**). There is radiographic evidence of joint space narrowing and early osteophyte formation. The joint is usually not clinically unstable. The clinical findings for stage II are similar to those for stage I except that they are more severe in degree.

The next stage of degenerative arthritis (stage III) involves complete loss of the joint articular cartilage, lateral and dorsal subluxation of the TMC joint, and joint instability (Fig. 20–1**C**). Attenuation with secondary calcification is found in the first intermetacarpal ligament, and osteophytes are present at ligament attachments around the joint. The radial facet of the trapezium has flattened. Osteophyte formation as a result of lateral joint subluxation has increased. Clinical instability of the joint is present. There is local joint tender-

ness and increased pain on axial compression of the joint.

The final stage of degenerative arthritis (stage IV) involves pantrapezial arthritis (Fig. 20–1**D**). Not only is the thumb TMC joint nearly devoid of normal articular cartilage, with lateral subluxation and excessive osteophyte formation, but the adjacent scaphotrapeziotrapezoidal (STT) joint is also involved in the degenerative process, with loss of articular joint cartilage. Radiographically, no normal joint space of the TMC joint remains, and the STT joint is significantly narrowed.

In both clinical stages III and IV of TMC arthritis, cystic degeneration may be present within the scaphoid and the trapezium as well as at the base of the first metacarpal. Clinical stages III and IV may also be associated with adduction contractures of the first metacarpal and hyperextension deformities of the MCP joint. In time, a fixed adduction contraction may develop, with inability to abduct the thumb for pinch or grasp and the functional use limited to key-type pinch.

Indications for Surgical Treatment

The primary indication for operative treatment of patients with TMC arthritis is failure to improve with conservative treatment. Each patient with this condition requires a time of splinting, nonsteroidal anti-inflammatory drugs (NSAIDs) and change of activities. Cortisone injections are also helpful, and we repeat such injections every 3 months if symptoms are relieved. Many patients, in fact, experience fewer symptoms, and usually one of five eventually requires surgical intervention.

The choice of surgical procedures is based on the clinical staging and radiographic classifications of Eaton-Littler (Table 20–1). Currently, we recommend the following practices based on the stages of arthritis:

Stage I: Conservative treatment (splinting, cortisone injection, and oral anti-inflammatory medications); limited surgical treatment with arthroscopic débridement and capsular shrinkage; or advanced surgical treatment with cheilectomy and capsular tightening; ligament reconstruction (Eaton-Littler technique); or metacarpal osteotomy.
Stage II: Cheilotomy and capsular tightening with ligament reconstruction (Eaton-Littler procedure); ligament reconstruction alone or with soft tissue interposition; total joint replacement.
Stage III: Partial trapezial resection with soft tissue interposition using the LRTI (Burton-Pelligrini) or Eaton-Littler ligament reconstruction. Weilby soft tissue interposition; Total Joint arthroplasty; Fusion
Stage IV: Trapezial excision with soft tissue interposition and ligament reconstruction (ligament reconstruction tendon interposition [LRTI], Eaton-Littler); Weilby suspensionplasty; trapezial excision alone.

Note that in the aforementioned options I do not list any indication for silicone replacement[2,34,54,59] of the trapezium or silicone condylar replacements of the base of the thumb metacarpal. With many excellent options, there is no longer any indication for silicone use as a thumb arthroplasty.

The most conservative of these procedures, for grade I or early grade II disease, includes a capsulotomy with a cheilectomy of arthritic bone (usually dorsal and radial) or arthrotomy with intermetacarpal ligament reconstruction (modified Eaton-Littler technique). More recent experience suggest that there is a role for arthrotomy and capsular shrinkage. Others suggest simple tenotomy of an accessory slip of the APL that inserts onto the trapezium. Zancolli and Zancolli reported on 18 patients who underwent APL tenotomy combined with retraining on pinch. Sixteen patients were pain free in activities of daily living, with an improved grip and range of motion.[65]

I believe that ligament reconstruction as proposed by Eaton and Littler is a quite reasonable procedure for stage I and early stage II symptomatic TMC arthritis. I have also used it for ligament laxity such as occurs in Ehlers-Danlos syndrome. Eaton reported the 7-year follow-up of patients undergoing ligament reconstruc-

tion.[24] Of 19 patients with stage I or stage II disease, 95 percent reported excellent or good results with respect to pain relief. The excellent and good results dropped to 74 percent in patients with stage III or stage IV disease. Freedman et al. reported a 15-year follow-up of results in 19 patients after ligament reconstruction alone.[28] Patients with stage I and stage II arthritis had 90 percent good to excellent results with no re-operations, whereas patients in stage III or stage IV had progression.

An alternative procedure to ligament reconstruction or arthroplasty in stage I and II disease is thumb metacarpal osteotomy. This was first described by Wilson in 1973.[64] This procedure corrects the adduction deformity of the first metacarpal. Wilson reported a complete relief of pain and improvement of grasp in all 8 patients. Molitor et al.[50] and Fujami et al.[29] have also reported good results with this procedure, demonstrating improvement of preoperative symptoms in 27 patients. These authors report good pain relief with pantrapezial arthritis as well as isolated basilar joint disease.

Soft tissue interposition alone with ligament reconstruction or a suspension arthroplasty without ligament reconstruction has many different options discussed in the following sections. For stage III, it is reasonable to resect the trapezial and metacarpal joint surfaces and preserve the scaphotrapezial joint. Soft tissue interposition with ligament reconstruction is a reasonable choice in many patients.[5,11,25,32,47] There is also the alternative of joint replacement with resurfacing joint arthroplasty.[1,5,6,19,33,41,43] For stage IV, resection of the entire trapezium with soft tissue interposition and ligament reconstruction or the suspension arthroplasties again appear best. Eaton has proposed the alternative of maintaining the trapezium with soft tissue interposition at both the TMC and STT joints.

Contraindications

There are few contraindications to basilar joint surgery. If a patient has an associated metacarpophalangeal hyperextension deformity (Fig. 20–5), I recommend that this condition be treated concurrently and not be considered a contraindication. In the rheumatoid patient, the extent of the disease of the hand and wrist must always be fully evaluated before treating an isolated joint. A failed silicone arthroplasty is not a contraindication for soft tissue arthroplasty and represents a good salvage procedure for silicone synovitis. Infection is also not a contraindication for soft tissue arthroplasty, although it is for total joint arthroplasty.

Operative Procedures for Trapeziometacarpal Arthritis

Ligament Reconstruction of the Trapeziometacarpal Joint

Ligament reconstruction of the TMC joint is recommend in patients with clinical stage I or early stage II. The

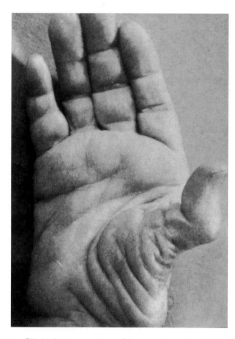

Figure 20–5. Clinical appearance of hyperextension deformity at the metacarpophalangeal joint associated with trapeziometacarpal arthritis.

patient should have a trial of splinting and cortisone injections. If there is evidence of instability without demonstrable arthritic signs, a ligament reconstruction alone can be very valuable. Studies have demonstrated both short- and long-term good results with this procedure.[24,28] Re-operation rates have been remarkably low with the exception of patients with advanced stage III or stage IV disease in whom soft tissue or total joint replacement is preferred.

Arthodesis (Fusion) of the Trapeziometacarpal Joint

When one is faced with stage III or IV TMC or pantrapezial arthritis in a young patient who needs a strong, stable, and pain-free thumb, fusion across the TMC or TMC-STT joints should be considered.[14] This operation is particularly preferred in industrial workers, either men or women, who are younger than 45 years of age and have potential for significant stress to their hands. Improved strength in both pinch and grasp results, although motion and dexterity are sacrificed. There are surgeons who advocate the use of TMC fusion in all stages of TMC arthritis, noting compensatory motion of the MCP and scaphotrapezial joints.[10] From the biomechanical standpoint, fusion of the TMC joint increases stress at the scaphotrapezial joint, and any evidence of pantrapezial arthritis is an absolute contraindication for fusion of the TMC joint alone.

Arthroplasty Soft Tissue Interposition Arthroplasty

Excision of the joint articular surfaces with interposition of soft tissue materials has been recommended for almost 30 years in the treatment of patients with thumb degenerative arthritis. The first procedures involved a simple interposition of soft tissue, such as fascia lata or tendon, between the joint articular surfaces. In the early papers dealing with this subject, ligament reconstruction was not described as part of the operative procedure. Silastic interposition arthroplasty then became popular, and soft tissue interposition was less commonly used.[4,13,20,30,53]

Prosthetic Replacement

Silastic Arthroplasty

Although less commonly chosen today, Silastic arthroplasty is considered by some for TMC arthritis in the presence of stage III disease.[2,34,59] A total trapezial silicone replacement is contraindicated today. A silicone space to resurface the trapeziometacarpal surface still has proponents. Silastic arthroplasty usually involves a condylar arthroplasty replacement of the thumb metacarpal, which is, in effect, a hemiarthroplasty. The joint surface of the trapezium is either ignored or shaved down to accept the convex surface of the condylar implant. I believe that there is a limited application for either a silicone or a metallic type of hemiarthroplasy (trapezial implant) for TMC arthritis and caution the reader to be very selective of low-demand patients if a spherical titanium ball or titanium trapezial implant is chosen. Instability of the implant and silicone or metallic synovitis suggests potential problems of wear and bone loss.

Joint Resurfacing Arthroplasty

A third alternative for treatment of stage II or III osteoarthritis of the TMC joint is a total joint resurfacing arthroplasty (Fig. 20–6). I believe that the implant design should duplicate the normal joint articular surface anatomy.[18,36] Ligament reconstruction for the intermetacarpal and anterior oblique may be necessary, combined with advancement of the TMC joint capsule. I have found that this is best performed through a dorsal rather than an anterior-volar approach. The procedure involves a dorsal capsular incision between the APL and extensor pollicis brevis (EPB) tendons. The resurfacing arthroplasty that we recommend consists of a metallic trapezial component and a polyethylene metacarpal component. The articular surfaces are biconcave to reflect TMC joint flexion-extension and abduction-adduction arcs of motion. The saddle-shaped reciprocal surfaces allow for a limited amount of axial rotation. The current arthroplasy has had limited use in the United States but relatively wider use in Europe and Great Britain. Several other designs from European investigators include convex-concave joint articular surface implants, ball-and-socket snap-fit joint replacements, and universal joint design replacement implants.[1–3,6,19,33,41]

OPERATIVE PROCEDURE

The surgical approach to the TMC joint is preferably dorsal for resurfacing TMC joint replacement in order to provide for accurate resection of the articular

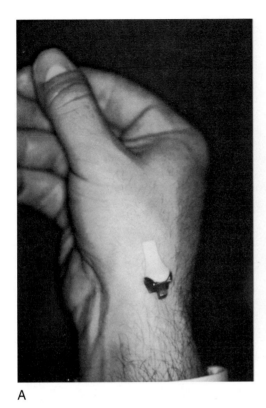

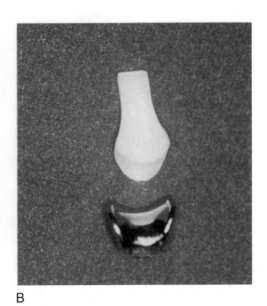

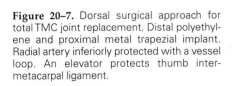

A   B

Figure 20–6. A, Resurfacing design for thumb TMC joint. Universal joint design has anatomic limits to provide constraint to rotation and separate axes for flexion-extension and abduction-adduction. **B,** Close-up appearance of resurfacing components for TMC joint.

surfaces (Fig. 20–7). This exposure also preserves intact the anterior oblique and volar collateral ligaments. Care must be taken to identify and protect the radial artery. With the dorsal approach, a longitudinal incision is performed between the APL and EPB. The dorsal capsule is incised and reflected to expose the entire dorsal base of the first metacarpal and dorsal aspects of the trapezium. It is necessary to undermine capsule attachments radially and ulnarly. With the thumb distracted, the depth of the necessary cut of the trapezial and thumb

metacarpal articular surface is determined and the surgery is then performed with a 3-mm blade on an oscillating saw. Rounding off the trapezial surface osteophytes with an special bur has benefits for proper seating of the trapezial component. For the trapezium implant, a small canal or retention cup is made within the trapezium with a bur and a curette.

For the distal component, the intramedullary canal of the thumb metacarpal is prepared with a bur, intermedullary reamers, sized intramedullary rasps. Trial

Figure 20–7. Dorsal surgical approach for total TMC joint replacement. Distal polyethylene and proximal metal trapezial implant. Radial artery inferiorly protected with a vessel loop. An elevator protects thumb intermetacarpal ligament.

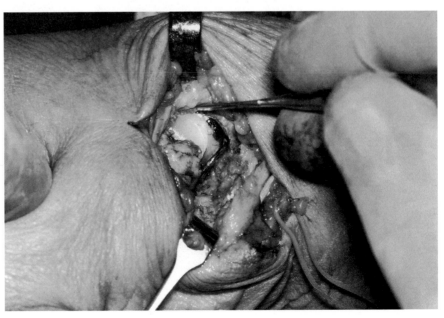

insertion of the two components is performed to assess ligament tension and joint motion. Additional bone may need to be removed from the base of the thumb metacarpal. The trapezium, which has a limited depth of 6 to 7 mm, should not be shortened more than 2 mm from the articular surface. Once the trial implants fit properly, the definitive implant components are inserted with bone cement within the intramedullary canals (Fig. 20–8). The joint should be articulated to induce proper joint surface contact, with moderate axial pressure maintained across the implant components until the bone cement cures.

Joint capsule closure is performed dorsally, with a reasonable tight capsule closure. The APL insertion may be advanced distally and radially to increase thumb abduction stance. If excess joint laxity is present, half of the flexor carpi radialis may be reflected from a proximal incision in the volar forearm, retrieved distally, and used to augment the radial-volar capsule before to definitive implant insertion.

Postoperative management is cast immbilization for 3 weeks followed by gradual thumb mobilization in a thumb spica splint. Good mobility can result from this early range of motion program (Fig. 20–8).

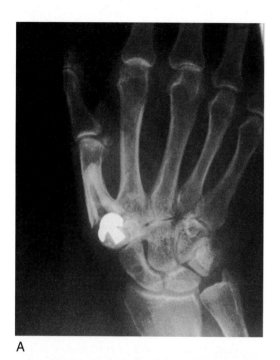

A

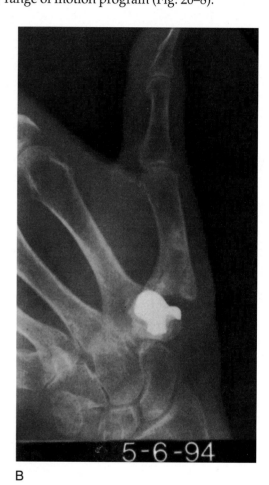

B

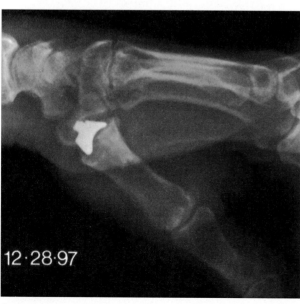

C

Figure 20–8. Motion after total TMC joint arthroplasty, showing 40 degrees of thumb TMC flexion-extension. **A**, Lateral view of TMC resurfacing arthroplasty. **B**, Oblique view of the thumb with extension-supination. **C**, Posteroanterior view of thumb abduction apposition.

Illustration continued on opposite page

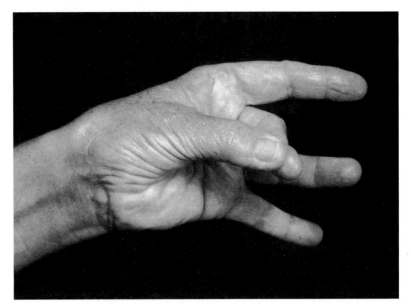

Figure 20–8. *Continued.* **D**, Thumb opposition after TMC arthroplasty.

D

Total Joint Arthroplasty Ball-and-Socket Designs

In selected patients (older than 50 years of age) who have TMC arthritis limited to stages II and III and who need firm pinch and prehensile grasp along with mobility, a ball-and-socket total joint replacement of the TMC joint may be considered (Fig. 20–9). There are

several current prostheses for total joint arthroplasty that use the ball-and-socket design.[1,6,19,33,45] With this prosthesis, the ball-and-stem unit is placed within the first metacarpal, whereas the cup portion is placed in the trapezium. Biomechanic studies have confirmed improved mechanics with the center of rotation in the trapezium. Ball-and-socket and resurfacing arthroplasty restore thumb TMC kinematics toward normal,

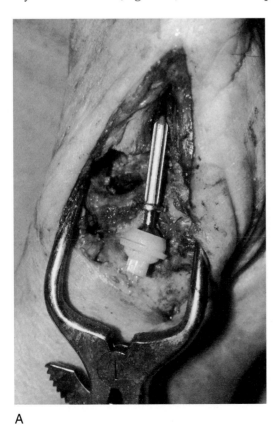

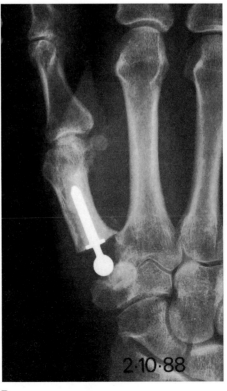

A

B

Figure 20–9. Total joint implants for the thumb TMC joint. De la Caffinière design with a trapezial cup and metacarpal ball. Components of each type are cemented in place with methylmethacrylate. **A**, De la Caffinière implant overlaying dorsal TMC joint incision. **B**, Lateral view of implanted De la Caffinière trapeziometacarpal, ball-and-socket total joint replacement.

in contrast to interposition arthroplasty. The trapezium cup has inherent stability plus a shorter lever arm, which may reduce the bending forces across the TMC joint. To date, all of the total joint arthroplasties require bone cement for fixation. The advantages of total joint arthroplasty are that it provides a fixed fulcrum to enhance joint stabilization and may not require as extensive an amount of ligament reconstruction as performed with the Silastic joint arthroplasties or interposition arthroplasty procedures.

OPERATIVE PROCEDURE

A volar or dorsal approach may be used for insertion of a total joint TMC arthroplasty. In the volar Wagner approach, the thenar muscle is reflected off the base of the first metacarpal and trapezium and the radial digital nerve is retracted dorsally along with the APL tendon, which is detached from its insertion to the base of the first metacarpal. The joint capsule is incised. It is necessary to resect the joint articular surface of the trapezium back a distance of 3 to 5 mm as well as to resect the base of the metacarpal a distance of 7 to 8 mm until a minimum space of 10 mm is present. Intramedullary canals, both the trapezial and first metacarpal, are prepared with use of appropriate burs and power reamers. The trapezial implant site is over-reamed so that a retaining cup of distal bone is created, which is larger than the neck of the opening into which the trapezial component is placed. Trial reductions are performed with uncemented implants to be sure the proper amount of bone has been resected. The implants manufactured today have both small and large sizes relative to the joint space. The implant chosen is usually a large size for men and a small size for women. After the trial reduction has been completed, bone cement is then inserted in a slightly wet stage. The trapezial and first metacarpal implants are implanted separately. Once the bone cement has matured, the joint can be articulated.

At the completion of implantation of the proximal and distal components and articulation of the joint, capsular repair and reattachment or advancement of the APL are performed. Mechanically, advancement of the APL increases its moment arm and tends to balance the thumb against a flexion or adduction force.

Postoperatively, splint immobilization is used for a period of 7 to 10 days, followed by mobilization of the TMC joint. As a result of inherent stability, motion can be started earlier than with interposition arthroplasty or silicone arthroplasty. I stress independent and combined flexion-extension, abduction-adduction, and circumduction motion. The final range of motion achieved with total joint implants is superior to that obtained with other types of joint arthroplasty.

Author's Preferred Method of Treatment (Mayo Clinic)

The preferred method of treatment of arthritis involving the thumb TMC joint is based on the stage of joint surface involvement. Using the classification system of

Eaton and co-workers, the treatment programs are defined as follows:

STAGE I: Normal or slight joint space narrowing without joint subluxation is noted. In this stage, there is no indication for joint arthroplasty, and conservative measures of splints and NSAIDs are recommended. By stabilizing the joint with a splint, the long-term problems of advancing osteoarthritis may be avoided.

With evidence of instability and failure to improve with conservative treatment, ligament reconstruction using the Eaton-Littler technique may be considered (Fig. 20–10A, B).[24] We also recommend this technique in patients who have had acute trauma involving the TMC joint or who are noted for excessive joint laxity (Ehlers-Danlos syndrome or other inherited collagen deficiency syndromes). This procedure augments or tightens the anterior oblique (volar), intermetacarpal, and dorsal radial ligaments. In patients with excessive adduction stance, an abduction wedge osteotomy[64] of the first metacarpal can also be considered in stage I or early stage II disease. Arthroscopy and débridement have had limited experience in my hands, but these procedures potential benefit provided the soft tissue can be stabilized and potentially aided by capsular shrinkage.

STAGE II: Loss of the joint cartilage space is noted, and there is usually lateral or radial joint subluxation. Calcification between the first and second metacarpals along the intermetacarpal ligament is present. In this stage of the disease, ligament reconstruction of the first intermetacarpal ligament may be considered with resection of osteophytes and joint débridement (Fig. 20–10A, B). The radial osteophytes can be removed and a good ligament reconstruction can still be performed based on remaining intact articular cartilage. If there is more than mild cartilage loss, the preferred surgical alternative in the elderly (>55 years) is soft tissue interposition[22,62] arthroplasty with ligament reconstruction (see Fig. 20–11).

In selected patients who need more pinch strength, joint arthroplasty can be considered. My preference is the resurfacing arthroplasty (see Fig. 20–8). As described earlier, resurfacing arthroplasty is a more anatomic procedure than a ball-and-socket joint. Bone resection is minimized, and joint capsule and ligament tension can be assessed. An alternative, in selected cases, is a corrective osteotomy of the trapezium, which can be performed if there is excessive trapezial tilt that is contributing to joint instability.[7] In an opening wedge osteotomy, a small bone graft can be taken from the distal radius and inserted laterally into the osteotomized trapezium. By leveling the joint articular surface, the lateral subluxing forces can be reduced and the degenerative process potentially abated. In general, interposition arthroplasty is preferred for stage II TMC arthritis.

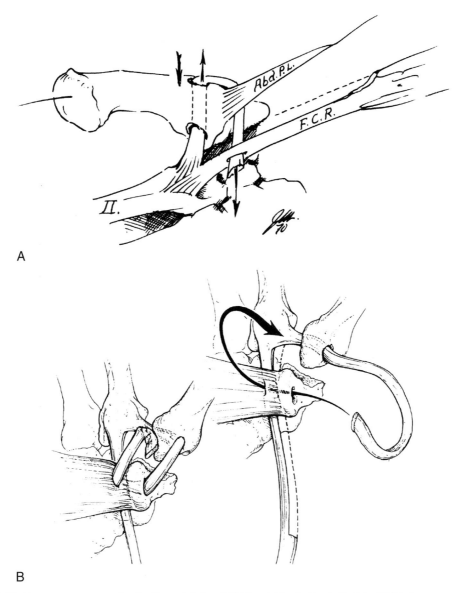

A

B

Figure 20–10. Ligament reconstruction for Stage I, II thumb TMC arthritis. **A,** One-half of the FCR is harvested proximally and brought distally to its insertion on metacarpal II. It is passed through metacarpal I, ulnar to radial, around the APL tendon and back to the FCR tendon. (From Eaton R, Lane L, Littler JW, et al: Ligament reconstruction for the painful thumb carpometacarpal joint: A long term assessment. J Hand Surg 9A:692, 1984.) **B,** Half of the FCR, after passing through the thumb metacarpal, is placed through the radial border of the transverse carpal ligament and then distal to the FCR.

STAGE III: Loss of the joint articular cartilage at the TMC joint is now complete and lateral subluxation of the first metacarpal is prominent with more than 50 percent of the joint surfaces displaced laterally. The osteoarthritis changes are limited to the TMC joint, with no radiologic changes visible at the scapho-trapezial joint. Increased density of the subchondral bone and prominent osteophytes at the ulnar border of the trapezium (intermetacarpal ligament) are usually present in addition to radial osteophytes and joint space narrowing.

In stage III TMC arthritis, soft tissue or total joint arthroplasty is required. We currently prefer a soft tissue interposition with excision of the trapezial articular surface in the elderly, low-demand patient

and resurfacing arthroplasty in other patients (similar to the options for stage II TMC arthritis) (Fig. 20–11A, B). In the soft tissue interposition arthroplasty, the distal third or half of the trapezium is excised and tendon or fascia is interposed.[12,25] Ligament reconstruction of the intermetacarpal ligament should be performed as described earlier.

The surgical approach that I prefer for soft tissue interposition resurfacing arthroplasty is the Wagner incision, in which the thenar muscles are lifted off the first metacarpal, the APL is released at its insertion, and the joint capsule is incised and sharply reflected off the trapezium and distal part of the first metacarpal. The joint surfaces are inspected, and radial and ulnar osteophytes are excised. The

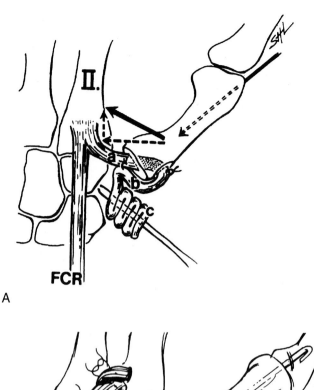

A

B

Figure 20–11. A, Soft tissue interposition of the TMC joint with ligament reconstruction (After Burton RI, Pellegrini VD: Surgical management of basal joint arthritis of the thumb. II. Ligament reconstruction with tendon interposition arthroplasty. J Hand Surg 11:324, 1986.) **B**, Ligament reconstruction using the abductor pollicis longus tendon. (After Thompson JS: Surgical treatment of trapeziometacarpal arthrosis. Adv Orthop Surg 2:105, 1988.)

distal third to half of the trapezium is removed with an osteotome or oscillating saw. The base of the first metacarpal is excised as appropriate for the interposition arthroplasty procedure selected. The support ligaments, however, must be preserved with a bur or oscillating saw.

The ulnar half of the flexor carpi radialis tendon is harvested through a proximal transverse incision. From the Wagner incision at the wrist, the palmaris longus tendon can also be harvested with a Brand tendon stripper with half of the flexor carpi radialis released proximally and reflected distally into the wound at the base of the thumb. There is adequate tendon for both ligament reconstructions and an interposition arthroplasty. Dividing the superficial fascia of the forearm helps to dissect out the flexor carpi radialis, as does flexion and extension of the wrist.

Joint reconstruction is performed by ligament reefing and soft tissue interposition (Fig. 20–11**A**). The ligament reconstruction involves placing drill or awl holes in the base of the first metacarpal, retrieving the proximal end of the flexor carpi radialis tendon previously harvested, and pulling the tendon graft through the first metacarpal, thereby bringing the base of the first and second metacarpals tightly together. For revision procedures, one can use the adductor pollicis longus and the extensor carpi radialis longus for the ligament reconstruction.

The TMC joint may be stabilized by insertion of Kirschner wires between the first and second metacarpals in a position of abduction and opposition. The radial capsule is repaired over the tendon interposition and the APL is advanced on the first metacarpal.

Total joint resurfacing arthroplasty may be considered in selected patients with excellent bone stock who have disease isolated to the TMC joint. I currently select patients younger than 55 years of age who wish a true joint replacement rather than a soft tissue interposition. Early results demonstrate better motion and strength with the resurfacing arthroplasty and with fewer tendencies toward prosthetic loosening than with total joint arthroplasty. More clinical trials are needed to determine the potential advantages of these procedures.

A dorsal operative approach is performed for resurfacing arthroplasty between the APL and extensor pollicis longus tendons. The radial artery is retracted ulnarly. The dorsal joint capsule is incised and reflected laterally and medially (see Fig. 20–7) to show the TMC joint. Bone is resected from the base of the metacarpal and trapezium, providing a joint space of 8 to 10 mm. The implant components are inserted as described earlier and held in place with bone cement.

This procedure has the advantage of a stable fulcrum (center of rotation) and is mechanically better than interposition arthroplasties. The inherent long-term risks of a cement joint arthroplasty in the hand may limit its widespread application and usefulness.

STAGE IV: Stage IV osteoarthritis of the TMC joint is advanced disease with total loss of the joint contour, radial and ulnar marginal osteophytes, and pantrapezial disease. When the osteoarthritis has progressed to this stage of the disease process, complete excision of the trapezium is recommended. The procedure may need to be combined with a capsular tightening at the MCP joint when adduction or hyperextension contractures of the MCP joint are present. I perform MCP capsulorrhaphy through a medial incision proximal to the adductor insertion on the thumb proximal phalanx and use a volar, ulnarly placed Mitek anchor to secure the volar-ulnar capsule in a tightened position.

The soft tissue interposition portion of the procedure is performed as described earlier, with use of both the palmaris longus and the remaining end of the flexor carpi radialis tendons as the interposed material. A tendon-weaving instrument is helpful in creating the tendon interposition. The rolled soft tissue mass is then sewn deep with nonresorbable sutures into the excised joint to the medial capsule adjacent to the trapezoid. The flexor carpi radialis tendon reinforces the anterior oblique and radial ligaments and can be sutured back onto itself. The APL is advanced and the capsule tightened and repaired with the thumb in abduction and opposition.

I have not used Gelfoam or other foreign allograft substances as the interposition material. One could choose fascia lata or a portion of the extensor retinaculum if the palmaris longus were absent. My experience with bovine tendon as an interposition material was not satisfactory. Silicone spacers would be a last choice in patients in whom adequate soft tissue for interposition material is not available. There appears to be little indication for a metallic or carbon material total trapezium replacement (Fig. 20–12).

Rehabilitation

Postoperatively, all patients are immobilized for a total of 3 to 4 weeks in a thumb spica cast after their swelling has resolved. A Kirschner wire is used in about half of the patients who show laxity of the TMC joint at the time of repair. The Kirschner wire is removed 3 weeks after surgery. For each patient, a forearm-based orthoplast thumb spica splint is recommended. The splint is worn full time at night for an additional 3 to 6 weeks. The patient removes the splint during the day for active range-of-motion exercises of the thumb, stressing flexion and circumduction as much as can be tolerated. Splint use is decreased over the next 3 weeks. At 6 weeks, the splint can be discarded unless the patient requries extra protection during heavy lifting. Patients are asked to refrain from forceful pinch and grasp for the first 3 months. Formal therapy is rarely required unless complications of local nerve pain or reflex sympathetic dystrophy develop. Up to 1 year is often required for patients to regain optimal postoperative motion.

Complications: Radial Nerve

Severe complications in basilar joint surgery are uncommon. The most serious complications are related to traction injury to the radial sensory or lateral antebrachial

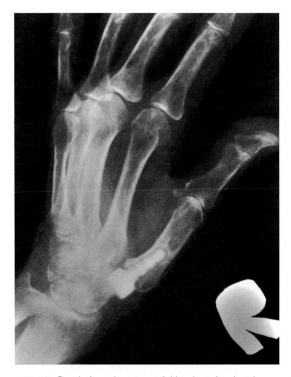

Figure 20–12. Pyrolytic carbon trapezial implant. Implant has eroded through the distal articular surface of the scaphoid. Note the loosening of the distal stem within the thumb metacarpal.

cutaneous nerves (Fig. 20–13). These nerves often pass directly across the surgical incision. Care must be taken to carefully protect these cutaneous nerves during the surgical procedure. If meticulous surgical dissection is carried out, intraoperative complications should be few. Branches of the palmar cutaneous branch of the median nerve, the lateral antebrachial cutaneous nerve, and, particularly, the radial sensory nerve should be dissected out in the early stages of the surgical procedure and protected throughout. The location of the radial artery should also be identified to avoid injury if the dorsal approach is performed as well during removal of the trapezium.

The second cause of complications is failure to diagnose comorbidities such as rheumatoid arthritis, lupus, or soft tissue laxity diseases (Ehlers-Danlos). Carpal tunnel syndrome, De Quervain's tenosynovitis, and wrist and finger flexor tenosynovitis may be present in patients with TMC degenerative arthritis. Scaphotrapezial arthritis may coexist in a certain percentage of patients. Procedures in which the trapezium is not completely removed should be avoided in this situation. Even if scaphotrapeziotrapezoidal joint disease is not suspected by physical examination or on radiographs of the thumb, the joint should always be examined intraoperatively before the definitive procedure is chosen.

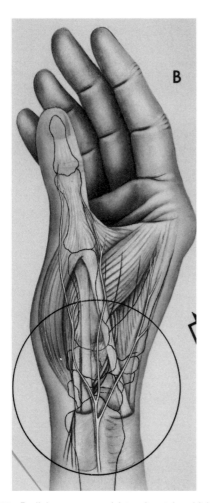

Figure 20–13. Radial sensory and lateral antebrachial cutaneous nerves.

Carpal tunnel syndrome has been reported to coexist with basilar joint arthritis in up to 43 percent of patients.[12] If operative treatment is required, we recommend an open carpal tunnel release at the same time through a separate palmar incision.

De Quervain's tenosynovitis is also included in the differential diagnosis of pain at the base of the thumb. Provocative maneuvers for De Quervain's tenosynovitis, especially the Finkelstein test, are often positive in both conditions. If there is uncertainty about the diagnosis, differential injections may be helpful. We prefer to treat De Quervain's disease conservatively before surgical treatment of the TMC joint.

In cases of implant arthroplasty, fracture or dislocation of the implant is always a potential complication.

In removing the trapezium, care must be taken to avoid damaging the flexor carpi radialis tendon in the base of the wound. Excising first the tuberosity of the trapezium and then the remainder of the trapezium piecemeal aids visualization and protect the flexor carpi radialis.

Reflex sympathetic dystrophy is a serious potential complication that has been observed after all forms of thumb arthroplasty. In a comparison of the results of both the Weilby suspensionplasty and the ligamentous reconstruction and tendinous interposition, incidence of serious comlications was similar. Patients, especially those who have trouble with rehabilitation, should be examined at bimonthly intervals or more often postoperatively for symptoms of reflex sympathetic dystrophy.

Residual pain from the first metacarpal articulating on the retained base of the trapezium has also been observed. For this reason, complete trapeziectomy is advocated and partial (distal) excision of the trapezoid is considered. Complications of surgery around the base of the thumb can be debilitating because of the high functional demands of this joint. A thorough preoperative examination to diagnose any comorbidities combined with careful surgical technique can help minimize this problem.

RHEUMATOID ARTHRITIS

Rheumatoid arthritis may include the thumb IP, MCP, or TMC joint individually or, more commonly, collectively.[28,29] With the latter, specific patterns of thumb collapse or instability result. Millender and Nalebuff[49] have classified the rheumatoid thumb into four different types that nicely describe the potential and actual deformity of each joint (Table 20–2). It is important to recognize the pattern of thumb instability because two or more joints often require simultaneous treatment.

The role of implant arthroplasty in the rheumatoid thumb is not completely developed. Fusion of the distal two joints (IP and MCP) has historically resulted in excellent thumb function and generally remains the treatment of choice. However, specific soft tissue reconstructions at the MCP and TMC joints can help maintain balance and strength for the thumb without the complete loss of motion associated with fusion. Total joint replace-

Table 20–2. NALEBUFF CLASSIFICATION OF THE RHEUMATOID THUMB

I. Boutonnière deformity—IP joint hyperextension, MCP joint flexion

II. IP hyperextension, MCP flexion dislocation of CMC joint

III. Swan-neck deformity—hyperextension of MCP and flexion of IP joint

IV. Gamekeeper thumb abduction deformity of MCP joint with secondary adduction of thumb metacarpal

CMC = carpometacarpal; IP = interphalangeal;
MCP = metacarpophalangeal.

ment has been advocated in selected patients for the IP and MCP joints (Figs. 20–14 and 20–15). The operative procedures for these joint arthroplasties are described in the following sections. It is important for each joint arthroplasty that soft tissue contractures, such as adduction of thumb metacarpal or flexion contracture of the MP joint be released at the same time as joint replacement if the operative procedure is to be successful.

Interphalangeal Joint Procedures

For hyperextension deformity of the IP joint (Nalebuff types I and II), instability at the MCP joint and erosive disease at the CMC joint are often present. Options for treatment include IP fusion with Kirschner wires or a Herbert screw or IP arthroplasty. Fusion is generally preferred because a stable IP joint does not limit thumb function and improves strength. Arthroplasty with a silicone or metal-polyethylene joint (proximal IP implant design) can be selected if the MCP joint is by nature stable or if MCP fusion is to be performed.

Surgical Technique

A dorsal longitudinal incision is made over the IP joint and the proximal phalanx (see Chapter 16, Figs. 16–18 and 16–19). The extensor tendon is split in the midline and retracted medially and laterally. The joint capsule is divided and the collateral ligaments are released from the proximal phalanx.

A dorsal extensor tendon splitting incision is then made, and the joint is exposed by division of the capsule; the radial and ulnar collateral ligaments are partially detached from the proximal phalanx and marked with a suture for later repair. The head of the proximal phalanx is removed with the oscillating saw, and the intramedullary canal is prepared with a leader (Swanson) bur or rasp. An osteotomy of the base of the distal phalanx is performed, and the intramedullary canal is similarly prepared. For a silicone implant, the appropriately sized implant is inserted and the collateral ligaments are reattached through pre-prepared drill holes at the end of the proximal phalanx. The divided extensor tendon is reapproximated. For a metal-polyethylene implant, the metal component, which duplicates the shape of the head of the proximal phalanx, and the polyethylene distal component are inserted and motion and stability are checked. If they are

satisfactory, the surgeon prepares for collateral ligament reattachment to the proximal phalanx through drill holes using a 4–0 Ticron suture. Bone cement is inserted into the intramedullary canal and the components are implanted. Reattachment of the collateral ligaments is completed, and the capsule and extensor tendon are closed in the midline. The thumb is immobilized for 2 weeks to allow for soft tissue healing before rehabilitation is started.

Metacarpophalangeal Joint Procedures

There are several options for treatment of the MCP joint in the rheumatoid thumb: synovectomy and reconstruction of the extensor tendon mechanism, transfer of extensor pollicis longus (EPL) to the base of the proximal phalanx, arthroplasty, and arthrodesis. For the flexion (boutonière) deformity (Nalebuff I), in which there is laxity of the extensor hood with displacement of the EPL ulnarward and volarly and collateral ligament laxity, soft tissue rebalancing procedures are recommended. Transfer of the EPL as the primary extensor of the MCP joint is the most valuable procedure in my experience for correcting thumb MP collapse deformity. Dorsal transfer of intrinsics may also be performed early in the disease process. For late presentation in which there is joint cartilage loss or fixed deformity of the MCP joint, joint arthrodesis is recommended. If the IP joint is quite stable and mobile, MCP arthroplasty of a resurfacing design could be considered. I have used both constrained and unconstrained MCP arthroplasties including ligament advancement (Figs. 20–14 and 20–15).

Arthroplasty of the thumb MCP joint can be performed by either a silicone or a polyethylene on metal implant. In my experience, the silicone implant does not provide sufficient stability in pinch for acceptable use. Using a semiconstrained MCP implant. We have had excellent results with demonstrated long-term success and survival of the implant (Fig. 20–15). McGovern et al. reported on the results of 54 primary thumb arthroplasties in 49 patients.[46] The majority of patients had rheumatoid arthritis. Thumb axis length and stability were maintained by use of the implant in 98 percent of the patients, and 87 percent reported improvement in grip and pinch strength. Periprosthetic loosening was not a major concern demonstrated, by 5-year survivorship of 93% and 10-year survivorship of 89%. Thumb MCP implants continue to be recommended in patients with rheumatoid arthritis, especially when there is advanced disease involving the distal interphalangeal and proximal thumb trapeziometacarpal joints.

For hyperextension deformity of the MCP joint (Nalebuff III), a volar capsulorrhaphy is an essential component of the reconstructive effort. The adductor contracture of the first metacarpal should also be released and the thumb pinned or splinted in abduction.

For thumb adduction (thumb metacarpal) contracture, often associated with lateral instability of the MCP joint (Nalebuff IV), release or lengthening

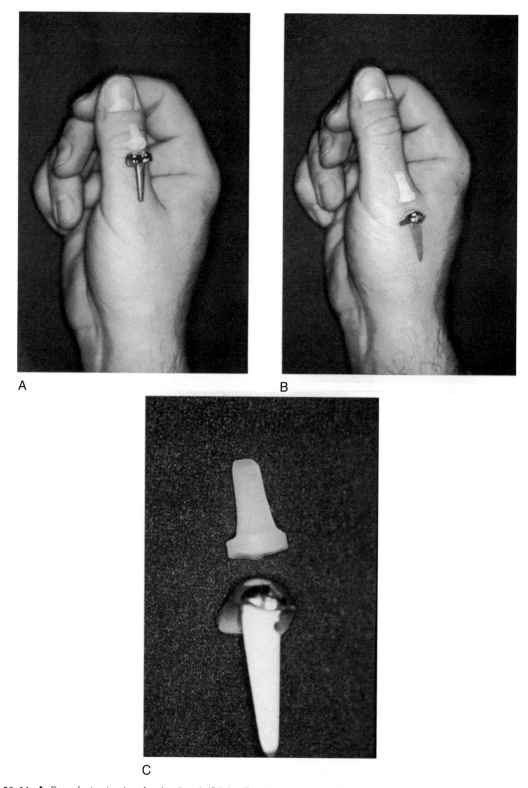

A

B

C

Figure 20–14. A, Resurfacing implant for the thumb IP joint. Distal compartment is polyethylene and proximal component is cobalt-chrome; bicondylar design. **B**, Resurfacing implant for thumb MCP joint. Convex proximal component with small palmar fins for ligament support. Distal concave polyethylene component. **C**, Close-up appearance of thumb MCP resurfacing implant.

of the adductor pollicis at its insertion and MCP fusion is usually required to provide a stable thumb.

Joint arthroplasty for the MCP joint is restricted to those circumstances in which the IP joint requires fusion and the TMC joint has limited motion. Here, the MCP joint becomes the primary area for thumb instability, and joint replacement is preferred to joint fusion.

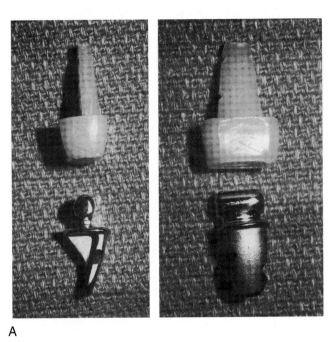
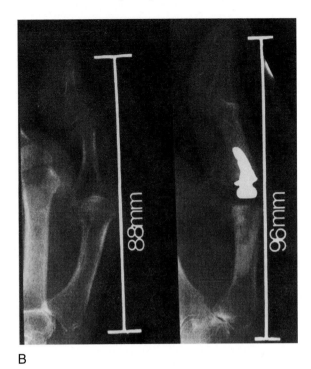

A   B

Figure 20–15. A, Dorsal and lateral views of the Steffee MCP joint implant, which is a two-part polyethylene and metal-hinged prosthesis. The proximal polyethylene component has a dorsally displaced stem to lower the center of rotation of the joint and a volar lip to block flexion at 40 degrees to prevent a flexion deformity. The distal component is snap-locked into the proximal component and allows for pure hinged flexion and extension. **B,** Thumb length increased after Steffee thumb arthroplasty. (From McGovern RM, Shin AY, Beckenbough RD, Linscheid RL; Long-term results of cemented Steffee arthroplasty. J Hand Surg 26A:115, 2001.)

Metacarpophalangeal Joint Arthroplasty

A dorsal curvilinear incision is made over the thumb MCP joint (Fig. 16–18). If there is deformity at the IP joint, the incision is extended distally. The extensor hood is divided between the EPL and extensor pollicis brevis (EPB) tendons, reflecting the medial and lateral extensor hoods. The capsule is divided in the midline (Fig. 16–19), a complete synovectomy is performed, and the proper collateral ligaments are released and tagged with a 3–0 mersilene (Ticron) suture. The two options for MCP arthroplasty are the semiconstrained implant (Steffee) and the resurfacing implant (Avanta) (Fig. 20–14). The Swanson MCP arthroplasty is too flexible to provide good MCP joint stability. The operative procedure is nearly identical for both implants, although the constrained implant does not require collateral ligament reattachment.

The trial implant is positioned over the joint to determine the amount of metacarpal head to resect. The base of the proximal phalanx may be removed up to 1 to 2 mm, preserving collateral ligament, volar plate, and extensor tendon attachments. The metacarpal head and base of the proximal phalanx are removed with an oscillating saw, and the intramedullary canals of the proximal phalanx and thumb metacarpal are reamed. The broach designed to match the prosthetic stem is used to prepare the intramedullary canal followed by insertion of trial components. The joint is articulated and range of motion tested. If the range of motion and joint stability are suitable, both components are inserted within the intramedullary canal with bone cement. A pressurized syringe is used for cement insertion, and pressure is maintained on the implants while the cement cures. (For resurfacing implants, reattachment of the collateral ligaments is necessary. One should pre-drill the metacarpal neck and place a 3–0 nonabsorbable suture into the bone before inserting the bone cement or prostheses.) After the cement has cured, the proper collateral ligaments are reattached under tension with the thumb in full extension. The capsule is repaired, and either the EPB is advanced or transfer of the EPL through the joint capsule is considered if a flexion deformity was present before surgery.

The thumb is immobilized for 2 weeks in a thumb spica cast, and then a controlled range-of-motion program is started.

Thumb Trapeziometacarpal Joint Procedures

Arthroplasty of the thumb TMC joint is often necessary to provide a stable thumb in the rheumatoid hand. Reconstruction may involve adductor release (Nalebuff type III or IV) and soft tissue stabilization or fusion at the MCP joint. Correcting distal joint deformity is important in any type of TMC joint arthroplasty if deformity forces are to be avoided.

The current preference for thumb TMC arthroplasty in rheumatoid arthritis is soft tissue interposition arthroplasty (see Fig. 20–11). Silicone resurfacing prostheses are contraindicated except in elderly patients. In a rheumatoid thumb, TMC joint metal on plastic replacement is not advocated because the bone stock is often deficient. Resection arthroplasty is a reasonable procedure with few associated complications and is my preference in the rheumatoid thumb. Future developments that would combine a total joint resurfacing implant with ligament reconstruction, however, offer a potential solution for a true joint replacement at the base of the rheumatoid thumb.

The operative procedure for the rheumatoid TMC joint is similar to that described for osteoarthritis. Hemiresection arthroplasty with ligament reconstruction is preferred to complete trapezium excision in an effort to maintain thumb length and stability. If there is pantrapezial disease, trapezium excision with soft tissue interposition should be performed. Release and balance of soft tissues (adduction contracture, APL distal transfer, capsule and volar plate lengthening at the MCP joint) usually accompany TMC joint arthroplasty. Silicone implants (condylar implants) may be considered in selected patients. Reactive silicone synovitis is less common in the rheumatoid thumb because stress loading is less. Total trapezium silicone replacement should be avoided, however, because it lengthens the thumb moment arm, leading to more instability and weakness. I have refrained from using silicone trapezium implants because of problems with implant instability (subluxation and dislocation).

RESULTS OF TREATMENT: TRAPEZIOMETACARPAL JOINT

Improvement in motion and pain relief can be expected after most types of arthroplasty for the thumb TMC joint. My personal experience is quite similar to that of studies reported by other hand surgeons. In the series of 91 patients of Dell et al.,[16] the majority had surgical treatment consisting of soft tissue interposition arthroplasty. Reconstruction of the ligaments was not performed. The patients uniformly had pain relief, although 9 of the 16 had mild pain with repetitive activities. Recession (subsidence) of the first metacarpal was noted (up to 3 mm) but was not thought to be clinically important. Thumb stability was good, and 50 degrees of abduction and 30 degrees of pronation were achieved; strength increased 147 percent from the preoperative measurement. I agree with Dell et al. that in patients with pantrapezial disease who have complete joint cartilage loss a total trapezial excision arthroplasty is required. I would not perform complete trapezial excision for stage II or stage III disease without evidence of involvement at the STT joint. Trapezial excision with soft tissue interposition is an excellent operation in most patients.

From a different viewpoint, Amadio and co-workers[4] studied the results of silicone arthroplasty versus interposition arthroplasty and found levels of pain relief

rates of 90 to 95 percent and motion with 42 degrees versus 46 degrees of abduction after both procedures. In their series of patients, the flexor carpi radialis was used to reinforce the joint, and Kirschner wire stabilization was performed. Subluxation was present after Silastic implants but not after the interposition procedures. Of importance, the strength of the thumb in patients without implants was as great as that in the implant group. Long-term relief of pain without late complications was achieved.

Burton and Pelligrini[12] have reported their extensive experience with interposition arthroplasty employing a ligament reconstruction with part of the flexor carpi radialis. In short- and long-term review of patients with advanced basal joint arthritis, they found consistently improved pinch and grip strength and a broader web space than after silicone arthroplasty. The procedure consisted of complete excision of the trapezium, tendon interposition, and reconstruction of the palmar oblique and intermetacarpal ligaments. In contrast to the technique described by Eaton and co-workers, the free end of the flexor carpi radialis is passed through the medullary canal of the thumb metacarpal rather than transversely through the base to create a sling to support the first metacarpal.

These same investigators reported their experience with 72 silicone arthroplasties of the thumb TMC joint in a retrospective study and detailed the problems of instability and prosthesis subsidence in approximately 25 percent of the patients reviewed. Dynamic tendon transfer did not prevent implant subluxation, whereas ligament reconstruction improved stability but did not prevent silicone wear or cold flow. They concluded that the forces across an osteoarthritic basal joint seemed to preclude a stable silicone implant arthroplasty in the absence of eventual silicone synovitis.

In a separate review of surgical treatment of TMC arthritis, Thompson[60] described a somewhat different type of suspensionplasty in which a dorsal slip of the APL or extensor carpi radialis longus tendon is passed through the base of the first metacarpal into the medullary canal of the first metacarpal and secured to the base of the second metacarpal, in effect replacing the intermetacarpal ligament. Weilby reported a reconstructive procedure of tendon interposition or suspension between the APL and flexor carpi radialis tendons.[62] Complete trapezium excision, ligament reconstruction, and tendon interposition is the pattern followed here, as in other interposition arthroplasties. Results of this procedure have been similar to those of Burton and Pelligrini, and the two techniques are quite similar except for the tendon used for the ligament reconstruction.[38,62]

COMPARISON OF RESULTS OF TRAPEZIOMETACARPAL ARTHROPLASTY

There continue to be varying opinions and controversy regarding the preferred procedures for the treatment of degenerative and rheumatoid arthritis of the thumb TMC joint. A wide variety of procedures have been described, but a lack of uniformity of evaluation and reporting makes comparative studies of different series of patients difficult. I have looked carefully at my own patients and the reports of others in an effort to draw meaningful conclusions regarding TMC arthroplasty. The following is a consensus of just a limited number of publications on the subject, which present some of the diversity of opinion and current thinking.

Hand surgeons, including Dell et al.,[20] Aune, Menon et al.,[48] Millender et al.,[49] and Belcher et al.[8] have reported 85 to 90 percent good to excellent (satisfactory) results after various types of interposition arthroplasty. In their research, ligament reconstruction has not been a part of the operative procedure, with the authors instead stressing total resection of the trapezium and the interposition of soft tissues. Ligament reconstruction, on the other hand, has been recommended as a necessary procedure in all but elderly women, who placed fewer demands on their hands according to most hand surgeons.[5,12,24,31,42] Most authors emphasize the importance of ligament reconstruction in restoring thumb alignment and strength. Reports on TMC arthroplasty have placed great emphasis on ligament reconstruction in addition to interposition arthroplasty. The overall return of strength and function appears to be better with this procedure than with soft tissue arthroplasty alone. Well-controlled, comparative series looking at the differences in patient satisfaction and clinical outcome between patients with and without ligament reconstruction are still needed.

Most recently, Rayan and Young reconfirmed the excellent results of tendon interposition with ligament reconstruction with the LRTI procedure. In 28 patients with Stage III and IV TMC arthritis, they reported 97% subjective improvement (40% excellent and 57% good results).[57] All patients had excellent pain relief and subsidence of the first metacarpal was minimal. They once again emphasized correction of the MP joint hyperextension deformity, which contributed to less than excellent results in 7 thumbs. Similarly, Lins et al. reported 89% satisfactory results in 27 LRTI procedures, with improvement in motion, strength and web space tightness.[42] More than 90 percent of patients had restoration of thumb extension-supination. The authors noted thumb metacarpal subsidence of a small degree in more than 50 percent of patients, but it was not clinically symptomatic. Finally, Eaton et al.[25] reported on 45 patients who had flexor carpi radialis tendon interposition with ligament reconstruction followed over 103 months. Pain relief was present in 93 percent, mobility equal to or greater than the opposite hand. Pinch strength was 86 percent and grasp 90 percent of the uninvolved extremity. They noted functional improvement and success in more than 94 percent of their patients.

Total arthroplasty of the TMC joint is a procedure limited to specific indications in which bone stock is good and the functional demands on the patient can be controlled. Motion and stability are desired by the patient. My patient selection has included a middle-aged surgeon who needed mobility to continue his practice and a more senior seamstress who had no evidence of osteoporosis and who wanted strong pinch for her home dressmaking avocation. The goal of prosthetic replacement is to establish a fixed fulcrum within the base of the thumb in order to provide inherent stability and avoid the need for ligament reconstruction. Of the four types of total joint arthroplasty currently performed, the results are quite similar with respect to motion, strength, and functional use of the thumb. In addition, the complications of prosthetic loosening and heterotopic bone formation appear nearly identical, with the possible exception of the French experience with the the de la Caffinière prosthesis.[19] In a series of 57 patients with 62 arthroplasties performed at the Mayo Clinic,[43] reasonable and often dramatic improvement in pinch and grip strength was noted in comparison with preoperative measurements. Motion, for example, improved to 40 degrees of flexion-extension and 50 degrees of palmar abduction, with nearly full thumb opposition. I measured the exact motion at the TMC joint in 30 patients and recorded motion close to that of a normal thumb. Using criteria established by Braun,[9] there were 21 excellent, 28 good, and 6 fair results. Seven poor results were associated with prosthetic loosening (11 percent). Heterotopic bone formation developed in 36 percent of my patients, limiting total motion but not producing pain or significant loss of function. Judicious use of cemented TMC arthroplasties continues, although recent trends are toward osseous integration with noncemented TMC prostheses that can be custom designed for each patient.

Arthrodesis of the thumb TMC joint can be an effective operation in selected cases in which stability of the thumb is more important than motion. Weinman and Lipscomb[63] reported their experience in 10 patients, and the procedure that they employed continues as the surgical technique of choice today. A solid fusion generally provides a pain-free, strong pinch, and the loss of motion is often compensated in adjacent joints. The main contraindication is pantrapezial arthritis. Muller[52] noted that there were several cases of advancing wrist arthritis after fusion of the TMC joint and Carroll and Hill[14] considered the presence of either MP joint or scaphotrapezial wrist joint arthritis as contraindications to the TMC fusion.

The actual benefit of thumb TMC fusion compared with other procedures was performed in a review of men with TMC disease from the Mayo Clinic.[5] In the series, which consisted of 47 patients with reconstruction for TMC arthritis, 16 had arthrodesis. Surprisingly, pinch strength and grip strength were not statistically better after arthrodesis than after silicone implant arthroplasty, interposition arthroplasty, or total joint replacement. Similarly, the ability to return to heavy or light labor was not influenced by the type of operative procedure. The conclusion drawn was that arthrodesis did not provide increased strength and stability over other reconstructive procedures as anticipated; therefore, if strength alone is the reason for a fusion, the decision should be reconsidered.

SUMMARY

Arthritis of the TMC joint is very common in the population, especially in women in their fifth and sixth decades. No prospective randomized studies have ever been done to compare the natural history of the disease with the results from surgical treatment by the Weilby suspensionplasty or the LRTI procedure. From my experience and that of others, these are the two preferred surgical procedures. Meticulous soft tissue dissection is required to prevent iatrogenic neuromas, which can be disabling to the patient. If done well, arthroplasty of the TMC joint can provide a strong, stable, and painless thumb that is very gratifying to the patient.[33]

Arthritis at the TMC joint is significantly disabling to the functional use of the hand. It is more common at this location than in any other area with the exception of the distal IP joints. Women have a greater predilection for TMC arthritis than men, but, fortunately, they may not be disabled enough to require surgical treatment.

To date, the most successful surgical procedure to treat thumb TMC arthritis is a resection/interposition arthroplasty either alone or with ligament-capsule reconstruction. In the experience of most hand surgeons, ligament reconstruction using a slip of the flexor carpi radialis, extensor carpi radialis, or abductor pollicis tendons provides improved strength without loss of motion and is associated with a low reoperation rate. The potential problem of subsidence (shortening) of the first metacarpal and impaction against the retained proximal half of the trapezium or against the scaphoid suggest the importance of ligament reconstruction as an essential part of the interposition arthroplasty procedure. Several authorities believe that a suspension arthroplasty procedure is ideal for the thumb TMC joint because it provides excellent motion, anatomic ligament reconstruction, and functional strength with a low rate of complications. I believe that these conclusions are correct and recommend this operation as the procedure of choice.

Silicone implant arthroplasty no longer has any specific indication in the treatment of TMC arthritis. Used alone, instability of the implant with subluxation or dislocation has persuaded most hand surgeons to seek alternative measures. With a ligament reconstruction procedure, the silicone condylar arthroplasty, as well as the trapezial replacement arthroplasty, can be considered, as is demonstrated by their continued popularity in Europe. However, the identification of silicone synovitis as an unwanted complication (approximately 20 percent) has lessened its reliability and safety.

Fusion of the thumb TMC joint is recommended when strength and stability are desired and motion can be sacrificed. It is generally preferred in men. Studies comparing strength and function, however, now suggest that fusion may not be better than arthroplasty and that stability alone in an individual performing heavy work may be the only reason to choose this operative procedure over an interposition or suspension-type arthroplasty.

Total joint replacement in the thumb TMC joint for the treatment of arthritis currently is limited to Eaton type II or III in selected patients needing strength and motion; musicians and surgeons are examples. We are working to perfect prosthesis design, cementing techniques, and soft tissue balance. I continue to use total joint arthroplasty when a fixed fulcrum is needed for stability and strength. Biomechanical studies[41,61] show the advantages of total joint replacement.[36] In the treatment of rheumatoid arthritis of the basal joint of the thumb, total joint arthroplasty is probably contraindicated because the bone is often too soft to support the compressive loads. Several young adults with excellent bone stock have had excellent results with total joint replacement, but loosening with time remains a significant concern. As technology progresses, however, many of the problems of implanting metal, polyethylene, or other materials, in bone will be overcome and a true "joint replacement" for the thumb TMC joint will be forthcoming.

For the rheumatoid thumb, most attention is placed on stabilizing the thumb MP joint. By soft tissue transfer (EPL transfer), deformity can be corrected and stability obtained. If soft tissue procedures would be ineffective, MP joint fusion or arthroplasty are recommended. We use arthroplasty if the thumb IP joint is to be fused and if fusion of the IP joint remains mobile. Thumb TMC joint in the patient with rheumatoid arthritis is best treated by liament reconstruction and soft tissue interposition combined with a volar plate-ulnar collateral ligament capsulodess of the thumb MCP joint.

References

1. Alnot JY, Beal D, Oberlin C, et al: Guepar total trapeziometacarpal prosthesis in the treatment of arthritis of the thumb. 36 case reports. Ann Chir Main 12:93, 1993.
2. Allieu Y, Peguignot JP, Asencio G, et al: Swanson trapezial implant in the treatment of peritrapezial arthrosis. A study of eighty cases. Ann Chir Main 3:113, 1984.
3. Alvat JY, Saint Laurent Y: Total trapeziometacarpal arthroplasty: Report on 17 cases of degenerative arthritis of the trapeziometacarpal. Ann Chir Main 4:11, 1985.
4. Amadio PC, Millender LH, Smith R: Silicone spacer or tendon spacer for trapezium resection arthroplasty comparison of results. J Hand Surg 7:237, 1982.
5. Amadio P, DeSilva SP: Comparison of the result of trapeziometacarpal arthrodesis and arthroplasty in men with osteoarthritis of the trapeziometacarpal. Ann Chir Main 9:358, 1990.
6. August AC, Coupland RM, Sandifer JP: Short-term review of the De La Caffiniere trapeziometacarpal arthroplasty. J Hand Surg 9B:185, 1984.
7. Bettinger PC, Smutz WP, Linscheid RL, et al: Material properties of the trapezial and trapeziometacarpal ligaments. J Hand Surg 25A:1085, 2000.
8. Belcher HJ, Nichall JE: A comparison of trapeziectomy with and without ligament reconstruction with tendon interposition. J Hand Surg 25B:350, 2000.
9. Braun RM: Total joint arthroplasty at the CMC joint of the thumb. Clin Orthop 195:161, 1985.
10. Brunelli G, Monini L, Brunelli F: Stabilization of the trapeziometacarpal joint. J Hand Surg 14B:209, 1989.
11. Burton RI: Basal joint arthritis. Fusion, implant or soft tissue reconstruction? Orthop Clin North Am 17:493, 1986.
12. Burton RI, Pellegrini VD: Surgical management of basal joint arthritis of the thumb. II. Ligament reconstruction with tendon interposition arthroplasty. J Hand Surg 11:324, 1986.
13. Carroll R: Fascial arthroplasty for the carpometacarpal joint of the thumbs. Orthop Trans 1:15, 1977.

14. Carroll R, Hill N: Arthrodesis of the carpometacarpal joint of the thumb. J Bone Joint Surg 55B:292, 1973.

15. Clayton ML: Surgery of the thumb in rheumatoid arthritis. J Bone Joint Surg 44A:1376, 1962.

16. Cooney WP, Chao EYS: Biomechanical analysis of static forces in the thumb during hand function. J Bone Joint Surg 59A:27, 1977.

17. Cooney WP, Lucca MJ, Chao EYS, Linscheid RL: The kinesiology of the thumb trapeziometacarpal joint. J Bone Joint Surg 63A:1371, 1981.

18. Cooney WP: Arthroplasty of the thumb axis. In Morrey BF (ed): Reconstructive Surgery of the Joints, 2nd ed. New York, Churchill Livingstone, 1996, pp 313–338.

19. de la Caffiniere J, Aucouturier P: Trapeziometacarpal arthroplasty by total prosthesis. Hand 11:41, 1979.

20. Dell P, Brushart T, Smith R: Treatment of trapeziometacarpal arthritis: Results of resection arthroplasty. J Hand Surg 3:243, 1978.

21. Eaton R, Littler JW: A study of the basal joint of the thumb. J Bone Joint Surg 51A:661, 1969.

22. Eaton R: Replacement of the trapezium for arthritis of the basal articulations: A new technique with stabilization by tenodesis. J Bone Joint Surg 61A:76, 1979.

23. Eaton RG, Glickel SZ: Trapeziometacarpal osteoarthritis: Staging as a rationale for treatment. Hand Clin 3:455, 1987.

24. Eaton R, Lane L, Littler JW, et al: Ligament reconstruction for the painful thumb carpometacarpal joint: A long term assessment. J Hand Surg 9A:692, 1984.

25. Eaton R, Glickel SZ, Littler JW: Tendon interposition arthroplasty for degenerative arthritis of the trapeziometacarpal joint of the thumb. J Hand Surg 10A:645, 1985.

26. Feldon P, Millender LH, Nalebuff EA: Rheumatoid arthritis in the hand and wrist. In Green DP (ed): Operative Hand Surgery, 3rd ed. New York, Churchill Livingstone, 1993, p 1678.

27. Flatt AE: The Care of the Rheumatoid Hand. St. Louis, CV Mosby, 1963.

28. Freedman DM, Eaton RG, Glickel SZ: Long-term results of volar ligament reconstruction for symptomatic basal joint laxity. J Hand Surg 25A:297, 2000.

29. Fujami T, Nakamura K, Shimajiri I: Osteotomy for trapeziometacarpal arthrosis. Acta Orthop Scan 63:462, 1992.

30. Gervis WH: Excision of the trapezium for osteoarthritis of the trapezium for osteoarthritis of the trapeziometacarpal joint. J Bone Joint Surg 31B:537, 1949.

31. Glickel SL, Eaton RG: Trapeziometacarpal osteoarthritis staging as a rationale for treatment. Hand Clin 3:455, 1987.

32. Glickel SZ, Kornstein AN, Eaton RG: Long-term follow-up of trapeziometacarpal arthroplasty with coexisting of scaphotrapezial disease. J Hand Surg 17A:612, 1992.

33. Hannula TT, Nahigian SH: A preliminary report: Cementless trapeziometacarpal arthroplasty. J Hand Surg 24A:92, 1999.

34. Howard FM, Simpson LA, Belsole RJ: Silastic condylar arthroplasty. Clin Orthop 195:144, 1985.

35. Imaeda T, An KN, Cooney WP III, Linscheid R: Anatomy of trapeziometacarpal ligaments. J Hand Surg 18:226, 1993.

36. Imaeda T, Cooney WP, Niebur GL, et al. Kinematics of the trapeziometacarpal joint. A biomechanical study comparing tendon interposition and total joint arthroplasty. J Hand Surg 21A:544, 1996.

37. Kauer JMG: Functional anatomy of the carpometacarpal joint of the thumb. Clin Orthop 220:7, 1987.

38. Kleinman WB, Eckenrade JF: Tendon suspension sling arthroplasty for thumb trapeziometacarpal arthritis. J Hand Surg 16A:983, 1991.

39. Kuczynski K: Carpometacarpal joint of the human thumb. J Anat 118:119, 1984.

40. Leach R, Bolton PE: Arthritis of the carpometacarpal joint of the thumb. Results of arthrodesis. J Bone Joint Surg 50A:1171, 1968.

41. Ledaux P: Cementless total trapeziometacarpal prostheses: Principle of anchorage. In Schuind F, An KN, Cooney WP, Garcia-Elias M (eds): Advances in the Biomechanics of the Hand and Wrist. NATO ASI Series. New York, Plenum Press, 1994.

42. Lins RE, Gelberman RH, McKeown L, et al: Basal joint arthritis: Trapeziectomy with ligament rconstruction and tendon interposition arthroplasty. J Hand Surg 21:202, 1996.

43. Linscheid RL, Cooney WP (eds): American Academy of Orthopaedic Surgeons Symposium on Total Joint Replacement of the Upper Extremity. St. Louis, CV Mosby, 1980.

44. Linscheid RL, Cooney WP, Dobyns JH: Metacarpotrapezial arthroplasty. In Inglis AE (ed): American Academy of Orthopaedic Surgeons Symposium on Total Joint Replacement of the Upper Extremity. St. Louis, CV Mosby, 1982, p 289.

45. Mautet F, Lignon J, Oberlm C, et al: Les prosthèses totales trapezio-metacarpiennes: Résultats de l'étude multicentrique (106 cas). Ann Chir Main Memb Super 9:189, 1996.

46. McGovern RM, Shin AY, Steffee Beckenbaugh RD, Linscheid RL: Long-term results of cemented arthroplasty of the thumb metacarpophalangeal joint. J Hand Surg 26A:115, 2001.

47. Menon J, Schoene H, Hohl J: Trapeziometacarpal arthritis: results of tendon interposition arthroplasty. J Hand Surg 6:442, 1981.

48. Menon J: Arthroscopic management of trapeziometacarpal joint arthritis of the thumb. Arthroscopy 12:581, 1996.

49. Millender LH, Nalebuff EA, Amadio PC, Philips C: Interpositional arthroplasty for rheumatoid carpometacarpal joint disease. J Hand Surg 3A:533, 1978.

50. Molitor P, Emory RJH, Meggit BF: First metacarpal osteotomy for carpometacarpal osteoarthritis. J Hand Surg 16B:424, 1991.

51. Muermans S, Coenen L: Interpositional arthroplasty with Gore-Tex, marlex or tendon for osteoarthritis of the trapeziometacarpal joint. A retrospective comparative study. J Hand Surg 23B:64, 1998.

52. Muller G: Arthrodesis of the trapeziometacarpal joint for osteoarthritis. J Bone Joint Surg 31B:540, 1949.

53. Murley A: Excision of the trapezium in osteoarthritis of the first carpometacarpal joint. J Bone Joint Surg 42B:502, 1960.

54. Peimer C, Jedige J, Eckert BS: Reactive synovitis after silicone arthroplasty. J Hand Surg 11:624, 1986.

55. Pellegrini VD: Osteoarthritis of the trapeziometacarpal joint. J Hand Surg 16A:975, 1991.

56. Pieron AP: The mechanism of the first carpometacarpal joint, an anatomical and mechanical analysis. Acta Orthop Scand 148(Suppl):1, 1973.

57. Rayan G, Young T: Ligament reconstruction arthroplasty for the TMC arthrosis. J Hand Surg 221:1067, 1997.

58. Sigfusson R, Lundborg G: Abductor pollicis longus tendon arthroplasty for treatment of arthrosis of the first carpometacarpal joint. Scand Plast Reconstr Hand Surg 25:73, 1991.

59. Swanson A, Swanson GD, Watermeire J: Trapezium implant arthroplasty: Long-term evaluation of 150 cases. J Hand Surg 6:125, 1981.

60. Thompson JS: Surgical treatment of trapeziometacarpal arthrosis. Adv Orthop Surg 2:105, 1988.

61. Uchiyama S, Cooney WP, Biebur G, et al: Biomechanical analysis of the TMC joint after surface replacement arthroplasty. J Hand Surg 24A:483, 1999.

62. Weilby A: Tendon interposition arthroplasty of the first carpometacarpal joint. J Hand Surg 13B:421, 1988.

63. Weinman DT, Lipscomb PR: Degenerative arthritis of the trapeziometacarpal joint: Arthrodesis or excision? Mayo Clin Proc 42:276, 1967.

64. Wilson J: Basal osteotomy of the first metacarpal in the treatment of arthritis of the carpometacarpal joint of the thumb. Br J Surg 60:854, 1973.

65. Zancolli EA, Ziadenberg C, Zancolli E Jr: Biomechanics of the trapeziometacarpal joint. Clin Orthop 220:14, 1987.

21

The Distal Radioulnar Joint

· WILLIAM P. COONEY III and RICHARD A. BERGER

Arthrosis of the distal radioulnar joint (DRUJ) is a common problem, which often leads to substantial disability from pain, weakness, and instability. Once degenerative changes in the articular surfaces of the DRUJ have developed, surgical options are limited, as there are, at the present time, no known procedures that can reconstitute the articular cartilage in this joint. Therefore, resection of one or both surfaces of the DRUJ is the current treatment of choice. This can take several forms, such as resection of the ulnar head, partial resection of the joint surfaces with or without interposition of connective soft tissue (matched resection arthroplasty, hemiresection interposition arthroplasty), or fusion of the distal radius and ulna with creation of a proximal pseudarthrosis such as the Kapandji-Sauvé procedure.

The most basic and time-honored method of resecting the arthritic surface of the DRUJ was introduced in 1912 by Darrach; however, it was first mentioned by Moore, in 1880, in the American literature for fresh injuries and in the German literature by Lauenstein in 1887. By convention, the term "Darrach resection" implies resection of the entire ulnar head. Although modifications of the technique have evolved, complications related to instability of the distal forearm resulting from loss of the ulnar head have remained the principal detractors from this procedure. The instability of the distal radius and wrist relative to the shortened ulna has been typically recognized as an anteroposterior (AP) instability. This has been thought to be related to the predictable weakness of grip strength and torsional strength of the forearm that occurs after the Darrach procedure. However, a convergence instability of the stump of the resected ulna toward the metaphysis of the radius has been identified as a common cause of progressive pain after the Darrach operation.

Stuart et al. reported that approximately 20 percent of the total constraint of the DRUJ is contributed by the articulation surface between the radius and ulna. Resecting the distal ulna, either partially or entirely, results in an enhanced tendency for convergence. Surprisingly, there is still a strong desire by clinicians to resect the arthrotic bone but this can result in pain and instability related to loss of the articular surfaces. To this end, an endoprosthesis has been developed at the Mayo Clinic to replace the ulnar head in patients who are undergoing or have undergone a Darrach resection. The device consists of a metallic stem, which inserts into the shaft of the ulna, and a polished metallic ulnar head, which has provisions for soft tissue attachments of the triangular fibrocartilage complex (TFCC) and the subsheath of the extensor carpi ulnaris. A similar device has been developed simultaneously, which uses a ceramic head and is currently available for use in Europe.

The DRUJ plays an important role in the integration of forearm-wrist-hand function, and disorders of this joint can cause considerable clinical impairment. Yet, as recently as 1984, problems of the DRUJ were considered both the new frontier as well as the "low back pain" of hand surgery and the forgotten joint in treatment of distal radius fractures and other associated carpal injuries.[22] However, interest and hence understanding continue to increase in all areas related to the DRUJ, and painful derangements of this complex area are now more commonly recognized and treated.

ANATOMY

The anatomy of DRUJ is important and is briefly discussed in the context of prosthetic design for joint replacement. The evolutionary process resulting in the loss of the ulnocarpal articulation and the development of a synovial distal radioulnar joint (DRUJ) provided for the development of pronation and supination of the forearm and, indirectly, the wrist. This was a distinct advantage not only in procurement of food but also in defense, in caring for young, and, later, in the efficient use of tools, which developed 2 million years ago. It is this mobility of the DRUJ, along with the prehensile thumb and cerebral development, that are the hallmarks of higher order primates.[1] The distal radioulnar joint, like the proximal radioulnar joint, is trochoid. It is an incongruous joint, however, because the radius of curvature of the concave sigmoid notch of the distal radius is 4 to 7 mm larger than the convex surface of the ulnar head[21] (Fig. 21–1A). The convex surface of the distal ulna, which is covered with articular cartilage over 270

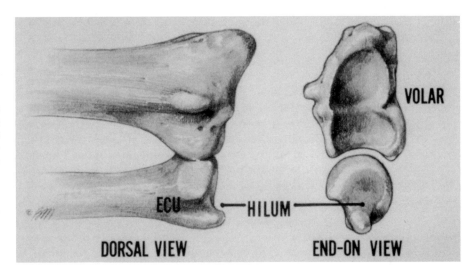

Figure 21–1. The radioulnar articulation in neutral or zero rotation as viewed from the dorsum and from end on. (From Bowers WH: Distal radioulnar joint arthroplasty. Current concepts. Clin Orthop 275:104, 1992.)

of its 360 degrees of circumference, is also correspondingly angled distally and ulnarly approximately 20 degrees relative to the shaft of the ulna.[15] A concave surface lies at the base of the ulnar styloid and is the attachment area for the TFCC and the ulnar collateral ligament (UCL) complex. The ulnar styloid provides an additional area of attachment for the ligamentous structures[8] and, proximally, a sulcus for the deep surface of the extensor carpi ulnaris (ECU) as well as the ECU subsheath[41] (Fig. 21–1).

The contribution of joint surface architecture to overall stability of the DRUJ is minimal, and, therefore, the ligamentous structures are of particular importance when implant replacement is considered. Biomechanical studies show that the most important stabilizer of the DRUJ is the TFCC.[31] The TFCC arises from the ulnar aspect of the lunate fossa of the distal radius and inserts into the ulnar head at the foveal region as well as into the base of the ulnar styloid. It extends distally and is joined by fibers of the UCL, which arise from the ulnar aspect of the ulnar styloid (Fig. 21–2). The fibrocartilage portion of the TFCC is triangular in shape, the peripheral borders serving to provide tension or constraint while the central portion resists compression loads. Its biconcave body stretches across the distal articular surface of the ulna and attaches to the concave region of the ulnar head and styloid. It is 1 to 2 mm thick at its base and may be as thick as 5 mm at the ulnar apex.[8] The TFCC functions not only as a major stabilizer of the DRUJ but also as a provider of continuous extension of the distal radius articular surface for wrist motion, a cushion for axial loads across the wrist, and a suspension and stabilization component of the ulnar carpus.[8,31] For prosthetic replacement of the distal ulna, the TFCC must be competent to resist the forces of both the wrist and DRUJ or be reconstructible by soft tissue ligament procedures to be described later.

In addition to the TFCC and the configuration of the sigmoid notch itself, other stabilizers of the DRUJ include the interosseous membrane, the extensor retinaculum and ECU subsheath, and the dorsal carpal ligament complex. Importantly, the dynamic forces of the extensor carpi ulnaris[41] and pronator quadratus[21] have also been shown to contribute to DRUJ stability.

BIOMECHANICS

The radius bears approximately 82 percent of axial loading with an intact TFCC, 94 percent when the TFCC is absent, and 100 percent after distal ulna excision.

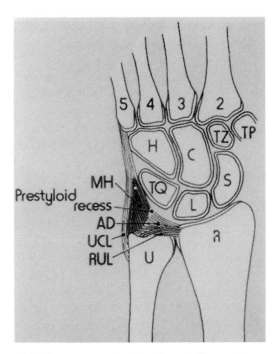

Figure 21–2. The components of the triangular fibrocartilage complex (MH, meniscus homologue; AD, articular disc; UCL, ulnar collateral ligament; RUL, dorsal and volar radioulnar ligaments). The extensor carpi ulnaris sheath (another component of the complex) is not shown. Other structures shown are the metacarpal bones (2, 3, 4, and 5); the carpal bones (S, styloid; L, lunate; TQ, triquetrum; H, hamate; C, capitate; TZ, trapezoid; TP, trapezium); and the radius (R) and the ulna (U). (From Palmer AK: The distal radioulnar joint. Orthop Clin North Am 15:321, 1984.)

Biomechanical studies that showed 17 percent ulna load in the controls found that this was decreased to 3.6 percent after silicone arthroplasty, to 2.4 percent after hemiresection arthroplasty, and to 1 percent after Darrach resection.[45]

Rotation is the primary function of the DRUJ. Forearm rotation of up to 150 degrees is possible at the DRUJ, with the distal radius and carpus rotating about the ulnar head in a 3:1 ratio of forearm to carpus motion.[24] Because of the incongruous nature of the DRUJ, forearm motion of pronation and supination must include sliding and translation as well as rotation. The ulnar head moves distally and dorsally in the sigmoid notch during pronation and proximally and volarly during supination.[33] In neutral rotation, approximately 60 to 80 degrees of the 130-degree convex articular surface of the ulna are in contact with the sigmoid notch, but this decreases to less than 10 percent in extreme rotation.[8] An intact TFCC and normal articular congruity are, therefore, necessary for normal joint function and stability. Unfortunately, neither are easily replicated with prosthetic replacement.

DRUJ include degenerative, rheumatoid, and post-traumatic types. It may be difficult to consider these disorders as a separate entity because they frequently are a result of, or coexist with, instability. As a group, however, they are characterized by painful rotation as a result of abnormal joint surfaces. Most pertinent to the topic of DRUJ arthroplasty is recognition of instability, ulnar impaction with the carpus, radioulnar impingement after resection arthroplasty, and arthritis.

Indications for distal ulna replacement can be considered either primary or secondary. Primary indications include comminuted distal ulna fracture, ulnocarpal abutment syndromes, post-traumatic arthritis, and rheumatoid arthritis. Secondary indications include failed distal ulna excision (Darrach procedure or Bowers hemiresection-interposition [HIT] procedure), failed silicone implants, chronic axial forearm instability (Essex-Lopresti lesion), and reconstruction of DRUJ instability associated with arthritis. For our purposes, the most common indication is failure of prior reconstructive procedures in which there is associated wrist and forearm instability.

CLASSIFICATION OF DISORDERS

Disorders of the distal radioulnar joint have been classified by Bowers (Table 21–1). Arthritic conditions of the

ETIOLOGY OF ARTHROSIS

Little information is available in the literature regarding the etiology and epidemiology of arthrosis of the distal

---

Table 21–1. DERANGEMENTS OF THE DISTAL RADIOULNAR JOINT

I. Acute Fractures
    A. *Fractures involving the sigmoid notch of the radius:* Colles', Barton's, distal radial metaphyseal fractures with comminution (Frykman's VBVIII), distal radial epiphyseal fractures or separations
    B. *Ulnar Articular Surface Fractures* (including chondral fractures)
    C. *Ulnar Styloid Fractures* (isolated or associated with fractures of the radius)
II. Acute Joint Disruption
    A. *TFCC disruption with dislocation or instability associated with fractures or other dislocations* (see I–C)
        1. Fracture separation of radial epiphysis
        2. Moore's fracture (Colles' fracture with disruption of distal radioulnar joint)
        3. Radial shaft or metaphysis fracture (Darrach, Galleazzi, Gughston, Milch, Smith)
        4. Radial head fractures (Essex-Lopresti)
        5. Isolated ulnar fractures
        6. Combined fractures of the radius and ulna
        7. Proximal radial-ulnar joint dislocations (traumatic or infantile)
        8. Radiocarpal joint dislocations
        9. Monteggia's injury (fracture of the ulna with proximal radioulnar dislocation)
    B. *Isolated TFCC Disruption with Instability*
    C. *Isolated TEC Disruption without Instability*
III. Chronic or Late-Appearing Joint Disruption Without Radiographic Arthritis
    A. *TFC injury, isolated without instability* (see II-C)
    B. *TFCC disruption with recurrent dislocation or instability*
        1. Isolated (see I-C, II-B)
        2. Associated with shaft deformity (see II–A)
IV. Joint Disorders
    A. *Ulnocarpal impaction syndrome length discrepancy with the ulna long relative to the radius*
        1. Premature closure of radial epiphysis secondary to trauma (acquired Madelung's deformity or premature wrist fusion)
        2. Excision or "settling" of radial head (or shaft) secondary to trauma, tumor, or infection
        3. Occupational overload of a "normal variant" long ulna
        4. Reconstruction of radial or ulnar shaft for trauma, tumor, or infection
    B. *Arthritis including osteoarthritis, arthritis after trauma, and articular chondromalacia with or without instability*
V. Other Disorders
    A. *Snapping or dislocating extensor carpi ulnaris*
    B. *Fixed rotational deformity*

Modified from Bowers WH: The distal radicular joint. *In* Green DP (ed): Operative Hand Surgery, 3rd ed. New York, Churchill Livingstone, 1993, p 973.

radioulnar joint. Inflammatory arthritides are probably the most completely documented causes of DRUJ arthrosis, particularly rheumatoid arthritis. This, no doubt, stems from an early pannus involvement of the DRUJ and ulnocarpal joint from the high degree of vascularity encountered in this region. This results in destruction of the articular surfaces of the ulnar head and the sigmoid notch, and subsequent loss of soft tissue integrity leads to further instability and pain. This often produces the condition known as *caput ulnae syndrome*, in which the radius subluxates from the ulna at the level of the DRUJ. This gives the appearance of a very prominent ulnar head, especially in pronation. Even with the inflammatory phase of the disease in quiescence, it is not unusual for patients with rheumatoid arthritis to continue to suffer from problems associated with residual degenerative disease and instability.

Post-traumatic causes for degenerative arthrosis no doubt exist but are poorly documented in the literature. These may be categorized as primary post-traumatic changes, largely resulting from malunited fractures of the distal radius involving the sigmoid notch, fractures of the ulnar head, or both. Even in the face of an anatomic union, the initial energy of the injury that causes a fracture may lead to chondrolysis and resulting degenerative changes. The second class of post-traumatic changes results from injuries to the soft tissues that stabilize the DRUJ. Such injuries may lead to chronic instability. This instability then, over time, predisposes the patient to premature destruction of the articular surfaces of the DRUJ.

The largest category of patients with definite degenerative changes in the DRUJ has no identifiable inciting event and is thus idiopathic. They may have minor congenital or developmental abnormalities of the geometry of the joint surfaces, laxity of the soft tissues, occupations that over time produce excessive torsional loads to the forearm, and so forth.

DIAGNOSIS

Disorders of the DRUJ are a particular challenge because of the compactness of anatomic structures in this region and their complexity of function. This is further complicated by a substantial number of disorders to be considered in the differential diagnosis of ulnar-sided wrist pain[44] (see Table 21–1).

In patients with arthritis, pathology related to the DRUJ is frequently significant and results in upper limb disability for functional activities of daily life. Patients complain of limited, painful rotation of the wrist; a sense of instability; snapping; clicking; or a weak, painful grip. Loss of motion is a sensitive indicator of intra-articular pathology.[14]

Numerous imaging modalities are useful to detect the full complement of pathology related to injury or disease at the DRUJ. These include plain films, stress views, tomograms, arthrography, arthrotomography, bone scan, computed tomography (CT), magnetic resonance imaging (MRI), and arthroscopy. However, a plain AP/lateral radiograph is usually adequate to diagnose arthritis and impingement after prior resection. True AP and lateral radiographs in neutral, radial, and ulnar deviation, and clenched-fist views are part of the initial assessment. The posteroanterior grip views should be taken in neutral forearm pronation-supination to avoid misinterpretation of positive or negative ulnar variance (Fig. 21–3). These radiographs should be studied for ulnar variance, radioulnar widening, subluxation, and degenerative changes and can be compared with radiographs of the contralateral side, when necessary. Subluxation of the ulna is best seen on a true lateral radiograph.[29] In addition, a semipronated view may help make dorsal-ulnar structures visible, and a semisupinated or ballcatcher view may show volar-ulnar structures. Clenched-fist or dynamic loaded views may allow more subtle instability or subluxation to be visualized. Dynamic axial CT of the wrist with stress loading is currently being studied as a more accurate method of measuring dorsal or volar instability.

CT has been shown to be clinically useful in the diagnosis of DRUJ disorders, including subluxation, dislocation, and joint surface abnormalities.[11,25,34]

DRUJ Arthroplasty

From a practical perspective, resection arthroplasty, with or without soft tissue interposition, has characterized the principal method of treatment of DRUJ arthritis. Within this broad category are included resection of the distal ulna (Darrach procedure) with its many variations, HIT (Bowers), matched distal ulna resection (Watson), and segmental resection of the ulna shaft with DRUJ arthrodesis (Sauvé-Kapandji). When there is isolated positive ulnar variance, mild arthritis, or both, ulna recession has traditionally been the procedure of choice.[12] These resection arthroplasties will be mentioned only very briefly because the failure of these procedures is the most common indication for distal ulna replacement.

Darrach. Darrach resection is essentially a complete excisional arthroplasty that does not restore load-bearing transmission along the ulnar column and depends on the development of postoperative scar tissue for stability and rotation (Fig. 21–4). Efforts to limit instability have prompted various partial resections. By limiting resection to a level just proximal to the sigmoid notch and by contouring the distal ulna so that no bony projections are likely to impinge on the distal radius, residual distal ulnar pain instability may be lessened. This is the theory behind the "matched" distal ulnar resection technique developed by Watson (Fig. 21–5).

Although Darrach resection has proven to be a useful procedure over the course of many decades,[9,19,23,30] there are reports suggesting that Darrach resections can result in serious disability, particularly in younger, active patients (Fig. 21–6).[2,3] At present, the general indications

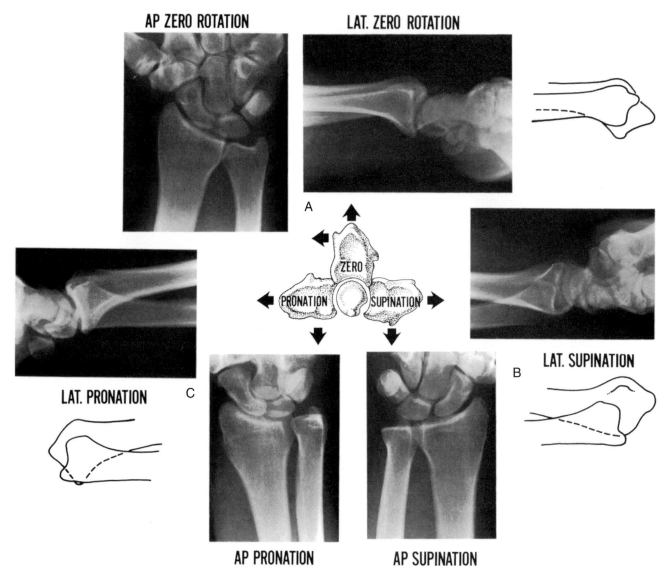

Figure 21–3. The determination of forearm rotation using the ulnar styloid as a reference point. **A,** Anteroposterior and lateral positions in zero rotation (the preferred standard position). **B,** Anteroposterior and lateral positions in full pronation. **C,** Anteroposterior and lateral positions in full supination. (From Bowers WH: The distal radioulnar joint. *In* Green DP [ed]: Operative Hand Surgery, 3rd ed. New York, Churchill Livingstone, 1993, p 973.)

for Darrach resection include disorders that cause derangement of the DRUJ resulting in painful, limited motion (e.g., rheumatoid, degenerative, and post-traumatic arthritis). This procedure is also frequently combined with radiolunate arthrodesis or total wrist arthroplasty in the advanced rheumatoid arthritis patient. Isolated instability and ulnocarpal impaction are controversial indications because instability is often worsened postoperatively, and better procedures exist for ulnocarpal impaction, such as ulnar shortening or wafer resection.

In cases in which there is instability of the resected distal ulna, a number of stabilization techniques using various configurations of tendons and soft tissue have been described by various authors. A distally based slip of flexor carpi ulnaris with a proximally based slip of

extensor carpi ulnaris through drill holes in the stump of resected ulna has been offered as a reliable and reproducible procedure.[10] A distally based slip of extensor carpi ulnaris (ECU) routed through a drill hole in the distal ulna and then bolstered by attaching the tendon to the remnant of the TFCC has also been described.[48] Other authors have described transfer of either a dorsal or volar flap of wrist capsule[5,42] or extensor retinaculum to help stabilize the distal ulna. Many surgeons currently recommend transfer of the pronator quadratus[35] from volar to dorsal imbricated to the distal stump of the ulna to prevent radioulnar impingement, dorsal subluxation, or both.

The concept of preservation of ulnar length by the wafer procedure has been described by Feldon et al. (Fig. 21–6).[16] This procedure shortens the ulnar load-

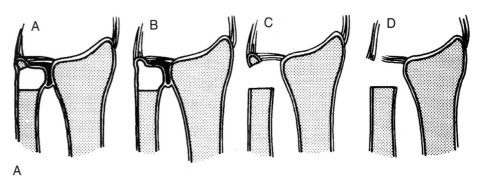

A

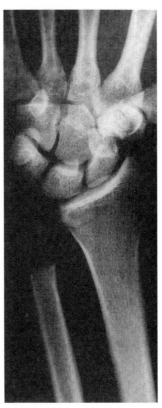

B

Figure 21–4. A, The Darrach procedure and its modifications as conceptualized by Dingman. (From Bowers WH: The distal radioulnar joint. *In* Green DP [ed]: Operative Hand Surgery, 3rd ed. New York, Churchill Livingstone, 1993, p 973. As adapted from Dingman PV: Resection of the distal end of the ulna [Darrach operation]. J Bone Joint Surg 34A:893, 1952.) **B**, Clinical example of the Darrach resection of the distal ulna (2 cm resection).

bearing column by resecting 2 to 4 mm of the distal articular surface, preserving the TFCC and sigmoid notch articulation, and is indicated for mild ulnocarpal impaction and as an adjunct in the treatment of TFCC tears. It does not, however, address instability or degenerative changes in the sigmoid notch, and, therefore, its indications should not be overextended.

Ulnar shortening osteotomy has been popularized by Milch[28] and has been referred to as the Milch osteotomy. It is indicated for the treatment of conditions related to positive ulnar variance, such as ulnocarpal impaction,[12] TFCC tears (in conjunction with repair),[4,6] and chondromalacia of the distal ulnar head.[12,26] It involves resection of a segment of distal ulnar diaphysis (range of 2.5 to 5 mm, with an average of 4 mm) with either transverse, step-cut, or oblique osteotomy and internal fixation (Fig. 21–7). Modern studies using dynamic compression plat-

ing report good results. An ulna recession provides for continuity between the wrist and the forearm, and, as such, is a much less destructive alternative to Darrach resection.[12]

In 1998, a hemiresection interposition arthroplasty technique was described that involved resection of only the articular portion of the ulnar head while preserving intact the ulnar styloid and ulnocarpal ligament complex, thereby maintaining a more normal anatomic relationship.[7] A soft tissue "anchovy" (capsule, tendon, or muscle) is interposed to minimize radioulnar contact. The procedure is indicated for early to midstage rheumatoid disease.[8]

The final procedure to stabilize the distal radioulnar joint that deserves to be discussed is the Sauvé-Kapandji procedure, or distal radioulnar fusion with surgical pseudarthrosis of the ulna (Fig. 21–8). First described in

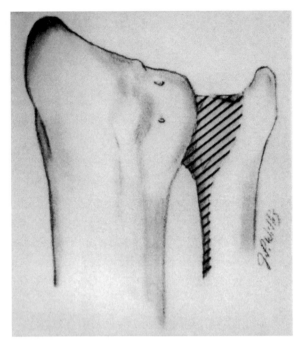

Figure 21–5. The ulna is resected in a convex fashion to match the concave radial metaphysis. Ulnar length and styloid process are preserved. (From Watson HK, Ryu J, Burgess RC: Matched distal ulnar resection. J Hand Surg 11A:812, 1986.)

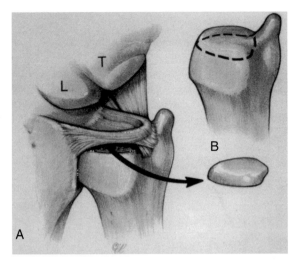

Figure 21–6. The Feldon "wafer" osteotomy. **A,** A 2- to 4-mm wafer of cartilage and bone is removed from the ulnar articular dome just under the triangular fibrocartilage complex. The radioulnar articulation is not disturbed. The procedure effectively shortens the ulnar load-bearing column. **B,** Magnified view of the area of bone resection. L = lunate; T = triquetrum. (From Bowers WH: The distal radioulnar joint. *In* Green DP [ed]: Operative Hand Surgery, 3rd ed. New York, Churchill Livingstone, 1993, p 973.)

1936[38] as an alternative to Darrach resection, the Sauvé-Kapandji procedure maintains a stable radioulnar surface for carpal motion while preserving forearm rotation, and, therefore, may be advantageous in a younger, more active population. The procedure provides normal transmission of axial loads across the wrist, preserves support and function of the extensor carpi ulnaris tendon, and preservation of the normal contour and appearance of the wrist.[44] It is indicated for degenerative arthritis of the DRUJ, ulnocarpal impingement with concomitant degenerative changes in the sigmoid notch, and younger rheumatoid arthritis patients with ulnar translocation of the carpus with DRUJ involvement.[8] The most common complication, proximal ulnar stump instability, has not been reported to be a significant problem (Fig. 21–9).[18] The procedure was noted to be consistently better than Darrach resection, but it is not perfect.[17,44] The Sauvé-Kapandji procedure has also been reported as a reliable salvage procedure for intractable disorders of the DRUJ that have been previously treated with other procedures.[37]

Arthrodesis

Arthrodesis of the DRUJ has been reported for forearm stabilization in paralytic and congenital disorders as

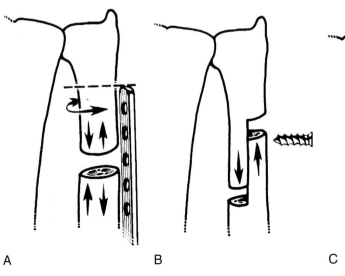

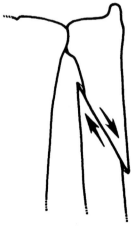

Figure 21–7. Ulnar osteotomy: transverse (**A**), step-cut (**B**), and oblique (**C**). The transverse osteotomy may be used for shortening, lengthening (with bone graft), or rotational corrections. The osteotomy should be planned so that the distal end of the plate does not impinge as the forearm rotates. Step-cut and oblique osteotomy techniques are most applicable for shortening. Compression screw or plate fixation may be used. (From Bowers WH: The distal radioulnar joint. *In* Green DP [ed]: Operative Hand Surgery, 3rd ed. New York, Churchill Livingstone, 1993, p 973.)

A   B   C

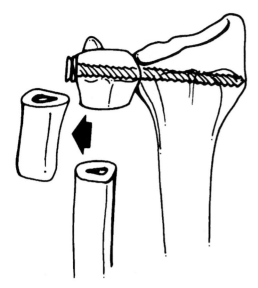

Figure 21–8. The Sauvé-Kapandji procedure involves a distal radioulnar arthrodesis and creation of a pseudarthrosis in the distal ulna. (From Sanders RA, Frederick HA, Hontas RB: The Sauvé-Kapandji procedure: A salvage operation for the distal radioulnar joint. J Hand Surg 16A:1125, 1991.)

well as for the treatment of bone loss as the result of trauma, infection, or tumor. In the setting of disorders of the DRUJ, arthrodesis is indicated as a salvage procedure when other motion-sparing options either have failed or are not possible.

REPLACEMENT ARTHROPLASTY

Replacement arthroplasty of the DRUJ is primarily used after previous failed distal ulna resection but has been used also in acute trauma and with wrist fusion to reconstruct the rheumatoid wrist. New anatomic design implants from both the United States and Germany have demonstrated reasonable results with distal ulna replacement with more than 3 years of follow-up.[46] Soft

tissue stabilization is an important component of any procedure that requires distal ulna replacement.

Implant Design

Two prosthetic design concepts have been developed to provide prosthetic replacement of the head of the distal ulna. They involve a ceramic head for the distal ulna and a titanium ingrown proximal stem (Martin-Herbert design) (Fig. 21–10) and a metal cobalt-chrome alloy ulnar head with soft tissue attachments (TFCC and ECU subsheath) (Fig. 21–11**A, B**) with a titanium ingrowth stem (Avanta Orthopedics). The implants are hemiarthroplasties and, as such, must align well with the sigmoid fossa of the distal radius. If an intact lesser sigmoid notch is not present or severely arthritic, distal ulnar replacement is contraindicated. Constrained implants for the DRUJ have been designed on a custom use basis only and have limited clinical experience. They have not been released within the United States by the Food and Drug Administration for clinical use.

Distal Ulnar Endoprosthetic Replacement

Silicone Ulna Prosthesis

In 1973, Swanson described the use of a silicone cap on the distal ulna after ulnar head resection (Fig. 21-10).[41] Subsequent concerns over implant fracture, displacement, and bone resorption secondary to silicone synovitis have limited its continued use.[27]

Martin-Herbert Distal Ulna Prosthesis

Herbert and co-workers in Germany developed a modular endoprosthetic replacement employing a metal stem and a ceramic cap (Fig. 21–10**A, B**). Their early results are

Figure 21–9. Radiographic and artistic illustration of the ulnar radial abutment: (1) a shortened ulna proximal to the sigmoid notch; (2) scalloping of the radius; and (3) radioulnar convergence. Proximal ulna stump impingement after distal ulna resection (1) occurs against the radius. Over time a groove (2) develops on the ulnar side of the radius as convergence (3) occurs between the radius and ulna. (From Bell MJ, Hill RJ, McMurtry RY: Ulnar impingement syndrome. J Bone Joint Surg 67B:126, 1985.)

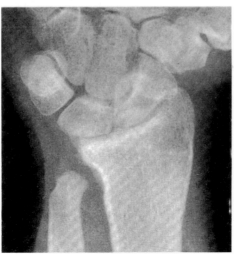
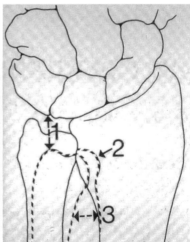

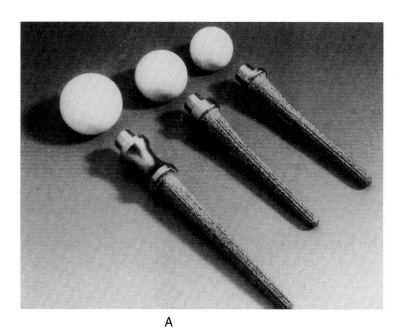

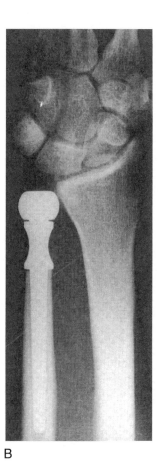

A   B

Figure 21–10. A, Ceramic modular ulna head replacement. **B,** Example of Herbert endoprosthesis implant with extended collar to replace the distal ulna.

reported in the literature and show great promise for this prosthesis.[46] With 23 patients with painful instability, they reported good results in 22 patients with 27 months of follow-up. The 1 failure was related to a low-grade infection. There were no cases of loosening, several instances of bone resorption at the bone prosthesis neck junction, and reactive bone at the sigmoid notch. These preliminary data suggest that this procedure has provided effective management for trauma and failed prior reconstructive efforts.

Technique. A dorsal incision is incorporated over the distal ulna. An ulnar-based capsular and retinacular flap is elevated, which includes the extensor carpi ulnaris and the ECU subsheath. The triangular fibrocartilage is preserved if at all possible at the time of the resection of the ulnar head so that a cuff of soft tissue is present that includes the TFCC, ECU subsheath, and dorsal-volar DRUJ capsule. If necessary, the sigmoid fossa is prepared to provide adequate seating for the ceramic ulnar head.

After proper preparation and insertion, the orientation may be assessed by intraoperative radiographs. The soft tissue closure of the preserved capsule is carefully performed to impart stability to the device and prevent subluxation during forearm rotation.

U-Head (Ulna) Prosthesis

Interest in the distal radioulnar joint has long existed at the Mayo Clinic as reflected by Linscheid's design of a custom implant for total joint replacement (see later).[26] More recently, an anatomic design based on cross-sectional CT of the wrist and cadaveric axial anatomy was designed by the Mayo wrist group for replacement of the distal ulna. This prosthesis, called "the U-Head" (Avanta Orthopaedic Inc., San Diego, CA), provides for replacement of the distal ulna with both standard and extended collar designs that allow primary and reconstruction replacement after previous DRUJ arthroplasties (Fig. 21–11). The essential feature of this modular endoprosthetic replacement is a series of variably sized titanium stems with a Morse taper to receive three cobalt-chrome head sizes. The elements are mutually interchangeable, allowing significant flexibility (Fig. 21–12). An important feature of the design is that it incorporates sutures to allow stabilization of the triangular cartilage and the extensor carpi ulnaris to help ensure stability of the implant. Importantly, significant basic science studies of the implant in a wrist simulator have demonstrated its ability to duplicate the normal kinematics of the distal radioulnar joint. In addition, these cadaver studies

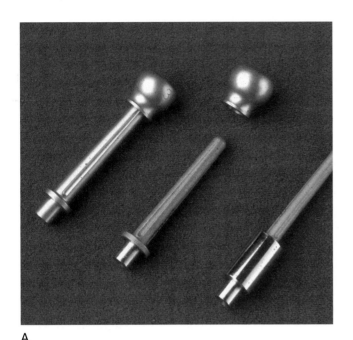

A

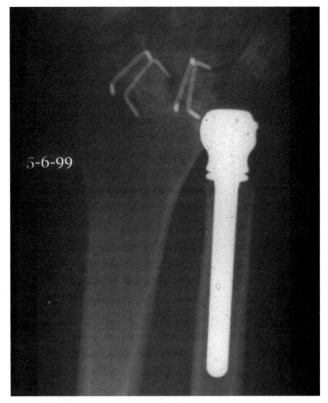

B

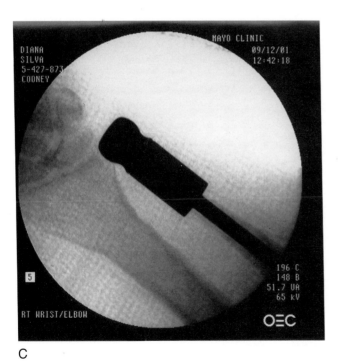

C

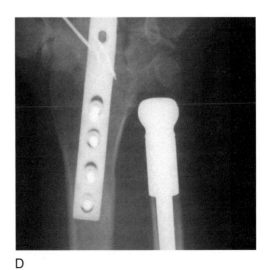

D

Figure 21-11. Avanta U-head prosthesis. **A,** Head at top and stem at the bottom. Shown are two sizes of the ulnar head (to the left), and extended collar (to the right). **B,** Clinical case of ulna head (U-head implant) associated with a partial wrist fusion. **C,** Clinical case of a failed Darrach resection with an extended collar and head prosthesis. **D,** Clinical case of ulna-radial impingement associated with a wrist fusion treated by an extended collar U-head.

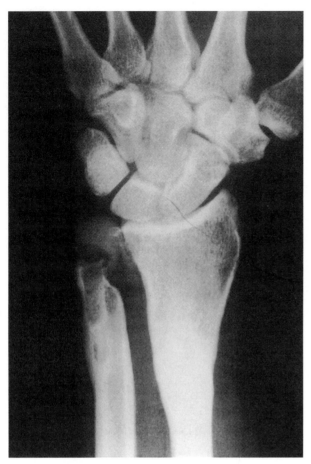

Figure 21–12. Swanson silicone implant.

with simulated active and passive loads have revealed close to normal transmission of forces across the radial ulnar joint, demonstrating enhanced stability of the DRUJ.

Technique (Fig. 21–13). The operative technique involves a dorsal or ulnar incision over the distal radioulnar joint. The extensor retinaculum is elevated ulnarly to the ECU subsheath so that a cuff of tissue including the ECU subsheath and the dorsal capsule of the DRUJ can be reflected as a unit. If the distal ulna is present, the TFC attachment is released at the base of the ulnar styloid or the ulnar styloid preserved and detached from the distal ulna. Using an alignment guide and measurement jig, the appropriate length of resection of the distal ulna is determined. If there is a previous Darrach resection (or other resection arthroplasty), the resection guide is used to determine the site of osteotomy of the distal ulna to match the extended collar U-head implant.

The distal ulna, after correct length and resection have been determined, is broached with anatomically designed instruments that match the circumference and length of the proximal stem component. Once the distal ulna is broached, a trial stem is inserted with the ulna head to determine whether proper articulation with the sigmoid fossa of the distal radius has occurred. If the length is correct, the proximal stem is inserted firmly into the medullary canal of the ulna and, once seated, the ulnar head is placed over the Morris taper and secured in place.

Soft tissues of the TFC and ECU subsheath are then attached to the head of the ulna through the holes provided. It is important that the holes face ulnarly in line with the posterior aspect of the olecranon process. A nonabsorbing heavy polyethylene suture is used for the soft tissue repair. The capsule is then imbricated

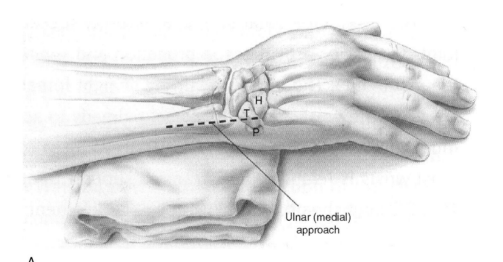

A

Figure 21–13. Surgical technique for insertion of a U-head implant. **A,** Dorsal ulnar incision outline on the right upper-extremity.

Illustration continued on opposite page

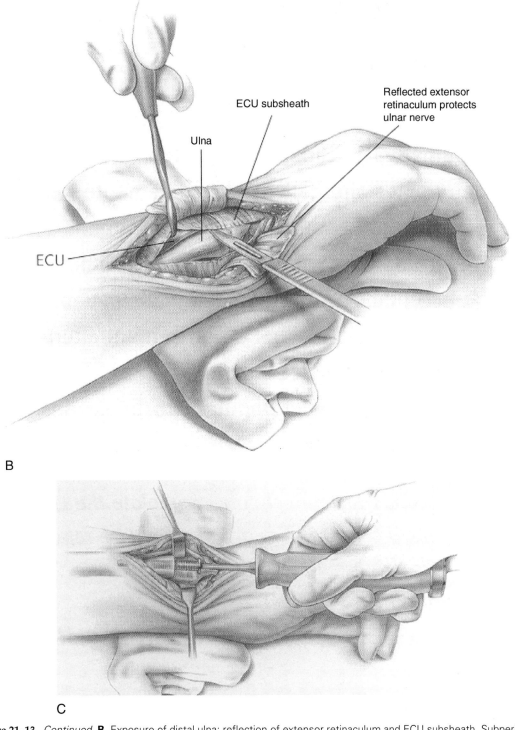

B

C

Figure 21–13. *Continued.* **B**, Exposure of distal ulna; reflection of extensor retinaculum and ECU subsheath. Subperiostial exposure of the ulna. **C**, After resecting of the distal ulna, the inframedullary coval is breached to fit one of three sizes of the prosthetic stems.

Illustration continued on following page

ulnarly with a Krackow-type suture. Stability of the implant within the DRUJ can be tested at this time.

Immobilization in a long-arm cast for 4 to 6 weeks is recommended to allow soft tissues to heal and to prevent instability. The length of immobilization is based on operative assessment of stability and the underlying diagnosis.[2]

Total Joint Replacement

To address the overarching issue of stability and impingement, efforts have been taken to replace both the radial and the ulnar elements of the joint. Kapandji used a screw and plate fixation for both proximal and

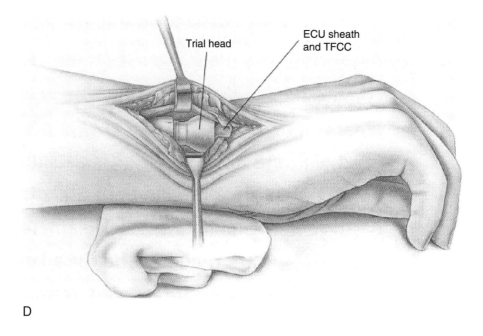

D

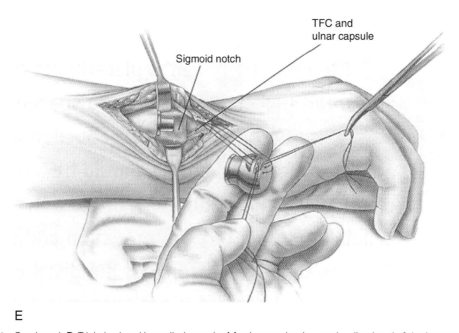

E

Figure 21–13. *Continued.* **D**, Trial ulna head is applied over the Morris taper busing on the distal end of the intramedullary ulna stem. **E**, The soft tissues (TFC and ECU subsheath) are attached to the permanent ulna head with nonresorbable 3-0 sutures.

Illustration continued on opposite page

distal components, incorporating a polyethylene-on-metal articular surface (Fig. 21–15). This design underscores the complexity of both the DRUJ. Linscheid developed a custom implant and inserted this in 3 patients (Fig. 21–16). There has been no reported long-term experience with either of these implants, and a review of 2 of the Linscheid implants demonstrated loosening in one and fracture of the ulnar stem in another.

Scheker Implant (Fig. 21–17). A third custom implant, which consists of a captured ulnar head and a fixed sigmoid notch radial component, has been designed by Scheker from Louisville, KY.[39] It is a true total joint replacement that is used in symptomatic patients with absent DRUJ, either from prior surgical procedure or from trauma. The implant is made of stainless steel with an ultra-high-molecular-weight polyethylene articulation. There are three sizes to facilitate the

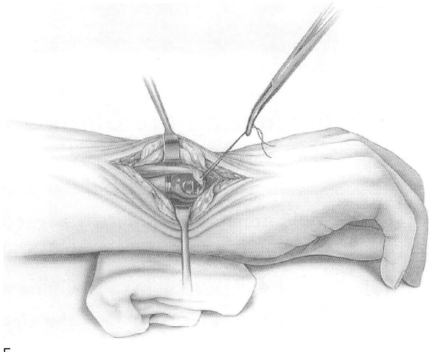

F

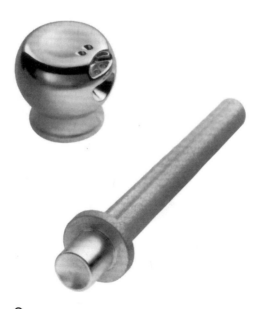

G

Figure 21-13. *Continued.* **F**, The ulnar head (U-head) is articulated onto the Morris taper brushing and the sutures attached to the ulnar head are tightened into place. **G**, The Avanta U-head prosthesis is designed for bone ingrowth to the titanium ulnar stem and the ulnar head is an endoprosthesis which articulates with the sigmoid form of the distal radius.

major purpose of improving strength of lifting. There have been no reports of prosthesis loosening, fracture, or joint wear to date.

Technique. An incision from the dorsal ulnar aspect of the distal forearm is extended radially to the ECU tendon. The ulna is approached between the ECU and the exten-

sor digiti quinti minimi. The ulna is immobilized and freed of surrounding tissues. The intraosseous membrane is released if it is extensively scarred, tight, or contracted, and the distal aspect of the ulna is resected to a level of healthy bone. The sigmoid notch is next identified, and the distal 7 cm of the distal radius from the sigmoid notch proximally is exposed to allow application of the template

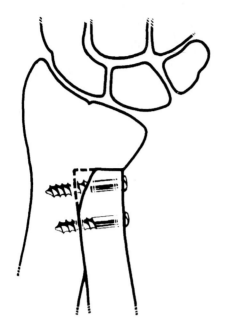

Figure 21–14. Distal radioulnar arthrodesis as described by Schneider and Imbriglia. (From Bowers WH: The distal radioulnar joint. *In* Green DP [ed]: Operative Hand Surgery, 3rd ed. New York, Churchill Livingstone, 1993, p 973.)

and the plate. Proper positioning of the distal aspect of the radial element is carefully assessed, and the plate is applied. The ulna is prepared to allow insertion of a stem down the medullary canal. A ball-and-socket mechanism allows a coupled articulation of the ulnar stem with the radial plate. The tissue is closed and the arm is placed in a splint for approximately 3 weeks.

Results

Silastic Implant. In a word, the Silastic endoprosthetic replacement of the distal ulna has been unreliable. Frequent mechanical failure of the implant from fracture or instability is well recognized as well as a synovitis generally associated with particulate debris from the rupture of the implant. Osseous resorption has also been described. Stanley and Herbert[20] assessed an experience with 20 Swanson Silastic implants for traumatic conditions and reported that 70 percent had acceptable clinical results; however, bone resorption was demonstrated in all cases. The implant was tilted or otherwise unstable in 40 percent of cases, and a frank implant failure occurred in 15 percent (1992). Similarly, Sagerman et al. reviewed 42 patients and noted some form of migration

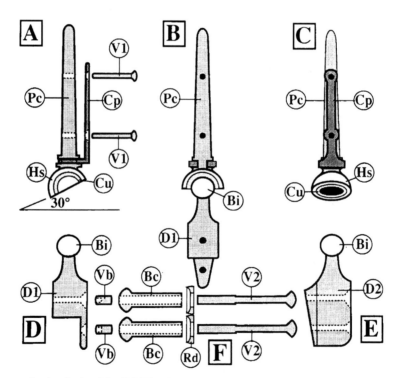

Figure 21–15. Custom distal radioulnar joint (DRUJ) arthroplasty prostheses as described by Kapandji. The DRUJ prosthesis with its two variants: on the left side, type A; on the right side, type B. **A,** Proximal part, front view (Pc, ulnar intramedullary pin; Cp, counterplate with two holes corresponding to two other threaded holes into the pin; V1, two screws, for the fixation of the proximal part, also including the two bony walls; Hs, hemispheric cup, fixed on the pin, with 30-degree tilt included; Cu, coating of the cup with HD polyethylene). **B,** Proximal part, side view (same captions, plus D1, distal part of the type A prosthesis, with a neck bearing a Bi: Ball, on metal sphere articulated with the cup. **C,** Proximal part, medial view, showing the indented form of the counterplate that bears, at its lower end, a 90-degree fork, well seen on **A** and **B. D,** Distal part of the type A prosthesis: This piece, D1, has a flap at its inferior and medial side. **E,** Distal part of the type B prosthesis: The left side of this distal piece, D2, is stronger and fits directly over the radius. **F,** The cylindrical nuts: The screws, V2, threaded only at their distal end, pass through the piece, D1 or D2, and the radius, and then are screwed inside the cylindrical nut, Bc, with a washer, Rd, on the radius wall. The counterscrew, or blocking screw, Vb, is screwed inside the cylindrical nut to avoid the unscrewing of V2. (From Kapandji AI: Prothàese radio-cubitale inféerieure. Ann Chir Main 11:320, 1992.)

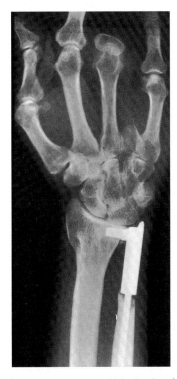

Figure 21–16. Custom constrained total joint implant for the distal ulna. (RL Linschied, MD, implant designer.)

or fracture of the implant in 63 percent.[36] They were not able to correlate the outcome with these changes; however, 1 patient did have histologically confirmed synovitis. In a comparative study of 18 patients with rheumatoid arthritis, no advantage was observed in those undergoing implant replacement with the Silastic implant compared with those in whom no implant was inserted at the time of resection.[49] Hence, we have little doubt that the Silastic implant offers no substantive advantage either in the rheumatoid or the traumatic condition to further justify its use.

Martin-Herbert implant. The single experience with this device is that provided by its designers. As mentioned earlier, the progress of 23 of the patients with this ceramic/metallic implant had been reported, with a limited follow-up averaging only 27 months.[46] The implant has not been approved for use in the United States except on a custom basis. Bowers reported result showing good experience with this implant, with the exception of patients who had had prior wrist fusion. New bone formation inferior to the sigmoid fossa has been noted related to the ceramic head articulation on cartilage and bone. It is too soon to tell whether this is a positive feature of the ceramic head. Further clinical experience is justified.

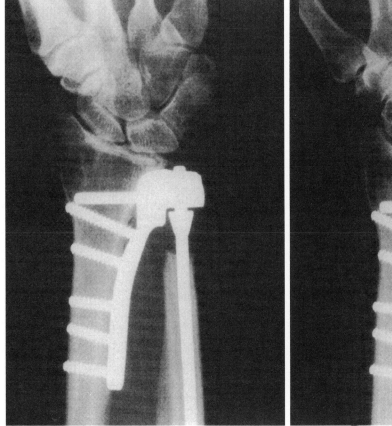
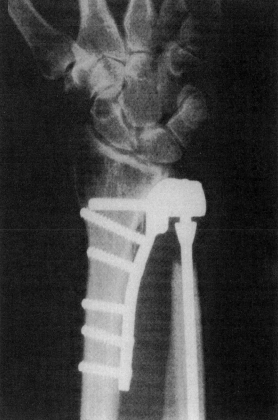

Figure 21-17. Custom constrained total joint implant for the distal ulna. (L Scheker, MD, designer.) Both custom implants are used on a limited basis with IRB institutional approval and are not commercially available.

U-Head implant. There are no reports in the literature regarding this device. There have been 22 U-head implants inserted at the Mayo Clinic and an additional 50 plus implants at selected hand centers in the United States and Europe. The results, in our experience, have been good to excellent. There have been 2 revisions in the Mayo series. One was for prosthetic loosening in a patient with osteoporosis. A second, larger stem was inserted with bone cement. A second patient had instability of the implant, and revision soft tissue procedures were performed. A referred patient with a failed U-head had revision with the custom Scheker inplant (Fig. 21–17). The mean follow-up of these implants is less than 2 years, however, and long-term loosening or instability remains a concern. Once again, this experience must be exposed to the test of time to enable a better understanding of its true role as a viable option for either rheumatoid or traumatic conditions or as a salvage procedure.

Shecker Total Replacement (Fig. 21–17). The designer reports 23 total DRUJ replacements for salvage of the DRUJ; all of these implants were inserted for severe instability and pain. There was at least one prior at the DRUJ in each patient. The mean surveillance once again is limited, averaging only 15 months, with the longest being 40 months. To date, the authors note that 22 of the 23 have had successful clinical outcomes, with a measurable improvement in grip and lifting strength. In addition, normal forearm pronation and supination is reported. It is noteworthy that 8 of the 13 who were out of work before the surgery have returned to some type of employment. One patient did undergo a resection for a deep infection.[39]

SUMMARY AND CONCLUSIONS

Without question, prosthetic replacement of the DRUJ is a procedure that is emerging and for which there is increased interest. The essential remaining impediment is difficulty in achieving stabilization of the implant because of the limited soft tissue in this region as well as the significant stresses placed on the articulation. The reports to date have been quite preliminary, and it would appear that there is a cautious degree of optimism. However the surveillance of outcomes is extremely limited and must be subjected to greater scrutiny over a significantly longer period of time before any of these prosthetic replacements can be offered or recommended with confidence.

References

1. Almquist EE: Evolution of the distal radioulnar joint. Clin Orthop 275:5, 1992.
2. Beiber EJ, Linscheid RL, Dobyns JH, Beckenbaugh RD: Failed distal ulna resections. J Hand Surg 13A:193, 1988.
3. Bell MJ, Hill RJ, McMurtry RY: Ulnar impingement syndrome. J Bone Joint Surg 67B:126, 1985.
4. Bilos ZJ, Chamberlain D: Distal ulnar head shortening for treatment of triangular fibrocartilage complex tears with ulna positive variance. J Hand Surg 16A:1115, 1991.
5. Blatt G, Ashworth CR: Volar capsule transfer for stabilization following resection of the distal end of the ulna. Orthop Trans 3:13, 1979.
6. Boulas HJ, Milak MA: Ulnar shortening for tears of the triangular fibrocartilaginous complex. J Hand Surg 15A:415, 1990.
7. Bowers WH: Distal radioulnar joint arthroplasty. Current concepts. Clin Orthop 275:104, 1992.
8. Bowers WH: The distal radioulnar joint. *In* Green DP (ed): Operative Hand Surgery, 3rd ed. New York, Churchill Livingstone, 1993, p 973.
9. Boyd HB, Stone MM: Resection of the distal end of the ulna. J Bone Joint Surg 26:313, 1944.
10. Breen TF, Jupiter JB: Extensor carpi ulnaris and flexor carpi ulnaris tenodesis of the unstable distal ulna. J Hand Surg 14A:612, 1989.
11. Burk DL, Karasick D, Wechsler RJ: Imaging of the distal radioulnar joint. Hand Clin 7:263, 1991.
12. Darrow JC, Linscheid RL, Dobyns JH, et al: Distal ulnar recession for disorders of the distal radioulnar joint. J Hand Surg 10A:482, 1985.
13. Dingman PV: Resection of the distal end of the ulna (Darrach operation). J Bone Joint Surg 34A:893, 1952.
14. Drobner WS, Hausman MR: The distal radioulnar joint. Hand Clin 8:631, 1992.
15. Ekenstam FA: Anatomy of the distal radioulnar joint. Clin Orthop 275:14, 1992.
16. Feldon P, Terrano AL, Belsky MR: The "wafer" procedure. Clin Orthop 275:124, 1992.
17. Goncalves D: Correction of disorders of the distal radio-ulnar joint by artificial pseudarthrosis of the ulna. J Bone Joint Surg 56B:462, 1974.
18. Gordon L, Levinsohn DG, Moore SV, et al: The Sauváe-Kapandji procedure for the treatment of posttraumatic distal radioulnar joint problems. Hand Clin 7:397, 1991.
19. Hartz CR, Beckenbaugh RD: Long-term results of resection of the distal ulna for post-traumatic conditions. J Trauma 19:219, 1979.
20. Stanley D, Herbet TJ: The Swanson ulna head prosthesis for posttraumatic disorders of the distal radio-ulna joint. J Hand Surg 17B:682–688, 1992.
21. Johnson RK, Shrewsbury MM: The pronator quadratus in motions and in stabilization of the radius and ulna at the distal radioulnar joint.
22. Kapandji AI: Prothèse radio-cubitale inféerieure. Ann Chir Main 11:320, 1992.
23. Kessler I, Hecht O: Present application of the Darrach procedure. Clin Orthop 72:254, 1970.
24. King GJ, McMurtry RY, Rubenstein JD, Gertzbein SD: Kinematics of the distal radioulnar joint. J Hand Surg 11A:798, 1986.
25. King GJ, McMurtry RY, Rubenstein JD, Ogston NG: Computerized tomography of the distal radioulnar joint: Correlation with ligamentous pathology in a cadaveric model. J Hand Surg 11A:711, 1986.
26. Linscheid RL: Ulnar lengthening and shortening. Hand Clin 3:69, 1987.
27. McMurtry RY, Paley D, Marks P, Axelrod T: A critical analysis of Swanson ulnar head replacement arthroplasty: Rheumatoid versus nonrheumatoid. J Hand Surg 15A:224, 1990.
28. Milch H: Cuff resection of the ulna for malunited Colles' fracture. J Bone Joint Surg 23:311, 1941.
29. Mino DE, Palmer AK, Levinsohn EM: The role of radiography and computerized tomography in the diagnosis of subluxation and dislocation of the distal radioulnar joint. J Hand Surg 8:23, 1983.
30. Nolan WB, Eaton RG: A Darrach procedure for distal ulnar pathology derangements. Clin Orthop 275:85, 1992.
31. Palmer AK: The triangular fibrocartilage complex of the wrist: Anatomy and function. J Hand Surg 6:153, 1981.
32. Palmer AK: The distal radioulnar joint. Orthop Clin North Am 15:321, 1984.
33. Palmer AK, Glisson RR, Werner FW: Ulnar variance determination. J Hand Surg 7:376, 1982.
34. Pirela-Cruz MA, Goll SR, Klug M, Windler D: Stress computed tomography analysis of the distal radioulnar joint: A diagnostic tool for determining translational motion. J Hand Surg 16A:75, 1991.
35. Ruby LK: Darrach procedure. *In* Gelberman RH (ed): Master Techniques in Orthopaedic Surgery: The Wrist. New York, Raven Press, 1994, p 279.

36. Sagerman SD, Seiler JG, Fleming LL, Lockerman E: Silicone rubber distal ulnar replacement arthroplasty. J Hand Surg 17B:689, 1992.

37. Sanders RA, Frederick HA, Hontas RB: The Sauvé-Kapandji procedure: A salvage operation for the distal radioulnar joint. J Hand Surg 16A:1125, 1991.

38. Sauvé K: Nouvelle technique traitement chirurical des luxations récidivantes isoléees de l'extremité inferieure du cubitus. J Chir 47:589, 1936.

39. Scheker LR, Babb BA, Killion PE: Distal ulnar prosthetic replacement. Orthop Clinics North Am 32:365, 2001.

40. Space TC, Louis DS, Francis I, Braunstein EM: CT findings in distal radioulnar dislocation. J Comput Assist Tomogr 10:689, 1986.

41. Spinner M, Kaplan EB: Extensor carpi ulnaris: Its relationship to the stability of the distal radio-ulnar joint. Clin Orthop 68:124, 1970.

42. Taleisnik J: The Wrist. New York, Churchill Livingstone, 1985.

43. Taleisnik J: Pain of the ulnar side of the wrist. Hand Clin 3:51, 1987.

44. Taleisnik J: The Sauvée-Kapandji procedure. Clin Orthop 275:110, 1992.

45. Trumble T, Glisson RR, Seaber AV, Urbaniak JR: Forearm force transmission after surgical treatment of distal radioulnar joint disorders. J Hand Surg 12A:196, 1987.

46. van Schoonhoven J, Fernandez DL, Bowers WH, Herbert TJ: Salvage of failed resection arthroplasties of the distal radioulnar joint using a new ulnar head prosthesis. J Hand Surg 25A:438, 2000.

47. Watson HK, Ryu J, Burgess RC: Matched distal ulnar resection. J Hand Surg 11A:812, 1986.

48. Webber JB, Maser SA: Stabilization of the distal ulna. Hand Clin 7:345, 1991.

49. White RE Jr: Resection of the distal ulna with and without implant arthroplasty in rheumatoid arthritis. J Hand Surg 11A:514, 1986.

22

Arthroplasty of the Wrist

· ROBERT D. BECKENBAUGH

The concept of performing fixed total joint arthroplasties of the wrist emerged quickly after the early dramatic success that was seen with total hip arthroplasty. Several designs of prostheses were developed in the early 1970s, using the same principles of plastic and metal articulation with cement fixation (Fig. 22–1) as had been used in hip arthroplasty.[29,30,50] Initial results demonstrating that pain relief and mobility were obtainable have encouraged continuous development in the field of fixed-fulcrum total joint arthroplasty of the wrist. Unlike the experience with the hip, however, the longevity of the initial good results was reduced, the number of complications was higher, and the need for reoperations was greater.[2,10,14] Because of the early failures, continued development and use of total wrist arthroplasties has been slower than in some other joints.

Other factors exist that have restricted the use of total wrist arthroplasties, including relative success with (1) limited soft tissue procedures (synovectomy and stabilization), (2) arthrodesis, and (3) silicone interposition arthroplasty.[10,11,34,39–46] All of these procedures are more conservative than total wrist replacement with a metal and plastic device because they require less bone resection, are more easily salvaged after failure, and have no inherent risk of loosening or adverse effect from a large foreign body (allergy, infection). After identifying significant problems with total wrist arthroplasty, the surgeon still must compare the increased potential benefits of total wrist arthroplasty and its complications with the benefits and complications of other, more conservative procedures.

ALTERNATIVE PROCEDURES

Synovectomy and Stabilization of the Wrist

Unlike synovectomy of many joints, the functional results in the wrist tend to be quite satisfactory and durable.[10,11,33,44] The primary indication for this procedure has been for patients who have pain with limited articular destruction and minimal deformity. Also, distal radioulnar disease that threatens the extensor tendons is an indication for synovectomy, which is often done in conjunction with repair of extensor tendon rup-

tures.[33,46] Despite the relative lack of logic for the procedure (all of the synovium cannot be removed), this operation reliably relieves pain and frequently provides functional stability.

As demonstrated by radiography, the disease process always progresses. However, in some instances, spontaneous intercarpal fusions occur, and in these instances, a painless, stable wrist is achieved. In other cases, progressive ulnar translation of the wrist occurs without much pain, but adverse mechanical effects can cause difficulties with finger function.[21,39] The procedure of radiolunate fusion has now been added to the basic procedure of synovectomy and stabilization to prevent this ulnar translation.[24,42] Although synovectomy and stabilization provide pain relief, reasonable function, and durability, the acceptable results are inferior to the best results of successful total wrist arthroplasty. Finally, failure of wrist synovectomy does typically allow subsequent wrist arthroplasty, provided the wrist extensor mechanism has been preserved.

Arthrodesis

Arthrodesis of the wrist is the most popular surgical procedure performed for wrist arthrosis at the current time.[32] In patients with rheumatoid arthritis, it is relatively easy to accomplish arthrodesis with minimal morbidity.[34,49] In patients with traumatic or degenerative arthritis, more complex techniques are used, but with modern plate fixation techniques, success rates are high.[30,34,49,52] The addition of bone graft substitutes appears to be a promising method for further simplification and decrease of techniques (Fig. 22–2A).

The advantages of wrist arthrodesis are obvious. The procedure is durable, provides pain relief, and, in many instances, is very functional.

The disadvantages of wrist arthrodesis are also obvious but often not emphasized. For example, it has been stated that arthrodesis provides more power as a result of stabilization and relief of pain, and this is correct. However, eliminating wrist motion *decreases* power grip, removing the mechanical advantage and excursion available to the finger flexors with wrist dorsiflexion. Stabilizing the wrist in a neutral fashion may help pre-

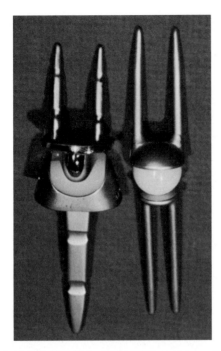

Figure 22–1. Volz *(left)* and Meuli *(right)* initial wrist prostheses. Note that both original prostheses were designed for insertion into the index and long metacarpals, and their proximal stems were structured over the prosthetic central axis.

vent ulnar deviation of the fingers secondary to radial deviation of the wrist. In contrast, eliminating the shock absorption of ulnar wrist motion increases the external ulnar deviation forces applied to the digits.

Absence of wrist motion in patients with rheumatoid arthritis can be functionally disabling. In patients with severe shoulder and elbow disease, eliminating wrist motion can make such functional tasks as eating, hair care, and personal hygiene *more* difficult. Total wrist arthroplasty has many practical and theoretical advan-

tages compared with wrist arthrodesis. In selecting a procedure for an individual patient, the potential benefits and complications and the need for reoperations must be compared to the relative ease and permanency of arthrodesis, and the patient must assist the surgeon in making the proper choice.[7] Preoperative rigid splinting of the wrist may assist the patient in making the decision for or against arthrodesis.

A functional arthrodesis is a relative contraindication to wrist arthroplasty unless it is bilateral or in a poor position. However, this can be converted to a wrist replacement provided the wrist extensors are intact.

Silicone Interposition Wrist Arthroplasty

In 1970, Swanson reported the development of a silicone rubber interposition arthroplasty similar to the design of his finger implant.[45] Conceptually, it is a true total wrist replacement in that both the radial carpal and midcarpal joint functions are replaced. The use of a pliable spacer, however, is very different mechanically and functionally from the solid metal and plastic prosthetic wrist arthroplasty device. With silicone devices, the forces across the prosthesis are dampened, greatly diminishing the chances of loosening, which is a common problem in most total wrist arthroplasties. There are potentials for prosthetic fracture, however, as well as subsidence of the prosthesis within bone.[8,13,40] In addition, with fixed fulcrum total wrist arthroplasty, restoration of wrist length is possible, whereas some shortening occurs with silicone arthroplasty. This may be associated with potential adverse effects on the extrinsic musculotendinous finger motors.

Silicone wrist arthroplasty is easily salvaged (by replacement or fusion). It has not been associated with the very high incidence of particulate synovitis seen in individual carpal implants.[36,41,43] However, continued

Figure 22–2. Special contoured wrist arthrodesis plate with bone graft. Note resorption and remodeling of bone graft in anteroposterior (**A**) and lateral projections (**B**).

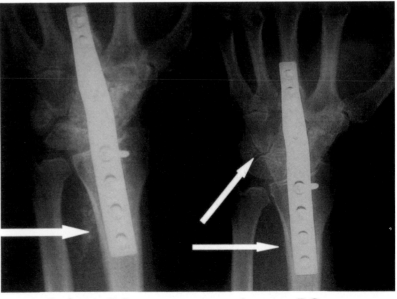

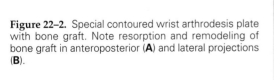

A   **2 days PO**   **1 year PO**

Illustration continued on following page

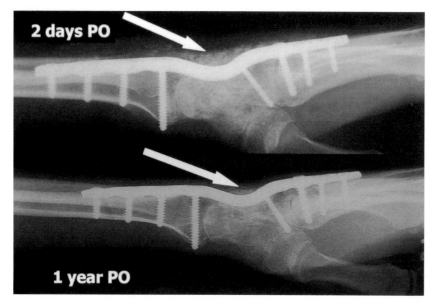

2 days PO

1 year PO

B

Figure 22–2. *Continued.*

problems with subsidence, recurrent deformity with fracture, and significant particulate synovitis in the long metacarpal have led to discontinuance of its use by most hand surgeons in the United States.[17,35,37] The decision to use the silicone implant is generally reserved for younger patients with weaker bone stock who may undergo reoperation in the future. The use of metal grommets and stronger silicone does not significantly improve the results of interposition arthroplasty (Fig. 22–3).[5]

INDICATIONS AND CONTRAINDICATIONS

The basic indication for total wrist arthroplasty is in patients with rheumatoid arthritis whose multiple upper extremity joints are involved and who have a distinct need for motion. In addition, to warrant this procedure, the patient should have pain or significant deformity. Patients with degenerative and post-traumatic arthritis of the wrist frequently have unilateral occurrence, which is most often associated with normal function of the shoulder, elbow, and hand; the more conservative approaches are generally indicated in these patients.

If there are special needs or desires for motion in these candidates, total wrist arthroplasty may be indicated. Patients in this category must be strongly advised of the limited use that is allowed postoperatively. For example, a patient may feel good enough and function well enough after total wrist arthroplasty with isolated wrist disease that he would wish to participate in sports such as golf or tennis or perform heavy labor such as carpentry. The devices and fixations available do not, however, allow these heavy impact activities without anticipated failure by loosening. A musician, however, with special needs for motion, anticipated light activities, and isolated wrist disease may be an excellent candidate for the procedure.

The paradox of treatment is that, in patients with traumatic and degenerative conditions, the bone stock and quality are better than in those with rheumatoid arthritis,

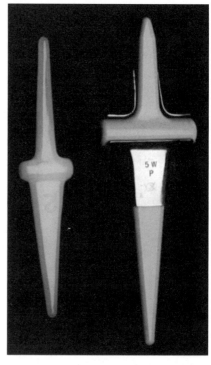

Figure 22–3. An early Swanson silicone wrist replacement *(left)*. A newer silicone device *(right)*. Note that the distal stem is shorter. The hub of the prosthesis is wider and broader, and the prosthetic surfaces are protected by a volar distal grommet and a proximal dorsal grommet. The prosthetic surface is from the bony image. Rectangular grommets are now used.

and the potential results and longevity are theoretically superior. The quality of bone in patients with rheumatoid arthritis is variable. In general, the disease results in decreased bone density and strength. The addition of steroid therapy or some of the newer immunologically oriented drugs may significantly weaken the bone. New distal component stem designs have been developed for use in these bone-deficient patients (Fig. 22–4). If marked osteoporosis is present (medullary canals with soft, fatty

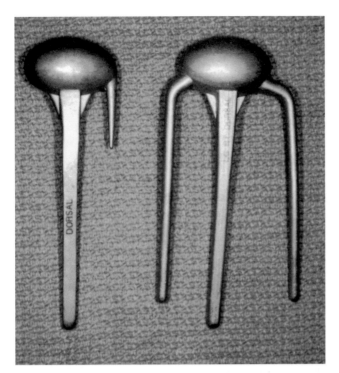

Figure 22–4. There are long-stemmed and triple-stemmed radial components (trial components) for use in bone-deficient and revision arthroplasty.

morrow), the procedure of total wrist arthroplasty may be relatively contraindicated.

A past history of sepsis is also a relative contraindication to total wrist arthroplasty. However, aggressive débridement and antibiotic therapy may allow consideration of the procedure in certain instances.

Absence of active radial wrist extensors is a contraindication to total wrist arthroplasty. This condition is actually rare, even in rheumatoid arthritis, but should be suspected if the wrist has a significant flexion deformity (not subluxation) preoperatively. If the radial wrist extensors cannot be repaired surgically, the procedure must be abandoned. Absence of the extensor carpi ulnaris (primarily an ulnar deviator of the wrist) is not a contraindication to total wrist arthroplasty, and, likewise, its presence is not sufficient to substitute for absent radial wrist extensors.

Excessive bone loss is not a contraindication to total wrist arthroplasty, and the procedure can be performed by direct distal implantation in the metacarpals. Retention of some portion of the distal carpal row improves fixation. Previous wrist procedures, including resection of the distal ulna or synovectomy, do not have adverse effects on wrist arthroplasty unless certain specific techniques have been used. If the extensor retinaculum has been placed volar to the extensor tendons in previous wrist reconstruction, some additional reconstruction is required to avoid tendon subluxation as motion is restored to the wrist. Deficiency of the extensor retinaculum can allow volar subluxation of the wrist extensors radially or of the digital extensors ulnarly, and this leads to deformity; therefore, the extensor retinaculum—or a

part of it—must be present or reconstructed for total wrist arthroplasty to be successful.

Previous wrist arthrodesis does not preclude total wrist arthroplasty, provided the wrist extensors are intact. The primary indication for taking down a wrist arthrodesis is to improve function in a patient who has not benefited by the arthrodesis but who has developed a need for motion as a result of increasing shoulder, elbow, or digit disease. An example is that of a patient with bilateral wrist fusions who can no longer care for his perineum because of absence of wrist flexion.

DESIGN DEVELOPMENT OF TOTAL WRIST ARTHROPLASTY

Fixed-fulcrum arthroplasties became available in the United States in the early 1970s. The majority of devices implanted were the designs created by Meuli or Volz (Fig. 22–1).[30,50]

The Meuli prosthesis is a ball-and-socket trunnion design with two malleable stems made of Protasul. The design allowed a range of motion in excess of normal and theoretically had minimal internal constraints. It was, however, difficult to balance wrist motion because the intrinsic center of motion of the prosthesis was not the same as that of the wrist.[23,53–55] As a result, the device allowed the wrist to develop an ulnar deviation deformity.[2] The prosthetic distal component was soon modified in several ways to correct this problem, with some success.[3,4,23] The major long-term problem with the ball-and-socket design has been loosening of the distal component.[14,25] This loosening occurs because in the functional mode the device is very constrained (i.e., pushing up from a chair or pushing open a door with the wrist in a fixed position transmits all forces to the distal component, resulting in loosening of the prosthesis).

The Volz design is minimally constrained, with a curved, anteroposteriorly grooved flexion-extension track (see Fig. 22–1). The device functions nicely but has a small contact point, which increases the radioulnar "teeter-totter" effect and, therefore, has also been causes problems of balance. Like Meuli, Volz redesigned the distal component to better balance the wrist, but the problem was not completely solved. The Volz design, because of its semiconstrained feature, has been associated with an acceptable rate of loosening and longevity. However, because of persistent balance problems the implant is not used today (R. Volz, personal communication).[6,16,26,51]

Both the Volz and Meuli devices were used cement fixation, as was suggested in the 1970s. The early clinical results were very encouraging, with pain relief, preservation of motion, and improved function. During this period, several other types of devices were developed. These various devices had limited success and were never extensively used. The concept of total wrist arthroplasty, however, was successful, and, in the 1980s, a second generation of prostheses was developed.

Five different varieties of new prosthetic designs were introduced: Clayton-Ferlic-Volz (CFV), Guepar,

Menon[27,28] (Fig. 22–5), Meuli[31] (Fig. 22–6) and Biaxial design (Fig. 22–7). These devices were designed to decrease the need for cement fixation, improve balance, and approach more normal wrist mechanics.[31] The Guepar device is no longer available secondary to abandonment by the manufacturer (Yves Alnot, May 2001, personal communication). The CFV wrist prosthesis has been abandoned secondary to instability and deformity associated with its distal point of articulation (Don Ferlic, M.D., May 1997, personal communication). The new Meuli prosthesis and the Menon prosthesis (now called the universal wrist prostheses) both make use of the concept of primary fixation of the implant in the carpal bones as opposed to metacarpal intramedullary stem fixation. Both device techniques now recommend formal carpal fusion with preservation of the distal carpal row. Fixation is achieved without cement through porous surfaced metal with the Meuli device and with screw fixation of a modular distal component in the universal wrist prosthesis (central screw replaced with cemented peg to satisfy United States Food and Drug Administration requirements). The biaxial technique has similarly been modified by Van Leeuwen to resect minimal carpal bones and achieve uncemented fixation in the carpal bones with the carpometacarpal joint of the long finger being the distal point of fixation.[48]

SURGICAL TECHNIQUE

The surgical technique for total wrist arthroplasty is basically the same regardless of the device used. Individual variations in techniques are limited to specific design parameters. The technique for biaxial wrist arthroplasty is described.

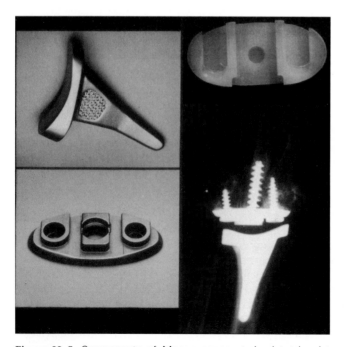

Figure 22–5. Components of Menon nonconstrained total wrist replacement.

Radiographic templates with 6 percent magnification are used to determine the appropriate prosthetic size (small, medium, or large [standard]). In general, the largest prosthesis possible should be used. The templates are also useful in estimating the amount of bone to be resected.

The incision is made straight longitudinally and centered over the dorsum of the wrist (Fig. 22–8**A**). A curved or angled incision is not necessary and may result in necrosis of skin edges. The skin and subcutaneous flaps are sharply elevated from the underlying extensor retinaculum. A longitudinal incision is made through the midportion of the fourth dorsal compartment (see Fig. 22–8**A**). With the scissors, the compartment of the extensor pollicis longus is opened ulnarly and the tendon retracted as the retinaculum is sharply incised radially to unroof the second dorsal compartment. Dissection is then carried further radially in a *subperiosteal* manner to expose the tendons of the first dorsal compartment in their course adjacent to the radial styloid. It is very important that these tendons be seen and carefully protected during the bony resection of the distal radius; otherwise, the saw may easily damage them. An extensor tenosynovectomy is then performed as appropriate.

Dissection is carried ulnarly to the fifth dorsal compartment, which is, however, not opened unless it is necessary to perform synovectomy. The common digital extensors are now retracted radially and an incision is made in the distal radioulnar joint capsule. A 1- to 2-mm rim of capsule is preserved on the radius and later used for repair. The capsule is then subperiosteally dissected ulnarly, leaving the fifth and sixth dorsal compartments intact and exposing the distal ulna. The ulna is resected with the sagittal saw just proximal to the sigmoid notch of the radius (see Fig. 22–8**B**). The distal ulna is *almost always* resected in total wrist arthroplasty to prevent abutment against the ulnar portion of the radial component. Failure to remove the distal ulna produces a bony prominence secondary to slight radial displacement of the hand, unless an undersized component is used.

A T-shaped incision is made in the dorsal wrist capsule, based transversely across the radial carpal joint, and extended longitudinally in the axis of the third metacarpal (see Fig. 22–8**C**). The capsule is then sharply dissected distally into two triangular flaps to the base of the metacarpals. Some of the synovium may be left during this portion of the procedure, because this tissue is used to cover the prosthesis during closure.

The distal end of the radius is then exposed subperiosteally. The radius is resected by means of a power sagittal saw into a plane perpendicular to its long axis. The amount of bone removed varies in accordance with the tension needed, but the initial cut should be the minimal width to allow a perpendicular distal surface of the radius and is generally at the level of the middle of the sigmoid notch (see Fig. 22–8**D**). The sagittal saw is then used to prepare a slightly concave (apex distal) resection of the carpus through the distal carpal row. In general, a 2.5-cm-wide space should be left for the prosthesis, and the volar capsule should be preserved if

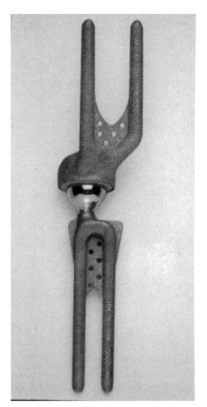

Figure 22–6. A, New Meuli prosthesis designed for use without cement fixation. **B**, Anteroposterior radiograph of properly balanced Meuli third-generation device.

A

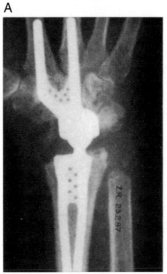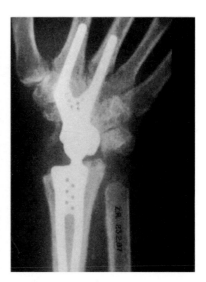

B

possible (not mandatory). After making the radial and carpal saw cuts, it is easy to remove the distal radius by sharp dissection from the adjacent soft tissues. Then, by flexing the wrist, the deformed carpal bones can be easily removed from the volar capsule or radius with a knife or rongeur.

Attention is turned to the preparation of the medullary canals for the prosthetic stems. A 1-cm longitudinal incision is made along the dorsal periosteum of the third metacarpal. The periosteum is elevated just distal to the metaphyseal plane to allow two Hohmann retractors to be placed. This maneuver aids immensely in the accurate identification and preparation of the medullary canal of the third metacarpal (see Fig. 22–8E).

Alternatively, the retractors may be bluntly passed beneath the interosseus and external to the periosteum. The wrist is flexed and, with use of a small, sharp awl, a canal is developed from the midportion of the neck of the capitate through to the third metacarpal medullary canal. A blunt awl is then passed down the canal until it strikes the distal firm end of the metacarpal head. The depth is noted with a finger and the awl is withdrawn. The length to the metacarpal head endpoint can then be checked along the dorsal metacarpal shaft to confirm the intramedullary position of the awl. Failure to reach an endpoint indicates that there may have been perforation of the metacarpal shaft. Once identified, the medullary canal is gradually expanded with awls,

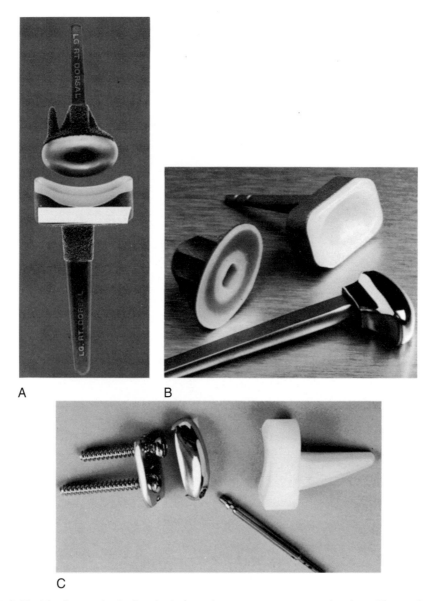

A

B

C

Figure 22–7. A, Biaxial wrist prosthesis. Prosthetic stems have some porous coated surfaces. The proximal articulating surface is offset ulnarly and palmarly, and the distal surface is designed for insertion of the third metacarpal with a stud into the trapezoid. **B**, Clayton-Ferlic-Volz prosthesis that uses variable sizes of shims on the proximal component, which has an ellipsoidal component and a distal concave, metal-backed polyethylene component. **C**, The Guepar wrist prosthesis. The distal component is ellipsoidal and metallic and is inserted on the index and long metacarpals with screws. The proximal polyethylene component is offset similar to the biaxial design and is a polyethylene non-metal-backed component.

presized reamers, and power burs to accept the stem of the prosthesis (see Fig. 22–8F). Using an awl, a separate hole is placed in the trapezoid or index metacarpal for the small prosthetic base stud. Medial and lateral burring is performed with the side-cutting power reamers to accept the wings of the prosthetic base, and careful adjustment allows a snug fit. Care is taken to orient the distal component in a plane parallel to the plane of the hand, avoiding any rotation. The distal trial component is then inserted and, if seating is satisfactory, attention is turned to the radial medullary canal. Further work on the distal bones is not necessary after the trial prosthesis is fitted except for the trapezoidal stud. Here, the canal must be enlarged 1 mm in diameter to accept the increased dimension of the porous coated stem. Some expansion

reaming may be necessary at the base of the long carpometacarpal subarticular cortices. The medullary canal bone is lightly cleared with side-cutting Swanson reamers and curettes to enhance cement fixation.

The trial prosthesis is removed and attention is turned to the proximal radius. A channel is prepared with an awl, starting at the midportion of the medullary canal of the radius. The radial reamers are then inserted, with a mallet to impact the medullary bone but not to remove it. It is easiest to start with the small reamer and progressively enlarge to the proper size. The reamer is placed to make the transverse plane parallel to the transverse plane of the radius. The reamer normally centers itself as it is driven proximally into the medullary canal unless the canal is exceptionally large (see Fig. 22–8G).

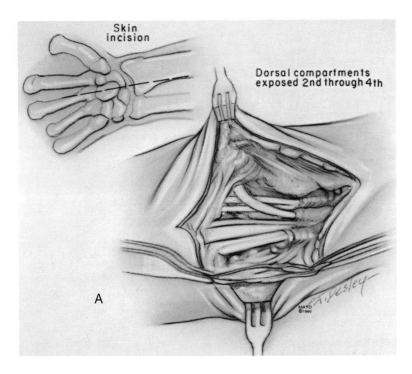

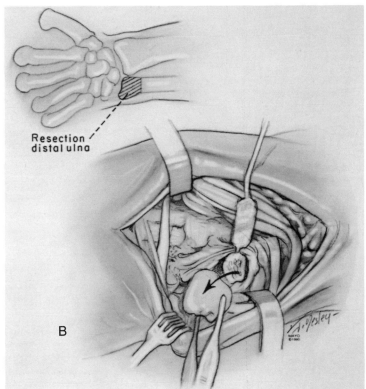

Figure 22–8. **A**, The tendons of the second through the fourth compartments are exposed through a longitudinal incision in the dorsal retinaculum. **B**, After subperiosteal exposure, enough distal ulna is resected to be just proximal to the level of the sigmoid notch or the level of the transverse excision of the radius.

Illustration continued on following page

The proximal trial component is inserted and the end of the radius is trimmed to allow a flat, surface-to-surface, contact fit. The distal trial prosthesis is then inserted and the wrist is put through a range of passive motion and tested for tension. The trial prosthesis is slightly looser than the real prosthesis, which has a 1-mm porous surface and a slightly thicker polyethylene bearing. Ideal or moderate tension is such that the

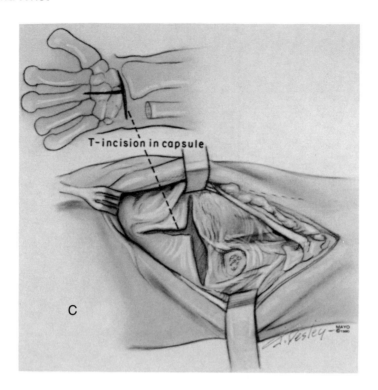

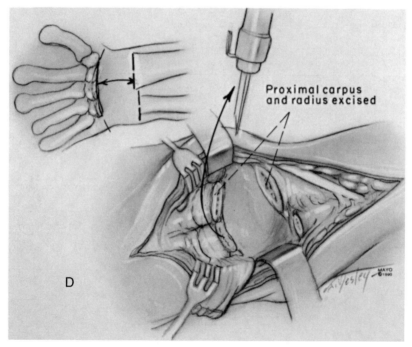

Figure 22–8. *Continued.* **C**, The T-shaped capsular incision is elevated distally by sharp dissection, preserving the synovium as necessary for later closure over the prosthesis. **D**, Enough of the carpus is sharply excised to allow the proper space for the prosthesis. It is desirable to leave the distal half of the distal carpal row intact if this bone stock is present.

Illustration continued on opposite page

prosthesis can distracted approximately 1 mm after reduction. Tight tension is present if seating (location) of the joint is just barely possible and no distraction is present (see Fig. 22–8H). The fit is considered loose if the distal component can be distracted beyond the distal

margins of the polyethylene on the sides of the proximal component. If the fit is too tight, more bone can be resected from the radius. If it is loose, increased attention is paid to capsular reconstruction, with longer periods of immobilization. It is not advisable to increase the

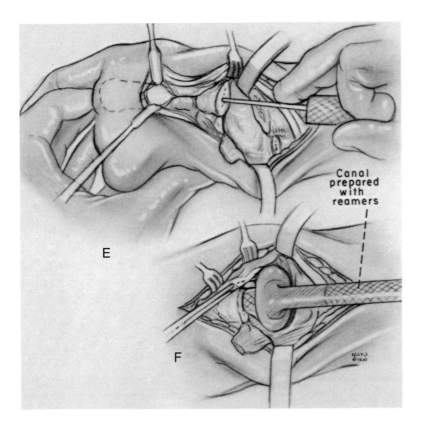

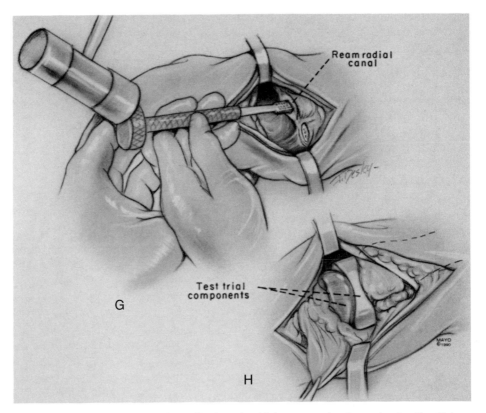

Figure 22–8. *Continued.* **E,** Extending the incision periosteally along the third metacarpal and exposing it with a Hohmann retractor greatly increases ease of identification and preparation of the canal of the third metacarpal. **F,** The impactor can be used to develop the proper shape for seating of the distal component, but, usually, some bone removal with a rongeur and power burr is also necessary. **G,** The proximal medullary canal bone is impacted rather than removed to increase the potential for fixation without cement. **H,** The hand is distracted to identify the amount of tension in the wrist. It should not be possible to distract the distal component beyond the polyethylene edge of the proximal component.

Illustration continued on following page

tension by incompletely seating the components. At this point, a survey radiograph may be taken to assess the correct position and alignment of the components.

A decision is then made as to whether methyl methacrylate cement should be used to supplement the fixation. In all situations except those involving previous medullary canal implants or excessive osteoporosis, the proximal component does not require cement, and cement is not desirable because of excessive stress shielding and resorption of the distal radius. The distal component is nearly always cemented. In patients with good bone stock and hardness, this may not be necessary.

The methyl methacrylate cement is mixed in a standard fashion (half a batch is enough). The cement may be mixed with 1 cc of methylene blue to assist in identification of any later revision. At 3 to 4 minutes, it is placed in a 12-ml plastic syringe, the tip of which has been widened by either an awl or a straight hemostat. A metallic syringe holder (available from a standard glass syringe) is necessary to provide adequate pressure to fill the medullary canal with cement (see Fig. 22–8I). Before injection of the cement in a liquid state, a small amount of cancellous bone is impacted distally in the medullary canal of the third metacarpal to act as a plug. Reinsertion of the metacarpal broach or trial component is necessary to ensure easy passage of the radial stem after the plug is built. Two to four milliliters of cement are injected distally, and the prosthesis is impacted (see Fig. 22–8J). Excess cement is trimmed

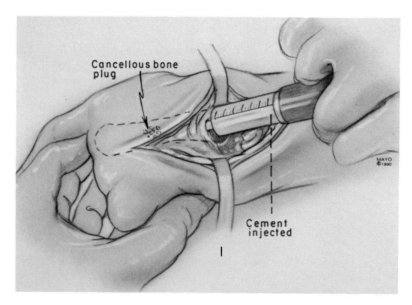

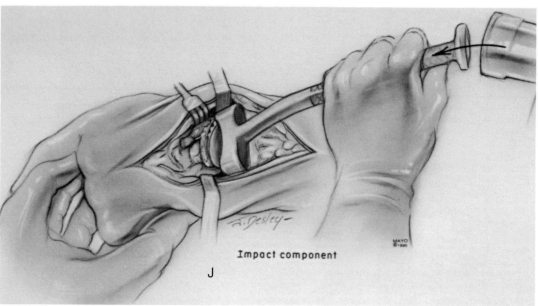

Figure 22–8. *Continued.* **I**, Cancellous bone may be used as a plug in the midportion of the metacarpal. The cement is injected in a semiliquid state under pressure. **J**, The distal component is firmly impacted and excess cement removed.

Illustration continued on opposite page

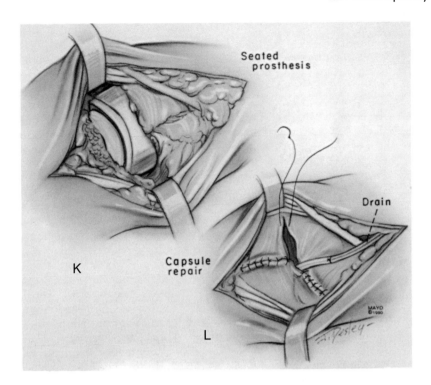

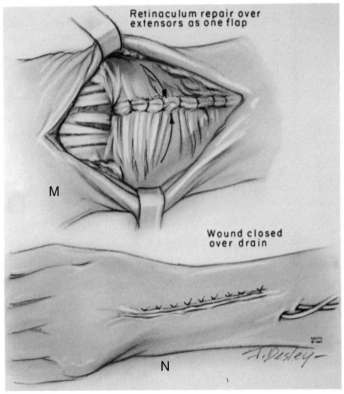

Figure 22–8. *Continued.* **K,** After the proximal component is seated, the wrist is put through a range of motion test and any abutting bone is resected. **L,** Capsular repair is important. It is accomplished with interrupted sutures over a deep suction drain. **M,** Retinacular tissues are closed in a single layer over the second through the fourth dorsal compartments. It is important to repair the retinaculum to prevent subluxation of the tendons volar to the prosthesis during palmar flexion of the wrist. **N,** A second subcutaneous drain is used and long-arm compression dressings are applied. (By permission of Mayo Foundation.)

and the cement allowed to set, maintaining distal pressure on the metacarpal component. The radial component is then seated with impaction and the prosthesis reduced.

Tension is tested and later noted in the operative notes for assistance in postoperative management. The passive range of motion is tested for impingement, usually observed in ulnar deviation when the radial component may abut against the ulnar carpal remnants, levering the components apart (see Fig. 22–8K). All impinging bone is resected. A check radiograph is taken to confirm proper positioning and to rule out cement extravasation.

The triangular capsular flaps are then closed over the prosthesis, and a suction drain sutures the tissues to each other on the midline and to capsular remnants or drill holes in the radius proximally (see Fig. 22–8L).

The capsular periosteal tissues over the resected stump of the distal ulna are then firmly imbricated and sutured to the capsular rim of the radius while an assistant pushes the ulna with an instrument in a volar direction. This repair is done with strong (2-0 or 1-0) polyglycol sutures and generally allows use of a short-arm cast postoperatively. The previously elevated flaps of the extensor retinaculum are then sutured to each other as a common layer over the second, third, and fourth dorsal compartments (see Fig. 22–8M). The skin and subcutaneous tissue are closed over suction drains and a long arm, bulky compression dressing with plaster splints is applied (see Fig. 22–8N).

The elbow is placed at 90 degrees and the forearm is placed in supination. The position of the wrist is variable. Excessive (greater than 30 degrees) extension should be avoided. If the wrist passively feels balanced in flexion and extension, 10 degrees of extension is used. If resting tension limits palmar flexion, a palmar-flexed position is preferred, and vice versa. The wrist is always placed in neutral radial and ulnar deviation.

As an alternative to distal intramedullary fixation with cement, Van Leeuwen has described cementless fixation with small components.[48] In this technique, the majority of the capitate is preserved and a small distal component is inserted so that its tip just crosses the subchondral bone of the carpometacarpal joint. Van Leeuwen, therefore, uses the strong subchondral bone for distal fixation and the intact carpus for proximal fixation in attempts to decrease dorsal breakout or migration of the distal component stem through the metacarpal. Cement is not used (Fig. 22–9). The results are satisfactory (see later), and the author has adopted this technique in younger patients. Trail has used this technique but also mismatches components when appropriate by using one size larger proximal components (Trail, Wrightington, England, August 2001: Personal communication). I have no experience with this modification.

POSTOPERATIVE CARE

After 2 to 4 days, the dressings are removed, and a long-arm plaster splint is applied to maintain the position.

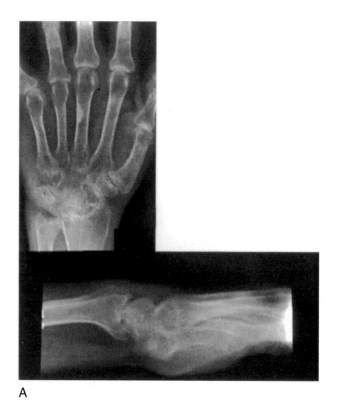

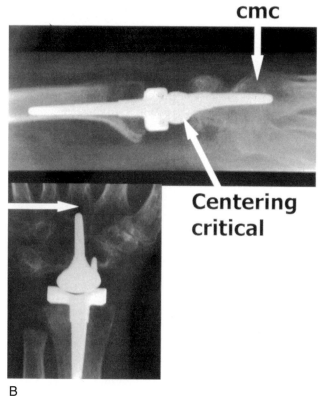

Figure 22–9. Severe rheumatoid involvement of the wrist (**A**). There is lack of cement and distal fixation at the base of the proximal metacarpal (**B**).

At 2 weeks, the splint and sutures are removed, and a variable management program is undertaken according to the tension of the fit as follows:

Loose fit: A short-arm cast is applied for 6 weeks and then a mobilization program as described under normal fit.
Tight fit: A motion program is begun, as described under normal fit, without any preliminary casting. If testing reveals that a tight fit has loosened at 2 weeks postoperatively, a cast is worn as for the normal fit.
Normal fit: At 2 weeks postoperatively, the patient should be able to generate 30 degrees of flexion and 30 degrees of extension, but without support, this motion may rapidly increase to excessive amounts; therefore, a short-arm cast is applied for 2 more weeks. At 4 weeks after surgery, the cast is removed and a resting splint is fabricated to support the wrist in 10 to 20 degrees of dorsiflexion and neutral radioulnar deviation. The patient is instructed in gentle active range of motion exercises and isometric strengthening techniques. Independent functional activities with the wrist out of the splint may be begun at 6 weeks and the patient may progress to free use of the wrist at 12 weeks postoperatively.

The goals of the procedure are to relieve pain and provide balanced wrist motion through a 60-degree flexion-extension arc. Excess mobility has led to prosthetic imbalance, subluxation, and loosening, and should be avoided. Common sense limitation of activities should be encouraged (see the earlier section describing indications and contraindications).[12]

RESULTS AND COMPLICATIONS

The published results of total wrist arthroplasty have been few because of the relatively limited use of these devices. Longer term results on the biaxial wrist and early data on the universal wrist are now available.[1,12] The following data summarize the generally reported clinical functions and complications of the most widely used devices as well as my interpretation of the findings.

Swanson Silicone Wrist Arthroplasty

In general, silicone arthroplasty provides pain relief and some motion. Late failure can occur with either subsidence of the device into the medullary canal or fracture of the components. Simmen and Gschwend believed the procedure was worthwhile but had the indications narrowed to patients with inactive arthritis and good ligaments.[40] Brase and Millender followed 21 patients for several years after an earlier study and showed that results deteriorated with time.[8,22] Fracture rates were 8 percent between 6 months and 5 years of follow-up and 20 percent after 5 years of follow-up. Both of these groups noted that fractures were associated with pain and that

they occurred in patients who achieved excess ranges of motion. Fracture was associated with pain and the necessity for reoperation in more than one half of patients.

In comparison, Comstock and associates identified a 65 percent fracture rate in a 6-year average follow-up study of silicone wrist implants.[13] They also noted high subsidence and deterioration of results with time, as did others.[16] Although the results vary somewhat in the various reported groups, in general, 25 degrees of dorsiflexion and 25 degrees of palmar flexion are achieved, with 5 degrees of radial deviation and 15 degrees of ulnar deviation. Some changes of erosion about the implant stem are seen. As mentioned earlier, this device is not now generally used.[15]

Meuli Wrist Prosthesis

The Meuli wrist prosthesis, including its original bendable Protasul stem and its subsequent offset stem device, demonstrated early dramatic improvement in function with pain relief and excellent range of motion.[29] Two significant problems with the device remained, however, and resulted in reoperation rates that were anticipated to reach nearly 35 percent at 5 years.[14] As time has gone by and experience has developed over more than 20 years with this original device, the complications and failures increased. Early problems included subluxation, which could generally be handled with casting. Problems of imbalance, however, are not correctable without surgery and tend to progress with time. Late complications have included loosening of the distal components with drift of the distal component into the carpal canal and secondary tendon and median nerve irritation requiring revision or, more commonly, removal. Excess polyethylene wear with reactive synovitis has been another occasional late serious feature with the original implants. The current Meuli device has been extensively revised to attempt to deal with these problems. The original designs are no longer used (HC Meuli, personal communication).[37]

Volz Wrist Prosthesis

The Volz design has a more "semiconstrained" articulating surface. This resulted in a lower loosening rate, but, because of the small contract area, significant balance problems remained with the "teeter-totter" effect. Dislocation was a problem, but distal component loosening was distinctly lessened.[6,16,42] Because of the balance problem, even though there were many acceptable longer term results, the Volz prosthesis was abandoned in favor of the current devices that have broader ellipsoidal articulating surfaces.

Trispherical Total Wrist Arthroplasty

This device is the only fixed articulating device with significant use. The constraints inherent in the hinge provides limitation of excess deformity and prevention of

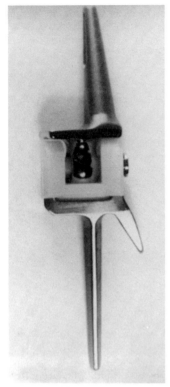

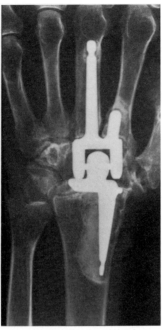

A   B

Figure 22–10. Trispherical total wrist device. **A,** The device is semi-constrained with a central axis pin. **B** and **C,** Anteroposterior and lateral radiographs of a patient 12 years after insertion. The patient has minimal motion but only slight pain and has had progressive loosening of the distal component, which has remained stable over the past several years.

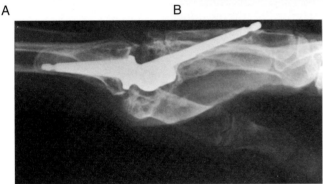

C

dislocation, but the inherent constraint can increase chances of failure at the bone-cement interface. Certain reports, however, suggest very satisfactory clinical function with few complications.[19] Some loosening and subsidence has occurred but not enough to necessarily require revision (Fig. 22–10).[1,20]

Biaxial and Universal Wrist Prosthesis

The results of the most recent generation of wrist prostheses with broader ellipsoidal articulating surfaces are satisfactory but limited.[12,15,28] Loosening of the distal component has been the major problem with the biaxial prosthesis, occurring in approximately 20 percent of patients with 6.5 years average follow-up.

The main problem with the universal prosthesis has been subluxation, occurring in approximately 15 percent of devices. Both biaxial and universal prosthetic arthroplasties have been associated with a physiologic and pain-free range of motion.[12,15,23,28]

NEW PROSTHETIC DESIGN

The distal component screw fixation with the universal wrist prosthesis has been very successful and has exhibited no loosening (Fig. 22–11). Similarly, Van Leeuwen has reported on three distal loosenings in 185 implants after 2 to 8 years of follow-up.[48] Currently, design modifications are being developed for both the biaxial and universal wrist prostheses (Brian Adams, June 2001, personal communication) in attempts to improve stability and fixation. Two new devices are being developed by Hubach (Fig. 22–12A) and Cooney (Fig. 22–12B, C).

Most new designs incorporate the concept of screw fixation of the distal component in the carpus as opposed to the metacarpal in conjunction with formal intercarpal fusion. Many surgeons believe that fusion of the carpometacarpal joints should be surgically performed if prosthetic stems cross them.[1,37] It is clear that an ellipsoidal or variant of this technique is appropriate whenever an articulating interface and modular components with precise instrumentation will be available for the devices.

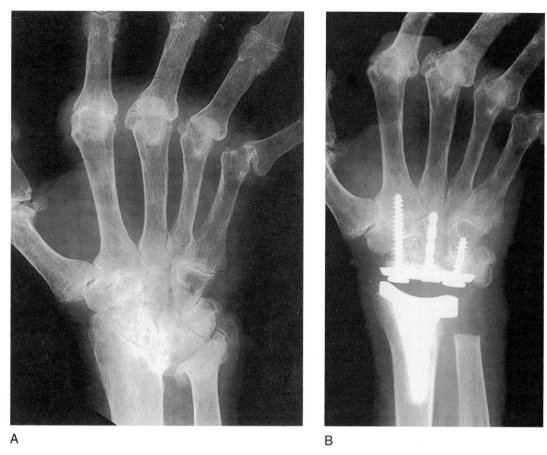

A

B

Figure 22–11. Severe rheumatoid wrist involvement with collapse (**A**). Distal screw fixation in the metacarpals has proven quite successful in clinical trials (**B**).

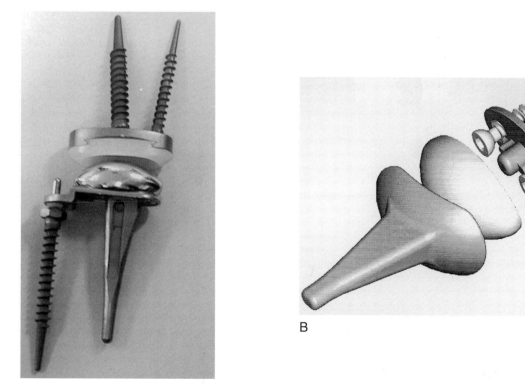

A

B

Figure 22–12. Newer designs feature fixation in the ulna as well as in the distal radius (**A**). An alternative includes an intercalary polyethylene element with distal screw fixation (**B**). This has proven very effective in the short term (**C**).

Illustration continued on following page

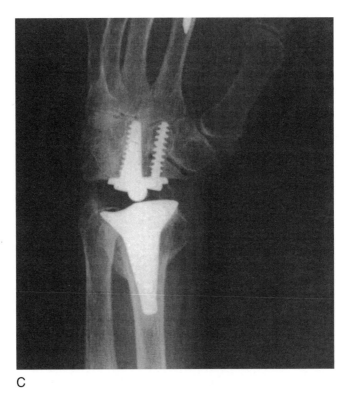

C

Figure 22–12. *Continued.*

Fixation of radial components is not a problem, but more anatomic sizing and shape will be incorporated.

REVISION AND SALVAGE

One of the important factors in consideration of total wrist arthroplasty as a reconstructive procedure is whether it can be salvaged. Experience has shown that total wrist arthroplasty may be salvaged in one of three ways:

1. Removal and casting with or without insertion of a spacer device to form a "pseudarthrosis"
2. Removal and fusion of the wrist
3. Revision with insertion of new standard or custom devices

In revision surgery, several technical points are significant. The capsule surrounding the device is very thick and must be extensively resected or released to allow wrist flexion and dislocation of the components for extraction. If only one component (distal) is to be revised, it may still be necessary to remove the proximal component to provide adequate exposure for reinsertion of a new component.

In removing cemented components, it may be helpful to split the dorsal cortex of the radius and/or the third metacarpal with a fine osteotome and then pry the cortex open like a book; the component and the cement mantle may then be disimpacted as a single unit (Fig. 22–13). If revision implant surgery is to be performed, it is better to extract the components and stems and slowly remove cement with a bur.

If the patient's bone is extremely osteoporotic or has multiple fractures after removal of components, simple closure of the pseudoprosthetic capsule may be performed. If it seems appropriate, a silicone wrist device may be inserted as a spacer. Postoperatively, the wrist is cast in a neutral position for 8 weeks and splinted for 6 more weeks. This generally results in a stable, painless pseudarthrosis, but there is obvious decrease in power (Fig. 22–14).

If the bone stock is satisfactory but the patient is not a candidate for revision to a new arthroplasty, arthrodesis is performed. In general, a cortical iliac graft is obtained and fashioned to fit in the medullary canal of the radius and base of the metacarpals (Fig. 22–15). Femoral head allograft with intramedullary rod fixation has also been reported.[9]

In patients loosening of the distal component, revision surgery is possible and can be successful with standard components.[18,38] In general, however, revision to a new arthroplasty should be accomplished with multiple pronged or long-stemmed components (see Fig. 22–4). Use of these implants allows stabilization with cement beyond and beside the area of weakened third metacarpal bone (Figs. 22–16 and 22–17).

AUTHOR'S PREFERRED METHOD

I prefer the use of the biaxial total wrist design. The technique of screw fixation of the distal component or limited penetration of the metacarpal (Van Leeuwen's technique) appears to be successful and logical. The concept of wrist replacement versus arthrodesis remains controversial.[47] In advising a patient with a painful dysfunctional wrist

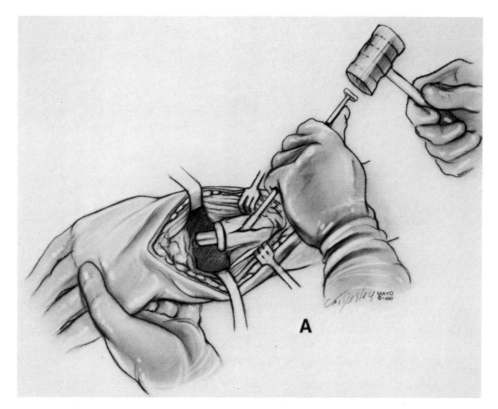

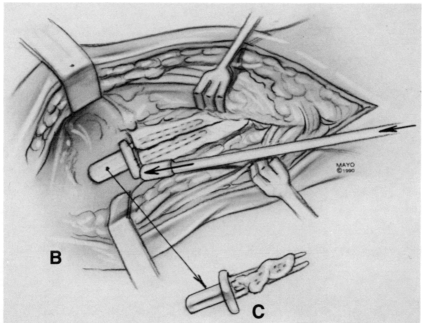

Figure 22–13. A, An osteotome is used to split the dorsal cortex of the radius from the proximal to the distal direction. **B** and **C,** After splitting the dorsal cortex, the radius can be pried open like a book and the component and its cement mantle are driven out of the medullary canal with an impactor and a mallet. This leaves a circle of cortical bone that can be easily stabilized to provide support for a fusion.

arthrosis on surgical alternatives, following several options are outlined in the following paragraphs.

An arthrodesis may be performed with the same amount of morbidity and the same recovery period as an arthroplasty.[7] The operation is permanent and relieves pain. There is no likelihood of reoperation. All motion is lost, but finger function may be enhanced. Certain activities of daily living may be difficult, such as reaching into narrow areas or cupboards and taking care of personal hygiene.

An arthroplasty provides a functional range of motion and some restoration of the length of the wrist.

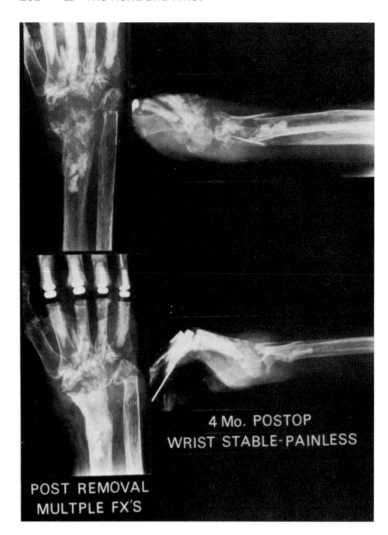

POST REMOVAL
MULTPLE FX'S

4 Mo. POSTOP
WRIST STABLE-PAINLESS

Figure 22–14. Anteroposterior and lateral views immediately after removal of the prosthesis in which the fragile bone was fractured in multiple planes *(top).* Four months after casting, the patient achieved a stable and painless pseudoarthrosis *(bottom).*

Figure 22–15. Thumb reconstruction 5 years after total wrist arthroplasty. **A,** The Kirschner wire and implant became infected.

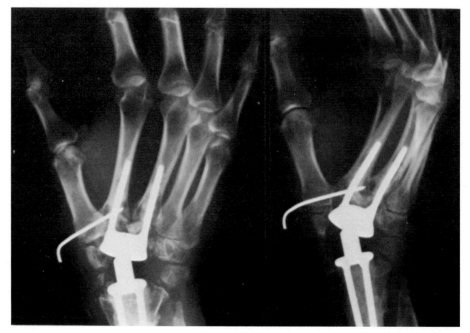

A

Illustration continued on opposite page

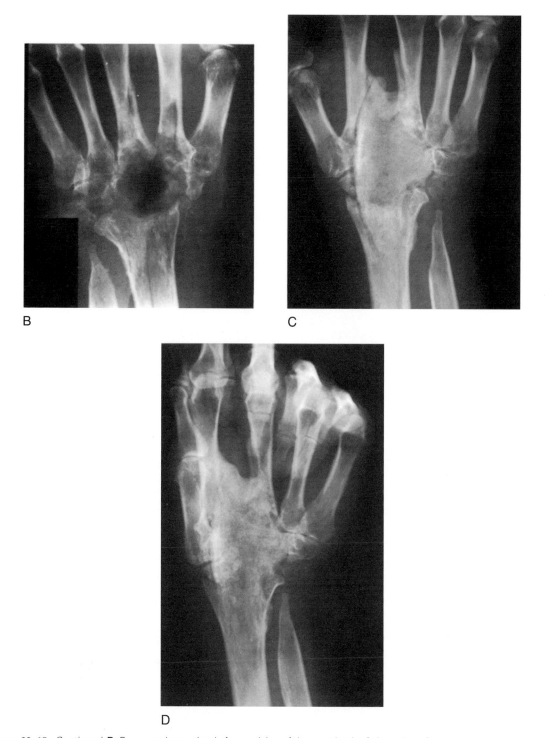

B

C

D

Figure 22–15. *Continued.* **B**, Bone stock remained after excision of the prosthesis. **C**, Insertion of large corticocancellous iliac bone graft. **D**, Fusion achieved 1 year after grafting.

Arthroplasty may increase power and function through automatic finger flexion with wrist extension. The procedure is likely to be associated with a one-in-five chance of need for revision in 5 years, and long-term results beyond that are not currently known. If the procedure fails, a fusion can typically be achieved but this procedure may be more difficult and may require iliac crest bone graft.

If a patient understands these facts and wishes to "gamble" on the arthroplasty option to preserve motion, I believe it is most appropriate to proceed with wrist arthroplasty. There is no question that the best results from total wrist arthroplasty are far superior to the results from wrist arthrodesis, and it is generally not possible to convince a patient with a successful wrist arthroplasty on one side to have a fusion on the other side.

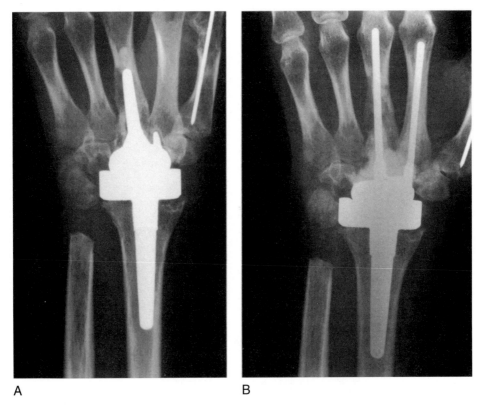

A   B

Figure 22–16. A, Loosening with cystic erosion of metacarpal shaft 2 years after biaxial implant. **B**, Revision with a two-pronged component and successful maintenance of fixation 4 years postoperatively.

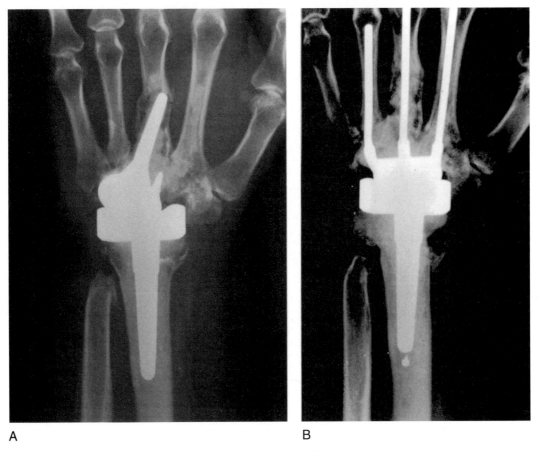

A   B

Figure 22–17. A, Loosening of the metacarpal component after a fall and fracture of the long metacarpal in a young rheumatoid patient who refused fusion. **B**, The patient is asymptomatic 4 years after revision with a custom three-pronged distal component.

References

1. Adams B: Total Wrist Arthrodesis: Universal total wrist arthroplasty. Presented at the Annual Meeting of the American Society for Surgery of the Hand, Baltimore, October 2001.
2. Beckenbaugh RD: Total joint arthroplasty: The wrist. Mayo Clin Proc 54:513, 1979.
3. Beckenbaugh RD: Implant arthroplasty in the rheumatoid hand and wrist: Current state of the art in the United States. J Hand Surg 8:676, 1983.
4. Beckenbaugh RD, Brown ML: Early experience with biaxial total wrist arthroplasty. Presented at the Annual Meeting of the American Society for Surgery of the Hand, Toronto, September 1990.
5. Beckenbaugh RD, Linscheid RL: Arthroplasty in the hand and wrist. *In* Green DP (ed): Surgery of the Hand, 2nd ed. New York, Churchill Livingstone, 1988, p 202.
6. Bosco JA III, Bynum DK, Bowers WH: Long-term outcome of Volz total wrist arthroplasties. J Arthroplasty 9:25, 1994.
7. Bracey DJ, McMurtry RY, Wallow D: Arthrodesis of the wrist using the AO technique. Orthop Rev 9:65, 1980.
8. Brase DW, Millender LH: Failure of silicone rubber wrist arthroplasty in rheumatoid arthritis. J Hand Surg 11A:175, 1989.
9. Carlson JR, Simmons BP: Wrist arthrodesis after failed wrist implant arthroplasty. J Hand Surg 23:893, 1998.
10. Clayton ML: Surgical treatment of the wrist in rheumatoid arthritis: A review of thirty-seven patients. J Bone Joint Surg 47A:741, 1965.
11. Clayton ML, Ferlic DC: Tendon transfer for radial rotation of the wrist in rheumatoid arthritis. Clin Orthop 100:176, 1974.
12. Cobb TK, Beckenbaugh RD: Biaxial total wrist arthroplasty. J Hand Surg 21A:1011, 1996.
13. Comstock CP, Louis DS, Eckenrode RJ: Silicone wrist implant: Long term follow-up study. J Hand Surg 13A:201, 1988.
14. Cooney WP, Beckenbaugh RD, Linscheid RL: Total wrist arthroplasty: Problems with implant failures. Clin Orthop 187:121, 1984.
15. Costi J, Krishnan J, Pearcy M: Total wrist arthroplasty. A quantitative review of the last 30 years. J Rheum 25:451, 1998.
16. Dennis DA, Ferlic DC, Clayton ML: Volz total wrist arthroplasty in rheumatoid arthritis: A long term review. J Hand Surg 11A:483, 1986.
17. Fatti JF, Palmer AK, Mosher JF: Long term results of silicone rubber arthroplasty of the wrist. J Hand Surg 11A:175, 1986.
18. Ferlic DC, Jolly SN, Clayton ML: Salvage for failed implant arthroplasty of the wrist. J Hand Surg 17:917, 1992.
19. Figgie HE, Ranawat CS, Inglis AE, et al: Preliminary results of total wrist arthroplasty in rheumatoid arthritis using the trispherical total wrist arthroplasty. J Arthroplasty 3:9, 1988.
20. Figgie HE, Ranawat CS, Inglis AE, et al: Trispherical total wrist arthroplasty in rheumatoid arthritis. J Hand Surg 15A:217, 1990.
21. Gellman H, Rankin G, Brumfield R, et al: Palmar shelf arthroplasty in rheumatoid wrist. J Bone Joint Surg 71A:223, 1989.
22. Goodman MJ, Millender LH, Nalebuff EA, Philips CA: Arthroplasty of the rheumatoid wrist with silicone rubber: An early evaluation. J Hand Surg 5:114, 1980.
23. Hamas RS: A quantitative approach to total wrist arthroplasty: Development of a precentered wrist prosthesis. Orthop Clin North Am 2:245, 1979.
24. Linscheid RL, Dobyns JH: Radiolunate arthrodesis. J Hand Surg 10A:821, 1985.
25. Lorei MP, Figgie MP, Ranawat CS, Inglis AE: Failed total wrist arthroplasty: Analysis of failures and results in operative management. Clin Orthop 342:84, 1997.
26. Menon J: Total wrist replacement using the modified Volz prosthesis. J Bone Joint Surg 69:998, 1987.
27. Menon J: Indications for total wrist arthroplasty. Presented at the Instructional Course of the American Society for Surgery of the Hand Annual Meeting, Phoenix, AZ, 1992.
28. Menon J: Universal total wrist implant: Experience with a carpal component fixed with three screws. J Arthroplasty 13:515, 1998.
29. Meuli HC: HCH arthroplasty du poignet. Ann Chir 27:527, 1973.
30. Meuli HC: Arthroplasty of the wrist. Clin Orthop 149:118, 1980.
31. Meuli HC: Uncemented total wrist arthroplasty. J Hand Surg 20A:115, 1995.
32. Millender LH, Nalebuff EA: Arthrodesis of the rheumatoid wrist. J Bone Joint Surg 55A:1026, 1973.
33. Millender LH, Nalebuff EA: Preventing surgery, tenosynovectomy and synovectomy. Orthop Clin North Am 6:765, 1975.
34. Millender LH, Nalebuff EA: Arthrodesis of the wrist joint in rheumatoid arthritis. Hand 12:149, 1980.
35. Palmer AK, Weimer FW, Murphy D, Glisson R: Functional wrist motion: A biomechanical study. J Hand Surg 10A:39, 1988.
36. Peimer CA, Medige J, Eckert BS, et al: Reactive synovitis after silicone arthroplasty. J Hand Surg 11A:624, 1986.
37. Report of Implant Committee, International Federation of Societies for Surgery of the Hand, Istanbul, June 2001.
38. Rettig ME, Beckenbaugh RD: Revision total wrist arthroplasty. J Hand Surg 18:798, 1993.
39. Shapiro JS: A new factor in the etiology of ulnar drift. Clin Orthop 68:34, 1970.
40. Simmen BR, Gschwend N: Swanson silicone rubber interpositional arthroplasty of the wrist and of the metacarpophalangeal joints in rheumatoid arthritis. Acta Orthop Belg 54:196, 1988.
41. Smith RJ, Atkinson RE, Jupiter JB: Silicone synovitis of the wrist. J Hand Surg 10A:47, 1985.
42. Stanley JK, Boot DA: Radio-lunate arthrodesis. J Hand Surg 14B:283, 1989.
43. Stanley JK, Tolat AR: Long-term results of Swanson Silastic arthroplasty in the rheumatoid wrist. J Hand Surg 18B:381, 1993.
44. Straub LR, Ranawat CS: The wrist in rheumatoid arthritis: Surgical treatment and results. J Bone Joint Surg 51A:1, 1969.
45. Swanson AB: Flexible implant arthroplasties for arthritic disabilities of the radial-carpal joint: A silicone rubber intramedullary stemmed flexible implant for the wrist joint. Orthop Clin North Am 4:383, 1973.
46. Taleisnik J: Rheumatoid arthritis of the wrist. Hand Clin 5:257, 1989.
47. Vicar AJ, Burton RI: Fusion versus arthroplasty. J Hand Surg 2A:790, 1986.
48. Van Leeuwen N: Biaxial Total Wrist Arthroplasty. Presented at the Anglo-Dutch "Amici Carpi" meeting, Amsterdam, June 1999.
49. Viegas SF, Rimoldi R, Patterson R: Modified technique of intramedullary fixation for wrist arthrodesis. J Hand Surg 14A:618, 1989.
50. Volz RG: The development of a total wrist arthroplasty. Clin Orthop 116:209, 1976.
51. Volz RG: Total wrist arthroplasty: A clinical review. Clin Orthop 187:112, 1984.
52. Wood MB: Wrist arthrodesis using radial bone graft. J Hand Surg 12A:208, 1987.
53. Youm Y, Flatt AE: Design of a total wrist prosthesis. Ann Biomed Eng 12:247, 1984.
54. Youm Y, McMurtry RY, Flatt AE: Kinematics of the wrist I. J Bone Joint Surg 60A:423, 1978.
55. Youm Y, McMurtry RY, Flatt AE: Kinematics of the wrist II. J Bone Joint Surg 60A:955, 1978.

III

The Elbow

BERNARD F. MORREY • SECTION EDITOR

23

Anatomy and Surgical Approaches

• BERNARD F. MORREY

ANATOMY

This chapter deals with relevant anatomy and the most helpful exposures for elbow joint replacement.

TOPICAL ANATOMY

The appropriate surgical approach to the elbow relies on the recognition of palpable landmarks: The tip of the olecranon, the medial and lateral epicondyles,[1] and the lateral column of the humerus. The medially based Mayo approach goes just to the medial aspect of the tip of the olecranon.[4] The lateral modified extensile Kocher approach crosses the lateral epicondyle,[12] the center of which serves as the attachment of the collateral ligament. The medial epicondyle is important to determine the location of the ulnar nerve and as a landmark for the insertion of the medial collateral ligament.

OSTEOLOGY AND JOINT STRUCTURE

A clear understanding of the normal anatomy of all three articular elements of the elbow joint is necessary to reliably perform the full spectrum of reconstructive procedures of this joint.

Humerus

The distal humerus consists of two supracondylar bony columns on which the trochlea and capitellum articular surfaces rest (Fig. 23–1). Just proximal to the trochlea, the prominent medial epicondyle serves both as attachment of the medial collateral ligament and the flexor pronator group and as the roof of the cubital tunnel protecting the ulnar nerve. The lateral collateral ligament originates from the flat and roughened surface of the middle of the lateral epicondyle.

Proximal to the articular surface of the trochlea, the coronoid fossa anteriorly and the olecranon fossa posteriorly receive the coronoid and olecranon processes during flexion and extension. These fossae develop spurs and are the source of impingement with degenerative arthritis of the elbow. The proximal aspect of the olecranon fossa is also an important landmark for identification of the intermedullary canal and to determine the depth of insertion and axis of rotation of some implants.[18]

The articular surface of the trochlea is offset in reference to the medullary canal, which is slightly lateral to the center of the trochlea. Therefore, removal of the trochlea and a portion of the capitellum is necessary to center an intramedullary device down the canal of the humerus. The lateral margin of the lateral column is the palpable landmark for proximal extension of the Kocher incision. This column is considerably larger and stronger than the medial column, thus allowing more removal of bone laterally than medially (Fig. 23–1). Proper axial rotation at the time of insertion of the humeral implant is best estimated by the plane formed by the posterior surfaces of the medial and lateral columns.[18]

On the lateral view, the anterior rotation of the articulation measures approximately 30 degrees, and joint replacement devices must be constructed in such a way as to allow replication of the axis of rotation (Fig. 23–2). The normal axis of rotation of the humerus is colinear with a line drawn from the anterior cortex of the distal humerus.

The orientation of the axis of rotation referable to the distal humerus in the anteroposterior plane is not at a right angle but rather has a valgus orientation referable to the long axis (Fig. 23–2). Hinged or captive joint replacements accommodate for the valgus disposition of the articular surface at the ulna.[17] The resurfacing mechanisms must accurately replicate the valgus tilt at the humerus because this is necessary to properly balance the ligaments and capsule. Hence, resurfacing designs may offer variable articular/stem angles of the implant.[26]

Radius

The articular surface is oriented on a 15-degree angle referable to the long axis of the radius, opposite in direction to the radial tuberosity (Fig. 23–3). Recognition of this poorly emphasized relationship allows proper placement of a radial component so that an accurate articulation with the capitellum occurs during pronation and supination.

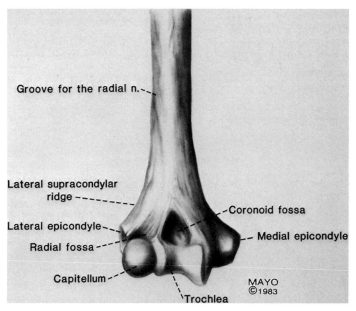

A

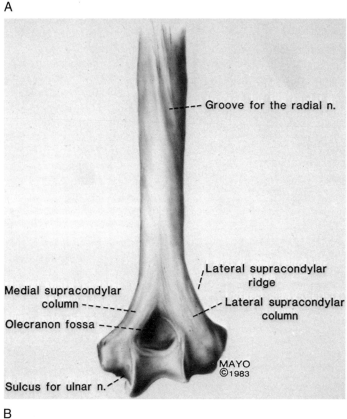

B

Figure 23–1. A, Osseous landmarks of the anterior aspect of the distal humerus. **B**, Posterior aspect of the distal humerus clearly shows the relationship of the all-important medial and lateral supracondylar bony columns.

Proximal Ulna

The proximal ulna has two subtle angular orientations. First is a slight valgus that averages about 4 to 5 degrees of the articulation referable to the proximal shaft. Most implants restore or replicate the carrying angle by allowing for the valgus angle at the ulnar component (Fig. 23–4).[2,14] On the lateral projection, the center of the articulation is located in the center of the greater sigmoid notch.[19]

LIGAMENTS AND CONSTRAINTS

A clear understanding of the anatomy and mechanics of the ligaments of the elbow is critically important for elbow joint replacement.

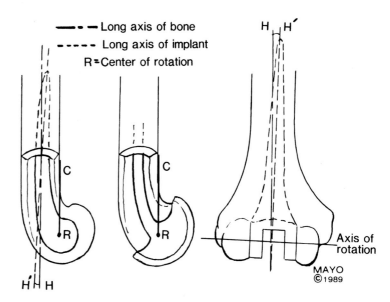

Figure 23–2. Center of rotation of both semiconstrained and resurfacing implants should be found on a line colinear with the anterior distal humeral cortex. The anterior tilt of the distal humeral articulation must be accounted for in the design of the implant. In the anteroposterior plane, the valgus tilt of the humeral articulation is accommodated by either the design of the implant or the technique of implantation.

Medial Ligament Complex

The medial lateral ligament complex consists primarily of the anterior and posterior bundles (Fig. 23–5). The anterior oblique bundle is the most discrete and functionally sufficient component.[13,20,25] The origin of this ligament is on the undersurface of the medial epicondyle, and on the lateral projection is on the axis of rotation at the anterior, inferior aspect of the medial epicondyle.[18] The insertion of the ligament is at the sublime tubercle of the coronoid process.

The posterior bundle of the medial collateral ligament is less well defined and can be released with impunity

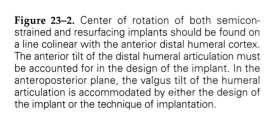

Figure 23–3. Proximal radius has a 15-degree angulation away from the radial tuberosity.

during joint replacement. However, the anterior portion should not be altered, if possible, when implanting a resurfacing device because this is necessary for stability of such implants.

Lateral Ligament Complex

The lateral ligament complex consists of the radial collateral ligament, the lateral ulnar collateral ligament, the less important accessory lateral collateral ligament, and the annular ligament (Fig. 23–6).[16] The latter two are of minimum relevance in the present context.

Lateral Ulnar Collateral Ligament

The lateral ulnar collateral ligament described only in the last decade of the 20th century[18,24] but recognition of its functional significance is now well accepted. It consists of the posterior portion of the radial collateral ligament and originates from the inferior aspect of the lateral epicondyle. It tends to be superficial to the angular ligament and inserts in a discrete location on the tubercle of the crista supinatoris. This ligament should be considered the analogue to the anterior bundle of the medial collateral ligament. It has a very similar orientation to the medial ligament and serves as a major stabilizer of the elbow joint. The lateral ulnar collateral ligament also tends to be isometric throughout the arc of elbow flexion (Fig. 23–7).[17] It is essential to repair or reconstruct this ligament when employing resurfacing implants.

MUSCLES ABOUT THE ELBOW

Relevant features with regard to elbow musculature are discussed with exposures about the elbow. Several important aspects referable to pathologic conditions or reconstructive procedures are discussed here.

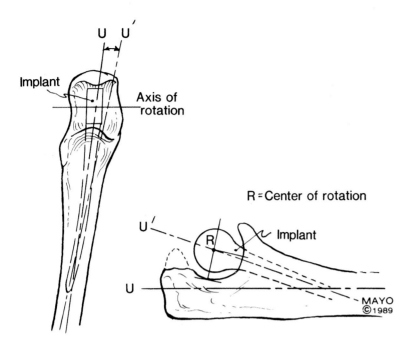

Figure 23–4. Valgus angulation of the proximal ulna is replicated by the design of ulnar implants. The center of rotation of the ulnar component is coincident with the center of rotation of the normal elbow lying in the projected center of the greater sigmoid notch.

Figure 23–5. Medial aspect of the joint. The anterior and posterior bundles of the medial collateral ligament are consistently present and identifiable.

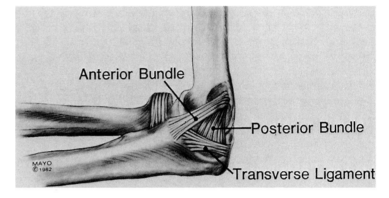

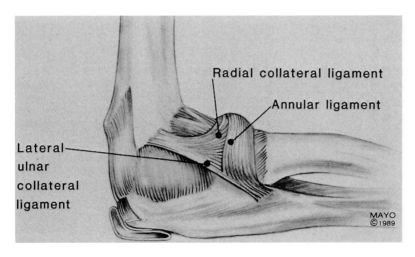

Figure 23–6. Lateral ligament complex is composed of the radial collateral ligament, the annular ligament, and the less well-recognized lateral ulnar collateral ligament.

Elbow Flexors

Biceps

The biceps tendon lies very close to the axis of rotation, inserting on the radial tuberosity. The biceps muscle is a reliable flexor even in the most extensively involved joints. Because of this, we tend to not insert but débride

the radial head[18] to increase the effectiveness of the biceps muscle to flex and supinate the elbow.

Brachialis

Because the insertion of the brachialis is distal to the tip of the coronoid process, osteophytic changes at the coronoid may be removed without compromising the insertion of

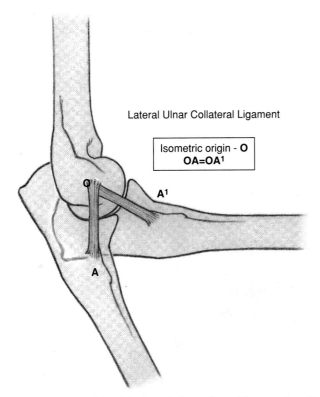

Lateral Ulnar Collateral Ligament

Isometric origin - **O**
OA=OA¹

Figure 23–7. The origin of the lateral ulnar collateral ligament is at the lateral tubercle, which is the isometric point of origin for the ligament and is coincident with the instant center of rotation.

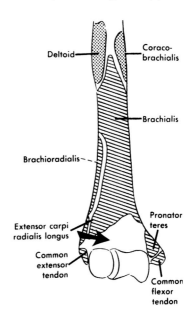

Figure 23–8. The brachialis inserts along the anterior aspect of the distal humerus, but the area immediately above the articulation is free of muscular origin, allowing placement of the flange of the Mayo-modified Coonrad implant. (From Hollinshead WH: The back and limbs. *In* Anatomy for Surgeons, vol 3. New York, Harper & Row, 1969, by permission of Mayo Foundation.)

the muscle. The origin of this muscle is from the entire anterior distal half of the humerus, which allows ready preparation of the anterior cortex proximal to the coronoid recess, thus accommodating the flange of the Coonrad-Morrey implant (Fig. 23–8). Furthermore, the entire anterior cortical surface of the distal humerus is available for the safe application of cortical struts (see Chapter 32).

Muscles Originating from the Lateral Epicondyle

The common extensor muscle group includes the extensor carpi radialis longus and brevis and the common extensor of the digits. This common origin is typically left inviolate during elbow joint replacement. Particular care should be taken to maintain the normal anatomic origin of the common extensors when inserting a resurfacing device because the dynamic element provided by these muscles may be important in stabilizing the elbow.

The collateral ligament may be scarred to and inseparable from the extensor muscle mass in some conditions. In this setting, the ligament and muscle may be released from the lateral epicondyle. However, care is taken to restore the complex after resurfacing procedures.

Elbow Extensors

Triceps Brachii

The triceps brachii comprises the entire posterior bulk of the musculature of the arm. The tendon attachment is

supplemented by medial fascial extensions and the anconeus muscle laterally, a feature employed in the Kocher and Mayo extensile exposures to the joint.[4,13] It is significant that the distal aspect of the muscle is comprised of a wide superficial fascial layer that blends with the triceps tendon distally. This anatomic feature is employed in the Campbell posterior surgical approaches to the joint.[1,5,6]

Anconeus

The anconeus muscle originates from a position at the posterior aspect of the lateral epicondyle and from the triceps fascia. It inserts in the lateral dorsal surface of the proximal ulna. The size of this muscle averages 9 × 3 cm and is of particular significance.[22] Its close approximation and association with the triceps mechanism allows reflection of this muscle with the triceps mechanism during the modified Kocher approach. Furthermore, the attachment to the triceps is useful, allowing mobilization for some cases of triceps insufficiency.

Flexor Pronator Group

The flexor pronator group of muscles consists of the pronator teres, flexor carpi radialis, flexor carpi ulnaris, palmaris longus, flexor digitorum superficialis, and flexor digitorum profundus. These all have a common origin at the medial epicondyle. The ulnar nerve enters the flexor carpi ulnaris, so this muscle is routinely split to expose the first motor branch when the nerve is translocated at the time of elbow replacement.

VASCULAR ANATOMY

The brachial artery serves as the major source of circulation to the elbow and is well protected by the brachialis posteriorly and biceps muscles anteriorly. It is rarely involved by pathologic processes or surgical exposures of the elbow. The position of the brachial artery at the elbow is demonstrated in Figure 23–9. Although the collateral circulation seems extensive, it may not be adequate to maintain a viable extremity if the artery is injured, ligated, or thrombosed, which sometimes occurs with elbow dislocation.

Radial Artery

In most instances, the radial artery originates at the level of the radial head and emerges from the anterior cubital space between the brachioradialis and the pronator teres muscles. It sends off a branch, the radial recurrent artery, ascending laterally through the supinator muscle to anastomose with the radial collateral artery. At the level of the lateral epicondyle, the radial recurrent artery is rarely observed during joint replacement because all exposures are from the posterior. However, the anastomoses can be a source of major bleeding in the elbow if violated during the procedure. The recurrent vessels are ligated during the extensile exposure of Henry.

Ulnar Artery

The ulnar artery is the largest of the two terminal branches of the brachial artery. Two recurrent branches originate distal to the origin of the artery, which arises distal to the coronoid. It ascends posterior to the medial epicondyle, and accompanies the ulnar nerve to anastomose with the superior ulnar collateral artery. Major branches of the ulnar recurrent artery may be encountered during a dissection that involves the ulnar nerve (Fig. 23–10).[29]

NERVES

All the major nerves, the musculocutaneous, median, radial, and ulnar, give off articular branches to innervate the elbow joint (Fig. 23–11).[10]

Median Nerve

The median nerve enters the anterior aspect of the brachium and crosses in front of the brachial artery as it

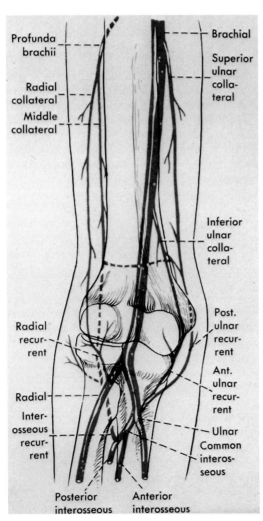

Figure 23–9. Anterior arterial circulatory pattern of the elbow. (From Hollinshead WH: The back and limbs. *In* Anatomy for Surgeons, vol 3. New York, Harper & Row, 1969, by permission of Mayo Foundation.)

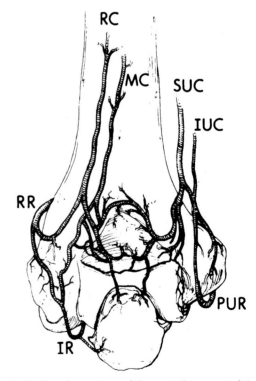

Figure 23–10. Vascular anatomy of the posterior aspect of the elbow. Branches of the ulnar recurrent artery are encountered with the medial Mayo approach as the ulnar nerve is dissected out of its bed. (From Yamaguchi K, Sweet FA, Bindra R, et al: The extraosseous and intraosseous arterial anatomy of the adult elbow. J Bone Joint Surg 79A:1653, 1997.)

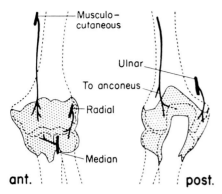

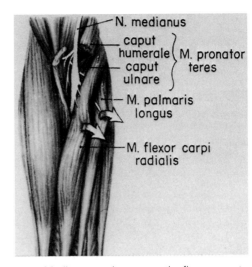

Figure 23–11. All the major nerves that cross the elbow contribute articular sensory branches to the joint. (From Gardner E: The innervation of the elbow joint. Anat Rec 162:161, 1948.)

Figure 23–12. Median nerve innervates the flexor pronator muscle groups, but there are no branches above the elbow joint. (From Hollinshead WH: The back and limbs. *In* Anatomy for Surgeons, vol 3. New York, Harper & Row, 1969, by permission of Mayo Foundation.)

passes across the intermuscular septum. It follows a straight course medial to the midline into the antecubital fossa and lies medial to the biceps tendon and brachial artery. It is rarely involved or injured as a result of elbow replacement. Because there are no branches of the median nerve to the arm, the first motor branches are to the pronator teres and flexor carpi radialis, but they are remote and thus not typically encountered during routine approaches to the elbow joint (Fig. 23–12).

Musculocutaneous Nerve

The cutaneous branch of this nerve emerges through the brachial fascia just at the lateral margin of the biceps tendon. It may rarely be entrapped here but more commonly is injured during anterior exposures of the joint.[3,9]

Radial Nerve

The radial nerve courses laterally to occupy the groove in the humerus that bears its name, emerging anteriorly and laterally to penetrate the lateral intermuscular septum before entering the anterior aspect of the arm. It is here that it is especially vulnerable during revision cement removal. It gives off motor branches above the spiral groove to the medial head of the triceps muscle. This branch continues distally through the medial head to terminate as the muscular branch to the anconeus muscle (Fig. 23–13). This anatomic relationship allows surgical approaches that reflect the anconeus and still preserve the innervation of this muscle.[4,12,22] In the antecubital space, the radial nerve penetrates the supinator

Figure 23–13. Continuation of the radial nerve serves as the innervation of the anconeus, allowing its viability during the Köcher exposure.

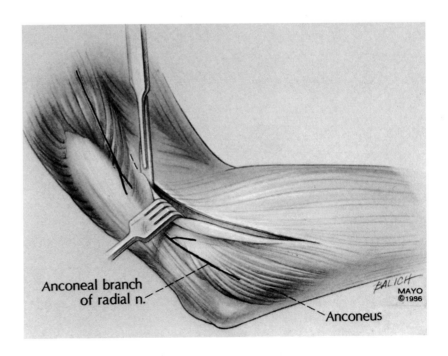

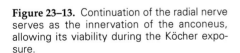

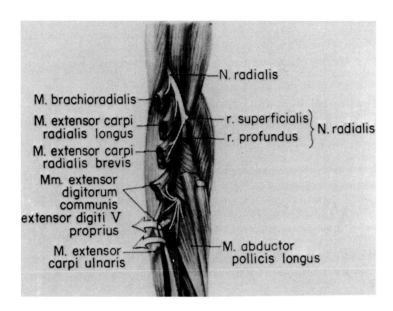

Figure 23–14. Muscles innervated by the radial nerve distal to the triceps. (From Hollinshead WH: The back and limbs. *In* Anatomy for Surgeons, vol 3. New York, Harper & Row, 1969, by permission of Mayo Foundation.)

muscle at the arcade of Frohse and continues distally into the forearm (Fig. 23–14). The radial nerve and posterior interosseous nerve are at risk of injury in this region, usually from retraction.[17,27] They may also be compromised by excessive hemorrhage or synovial distension.

Ulnar Nerve

The ulnar nerve is by far the most important nerve when one is dealing with reconstructive procedures about the elbow joint. The ulnar nerve appears in the distal humerus along the medial margin of the triceps muscle and accompanies the superior ulnar collateral branch of the brachial artery and the ulnar collateral branch of the ulnar artery. Because there are no motor branches of this nerve in the brachium, it is readily translocated or moved from its bed. In the distal humerus, it passes into

the cubital tunnel behind the medial epicondyle and under the cubital tunnel retinaculum[23] to rest against the posterior aspect of the medial collateral ligament (Fig. 23–15). The close proximity of the ulnar nerve to the ulnar collateral ligament accounts, in part, for its vulnerability to nerve compression, entrapment, and stretch. Variably sized joint articular branches may be seen to emerge just proximal to the cubital tunnel or at the cubital tunnel, but the first motor branch to the flexor carpi ulnaris usually is 1 to 2 cm distal to the medial epicondyle.

NEUROVASCULAR RELATIONSHIPS

A clear understanding of the neural and vascular relationships in the region of the elbow joint is an absolute necessity before elbow joint reconstruction can be per-

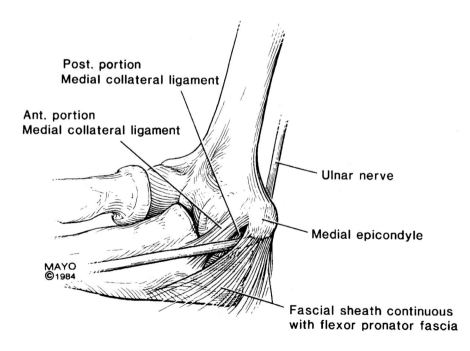

Figure 23–15. Ulnar nerve is vulnerable to injury with extensile elbow exposure from the medial direction to perform elbow joint replacement.

formed.[9,11] Of particular note is the vulnerability of the ulnar nerve to stretch with a valgus stress that might occur with some procedures. The anterior neurovascular structures are generally well protected by the brachialis muscle.[9]

SURGICAL APPROACHES

The "Family" of Posterior Exposures

I have found virtually all reconstructive procedures can be done through a posterior skin incision (Fig. 23–16). The elbow tolerates subcutaneous dissection through either the medial or the lateral aspects of the joint (Fig. 23–17). In this section, emphasis is placed on those exposures that are employed for elbow replacement. Of course, they may be adapted for the treatment of other conditions as well.[8,15,21]

Extensile Köcher[12]

Indications

The extensile Köcher approach may be used for joint arthroplasty, ankylosis, complex fractures of the distal

humerus, synovectomy, radial head excision, and débridement for infection.

Description of Technique

The skin incisions begins 8 cm proximal to the joint just posterior to the supracondylar bony ridge and continues distally over the subcutaneous border of the ulna (Fig. 23–18A) approximately 6 cm distal to the tip of the olecranon. The subcutaneous flap is elevated and the triceps is identified and freed from the brachioradialis and extensor carpi radialis longus along the posterior aspect of the lateral column to the level of the joint capsule. The interval between the extensor carpi ulnaris and anconeus is identified distally and are developed to expose the capsule of the radiohumeral joint. The anconeus is reflected subperiosteally from the proximal ulna (Fig. 23–18B). Sharp dissection frees the bony attachment of the triceps expansion of the anconeus at the lateral epicondyle. The extensor carpiulnaris is elevated distally, the common extensor is elevated from the epicondyle, and the extensor carpi radialis longus is released from the distal aspect of the anterior lateral column (Fig. 23–18C). After the subperiosteal release of the radial collateral ligament from the humerus, the joint may be dislocated with varus stress, providing generous exposure (Fig. 23–18D).

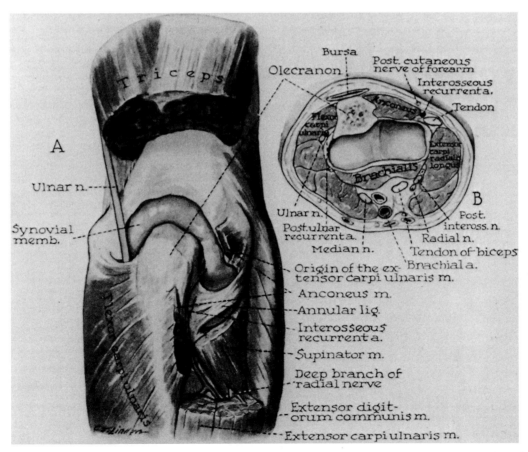

Figure 23–16. Posterior and cross-sectional view of the elbow joint showing the ulnar nerve and other muscular and neurovascular relationships. (From Thorek P: Anatomy in Surgery. Philadelphia, JB Lippincott, 1962.)

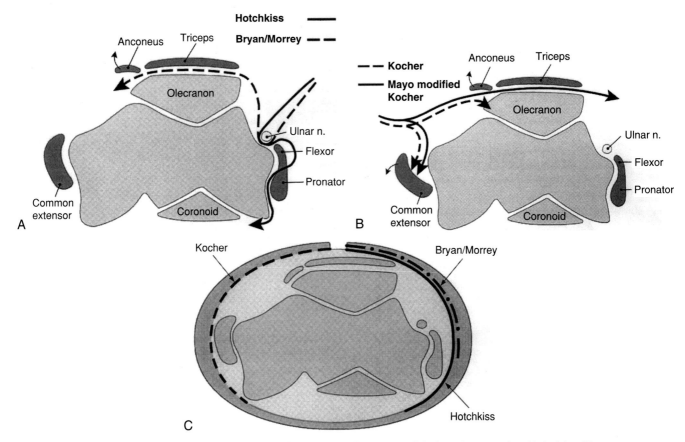

Figure 23–17. Both medial (**A**) and lateral (**B**) deep intervals are accessible through a posterior skin incision (**C**).

Mayo Modified Extensile Köcher[18,19]

Indications

The modified Mayo extensile Köcher approach is used for release of ankylosed joints, interposition replacement arthroplasty, and resurfacing total elbow replacement.

Description of Technique

The Mayo modification and extension of the Köcher extensile approach shown in Figure 23–17 consists of reflecting the triceps insertion from the tip of the olecranon by sharp dissection, as with the Mayo approach (Fig. 23–19). In this way, the entire extensor mechanism may be reflected medially, allowing the elbow to be more readily opened with varus stress than is possible when the joint is tightly contracted. The triceps is reattached in a fashion identical to that described for the Mayo approach. Routine closure in layers is performed, but the radial collateral ligament should be reattached to the bone through holes placed in the lateral epicondyle.

Triceps Splitting[5]

Indications

The triceps-splitting approach is used for elbow arthroplasty, unreduced elbow dislocation, distal humeral frac-

ture, posterior exposure of the joint for ankylosis, sepsis, degenerative arthritis, and synovectomy. We prefer this for the multiple reoperated revision elbow (Fig. 23–20).

Description of Technique

The skin incision begins in the midline over the triceps, approximately 10 cm above the joint line, curves gently laterally or medially at the tip of the olecranon, and continues distally over the lateral aspect of the subcutaneous border of the proximal ulna for a distance of approximately 5 to 6 cm. If the incision is curved medially at the olecranon, the scar may have less tendency to contract.[13]

The triceps is exposed along with the proximal 4 cm of the ulna. A midline incision is made through the triceps, fascia, and tendon and is continued distally across the insertion of the triceps tendon at the tip of the olecranon and down the subcutaneous crest of the ulna (Fig. 23–20). The triceps tendon and muscle are split longitudinally, exposing the distal humerus. The anconeus is then reflected subperiosteally laterally, whereas the flexor carpi ulnaris is similarly retracted medially. The insertion of the triceps is carefully released from the olecranon, leaving the extensor mechanism in continuity with the forearm fascia and muscles medially and laterally. The ulnar nerve is visualized and protected in the cubital tunnel. Closure of the triceps fascia only is required proximally, but the insertion may be supplemented with a suture passed through the tip of the olecranon. The wound is then closed in layers.

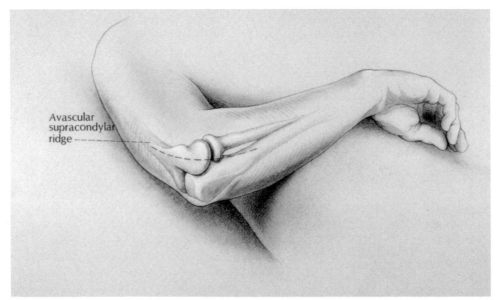

A

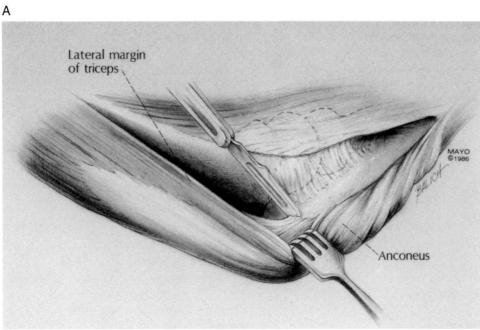

B

Figure 23–18. **A,** The extensile Köcher exposure is performed by an incision extended 8 cm proximal to the joint just posterior to the supracondylar bony ridge and distally over the anconeus for approximately 6 cm. **B,** The interval between the anconeus and the extensor carpi ulnaris is entered. **C,** The anconeus is reflected subperiosteally from the proximal ulna along with its fascial attachment to the triceps. The triceps is elevated from the humerus, the capsule is released posteriorly, and, optionally, the tip of the olecranon is removed. The common extensor tendon is released from the lateral epicondyle of the humerus as necessary to expose the capsule, which is entered with a longitudinal incision and released with a transverse incision.

Illustration continued on following page

Oblique Osteotomy: Mayo Posteromedial Exposure (Bryan, Morrey)[4,19]

Indications

The Mayo posteromedial approach is used for joint arthroplasty, elbow dislocation, T and Y and medial condylar fractures, synovial disease, and infection.

Description of Technique

The patient is placed in the lateral decubitus or supine position, with a sandbag under the scapula. A nonsterile pneumatic tourniquet is applied high on the arm and the forearm is brought across the chest (Fig. 23–21). A straight posterior incision is made medial to the midline, approximately 10 cm proximal and 7 cm distal to the tip of the olecranon. The ulnar nerve is

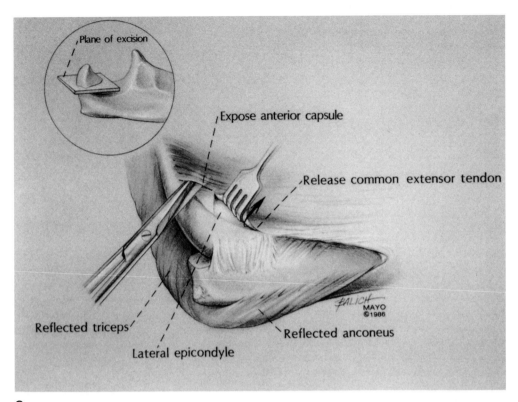

C

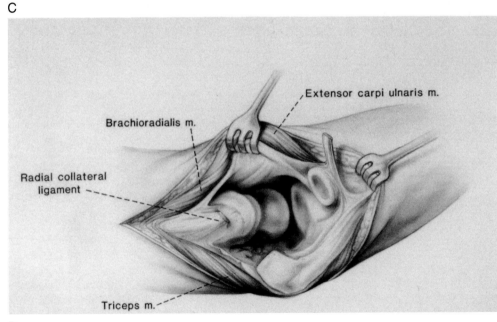

D

Figure 23–18. *Continued.* **D**, Release of the radial collateral ligament at its humeral origin allows the joint to sublux, exposing the entire distal humeral articulation. (From Morrey BF, Schneeberger A: Anconeus arthroplasty. J Bone Joint Surg 84A, 2002.)

identified proximally in the epineural fat at the margin of the medial head of the triceps and, depending on the procedure, is either protected or carefully dissected free of the cubital tunnel to its first motor branch.

The medial aspect of the triceps is elevated from the humerus and the posterior capsule is incised. The superficial fascia of the forearm is then incised distally for about 6 cm, to the periosteum just to the medial aspect of the crest of the proximal ulna. The periosteum and fascia complex is carefully reflected laterally. The medial part of the ulnar tissue complex is the weakest portion of the reflected tissue; therefore, care must be exerted to maintain continuity of the triceps mechanism at this point. The remaining portion of the triceps mechanism then is reflected by releasing its attachment to the olecranon. The anconeus is elevated subperiosteally from the proximal ulna, and the remaining fibers of the triceps are freed from the posterior aspect of the lateral column, thus widely exposing the entire joint, including the radial head.

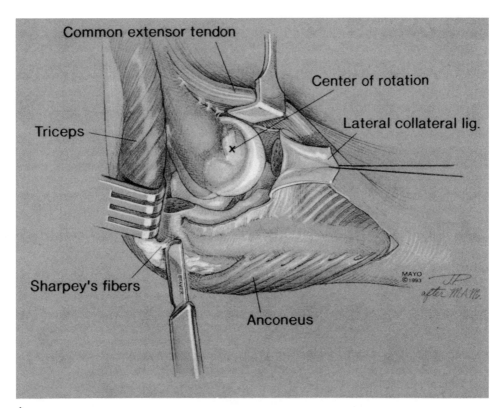

A

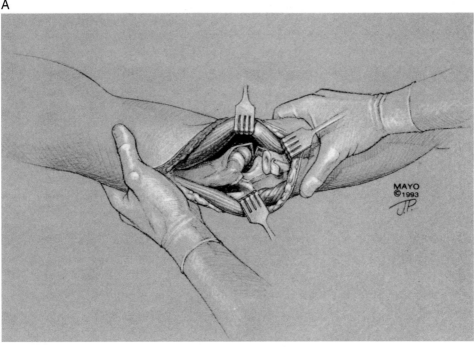

B

Figure 23–19. The Mayo modified extensile Köcher approach. The triceps attachment to the tip of the olecranon may be released by sharp dissection (**A**), allowing complete translation of the extensor mechanism medially and providing more extensile exposure to the joint (**B**).

The tip of the olecranon is removed for clear visualization of the trochlea. The ligaments are released medially and laterally from the humerus. In cases of semiconstrained joint replacement, repair of these ligaments is not necessary. The triceps is returned to its anatomic position and sutured directly to the bone of the proximal end of the ulna. The periosteum then is sutured to the superficial forearm fascia as far as the margin of the flexor carpi ulnaris. The tourniquet is deflated, hemostasis is secured, and the wound is drained and closed in layers.

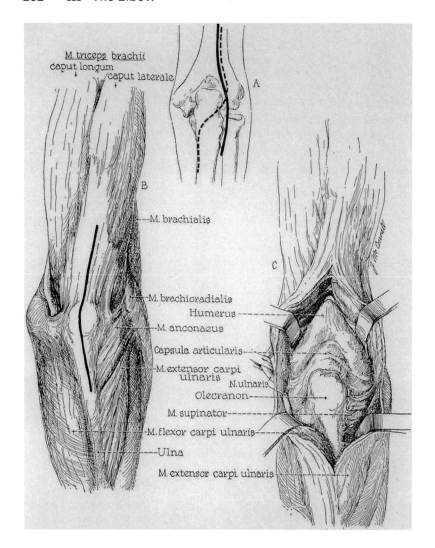

Figure 23–20. The original description of the Campbell posterior muscle-splitting approach calls for a curved incision, but I prefer a straight one just lateral to the tip of the olecranon and the subcutaneous border of the ulna. (From Anson BJ, McVaya CR: Surgical Anatomy, 5th ed, vol 2. Philadelphia, WB Saunders, 1971.)

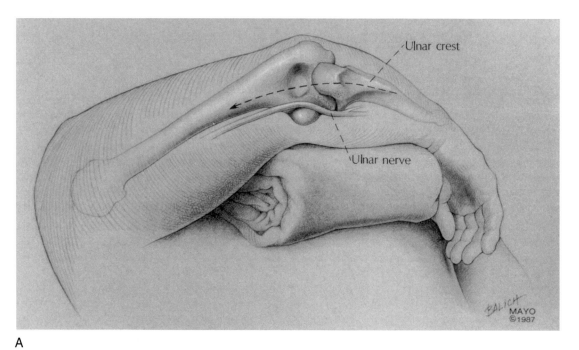

Figure 23–21. The Bryan-Morrey posterior approach. **A**, A straight posterior skin incision (approximately 14 cm) is made.

Illustration continued on opposite page

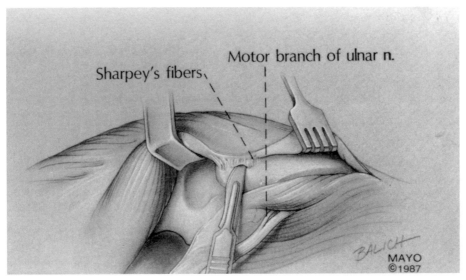

B

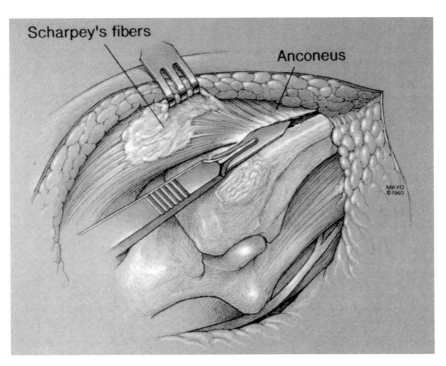

C

Figure 23–21. *Continued.* **B,** The medial border of the triceps is identified and released, and the superficial forearm fascia is sharply incised to allow reflection of the fascia and periosteum from the proximal ulna. The ulnar nerve has been translocated anteriorly to subcutaneous tissue. **C,** The extensor mechanism is being reflected laterally, and the anconeus is being subperiosteally released from the ulna, allowing exposure of the radial head. The junction of the ulna, periosteum, and fascia with the insertion site of Sharpey's fibers is the most tenuous portion of the reflected mechanism. The proximal olecranon is removed for joint exposure.

Illustration continued on following page

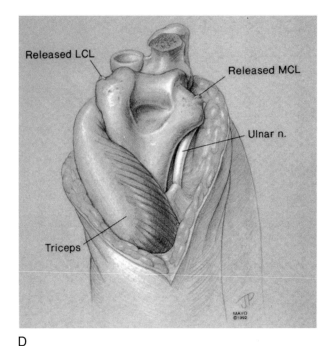

D

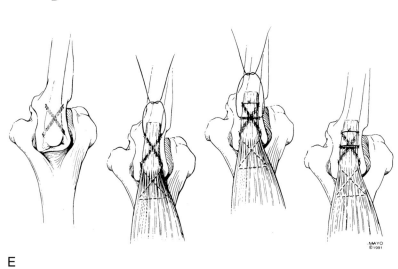

E

Figure 23–21. *Continued.* **D**, The shoulder is externally rotated and the forearm is hyperflexed. Release of the collateral ligaments allows the ulna to separate from the humerus, providing excellent exposure. **E**, The triceps is reattached by a heavy (No. 5), nonabsorbable suture placed through crossed holes in the ulna with a criss-cross stitch in the triceps tendon. An additional transverse suture secures the triceps to the tip of the olecranon. (From Morrey BF [ed]: The Elbow. Philadelphia, Lippincott Williams & Wilkins, 1994, by permission of Mayo Foundation.)

A variation of this exposure releases the triceps with its osseous attachment as a wafer of bone instead of reflecting the tendon sharply from the ulna.[28]

References

1. Anson BJ, McVaya CR: Surgical Anatomy, 5th ed, vol 2. Philadelphia, WB Saunders, 1971.
2. Atkinson WB, Elftman H: The carrying angle of the human arm as a secondary sex character. Anat Rec 91:46, 1945.
3. Banks SW, Laufman H: An Atlas of Surgical Exposures of the Extremities, 2nd ed. Philadelphia, WB Saunders, 1987.
4. Bryan RS, Morrey BF: Extensive posterior exposure of the elbow, a triceps-sparing approach. Clin Orthop 166:188, 1982.
5. Campbell WC: Incision for exposure of the elbow joint. Am J Surg 15:65, 1932.
6. Campbell WC: Surgical approaches. *In* Edmonson AS, Crehnshaw AH (eds): Campbell's Operative Orthopedics, 6th Ed, Vol 1. St. Louis, CV Mosby, 1971, p 119.
7. Capener N: The vulnerability of the posterior interosseous nerve of the forearm, a case report and anatomic study. J Bone Joint Surg 48B:770, 1966.

8. Ebraheim NA, Andreshak TG, Yeasting RA, et al: Posterior extensible approach to the elbow joint and distal humerus. Orthop Rev 22:578, 1993.

9. Eycleshymer AC, Schoemaker DM: A Cross-Section Anatomy. New York, D Appleton, 1930.

10. Gardner E: The innervation of the elbow joint. Anat Rec 102:161, 1948.

11. Hollinshead WH: The back and limbs. In Anatomy for Surgeons, vol 3. New York, Harper & Row, 1969.

12. Kocher T: Textbook of Operative Surgery, 3rd ed. Translated by H. J. Stiles and C. B. Paul. London, A&C Black, 1911.

13. Langman J, Woerdeman MW: Atlas of Medical Anatomy. Philadelphia, WB Saunders, 1976.

14. Lanz T, Wachsmuth W: Praktische Anatomie. Berlin, ARM, Springer-Verlag, 1959.

15. MacAusland WR: Ankylosis of the elbow: With report of four cases treated by arthroplasty. JAMA 64:312, 1915.

16. Martin BF: The annular ligament of the superior radial ulnar joint. J Anat 52:473, 1956.

17. Morrey BF: Applied anatomy and biomechanics of the elbow joint. Instr Course 35:59, 1986.

18. Morrey BF (ed): The Elbow and Its Disorders, 3rd ed. Philadelphia, WB Saunders Company, 2000.

19. Morrey BF: Elbow exposures. In Morrey BF (ed): Master Techniques in Orthopedic Surgery: The Elbow. New York, Raven Press, 1994, p 59.

20. Morrey BF, An KN: Functional anatomy of the ligaments of the elbow. Clin Orthop 201:84, 1985.

21. Morrey BF, Ho E: Surgical correction for triceps insufficiency. J Bone Joint Surg 69A:523–532, 1987.

22. Morrey BF, Schneeberger A: Anconeus arthroplasty. J Bone Joint Surg 84A, 2002.

23. O'Driscoll SW, Horii E, Carmichael SW, Morrey BF: The cubital tunnel and ulnar neuropathy. J Bone Joint Surg 73B:613, 1991.

24. O'Driscoll SW, Horii E, Morrey BF, Carmichael SW: Anatomy of the ulnar part of the lateral collateral ligament of the elbow. Clin Anat 5:296, 1992.

25. Schwab GH, Bennett JB, Woods GW, Tullos HS: The biomechanics of elbow stability, the role of the medial collateral ligament. Clin Orthop 146:42, 1980.

26. Wevers HW, Siu DW, Brookhoven LH, Sorbie C: Resurfacing elbow prosthesis: Shape and sizing of the humerus component. J Biomech Surg 7:241, 1985.

27. Witt JD, Kamineni S: The posterior interosseous nerve and the posterolateral approach to the proximal radius. J Bone Joint Surg 80B:240, 1998.

28. Wolfe SW, Ranawat CS: The osteo-anconeus flap: An approach for total elbow arthroplasty. J Bone Joint Surg 72A:684, 1990.

29. Yamaguchi K, Sweet FA, Bindra R, et al: The extraosseous and intraosseous arterial anatomy of the adult elbow. J Bone Joint Surg 79A:1653, 1997.

24

Relevant Biomechanics

• KAI-NAN AN and BERNARD F. MORREY

As with any joint reconstructive procedure, a clear and detailed understanding of the relevant biomechanics of the joint is essential. Although the mechanics of the elbow have traditionally been considered somewhat complex, the understanding may be simplified if the discussion is arbitrarily divided into the main joint functions: motion, stability (constraints), and strength (forces).[17] These features are briefly discussed in the context of joint reconstructive surgery.

MOTION

The elbow is classified as a trochleoginglymoid joint; that is, it has two degrees of freedom: flexion-extension and axial rotation. Technically, this motion is considered both rolling and spinning.

Characteristics

Axis of Rotation

The axis of rotation of flexion-extension has been defined as occurring about a tight locus of points measuring only 2 to 3 mm in the broadest dimension (Fig. 24–1).[26] This locus is positioned at the center of the projected center of the trochlea and at the center of the capitellum.[16] This is one of the most important features of the biomechanics of this joint, because replication of this axis is essential for the proper balancing of soft tissue, particularly necessary in resurfacing joint replacement,[6,8] distraction arthroplasty,[18] and ligament reconstruction[27] and for optimum strength after replacement.[23]

Carrying Angle

The carrying angle of the elbow joint is replicated by all joint replacement implants by angular changes either at the humerus, the ulna, or both. Any of these design approaches may be considered biomechanically sound,[2,7] and this characteristic is of importance primarily to balance the collateral ligaments in resurfacing joint replacement.

Functional Motion

Although the elbow has a normal arc of flexion-extension of 0 to 150 to 160 degrees and pronation-supination of 75 to 85 degrees,[5] the full arc of motion is not generally used for most activities of daily living. Most such activities can be carried out with an arc of motion of 30 to 130 degrees of flexion-extension (Fig. 24–2) and by 50 degrees of pronation and 50 degrees of supination.[24]

CONSTRAINTS

Understanding the constraints of the elbow is simplified by dividing these elements into static and dynamic contributions. The static contribution to elbow stability is

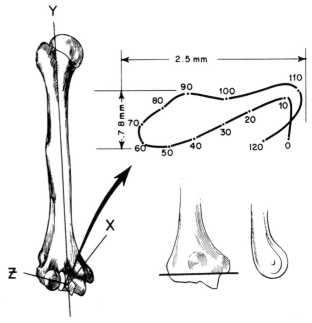

Figure 24–1. Very small locus of instant center of rotation for the elbow joint demonstrates that the axis may be replicated by a single line drawn from the inferior aspect of the medial epicondyle through the center of the lateral epicondyle, which is in the center of the lateral projected curvature of the trochlea and capitellum. (Modified from Morrey BF, Chao EY: Passive motion of the elbow joint. J Bone Joint Surg Am 58:501, 1976.)

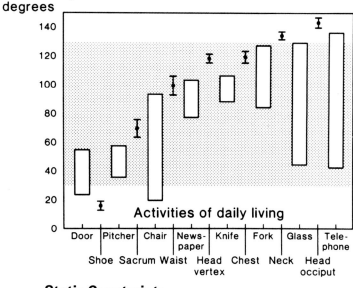

Elbow flexion, degrees

Activities of daily living

Door Shoe | Pitcher Sacrum | Chair Waist | News-paper | Knife Head vertex | Fork Chest | Glass Neck | Tele-phone Head occiput

Figure 24–2. Functional arc of elbow motion for activities of daily living is approximately 100 degrees (between 30 and 103 degrees). (Adapted from Morrey BF, Askew LJ, An KN, Chao EY: A biomechanical study of functional elbow motion. J Bone Joint Surg Am 63:872, 1981.)

Table 24–1. PERCENT CONTRIBUTION OF RESTRAINING VARUS-VALGUS DISPLACEMENT

Position	Component*	Percent Contribution	
		Varus	*Valgus*
Extension	MCL	—	30
	LCL	15	—
	Capsule	30	40
	Articulation	55	30
Flexion	MCL	—	55
	LCL	10	—
	Articulation	75	35

*MCL, medial collateral ligament complex; LCL, lateral collateral ligament complex.

further subdivided into articular and ligamentous capsular features. In general, it may be concluded that the articular and ligamentous components to joint stability are about equally divided[19] (Table 24–1). The articular contribution is further subdivided into the radiohumeral and ulnohumeral joints.

Static Constraints

Articular Contribution

RADIOHUMERAL JOINT

The role of the radial head in preventing valgus instability of the elbow has been a source of speculation for many years. The three-dimensional displacement characteristics of the elbow following medial collateral ligament and radial head removal have been studied with a magnetic field–generating telemetry system.[1] When the radial head is removed first, virtually no change in valgus or axial stability of the joint is demonstrated.[22] However, when the medial collateral ligament is removed, the elbow becomes unstable and subluxes. Conversely, when the anterior bundle of the medial collateral ligament is removed first, a modest but definite and consistent instability to valgus and axial rotation is present (Fig. 24–3). However, with subsequent removal of the radial head, dramatic instability ensues.

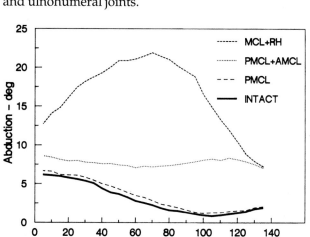

A

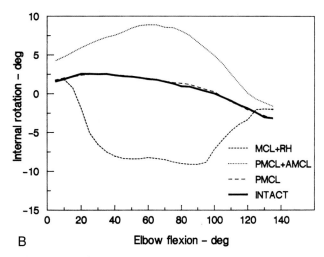

B

Figure 24–3. A, The valgus stability of the elbow is slightly altered by release of both elements of the medial collateral ligament, with dramatic instability and subluxation if the radial head is then removed. **B,** Axial rotation of the elbow is changed moderately when both elements of the medial ligament are removed. When the radial head is removed last, the elbow becomes unstable and subluxes.

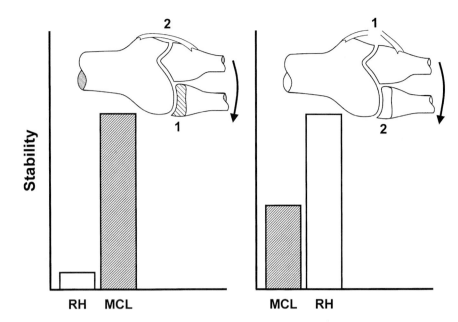

Figure 24–4. Diagrammatic representation demonstrating that the radial head is a secondary stabilizer to the elbow in valgus stress, whereas the medial collateral ligament should be considered a primary stabilizer.

The interpretation leaves one to conclude that the radial head should be considered a secondary stabilizer of the joint. The implications are obvious: The radial head must be preserved or its function replicated if there is medial collateral ligament dysfunction (Fig. 24–4).

The kinematics and stability of the elbow joint after implant replacement have been evaluated using the same model. The motion pattern depends on the articular geometry of the implant and the compressive force across the joint. The maximum valgus-varus laxity of the Souter-Strathclyde implant was 6.5 degrees, which was slightly greater than that of the intact elbow at 4.3 degrees, whereas the rotatory laxity was similar to that of the intact elbow.[31] The maximum valgus-varus laxity was reduced to 4.8 degrees with increased muscle load-ing. The maximum valgus-varus laxity are 9.6, 9.7, and 10.8 degrees for the Norway, the Capitellocondylar, and the Coonrad-Morrey prostheses, respectively.

ULNOHUMERAL JOINT

The elbow joint is one of the most congruent joints of the body. The contact area of the ulna with respect to the trochlea may be considered to consist of two anterior and two posterior articulating surfaces on the coronoid and olecranon, respectively (Fig. 24–5).[11,12,34] Loss of the olecranon is unimportant for stability,[3] but loss of the coronoid allows posterior ulnar displacement that is difficult or impossible to reconstruct effectively.[30]

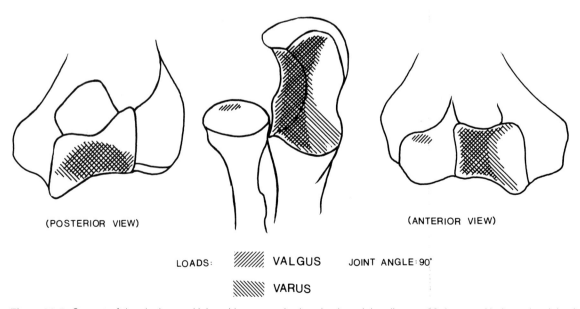

Figure 24–5. Contact of the ulnohumeral joint with varus and valgus loads and the elbow at 90 degrees. Notice only minimal radiohumeral contact in this loading condition. (From Stormont TJ, An KN, Morrey BF, Chao EY: Elbow joint contact study: comparison of techniques. J Biomech 18:329, 1985.)

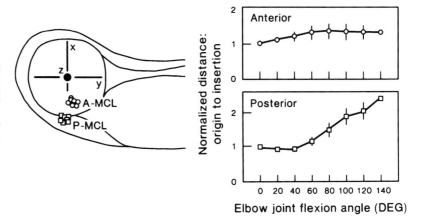

Figure 24–6. The medial collateral ligament does not originate from the axis of rotation. Thus slight changes in length relationship as a function of elbow flexion are observed. Of the two elements, the anterior bundle of the medial collateral ligament is most isometric. (Modified from Morrey BF, An RN: Functional anatomy of the ligaments of the elbow. Clin Orthop 201:84, 1985.)

Ligaments

The anatomy of the medial and lateral collateral ligament complexes has been discussed in detail in Chapter 23. The origin of the medial ulnar collateral components does not coincide with the axis of flexion, although the anterior bundle of the complex is almost isometric during flexion (Fig. 24–6).[20] In contrast, the lateral collateral complex originates at the axis of rotation. Hence, this ligament is isometric during elbow flexion (Fig. 24–7). The anterior bundle of the ulnar collateral ligament has been shown to be the prime valgus stabilizer of the elbow.[10,33] The lateral ulnar collateral ligament has been demonstrated to play a similar role in varus and rotatory stability of the joint.[28] Advanced measurement techniques also have been used to study the role of soft tissue constraints after semiconstrained arthroplasty. The typical motion pattern is within the balance of the articulation, implying that the out-of-plane forces are absorbed by soft tissue constraints before being transmitted to the bone-cement interface[29] (Fig. 24–8). Sectioning of the lateral collateral ligament or the medial collateral ligament significant increased the joint laxity of the elbow joint after implant replacement (Fig. 24–9).[15]

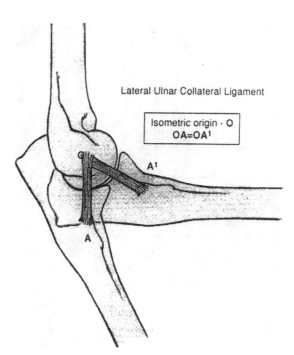

Figure 24–7. The lateral collateral ligament originates right at the axis of rotation. Thus there is little change in the length of this ligament as a function of elbow flexion.

Figure 24–8. Semiconstrained Mayo-modified Coonrad implant demonstrates an amplitude of varus-valgus rotation during elbow flexion that is less than that provided by the articulation. This suggests that the soft tissue partially stabilizes the implant.

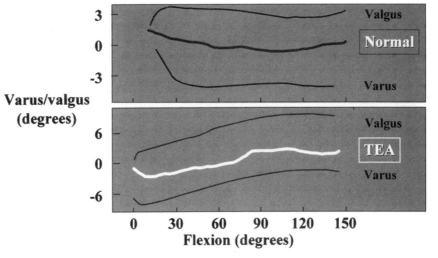

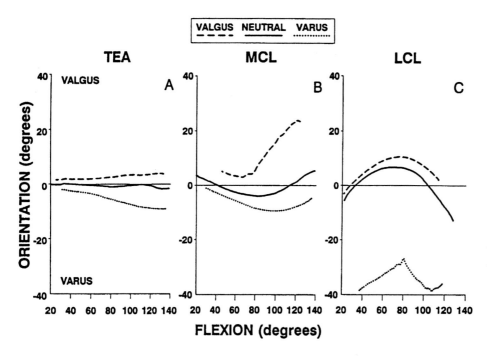

Figure 24–9. The motion patterns of the capitellocondylar elbow prostheses after lateral collateral ligament (LCL) sectioning. **A**, The motion after arthroplasty with the ligament still intact. **B**, After sectioning of the medial collateral ligament (MCL). The elbow became markedly unstable with valgus loading. **C**, After sectioning of the LCL. Gross varus instability occurred after the lateral ulnar and radial collateral ligaments were removed. (From King GJW, Itoi E, Nieber GL, et al: Motion and laxity of the capitellocondylar total elbow prosthesis. J Bone Joint Surg Am 76:1000–1008, 1994.)

Dynamic Effect

What few studies have been done on the dynamic stabilizers of the elbow suggest a minimal to modest influence on varus-valgus stability.[9] The flexor and extensor motors tend to posteriorly displace the ulnohumeral joint, but they do provide a slight varus-valgus stabilizing effect.[22] The overall dynamic effect of the flexors and extensors is well known to posteriorly displace the forearm referable to the humerus at 90 degrees of flexion. It is for this reason that the resurfacing implants tend to dislocate in this position. Fractures of the coronoid also demonstrate this dynamic effect, with the tendency for posterior displacement of the ulna referable to the humerus at 90 degrees.

JOINT FORCES

Radiohumeral Joint

Static axial load of the extended joint has revealed that about 40 percent of forces are transmitted through the radiohumeral joint and 60 percent through the ulnohumeral articulation,[12,13,35] and that the absolute force through the radial head exceeds several times body weight.[21]

The force transmission across the radiohumeral joint also decreases in supination and increases in pronation (Fig. 24–10). This apparently is due to a screw-home mechanism of the radius with respect to the ulna,[21] with slight proximal migration occurring in pronation and slight distal translation occurring in supination. This observation is important in designing rehabilitation programs that protect the radiohumeral joint for such conditions as osteochondritis dissecans and radial head fracture and • prosthetic replacement.[25]

Ulnohumeral Joint

The force across a joint is dependent on the efficiency of the muscle(s) that are recruited. For the elbow, the least efficiency is in extension (the shortest moment arm) and the greatest efficiency is at 90 degrees of flexion (Fig. 24–11). When lifting weight, the maximum flexion strengths for an average normal person range from 100 N with the elbow in the extended position to 400 N with the elbow at the 90-degree flexed position.[4,14] The placement of the implant could influence the kinematics and the muscle moment arms of the elbow joint and, eventually, the muscle and joint forces.[32]

Calculations under these loading conditions suggest that the resultant joint force through the ulnohumeral

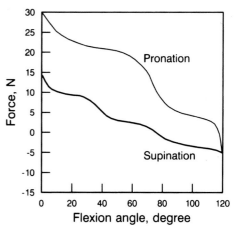

Figure 24–10. During all flexion angles of the elbow, pronation is associated with greater force transmission across the radiohumeral joint than is supination. (Modified from Morrey BF, An KN, Stormont TJ: Force transmission through the radial head. J Bone Joint Surg Am 70:250, 1988.)

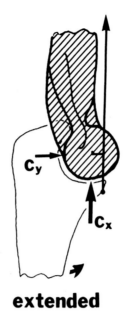
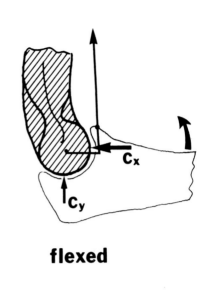

Figure 24–11. The mechanical advantage of elbow flexors changes depending on the position of the forearm. As the lever arm increases at 90 degrees of flexion, greater torque can be generated even though the resultant force across the elbow does not increase.

extended

flexed

joint can range from one to three times body weight (Fig. 24–12). When the elbow is in the extended position, the resultant joint force points anteriorly. When the elbow is in a more flexed position, the resultant force points posteriorly. The cyclic, high-grade load applied to the elbow justifies consideration of the elbow as a weight-bearing joint and further accounts for the high loosening rate seen in the early constrained joints in which motion transmitted across the

articulation was directed to the bone-cement interface (Fig. 24–13).

DESIGN CONSIDERATIONS

Based on the above review of the biomechanics of the joint, the optimum replacement elbow joint should be adequately designed so that it can be reliably implanted

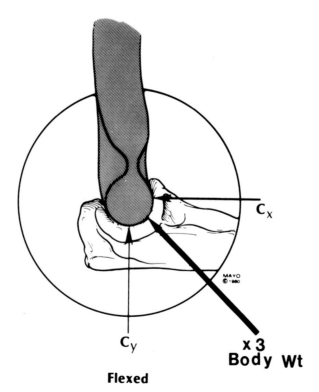

Flexed

Figure 24–12. Under strenuous lifting of weight in the hand, up to three times body weight can be transmitted across the elbow joint. The direction of these resultant forces changes with joint angle.

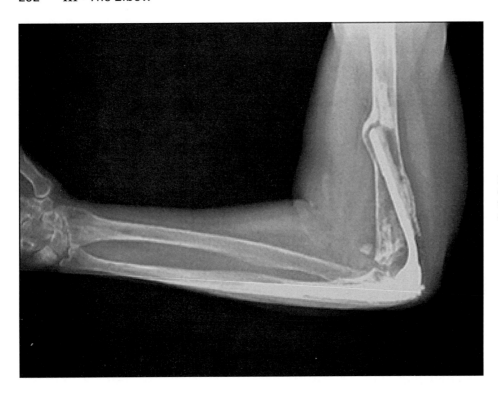

Figure 24–13. Typical loosening pattern of a fixed hinge implant, with the tip of the prosthesis eroding superiorly and anteriorly through the humerus.

in a manner to replicate the axis of rotation. The surgical technique should be designed to preserve as much as possible of the soft tissue ligamentous constraints; if violated, these must be anatomically repaired when using the resurfacing options. Anatomic placement of the axis of rotation provides the proper mechanical advantage of flexors and extensors that allows the patient to have the best possible restoration of strength function. The intramedullary stem fixation is probably not adequate to resist the stresses imparted to the system. A supplementary flange placed in the distal aspect of the humerus tends to resist the adverse effects of the posterosuperior force as the elbow initiates and completes the flexion movement (Fig. 24–14). In addition, this design characteristic resists axial rotation of the implant as well, thus lessening the overall complication rate of loosening.

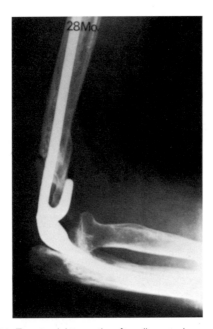

Figure 24–14. Twenty-eight months after elbow replacement for post-traumatic arthritis with the new Mayo-modified Coonrad implant. The anterior or distal humeral cortex has hypertrophied because it has been in close approximation to the flange.

References

1. An KN, Jacobsen MC, Berglund LJ, Chao EYS: Application of a magnetic tracking device to kinesiologic studies. J Biomech 21:613, 1988.
2. An KN, Morrey BF, Chao EYS: Carrying angle of the human elbow joint. J Orthop Res 1:369, 1984.
3. An KN, Morrey BF, Chao EYS: The effect of partial removal of the proximal ulna on elbow constraint. Clin Orthop 209:270, 1986.
4. Askew LJ, An KN, Morrey BF, Chao EYS: Isometric elbow strength in normal individuals. Clin Orthop 222:261, 1987.
5. Boone DC, Azen SP: Normal range of motion of joints in male subjects. J Bone Joint Surg Am 61:756, 1979.
6. Evans GB, Daniels AU, Serbousek JC, Mann RJ: A comparison of the mechanical designs of articulating total elbow prostheses. Clin Mater 3:235, 1988.
7. Figgie HE III, Inglis AE, Gordan NH, et al: A critical analysis of mechanical factors correlated with bone remodeling following total elbow arthroplasty. J Arthroplasty 1:175, 1986.
8. Figgie HE III, Inglis AE, Mow C: A critical analysis of alignment factors affecting functional outcome in total elbow arthroplasty. J Arthroplasty 1:169, 1986.
9. Funk DA, An KN, Morrey BF, Daube JR: Electromyographic analysis of muscles across the elbow joint. J Orthop Res 5:529, 1987.
10. Fuss FK: The ulnar collateral ligament of the human elbow joint: anatomy, function and biomechanics. J Anat 175:203, 1991.
11. Goel VK, Smith D, Bijlani V: Contact areas in human elbow joints. J Biomech 104:169, 1982.
12. Hall AA, Travill R: Transmission of pressures across the elbow joint. Anat Rec 150:243, 1964.

13. Hotchkiss RN, An KN, Sowa DT, et al: An anatomic and mechanical study of the interosseous membrane of the forearm: pathomechanics of proximal migration of the radius. J Hand Surg 14:256, 1989.
14. Jorgensen K, Bankov S: Maximum strength of elbow flexors with pronated supinated forearm. Med Sport Biomech 6:174, 1971.
15. King GJW, Itoi E, Neibur GL, et al: Motion and laxity of the capitellocondylar total elbow prosthesis. J Bone Joint Surg Am 76:1000–1008, 1994.
16. London JT: Kinematics of the elbow. J Bone Joint Surg Am 63:529, 1981.
17. Morrey BF: Applied anatomy and biomechanics of the elbow joint. Instr Course Lect 35:59, 1986.
18. Morrey BF: Posttraumatic contracture of the elbow: operative treatment including distraction arthroplasty. J Bone Joint Surg Am 72:601, 1990.
19. Morrey BF, An KN: Articular ligamentous contributions to the stability of the elbow joint. Am J Sports Med 11:315, 1983.
20. Morrey BF, An KN: Functional anatomy of the ligaments of the elbow. Clin Orthop 201:84, 1985.
21. Morrey BF, An KN, Stormont TJ: Force transmission through the radial head. J Bone Joint Surg Am 70:250, 1988.
22. Morrey BF, An KN, Tanaka S: Valgus stability of the elbow: a definition of primary and secondary constraints. Clin Orthop 265:187, 1991.
23. Morrey BF, Askew LJ, An KN: Strength function after elbow arthroplasty. Clin Orthop 234:43, 1988.
24. Morrey BF, Askew LJ, An KN, Chao EY: A biomechanical study of functional elbow motion. J Bone Joint Surg Am 63:872, 1981.
25. Morrey BF, Askew LJ, Chao EY: Silastic prosthetic replacement of the radial head. J Bone Joint Surg Am 63A:454, 1981.
26. Morrey BF, Chao EY: Passive motion of the elbow joint. J Bone Joint Surg Am 58:501, 1976.
27. Nestor BJ, O'Driscoll SW, Morrey BF: Ligamentous reconstruction for posterolateral rotatory instability of the elbow. J Bone Joint Surg Am 74:1235, 1992.
28. O'Driscoll SW, Bell DF, Morrey BF: Posterolateral rotatory instability of the elbow. J Bone Joint Surg Am 73:440, 1991.
29. O'Driscoll SW, Tanaka S, An KN, Morrey BF: The kinematics of the semiconstrained total elbow prosthesis. J Bone Joint Surg Br 74:297, 1992.
30. Regan W, Morrey BF: Fractures of the coronoid process of the ulna. J Bone Joint Surg Am 71:1348, 1989.
31. Schneeberger AG, King GJW, Song SW, et al: Kinematics and laxity of the Souter-Strathclyde total elbow prosthesis. J Shoulder Elbow Surg 9:127–134, 2000.
32. Schuind F, O'Driscoll SW, Korinek S, et al: Changes of elbow muscle moment arms after total elbow arthroplasty. J Shoulder Elbow Surg 3:191–199, 1994.
33. Schwab GH, Bennett JB, Woods GW, Tullos HS: Biomechanics of elbow instability: the role of the medial collateral ligament. Clin Orthop 146:42, 1980.
34. Stormont TJ, An KN, Morrey BF, Chao EY: Elbow joint contact study: comparison of techniques. J Biomech 18:329, 1985.
35. Walker PS: Human Joints and Their Artificial Replacements Springfield, IL: Charles C Thomas, 1977, p 182.

25

Radial Head Prosthetic Replacement

• BERNARD F. MORREY

The first English-language reference we can find to prosthetic replacement of the radial head is that of Speed in 1941[19] describing a Vitallium implant employed in three patients. Cherry[3] discussed limited experience with an acrylic implant a decade later, and the modern use of a silicone radial head implant was popularized by Swanson.[20] The logical basic reason to use a radial head implant is to enhance function, and success is measured by the ability to restore axial or angular (valgus) stability. Morrey et al. have shown that the medial head is an important stabilizer of the elbow if the medial collateral ligament is deficient.[17] King et al. subsequently demonstrated that the deficiency can be effectively compensated by metallic but not Silastic radial head implant.[11]

INDICATIONS

A "complicated" radial head fracture is considered the indication for the use of the prosthesis. Such a fracture is seen in six clinical settings[7,8]:

1. Dislocation of the elbow with radial head fracture (type IV fracture)
2. Concurrent medial collateral ligament disruption
3. Concurrent or residual lateral ulnar collateral ligament dysfunction
4. Monteggia variant with olecranon and radial head fracture
5. Fracture of the coronoid
6. As a reconstruction option

If the elbow dislocates, the medial collateral ligament is torn and, if the radial head is excised, the elbow is grossly unstable. In this setting replacement with a radial head prosthesis will enhance stability and allow early motion (Fig. 25–1). Increased valgus angulation, probably resulting from concurrent medial ligament injury,[8,9,17,18] may also be addressed with use of a prosthetic radial head.[12,20] Instability of the proximal radius associated with severe fractures or excessive excision[12,19,22] may be lessened with use of an implant. With large type II coronoid fractures, considerably enhanced stability is offered by the radial head, hence the prosthesis may provide some element of stability in this clinical setting

(Fig. 25–2). Finally, the implant stabilizes the radius if the head is removed in the presence of interosseous membrane and distal radioulnar joint disruption.

PROSTHETIC DESIGN

The early prostheses were made of Vitallium[19,22] or acrylic,[3] but the Silastic Swanson was certainly the most commonly used in this country[14,15,21] and abroad.[12,13] However, the host of complications coupled with the poor mechanical properties of Silastic to withstand axial load have dramatically lessened the use of this material as a prosthetic radial head replacement. Gupta and colleagues have recently assessed the mechanical properties of cobalt/chrome, titanium alloy, alumina ceramic, and ultra-high-molecular-weight polyethylene.[6] Any of the rigid implants were shown to be clearly superior to the Silastic device, and several are now commercially available (Fig. 25–3).

The bipolar design of Judet is a real advance in design concept[10] (Fig. 25–4). However, concern does exist regarding the extent of the exposure necessary to implant the device as a result of the length of the stem and the fact that the relatively thick radial head implant requires excision of considerable bone. Because of the increasing recognition of the "complex instability" of fracture-dislocation, and because of the theoretical advantages of radial head replacement in this setting, renewed interest has been generated in prosthetic replacement and hence in an improved implant design. The newer designs have several size options, flexibility at the articulation, and enhanced instrumentation to allow accurate and reproducible implantation. At the Mayo Clinic, we have developed a replacement that is designed to be more easily inserted and provides the flexibility of surgery options necessary to treat the pathology that occurs at this joint (Fig. 25–3C).

TECHNIQUE (rHEAD, AVANTA)

Exposure

A supine position and capsular exposure through Köcher's interval is employed (Fig. 25–5). The lateral

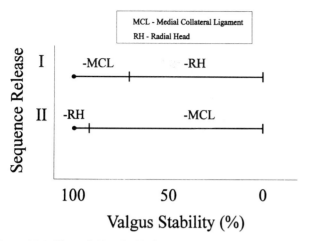

Figure 25–1. The radial head adds little stability if the medial collateral ligament (MCL) is intact. If the MCL is torn, the radial head assumes an important secondary stabilizing role. (Copyright Mayo Foundation.)

capsule is entered slightly anterior to the collateral ligament, and the annular ligament and capsule are reflected anteriorly and posteriorly to expose the radial head. A portion of the lateral collateral ligament and anterior capsule can be reflected from the lateral epicondyle and anterior humerus to facilitate exposure if necessary. Efforts are made not to detach the lateral ulnohumeral ligament, but, if greater exposure is required, the ligament is reflected from its humeral origin. If the ligament has been disrupted, then the exposure progresses through the site of disruption to expose the radiohumeral joint. The common extensor tendon and anterior capsule are retracted as needed for adequate exposure (Fig. 25–6).

Resection Guide

Congruous prosthetic articulation requires an accurate resection that provides precise implant placement. A resection guide has thus been developed to replicate the anatomic axis of forearm rotation using the capitellum and ulnar styloid as landmarks. The cutting guide is adjusted proximally or distally for the desired amount of radial head resection.

Resecting the Radial Head

During resection, forearm rotation should be assessed to ensure resection perpendicular to the axis of rotation (Fig. 25–7). The distal extent of resection is the minimal amount that is consistent with the restoration of function as dictated by the fracture line or previous radial head resection but still compatible with implant insertion and length restoration options for the design being used.

Intramedullary Preparation

Varus stress and rotation of the forearm allows exposure of the medullary canal, especially if the elbow is unstable. If the stability does not allow exposure of the proximal radius, careful reflection of the origin of the collateral ligament from the lateral epicondyle may be necessary to permit adequate exposure to the medullary canal. The canal is entered with a starter awl using a twisting motion, followed by the curved broach (Fig. 25–8).

Trial Reduction

The appropriate-sized trial stem is inserted with a rotating motion, placing the stem down the canal (Fig. 25–9). The appropriate-sized trial head is then applied (Fig. 25–10). Tracking, both in flexion and extension and in forearm rotation, should be carefully assessed. If the collateral ligament has been released, that is compensated for during the trial reduction. Malalignment of the radial osteotomy cut will cause malseating of the implant and hence abnormal tracking during flexion-extension and/or forearm pronation and supination.

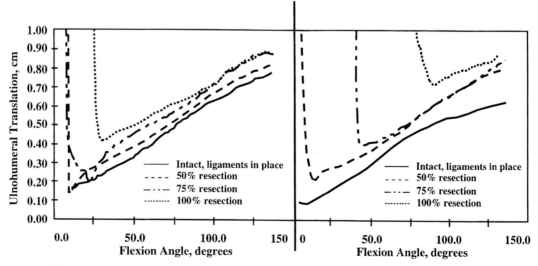

Figure 25–2. When approximately 50% of the coronoid is absent, the radial head assumes an important role in elbow stability.

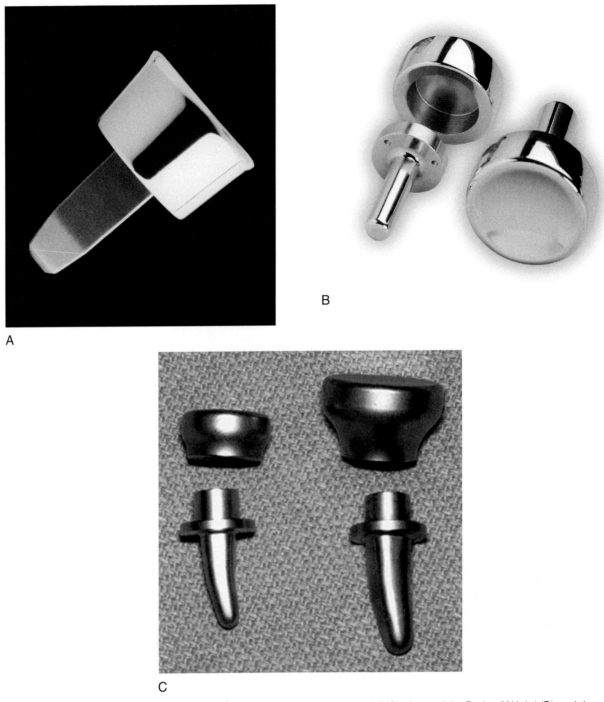

Figure 25–3. Metallic implants are now available as the monoblock (Wright) (**A**), the modular Evolve (Wright) (**B**), and the rHead (Avanta) (**C**).

Implanting the Final Components

Once proper size, alignment, and positioning of the implant have been determined, the prosthetic radial stem is inserted with a rotational motion down the medullary canal and tapped in place with the impactor. Bone cement (polymethylmethacrylate [PMMA]) may occasionally be used if secure press-fit fixation is not attainable, but I try to avoid the use of PMMA in all settings. The modular head is next placed over the taper

using longitudinal distraction and/or varus stress to distract the radiocapitellar interface sufficiently to permit the radial head to be inserted. The radial head implant is secured using the impactor. Alignment is again assessed.

Closure

Reconstitution of the lateral ulnar collateral ligament (LUCL) is essential at closure. If the ligamentous tissue

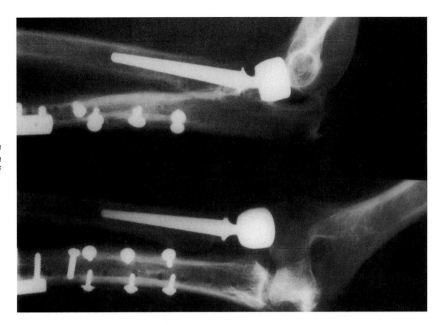

Figure 25–4. The articulated "bipolar" device designed by Judet represents a real advance in the concept of radial head replacement. (Courtesy of Tornier SA, Saint-Ismier, France.)

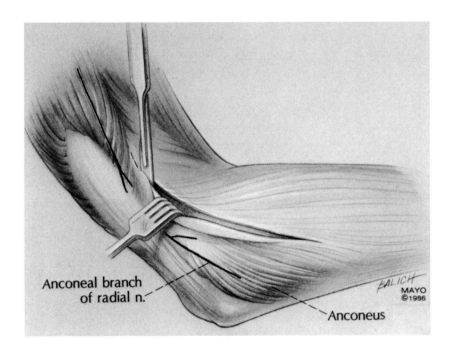

Figure 25–5. The patient is placed in a supine position with the arm brought across the chest. A Köcher incision is made and the interval between the anconeus and extensor carpi ulnaris is developed.

appears inadequate, it should be reinforced with a No. 5 nonabsorbable Bunnell or Krackow suture (Fig. 25–11). For reconstruction applications, a formal LUCL substitute with tendon allograft (palmaris) or autograft (plantaris) may be necessary.

Aftercare

Passive flexion and extension is allowed on the second day, assuming the elbow is stable. The goal of radial head replacement and soft tissue repair/reconstruction is to achieve elbow stability. Both flexion-extension and pronation-supination arcs are allowed without restriction. Active motion can begin by day 5.

Long-term aftercare requires surveillance, as is the case with any prosthetic replacement. If the implant is asymptomatic and tracks well, routine implant removal is not necessary.

RESULTS

The use of the Silastic implant is plagued with complications ranging from mechanical inadequacy to adverse response from particulate debris, so this implant is no longer used to any extent.[1,22] The Vitallium metallic replacement did provide satisfactory results in a limited number of uncomplicated radial head fractures.[2] An early careful and detailed description by Harrington et al. of the

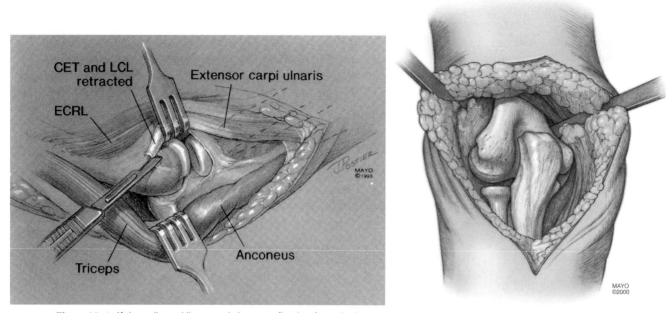

Figure 25–6. If the collateral ligament is intact, reflection from the humeral attachment to a variable extent may be necessary for adequate exposure and implant insertion.

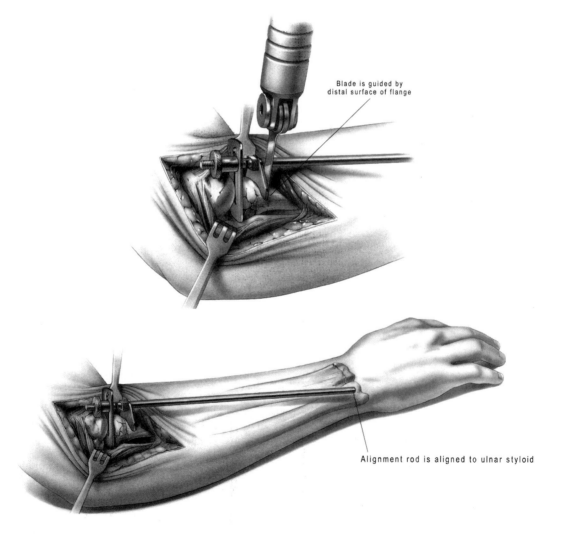

Figure 25–7. The alignment device is inserted in the joint. The distal portion is placed over the ulnar styloid and the proximal portion rests against the capitellum. An oscillating saw is used to resect the neck perpendicular to the axis of rotation (*inset*).

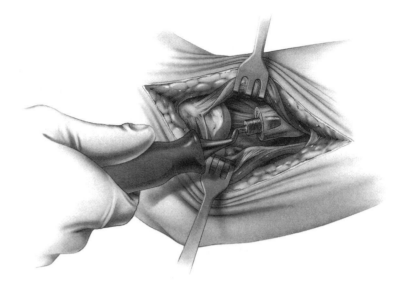

Figure 25–8. Insertion of the broach down the canal is facilitated by the curvature, which matches the stem of the implant.

use of 15 Vitallium and 2 Silastic replacements for unstable elbow joints documented 8 excellent, 6 good, 2 fair, and 1 poor result.[7] These investigators wisely recommend use of the implant specifically in complicated fractures.

Edwards et al. compared 14 patients with simple radial head fractures treated by excision to 11 patients given metallic prosthetic replacements.[4] They showed satisfactory results in 76% of those with the device. Judet et al. reported on 12 patients followed for at least 2 years; 5 had a prosthesis inserted for acute fractures and all had a satisfactory outcome.[10] We must await results of the clinical experience with the current generation of implants (Fig. 25–12).

In summary, the available data suggest that a radial head prosthesis is useful in fractures associated with elbow or wrist instability. The recent introduction of several modular metallic implants has filled a significant void. However, concern exists over the continued absence of a design that addresses the problems of an extensive resection and of implant alignment and stability.

COMPLICATIONS

Numerous adverse effects have been associated with radial head implants. Fatigue failure has occurred with both the acrylic[4] and the Silastic[14,16] prostheses. Fatigue failure of implants made of Silastic appears to account for most of the poor results. The inadequate material properties of the Silastic device for use at the radial head are generally accepted and have been confirmed by recent studies.[1,23] Furthermore, the synovitis reported with Silastic finger implants also occurs at the elbow.[5,25] Worsing and colleagues observed clinical and experimental evidence of foreign-body giant cell reaction elicited by particulate Silastic debris.[24] We have

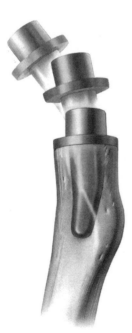

Figure 25–9. The curved trial stem of the implant is readily inserted down the canal.

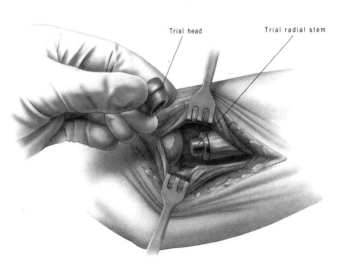

Trial head   Trial radial stem

Figure 25–10. The appropriate sized head is applied.

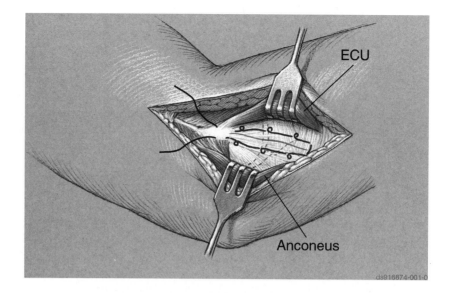

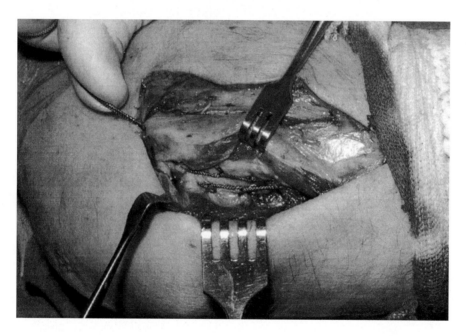

Figure 25–11. Formal repair/reconstruction of the LUCL is necessary to assure proper stability in those clinical instances in which the radial head implant is inserted.

observed an articular reaction from Silastic identical to that seen in rheumatoid arthritis.[24] Thus, because of their inadequate material properties and demonstrable adverse biologic characteristics, Silastic replacements should not be used at the elbow.

Metallic implants have gained considerable popularity in recent years. Malalignment and dislocation are possible with all radial head devices.[7] The greatest current concern to the author is that of the long-term effect of the metal-capitellar articulation. As we await the long-term outcome data of the current generation of modular/metallic radial head implants, incongruity and articular compatibility are of greatest concern. Design is of great interest to help address these concerns.

AUTHOR'S PREFERENCE

We use the radial head prosthesis for acute fractures according to the indications set forth above:

1. Medial collateral deficiency (see Fig. 25–12)
2. Coronoid deficiency
3. Lateral collateral deficiency in selected cases
4. Axial instability from Essex Lopresti lesions

For revision or reconstructive intervention, the same general indications apply. Technically, assessing the alignment of the implant in rotation and flexion and restoration of the LUCL are the most important considerations. If the device is not well aligned, the decision to

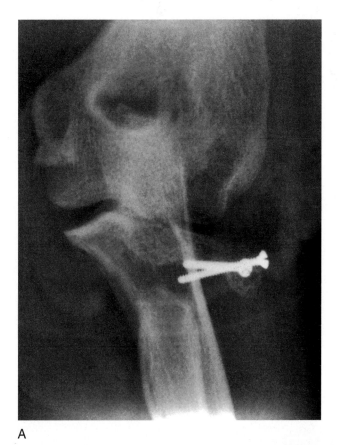

A

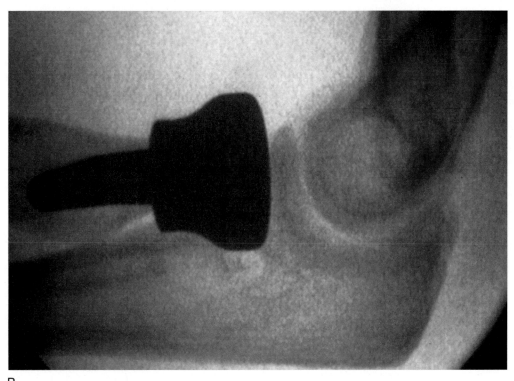

B

Figure 25–12. Fracture-dislocation (**A**) treated by Evolve radial head replacements (**B** and **C**).

Illustration continued on following page

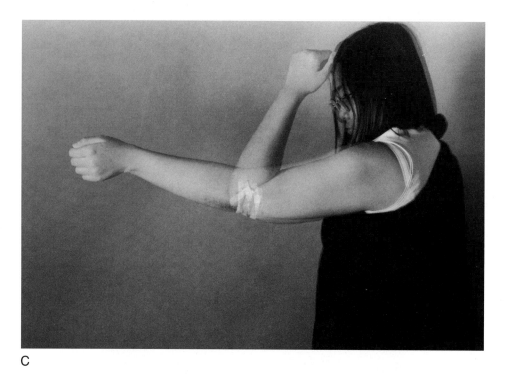

C

Figure 25–12. *Continued.*

have the device recut the radius or to employ an alternate solution, such as an anconeus insertion into the radiohumeral joint, is made. Our implant of choice is the rHead because we prefer the stem to fill the canal rather than be allowed to move freely within it.

References

1. Carn RM, Medige J, Curtain D, Koenig A: Silicone rubber replacement of the severely fractured radial head. Clin Orthop 209:259, 1986.
2. Carr CR, Howard JW: Metallic cap replacement of radial head following fracture. West J Surg 59:539, 1951.
3. Cherry JC: Use of acrylic prosthesis in the treatment of fracture of the head of the radius. J Bone Joint Surg Br 35:70, 1953.
4. Edwards GE, Rostrup O: Radial head prosthesis in the management of radial head fractures. Can J Surg 3:163, 1960.
5. Gordon M, Bullough PG: Synovial and osseous inflammation in failed silicone-rubber prostheses. J Bone Joint Surg Am 64:574, 1982.
6. Gupta GG, Lucas G, Hahn DL: Biomechanical and computer analysis of radial head prostheses. J Shoulder Elbow Surg 6:37–48, 1997.
7. Harrington IJ, Tountas AA: Replacement of the radial head in the treatment of unstable elbow fractures. Injury 12:405, 1981.
8. Hotchkiss RN: Displaced fractures of the radial head: internal fixation or excision? J Am Acad Orthop Surg 5:1–10, 1997.
9. Johansson O: Capsular and ligament injuries of the elbow joint. Acta Chir Scand (Stockh) Suppl 287, 1962.
10. Judet T, de Loubresse CG, Piriou P, Charnley G: A floating prosthesis for radial-head fractures. J Bone Joint Surg Br 78:244–249, 1996.
11. King GJW, Zarzour ZDS, Rath DA, et al: Metallic radial head arthroplasty improves valgus stability of the elbow. Clin Orthop 368:114–125, 1999.
12. Mackay I, Fitzgerald B, Miller JH: Silastic replacement of the head of the radius in trauma. J Bone Joint Surg Br 61:494, 1979.
13. Martinelli B: Fractures of the radial head treated by substitution with the Silastic prosthesis. Bull Hosp Joint Dis 36:61, 1975.
14. Mayhall WST, Tiley FT, Paluska DJ: Fractures of the Silastic radial head prosthesis. J Bone Joint Surg Am 53:459, 1981.
15. Morrey BF, Askew L, Chao EY: Silastic prosthetic replacement for the radial head. J Bone Joint Surg Am 53:454, 1981.
16. Morrey BF, Chao EY, Hui FC: Biomechanical study of the elbow following excision of the radial head. J Bone Joint Surg Am 61:63, 1979.
17. Morrey BF, Tanaka S, An KN: Valgus stability of the elbow: a definition of primary and secondary constraints. Clin Orthop 265:187–195, 1991.
18. Schwab GH, Bennett JB, Woods GW, Tulloos HS: The biomechanics of elbow instability: the role of the medial collateral ligament. Clin Orthop 146:42, 1980.
19. Speed K: Ferrule caps for the head of the radius. Surg Gynecol Obstet 73:845, 1941.
20. Swanson AB: Flexible Implant Resection Arthroplasty in the Hand and Extremities. St. Louis: CV Mosby, 1973.
21. Swanson AB, Jaeger SH, LaRochelle D: Comminuted fractures of the radial head: the role of silicone-implant replacement arthroplasty. J Bone Joint Surg Am 63:1039, 1981.
22. Taylor TKF, O'Connor BT: The effect of the radius in adults. J Bone Joint Surg Br 46:83, 1964.
23. Trepman E, Ewald FC: Early failure of silicone radial head implants in the rheumatoid elbow. J Arthroplasty 6:59, 1991.
24. VanderWilde RS, Morrey BF, Melberg MW, Vinh TN: Inflammatory arthrosis of the ulno-humeral joint after failed Silicone radial head implant. J Bone Joint Surg Br 76:78–81, 1994.
25. Worsing RA, Engber WD, Lange TA: Reactive synovitis from particulate Silastic. J Bone Joint Surg Am 64:581, 1982.

26

Resurfacing Elbow Replacement Arthroplasty

• RONALD L. LINSCHEID and BERNARD F. MORREY

Over the years, a number of design improvements have been made in elbow replacement prostheses, bringing the status of the replacement of this joint to that of reliable intervention.[11,13,14,17] The decision to choose a semiconstrained or surface replacement prosthesis is based on the underlying diagnosis and the extent of the pathology. Two design philosophies have developed over the years that have in the past been termed *unconstrained* and *semiconstrained*. However, because these terms refer to the degree of congruity at the acetabular surface, the use of "unconstrained" for several unlinked implants, such as the Souter, is highly inappropriate because this particular design is very tightly constrained. In the past we have used the term *resurfacing* to characterize the design. This term is not accurate, however, because, although it describes the Kudo and capitellocondylar prostheses, it does not accurately describe the Souter implants. Nonetheless, we use this term in this chapter, although "linked versus unlinked" is probably a more accurate, all-encompassing phrase to describe the basic differences in the design philosophy.

THE CONCEPT

Resurfacing elbow replacement has been developed largely because the concept of replicating normal activity makes intuitive sense, and because of the poor results with the early replacement models of more constrained implants. It goes without saying that, if one accepts this concept of an anatomic replacement, there must be sufficient bone stock, capsular integrity, and muscle strength to validate the use of a surface replacement prosthesis. Most early designs originally lacked stems for a more conservative and possibly easier insertion with more limited exposures.[15,19,29,42,53,57] However, such implant designs have shown a consistent tendency to fixation failure (Fig. 26–1). Kudo and Kunio, for example, reported 5 of 37 patients with posterior displacement of the nonstemmed humeral implant.[25] Hence, all resurfacing devices now include both humeral and ulnar intramedullary stems of variable length.

A variety of resurfacing design strategies to cope with the complex anatomy of the elbow have been

used.[8,42,45,48,57] Options are available from North America (Fig. 26–2) and from Asia and Europe (Fig. 26–3). The simplest concept is to align the ulnar and humeral shafts using the stems of the components.[16,18] The slight translation that occurs requires the assumption that the radial head is absent. Normal anatomic relationships are respected. The normal 5- to 7-degree valgus inclination of the trochlea relative to the anatomic axis of the humerus is generally incorporated in the humeral design.[7,10,28] The normal external rotation of the articulation with respect to the transepicondylar axis is accommodated by design or technique. The design universally incorporates an angulation of the humeral articulation of approximately 30 degrees to replicate the normal articular anterior disposition.[10,38,40,48]

The evolution of the ulnar implant design has resulted in variable stem designs and lengths. In addition, clinical experience has increasingly supported a metallic backing or "tray" to aid implantation and inhibit cold flow deformation of the softer material.[11,38] The articulation and stem will variably replicate the normal 5- to 7-degree valgus angulation.

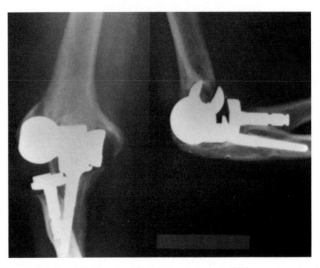

Figure 26–1. At 5.5 years after insertion of an ERS nonstemmed humeral component, the distal humerus fractured and the implant displaced posteriorly.

303

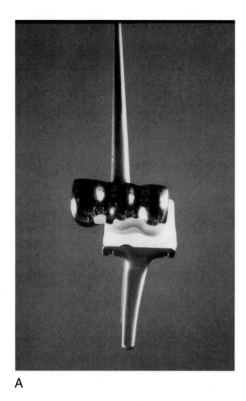

A

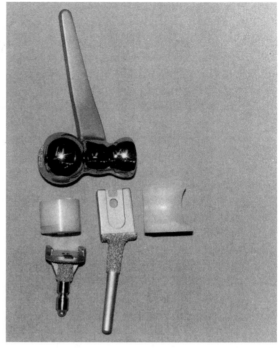

B

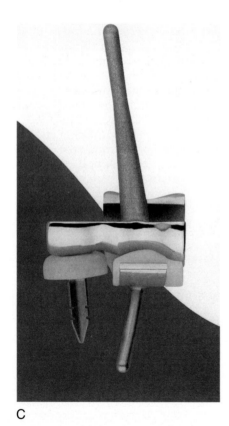

C

Figure 26–2. Resurfacing implants used in the United States. **A,** The capitellocondylar implant employed several thicknesses of high-density polyethylene with varying humeral and ulnar angles to accommodate anatomic variation. **B,** The ERS implant allows for the replacement of the radial head with a modular system, providing for some flexibility with regard to thickness of the implant. **C,** The Sorbie device is a three-component implant.

Stringent technical considerations must be followed to ensure alignment and accurate component orientation and tension in all three planes to resist the eccentric motions that would impose additional shear across the bone-prosthesis interfaces.[15] Several recent studies have demonstrated the sensitivity of surgical technique to the specific design type. The Souter-Strathclyde is a highly conforming implant but demonstrates a tendency to internal rotation of the ulna during flexion. This intrinsic tendency was linked to a propensity to insert the humeral component in slight (5-degree) external rotation.[46] In contrast, internal/external rotational malposition of the capitellocondylar implant tends to cause maltracking but does not increase the tendency for instability.[20] King et al. demonstrated an increased varus-valgus laxity of this device with flexion exceeding 90 degrees.[22] This, coupled with the increased posterior deforming forces at 90 degrees, may account for some of the instability seen with this implant. Further studies have emphasized the need for careful soft tissue balancing.[21] The role of the radial head is speculated to enhance force transmission and impart increased stability. In the ERS design, the radial head has been clearly demonstrated to enhance stability.[36] Clinically, a radial head component was shown to be of no value in the capitellocondylar design.[56]

PATIENT SELECTION

Because of the requisite of bone stock and ligament integrity, resurfacing is largely reserved for the patient with rheumatoid arthritis. In the radiographic classification system used at the Mayo Clinic, this limits the use to type II or IIIA involvement,[33] that is, limited osseous involvement. In addition to osseous integrity, adequate

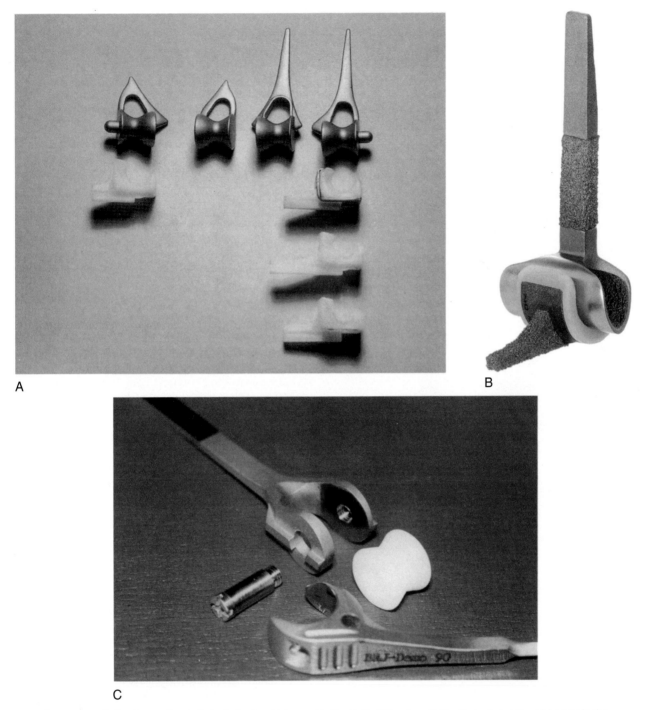

Figure 26–3. A, The Souter-Strathclyde device is widely used in the United Kingdom. **B**, The Kudo design is well known in the Orient. **C**, The innovative design of Risung from Norway has been particularly successful clinically.

ligamentous and muscular function are prerequisites for this type of implant. More recently, the need to revise some of these devices has resulted in longer stemmed revision designs with more stable snap-fit articulations, such as is now available with the Souter design.

Indications

As with all implants, relentless pain constitutes the best indication for elbow joint replacement. Adequate motion (40 to 100 degrees) is desirable because stiff joints require extensive dissection, increasing the likelihood of instability. As with any prosthetic replacement, absence of infection is a prerequisite. Ideally the patient should be over 50 years, but, realistically, the technique is used for rheumatoid arthritis at all ages. Most surgeons consider resurfacing more conservative than semiconstrained implants, and thus one may prefer the surface replacement prosthesis for the younger patient.

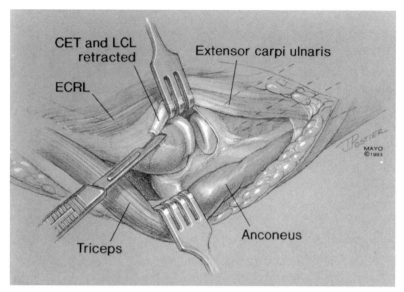

CET and LCL retracted
ECRL
Extensor carpi ulnaris
Triceps
Anconeus

Figure 26–4. Exposure of the elbow joint. **A**, A modified extensile Köcher approach releases a portion of the triceps tendon from the tip of the olecranon and releases the collateral ligament and extensor mechanism as a sleeve from its humeral origin. **B**, Alternatively, triceps-splitting exposure is used.

A

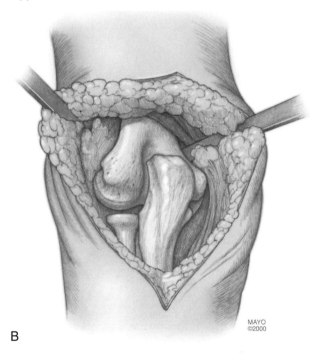

B

Contraindications

Active or recent (<1 year) infection is a firm contraindication for the surface replacement prosthesis. Absence of either supracondylar bony column and severe deficiency of either ligament also mitigate against the use of resurfacing devices. Alternative procedures such as synovectomy should also be considered in young patients (<40 years) prior to arthroplasty.

IMPLANT SELECTION

Of the several devices available, choice largely depends on surgeon preference. To date, all have humeral and ulnar stems. Replacement of the radial head is done on theoretical grounds and is available but considered optimal on some implants, such as that recently designed by Sorbie. Our laboratory data do support the value of the radial head in the Pritchard ERS design.[36] However, the inclusion of this articulation adds an additional variable and complexity to the technique and is another source of potential wear. In the final analysis, reproducibility and simplicity of technique, as well as demonstrated reliable outcomes, should drive surgeon preference. Because the Kudo implant is the most commonly used resurfacing design worldwide, we will demonstrate this surgical technique.

SURGICAL TECHNIQUE

Exposure

Some surgeons prefer a midline triceps-splitting approach. The Köcher exposure to the elbow joint preserves the medial collateral ligament and the triceps insertion and is modified to provide sufficient exposure for implantation of the resurfacing components (Fig. 26–4). The release minimizes dead space and preserves most of the blood supply to the elbow because all of the soft tissue dissection is lateral rather than medial. The ulnar nerve is exposed and decompressed into the flexor carpi ulnaris as needed to prevent excessive bending or kinking when the elbow joint is dislocated.[4] Furthermore, the elbow joint should be relocated regularly during the operation to avoid prolonged excessive tension on the ulnar nerve.

After dislocation of the elbow joint, additional exposure can be obtained by incision of the fibers of the triceps that insert on the tip of the olecranon. Further distraction of the humerus from the ulna is obtained by releasing the anterior and posterior capsule to the attachment of the ulnar collateral ligament. Care must be taken to protect the ulnar nerve, which is directly

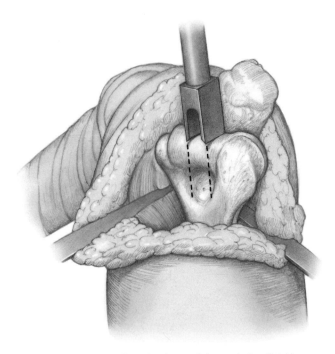

Figure 26–5. After the elbow has been dislocated, the distal humerus is prepared in such a way as to receive the humeral implant.

medial to the medial aspect of the capsule and the medial ligament.

Bone Preparation

Humeral bone resection is performed to allow restoration of the normal elbow kinematics (Fig. 26–5). The center of rotation of the humeral component in the transverse plane is determined by rotation of the humeral compo-

nent 5 degrees external to an imaginary line between the epicondyles.[10] This places the center of the capitellum approximately 1 cm anterior to the lateral epicondyle, which replicates the plane of motion for the distal humeral articular surfaces and helps to prevent rotatory dislocation. In the lateral plane, the center of rotation of the humeral component should intersect a line drawn along the anterior cortex of the humerus. However, each implant has unique design features, so the preparation and insertion must recognize this as well. Although all systems are different, identification of the medullary canal is required in all. Newer designs, such as that of Sorbie, are very carefully instrumented to assure accurate placement. Others have a trial-and-error philosophy of insertion (Fig. 26–6).

The medullary canal of the ulna is identified and prepared with a rasp. Olecranon bone preparation is carefully done to avoid fracture, to avoid improper axial rotation, and to ensure proper placement of the axis of rotation (Fig. 26–7). Another common error of many systems is not to place the ulnar implant far enough dorsally. If the stem is directed from anterior to posterior, the balance of the ligaments is affected and proper tracking can be a problem.

Trial Reduction

Once the trial components are in place, the prosthetic elbow is flexed and extended, with the forearm in full pronation for the lateral exposure. The device should track smoothly with no tendency to dislocate. The joint should be stable at 90 degrees of flexion and resist varus-valgus and posterior forces. If the articulation is too loose, most designs provide an ulnar component with thicker ultra-high-molecular-weight polyethylene

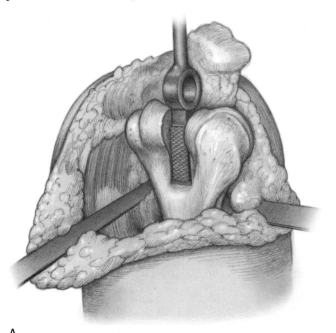

A

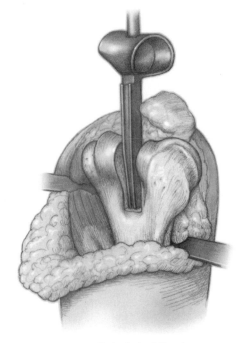

B

Figure 26–6. A, A trial-and-error method must be used to fit some implants, in this instance, a Kudo. **B,** A trial implant assures adequate preparation of the humerus.

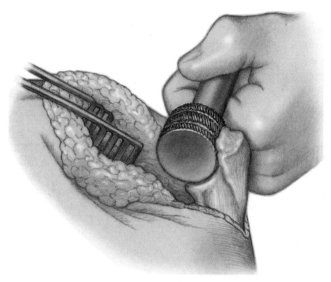

Figure 26–7. The ulnar canal is prepared with a rasp designed for this purpose. The articular portion of the olecranon is further prepared with a burr situated so as to accurately allow insertion of the ulnar component.

(UHMWPE). A common problem for many devices is that the medial (trochlear) side is too tight. This is usually corrected at the humeral level, and may involve soft tissue release. Proper balance and stability should be obtained at this time because successful revision for an unstable implant using soft tissue procedures is unpredictable.

Closure

It is important to restore the integrity of the soft tissue envelope on the lateral aspect of the elbow joint by suture of the lateral extensor-tendon mass and the remnants of the lateral ligament to the lateral epicondyle. The tendon of the origin of the anconeus is replaced. The triceps is reattached with a heavy (No. 5) nonabsorbable suture, and the superficial fascia is closed completely.

Postoperative Management

This varies widely from surgeon to surgeon based on the philosophy of 2 to 3 weeks' protection to 2 to 3 days' early motion. In our practice, flexion-extension exercises as well as rotation of the forearm, with the elbow held at the side, are usually started on the third postoperative day. The patient is advised not to reach out laterally for 6 weeks to avoid vertical shear forces across the lateral repair. Six weeks after the operation, the patient is allowed to return to normal activities but is advised not to lift anything heavier than 10 to 15 pounds (5 to 7 kg). If the elbow is unstable, we protect it in a splint for 3 weeks.

RESULTS

Intermittent to long-term results are emerging for several device designs used for rheumatoid arthritis.[3,6,12,19,27,29,34,35,39,43,45] Pain relief is over 90 percent if complications are avoided. The range of motion averages about 35 to 135 degrees. The complication rates remain relatively high.[11,15,25,37,40,44,52,55,60] We have summarized the recent experience with resurfacing over the last 10 years in Table 26–1. Almost all patients (98 percent) had rheumatoid arthritis.

Outcomes in the Literature

Souter-Strathclyde Implant

The basis for discussion starts with Souter's own series of about 250 procedures followed for variable periods over a 10-year time frame (Fig. 26–8). Although overall about 85 percent did well, fracture and instability occurred in 5 percent and radiographic loosening was present in 12 percent. Others have reported survival free of revision at 87 percent with maximum follow-up of 12 years.[47] If definite loosening is the end point, the survival falls to 80 percent.[54] One Swedish experience with 19 devices revealed 5 (26 percent) to be loose at 6 years.[50] An additional study from Sweden of 30 procedures assessed at a mean of 5 (range 2 to 10) years revealed a 20 percent revision rate and an 80 percent loosening rate at the humerus. This implant was abandoned by those investigators.[2]

Kudo Implant

In Japan, Kudo et al. reported an overall acceptable rate of 78 percent among 37 patients followed a mean of 9.5

Table 26–1. OUTCOMES OF RESURFACING IMPLANTS REPORTED IN LAST 10 YEARS

Study	Year	Implant	Cases	% Satisfactory	% Instability	% Revision	Follow-up Time (yr)
Pöll and Rozing[37]	1991	Souter	34	80	10	15	4
Burnett and Fyfe[5]	1991	Souter	23	88	9	12	3
Lyall et al.[30]	1994	Souter	19	90	15	10	3.5
Sjoden et al.[50]	1995	Souter	19	80	5	—	5
Andreassen and Solheim[2]	1997	Souter	30	40	—	20	5 (2–10)
Allieu et al.[1]	1998	Roper-Tuke	12	84	8	16	9 (8–13)
Yanni et al.[61]	2000	Roper-Tuke	59	84	4	4	6.5 (4–10)
Verstreken et al.[58]	1998	Kudo	15	85	15	—	3
Ewald et al.[11]	1993	Capitellocondylar	202	95	4	2	6 (2–15)
Ljung et al.[26]	1995	Capitellocondylar	50	96	2	2	3
Risung[41]	1997	"Norway"	118	—	—	3	4

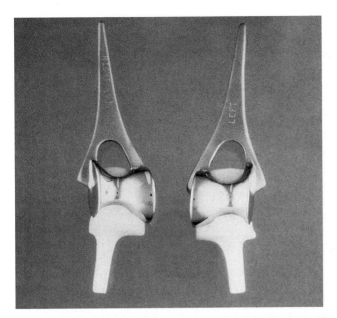

Figure 26–8. The Souter is a tightly constrained unlinked implant with greater emphasis on stem length and size in the current design.

years[24] (Fig. 26–9). Of interest, these investigators also reported the only experience with an uncemented application in 32 elbows, all with rheumatoid arthritis. After a mean surveillance of 3 years, a good (25 elbows)

or fair (2 elbows) result occurred in 85 percent of this series.[25] In fact, satisfactory outcomes were also reported in all six patients with the so-called mutilans deformity.[23] Others have reported an 87 percent satisfactory rate at 3 years with the Kudo device.[58]

Capitellocondylar Implant

The largest experience of resurfacing elbow arthroplasty in this country is with the capitellocondylar prosthesis.[11,13,55,56] The capitellar aspect of the humeral component is fashioned to accept articulation with a radial prosthesis, but recent recommendations of Trepwald et al. are to delete this component.[56] The most definitive results have been reported by Ewald and colleagues in four series: (1) 56 cases with an all-plastic ulnar component inserted through a posterior approach[10]; (2) 26 cases with a metal-backed ulnar component inserted posteriorly[8]; and (3) 120 cases inserted through a Köcher midlateral approach.[9] The definitive series was that reported by Ewald et al. in 1993.[11] An experience of 202 replacements for rheumatoid arthritis with a mean surveillance of 6 years (range 2 to 15) was reported to have resulted in 92 percent satisfactory outcomes. The arc of motion was in the functional range, 30 to 138 degrees. Although the complication rate was 30 percent, most complications were not such as to alter the outcome. Only 8 percent of patients had a reoperation, half

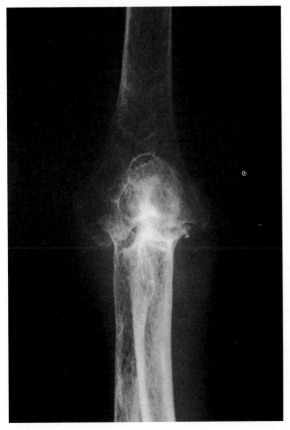

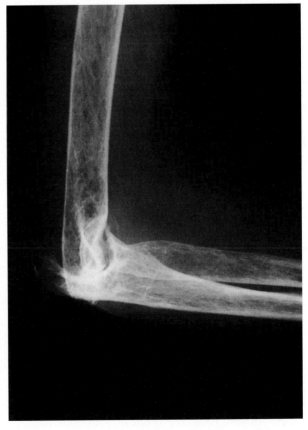

A

Figure 26–9. A, Mayo type II classification of radiographic involvement of the elbow with rheumatoid arthritis.

Illustration continued on following page

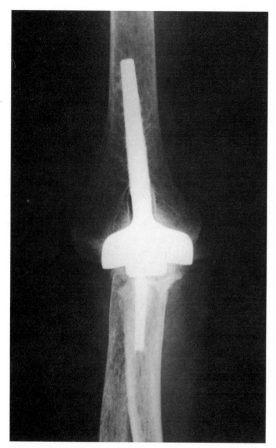
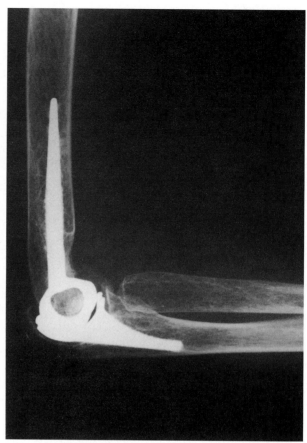

B

Figure 26–9. *Continued.* **B**, Effective 5-year outcome with Kudo device.

the reoperation rate reported by Ljung et al.[26] The functional rating score increased from 26 to 91 points. Unfortunately, this device is no longer available from the manufacturer.

Other Devices

In Norway, the novel and innovative design of Risung, Teigland, and Pahle has also been described along with clinical outcomes.[40] Results after 12 years show a satisfactory outcome in over 90 percent of cases (see Table 26–1). Yanni et al. have reported 84 percent satisfactory outcomes at 6 years (range 4 to 10) after inserting 59 Roper-Tuke devices. Radiographic loosening was recorded in 35 percent of humeral and 25 percent of ulnar components.[61] Allieu et al. have reported the 10-year outcome of 12 Roper-Tuke implants, with pain relief in 8 cases; revision for loosening was required in 2 (16 percent).[1]

Mayo Clinic Results

The Mayo Clinic experience with resurfacing includes 52 capitellocondylar and 35 SRS devices, 90 percent of which were inserted for rheumatoid arthritis. Pain, crepitus, and decreased range of motion were indications for surgery. Adequate bone stock apparent radiographically was also a prerequisite. This required the

presence of both condyles and epicondyles as well as the olecranon. Moderate erosive changes with the previous excision of the radial head were present in 15 percent of cases.

Capitellocondylar Implant

Overall relief of pain and restoration of elbow flexion were reliably obtained with this implant (Fig. 26–10). Unfortunately, as reported by others,[55,60] postoperative dislocation was a disconcerting problem that did not easily resolve with relocation and immobilization in several instances. Of a total of 52 cases, posterior dislocation occurred in 6 (12 percent). Three of these were eventually replaced with hinged prostheses and two became secondarily infected, with wound dehiscence. This experience prompted the senior author (R.L.L.) to assess the three-component SRS system designed by Roland Pritchard.

Resurfacing Elbow Prosthesis

In the SRS series of 35 elbows, follow-up ranged from 6 to 67 months, with an average of 40 months. The flexion arc improved from 39 to 124 to 24 to 135 degrees. Pronosupination improved moderately from preoperative values. We determined results based on the Ewald scoring system,[11] with a 100-point scale. Pain was assigned 50, function 30, motion 10, flexion

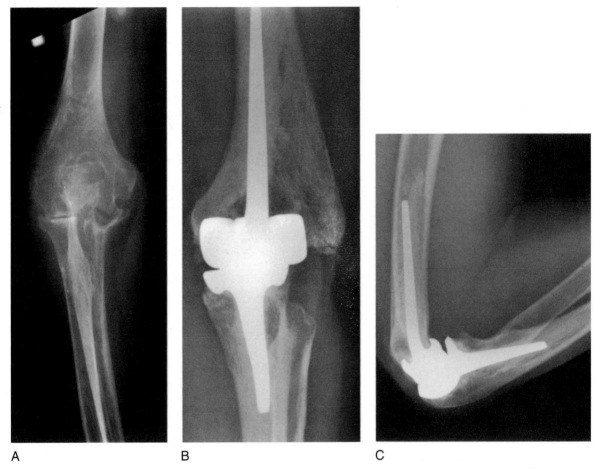

A   B   C

Figure 26–10. Moderate type II rheumatoid arthritis (**A**) successfully treated by capitellocondylar device 5 years after surgery (**B** and **C**).

contracture 5, and deformity 5 points. Based on this standard, there were 24 (69 percent) good, 8 (23 percent) fair, and 3 (9 percent) poor outcomes (Fig. 26–11).

This device is no longer being used at our institution. However, because there continues to be interest in the concept of resurfacing arthroplasty, some of our partners are investigating the Sorbie device.

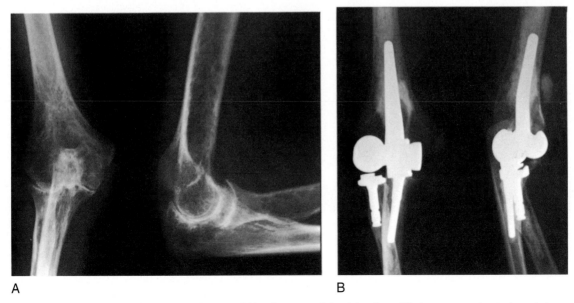

A   B

Figure 26–11. A 44-year-old female with rheumatoid involvement of the right elbow (**A**) demonstrated no pain and almost normal range of motion 1 year after an ERS implant (**B**).

Inadequate experience exists to date to render a comment, other than it is technically challenging to insert.

COMPLICATIONS

This topic is covered in detail in Chapter 30. Gschwend et al. have summarized the world's literature of elbow replacement complications in a review article.[17] Most series place the complication rate between 15 and 30 percent.

Problems with mechanical failure were well described in the early literature. Sepsis and loosening occurred in the nonstemmed humeral component in 8 of 13 Wadsworth implants an average of 5.7 years after surgery.[27] A loose component was also observed in 2 of 22 nonstemmed Liverpool implants.[52] A comprehensive review of the Souter implant from the Netherlands reported instability in 3 of 34 cases (9 percent).[50] Kudo and Kunio also reported posterior displacement of the articulation (14 percent) because of the lack of a stem on the early version of the humeral device.[25] That several recent reports have shown poor outcomes with the Souter implant, largely as a result of loosening of one or the other components, emphasizes (1) the impact of a highly constrained device and (2) the need for longer than 5-year average follow-up to fully assess durability.

Weiland et al. noted malposition of the ulna referable to the humeral component as it displaced into the groove between the trochlea and capitellar condyles in 20 percent of their patients with a capitellocondylar implant.[60] These complications to some extent are explained by the problems inherent in learning a new system, the so-called learning curve. The report of Ruth and Wilde[44] and most other experiences are similar, with a comparable or even higher incidence of instability.[19,27,29,31,37,45,51,52,59]

Mayo Experience with Complications

Infection. There were two cases of deep infections (6 percent) among 35 cases; each was associated with a partial triceps disruption. One eventually was revised to a hinged prosthesis, and one was converted to a fibrous arthroplasty.

Neuropathy. Ulnar paresthesias occurred in five patients (15 percent), one of whom required release of the nerve at 24 hours. The others recovered rapidly without further treatment. One instance of transient plexopathy occurred as well.

Loosening. Loosening, as implied by a lucent line on either side of the bone-cement junction of 1 mm or more, was noted on follow-up radiographs around two ulnar, one humeral, and two radial components.

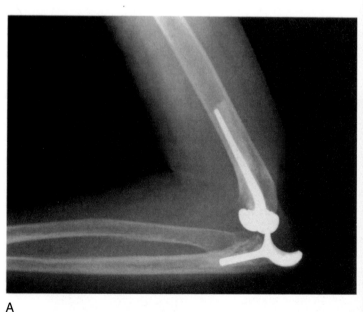

A

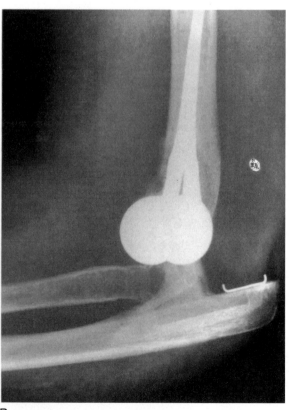

B

Figure 26–12. Instability is a concern with all unconstrained devices, including the capitellocondylar (**A**), the Souter-Strathclyde (**B**), the London (**C**), and the ERS (**D**).

Illustration continued on following page

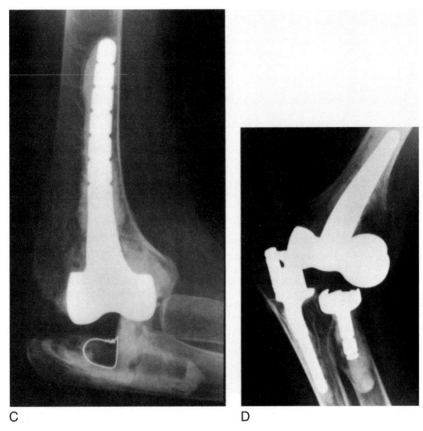

C   D

Figure 26–12. *Continued.*

Instability. As with most reports, instability continues to be a concern in our practice (Fig. 26–12). There was one (3 percent) immediate dislocation associated with a brachial plexopathy that required 4 weeks of external fixator support. There was eventual recovery of muscle function and a good result. There were two subluxations that required manipulation and casting (6 percent). One additional patient dislocated at 10 months and a hinged prosthetic replacement was performed. The overall rate of instability was thus 12 percent. One case of instability was due to a dislocated ulnar UHMWPE insert.

Probability of Reoperation. Using the Kaplan-Meier method, the probability of reoperation for any reason was estimated as 8 percent at 1 year and 28 percent at 3 years.

Prevention

Avoidance of complications is best achieved by careful planning and meticulous technique. Exposure and gentle retraction of the ulnar nerve will help prevent postoperative palsies. Better tissue balance and identifying and tagging the collateral ligaments will improve the ability to restore stability during closure.[9,38] Completion of the synovectomy aids exposure. Examination of the position and movement of the components before cementing allows identification and correction of malposition. Immobilization of the elbow for 4 weeks in slight flexion will allow the triceps to heal and helps prevent late disruption and hurried mobilization.[32]

Treatment

The treatment of the more severe complications can be very challenging for both patient and surgeon. Dislocations are reduced immediately. Immobilization for a protracted period to allow the capsule to tighten must be monitored with frequent radiographs to be sure redislocation does not occur within the cast. Occasionally secondary repair of the collateral ligaments or triceps may be successful. Loosening, fracture, or malalignment during movement may necessitate revision (see Chapter 32).

Infection is treated by an aggressive débridement protocol if the proper solution factors are met, or by component removal in the remainder of cases (see Chapter 31).

AUTHORS' PREFERENCE

Currently, the second author (B.F.M.) has abandoned the use of this type implant in his practice. The reasons are unpredictable instability, technical difficulty and limited indications. He is nonetheless supportive of ongoing efforts to improve the design and outcomes of this class of devices.

References

1. Allieu Y, zu Reckendorf GM, Daude O: Long-term results of unconstrained Roper-Tuke total elbow arthroplasty in patients with rheumatoid arthritis. J Shoulder Elbow Surg 7:560–564, 1998.
2. Andreassen G, Solheim LF: Follow-up of Souter elbow prostheses. Tidsskr Nor Laegeforen 117:940–942, 1997.
3. Bayley JIL: Elbow replacement in rheumatoid arthritis. Reconstr Surg Traumatol 18:70, 1981.
4. Bryan RS, Morrey BF: Extensive posterior exposure of the elbow: a triceps sparing approach. Clin Orthop 166:199, 1982.
5. Burnett R, Fyfe IS: Souter-Strathclyde arthroplasty of the rheumatoid elbow: 23 cases followed for 3 years. Acta Orthop Scand 62:52–54, 1991.
6. Davis RF, Weiland AJ, Hungerford DS, et al: Nonconstrained total elbow arthroplasty. Clin Orthop 171:156, 1982.
7. Evans BG, Daniels AU, Serbousek JC, Mann RJ: A comparison of the mechanical designs of articulating total elbow prostheses. Clin Materials 3:235, 1988.
8. Ewald FC: Nonconstrained metal to plastic total elbow arthroplasty. In Inglis AE (ed): Symposium on Total Joint Replacement of the Upper Extremity. St. Louis, CV Mosby, 1982, p 141.
9. Ewald FC, Jacobs MA: Total elbow arthroplasty. Clin Orthop 182:137, 1984.
10. Ewald FC, Scheinberg RD, Poss R, et al: Capitellocondylar total elbow arthroplasty: two to five year follow-up in rheumatoid arthritis. J Bone Joint Surg Am 63:1259, 1980.
11. Ewald FC, Simmons ED Jr, Sullivan JA, et al: Capitellocondylar total elbow replacement in rheumatoid arthritis: long term results. J Bone Joint Surg Am 75:498–507, 1993.
12. Ferlic DC, Clayton ML, Parr CL: Surgery of the elbow in rheumatoid arthritis. J Bone Joint Surg Am 58:726, 1987.
13. Friedman RJ, Lee DE, Ewald FC: Nonconstrained total elbow arthroplasty. J Arthroplasty 4:31, 1989.
14. Gill DRJ, Morrey BF: The Coonrad-Morrey total elbow arthroplasty in patients who have rheumatoid arthritis: a ten to fifteen year follow-up study. J Bone Joint Surg Am 80:1327–1335, 1998.
15. Goldberg VM, Figgie HE III, Inglis AF, Figgie MP: Total elbow arthroplasty. J Bone Joint Surg Am 70:778, 1988.
16. Gschwend N, Loehr J, Ovosevic-Radovanovic D, Scheler H: Semiconstrained elbow prostheses with special reference to the GBS III prosthesis. Clin Orthop 232:104, 1988.
17. Gschwend N, Simmen BR, Matejovsky Z: Late complications in elbow arthroplasty. J Shoulder Elbow Surg 5(2, Pt 1):86–96, 1996.
18. Inglis AE, Pellici PM: Total elbow replacement. J Bone Joint Surg Am 62:1252, 1980.
19. Ishizuki M, Nagatzuka Y, Arai T, et al: Preliminary experiences with a hingeless total elbow arthroplasty. Ryumachi 17:4, 1977.
20. Itoi E, King GJW, Niebur GL, et al: Malrotation of the humeral component of the capitellocondylar total elbow replacement is not the sole cause of dislocation. J Orthop Res 12:665–671, 1994.
21. King GJW, Glauser SJ, Westreich A, et al: In vitro stability of an unconstrained total elbow prosthesis. J Arthroplasty 8:291–298, 1993.
22. King GJW, Itoi E, Niebur GL, et al: Motion and laxity of the capitellocondylar total elbow prosthesis. J Bone Joint Surg Am 76:1000, 1994.
23. Kudo H: Non-constrained elbow arthroplasty for mutilans deformity in rheumatoid arthritis: a report of six cases. J Bone Joint Surg Br 80:234–239, 1998.
24. Kudo H, Iwano K, Nishino J: Cementless or hybrid total elbow arthroplasty with titanium-alloy implants: a study of interim clinical results and specific complications. J Arthroplasty 9:269–278, 1994.
25. Kudo H, Kunio I: Total elbow arthroplasty with a non-constrained surface replacement prosthesis in patients who have rheumatoid arthritis: a long-term follow-up study. J Bone Joint Surg Am 72A:355–362, 1990.
26. Ljung P, Jonsson K, Rydholm U: Short-term complications of the lateral approach for non-constrained elbow replacement: follow-up of 50 rheumatoid elbows. J Bone Joint Surg Br 77:937–942, 1995.
27. Ljung P, Lidgren L, Rydholm U: Failure of the Wadsworth elbow: nineteen cases of rheumatoid arthritis followed for five years. Acta Orthop Scand 60:254, 1989.
28. London JT: Kinematics of the elbow. J Bone Joint Surg Am 63:529, 1981.
29. Lowe LW, Miller AJ, Alum RL, Higgison DW: The development of an unconstrained elbow arthroplasty. J Bone Joint Surg Br 66:243, 1984.
30. Lyall HA, Cohen B, Clatworthy M, Constant CR: Results of the Souter-Strathclyde total elbow arthroplasty in patients with rheumatoid arthritis: a preliminary report. J Arthroplasty 9:279–284, 1994.
31. Madsen F, Gudmundson GH, Söjbjerg JO, Sneppen O: The Pritchard Mark II elbow prostheses in rheumatoid arthritis. Acta Orthop Scand 60:249, 1989.
32. Maloney WJ, Schurman DJ: Cast immobilization after total elbow arthroplasty. Clin Orthop 245:117, 1989.
33. Morrey BF, Adams RA: Semiconstrained arthroplasty for the treatment of rheumatoid arthritis of the elbow. J Bone Joint Surg Am 74:479–490, 1992.
34. Morrey BF, Askew LJ, An K-N, Chao EYS: A biomechanical study of normal functional elbow motion. J Bone Joint Surg Am 63:872–877, 1981.
35. Morrey BF, Bryan RS: Total joint replacement. In Morrey BF (ed): The Elbow and Its Disorders. Philadelphia, WB Saunders, 1985, p 774.
36. Neale PG, Chou P, Ramsey M, et al: Kinematics and stability of the Pritchard ERS total elbow. Presented at the 44th Annual Meeting of the Orthopedic Research Society, March 16–19, 1998, New Orleans, LA.
37. Pöll RG, Rozing PM: Use of the Souter-Strathcylde total elbow prosthesis in patients who have rheumatoid arthritis. J Bone Joint Surg Am 73:1227–1233, 1991.
38. Pritchard RW: Anatomic surface elbow arthroplasty: a preliminary report. Clin Orthop 179:223, 1983.
39. Redfern DRM, Dunkley AB, Trail IA, Stanley JK: Revision total elbow replacement using the Souter-Strathclyde prosthesis. J Bone Joint Surg Br 83:635–639, 2001.
40. Risung F: Characteristics, design and preliminary results of the "Norway Elbow System." In Hämäläinen M, Hagena F-W (eds): Rheumatoid Arthritis Surgery of the Elbow, vol 15: Rheumatology. Basel, Karger, 1991, pp 68–72.
41. Risung F: The Norway elbow replacement: design, technique and results after nine years. J Bone Joint Surg Br 79:394–402, 1997.
42. Roper BA, Tuke M, O'Riordan SM, Bulstrode CJ: A new unconstrained elbow. J Bone Joint Surg 68:566, 1986.
43. Rosenberg GM, Turner RH: Nonconstrained total elbow arthroplasty. Clin Orthop 187:154, 1984.
44. Ruth JT, Wilde AH: Capitellocondylar total elbow replacement: a long-term follow-up study. J Bone Joint Surg Am 74:95, 1992.
45. Rydholm U, TJ'Ornstrand B, Pettersson H, Lidgren L: Surface replacement of the elbow in rheumatoid arthritis. J Bone Joint Surg Br 66:737, 1984.
46. Schneeberger AG, King GJW, Song S-W, et al: Kinematics and laxity of the Souter-Strathclyde total elbow prosthesis. J Shoulder Elbow Surg 9:127–134, 2000.
47. Shah BM, Trail IA, Nuttall D, Stanley JK: The effect of epidemiologic and intraoperative factors on survival of the standard Souter-Strathcylde total elbow arthroplasty. J Arthroplasty 15:994–998, 2000.
48. Shiba R, Sorbie C, Siu DW, et al: Geometry of the humeroulnar joint. J Orthop Res 6:897, 1988.
49. Sjoden G, Blomgren G: The Souter-Strathclyde elbow replacement in rheumatoid arthritis: 13 patients followed for 5 (1–9) years. Acta Orthop Scand 63:315–317, 1992.
50. Sjoden GO, Lundberg A, Blomgren GA: Late results of the Souter-Strathcylde total elbow prosthesis in rheumatoid arthritis: 6/19 implants loose after five years. Acta Orthop Scand 66:391–394, 1995.
51. Soni RK, Cavendish ME: A review of the Liverpool elbow prosthesis from 1974 to 1982. J Bone Joint Surg Br 66:248, 1984.
52. Sourmelis GS, Burke FD, Varian JPW: A review of total elbow arthroplasty and an early assessment of the Liverpool elbow prosthesis. J Hand Surg 11B:407, 1986.
53. Souter WA: Anatomical trochlear stirrup arthroplasty of the rheumatoid elbow. In Kashiwagi D (ed): Elbow Joint: Proceedings of the International Seminar, Kobe, Japan, February 22–24, 1985. International Congress Series No. 678. New York, Elsevier Science, 1985, p 305.

54. Trail IA, Nuttall D, Stanley JK: Survivorship and radiological analysis of the standard Souter-Strathclyde total elbow arthroplasty. J Bone Joint Surg Br 81:80–84, 1999.

55. Trancik T, Wilde AH, Borden LS: Capitellocondylar total elbow arthroplasty: two to eight year experience. Clin Orthop 223:175, 1987.

56. Trepman E, Vella IM, Ewald FC: Radial head replacement in capitellocondylar total elbow arthroplasty: 2 to 6 year follow-up evaluation in rheumatoid arthritis. J Arthroplasty 6:67–77, 1991.

57. Venable CS: An elbow and an elbow prosthesis: case of complete loss of the lower third of the humerus. Am J Surg 83:271, 1952.

58. Verstreken F, De Smet L, Westhovens R, Fabry G: Results of the Kudo elbow prosthesis in patients with rheumatoid arthritis: a preliminary report. Clin Rheumatol 17:325–328, 1998.

59. Wadsworth TG: A new technique of total elbow arthroplasty. Eng Med 10:69, 1980.

60. Weiland AJ, Weiss APC, Wills RP, Moore JR: Capitellocondylar total elbow replacement. J Bone Joint Surg Am 71:217, 1989.

61. Yanni ON, Bearn CBDA, Gallannaugh SC, Joshi R: The Roper-Tuke total elbow arthroplasty. J Bone Joint Surg Br 82:705–710, 2000.

27

Semiconstrained Total Elbow Replacement: Indications and Surgical Technique

• BERNARD F. MORREY

The value of—and rationale for—the semiconstrained joint replacement has been well established since the first editions of this text. The major development has been the broadening of the indications beyond rheumatoid arthritis to include a host of traumatic conditions. Improved stability from the articular design and lessened stress to the bone cement interface realized by the laxity, or play, that occurs at the ulnohumeral articulation have been major advances in elbow replacement.[13] The fixation attained by the bone graft behind the flange of the Coonrad-Morrey implant further enhances fixation and lessens stress at the bone cement interface. Although there are several semiconstrained designs available, I describe in detail the surgical procedure for the insertion of a Mayo modified Coonrad total elbow arthroplasty (Coonrad-Morrey) with which I have the greatest level of experience and which has been used almost exclusively at the Mayo Clinic since 1981.

INDICATIONS

The indications for total elbow arthroplasty are similar to those of other joints, the most common being pain that significantly alters activities of daily living. This is typically seen in patients with rheumatoid arthritis and in those with certain traumatic conditions.

The second most frequent indication for joint replacement is dysfunctional instability. This presentation is seen in the very severe grade IV type of rheumatoid arthritic elbow as well as with post-traumatic arthrosis resulting from distal humeral nonunion or joint resection.

The third and least common indication for elbow joint replacement is that of the ankylosed elbow; this may be seen in several circumstances, including juvenile rheumatoid arthritis, some forms of adult onset rheumatoid arthritis, post-traumatic arthritis, and other inflammatory conditions that cause ankylosis of this joint.

The specific techniques for each of these indications are illustrated and discussed in subsequent chapters. I discuss stiffness with the rheumatoid technique and incorporate instability into the discussion of management of traumatic elbow condition. Here, I discuss the generic implantation most appropriate for an uncomplicated form of rheumatoid arthritis.

CONTRAINDICATIONS

Absolute contraindications are (1) an active or subacute infection and (2) neuromuscular deficiency of the elbow joint flexors.

A history of previous infection is a relative contraindication. Replacement may proceed in the absence of an active infection.

Severe soft tissue scarring and poor tissue coverage are relative contraindications to replacement. However, such situations can usually be converted to an acceptable setting with a soft tissue surgical procedure that is performed before or, occasionally, concurrent with joint replacement.

Deficiency or absence of the triceps musculature markedly decreases the effectiveness of elbow extension and the ability to work overhead but is not an absolute contraindication. In some instances, active flexion and relief of pain justify joint replacement, even if active extension is not possible.

PREOPERATIVE PLANNING

Routine anteroposterior (AP) and lateral radiographs are the only imaging studies needed for this procedure. The most important considerations in this process are (1) to assess humeral bow or angular deviation and medullary canal size in the lateral projection and (2) to note the size of the ulnar medullary canal in both projections and the bow in the AP view. In patients with juve-

316

nile rheumatoid arthritis, the medullary canal may be extremely small. In such cases, the special small ulnar implant should be used.

SURGERY

Although some surgeons use an arm board, I prefer to position the patient in a supine position with a sandbag under the scapula. The arm is draped free and the table is rotated approximately 10 degrees away from the operated extremity to further elevate the elbow and the limb (Fig. 27–1). A general anesthesia is used in almost all intances.

Technique: Rheumatoid Arthritis

Any one of a number of approaches may be used. I prefer the Bryan-Morrey approach.[1] A straight incision is made just medial to the tip of the olecranon between the medial epicondyle. The incision extends approximately 5 to 7 cm distal and 7 to 10 cm proximal to the tip of the olecranon. The subcutaneous tissue over the medial aspect of the triceps is elevated, exposing the medial margin of the triceps and the ulnar nerve. I always identify and translocate the ulnar nerve that has not been previously moved. The nerve is isolated at the medial margin of the triceps proximally. The dissection is carried distally to the cubital tunnel retinaculum, which is split, and carried further distally to the first motor branch of the flexor carpi ulnaris. If there are adhesions to the capsule, as sometimes occur with rheumatoid arthritis or scarring from a traumatic cause, the use of magnification loops may be effective. Bipolar cautery is used and the nerve is translocated into a subcutaneous pocket.

An incision is next made just to the medial aspect of the crest of the ulna, which releases the forearm fascia and the periosteum over the ulna. The medial aspect of the triceps is then elevated from the posterior aspect of the humerus and from the posterior capsule, and the tissue is reflected proximally and distally to the triceps insertion. The discrete insertion of the triceps to the tip of the olecranon by Sharpey's fibers is released by a sharp dissection (Fig. 27–2), allowing a flap of tissue to be raised, including the triceps, the forearm fascia and ulnar periosteum, and, when the anconeus is exposed, it is reflected to the lateral aspect of the proximal ulna (Fig. 27–3). Continued release of the extensor mechanism from the lateral epicondyle allows complete exposure of the posterior aspect of the joint. The lateral and medial collateral ligaments are then released from their humeral attachment, providing excellent exposure of the distal humerus and proximal ulna (Fig. 27–4). The humerus is externally rotated and the elbow is fully flexed.

The midportion of the trochlea is removed with a rongeur or a saw depending on the quality of the bone (Fig. 27–5). The medial and lateral columns are identified and the roof of the olecranon is entered by means of either a bur or a rongeur, again depending on the bone quality. The medullary canal of the humerus is then identified with a long twist reamer which serves as the alignment stem. The humeral canal is typically very spacious in the rheumatoid patient, allowing easy access to this instrument (Fig. 27–6).

Placement of the alignment stem down the full length of the humeral canal accurately centers the distal cutting block (Fig. 27–7), the side arm of which rests on the capitellum. The flat of the template is oriented to the plane of the posterior columns to ensure accurate rotatory alignment (Fig. 27–8). With an oscillating saw, the trochlea is removed (Fig. 27–9). A small-diameter rasp is initially used to access the canal and ensure that the rasp can be centered on the resected distal humerus. The appropriate rasp (standard, small, extra small) is then used, depending on the size of the canal (Fig. 27–10). The small 4-inch implant is most commonly used in the rheumatoid elbow. This size implant prevents problems with future replacement if there is shoulder pathology. In most traumatic problems, the 6-inch stem is used. An

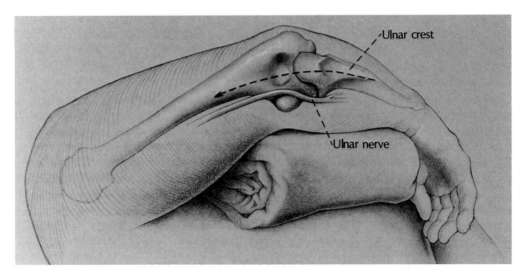

Figure 27–1. The patient is supine and the arm brought across the chest. The ulnar nerve is identified at the medial margins of the triceps and dissected to the first motor branch. (Mayo © 1987. By permission of Mayo Foundation for Medical Education and Research.)

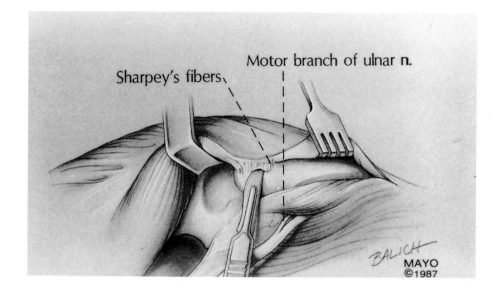

Figure 27–2. The soft tissue is elevated from the subcutaneous border of the ulna and the medial margin of the triceps from the posterior aspect of the humerus. (By permission of Mayo Foundation for Medical Education and Research.)

Figure 27–3. The anconeus is elevated and maintains the continuity of the extensor mechanism. (By permission of Mayo Foundation for Medical Education and Research.)

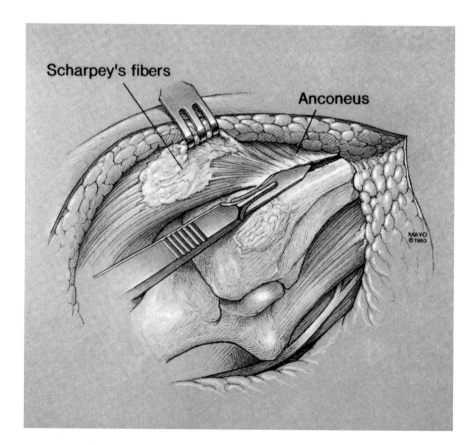

extra-small device is also available for the elbows of Asian and juvenile rheumatoid patients.

The brachialis muscle is released from the anterior cortex of the humerus with a curved elevator to accommodate the flange of the device (Fig. 27–11). The articulation of the trial humeral component is placed within the resected trochlea. If enough bone has been removed to accommodate the width of the implant articulation, a trial insertion is carried out.

The medullary canal of the ulna is easily identified because the proximal ulna has had soft tissue released. The canal is most easily entered with a high-speed bur placed approximately at a 45-degree angle to the long axis at the base of the coronoid (Fig. 27–12). The canal is then entered with a small awl. To ensure longitudinal access down the ulna, the olecranon is notched in line with the awl (Fig. 27–13). Serial rasps are introduced with a twisting motion. Complete seating often requires

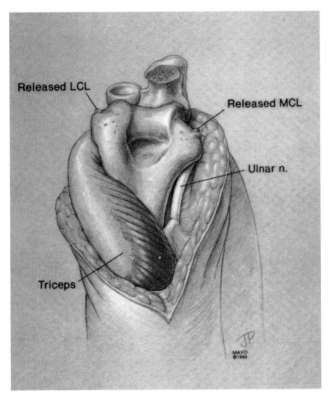

Figure 27–4. Release of the medial-lateral collateral ligaments and flexion of the elbow. (By permission of Mayo Foundation for Medical Education and Research.)

the use of a mallet, and care is taken to ensure that rotation of the ulnar component is at a right angle with the flat portion of the implanted olecranon (Fig. 27–14).

The depth of the insertion is such that the center of the olecranon component is coincident with the center of curvature of the greater sigmoid fossa; that is, halfway between the tip of the olecranon and the coronoid

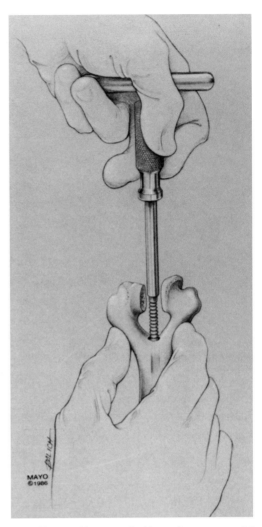

Figure 27–6. The canal is entered with a twist reamer and the alignment guide is centered in the canal.

Figure 27–5. A rongeur for soft bone or oscillating saw for more sclerotic bone is used to remove the midportion of the trochlea.

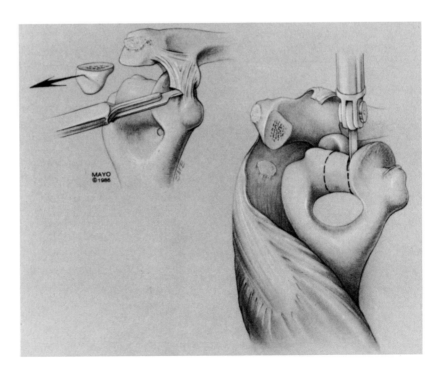

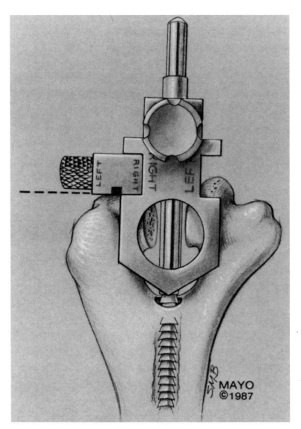

Figure 27–7. The handle is removed and the humeral cutting block is in place, the side arm resting on the capitellum. (By permission of Mayo Foundation for Medical Education and Research.)

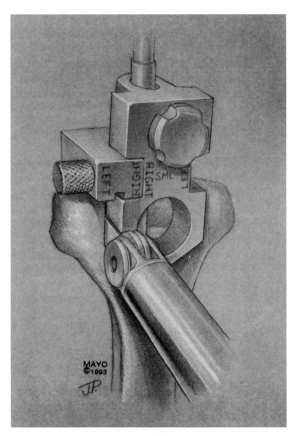

Figure 27–9. Accurate removal of bone with the oscillating saw. (By permission of Mayo Foundation for Medical Education and Research.)

(Fig. 27–15). It is wise then to insert the humeral component and to perform a trial reduction to make certain that there is no residual flexion contracture and to identify and remove any impingement.

Medullary canals of both the bones are cleansed with a pulsating lavage system and dried. For surgeons who have less experience with the procedure, it is safest to cement the implants separately. If this is done, the ulnar component is first cemented with the injection gun and the stem that is cut to the length of the ulnar component. The ulnar component is inserted into the cemented medullary canal and impacted into proper position as noted earlier.

For the humerus, a cement restrictor is displayed, and a bone graft is prepared from the excised trochlea, which measures approximately 2 cm by 2 cm and is

from 2 mm to 4 mm thick. The injector nozzle is cut to the proper humeral stem length, 10 or 15 cm, and placed down the medullary canal to deliver the cement to the appropriate depth (Fig. 27–16).

The bone graft is placed at the anterior aspect of the humerus, just proximal to the cut in the distal humerus, before insertion of the humeral component (Fig. 27–17). The humeral component is inserted to the depth at which articulation with the ulna is possible. The previously placed bone graft engages the flange at the time of implant coupling. The ulnar component is then articulated by placement of the hollow pin across the humerus and through the ulna. It is secured with a second pin inserted into the hollow one until a snapping sound is heard (Fig. 27–18).

After the prosthesis has been coupled, the ulna is placed at a 90-degree angle and the humeral component is impacted down the medullary canal. The humeral component is usually inserted so that the distal aspect of the component is at the level of, or slightly proximal (1 or 2 mm) to, the contour of the distal capitellum.

The elbow is placed through a range of motion to ensure full extension and flexion. Usually an arc of 10 degrees to 140 degrees is obtainable at the time of surgery. The radial head need not be removed for proper functioning of the device, but it should be excised if the pathology so dictates. The triceps is reattached through drill holes placed in a cruciate and transverse fashion (Fig. 27–19). A heavy, nonabsorbable (No. 5)

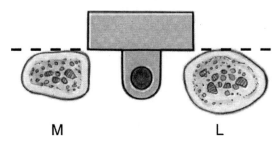

M   L

Figure 27–8. The humeral cutting block is oriented co-planar with the plane of the posterior aspect of the medial and lateral humeral columns.

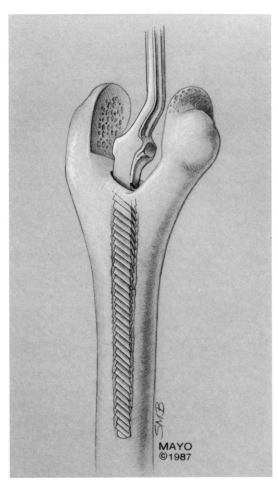

Figure 27–10. The humeral canal is rasped to the appropriate size.

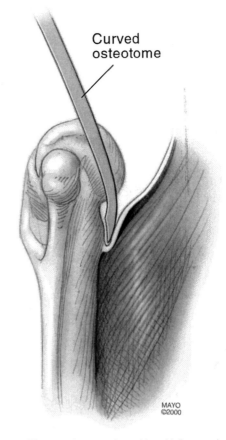

Figure 27–11. The anterior capsule and brachialis muscle insertion is released from the anterior humeral cortex with a curved osteotome.

suture is then brought through the distal medial hole with a Keith needle. The elbow is placed in a 90-degree angle, and the triceps is reduced over the tip of the olecranon. The needle pierces the triceps and a criss-cross, or Krachow, stitch is placed in the triceps

tendon. A transverse suture is then placed across the ulna and through the tendon to further stabilize the attachment.

The ulnar nerve is moved into the subcutaneous pocket and stabilized by a stitch. A drain is optional, but

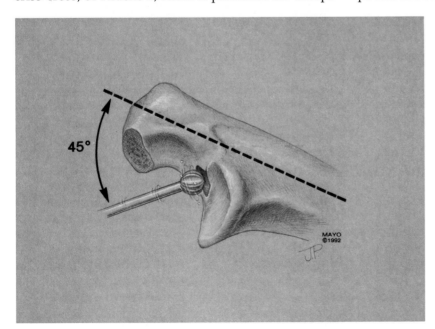

Figure 27–12. Medullary canal of the ulna is identified with a high-speed bur. If the bone is soft, a rongeur can be used.

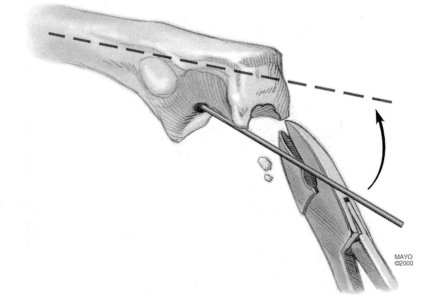

Figure 27–13. To assist in proper alignment, the olecranon is notched with a rongeur in line with the awl.

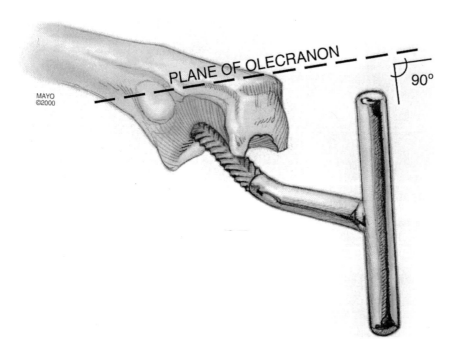

PLANE OF OLECRANON

90°

Figure 27–14. Proper orientation of the rasp is with the handle perpendicular to the flat of the proximal ulna.

Figure 27–15. A trial reduction of the ulna ensures axial rotation as well as proper depth of insertion, replicating the center of the normal articular contour. (By permission of Mayo Foundation for Medical Education and Research.)

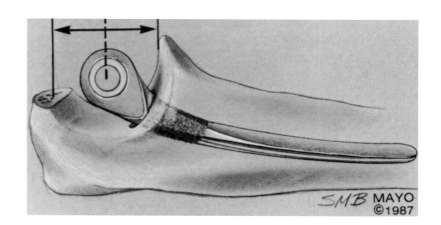

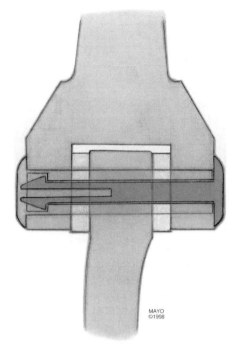

Figure 27–18. The pin-within-the-pin articulating mechanism couples the device.

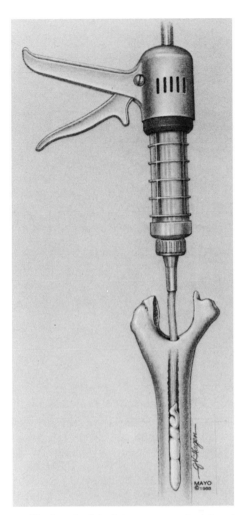

Figure 27–16. The length of the injector system is determined by the anticipated length of the appropriately sized humeral component to be used.

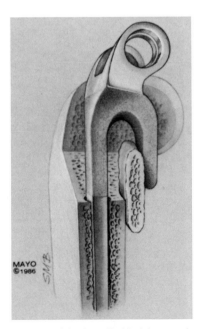

Figure 27–17. A bone graft is placed behind the anterior cortex of the distal humerus, against which the flange of the implant articulates.

care is taken to avoid any suture knots in the subcutaneous border of the ulna. In patients with rheumatoid arthritis, a 3–0 monofilament running suture is used if the skin is thin or atrophic.

POSTOPERATIVE MANAGEMENT

The arm is wrapped in full extension. If there has been a significant flexion contracture, an anterior splint is used. The arm is elevated overnight and during the second day. If drains are used, they are removed the following day. The patient is then allowed to move the elbow as tolerated. A collar and cuff are helpful to keep the patient comfortable. No formal physical therapy is required or employed. Occupational therapy may be helpful for very debilitated patients, but I have not found this necessary over the past several years. Occasionally, if a flexion contracture of greater than 40 degrees persists at discharge, an adjustable splint is used for 8 to 12 weeks to try to resolve this problem.

Functional Limits

Patients are advised before surgery that after the procedure that they are not to lift 1 to 2 pounds repetitively and that they cannot lift more than 5 to 10 pounds in a single event.

RESULTS

This semiconstrained implant was first used in the latter part of 1981, and I have used it almost exclusively

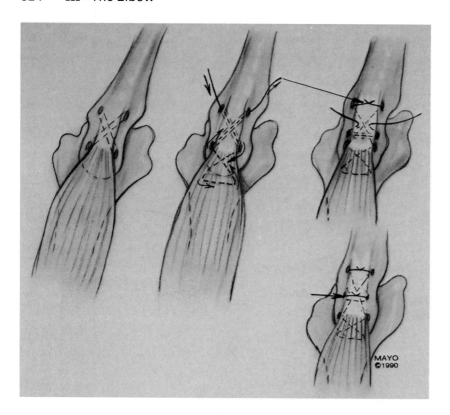

Figure 27–19. Cruciate and transverse drill holes are placed in the proximal ulna. Sutures are then placed through the ulna and in a criss-cross fashion in the tendon. The elbow is at 90 degrees of flexion when these sutures are tied. Alternatively, a locked (Krachow) stitch may be employed.

since then with few modifications. This implant, the Coonrad-Morrey device, has been used in almost 1000 patients in our Mayo practice. The trends in use and indications are shown in Table 27–1. Current indications in our practice are for patients with rheumatoid arthritis (37 percent), posttraumatic injury (30 percent), and revision total elbow replacement surgery (26 percent). The results for the spectrum of indications are summarized in Table

27–2. The outcome for patients with rheumatoid arthritis is particularly gratifying because the survival rate now rivals that of hip replacement (93 percent at 12.5 years[3]) (Fig. 27–20). Good long-term results have also been observed after treatment of patients with post-traumatic arthrosis (Fig. 27–21) and of those with post-traumatic nonunion of the distal humerus (Fig. 27–22). Good early results have also been reported in patients who have undergone the semiconstrained procedure.[4,11] Details of the use of implants for patients with rheumatoid and traumatic conditions are discussed in detail in Chapters 28 and 29.

COMPLICATIONS

The complications following elbow arthroplasty have been nicely reviewed by Gschwend[5] and are discussed in detail in Chapter 30, but a few comments are appropriate here. It is now well known that semiconstrained implants have a lower incidence of loosening than the earlier, more rigidly constrained articulated devices.[4,11]

Table 27–1. CHANGING TRENDS AND INDICATIONS FOR THE USE OF ELBOW REPLACEMENT IN THE MAYO PRACTICE

Year Number	1992 500	2000 920
Diagnoses	Percent	Percent
Rheumatoid	47	37
Traumatic*	23	30
Revision	22	26
Other	8	7

*Includes acute fracture, post-traumatic arthrosis, and nonunion.

Table 27–2. MAYO EXPERIENCE WITH SEMI-CONSTRAINED ELBOW REPLACEMENT FOR A SPECTRUM OF CONDITIONS

Diagnosis	Procedures	Surveillance (mean, yr)	Outcome Satisfactory MEPS	Outcome Satisfactory Subjective
Rheumatoid[3]	78	12.5	88	92
Traumatic arthritis[13]	41	6.5	86	91
Humeral non-union[7]	39	4.5	88	91
Acute fracture[2]	21	5.0	87	92
Resection[12]	19	6.0	86	84
Ankylosis[6]	14	5.3	66	78

Data from references 2, 3, 6, 7, 12, and 13.

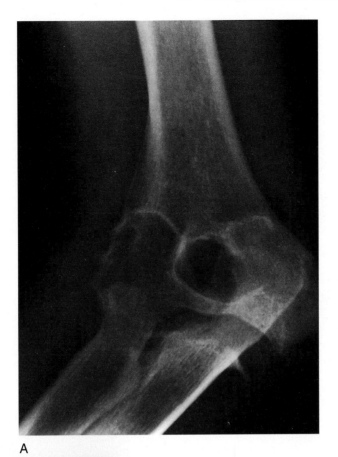

A

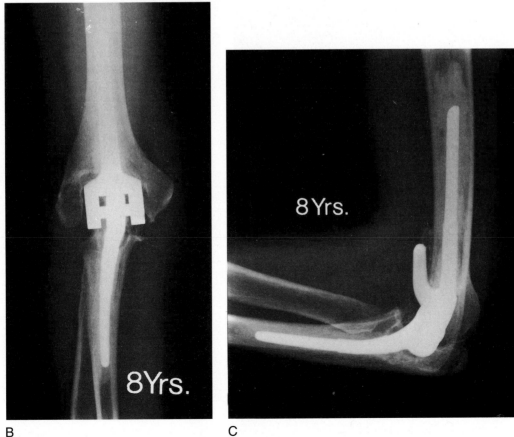

B   C

Figure 27–20. Patient with severe type III rheumatoid arthritis (**A**) effectively treated with the semiconstrained implant (**B** and **C**).

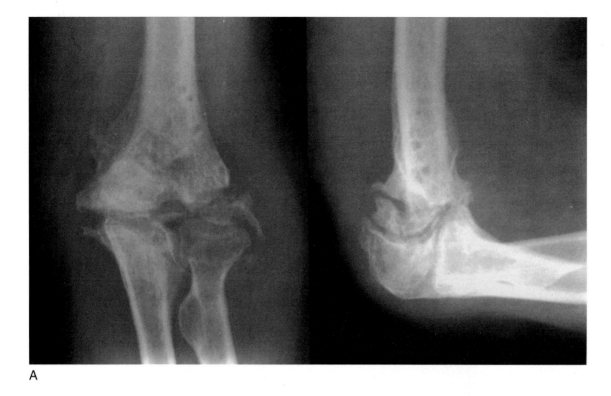

A

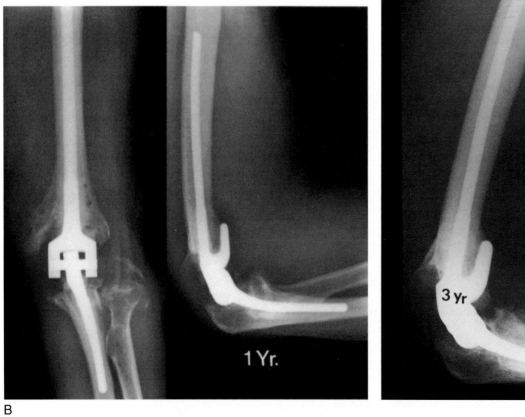

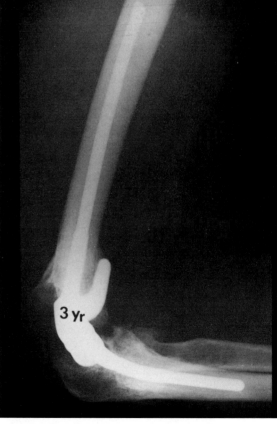

B

Figure 27–21. Post-traumatic arthrosis in a 68-year-old man after failed open reduction with internal fixation (**A**). Excellent radiographic (**B**) and functional result observed 3 years after treatment (**C**).

Illustration continued on opposite page

In the past, experience with loosening at the Mayo Clinic was almost nonexistent.[9] Since 1997, an increased incidence in ulnar osteolysis has prompted the change from a polymethylmethacrylate precoat to a plasma spray surface finish for the ulnar component. The treatment of choice for patients with loose or unstable implants is revision/reimplantation, if possible, and this procedure is discussed in Chapter 32.

Mechanical failure is an uncommon problem with most elbow replacements. I have observed 12 patients with fractured components: 8 (1 percent) of the ulna and 4 (.5 percent) of the humeral component over the last 10 years. In all but four instances, the patient had sustained a significant injury or was using the elbow in an aggressive manner (e.g., lifting 100-pound bags of feed). Reimplantation has been successful in all patients to date.[13] To my knowledge, there have been no ulnar fractures since the ulnar component was surfaced the precoat.

Injury to the ulnar nerve is a well-recognized complication of total elbow arthroplasty, cited in the literature as a complication with a 2 percent to 26 percent incidence,[8] averaging about 5 percent.[2,9] My personal experience is that .5 percent of patients have motor deficiency and about 5 percent have permanent paresthesias. In my opinion, this complication is lessened by exposing, protecting, and translocating the ulnar nerve.

Notable weakness of the triceps is observed in less than 10 percent of patients. Triceps deficiency has required reoperation in 2 percent and was considered successful in 50 percent either from reattachment of the implant or with reoperation using an anconeus rotational reconstruction.

Although wound healing was a major problem in the early experience with total elbow arthroplasty, in my

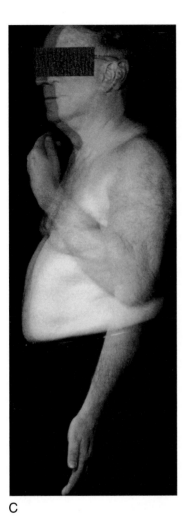

C

Figure 27–21. *Continued.*

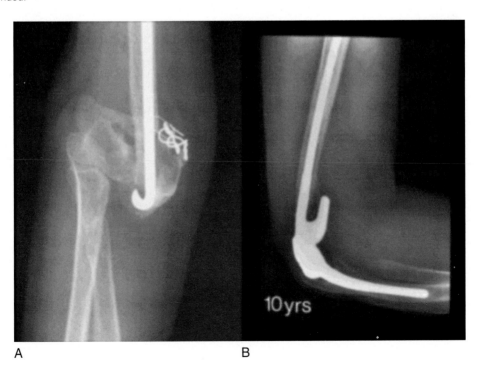

A   B

Figure 27–22. A, A long-established nonunion rendered this extremity useless in a 65-year-old female. **B**, The patient reported nearly normal function 10 years after implantation of semiconstrained implant.

personal experience, the incidence is currently just over 1 percent. Since 1992, there have been five significant wound problems occurring in 300 procedures.

In patients with very thin boneses, in those with rheumatoid arthritis, fracture of the medial supracondylar column is not uncommon and is not considered a significant event. This has occurred in approximately 5 percent of my patients. If the column is extremely thin, I simply excise the fragment. Otherwise, the fragment is secured to the implant with a No. 5 Mersilene suture. I do not alter the postoperative course in response to this occurrence because, to date, no adverse effects have been appreciated as a result of this type of fracture.

References

1. Bryan RS, Morrey BF: Extensive posterior exposure of the elbow. A triceps-sparing approach. Clin Orthop 166:188, 1982.
2. Cobb TK, Morrey BF: Total elbow arthroplasty as primary treatment for distal humeral fracture in elderly patients. J Bone Joint Surg 79A:826, 1997.
3. Gill DRJ, Morrey BF: The Coonrad-Morrey total elbow arthroplasty in patients who have rheumatoid arthritis. A ten to fifteen year follow-up study. J Bone Joint Surg 80A:1327, 1998.
4. Gschwend N, Loehr J, Ivosevic-Radovanovic D, et al: Semiconstrained elbow prostheses with special reference to the GSB III prosthesis. Clin Orthop 232:104, 1988.
5. Gschwend N, Simmen BR, Matejovsky Z: Late complications in elbow arthroplasty. J Shoulder Elbow Surg 5:86, 1996.
6. Mansat P, Morrey BF: Semiconstrained total elbow arthroplasty for ankylosed and stiff elbows. J Bone Joint Surg 82A: 1261, 2000.
7. Morrey BF, Adams RA: Semiconstrained joint replacement arthroplasty for distal humeral nonunion. J Bone Joint Surg 77B: 67, 1995.
8. Morrey BF: Complications of total elbow arthroplasty. *In* Morrey BF (ed): The Elbow and Its Disorders, 3rd ed. Philadelphia, WB Saunders, 2000.
9. Morrey BF, Bryan RS: Complications after total elbow arthroplasty. Clin Orthop 170:202, 1982.
10. O'Driscoll S, An K, Morrey BF: The kinematics of elbow semiconstrained joint replacement. J Bone Joint Surg 74B:297, 1992.
11. Pritchard RW: Long-term follow-up study: Semiconstrained elbow prosthesis. Orthopedics 4:151, 1981.
12. Ramsey ML, Adams RA, Morrey BF: Instability of the elbow treated with semiconstrained total elbow arthroplasty. J Bone Joint Surg 81A:38, 1999.
13. Schneeberger AG, Adams R, Morrey BF: Semiconstrained total elbow replacement for the treatment of posttraumatic arthritis and dysfunction. J Bone Joint Surg 79A:1211, 1997.

28

Results of Semiconstrained Replacement for Rheumatoid Arthritis

•BERNARD F. MORREY and R. A. ADAMS

In this chapter, we discuss the management of rheumatoid involvement of the elbow by semiconstrained joint replacement.

We have classified the radiographic appearance of rheumatoid arthritis of the elbow into five stages. Characterization based on the inflammatory and destructive features has provided a staging system that is used to direct our treatment logic (Table 28–1).[3,11]

GENERAL INDICATIONS

As with all implant options, the best and most commonly employed reason for prosthetic replacement is to relieve pain. Stiffness can be included as an indication in older patients, especially those with bilateral involvement and joint distraction, because this group has few reliable alternatives. Gross instability is also an indication in some patients with the Stage IV "mutalans" version of the disease (Fig. 28–1).

Synovectomy is ideally reserved for the early radiographic stages of the disease (types I and II) when the joint architecture is still intact[8,10] (Fig. 28–2).

SPECIFIC INDIATIONS: SEMICONSTRAINED ARTHROPLASTY

As noted in the previous chapter, the term semiconstrained refers to a coupled articulation with some laxity, or play, at the articulation. In contrast to resurfacing implants, the indications for the semiconstrained implant in general terms represent the full spectrum of elbow pathology. Hence, patients with rheumatoid arthritis can be managed regardless of the amount of bone or soft tissue that has been destroyed. Currently, in our practice, patients of all ages are treated with the semiconstrained device, because the reliability of resurfacing implants has not been demonstrated in our experience. The juvenile rheumatoid patient or the patient with any elbow stiffness that requires an extensive dissection and soft tissue release is readily addressed by the coupled implant, without concern for dislocation.

CONTRAINDICATIONS

There are no unique contraindications to the semiconstrained devices. In the rheumatoid patient, a longer stemmed (15 cm) device is contraindicated if there is or may be consideration of a shoulder replacement. Sepsis and motor dysfunction are contraindications with this device as with other implants.

RESULTS

Several semiconstrained implants have been used in the United States and Europe for more than two decades (Fig. 28–3). The results are reported in Table 28–2.

Triaxial. There is limited up-to-date information about this device. Most of the reports have emanated from the designers, the most comprehensive being that of Kraay et al.[7] This snap-fit design was used in 113 cases: 86 for patients with rheumatoid arthritis and 27 for those with traumatic or "other" etiologies. The outcome varied greatly between the two groups, with variable surveillance up to 99 months. A 6-percent incidence of infection was reported. Loosening was less common in the rheumatoid group (2 percent), compared with the post-traumatic group (22 percent). The survival at 3 years for rheumatoid and traumatic patients was 92 percent and 73 percent, respectively. Over time, the outcome deteriorated for the post-traumatic group. At 5 years, the survival was 90 percent and 53 percent for the two groups, respectively.

The GSB. This Swiss implant is particularly popular in Europe, as a primary implant for rheumatoid arthritis and for trauma and revision situations. Possibly the best and most recent insight as to its effectiveness is gleaned from a review article on complications of elbow replacement by Gschwend et al.[6] In this paper, 133 procedures

Table 28–1. RADIOGRAPHIC APPEARANCE AND TREATMENT OPTIONS

	Radiographic Appearance	Treatment
Type I	Synovitis with a normal appearing joint	Synovectomy
Type II	Loss of joint space	Synovectomy
	Maintenance of subchondral architecture	TEA: Resurfacing/semiconstrained
Type IIIA	Alteration of the subchondral architecture	TEA: Resurfacing/semiconstrained
Type IIIB	Alteration of the architecture with deformity	TEA: Semiconstrained
Type IV	Gross deformity	TEA: Semiconstrained
Type V	Ankylosis[3]	TEA: Semiconstrained

TEA = total elbow arthroplasty.

are discussed. In 48 patients with severe rheumatoid disease, 4 (8 percent) were radiographically loose at 10 to 15 years. The authors report an overall rate of revision for loosening in the rheumatoid group of 2.8 percent and in the post-traumatic group of 6.5 percent. Because of the unique design, the most common problem is that of articular disassembly, which occurs in 3.5 percent of rheumatoid patients and in 15.6 percent of post-traumatic patients through the years (Fig. 28–4). The authors conclude that elbow replacement performed by

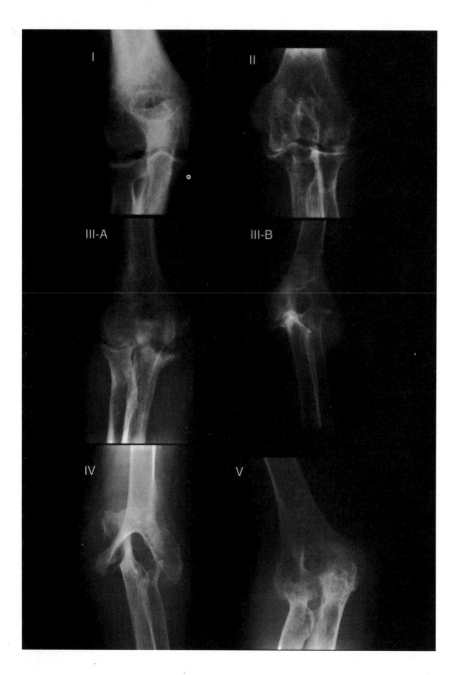

Figure 28–1. Mayo Radiographic Classification of rheumatoid arthritis (see text for definitions). The type V classification was recently added by Connor and Morrey to account for ankylosis.

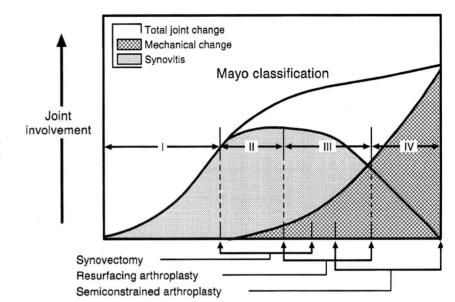

Figure 28–2. Schema relating the inflammatory and structure changes to radiographic appearance and treatment options.

experienced surgeons in selected patients approaches the success of hip or knee replacement (Fig. 28–5).

More recently, a report of the experience was updated by Simmen et al.[16] The 10- to 20-year (mean, 13.5 years) outcomes of 66 cases reveal that the 10-year success rate is 90 percent. Loosening and infection each occurred in 3 patients (5 percent). The revision rate was 8.4 percent. Disassembly remains the most common problem.[16]

Not all have had such impressive results. Schneeberger et al. reported a 60-percent unsatisfactory rate among 14 patients, with follow-up from 2 to 10 years.[15]

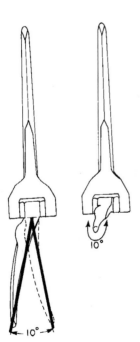

Figure 28–3. The concept of a semiconstrained implant is one that allows some motion or laxity at the ulnohumeral articulation but yet is constrained with regard to the coupling of the components, usually by a pin or axes.

Complications were frequent owing to articular uncoupling in 2 patients and loosening in 4. The loosening was attributed to poor cement technique. On the other hand, Canovas et al. recently reported a 95-percent satisfactory result in 20 patients with the GSBIII at a mean of 3 years after surgery.[2] Hence, the outcome appears to be particularly sensitive to surgical technique.

Mayo Experience

Coonrad-Morrey. The device is characterized by a flange to absorb posterior and torsional forces and a "loose hinge" to absorb axial and rotating forces transmitted to the bone cement interface (Fig. 28–6). Since 1982, our personal experience has been limited to this specific semiconstrained implant. Using the Mayo Elbow Performance Score to document outcome, we have reviewed our experience with both adult rheumatoid patients and juvenile rheumatoid or arthritic patients.[11] Since 1982, experience at our clinic with 927 procedures includes 330 patients (35 percent) with rheumatoid arthritis. In 1998, Gill presented the 10- to 15-year results of 78 consecutive elbows that received the Coonrad-Morrey semiconstrained total elbow arthroplasty.[4] At latest follow-up, 97 percent had no pain or only mild pain (Fig. 28–7). The mean arc of flexion was 28 degrees to 131 degrees. Pronation averaged 68 degrees and supination 62 degrees. In the 76 patients who had long-term radiographic evaluation, there were 2 loose ulnar components, 1 of which was associated with an infection. The other did not require revision at the time of follow-up. However, 5 devices had worn bushings (7 percent) but were not revised (see Chapter 30).

Serious complications occurred in 11 elbows (14 percent), requiring reoperations in 10 patients (13 percent). Delayed complications include avulsion of the triceps in 3, 2 deep infections, 2 ulnar fractures and 1 fracture of an

Table 28–2. SEMICONSTRAINED ELBOW REPLACEMENT FOR RHEUMATOID ARTHRITIS (12 REPORTS, 6 IMPLANTS)

Author	Implant	No.	Rheumatoid Arthritis (%)	Follow-up (yr)	Extension-flexion	Pronation-supination	Pain Relief	Comp (%)	Revised Loose	Satisfied (%)
Inglis, 1978	Triaxial	44	64	3.5	—	—	89	36	2	—
Pritchard, 1981	Pritchard II	92	60	2.5	—	—	98	15	2	85
Rosenfeld, 1982	Pritchard I and II	14	100	2.6	—	—	100	53	—	94
Gschwend, 1988	GSB III	71	72	4	29–140	69–64	93	27	—	91
Canovas, 1999	GSB III	20	20	3	30–139	68–71	95	15	—	95
Leber, 1988	Triaxial	11	100	4 (est)	30–132	75–75	91	36	—	91
Morrey, 1989	Pritchard II	47	48	>5	30–135	60–65	90	32	4	80
Morrey, 1989	Coonrad-Morrey	237	40	>5	29–132	64–62	92	15	2	88
Madsen, 1989	Pritchard II	25	100	3	28–130	65–62	100	8	1	92
Kraay, 1994	Triaxial	86	100	5					3	92
		27	(P.T.)	5	—	—	—	—	22	53
Risung, 1997	Norway	118	100	4.3	—	—	—	—	4	—
Gill, 1998	Coonrad-Morrey	78	100	12.5	31–136	61–62	92	24	1	93
TOTAL		843		5	29–133	65–63	91	26	2	89

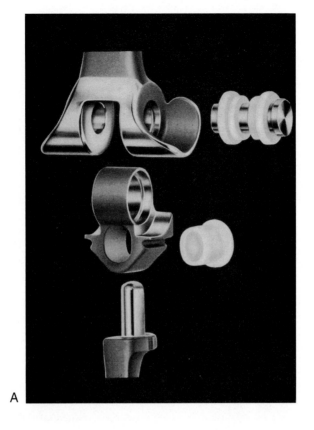

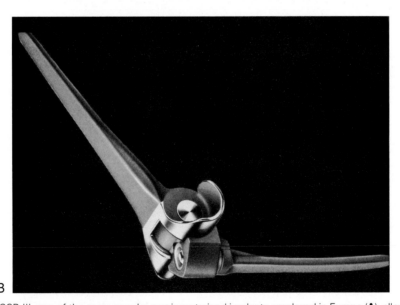

Figure 28–4. The GSB-III, one of the more popular semiconstrained implants employed in Europe (**A**), allows axial rotation of the ulna (**B**). (Courtesy of B. R. Simmen.)

ulnar component. A fracture of the epicondyle is considered unimportant from a functional perspective, but it does reflect the surgeon's technique or the pathology being addressed. Two elbows (2 percent) were revised for aseptic loosening.

The overall 12-year Kaplan-Meier survival rate of this implant was 92.4 percent (Fig. 28–8). An 86-percent good or excellent rating was achieved according to the Mayo

Elbow Performance Score,[11] and 91 percent subjective satisfactory results were present at 12 years of follow-up.

JUVENILE RHEUMATOID ARTHRITIS

The patient with so-called juvenile rheumatoid arthritis poses real problems. Concern about the young age,

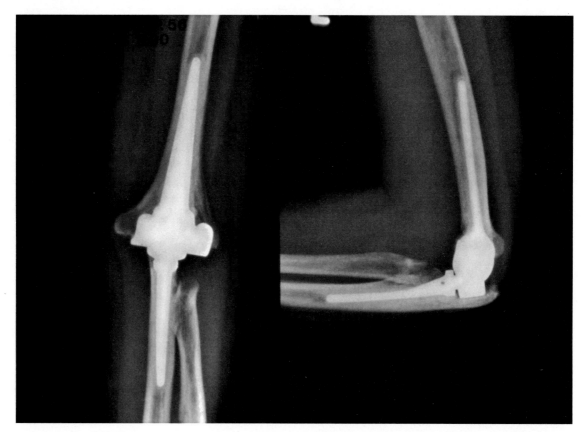

Figure 28–5. The GSB III allows replacement for rheumatoid for rheumatoid arthritis. (Courtesy of B. R. Simmen.)

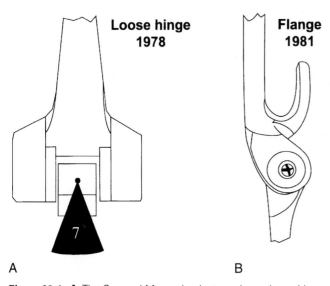

Figure 28-6. A, The Coonrad-Morrey implant employs a loose hinge articulation (1978) and (**B**) a flange (1981) to resist posterior and torsional stresses at the humerus.

frequent stiffness, and small bones make this a difficult management problem. Because these patients have a burnt-out inflammatory process, and because the disease is present during growth, the bones are extremely small and the joint is stiff. These joints are not amenable to synovectomy and do poorly with interposition arthroplasty. Hence, replacement is often performed even in the young patient.

Technique. The most important consideration is an extensive release of soft tissue. This often includes release of the flexor and extensor muscle masses from the humeral condyles as well as a complete resection of the anterior capsule (Fig. 28–9).

RESULTS

Unfortunately, there are few reports regarding the technique or outcome of replacement or any other surgical intervention for that matter. Conner et al. reviewed 24 procedures for juvenile rheumatoid arthritis at the Mayo Clinic a mean of 7.3 years after surgery. Although 96 percent had dramatic relief of pain and the Mayo Elbow Performance Score functional score improved from 9 to 23, flexion improved only 17 degrees, from 73 to 90 degrees. As noted, the major technical problems are articular stiffness and extremely small bones that require equally extremely small implants (Fig. 28–10).

CONCLUSIONS

The current prosthetic options available to manage the patient with rheumatoid arthritis provide predictable

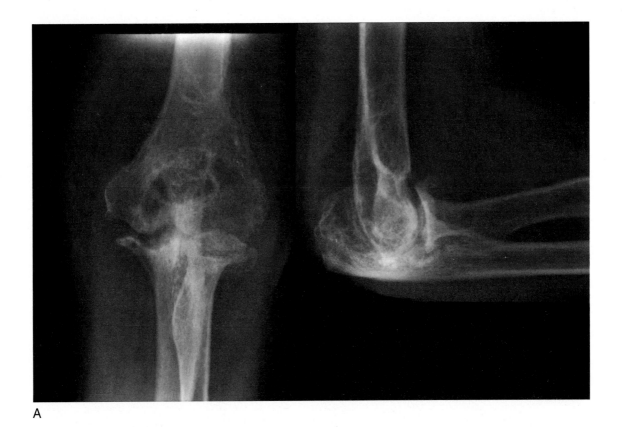

A

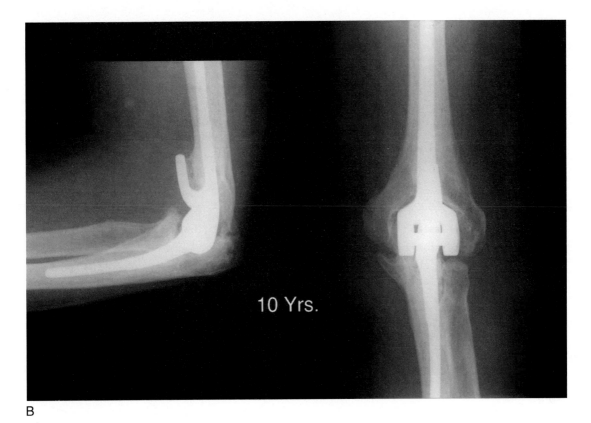

10 Yrs.

B

Figure 28–7. A, Grade III rheumatoid arthritis. **B**, Ten year result with the Coonrad/Morrey implant.

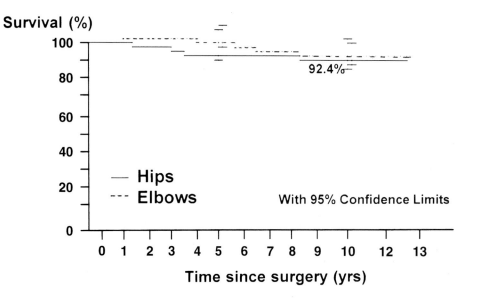

Survival (%)

— Hips
--- Elbows

92.4%

With 95% Confidence Limits

Time since surgery (yrs)

Figure 28–8. The Coonrad-Morrey Kaplan-Meier Survival Curve for revision at 10 to 15 years is similar to that of hip replacement for rheumatoid arthritis.

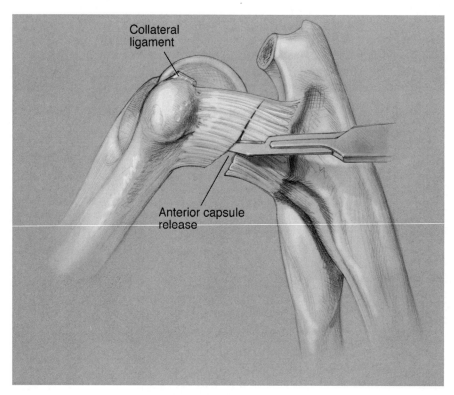

Collateral ligament

Anterior capsule release

Figure 28–9. Aggressive release of the capsule and flexor/extensor muscle attachment at the humerus is often required to address the stiffness seen in the patient with juvenile rheumatoid arthritis.

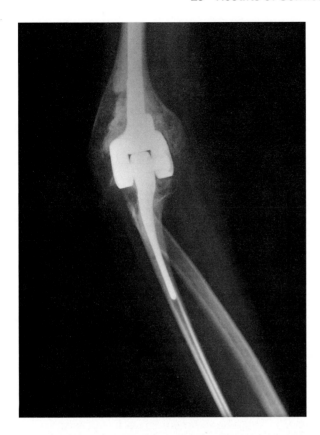

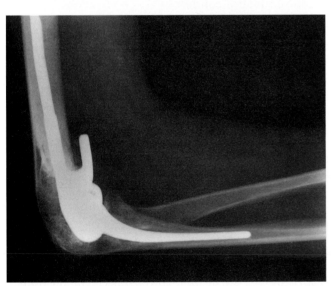

Figure 28–10. The medullary canal of the juvenile rheumatoid patient is extremely small in some instances. Extra-small stems are required to effectively manage these patients.

outcomes. Joint replacement is emerging as a reliable and predictable procedure in the hands of an experienced surgeon. The semiconstrained implant predictably yields these outcomes, even with the broad spectrum of pathology. The complication rate remains high (see Chapter 30).

References

1. Bayley JIL: Elbow replacement in rheumatoid arthritis. Reconstr Surg Traumatol 18:70, 1981.
2. Canovas F, Ledoux D, Bonnel F: Total elbow arthroplasty in rheumatoid arthritis. 20 GSBIII prosthesis followed 2–5 years. Acta Orthop Scand 70:564–568, 1999.
3. Connor PM, Morrey BF: Total elbow arthroplasty in patients who have juvenile rheumatoid arthritis. J Bone Joint Surg 80:678–688, 1998.
4. Gill DRJ, Morrey BF: The Coonrad-Morrey total elbow arthroplasty in patients who have rheumatoid arthritis. A 10 to 15 year follow-up study. J Bone Joint Surg 80A:1327–1335, 1998.
5. Gschwend N, Loehr J, Ivosevic-Radovanovic D, et al: Semiconstrained elbow prosthesis with special reference to the GSB III prosthesis. Clin Orthop 232:104, 1988.
6. Gschwend N, Simmen BR, Matejovsky Z: Late complications in elbow arthroplasty. J Shoulder Elbow Surg 5(2)Pt. 1:86–96, 1996.
7. Kraay MJ, Figgie MP, Inglis AE, et al: Primary semiconstrained total elbow arthroplasty. Survival analysis of 113 consecutive cases. J Bone Joint Surg 76B:636–640, 1994.
8. Lee BPH, Morrey BF: Arthroscopic synovectomy of the elbow for rheumatoid arthritis. A prospective study. J Bone Joint Surg 79B:770, 1997.
9. Madsen F, Gudmundson GH, Sjbjerg JO, Sneppen O: Pritchard Mark II elbow prosthesis in rheumatoid arthritis. Acta Orthop Scand 60:249–253, 1989.
10. Morrey BF: The elbow: Semiconstrained devices. In Morrey BF (ed): Joint Replacement Arthroplasty, 3rd ed. Philadelphia, Churchill Livingstone, 2000.
11. Morrey BF, Adams RA: Semiconstrained arthroplasty for the treatment of rheumatoid arthritis of the elbow. J Bone Joint Surg 74A:479–490, 1992.
12. Pritchard RW: Long-term follow-up study: Semiconstrained elbow prosthesis. Orthopaedics 4:151, 1981.
13. Risung F: The Norway elbow replacement. Design, technique and results after nine years. J Bone Joint Surg 79B:394–402, 1997.
14. Rosenfeld SR, Ansel SH: Evaluation of the Pritchard total elbow arthroplasty. Orthopedics 5:713, 1982.
15. Schneeberger AG, Hertel R, Gerber C: Total elbow replacement with the GSB III prosthesis. J Shoulder Elbow Surg 9:135–139, 2000.
16. Simmen BR, Schwyzer HK, Loehr J, Gschwend N: Joint Replacement in Rheumatoid Arthritis. 8th ICSS April 23-26, 2001, Cape Town, South Africa.

29

Semiconstrained Elbow Replacement: Results in Traumatic Conditions

• BERNARD F. MORREY

For elbow trauma, prosthetic replacement may be indicated and is effective in both acute and reconstructive settings (Table 29–1).

ACUTE DISTAL HUMERAL FRACTURE

Indications for Replacement

The treatment of choice for most displaced intra-articular fractures of the elbow joint is open reduction and internal fixation.[13,16,17] However, in a review of nine studies of osteosynthesis of distal humerus fractures, fair to poor outcomes were reported in 25 percent, with a high complication rate requiring secondary procedures in 70 percent.[13] In the elderly, problems of fixation are exaggerated as a result of marked osteoporosis and extensive comminution.[13,16,34]

Hence the indication for semiconstrained total joint replacement for acute fractures of the distal humerus is limited to patients older than about 65 years with an extensively comminuted fracture that is not amenable to an adequate and stable osteosynthesis. The usual findings are (1) a large number of small fragments, (2) poor-quality osteoporotic bone, (3) significant loss of joint fragments in open injuries, and (4) pre-existing joint damage in patients with rheumatoid arthritis or other inflammatory joint diseases. The fact that, at the Mayo Clinic, only 21 acute distal humerus fractures (10 of them having associated rheumatoid arthritis) were treated by total joint replacement during a 10-year period emphasizes our strict selection criteria.[4]

Technique

The operative technique for implantation of the semiconstrained Coonrad-Morrey prosthesis is described in Chapter 27, but the specific features that are characteristic of the procedure for acute fracture should be emphasized. A type II or III compound fracture should first be irrigated and débrided to avoid wound infection. Total elbow replacement is then performed in a second stage.

A type I wound may be treated in a single stage after careful and thorough débridement.

A posterior midline incision is used after the hematoma is evacuated, and the exposure is generally initiated from the medial aspect. Fracture fragments are excised. The ulnar nerve is always identified and transposed anteriorly in a subcutaneous pocket after translocating the nerve by releasing the flexor/pronator muscle group from the fractured medial epicondyle (Fig. 29–1A). The extensor mass is released from the fractured lateral condyle (Fig. 29–1B). Working from both sides of the triceps attachment, all remaining fracture fragments are excised. A portion of bone is preserved to prepare the bone graft to be placed behind the flange of the humeral implant. The triceps attachment is left intact, which allows for rapid functional recovery.

Significant bone stock deficiencies with lack of one or both epicondyles does not change or complicate the implantation of the humeral component. This device requires only the humeral diaphysis to obtain secure fixation. Therefore, the reconstruction of the condyles is not required or recommended (Fig. 29–2).

The humeral device is available in three lengths—10, 15, and 20 cm—and in three diameters—standard, small, and extra small. It has an extended flange option useful in treating distal humeral deficiency (Fig. 29–3). In cases of acute fracture, we normally use the 15-cm (6-inch) stem. The extended flange is used for fractures occurring proximal to the roof of the olecranon fossa. The standard long flange implant can be used for fractures involving 6 cm of distal humerus. By allowing 2 cm of shortening, which does not cause measureable strength loss, up to 8 cm of distal humerus may be reconstructed with this system (Fig. 29–4). A trial reduction is carried out, and proper depth of humeral insertion is determined.[14]

The humerus is easily prepared with the appropriate-sized rasp. For the ulna preparation, the forearm is internally rotated and a small portion of triceps attachment is released from the medial corner of the olecranon. This allows better exposure of the olecranon, which is removed to allow access down the canal. The subcutaneous portion of the proximal ulna is palpated and the ulna is entered with a high-speed burr at the base of the

Table 29–1. MAJOR COMPLICATIONS WITH TOTAL ELBOW ARTHROPLASTY AFTER ACUTE FRACTURE AND TRAUMATIC ARTHROSIS

Orthopedic Complication	Acute[4] (N = 21)	Arthrosis[29] (N = 41)	Ankylosis[22] (N = 14)	Nonunion[25] (N = 39)	Gross Instability[28] (N = 19)
Loosening	0	0	2*	0	1
Infection	0	2*	2*	2	0
Wear	0	2*	0	3	0
Fracture of ulnar component	1*	5*	1*	0	2
Other	1	4	2	2	1
Total (%)	10	32	50	18	21

*Required revision/reoperation.

coronoid. The ulnar canal in older patients is usually atrophic, and the canal requires relatively little preparation. Care must be taken, however, to assure that the rasp is down the canal.

A trial reduction is performed. The standard-length ulnar component is usually used. The small- and standard-diameter sizes of the humeral and ulnar components are interchangeable, so either element can be used depending on the best fit for each bone. Proper depth of humeral insertion is determined by placing axial traction on the forearm when flexed 90 degrees. The position of the humeral component is noted and is thus determined to be the proper depth of insertion (Fig. 29–5).

The cement injector system is used because the components are usually inserted simultaneously. Absence of the distal humerus facilitates coupling the implant with the interlocking axes.

At the end of the procedure, if the triceps has been reflected, it is reattached to the olecranon with two No. 5 nonabsorbable sutures, allowing immediate use of the joint. Compression dressings and elevation of the extremity are recommended for about 2 days, followed by gentle active range of motion as tolerated. Formal physical therapy is not necessary.

Results with the Coonrad-Morrey Prosthesis

The Mayo experience of 21 semiconstrained Coonrad-Morrey total elbow replacements in 20 patients with distal humeral fracture was reported by Cobb and Morrey in 1997[4] and remains the only report of total elbow replacement for acute fractures in the literature to date. The specific indication for total elbow arthroplasty was an extensively comminuted intra-articular fracture in 11 patients who were more than 65 years old, and a comminuted acute fracture of the distal aspect of the

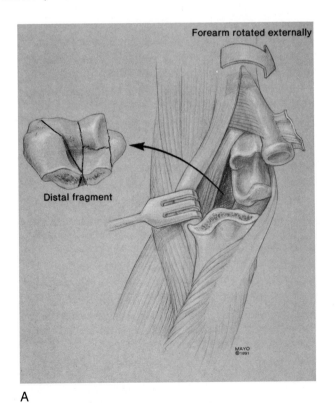

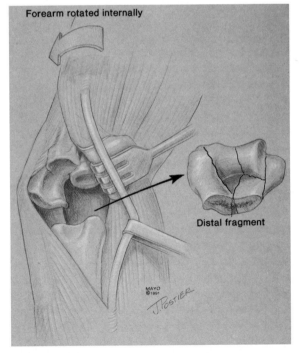

A

B

Figure 29–1. For acute fractures and distal humeral nonunion, the fracture fragments are completely excised, releasing all tissue both medially (**A**) and laterally (**B**), thus allowing implantation without removal of the triceps. The ulna is best prepared by releasing the medial aspect of the triceps attachment, rotating the ulna, and approaching the canal from the medial aspect of the ulna. (By permission of Mayo Foundation for Medical Education and Research.)

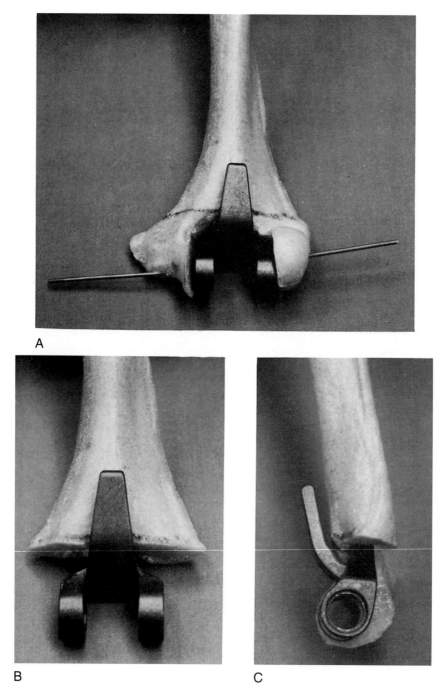

Figure 29–2. With bone loss at the level of the roof of the olecranon fossa (**A**) the axis of rotation remains at the anatomic level (**B** and **C**).

humerus in 9 patients (10 elbows) who also had destruction of the articular surface secondary to rheumatoid arthritis. The mean age of the patients at the time of injury was 72 years (range 48 to 92). Follow-up averaged 4 years. Subjectively, all 21 patients were satisfied (Fig. 29–6). On the basis of the Mayo Elbow Performance Score (MEPS), 15 elbows had an excellent and 5 had a good result. Pain relief was reliably obtained, with 17 patients having no pain and 3 patients having mild pain. The mean arc of flexion-extension was 25 to 130 degrees, and the mean arc of pronation-supination was 74 to 73

degrees. With a maximum follow-up of 10.5 years, no implant was loose. Severe osteoporosis was common but did not appear to influence the functional result.

Complications/Reoperations

There were two cases of temporary ulnar nerve neurapraxis. One patient fell on the outstrethced hand 3 years after surgery, fracturing the ulnar component of the implant. Ten years after revision, at age 85, a MEPS score of 90 was calculated.

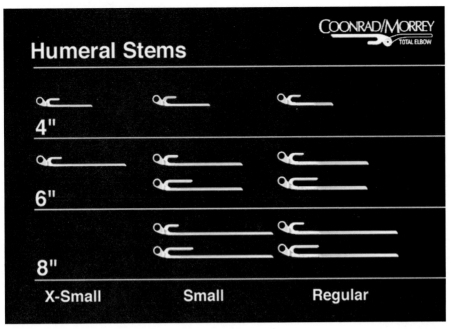

Figure 29–3. Three lengths and three diameters of humeral implants are available. The extended flange is available in 150- and 200-cm stem lengths.

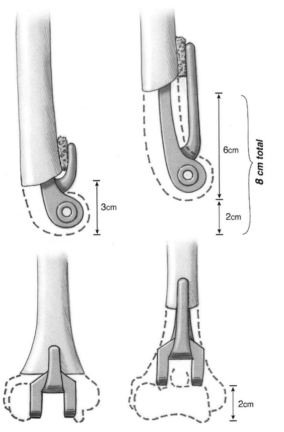

Figure 29–4. Using an extended flange and allowing 2 cm of shortening, up to 8 cm of distal humeral bone loss is addressed by this system.

Conclusion

Semiconstrained Coonrad-Morrey total elbow replacement for acute fractures of the distal aspect of the humerus can be a very reliable treatment in a specific group of elderly patients but is not an alternative procedure to osteosynthesis in younger patients.

FRACTURE OF THE OLECRANON

This is a rare indication for elbow replacement. We reserve the prosthesis for severely comminuted Mayo IIIB fractures when osteosynthesis and stability are not considered attainable.

TRAUMATIC ARTHRITIS

Post-traumatic osteoarthrosis differs from acute traumatic conditions in several aspects and poses greater treatment difficulties. This chronic painful condition is usually characterized by stiffness, joint and bone deformity with extensive soft tissue contractures, bone loss, and instability. Typically one or more previous procedures have resulted in a poor soft tissue envelope, infection, and nerve injury.[29]

Nonreplacement Options

Few options exist to salvage severe post-traumatic osteoarthrosis. Arthrodesis reliably relieves pain[23] but results in great functional impairment,[27] and hence is

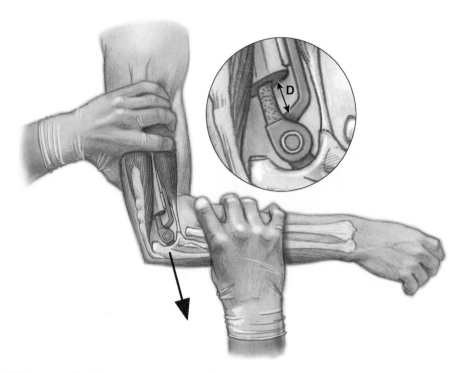

Figure 29–5. With severe distal humerus bone loss, traction is applied to the forearm at 90 degrees of flexion. The resulting position of the humerus (*D*) is defined as the optimum position of insertion.

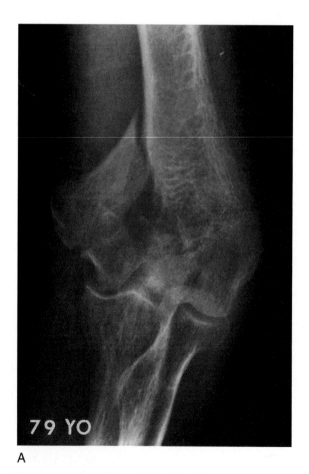

A

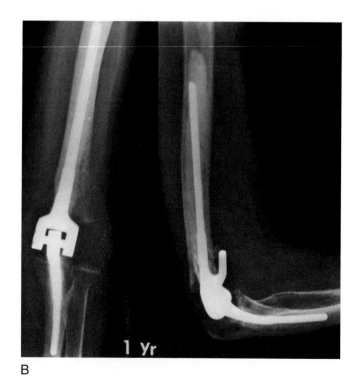

B

Figure 29–6. A, A 79-year-old female with a comminuted distal humeral fracture. **B,** Patient is asymptomatic with essentially normal function at 1 year after joint replacement.

rarely considered a viable option.[6,26] Interposition arthroplasty may be considered for a young patient, particularly one who has stiffness. Restoration of motion and relief of pain can be achieved with a reasonable (70 percent) but unpredictable rate of success.[7,9,19,24,32] However, interposition arthroplasty has an even higher rate of complication than that associated with semiconstrained total elbow replacement.[7,19] Interposition arthroplasty also is not considered suitable for patients who perform strenuous physical labor.[3,19] Varying results have been reported for allograft replacement of the entire elbow joint.[5,33] Concern regarding the high complication rate (30 percent), continued degenerative changes, and neurotrophic changes of the allograft explain why this procedure has not found wide acceptance.

Prosthetic Replacement Selection

For post-traumatic osteoarthrosis, total joint replacement using the semiconstrained Coonrad-Morrey prosthesis is in our hands the treatment of choice in selected elderly patients. Advanced destruction of the ulnohumeral joint with marked narrowing or loss of the joint space is thought to preclude other reliable treatment modalities such as débridement or ulnohumeral arthroplasty for those patients who are older than 60 years. For patients younger than 60 years, total elbow replacement should be performed only with reservation, if no other suitable alternatives of operative treatment are available or for those who have failed other reconstructive procedures, such as interposition arthroplasty. Furthermore, replacement is reserved only for those patients who do not perform strenuous physical activities.

Activity

Concerns about excessive use and wear are significant. We always advise the patients after a total elbow replacement to avoid single-event lifting of objects that weight more than 5 kg as well as repetitive loads of more than 1 kg. We discourage playing golf. Patients unwilling to accept these restrictions are not operated on or are offered an interposition arthroplasty.

Deformity and Stiffness

The pathologic presentation post-trauma can vary from gross instability to ankylosis. Instability is discussed below. Here we deal with deformity and stiffness. Deformity, a feature often encountered in post-traumatic osteoarthrosis, is expressed as angular abnormalities of more than 30 degrees or fixed subluxation (Fig. 29–7).[29] Longstanding deformity, extensive soft tissue contraction, prior treatment, or sepsis also potentiate soft tissue contractures. Unlinked resurfacing total elbow prostheses usually do not allow the extensive releases required to correct this pathology without causing instability. Although hinged semiconstrained prostheses have the major advantage of being able to correct deformity and

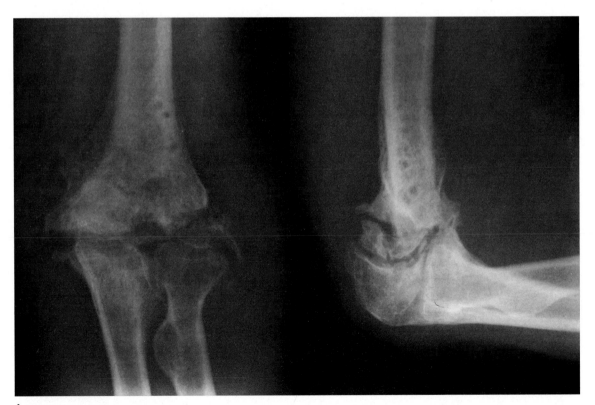

A

Figure 29–7. **A**, Severe arthrosis with posterior subluxation after open reduction and internal fixation (ORIF) and hardware removal. **B**, Excellent result at 3 years.

Illustration continued on following page

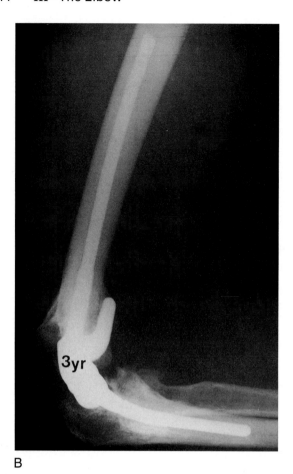

B

Figure 29–7. *Continued.*

tolerate extensive releases, this correction may be at the expense of persistent or increased asymmetric loads imparted by the distorted soft tissues, causing increased wear of the prosthesis. Overall, a marked preoperative deformity of the elbows was associated in our experience with a significantly higher rate of complication ($P = 0.02$).[28] The final arc of motion in the ankylosed joint is also considerably less than the norm.[28]

Technique

Special technical considerations for the management of the various expressions of the traumatic elbow are important to review.

Incision

A midline posterior incision is preferred. Prior skin incisions are used if they allow exposure of both medial and lateral aspects of the joint. If prior incisions are poorly placed, they are ignored if they are at least 1 year old.

Ulnar Nerve

The ulnar nerve is identified and isolated. If asymptomatic and previously translocated, it is left alone after

noting its course. If the nerve is in its anatomic location, it is released proximal to Struthers' ligament and distally to the first motor branch and brought into a subcutaneous pocket anteriorly.

Triceps

For most presentations, the Mayo approach is used and the triceps is reflected from medial to lateral. With gross instability from lack of a distal humerus, the triceps is left intact and the posterior aspect of the humerus is identified medially. The extensor mechanism is freed proximally and distally to its site of attachment. The end of the humerus is delivered from the side of the triceps most easily accomplished based on the pre-existing deformity. If no tendency exists, we expose the humerus from the medial margin of the humerus but take special care to protect the ulnar nerve.

Tissue Release

If unstable, the humerus is exposed as described above. The ulna is prepared by rotating the forearm, releasing a portion of the medial triceps attachment and removing the olecranon tip. This allows entry of the canal from the medial aspect by a burr through the base of the coronoid.

If the joint is ankylosed or stiff, exposure is the most difficult but important part of the procedure. The tip of the olecranon is removed after the triceps is reflected laterally with the Mayo approach. By flexing the forearm, the joint can be identified, and adhesions are removed by sharp dissection. The collateral ligaments are released from the humerus, and the elbow is further flexed. With stiff joints, the anterior capsule is contracted so the capsule is sharply excised, being careful anterior to the radial head. If the stiffness is severe, we release both flexion and extension muscle origins from the humeral condyles (Fig. 29–8).

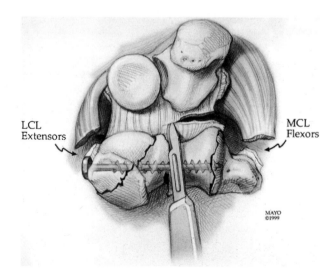

LCL
Extensors

MCL
Flexors

MAYO
©1999

Figure 29–8. If the traumatic arthritis is associated with marked fibrosis, capsular and possibly epicondylar attachment releases are required to enhance motion. (By permission of Mayo Foundation for Medical Education and Research.)

Preparation and Implantation

For the unstable joint with absent distal humerus, a most important technical step is trial reduction and tensioning the elbow distally at 90 degrees' flexion (see Fig. 29–5). This determines the proper depth of insertion of the humeral component when the bone loss exceeds 5 to 6 cm.

For the stiff joint, if trial reduction reveals persistent contracture exceeding 30 degrees in flexion or extension, the humeral component is set more proximally. The limiting factor is the medial column, which will fracture if the device is placed too proximal. In severe contracture, an acceptable tactic is to osteotomize the medial column, removing it if necessary.

Final rotational placement of the implant follows the guidelines noted above. If the distal humerus is absent, the anterior triangular orientation of the humeral cortex, the intermuscular septum, and even the location of the radial nerve can all be used to properly orient the humeral component in internal-external rotation.

Closure

Prior to closure for post-traumatic arthritis, we always release the tourniquet and obtain hemostasis. For the patient with an intact triceps, the closure is routine. In the ankylosed elbow the triceps is brought back over the ulna and motion tested. If the triceps is so contracted as to restrict flexion past 100 to 110 degrees, the anconeus is mobilized by releasing the interval between it and the extensor carpi ulnaris. The muscle is elevated and rotated over the ulna. If the triceps remains a problem, the anconeus is elevated from its bed and brought over the proximal ulna. The elbow is flexed to about 110 to 120 degrees and the triceps and anconeus are attached through drill holes to the ulna in the recessed position (Fig. 29–9).

Aftercare

For the unstable elbow, no specific restrictions are required. For the stiff joint, adjustable night splints are used, especially to address flexion contracture.

Results

Traumatic Arthrosis: Results in the Literature

Little exists in the literature regarding outcomes of elbow replacement for trauma. What has been described is rather implant specific and pessimistic,[10,18,20,21,30] and does not distinguish the results based on the pathology being treated.[2,18,20,21,30]

Inglis and Pellicci,[15] in 1980, reported little improvement in nine patients who had been managed with a semiconstrained Pritchard-Walker triaxial implant. Lowe et al.[21] reported a satisfactory result in only one of seven trauma patients who had an unconstrained device. In 1984, Soni and Cavendish[30] reported a good or excellent result for only three of eight patients who had an unconstrained implant. Apart from our own experience, Figgie et al.[8] published the only other report suggesting a favorable experience with a semiconstrained (triaxial) prosthesis. This report, however, was on custom-designed stems with variable lengths as well as fixation with or without cement for the treatment of post-traumatic conditions not well characterized. Eight of their nine patients were reported as having a satisfactory result.[8] In 1994, Kraay et al.,[20] from the same institution, reported their experience with a linked semiconstrained implant. Of 113 patients, only 18 had been managed for post-traumatic osteoarthrosis, nonunion, or fracture. The results of these patients were disappointing, with a 5-year rate of survival of the implants of only 53 percent. There were five loose humeral components and two infections among the 18 patients.

In 1996, Gschwend et al.[12] reported their experience with 26 patients with post-traumatic osteoarthrosis of the elbow treated with total joint replacement using the semiconstrained GSB III implant. The mean follow-up was 4.3 years (maximum 14 years). Pain relief was obtained in 82 percent of cases; the mean arc of flexion was 34 to 126 degrees. However, the revision rate was 31 percent as a result of aseptic loosening in two, disassembly in four, and ectopic bone formation in two elbows. By far the largest experience with joint replacement for post-traumatic stiffness is from India. Baksi reported outcomes of 68 stiff elbows treated by his design of a semiconstrained implant.[1] Although the mean age was only 29 years, he reported 80 percent satisfactory outcomes at 10 years. The mean arc of motion in 87 percent was reported at 27 to 115 degrees. Complications occurred in 14 (20 percent) and infection was present in 7 (10 percent). The radiographic status of these patients is unclear.

Mayo Clinic Experience

An in-depth review of the Mayo experience with repair of traumatic conditions has been reported.

TRAUMATIC ARTHRITIS

In 1997, Schneeberger et al. reviewed 41 consecutive cases of traumatic arthritis treated from 1981 to 1993 by semiconstrained Coonrad-Morrey elbow replacement and followed an average of 6 years.[29] The mean age of the patients was 57 years (range 32 to 82). The indication for joint replacement was pain for 36 patients; reduced, painful range of motion for 2 patients; and dysfunction with a flail elbow for 3 patients. The average time from the original fracture to the joint replacement was 16 years (range 3 months to 64 years).

This is a very difficult group of patients to manage. All but two patients (95%) had had previous surgery, with the average being 2.3 procedures (range 0 to 7). Significant bone stock deficiency with loss of at least one condyle was present in 13 patients, and 14 patients had a significant joint or bone deformity. Ten of 41 elbow joints were preoperatively subluxed and 7 were dislocated (Fig. 29–10). Additional complications from prior surgery included mild to moderate ulnar neuropathy in

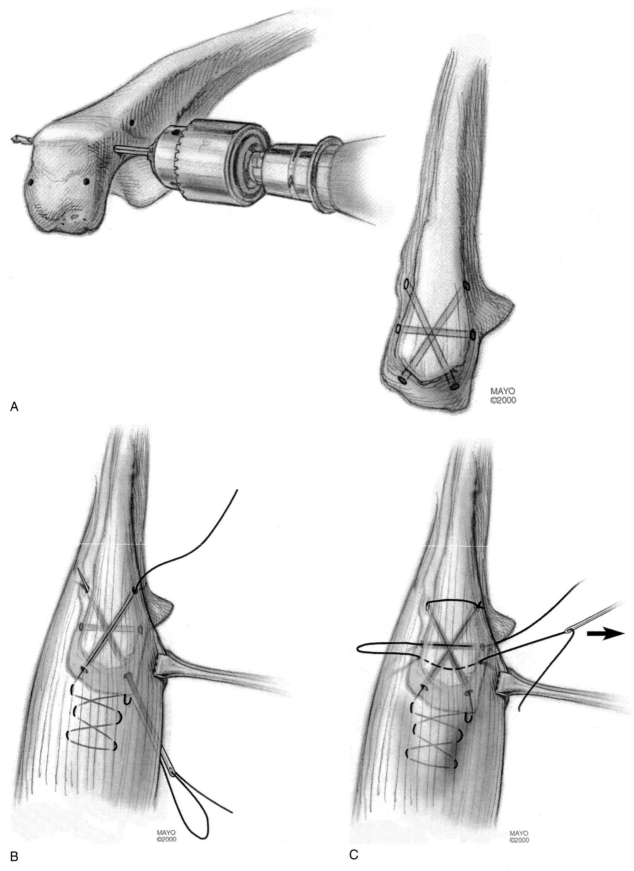

A

B

C

Figure 29–9. Secure reattachment of the triceps is accomplished with crossing drill holes in the olecranon (**A**) and the use of No. 5 nonabsorbable suture in a criss-cross (**B**) and transverse (**C**) pattern. (By permission of Mayo Foundation for Medical Education and Research.)

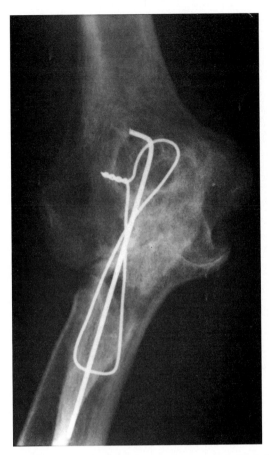

Figure 29–10. A 58-year-old farmer showing preoperative deformity and stiffness. The patient had moderate pain and marked loss of motion.

six patients and radial nerve palsy caused by a complete traumatic laceration in one patient.

At the latest follow-up, objectively 40 percent of outcomes were rated excellent and 43 percent were considered good, for an overall rate of 83 percent satisfactory objective outcome. Subjectively, 95 percent of the patients with a functioning implant expressed satisfaction with the operation. Although the rate of pain relief (76 percent) was considered to be rather high, it was not as high as that reported after the treatment of rheumatoid arthritis (93 percent).[25] At follow-up, the mean arc of flexion-extension was 27 to 131 degrees, and the mean arc of pronation-supination was 60 to 66 degrees (Fig. 29–11). An average of 4.8 of the 5 activities of daily living could be performed by the patients, and strength improvement averaged approximately 30 percent.

The radiologic analysis showed all grafts behind the flange to have incorporated. There was not one case of aseptic loosening within the 12 years of follow-up.

Stiffness. As a special subset, Mansat and Morrey[22] reported 14 cases of post-traumatic arthritis with no or less than 30 degrees of motion treated by the Coonrad-Morrey implant. Patients were followed for a mean of 63 months. The average preoperative MEPS was 39 points (range, 5 to 64 points), and the mean postoperative score was 73 points (range, 45 to 100 points).

Pain. At the most recent follow-up evaluation, none of the elbows was severely painful, and 6 of 14 were free of all pain.

Range of Motion. The mean total preoperative arc of flexion was 7 degrees, representing a mean arc ranging from 69 to 76 degrees. Postoperatively, total arc of flexion was 67 degrees (range 42 to 109 degrees). Hence, the mean increase in the arc of flexion was 60 degrees, 33 degrees in flexion and 27 degrees in extension.

Complications. The majority of the complications were of a mechanical cause. Fracture of the ulnar component occurred in one prosthesis in the acute fracture group and in five prostheses in the post-traumatic group 2 to 9 years (average, 4.3 years) postoperatively. Before breakage, all six patients had an excellent result with an asymptomatic, essentially normal elbow. The cause of failure were severe noncompliance, such as

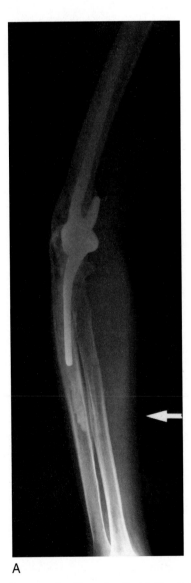

A

Figure 29–11. Postoperative films of patient in Figure 29–10 showing excellent range of motion.

Illustration continued on following page

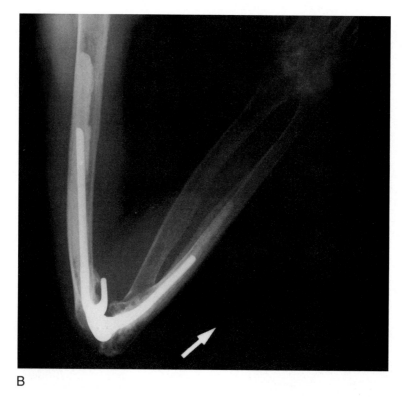

B

Figure 29–11. *Continued.*

regular lifting of weights of more than 50 kg in two patients. The revisions involved an average of less than 70 minutes of tourniquet time. There were no operative or delayed complications from the reoperation.

The fractures of the ulnar component always occurred at the site of sintered beads. The current implant has a plasma-titanium spray, and no fractures of the ulnar component have occurred with this implant to date.

Because the total elbow prosthesis is a mechanical device, it is subject to wear, particularly of the polyethylene bushings. Those patients with post-traumatic osteoarthrosis in our series who were younger than 60 years had a higher rate of complication (35 vs. 17 percent) and, accordingly, a lower proportion of satisfactory results (78 compared to 89 percent) (Fig. 29–12).

Despite the use of semiconstrained devices, most series of post-traumatic osteoarthrosis are still complicated by a certain rate of loosening.[20] However, no loosening was observed by Figgie et al.[8] in their series of nine semiconstrained triaxial prosthesis with custom-designed stems. Gschwend et al.[12] reported that, after a mean of 4.3 years (maximum 14 years), loosening occurred in 2 of 26 patients. That only 1 of the 62 cases reported at the Mayo Clinic have loosened indicates the great improvement in total elbow replacement, particularly in this very difficult group of patients.

ANKYLOSIS

This group has the greatest incidence of complications. Mansat and Morrey reported 7 of 14 patients with complications in the Mayo Clinic experience.[22] Of even greater concern is that four of the seven patients had a

reoperation. Infection occurred in two of these patients; one was salvaged with a fair result and one had a resection arthroplasty with a poor outcome. A proximal ulnar fracture required revision at 1 year. The revision was effective for 9 years, but the current radiograph shows a loose ulnar component, and the patient will likely require additional surgery.

Distal Humeral Nonunion and Gross Instability

Post-traumatic instability from bone loss and nonunion are special cases well managed with the Coonrad-Morrey device.[29] Because of its hinge design, this implant yields immediate and durable stability. In contrast to certain other semiconstrained implants,[12] the Coonrad-Morrey device provides valgus-varus and axial stability without a tendency of disassembling of the components. In fact, significant bone stock deficiency was present in approximately 33 percent of patients in our series with posttraumatic osteoarthrosis. Only the humeral diaphysis is required to obtain secure fixation of the Coonrad-Morrey prosthesis. Rotational and anteroposterior stability is maintained by the anterior flange and bone graft. Thus this implant does not require the condyles for mechanical support. In post-traumatic osteoarthrosis, as in acute fracture, loss of the condyles does not require their reconstruction. This enormously facilitates total elbow replacement and constitutes a great advantage over those total elbow prostheses that need the condyles for stability.[11,12,31] If the bone loss extends into the supracondylar area, this is accommodated as

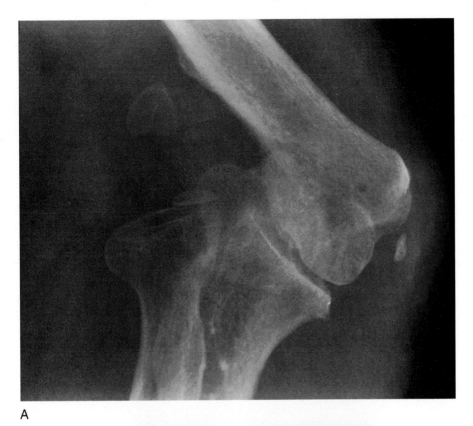

A

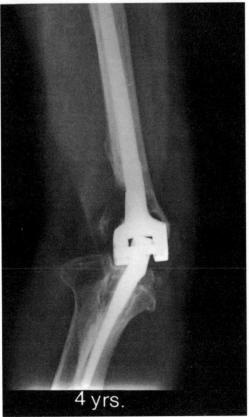

B

Figure 29–12. A, Preoperative radiograph showing marked osseous deformity in a 41-year-old man who had sustained a supracondylar fracture in his childhood. He had severe pain and moderate instability. **B,** Anteroposterior radiograph, made 4 years postoperatively, showing worn bushings with valgus angulation. The patient had returned to his previous job as a construction worker, which involved lifting as much as 150 kg on a regular basis, against the advice of the surgeon.

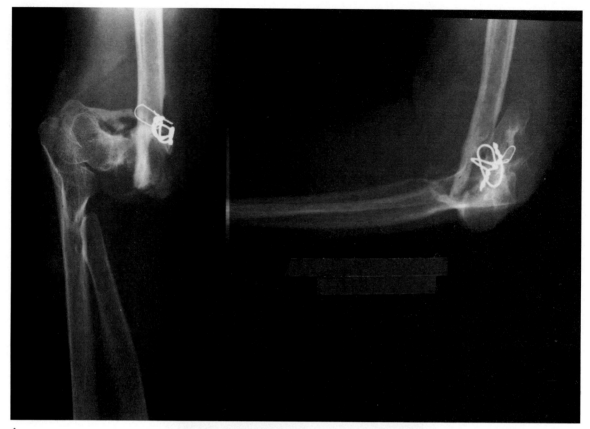

A

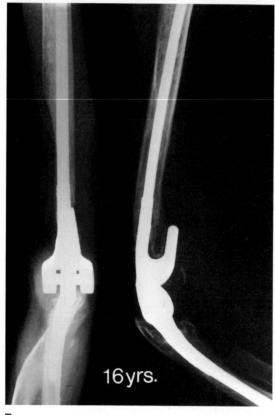

B

Figure 29–13. A, Marked deformity with gross instability in a 70-year-old patient with distal humeral nonunion. **B**, At 16 years postimplant, the patient is without pain and the bushings show little wear.

descried above (see Figs. 29–3 and 29–4). In chronic situations, weakness after surgery, even with shortening of the extremity, is not appreciated by patients as a result of muscle contracture or preoperative weakness from pain.

Mayo Clinic Experience

Assessment of 39 distal humeral nonunions treated by the Coonrad-Morrey replacement was reported by Morrey and Adams in 1995, with a mean surveillance of over 4 years.[25] Of these, 86 percent were rated by the MEPS as satisfactory. Ramsey et al. have reported the intermediate to long-term results of Coonrad-Morrey prosthetic replacement for gross instability. With surveillance of between 2 and 12 years, 16 of 19 patients (84 percent) had a satisfactory outcome based on the MEPS[28] (Fig. 29–13). Most problems were of a "mechanical" nature, with more than half of patients having problems with wear debris and ulnar nerve irritation. The complication rates in the two studies were 21 and 18 percent, respectively. Reoperation was required in 8 of the combined group of 58 patients (14 percent).

Improvement in useful motion of the elbow is dramatic following surgery done primarily for the restoration of stability. The limitations of a patient with dysfunctional instability are obvious. The inability to position the hand in space compromises the ability to perform daily activities. Re-establishing a stable fulcrum for elbow motion significantly improves functional activities. Postoperatively, a functional range of motion is re-established with an average flexion arc of approximately 100 degrees.

Revision

A revision with a Coonrad-Morrey semiconstrained total elbow arthroplasty was performed 15 years after the first procedure for loosening. The patient had a satisfactory result 2 years after the revision. The elbows of two other patients had a complete radiolucent line around both the humeral and the ulnar component, and one was revised because of ulnar component loosening 1 year after the first procedure.

References

1. Baksi DP: Sloppy hinge prosthetic elbow replacement for post-traumatic ankylosis or instability. J Bone Joint Surg Br 80:614–619, 1998.
2. Brumfield RH Jr, Kuschner SH, Gellman H, et al: Total elbow arthroplasty. J Arthroplasty 5:359–363, 1990.
3. Cheng SL, Morrey BF: Treatment of the mobile, painful arthritic elbow by distraction interposition arthroplasty. J Bone Joint Surg Br 82:233–238, 2000.
4. Cobb TK, Morrey BF: Total elbow replacement as primary treatment for distal humeral fractures in elderly patients. J Bone Joint Surg Am 79:826–832, 1997.
5. Dee R: Total replacement arthroplasty of the elbow for rheumatoid arthritis. J Bone Joint Surg Br 54:88–95, 1972.
6. Ewald FC, Jacobs MA: Total elbow arthroplasty. Clin Orthop 182:137–142, 1984.
7. Figgie HED, Inglis AE, Mow C: Total elbow arthroplasty in the face of significant bone stock or soft tissue losses: Preliminary results of custom-fit arthroplasty. J Arthroplasty 1:71–81, 1986.
8. Figgie HE III, Inglis AE, Ranawat CS, Rosenberg GM: Results of total elbow arthroplasty as a salvage procedure for failed elbow reconstructive operations. Clin Orthop 219:185–193, 1987.
9. Froimson AI, Silva JE, Richey D: Cutis arthroplasty of the elbow joint. J Bone Joint Surg Am 58:863–865, 1976.
10. Garrett JC, Ewald FC, Thomas WH, Sledge CB: Loosening associated with GSB hinge total elbow replacement in patients with rheumatoid arthritis. Clin Orthop 127:170–174, 1977.
11. Gschwend N, Loehr J, Ivosevic-Radovanovic D, et al: Semiconstrained elbow prosthesis with special reference to the GSB III prosthesis. Clin Orthop 232:104–111, 1988.
12. Gschwend N, Scheier H, Bähler A, Simmen B: GSB III elbow. In Rüther W (ed): The Elbow: Endoprosthetic Replacement and Non-endoprosthetic Procedures. Berlin, Springer-Verlag, 1996, pp 83–98.
13. Helfet DL, Schmerling GJ: Bicondylar intra-articular fractures of the distal humerus in adults. Clin Orthop 292:26–36, 1993.
14. Hughes RE, Schneeberger AG, An K-N, et al: Reduction of triceps muscle force after shortening of the distal humerus: a computational model. J Shoulder Elbow Surg 6:444–448, 1997.
15. Inglis AE, Pellicci PM: Total elbow replacement. J Bone Joint Surg Am 62:1252–1258, 1980.
16. John H, Rosso R, Neff U, et al: Operative treatment of distal humeral fractures in the elderly. J Bone Joint Surg Br 76:793–796, 1994.
17. Jupiter JB, Neff U, Holzach P, Allgöwer M: Intercondylar fractures of the humerus. J Bone Joint Surg Am 67:226, 1985.
18. Kasten MD, Skinner HB: Total elbow arthroplasty. Clin Orthop 290:177–188, 1993.
19. Knight RA, Zandt LV: Arthroplasty of the elbow. J Bone Joint Surg Am 34:610–618, 1952.
20. Kraay MJ, Figgie MP, Inglis AE, et al: Primary semi-constrained total elbow arthroplasty. J Bone Joint Surg Br 76:636–640, 1994.
21. Lowe LW, Miller AJ, Allum RL, Higginson DW: The development of an unconstrained elbow arthroplasty. J Bone Joint Surg Br 66:243–247, 1984.
22. Mansat P, Morrey BF: Semiconstrained total elbow arthroplasty for ankylosed and stiff elbows. J Bone Joint Surg Am 82:1260–1268, 2000.
23. McAuliffe JA, Burkhalter WE, Ouellette EA, Carneiro RS: Compression plate arthrodesis of the elbow. J Bone Joint Surg Br 74:300–304, 1992.
24. Morrey BF: Post-traumatic contracture of the elbow: Operative treatment including distraction arthroplasty. J Bone Joint Surg Am 72:601–618, 1990.
25. Morrey BF, Adams RA: Semi-constrained elbow replacement for distal humeral nonunion. J Bone Joint Surg Br 77:67–72, 1995.
26. Morrey BF, Adams RA, Bryan RS: Total replacement for post-traumatic arthritis of the elbow. J Bone Joint Surg Br 73:607–612, 1991.
27. O'Neill OR, Morrey BF, Tanaka S, An K-N: Compensatory motion in the upper extremity after elbow arthrodesis. Clin Orthop 281:89–96, 1992.
28. Ramsey ML, Adajs RA, Morrey BF: Instability of the elbow treated with semiconstrained total elbow arthroplasty. J Bone Joint Surg Am 81:38–47, 1999.
29. Schneeberger AG, Adams R, Morrey BF: Semiconstrained total elbow replacement for the treatment of post-traumatic osteoarthrosis. J Bone Joint Surg Am 79:1211–1222, 1997.
30. Soni RK, Cavendish ME: A review of the Liverpool elbow prosthesis from 1974 to 1982. J Bone Joint Surg Br 66:248–253, 1984.
31. Souter WA, Nicol AC, Paul JP: Anatomical trochlear stirrup arthroplasty of the rheumatoid elbow. J Bone Joint Surg Br 67:676, 1985.
32. Tsuge K, Murakami T, Yasunaga Y, Kanaujia RR: Arthroplasty of the elbow. J Bone Joint Surg Br 69:116–120, 1987.
33. Urbaniak JR, Black KE Jr: Cadaveric elbow allografts: a six year experience. Clin Orthop 197:131–140, 1985.
34. Zuckerman JD, Lubliner JA: Arm, elbow and forearm injuries. In Zuckerman JD (ed): Orthopaedic Injuries in the Elderly. Edited by Baltimore: Urban & Schwarzenberg, 1990, pp 345–407.

30

Complications of Total Elbow Arthroplasty

• SHAWN W. O'DRISCOLL

Complications have been reported with varying frequency after total elbow arthroplasty and have been categorized according to severity and whether or not reoperation has been required. The specific nature of the complications can be general, or specific to the type of prosthesis or the surgical approach used. In addition, preoperative factors strongly influence the incidence and nature of the complications.

As with many surgical procedures, it can be helpful to categorize complications as operative or postoperative, with the postoperative complications considered as early or late. Table 30–1 lists the complications, according to this categorization, which have been reported with some degree of frequency to the Mayo Clinic or those that have occurred there.

FRACTURES

Little has been written about intraoperative fractures, or about periprosthetic fractures in general, in the area of the elbow.[1,3,24,43] The classification of these fractures is similar to that of periprosthetic fractures in the knee, according to the region and the status of the bone stock and the fixation of the stem, as the following outline indicates[43]:

I. Region
   A. Periarticular: Humerus ∏ condyle, epicondyle; ulna ∏ olecranon, coronoid
   B. Shaft—around or at the tip of the stem
   C. Shaft—beyond the tip of the stem

II. Status of stem and bone stock
   A. Well-fixed, adequate bone quality
   B. Loose, adequate bone quality
   C. Severe bone loss or osteolysis

Intraoperative fractures typically involve the humeral condyles (Fig. 30–1A). These are predisposed to fracture by thinning of the cortex and by the creation of bone cuts that leave too narrow a bridge of bone between the epicondyle and the shaft. Stress risers can occur in this area owing to the shape of the bone cuts. Certain prostheses leave angular defects, whereas others have more rounded contours. In addition, if the space available for the prosthesis between the epicondyles is too narrow, the epicondyle can fracture during component insertion.

Humeral stem fractures can also occur during component insertion. They can occur either because placement of a cement restrictor is too tight (see Fig. 30–1B) or because a component is either too tight or is not the same shape as the canal. Such fractures typically cause only minimally displaced cracks in the cortex and can be managed by cerclage wiring. It is important that the twist in the wires and the ends of the wires are placed well away from the radial or ulnar nerves (see Fig. 30–1B). Fractures at the tip of the stem can occur because of proximal alteration in the shape of the cortex. Occasionally, a prosthesis has to be contoured to avoid a proximal fracture at the tip (see Fig. 30–1C). Shaft fractures often cause displacement and require internal fixation with plates and/or strut grafts with screw fixation and/or cerclage wiring. A combination of these techniques may be used.

Intraoperative periprosthetic fractures of the olecranon are rather common, but shaft fractures of the ulna are not as common as fractures in the humerus. The rheumatoid patient is at risk of having the rasp or the stem of the prosthesis driven out through the subcutaneous or medial border of the ulna. This is especially common with long-stemmed ulnar components in the face of a radially deviated proximal ulna. This may result from cortical remodeling of the anterior aspect of the intramedullary canal resulting from chronic impingement of the bicipital tuberosity against the ulna (see Fig. 30–1D). Such fractures can be managed intraoperatively by cerclage wiring, usually with strut grafting to unload the area.

COMPONENT MALPOSITION

As with any prosthesis, component malposition is possible. Humeral stem malposition can be slight (valgus, varus, or rotational), and these disturbances may cause

Table 30–1. COMPLICATIONS OF TOTAL ELBOW ARTHROPLASTY

Operative

Fractures
Component malposition
Ulnar nerve injury

Early Postoperative

Wound slough or necrosis
Instability
Infection
Triceps deficiency

Late Postoperative

Instability
Triceps deficiency
Infection
Periprosthetic fracture
Loosening
Bushing wear
Osteolysis
Partial or complete component disengagement
Component fracture

kinematic alterations in the function of the elbow.[27,28] Ulnar component malposition is almost always rotational and predisposes the patient to either instability or wear of the prosthesis.[49] Severe component malposition can occur if the stem of the prosthesis is placed outside the bone (Fig. 30–2**A**, **B**). If humeral components are placed outside the humerus, revision is usually required. As the components may be stable or unstable, the decision to revise is based on the likelihood that the prosthesis will be unable to function in situ.

ULNAR NERVE

Ulnar nerve injuries have been reported with tremendous variation in nature and frequency.[37,40,51] Much of the early literature concerning ulnar nerve injuries may have been influenced by the surgical approach[31,50]; however, it is increasingly common to identify and isolate the ulnar nerve and then transpose it. This method has the advantage of lessening the likelihood of intraoperative compression or postoperative entrapment of the nerve in the new articulation. However, there is a possibility of iatrogenic complications. Nerve lacerations can occur, most commonly in a revision situation. Two important guidelines, which are functions of underlying pathology in the ulnar nerve of elbows that have been previously reoperated, are as follows: (1) the location of the ulnar nerve cannot be assumed based on the previous surgery, regardless of whether it had or had not apparently been transposed; (2) the ulnar nerve can take a sudden S-shaped or Z-shaped change in direction from a proximal to a distal direction, making it possible to traverse the nerve with the dissecting instruments during exposure (Fig. 30–3).

Temporary mild nerve palsies are very common and are managed expectantly. Complete nerve lesions whose nerves are known to be structurally intact and apparently undamaged during surgery are managed by observation. Those that potentially have structural lesions are managed by re-exploration.

POSTOPERATIVE COMPLICATIONS

Early Postoperative Complications

Wound Healing

The surgical approach to the elbow has varied in the past and still varies somewhat from institution to institution. I generally use a universal posterior skin incision.[42] This allows access to the medial and lateral sides of the elbow. Ulnar nerve exploration and transposition can be performed conveniently through this exposure. The main complication with this surgical incision is the possibility of partial or complete wound slough or necrosis (Fig. 30–4). Severe wound slough is possible but very unlikely in the setting of total elbow arthroplasty; it is more likely in the presence of severe trauma or reconstruction after severe post-traumatic deficits. Decreased vascularity requires the creation of skin flaps, and swelling occurs postoperatively. The likelihood of necrosis is minimized if full-thickness skin flaps are taken down to the deep fascia, if the soft tissues are handled carefully, and, most importantly, if postoperative swelling is minimized. Prevention of necrosis is most effectively achieved by (1) ensuring that hemostasis is maintained during surgery, and (2) by keeping the patient's arm extended and elevated postoperatively in either a padded Jones bandage or a cryotherapeutic device until the acute risk of severe swelling has diminished. The usual time frame is about 36 hours, depending on the circumstances. In cases of increased likelihood of swelling or compromised soft tissues, one might even consider keeping the arm in this position for 5 days or, occasionally, even longer.

Instability

There are two broad classes of total elbow arthroplasty in current use—linked[2,16,20,21] and unlinked[1,3,8,10,14,30,32] (the latter are also called resurfacing). Etiologic factors include the implant design, surgical approach, surgeon, patient, and postoperative management. The stability intrinsic to the articular geometry of an unlinked prosthesis may not replicate the stability provided by the normal elbow. Any elbow prosthesis must reproduce, or compensate for not reproducing, the axis of rotation of the elbow and the valgus carrying angle in both the humerus and the ulna. Bone preparation must be performed reproducibly so that the final position and orientation of the components are correct. For hip and knee surgery, such instrumentation has advanced greatly, but it is severely lacking for elbow replacement. Many implants are inserted through a lateral surgical approach. An inadequate or failed repair of the lateral collateral ligament may result in posterolateral,

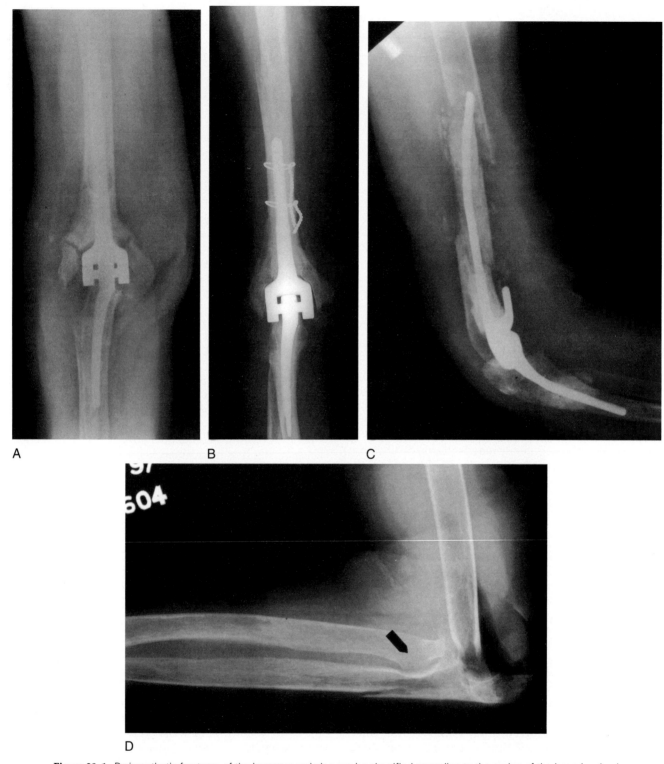

A

B

C

D

Figure 30–1. Periprosthetic fractures of the humerus and ulna can be classified according to the region of the bone involved (**A** = periarticular; **B** = shaft around or at the tip of the stem; **C** = shaft beyond the tip of the stem) as well as the status of the stem and bone stock (**D**).

rotational, and varus instability of the elbow.[44,45] Experience in the laboratory has revealed that an improperly aligned ulnar component limits the elbow to either restricted motion or mandatory subluxation.[49] Patients with significant loss of bone structure, ligament deficiency, or tendon deficiency around the elbow are at increased risk of instability after total elbow arthroplasty.[13] The patient's capacity to protect the elbow from unbalanced forces in the postoperative period may be impaired. Of most concern is the repeated varus stress that the elbow experiences each time it is moved in a plane that is not vertical. The management of an unstable

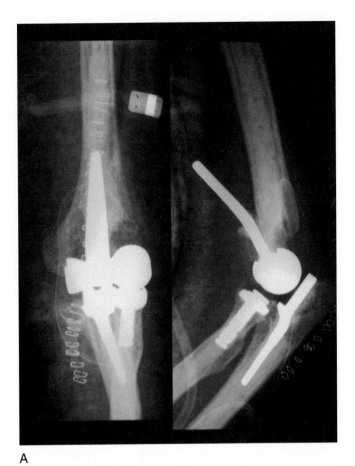

A

B

Figure 30–2. Component malposition. Examples of components placed entirely (**A**) or partially (**B**) outside the canal. If a partially extruded stem is well fixed in place, as in example **B**, intraoperative revision may not be necessary. The malpositioned ulnar component was still functioning well 12 years after implantation.

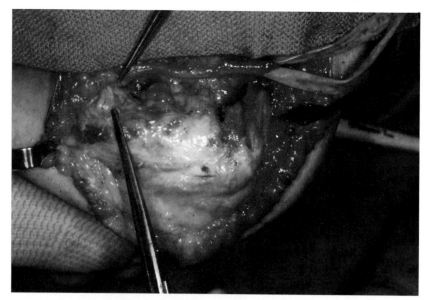

Figure 30–3. The ulnar nerve is at significant risk of injury during revision surgery. The exact course and location of the nerve are unpredictable, despite prior treatment or documentation of transposition. In this case, the nerve took a sudden Z-shaped turn and was at risk of being transected.

elbow arthroplasty depends on the pathoanatomy and temporal relationship to the replacement surgery. Closed reduction and immobilization of the elbow may correct subluxation or dislocation of an unlinked total elbow in the early postoperative period but is not usually successful later.[34] Chronic or recurrent instability of an unlinked total elbow arthroplasty that has well-positioned components is an indication for ligament reconstruction and correction of any deficiency in the healing of the triceps and other tendons around the elbow.[4] Malpositioned components cause abnormal soft tissue balance and maltracking; therefore, they require revision. Unfortunately, correction is often unsuccessful, and conversion to a linked total elbow arthroplasty is then required.[48] Patients who have multifactorial causes of instability, such as combined soft tissue insufficiency, bony deficits, and component malposition, should be

considered for revision to a linked total elbow arthroplasty. It is anticipated that the future of total elbow arthroplasty will bring major improvements in surgical instruments, including cutting and alignment jigs. Prosthetic designs must have intrinsic features that permit patients to have latitude in motion and stability. Finally, the importance of eliminating any unbalanced forces through proper component selection, insertion, and soft tissue tensioning, regardless of whether a linked or unlinked prosthesis is used, cannot be overstated. One must realize that the same unbalanced forces that cause instability in a device that permits uncoupling also cause eccentric wear on the polyethylene articulation in a device that does not permit uncoupling. Such wear predisposes the patient to osteolysis, which is the major current concern in replacement arthroplasty.

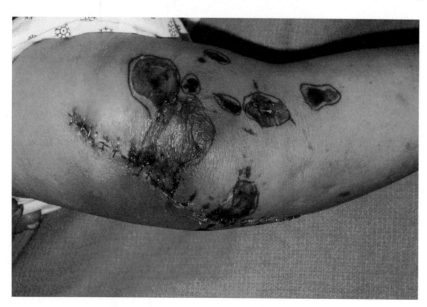

Figure 30–4. Wound complications can occur and are principally caused by elevation of the skin flaps and postoperative swelling. Areas of partial necrosis such as this can usually be managed nonsurgically by extending the elbow in a well-padded splint and elevating it for several days.

Management of the unstable elbow in the early postoperative period is nonsurgical if the integrity of the periarticular soft tissues was thought to be good at the time of surgery and if there was a reasonable degree of certainty regarding the correct orientation of the components. The elbow can be immobilized for 3 weeks in a cast in a stable position, which usually includes a moderate degree of flexion and a specific position of forearm rotation, depending on which soft tissues were released during the surgery. Negative prognostic indicators of the failure of nonsurgical treatment include persistent subluxation in the flexed position (Fig. 30–5**A**) and persistent postoperative subluxation or dislocation in a cast (Fig. 30–5**B**). It is noteworthy that the use of a radial head component has not been clearly shown to alter the incidence of instability (Fig. 30–5**C**). However, key factors in this regard have been that the orientation and positioning of the radial head component have been left to the judgment of the surgeon, without provision of any specific guidelines or instruments, and without any scientific data describing how these procedures should be done.

Unlinked arthroplasties are not suitable in certain circumstances, such as in patients with severe soft tissue or bone loss, or with flail elbow (Fig. 30–6). In patients with profound preoperative instability, it is unlikely that stability can be attained or maintained with anything other than a linked prosthesis.

Infection

Infection remains one of the major problems and concerns after total elbow arthroplasty and is discussed in this chapter under late postoperative infections and in Chapter 31.

Triceps Deficiency

Most total elbow replacement procedures involve some form of reflection or detachment of the triceps tendon from the olecranon. This detachment puts the tendon at risk of failure to heal. This risk is further increased by any deterioration in the quality of the tissue, such as occurs in patients with rheumatoid arthritis, whose tissue in the region of the olecranon is markedly thinned. Attempts have been made to preserve the triceps attachment.[46,51]

Partial or complete triceps detachment is probably much more common than recognized.[5,6,20,24,46] With the current Bryan-Morrey triceps-reflecting approach of, the triceps anconeus sleeve can detach laterally without being fully disrupted. This results in weakness, particularly in terminal extension. The key physical finding in patients with partial triceps detachment is weakness in the terminal portion of the extension arc. One can be easily fooled by apparently good strength in the flexion portion of the extension arc. The defect in the tendon is not always palpable at the olecranon, but, if it is, the diagnosis is clear.

Attempts to prevent partial or complete triceps tendon detachments have included variations in the method for detaching or repairing it. The Bryan-Morrey approach involves reflecting the triceps from a medial to

a lateral direction from the ulna in continuity with the anconeus and its overlying fascia and periosteum. In patients with good quality soft tissues, this reflection provides a significant increase in the ability of the reattached tendon to tolerate tensile loads. However, in patients with rheumatoid arthritis, there may be little continuity between the triceps tendon fibers at the insertion on the olecranon and the distal lateral anconeus sleeve. In such patients, the tendon can be reattached more medially than normally, with the anconeus brought up over the olecranon. The primary repair is performed with use of heavy, nonabsorbable sutures, which compress the tendon right against the bone and then weave the sutures up into the triceps tendon to unload the attachment side of the bone.

Repair of ruptures should be performed as early as possible to prevent problems relating to chronic retraction. The tendon and bone ends are freshened, and then the tendon is reattached with No. 5 nonabsorbable sutures. The elbow is protected postoperatively from flexing beyond the point of tension in the repair for 6 weeks. Otherwise, gentle motion is permitted. For detachments that are chronic and severely retracted, or those associated with marked loss of tendon substance, a reconstruction with an Achilles tendon allograft is my currently preferred method. However, experience at the Mayo Clinic with using Achilles tendon allografts has principally been in patients who have had triceps ruptures but have not had a joint replacement. Attachment to the often thin and otherwise altered olecranon can be a challenge in the patient with rheumatoid arthritis.

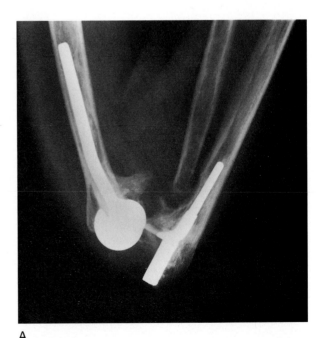

A

Figure 30–5. Instability in the first few days or weeks postoperatively usually represents significant component malposition or soft tissue deficiency or disruption. In such cases, flexion (**A**) of the elbow does not necessarily provide stability nor does the elbow necessarily stay reduced in a cast (**B**).

Illustration continued on following page

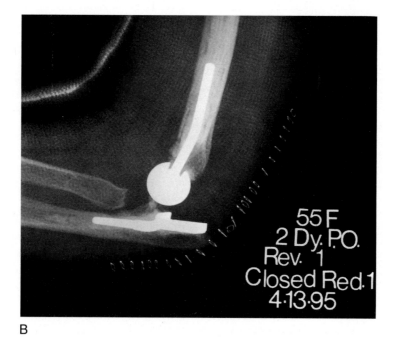

B

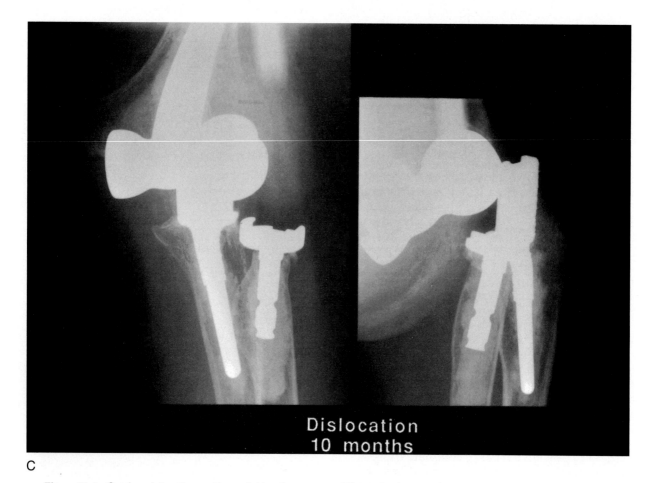

C

Figure 30–5. *Continued.* An elbow with a radial head component (**C**) can also be unstable, because component position and soft tissue balance are essential, whether or not there is a radial head component.

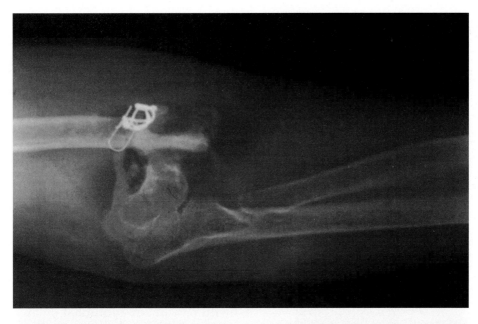

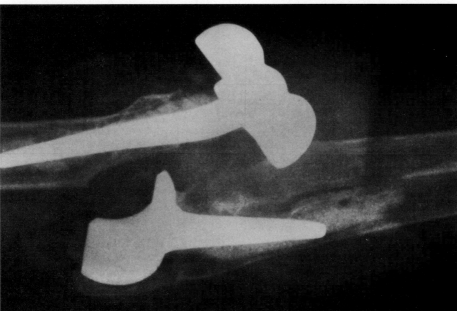

Figure 30–6. Unlinked prostheses are contraindicated in certain circumstances. In this case, a patient with a supracondylar nonunion was treated by resection of the distal humeral fragments and implantation of an unlinked prosthesis. It should not be surprising that gross instability resulted after complete loss of the origins of the collateral ligaments and common extensor and flexor tendons.

Late Postoperative Complications

Infection

Infection can occur early or late, but in either case, it represents a potentially devastating complication (Fig. 30–7A, B).[23] This subject is discussed in detail in Chapter 31.

Periprosthetic Fracture

As mentioned earlier, under operative complications, periprosthetic fractures in the elbow are classified according to the factors that determine their prognosis and treatment: the location of the fracture in relation to the stem, the security of the fixation, and the quality of the bone.[43] These factors are similar to those in the classification system devised by Duncan and Masri for periprosthetic femoral fractures after total hip replacement.[12] At the Mayo Clinic, experience has been gained from more than 1000 total elbow arthroplasties, of which about 80 percent were primary and 20 percent were revisions. Among the primary procedures, our incidence of periprosthetic fractures has been approximately 5 percent.

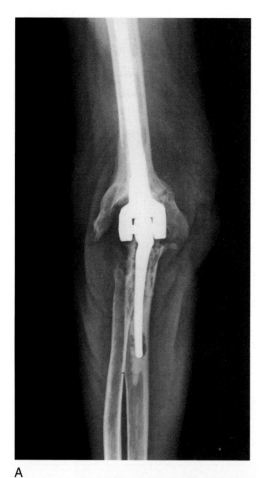

A

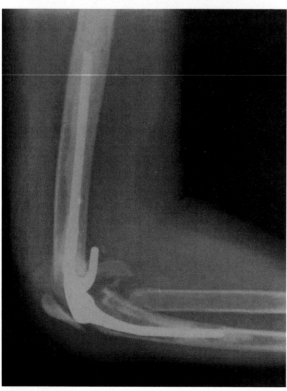

B

Figure 30–7. Infection can occur with significant bony resorption (**A**) and even periprosthetic fracture (**B**).

Humeral Fractures

PERIARTICULAR (TYPE A)

Fractures of the condyles often occur intraoperatively but can also occur as a result of stress or fatigue failure postoperatively (Fig. 30–8**A**). Patients with late fractures are managed nonsurgically because they usually become asymptomatic. The main concern regarding these fractures is that if the prosthesis is removed because of infection, the condyles are required to "contain" the ulna for a satisfactory resection arthroplasty.[17] If the condyles are not intact, the elbow remains flail and virtually functionless.

Humeral shaft fractures around the stem or at its tip (type B [Fig 30–8**B**, **C**, and **D**]) typically occur as a result of trauma or pathologic fracture occasioned by loosening or osteolysis around the component. Depending on the quality of the bone and the etiology, the treatment varies, but it usually requires open reduction and internal fixation with cerclage wires, with or without additional onlay allograft struts or plates. If the fracture occurs intraoperatively before stem insertion, it is held reduced, and a stem long enough to bypass and stabilize it is used. If this is not possible, or if the stem would be unreasonably long, the fracture is plated.

Fractures around a well-fixed stem (type B1) are usually at the tip of the prosthesis. They are treated by open reduction and internal fixation.

Fractures around a loose stem (types B2 and B3) usually occur in the presence of osteolysis. Revision is almost always required. Revision techniques and logic are discussed in Chapter 31, but these can be very difficult operations. The surgeon must have the skills and tools required for cement removal from a small canal, familiarity with the neural anatomy at all levels of the arm, and availability of allograft humeral bones and a range of prostheses. Occasionally, internal fixation with a plate placed posteriorly along the lateral side of the prosthesis is also necessary. An allograft strut can also been used. If osteolysis is severe, impaction bone grafting is usually performed.

Fractures beyond the tip of the stem (type C) are considered as routine humeral shaft fractures, and patients are treated with immobilization and functional bracing.

Ulnar Periprosthetic Fractures

Periarticular fractures of the ulna (type A) usually involve the olecranon, because the coronoid is rarely fractured. The olecranon is probably the second most common fracture requiring total elbow arthroplasty. The olecranon is particularly prone to fracture in patients with rheumatoid arthritis, owing to erosive thinning of the semilunar notch of the ulna, and, most commonly, the fracture exists before the arthroplasty is performed. Fractures can occur postoperatively as a result of forceful triceps contraction or as a stress fracture. In the latter cases, the bone is usually thin and unsupported by the prosthesis or by cement. The long lever arm, combined with the bending moment arm of the triceps, causes fatigue failure of the bone (Fig. 30–9**C**).

The patient's treatment is usually determined by whether or not the olecranon fragment is displaced. If not, a period of immobilization is recommended. This usually permits a stable fibrous nonunion to develop. If there is significant displacement, the triceps is weakened, and open reduction is preferred. If the bone is thin, as is usually the case, it is simply reduced and held with heavy (No. 5) nonabsorbable suture through drill holes in the ulna (and into the cement). If the bone fragment is substantial, internal fixation is performed either with tension band wiring or with a plate. One must be prepared, however, to deal with wound complications caused by the hardware. If the fracture does not displace, the functional outcome is similar to that of an osseous and stable fibrous union (G. Mara, Olecranon Fractures and to the Elbow Arthroplasty, unpublished data).

Fractures around a well-fixed stem (type B1) usually occur right at the tip of the stem. If they are displaced, patients are treated by open reduction and internal fix-

ation (see Fig. 30–9**D**); if they are undisplaced, oblique and stable, they are managed by a period of immobilization. Transverse fractures tend not to heal.

Fractures around a loose stem (types B2 and B3) usually occur through a portion of the ulna that is weakened as a result of erosion from loosening or osteolysis (see Fig. 30–9**E**, **F**). Some of these patients may have minimally displaced fractures, but revision is required for two reasons. First, the fracture is not likely to unite. Second, the loose stem remains symptomatic, causing further endosteal erosion, and the fracture is likely to displace principles similar to those described previously for humeral shaft revisions are employed. Distal removal of cement from the canal is challenging, usually requiring the use of an ultrasonic cement removal device. The primary objective is to bypass the fracture with a longer stem and thereby stabilize it.

Allograft struts, with or without impaction bone grafting, are employed to permit bypass of the fracture with a long-stem ulnar component. This component may need to be custom ordered, but it is available with at least one semiconstrained prosthesis. Allograft-prosthetic composites have been used when the bone is destroyed. If the bone is of adequate quality, it can be fixed by placing a

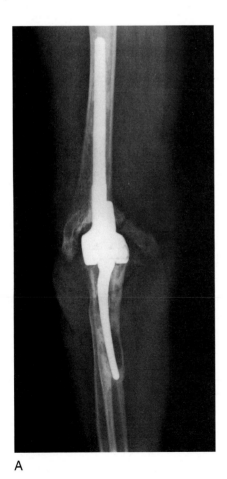

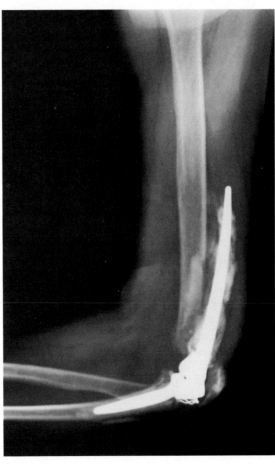

A

B

Figure 30–8. Periprosthetic humeral fractures. Late periprosthetic fractures can be traumatic or pathological. **A,** Humeral type A periarticular fracture of the medial condyle. This can also occur as a fatigue fracture as a result of weakened bone being pulled on by the common flexor pronator tendon (or the common extensor tendon on the lateral side). **B,** Humeral type B fracture around the stem.

Illustration continued on following page

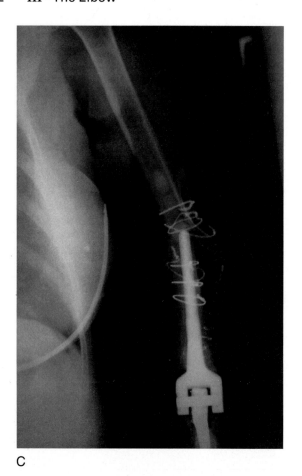

C

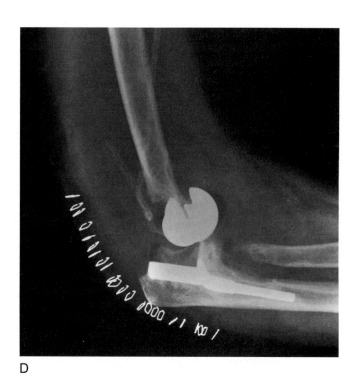

D

Figure 30–8. *Continued.* **C,** Humeral type B fracture at the tip of a stem that has failed treatment with an allograft strut. **D,** Humeral fracture specific to components placed without a stem. Such components are no longer used because of the frequency with which this complication occurred.

3.5 DC plate along the posterior surface of the ulna to bridge the fracture site. Screws can be inserted in a unicortical fashion along the side of the prosthesis.

Patients with fractures of the ulnar shaft beyond the tip (type C) are treated the same as those who have any routine ulnar shaft fracture.

Loosening

Aseptic loosening has not been commonly reported[5,6,14,19,20,25,26,37,38,47,50] since the introduction of the fully constrained hinged prosthesis; however, it does occur with unlinked and linked prostheses (Figs. 30–10 and 30–11). It was reasoned for many years that unlinked prostheses would have a lower rate of mechanical loosening than linked prostheses, but whether or not this is true still remains questionable. With unlinked prostheses, loosening can occur around each of the components—radial, ulnar, and humeral (see Fig. 30–10A to C). It is my opinion that loosening around the radial component can be explained, to a great extent, by malposition or malorientation of the components (see Fig. 30–10A).

Mechanical loosening of linked prostheses has been less frequent than might have been originally expected.[20,22] Advances in cementing techniques may improve this even further.[7] In the design used here, ulnar component loosening has been noticed to have become much more common since the titanium bead coat on the component was changed to a cement precoat (Figs. 30–11 and 30–12).[24]

Pistoning of the ulnar component may not be apparent on static radiographs. Patients experiencing pistoning may be aware of a mechanical friction sensation inside the ulna during flexion and extension of the elbow. Radiographs taken in flexion and extension may show axial displacement or pistoning of the ulnar component within the ulna (see Fig. 30–12A).

Revision of mechanically loose components should be performed before there is substantial bone loss, which can arise simply from mechanical abrasion, but which may also be caused by osteolysis secondary to the abrasion or secondary to what has been interpreted as debonding of the ulnar precoat (see Fig. 30–12B, C, and D). Revision techniques are discussed elsewhere[9,11,15,16,18,35,36,41] and in Chapter 32.

Bushing Wear

The main complication seen in medium to long-term follow-up of the Coonrad-Morrey linked total elbow prosthesis relates to wear of the bushing that links the ulnar and humeral components (Fig. 30–13). Although this linkage mechanism functions very well in the short term, long-term wear is not surprising. The polyethylene component is thin, and the moment arms resisting varus and valgus as well as rotational stresses across the elbow are greatly reduced compared with those in the intact elbow.

There is an additional biomechanical reason for bushing wear that is relevant to elbow replacements in general, although perhaps more so for the Coonrad-Morrey device, because of its small bushing. Approximately 60 percent of the axial load across the elbow is transmitted through the radiohumeral articulation.[39] However, if the radiohumeral articulation is not replaced, this force must be transmitted to the ulna, which produces a very significant valgus torque across the elbow during axial loading (Fig. 30–14).

The danger of bushing wear is that it can predispose the patient to osteolysis, a complication that is seen with

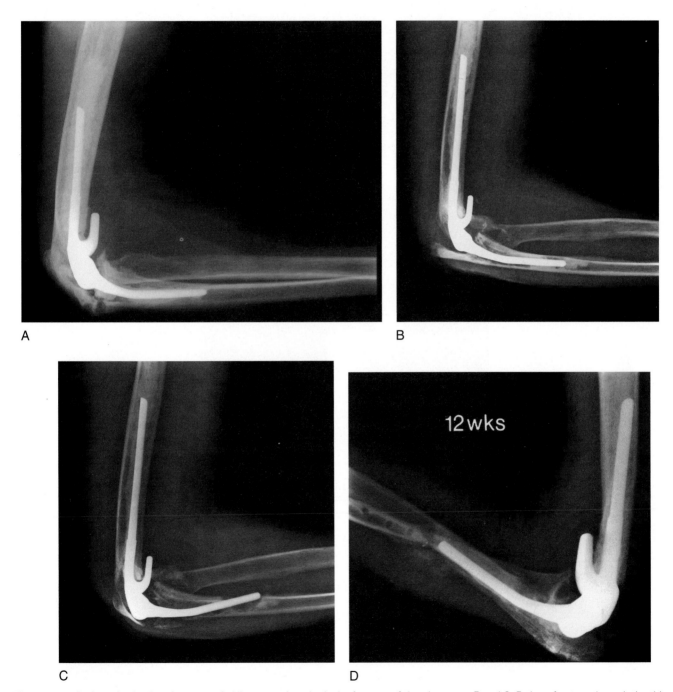

A

B

C

D

Figure 30–9. Periprosthetic ulnar fractures. **A**, Ulnar type A periarticular fracture of the olecranon. **B** and **C**, Fatigue fracture through the thin, unsupported region of the olecranon. **D**, Ulnar type B fracture at the tip of the stem. This patient was unsuccessfully managed by nonoperative treatment and required internal fixation.

Illustration continued on following page

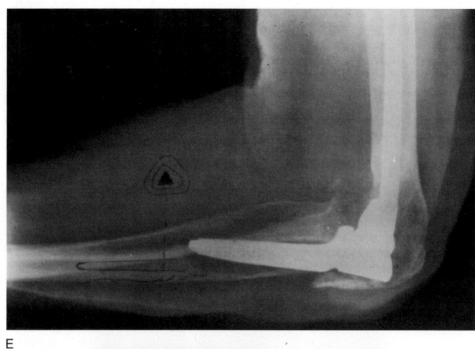

E

F

Figure 30–9. *Continued.* **E** and **F**, Type B fractures around the stem with a loose component require revision to prevent further displacement and bone damage.

increasing frequency as the follow-up time on these prostheses becomes longer (Figs. 30–15 to 30–17). This is discussed in the section on osteolysis that follows.

Osteolysis

Just as the dominant current concern in hip and knee replacement is osteolysis, there is now recognition that this same complication occurs in elbow replacement. As

the duration of follow-up increases, more cases of osteolysis are being seen. There are basically two patterns of osteolysis. The first, as mentioned earlier, seems to be specific to the use of a polymethylmethacrylate (PMMA) precoat on the ulnar components of the Coonrad-Morrey prosthesis (see Fig. 30–12). Osteolysis around these components can occur at the tip of the prosthesis, part way along it, or proximally. However, the specific pattern of osteolysis at the tip may be unique to this component and has been reported in the peer review literature by

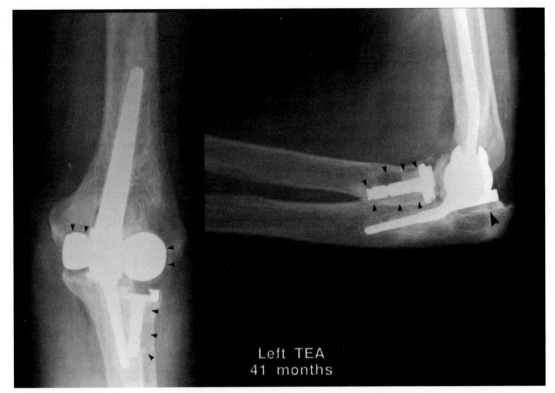

A

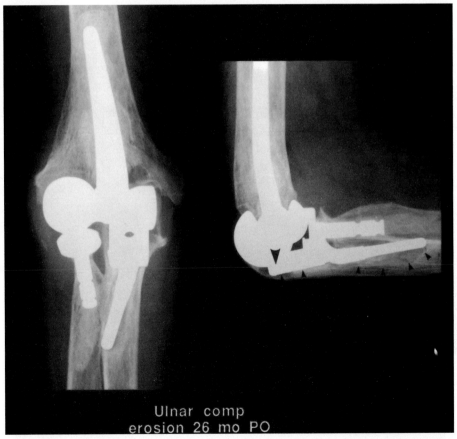

B

Figure 30–10. Loosening around an unlinked prosthesis. **A**, Loosening of the radial component, which is somewhat malpositioned. **B**, Ulnar component loosening with displacement of the tip of the prosthesis causing endosteal erosion.

Illustration continued on following page

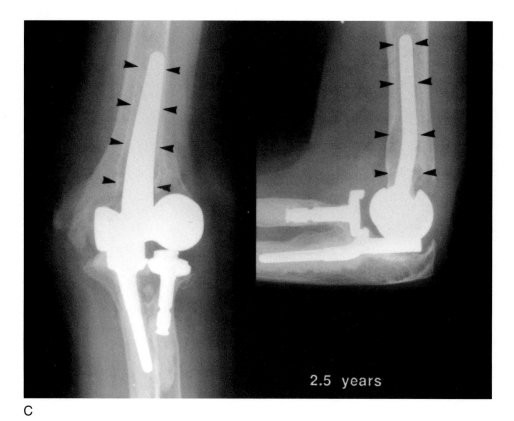

C

Figure 30–10. *Continued.* **C,** Humeral component loosening with a complete lucent line.

Hildebrand et al.[24] This PMMA precoat is no longer recommended nor should it be used.

The type of osteolysis that causes more concern is periarticular osteolysis, which involves the proximal ulna, the distal humerus, or both, secondary to wear of the bushing (see Fig. 30–15A to F). Once the polyethylene bushing has worn sufficiently, metal-on-metal contact occurs, and particulate debris from the titanium prosthesis can cause a severe metallosis reaction, with black staining of the tissues and bone erosion (see Fig. 30–15C to F). This particulate debris can cause an intense reaction, with enzymatic digestion of bone not only in the periarticular region but also along the course of the prosthesis (see Figs. 30–16 and 30–17). The pattern

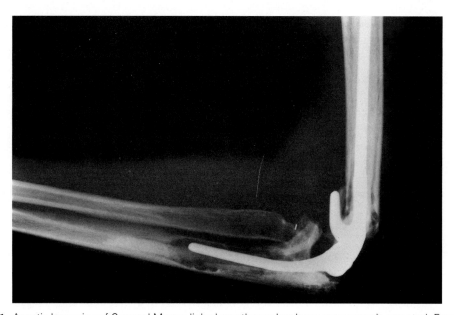

Figure 30–11. Aseptic loosening of Coonrad-Morrey linked prostheses has been uncommonly reported. Experience with loosening of the ulnar component seems to relate to the PMMA precoat.

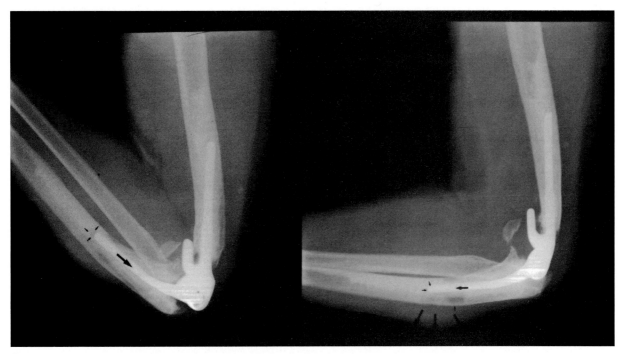

A

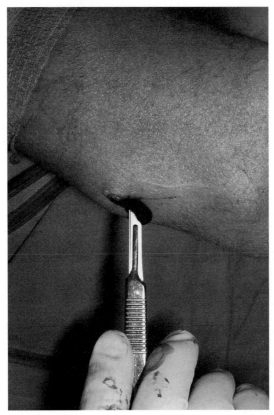

B

Figure 30–12. Significant bony resorption around a loose ulnar component. **A,** Early distal osteolysis 3 years postoperatively in a patient whose ulnar component is pistoning back and forth in the cement mantle. **B,** Incision of the fluctuant area near the tip of the ulnar stem reveals black fluid.

Illustration continued on following page

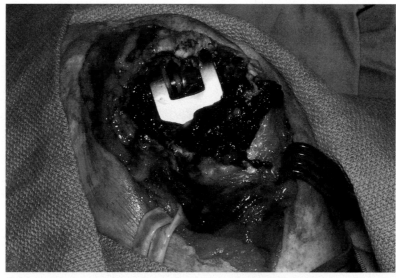

C

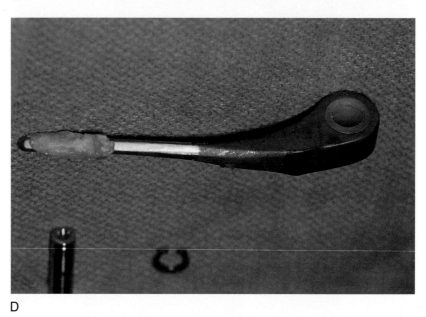

D

Figure 30–12. *Continued.* **C**, Arthrotomy reveals black titanium particulate debris. **D**, Burnishing of the PMMA precoat on an ulnar component that has been in place for only 3 years. This ulnar precoat is no longer being recommended or used.

of bone destruction can be so extensive as to suggest the possibility of infection, and the bone scan may even resemble that seen with infection (see Fig. 30–17**B**).

Osteolysis can occur with all prosthetic designs, including unlinked surface replacements (Fig. 30–18). In such cases, the osteolysis typically relates to wear of the polyethylene components (see Fig. 30–18**B**). If there is no metal contact, the particulate debris tissue reaction tends to be a pale color rather than black (see Fig. 30–18**B**).

Revision is indicated for progressive osteolysis to prevent the potential complications of extensive bone loss leading to periprosthetic fracture (see the earlier discussion of periprosthetic fractures), or component fracture (see the later discussion of component fracture). All of the osteolytic material must be débrided, which requires very extensive soft tissue dissection. This material can

extend well beyond the apparent area of bone resorption, including the area in and around nerves and even out to the skin (see Fig. 30–15**B**). The need for removing osteolytic material completely relates to the fact that its enzymatic properties permit ongoing resorption of bone. If bone destruction has been significant, impaction bone grafting is used to restore bone. I have been very pleased with the early results of this technique.

Component Disengagement

Linked prostheses were designed to overcome the problem of instability seen with unlinked prostheses. However, depending on the design of the linked prosthesis, disengagement is still theoretically or actually

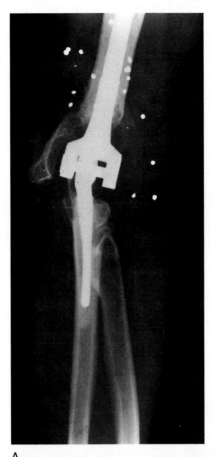

A

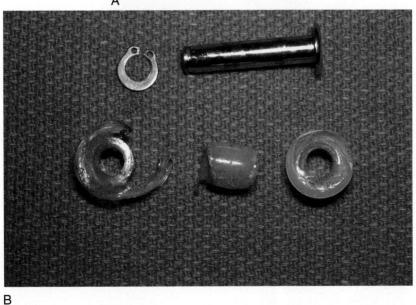

B

Figure 30–13. Bushing wear is a potential long-term complication of the Coonrad-Morrey linked prosthesis. **A**, Radiographs reveal asymmetric distance between the ulnar and humeral components, indicating wear of the polyethylene bushing. This appears to be more common in patients with loss of distal humeral bone. **B**, The bushing is worn asymmetrically, and, in some places, the plastic is worn right through. It is important that these bushings be exchanged before the wear advances through to the point where metal-on-metal contact occurs, such as in Figure 30–15.

possible. Snap-fit prostheses can disengage owing to significant stress or after a period of wear of the polyethylene, which loosens the snap fit. Prostheses such as the Pritchard Mark II, that rely on polyethylene for the linkage mechanism, can be catastrophically disengaged if the polyethylene fails.[33,52] The Coonrad-Morrey prosthesis, which has a bolt across the articulation, has not been reported to dissociate completely, but the original C-ring design, which was used to hold the bolt in place, has been observed to disengage (Fig. 30–19). Anecdotally,

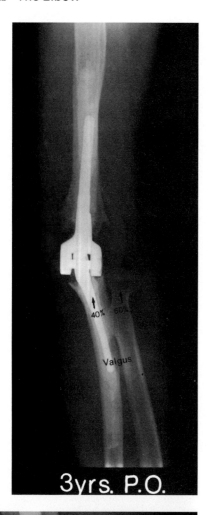

Figure 30–14. When the radiohumeral articulation is removed, the axial forces across the elbow are unbalanced into the valgus. With a short moment arm through the bushing, the bearing stresses are greatly increased, predisposing the bushing to wear, particularly in patients who lack periarticular soft tissue support after distal humeral bone resection.

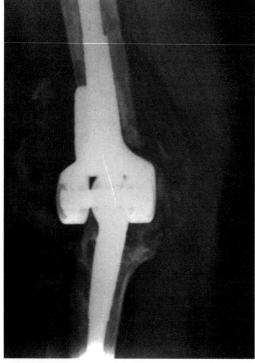

A

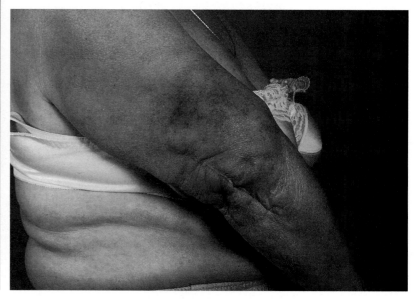

B

Figure 30–15. The major long-term concern is osteolysis. **A,** Extensive bony resorption in the periarticular region. **B,** Black stain has extended to the subcutanaeous tissues.

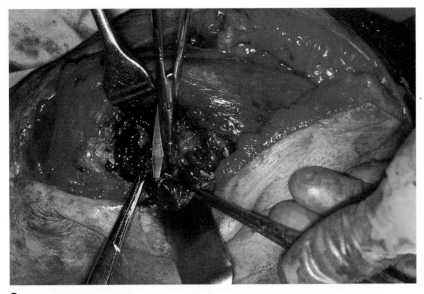

C

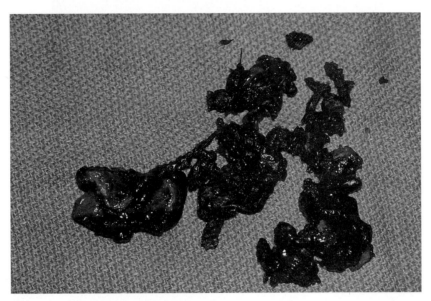

D

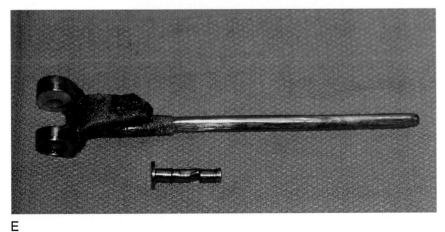

E

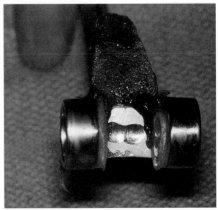

F

Figure 30–15. *Continued.* **C** and **D**, Arthrotomy reveals extensive black titanium particulate debris. **E** and **F**, The asymmetric wear on the bushing has permitted erosion into the metal bolt (which was titanium in the earlier prostheses and was changed to cobalt chrome in the early 1990s). Loss of the bushing permits metal contact between the ulnar and humeral components, which initiates a titanium particulate debris reaction.

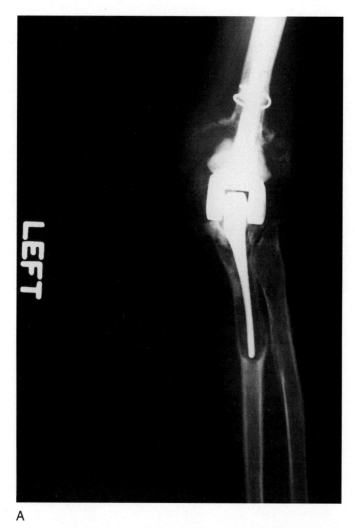

A

Figure 30–16. **A** and **B**, Advanced endosteal erosion and bony resorption around the tip of a loose ulnar component with irregular proximal resorption as well as complete loss of the humeral condyles as a result of osteolysis. The ulnar bone loss in a case such as this is currently managed by impaction bone grafting.

Illustration continued on opposite page

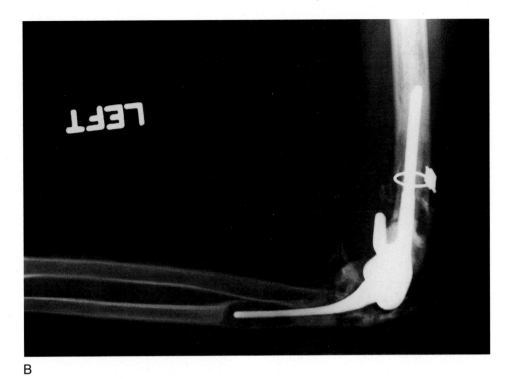

B

Figure 30–16. *Continued.*

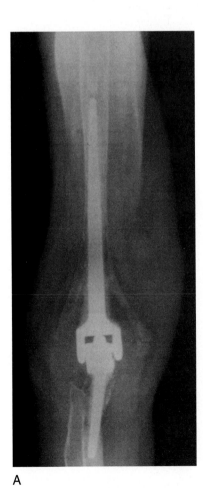

A

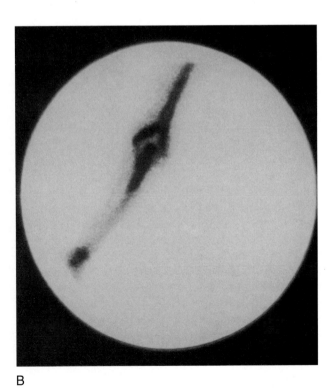

B

Figure 30–17. A, The bony erosion in osteolysis can be irregular and resemble infection. **B**, A bone scan can also resemble that of an infection.

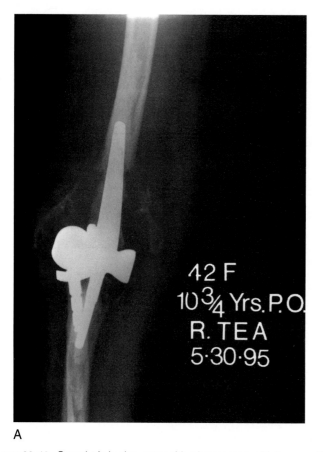

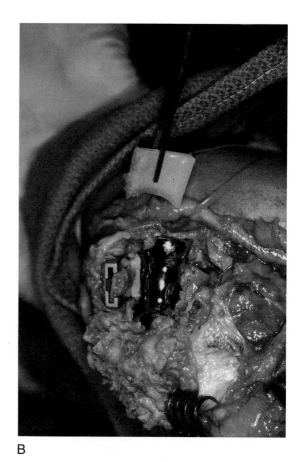

A   B

Figure 30–18. Osteolysis is also seen with a longer term of follow-up after insertion of unlinked prostheses. **A,** Extensive erosion of the distal humerus. The components remain well fixed. **B,** Operative findings include extensive particulate debris reaction (pale tissue). The ulnar polyethylene component has worn through and fractured.

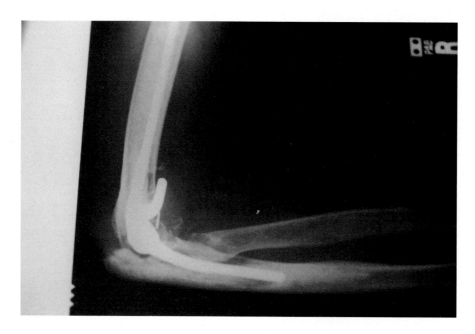

Figure 30–19. Although no true dislocations or complete disengagements of the Coonrad-Morrey prosthesis have been reported, a number of cases of C-ring disengagement have been seen. In this case, the C-ring is sitting just anterior and inferior to the humeral flange. This may be more common if the prosthesis has been used for distal humeral fractures and nonunions (in which the fragments have been excised) or if there is osteolysis.

it has been my experience that this is usually seen in the presence of periarticular osteolysis, and perhaps more commonly when the prosthesis is used after distal humerus fracture or nonunion.

Component Fracture

Component fracture can occur, typically involving either the ulnar or humeral stem. Apart from one model of the

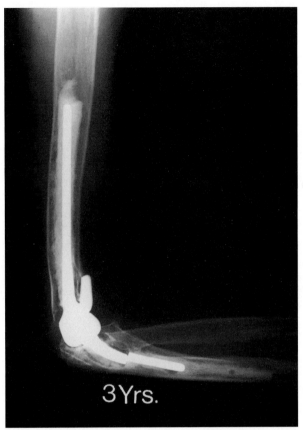

A

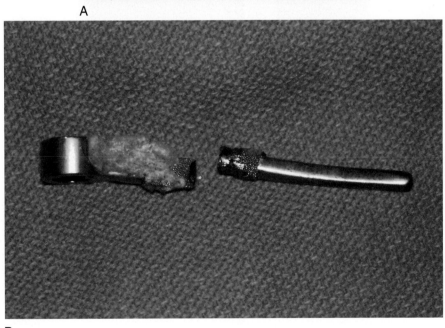

B

Figure 30–20. Ulnar component fracture. **A,** Fracture of the ulnar component of a Coonrad-Morrey prosthesis 3 years postoperatively. The distal half of the component is well fixed, but the component failed at the distal margin of the proximal osteolysis. **B,** Ulnar component fractures have generally occurred through the region of the titanium bead coat. Although this region may be weakened by the process, a stress riser is likely present because of the proximal osteolysis.

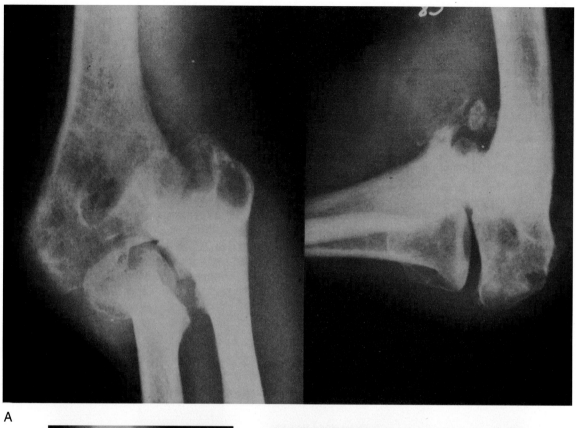

A

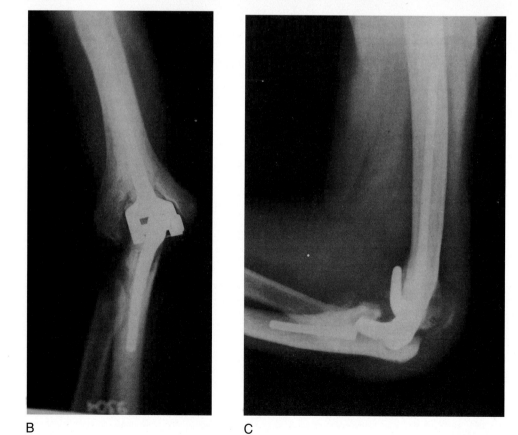

B   C

Figure 30–21. Ulnar component fracture in a patient with malalignment. **A,** Preoperative radiographs reveal severe malalignment. **B,** With continuing force imbalance across the elbow, the bushing wears asymmetrically (note nonparallel spaces between the ulnar and humeral components). **C,** Proximal osteolysis, in combination with a well fixed distal stem, permits the ulnar component to fracture because of fatigue failure.

Kudo prosthesis that demonstrated a propensity for fracture at the junction between the stem and the articulation, unlinked resurfacing designs with short intramedullary stems do not appear to be susceptible to fracture.[29] Experience at the Mayo Clinic, and reports by Schneeberger et al.[49] have revealed that fracture of the stem of the ulnar component is the more common failure. Ulnar stem components typically fracture in the proximal portion of the stem where the bead coat had been used (Fig. 30–20). This fracture location has been thought to be caused by the manufacturing process, which involves the application of the bead coat. However, my own observations have revealed a consistent finding of proximal osteolysis where there is a well-fixed distal stem, with the fracture occurring at the junction of the well-fixed stem and the proximal osteolysis (see Fig. 30–20A). I believe these ulnar component prosthetic fractures represent fatigue failure of the component resulting from abnormal stress across the component caused by unbalanced loading across the articulation as described in Figure 30–14. This unbalanced loading leads to wear of the bushing and subsequent osteolysis, with stress concentration in the proximal half of the ulnar stem. If unbalanced loading is indeed important, it is understandable that implantation of a prosthesis in an elbow that is unbalanced preoperatively and remains malaligned, would predispose the patient to fracture of the ulnar component as well. Moreover, this sequence of events has been observed (Fig. 30–21).

The section editor has a somewhat different view. It has been observed that the osteolysis progresses after the fracture due to fretting of the fracture surfaces.

Humeral stem component fracture has been less commonly seen. I have one of my own patients and one who was referred to me with humeral stem fractures at the lower portion of the stem. Both cases appeared to be fatigue failure resulting from distal local bone resorption in the presence of a proximal well-fixed stem (Fig. 30–22).

Treatment of a patient with a fractured stem requires revision of the prosthesis. The removal of the well-fixed portion of the stem is facilitated by the use of tiny burs that work around the stem. In one case of a patient with juvenile rheumatoid arthritis, there was not enough space to work around the stem, making removal exceedingly difficult. This eventually required driving the stem out with a special instrument that was placed through a window distal to the tip of the stem. Addressing the underlying cause is most important. In cases of significant imbalance across the elbow, a custom designed Triphalange Outrigger component has been used in a few cases, but the follow-up is too limited to confirm whether this will work well.

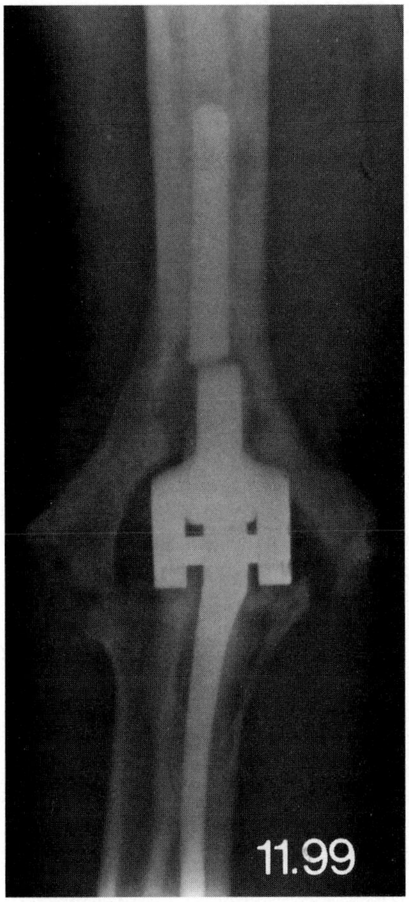

SUMMARY

Complications after total elbow arthroplasty are relatively common and represent a wide spectrum of conditions. Fortunately, many of these complications do not compromise the final result, and most of those that are serious can be reliably corrected with revision surgery. However, surgeons must be prepared to face significant challenges in dealing with these complications.

Figure 30–22. Fatigue failure of a humeral component at the junction between an area of distal osteolysis and a well-fixed proximal stem.

References

1. Allieu Y, Meyer zu Reckendorf G, Daude O: Long-term results of unconstrained Roper-Tuke total elbow arthroplasty in patients with rheumatoid arthritis. J Shoulder Elbow Surg 7:560–564, 1998.
2. Baksi DP: Sloppy hinge prosthetic elbow replacement for post-traumatic ankylosis or instability. J Bone Joint Surg Br 80:614–619, 1998.
3. Brumfield RH, Kuschner SH, Gellman H, et al: Total elbow arthroplasty. J Arthroplasty 5:359–363, 1990.
4. Chiodo CP, Terry CL, Koris MJ: Reconstruction of the medial collateral ligament with flexor carpi radialis tendon graft for instability after capitellocondylar total elbow arthroplasty. J Shoulder Elbow Surg 8:284–286, 1999.
5. Cobb TK, Morrey BF: Total elbow arthroplasty as primary treatment for distal humeral fractures in ederly patients. J Bone Joint Surg 79:826–832, 1997.
6. Connor PM, Morrey BF: Total elbow arthroplasty in patients who have juvenile rheumatoid arthritis. J Bone Joint Surg Am 80: 678–688, 1998.
7. Danter MR, King GJ, Chess DG, et al: The effect of cement restrictors on the occlusion of the humeral canal: An in vitro comparative study of 2 devices. J Arthroplasty 15:113–119, 2000.
8. Davis RF, Weiland AJ, Hungerford SD, et al: Nonconstrainded total elbow arthroplasty. Clin Orthop 171:156–160, 1982.
9. Dean GS, Holliger EH IV, Urbaniak JR: Elbow allograft for reconstruction of the elbow with massive bone loss. Long term results. Clin Orthop 341:12–22, 1997.

10. Dennis DA, Clayton ML, Ferlic DC, et al: Capitello- condylar total elbow arthroplasty for rheumatoid arthritis. J Arthroplasty 5:S83–S88, 1990.

11. Dent CM, Hoy G, Stanley JK: Revision of failed total elbow arthroplasty. J Bone Joint Surg 77–B:691–695, 1995.

12. Duncan CP, Masri BA: Fractures of the femur after hip replacement. Instr Course Lect 44:293–304, 1995.

13. Ewald FC: Capitellocondylar total elbow arthroplasty. In Morrey BF (ed): Master Techniques in Orthopaedic Surgery: The Elbow. New York, Raven Press, 1994, pp 209–230.

14. Ewald FC, Simmons ED, Sullivan JA, et al: Capitellocondylar total elbow replacement in rheumatoid arthritis. J Bone Joint Surg 75A:498–507, 1993.

15. Ferlic DC, Clayton ML: Salvage of failed total elbow arthroplasty. J Shoulder Elbow Surg 4:290–297, 1995.

16. Figgie HE, Inglis AE, Mow C: A critical analysis of alignment factors affecting functional outcome in total elbow arthroplasty. J Arthroplasty 1:169–173, 1986.

17. Figgie MP, Inglis AE, Mow CS, et al: Results of reconstruction for failed total elbow arthroplasty. Clin Orthop 253:123–132, 1990.

18. Foulkes GD, Mitsunaga MM: Allograft salvage of failed total elbow arthroplasty. A report of two cases. Clin Orthop 296:113–117, 1993.

19. Gill DR, Cofield RH, Morrey BF: Ipsilateral total shoulder and elbow arthroplasties in patients who have rheumatoid arthritis. J Bone Joint Surg Am 81:1128–1137, 1999.

20. Gill DR, Morrey BF: The Coonrad-Morrey total elbow arthroplasty in patients who have rheumatoid arthritis. A ten to fifteen-year follow-up study. J Bone Joint Surg Am 80:1327–1335, 1998.

21. Gschwend N, Scheier NH, Baehler AR: Long-term results of the GSB III elbow arthroplasty. J Bone Joint Surg Br 81:1005–1012, 1999.

22. Gschwend N, Simmen BR, Matejovsky Z: Late complications in elbow arthroplasty. J Shoulder Elbow Surg 5:86–96, 1996.

23. Gutow AP, Wolfe SW: Infection following total elbow arthroplasty. In Hand Clinics: Difficult Disorders of the Elbow and Forearm. Philadelphia, WB Saunders, 1994, pp 521–529.

24. Hildebrand KA, Patterson SD, Regan WD, et al: Functional outcome of semiconstrained total elbow arthroplasty. J Bone Joint Surg 82A:1379–1386, 2000.

25. Inglis AE: Revision surgery following a failed total elbow arthroplasty. Clin Orthop 170:213–218, 1982.

26. King GJ, Adams RA, Morrey BF: Total elbow arthroplasty: Revision with use of a non-custom semiconstrained prosthesis. J Bone Joint Surg Am 79:394–400, 1997.

27. King GJW, Glauser SJ, Westreich A, et al: In vitro stability of an unconstrained total elbow prosthesis. Influence of axial loading and joint flexion angle. J Arthroplasty 8:291–298, 1993.

28. King GJW, Itoi E, Niebur GL, et al: Motion and laxity of the capitellocondylar total elbow prosthesis. J Bone Joint Surg 76A: 1000–1008, 1994.

29. Kudo H, Iwano K, Nishino J: Cementless or hybrid total elbow arthroplasty with titanium-alloy implants. A study of interim clinical results and specific complications. J Arthroplasty 9:269–278, 1994.

30. Kudo H, Iwano K, Nishino J: Total elbow arthroplasty with use of a nonconstrained humeral component inserted without cement in patients who have rheumatoid arthritis. J Bone Joint Surg Am 81:1268–1280, 1999.

31. Liung P, Jonsson K, Rydholm U: Short-term complications of the lateral approach for non-constrained elbow replacement. J Bone Joint Surg 77B:937–942, 1995.

32. Lyall HA, Cohen B, Clatworthy M, Constant CR: Results of the Souter-Strathclyde total elbow arthroplasty in patients with rheumatoid arthritis. A preliminary report. J Arthroplasty 9:279–284, 1994.

33. Madsen F, Sojbjerg JO, Sneppen O: Late complications with the Pritchard Mark II elbow prosthesis. J Shoulder Elbow Surg 3:17–23, 1994.

34. Maloney W, Schurman DJ: Cast immobilization after total elbow arthroplasty. Clin Orthop 245:117–122, 1989.

35. Morrey BF: Revision of failed total elbow arthroplasty. In Morrey BF (ed): The Elbow and Its Disorders. Philadelphia, WB Saunders, 1993, pp 676–689.

36. Morrey BF: Revision of total elbow arthroplasty. In Morrey BF (ed): Master Techniques in Orthopaedic Surgery: The Elbow. New York, Raven Press, 1994, pp 257–275.

37. Morrey BF, Adams RA: Semiconstrained arthroplasty for the treatment of rheumatoid arthritis of the elbow. J Bone Joint Surg 74A:479–490, 1992.

38. Morrey BF, Adams RA, Bryan RS: Total replacement for post–traumatic arthritis of the elbow. J Bone Joint Surg 73B:607–612, 1991.

39. Morrey BF, An K-N, Stormont TJ: Force transmission through the radial head. J Bone Joint Surg 70A:250–256, 1988.

40. Morrey BF, Bryan RS: Complications of total elbow arthroplasty. Clin Orthop 170:204–212, 1982.

41. Morrey BF, Bryan RS: Revision total elbow arthroplasty. J Bone Joint Surg 69A:523–532, 1987.

42. O'Driscoll S: Elbow: Reconstruction. In Kasser J (ed): Orthopaedic Knowledge Update 5. Rosemont, IL, American Academy of Orthopaedic Surgeons, pp 283–294.

43. O'Driscoll S, Morrey B: Periprosthetic fractures about the elbow. Orthop Clin North Am 30:319–325, 1999.

44. O'Driscoll SW, Horii E, Morrey BF, Carmichael SW: Anatomy of the ulnar part of the lateral collateral ligament of the elbow. Clin Anat 5:296–303, 1992.

45. O'Driscoll SW, Morrey BF: Surgical reconstruction of the lateral collateral ligament. In Morrey BF (ed): Master Techniques in Orthopedic Surgery: The Elbow. New York, Raven Press, 1994, pp 169–182.

46. Pierce TD, Herndon JH: The triceps preserving approach to total elbow arthroplasty. Clin Orthop 354:144–152, 1998.

47. Ramsey ML, Adams RA, Morrey BF: Instability of the elbow treated with semiconstrained total elbow arthroplasty. J Bone Joint Surg Am 81:38–47, 1999.

48. Ring D, Kocher M, Koris M: Revison of Unstable Total Elbow Arthroplasty. San Francisco, American Shoulder and Elbow Surgeons, 2001.

49. Schneeberger A, King G, Song S-W, et al: Kinematics and laxity of the Souter-Strathclyde total elbow prosthesis. J Shoulder Elbow Surg 9:127–134, 2000.

50. Trancik T, Wilde AH, Borden LS: Capitellocondylar total elbow arthroplasty. Two to eight year experience. Clin Orthop 223: 175–180, 1987.

51. Wolfe SW, Ranawat CS: The osteo-anconeus flap. An approach for total elbow arthroplasty. J Bone Joint Surg 72A:684–688, 1990.

52. Wretenberg PF, Mikhail WE: Late dislocation after total elbow arthroplasty. J Shoulder Elbow Surg 8:178–80, 1999.

31

The Treatment of the Infected Total Elbow Arthroplasty

• KEN YAMAGUCHI and BERNARD F. MORREY

Improvements in both surgical technique and prosthetic design have significantly reduced the complication rates of total elbow arthroplasty. However, infection has remained a relatively common and potentially catastrophic complication, with reported rates as high as 1.5 percent to 11 percent.[2,4,5,7–13,16,17,21,23,24] Although the most recent clinical trails have reflected an improvement in infection rates, the prevalence has remained alarmingly high. It was not long ago that most reports focused only on identification and characterization of infections.[8,12,13,24] With little information on which to base treatment decisions, poorly functioning and sometimes painful excisional arthroplasty was the procedure of choice.[8,13,24] More recently, treatment options that have allowed concurrent eradication of the infection with either prosthetic retention or reimplantation have been explored with relatively good results.[19,25,26] The objective of this chapter is to review the evaluation and treatment of the infected total elbow arthroplasty. In particular, patient presentation, including health profile, duration of symptoms, fixation of components, and the bacteriology are related to indications for various treatment strategies for the infected elbow arthroplasty.

ETIOLOGY AND INCIDENCE

Since initial reports were made on infections of total elbow arthroplasties, the clinical presentation of these prosthetic infections has changed. Increased awareness of this complication has led to a high index of suspicion and hence earlier recognition.[8] However, the rate of infection for elbow arthroplasties remains well above that for the lower extremity arthroplasties, in part because of the high prevalence of severe rheumatoid arthritis (RA) or post-traumatic arthritis.[8,13,24] In addition to being immunocompromised, those with rheumatoid arthritis often place a great deal of pressure over this subcutaneous joint. Those with post-traumatic arthritis frequently have undergone multiple operations that compromise the vascularity of the soft tissues and thus increase the risk of wound-healing complications.[8,24] Risk factors for total elbow infections include rheumatoid arthritis, previous surgical procedures,[13] and previous local infections.[24] Delayed wound healing, wound drainage lasting longer than 10 days postoperatively, and reoperation are prognostic factors associated with increased infection rates.[24]

The incidence of infections after total elbow arthroplasties appears to have declined with improvements in surgical techniques. In a literature search of total elbow clinical trials published after the mid-1990s, there were 15 series reported in the literature. These comprise 457 total joints, among which there were 12 infections reported for an overall prevalence of 2.6 percent. It is interesting to note that among the 15 studies, 10 reported a zero percent incidence of infections. The complete lack of infections seen in these studies may have reflected the routine use of antibiotic-impregnated cement to implant total elbow components. It appears that the use of antibiotic-impregnated cement to implant the components, as well as meticulous postoperative hematoma control, has been helpful in lowering the incidence of infections. By protocol at the Mayo Clinic, postoperative elbows are kept in full extension for a period of 2 days, with the arm elevated before the institution of range of motion exercises. Experience at the Mayo Clinic has shown a decrease in infection rate from initial report of 8 percent to a more recent incidence of 3 percent.[13,25]

Now available are the results of a long-term clinical trial of total elbows performed at the Mayo Clinic, in which there was at least 10 years of follow-up, with a range of 10 to 15 years. There were 2 infections seen among 78 elbows, for a rate of 2.6 percent, which exactly mirrors the incidence seen from the previously identified clinical trials after the mid-1990s.

PATIENT PROFILE

Perhaps the most important consideration in treating a patient with an infected total elbow arthroplasty is overall health status, which comprises the medical condition as well as functional needs and expectations. Many patients with rheumatoid arthritis are medically debilitated as a result of immunosuppressive medications, anemia of chronic disease, and, sometimes, poor nutrition. For these patients, the only goal for surgery may be a noninfected, pain-free elbow. The most appropriate treatment for these individuals may be resection arthroplasty. For others in relatively good health, preservation of function remains an important goal. Treatment of infection with arthroplasty preservation requires multiple surgical procedures and aggressive treatment associated with a high risk of complications. Thus, any treatment plan should be placed in the context of the patient's needs and the ability to withstand this treatment.

The clinical presentation of an infected total elbow arthroplasty is often subtle and only recognized if a high index of suspicion is maintained.[24] In many (e.g., patients with RA), the systemic signs of sepsis (fever and tachycardia) are absent,[13] but the patient usually complains of increased pain or pain at rest. Acute inflammation is usually detectable by local signs such as the presence of warmth, erythema, and tenderness. In many, there may be drainage from the wound or soft tissues.[8,13,24] These points become important in determining the onset and, thus, chronicity of an infection.

Preoperative evaluation is critical in establishing range of motion, stability of the elbow, neurologic status, and the function of the biceps and triceps muscles. Laboratory data may be of limited value because most patients have a normal leukocyte count but an elevated neutrophil count on differential analysis.[13] The erythrocyte sedimentation rate (ESR) is often elevated but not specific because many have systemic inflammatory disease. The use of nuclear medicine modalities may increase the accuracy of preoperative diagnosis of prosthetic joint infection. A study evaluating the utility of Tc-99m labeled leukocytes showed a sensitivity of 70 percent, a specificity of 100 percent, and an overall diagnostic accuracy of 93 percent. The use of leukocyte scintigraphy dramatically improved the specificity of a bone scan in the assessment of a painful prosthetic joint. In contrast, the use of indium-111 labeled leukocytes in another series was not shown to be highly accurate, with a positive scintigraph increasing the likelihood of finding an infection to only 30 percent. The authors concluded that use of sequential technetium-99-hydroxymethyl diphosphonate and indium-111 leukocyte imaging cannot be advocated for differentiating a cold infection from mechanical failure in painful total joint arthroplasties. The use of cultures was similarly found to be inaccurate. In one study, preoperative aspirate levels were only 28 percent sensitive. In particular, a negative culture must be viewed with high suspicion. A study investigating the presence of bacterial infection by the use of immunofluorescence microscopy and PCR amplification of the bacterial 16-S rRNA gene showed that the incidence of prosthetic joint reinfection in revision surgery is grossly underestimated by current culture detection methods. In light of this information, making the diagnosis of infection can be exceedingly difficult in the context of a failed arthroplasty. In general, patients are considered infected when there are positive cultures and/or strong clinical suspicion (based on high white blood count, ESR, operative observations, and so forth) in the context of supportive microscopic pathology.

DURATION OF SYMPTOMS

Classically, infections have been categorized according to length of time from surgery. An infection is considered acute if it develops within 3 months of operation, subacute if onset is between 3 months and 1 year, and late if recognition occurs 1 year after surgery.[13,24] However, the time interval from the index procedure to the development of infection has not been shown to correlate with infection results.[15,25] The duration of symptoms, as in the experience with total knee arthroplasty, has demonstrated a correlation with successful treatment by irrigation and débridement.[18] Therefore, delineating the onset of symptoms has correlated better with the onset of infection and has direct implications on the treatment strategy.

FIXATION OF COMPONENTS

The determination of component fixation in the context of infection is based on the initial radiographic assessment in conjunction with intraoperative findings. The quality of the fixation is critical in deciding which treatment protocol to undertake. High-quality radiographs are necessary for the detection of radiolucent lines, cortical erosions, and osteolysis consistent with septic loosening of the prosthesis. Comparison with previous radiographs offers invaluable information. Loose or poorly fixed components obviate treatment with component retention.

BACTERIOLOGY

As opposed to soft tissue infections, the microorganisms of implant infections are often difficult to eradicate and continue to be a significant problem. This has been demonstrated in total elbow infections, in which the type of organism has had a profound impact on the treatment methods.[25] Organisms vary in virulence, adherence, and the elaboration of extracellular components. Many factors influence the adherence of bacteria to the prosthesis, including alterations in host immune competence and the ability of bacteria to produce an extracellular matrix.[3,7] Studies of infected orthopedic implants have shown that up to 76 percent of the infectious microorganisms produce a significant biofilm extracellular matrix that improves adherence to the implant.[3] Of these, coagulase-negative staphylococci have been the most common and the most problematic biofilm producers.[3,22] Unlike total hip and total knee replacements, the infection rate of elbow replacements with gram-negative microorganisms has been less common.[25]

Coagulase-positive staphylococci (i.e., *Staphylococcus aureus*), which are more virulent microorganisms with the capacity to invade and infect healthy tissues, have less of an ability to form a significant biofilm. Coagulase-negative staphylococcal organisms, particularly *Staphylococcus epidermidis*, have been recognized as the primary pathogen of orthopedic device infections because of their unusual capacity to attach to and to colonize orthopedic implants.[1,7] Although a relatively nonvirulent pathogen that normally lives in harmony on our skin, *S. epidermidis* can form a tenacious bacterial biofilm ("slime")—a polysaccharide glycocalyx (protein plus carbohydrate) that envelopes the bacteria. This promotes colonization and adherence and protects the bacteria from desiccation and host defense mechanisms.[3] It also protects them from antibiotic penetration and can even permit adherence to antibiotic-impregnated cement. This accounts for persistence and resistance to treatment of *S. epidermidis*.[7] Not surprisingly, the presence of *S. epidermidis* has thus been associated with a high incidence of failure if prosthetic retention is attempted with irrigation and débridement.[25]

TREATMENT OPTIONS

Once the diagnosis of an infected total elbow arthroplasty is suspected or confirmed, the treatment is focused on the surgical intervention. Consideration of a particular treatment plan must place strong emphasis on (1) duration of symptoms, (2) component fixation, (3) bacteriology, and (4) patient's health status (Fig. 31–1). Debilitated patients who are unable to withstand the rigors of multiple surgical procedures are best served with an excisional arthroplasty. Irrespective of treatment chosen, the primary objective remains a long-term infection cure, which is dependent on the complete removal of the bacteria and their glycocalyx. A secondary concern is restoration of function. All treatment plans require a minimum 6-week course of intravenous antibiotics.

Irrigation and Débridement with Retention of the Components

The initial experience with irrigation and débridement with retention of the components resulted in poor outcomes, with most patients failing to respond to this treatment. Wolfe et al. reported 8 failures in 11 patients with this technique; the other 3 elbows were deemed successes despite intermittent wound drainage.[24] The Mayo Clinic's initial experience was similar, with only 1 of 9 patients treated successfully. However, with increased awareness and earlier detection of infection, patients are now often seen with well-fixed components and without apparent bone involvement.

Experience with infected total knee arthroplasty has demonstrated a high correlation between the duration of symptoms of infection (21 days or less) and outcome with component retention.[18] Using this principle of less than 30 days of symptom duration, a study reported a 50 percent long-term success rate for irrigation and débridement of infected total elbows (at a mean 71-

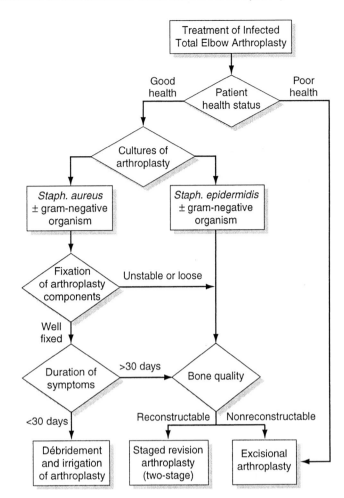

Figure 31–1. Treatment algorithm for the infected total elbow.

month follow-up).[25] Furthermore, the bacteriology played a significant role with all 4 patients infected by *S. epidermidis* who failed to respond to this treatment protocol, whereas in 6 of 8 patients who had a *S. aureus* infection, the disease was successfully eradicated.[25] Therefore, treatment with débridement and component retention is dependent on both symptom duration and bacteriology.

The relative success seen with irrigation débridement of components that are detected early must also be weighed with the consequence of performing a revision arthroplasty when components are well fixated. In general, when an infection is detected early, the components remain securely implanted in bone. In the series by Wolfe et al., 3 of 8 patients sustained fractures of the humerus or ulna with component removal.[24] In aseptic revisions, Morrey noted fractures in 11 of 33 subjects. These results exemplify the difficulty in removing the components without compromising the bone structure[14] and have renewed the interest in component retention. Clearly, removal of well-fixed components can result in serious complications that can be avoided by an initial attempt at irrigation and débridement.

The indications for this treatment include (1) the presence of well-fixed surgical components by both radiographic and intraoperative examination; (2) bacteriology that suggests *S. aureus* or other pathogen amenable to this form of treatment; (3) a suitable soft tissue envelope with or without the use of flaps; (4) a patient who is medically fit to withstand the required multiple surgical procedures; and (5) duration of symptoms less than 30 days. A contraindication to component retention is an infection caused by *S. epidermidis*.

Surgical Technique

The technique for irrigation and débridement with component retention is through a posterior approach that uses the previous incision.[25] A standard extensile triceps-sparing approach is used as previously described for primary total elbow arthroplasties. Care should be taken to preserve the triceps insertion in continuity with the distal forearm fascia. Triceps evulsion is a significant complication of revision surgery. Once the distal humerus is exposed, removal of the medial and lateral condyles is generally necessary to obtain exposure to the articulating pin. With semiconstrained implants, removal of the medial and lateral condyles usually does not result in perceptible loss of forearm strength. The stability of the component fixation in bone is confirmed after complete disarticulation of the components, including removal of the bushings (Fig. 31–2). This is an essential component of the procedure. The joint is débrided of all necrotic debris and copiously irrigated with pulsatile saline lavage. Antibiotic-impregnated polymethylmethacrylate (PMMA) beads, with a concentration of 1 g of tobramycin per package of cement, are placed in the wound before closure. Patients return to the operating room every fourth day for repeat irrigation and débridement with antibiotic PMMA bead exchange. The number of repeat irrigation and débridement procedures is variable, but, usually, 3 or 4 are required. The patient concurrently receives bacteria-sensitive intravenous antibiotics for a minimum period of 6 weeks (based on serum minimal inhibitory and bactericidal concentrations).[25] The use of chronic suppressive antibiotics is controversial and depends on the surgeon's preference.

Overall success rate of the series of Yamaguchi et al. was 50 percent, but it was increased to 70 percent when those infected with *S. epidermidis* were eliminated.[25] Outcomes produced good functional results but carried a 43 percent incidence of complications, including 21 percent incidence of wound breakdown or triceps avulsion and 21 percent incidence of peripheral nerve injury.

Staged Exchange Arthroplasty

As seen with staged exchange arthroplasty for lower extremity infections, the technique has also been successfully used for infected total elbow arthroplasties. Yamaguchi et al. reported an 80 percent success rate with staged revision; the only failures occurred in patients infected with *S. epidermidis*.[25] Moreover, the mean increase in Mayo Elbow score was from 21 to 79, demonstrating good functional improvement. The

procedure's success was dependent on the complete eradication of the pathogenic microorganism, which necessitated the complete removal of all prosthetic components, including PMMA.

Although not yet well defined, the most common indications for staged exchange arthroplasty are (1) radiographic or intraoperative evidence of loose components with sufficient bone stock for reconstruction, (2) duration of symptoms longer than 30 days, and (3) a medically fit patient. A relative contraindication, depending on the decision of the surgeon and the patient, is an infection caused by *S. epidermidis*.

Surgical Technique

The surgical technique uses the previous posterior incision to expose the joint, with consideration of flaps for soft tissue coverage. When possible, the triceps insertion to the olecranon is removed in continuity with the distal forearm fascia to better preserve extension strength and enhance bone tendon healing. The exposure should be extended proximally as necessary to find the ulnar nerve in undisturbed tissue. This allows distal dissec-

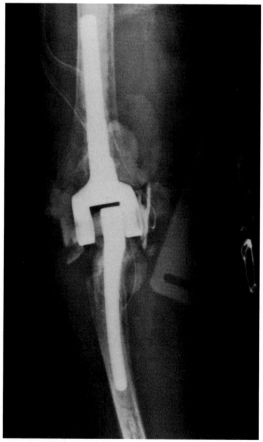

A

Figure 31–2. A and **B,** Intraoperative radiograph from a representative patient who underwent successful irrigation and débridement. The patient had well-fixed components and 1 day of infection symptoms. The component was disarticulated with bushings and pin removal as an essential portion of the débridement procedure.

Illustration continued on opposite page

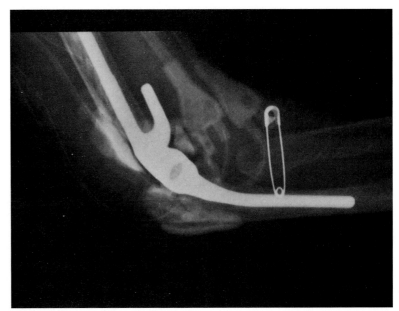

Figure 31–2. *Continued.*

B

tion to be performed along the nerve and in a more accurate fashion. Often, the radial nerve should also be identified. Once exposure to the joint is obtained, the distal portions of the mediolateral columns need to be removed to obtain access to the prosthetic articulating pin. Conversely, if the humeral component is grossly loose, it can be pulled distally to gain access to the disarticulating pin. Generally, both the humeral and ulnar components should be loose to some extent as an indication for proceeding with resection arthroplasty. In the context, well-fixed components, irrigation, and débridement may be preferred. Once both the humeral and ulnar components are removed, a meticulous removal of any polyethylene metal debris and cement is performed. It is vitally important to comprehensively remove all nonviable tissue while preserving as much bone stock as possible. This is particularly important on the ulnar side, where the available bone stock can be quite limited.

Preparation and débridement of the ulna can be enhanced by making an osteotomy of the ulnar shaft distal to the tip of the ulnar component. This allows easy access to the distal portion of the ulna as well as allowing a distal and proximal exposure to intramedullary retained cement. The osteotomy site can then be bridged by a long-stemmed ulnar component on final implantation (Fig. 31–3).

Once components are removed and all nonviable tissues or components débrided, an antibiotic-impregnated PMMA (tobramycin 1 g per package of PMMA) is then used as a spacer between the humerus and the ulna to maintain soft tissue tension (Fig. 31–4). The wound is closed and the limb is placed in a cast or hinged orthosis for 4 weeks. Alternatively, as needed, another open débridement can be performed 3 days later before closure and cast placement. A concurrent 6-week treatment with directed intravenous antibiotics is initiated.

Consideration of longer staging intervals and repeat irrigation débridement can be given to more resistant infections such as *S. epidermidis.*

Two weeks after the cessation of intravenous antibiotics, repeat cultures are performed in planning for reimplantation. If there are any concerns about persistent infection, an open irrigation and débridement is performed again, including an exchange of antibiotic-impregnated cement spacer.

Reimplantation is performed along the same lines as revision total elbow arthroplasty. Long-stemmed humeral and ulnar components are generally preferred. In cases in which significant bone stock has been lost, a modified Ling-type construct is employed (Fig. 31–5). In this procedure, cancellous allograft bone is morcellized into relatively small fragments and then inserted into both the humeral and ulnar canals. Trial components are then used to impact the bone graft radially away from the prosthesis, which creates a canal within the bone graft for implantation. The relatively tapered forms of the humeral and ulnar components allow this impaction to be done effectively. After impaction of the cancellous bone graft, the components are then implanted with use of antibiotic-impregnated PMMA.

Immediate Exchange Arthroplasty

There has been very minimal information regarding immediate exchange for infection in total elbows. To date, there has been only 1 case reported.[25] This case resulted in a failure to eradicate the infection.

The majority of experience with the lower extremity has occurred in Europe, with only anecdotal and early reports in North America. Success rates with immediate exchange arthroplasty for infected total knee replacements vary from 35 percent to 75 percent; suggested improved

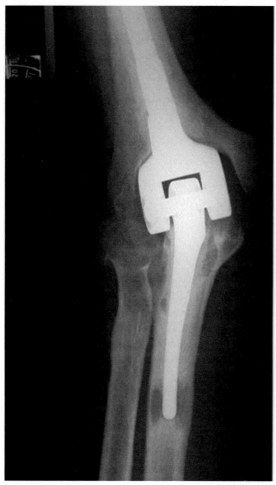
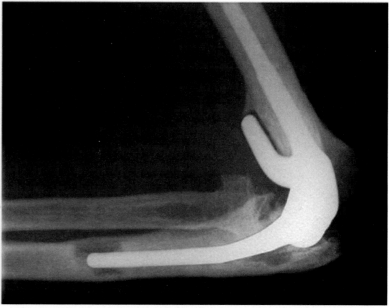

A

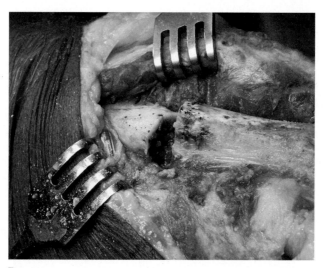

B

Figure 31–3. A, Radiographs from a patient with an infection and distal ulnar osteolysis. Revision of this component would require removal of the ulnar stem, a cement mantle, and débridement of the distal lesion. **B**, Component and cement removal as well as débridement of the distal ulna was facilitated by performing and osteotomy at the osteolysis site. The two ulna shaft pieces were then sequentially delivered so that a débridement could be performed and later bridged by a long-stemmed ulnar component.

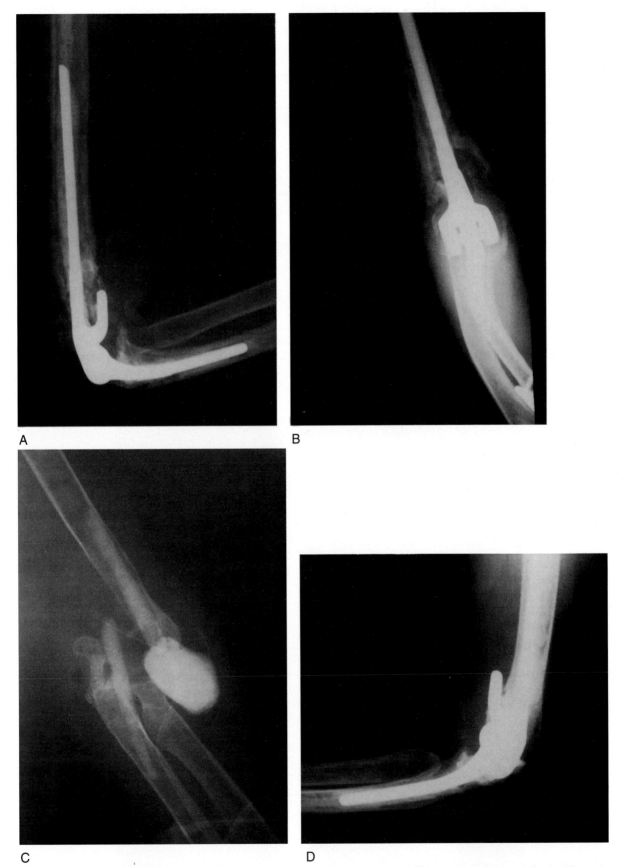

A

B

C

D

Figure 31–4. This is a 45-year-old man who underwent staged exchange arthroplasty. This man had a *S. aureus* infection 68 months from the primary procedure. He had had 56 days of symptoms before presentation. **A** and **B**, Anteroposterior and lateral radiographs of the elbow, with scalloping of the cortical bone and prosthetic loosening consistent with infection. **C**, The component was removed and antibiotic-impregnated cement was placed. Seven weeks later, the patient underwent reimplantation of a semi-constrained prosthesis with antibiotic-impregnated cement. **D**, At 64 months of follow-up, there are no signs of persistent infection.

results may occur with gram-positive non-glycocalyx producing organisms.[6,20]

The indications for immediate exchange arthroplasty are probably very limited and, at this time, undetermined. The principles of surgical treatment are similar to those used for the staged revision, with aggressive débridement with removal of all foreign material, antibiotic-impregnated cement fixation, and a concomitant 6 to 12 weeks of intravenous antibiotic therapy.

Resection Arthroplasty

Resection arthroplasty has been the standard of treatment for infected elbow arthroplasty and constitutes the largest treatment experience. Functional results are usually limited but can be associated with a high satisfaction rate. Moreover, because many of these patients are debilitated, it is considered the treatment of choice for those who are medically frail and unfit for extensive or multiple surgical procedures. If the arthroplasty is successful, it often provides a relatively pain-free satisfactory range of active motion with reasonable stability. This is more likely to occur when the medial and lateral columns of the distal humerus are intact. If the elbow is flail or grossly unstable, it is usually nonfunctional and often painful.

The technique of elbow resection arthroplasty involves removal of the implant components through the previous incision followed by complete removal of the PMMA. All necrotic and contaminated tissue is excised. If the condyles of the distal humerus remain intact, they are then contoured and deepened to encircle the ulna. The soft tissue coverage is established by primary closure or local rotation flaps. Concurrent treatment with 4 to 6 weeks of appropriate antibiotic therapy is used. The limb is placed in a cast or external fixator for 3 to 4 weeks to obtain soft tissue stability.

Complications

Treatment strategies aimed at prosthetic retention either with irrigation and débridement or with reimplantation in a staged or immediate fashion have been associated with a high complication rate. In a study regarding infected elbow treatment options, multiple irrigation and débridements were associated with triceps insufficiencies, nerve injuries, and skin or wound breakdown.

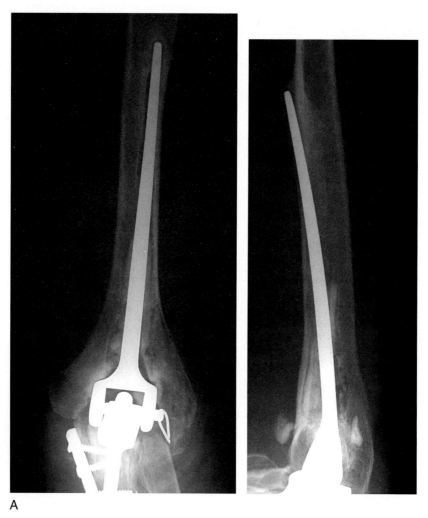

A

Figure 31–5. A, Radiographs of a loose humeral component with profound osteopenia at the distal humerus.

Illustration continued on opposite page

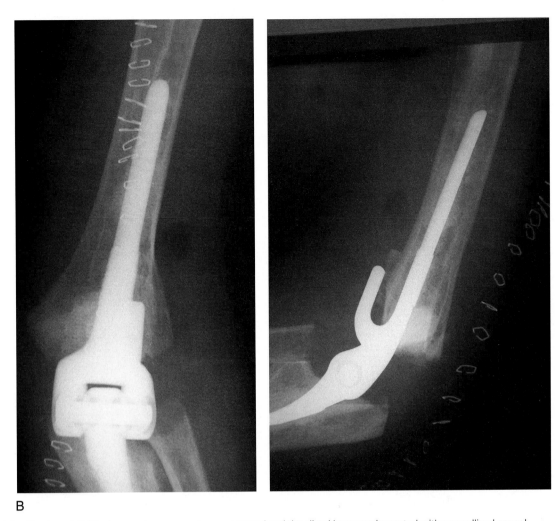

B

Figure 31–5. *Continued.* **B,** The humeral component was removed and the distal humerus impacted with morcellized cancellous allograft. A new humeral component was then cemented into place within the impacted cancellous bone graft bed.

Additionally, procedures aimed at reimplantation in either a staged or immediate fashion were associated with similar complications. Thus, special attention needs to be given to protecting surrounding neurovascular structures as well as the triceps insertion and operative wound. The multiple irrigation and débridements associated with infection eradication appear to put all of these structures at significant risk. Hence, in the treatment of the infected total elbow arthroplasty, special consideration should be taken in using triceps-on approaches, and proactive planning for possible soft tissue coverage procedures should be done. Of course, the high risk of complications and the associated morbidity are significant considerations that have to be discussed with the patient before an attempt is made to perform any prosthetic salvage strategy in the context of infected elbow arthroplasty.

CONCLUSION

Infection remains a significant and severe complication of total elbow arthroplasty, with an incidence above that of lower extremity joint replacements. Previously, the only treatment option was excisional arthroplasty. Newer reports of this problem suggest that both irrigation and débridement and staged exchange arthroplasty can be successful treatment modalities given the appropriate indications (see Fig. 31–1). As such, selected treatment methods may improve both function and satisfaction after this most devastating complication.

References

1. Blanchard CR, Sanford BA, Lankford J, Railsback R: *Staphylococcus epidermidis* biofilm formation on orthopaedic implant materials. Orthop Trans 1997.
2. Brumfield RH Jr, Kuschner SH, Gellman H, et al: Total elbow arthroplasty. J Arthroplasty 5:359–363, 1990.
3. Christensen GD, Baldassarri L, Simpson WA: Colonization of medical devices. *In* Bisno AL, Waldvogel FA (eds): Infections Associated with Indwelling Medical Devices, 2nd ed. Washington, DC, American Society for Microbiology, 1994, pp 45–78.
4. Davis RF, Weiland AJ, Hungerford DS, et al: Nonconstrained total elbow arthroplasty. Clin Orthop 171:156–160, 1982.
5. Ewald FC, Simmons ED Jr, Sullivan JA, et al: Capitellocondylar total elbow replacement in rheumatoid arthritis. Long-term results

[published erratum appears in J Bone Joint Surg Am 75:1881, 1993]. J Bone Joint Surg Am 1993 75A:498, 1993.

6. Fitzgerald RH, Nasser S: Infections following total hop arthroplasty. *In* Callaghan JJ, Dennis DA, Paprosky WG, Rosenbery AG (eds): Hip and Knee Reconstructon. Rosemont, IL, American Academy of Orthopaedic Surgeons, 1995, pp 157–162.

7. Gristina AG: Microbial adhesion versus tissue integration. Science 237:1588–1595, 1987.

8. Gutow AP, Wolfe SW: Infection following total elbow arthroplasty. Hand Clinics 10:521–529, 1994.

9. Kasten MD, Skinner HB: Total elbow arthroplasty. An 18-year experience. Clin Orthop 290:177–188, 1993.

10. Kraay MJ, Figgie MP, Inglis AE, et al: Primary semiconstrained total elbow arthroplasty. Survival analysis of 113 consecutive cases. J Bone Joint Surg 76B:636–640, 1994.

11. Morrey BF, Adams RA: Semiconstrained arthroplasty for the treatment of rheumatoid arthritis of the elbow. J Bone Joint Surg 74A:479–490, 1992.

12. Morrey BF, Bryan RS: Complications of total elbow arthroplasty. Clin Orthop 170:204–212, 1982.

13. Morrey BF, Bryan RS: Infection after total elbow arthroplasty. J Bone Joint Surg 65A:330–338, 1983.

14. Morrey BF, Bryan RS: Revision total elbow arthroplasty. J Bone Joint Surg 69A:523–532, 1987.

15. Poss R, Thornhill TS, Ewald FC, et al: Factors influencing the incidence and outcome of infection following total joint arthroplasty. Clin Orthop 182:117–126, 1984.

16. Rosenberg GM, Turner RH: Nonconstrained total elbow arthroplasty. Clin Orthop 187:154–162, 1984.

17. Ruth JT, Wilde AH: Capitellocondylar total elbow replacement. A long-term follow-up study. J Bone Joint Surg 74A:95–100, 1992.

18. Schoifet SD, Morrey BF: Treatment of infection after total knee arthroplasty by débridement with retention of the components. J Bone Joint Surg 72A:1383–1390, 1990.

19. Tetro AM, Yamaguchi K: Treatment of the infected total elbow arthroplasty. *In* Williams GR Jr (ed): Seminars in Arthroplasty. Philadelphia, WB Saunders, 1998, pp 80–87.

20. Thornhill TS: Total knee infections. *In* Callaghan JJ, Dennis DA, Paprosky WG, Rosemont AG (eds): Hip and Knee Reconstruction. Rosemont, IL, American Academy of Orthopaedic Surgeons, 1995, pp 297–300.

21. Trancik T, Wilde AH, Borden LS: Capitellocondylar total elbow arthroplasty. Two-to eight-year experience. Clin Orthop 223: 175–180, 1987.

22. Van Pett K, Schurman DJ, Smith RL: Quantitation and relative distribution of extracellular matrix in *Staphylococcus epidermidis* biofilm. J Orthop Res 8:321–327, 1990.

23. Weiland AJ, Weiss AP, Wills RP, Moore JR: Capitellocondylar total elbow replacement. A long-term follow-up study. J Bone Joint Surg 71A:217–222, 1989.

24. Wolfe SW, Figgie MP, Inglis AE, et al: Management of infection about total elbow prostheses. J Bone Joint Surg 72A:198–212, 1990.

25. Yamaguchi K, Adams RA, Morrey BF: Infection after total elbow arthroplasty. J Bone Joint Surg 80A:481–491, 1998.

26. Yamaguchi K, Adams RA, Morrey BF: Semiconstrained total elbow arthroplasty in the context of treated previous infection. J Shoulder Elbow Surg 8:461–465,1999.

32

Revision/Salvage Total Elbow Arthroplasty

BERNARD F. MORREY

Over the last few years, the understanding and techniques needed to successfully revise the failed arthroplasty have expanded considerably. The management of sepsis after total elbow arthroplasty is discussed in Chapter 30. Comments in this chapter are thus limited to the nonseptic failed implant arthroplasty. The issue of revision elbow reconstruction has not been extensively discussed in the literature, either after failed implant or interposition techniques.[4-6,8-10,14] The array of salvage options are shown in Table 32–1 and were discussed in detail in the second edition of this text. The only real goal is functional restoration, and advances in this surgery have been in the realm of reimplantation; hence, the focus of this chapter.

FAILED ARTHROPLASTY WITHOUT PRIOR JOINT REPLACEMENT

I have only occasionally revised a failed interposition arthroplasty with a second interposition procedure. The aseptic failed nonimplant arthroplasty (i.e., the unsuccessful interposition or resection procedure) is most often treated best with total elbow replacement. In my experience, resurfacing prostheses are not reliable in this setting because of instability, and, hence, I favor a stemmed, semiconstrained design such as the Coonrad-Morrey device.

Technique. The most important technique considerations are the management of the ulnar nerve and triceps attachment. Adequate release of pericapsular scar tissue is important in many cases. Otherwise, the technique is similar to that for prosthetic replacement for posttrauma arthritis.

Results

My experience with prosthetic replacement for failed interposition arthroplasty has been reported by Blaine et al.[1] The outcome after 13 interposition arthroplasty procedures was quite reliable and comparable with that seen after primary replacement for traumatic conditions at a mean of 9 years after surgery; relief of pain and restoration of stability was observed in 85 percent of cases. I conclude that prior interposition arthroplasty does not compromise the outcome of joint replacement, so it should continue to be considered in the young (younger than 55 to 65 years of age) patient with traumatic arthrosis or stiffness.

FAILED PROSTHETIC REPLACEMENT

Presentation

A broad spectrum of clinical and pathologic states is encountered with failed total elbow arthroplasty. Several specific features of the presentation are considered as the management plan is formulated.

1. A failed prosthesis manifests either with or without a periprosthetic fracture.
2. If the integrity of the bone is not compromised, scarring by fracture, osteolysis, or osteoporosis is present.
3. Stiffness, scarring, and contracture of the soft tissue are common in the triceps, ulnar nerve, static deformity, and skin. In this chapter, the focus is on the reliability of implant options that allow the full spectrum of failure types to be addressed.

The nature of the failure is very much a function of the specific type of implant used. Some designs are more prone to loosening, others to instability, and still others to dissociation of the articulation.[4,7,9,10] Third-body wear can be devastating if this causes extensive osteolysis (Fig. 32–1). Loose implants may not be painful; there-

---

Table 32–1. SURGICAL OPTIONS FOR THE FAILED TOTAL ELBOW ARTHROPLASTY ARE CONSIDERED AS FUNCTION OR AS SALVAGE PROCEDURES

Nonimplant salvage
  Fusion
  Resection
Functional restoration
  Prosthetic articulation
  Allograft replacement
  Implant insertion

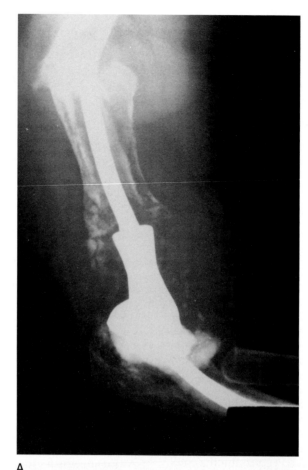

A

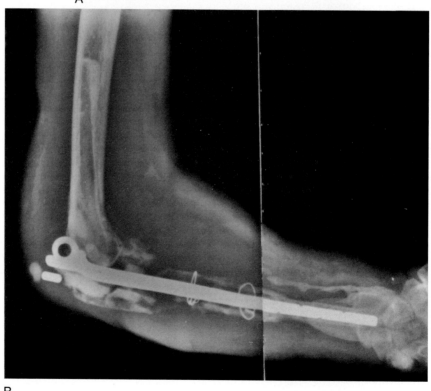

B

Figure 32–1. Extensive osteolysis can be devastating, causing fracture (**A**), and can be so extensive as to resolve virtually the entire bone (**B**).

fore, they should be followed carefully. Revision is offered, even if the patient does not have pain, because extensive osteolysis can lead to fracture, making revision even more difficult.

History

The most important historical information is the duration of implantation and the function early after implantation. An earlier than expected failure may be caused by sepsis. Hence, assessment for—and excluding the possibility of—sepsis is a most important consideration before any revision procedure, but especially in those with early unexplained or unanticipated failure.[18]

Evaluation

Laboratory. The sedimentation rate and C-reactive protein studies are regularly employed, along with aspiration of the joint, if there is any question of sepsis.

Radiographic. The radiograph is, of course, most helpful evidence for defining the exact cause of failure. Based on the radiographic appearance of the failure, the appropriate preoperative plan is formulated depending primarily on the quality of the bone. In our practice, my colleagues and I do not offer surgery for radiolucent lines that are not painful, although we do offer surgery if there is progressive resorption, bone loss, or impending fracture.

SURGICAL OPTIONS AND DETERMINANTS

Our current practice recognizes and employs several strategies to revise the noninfected failed implant, predicated on the status of the implant articulation and fixation, the quality of bone and presence or absence of fracture (Table 32–2). Since 1982, 26 percent of 920 elbow

Table 32–2. SURGICAL OPTIONS FOR FUNCTIONAL RESTORATION BY IMPLANT INSERTION

Functional Salvage

Implant reinsertion
  Osseous integrity
    Intact cement
    Intact bone
  Osseous deficiency
    Enhancement
      Cancellous infection
      Strut
      Combination

replacements that used the Coonrad-Morrey implant have had revisions.

Articular Revision

This is a simple procedure that addresses articular coupling failure or polyethylene wear (Fig. 32–2). If the design has proved reliable and stable, replacement of the polyethylene bushings is all that is required. If the design has demonstrable and recurrent problems of articular failure, consideration of a complete revision to a new design should be considered.

Technique. Depending on the design, revision of the bushing is relatively straightforward. Care is taken to débride all reactive debris-laden tissue to eliminate ongoing lysis. A secure triceps repair is very important. Assessment of olecranon resorption is important because lysis can decrease the mechanical advantage offered by this bone. In some instances, the olecranon is reconstructed with a strut graft.

Implant Revision

The various options for reinsertion are predicated on the status and quality of bone and the presence or absence of fracture.

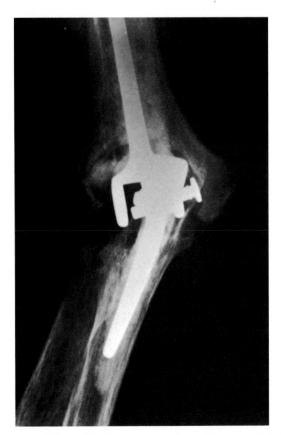

Figure 32–2. Failure of the locking mechanism is the most predictable of all revision types.

If bone stock is adequate, salvage options consist of arthrodesis or resection. Functional restoration is obtained by interposition or total elbow replacement. If adequate bone is not present, total elbow replacement with a semiconstrained or custom implant used alone or with graft augmentation clearly provides the most functional outcome.

Periprosthetic Fracture. With increased longevity and expanded use of elbow replacements by the orthopedic community, a growing number of periprosthetic fractures are being seen. We have found it helpful to classify these according to site of involvement: type I—metaphyseal; type II—stem involvement; type III—proximal or distal to the stem tip (Fig. 32–3). Management strategies are discussed later based on this classification.

Functional Restoration Revision Options

We consider reinsertion revision procedures in six circumstances depending on the aforementioned features of osseous competency. These options include:

1. Reinsertion into intact cement
2. Reinsertion into the host bone
3. Reimplantation into cancellous augmented host bone reinsertion
4. Reimplantation into strut-graft–augmented host bone
5. Use of a "composite" allograft
6. Custom device reconstruction

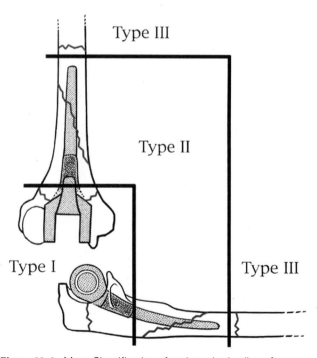

Figure 32–3. Mayo Classification of periprosthetic elbow fractures. Type I, metaphyseal; Type II, involves stem; Type III, beyond stem. (With permission, Mayo Foundation.)

TECHNIQUE OF REIMPLANTATION REVISION

General Considerations

Preoperative Planning and Implant Selection

The loose elbow implant may cause bone resorption. This may cause weak or absent triceps function because of resorption of the olecranon. The most important consideration is whether adequate fixation can be obtained with another stemmed implant given the amount and quality of the intact cement mantle or of bone. Hence, the most common special implant need is adequate stem length. The largest stemmed implant that comfortably fits into the bone stock is preferable. For humeral revisions, we use either the 15- or 20-cm humeral stem of the Coonrad-Morrey device. Special long-stemmed ulnar components are also routinely available. The extended flange is especially helpful for deficient distal humeral bone stock (Fig. 32–4). Custom devices are, therefore, rarely needed with this system.

Surgical Procedure

General Considerations and Prior Surgery

The surgical exposure is modified according to the patient's presentation.[2] Previous skin incisions are used as much as possible. The ulnar nerve is identified and decompressed if it is symptomatic or simply protected if it is not symptomatic. The management of the triceps is according to one of three methods: (1) the triceps is reflected (Mayo) (Fig. 32–5); (2) the triceps is split, particularly in patients in whom there have been multiple procedures with poor triceps tissue; or (3) the triceps is left attached to the ulna; after the joint or pseudarthrosis is resected and the ulna is rotated and displaced, adequate exposure is often attained even while leaving the triceps attached (Fig. 32–6).

SPECIFIC TECHNICAL CONSIDERATIONS

Preservation of Cement Mantle

If the bone-cement interface is intact, the cement may be left and a new device recemented in the existing polymethylmethacrylate mantle.

A high-speed bone bur with a 2-mm head and long extension is helpful to remove cement between implant and bone (Fig. 32–7). Furthermore, if the bone-cement interface is secure, the cement cavity is expanded with the 4-mm "olive" bur to receive the revision implant stem. The wall of the bone cement component is left alone. Cement injection systems are used to inject the cement down into the canal. Typically, for revision surgery, each component is cemented

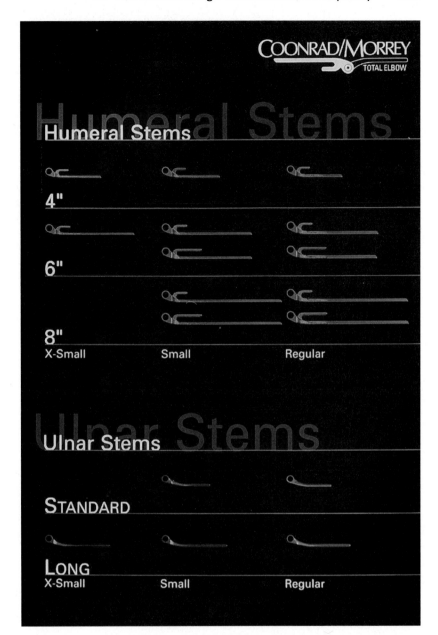

Figure 32–4. Standard humeral and ulnar implants have considerable dimensional variety. The availability of the extended flange virtually eliminates the need for custom devices.

separately to minimize technical complications. Great care must be taken to avoid injury to the nerves. We graft large cortical defects with autogenous cancellous bone to avoid extravasation of cement and to prevent fracture.

Cement Removal and Reinsertion

If the cement is not intact, the medullary canal must be identified for a long implant to be inserted after removal of the cement. We use an Esmarch technique to expose the humerus as proximally as necessary. Exposure or location and palpation of the radial nerve are necessary to avoid injury to the radial nerve (see Fig. 32–8). The humerus is then palpated to avoid violation of the cortex at the time of cement removal.

The ulna is extensively exposed in a subcutaneous fashion for as great a distance as necessary to have adequate exposure and to avoid violation of the ulnar cortex. If there is thinning at the tip of the implant, if a fracture has occurred, or if specific attention must be given to more distal insertion of the stem down into the canal, the entire subcutaneous border of the ulna may be exposed to the extent necessary to avoid penetration.

Closure is carefully done, and special care is taken to ensure triceps function. After revision procedures, if an allograft has been used, or if there has been extensive bone loss and excessive motion is of concern, the elbow is placed in a splint in extension. After 4 to 6 weeks, the splint is removed and motion is begun. Because the range of motion after revision elbow replacement is virtually the same as that after primary joint replacement,

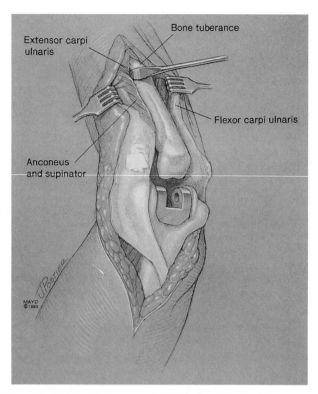

Figure 32–5. If the distal humeral condyles are intact, a Mayo triceps reflection approach is preferred.

early mobilization of the revision implant is not particularly important.

RESULTS

Reimplantation

There is very little information with regard to the reimplantation of an artificial device for a previously failed joint replacement.[14] Our experience has been updated with 41 patients followed for an average of 5 years (range, 2 to 11 years).[10] Approximately half of these patients had rheumatoid arthritis, and the other half had post-traumatic arthritis as their underlying diagnosis. Pain relief was gratifying in 90 percent of patients, but 4 of the 41 continue to have pain because of component loosening or residual nerve irritation. The revision-free rate for the overall group of 41 patients was 92 percent. Those with rheumatoid arthritis had a 96-percent revision-free rate, whereas those with post-traumatic arthritis had an 86 percent revision-free rate. The average arc of motion was from 28 to 130 degrees of flexion, 55 degrees of pronation, and 60 degrees of supination. Loosening has not been a problem (Fig. 32–9).

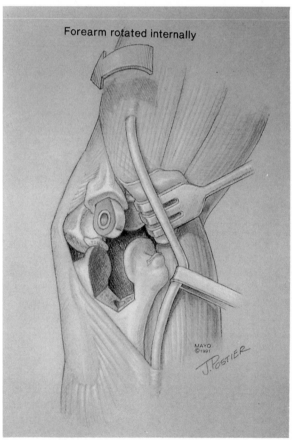

A

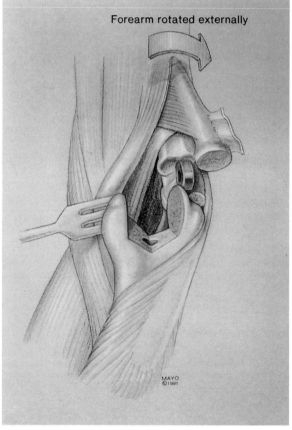

B

Figure 32–6. In patients with loss of the distal humerus, the triceps can sometimes remain attached to the proximal ulna. The articulation is released and the ulna can simply be rolled out of the way, leaving the triceps attached medially (**A**) or laterally (**B**).

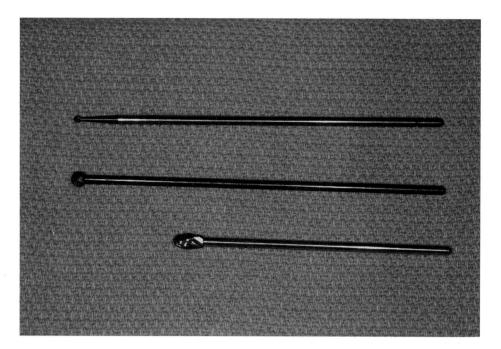

Figure 32–7. Simple bone burs with head diameters of 1 to 4 mm are effective in addressing the bone/cement interface and in expanding the intact cement mantle.

Complications

Significant complications occurred in 7 (16 percent) of the 41 patients. Three had radial nerve injuries, 1 caused by perforation of the cortex by a high-speed bur, and 1 was left with an excisional arthroplasty as a result of titanium synovitis. The bushings were worn and required replacement 6 years after the original surgery in 1 patient because of excessive use, and 1 patient

fell on the outstretched hand and sustained a periprosthetic fracture. There were no infections in this experience.

Our experience, therefore, suggests that prosthetic reimplantation is probably the most viable option for revision of total elbow arthroplasty. If the patient is young, more than one revision may be required, and other options, such as resection or fusion, should be considered.

OSSEOUS ENHANCEMENT OPTIONS

If the process has caused resorption, osteolysis, or a periprosthetic fracture, an "augmentation" procedure is indicated in the form of impaction grafting or strut augmentation.

IMPACTION GRAFTING

Indication. Impaction grafting is warranted if the patient has expanded cortical bone of inadequate quality to securely re-cement a stemmed implant.

Procedure. The extent of the expanded lytic bone is determined. The distance "D" of stem fixation that is attainable in the uninvolved bone is also determined. A rigid tube is placed in the expanded cortical portion of the bone. The elbow cement injector tube is cut at a distance "D" plus the length of the cortical expansion. Cancellous bone or bone substitute is firmly packed around the outer tube (Fig. 32–10). Cement is injected into the intact canal through an inner tube and withdrawn for the distance "D," after which the two tubes are withdrawn simultaneously while cement is injected in the region of the expanded cortex. The implant is then inserted (Fig. 32–11). This

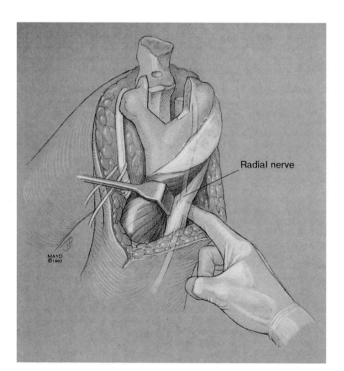

Figure 32–8. The humeral shaft is exposed sufficiently to palpate the radial nerve and to lessen the likelihood of penetration.

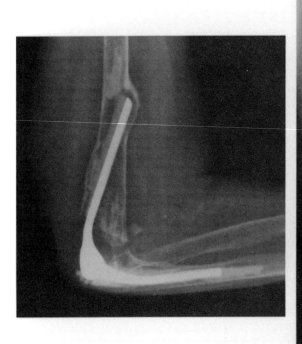
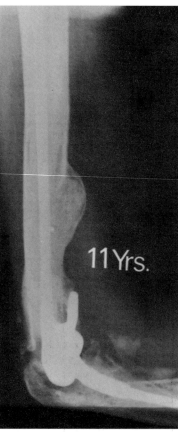

Figure 32–9. Reinsertion into osseous envelope after cortical penetration of a loose humeral stem shows no evidence of loosening or lucency 11 years after 150-cm implant revision.

technique may be used both for the humerus and the ulna.

Results

We have reviewed experience with 12 instances of impaction grafting since 1993, 8 of the humerus and 6 of the ulna.[11] After a mean of 3 years follow-up (range, 2 to 6 years), 1 has been re-revised. A subjective satisfactory result is present in 10 of the 12 patients (84 percent) (Fig. 32–12). One patient became infected and required removal of the implant.

STRUT GRAFTING

This technique is especially useful for type II and type III periprosthetic fractures and for distal humeral bone loss. The most effective application is that of an anterior strut that transverses the osteolysis or fracture and captures the flange anteriorly. A posterior strut is employed in part to prevent the wire from cutting through the host bone. The radial nerve is exposed for humeral applications, and at least two circumferential wire fixation points are required around the normal host bone or proximal to the fracture, and two around the osteolysis or expanded periarticular bone distal to the fracture (Fig. 32–13). The design of the Coonrad-

Morrey implant allows restoration of the axis of rotation with a deficient humerus from the level of the olecranon fossa (Fig. 32–14). The use of the extended flange and an anterior strut graft allows management of distal humeral deficiencies up to 8 cm. If greater than 2 cm of bone loss occurs proximal to the olecranon fossa, the length is accommodated by the extended flange (Fig. 32–15). The implant is simply inserted to the desired depth, and the deficient bone is bridged by the flange and graft. If up to 5 cm bone loss is present proximal to the fossa, 3 cm is accommodated by the flange and strut graft and 2 cm of shortening is accepted. The proper depth of insertion is determined by flexing the articulated trial prostheses, and, with the elbow at 90 degrees of flexion, displacing the ulna distally until tension limits further displacement and observing the depth of insertion of the humeral component at that point (Fig. 32–16).

Results

We have reviewed our experience with 13 patients treated with humeral strut grafts.[16,17] Of these, 12 are considered satisfactory (93 percent) a mean of 5 years after surgery. The grafts appear to have been incorporated in all the patients. Patient satisfaction parallels the 93 percent radiographic satisfaction rate (see Fig. 32–12).

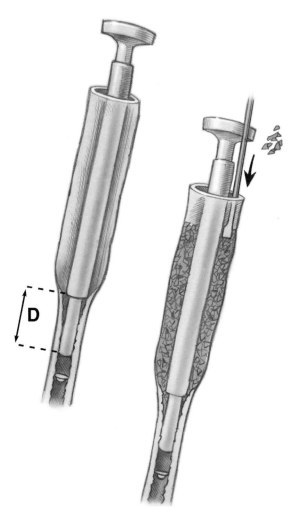

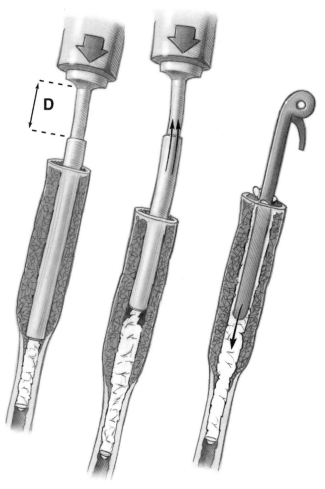

Figure 32–10. For impaction grafting, a semirigid tube is inserted across the expanded osteolytic segment. The cement injector nozzle passes through the outer tube for a distance "D" into normal bone. Cancellous bone is firmly impacted around the tube. (Mayo © 2000. By permission of Mayo Foundation for Medical Education and Research.)

Figure 32–11. Cement is delivered to the intact bone for a distance "D." When the injector gun is withdrawn to the level of the outer tubes, they are withdrawn together while the cement continues to be injected into the void. The implant is then inserted. (Mayo © 2000. By permission of Mayo Foundation for Medical Education and Research.)

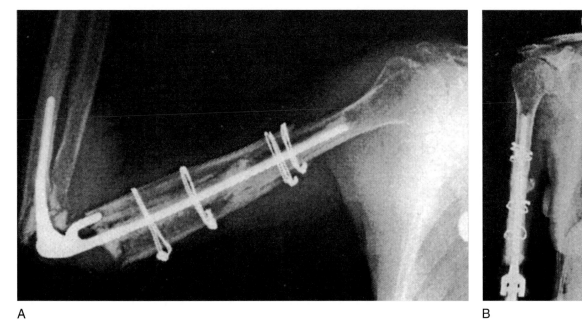

A

B

Figure 32–12. Patient with severe bone loss and fracture after failed Coonrad-Morrey implant (**A**). After 2 years, the impaction graft with struts is still successful both clinically and radiographically (**B**).

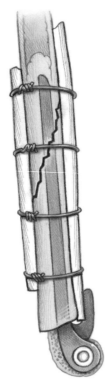

Figure 32–13. Concept of strut grafting for fracture or bone deficiency. The strut graft is applied anteriorly to engage flange; posteriorly, the strut supports the wire fixation.

Allograft Prosthetic Composite Reconstruction

In the past we have employed allograft prosthesis composites on both the humerus and ulna. Overall, the problem with interface union has prompted us to limit the use of this surgical technique. However, it was successful in the majority of patients in whom it was used (Fig. 32–17). In some instances of expanded bone, an allograft composite may be inserted into a shell of bone. We are currently assessing our experience with this surgery. Thus far, experience with 16 cases reveals that humeral and ulnar composites have been employed. We were surprised to learn that as a group these patients did rather well. Only 2 have been revised, leaving 88 percent still functioning a mean of 6 years after surgery.[12]

Custom Implant

The distinguishing feature of a custom implant today is that of extra stem length, which is most helpful for proximal ulnar deficiencies. Length is of greater value than bulk. Some have continued to advocate custom replacements for most instances requiring revision.[7,8,16] This option is less attractive today, and an allograft reconstruction in conjunction with the joint replacement is more often considered. Nonetheless, some excellent long-term results have been reported even with earlier designs.

Currently, the most common use of a custom design is for special-length stems to bypass defects caused by a loose stem and to secure fixation into more normal bone (Fig. 32–18).

The use of custom implants is limited by the extreme cost, delays in manufacture, and the occasional misfit, rendering them unsuitable in many applications. The current implant array has the 20-cm stem length and expanded flange readily available, making the need for custom implants very uncommon (see Fig. 32–4).

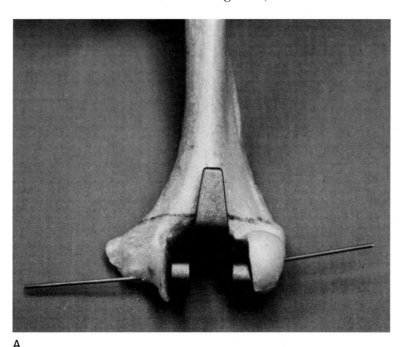

A

Figure 32–14. Normal axis of rotation (**A**). With removal of the condyles, the axis is maintained with a flanged implant, as noted in the anteroposterior (**B**) and lateral (**C**) planes.

Illustration continued on opposite page

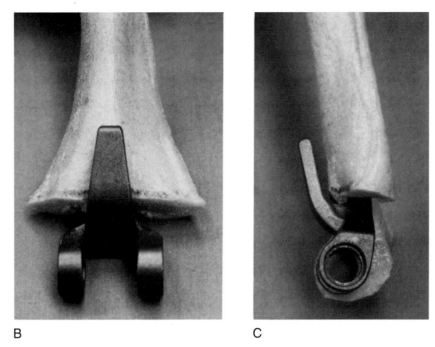

B   C

Figure 32–14. *Continued.*

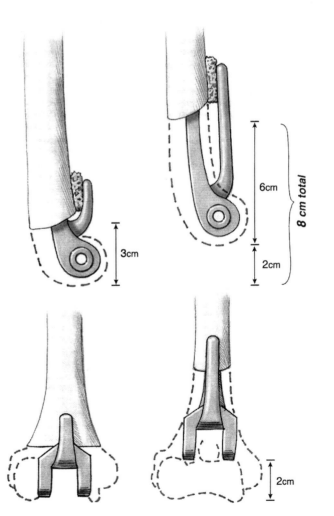

Figure 32–15. The implant is routinely seated such that the distal 3 cm of humeral bone is not required for fixation of the implant (**A**). The extended flange allows an additional 3-cm bone loss, and 2 cm of host bone is still covered by the flange (**B**). If an additional 2 cm of bone is lost, the implant may be inserted further up into the canal for about 2 cm. Hence, 8 cm of deficiency can be treated (**C**).

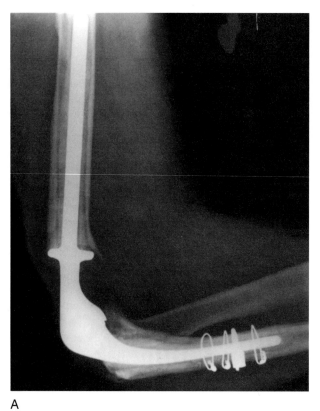

A

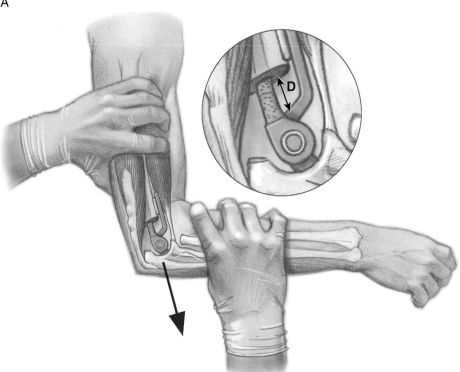

B

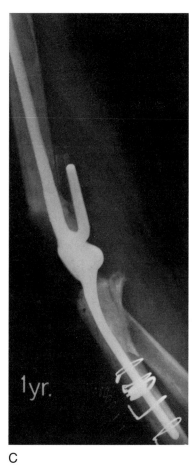

C

Figure 32–16. A loose custom implant and a resected distal humerus (**A**). Proper tensioning of the extended flanged implant can be achieved by observing the flange position as the elbow is flexed 90 degrees while distal pressure places flexors and extensors under tension (**B**). The complex revision is simplified by the properly inserted extended flange device (**C**).

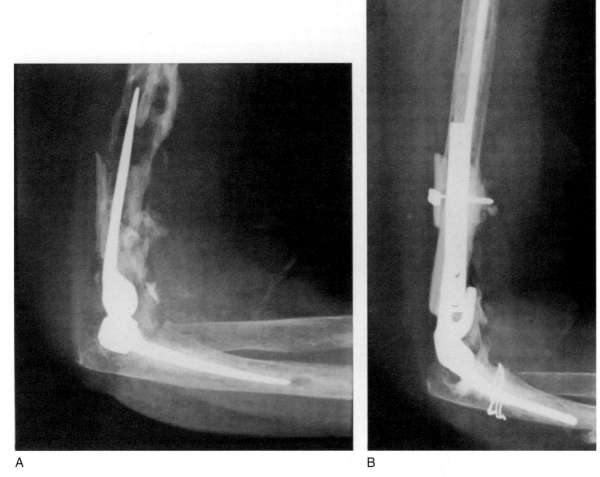

Figure 32–17. A, Massive osteolysis of the distal humerus, completely resorbing the distal third of the bone. **B**, Composite allograft with plate fixation to control rotatory stability until the bone graft heals.

AUTHOR'S PREFERRED TECHNIQUE

Of the various options for the noninfected salvage, the most logical, in my opinion, is some form of reinsertion.

Reimplantation

The semiconstrained implant is used in virtually all instances and all presentations. The procedure may be staged if there is concern about infection or if bone graft is needed. Because a 20-cm humeral stem, an extended flange, and a long ulnar stem are all available as standard options, a custom implant is rarely needed.

Reinsertion into Cement

This procedure is most often performed after a fractured implant, especially in the ulna. This technique is a very effective option with a modest complication rate and is preferred if the cement mantle is intact.

Reinsertion into Bone

This procedure is clearly the treatment of choice if adequate bone is present at the site of the prior implant, or if it can be attained with a larger/longer implant.

Cancellous Augmentation

Using a longer stem to secure fixation into the intact canal, impaction grafting is used if the osteolysis expands the host bone to approximately twice its original diameter.

Strut Grafting

This type of grafting is used to reinforce the expanded osteolytic bone or to bridge periprosthetic fracture. If used for the ulna, proximal extension allows reconstruction of the lever arm of the olecranon to enhance the mechanical advantage of the triceps tendon.

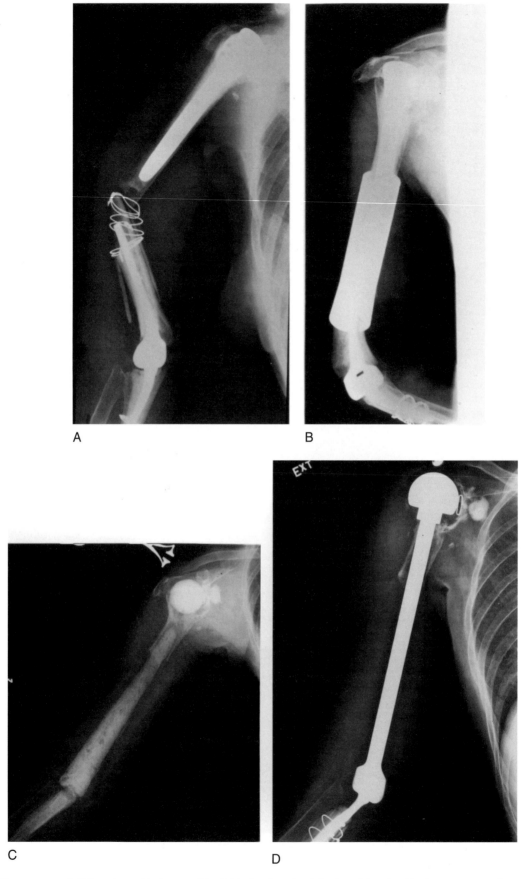

A   B

C   D

Figure 32–18. A, This patient with rheumatoid arthritis developed an infection of the shoulder, humerus, and elbow after four procedures to reconstruct arthritic shoulder and elbow joints. **B,** Most recently, she developed an infection after a custom replacement of the elbow and humerus. Reconstruction consisted of resecting virtually the entire humerus and, after a series of débridements, use of methyl-methacrylate-impregnated cement to maintain length (**C**). A custom humeral replacement with a shoulder and elbow articulation was implanted (**D**). The patient was doing well 1 year after surgery.

References

1. Blaine T, Adams R, Morrey BF: Conversion of interposition arthroplasty to semiconstrained total elbow arthroplasty. San Francisco, CA, AAOS, March 2001.
2. Bryan RS, Morrey BF: Extensive posterior exposure of the elbow: A triceps-sparing approach. Clin Orthop 166:188, 1982.
3. Dean GS, Holliger EH, Urbaniak JR: Elbow allograft for reconstruction of the elbow with massive bone loss. Long term results. Clin Orthop 341:12, 1997.
4. Dent CM, Hoy G, Stanley JK: Revision of failed total elbow arthroplasty. Adv Orthop Surg 20:172, 1996.
5. Dee R: Reconstructive surgery following total elbow endoprosthesis. Clin Orthop 170:196, 1982.
6. Ferlic DC, Clayton ML: Salvage of failed total elbow arthroplasty. J Shoulder Elbow Surg 4:290, 1995.
7. Figgie HE, Inglis AE, Mow C: Total elbow arthroplasty in the face of significant bone stock or soft tissue losses: Preliminary results of custom-fit arthroplasty. J Arthroplasty 1:71, 1986.
8. Figgie HE, Inglis AE, Ranawat CS, Rosenberg GM: Results of total elbow arthroplasty as a salvage procedure for failed elbow reconstructive operations. Clin Orthop 219:185, 1987.
9. Gschwend N: Salvage procedure in failed elbow prosthesis. Arch Orthop Trauma Surg 101:95, 1983.
10. King G, Adams R, Morrey BF: Revision of failed elbow arthroplasty with a semiconstrained device: 5 year results [in press].
11. Lobenberg MI, Morrey BF, O'Driscoll SW: Use of impaction grafting for revision total elbow arthroplasty. San Francisco, American Academy of Orthopaedic Surgeons, March 2001.
12. Mansat P, Morrey BF: Allograft/prosthetic composites as a salvage for failed total elbow arthroplasty. Dallas, American Shoulder and Elbow Surgeons, Feb, 2002.
13. Morrey BF, Adams RA: Semiconstrained joint replacement arthroplasty for distal humeral nonunion. J Bone Joint Surg 77B:67, 1995.
14. Morrey BF, Bryan RS: Revision total elbow arthroplasty. J Bone Joint Surg 69A:523, 1987.
15. O'Driscoll SW, Morrey BF: Periprosthetic fractures about the elbow. Orthop Clinics NA 30:319, 1999.
16. Ross AC, Sneath RS, Scales JT: Endoprosthetic replacement of the humerus and elbow joint. J Bone Joint Surg 69B:652, 1987.
17. Sanchez Sotelo J, Morrey BF, O'Driscoll SW: Use of cortical struts for periprosthetic fractures and revision total elbow arthroplasty. San Francisco, American Academy of Orthopaedic Surgeons, March 2001.
18. Yamaguchi K, Adams RA, Morrey BF: Infection after total elbow arthroplasty. J Bone Joint Surg 80A:481, 1998.

IV

The Shoulder

ROBERT H. COFIELD • SECTION EDITOR

33

Shoulder Arthroplasty: Anatomy and Surgical Approaches

•JOHN W. SPERLING and ROBERT H. COFIELD

Successful shoulder arthroplasty is dependent on a thorough knowledge of the shoulder's detailed anatomy and function. Understanding the anatomic basis of surgical approaches used for shoulder arthroplasty allows the surgeon to address associated shoulder pathology and safely perform extensile measures when necessary. Additionally, research has improved our understanding of the variability of osseous shoulder anatomy. This information has driven the trend toward the development of shoulder arthroplasty components that facilitate more anatomic reconstruction. The purpose of this chapter is to present a focused discussion of shoulder anatomy that is relevant to surgical approaches for shoulder arthroplasty and prosthetic design.

OSTEOLOGY

Clavicle

The clavicle acts as a strut and represents the only direct osseous attachment of the upper extremity to the appendicular skeleton. It contains a double curve, with the medial half bowing anteriorly and the lateral half shaped posteriorly. The medial end is rounded and forms a synovial articulation with the sternum, which is further stabilized by ligamentous attachments to the first rib. Laterally, the clavicle is flattened, and it forms a synovial articulation with the acromion. During shoulder elevation, the clavicle elevates up to 35 degrees and rotates up to 50 degrees.[15] When it is examined in cross-section, the clavicle has an expanded medial end that transitions into a round midportion and gradually widens and becomes progressively flat laterally.[9]

Sternoclavicular Joint

The sternoclavicular joint is formed by the medial end of the clavicle and the posterolateral facet of the manubrium sterni. The chondral portion of the first rib forms the inferior portion of this synovial joint. The overall shape of the articulation is incongruous. Interposed in the joint

is a thick fibrocartilaginous disc that is concave laterally and convex medially. Joint stability results from the articular disc as well as the capsule, the anterior and posterior sternoclavicular ligaments, the costoclavicular ligaments, and the interclavicular ligament (Fig. 33–1). The sternoclavicular joint is an extremely stable articulation with a total cephalad and caudal excursion of up to 60 degrees.[18]

Acromioclavicular Joint

The acromioclavicular joint is formed by the articulation of the flattened lateral end of the clavicle with the medial end of the acromion. Interposed is a meniscoid disc that is surrounded by a relatively lax joint capsule. Stability of the joint results from the superior and inferior acromioclavicular ligaments and the coracoclavicular ligaments. The superior acromioclavicular ligament is stronger than the inferior; however, the prime stabilizers of this articulation are the conoid and trapezoid components of the coracoclavicular ligament (Fig. 33–2). The conoid ligament is medial to the trapezoid and appears to be the major component in joint stability.[7] During scapular rotation, displacement of the acromioclavicular joint can be from 5 to 20 degrees.[15,18]

Scapula

The scapula body is broad and flat and serves as a site for multiple muscle attachments. The coracoid process projects anteriorly and laterally. Medial to the coracoid base is the scapular notch, which is covered by the superior transverse scapular ligament, forming a tunnel for passage of the suprascapular nerve (Fig. 33–3A). On the posterior surface of the scapula is the scapular spine, which projects in a cephalad and lateral direction. The scapular spine divides the posterior surface of the scapula into the supraspinatus fossa above and the infraspinatus fossa below. The scapular spine broadens and diverges from the scapular body, forming the acromion process with its medial articulation to the clavicle. The lateral aspect of

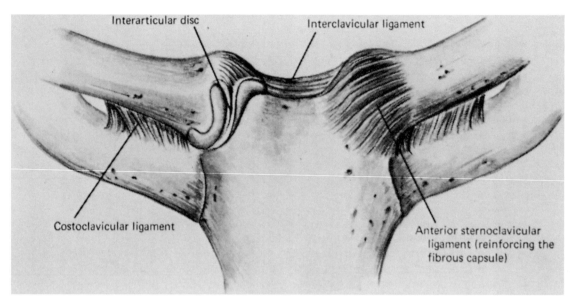

Figure 33–1. Anterior view of the sternoclavicular joint. (From DePalma AF: Surgery of the Shoulder, 3rd ed. Philadelphia, JB Lippincott, 1983.)

the scapula narrows in the form of a triangle with its apex at the glenoid fossa (see Fig. 33–3**B**).

Coracoacromial Arch

The coracoacromial arch is formed by the acromion process, the coracoid process, and the coracoacromial ligament. The acromion is flat and broad as it projects from the scapular spine over the humeral head. The undersurface slants in a posterior and inferior direction. Its anterior margin is level with the anterior surface of the distal clavicle but may extend slightly farther (see Fig. 33–2). The acromion serves as a mobile attachment site for the anterior and lateral deltoid. When the shoulder is abducted, the humeral head passes beneath the

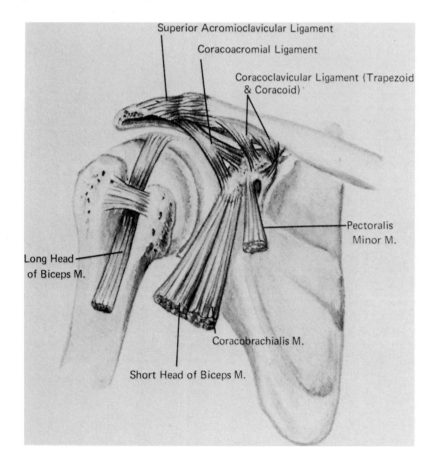

Figure 33–2. Anterior view of the acromioclavicular joint, coracoacromial arch, and proximal humerus. (From DePalma AF: Surgery of the Shoulder, 3rd ed. Philadelphia, JB Lippincott, 1983.)

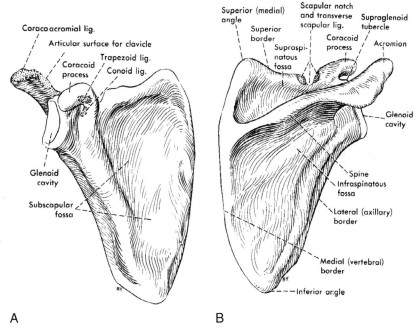

Figure 33–3. A, Anterior view of the scapula. **B,** Posterior view of the scapula.

acromion, and the greater tuberosity must be externally rotated to clear the undersurface of the acromion to achieve full shoulder elevation.

The coracoacromial ligament arises from the lateral edge of the coracoid process and attaches to the undersurface of the acromion. An anatomic and histologic study of the coracoacromial ligament in 50 shoulders performed by Holt and Allibone revealed three primary shapes of the ligament: quadrangular, Y-shaped, and broad banded.[11] The authors note that the quadrangular and Y-shaped ligaments accounted for 90 percent of those observed. This ligament serves as a boundary between the rotator cuff and the overlying deltoid.

Proximal Humerus

The proximal humerus consists of the lesser tuberosity, greater tuberosity, humeral head, and proximal humeral shaft (Fig. 33–4). At the junction of the tuberosities and humeral head is the anatomic neck. The surgical neck is located below the level of the tuberosities. The greater tuberosity serves as the attachment site for the supraspinatus, infraspinatus, and teres minor. The lesser tuberosity is the attachment location for the subscapularis tendon. The bicipital groove, located between the tuberosities, contains the long head of the biceps tendon. Some authors report that the bicipital groove can be a reliable guide in determining the angle of osteotomy during shoulder arthroplasty. Doyle and Burks reported that placing the fin of a humeral head implant 12 mm posterior to the bicipital groove more accurately reproduces normal anatomy than using 30 to 40 degrees of retroversion.[6]

Proximal humerus anatomy varies significantly, depending on the individual.[14,23,24] Investigation has revealed that there are four geometrical variations present in regard to the humeral head: inclination, retro-

version, medial offset, and posterior offset.[2] The inclination, defined as the angle between the shaft and the base of the articular surface, varies between 25 and 55 degrees.[2,4,14,19,24] The reported range of retroversion varies greatly, from 10 degrees of anteversion to more than 50 degrees of retroversion.[2,4,25]

Additionally, the center of rotation of the humeral head is noted to be medial and posterior to the center of the humeral canal.[2,14,19,24,26] In a study by Boileau and Walch of the three dimensional anatomy of 65 humeri, the mean posterior offset was 2.6 mm and the mean

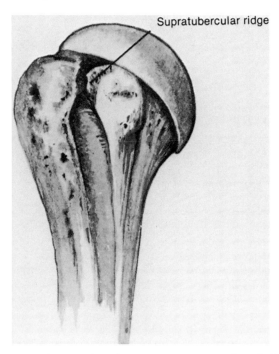

Figure 33–4. Anterior view of the proximal humerus. (From DePalma AF: Surgery of the Shoulder, 3rd ed. Philadelphia, JB Lippincott, 1983.)

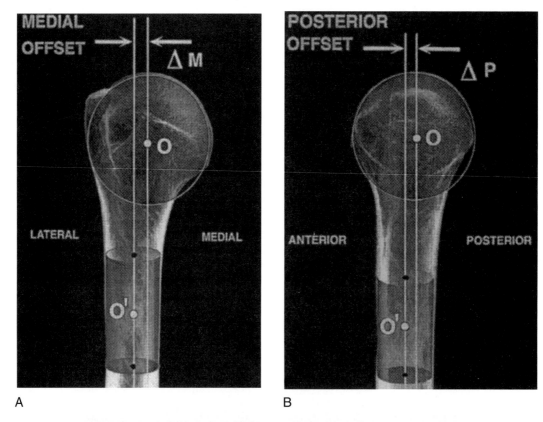

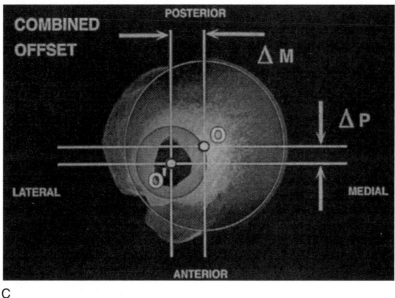

Figure 33–5. The figure demonstrates the translation of the articular head surface in relation to the theoretical stem axis: (**A**) medial offset; (**B**) posterior offset; (**C**) combined offset. (From Boileau P, Walch G: The three-dimensional geometry of the proximal humerus. Implications for surgical technique and prosthetic design. J Bone Joint Surg 79B:857-865, 1997.)

medial offset was 6.9 mm^2 (Fig. 33–5). Roberts reported a mean posterior offset of 4.7 mm in a study of 39 humeri.[26] The radius of curvature of the humeral head has also been shown to vary from approximately 18 to 30 mm.[2,14,19,24]

These anatomic studies have implications in regard to prosthetic design. One theory is that restoration of normal geometry should result in improved motion after

shoulder arthroplasty. Anatomic replacement of the joint, in theory, should give back normal soft tissue tension with a restored center of rotation. Previous work has demonstrated that small changes in glenohumeral anatomy result in altered glenohumeral kinematics.[1,10] Pearl and Kurutz performed a geometric analysis of four commonly used prosthetic systems.[22] Their study demonstrated that none of the prosthetic systems replicated the articular surface. On average, the center of rotation was displaced by 14.7 mm from its original position. Additionally, the prosthesis resulted in a lateral and superior shift of the center of rotation. The authors note that this change in the center of rotation may effect late complications of shoulder arthroplasty including superior humeral migration, glenoid component loosening, and rotator cuff tendinopathy.

This anatomic information has resulted in the evolution of shoulder arthroplasty designs that permit modification to the individual bony anatomy.[2,28] Boileau and Walch have reported on the use of a system that allows modularity in regard to inclination with variably angled neck components. Retroversion is obtained by performance of osteotomy of the articular surface. Lastly, posterior and medial offset is achieved by eccentric indexing. At this time, insufficient long-term data are available to determine whether this new prosthetic design results in improved results.

Glenoid

The glenoid is a shallow fossa that is in the form of an inverted comma (Fig. 33–6). The supraglenoid tubercle defines the upper border of the glenoid. Moving inferiorly, the glenoid fossa becomes progressively broader. The ratio of the lower half to the upper half is approximately 1.0:0.8. The glenoid surface is directed laterally, anteriorly, and superiorly. The mean glenoid retroversion measures 7.5 degrees plus 5 degrees from the plane of the scapula.[4,5] Its radius of curvature may be flat, slightly curved, or socket-like. In the study by Iannotti,

the average dimension of the glenoid in the superior-inferior direction was 39 mm and 29 mm millimeters in the anterior-posterior direction.[14]

Finite element analysis has demonstrated the anatomic variation of the mechanical properties of the glenoid.[17] The authors reported that the mechanical properties were significantly higher at the posterior edge and at the center of the glenoid. This report has implications for the quality of glenoid bone available at the time of shoulder arthroplasty.

SOFT TISSUE SUPPORT AND FUNCTION

The complex synchronous interaction between the static and dynamic stabilizers permits a wide range of shoulder motion with little inherent stability. These structures include the glenoid labrum, capsule, ligaments, rotator cuff, long head of the biceps tendon, bursas, and superficial muscles of the shoulder girdle.

Labrum, Capsule, and Glenohumeral Ligaments

Although the actual size of the glenoid is quite small, the labrum has been shown to deepen the glenoid socket by approximately 50 percent.[13] Composed of dense fibrous tissue, the labrum is triangular in shape and approximately 0.5 cm wide. Lippett has shown that removal of the labrum results in a 20 percent decrease in the glenohumeral joint's stability under shear stress. The joint capsule may be either

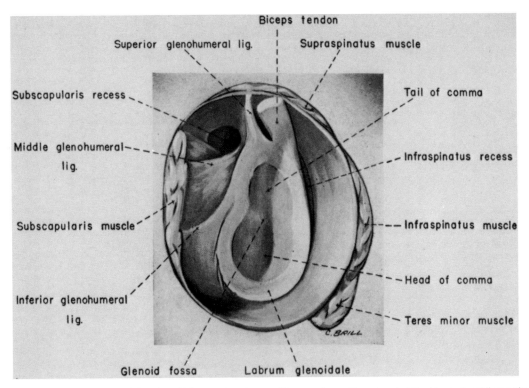

Figure 33–6. Lateral view of the glenoid fossa, glenohumeral ligaments, and long head of the biceps brachii muscle. (From DePalma AF: Surgery of the Shoulder, 3rd ed. Philadelphia, JB Lippincott, 1983.)

circumferentially attached to the labrum or interrupted by smooth synovial recesses, the most common one originating between the superior and middle glenohumeral ligaments.

The glenohumeral ligaments themselves are quite variable. These ligaments represent capsular thickenings in various positions of shoulder elevation and rotation. The superior glenohumeral ligament originates at the upper end of the glenoid fossa and inserts near the lesser tuberosity. It has attachments to the coracoid, the middle glenohumeral ligament, and the long head of the biceps. Most variable in appearance, the middle glenohumeral ligament arises from the labrum anteriorly and attaches to the lesser tuberosity.

The inferior glenohumeral ligament passes from the middle of the anterior labrum to an inferior and medial location on the neck of the humerus. O'Brien and colleagues have described the inferior glenohumeral ligament as composed of an anterior and a posterior band with an intervening axillary pouch.[21] The anterior band becomes progressively wider with abduction and external rotation, preventing anterior displacement of the humeral head. Internal rotation of the shoulder results in widening of the posterior band and prevention of posterior displacement of the humeral head.

The long head of the biceps tendon passes in the intertubercular groove beneath the capsule and attaches to the supraglenoid tubercle (see Fig. 33-6). The transverse humeral ligament covers and stabilizes the tendon in its groove and a firm synovial sheath covers the extra-articular portion of the tendon. The long head of the biceps seems to play a role in humeral head stability.[16,27]

Rotator Cuff

The rotator cuff is composed of the supraspinatus, subscapularis, infraspinatus, and teres minor muscles (Fig. 33-7). The subscapularis muscle arises from the ventral surface of the scapula, whereas the supraspinatus and infraspinatus muscles originate from the supraspinatus and infraspinatus fossae, respectively. The supraspinatus, infraspinatus, and teres minor insert into the greater tuberosity. The subscapularis inserts into the lesser tuberosity. The supraspinatus and infraspinatus muscles are innervated by the suprascapular nerve and the teres minor tendon receives its innervation from a branch of the axillary nerve. The subscapularis muscle receives innervation from the upper and lower subscapular nerves.

The coracohumeral ligament originates on the lateral border of the coracoid process and traverses between the supraspinatus and subscapularis tendons. It blends with the anterior joint capsule and bridges the bicipital groove. This important structure acts as a passive stabilizer to prevent inferior subluxation and resists excessive external rotation.

Bursae

Overlying the rotator cuff is the subacromial bursa. It extends from the greater tuberosity to the undersurface of the acromion and the coracoacromial ligament (Fig. 33-8). It is firmly adherent to the acromion and outer surface of the rotator cuff tendons. This is an extremely important structure in that it allows two adjacent

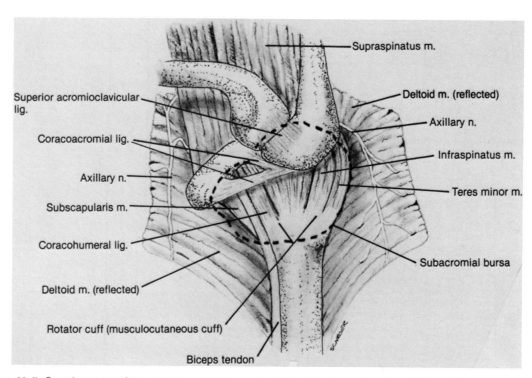

Figure 33-7. Superior aspect of the acromion and rotator cuff with the deltoid muscle reflected. (From DePalma AF: Surgery of the Shoulder, 3rd ed. Philadelphia, JB Lippincott, 1983.)

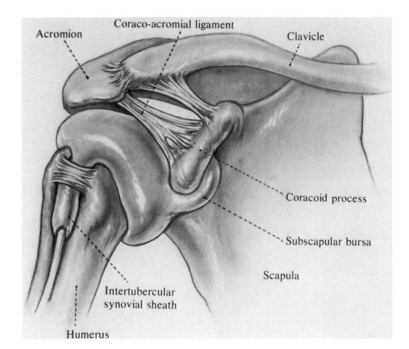

Figure 33–8. Anterior view of the subacromial bursa and surrounding structures. (From Polley HF, Hunder GG: Physical Examination of the Joints. Philadelphia, WB Saunders, 1978.)

muscle groups, the rotator cuff below and deltoid above, to glide past each other with minimal friction and negates the effect of their differing excursions.

The subscapularis bursa lies deep to the subscapularis muscle. It communicates with the joint through the recess between the superior and middle glenohumeral ligaments. This bursa normally does not communicate with the subacromial bursa.

Other bursas include those of the pectoralis major, the latissimus dorsi, and teres major, which are interposed between each of these tendons and the proximal humerus. A subscapular bursa is located between the proximal aspect of the scapula and the upper three ribs.

Muscles

Shoulder motion is dependent on the synchronous rhythm of the proximal humerus and the scapula. In 180 degrees of total shoulder elevation, approximately 120 degrees is derived from the glenohumeral joint and 60 degrees is accomplished through the scapulothoracic articulation, making an overall glenohumeral to scapulothoracic motion ratio of 2:1.[15] The initial 30 degrees of elevation are almost purely glenohumeral motion, and the remaining glenohumeral to scapulothoracic motion ratio is 5:4. During the first 30 to 60 degrees of elevation, the center of rotation of the glenohumeral joint moves upward from its resting position approximately 3 mm but moves very little, if any, thereafter.[20]

The muscle groups that control shoulder motion and their innervations are summarized in Table 33–1. A brief description of regional anterior and posterior glenohumeral anatomy follows.

Anterior. The deltoid, a superficial muscle covering the rotator cuff, has three parts: anterior, middle (lateral), and posterior. It originates from the lateral third of the clavicle, the acromion, and the scapular spine and inserts into the deltoid tuberosity of the humerus. The axillary nerve, which innervates the deltoid, leaves the posterior cord of the brachial plexus and passes through the quadrangular space with the posterior circumflex vessels and pierces the muscle posteriorly. A frequently cited number, the axillary nerve has been reported to traverse the deltoid approximately 4 to 5 cm inferior to the acromion process. However, Burkhead and colleagues have reported that the axillary nerve can be as close as 3.1 cm from the lateral tip of the acromion.[3] Additionally, the nerve was less than 5 centimeters from the acromion edge in 20 percent of the specimens.

Pectoralis Major. Covering the coracobrachialis muscle is the tendon of the pectoralis major. It inserts on the lateral side of the intertubercular groove. Because the long head of the biceps tendon lies directly beneath the insertion site, one must be careful when releasing the pectoralis major so as not to damage the tendon of the long head of the biceps. The teres major and latissimus dorsi tendons attach just medial and inferior to the pectoralis major tendon on the medial side of the intertubercular groove.

Conjoined Tendons. Three conjoined tendons attach to the coracoid process. Most superficial is the short head of the biceps brachii. Beneath it is the coracobrachialis tendon and deepest is the pectoralis minor tendon. The biceps and coracobrachialis are innervated by the musculocutaneous nerve, which arises from the lateral cord of the brachial plexus. In an average arm, the musculocutaneous nerve enters the coracobrachialis

Table 33–1. MUSCLES CONTROLLING SHOULDER MOTION AND THEIR INNERVATIONS

Motion	Primary Muscles	Innervation
Shoulder		
Abduction	Deltoid	Axillary nerve
		Supraspinatus
		Suprascapular nerve
Forward flexion	Deltoid	Axillary nerve
	Pectoralis major	Pectoral nerves
	Coracobrachialis	Musculocutaneous nerve
	Biceps	Musculocutaneous nerve
Adduction	Pectoralis major	Pectoral nerves
	Latissimus dorsi	Thoracodorsal nerve
	Teres major	Lower subscapular nerve
External rotation	Infraspinatus	Suprascapular nerve
	Teres minor	Axillary nerve
Internal rotation	Subscapularis	Subscapular nerve
Scapula		
Elevation	Trapezius (middle)	Accessory nerve
	Levator scapulae	Nerve to levator scapulae
	Rhomboid major and minor	Dorsal scapular nerve
Depression	Latissimus dorsi	Thoracodorsal nerve
	Pectoralis major (lower)	Pectoral nerves
Upward rotation	Trapezius (middle)	Accessory nerve
	Serratus anterior	Long thoracic nerve
Downward rotation	Levator scapulae	Nerve to levator scapulae
	Rhomboid major and minor	Dorsal scapular nerve
Abduction (protraction)	Serratus anterior	Long thoracic nerve
	Pectoralis minor	Pectoral nerves
Adduction (retraction)	Trapezius	Accessory nerve
	Rhomboid major and minor	Dorsal scapular nerve

Adapted from Hollinshead WH: Anatomy for Surgeons: The Back and Limbs, 3rd ed. Philadelphia, Harper & Row, 1982.

and biceps brachii between 4 and 8 cm from the tip of the coracoid process or approximately 7 cm from the tip of the acromion.[12] This relationship can be affected by previous surgery, especially previous transfer of the coracoid process, as in the Bristow anterior shoulder capsule repair. One must be careful when retracting the conjoined group medially during anterior exposure of the glenohumeral joint to avoid musculocutaneous nerve neuropraxia.

Superior. The trapezius drapes over the superior aspect of the shoulder and is innervated by the accessory cranial nerve. It has a tendinous insertion in the posterior clavicle, medial acromion, and superior portion of the scapular spine. Directly beneath it lies the supraspinatus muscle.

Posterior. The posterior third of the deltoid, the most superficial posterior muscle, originates from the scapular spine. Deep to the deltoid lie the infraspinatus and teres minor muscles of the rotator cuff. The long head of the triceps attaches to the inferior neck of the scapula.

NEUROVASCULAR STRUCTURES

In reconstructive shoulder surgery, such as total shoulder arthroplasty, a thorough knowledge of neurovascular anatomy is mandatory because of the proximity of these structures in any exposure of the glenohumeral joint.

Vascular Anatomy

The shoulder region enjoys a rich and intricate blood supply. After the subclavian artery crosses the first rib, it emerges as the axillary artery, which is divided into three parts. After giving off six main branches, the axillary artery becomes the brachial artery in the upper arm. The axillary artery enters the axilla above the pectoralis minor muscle, resting on the serratus anterior with the axillary vein medial to it. It continues distally and laterally, resting on connective tissue covering the subscapularis and teres major muscles. Its six branches, in order, are the supreme thoracic, thoracoacromial, lateral thoracic, subscapular, and the anterior and posterior humeral circumflex arteries.

The thoracoacromial artery promptly divides into the pectoral and deltoid artery. The pectoral branch courses down between the pectoralis major and minor muscles, supplying both, and anastomoses with the lateral thoracic artery (Fig. 33–9). The deltoid branch descends adjacent to the cephalic vein in the deltopectoral interval, giving branches to both of these muscles. It gives off an acromial branch and ends near the deltoid insertion.

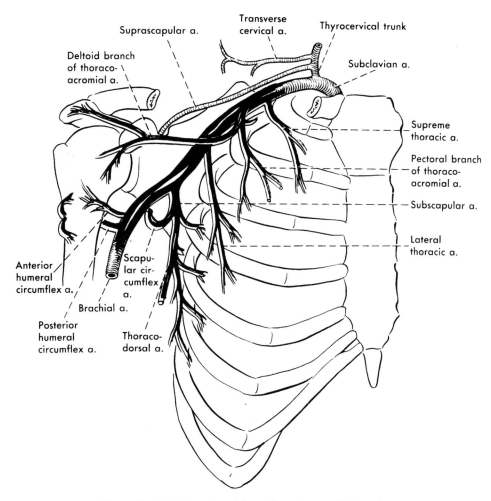

Figure 33–9. Anterior view of the axillary artery and its branches.

The acromial branch, which originates at about the level of the tip of the coracoid process, continues upward and laterally over the acromial process. A small clavicular branch often comes off the deltoid branch with the acromial branch and supplies the acromioclavicular joint. During total shoulder arthroplasty through the deltopectoral interval, the deltoid, acromial, clavicular, and anterior humeral circumflex arteries must be isolated and cauterized to avoid excessive bleeding and to gain adequate exposure.

The anterior and posterior humeral circumflex arteries are usually the last branches of the axillary artery. The anterior circumflex arises just inferior to the subscapularis tendon insertion into the humerus, deep to the coracobrachialis and the long head of the biceps tendon. It encircles the anterior half of the humerus deep to the deltoid and anastomoses with the posterior humeral circumflex artery. The posterior humeral circumflex artery joins the axillary nerve passing through the quadrangular space and encircles the humerus posteriorly before anastomosing with the anterior humeral circumflex artery. A posterior branch also enters the joint, and together with the anterior humeral circumflex, it supplies the overlying deltoid muscle. Gerber and colleagues reported that the humeral head is consistently perfused by the anterolateral ascending branch of the anterior circumflex artery.[8] This vessel runs parallel to the lateral aspect of the long head of the biceps tendon and enters the humeral head at the junction of the intertubercular groove and the greater tuberosity.[8]

Neuroanatomy

During shoulder reconstruction, through an anterior approach, the lateral and posterior cords of the brachial plexus are susceptible to traction neuropraxia (Fig. 33–10). The musculocutaneous nerve becomes the most prominent nerve in the brachial plexus when the arm is abducted, making it especially susceptible to neuropraxia if excessive traction is applied. It enters the coracobrachialis muscle between 4 and 8 cm from the tip of the coracoid process.

Innervation to the major muscle groups of the shoulder girdle is included in Table 33–1. The axillary and suprascapular nerves have special importance in glenohumeral reconstructive surgery. The axillary nerve comes off the posterior cord of the brachial plexus and rests on the anterior surface of the subscapularis muscle. It continues posteriorly around the

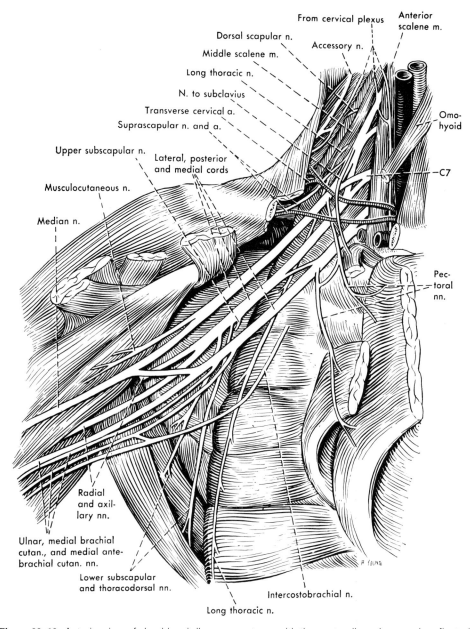

Figure 33–10. Anterior view of shoulder girdle neuroanatomy with the pectoralis major muscle reflected.

inferior border of the subscapularis and joins the posterior humeral circumflex artery and vein passing through the quadrangular space (Fig. 33–11). Anteriorly, this space is defined by the subscapularis superiorly, the surgical neck of the humerus laterally, the long head of the triceps medially, and the upper border of the teres major inferiorly. Posteriorly, the superior border is formed by the teres minor muscle. The axillary nerve gives a branch to the teres minor muscle after passing through the quadrangular space and continues on to innervate the deltoid. On the undersurface of the deltoid, the axillary nerve can be palpated deep to a thick protective fascial covering. One must be careful when placing a retractor under the deltoid so as not to put excessive pressure directly on the nerve.

The suprascapular nerve runs with the suprascapular artery to the superior border of the scapula. The nerve passes beneath the superior transverse scapular ligament, whereas the artery passes above it. They rejoin and continue beneath the supraspinatus muscle, then progress into the infraspinatus fossa and supply both of these muscles. The location of this nerve limits the amount of stripping of the glenoid neck that can be accomplished when these tendons are mobilized.

SURGICAL APPROACHES

In prosthetic arthroplasty of the shoulder, the deltopectoral and anteromedial exposures are the most useful approaches. Proper exposure sets the stage for correct

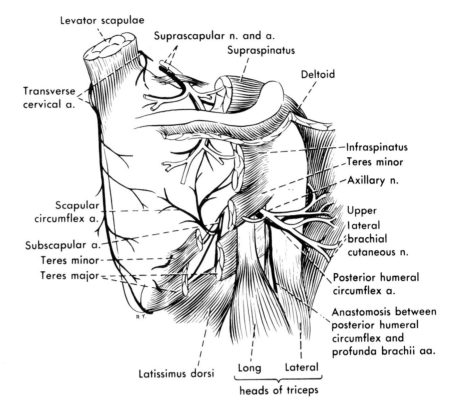

Figure 33–11. Posterior view of shoulder girdle neurovascular anatomy with the deltoid muscle reflected.

prosthetic component placement and soft tissue reconstruction.

Deltopectoral Approach

After general anesthesia is induced, the patient is placed in a beach chair (semi-sitting) position with the affected shoulder and the lateral half of the scapula extending over the edge of the table. A towel is placed beneath the medial half of the scapula. The head is tilted slightly in the opposite direction and is secured with tape that is fastened to the table or a head rest and to a towel on the patient's forehead. A chest strap secures the upper torso. A pole holds the wrist of the affected extremity and a sterile skin preparation is performed from approximately the lateral half of the hemithorax anteriorly and posteriorly, and distally to the wrist. Draping is accomplished so that the entire shoulder girdle is accessible, and the drapes are secured with a large plastic adhesive film. The hand is wrapped in a towel, stocking, and elastic wrap is applied to the lower arm (Fig. 33–12).

With the wrapped hand clamped across the chest, a 12- to 15-cm incision is made beginning 1 cm medial to the acromioclavicular joint and extended distally and laterally (Fig. 33–13). Dissection continues to the level of the deltoid fascia, and the skin is undermined medially so that the deltopectoral interval, which is identified by its overlying areolar tissue, can be reached. The interval is bluntly separated while the deltoid is retracted laterally. The surgeon begins proximally and works distally to identify and cauterize the acromial and deltoid branches of the thoracoacromial arteries. Midway

through the depth of the interval, the cephalic vein is identified and is gently retracted medially (Fig. 33–14). Venous branches from the deltoid to the cephalic vein can then be isolated and cauterized. Often, a large venous plexus exits the midportion of the undersurface of the deltoid to anastomose with the humeral circumflex vessels. This plexus should be identified and cauterized completely before the deltoid muscle is mobilized

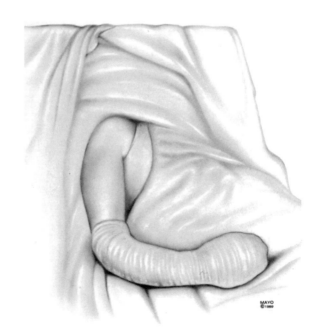

Figure 33–12. Draping for total shoulder arthroplasty.

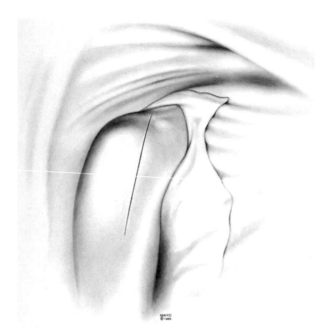

Figure 33–13. Total shoulder arthroplasty skin incision.

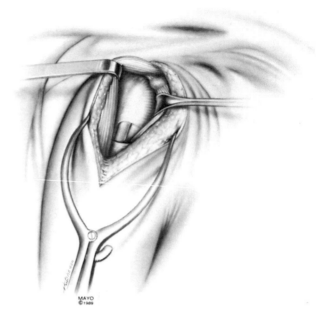

Figure 33–15. Dissection to the level of the clavipectoral fascia.

laterally (Fig. 33–15). The arm is then placed in 30 degrees of abduction on a padded Mayo stand adjusted to the height of the elbow. With a medium-sized Richardson retractor medially beneath the pectoralis major and a large one retracting the deltoid laterally, the clavipectoral fascia just lateral to the conjoined tendons is vertically incised to the level of the inferior border of the coracoacromial ligament. The subdeltoid space is mobilized bluntly, with avoidance of pressure on the nearby brachial plexus. A small, 1-inch-long knee retractor is placed under the conjoined tendons 2 cm distal to the coracoid process, thereby avoiding forceful medial retraction trauma to the musculocutaneous nerve.

The arthrotomy incision is made in the subscapularis tendon, 2 cm medial to the long head of the biceps tendon or 1 cm medial to the lesser tuberosity, with the arm externally rotated (Fig. 33–16). At the superior margin, the incision is directed medially toward the coracoid process to avoid transecting the long head of the biceps tendon. Inferiorly, the anterior humeral circumflex vessels must be ligated. The capsule is incised in line with the subscapularis incision and stay sutures are placed through both. The arm should be placed in an adducted

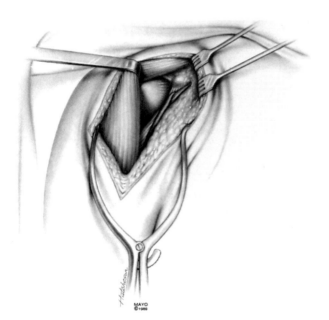

Figure 33–14. The deltopectoral interval is identified with the cephalic vein retracted medially.

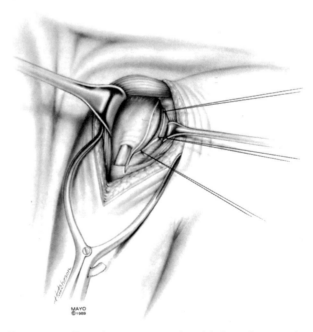

Figure 33–16. Retention sutures are placed during arthrotomy through the subscapularis and anterior capsule.

and externally rotated position during release of the inferior capsule to minimize risk to the axillary nerve. When releasing the inferior capsule, one must be cognizant of the position of the axillary nerve and the proximity to this structure. After adequate release of the subscapularis tendon and the anterior inferior capsule, a Darrach retractor is placed behind the humeral head and in front of the glenoid. The humeral head is dislocated anteriorly with external rotation, extension, adduction, and gentle upward force on the elbow (Fig. 33–17). When a rotator cuff tear exists alone or in conjunction with acute or chronic fractures, the arthrotomy incision incorporates the tendon defect. The long head of the biceps tendon serves as a landmark when the anatomy is grossly distorted and arthrotomy proceeds adjacent to it.

Extensile Measures

In most patients, the technique described in the preceding section is adequate; however, a significant number of patients require additional exposure for proper component placement and soft tissue repair. This is most likely in muscular individuals, in those with post-traumatic deformities with degenerative joint disease, and in those with large rotator cuff tears. Additional exposure can be obtained by one of six methods: (1) release of the superior 1 to 2 cm of the pectoralis major insertion; (2) division of the coracoacromial ligament; (3) partial release of the deltoid insertion into the deltoid tuberosity; (4) partial or complete release of the anterior deltoid from the clavicle and anterior acromion (anteromedial exposure); or (5) extended capsular release. Partial or complete release of the conjoined tendon group may also be performed (6); however, this is not recommended. Many patients with post-traumatic deformities and large repairable rotator cuff tears require some release of the anterior deltoid. Preservation of the coracoacromial ligament is especially useful in patients with rheumatoid arthritis to help provide superior stability in the face of significant rotator

cuff thinning or tearing. When an extended capsular release is performed after humeral head resection, the axillary nerve must first be isolated and protected. The capsular incision is extended inferiorly along the humeral neck and then directed medially toward the glenoid as the incision proceeds posteriorly. Most patients with osteoarthritis have a large inferior osteophyte, which, when resected, creates a voluminous inferior capsule, obviating the need for additional capsular release.

Dangers

The musculocutaneous nerve enters the coracobrachialis muscle 4 to 8 cm distal to the tip of the coracoid process. Medial retraction of the conjoined group must be gentle to prevent neurapraxia.

The axillary nerve is at risk of injury during capsular release. It passes inferior to the subscapularis tendon through the quadrangular space and can be palpated just below and posterior to the subscapularis tendon. A retractor should be used to protect the nerve when additional inferior and posterior capsular release is performed.

Glenoid preparation requires posterior displacement of the humeral head with the arm abducted and externally rotated. This position stretches the brachial plexus, particularly the posterior cord and the musculocutaneous nerve (Fig. 33–18). An effort should be made not to allow excessive retraction force to be applied at any time to prevent neurapraxia of these structures.

Special Reconstructive Problems

The techniques described in the previous section apply to the management of most patients who require hemiarthroplasty or total shoulder arthroplasty. However, additional methods may be required to manage patients with anterior capsular-cuff contracture and acute or chronic proximal humeral fractures.

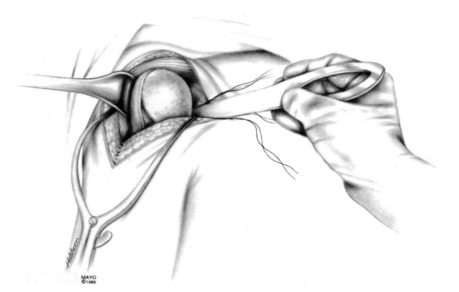

Figure 33–17. The humeral head is dislocated anteriorly.

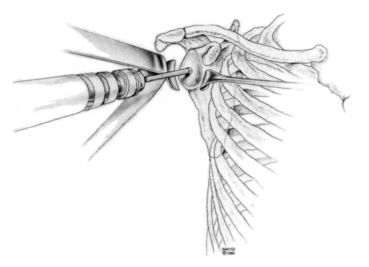

Figure 33–18. Retractors in place during glenoid preparation.

Anterior capsular and rotator cuff scarring can result from previous trauma or may be present in patients with osteoarthritis, osteonecrosis, or rheumatoid arthritis. If contracture is severe, we prefer to incise the subscapularis directly off the lesser tuberosity. At the completion of the procedure, the subscapularis is repaired along the anterior aspect of the humerus at the osteotomy site. Drill holes should be created in the sutures passed before implantation of the prosthesis. For every 1 cm that the subscapularis is advanced, approximately 20 to 30 degrees of external rotation is gained. Another option to increase external rotation is to perform a Z lengthening of the subscapularis (Fig. 33–19). Additional lengthening is achieved by dissecting the anterior capsule from the glenoid neck.

As mentioned, the arthrotomy incision in four-part proximal humeral fractures or chronic malunited fractures requiring tuberosity osteotomy is made superiorly along the long head of the biceps tendon. In chronic fractures with tuberosity malunion, the greater and/or lesser tuberosity is then osteotomized. Because of the bone loss that usually occurs at the level of the surgical neck in patients with acute

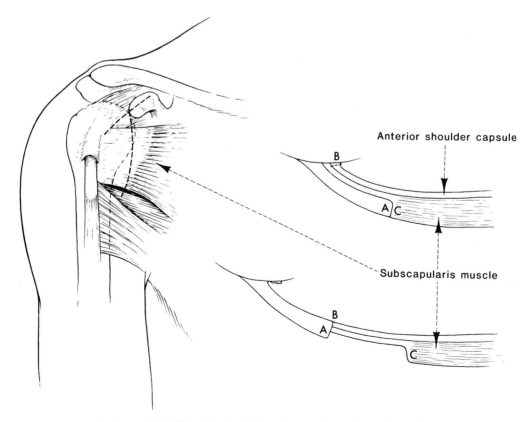

Anterior shoulder capsule

Subscapularis muscle

Figure 33–19. Z-lengthening of the subscapularis may be performed.

fractures, and in many with chronic fractures, care must be taken to restore proper height and retroversion to the humeral component. After the humeral component is cemented at the correct level in an appropriate amount of retroversion, as described earlier, the area between the humeral shaft and the head of the humeral component is bone grafted (Fig. 33–20). The tuberosities are positioned below the level of the prosthetic humeral head with nonabsorbable No. 5 Mersilene sutures through both fin holes, the cuff and tuberosities, and the humeral shaft. Stable tuberosity repair is a critical component of maximizing outcome.

Anteromedial Approach

Occasionally, the deltopectoral approach is not adequate to perform surgery for complex fractures or shoulder arthroplasty. This is particularly true when there has been previous scarring or when work needs to be done not only on the anterior but also on the posterior aspect of the shoulder. Incising the deltoid origin from the clavicle and anterior acromion has evolved to be called the anteromedial surgical exposure. Initially, incisions to accomplish this were curved or angulated, following the course of the deltopectoral groove and the outline of the lateral portion of the clavicle and acromion. The shoulder strap incision was then introduced, and the modern variations of this approach are essentially identical to the incision used for the deltopectoral approach (see Fig. 33–13). However, after the deltopectoral groove is cre-

ated, limited skin flaps are developed superiorly to expose the origin of the deltoid and the insertion of the trapezius. An incision is then made across the top of the clavicle, the anterior third of the acromioclavicular joint, and the anterosuperior margin of the anterior acromion. The origin of the deltoid on the clavicle is J-shaped, extending from near the midline on the superior aspect of the clavicle around the front of the clavicle and, to some degree, on the inferior portion of the anterior aspect of the clavicle. The fibrous attachments of the deltoid to the clavicle are then stripped from the clavicle with all fibrous tissue possible taken with the deltoid muscle to facilitate later repair. A portion of the anterior capsule of the acromioclavicular joint is in a similar fashion incised with the deltoid to allow more firm attachment of the muscle later. Laterally, on the anterior acromion, all fibers again are incised from this bone to strengthen the later repair (Fig. 33–21).

As one can recognize, this method allows one to carefully dissect the interval between the deltoid and the underlying humeral head and rotator cuff. When extensive scar formation is present, this dissection may be quite difficult; it is, however, important to be exacting in the dissection because the branches of the axillary nerve to the deltoid lie on the undersurface of the deltoid muscle, and any transgression into the deltoid muscle will endanger its innervation. This approach also allows one to retract the deltoid laterally and the humeral head anteriorly and to effectively work on the lateral aspect and, to a lesser extent, the posterior aspect of the proximal humerus. It is, of course, possible to release more deltoid from the acromion process, extending the release along the lateral aspect of the acromion, thereby making this a very extensile exposure. However, that degree of exposure is seldom necessary for reconstructive shoulder procedures.

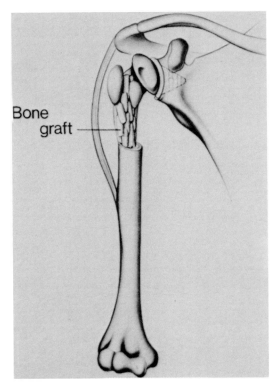

Figure 33–20. Proper humeral height and retroversion are restored. Bone graft is placed to compensate for bone deficiency. (From Neer CS, Watson KL, Stanton FJ: Recent experience in total shoulder replacement. J Bone Joint Surg 64A:319, 1982.)

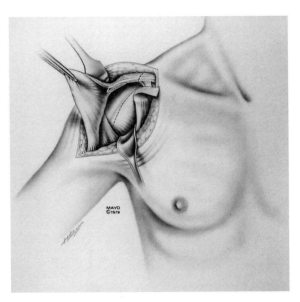

Figure 33–21. The anteromedial approach to shoulder surgery entering through the deltopectoral groove and associated with release of the deltoid origin from the clavicle and anterior acromion (SP-63915-D).   [AU] OK?

SUMMARY

Knowledge of the shoulder girdle osteology, soft tissue envelope, and neurovascular anatomy provides the basis for safe and adequate exposure and allows for soft tissue repair and reconstruction during shoulder arthroplasty. Additionally, a solid understanding of the shoulder anatomy allows one to safely perform extensile exposures when necessary. With proper exposure, soft tissue balancing, and placement of components, shoulder arthroplasty can consistently relieve pain and improve shoulder function.

References

1. Ballmer FT, Sidles JA, Lippitt SB, Matsen FA: Humeral prosthetic arthroplasty: Surgically relevant considerations. J Shoulder Elbow Surg 2:296–306, 1993.
2. Boileau P, Walch G: The three-dimensional geometry of the proximal humerus. Implications for surgical technique and prosthetic design. J Bone Joint Surg Br 79:857–865, 1997.
3. Burkhead WZ, Scheinberg RR: Surgical anatomy of the axillary nerve. J Shoulder Elbow Surg 1:31–36, 1992.
4. Cyprien JM, Vasey HM, Burdet A, et al: Humeral retrotorsion and glenohumeral relationship in the normal shoulder and in recurrent anterior dislocation (scapulometry). Clin Orthop 175:8–17, 1983.
5. Das SP, Saha AK, Roy GS: Observations on the tilt of the glenoid cavity of scapula. J Anat Soc India 15:114, 1966.
6. Doyle AJ, Burks RT: Comparison of humeral head retroversion with the humeral axis/biceps groove relationship: A study in live subjects and cadavers. J Shoulder Elbow Surg 7:453–457, 1998.
7. Fukuda K, Craig EV, An KN, et al: Biomechanical study of the ligamentous system of the acromioclavicular joint. J Bone Joint Surg Am 68:434–440, 1986.
8. Gerber C, Schneeberger AG, Vinh TS: The arterial vascularization of the humeral head. An anatomical study. J Bone Joint Surg Am 72:1486–1494, 1990.
9. Harrington MA Jr, Keller TS, Seiler JGD, et al: Geometric properties and the predicted mechanical behavior of adult human clavicles. J Biomech 26:417–426, 1993.
10. Harryman DT, Sidles JA, Harris SL, et al: The effect of articular conformity and the size of the humeral head component on laxity and motion after glenohumeral arthroplasty. A study in cadavers. J Bone Joint Surg Am 77:555–563, 1995.
11. Holt EM, Allibone RO: Anatomic variants of the coracoacromial ligament. J Shoulder Elbow Surg 4:370–375, 1995.
12. Hoppenfeld S, DeBoer P: Surgical Exposures in Orthopaedics. The Anatomic Approach. Philadelphia, JB Lippincott, 1982.
13. Howell SM, Galinat BJ: The glenoid–labral socket. A constrained articular surface. Clin Orthop 243:122–125, 1989.
14. Iannotti JP, Gabriel JP, Schneck SL, et al: The normal glenohumeral relationships. An anatomical study of one hundred and forty shoulders. J Bone Joint Surg Am 74:491–500, 1992.
15. Inman VT, Saunders JB, Abbot LC: Observations on the function of the shoulder joint. J Bone Joint Surg 26:1, 1944.
16. Kumar VP, Satku K, Balasubramaniam P: The role of the long head of biceps brachii in the stabilization of the head of the humerus. Clin Orthop 244:172–175, 1989.
17. Mansat P, Barea C, Hobatho MC, et al: Anatomic variation of the mechanical properties of the glenoid. J Shoulder Elbow Surg 7:109–115, 1998.
18. Matsen FAI, Thomas SC: Glenohumeral instability. In Evarts CM (ed): Surgery of the Musculoskeletal System, 2nd ed. New York, Churchill Livingstone, 1990, p 1439.
19. McPherson EJ, Friedman RJ, An YH, et al: Anthropometric study of normal glenohumeral relationships. J Shoulder Elbow Surg 6:105–112, 1997.
20. Neer CS, Rockwood CA: Fractures and dislocations of the shoulder. In Rockwood CA, Green DP (eds): Fractures. Philadelphia, JB Lippincott, 1984, p 675.
21. O'Brien SJ, Neves MC, Arnoczky SP, et al: The anatomy and histology of the inferior glenohumeral ligament complex of the shoulder. Am J Sports Med 18:449–456, 1990.
22. Pearl ML, Kurutz S: Geometric analysis of commonly used prosthetic systems for proximal humeral replacement. J Bone Joint Surg Am 81:660–671, 1999.
23. Pearl ML, Volk AG: Retroversion of the proximal humerus in relationship to prosthetic replacement arthroplasty. J Shoulder Elbow Surg 4:286–289, 1995.
24. Pearl ML, Volk AG: Coronal plane geometry of the proximal humerus relevant to prosthetic arthroplasty. J Shoulder Elbow Surg 5:320–326, 1996.
25. Poppen NK, Walker PS: Normal and abnormal motion of the shoulder. J Bone Joint Surg Am 58:195–201, 1976.
26. Roberts SN, Foley AP, Swallow HM, et al: The geometry of the humeral head and the design of prostheses. J Bone Joint Surg Br 73:647–650, 1991.
27. Rodosky MW, Harner CD, Fu FH: The role of the long head of the biceps muscle and superior glenoid labrum in anterior stability of the shoulder. Am J Sports Med 22:121–130, 1994.
28. Walch G, Boileau P: Prosthetic adaptability: A new concept for shoulder arthroplasty. J Shoulder Elbow Surg 8:443–451, 1999.

34

Relevant Biomechanics

•KAI-NAN AN and BERNARD F. MORREY

To make the subject of biomechanics of the gleno-humeral joint both comprehensive and relevant, the material in this chapter is discussed in three parts, according to the concept of joint function that is familiar to clinicians: motion, constraints, and forces across the joint. Although this organization is somewhat arbitrary, it does allow discussion of reconstruction considerations in an orderly and clinically familiar fashion.

MOTION

Articular Surface

The articular surface of the humerus composes just over one third of the surface of the sphere, with an arc of about 150 degrees. The articular surface is oriented with an upward tilt of approximately 45 degrees and retroverted 30 to 40 degrees referable to the condylar line of the distal humerus (Fig. 34–1).[3,4,23]

In the frontal plane, the articular surface of the glenoid composes an arc of approximately 75 degrees that is in the shape of an inverted comma. The long axis dimension averages about 3.5 to 4 cm. In the sagittal plane, the arc of curvature of the glenoid is only about 50 degrees, with a dimension of 2.5 to 3 cm (Fig. 34–2).[23] The slight upward tilt and retroverted orientation of the glenoid normally is not particularly significant in joint replacement because the glenoid is frequently deformed, and surgical reconstruction is limited by the bone and the architecture that are present.

Arm Elevation

The most important function of the shoulder, arm elevation, has been extensively studied to determine the relationship and contribution of the glenohumeral and scapulothoracic joints, the so-called scapulothoracic rhythm.[3,5,6,13,19] The various studies can be simply summarized. Although variation exists during the first 30 degrees of elevation, the overall ratio throughout the entire arc of arm elevation is about 2:1 (glenohumeral contribution, 2; scapulothoracic contribution,

1) (Fig. 34–3). It has been long recognized that maximum arm elevation occurs only with external rotation of the humerus. This obligatory axial rotation is necessary to clear the glenoid tuberosity from the acromial arch and to accommodate movement of the retroverted articular surface into an optimal position for glenoid contact.[2,25] The plane of maximal glenohumeral elevation has been found to be 23 degrees anterior to the plane of the scapula.[2]

A great amount of the motion that is normally present in the shoulder joint is possible only with the implant that replicates the normal curvatures. Hence, the prototype of successful implants, such as that of Neer,[17] has 75 degrees of replaced glenohumeral articulation, which allows essentially normal motion. However, in vivo, the soft tissue dictates the arc of motion commonly shared between the glenohumeral and scaphothoracic joints. Furthermore, if the supporting soft tissue structures are inadequate, the implant is potentially unstable, because the normal glenohumeral articulation is inherently unstable. In this setting, a more constrained implant may be considered. Greater constraint is brought about by increasing the contact of the glenoid on the humerus, thereby increasing the arc of curvature of the glenoid component. However, a more stable implant requires a greater capture of the humeral head and thus results in a decreased arc of motion and a mechanical impingement at the extremes of motion. This type of design inherently decreases the range of motion and naturally increases the potential for glenoid component loosening.

Joint Contact and Center of Rotation

The center of rotation of the glenohumeral joint has been defined as a locus of points situated within 6 mm of the geometric center of the humeral anatomic head.[19] The relatively small dimension of this locus and its position in the geometric center of the humeral head suggest that only a small amount of translation normally occurs at this joint. Under normal circumstances, shoulder motion is defined as sliding—which is the translation of the humeral head on the glenoid—and rolling—which is the motion of one fixed segment of the humeral head on a corresponding surface of the glenoid (Fig. 34–4).

423

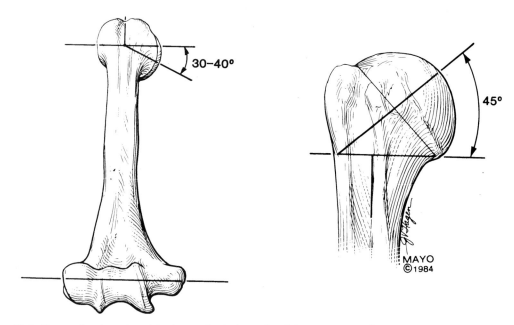

Figure 34–1. Geometric orientation of the humeral articular surface is important to replicate to provide prosthetic stability.

Finally, spinning motion is that in which one segment moves about an axis of rotation with a constant contact point on the opposite surface. For shoulder motion, all three elements are thought to exist. The normal contact locus of the humeral head on the face of the glenoid has been mapped by Nobuhara,[18] as shown in Figure 34–5.

CONSTRAINTS

It is convenient to assume that any constraint consists in part of static and dynamic elements. The static factors include articular, capsular ligamentous, and negative pressure elements. Dynamic stability is brought about by muscle activity, which, for the shoulder, consists

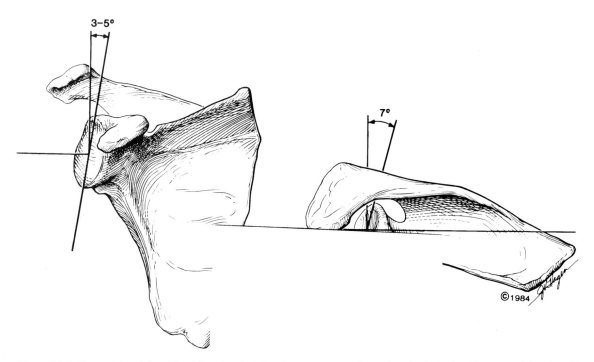

Figure 34–2. Geometric relationship of the glenoid is less important to replicate, but the limited architecture of the glenoid should be recognized.

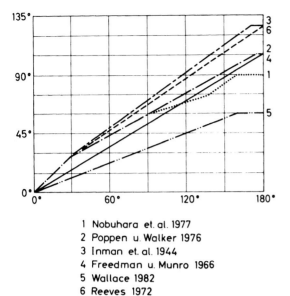

1 Nobuhara et. al. 1977
2 Poppen u. Walker 1976
3 Inman et. al. 1944
4 Freedman u. Munro 1966
5 Wallace 1982
6 Reeves 1972

Figure 34–3. In general, there is a 2:1 ratio of glenohumeral-to-scapulothoracic motion in the normal shoulder during arm elevation. (From Bergmann G: Biomechanics and pathomechanics of the shoulder joint with reference to prosthetic joint replacement. *In* Kölbel R, Helbig B, Blauth W [eds]: Shoulder Replacement. Berlin, Springer-Verlag, 1987, p 33.)

primarily of the rotator cuff components. For a total shoulder replacement, stability is predicated on the accuracy of the articular design as well as on the presence and function of the rotator cuff musculature.[21] For

most reconstructive procedures, restoration of dynamic stabilizers is essential for proper joint function.

Static Constraints

In the normal shoulder, the articular contribution to stability is minimal, because the glenoid component is essentially flat.[22] However, slight glenoid concavity and dynamic compression still provide significant joint stability in the midrange of glenohumeral motion, where the capsule and ligaments are lax.[15] In laboratory tests, relative translations between the glenoid and the humeral head and the forces resisting translation were recorded and the stability ratio, defined as the peak translation force divided by the applied compressive force, was calculated.[14] The average stability ratio was higher in the hanging arm position than in glenohumeral abduction (Fig. 34–6). With an intact labrum, the highest stability ratio was detected in the inferior direction. In the absence of a labrum, the greatest stability was in the superior direction. In both conditions, the anterior direction showed the lowest stability ratio. Resection of the glenoid labrum resulted in an average decrease of 10 percent in the stability ratio. In joint replacement surgery, substitution of a more constrained articular surface to accommodate muscle and capsular deficiencies has not been proved successful.

The shoulder capsule itself is thin and redundant. In some, this redundancy may be a congenital variation of a normal[24] capsule, or it may be secondary to rheumatoid

Figure 34–4. All three types of motion (sliding, rolling, spinning) occur at the glenohumeral articulation.

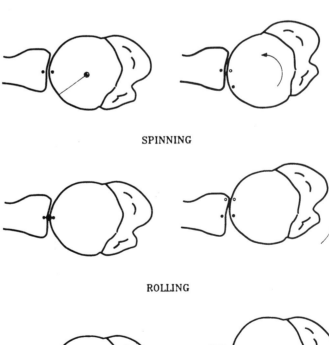

SPINNING

ROLLING

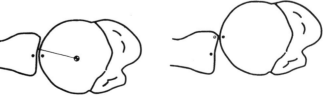

SLIDING

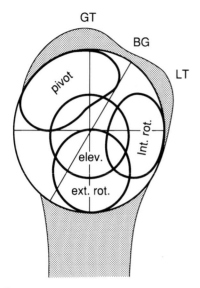

Figure 34–5. Contact area of the humerus on the glenoid is depicted for various positions and motions. (From Nobuhara K: The Shoulder: Its Function and Clinical Aspects. Tokyo, Igaku-Shoin, 1987.)

or other inflammatory or pathologic processes. Conversely, if the pathologic process has caused joint capsule contracture, this must be addressed with most reconstructive procedures, and it is critical to correct the contracture with prosthetic replacement.

Understanding the concept of load sharing of the constraining elements of the joint is probably nowhere more important than in the shoulder. A basic premise is that the capsule may function in a coordinated manner to resist joint translation. Primarily, displacement generates resistance by its very presence, but, secondarily,

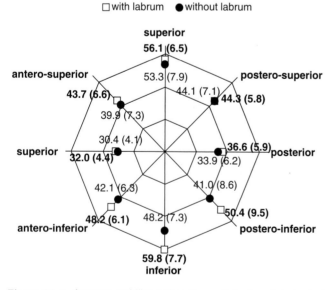

Figure 34–6. Average stability ratios (percent) in the eight tested directions with and without labrum. Values represent mean and standard deviation. (From Halder AM, Kuhl SG, Zobitz ME, et al: Effects of glenoid labrum and glenohumeral abduction on shoulder joint stability through concavity compression: An in vitro study. J Bone Joint Surg 83A:1062, 2001.)

resistance occurs because of increased joint contact pressure in the direction opposite to the displacement. This resistance also increases joint stability. In fact, the relationship between increased joint contact pressure and resistance to translation has been studied and is described later (Fig. 34–7).

The influence of atmospheric or intra-articular pressure on stability of the shoulder has been assessed by experimental and analytic investigations.[12] The shoulder was seen to undergo subluxation inferiorly by as much as 2 cm after capsular puncture, with marked alteration in joint constraint while passive motion exercises were performed. Intra-articular pressure up to -82 cm H_2O was observed with the arm loaded.

Dynamic Stability

Of the 26 muscles that cross the shoulder joint, only the four components of the rotator cuff are thought to play any significant role in the dynamic stability of the shoulder joint itself. The clinical implications and the paramount importance of the rotator cuff in maintaining proper function of the shoulder have been recognized by all.

It has been demonstrated that the humeral head is positioned in the center of the glenoid in the horizontal plane by a mechanism that is independent of the specific muscles stimulated.[9] Thus, even without equal muscle contracture from the anterior or posterior cuff components (i.e., a dynamic imbalance), the activity of the remaining cuff still centers the humerus on the glenoid surface. The role of the rotator cuff in stabilizing the shoulder joint has been well recognized. To represent more realistically the biomechanical role of the force vectors providing dynamic glenohumeral stability, Lee et al.[14] defined a new biomechanical parameter, the dynamic stability index (DSI). The DSI of a muscle in a specific glenohumeral position included both the effects resulting from the shear force generated by the muscle itself and by the concavity-compression mechanism of the compressive force. The DSI in the anterior direction of the four muscles of the rotator cuff and the three heads of the deltoid for the glenohumeral joint varied with the position of the joint (Fig. 34–8).

The central role of the deltoid muscle in elevating the arm is also known to be countered by the depressive action of the anterior and posterior rotator cuff musculature. Thus, the short rotators stabilize the joint by increasing the compressive force between the glenohumeral articular surfaces. An intact rotator cuff plays an additional, secondary role in glenohumeral stability. As excursion increases because of the activity of the cuff musculature, a secondary tightening of the static constraints occurs to the extent that the capsule is surgically or spontaneously reconstituted. This produces an additional element of static constraint that is not present if active motion has not occurred.

The subscapularis has been shown to be important, if not essential, as an anterior barrier to resist anteroinferior humeral head displacement with abduction and external rotation. Because the cross-sectional areas of the

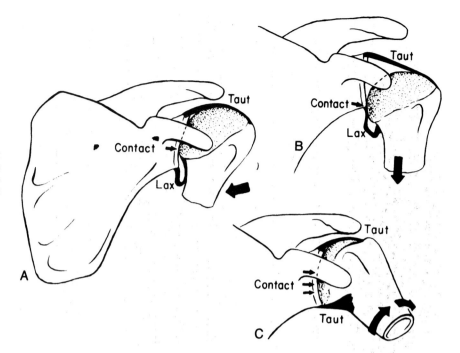

Figure 34–7. Dempster's theory[4] is that joint stability is provided by increased contact forces resulting from tautness of the soft tissue constraints as well as the barrier effect of the soft tissue constraints themselves.

rotator cuff musculature anteriorly and posteriorly are essentially equal, the torque generated by these groups is balanced with respect to a force coupling that resists both anterior and posterior humeral head translation. The role of the biceps tendon in glenohumeral joint constraint has also been studied.[11] Contractions of both the long and short heads of the biceps provide compressive forces on the joint surface and also exert a sling effect on the movement of the humeral head. This is especially true in patients with deficient rotator cuff function.

Surgical Considerations

An intact or restored rotator cuff function is the obvious and long recognized prerequisite that ensures shoulder

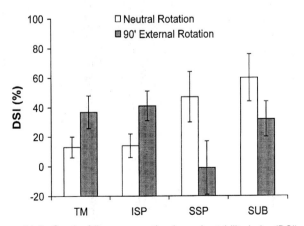

Figure 34–8. Graph of the mean on the dynamic stability index (DSI) of the four rotator cuff muscles and the three heads of the deltoid muscle in the anterior direction. The DSI is a percent ratio of the magnitude of maximum anterior dislocating shear force that can be stabilized by the rotator cuff muscle to the magnitude of rotator cuff muscle force. The I-bars indicate the standard deviation.

stability and motion. Technically, the scarred cuff muscle and capsule should be released to allow equal tension anterior and posterior to the joint. Restoration of a torn or deficient cuff is desirable for proper shoulder stability as well as rehabilitation and return of functional motion. Hemorrhage or effusion associated with surgical treatment of a fracture or reconstructive joint replacement may nullify the negative intra-articular pressure in the dependent shoulder and allow the humeral head to translate inferiorly. In this position of subluxation, or dislocated position, the humeral head should be spontaneously reduced, with resorption of the intra-articular fluid.

Increasing the conformity of the glenoid and humeral articular surfaces as an additional means of enhancing stability is well recognized. This design feature has several consequences. The amount of motion that is present in the prosthetic system is directly influenced by its inherent articular stability. The more constrained the glenohumeral articulation, the less motion. Furthermore, at extremes of elevation, the humeral components abut against the more pronounced constrained glenoid margin, causing compression at the superior margin and tension at the inferior bone-cement interface. The force transmission associated with varieties of glenohumeral design is discussed later.

FORCE TRANSMISSION

Normal force transmission across the shoulder joint has been studied by several investigators.[1,10,16,25] With simple arm elevation, a force of approximately one times the body weight is generated across the glenohumeral joint, occurring at about 90 degrees of abduction. When as small a weight as 50 N is lifted, the generated force is approximately 2.5 times that of the body weight.[1] Of equal or greater importance is the changing direction of

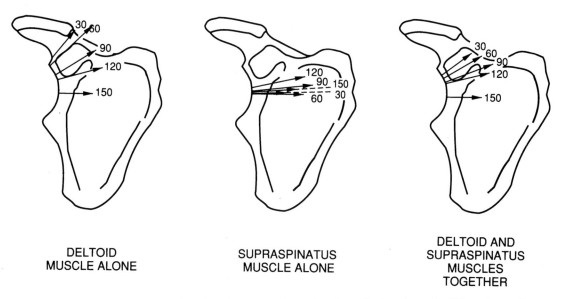

Figure 34–9. Direction and magnitude of resultant joint forces depend on the activation of muscles. When the resultant vector is at the superior margin, the tendency is for an unstable joint and a disadvantageous means of force transmission.

the resultant vector during different degrees of arm elevation. The direction and magnitude of this resultant vector have been studied by Poppen and Walker,[20] who related the orientation of this resultant vector to the glenoid surface. With arm elevation up to 60 degrees, the direction of the resultant vector remains extrinsic to the glenoid surface, and this position is at the superior margin of the glenoid rim (Fig. 34–9). If the resultant vector is not directed through the glenoid surface, the joint is considered to be in an unstable mode. Resolution of the component forces demonstrates that a significant superior shear force or subluxation force therefore exists up to about 60 degrees of arm elevation. If the glenohumeral angle is greater than 60 degrees, the resultant vector is directed within the confines of the glenoid surface. This is an inherently stable configuration.

If the supraspinatus is not functioning, the deltoid is responsible for shoulder elevation. The initiation of abduction in this instance is associated with a poor mechanical advantage; thus, a large initial resultant vector is directed superiorly, away from the articular confines of the glenoid. This is a poor mechanical arrangement because the muscle force tends toward subluxation of the shoulder superiorly. With the arm elevated beyond 60 degrees, this muscle becomes more efficient, resulting in less joint force. However, the direction of the resultant force is not ideally situated toward the center of the glenoid surface. Coordination of these two muscles seems to provide the best condition for joint resultant force and thus stability (see Fig. 34–9).

Surgical Considerations

The biomechanical data clearly explain the essential role of the rotator cuff in shoulder replacement. It is certain that a functioning cuff provides essential stability as well as arm elevation with forces of lower magnitude

and more advantageous distribution. In individuals who are unable to abduct the glenohumeral joint more than 60 degrees, an unfavorable loading pattern at the superior aspect of the glenoid occurs, and this is associated with potential increased wear and loosening of prosthetic implants. The major implication of these data, therefore, relates to the design of the glenoid and its fixation.

Various glenoid design configurations have been studied with regard to their biomechanical implication. Walker[26] has provided a theoretical analysis of the effect of changing glenoid thickness associated with the force moments acting on the fixation of the device. For every increase of 1 mm in component thickness, an approximate 5-percent increase of 5 percent in loosening moment was calculated. In contrast, if the radius of curvature was decreased, the moment was decreased proportionally. Considering that the resultant vector was at the superior margin at 60 degrees of abduction, the effect of muscle force on the glenoid was lessened by a thinner glenoid component with a small arc of curvature.

Fixation

The inter-relationship of glenoid design and fixation has also been investigated in the laboratory. Fukuda et al.[7] have shown that the stability of the joint is directly related to the magnitude of axial compression applied. This relationship was, as expected, greater in the more constrained designs (Fig. 34–10). However, as greater stability was designed into the implant interface, a greater incidence of failure was anticipated because of the associated increase of stresses on the high-density polyethylene. It was observed that high forces (greater than 200 N) cause plastic deformation as the humeral head dislocates over the rim. However, lower stresses, such as 90 N, cause no such deformation. Furthermore, a combination of shear and compressive forces tends to

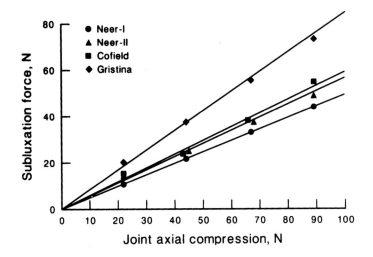

Figure 34–10. Anteroposterior subluxation forces of the humeral component of different glenoid designs using different joint compressive loads.

cause a shearing force that may dissociate the high-density polyethylene from its metal back support. It is also reasonable to extrapolate these findings to determine the effect on the bone-cement interface.

Finally, the concept of fixation as a function of glenoid design has been a cause of major concern with regard to the shoulder joint. Glenoid loosening remains a major concern for the long-term prognosis of the joint. When a standardized technique was used, the pullout force of four currently available implants was studied with or without pretest fatigue loading. Fatigue loading did not alter the results of the experiment, which demonstrated that component fixation strength was greatest in a three-pronged implant followed by the asymmetric keel; finally, the symmetric keeled implant demonstrated the least resistance to axial displacement. This is not a physiologic means of loading this implant; so these data can be interpreted only as experimental.

References

1. Bergmann G: Biomechanics and pathomechanics of the shoulder joint with reference to prosthetic joint replacement. *In* Kölbel R, Helbig B, Blauth W (eds): Shoulder Replacement. Berlin, Springer-Verlag, 1987, p 33.
2. Browne AO, Morrey BF, Hoffmeymer P, et al: Elevation of the arm in the plane of the scapula. J Bone Joint Surg 72B:843, 1990.
3. Codman EA: The Shoulder. Malabar, FL, Krieger, 1934.
4. Dempster WT: Mechanisms of shoulder movement. Arch Phys Med Rehabil 46A:49, 1965.
5. Doddy SG, Waterland JC, Freedman L: Scapulohumeral goniometer. Arch Phys Med Rehabil 51:711, 1970.
6. Freedman L, Munro RH: Abduction of the arm in scapular plane: Scapular and glenohumeral movements. J Bone Joint Surg 18A:1503, 1966.
7. Fukuda K, Chen CM, Cofield RH, Chao EY: Biomechanical analysis of stability and fixation strength of total shoulder prostheses. Orthopedics 11:141, 1988.
8. Halder, AM, Kuhl, SG, Zobitz ME, et al: Effects of glenoid labrum and glenohumeral abduction on shoulder joint stability through concavity compression: an in vitro study. J Bone Joint Surg 83A:1062, 2001.
9. Howell SM, Galinat BJ, Renzi AJ, Marone PJ: Normal and abnormal mechanics of the glenohumeral joint in the horizontal plane. J Bone Joint Surg 70A:227,1988.
10. Inman VT, Saunders M, Abbot LC: Observations on the function of the shoulder joint. J Bone Joint Surg 26:1, 1944.
11. Itoi E, Kuechle DK, Newman SR, et al: Stabilizing function of the biceps in stable and unstable shoulders. J Bone Joint Surg 75B:546, 1993.
12. Itoi E, Motzkin NE, Brown AD, et al: Intraarticular pressure of the shoulder. Arthroscopy 9:406, 1993.
13. Laumann U: Kinesiology of the shoulder joint. *In* Kölbel R, Helbig B, Blauth W (eds): Shoulder Replacement. Berlin, Springer-Verlag, 1987.
14. Lee SB, Kim KJ, O'Driscoll SW, et al: Dynamic glenohumeral stability provided by the rotator cuff muscles in the mid-range and end-range of motion. A study in cadaver. J Bone Joint Surg 82A:849, 2000.
15. Lippitt SB, Vanderhooft JE, Harris SL, et al: Glenohumeral stability from concavity-compression: A quantitative analysis. J Shoulder Elbow Surg 2:27, 1993.
16. Morrey BF, An KN: Biomechanics of the shoulder. *In* Rockwood C, Matsen R (eds): Shoulder. Philadelphia, WB Saunders, 1990.
17. Neers CS II: Articular replacement of the humeral head. J Bone Joint Surg 37A:215, 1955.
18. Nobuhara K: The Shoulder: Its Function and Clinical Aspects. Tokyo, Igaku-Shoin, 1987.
19. Poppen NK, Walker PS: Normal and abnormal motion of the shoulder. J Bone Joint Surg 58A:195, 1976.
20. Poppen NK, Walker PS: Forces at the glenohumeral joint in abduction. Clin Orthop 58:165, 1978.
21. Reeves B, Jobbins B, Flowers M: Biomechanical problems in the development of a total shoulder endoprosthesis. J Bone Joint Surg 54B:193, 1972.
22. Saha AK: Dynamic stability of the glenohumeral joint. Acta Orthop Scand 42:491, 1971.
23. Steindler A: Kinesiology of the Human Body Under Normal and Pathological Conditions. Springfield, IL, Charles C Thomas, 1955.
24. Uhthoff H, Piscopo M: Anterior capsular redundancy of the shoulder: Congenital or traumatic? J Bone Joint Surg 67B:363, 1985
25. Walker PS: Human Joints and Their Artificial Replacements. Springfield, IL, Charles C Thomas, 1977.
26. Walker PS: Some bioengineering considerations of prosthetic replacement for the glenohumeral joint. *In* Inglis AE (ed): Symposium on Total Joint Replacement of the Upper Extremity. St. Louis, CV Mosby, 1982, p 25.

35

Arthroplasty for Acute Fractures of the Proximal Humerus

• MICHAEL E. TORCHIA, FRANCISCO LOPEZ-GONZALEZ, and GUIDO HEERS

In 1970, Neer published classic articles on fractures of the proximal humerus. In part II of the series, the results of treatment of four-part displacements were reported. With this severe pattern of injury, both nonoperative treatment and open reductions led to dismal results in every case. Only humeral head replacement (HHR) produced a satisfactory outcome consistently.[25] Although others have published their experience,[1,5,9,15,19,21,32,35,37] Neer's work has remained influential and has directed treatment for the past 30 years.

During the past two decades, most patients with four-part fractures requiring HHR have been treated with implants designed to treat those with glenohumeral arthritis. The results have been variable. More recently, implants specifically designed to treat patients with fractures have been developed with the hope of improving clinical results.

PATIENT EVALUATION

Although the definitive diagnosis is made based on radiographs, the history and examination remain important. The history often reveals a low-energy mechanism of injury (fall) in an elderly patient. Many patients who are treated with HHR for acute fractures have cognitive deficits and few remaining social supports. These factors may inhibit their ability to protect the tuberosity repair postoperatively.

The initial physical examination typically focuses on the general health of the patient, the condition of the skin, and the neurovascular integrity of the extremity. Even with low-energy fractures, nerve and vessel injuries do occur. These findings are best recognized preoperatively and treated appropriately.

The radiographic evaluation is critical. In managing fractures of the proximal humerus, good treatment decisions depend on good-quality radiographs. An anteroposterior view in the plane of the scapula and an axillary view are the two most important images. In the setting of an acute fracture, high-quality films can be difficult to obtain. It is often helpful for the surgeon to assist with patient positioning, arm support (for the axillary view), and confirmation of the appropriate trajectory of the x-ray beam. In most cases, good quality radiographs allow the fracture patterns to be understood and classified. If radiographs do not provide this information, computed tomography scanning can be performed.

It is important to be aware of the so-called valgus impacted four-part pattern.[16] Although all four segments are fractured, the displacement is not typical enough to qualify as a true four-part pattern according to Neer's criteria. The lack of severe displacement lessens the chance of post-traumatic avascular necrosis and allows the fracture to be treated with reduction and fixation rather than replacement of the humeral head.

INDICATIONS FOR HUMERAL HEAD REPLACEMENT IN ACUTE FRACTURES

The indications for HHR in the setting of acute trauma have become more refined. In general, the use of HHR is reserved for the elderly with poor bone quality and fracture patterns that preclude salvage of the humeral head or stable internal fixation. These would include head splitting fractures (Fig. 35–1), Neer four-part fractures, selected Neer three-part fractures and fracture dislocations in patients with poor bone quality and a very small head fragment, selected severe impression fractures in elderly patients involving more than 40 percent of the articular surface, and selected anatomic neck fractures in which internal fixation is not possible. Generally in patients younger than 60 years of age, an attempt is often made to salvage the proximal humerus rather than replace it.

This trend away from HHR and toward internal fixation reflects the advent of improved implants for internal fixation (Fig. 35–2), a new understanding of the clinical

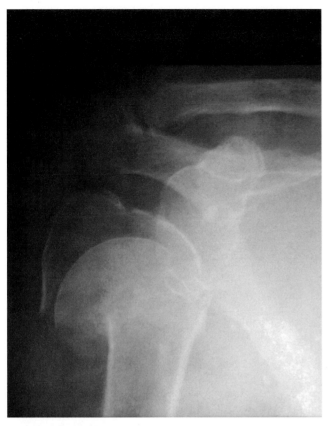

Figure 35–1. An example of a head-splitting fracture. Note that the majority of the humeral head is pointing away from the glenoid.

significance of post-traumatic avascular necrosis,[14] and the relatively high rate of complications reported with HHR for trauma.[2,22] Of interest, a group from Paris has developed a new implant, the Bilboquet device, which may further limit the indications of HHR for patients with acute fractures, even in the setting of poor bone quality.[10]

SURGICAL TECHNIQUE

If humeral head replacement is undertaken, the objective should be anatomic reconstruction of the proximal humerus. The importance of prosthetic head size, implant position, and tuberosity position have been emphasized by several authors.[3,8,12,27,34] These studies suggest that HHR has little chance of restoring satisfactory function of the shoulder unless the height of the humeral head, degree of retroversion, head size, and tuberosity position are anatomic or near anatomic within a few millimeters or degrees. Achieving this goal consistently requires good planning and, suitable instruments, and skillful surgical technique.

Preoperative Planning

This step is essential. A high-quality radiograph of the opposite shoulder is useful. The single best view is an anteroposterior image in the scapular plane with the arm held in external rotation. Because the goal of surgery is to recreate normal anatomy, making a template of the opposite, uninjured, proximal humerus helps determine appropriate stem size, head size, head offset, and position of tuberosity (Fig. 35–3). Preoperative construction of a template complements intraoperative guidelines such as checking "soft tissue tension." A full-length view of the humerus with radiographic markers also can be used to assist in determining true arm length.

Patient Positioning

The beach chair position is recommended. Several details are worthy of emphasis. The legs and feet are elevated, hip flexion is limited to 90 degrees or less, and the table is placed in the slight Trendelenburg position. This approach minimizes lower extremity venous stasis and reduces the tendency for larger patients to slide down the table during the procedure. The cervical spine is positioned neutrally to minimize the risk of stretch injury to the cervical cord and brachial plexus. Lateral positioning of the shoulder allows surgical access to the humeral canal and improved fluoroscopic imaging.

Skin Preparation

Particular attention should be directed to the cleansing of the skin. Many fractures are operated several days after injury, and most patients find maintenance of axillary hygiene impossible during this time interval. Subsequently, microbial growth in this region can become substantial and may contribute to a postoperative deep infection.[22] For this reason, after anesthesia is induced, pre-scrubbing of the axilla with alcohol is recommended the standard surgical preparation is done.

Exposure

A modification of the deltopectoral approach is used. The entire deltopectoral interval from the clavicle to the humerus is developed. Specifically, all veins draining the deltoid (between the medial border of the muscle and the cephalic vein) are cauterized or ligated. Leaving the cephalic vein with the pectoralis major muscle intact allows better mobility of the deltoid and greater ease in exposing the posterior aspect of the greater tuberosity and shaft. The clavipectoral fascia is incised and the subacromial/subdeltoid bursa is entered. Slight abduction of the arm at this point relaxes the deltoid muscle and protects the terminal branches of the axillary nerve. Periosteal attachments of the shaft and greater tuberosity are preserved to enhance healing after the repair.

Deeper exposure of the dislocated head fragment is typically achieved by working through a longitudinal fracture line in the greater tuberosity. This is most often associated with a small, longitudinally split supraspinatus

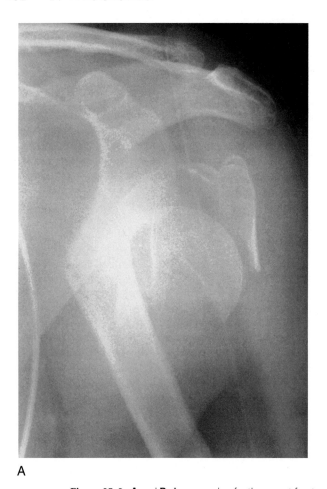

A

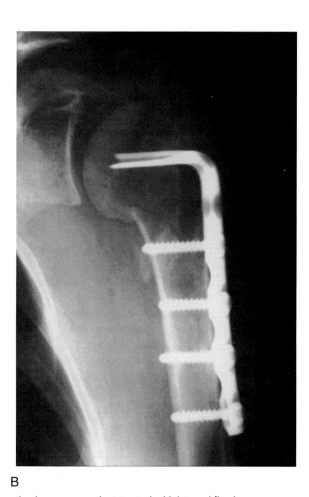

B

Figure 35–2. A and **B**, An example of a three-part fracture dislocation in a young patient treated with internal fixation.

tendon, which can be surgically enlarged toward the superior glenoid labrum as needed to gain access to the head fragment, the glenoid, and the upper portion of the humeral shaft. Although many texts illustrate four-part fractures as occurring through the bicipital groove, most often the hard bone of the groove remains intact and the coronal fracture line occurs just posterior to this area (Fig. 35–4).

Once exposed, the glenoid articular surface is assessed. Unless the patient suffers from associated disease such as inflammatory arthritis, the glenoid cartilage is usually well preserved and does not need to be replaced. Next, the shaft of the humerus is gently exposed with care to avoid iatrogenic stripping of the periosteum. At this point, it is convenient to drill holes in the upper portion of the shaft and place sutures in anticipation of tuberosity repair after cementation.

TRIAL REDUCTION

The trial reduction process can be divided into at least three steps: (1) restoration of humeral length, (2) restoration of appropriate humeral head retroversion, and (3) restoration of humeral head offset or size.

The length of the arm is determined by the height of the prosthesis. If the humeral head is positioned too low,

permanent inferior subluxation can occur. If the implant position is too high, the tuberosity and rotator cuff repair will be subjected to excessive tension and may fail.

Perhaps the most accurate tool for restoring humeral length is a ruler. To this end, Boileau has developed an external fracture jig that has enabled surgeons to restore the length of the humerus more consistently during arthroplasty for fractures.[3] Williams and Rockwood[34] have developed an internal jig that clamps to the diaphysis. Both jigs hold the trial implant in place during trial reduction and allow clinical assessment of height, version, and tension of the rotator cuff with the tuberosities reduced. A similar concept was conceived by Frankle,[12] who developed a modular system that allows the trial stem to be press fitted for stability. The trial implant bodies are etched in 5-mm increments. Based on the preoperative plan, the surgeon can calculate how far above the shaft fragment to set the head.

Several intraoperative guidelines can also be used to assess humeral height: (1) the tension in the long head biceps, (2) the tension of the reduced tuberosities, and (3) the distance between the supraspinatus tendon and the coracoacromial ligament. Perhaps the most useful landmark is the upper border of the anatomically reduced greater tuberosity. In most shoulders, the apex of the humeral head rests just above the greater tuberosity. This relationship and its variations can be appreciated

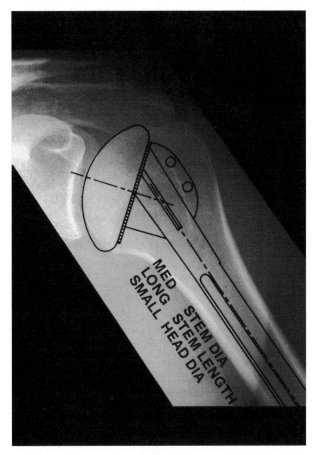

Figure 35–3. An example of preoperative construction of a template using a radiograph of the opposite shoulder.

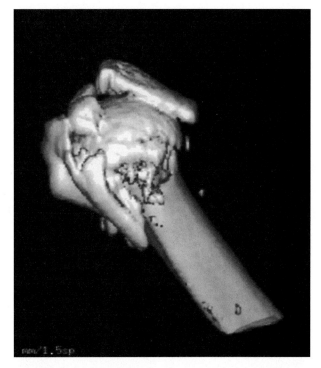

Figure 35–4. A three-dimensional computed tomography scan demonstrating the typical fracture pattern, with a slit in the coronal plane of the greater tuberosity.

on the radiograph of the opposite shoulder used to create the template. At surgery, with the trial implant in place and the greater tuberosity reduced and provisionally fixed, a radiograph or fluoroscopic image of the shoulder can be made to confirm the clinical impressions concerning the position of the implant and tuberosities. If these newer systems are not available, the trial implant is either held in place with a clamp or a press fit is achieved with a sponge. The height and version are then marked.

Retroversion

In the setting of an acute fracture, reliable landmarks are often absent, and there is a tendency for the surgeon to malrotate the humeral component. It should be recognized that there exists great variability in the degree of retroversion of the humerus,[3,17,23,29,33] with the average value measuring 20 degrees relative to the epicondylar axis.[3,23] If the forearm is used as a reference point approximately 25 degrees to 30 degrees of retroversion are appropriate in most cases. LeHeuc has pointed out the negative impact of excessive retroversion.[18] If the greater tuberosity is reduced and repaired a prosthetic head that has been placed in too great a degree of retroversion, the repair will come under excessive tension

when the arm is brought into internal rotation against the abdomen. The posterior tuberosity displacement cannot always be appreciated on radiographs and may be one cause of "tuberosity resorption." Perhaps a more common cause of tuberosity migration is the failure of the shaft of the humerus to heal.

Cementation

Cement is used to gain immediate stability of the implant. It is advisable to avoid filling the proximal metaphysis with cement because this is the only area available for tuberosity healing (Fig. 35–5). Given the relatively high risk of infection, the use of antibiotics in the cement is reasonable.

Tuberosity Repair

Conditions for healing of the tuberosity to the shaft may be optimized by avoiding the tendency to overtrim or thin the tuberosity, by not filling the metaphysis with metal and cement, and by selecting a humeral head size similar to that of the fractured head or the opposite side (see Fig. 35–5). Adjunctive cancellous bone grafting from the resected humeral head is advisable, and secure repair of the tuberosities is essential. The heavy suture placed in the configuration described by Hawkins typically provides satisfactory stability. Additional fixation in compression can be achieved by placing "cerclage" sutures or wires around the medial neck of the implant and the tuberosities.[18]

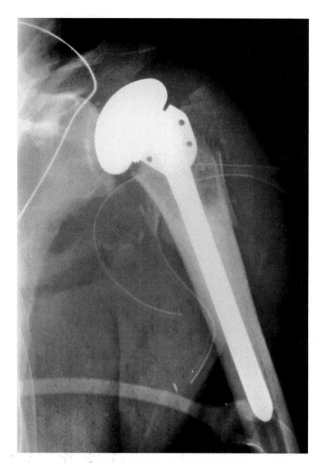

Figure 35–5. Demonstration of the preferred cement technique. Little if any cement is left in the proximal metaphysis to allow room for autogenous bone graft and the native greater tuberosity.

REHABILITATION

If a true anatomic reconstruction has been achieved (i.e., appropriate length of arm, head size, and version), the tuberosity position is correct and the osteosynthesis is secure, nearly full passive range of motion should be possible.

In practice, rehabilitation in each case is individualized because of variations in bone quality and patient understanding. After repair of the tuberosities, the arm is taken through a passive range of motion while the osteosynthesis site is directly examined. The limit at which passive motion brings the repair under stress is recorded. Postoperatively, supine passive elevation and external rotation are prescribed to a limit of 5 to 10 degrees less than the intraoperative measurements. Occasionally, the tuberosity is comminuted to such an extent that a secure repair cannot be achieved, and a limited goals rehabilitation program[25,26] is prescribed.

RESULTS

Many grading systems have been used to assess the outcome of shoulder arthroplasty for proximal humerus fractures. Although this variability precludes a highly accurate comparison of results, most authors do report shoulder

range of motion and comfort. In our review of published series (Table 35–1), there was a wide range in the values reported for mean elevation (from 58 to 131 degrees).[12,21] The degree of pain experienced by patients following HHR was also variable. The percentage of patients with no pain or mild pain ranged from 60 percent to 95 percent.

Mayo Clinic Experience

We have updated the review of our experience with HHR for acute fractures at Mayo. Including the cases from the two previously published series,[22,32] 75 cases were performed between 1970 and 1998. The average follow up interval was 40 months. Sixty-six of the 75 patients (88 percent) reported mild or no pain. Active elevation and external rotation averaged 101 degrees and 38 degrees, respectively.

These data and those of others,[13,15] suggest that patients treated with humeral head replacement for acute fractures are usually free of severe pain. The functional outcome seems to be less predictable. Many patients are left with a restricted range of motion, especially for active arm elevation. Newer implants and techniques[12] may allow the average result to reach the relatively high standard set by Neer some 30 years ago.

The factors affecting outcome have been extensively discussed in the literature and include the fracture pattern, timing of surgery, patient's age, position of the implant, and aftercare.[1,3,7,9,15]

Fracture Pattern

Two reports suggested that functional outcome of three-part fractures treated primarily with HHR was better than for four-part fractures.[15,37] This outcome would not be entirely unexpected because of the larger fragments of tuberosity available for repair in this setting.

Timing of Surgery

There is some rationale for early treatment before the development of unwanted scar, contracture, and bone deformity. Tanner and Cofield compared the results of humeral head replacement in acute and chronic fractures, in which they included patients with malunion: the complication rate was higher for the delayed cases.[32] In a study done by Bosch,[4] the length of time between injury and hemiarthroplasty was the best predictor of the outcome of the case. The outcome was inversely proportional to the time interval between injury and hemiarthroplasty. The results were significantly better after early operation, despite the fact that the fracture pattern was more severe in this group.[4]

Age

Advanced age (older than 70 years) has also been associated with less satisfactory results.[15] This finding was

Table 35–1. SHOULDER ARTHROPLASTY: REVIEW OF PUBLISHED SERIES

Year	Author	No. of Patients	Mean Age	Fracture Type (Neer System)	Prosthesis Type	Follow-up Time (mo)	No (mild) pain/ moderate pain/ severe pain	ROM Active Elevation Rotation	ROM External Rotation	ROM Internal Rotation
1970	Neer[25]	43	55	3, 4 part	Neer I	56	NA/NA/3	5>140 degrees, 34: 90–135°, 4<90 degrees	NA	NA
1983	Tanner[32]	16	69	3, 4 part	Neer	38	12/4/2	101	P:32	P:L1
1984	Stableforth[31]	16	66	4 part	Neer II	18 mo–12 yr	11/0/2	11>90 1<45	8>25 2<5	15 =T12
1988	Rietveld[28]	14	65	4 part	Neer II	38	2/12/2	9>90 5<90	11>25 3<25	NA
1991	Frich[13]	15		2, 3, 4 part	Neer II	2 yr (1–5)	NA	P:77	P:17	NA
1992	Moeckel[19]	22	70	3, 4 part	Modular Biomet	36	19/1/2	119	40	T12
1994	Compito[7]	64	62	3, 4 part	NA	33	47/15/2	127 22>30	31>50	NA
1995	Goldman[15]	22	67	3, 4 part	Neer II/Cofield	30	16/6/0	107	31	1,2
1997	Wretenberg[35]	18	82	3, 4 part	Neer	3, 5 yr	NA/17/1 II/NA/NA	NA	NA	NA
1998	Zyto[37]	27	71	17–3 part 10—4 part	Neer II Biomet	39	18/7/2	70	45	50
1998	Bosch[4]	22	64.5	3, 4 part	Neer II	42	21/NA/NA	93	NA	NA
1998	Movin[21]	18	71	NA	10 Neer 8 Global	36	NA	58	NA	NA
1998	Skutek[30]	13	62	3–3 part 10–4 part	Neer II	50	12/1/0	NA	NA	NA
1999	Boss[5]	20	77	NA	Neer II	32.5	12/8/2	99	NA	NA
1999	Boileau[3]	66	66	7–3 part 59–4 part	Aequalis	19	58/7/1	17≤90 45>90 4≥150	NA	NA
2000	Ambacher[1]	27	na	23—4 part 4–3 part	15 Neer 12 Aequalis	3.5 yr	22/NA/NA	94	27	84
2001	Frankle[12]	68	65	45—4 part 26—3 part 9 – head split 1 impacted head fx	38 Encore 35 Sutter 9 Global	30	59/NA/NA	131	43	L5

Data from references 1, 3–5, 7, 12, 13, 15, 19, 21, 25, 28, 30–32, 35, 37.
Fx = fracture; NA = not applicable; ROM = range of motion.

attributed to the possibility that these patients may be less determined to pursue a rigorous rehabilitation program after HHR because of their limited functional needs. Wretenberg[35] also noted inferior results in his series in which patients averaged 82 years of age and only obtained 55 degrees average elevation. He added that these patients usually have decreased elevation present in their contralateral nonoperated shoulder as well, making this decreased range of motion somewhat related to physiologic age changes. Finally, in the older patient, the tuberosity fragments are more comminuted and osteoporotic, making fixation and union less predictable. Poor functional results for arthroplasty in the elderly patient are typically offset by a high satisfaction rate among these patients, because pain relief plays a much greater role than the demand for physical performance. It is noteworthy that the mean age of Dr. Neer's patients was 55 years. This factor may be responsible for his high rate of satisfactory results.

Prosthesis Malposition

Perhaps the most common reason for failure in HHR is prosthetic malposition. Boileau[3] found that differences between the original anatomy and the prosthetic design led to altered biomechanics. In his clinical series, the most significant factor associated with a poor functional outcome was malposition of the prosthesis, especially when placement of the prosthesis was too proud or in excessive retroversion. Also found in this series was a clear correlation between prosthesis positioning and greater tuberosity migration leading to nonunion, malunion, and late bone resorption.

In a study by Frankle (unpublished data, AAOS 2001), a correlation between head-to-tuberosity distance and patient functional outcome and satisfaction was found. A distance of 13 mm or greater was associated with poorer results.

COMPLICATIONS

Many authors have recognized the challenges achieving a good result with HHR for acute trauma. An analysis of a series of 30 failed prosthetic replacements for displaced proximal humerus fractures showed that the single greatest cause of failure was detachment of the greater tuberosity. Loosening of the humeral prosthesis occurred in 13 shoulders, 2 of which were also infected. Nerve injury was diagnosed in 30 percent; glenoid erosion and malposition of the humeral prosthesis occurred in 23 percent. Ectopic bone formation was present in 16 percent of these failures.[2]

In a review done by Muldoon and Cofield,[22] complications were diverse, wound healing problems, infection, nerve injury, humeral fracture, component malposition, instability, tuberosity healing problems, rotator cuff tearing, reflex sympathetic dystrophy, heterotopic ossi-

fication, periarticular fibrosis, component loosening and glenoid arthritis with instability, tuberosity malunion or nonunion, and heterotopic bone formation were the most frequently occurring problems.

In our combined series of 75 cases done between 1970 and 1998, complications occurred in 25 patients (33 percent), and centered around tuberosity and rotator cuff healing. These included 6 nonunions of one or both tuberosities, 13 cases that had mild to moderate anterosuperior instability related to rotator cuff insufficiency, 4 infections (1 superficial and 3 deep), 1 wound hematoma, and 1 reflex sympathetic dystrophy. Five reoperations were necessary, 3 to treat infections, 1 for tuberosity repair, and 1 for drainage of a hematoma.

CONCLUSIONS

Humeral head replacement for acute fractures of the proximal humerus is a challenging procedure with the potential for frequent complications. Optimal function of the shoulder after this procedure requires anatomic or near anatomic reconstruction and secure healing of the tuberosities. Newer techniques, instruments, and implants may improve clinical results.

References

1. Ambacher T, Erli H, Parr O: Significance of rehabilitation to the functional outcome after primary hemiarthroplasty of the humeral head fractures. Acktuelle Traumatol 30:20–25, 2000.
2. Bigliani LU, Flatow EL, McCluskey GM, Fischer RA: Failed prosthetic replacement in displaced proximal humerus fractures. Orthop Transpl 15:747–748, 1991.
3. Boileau P, Walch G: Shoulder arthroplasty for proximal humeral fractures: problems and solutions. *In* Walch G, Boileau P (eds): Shoulder Arthroplasty. Berlin, Springer Verlag, 1999, pp 297–314.
4. Bosch U, Skutek M, Fremerey RW, Tscherne H: Outcome after primary and secondary hemiarthroplasty in elderly patients with fractures of the proximal humerus. J Shoulder Elbow Surg 7:479–484, 1998.
5. Boss AP, Hintermann B: Primary endoprosthesis in comminuted humeral head fractures in patients over 60 years of age. Int Orthop 23:172–174, 1999.
6. Brown TD, Bigliani, LU: Complications with humeral head replacement. Orthop Clin North Am 31:2000.
7. Compito CA, Self EB, Bigliani LU: Arthroplasty and acute shoulder trauma. Reasons for success and failure. Clin Orthop 307:27–36, 1994.
8. Coumo F, Lodenberg, M, Jones D, Zuckerman JD: The Effect of Greater Tuberosity Placement on Active Range of Motion after Hemiarthroplasty for Acute Fractures of the Proximal Humerus. Presented at the 16th Open Meeting of the ASES, Orlando, Fla, 2000.
9. Dines DM, Warren RF: Modular shoulder hemiarthroplasty for acute fractures. Surgical considerations. Clin Orthop 307:18–26, 1994.
10. Doursounian L, Grimberg J, Cazeau C, et al: A new internal fixation technique for fractures of the proximal humerus—the Bilboquet device: A report of 26 cases. JSES 9:279–288, 2000.
11. Frankle M, Greenwald D, Markee B, Ondrovic L: The Biomechanical Effects of Malposition of Tuberosity Fragments on the Humeral Prosthetic Reconstruction for Four-Part Proximal Humeral Fractures. Presented at the 17th Open Meeting of the ASES, San Fancisco, 2001.
12. Frankle M: Outcomes of Prosthetic Replacements for Acute Fractures of the Proximal Humerus. Presented at the 17th Open meeting of the ASES, San Francisco, 2001.

13. Frich LH, Sojbjerg JO, Sneppen O: Shoulder Arthroplasty in Complex Acute and Chronic Proximal Humeral Fractures. Orthopedics 14:949–954, 1991.
14. Gerber C, Hersche O, Berberat C: The clinical relevance of post-traumatic avascular necrosis of the humeral head. Shoulder Elbow Surg 7:586–90, 1998.
15. Goldman RT, Koval KJ, Cuomo F, et al: Functional outcome after humeral head replacement for acute three- and four-part proximal humeral fractures. J Shoulder Elbow Surg 4:81–86, 1995.
16. Jakob P, Miniaci A, Anson PS, et al: Four-part valgus impacted fractures of the proximal humerus. J Bone Joint Surg 73B:295–298, 1991.
17. Krahl VE, Evans FG: Humeral torsion in man. Am J Phys Anthropol 3:229–253, 1945.
18. LeHeuc JC, Boileu P, Sinnerton R, Hovroka I: Tuberosity osteosynthesis. In Walch G, Boileau P (eds): Shoulder Arthroplasty. Berlin, Springer Verlag, 1999, pp 323–329.
19. Moeckel BH, Dines DM, Warren RF, Altchek DW: Modular hemiarthroplasty for fractures of the proximal part of the humerus. J Bone Joint Surg 74A:884–999, 1992.
20. Moda SK, Chada NS, Sangwan SS, et al: Open reduction and fixation of proximal humerus fractures and fracture dislocation. J Bone Joint Surg 72B:1050–1052, 1999.
21. Movin T, Sjoden O, Ahregart L: Poor function after shoulder replacement in fracture patients. Acta Orthop Scand 69:392–396, 1998.
22. Muldoon MP, Cofield RH: Complications of Humeral Head Replacement for Proximal Humeral Fractures [review]. Instr Course Lect 46: 15–24, 1997.
23. Neer CS: Articular replacement for the humeral head. J Bone Joint Surg 37A:215–228, 1955.
24. Neer CS: Follow-up notes on articles previously published in the journal: Articular replacement for the humeral head. J Bone Joint Surg 46A:1607–1610, 1964.
25. Neer CS II: Displaced proximal humerus fractures. Part I. Classification and evaluation. J Bone Joint Surg 52A:1077–1089, 1970.
26. Neer CS II: Displaced proximal humerus fractures. Part II. Treatment of three-part and four-part displacement. J Bone Joint Surg 52A:1090–1093, 1970.
27. Nicholoson GP, Duckworth, MA: Operative Treatment of Proximal Humeral Malunions: Radiographic and Clinical Assessment Presented at the 15th Open Meeting of the ASES. Anaheim, Ca 1999.
28. Rietveld AB, Daanen HA, Rozing PM, Obermann WR: The lever arm in glenohumeral abduction after hemiarthroplasty. J Bone Joint Surg 70B:561–565, 1988.
29. Roberts S, Foley A, Swallow H, et al: The Geometry of the humeral head and the design of prostheses. J Bone Joint Surg Br 73:647–650, 1991.
30. Skutek M, Fremerey RW, Bosch U: Level of physical activity in elderly patients after hemiarthroplasty for three- and four-part fractures of the proximal humerus. Arch Orthop Trauma Surg 117:252–255, 1998.
31. Stableforth PG: Four-part fractures of the neck of the humerus. J Bone Joint Surg Br 66:104–108, 1984.
32. Tanner MW, Cofield RH: Prosthetic arthroplasty for fractures and fracture dislocation of the proximal humerus. Clin Orthop 179:116–128, 1983.
33. Walch G, Boileau P: Morphological study of the proximal humerus. J Bone Joint Surg Br 74 (Suppl I):14, 1991.
34. Williams GR, Wong K, Pepe M, et al: Effect of humeral articular malposition after total shoulder arthroplasty on impingement, range of motion, and translation. Presented at the 15th Open Meeting of the ASES, Anaheim, Ca, 1999.
35. Wretenberg P, Ekelund A: Acute hemiarthroplasty after proximal humerus fracture in old patients. A retrospective evaluation of 18 patients followed for 2-7 years. Acta Orthop Scand 68:121–123, 1997.
36. Zuckerman JD, Cuomo F, Koval KJ: Proximal humeral replacement for complex fractures. Indications and surgical technique. Instr Course Lect 46:7–14, 1997.
37. Zyto K, Wallace WA, Frostick SP, Preston BJ: Outcome after hemiarthroplasty for three-and four-part fractures of the proximal humerus. J Shoulder Elbow Surg. 7:85–89, 1998.

36A

Shoulder Arthroplasty for Arthritis

• ROBERT H. COFIELD, STEVEN J. HATTRUP,
JOAQUIN SANCHEZ-SOTELO, and SCOTT P. STEINMANN

This chapter displays basic information about the common diagnostic categories for which shoulder arthroplasty is performed.[3–5] These include primary and secondary osteoarthritis, rheumatoid arthritis, arthritis secondary to old trauma, osteonecrosis, and cuff tear arthritis. Another chapter in this section focuses on shoulder arthroplasty for trauma. There is also a separate chapter outlining the results of revision shoulder arthroplasty, and in the chapter on complications of shoulder arthroplasty, stiffness and contractures are addressed. This chapter concludes with segments addressing rotator cuff tears and handling bone deficiencies.

In the early 1950s, Neer introduced the humeral head prosthesis, with the initial plan of using this device for complex shoulder fractures.[16,17] In 1964, he tabulated the indications for humeral head replacement that had occurred up to that point in time.[18] These included 56 shoulder replacements and 42 procedures that had been done for acute or delayed trauma. In Neer's large 1982 series of patients undergoing total shoulder arthroplasty, the distribution of indications had changed.[21] Rheumatoid arthritis, osteoarthritis, and arthritis related to old trauma were the most common diagnostic categories. Somewhat less frequent indications were prosthetic revision, arthritis of recurrent dislocation, cuff tear arthropathy, and a miscellaneous group. In reporting our experience from 1975 to 1992, osteoarthritis, rheumatoid arthritis, and traumatic arthritis were also the three large diagnostic categories; revision surgery, osteonecrosis, and cuff tear arthropathy represented the other three diagnostic groups with only a small miscellaneous group.[4] Table 36A–1 depicts the diagnoses in shoulder arthroplasty for which surgery was performed between 1990 and 1999. It can be seen that osteoarthritis dominated this list of surgical indications, with the other categories having lesser numbers. Revision surgery had become the second most common surgical indication, with rheumatoid arthritis third, cuff tear arthritis fourth, acute trauma and traumatic-induced arthritis fifth, and osteonecrosis sixth. Understanding the characteristics of these forms of arthritis should lead to a much more complete ability to address the structur-

al abnormalities encountered during surgery and hence result in superior outcomes for the patients so treated.

OSTEOARTHRITIS

Osteoarthritis in the shoulder, as in other joints, can be primary or secondary. The primary group is the largest group by far. The characteristics of osteoarthritis have been accurately defined by Neer, and understanding has expanded with greater experience.[20,21] This category of arthritis is the most stereotypical, with many patients having almost identical changes in the joint and the surrounding structures (Fig. 36A–1).

The humeral head exhibits flattening and, seemingly, enlargement. There is notable subchondral sclerosis. There may be subchondral cysts, but these are usually not prominent. The cartilage loss on the humeral head is superior and central, spreading toward the periphery. There are peripheral osteophytes that are especially prominent inferiorly, and these contribute to the limitation of overhead movement. On the glenoid, there may be cartilage loss over the entire surface, or over just the posterior one half to two thirds of the surface. This cartilage loss is often associated with bone erosion. It can be central but is more commonly posterior, again associated with flattening of the joint surface. Subchondral plate sclerosis is often present. Cysts may also be present, particularly posteriorly. They are often not large, but they can be quite troublesome because of the small amount of bone typically present in the glenoid neck. There are peripheral osteophytes surrounding the glenoid. Occasionally, these are clearly visible within the joint at the time of surgery, but often they are hidden by the surrounding capsule.[20]

Joint position is often altered.[1] It certainly can be concentric, with the humeral head sitting directly over the glenoid, but, more often, there is posterior humeral subluxation that on radiographs often appears as if there is also superior subluxation (Fig. 36A–2). The joint position changes are associated with capsule changes. The capsular volume is usually enlarged posteriorly. When there are large osteophytes present, capsular volume may be

Table 36A–1. DIAGNOSES IN SHOULDER ARTHROPLASTY: 1990–1999

	Total Shoulder Arthroplasty	Humeral Head Replacement	Total
Osteoarthritis	381	32	413
Rheumatoid arthritis	108	50	158
Trauma/traumatic arthritis	64	26	90
Cuff tear arthropathy	37	77	114
Osteonecrosis	17	20	37
Revision surgery	140	37	177
	747	242	989

enlarged inferiorly but typically has a somewhat contracture-limiting overhead movement. The superior aspect of the capsule is usually of normal length, whereas the anterior aspect is usually somewhat contracted. Loose bodies can be present. They can be attached to the synovium, be located in the axillary recess, or be resting posteriorly or anteriorly in the subscapularis recess.

Tears of the rotator cuff in association with osteoarthritis are uncommon, although they do exist in 5 to 10 percent of patients.[6,21,35] Usually, they are small to medium-sized, involving the supraspinatus or the supraspinatus and the anterior aspect of the infraspinatus. Interestingly, because magnetic resonance imaging scans are now obtained on a number of shoulders, it is evident that there is often extensive degenerative change within the rotator cuff tendons in these patients—in the absence of frank tendon tearing. Perhaps this is a concomitant associated feature of the degenerative joint disease; perhaps it is secondary to joint instability with subluxation and tendon wear; or, possibly, these degenerative changes initiate subluxation, which in turn leads to joint instability, cartilage wear, and osteoarthritic changes.

When surgical technique is considered, the long deltopectoral approach is almost always all that is needed for adequate surgical exposure.[21] Typically, there is a limited amount of scarring in the subacromial-subdeltoid region. When the rotator cuff interval is incised, a large amount of clear, watery, synovial fluid may escape. If there is greater than 30 degrees of external rotation, the rotator cuff and capsule incision can be made through the subscapularis tendon overlying the usual insertion site of the capsule on the humeral head. This incision is then continued inferiorly and somewhat laterally as the subscapularis attachment becomes more muscular. The anteroinferior capsule is incised from the bone of the humerus, and, with external rotation, the inferior aspect of the shoulder capsule is progressively brought into view. If osteophytes are present inferiorly on the humeral head, these are removed to expose the capsule more fully. If there has been limitation of passive overhead movement (as is usually the case), the inferior capsule is carefully incised from the neck of the humerus.

We typically prepare the humeral canal before doing the humeral osteotomy. This allows us a firm reference to the axis of the humerus against which we can refer-

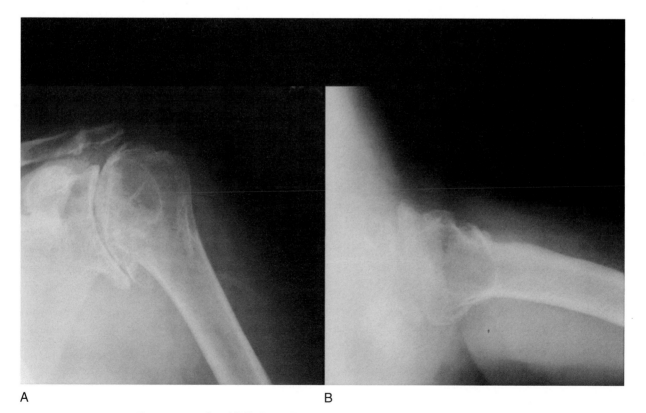

A   B

Figure 36A–1. **A** and **B**, Typical radiographic appearance of osteoarthritis. See text.

Illustration continued on following page

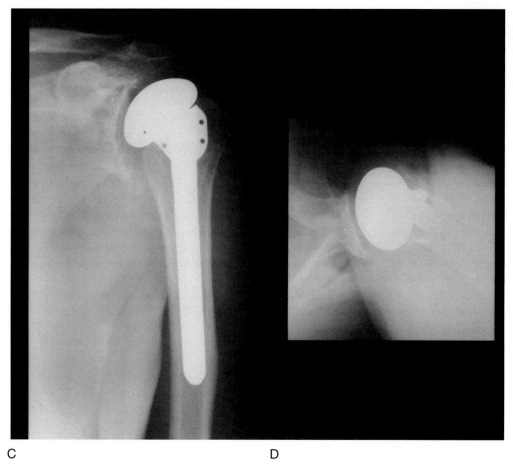

C   D

Figure 36A–1. *Continued.* **C** and **D**, After total shoulder arthroplasty.

ence the humeral osteotomy cut. We prefer to use a cutting guide that has both intramedullary and extramedullary reference points. The major extramedullary reference point is to the axis of the forearm with the elbow flexed 90 degrees. The osteotomy cut is then indexed against the junction of the rotator cuff with the humeral head superiorly, cutting perhaps 1 mm above that junction so as to not disturb rotator cuff attachments laterally. With the cutting guide set at 30 degrees, observation of the posterior cuff attachments is then performed to ensure that the 30 degree cut is reasonable. In shoulders without posterior humeral subluxation or posterior glenoid wear and slightly more inherent retrotorsion, the angle of the cut may be increased to 35 degrees. On the other hand, if there is posterior humeral subluxation and posterior glenoid wear, the angle of the cut may be decreased to approximately 20 degrees, thus varying somewhat the length of bone remaining on the posterior aspect of the humeral head and affecting the tightness of the posterior capsule and rotator cuff. After humeral osteotomy, a humeral trial prosthesis is placed, and the humeral metaphysis is trimmed anteriorly, medially, and laterally so that bone does not extend beyond the arc of the prosthesis, thus avoiding later impingement against the glenoid or a glenoid component. A trial reduction is then performed,

and motion is assessed. If overhead motion is limited, the extent of inferior capsule release is assessed and may be extended somewhat more posteriorly, again placing the cut on the humerus to avoid injury to the axillary nerve.

The humeral trial device is removed, and, in the presence of anterior contracture, an incision is made along the anterosuperior glenoid rim, incising the capsule attachments there. This incision then continues laterally along the superior band of the inferior glenohumeral ligament. The subscapularis and this attached segment of anterosuperior shoulder capsule can then be elevated somewhat from the subscapularis fossa to allow much more flexibility of the anterior structures.

Glenoid exposure is now possible if the humerus is abducted approximately 70 degrees, which pushes the proximal humerus in a posterior direction. A Fukuda retractor, a humeral neck retractor (a modified Hohmann), or a Darrach retractor is placed across the front of the proximal humerus and behind the posterior lip of the glenoid. The anterior structures are held out of the way by a long knee retractor. Soft tissues overhanging the rim of the glenoid are excised, and, typically, there is a full exposure of the glenoid, with direct and not angular visibility. If there is any cartilage remaining on the anterior aspect of the glenoid, this is removed

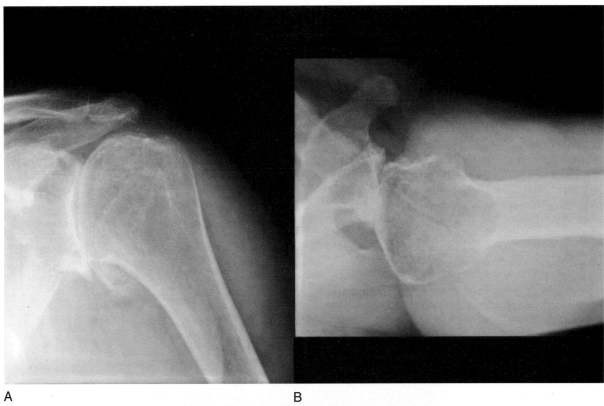

A   B

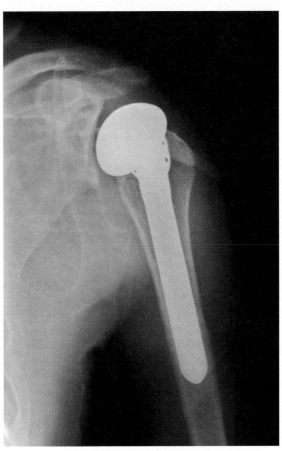

C

Figure 36A–2. A and **B**, Osteoarthritis associated with posterior humeral subluxation. **C**, After total shoulder arthroplasty. A larger head size was used tighten the posterior capsule.

with a curette. Removal of the cartilage exposes the normal subchondral plate with which worn areas, particularly those caused by posterior wearing, can be compared. It is not unusual for the front quarter to one third of the glenoid to have this cartilage covering and to have a normal subchondral plate. When the covering is removed, it is apparent that there has been central and posterior erosion of the posterior two thirds to three quarters of the glenoid. This erosion is present to a varying depth. When there is a small amount of erosion it can almost be ignored, with reaming of the glenoid in the usual plane of the glenoid as denoted by the remaining subchondral plate. If there is slightly more wear, the facing reamer is directed just a few degrees posteriorly to accommodate this small amount of wear yet obtain a firm seating of the glenoid component. If there is a larger amount of posterior wear, the glenoid can be reamed normally or with only a slight posterior tilt if there is ample glenoid neck present to seat a component. If there is not, only a small amount of anterior reaming is possible, and bone graft is added to the deficient area posteriorly after holes have been prepared in the keel or column in the glenoid neck. The glenoid is then fixed in position. Trial is then made of various sizes of humeral heads. The real humeral component is fixed in position, and the subscapularis and anterior shoulder capsule are repaired. After this is done, the shoulder is taken through a range of motion, and the amount of external rotation, internal rotation, and elevation are recorded. This record serves as a guide in planning the physiotherapy in the early postoperative period.

The preceding discussion describes the common and quite typical surgical approach to shoulder arthroplasty, because osteoarthritis represents the largest patient group and the group against which variations in surgical technique from other disease processes are indexed. It is important to note that a change in outcome has occurred for osteoarthritis since the early 1990s. Because of the more extensive capsule releases that are done, the great attention to care in bone work, the presence of adjunctive instruments to prepare the humerus and the glenoid, and the variation in implant sizes, obtain stability of the joint can be achieved in almost all patients, with anticipation of 75 percent normal active motion. There is still some debate about whether or not to place a glenoid component in a patient with osteoarthritis. Our results indicate the pain relief is more consistent when a glenoid is placed.[10] No doubt, this is yet again a standard with which other disease processes need to be compared.[15]

RHEUMATOID ARTHRITIS

Of course, we all wish we had a better understanding of the cause of rheumatoid arthritis. It has protean manifestations and a highly variable course. It can begin and progress slowly but relentlessly. It can begin and then stop, apparently becoming inactive. It can have a recurring course. The usefulness of surgical procedures for rheumatoid arthritis was identified quite early in the orthopedic history in North America.[28] In Scandinavia,

there has been an intense interest in rheumatoid arthritis of the shoulder.[23] In the Finnish reviews of large numbers of rheumatoid patients, involvement of the shoulder has been identified as being quite common.[14,34] The rheumatoid disease may involve the glenohumeral joint, the acromioclavicular joint, the rotator cuff tendons, the biceps tendon, and the scapulocostal junction. It sometimes just causes arthralgias; at other times, the radiographic appearance is that of osteoarthritis. There can be a greatly enlarged subdeltoid bursa with rice body formation.[31] The patient may seem if he or she has a frozen shoulder. Some patients develop calcific tendinitis, reflex sympathetic dystrophy, or cervical spine radiculopathy. All of these things can lead to a complex and sometimes confusing presentation. Certainly, the more widespread and severe the rheumatoid arthritis is in an individual, the more likely the shoulder is to be involved. Also, the longer rheumatoid arthritis is present, the more common it is for the shoulder to become involved, but it is not possible to predict shoulder involvement, nor is it certain that involvement will worsen over time.[7]

There have been a number of classifications developed for patients with rheumatoid arthritis and rheumatoid joint involvement. These include functional capacity, stages of rheumatoid arthritis radiographically, and patterns of involvement. In 1971, Neer suggested consideration of the dry type of rheumatoid arthritis; the wet type of rheumatoid arthritis, with abundant synovium and synovially generated changes (Fig. 36A–3), and the resorptive type of arthritis, with an excessive amount of bone resorption as a part of the destructive process.[13,19] It is worthwhile to consider the complexity of rheumatoid disease and the extensive amount of thinking that has gone into attempting to understand shoulder involvement. It is probably best to analyze each tissue in the shoulder for each patient who has this diagnosis. Certainly, there may be varying degrees of cartilage loss. This is usually best appreciated on an axillary view or on a 40-degree posterior oblique view of the shoulder joint. The bone about the shoulder is typically osteopenic, and there is serious concern about humeral fracturing at the time of shoulder arthroplasty. This may prompt an anteromedial approach, releasing the anterior deltoid origin from the clavicle and anterior acromion in certain patients with extreme osteopenia who should have no torsional forces on the humeral shaft. There may be a varying amount of erosive change at the margin of the joint. This is most strikingly seen along the superior aspect of the humeral head, but it occurs in other locations too. There may be extensive subchondral cyst formation replacing a portion or almost the entirety of the humeral head and, unfortunately, replacing much of the bone of the glenoid neck. Often, these latter changes are not readily apparent on standard images. In addition, once the cartilage is lost, there may be extensive resorption or erosion of the subchondral bone surfaces. This is particularly true on the glenoid side of the joint, where the wear is often central and can be extreme, extending to near the base of the glenoid neck. In this latter situation, there is often

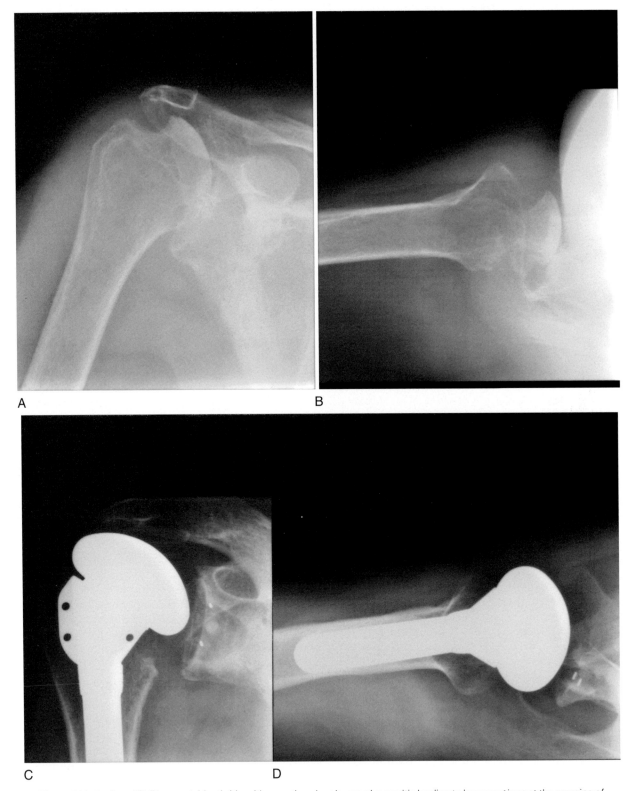

A

B

C

D

Figure 36A–3. A and **B**, Rheumatoid arthritis with an active glenohumeral synovitis leading to large erosions at the margins of the joint in addition to cyst formation, cartilage loss, and weakening of the rotator cuff tendons. **C** and **D**, After total shoulder arthroplasty. The rotator cuff was thin but not torn.

not enough bone remaining to support a glenoid component; in such cases, a humeral head replacement alone seems to be the better choice (Fig. 36A–4).

At surgery, the subdeltoid bursa may be scarred or there may be a very hypertrophic bursitis. The abnormal bursa is removed. There may be extensive rice body formation, and these bodies are evacuated. Of course, as in all shoulder arthroplasty surgery, if fibrosis is present, this is divided so that one has the hope of obtaining more ample motion after surgery.

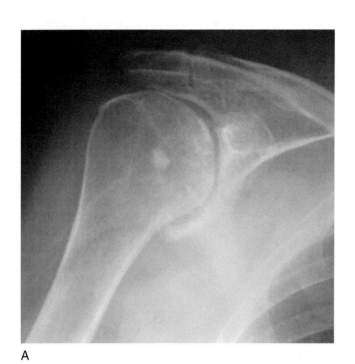

A

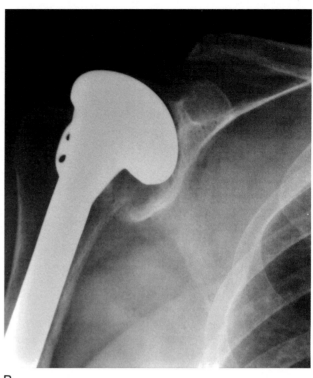

B

Figure 36A–4. A, Rheumatoid arthritis of the shoulder with extreme central erosion of the glenoid. **B,** After humeral head replacement. Not enough bone remained to securely fix a glenoid component in place.

Interestingly, the changes in the rotator cuff vary by location. Anteriorly, the subscapularis is often spared from much involvement. The superior aspect of the rotator cuff may be normal. It is more commonly thought to be somewhat thin, with fibrosis interposted between the usual tendon fibers. In one large radiographic study of rotator cuff tendons in rheumatoid patients with a painful shoulder, arthrograms showed approximately one quarter of the patients as having full-thickness rotator cuff tears.[8] At the time of surgery, full-thickness rotator cuff tears have been identified in one quarter to one half of patients undergoing shoulder arthroplasty.[6,21,26] These tears are usually superior, and the tissues adjacent to the tear may be moderately to severely affected, depending on the state of advancement of the disease process in this tissue. At surgery, the coracoacromial arch is assessed. Irregularities on the undersurface of the acromion are smoothed, and, typically, attempts are made to preserve the coracoacromial arch intact, including the coracoacromial ligament—as an aid to supporting the weakened rotator cuff tissue.[29,33]

As in osteoarthritis, if there is more than 30 degrees of external rotation with the arm at the side, the anterior arthrotomy is made through the interval area and through the subscapularis tendon. This is deepened to the level of the capsule insertion, and the capsule is released from the humerus anteriorly, anteroinferiorly, and inferiorly. The humeral canal and humerus are prepared as in osteoarthritis. The joint is distracted, and a synovectomy is performed. Typically, the anterorsuperior shoulder capsule is released from the glenoid, and, in contracted joints, it may be necessary to release the capsule superiorly above the anchor of the long head of the biceps tendon and posteriorly along the glenoid rim. After release of the contractures, the rotator cuff is again inspected, and if there is any full-thickness rotator cuff tearing, plans are laid for tendon repair in a rather typical fashion, tendon to tendon and tendon to bone, as needed. It is important to recognize that the standard preoperative radiographs may show superior subluxation of a moderate degree. This is, of course, associated with thinning of the rotator cuff tendons but may or may not be associated with full-thickness rotator cuff tearing.

The glenoid is exposed with use of the same arm position as in osteoarthritis. Care must be taken not to lever forcefully on the glenoid rim because of the osteopenia and erosions that are present. The central portion of the glenoid is identified, and a drill or bur hole is made to assess the depth of the glenoid neck. If there is greater than 1½ cm of depth, it is certainly possible to place a glenoid component. If the depth of the glenoid neck is 1 cm or less, it is easily understandable that security of glenoid fixation will be compromised; therefore, consideration is given to humeral head replacement alone.

After the glenoid situation has been addressed, there are some issues concerning humeral component fixation.[11] We continue to use a tissue ingrowth humeral component if there is reasonably strong metaphyseal bone and good cortical support distally. If either of these is not present, we cement the humeral component in place. Consideration must be given to the ipsilateral elbow. If there is a moderate or strong likelihood of future total elbow arthroplasty, the decision may be to shorten the humeral component to approximately 115 mm rather than use the 145 mm stem. A plug is placed just distal to the stem, and the humeral component is secured with bone cement. This then allows ample space for placement of the humeral component of the total elbow arthroplasty. On the other hand, if a total elbow arthroplasty is already present, it would seem reasonable to consider the use of bone cement proximally to join the two cement columns and eliminate a stress-rising effect in the central portion of an extremely osteoporotic humeral shaft.

Some have placed great importance on involvement of the acromioclavicular joint.[13] We have personally not found this to be much of an issue in these patients. If such involvement does occur, it usually responds to a corticosteroid injection. At the time of implant surgery, we have usually elected not to address acromioclavicular pathology and have not been disappointed in surgical outcome, because later acromioclavicular joint symptoms have not become apparent. We have noted, as have others, that the scapulothoracic junction is somewhat affected in these patients, and even with complete tissue releases surrounding the glenohumeral joint, the patient may still have deficiency of passive overhead movement related to stiffness at the scapulothoracic junction and fibrosis of the muscles extending from the chest wall to the scapula or the humerus.

Two additional variations should be mentioned. The first is the group of patients with juvenile rheumatoid arthritis. These patients often have severe rheumatoid disease with relatively long-standing, intense inflammation and, correspondingly, a rather intense fibrotic response. The tissues tend to be frail yet stiff. Additionally, bone size is much reduced, and consideration needs to be given to extra-small or custom components. It has been disappointing in this patient group that at surgery, even after extensive release, full or nearly full passive motion often cannot be obtained; moreover, after surgery, despite full and long-standing rehabilitation, the gains achieved at surgery cannot usually be maintained.[30] The second special, group includes middle-aged or elderly patients, often women, who have unilateral or bilateral shoulder disease. The radiographic picture is one of cartilage loss associated with osteopenia. The secondary features of osteoarthritis are absent. The rheumatoid factor may be negative or borderline, and there are no other—or few other—signs of an inflammatory arthritic process. On the other hand, there are usually no other areas of osteoarthritic joint involvement. One would speculate that this might well have been a rheumatoid arthritis or another inflammatory arthritis that appeared, destroyed the joint, and became inactive. Neer has termed this picture "the syndrome" for want of a better definition of this variation of the inflammatory arthritic process.[19]

TRAUMATIC ARTHRITIS

Patients with arthritis secondary to trauma are a variable group.[9] Arthritis can develop as a complication from the use of metallic internal fixation, whether from previous fracture treatment or from, for example, treatment for recurrent dislocations that included use of suture anchors that intruded into the joint. Arthritis from recurrent dislocations is uncommon, but, indeed, it does occur,[27] and, of course, arthritis does develop after chronic unreduced dislocations and fracture malunions; on occasion, it is associated with fracture nonunions.[32] There is the specter of osteonecrosis, which can occur after a number of types of proximal humeral traumatic events. There are direct injuries to the articular surface caused by head-splitting or impaction fractures. Sometimes, direct injury can occur just from impaction of the cartilage itself, which can occasionally lead to subtle osteochondral injuries.[30] Also, between 5 percent and 10 percent of patients who have had complex proximal humeral fractures treated with humeral head hemiarthroplasty develop glenoid arthritis and require revision to total shoulder arthroplasty.

When there is trauma, many of the adjacent tissues may suffer the effects in addition to the cartilage itself. Certainly, there is bone deformity, and, in fact, there may be bone loss. The surrounding shoulder capsule is often scarred and stiff. The rotator cuff may be damaged by fibrosis, or the attachments may be altered by tuberosity fractures with malunion or nonunion. In addition, there may be muscle atrophy from disuse and intrinsic muscle contracture resulting from lack of motion at the glenohumeral joint. Nerve injury may be associated with musculoskeletal injury and it sometimes eludes diagnosis because a joint and its surrounding muscles cannot be examined carefully. Electromyelography can be a useful adjunct to diagnosis in this patient group.

After recurrent dislocations, it is most common to see secondary osteoarthritis in patients who have had earlier surgery to control the dislocations. At the time the patient manifests arthritis, there is often posterior humeral subluxation and anterior shoulder capsule tightness. This is not unlike the picture seen in patients with typical osteoarthritis, except that the changes may be more extensive. Treatment includes anterior capsule and subscapularis lengthening, careful attention to component position during surgery, and, on occasion, tightening of the posterior shoulder capsule. An excellent to satisfactory outcome is to be expected but will not be quite as good as that of the typical osteoarthritic patient who has not experienced trauma and earlier surgery.

Chronic, unreduced dislocations are typically posterior but can be anterior or inferior. If the chronic, unreduced posterior dislocations are only several months old and 50 percent or more of the articular surface of the humeral head remains, open reduction and transfer of the lesser tuberosity or subscapularis into the defect suffice. However, if the dislocation is of 6 months' duration or longer, the size of the humeral head impression defect is greater than 50 percent, or the remaining bone is extremely osteopenic, it is highly likely that prosthetic arthroplasty will be necessary.[2,12,24,25] Usually, the outcome in this group of patients is also expected to be quite good, because the amount of posterior capsule stretching in a posterior direction is often compensated for by the medial position of the humeral head, and when the humeral head is brought back into the joint, the posterior capsule has normal or nearly normal tissue tightness. The superior aspect of the rotator cuff also is nearly normal. The inferior capsule is typically released as a part of the exposure for open reduction, and the anterior capsule and subscapularis are lengthened.

A number of types of malunion exist, reflecting the large spectrum of proximal humeral fractures. There can be a two-part malunion involving the articular surface fragment, a three-part malunion involving the humeral head and the greater or (less commonly) lesser tuberosity, or a four-part malunion. Additionally, osteonecrosis of the head fragment may be present (Fig. 36A–5). When there is malunion between the head and the shaft, it may be necessary to be creative in positioning the prosthetic humeral head and fixing the stem in the humerus. Usually, however, this can be accomplished without osteotomy of the head-shaft junction. In malunion of the lesser tuberosity, an osteotomy can be done by repositioning the lesser tuberosity, or the majority of the bone of the lesser tuberosity can be excised with the remaining bone fixed to an appropriate position on the anterior aspect of the joint. In malunion of the greater tuberosity, it is occasionally possible to slightly malposition the humeral head implant to match this without osteotomy of the greater tuberosity per se. If this can be accomplished, it is preferable, because the outcome after reconstructive surgery is better if the tuberosities are not repositioned and do not need to heal. However, when the tuberosity is severely malpositioned superiorly, posteriorly, or both superiorly and posteriorly, a portion of the tuberosity may need to be osteotomized and repositioned, or the whole tuberosity may need to be osteotomized in a biplanar or triplanar fashion and be repositioned behind the prosthetic humeral head. Fixation is then undertaken both to the prosthesis and to the humeral shaft, and, typically, bone graft is applied surrounding the junctions of these bones to help promote healing. In spite of this, tuberosity nonunion occurs in at least one quarter of the patients so treated.

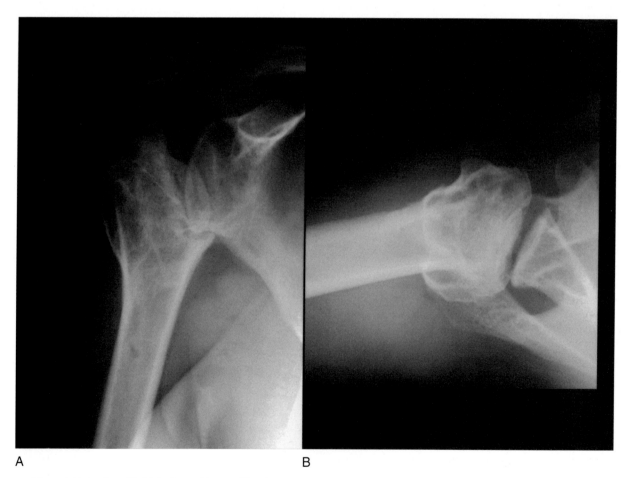

A   B

Figure 36A–5. **A** and **B**, Malunion and humeral head osteonecrosis secondary to a comminuted proximal humeral fracture.

Illustration continued on opposite page

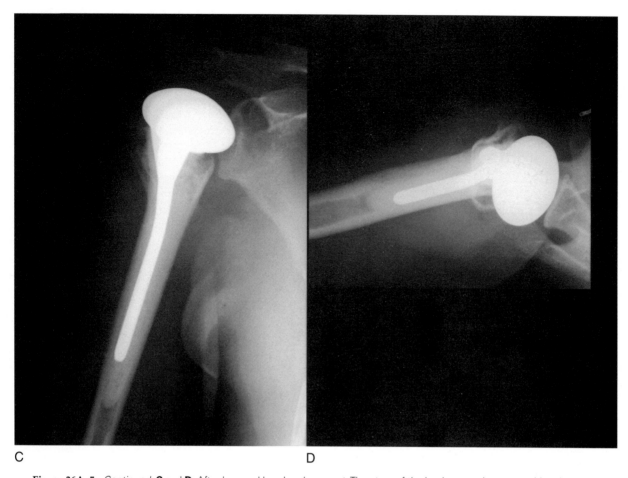

C   D

Figure 36A–5. *Continued.* **C** and **D**, After humeral head replacement. The stem of the implant was bent to position the prosthetic humeral head accurately in relationship to the malunited humeral tuberosities and to fit the prosthetic stem within the humeral canal.

When traumatically induced osteonecrosis occurs, the results are better if there is not accompanying malunion of adjacent tuberosity fragments. However, the outcome is not as good as in patients who develop osteonecrosis after the use of corticosteroids. This is true because of the associated soft tissue changes that have occurred as a result of the traumatic event. However, when this procedure is performed, the best attempt possible is made to release contractures and to excise excessive scar in order to gain more movement and function after prosthetic replacement. It has been our practice to replace the glenoid if it has undergone substantial changes. If the glenoid is entirely covered with cartilage, or if there is only a minimal amount of exposed bone, we typically place the humeral head implant alone.

There are some patients with nonunion of the proximal humerus involving the humeral head fragment or the humeral head fragment with one or more tuberosities attached. This ununited fragment may be extremely osteopenic, and it may be cavitated so that only a shell of bone remains (Fig. 36A–6). In these circumstances, prosthetic arthroplasty seems reasonable, whereas, for the typical nonunion of the proximal humerus, we prefer internal fixation and bone grafting rather than prosthetic arthroplasty.

One can easily see that there is a great deal of variation within this patient subgroup. It is extremely important to understand the bony deformity that is present. If standard radiographs do not allow this to be done, computed tomography scanning can be a useful adjunct to establishing a precise diagnosis for the bony deformity. The newer, thin-slice computed tomography scanners with three-dimensional reconstructions are now becoming particularly valuable for this patient group.

Treating patients in this diagnostic subgroup, it is important to recall the admonition that pain relief may be somewhat less predictable than one would ordinarily wish, and particularly less predictable than in those who have been treated primarily with an arthroplasty for complex proximal humeral fractures. It is also important to recall that the surgery may be much more technically difficult than the radiographs imply—because of all the associated bony and soft tissue problems.[22]

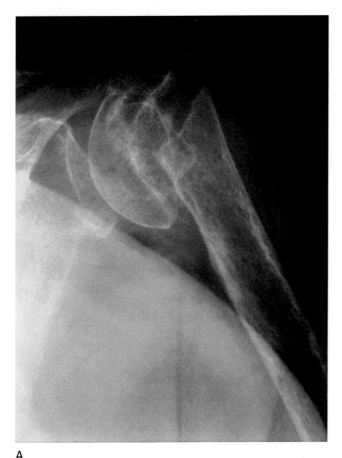

A

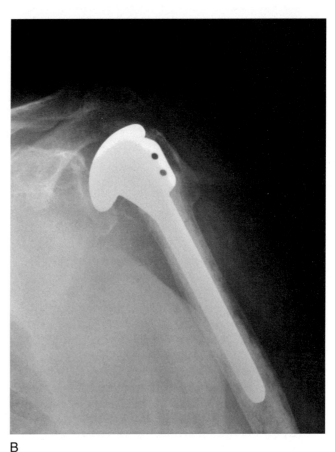

B

Figure 36A–6. A, Long-standing nonunion of the proximal humerus in an elderly woman. At surgery, the humeral head was cavitated with sclerosis at the fracture site. The remaining bone of the humeral head was extremely osteopenic. **B,** After humeral head replacement. The tuberosities were fixed with No. 5 suture, bone graft from the humeral head was added at the tuberosity-humeral shaft junction and healing occurred.

References

1. Badet R, Boulahia A, Walch G: Computerized tomography measurement of anteroposterior humeral dislocation. Proposing a method. Application to centered osteoarthritis. Rev Chir Orthop Reparatrice de 1 Appar Mot 84:508, 1998.
2. Checchia SL, Santos PD, Miyazaki AN: Surgical treatment of acute and chronic posterior fracture-dislocation of the shoulder. J Shoulder Elbow Surg 7:53, 1998.
3. Cofield RH: The shoulder. *In* Kelly WN, Haris ED Jr, Ruddy S, Sledge CB (eds): Textbook of Rheumatology 5th ed. Philadelphia, WB Saunders, 1997, p 1696.
4. Cofield RH, Becker DA: Shoulder arthroplasty. *In* Morrey BF (ed): Reconstructive Surgery of the Joints, 2nd ed. New York, Churchill Livingstone, 1996, p 753.
5. Cofield RH: Degenerative and arthritic problems of the glenohumeral joint. *In* Rockwood CA Jr, Matsen FA III (eds): The Shoulder. Philadelphia, WB Saunders, 1990, p 678.
6. Cofield RH: Unconstrained total shoulder prostheses. Clin Orthop 173:97, 1983.
7. Dijkstra J, Dijkstra PF, Klundert WVD: Rheumatoid arthritis of the shoulder. Fortschr Rontgenstr 142:179, 1985.
8. Ennevaara K: Painful shoulder joint in rheumatoid arthritis: A clinical and radiological study of 200 cases with special reference to arthrography of the glenohumeral joint. Acta Rheum Scand (Suppl 11):1, 1967.
9. Frich LH, Sojbjerg JO, Sneppen O: Shoulder arthroplasty in complex acute and chronic proximal humeral fractures. Orthopedics 14:949, 1991.
10. Gartsman GM, Roddey TS, Hammerman SM: Shoulder arthroplasty with or without resurfacing of the glenoid in patients who have osteoarthritis. J Bone Joint Surg 82A:26, 2000.
11. Gill DR, Cofield RH, Morrey BF: Ipsilateral total shoulder and elbow arthroplasties in patients who have rheumatoid arthritis. J Bone Joint Surg 81A:1128, 1999.
12. Hawkins RJ, Neer CS II, Pianta RM, Mendoza FX: Locked posterior dislocation of the shoulder. J Bone Joint Surg 69A:9, 1987.
13. Kelly IG: Unconstrained shoulder arthroplasty in rheumatoid arthritis. Clin Orthop 307:94, 1994.
14. Laine VAI, Vainio KJ, Pekanmaki K: Shoulder affections in rheumatoid arthritis. Ann Rheum Dis 13:157, 1954.
15. Matsen FA III: Early effectiveness of shoulder arthroplasty for patients who have primary glenohumeral degenerative joint disease. J Bone Joint Surg 78A:260, 1996.
16. Neer CS, Brown TH Jr, McLaughlin HL: Fracture of the neck of the humerus with dislocation of the head fragment. Am J Surg 85:252, 1953.
17. Neer CS II: Articular replacement for the humeral head. J Bone Joint Surg 37A:215, 1955.
18. Neer CS II: Follow-up notes on articles previously published in the journal. Articular replacement for the humeral head. J Bone Joint Surg 46A:1607, 1964.
19. Neer CS II: The rheumatoid shoulder. *In* Cruess RR, Mitchell NS (eds): Surgery of Rheumatoid Arthritis. Philadelphia, JB Lippincott, 1971, p 117.
20. Neer CS II: Replacement arthroplasty for glenohumeral osteoarthritis. J Bone Joint Surg 56A:1, 1974.
21. Neer CS II, Watson KC, Stanton FJ: Recent experience in total shoulder replacement. J Bone Joint Surg 64A:319, 1982.

22. Norris TR, Green A, McGuigan FX: Late prosthetic shoulder arthroplasty for displaced proximal humeral fractures. J Shoulder Elbow Surg 4:271, 1995.
23. Petersson CJ: Painful shoulders in patients with rheumatoid arthritis. Scand J Rheum 15:275, 1986.
24. Pritchett JW, Clark JM: Prosthetic replacement for chronic un reduced dislocations of the shoulder. Clin Orthop 216:89, 1987.
25. Rowe CR, Zarins B: Chronic unreduced dislocations of the shoulder. J Bone Joint Surg 64A:494, 1982.
26. Rozing PM, Brand R: Rotator cuff repair during shoulder arthroplasty in rheumatoid arthritis. J Arthroplasty 13:311, 1998.
27. Samilson RL, Prieto V: Dislocation arthropathy of the shoulder. J Bone Joint Surg 65A:456, 1983.
28. Smith-Peterson MN, Aufranc OE, Larson CB: Useful surgical procedures for rheumatoid arthritis involving joints of the upper extremity. Arch Surg 46:764, 1943.
29. Sojbjerg JO, Frich LH, Johannsen HV, Sneppen O: Late results of total shoulder replacement in patients with rheumatoid arthritis. Clin Orthop 366:39, 1999.
30. Sperling JW, Cofield RH, Rowland CM: Neer hemiarthroplasty and Neer total shoulder arthroplasty in patients fifty years old or less. Long-term results. J Bone Joint Surg 80A:464, 1998.
31. Steinfeld R, Rock MG, Younge DA, Cofield RH: Massive subacromial bursitis with rice bodies. Clin Orthop 301:185, 1994.
32. Tanner MW, Cofield RH: Prosthetic arthroplasty for treatments and fracture-dislocations of the proximal humerus. Clin Orthop 179:116, 1983.
33. Thomas BJ, Amstutz HC, Cracchiolo A: Shoulder arthroplasty for rheumatoid arthritis. Clin Orthop 265:125, 1991.
34. Vainio K: Orthopaedic surgery in the treatment of rheumatoid arthritis. Ann Clin Res 7:216, 1975.
35. Walch G, Boulahia A, Boileau P, Kempf JF: Primary glenohumeral osteoarthritis: Clinical and radiographic classification. The Aequalis group. Acta Orthop Belg 2(Suppl. 64):46, 1998.

36B

Shoulder Arthroplasty for Osteonecrosis

• STEVEN J. HATTRUP

Osteonecrosis of the humeral head can be associated with a number of etiologic agents, the most common of which are trauma and corticosteroid use.[13] Other potential causes include alcohol abuse, dysbaric disease, Gaucher's disease, sickle cell disease, radiation, and systemic lupus erythematosus. Frequently, the cause cannot be identified. Ultimately, osteonecrosis can lead to painful collapse of the articular surface of the humeral head and require prosthetic reconstruction. The diverse etiologies, however, can lead to different natural histories and results after surgery.

ETIOLOGY

Trauma produces osteonecrosis through disruption of the blood supply of the humeral head. The anterolateral ascending branch of the anterior humeral circumflex artery travels along the lateral aspect of the bicipital tendon and becomes intraosseous at the upper end of the bicipital groove.[11,16] Laing termed this intraosseous extension the arcuate artery.[16] Although he found a rich periosteal vascular network on the proximal humerus, there were few intraosseous anastomoses with the arcuate artery. Gerber elegantly confirmed the importance of the anterolateral ascending artery as the prime vascular supply to the humeral head[11] (Fig. 36B–1). He also demonstrated that the posterior humeral circumflex artery supplied only the posterior-inferior head and posterior greater tuberosity. More recently, Brooks and colleagues re-examined this issue in 16 cadaver shoulders.[5] They found more significant intraosseous anastomoses between the arcuate artery and posterior humeral circumflex artery, metaphyseal vessels, and vessels in the greater and lesser tuberosities. These allowed some perfusion to persist in fractures including the upper part of the neck with the head fragment.

Laceration of the anterolateral ascending artery from fracture fragments or surgical dissection can potentially produce osteonecrosis. Risk factors include increasing comminution and displacement as well as level of the fracture. The more proximal the fracture, the more likely the vascular supply will be disrupted distal to any anastomoses. Schai et al. documented the increased incidence of osteonecrosis with increased comminution.[23] In a study of serial proximal humeral fractures, 13 in 48 three-part and 20 in 23 four-part fractures evidenced partial or complete osteonecrosis. The potential also exists for the dissection attendant on internal fixation to disrupt the vascular supply. The trauma necessary to produce these fractures and the injury incurred during surgical treatment can produce scarring and other anatomic changes that can adversely affect the natural history and surgical outcome of the avascular necrosis. The mechanism by which osteonecrosis is induced by corticosteroids is thought to involve alterations in fat metabolism, with fatty hypertrophy occurring in the marrow.[6] This results in vascular occlusion, and, ultimately, in avascular necrosis. An alternative theory involves the formation of fatty emboli from hyperlipidemia, which cause vascular occlusion and then osteonecrosis. Other agents of fatty hypertrophy, including alcoholism or an embolic phenomenon such as sickle cell disease, can result in osteonecrosis as well. The different pathways to osteonecrosis can run different courses and have varying influence on surgical outcomes.

CLASSIFICATION

Osteonecrosis of the humeral head is classified by Cruess with a staging system similar to that devised for the femoral head by Ficat and Arlet[6,10] (Fig. 36B–2). The appropriate stage is best determined by a complete set of shoulder radiographs, including 40-degree posterior oblique views in internal and external rotation as well as an axillary lateral view. Stage I is preradiographic, with the disease typically diagnosed on magnetic resonance imaging. Mottled sclerosis is present on the plain radiographs in stage II disease. The sclerosis is generally found in the subarticular segment of the superocentral humeral head, and the articular surface remains intact. Progression to fracture of the subchon-

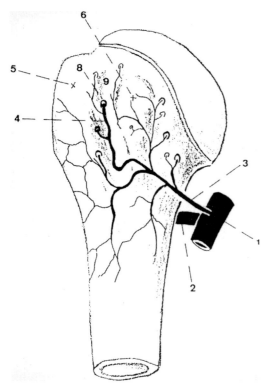

Figure 36B–1. Vascular supply to the humerus head. 1, axillary artery; 2, posterior humeral circumflex artery; 3, anterior humeral circumflex artery; 4, anterolateral ascending artery; 5, greater tuberosity; 6, lesser tuberosity; 8, entry point of the anterolateral branch into bone; 9, intertubercular groove. (From Gerber C, Hersche O, Berberat C: The clinical relevance of posttraumatic avascularnecrosis of the humeral head. J Shoulder Elbow Surg 7:586–590, 1998.)

dral bone is indicated by the presence of a crescent sign, which marks stage III disease. The articular surface may have mild flattening in this stage. Overt collapse and incongruity of the articular surface denotes stage IV, and stage V is found when secondary degenerative changes set in.

NATURAL HISTORY

The severity of the clinical course is dependent on the etiologic mechanism. The process appears to be particularly benign in sickle cell disease. Milner studied more than 2500 patients with sickle cell disease, finding an overall incidence of osteonecrosis in the humeral head of 5.6 percent.[18] The prevalence was age related, with an incidence of 2.7 percent in those patients younger than 25 years of age and increasing to 19.8 percent after age 35 years. Symptoms of pain and limitation of motion were found in just 21 percent of the study group, and only a single patient underwent replacement. David described a somewhat less favorable but still positive course in his series of 276 shoulders.[8] The incidence of osteonecrosis was 14.8 percent at an average age of 25 years, and only two joint replacements were reported.

Cruess, in 1976, described the outcome in 18 patients with steroid-induced osteonecrosis.[7] There were 8 patients who had minimal deformity and only mild symptoms. Six other patients had more extensive deformity and more substantial pain. These patients required limitation of activities. There were 5 shoulders in 4 patients that required humeral head replacement for severe pain. All had successful results.

L'Insalata and colleagues, in a series of 65 shoulders in 42 patients, also reported mixed results.[17] The most common etiology was steroid use, found in 52 shoulders. At an average of 2 years after initial presentation, 35 shoulders underwent replacement. The remaining 30 shoulders, treated nonoperatively, were reviewed at an average of 10 years. Fifteen shoulders had substantial symptoms and the other 15 were thought to have a satisfactory outcome. Thus, 10 years after diagnosis, the success rate was less than 1 of 4 patients. Poorer results were significantly related to more advanced disease (stage III or higher). A trend toward better results in shoulders with a steroid etiology was not statistically significant.

Gerber and colleagues have examined the issue of post-traumatic osteonecrosis.[12] At an average of 7.5 years after fracture, 25 shoulders were radiographically and clinically evaluated. Osteonecrosis was always associated with disability, but a significant relationship was found between outcome and anatomic reduction. Thirteen patients who had reduction within 2 mm were compared with 12 patients who had proximal humeral malunion. Subjective outcome, pain, and range of motion were all superior in patients with more anatomic reduction. The authors believed that the end result for shoulders with osteonecrosis was equivalent to that of humeral head replacement (HHR) for fracture treatment, provided anatomic reduction was initially obtained. Failure to achieve reduction increases the potential need for arthroplasty.

The experience at the Mayo Clinic recently examined several years ago.[13] In 151 patients with 200 affected shoulders, the most common etiologies were corticosteroid use in 112, trauma in 37, and unknown in 44. Ninety-seven shoulders required replacement at an average of 0.9 years after replacement. The need for arthroplasty was significantly more common with increased extent of head involvement, advancing stage of disease, and traumatic etiology (Fig. 36B–3). By 3 years after diagnosis, 77.8 percent of shoulders with traumatic osteonecrosis had been replaced compared with 43.7 percent of those with a steroid etiology. Of those shoulders not replaced, 60 were followed an average of 8.6 years. There was no pain to occasional moderate pain in 46, and moderate to severe pain in 14 patients. Motion in these shoulders was well preserved, with mean values of 153 degrees of flexion, 134 degrees of abduction, and 63 degrees of external rotation. The majority of patients were able to maintain basic activities of daily living such as toileting and dressing, but more advanced activities such as overhead lifting and sports were generally impossible.

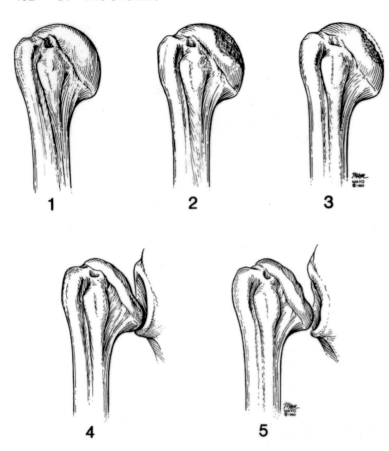

1   2   3

Figure 36B–2. The five stages of osteonecrosis of the proximal humerus as described by Cruess.[6] See text for detailed explanation.

4   5

TREATMENT OPTIONS

The favorable natural history for many patients makes it reasonable initially to treat patients conservatively, especially in steroid-induced osteonecrosis. Analgesic medication, activity modification, and gentle physical modalities are appropriate. Many patients have relatively mild symptoms and prolonged function of the shoulder, even in more advanced stages of disease. However, if conservative methods are unsuccessful, shoulder replacement is indicated (Figs. 36B–4 and 36B–5). In stage III disease, radiographic findings may be subtle, but symptoms may be severe and may be relieved only by arthroplasty. Careful scrutiny of radiographic studies is essential. The crescent sign indicative of subchondral collapse and a cartilage flap detached from the underlying necrotic bone may be evident on only a single radiographic view or on computed tomography. With more extensive head involvement, advanced stage of disease, and a history of trauma, the prognosis becomes poorer and the threshold to proceeding to replacement lower.

The most common contraindications to replacement are active infection and the combination of rotator cuff and deltoid loss. Infection can be extremely subtle, and the possibility must be considered whenever there has been prior surgery, especially if there has been a recent and failed procedure. Depending on the clinical circumstances, evaluation may include erythrocyte sedimentation rate and C-reactive protein levels, indium-111 scanning, and joint aspiration. The ultimate diagnosis

may await intraoperative histology reports and cultures. The combination of deltoid loss with an irreparable rotator cuff is an indication for consideration of arthrodesis. Prosthetic replacement in this situation is not practical.

A more challenging decision arises with a younger patient. Because of the incidence of trauma, the use of steroids for many medical disorders, and the prevalence of other related problems, such as alcoholism, osteonecrosis frequently occurs earlier in life than degenerative problems. In patients seen at the Mayo Clinic for osteonecrosis between 1981 and 1991, the average age was 57 years and ranged from 21 to 84 years.[13] Youth is not an absolute contraindication for arthroplasty, but careful consideration must be given to the patient's situation and expectations. The patient needs to be aware of the long-term consequences of replacement, the importance of activity restrictions, and the potential, or even probability, of revision surgery. To avoid the stresses on a glenoid component, HHR may need to be considered over total shoulder arthroplasty (TSA) in individuals who cannot adequately restrict their activities because of their livelihood and poor work alternatives. Arthrodesis remains a poor treatment option because it provides power only at low angles of elevation.

Some authors have suggested core decompression as an option for earlier stages of the disease. The literature is mixed and limited concerning this procedure. Neer had poor results with core decompression and bone grafting in 2 patients.[20] L'Insalata similarly had uniformly poor results in 5 shoulders.[17] Four shoulders had stage III disease and the fifth was unspecified. Replacement was necessary for all patients. Mont and associates described more extensive experience in a series of 30 shoulders.[19] Using the University of California, Los Angeles score, all

14 shoulders with stage I or II disease had excellent or good outcomes. Of the 10 shoulders with stage III disease, 7 had excellent and 3 had poor outcomes. Their experience needs to be weighed against the frequently benign natural history of osteonecrosis.

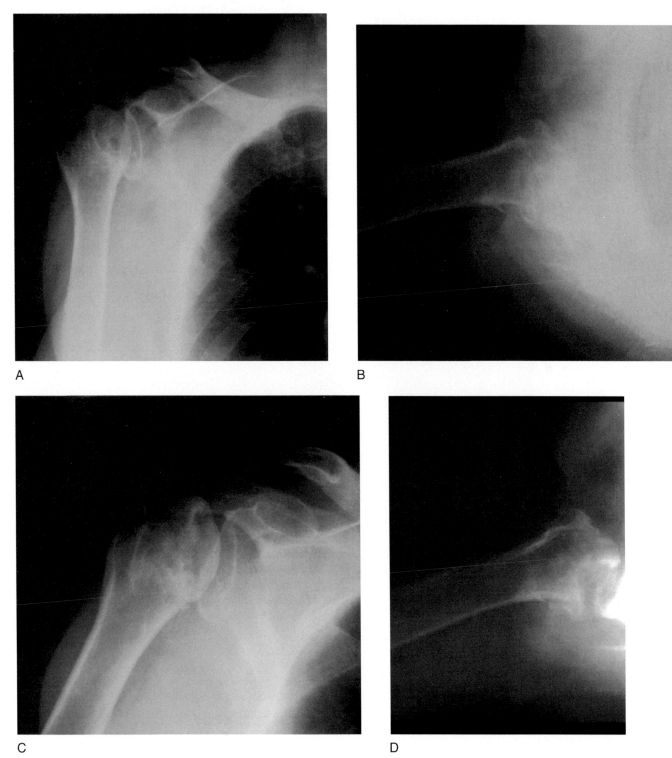

A

B

C

D

Figure 36B–3. A–D, This patient had an initial evaluation of shoulder pain on 11/12/86. Radiographs revealed a large area of stage II osteonecrosis (see **A** and **B**). Conservative treatment was elected, but the patient, less than a year later, had worsening pain. Repeat radiographs revealed collapse of the articular surface and stage IV disease (**C** and **D**).

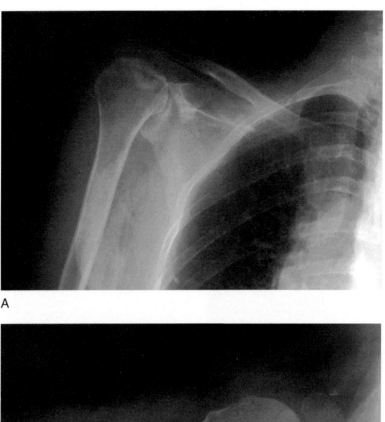

A

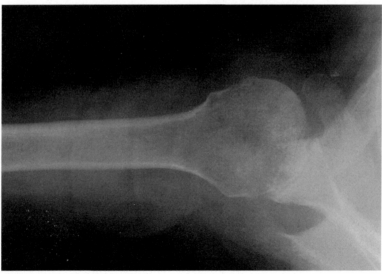

B

Figure 36B–4. A–D, This 71-year-old patient suffered from long-standing chronic obstructive pulmonary disease, with prior steroid treatment. Preoperative radiographs revealed joint space narrowing, superior subluxation of the humeral head, superior glenoid erosion, and osteonecrosis of the humeral head (**A** and **B**).

Illustration continued on opposite page

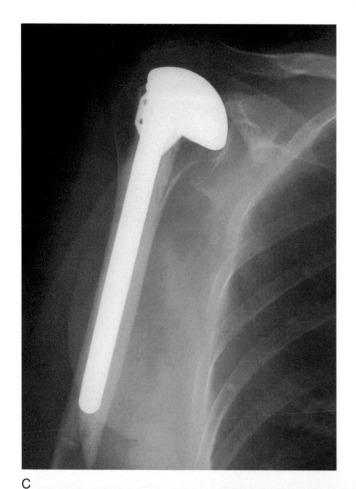

C

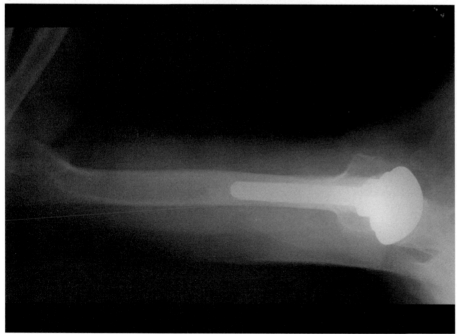

D

Figure 36B–4. *Continued.* Because of substantial rotator cuff damage, humeral head replacement was elected for reconstruction (**C** and **D**).

RESULTS OF REPLACEMENT

Often, the outcome of replacement for osteonecrosis is hidden in the results for more common disorders such as osteoarthritis and traumatic arthritis. However, a number of authors have written of their results, gener-ally reporting a limited number of cases. In 47 cases scat-tered through nine articles, pain relief was near uniform and range of motion varied from two thirds to nearly normal.[1–4,7,9,15,21,24] Rutherford and Cofield evaluated 17 shoulders at follow-up of 2 to 6.5 years.[22] HHR was per-formed in 11 shoulders and TSA in 6 shoulders. Pain relief was nearly uniform at 94 percent. Range of motion was similarly excellent, with active abduction of 161 degrees in HHR and 150 degrees after TSA.

In a more extensive study, the results of replacement for osteonecrosis at the Mayo Clinic were reported.[14] In 114 patients, 71 HHRs and 56 TSAs were performed over the study period of 1974 to 1992. Thirty-six shoulders were lost to follow-up because of the death of the patients, and an additional 3 patients declined study participation. At average follow-up of almost 9 years,

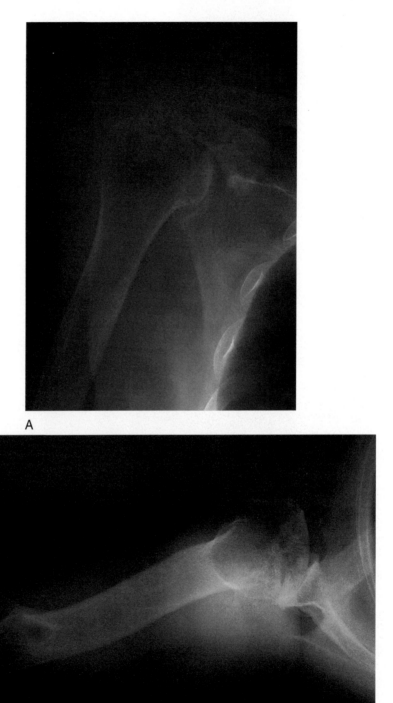

A

B

Figure 36B–5. A–D, This is another example of osteonecrosis complicating chronic pulmonary disease after treatment with steroids in a 71-year-old woman (**A** and **B**). In this situation, the rotator cuff was sufficiently intact to allow glenoid resurfacing during reconstruction (**C** and **D**).

Illustration continued on opposite page

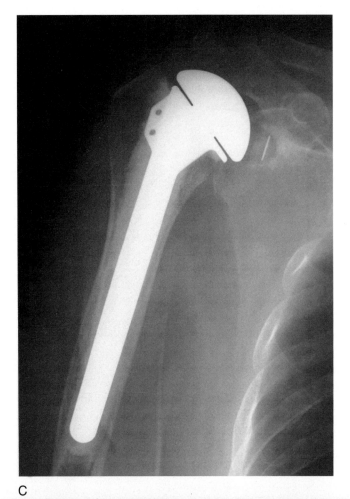

C

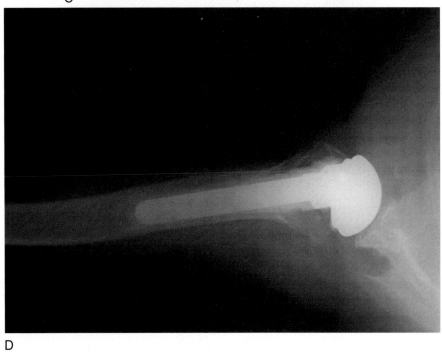

D

Figure 36B–5. *Continued.*

subjective improvement was expressed for 70 of the remaining 88 shoulders (79.5 percent) and no pain to occasional moderate pain in 68 (77.3 percent). The American Shoulder and Elbow Surgeon (ASES) score was used for evaluation, with mean outcome of 63. A substantial difference in results became evident when the outcome was evaluated by etiology. Inferior results in both range of motion and ASES score were found in post-traumatic osteonecrosis, with improved outcome in patients with a steroid-induced disease. The mean ASES score in shoulders with a steroid etiology was 69 compared with 55 in those with post-traumatic disease. A similar difference in range of motion was evident, with mean flexion of 138 degrees and external rotation of 66 degrees in steroid-induced disease versus 107 degrees flexion and 49 degrees external rotation in traumatic osteonecrosis. These differences were statistically significant. Reconstruction in post-traumatic osteonecrosis can be complicated by the sequelae of the fracture injury and possible internal fixation, including scarring and stiffness of the rotator cuff and bony deformity. In other causes of osteonecrosis, the rotator cuff and capsule are essentially normal until late in the process when secondary degenerative changes develop.

In this series, each physician chose glenoid resurfacing after evaluation of the degree of pathologic involvement. There was no randomization. Little variation was discovered in the outcomes of HHR and TSA. Mean ASES scores were 63 after HHR and 62 after TSA. Range of motion likewise differed minimally. Interestingly, though, there was a tendency for the patients' assessment of their condition to be downgraded after HHR. Almost 14 percent of patients complained they were worse after HHR compared with a single patient (2.8 percent) after TSA. It remains our practice to resurface the glenoid if there is any significant articular cartilage damage.

SUMMARY

Numerous etiologic agents can result in a common disorder of the shoulder, which is osteonecrosis. These agents have differing clinical courses, which is particularly benign in sickle cell disease, moderate in steroid-induced disease, and poor in post-trauma osteonecrosis. There is a similar difference in the outcome from arthroplasty, with substantially better clinical scores and range of motion found in reconstruction for steroid-induced disease compared with those who have post-traumatic disorders. Most patients in all diagnostic groups had lessening of their pain. HHR is chosen over TSA when the articular cartilage is well preserved on the glenoid.

References

1. Amstutz HC, Thomas BJ, Kabo JM, et al: The DANA total shoulder arthroplasty. J Bone Joint Surg 70A:1174–1182, 1988.
2. Bade HA, Warren RF, Ranawat CS, Inglis AE: Long term results of Neer total shoulder replacement. *In* Bateman JE, Welsh RP (eds): Surgery of the Shoulder. Philadelphia, BC Decker, 1984, p 294.
3. Boyd AD, Aliabadi P, Thornhill TS: Postoperative proximal migration in total shoulder arthroplasty. Incidence and significance. J Arthroplasty 6:31–37, 1991.
4. Boyd AD, Thomas WH, Scott RD, et al: Total shoulder arthroplasty versus hemiarthroplasty. Indications for glenoid resurfacing. J Arthroplasty 5:329–336, 1990.
5. Brooks CH, Revell WJ, Heatley FW: Vascularity of the humeral head after proximal humeral fractures. J Bone Joint Surg 73B:132–136, 1993.
6. Cruess RL: Experience with steroid-induced avascular necrosis of the shoulder and etiologic considerations regarding osteonecrosis of the hip. Clin Orthop 130:86–93, 1978
7. Cruess RL: Steroid-induced avascular necrosis of the head of the humerus. Natural history and management. J Bone Joint Surg 58B:313–317, 1976.
8. David HG, Bridgman SA, Davies SG, et al: The shoulder in sickle-cell disease. J Bone Joint Surg 75B:538–545, 1993.
9. Dines DM, Warren RF, Altcheck DW, Moeckel B: Post-traumatic changes of the proximal humerus: Malunion, nonunion, and osteonecrosis. Treatment with modular hemiarthroplasty or total shoulder arthroplasty. J Shoulder Elbow Surg 2:11–21, 1993.
10. Ficat RP: Idiopathic bone necrosis of the femoral head. Early diagnosis and treatment. J Bone Joint Surg 67B:3–9, 1985.
11. Gerber C: The arterial vascularization of the humeral head. J Bone Joint Surg 72A:1486–1494, 1990.
12. Gerber C, Hersche O, Berberat C: The clinical relevance of post-traumatic avascular necrosis of the humeral head. J Shoulder Elbow Surg 7:586–590, 1998.
13. Hattrup SJ, Cofield RH: Osteonecrosis of the humeral head: Relationship of disease stage, extent, and cause to natural history. J Shoulder Elbow Surg 8:559–564, 1999.
14. Hattrup SJ, Cofield RH: Osteonecrosis of the humeral head: Results of replacement. J Shoulder Elbow Surg 9:177–182, 2000.
15. Kay SP, Amstutz HC: Shoulder hemiarthroplasty at UCLA. Clin Orthop 228:42–8, 1988
16. Laing PG: The arterial supply of the adult humerus. J Bone Joint Surg 38A:1105–1116, 1956.
17. L'Insalata JC, Pagnani MJ, Warren RF, Dines DM: Humeral head osteonecrosis: Clinical course and radiographic predictors of outcome. J Shoulder Elbow Surg 5:355–361, 1996.
18. Milner PF, Kraus AP, Sebes JI, et al: Osteonecrosis of the humeral head in sickle cell disease. Clin Orthop 289:136–143, 1993.
19. Mont MA, Maar DC, Urquhart MW, et al: Avascular necrosis of the humeral head treated by core decompression. J Bone Joint Surg 75B:785–788, 1993.
20. Neer CS II: Shoulder Reconstruction. Philadelphia, WB Saunders Co, 1990.
21. Neer CS II, Watson KC, Stanton FJ: Recent experience in total shoulder replacement. J Bone Joint Surg 64A:319–337, 1982.
22. Rutherford CS, Cofield RH: Osteonecrosis of the shoulder [abstract]. Orthop Transpl 11:239, 1987.
23. Schai P, Imhoff A, Preiss S: Comminuted humeral head fractures: A multicenter study. J Shoulder Elbow Surg 4:319–330, 1995.
24. Warren RF, Ranawat CS, Inglis AE: Total shoulder replacement. Indications and results of the Neer nonconstrained prosthesis. *In* Inglis AE (ed): American Academy of Orthopedic Surgeons Symposium: Total Joint Replacement of the Upper Extremity. St. Louis, CV Mosby, 1982, p 56.

36C

Shoulder Arthroplasty for Cuff-tear Arthropathy

• JOAQUIN SANCHEZ-SOTELO

Cuff-tear arthropathy was first described in detail by Neer[11] in 1983 as a clinical entity consisting of severe disorganization of the glenohumeral joint after some massive tears of the rotator cuff. Two years before, McCarthy and co-workers had reported similar pathologic changes under the term "Milwaukee shoulder."[10] They had hypothesized that the bone and soft tissue destruction resulted from the production of basic calcium phosphate crystals and that the associated release of proteases into the joint occurred as in other crystal-induced arthritides. Cuff-tear arthropathy and the Milwaukee shoulder possibly are a single pathologic entity whose etiology has not been completely elucidated.

Rotator cuff-tear arthropathy (RCTA) should be distinguished from other conditions that may combine degenerative changes of the glenohumeral joint and a tear of the rotator cuff. The diagnosis of RCTA requires the association of a massive and irreparable rotator cuff tear with glenohumeral cartilage loss and progressive bone loss of the humeral head, the glenoid, and either the coracoacromial arch or the distal clavicle, or both.

CLINICAL PRESENTATION

Patients with RCTA are typically elderly and have a history of long-standing shoulder pain, decreased active motion, and limited function.[1,11,15,16] Some complain of recurrent episodes of shoulder swelling.[11,15] They have commonly received multiple corticosteroid injections and may have undergone one or more operations, most frequently acromioplasty and rotator cuff débridement or repair.[1,15,16]

Physical examination usually reveals swelling of the shoulder involving the subacromial bursa and glenohumeral joint as well as atrophy in the supraspinous and infraspinous fossae. Glenohumeral motion may be accompanied by crepitus and is usually painful. Active and passive ranges of motion are decreased and there is weakness, especially in abduction and external rotation. The status of the deltoid muscle should be evaluated,

especially in patients with a history of prior surgery; deltoid weakness may severely compromise the function of shoulder arthroplasty. Anterosuperior glenohumeral instability is also common in severely affected shoulders.

The radiographic findings in RCTA are characteristic (Fig. 36C–1**A**). In addition to the glenohumeral joint space narrowing present in other forms of shoulder arthritis, the humeral head migrates superiorly to contact the coracoacromial arch. There are variable degrees of bone loss secondary to erosion of the acromion, the distal clavicle, and the glenoid and coracoid process. The humeral head may collapse, and the inferior rim of the glenoid may create a humeral notch medially. RCTA should be distinguished from inflammatory arthritis, infections, old post-traumatic arthritis, avascular necrosis, metabolic diseases, and neuropathic arthropathy.[11] If alternative diagnoses can be excluded, no further laboratory or imaging studies are necessary.

TREATMENT OPTIONS

When conservative treatment fails to control patient symptoms, several surgical options have been proposed. Arthroscopic débridement may improve some patients temporarily.[4] Glenohumeral arthrodesis may be considered for patients who have a nonfunctional deltoid muscle.[2] Constrained and semiconstrained total shoulder arthroplasties have been accompanied in the past by high rates of mechanical failure,[14] and nonconstrained total shoulder arthroplasty has been associated with a substantial rate of glenoid component failure.[3,9] The "Delta" or "reversed prosthesis" (Johnson and Johnson), specifically designed for a shoulder with a deficient cuff, has renewed interest in the use of more constrained implants in RCTA.[7] In this design, the articular surface of the humeral component is concave to articulate with a convex glenoid articular surface. Good functional results and substantial improvement in active range of motion have been reported in Europe with use of the Delta prosthesis. However, longer follow-up is needed to determine whether this particular design is more durable than other constrained prosthesis used previously. I have no personal experience with the use of this implant. For all these reasons, at the present time, I consider shoulder hemiarthroplasty the procedure of choice for patients with RCTA and adequate deltoid function.[1,13,14,16]

TECHNICAL ASPECTS OF SHOULDER HEMIARTHROPLASTY FOR RCTA

The main challenges of shoulder hemiarthroplasty for this condition are to improve range of motion and to achieve a well-balanced and stable reconstruction. The shoulder is approached through the deltopectoral interval. The subdeltoid bursa is incised vertically from the inferior edge of the coracoacromial ligament distalward, lateral to the conjoined tendons. The fibrous tissue adjacent to the coracoacromial ligament at the upper portion of the subscapularis tendon is left intact. When passive external rotation is greater than 30 degrees, any remaining subscapularis is incised through tendon; otherwise, it is released from the humerus. The anteroinferior shoulder capsule is released from the humerus, and the humeral head is dislocated forward. The humeral head is resected in 35 degrees of retroversion at the level of the previous insertion site of the supraspinatus tendon.

The glenoid may not require any specific preparation, but, occasionally, it is smoothed or reshaped with the use of a bur or reamer. Some authors have recommended the use of small heads to decrease tension on any repaired cuff tissue; others use large heads, thinking that a larger head may provide more joint stability. I have found that, generally, a medium-sized head fits best (see Fig. 36C–1B). Small heads tend to be unstable, and very large heads overstuff the joint.

Postoperatively, the limb is placed in a shoulder immobilizer that is used during the daytime and at night for 1 month. Passive range of motion exercises are started the day after surgery, with elevation limited to 120 degrees and external rotation to 20 degrees. Pulley exercises for flexion, self-assisted wand exercises, and isometrics are started after 5 to 6 weeks. Elastic strap strengthening is added at 8 to 10 weeks after surgery.

RESULTS

The results of shoulder hemiarthroplasty at the Mayo Clinic in a series of 33 shoulders followed for an average of 5 years (range, 2 to 11 years) have been reviewed. The average age of the patients at the time of surgery was 69 years (range, 50 to 87 years), and 11 shoulders had undergone between one and four previous procedures, including an acromioplasty in 8 of them.

Shoulder hemiarthroplasty was significantly associated with pain relief. However, at the most recent evaluation, 9 patients (27 percent) had moderate pain at rest or pain with activity. Mean active elevation improved from 72 to 91 degrees (P=0.008), mean internal rotation

improved from L3 to L1 (P=0.02), and mean active external rotation improved from 36 to 41 degrees (not significant). Strength improved significantly only in external rotation. Using Neer[12] limited goals criteria, successful results were achieved in 22 cases (67 percent). However,

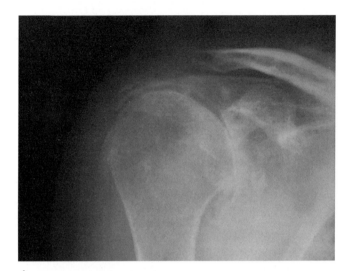

A

B

Figure 36C–1. A, Preoperative radiograph of a 76-year-old patient with rotator cuff-tear arthropathy of the right shoulder. Note the superiorly migrated humeral head with erosion of the undersurface of the acromion. **B,** Radiographic evaluation of the same patient 2 years after shoulder hemiarthroplasty shows a stable reconstruction with no further bone loss.

most patients were satisfied with the outcome of the surgery and only 4 shoulders were subjectively considered to be the same or worse than before the operation. Two factors were associated with a less satisfactory outcome: prior subacromial decompression and the extent of proximal migration of the humeral head.

At the most recent radiographic evaluation, progression of anterior or superior subluxation was appreciated in 9 of the 31 cases that had complete radiographic follow-up. Eight shoulders had progressive superior erosion of the glenoid, 14 had progressive erosion of the acromion, and 2 developed an acromial fracture (Fig. 36C–2). In addition, 8 shoulders developed notching of the medial aspect of the proximal humerus at the level of the inferior rim of the glenoid. None of the components was considered to be radiographically loose or was revised. With the numbers available, neither the humeral head size used nor progression of bone loss were found to influence the outcome of surgery.

Table 36C–1 summarizes the Mayo Clinic results as well as those reported by other authors. The percentage of patients with no pain or mild pain at most recent follow-up after hemiarthroplasty has ranged from 47 percent to 86 percent, although subjective satisfaction has been generally higher.[1,5,15,16] Shoulder hemiarthroplasty has also provided moderate gains in motion and strength. The main complications observed have included instability and symptomatic glenoid erosion.[6,9]

In my experience, shoulder hemiarthroplasty provides marked pain relief in about three quarters of the patients with RCTA and modest improvements in range of motion and strength. Persistent pain, anterosuperior instability, and progressive bone loss may complicate the procedure. A less satisfactory outcome should be expected in patients with prior violation of the coracoacromial arch. The use of either small humeral head sizes in an attempt to facilitate reconstruction of the cuff or large sizes to maximize joint stability does not seem to be justified. Although shoulder hemiarthroplasty is not a perfect answer for patients with RCTA, it probably represents the best available reconstructive option for this difficult problem at the present time.

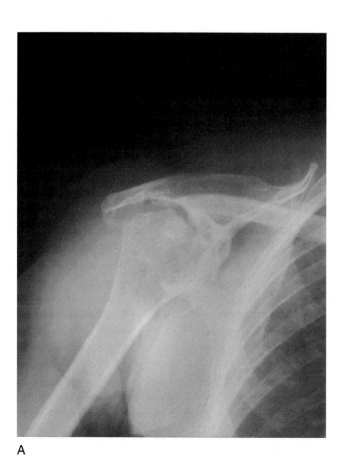

A

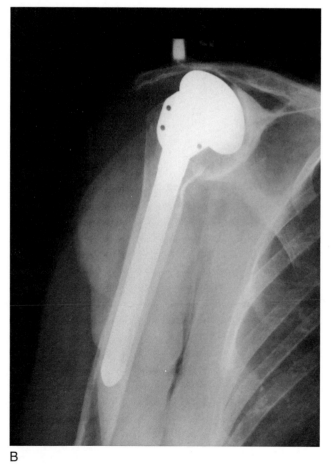

B

Figure 36C–2. **A**, Preoperative radiograph of an 87-year-old patient with RCTA. **B**, Radiograph taken 3 years after hemiarthroplasty demonstrates bone loss at the superior aspect of the glenoid and of the undersurfaces of the distal clavicle and acromion.

Table 36C-1.   REPORTED RESULTS OF SHOULDER HEMIARTHROPLASTY FOR RCTA

Study	N	Age Mean (range)	Follow-up Yr Mean (range)	No Pain or Mild Postoperative pain (percent)	Active Elevation Preoperative/Postoperative Degrees Mean (range)	Successful Results*	Comments
Arntz et al.[1] (1993)	18	71 (54–84)	3 (2–10)†	11 (61)	66 (44–90) / 112 (70–160)	NR	Two reoperations for symptomatic glenoid erosion, 1 for symptomatic instability and 1 for postoperative traumatic fracture of the acromion.
Williams and Rockwood[15] (1996)	21	72 (59–80)	4 (2–7)	18 (86)	70 (0–155) / 120 (15–160)	18 (86 percent)	No cases of instability or reoperation were reported.
Field et al.[5] (1997)	16	74 (62–83)	3 (2–5)	13 (81)	60 (40–80) / 100 (80–130)	10 (62 percent)	There was 1 intraoperative humeral shaft fracture. Four cases of instability, 2 of requiring reoperation for subscapularis advancement (1 case) and resection arthroplasty (1 case).
Zuckerman et al.[16] (2000)	15	73 (65–81)	2 (1–5)	7 (47)	69 (20–140) / 86 (45–140)	NR	Eleven patients (87 percent) were satisfied with the operation. There was 1 case of anterior instability.
Mayo Clinic series	33	69 (50–87)	5 (2–11)	24 (73)	72 (30–150) / 91 (40–165)	22 (67 percent)	One intraoperative humeral shaft fracture. Seven cases of anterosuperior instability.

Data from references 1, 5, and 16.
* According to Neer's limited goals criteria.[10]
† For shoulders not revised.
N = number of shoulders with rotator cuff-tear arthropathy; NR = not reported.

References

1. Arntz CT, Jackins S, Matsen FA: Prosthetic replacement of the shoulder for the treatment of defects in the rotator cuff and the surface of the glenohumeral joint. J Bone Joint Surg 75A:485–491, 1993.
2. Arntz CT, Matsen FA, Jackins S: Surgical management of complex irreparable rotator cuff deficiency. J Arthroplasty 6:363–370, 1991.
3. Brownlee RC, Cofield RH: Shoulder replacement in cuff tear arthropathy. Orthop Transpl 10:230, 1986.
4. Ellman H, Kay SP, Wirth M: Arthroscopic treatment of full-thickness rotator cuff tears: 2- to 7-year follow-up study. Arthroscopy 9: 195–200, 1993.
5. Field LD, Dines DM, Zabinski SJ, Warren RF: Hemiarthroplasty of the shoulder for rotator cuff arthropathy. J Shoulder Elbow Surg 6:18–23, 1997.
6. Franklin J, Barret W, Jackins SE, Matsen FA: Glenoid loosening in total shoulder arthroplasty. Association with rotator cuff deficiency. J Arthroplasty 3:39–46, 1988.
7. Grammont PM, Baulot E: Delta shoulder prosthesis for rotator cuff rupture. Orthopedics 16:65–68, 1993.
8. Laurence M: Replacement arthroplasty of the rotator cuff deficient shoulder. J Bone Joint Surg 73B: 916–919, 1991.
9. Lohr JF, Cofield RH, Uhthoff HK: Glenoid component loosening in cuff tear arthropathy. J Bone Joint Surg 73B(Suppl II):106, 1991.
10. McCarthy DJ, Halverson PB, et al: "Milwaukee shoulder"—association of microspheroids containing hydroxyapatite crystals, active collagenase, and neutral protease with rotator cuff defects. I. Clinical aspects. Arthritis Rheum 24:464–473, 1981.
11. Neer CS, Craig EV, Fukuda H: Cuff-tear arthropathy. J Bone Joint Surg 65A:1232–1244, 1983.
12. Neer CS, Watson KC, Stanton FJ: Recent experience in total shoulder replacement. J Bone Joint Surg 64A:319–337, 1982.
13. Pollock RG, Deliz ED, McIlveen SJ, et al: Prosthetic replacement in rotator cuff-deficient shoulders. J Shoulder Elbow Surg 1:173–186, 1992.
14. Post M, Haskell SS, Jablon M: Total soulder replacement with a constrained prosthesis. J Bone Joint Surg 62A:327–335, 1980.
15. Williams GR, Rockwood CA: Hemiarthroplasty in rotator cuff-deficient shoulders. J Shoulder Elbow Surg 5:362–367, 1996.
16. Zuckerman JD, Scott AJ, Gallagher MA: Hemiarthroplasty for cuff tear arthropathy. J Shoulder Elbow Surg 9:169–172, 2000.

36D

Rotator Cuff Deficiency

• STEVEN J. HATTRUP

Rotator cuff deficiency, is diagnosis related. It is distinctly uncommon in osteoarthritis and, when present, tends to be small.[5,10,15,16] Neer pointed out that in osteoarthritis, "the forces necessary to generate this type of wear logically require the rotator cuff to be intact."[9] In a consecutive series of 273 total shoulder arthroplasties, he noted that the rotator cuff was intact in 59 of 62 shoulders with osteoarthritis. It was torn only in 3 all were paraplegic patients who used their shoulder in a weight-bearing manner. Cofield noted similar findings in his series at the Mayo Clinic.[5] He found the incidence of rotator cuff tearing was 6 in 53 (11 percent) shoulders with osteoarthritis. Walch, in a study evaluating 84 shoulders with osteoarthritis by arthrograms, found tearing of the supraspinatus tendon in 10 percent and extension into the infraspinatus in only 2.6 percent.[16] In comparison, shoulders with rheumatoid arthritis typically do suffer from damage to the rotator cuff consisting of tearing or attenuation, or both.[5,7,9,15] Neer found that attenuation of the rotator cuff was generally present and complete tearing was found in 29 of 69 shoulders.[9] Cofield reported thinning of the cuff in 37 of 66 shoulders and tears in 18 (27 percent).[5] Friedman determined the rotator cuff was normal in only 25 percent of 24 shoulders and Walch noted complete tearing in 40 percent.[2,16] The status of the rotator cuff in turn influences the method and results of reconstructive surgery.[4,8,15,16]

In the 46 shoulders with osteoarthritis replaced by Walch and Boileau, all 4 tears found were considered minor and easily managed.[15] Cofield reported 4 small and 2 medium tears in 53 shoulders with osteoarthritis.[5] Of the overall series of 176 shoulders, 48 had rotator cuff tearing. Thirty-one of the 48 tears were reparable with standard techniques involving direct suture to tendon or bone in 14 cases and adjunctive subscapularis transposition in an additional 17 shoulders. Fourteen of the remaining 17 shoulders had the massive tearing associated with cuff tear arthropathy. Thus, Cofield's experience suggests that, with the exception of cuff tear arthropathy, when rotator cuff tearing is encountered during the course of arthroplasty, it is typically a reparable lesion. In contrast, the inflammatory process in the rheumatoid shoulder produces damage to the rotator cuff of thinning and secondary dysfunction as well as cuff tearing. This is commonly recognized on radiographs by superior migration of humeral head with respect to the glenoid. However, Boyd has shown in the replaced shoulder that factors other than rotator cuff tearing can produce superior subluxation of the humeral head.[2] These include dynamic imbalance between a strong deltoid and an attenuated rotator cuff, a superior facing glenoid, and a proud humeral component. An attenuated and dysfunctional rotator cuff is not a reparable lesion. It is, therefore, worthwhile to preserve the coracoacromial ligament routinely in reconstruction of the rheumatoid shoulder to reduce the risk of superior instability of the replacement.

Intuitively, one would anticipate the status of the rotator cuff to be important to the outcome of shoulder arthroplasty. Cofield wrote in 1984 that postoperative range of motion was clearly related to the condition of the rotator cuff at the time of surgery.[4] He found that the average abduction after surgery was 143 degrees with a normal rotator cuff, compared with 102 degrees if it was thin, and only 63 degrees if a major repair was necessary. Similarly, Hawkins found that although pain relief was not affected by rotator cuff repair, range of motion was.[8] Average forward flexion was 88 degrees with repair versus 120 degrees if repair was not necessary. A few surgeons have thought that the actual integrity of the rotator cuff was not highly significant.[3,7] Friedman analyzed the results in 24 total shoulder arthroplasties in 1989.[7] He found motion, pain relief, and function no better in patients with an intact rotator cuff. Likewise, Boyd found the presence of a major rotator cuff tear was not associated with a significant reduction in the average postoperative range of motion.[3] Yet both Friedman and Boyd dealt with either an exclusively or primarily rheumatoid population. There are a number of issues that interfere with the outcome of arthroplasty in the rheumatoid shoulder in addition to cuff tearing.[6] These include general debility, poor quality of the soft tissue, deficient muscle strength, and poor bone stock. It thus becomes more difficult to isolate the influence from purely the rotator cuff tear.

Figgie and Rozing separately looked at the issue of the quality of the tendon tissue and resultant repair of the rotator cuff in cases of inflammatory arthritis.[6,11] Figgie classified the status of the rotator cuff into 3 groups.[6,11] Group I, with 6 shoulders, included shoulders with either allograft repair or marked fibrosis. Group II consisted of 30 shoulders with attenuated cuffs or reparable tears. The 14 shoulders with normal cuffs constituted group III. Outcome was significantly related to the status of the rotator cuff as evaluated by the Department of Health and Human Services (HHS) score. The scores were 65 for group I, 84 for group II, and 95 for group III. Rozing studied 40 shoulders, all involved with rheumatoid arthritis.[11] After evaluating the results with the HHS score, he found that there were statistically significant higher scores with improved status of the cuff. The HHS scores were superior in shoulders with intact cuffs compared with shoulders with a good repair of torn tendon, and in turn those scores were better than those in shoulders with an insufficient or incomplete repair. In addition, Rozing found that the HHS scores in shoulders with a good repair continued to improve over time, whereas shoulders with an insufficient repair or irreparable lesion plateaued at 6 to 12 months and remained static.

The status of the rotator cuff has important long-term implications for the survival of the replacement as well. Sperling found there was a substantially increased risk of revision of shoulder arthroplasty if there was a rotator cuff tear present at the time of the primary procedure.[13] The influence of the incompetent rotator cuff on the durability of the glenoid component has been well recognized. Stewart found that all the patients with loose components in his series had a thinned or torn rotator cuff.[14] With a similar experience, Barrett suggested that the mechanism related to superior subluxation of the humeral head secondary to the cuff deficiency.[1] This produced eccentric loading on the glenoid and ultimately resulted in loosening. Søjbjerg showed that the degree of proximal humeral migration was related to the preoperative status of the rotator cuff, and glenoid loosening in turn was associated with the resultant eccentric loading.[12] It seems clear that the status of the rotator cuff has important implications for the outcome of a shoulder arthroplasty, and every attempt should be made to achieve a secure repair.

Preoperative radiographic evaluation of the shoulder invariably includes plain radiographs. As noted earlier, there can be superior subluxation of the humeral head with respect to the glenoid and narrowing of the acromiohumeral distance in shoulders with rotator cuff tearing. These findings are also frequent in shoulders with rheumatoid arthritis in which the rotator cuff is attenuated and not torn. However, they can be found in shoulders with osteoarthritis as well, and these findings may be misleading. The axillary lateral in these situations often indicates posterior glenoid erosion with subsequent posterior glenohumeral subluxation. The incongruency in the joint may falsely suggest the presence of rotator cuff tear. Because rotator cuff problems are uncommon and typically small enough in osteoarthritis as not to be an issue, preoperative evaluation with magnetic resonance imaging is not routinely indicated. It is more commonly reserved for special circumstances such as prior cuff surgery, trauma to the proximal humerus and tuberosities, and, perhaps, in rheumatoid arthritis.

The surgical technique involved in addressing rotator cuff tears entails a combination of the standard methods used in shoulder replacement and tendon repair procedures. Even if a cuff tear is known or suspected, the same initial deltopectoral approach is used. In disease processes such as rheumatoid arthritis, in which rotator cuff damage is anticipated, the coracoacromial arch and ligament should be preserved. The anterior capsule and subscapularis are taken down together unless an extreme internal rotation contracture or prior subscapularis shortening is present. Lengthening via a Z-plasty then is necessary (Fig. 36D–1). Superiorly, the arthrotomy is directed into the cuff defect. This allows the possibility of transposing the subscapularis superiorly into the tear for better coverage (Fig. 36D–2). A routine osteotomy can be performed, but if a tear is known or discovered, a more aggressive humeral cut should be considered. In combination with the choice of a smaller humeral head, removal of more bone diminishes the volume of the glenohumeral joint to be covered. In electing a more a distal osteotomy, though, it is essential to avoid transecting the cuff attachment, especially posteriorly, where exposure may be limited. In every arthroplasty, it is important to carefully inspect the rotator cuff after the osteotomy. This is the best time to define the extent of any cuff tearing. If a small tear in the supraspinatus tendon is present, this can be handled simply by creating an appropriate bony bed along the greater tuberosity and prepositioning sutures through the tuberosity. The repair can then be easily accomplished after component selection and insertion. On the other hand, if a more substantial tear is identified superiorly or posteriorly, better exposure becomes necessary. This is provided by developing a lateral skin flap and by creating a deltoid splitting incision off the anterolateral acromion edge. The same excellent exposure familiar to any experienced shoulder surgeon is then available, and standard techniques are used for tendon mobilization and repair.

After the margins of the tear are delineated, the flexibility and quality of the tendon substance are evaluated. In combination with the security of the repair, these factors determine the aggressiveness of the rehabilitation program. As in any repair, the tendons are mobilized to minimize tension across the suture line. All bursal adhesions are resected extra-articularly, and the coracohumeral ligament is released. It can be difficult on occasion to differentiate thickened bursa from attenuated tendon substance. The key is to follow the tendon down to its insertion on the tuberosity. Intra-articularly, the tendons can be tethered along the glenoid margin. Anteriorly, the subscapularis is freed by creation of a Bankart type of lesion. A finger, or Darrach, retractor can be slid medially on the glenoid neck to finish the mobilization. This does not lead to anterior instability as in

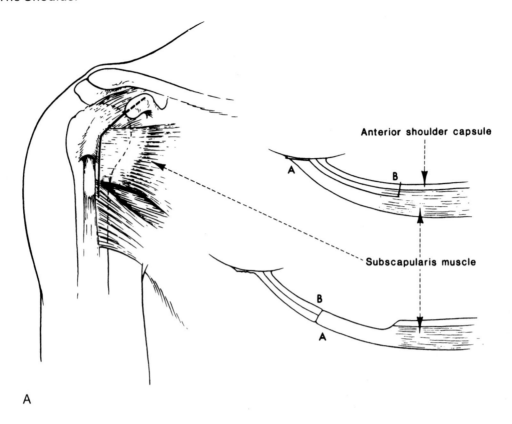

A

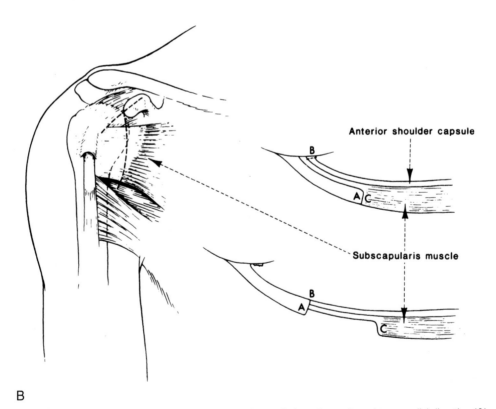

B

Figure 36D–1. Z-lengthening of the subscapularis tendon can be carried out from a lateral to a medial direction (**A**) or from a medial to a lateral direction (**B**).

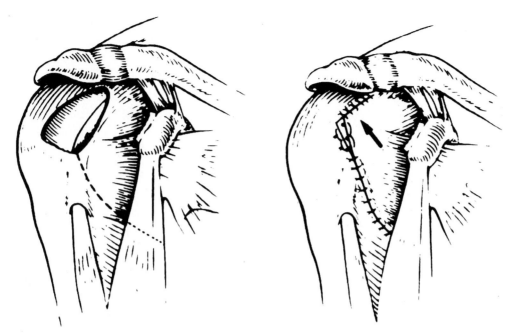

Figure 36D–2. The subscapularis can be transposed superiorly into a cuff defect to aid in closure.

the youthful shoulder. Rather, it allows the ability to advance the subscapularis laterally and superiorly as necessary. At times the subscapularis is best repositioned medially along the humeral osteotomy. This eases the repair but tends to cause weakness in internal rotation and a positive liftoff sign. Depending on the tear pattern, the capsular release along the glenoid margin can be extended superiorly and posteriorly as needed (Figs. 36D–3 and 36D–4). Once the cuff is mobilized to the extent possible, the ability to accomplish a repair is assessed and a decision on glenoid resurfacing is made (Fig. 36D–5). Resurfacing of the glenoid is reason-

able if a functional reconstruction of the rotator cuff is anticipated. Once the glenoid has been addressed, attention is directed back to the humerus. A 1-cm-wide bed of freshened bone is prepared along the greater tuberosity at the site of the planned repair, and heavy, nonabsorbable sutures are positioned (Figs. 36D–6 and 36D–7). Posteriorly, these are tied, but they are tagged more superiorly and anteriorly until after implant insertion. As noted earlier, the choice of a relatively small humeral head trial can be useful to ease the repair. The head size is chosen that allows maintenance of stability yet eases the stress on the cuff over the head. The

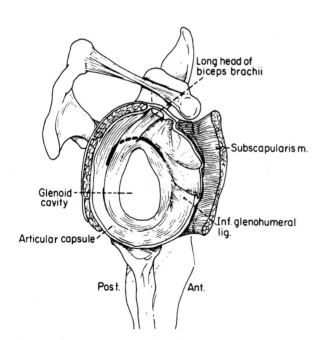

Figure 36D–3. A posterior release is done along the glenoid rim.

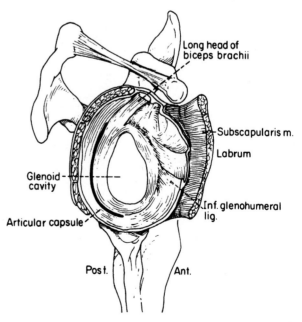

Figure 36D–4. A superior release is preformed along the glenoid rim just above the biceps tendon.

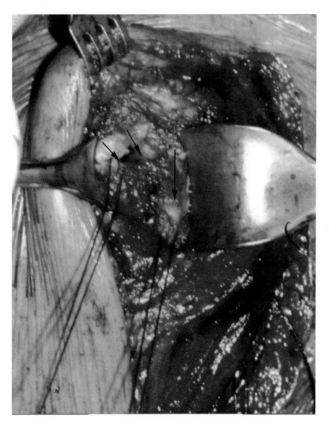

Figure 36D–5. The rotator cuff tendons have been mobilized and flexibility is assessed through the adjunctive deltoid splitting incision. The tendons are marked *(small arrows)* and the tendon defect, which overlies the greater tuberosity, is also marked *(large arrow).*

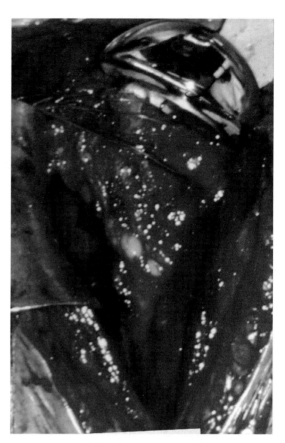

Figure 36D–7. Implant insertion is carried out before the sutures are tied. Reduction of the joint and cuff repair is then carried out.

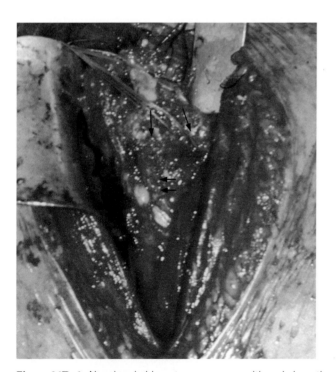

Figure 36D–6. Nonabsorbable sutures are prepositioned along the greater and lessor tuberosities as seen through the deltopectoral incision. The tuberosities with sutures are marked *(large arrows)* as is the humeral shaft *(two small arrows).*

amount, if any, of superior subscapularis transposition can be determined as the final repair pattern is chosen. Insertion of the real head implant and completion of the supraspinatus and subscapularis sutures follow. Ideally, the repair will be tension free, with the arm at the side of the patient's body. Although an abduction orthosis diminishes stress along the supraspinatus repair, such orthoses tend to rotate posteriorly and place excessive strain anteriorly on the subscapularis repair. It is, therefore, quite rare for an abduction brace to be used. The final step is to determine the degree of motion and aggressiveness allowed in postoperative physical therapy. Those limits must be conveyed to the patient and the physical therapist. It is not a success to achieve full passive range of motion at the cost of active motion. Surgery, much like politics, is the art of the possible; adequate, not full, active range of motion may be the most realistic goal.

The work by both Figgie and Rozing indicates that the results of surgery, even if a repair is accomplished, are inferior to those reconstructions in shoulders with normal rotator cuffs.[6,11] In addition, the degenerated tendon tissue is subject to re-rupture. Cofield, in his series of 60 shoulders with 13 tears, found that 5 recurred.[7] Attempts have been made to use a subacromial spacer to compensate for the deficient rotator cuff, and Neer did design a hooded glenoid component to resist the superior migration of the humeral head.[9] Nwakama described the shoulders of 7 patients treated at the Mayo Clinic with the Neer 600 percent glenoid component.[10] All shoulders but 1 had an unsuccessful or unsatisfactory result, and 5 continued to demonstrate anterosuperior subluxation. Two shoulders had required revision surgery at average follow-up of 69 months. This method of treatment cannot be recommended. Treatment of rotator cuff disease in shoulder replacement surgery requires instead recognition of the combination of arthritis and cuff disease, use of fairly standard techniques and prostheses, a decision regarding the appropriateness of glenoid resurfacing in the particular case, and an appropriate rehabilitation program.

References

1. Barrett WP, Franklin JL, Jackins S, et al: Total shoulder arthroplasty. J Bone Joint Surg 69A:865–872, 1987.
2. Boyd AD Jr, Aliabadi P, Thornhill TS: Postoperative proximal migration in total shoulder arthroplasty. Incidence and significance. J Arthroplasty 6:31–37, 1991.
3. Boyd AD, Thomas WH, Scott RD, et al: Total shoulder arthroplasty versus hemiarthroplasty. Indications for glenoid resurfacing. J Arthroplasty 5:329–336, 1990.
4. Cofield RH: Total shoulder arthroplasty with the Neer prosthesis. J Bone Joint Surg 66A:899–906, 1984.
5. Cofield RH: Unconstrained total shoulder prostheses. Clin Orthop 173:97–108, 1983.
6. Figgie HE III, Inglis AE, Goldberg VM, et al: An analysis of factors affecting the long-term results of total shoulder arthroplasty in inflammatory arthritis. J Arthroplasty 3:123–130, 1988.
7. Friedman RJ, Thornhill TS, Thomas WH, Sledge CB: Nonconstrained total shoulder replacement in patients who have rheumatoid arthritis and class IV function. J Bone Joint Surg 71A:494–498, 1989.
8. Hawkins RJ, Bell RH, Jallay B: Total shoulder arthroplasty. Clin Orthop 242:188–194, 1989.
9. Neer CS II, Watson KC, Stanton FJ: Recent experience in total shoulder replacement. J Bone Joint Surg 64A:319–337, 1982.
10. Nwakama AC, Cofield RH, Kavanagh BF, Loehr JF: Semiconstrained total shoulder arthroplasty for glenohumeral arthritis and massive rotator cuff tearing. J Shoulder Elbow Surg 9:302–307, 2000.
11. Rozing PM, Brand R: Rotator cuff repair during shoulder arthroplasty in rheumatoid arthritis. J Arthroplasty 13:311–319, 1998.
12. Søjbjerg JO, Frich LH, Johannsen HV, Sneppen O: Late results of total shoulder replacement in patients with rheumatoid arthritis. Clin Orthop 366:39–45, 1999.
13. Sperling JW, Cofield RH, Rowland CM: Neer hemiarthroplasty and Neer total shoulder arthroplasty in patients fifty years old or less. J Bone Joint Surg 80A:464–473, 1998.
14. Stewart MPM, Kelly IG: Total shoulder replacement in rheumatoid disease. J Bone Joint Surg 79B:68–72, 1997.
15. Walch G, Boileau P: Prosthetic adaptability: A new concept for shoulder arthroplasty. J Shoulder Elbow Surg 8:443–451, 1999.
16. Walch G, Boulahia A, Boileau P, Kempf JF: Primary glenohumeral osteoarthritis: Clinical and radiographic classification. The Aequalis Group. Acta Orthop Belg 64(Suppl 2):46–52, 1998.

36E

Bone Deficiency in Total Shoulder Arthroplasty

• SCOTT P. STEINMANN

Glenoid bone stock deficiency is one of the more difficult problems associated with total shoulder arthroplasty. Many different clinical diagnoses can appear with significant degeneration of the glenoid. Because of the relatively small amount of bone in the native glenoid, bone loss can severely affect prosthesis fixation and, ultimately, joint stability. Understanding the natural anatomy of the glenoid and scapula is helpful in determining the significance of bone loss encountered at surgery.

ANATOMY

The glenoid is wider in the superoinferior direction than in the anteroposterior direction, averaging 35 to 40 mm versus 25 to 30 mm.[15] The glenoid can be either anteverted or retroverted with respect to the plane of the scapula. In most instances, the glenoid is slightly retroverted an average of –2 degrees to –8 degrees.[4,7,11,24] However, in 25 percent of scapulae, there can be slight anteversion averaging between 2 and 10 degrees.[24]

Depending on the pathology of the arthritic shoulder, the glenoid version can be altered in either the anteroposterior or superoinferior directions. Computed tomography (CT) scan studies[11,18] have shown the amount of retroversion to increase in arthritic shoulders. The glenoid was found to be anteverted 2 degrees in a control group of patients, whereas the mean retroversion was –14 degrees in patients with osteoarthritis and –7 degrees in patients with inflammatory arthritis.[11] Another study found the mean retroversion of control shoulders to be –3 degrees and the mean retroversion to be –7.6 degrees in rheumatoid arthritis (–15.1 to 8.2 degrees) and –12.5 degrees in osteoarthritis (–14.1 to 3 degrees).[18] Both studies confirm the clinical observation that arthritis is primarily a posterior wear phenomenon.

The vertical inclination of the glenoid can also vary with an associated pathologic process. Typically, the glenoid surface is superiorly oriented 3 to 5 degrees on average, although there is a wide variation in the literature.[1,5,8,9,12,22,26,28] This superior angulation is thought to help inhibit inferior subluxation of the glenohumeral joint. It is difficult to apply a precise angle of orientation to the glenoid because it is highly mobile in the plane of the scapula. In rheumatoid arthritis, a superior inclination of the glenoid is increased, and in osteoarthritis, the wear pattern typically causes a more inferior inclination.

PATHOLOGIC CONDITIONS

Glenoid bone deficiency can result from a number of pathologic conditions including osteoarthritis, arthritis of dislocation, inflammatory arthritis (rheumatoid arthritis), skeletal underdevelopment (congenital hypoplasia), pressure erosion from long-standing dislocation (trauma, Erb's palsy) or extreme glenohumeral instability such as cuff tear arthropathy.

Most commonly, glenoid bone loss is encountered in patients with either osteoarthritis or rheumatoid arthritis. Understanding the wear patterns of the glenoid can be helpful in analyzing these patients. In a CT scan study looking at glenoid wear patterns in osteoarthritis, three types of wear were described: Type A (53.5 percent), with primarily central wear; type B (39.5 percent), with primarily posterior wear with a biconcave glenoid, and type C (5 percent), with severe glenoid retroversion greater than 25 percent.[27] In rheumatoid arthritis, the wear pattern tends to be more central and superior, with formation of large subchondral cysts and erosion of the glenoid neck. This can often be quite dramatic, with central erosion of the bone to the level of the coracoid. In extreme cases of rheumatoid arthritis, significant medial erosion can make placement of a glenoid component quite difficult.

The majority of patients with osteoarthritis have primarily a central wear pattern, with a minority of patients having severe posterior wear. It is extremely rare in patients with primary osteoarthritis to have an anterior glenoid wear pattern. In a normal glenoid, the depth of available cancellous bone for prosthetic fixation is relatively shallow, averaging 31.5 mm (range 26 to 40 mm).[16] In cases of rheumatoid arthritis with severe erosion, this available cancellous bone may be less than

10 to 15 mm in depth, compromising the fixation of the glenoid prosthesis.

The wear pattern associated with chronic dislocation or trauma can affect either the anterior or posterior glenoid rim. A fracture of the glenoid rim can be associated with a traumatic dislocation and be a cause of recurrent instability. With small anterior rim fractures, stability can be achieved with repair of the capsule to the glenoid rim.[3] Cadaveric biomechanical studies have suggested that a loss of 25 percent of the posterior glenoid does not significantly increase displacement of the glenoid component in response to a posteriorly directed load.[6] In practice, though, the entire glenoid prosthesis should be supported by glenoid bone stock to minimize stress on the component.

In cases with chronic dislocation, in addition to addressing the problem of glenoid bone loss, often the capsule is stretched by the displaced humeral head. This accompanying redundancy of the capsule can lead to postoperative instability of the humeral prosthesis.[13] In such patients, careful attention must be given to soft tissue tensioning, and version of the components is crucial to glenohumeral stability.

PREOPERATIVE EVALUATION

Before surgery, patients should be evaluated with standard shoulder radiographs. This includes 40-degree posterior oblique, scapular lateral, and axillary views. The 40-degree posterior oblique view provides a true anteroposterior view of the glenoid. If significant erosion is present on the plain radiographs, a CT scan is obtained. Axial CT can demonstrate the pattern of glenoid bone loss. Glenoid version can be measured from an axial CT scan; however, if the patient is positioned obliquely in the scanner, the degree of posterior wear and the amount of glenoid tilt are altered.[16,23] The glenoid version is calculated by drawing a line across the glenoid connecting the anterior and posterior edges. If the patient has significant posterior erosion and a biconcave glenoid, the correct version is measured from the anterior and posterior edges of the posterior concavity. A line is then drawn from the midpoint of the articular surface to the medial border of the scapula. The resultant angle determines the glenoid version (Fig. 36E–1). The humeral version is not typically calculated preoperatively but is determined at the time of surgery. The humeral version can be calculated if desired by a technique involving CT scanning at the proximal humerus and at the distal humerus.[14] The desired humeral version is relatively easy to establish at surgery by altering the cut of the humeral head. However, it is important to realize the great variability in humeral retroversion in the general population.[21]

Three-dimensional CT and magnetic resonance imaging (MRI) reconstruction are now technically possible to aid in determining the extent of glenoid bone loss. Both techniques, however, do not add much to the information obtained from plain radiographs and CT scans. MRI can give information on the extent of soft tissue disease, can determine the general condition of the rotator cuff tendon, and can provide identification of bone cysts that may require bone grafting. MRI, however, is not necessary to determine the extent of glenoid bone loss.

SURGICAL TECHNIQUE

Glenoid bone loss is not a contraindication to total shoulder arthroplasty. The decision to implant a glenoid prosthesis, however, should be based on the amount of remaining glenoid bone stock; the condition of the soft tissues and, particularly, the status of the rotator cuff; and the demands of the patient. Diagnosis is also of importance in determining whether the glenoid

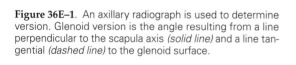

Figure 36E–1. An axillary radiograph is used to determine version. Glenoid version is the angle resulting from a line perpendicular to the scapula axis (solid line) and a line tangential (dashed line) to the glenoid surface.

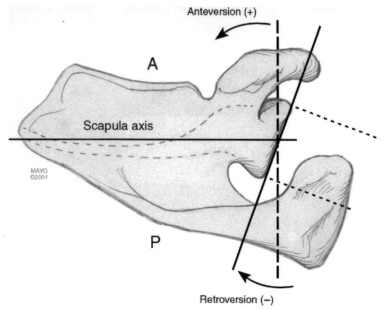

component should be implanted. A rheumatoid arthritis patient with a markedly attenuated rotator cuff should probably not have a prosthesis placed even in the face of relatively mild glenoid bone loss. Such situations have been noted to result in glenoid component loosening, the so-called rocking horse phenomenon.[10]

After the condition of the soft tissues and bony component of the glenohumeral joint is assessed and the decision is made to implant a glenoid prosthesis, there are several different techniques that could be used to address bone deficiency of the glenoid. These include use of a custom glenoid component, cement augmentation, high coracoid placement, altering the glenoid version, asymmetrical reaming, and bone grafting.[3]

The two types of bone loss commonly seen are cavity and peripheral segmental deficiency. In a cavity defect, the cortical rim of the glenoid is intact and the version is minimally changed. This is usually seen in rheumatoid arthritis. Cavity lesions can be filled with cancellous bone graft from the resected humeral head. After the soft tissue component of the cyst is curetted to bone, morcellized bone from the humeral head is impacted into the glenoid defect. After the glenoid impaction is completed, the keel slot or peg holes are fashioned in the glenoid to receive the prosthesis. This type of fixation usually results in a secure glenoid component. Use of a cemented or uncemented glenoid component can be used in this situation.

A peripheral segmental deficiency is a more problematic concern, and different options exist for glenoid component fixation. Placement of bone cement behind the glenoid to augment version should be avoided. Although the initial fixation may seem adequate, the stresses on the glenoid will tend to break loose the block of cement and lead to toggle motion and potential keel or peg breakage (Fig. 36E–2).

A customized glenoid component may seem to be an attractive method of restoring glenoid version. However, there is increased stress on the fixation because of the higher constraint of such components.[17,19] This increased stress may potentially lead to a higher loosening rate of the glenoid component. An additional concern is that custom components sometimes require custom instruments for implantation, which can increase the cost of shoulder arthroplasty.

High placement of the glenoid component in the coracoid can be helpful in cases of cuff tear arthropathy or in cases of severe rheumatoid arthritis with superior wear. With significant superior and medial erosion, the ebernated articular surface becomes continuous with the base of the coracoid. The component slot or peg holes can be made high in the cancellous bone of the coracoid. This is usually the best option in cases of superior humeral migration rather than attempting to lower the humerus (Fig. 36E–3). Maintaining a formerly superiorly migrated humerus in a reduced anatomic location has not been successful.

Another approach to glenoid bone loss is to accept the altered version of the worn glenoid and alter the humeral version. This technique is possible if there is no subluxation of the humerus and if the wear of the glenoid is uniform and does not demonstrate a biconcave surface. When implanting the glenoid in mild retroversion or anteversion, the version of the humerus should be altered so that the total combined retroversion of both the humerus and glenoid components does not exceed 40 degrees.[19] For example, if the glenoid which is normally assumed to be in neutral version, is placed in 30 degrees of retroversion because of posterior wear, the humeral component should be placed in no more than 10 degrees of retroversion (Fig. 36E–4). Care should be taken when implanting the glenoid not to penetrate the

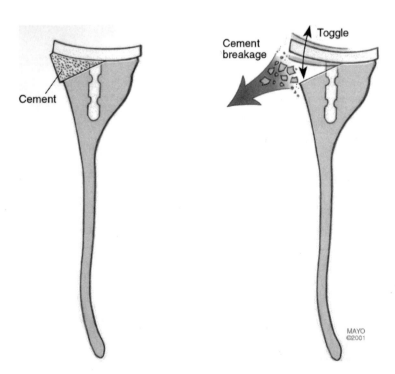

Figure 36E–2. Cement placed behind a prosthesis will tend to loosen and dislodge. The resulting toggle of the prosthesis can result in failure.

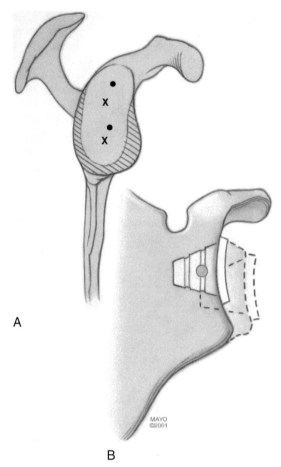

A

B

Figure 36E–3. A, The letter "X" marks the superior and inferior borders of a typical keel placement site. Dark circles mark a more superior placement site. **B**, Dotted lines represent standard glenoid placement. Medial wear allows superior glenoid placement.

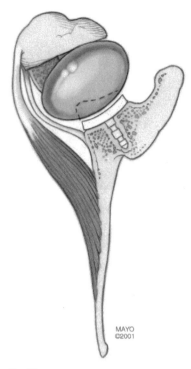

Figure 36E–4. Significant posterior wear. Humeral component placed in minimal retroversion.

This solution is appealing because it is technically simple and avoids overtensioning of the rotator cuff. Theoretically, if the rotator cuff is under increased tension, the polyethylene surface of the glenoid will have increased wear. The technique is probably the most commonly used procedure to address glenoid bone loss and is applicable to many arthritic conditions (Fig. 36E–7).

anterior cortex of the scapula with the keel of the component. In such cases, the keel may need to be shortened or the most anterior peg trimmed.

This technique is not recommended if the version of the glenoid is significantly altered. However, in cases of chronic dislocation or arthritis of Erb's palsy, in which there is unusually severe wear of the glenoid accompanied by shortened and contracted external rotators of the rotator cuff, this may be the best option. In cases of Erb's palsy, if an attempt is made to restore the normal version of the glenoid, the already contracted external rotators come under increased tension with the potential for an avulsion of the rotator cuff or fracture of the greater tuberosity. In the rare case of arthritis of Erb's palsy, it is usually best to accept the altered version of the glenohumeral joint and implant the prosthetic component without major alterations to the soft tissues (Fig. 36E–5).

The simplest technique to consider if there is glenoid bone loss is to preferentially ream the "high" side of the glenoid. For instance, if there is significant posterior glenoid erosion, the anterior high side can be asymmetrically reamed to reorient the articular surface (Fig. 36E–6). Likewise, if there is a superior tilt in rheumatoid arthritis, the inferior glenoid can be reamed to recontour the joint.

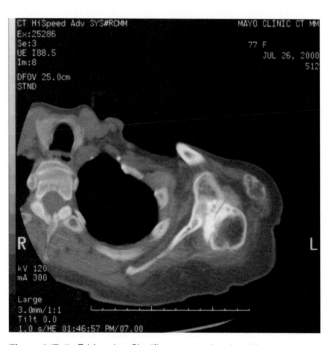

Figure 36E–5. Erb's palsy. Significant posterior glenoid wear and subluxation seen on computed tomography scan.

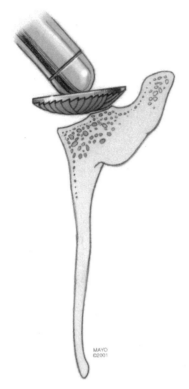

Figure 36E–6. Asymmetrical reaming. The "high" anterior side can be reamed to reorient the articular surface.

Bone grafting of the glenoid can be used if there is significant bone loss. This technique can be used if there is posterior wear from osteoarthritis, anterior wear from a dislocation, superior wear from rheumatoid arthritis, or an associated fracture. It should be recognized, however, that when bone graft is added to the deformed medialized glenoid, the capsule and rotator cuff can become overtightened and potentially limit joint mobility. In one series, this technique was used in only 3.3 percent of all total shoulder arthroplasties.[25]

TECHNIQUE OF GLENOID BONE GRAFTING

The initial steps of preparing a glenoid for bone grafting are identical to those used for the technique of exposing the glenoid for standard total shoulder arthroplasty. After adequate visualization of the glenoid articular surface is achieved, the high side is contoured with standard glenoid reamers to match the medial surface of the glenoid component. The keel slot or column holes are then made. A bone graft is obtained ideally from the resected humeral head. It is best to use the firmer subchondral bone of the humeral head because screw thread purchase is best in this denser bone. A wedge graft is then fashioned and held in place with K-wires or drill bits. Two countersunk 3.5-mm screws are then used to secure the graft to the glenoid. It is safest to recontour the graft to match the back surface of the glenoid component with a bur

rather than a reamer because the larger torque of a reamer can potentially dislodge the fragile graft. After contouring the graft, the glenoid component is then cemented or screwed into place (Fig. 36E–8).

An alternative to this technique is to not use screws to secure the graft but rather to use the glenoid component to hold the graft in place. This is possible if a noncemented glenoid component is used. The screws in the prosthesis tend to provide compression that can capture and hold the graft in place.

RESULTS OF GLENOID BONE GRAFTING

One study reported on 28 patients who had glenoid bone grafting, the majority for osteoarthritis.[25] The bone graft was held in place in the majority with 3.5-mm screws. Both cemented and uncemented prostheses were used. At 5.3 year average follow-up, all bone grafts had healed by radiographic evaluation. Three prostheses had complete radiographic lucencies greater than 1.5 mm in width and were thought to represent loose glenoid components. Two patients underwent reoperation. One patient had an anterior dislocation 1 month after arthroplasty and

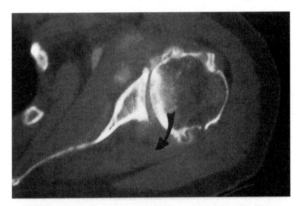

A

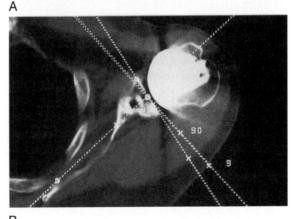

B

Figure 36E–7. **A,** Correcting posterior glenoid wear by decreasing the bone anteriorly with purposeful eccentric reaming of the glenoid articular surface. **B,** Postoperatively, the glenoid component is grossly perpendicular to the scapula. (From Walch G, Boileau P: Primary glenohumeral osteoarthritis. Clinical and radiographic classification. In Walch G, Boileau P [eds]: Shoulder arthroplasty. Berlin, Springer-Verlag, 1999, with permission.)

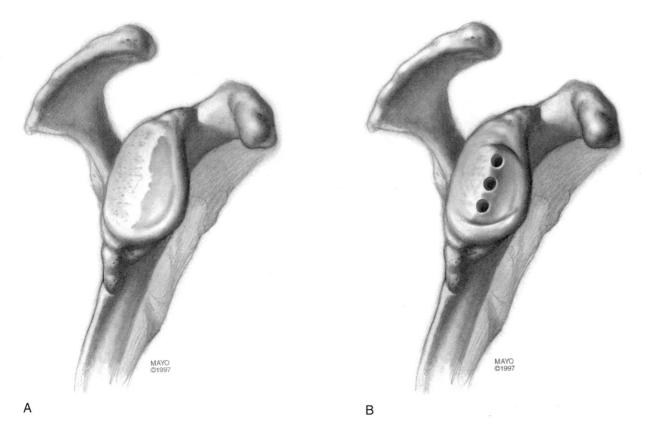

A

B

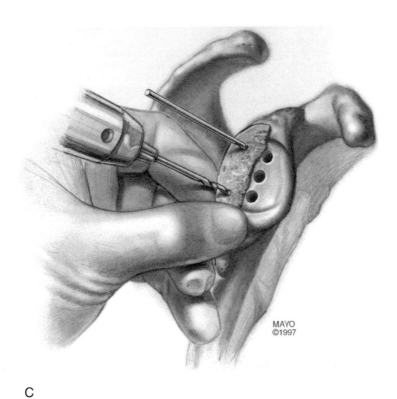

C

Figure 36E–8. Steps in placement of glenoid bone graft. **A,** Segmental erosion of posterior half of bony glenoid. **B,** Preparation of anterior portion of glenoid subchondral bone and placement of column holes. **C,** Placement of humeral head graft in deficient area of glenoid; it is held in place with drill bits to be followed by final screw placement.

underwent successful anterior soft tissue reconstruction. The other patient developed posterior subluxation and required surgical tightening of the posterior capsule. Both patients had well-healed posterior bone grafts. With use of Neer's evaluation system,[25] 82 percent were rated as either excellent or satisfactory (Fig. 36E–9).

These results are similar to those of Neer and Morrison,[20] who reported on 19 patients at 4.4 years of follow-up. They reported 89 percent excellent or satisfactory results using an identical rating system. All bone grafts had healed with no loosening or shifting in position of the glenoid prosthesis; no revision surgery was necessary.

Hill and Norris[14] presented data on 17 patients undergoing glenoid bone grafting. Using the same rating system, there were only 53 excellent and satisfactory results. Three patients developed graft related problems which included nonunion, shift in component position, and resorption of the graft. Five patients required revision surgery for glenoid failure (29 percent). Shoulder instability appears to be a very significant factor associated with failure of a glenoid component. In both the series reported by Steinmann and Cofield[25] and that of Hill and Norris,[14] the majority of reoperations were for recurrent instability.

In conclusion, the need for this segmental type of bone grafting is uncommon. There are now more options among glenoid components, including a choice of columns or keels, thicker size, implants with a slight angle, and cemented or noncemented design. However, there will be the occasional patient in whom bone grafting will be appropriate. This would be a patient who shows not only glenoid wear but also preexisting subluxation of the humeral head in the direction of the wear and a lax shoulder capsule. Intraoperatively, the decision to bone graft will be considered if: (1) a limited amount of reaming of the high side does not allow correction of the glenoid version, and (2) for patients in whom significant glenoid wear exists in the presence of humeral head subluxation and capsular laxity.

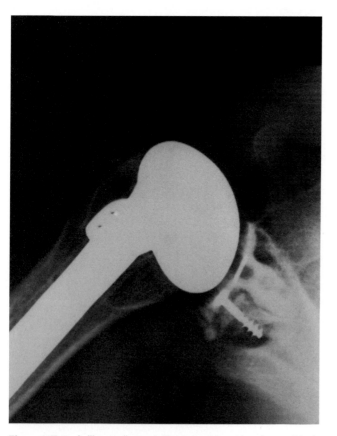

Figure 36E–9. Axillary radiograph. Total shoulder arthroplasty with single screw securing posterior bone graft. Cemented glenoid prosthesis.

References

1. Basmajian JV, Bazant FJ: Factors preventing downward dislocation of the adducted shoulder joint: An electromyographic and morphological study. J Bone Joint Surg 41A:1182, 1959.
2. Bell RH, Noble JS: The management of significant glenoid deficiency in total shoulder arthroplasty. J Shoulder Elbow Surg 9:248–256, 2000.
3. Bigliani LU, Newton PM, Steinmann SP, et al: Glenoid rim lesions associated with recurrent anterior dislocation of the shoulder. Am J Sports Med 26:41–45, 1998.
4. Brewer BJ, Wubben RC, Carrera GF: Excessive retroversion of the glenoid cavity. A cause of nontraumatic posterior instability of the shoulder. J Bone Joint Surg 68A:724–731, 1986.
5. Buechel FF: Glenohumeral joint in the chimpanzee: Comparative anatomical analysis for use in endoprosthetic replacement. J Med Primatol 6:108–113, 1977.
6. Collins D, Tencer A, Sidles J, Matsen FA III: Edge displacement and deformation of glenoid components in response to eccentric loading. The effect of preparation of the glenoid bone. J Bone Joint Surg 74A:501–507, 1992.
7. Cyprien JM, Vasey HM, Burdet A, et al: Humeral retrotorsion and glenohumeral relationship in the normal shoulder and in recurrent anterior dislocation (scapulometry). Clin Orthop 175:8–17, 1983.
8. Edelson JG: Patterns of degenerative change in the glenohumeral joint. J Bone Joint Surg 77B:288–292, 1995.
9. Engelbrecht E, Heinert: More than ten years' experience with unconstrained shoulder replacement. *In* Kolbel R, Helbig B, Blauth W (eds): Shoulder Replacement. New York, Springer-Verlag, 1987, pp 85–91.
10. Franklin JL, Barrett WP, Jackins SE, Matsen FA: Glenoid loosening in total shoulder arthroplasty. J Arthroplasty 3:39–46, 1988.
11. Friedman RJ, Hawthorne KB, Genez BM: The use of computerized tomography in the measurement of glenoid version. J Bone Joint Surg 74:1032–1037, 1992.
12. Gouaze A, Castaing J, Soutoul JH, Chantepie G: Sur l'orientation de l'omoplate et de sa cavité glénoide. Arch Anat Pathol 10:175–181, 1962.
13. Hill JA, Tkach L, Henddx RW: A study of glenohumeral orientation in patients with anterior recurrent shoulder dislocations using computerized axial tomography. Orthop Rev 18:84–91, 1989.
14. Hill JM, Norris TR: Long-term results of bone grafting for glenoid deficiency in total shoulder arthroplasty. Orthop Trans 20:58, 1996.
15. Ianotti JP, Gabriel JP, Schneck SL, et al: The normal glenohumeral relationships: An anatomical study of 140 shoulders. J Bone Joint Surg 74A:491–500, 1992.
16. Mallon WJ, Brown HR, Vogher JB III, Martinez S: Radiographic and geometric anatomy of the scapula. Clin Orthop 277:142–154, 1992.
17. Morrison DS: Glenoid deficiency in total shoulder arthroplasty: *In* Bigliani LU (ed): Complications in shoulder surgery. Baltimore, Williams and Wilkins, 1993, pp 73–80.
18. Muladji AB, Beddow FH, Lamb GHR: CT-measurement of glenoid erosion in arthritis. J Bone Joint Surg 76B:384–388, 1994.
19. Neer CS: Glenohumeral arthroplasty. *In* Neer CS (ed): Shoulder Reconstruction. Philadelphia, WB Saunders, 1990, pp 146–271.
20. Neer CS, Morrison D: Glenoid bone grafting in total shoulder arthroplasty. J Bone Joint Surg 70A:1154–1162, 1988.

21. Pearl MI, Volk AG: Retroversion of the proximal humerus in relationship to prosthetic replacement arthroplasty. J Shoulder Elbow Surg 4:286–289, 1995.
22. Pizon P: Osteometrie scapho-humérale. Presse Med 67:1531–1533, 1959.
23. Randelli M, Gambrioli PL: Glenohumeral osteometry by computed tomography in normal and unstable shoulders. Clin Orthop 208:151–156, 1986.
24. Saha AK: Dynamic stability of the glenohumeral joint. Acta Orthop Scand 44:668–678, 1973.
25. Steinmann SP, Cofield RH: Bone grafting for glenoid deficiency in total shoulder replacement. J Shoulder Elbow Surg 9:361–367, 2000.
26. Toris T: Roentgenographical examination of the tilted angle of the scapula in the resting position. Jpn Orthop Assoc 55:395, 1981.
27. Walch G, Boileau P: Primary glenohumeral osteoarthritis. Clinical and radiographic classification. *In* Walch G, Boileau P (eds): Shoulder Arthroplasty. Berlin, Springer-Verlag, 1999.
28. Wirth MA, Lyons FR, Rockwood CA Jr: Hypoplasia of the glenoid. J Bone Joint Surg 75A:1175–1184, 1993.

37

Arthroscopy for Shoulder Arthritis and Applications to Shoulder Arthroplasty

• SHAWN W. O'DRISCOLL

Although arthroscopy has been used extensively for alleviation of pain caused by osteoarthritis of the knee, little has been written concerning its use for shoulder arthritis.[22] On the other hand, experience in my own practice has greatly expanded the indications for arthroscopic treatment of elbow arthritis. Compared with the knee, both the shoulder and the elbow can meet many functional demands without bearing high compressive or shear stresses across the joint surface. By contrast, the knee must bear the full weight of the body in order to function. In this regard, the possibility exists that arthroscopic intervention in the shoulder might be more successful than in the knee and therefore merits consideration.

The role of arthroscopy in shoulder arthritis can be considered in the context of osteoarthritis, rheumatoid arthritis, cuff tear arthropathy, post-traumatic arthritis, and postsurgical shoulder arthroplasty.

OSTEOARTHRITIS

The Unresolved Clinical Problem

Although total shoulder arthroplasty is highly successful in relieving pain and restoring function, there exist at least two populations of patients with severe glenohumeral arthritis for whom shoulder replacement is not ideal. These include (1) young and middle-aged patients whose longevity makes it likely that prosthetic failure will occur in the future, and (2) older patients who subject their shoulders to very high loads or impact, such as experienced while performing carpentry, masonry, metalwork, woodchopping, or hunting big game. Such patients often choose—or are advised—to delay having a shoulder replacement; therefore, they may suffer severe pain until they are no longer able to perform such activities. Nonsurgical treatment often provides little help. Some surgeons recommend hemiarthroplasty as a more conservative option, but even this is not a suitable choice

for patients with posterior glenoid erosion resulting from static posterior subluxation of the humeral head, which is common in glenohumeral osteoarthritis (Fig. 37–1). If a relatively risk-free, minimally invasive surgical procedure could provide pain relief or lessening of pain, it would unquestionably be of great value to such patients.

Causes for Pain in Glenohumeral Osteoarthritis

Normally, implicit in our recommendation for joint replacement is the assumption that the patient's pain arises from the damaged joint surface (assuming that pain is the dominant indication for surgery). However, it is well recognized that a patient may have radiographic evidence of advanced osteoarthritis of the glenohumeral joint yet have no pain at all.

There are essentially three origins of the pain experienced by patients with glenohumeral osteoarthritis: (1) rest pain, (2) pain at the endrange of motion, and (3) pain with use in the midrange of motion. Night pain may represent rest pain, but it can also be positional (usually at the endrange of motion or because of joint subluxation).

Rest pain is probably caused by synovitis or inflamed periarticular soft tissues. Pain at the endrange of motion is typically caused by impingement (related to osteophytes), pinching of synovitic tissues, or stretching of the inflamed periarticular soft tissues. Neither of these types of pain necessarily requires elimination by joint replacement. Finally, pain with use in the midrange of motion, is usually (and appropriately) thought to arise from the damaged articular surface, which necessitates a joint replacement. However, in some patients, even this pain with use in the midrange of motion may arise from the inflamed soft tissues rather than, or in addition to, the damaged joint surface. Compressive, tensile, and shear stresses occur in the periarticular soft tissues as they are compressed against the articulation by the force

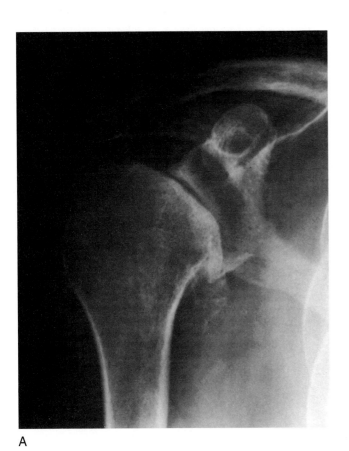

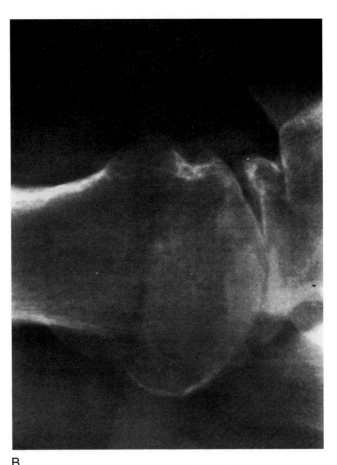

A

B

Figure 37–1. Anteroposterior (AP) and axillary radiographs of a typical patient with advanced glenohumeral osteoarthritis. The AP view shows cartilage loss with hypertrophic changes including inferior osteophytes. The axillary view shows the typical posterior glenoid erosion and subluxation, with a biconcave glenoid surface. The humeral head is sitting in the static posterior subluxation position.

of muscle contraction or as they glide over the joint with motion. Hypertrophic synovium can potentially be pinched in the articulation.

By deduction, it should be possible for a patient with radiographic evidence of advanced glenohumeral osteoarthritis to have severe pain that does not arise from, nor require replacement of, the damaged joint surfaces themselves.

Concept of Glenoidplasty

In our experience with shoulder arthroplasty, almost 40 percent of patients with glenohumeral osteoarthritis have posterior subluxation of the humeral head, which leads to posterior glenoid erosion (Fig. 37–2). This erosion decreases the contact area, increasing the contact pressure. The posterior erosion leaves a vertical ridge near the center of the glenoid, over which the humeral head may experience subluxation and reduction, causing symptoms of instability. Eventually, patients may develop what appears to be static posterior subluxation.

Glenoidplasty involves removal of the central ridge and recontouring of the glenoid to match the curvature of the humeral head. This matching process permits

the humeral head to reduce, relaxing the anterior soft tissues and increasing the joint contact area, which decreases the contact pressure (Fig. 37–3). The concept shares some biomechanical principles with that of varus or valgus femoral osteotomy for osteoarthritis of the hip.

Rationale for Osteocapsular Arthroplasty

Treating patients with advanced osteoarthritis of the elbow by means of osteocapsular arthroplasty (removal of osteophytes, synovectomy, and capsulectomy) relieves them of both impingement pain at the limits of motion and rest pain. On the basis of that experience and considering the causes of pain described earlier, we reasoned that the same might be true of patients with glenohumeral osteoarthritis.

Indications for Osteocapsular Arthroplasty

To be considered for this operation, a patient has to be a candidate for total shoulder arthroplasty (TSA) and meet *all of the following* criteria:

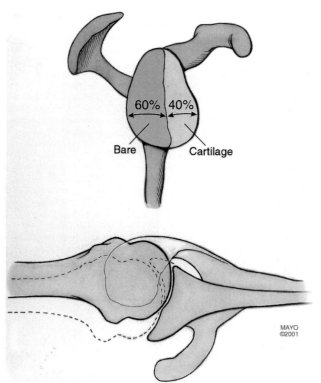

Figure 37–2. Schematic illustration representing the biomechanical consequences of static posterior subluxation and glenoid erosion, as would be viewed on the axillary radiograph. Three features are seen. (1) Posterior subluxation of the humeral head on the glenoid (*the original position indicated by the dotted lines*). (2) Decreased contact area on the glenoid, which increases the contact pressure in the joint surface. In our patient, the contact area averaged 60 percent of the total glenoid, with the anterior 40 percent of the glenoid not in contact with the humeral head. (By permission of Mayo Foundation for Medical Education and Research.)

- Moderate to advanced glenohumeral osteoarthritis
- Moderate to severe pain that caused functional impairment unresponsive to nonsurgical treatment
- Painless crepitus during glenohumeral motion with joint compression

In addition, candidates must have *at least one* of the following relative contraindications to TSA:

- Age younger than 50 years
- Heavy physical demands on the shoulder
- Refusal of joint replacement

Contraindications

- Failure to meet the inclusion criteria
- On physical examination, pain in response to passive motion in the midrange during compression of the glenohumeral joint
- Irregular erosion of the glenoid or humeral articular surfaces

Indications for Glenoidplasty

In addition to the indications for osteocapsular arthroplasty, for this study, it was also required that the patient have a biconcave glenoid resulting from posterior erosion by the humeral head. Neither age nor a history of a prior successful TSA on the contralateral shoulder was a contraindication.

Surgical Technique

Setup, Equipment, and Portals

The patient is placed in the beach chair position after general anesthesia is obtained. The three main arthroscopic portals are established and include a high and midposterior portal as well as the standard anterior portal. Frequently, a fourth portal is added at the midlevel anteriorly. A third posteromedial portal can be used for the placement of a retractor to hold the axillary pouch away from the humeral head and neck.

The flow is maintained through a modified pulsatile lavage system that is used to wash the canal during joint replacement and to irrigate open fractures. The spray nozzle is cut off from its connecting tubing and then connected to the arthroscope via a standard intravenous line. The driving pressure is set at 50 mm Hg and flow is controlled by the assistant, who uses the flow control valve. The auditory feedback ("putt-putt") of the pulsatile lavage system is invaluable in permitting the surgeon to monitor the fluid flow into the joint without having to question others or consult a display panel.

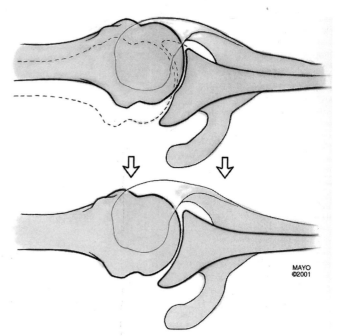

Figure 37–3. Concept and goals of glenoidplasty. Preoperatively, the posterior glenoid erosion creates a biconcave glenoid with a central ridge over which the humeral head can exhibit subluxation and reduction (giving the patient symptoms of instability) or behind which the humeral head can sit in a fixed static subluxation position (*top view*). By removing this central ridge and deepening the glenoid, a single concavity is recreated, increasing congruity and permitting concentric reduction of the humeral head in the glenoid (*bottom view*). This increases contact area and decreases contact pressure at the joint surface. The cartilage on the anterior 40 percent of the glenoid does not articulate with the humeral head, and therefore is not being used. This obviates any concern about removal of this cartilage. (By permission of Mayo Foundation for Medical Education and Research.)

Edema is controlled by constantly maintaining direct outflow through one or more portals and also through the shaver device. No drainage tubing is connected to the outflow cannulas.

Osteocapsular Arthroplasty

Osteocapsular arthroplasty includes synovectomy, removal of osteophytes, and partial capsulectomy. Of course, loose bodies or debris are also removed. Once the joint has been evaluated, the next step is to perform a complete, systematic synovectomy (a significant degree of synovitis was usually seen in our patients) (Fig. 37–4). We use a 4.8- or 5.5-mm shaver (gator blade) and begin with the anterosuperior aspect of the joint, moving posteriorly and then inferiorly into the axillary recess and finally removing the posterior inferior synovium. The aim is to clear away all traces of synovitis. The midposterior portal is used for cleaning the axillary pouch, but it is imperative to recognize the proximity of the axillary nerve beneath the axillary capsule.

After the synovitis has been removed, an osteocapsular arthroplasty can be performed as needed. This procedure includes removal of any inferior osteophyte from the humeral head and release of the entire capsule to improve range of motion and alleviate impingement pain (Fig. 37–5). This step requires that the surgeon have a thorough understanding of the three-dimensional anatomy of the shoulder joint, for the purpose of differentiating between osteophyte and normal bone or articular surface. The procedure requires the surgeon to "sculpt" the bone to permit a greater range of motion. During the operation through the posterior portals, the inferior humeral osteophyte is removed first with a hooded 4.0-mm (slap) bur, which protects the inferior capsule and the axillary nerve. The goal is to begin posteriorly and move anteriorly with the bur. The humerus

may be moved to optimize the visibility of the osteophyte and the positioning of the instrument. When the inferior capsular attachment to the humeral head is identified, the normal architecture of the humerus can be recreated. The bur can be alternated with the 5.5-mm gator blade, which débrides any loose bony fragments and soft tissues left behind by the bur. We routinely avoid using suction on our instruments but instead allow free flow out to the floor. This practice decreases the likelihood that soft issue may unintentionally be drawn into the instrument with potential resultant damage to the axillary nerve. The most difficult part of the procedure is the removal of the anterior aspect of the inferior osteophyte. It may be necessary to use a curved curette to reach around and remove the remaining osteophyte. Remaining loose fragments of bone may be removed with a grasper or shaver, and fine contouring may be done with the shaver or hand rasps as necessary.

Removal of the inferior osteophyte, greatly increases the space workspace in the inferior axillary pouch. This greater area enhances visibility of the inferior capsule and ensures a safer performance of a partial capsulectomy. Through the posterior portals, a capsulotomy is made by using a motorized shaver in the posterior aspect of the inferior capsule, well away from the axillary nerve. In the right shoulder, this is at about the 7 o'clock position, adjacent to the glenoid rim. Through this opening, the plane between the inferior capsule and the extra-articular soft tissues can be developed with a wide duckling basket punch. The surgeon can then resect the capsule by moving from a posterior to an anterior direction with the duckling, clearly viewing the capsule and the underlying soft tissues. The duckling is used to lift the capsule off the triceps and subscapularis, with care taken to have only capsular tissue in each bite. The shaver is used to widen the resection.

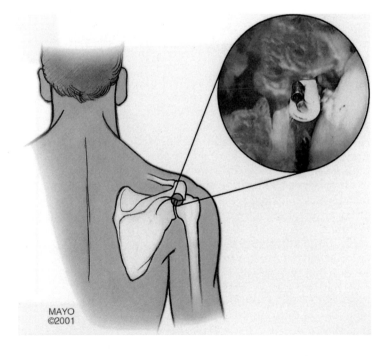

Figure 37–4. A typical feature in these patients is a proliferative inflammatory villonodular synovitis. This is usually present throughout the shoulder and is the likely and important contributor to pain. Total synovectomy is an important part of the treatment, and the first part of the operation. (By permission of Mayo Foundation for Medical Education and Research.)

MAYO
©2001

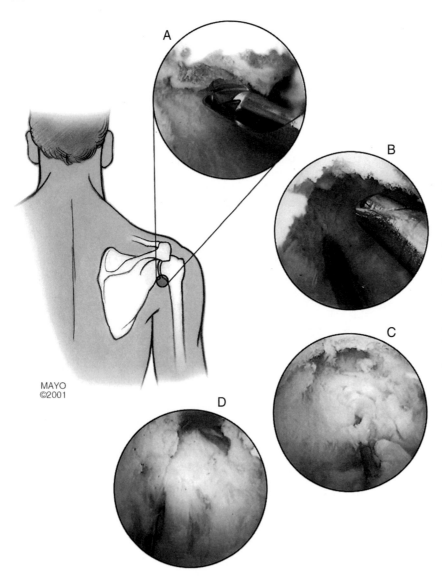

A

B

C

MAYO
©2001

D

Figure 37–5. Osteocapsular arthroplasty. **A**, Marginal humeral head osteophytes, particularly on the inferior aspect of the humeral head, impinge against the glenoid. The osteophytes are excised. **B**, Anterior and inferior capsular contractures. The capsule is released, which relieves tension on the tight soft tissues and contributes to improvement and motion. The probe indicates the location of the axillary nerve beneath the capsule. **C**, Inferior and anterior capsulotomy is performed. Visual identification of the axillary nerve permits one to dissect and cut the capsule while the nerve is under direct observation. In this case, the nerve is being gently probed and lifted up into the capsulotomy site. **D**, Close-up view of the axillary nerve after partial capsulectomy. (By permission of Mayo Foundation for Medical Education and Research.)

After the 6 o'clock position is reached, the axillary nerve can be exposed. On the right shoulder, it passes from the 11 o'clock position to the 5 o'clock position, appearing from beneath the subscapularis muscle and disappearing beneath the triceps tendon (see Fig. 37–5). At that point, the axillary nerve may already have arborized. It is safest to perform the capsulectomy as close to the inferior glenoid rim as possible, because the nerve lies closest to the capsule midway between the glenoid and capsular insertion on the humerus. The axillary nerve can be identified with a probe and protected. Once it has been seen, the remainder of the anteroinferior capsule can be safely and confidently resected.

Next, the anterior osteophytes are removed, and an anterior partial capsulectomy is performed. The biceps tendon can be held inferiorly with a probe or grasper, and the capsule around the rotator interval can be removed. Any remaining anteroinferior capsule can be removed through the anterior portals, connecting to the inferior extent of the capsulectomy.

Glenoidplasty

After the capsule has been released anteriorly and inferiorly, a glenoidplasty is performed if there is a biconcave glenoid as a result of posterior erosion. Performance of the glenoidplasty after the capsulotomy permits greater access to what would otherwise be a very tight articulation. The biconcave shape of the glenoid can best be appreciated by looking inferiorly through the anterior portal (Fig. 37–6). The cartilage is removed from the anterior glenoid facet by means of shaver. This leaves behind a central bony ridge, which must then be removed with the bur. The goal is to recreate a single concave surface of the glenoid. By viewing the glenoid from multiple portals and progressing from a small to a large bur and eventually to a large hemispherical hand rasp, the glenoid can be deepened and the concave surface restored. Any obvious irregularities of the humeral head may also be removed. The completeness and adequacy of the glenoidplasty can be assessed intraoperatively by compressing the humeral head against the glenoid and rotating the humerus while palpating for crepitus. The humeral head should ideally

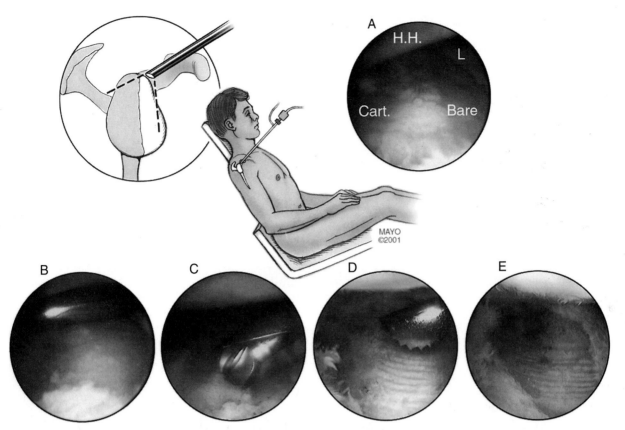

Figure 37–6. Technique of glenoidplasty. All arthroscopic views are as seen with the arthroscope in the anterosuperior portal, looking inferiorly on the glenoid (*glenoid oriented horizontally in the photos*). **A**, Arthroscopic view of the osteoarthritic glenoid before glenoidplasty. The posterior half of the glenoid is eroded down to bare bone (bare), whereas the anterior half has a layer of fibrillated cartilage (Cart) and labrum (L) remaining on it. The humeral head (H.H.) has been retracted inferiorly, which has been made possible by the previous capsulotomy and debulking of the osteophytes around the humeral head. **B**, The fibrillated cartilage remaining on the anterior portion of the glenoid is removed with a motorized shaver. This exposes the vertical bony ridge seen on the axillary radiograph, which delineates the eroded posterior glenoid from the normal contour of the anterior glenoid. **C**, A bur is used to recontour the glenoid and restore the concave shape to match that of the humeral head. **D**, The final "grading" or contouring of the surface of the glenoid is performed with a large rasp. **E**, Arthroscopic view of the recontoured glenoid, which now has a concave shape that matches the humeral head in the transverse and coronal planes. (By permission of Mayo Foundation for Medical Education and Research.)

rotate smoothly on the new glenoid surface. Once all pathology has been appropriately addressed, the joint is injected with a solution of bupivicaine and morphine for pain control. Celestone injection was given to only one patient at the end of the procedure.

Postoperative Management

In the postoperative period, after the patient has recovered from anesthesia and a satisfactory neurovascular exam has been performed, an intrascalene catheter is placed to provide postoperative analgesia. The patient can then be placed in a continuous passive motion shoulder device for 3 days. Active and passive range of motion exercises are started immediately postoperatively. The patient is discharged from the hospital on postoperative day number four, with instructions for how to use the continuous passive motion machine for 1 month. The patient begins to practice isometric strengthening immediately and progresses to isotonic exercises as tolerated. No restrictions are imposed, and the patient is instructed to use the shoulders as pain permits.

Operative Findings

At the time of arthroscopy, four patients in the study group were noted to have a partial tear of the rotator cuff; none of these tears had been repaired. Three patients had complete disruptions of the intra-articular portion of the biceps tendon. An average of 58 percent of the glenoid was noted to be devoid of articular cartilage (range 40 percent to 90 percent) at the time of arthroscopy (see Fig. 37–2). The subacromial space is usually not even entered unless there is a suspicion that subacromial pathology is causing symptoms. In other words, the focus of this operation is specifically the osteoarthritis and not a constellation of pathologies involving the cuff and subacromial space.

RESULTS TO BE EXPECTED

Clinical Outcomes

Although this experience is still somewhat preliminary, half of the patients who have been followed for up to 5 years have experienced complete elimination of their pain and are capable of heavy demands on the shoulder, whereas a total of 85 percent have experienced sufficient lessening of pain to have made the operation quite worthwhile both objectively and subjectively. Two patients required total shoulder arthroplasty for persistent severe pain. Improvement in motion has been satisfactory in external rotation but less predictable in elevation. Average gains in external rotation have been about 25 degrees, but elevation gains have been only about 5 degrees. Thus far, there have been no permanent serious complications.

Radiographic Outcomes

Radiographic examination revealed that the biconcave glenoid had been changed back to a single concavity and that the radius of curvature of the glenoid approximated that of the humeral head (Figs. 37–7 and 37–8). In addition, all cases showed concentric reduction of the humeral head in the glenoid fossa (see Figs. 37–7 and 37–8). Measurements made on the axillary radiographs demonstrated the average glenoid depth to have increased between 3.25 mm and 4.0 mm (plus or minus 2.6 mm) postoperatively (Fig. 37–9).

Prior Literature on Arthroscopic Treatment of Glenohumeral Osteoarthritis

Although a substantial body of literature has reported the role of arthroscopy in osteoarthritis of the knee, little has been written regarding arthroscopic treatment of glenohumeral osteoarthritis. Weinstein et al. reported 80 percent satisfactory improvement in 25 patients with *early* osteoarthritis who were treated by arthroscopic débridement.[22] They recommend such débridement only for "early osteoarthritis in which there remains concentric glenohumeral articulation with a visible joint space on the axillary radiograph." They state that it is "not recommended when there is severe joint incongruity or large osteophytes." Clearly, our patients represent a very different population from those reported by Weinstein et al. In fact, there is no reason to believe that their recommendations are anything but accurate, and I would concur with them. In other words, I believe that for moderate or advanced glenohumeral osteoarthritis with posterior glenoid erosion and joint incongruity, glenoidplasty and osteocapsular arthroplasty are logically required to obtain clinical benefit.

Cameron et al.[22a] reported at the meeting of the American Academy of Orthopaedic Surgeons in 2000 a similar experience in arthroscopically treating patients with grade IV chondral lesions of the shoulder. They treated 61 patients with débridement with or without arthroscopic capsular release, with 88% satisfactory improvement. However, their patients also had only early osteoarthritis.

Possible Explanations for Pain Relief

It has become apparent that what might seem surprising concerning pain relief should perhaps not be so unexpected. From rather extensive experience treating patients with osteoarthritis of the elbow by means of arthroscopic osteocapsular arthroplasty, I can say with

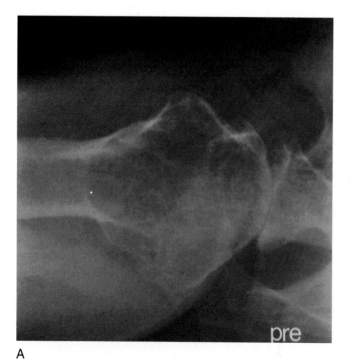
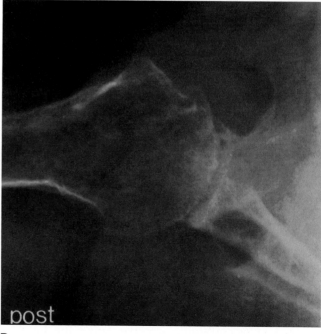

A   B

Figure 37–7. Axillary radiographs of a patient with advanced primary glenohumeral osteoarthritis before and after glenoidplasty. **A,** The preoperative axillary view shows the typical posterior glenoid erosion and subluxation, with a biconcave glenoid surface. The humeral head is sitting in the posterior static subluxation position. **B,** The postoperative axillary radiograph shows the restoration of a concave glenoid and a concentric glenohumeral articulation.

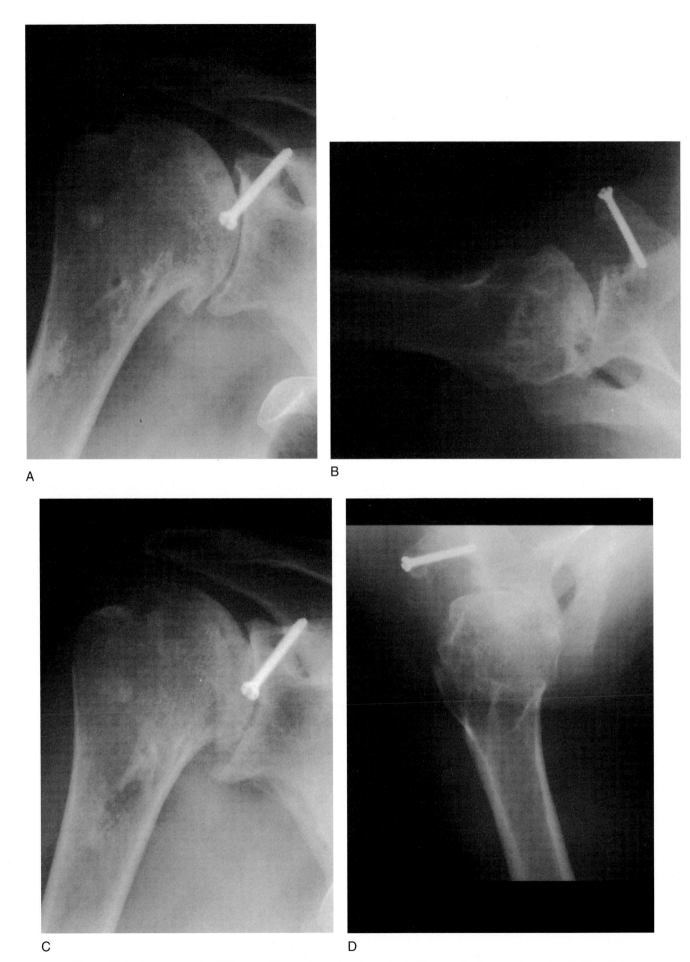

A

B

C

D

Figure 37–8. Anteroposterior (AP) and axillary radiographs of a patient with capsulorrhaphy arthropathy. **A**, The AP view shows cartilage loss with large osteophytes. **B**, The axillary view reveals static posterior subluxation of the humeral head and posterior glenoid erosion, which has caused a biconcave glenoid surface. (**C** and **D**) The postoperative radiographs show the restoration of a concave glenoid, a concentric glenohumeral articulation, and reduction in the osteophytes.

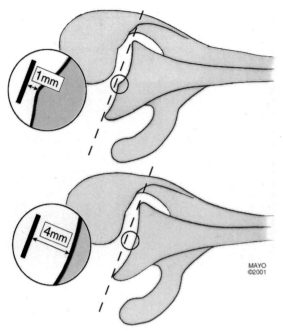

Figure 37–9. Schematic representation of the glenoid in the transverse plane (comparable with the axillary radiographic view). Glenoidplasty removes the central bony ridge, converts the biconcave glenoid back to a single concavity, and increases the depth of the glenoid. In this study, the average glenoid depth increased from 1 mm preoperatively to 4 mm postoperatively. (By permission of Mayo Foundation for Medical Education and Research.)

confidence that relief of the pain at the endrange of motion probably occurs because of osteophyte removal, soft tissue débridement, and capsular release. In the shoulder, restoration of a concentric glenohumeral articulation is important in relieving impingement, but it also permits stability and relaxes the anterior soft tissues. It is possible that synovectomy also eliminates pinching of inflamed tissue in the articulation. Relief from rest pain is likely due to the synovectomy. This has also been found to be predictable in patients with rheumatoid shoulders and elbows.

Pain with use in the midrange of motion, although not predictably relieved, was decreased in some. Many of the patients who have pain in the midrange of motion do have pain with resisted motion but not with passive motion when the glenohumeral joint is compressed. In fact, many of these patients also have painless crepitus with passive motion during glenohumeral compression. Relief of midrange pain in such patients may be explained on the basis of release of the capsule and removal of the inflamed synovium, because these structures are squeezed, stretched, and sheared by the force of muscle contraction or as they glide over the joint with motion. Synovectomy also prevents any hypertrophic inflamed synovium from being pinched in the articulation. Thus, painless crepitus during glenohumeral rotation with joint compression is a critical predictor of success of this procedure.

There are no data to distinguish the benefits arising from glenoidplasty from those derived from osteocapsular arthroplasty. However, at our institution, we initially performed only glenoidplasty with some success. Potential reasons for pain relief from the glenoidplasty are several.

The increase in joint contact area decreases the joint contact pressures, essentially unloading the joint. Further unloading follows restoration of concentricity because of improved balance of forces across the joint. Harryman et al. showed that posterior subluxation that causes increased posterior glenohumeral joint contact stresses is associated with tightening of the anterior soft tissues.[9] Hawkins and Angelo documented that with such long-standing imbalance caused by overtightening of the anterior capsule and subscapularis tendon, posterior glenoid erosion and eventually osteoarthritis develop.[10] Four of our patients had such capsulorrhaphy arthropathy. Also, proper alignment at least partially relaxes the tight anterior soft tissues. One patient, treated only by glenoidplasty, experienced substantial improvement in external rotation.

Finally, it is noteworthy that some patients with radiographic evidence of moderate or advanced osteoarthritis do not have pain. If it is possible to have radiographic evidence of arthritis and have no pain, it should be theoretically possible to start with radiographic evidence of arthritis and pain, and after being treated, have arthritis but no pain.

Recommendations

Our current indications for arthroscopic glenoidplasty with osteocapsular arthroplasty are in patients with advanced glenohumeral osteoarthritis, a biconcave glenoid resulting from posterior erosion by the humeral head, *and* moderate to severe pain causing functional impairment that has failed to respond to nonsurgical treatment *and* painless crepitus with glenohumeral motion during joint compression. In addition, the patients must have a relative contraindication to TSA such as age younger than 50 years, excessive physical demands on the shoulder, or, simply, unwillingness to consider joint replacement. Some patients insist on exhausting any possible minimally invasive treatment options before electing major surgery.

The main contraindication is, on physical examination, the presence of pain during passive motion in the midrange while the glenohumeral joint is compressed. Age is not necessarily a contraindication, and we have performed this procedure in patients up to the age of 78 years. A prior successful TSA on the contralateral shoulder is not a contraindication either, because the earlier procedure was probably done when there were thought to be no other options to offer the patient.

Prognostic Factors

Although further experience will be required to determine and confirm those factors that are useful prognostically, we have gained the impression that the following might be good or poor prognostic factors (Table 37–1).

Potential Problems and Future Concerns

It is prudent to consider the possible negative side effects of removing either the remaining articular cartil-

Table 37–1. PROGNOSTIC FACTORS

	Good Prognostic Factor	Poor Prognostic Factor
History	Impingement pain at endrange of motion Rest pain	Pain in the midrange of motion
Physical Examination	Painless crepitus Absence of pain with G-H compression during humeral rotation	Painful crepitus Pain with G-H compression during humeral rotation
Radiographs	Prominent central ridge owing to posterior wear Large inferior humeral osteophyte Large loose bodies	Nearly concentric G-H articulation Minimal osteophytes Subchondral erosive changes

G-H = glenohumeral.

age from the anterior glenoid or any of the subchondral bone from the glenoid. Owing to posterior subluxation, the cartilage that remains on the anterior glenoid is usually not being used, so it is unlikely that its removal should cause undesirable effects. However, restoring the concave contour of the glenoid does involve removing up to about 4 mm of subchondral bone from the central glenoid, and less from the rest of the glenoid. This could cause accelerated erosion of the glenoid. Although we have not yet seen this erosion, we are concerned about it. As a consequence, glenoid component replacement may not be possible at a later stage if TSA is required. The glenoid remains retroverted after glenoidplasty; concentricity but not version is restored, which could permit recurrence of the posterior subluxation and further wear. Because the sclerotic subchondral bone is partially removed, such wear could be accelerated. Further follow-up will be required to determine the likelihood of development of these complications. It is for these reasons that glenoidplasty is to be considered in its preliminary stage of development.

Summary

In summary, arthroscopic glenoidplasty appears to be a valuable option to offer certain patients with advanced glenohumeral osteoarthritis. The ideal patient is one whose only other reasonable option is a total shoulder replacement but who has a relative contraindication to replacement of the joint or who may simply be unwilling to undergo joint replacement. The results of arthroscopic glenoidplasty do not appear to be equivalent to those of TSA. Thus, glenoidplasty is meant to serve not as a substitute for TSA but as an alternative when TSA is not a desirable option. With strict adherence to indications and contraindications, the majority of patients can expect partial or complete pain relief, although improvement in motion is not as reliable. With further experience, particularly from others, advances may possibly improve functional gains as well.

RHEUMATOID ARTHRITIS AND CUFF TEAR ARTHROPATHY

There is really no information in the literature to guide the surgeon concerning the role of arthroscopy in managing the patient with rheumatoid arthritis of the

shoulder. In fact, over the past few years, techniques have been developed for arthroscopic total synovectomy and capsular release of the shoulder. Our approach has been to base indications for arthroscopy on principles similar to those outlined for osteoarthritis in terms of palliative intervention for pain control in patients with relative contraindications to shoulder replacement, and also as an intermediate stage of surgical intervention for early stages of arthritis with incomplete cartilage loss and minimal or no bone destruction. Arthroscopic total synovectomy, with capsular release as necessary, has provided satisfactory pain relief and obviated joint replacement in 12 consecutive patients with rheumatoid arthritis managed by this approach.

Our impression is that capsular contracture is not only common in patients with rheumatoid arthritis affecting the glenohumeral joint but that release of such contracture is an important component of surgical intervention. Patients typically experience pain at the limits of motion, and such limitation increases the contact stresses on the already damaged joint surfaces. Furthermore, the resistance to motion owing to the contracture generates painful tension in the inflamed periarticular soft tissues. An additional indication for contracture release is to excise the impinging osteophytes at the margins of the joint.

In many centers, cuff tear arthropathy is traditionally managed by hemiarthroplasty. However, when one considers that the results are not highly predictable with hemiarthroplasty and that the outlook is rather bleak for a patient who has failed to respond to hemiarthroplasty for cuff tear arthropathy, our approach is to perform an arthroscopic synovectomy and débridement of the cuff with minimal acromioplasty (retaining any superior coracoacromial structures). An important part of arthroscopic management of cuff tear arthropathy is to remove inflamed tissue from the subacromial bursa and to remove fragments of soft tissue that can potentially give rise to mechanical irritation, such as flaps. We have used the same approach in patients with massive cuff tears associated with arthritis, whose radiographic picture is slightly different from that typically seen in cuff tear arthropathy. The outcomes have been relatively satisfactory from a palliative perspective. Thirteen patients with massive cuff tears were treated with cuff tear arthropathy in the manner described. Each patient experienced some degree of pain relief, and several of the patients had complete or near complete relief of pain. Conversion to hemiarthroplasty was not performed, and no complications have been experienced to date.

AFTER SHOULDER ARTHROPLASTY

Arthroscopy has been found to have potential diagnostic and therapeutic applications after shoulder arthroplasty. The concept of visualizing a joint after replacement is not new, because it has been used in the knee for several indications.[1,3,5,7,11,15,17,21]

Bonutti et al., who used arthroscopy to evaluate glenoid component loosening in nine patients, found it to be a valuable technique for assessing glenoid stability.[4] They confirmed their arthroscopic findings with a subsequent open procedure, at which time they addressed the glenoid component's instability.

Hersch and Dines reported diagnostic arthroscopy in 10 patients with 12 failed TSAs. Arthroscopic treatment included acromioplasty, débridement of the biceps tendon, capsular release, and removal of loose bodies including cement fragments. They found arthroscopy to be useful not just diagnostically but also therapeutically.

Arthroscopic Removal of Painful Loose Glenoid Component

Although TSA enjoys a successful clinical track record for pain relief and improvement of function, there are significant concerns regarding the prevalence of glenoid lucent lines and, therefore, the possibility of glenoid component loosening over the long term.[20,24] Treatment options for symptomatic glenoid loosening include revision of the component or conversion to hemiarthroplasty by removal of the loose glenoid component, with or without bone grafting the glenoid.[18,24] Currently absent from the literature are data regarding the efficacy of these or other treatments for the problem. The philosophy of glenoid removal is based on reports of humeral hemiarthroplasty without a glenoid component, which has been reasonably successful in the treatment of glenohumeral arthritis.[2,5,6,8,12-14,16,23] We have found that it is possible to arthroscopically remove a symptomatic loose glenoid component and underlying cement.

Five patients, aged 66 to 78 years, with painful failed total shoulder arthroplasties secondary to glenoid loosening, have been revised to hemiarthroplasties by arthroscopic removal of the loose glenoid components and cement. The shoulder arthroplasties were initially indicated for the treatment of primary osteoarthritis (OA) in four patients, and for OA that was secondary to synovial osteochondromatosis in one patient. The first patient had had two prior revisions for recurrent instability of his TSA—one soft tissue repair and one complete component revision with soft tissue repair anteriorly and posteriorly. Another patient had had four prior revisions for infection.

The glenoids had all been cemented with modern cementing techniques, including reaming of the glenoid face, instrumented preparation of the glenoid cavity for the keel, water-pik lavage followed by pressure packing of the glenoid cavity with epinephrine-soaked sponges, and pressurization of the glenoid cement.

The indication for revision surgery in each case was severe pain and progressive radiolucent lines around the glenoid component that had been inserted 10 to 144 months before arthroscopic removal. The reason for considering glenoid removal and conversion to hemiarthroplasty was primarily to obviate the need for difficult open revision of the glenoid component. In the first case, there was little reason to believe that another revision could be successful. Because the patient was frail, the goal in his case was to attempt to do as minimal a surgery as possible to help control his pain.

Surgical Technique

Standard posterior and anterior portals are used to start, and accessory anterior and/or posterior portals are made as recommended. A 7-mm cannula is placed in the high anterior portal. A standard 30-degree, 4-mm arthroscope was used in all cases. Orientation can be difficult because of distorted reflections of the polished metal humeral head. The first step is to perform a local synovectomy and débridement around the anterior, superior, and posterior margins of the glenoid component and to confirm glenoid component looseness with a probe. Next, a curved osteotome (4 to 6 mm) through the anterior portal is used to make three sets of cuts (Fig. 37–10) so that the prosthesis can be removed in four pieces. The first cut (1a) transects the glenoid prosthesis diagonally in an anterosuperior to posteroinferior direction (Fig. 37–11). The second part (1b) of that set divides the remaining intact polyethylene between the cut portion of the face plate and the underlying keel (see Fig. 37–11). The superior third of the glenoid face plate can be withdrawn through the anterior portal by grasping it at the tip and taking advantage of the "aerodynamic" shape created by the diagonal cut (Figs. 37–11 and 37–12). The second set of similar cuts (2a and 2b) detaches the inferior third of the glenoid face plate from the middle portion and from the keel (see Fig. 37–12). The osteotome is then passed beneath the remaining middle part of the face plate (cut 3), separating it from the keel (Fig. 37–13**A**, **B**). The keel is removed by backing it out with a twisting motion, apex first. Strong graspers are recommended because the soft tissues around the portal needs to stretch to permit component extraction. A Ferris-Smith grasper, normally used to extract an intervertebral disc or intramedullary cement, is useful. The cement is then removed in pieces, breaking it up with a curved osteotome as necessary. A curette is used to clean the glenoid cavity. A total synovectomy is performed if there is significant synovitis present. Finally, a capsulotomy can be performed to improve motion, if necessary.

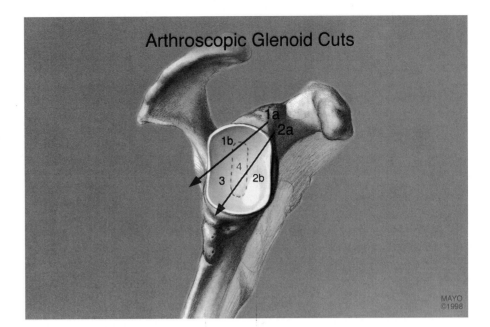

Figure 37–10. The glenoid is cut into four pieces with three sets of cuts, designed to create "aerodynamically" shaped pieces and to take advantage of the keel to hold the component in place until the final cut has been made. Each of the cuts is made using a 4- to 6-mm osteotome through the anterior portal. (By permission of Mayo Foundation for Medical Education and Research.)

Techniques that have not been found helpful include grinding the glenoid with a bur or cutting it into small pieces with bone-biting instruments. In one case, the unwise decision was made to fully amputate the keel, but that rendered the remainder of the glenoid component unstable and difficult to cut.

Postoperatively, the patients were given a sling for comfort for the first few days, but they were encouraged to start moving the limb right away and to pursue activities as tolerated. The procedure is generally performed on an outpatient basis unless there is concern about the preoperative general medical status.

RESULTS TO BE EXPECTED

From a technical perspective, this operation is likely to be successful in the hands of an experienced arthroscopist. Glenoid loosening can be confirmed by using a probe to lift the component away from the underlying bone.

Our five patients have been followed for 27 months (range, 13 to 41 months) (Fig. 37–14**A**, **B**). From a clinical perspective, the procedures have been helpful. Each of the patients feels better than before the glenoid removal, and each one is glad it was done and would choose to do

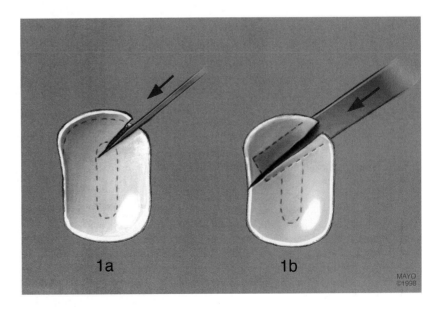

Figure 37–11. Cut 1a separates the superoposterior third of the glenoid face plate from the remainder of the face plate, leaving a small attachment to the underlying keel. Cut 1b separates the component fragment from the keel to permit removal. (By permission of Mayo Foundation for Medical Education and Research.)

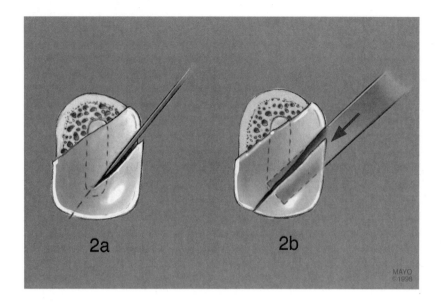

Figure 37–12. Cuts 2a and 2b, similar to cuts 1a and 1b noted earlier, separate the anteroinferior third of the face plate from the middle portion and from the keel. (By permission of Mayo Foundation for Medical Education and Research.)

the same again if faced with that decision. No further surgeries have been performed in any of the five patients. Pain relief was partial (40 percent to 50 percent) in three patients, and complete (100 percent) in two patients. Functional improvement, not surprisingly, paralleled pain relief; the two patients with complete pain relief gained 55 degrees of elevation each and 35 degrees to 45 degrees of external rotation. The other three patients, who had partial pain relief, did not gain motion.

Strength improvements were noted, but they were undoubtedly related to pain relief. No complications were encountered. Each patient is convinced that the operation was worthwhile and would undergo the same in the future if faced with a similar decision.

RECOMMENDATIONS

Arthroscopic removal of a loose glenoid component and its cement represents an appealing alternative to open revision surgery for failed total shoulder arthroplasty caused by symptomatic glenoid loosening. The concept is practicable, and the questions that remain to be answered concern its predictability, success, and the determination of what indications, contraindications, and complications. A larger series with longer follow-up will be needed to answer those questions.

In addition, there are some limitations and potential pitfalls to this technique. Only all-polyethylene components and associated PMMA can be removed; removal of metal components is unrealistic. It is difficult to bone graft glenoid defects should this be deemed necessary.

Damage to the surface of the humeral head can occur as a result of scuffing by the instruments, and this could theoretically lead to component wear.[19]

The issue of total arthroplasty component damage from the arthroscopic instruments has received scant attention in the literature. We observed that the humeral component was marked following this procedure. We suspect that it is highly unlikely that the procedure

could be performed without contacting and marking the humeral component. The issue of how this relates to the longevity of the implant is unknown at this time. This may be an important consideration if in the future a revision glenoid component was implanted. The result would be a scuffed/roughened humeral component articulating on a polyethylene component, which could potentially lead to increased polyethylene wear and early failure of the prosthesis. Therefore, we do not recommend this technique if implantation of a revision glenoid component is a likely possibility. At the current time, there are no plans to reimplant a glenoid component in our patients.

There are alternatives that were not employed in these patients, including bone grafting the glenoid cavity; such an alternative could be considered in future clinical applications. In fact, arthroscopic removal of a loose glenoid component (and cement) combined with bone grafting of the defect could theoretically be used as an interim procedure to restore glenoid bone stock in preparation for reimplantation of a glenoid component. Synovectomy, potentially an important part of the procedure, was performed in each patient in this series and may have contributed to pain relief.

Summary

Arthroscopic removal of a loose glenoid component along with its cement can be considered for patients who have a painful, loose polyethylene glenoid component without rotator cuff deficiency and without other evidence to suggest a cause for failure of the total shoulder arthroplasty. It should be considered in elderly or frail patients for whom the need to minimize further surgery is even more important. Contraindications would be the presence of a metal-backed glenoid component or severe bone loss that would compromise the bony rim of the glenoid so that containment of the humerus in the glenoid is not likely to be possible after removal of the glenoid component.

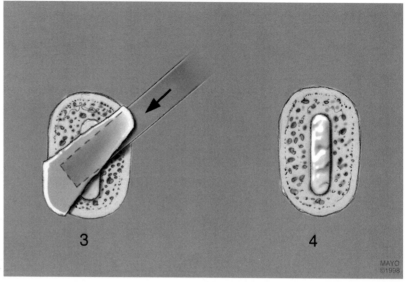

Figure 37–13. A and **B**, The third and fourth segments of the glenoid component (*middle portion of faceplate and keel respectively*) are separated by cut number three with the osteotome. The technique shows the osteotome coming from the anterior portal in this combined segmatic/arthroscopic view. (By permission of Mayo Foundation for Medical Education and Research.)

A

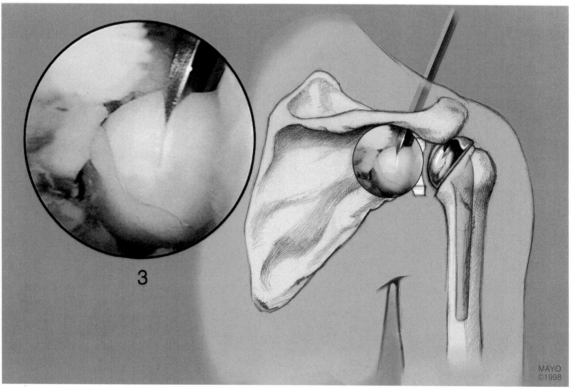

B

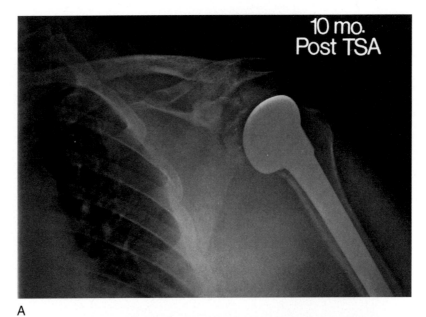

Figure 37–14. A, Preoperative radiograph showing a wide, complete, progressive radiolucent line around a cemented glenoid component. **B,** Radiograph taken 17 months after arthroscopic glenoid component removal shows concentric remodeling of the remaining glenoid bone stock. This patient had essentially complete relief from pain.

References

1. Allardyce TJ, Scuderi GR, Insall JN: Arthroscopic treatment of popliteus tendon dysfunction following total knee arthroplasty. J Arthroplasty 12:353–355, 1997.
2. Bell SN, Gschwend N: Clinical experience with total arthroplasty and hemiarthroplasty of the shoulder using the Neer prosthesis. Int Orthop 10:217–222, 1986.
3. Bocell JR, Thorpe CD, Tullos HS: Arthroscopic treatment of symptomatic total knee arthroplasty. Clin Orthop 125–134, 1991.
4. Bonutti PM, Hawkins RJ, Saddemi S: Arthroscopic assessment of glenoid component loosening after total shoulder arthroplasty. Arthroscopy 9:272–276, 1993.
5. Boyd AD Jr, Thomas WH, Scott RD, et al: Total shoulder arthroplasty versus hemiarthroplasty. Indications for glenoid resurfacing. J Arthroplasty 5:329–336, 1990.
6. Field LD, Dines DM, Zabinski SJ, Warren RF: Hemiarthroplasty of the shoulder for rotator cuff arthropathy. J Shoulder Elbow Surg 6:18–23, 1997.
7. Flood JN, Kolarik DB: Arthroscopic irrigation and débridement of infected total knee arthroplasty: Report of two cases. Arthroscopy 4:182–186, 1988.
8. Groh GI, Badwey TM, Rockwood CA: Treatment of cysts of the acromioclavicular joint with shoulder hemiarthroplasty. J Bone Joint Surg 75A:1790–1794, 1993.
9. Harryman DT, Sidles JA, Clark JM, et al: Translation of the humeral head on the glenoid with passive glenohumeral motion. J Bone Joint Surg 72A:1334–1343, 1990.
10. Hawkins RJ, Angelo RL: Glenohumeral osteoarthrosis. A late complication of the Putti-Platt repair. J Bone Joint Surg 72A:1193–1197, 1990.
11. Johnson DR, Friedman RJ, McGinty JB, et al: The role of arthroscopy in the problem of total knee replacement. Arthroscopy 6:30–32, 1990.

12. Jonsson E, Brattstrom M, Lidgren L: Evaluation of the rheumatoid shoulder function after hemiarthroplasty and arthrodesis. Scand J Rheum 17:17–26, 1988.
13. Kay SP, Amstutz HC: Shoulder hemiarthroplasty at UCLA. Clin Orthop 228:42–48, 1988.
14. Levine WN, Djurasovic M, Glasson J-M, et al: Hemiarthroplasty for glenohumeral osteoarthritis: Results correlated to degree of glenoid wear. J Shoulder Elbow 6:449–454, 1997.
15. Markel DC, Luessenhop CP, Windsor RE, Sculco TA: Arthroscopic treatment of peripatellar fibrosis after total knee arthroplasty. J Arthroplasty 11:293–297, 1996.
16. Marmor L: Hemiarthroplasty for the rheumatoid shoulder joint. Clin Orthop 122:201–203, 1977.
17. Nordt W, Giangarra CE, Levy IM, Habermann ET: Arthroscopic removal of entrapped debris following dislocation of a total hip arthroplasty. Arthroscopy 3:196–198, 1987.
18. Petersen SA, Hawkins RJ: Revision of failed total shoulder arthroplasty. Orthop Clin North Am 29:519–33, 1998.
19. Raab GE, Jobe CM, Williams PA, Dai QG: Damage to cobalt-chromium surfaces during arthroscopy of total knee replacements. J Bone Joint Surg Am 83A:46–52, 2001.
20. Torchia ME, Cofield RH, Settergren CR: Total shoulder arthroplasty with the Neer prosthesis: Long-term results. J Shoulder Elbow Surg 6:495–505, 1997.
21. Wasilewski SA, Frankl U: Arthroscopy of the painful dysfunctional total knee replacement. Arthroscopy 5:294–297, 1989.
22. Weinstein DM, Bucchieri JS, Pollock RG, et al: Arthroscopic débridement of the shoulder for osteoarthritis. Arthroscopy 16:471–746, 2000.
22a. Cameron BD, Galatz LM, Ramsey ML, et al: Non-prosthetic management of grade IV osteochondral lesions of the glenohumeral joint. J Shoulder Elbow Surg 11:25-32, 2002.
23. Williams GR, Rockwood CA: Hemiarthroplasty in rotator cuff-deficient shoulders. J Shoulder Elbow Surg 5:362–367, 1996.
24. Wirth MA, Rockwood CA Jr: Complications of shoulder arthroplasty. Clin Orthop 307:47–69, 1994.

38

Shoulder Component Design and Fixation

• ROBERT H. COFIELD

IMPLANT DESIGN

Shoulder implant design is a complex interplay among replacing cartilage surfaces, restoring anatomy, taking into account biomechanical testing and theory, recognizing the benefits and limitations of various materials, considering the manufacturing processes, perceiving marketing issues, and heeding surgeons' needs for relative ease of insertion leading to reproducibility in surgery and consistency in outcome.

Much of the scientific focus on implant design for the shoulder has centered around a better understanding of the variations in anatomy of the upper end of the humerus. Multiple studies have used direct measurements of bones and, often, various means of adjunctive imaging. A number of studies have shown the humeral head to be not quite spherical but very close to being so, with the humeral head radius varying between 19 and 32 mm and averaging 22 to 25 mm.[2,5,20,36,37,46] The thickness of the humeral head in various investigations has ranged from 12 to 24 mm, with averages from 15 to 20 mm.[5,20,36,37,46] The humeral head inclination relative to the axis of the humerus has varied between 120 and 145 degrees, with averages of 130 to 35 degrees.[5,20,35,37,46] Assessment of humeral head retroversion has been more complicated as the angle has been measured in comparison with the transepicondylar axis, a tangent to the trochlea, a tangent to the elbow, or with reference to the forearm. Retrotorsion relative to the transepicondylar axis in various series has ranged from –5 to 60 degrees, with averages from 18 to 22 degrees.[5,36,37,46] In surgery, the most applicable of these references for humeral retrotorsion is to the axis of the forearm, and in the one study in which this was assessed, the average was 41 degrees.[19] In relation to the top of the greater tuberosity, the uppermost point of the humeral head rests above the level of the tuberosity by a range of 3 to 20 mm, averaging 8 to 8.7 mm.[20,34]

As a number of prosthetic systems have developed a fixed relationship between the central axis of the humeral shaft and the center of the humeral head, "new" additional anatomic parameters have also been identified. The anteroposterior offset of the humeral head relative to the central axis of the humerus has ranged from 3 mm of anterior offset to 11 mm of posterior offset and has averaged between 2 and 5 mm of posterior offset.[2,5,36,46] The medial-lateral offset of the humeral head center relative to the central axis of the humeral shaft has ranged between 3 and 14 mm of medial offset, with averages between 7 and 11 mm.[5,28,35]

The internal humeral canal diameter has been less commonly measured. In two studies, this ranged between 8 and 14 mm and averaged 11 to 12 mm.[2,35]

Considering all these various parameters, it is easy to understand that prosthetic systems replacing the humeral head may alter joint kinematics, and, in this setting, that has been assessed by measuring the effect of various implants on the center of rotation of the humeral head.[26] Typically, in implant systems, the center of rotation is shifted upward and laterally.[34]

Glenoid size has been measured in four studies.[12,20,21,27] The superior-to-inferior dimension ranges between 26 and 48 mm with averages between 34 and 40 mm. The anteroposterior dimension is highly variable, depending on where the measurement is taken. The largest measurements have varied between 16 and 35 mm, with averages between 24 and 29 mm.

Saha recognized that the radius of curvature of the humeral head and the radius of curvature of the glenoid in a shoulder joint may vary somewhat, leading to a lack of complete conformity between the articular surfaces.[38] In one study, the radius of curvature of the glenoid was on average 2.3 mm greater than the radius of curvature of the humeral head.[20] These differences in radius of curvature have been particularly apparent when the respective bones are assessed. When the actual articular cartilage surfaces are analyzed, the surfaces are quite conforming.[42] Biomechanical studies have indicated that the translations seen in a natural shoulder joint are best reproduced in reconstructed joints that have somewhat less conforming articulations.[23] A higher degree of conformity and constraint directly affects the forces generated during testing of translation and rotation of the humeral head.[1,41] Also, during translation, higher forces are recognized at the glenoid component as joint conformity increases.[22] However, when assessing kinematics of the glenohumeral joint in a cadaveric model with an intact capsule and rotator cuff tendons, alterations in motion patterns were minimally affected by a reduction in congruity between the articular surface prosthetic components—the sizes of the components inserted had a much more dominant effect on altering the joint kinematics.[17]

The material properties of polyethylene must also be considered when the curvature of the glenoid is altered relative to the humerus. An increasing amount of "mismatch" decreases contact area and increases contact pressure. For a load approximating body weight, contact stress exceeds yield stress for polyethylene when the radial mismatch is greater than 3 mm.[28]

One can see from the preceding paragraphs that there are a great variety of anatomic and biomechanical factors to be considered. This may lead to consideration of quite complex implant systems; however, the complexity of design may generate additional unanticipated problems, and the general admonition is to avoid components with multiple parts, if at all possible. For example, modularity of implant systems has been well accepted in the orthopedic community to facilitate implant insertion, to aid in revision surgery, and to engender a manageable amount of implant inventory. A number of studies have been reported attesting to the safety and efficacy of modular humeral components.[10,14,16] However, in spite of great care taken in prosthetic design, there are occasional dissociations of modular humeral head or glenoid components, and such dissociations have been reported.[3,9,11]

A SHOULDER ARTHROPLASTY SYSTEM

For more than 20 years, the various components of shoulder implant design (Smith and Nephew, Memphis, TN) have been carefully studied. Many things must be considered as outlined in Table 38–1. These must balance the many factors contributing to implant design. The surfaces must be replaced with materials that have acceptable wear characteristics. Anatomy must be respected as must biomechanical theory and testing. Competing ideas that simplicity versus complexity must be mated to create the ease of insertion that leads to reproducibility during surgery. This implies that some portions of the design will be near the mean of humeral variability, whereas others will vary in size or shape to match the spectrum of human dimensions.

A consideration of the humeral head reveals that the radius of curvature varies somewhat between anatomic specimens but not dramatically. To avoid undue complexity, we have selected a constant radius of curvature for the humeral head that is in the midrange of anatomic values. By treating the glenoid in the same manner, it is possible to match any humeral head with any glenoid. Additionally, to aid in the potential need for revision surgery, the radius is also equal to that of the implant that has been used most commonly over time (Neer II, 3M, St. Paul, MN). On the other hand, humeral

Table 38–1. CONSIDERATIONS IN SHOULDER IMPLANT DESIGN

Humeral head
    Radius of curvature
    Thickness and width
    Offsets
    Head-stem fixation
    Extraction capability
Humeral stem
    Shape
    Length(s)
    Width(s)
    Fins
    Suture holes
    Surface finish/fixation methods
Humeral instrumentation
    Resection guide
    Drills, reamers
    Trials
    Impaction, distraction device
Humeral component materials
Glenoid component
    Shape
    Sizes (height and width)
    Thickness
    Surface curvature
    Pegs/keel
    Surface finish/fixation methods
Glenoid instrumentation
    Guides
    Drills
    Reamers
    Router
    Rasps/sizers
    Trials
    Pusher
Glenoid component materials
Instrument cases
    Organized
    Sequenced (Charnley)

head sizes vary considerably, and to obtain the best tension in the soft tissues and to address ample mobility while respecting stability, head sizes should vary, and their variability should be intuitively understandable. The system has included a proportionate increase in thickness and width of the humeral heads, increasing by 2-mm increments in diameter and height for each larger implant size within the normal range of humeral head sizes. The system has always included a medial offset relative to the axis of the humeral shaft. Over time, it has not included a means to address anterior or posterior offset unless the humeral stem is eccentrically cemented in the humeral canal. Although I believe that these issues are seldom important in shoulder arthroplasty, additional sets of humeral heads have been developed to make it possible to have additional anterior, posterior, or medial offset in selected cases. In a modular humeral head system, the tapered junction must be secure, and it seems reasonable to use a taper design that has been proved in large numbers of hip joint replacements. There must be a simple means to separate the humeral head from the stem. Extraction slots on the undersurface of the humeral head were selected to accomplish this, and a simple wedge-shaped removal tool can do the job.

The design of the humeral stem is critical. A single angle of inclination of the humeral head relative to the shaft has been selected, approaching the mean of this angle in human studies. This angle is slightly greater than that of the anatomic neck relative to the shaft and has the added positive effects of preserving humeral metaphyseal bone, creating the opportunity for tissue ingrowth fixation rather than cement fixation alone, and eliminating the potential for filling the inferior aspect of the glenohumeral joint with the prosthetic humeral head and thereby limiting overhead movement. A rather narrow, cylindrical stem preserves bone of the proximal humerus, saves space for tuberosity positioning and adjunctive bone grafting, and facilitates bone preparation with cylindrical cutting tools. The standard length implant must be long enough to reach the proximal end of the cylindrical humeral isthmus with its strong cortical bone. Longer stem lengths should be available to address distally extending fractures or oncologic problems. There should be only a minimal proximal expansion of the humeral stem to preserve the metaphyseal humeral bone and to allow off-axis insertion in cases of old trauma with malunion and other more unusual situations. The proximal portion of the stem contains four fins for rotational stability, with suture holes in all fins for additional security in tuberosity attachment. The stem diameter should vary in understandable amounts, and this system increases 2 mm in diameter for each larger component. For the surface finish, it is important to limit texturing to the metaphyseal region, and, if possible, take advantage of tissue ingrowth instead of simple texturing in this region. The more distal aspect of the stem should be smooth, preferably polished, as in this implant, for use with cement and for easy extraction in implants inserted with or without cement.

The humeral instruments should allow carpenter-like fitting for the implant. This includes a resection guide that uses both intramedullary and extramedullary referencing, cylindrical humeral reamers, and adjunctive drills for preparation of harder bone. The reamers and drills should exactly equal implant size and have clear depth markings. Trial components should exactly reproduce the implants, and stem extensions should be available for trials of longer humeral stems. There should be a strong impaction and distraction device for the trial and real implants. The trial implants should have a metaphyseal plate to protect the exposed cancellous bone during glenoid preparation. Humeral head trials should fit the stem trials and the real implant stems (Fig. 38–1).

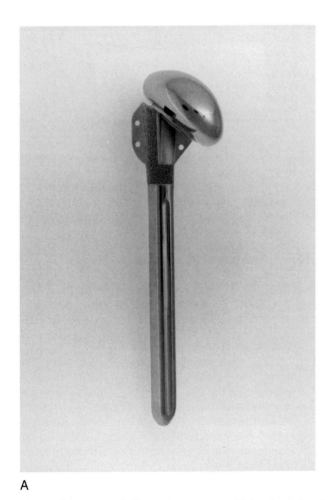

A

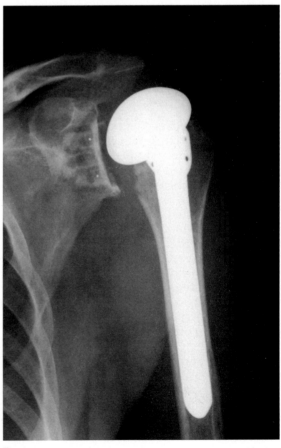

B

Figure 38–1. A, Humeral component with head and stem impacted together. **B**, Radiograph of humeral component in place as a part of total shoulder arthroplasty.

There are several materials that can be considered to construct the various parts of a humeral component. These include stainless steel, chrome-cobalt, titanium, and ceramics. For this system, chrome-cobalt has been selected for the both the humeral heads and the stems.

The glenoid component should also include a variety of options. The most useful glenoid component is made of all high-density polyethylene, and, in this system, comes in three sizes. Each of these sizes has two thicknesses, 4 mm and 6 mm. To reduce forces across the glenoid and improve joint kinematics, the glenoid radius of curvature is 2 mm greater than the humeral component radius of curvature and is constant throughout system sizes. The undersurface of the component is textured, and there are limited numbers of slots and holes to improve glenoid keel fixation in the bone cement. Additionally, pegged polyethylene components are available. The pegs maintain the area of contact between the implant and the cement. They do allow an easier and more reproducible insertion technique; however, there is a reduction in the mass of polyethylene and some lingering concern about glenoid component strength (Fig. 38–2).

Using similar instruments, there is also a pegged, metal-backed tissue ingrowth glenoid component in standard

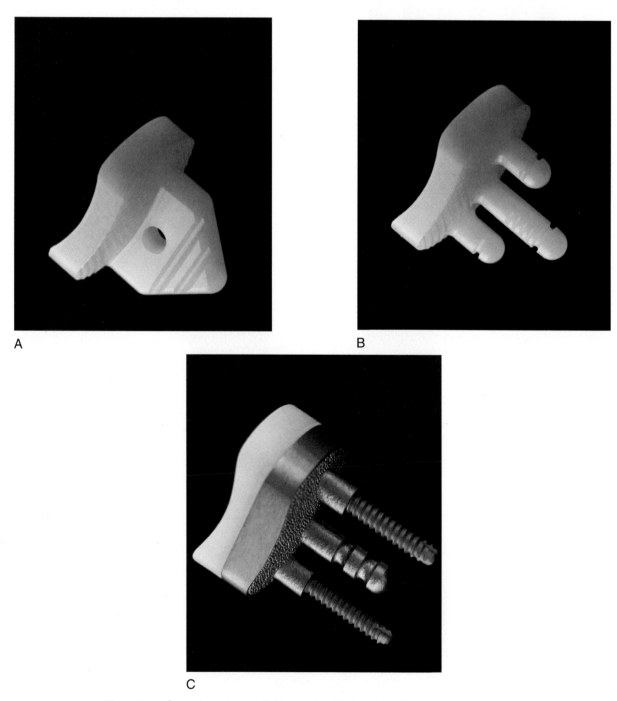

A

B

C

Figure 38–2. Glenoid component. **A**, Keel design. **B**, Peg design. **C**, Tissue ingrowth design.

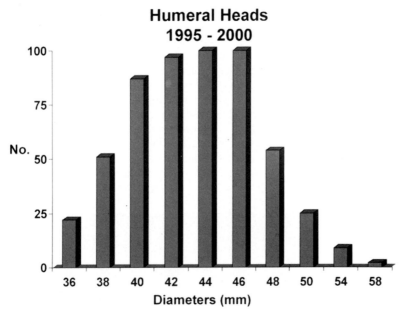

Figure 38–3. The various humeral head sizes implanted in 562 shoulders.

and small sizes for use in special situations, currently limited to shoulders in which there is a moderate amount of medial glenoid bone erosion that would preclude secure fixation with all-polyethylene keel or peg designs.

Glenoid instruments include guides for preparation of the pegs or keel, three sizes of reamers to precisely prepare the subchondral plate, drills to prepare the holes for the pegs, a router to prepare the slot for the keel, and keel and peg rasps/sizers to finish the preparation of the bone within the glenoid neck. A pusher is available to firmly seat the glenoid component and to hold it in position while the bone cement is hardening.

The system includes well-organized instrument cases: a case for humeral preparation, a case containing humeral trials, a case containing extra humeral preparation items for longer stems or extra-large heads, an instrument tray with added retractors, and a glenoid tray.

As can be seen from the preceding discussion, in constructing an implant sytem, many points are considered; in total approximately 40 or 50 items need in-depth consideration humeral and glenoid implants and the adjunctive instruments are being designed.

The graphs display the distribution of humeral head sizes, humeral stem sizes, and the sizes of glenoid components that have been used during the past six years (Figs. 38–3 through 38–5). It can be easily seen, as would be anticipated with variations in humeral size and anatomy, that a variety of component sizes have been used, with the most commonly used components in the midranges of bone size.

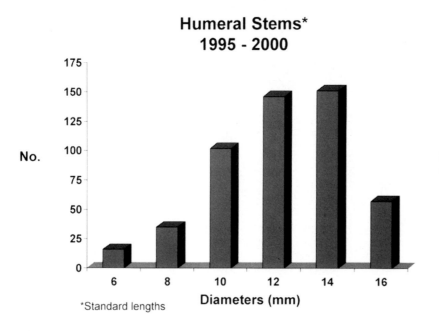

Figure 38–4. The various humeral stem sizes implanted in 507 shoulders.

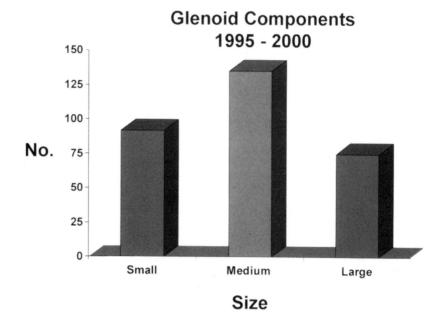

Figure 38–5. The various glenoid sizes implanted in 302 shoulders.

COMPONENT FIXATION

There are a number of areas that should be considered on this topic. These include finite element modeling and analysis, mechanical pullout testing, results of clinical series, reports on implantation technique, and radiographic analysis of implant security.

Several authors have undertaken finite element analysis of the glenoid and the humerus.[13,25,32,33,44] Of importance to component fixation, the analysis of the glenoid clearly indicates that a cemented polyethylene component should most closely replicate the stress distribution seen in a normal glenoid. If metallic materials are introduced, the analysis is greatly distorted by the presence of the metal, particularly when the metal contacts the cortical bone.

Mechanical pullout tests have been done with bone or bone simulated by various materials such as variable densities of polyurethane.[15,48] Although one would initially believe that this form of testing might have strong relevance to implant design and fixation, this has not been proved to be the case. The forces and displacements determined before and after many cycles of loading show very little difference, and the force to displacement (distraction) is most dependent upon the material properties of the implant system. Results are most notably affected by having metal as a part of the fixation for the implanted glenoid—the metal, of course, being much more resistant to distraction than polyethylene.

Many clinical series have, as an adjunct to reporting results, assessed the relatively high frequency of glenoid lucent lines, and the quite low necessity for revision surgery for component loosening.[6] In a similar fashion, my colleagues and I assessed 89 shoulders with an average 9.7 years of follow-up (range, 5 to 17 years).[45] These patients had surgery between 1975 and 1981 that included the diagnoses of osteoarthritis, rheumatoid arthritis, and post-traumatic arthritis. The survival curve illustrated the need for revision surgery to be quite low.

Notably, over this approximately 10-year average follow-up period, only 5.6 percent of the glenoids had clinical loosening, and 1.8 percent of the humeral components had clinical loosening. We did, however, notice in the assessment of our series that there was a significant frequency of radiographic change surrounding both components. We were of the opinion that 44 percent of the glenoid components were radiographically loose; of the humeral components, 45 percent, almost all of which were press-fitted, were radiographically loose. This and other studies have led us to the conclusion that assessment of radiographic characteristics of components is most sensitive in distinguishing between components that behave favorably and those that may be predisposed to clinical loosening.[7,8,18,24,29,47]

To further this end, we developed a system for radiographic assessment of glenoid and humeral components, and then applied it in four clinical series. The basic format was to have comparative radiographic views done early (within 2 months of surgery) and late (those done at most recent follow-up). Radiographic analysis would include a zonal analysis surrounding the glenoid component. We currently favor five zones for pegged components and six zones for keeled components. The humeral interface is divided into eight zones, very similar to the system used for the femoral component in hip arthroplasty. The locations of the lucent lines are noted, and their thickness is measured to 0.5 mm. Three observers then assess the early and late radiographs and offer their opinion about whether or not there has been a shift in component position for either the glenoid or the humeral component. Earlier, measurements of radiographs were done to determine whether a change in position had occurred. These measurements correlated closely with the opinions of the independent observers, and the measurements have been discontinued.

In addition to collecting the raw data, we then developed empirical criteria when a component might be radiographically "at risk" for clinical problems. These

Table 38–2. RADIOGRAPHIC ASSESSMENT OF SHOULDER ARTHROPLASTY

Studies	No. Shoulders	Mean Follow-up (yr.)
Cemented Neer II glenoid	81	4.1
Press-fitted humerus	72	4.1
Cemented humerus	43	6.6
Ingrowth glenoid	62	4.6
Ingrowth humerus	62	4.6
Second generation, cemented glenoid	88	3.5
Ingrowth humerus	73	3.5

included a glenoid component that had a complete lucent line surrounding the implant, some part of which was 1.5 mm or greater in thickness, or a glenoid component that was judged to have shifted in position by two in three or three in three of observers. Similarly, a humeral component was judged to be at risk for clinical problems if lucent lines were in three or more zones and were greater than 2 mm in width, or if two in three or three in three independent observers saw a shift in humeral component position.

The four clinical studies are outlined in Table 38–2. The first study on the cemented Neer II glenoid component and the press-fit humeral component occurred in patients operated on between 1981 and 1985.[31] There was one surgeon and a consistent surgical technique. This included power burring for surface preparation on the glenoid, burring the keel slot without guides, partially preserving the subchondral plate and undermining it with bulb lavage and sponge packing for cleaning the glenoid, placing the cement in the glenoid and packing it for three to four pressure cycles, and then placing a component in the bone and holding it in position with the thumb. In this group of patients, 72 humeral components were press-fitted and 9 were cemented in place. On radiographic analysis, 31 percent of the glenoid components were judged to be at risk by these criteria, and, surprisingly, 56 percent of the press-fitted humeral components were judged to be at risk.[40]

The second study included a clinical group, operated on between 1976 and 1987, who had a cemented humeral component as a part of hemiarthroplasty or total shoulder replacement.[39] Only 1 humeral component (2 percent) exhibited radiographic features of at-risk magnitude.

Shoulders undergoing placement of an ingrowth total shoulder arthroplasty between 1989 and 1992 were assessed.[43] Strikingly, only 4 glenoid components (6.5 percent) and 6 humeral components (9.7 percent) were judged to be radiographically at risk.

Most recently, we radiographically assessed the second generation of total shoulder arthroplasty.[4] These procedures were done between 1990 and 1995. The improved techniques included the availability of a variety of glenoid component sizes and variations, glenoid instruments, use of pulsatile lavage for cleansing the glenoid neck, direct use of cement pressurization into the glenoid keel slot, component impaction and holding with an insertion device,[30] and better balanc-

ing of the joint by using various soft tissue releases and tightening procedures. In this patient group, 12 (14 percent) exhibited at-risk changes of the glenoid component, and 3 in 73 tissue ingrowth humeral components (4 percent) exhibited radiographic changes of at-risk level.

Thus, for this more complex and systemic radiographic assessment of total shoulder arthroplasty, we were able to conclude that the radiographic changes surrounding the earlier implant design and the earlier implant technique are potentially problematic for later clinical problems. Tissue ingrowth surfaces for the glenoid are promising for component fixation of bone, but, of course, are currently questionable because of accelerated polyethylene wear in a few patients. The radiographic changes surrounding the second-generation cemented glenoid components are less than half of those seen in the early series, but they still cause concern. When we have 2 more years of follow-up, we may be able to assess the radiographic features of total shoulder arthroplasties with a mismatch of the humeral and glenoid radii of curvatures, and we may then be able to judge the effect of humeral modularity on joint kinematics—as reflected in the radiographic changes seen. Three or four years after that, cemented pegged glenoid components can be assessed.

Assessment of the humeral components has led us to conclude that surgeons should be wary of the use of press-fit stems. The incorporation of tissue ingrowth (perhaps more substantial texturing) has much improved the radiographic features surrounding the humeral component. However, it is clearly recognizable that cementing the humeral component yields the best radiographic features and, quite likely, the most durable fixation for the humeral component.

Having assessed these things for a typical arthritic shoulder undergoing shoulder arthroplasty, we currently recommend an all-polyethylene cemented glenoid component whenever practically possible, with use of advanced surgical techniques. We currently also continue to use the tissue ingrowth humeral component with the tissue ingrowth surfaces limited to the undersurface of the plate for the trunion and on the upper few centimeters of the stem, contacting only the humeral metaphysis and not diaphyseal bone.

References

1. Anglin C, Wyss UP, Pichora DR: Shoulder prosthesis subluxation: Theory and experiment. J Shoulder Elbow Surg 9:104, 2000.
2. Ballmer FT, Sidles JA, Lippitt SB, Matsen FA: Humeral prosthetic arthroplasty: Surgically relevant considerations. J Shoulder Elbow Surg 2:296, 1993.
3. Blevins FT, Deng X, Torzilli PA, et al: Dissociation of modular humeral head components: A biomechanical and implant retrieval study. J Shoulder Elbow Surg 6:113, 1997.
4. Boardman ND III, Cofield RH, Torchia ME, et al: Radiographic analysis of second generation total shoulder arthroplasty [in press].
5. Boileau P, Walch G: The three-dimensional geometry of the proximal humerus. Implications for surgical technique and prosthetic design. J Bone Joint Surg 79B:857, 1997.

6. Brems J: The glenoid component in total shoulder arthroplasty. J Shoulder Elbow Surg 2:47, 1993.
7. Brostrom LA, Kronberg M, Wallensten R: Should the glenoid be replaced in shoulder arthroplasty with an unconstrained Dana or St. Georg prosthesis? Ann Chir Gynaecol 81:54, 1992.
8. Cofield RH: Uncemented total shoulder arthroplasty. Clin Orthop 307:86, 1994.
9. Cooper RA, Brems JJ: Recurrent dissembly of a modular humeral prosthesis. J Arthroplasty 6:375, 1991.
10. Dines DM, Warren RF: Modular shoulder hemiarthroplasty for acute fractures. Clin Orthop 307:18, 1994.
11. Driessnack RP, Ferlic DC, Wiedel JD: Dissociation of the glenoid component in the Macnab/English total shoulder arthroplasty. J Arthroplasty 5:15, 1990.
12. Ebraheim NA, Xu R, Haman SP, et al: Quantitative anatomy of the scapula. Am J Orthop 29:287, 2000.
13. Ehnes DL, Stone JJ, Cofield RH, An KN: Analysis of the shoulder implant. Biomed Sci Instrum 36:129, 2000.
14. Fenlin JM, Ramsey ML, Allardyce TJ, Brierman BG: Modular total shoulder replacement: Design rationale, indications and results. Clin Orthop 7:37, 1994.
15. Fukuda K, Chen CM, Cofield, RH, Chao EYS: Biomechanical analysis of stability and fixation strength of total shoulder prostheses. Orthopedics 11:141, 1988.
16. Gartsman GM, Russell JA, Gaenslen E: Modular shoulder arthroplasty. J Shoulder Elbow Surg 6:333, 1997.
17. Harryman DT, Sidles JA, Harris SL, et al: The effect of articular conformity and the size of the humeral head component on laxity and motion after glenohumeral arthroplasty. A study in cadavera. J Bone Joint Surg 77A:555, 1995.
18. Havig MT, Kumar A, Carpenter W, Seiler JG: Assessment of radiolucent lines about the glenoid. J Bone Joint Surg 70A:428, 1997.
19. Hernigou P, Duparc F, Filali C: Humeral retroversion and shoulder prosthesis. Rev Chir Orthop Reparatrice Appar Mot 81:419, 1995.
20. Iannotti JP, Gabriel JP, Schneck SL, et al: The normal glenohumeral relationships. An anatomical study of 140 shoulders. J Bone Joint Surg 74A:491, 1992.
21. Jobe CM, Iannotti JP: Limits imposed on glenohumeral motion by joint geometry. J Shoulder Elbow Surg 4:281, 1995.
22. Karduna AR, Williams GR, Iannotti JP, Williams JL: Total shoulder arthroplasty biomechanics: A study of the forces and strains at the glenoid component. J Biomech Eng 120:92, 1998.
23. Karduna AR, Williams GR, Williams JL, Iannotti JP: Glenohumeral joint translations before and after total shoulder arthroplasty. J Bone Joint Surg 70A:1166, 1997.
24. Kelleher IM, Cofield RH, Becker DA, Beabout JW: Fluoroscopically positioned radiographs of total shoulder arthroplasty. J Shoulder Elbow Surg 1:306, 1992.
25. Lacroix D, Prendergast PJ: Stress analysis of glenoid component designs for shoulder arthroplasty. Proc Inst Mechanical Eng (H) 211:467, 1997.
26. de Leest O, Rozing PM, Rozendaal LA, van der Helm FCT: Influence of glenohumeral prosthesis geometry and placement on shoulder muscle forces. Clin Orthop 330:222, 1996.
27. Mallon WJ, Brown HR, Vogler JB III, Martinez S: Radiographic and geometric anatomy of the scapula. Clin Orthop 277:142, 1992.
28. Matsen FA III, Lippitt SB, Sidles JA, Harryman DT II: Practical Evaluation and Management of the Shoulder. Philadelphia, WB Saunders Company, 1994, pp 181–198.
29. Maynou C, Petroff E, Mestdagh F, et al: Devenir clinique et radiologique des implants humeraux des arthroplasties d'épaule. Acta Orthop Belg 65:57, 1999.
30. Norris BL, Lachiewicz PF: Modern cement technique and the survivorship of total shoulder arthroplasty. Clin Orthop 328:76, 1996.
31. O'Driscoll, SW, Wright TW, Cofield RH, Ilstrup D, Mansat P: The glenoid problem. Radiographic assessment of the glenoid component in total shoulder arthroplasty. In Mansat P (ed): Prothèses d'épaule. Toulouse, Expansion Scientifique Publication, 1999, p 337.
32. Orr TE, Carter DR: Stress analyses of joint arthroplasty in the proximal humerus. J Orthop Res 3:360, 1985.
33. Orr TE, Carter DR, Schurman DJ: Stress analyses of glenoid component designs. Clin Orthop 232:217, 1988.
34. Pearl ML, Kurutz S: Geometric analysis of commonly used prosthetic systems for proximal humerus replacement. J Bone Joint Surg 81A:660, 1999.
35. Pearl ML, Volk AG: Coronal plane geometry of the proximal humerus relevant to prosthetic arthroplasty. J Shoulder Elbow Surg 5:320, 1996.
36. Roberts SN, Foley AP, Swallow HM, et al: The geometry of the humeral head and the design of prostheses. J Bone Joint Surg 73B:647, 1991.
37. Robertson DD, Yuan J, Bigliani LU, et al: Three-dimensional analysis of the proximal part of the humerus: Relevance to arthroplasty. J Bone Joint Surg 82A:1594, 2000.
38. Saha AK: Recurrent anterior dislocation of the shoulder. A new concept. Calcutta, Academic Publishers, 1969, pp 9–10.
39. Sanchez-Sotelo J, O'Driscoll SW, Torchia ME, et al: Radiographic assessment of cemented humeral components in shoulder arthroplasty [in press].
40. Sanchez-Sotelo J, Wright TW, O'Driscoll SW, et al: Radiographic assessment of uncemented humeral components in total shoulder arthroplasty [in press].
41. Severt R, Thomas BJ, Tsenter MJ, et al: The influence of conformity and constraint on translational forces and frictional torque in total shoulder arthroplasty. Clin Orthop 292:151, 1993.
42. Soslowsky LJ, Flatow EL, Bigliani LU, Mow VC: Articular geometry of the glenohumeral joint. Clin Orthop 285:181, 1992.
43. Sperling JW, Cofield RH, O'Driscoll SW, et al: Radiographic assessment of ingrowth total shoulder arthroplasty. J Shoulder Elbow Surg 9:507, 2000.
44. Stone KD, Grabowski JJ, Cofield RH, et al: Stress analyses of glenoid components in total shoulder arthroplasty. J Shoulder Elbow Surg 8:151, 1999.
45. Torchia ME, Cofield RH, Settergren CR: Total shoulder arthroplasty with the Neer prosthesis: Long-term results. J Shoulder Elbow Surg 6:495, 1997.
46. Walch G, Boileau P: Morphological study of the humeral proximal epiphysis. In Proceedings of the European Society for Surgery of the Shoulder and Elbow. J Shoulder Elbow Surg 74B(Suppl I):14, 1992.
47. Wallace AL, Phillips RL, MacDougal J: Resurfacing of the glenoid in total shoulder arthroplasty. A comparison, at a mean of five years, of prostheses inserted with and without cement. J Bone Joint Surg 81A:510, 1999.
48. Walker PS: Human joints and their artificial replacements. Springfield, Il, Charles C. Thomas Publishers, 1977, p 351.

39

Rehabilitation and Activities After Shoulder Arthroplasty

• DIANE L. DAHM and JAY SMITH

The goal of rehabilitation is to restore optimal, pain-free function within the anatomic, physiologic, and biomechanical constraints of the patient. Rehabilitation success is predicated on several principles that are reviewed in this chapter (Table 39–1). An understanding of the principles of shoulder arthroplasty rehabilitation allows clinicians to develop rational treatment protocols and yet allow deviation from these protocols when necessary to meet the needs of the individual patient.

COMPLETE PREOPERATIVE COUNSELING

Ideally, the rehabilitation process begins with preoperative counseling for the patient, the family, and other caregivers. Realistic goal setting is encouraged, based on clinical and radiographic data. Modified or limited goals may be warranted in patients with excessive bone loss, rheumatoid arthritis, failed cuff repair, cuff arthropathy, post-traumatic arthritis, neurologic dysfunction, or previously failed shoulder arthroplasty.[1] In such cases, pain control is the primary surgical indication, with motion and functional restoration as secondary goals.

The patient should be identified as the primary active participant in the recovery process, receiving support from caregivers who should be identified preoperatively.[2] The patient and caregivers are counseled regarding the surgery, the early postoperative recovery period, anticipated pain and stiffness, the postoperative rehabilitation process, and the likelihood that up to a year may be required to realize an optimal outcome after the surgical procedure.[2] Identified caregivers need to agree to assist the patient with daily activities and to possibly transport the patient to physical therapy if necessary.

When appropriate, a preoperative exercise program may be implemented to optimize shoulder girdle motion, to strengthen the rotator cuff and scapular stabilizer muscles, and to condition the contralateral arm.

OBTAIN ADEQUATE PAIN CONTROL

Postoperative pain not only causes the patient and family anxiety and suffering but also reflexively inhibits the shoulder girdle musculature and impedes range of motion, strengthening, and functional gains. Pain relief is the primary indication for shoulder arthroplasty in most cases and should take precedence over functional gains.[1] Postoperative pain control can be facilitated by judicious analgesic use, including the coordination of analgesic administration with physical therapy sessions to provide optimal pain control when needed. Cryotherapy may be applied acutely postoperatively as needed, as well as after exercise to reduce pain and inflammation. It is also important to counsel patients that motion itself assists in providing pain control by increasing regional blood flow, removing toxic metabolites from the surgical site, and providing pain-modulating proprioceptive feedback to the central nervous system.[3]

INITIATE EARLY NONTRAUMATIC MOTION

Early mobilization promotes physiologic collagen formation, minimizes the adverse effects of immobility, and provides the foundation for functional restoration.[4,5] As previously stated, range of motion (ROM) also facilitates pain control via proprioceptive mechanisms.[3]

ROM goals are typically 150 degrees of elevation (ELE), 50 degrees of external rotation (ER) and T9 internal rotation (IR) for patients with osteoarthritis (OA) who have intact rotator cuffs, and 20 to 40 degrees less in all directions in OA patients who have cuff tears or patients with rheumatoid arthritis (RA) who often have some degree of rotator cuff insufficiency.[6,7] Most daily activities can be performed with approximately 20 to 40 degrees of ELE, ER, and IR.[6]

Early ROM must be balanced against the risks of tissue damage, increased pain, and instability. Maintaining stability is a primary concern for functional restoration

Table 39–1. PRINCIPLES OF REHABILITATION FOR SHOULDER ARTHROPLASTY

1. Complete Pre-operative Counseling
2. Obtain Adequate Pain Control
3. Initiate Early Non-Traumatic Motion
4. Restore Function
5. Protect the Prosthesis
6. Provide Counseling Regarding Activities

after arthroplasty.[8–10] Although deltoid preservation, restoration of myofascial sleeve tension, and improved component design and fixation have facilitated early ROM, clinicians must consider several patient and surgical factors when implementing postoperative ROM programs.

Patients with OA may have persistent glenoid retroversion despite attempts at surgical correction, thus increasing the risk of posterior instability during sagittal plane ELE and horizontal adduction.[1,11] Persistent acromioclavicular joint disease may also be aggravated by horizontal adduction motions. Rotator cuff contractures requiring extensive soft tissue releases such as subscapularis Z-plasty lengthening limit the safe range of available ER until tissue healing occurs.[12] Unlike typical OA patients, RA and post-traumatic OA patients are more likely to have rotator cuff or capsuloligamentous insufficiency, and thus the potential for multidirectional instabilities. Intraoperative ROM assessment is essential in these patients to determine the safe and stable arcs of motion for postoperative rehabilitation.

Surgical factors to be considered include component design and placement, fixation, and soft tissue integrity. The risk of anterior instability may be increased by component anteversion, subscapularis or capsule insufficiency, or coracoacromial arch insufficiency in the setting of a rotator cuff tear.[9] Posterior instability is common with excessive component retroversion or generalized soft tissue insufficiency.[8,9] Standard nonconstrained components offer potentially more ROM than more constrained designs but rely on soft tissue integrity for stability. Semiconstrained or fully constrained designs are used only in special circumstances and maintain stability by markedly sacrificing ROM.[14] If the humeral head is oversized, the joint may become "overstuffed," increasing rotator cuff tension and thus restricting motion.[13] On the contrary, use of an undersized humeral head or failure to restore the normal humeral offset (lateral coracoid to lateral tuberosity distance of 1.5 to 2.0 cm) compromises the length-tension relationship and mechanical properties of the cuff muscles, thereby reducing the ability to actively elevate the arm.[15] Early ROM may be safely initiated with either cemented or uncemented components.

In practice, ROM programs are implemented as soon as possible after surgery. Contralateral upper limb conditioning should begin immediately. Prolonged sling or splint immobilization of the affected shoulder is avoided unless concomitant rotator cuff repair or reconstruction has been performed. ROM guidelines are determined by considering the intraoperative examination and the patient and surgical factors previously discussed. The intraoperative ROM is typically not exceeded for 2 to 6 weeks.

ROM programs should focus on early restoration in a controlled manner of the primary motions of ELE and ER. Three to five exercise sessions of short duration (5 to 10 minutes) are performed each day.[1,2] Advantages include simplicity for improved compliance, frequent sessions to avoid prolonged inactivity, and short duration to avoid overwork and stiffness. Analgesics and modalities (heat, cryotherapy, and electrical stimulation) are coordinated with exercise sessions to optimize efficacy. Early exercise sessions are performed by physical therapists, with a gradual shift to patient and caregiver. Intraoperative photographs may be used to demonstrate the available ROM.[2] Postoperative interscalene blocks may be used to assist in reducing anxiety and pain. Continuous passive motion in shoulder arthroplasty patients has not been formally validated and poses some technical challenges for those unfamiliar with this application.

Pendulum (Codman's) exercises are useful to facilitate relaxation and pain control, to promote scapulothoracic mobility and stability, and to initiate early nontraumatic glenohumeral joint motion.[16–18] It is important to ensure relaxation in order to protect the cervical spine and the contralateral arm. In the right arm, forearm pronation (and shoulder internal rotation) can be coupled with counterclockwise pendulums, and forearm supination (and shoulder external rotation) can be coupled with clockwise pendulums to take advantage of upper limb proprioceptive neuromuscular facilitation (PNF) patterns that simulate functional movement patterns (Fig. 39–1). Caution may be needed in patients with generalized soft tissue laxity who may find the distraction of the hanging upper limb (14 percent of body weight) to be too painful.

Restoring ELE is an early priority. Exercises are begun in the supine position to offset gravity and facilitate assisted motion provided by the patient or therapist. If possible, ELE should be performed in the scapular plane (30 to 40 degrees anterior to the coronal plane) to allow the greatest impingement-free arc of motion with minimal soft tissue stress.[19,20] Biomechanically, the scapular plane is preferred for daily activities, and motion in this plane functionally transfers to both the sagittal and coronal planes without increasing glenohumeral joint reaction forces.[21,22] Pillows may be used to move the scapula into the scapular plane during supine exercises, but caution must be exercised to avoid anteriorly tilting or excessive internal rotation of the scapula (Fig. 39–2).[1] This malpositioning increases glenohumeral extension and anterior tensile forces. Although passive ROM (PROM) may be used early, a transition to active assisted ROM (AAROM) is made as soon as possible to activate the shoulder girdle musculature. During performance of therapist-assisted motions, a more proximal humeral grasp reduces patient apprehension and muscle co-contraction and also allows the therapist to apply gentle traction to the shoulder as necessary to improve pain-free mobility.[1,2] Supine PROM and

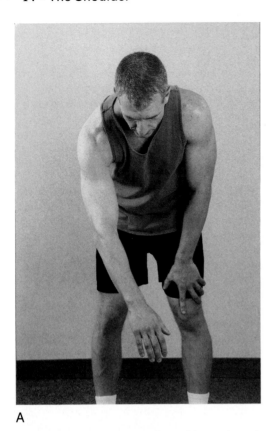

A

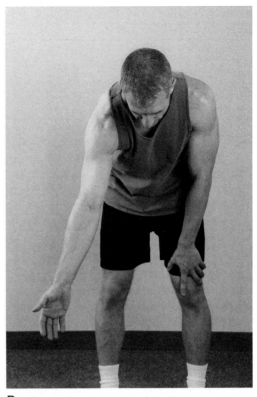

B

Figure 39–1. Pendulum exercises with proprioceptive neuromuscular facilitation (PNF) (**A**) clockwise in pronation and (**B**) counterclockwise in supination.

AAROM ELE exercises produce rotator cuff electromyography (EMG) activity equivalent to 10 percent to 20 percent of a maximal voluntary contraction.[17,18]

ER is often the most difficult and painful motion to restore. However, significant functional losses occur if ER ROM is less than 40 to 45 degrees. Patients who have had anterior soft tissue rebalancing may be at risk for compromising the repair or reconstruction if overstressed. In these patients, as well as in those with risk factors for anterior instability, the intraoperative ROM assessment determines the safe range of ER in the early postoperative period. ER exercises are also started supine and progress from PROM to AAROM and eventually to active ROM (AROM) exercises. During performance of supine ER exercises, maintaining the arm in slight abduction (4 to 6 cm), and in the scapular plane if possible, provides optimal tension-free ROM.[2] Active assisted ROM exercises should be performed with the elbow flexed to 90 degrees and the ER motion applied perpendicular to the long axis of the humerus. Patients commonly extend the elbow instead of externally rotating the shoulder, thereby decreasing the effectiveness of the exercise (Fig. 39–3). In patients with cuff repairs, patient AAROM with a cane or wand may be preferable to therapist AAROM for ER, because studies have demonstrated higher EMG activity in cuff muscles during the latter exercise.[18]

As pain is reduced and patients demonstrate adequate shoulder girdle control during supine exercises, the patients progress to more functional upright activities.

Under the influence of gravity, AAROM and AROM exercises also serve to initiate the strengthening process for the shoulder girdle. Studies have demonstrated that EMG activity (as a percentage of a maximal voluntary contraction) increases by 10 percent to 30 percent during the transition from supine to upright exercise.[17,18] Caution must be taken if rotator cuff integrity is a concern.

Upright exercises include AAROM and AROM exercises in ELE and ER. Elevation is initially performed in the scapular plane and can be assisted by another person, a wand or cane, wall climbing, or pulleys. Use of the wall or of a cane or wand appears to be tolerated best by patients (Fig. 39–4). Many patients find pulleys difficult to use initially, and relatively high EMG signals have been recorded in the cuff muscles during pulley assisted ELE compared ELE assisted by wand or cane.[18] Therefore, pulleys are initiated subsequent to wand, cane, and/or wall walking exercises. To reduce anxiety, patients initially face the suspended pulley. After they become comfortable with the technique, they turn away from the pulley to increase the efficacy of the exercise.[23] As acceptable shoulder control is established, AROM ELE motions are implemented. The elbow is initially flexed to reduce the gravitational moment arm and glenohumeral joint forces.

Standing ER is less dependent on gravity than ELE. While the patient is standing, PROM ER exercise can be performed by means of a doorway stretch (Fig. 39–5). Unless contraindicated, this stretch may be facilitated

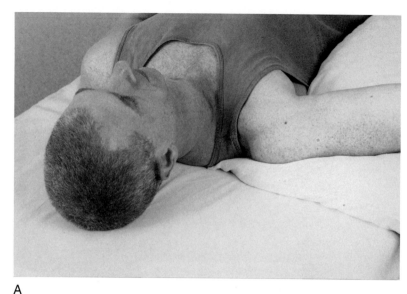

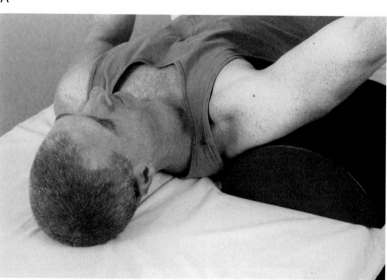

Figure 39–2. A, Proper positioning of the scapula. **B**, Improper positioning of the scapula.

A

B

by contract-relax techniques. An example of an upright functional AROM ER exercise is an integrated scapular retraction–shoulder ER motion without external resistance (Fig. 39–6).

Internal rotation exercises are generally limited to PROM to the level of the chest for the first 4 to 6 weeks and may be performed with the patient standing or supine. Progression from PROM to AAROM and AROM is performed as tolerated at 4 to 6 weeks. This allows protection of the subscapularis repair during the early weeks after surgery.

RESTORE FUNCTION AND PROTECT THE PROSTHESIS

Once pain control is achieved and acceptable AROM is established, the rehabilitation program begins to emphasize functional strengthening of the scapular stabilizer and rotator cuff musculature. The tolerance limits of current prosthesis designs with respect to com-

pression and shear forces are unknown. Resultant glenohumeral joint (GHJ) reaction forces gradually increase during ELE, reaching values equal to 90 percent of body weight at 90 degrees.[21] It has been postulated that the shear component of the resultant joint reaction force is most damaging, and excessive GHJ shear forces have been implicated as a primary cause of glenoid loosening in shoulder arthroplasty patients.[24,25]

The importance of the rotator cuff in minimizing GHJ shear cannot be overemphasized. During upper limb elevation, the rotator cuff maintains a stable locus of rotation so that the GHJ exhibits ball-and-socket kinematics.[26] With cuff insufficiency, this kinematic behavior is disrupted and excessive translation of the humeral head may occur with respect to the glenoid.[26] A similar pattern has been observed in the structurally intact rotator cuff after fatiguing exercise.[27] In both situations, GHJ shear forces can be expected to increase. Excessive humeral head translation produces eccentric edge loading of the glenoid, creating a "rocking horse glenoid," which has been documented as a cause of glenoid component failure.[24,25]

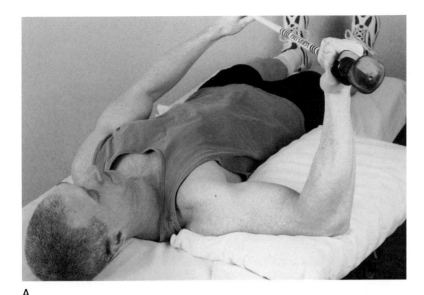

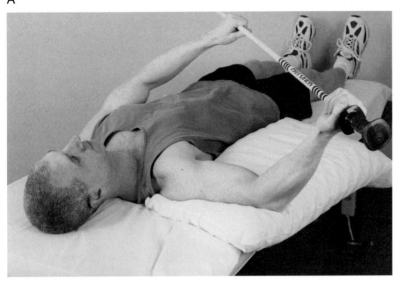

Figure 39–3. A, Correct position with elbow flexed to 90 degrees. **B,** Incorrect position with elbow extended.

In general, patients with intact rotator cuffs tolerate more aggressive rehabilitation and have better functional outcomes compared with those who have rotator cuff insufficiency.[28] Patients with rotator cuff insufficiency not repaired surgically often require a modified or limited goals program in which pain control is the primary desired outcome and motion and functional gains are secondary.[1] For those with rotator cuff repairs, the active rehabilitation process is generally delayed 4 to 6 weeks to allow adequate tissue healing.

Strengthening and conditioning exercises for the shoulder girdle begin with the ROM program previously described. Contralateral upper limb conditioning is recommended to avoid overuse injury while the affected shoulder is healing. On the affected side, isometric contractions are initiated early in the directions of ELE, ER, and IR. However, in the setting of cuff repair, strengthening may be delayed 6 to 12 weeks, depending on the size of the tear and the integrity of the repair. Isometric contractions are generally safe and can maintain strength when performed for three to six brief (5 to 6-second) repetitions multiple times per day.[29] Shear and capsuloligamentous strain are reduced because joint motion is minimized. Because isometric strengthening is angle specific, if patients perform isometric contractions about every 30 degrees in a motion arc, they can achieve better functional carryover to isotonic activities. Painful arcs of motion can be avoided. In many cases, isometric strengthening and AROM exercises can be combined so that the patient stops every 30 degrees during an AROM exercise and performs several isometric contractions in that position. The patient who performs this exercise can then progress to an AROM exercise with manual resistance applied by the therapist as described later.

The patient's progression to isotonic resistance exercise occurs as soon as tolerated because of better functional carryover. Initiation may take 6 to 12 weeks postoperatively in rotator cuff intact patients, and up to 3 to 6 months postoperatively for patients with rotator cuff repairs. Elevation is initially performed with the elbow flexed to reduce the upper limb moment arm.[21] It must be remem-

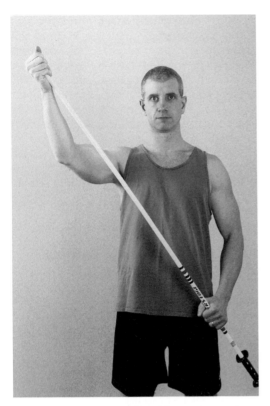

Figure 39–4. Scapular plane elevation with use of a wand.

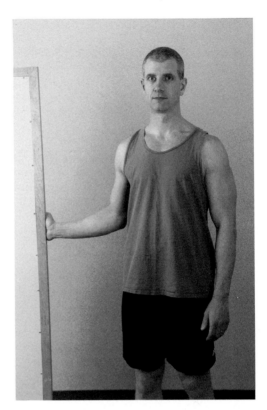

Figure 39–5. Doorway stretch in external rotation.

bered that the shoulder musculature only requires enough strength to move the upper limb when loaded within the weight restrictions determined by the surgeon. The underlying principle for the strengthening phase is to consider the position and magnitude of load that the patient's shoulder will experience during the functional movements for daily activities. Resistance exercises are usually done twice daily, starting with a resistance at which patients can complete 8 to 12 high-quality repetitions.

The choice of exercise mode is variable, and no controlled studies have been completed on patients after

arthroplasty. Patients are trained to accomplish functional arcs of motion in ELE and rotation. Resistance can be applied manually by handheld weights or with the use of elastic bands or aquatic therapy. Elastic resistance increases in the terminal arcs of motion. This is nonphysiologic and has caused excessive muscle soreness in some patients. Close monitoring is necessary. Aquatic therapy offers the benefits of isokinetic-type resistance, buoyancy, and warmth. This treatment is a reasonable option for a patient whose wound is healed and who has access to a therapeutic pool. Although manual

Figure 39–6. Active range of motion in external rotation with scapular retraction.

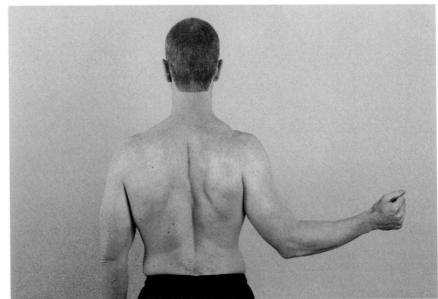

resistance provided by the therapist or caregiver is relatively labor intensive, it provides the benefits of finely tuned resistance, immediate feedback, and unrestricted directions of motion. It is preferable to initiate isotonic resistance training with AROM coupled with therapist-applied manual resistance (Fig. 39–7), followed by transition to an unassisted handheld weight strengthening program. Weights are increased in small increments. Specific exercises essentially reflect the Neer phase I shoulder rehabilitation program, which has been documented to produce greater than 20 percent of a maximal voluntary contraction EMG activity in the rotator cuff musculature.[17,18,30] Patients are encouraged to maintain a long-term conditioning program for both shoulders to counteract the effects of aging and to maintain optimal rotator cuff and shoulder girdle function.

During the strengthening phase, several measures can be taken to minimize shear forces across the GHJ, such as flexing the elbow to reduce the effective moment arm.[21] A 5-kg weight elevated with the elbow extended increases GHJ reaction forces by 200 percent to 300 percent; this can be reduced by about 50 percent simply by flexing the elbow.[21] Maximum GHJ shear occurs at 60 degrees of scapular plane elevation, decreasing rapidly above and below this position.[21] Consequently, patients should avoid unsupported ELE in the 40- to 70-degree motion arc until cuff function is optimized through ER and IR strengthening. Alternatively, closed kinetic chain exercises such as the scapular clock exercise can be used to exercise in this motion arc. During this exercise, the axial force imparted through the upper limb by the wall theoretically reduces deltoid activity and superior shear forces, thereby controlling the eccentric edge-loading phenomenon in the setting of rotator cuff insufficiency (Fig. 39–8).[26,31] Additionally, patients should avoid exercising to fatigue because cuff fatigue may also result in excessive humeral head translation and potentially increase GHJ shear.[27]

Scapulothoracic conditioning should also start early with ROM and strengthening of the scapular stabilizers with shrugs, rowing, serratus anterior strengthening exercises, and closed chain exercises including table top weight shifts and scapular clock exercises.[26,31,32] If the anterior soft tissues are repaired or insufficient, rowing past the midcoronal plane should be avoided. If inferior laxity is a concern, resisted shrugs should be avoided with handheld weights or elastic resistance. Serratus exercises can include punching motions, close chain exercises on the table or wall, or "bear hug" exercises.[26,31,33] Patients with posterior instability should avoid posterior apprehension positions during these exercises.

PROVIDE COUNSELING REGARDING ACTIVITIES

A common concern for the arthroplasty patient is the ability to return to recreational and sporting activities. As techniques and results of shoulder arthroplasty continue to improve, it is likely that arthroplasty will be performed in an increasing number of physiologically younger, active patients.

A survey of 100 experienced shoulder surgeons generated a list of recommended sports after shoulder arthroplasty.[34] Highly recommended are bicycling, croquet, golf, hiking, throwing horseshoes, knitting, running, shuffleboard, swimming, and walking. Sports specifically not recommended include baseball, boxing, football, and motocross. Recommendations were based solely on preferences and experiences of individual surgeons.

Golf is one sport that has been specifically studied in the shoulder arthroplasty patient. At an average follow-up of 53.4 months, 23 of 24 patients had been able to resume playing golf after surgery.[35] The average length

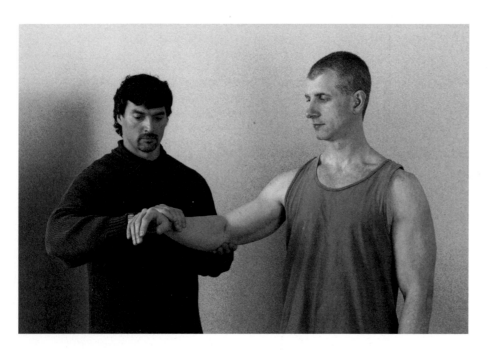

Figure 39–7. Isotonic exercise with manual resistance.

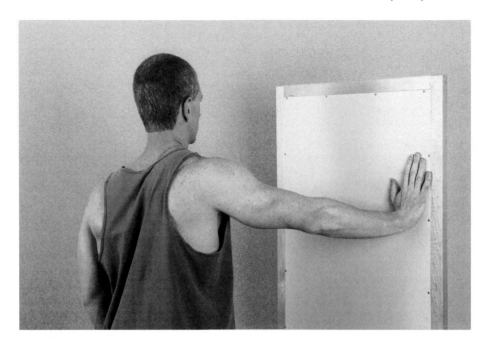

Figure 39–8. Scapular clock exercise demonstrating elevation of the scapula.

of time from shoulder arthroplasty to return to playing golf was 4.5 months, and most patients reported that they had achieved their preoperative handicap. In this series of 20 total shoulder arthroplasties and 6 hemiarthroplasties, playing golf was not found to result in increased radiographic evidence of component loosening. Specifically, the incidence of radiolucent lines in patients who resumed playing golf was not increased significantly when compared with those in the control group.[35] A survey of the members of The American Shoulder and Elbow Society revealed that 91 percent of shoulder surgeons would encourage patients with shoulder arthroplasty to resume playing golf. Most reported surgeons placing no limits on the number of golf rounds played weekly; however, nearly one third of the surgeons surveyed recommended hemiarthroplasty for active golfers because of concerns regarding potential complications related to the glenoid component.

In keeping with the basic rehabilitation principles discussed earlier in this chapter, some general recommendations for return to sport after total shoulder arthroplasty apply. Patients should be counseled that the particular activity or sport in which they are participating should be performed with little or no pain. Functional motion should be regained before resuming the activity. Activities placing the patient at risk of falling or jarring the shoulder (including contact sports) should be avoided. Sports or activities requiring the shoulder to be placed frequently at extremes of motion should also be avoided. Finally, patients should start a given activity gradually and learn the proper form and technique before participation. The time line for return to play has been recommended to be 2 weeks after arthroplasty, return to chipping after 4 to 6 weeks, and use of medium and longer irons 6 to 8 weeks after arthroplasty. These authors do not recommend full play for at least 3 to 4 months after arthroplasty.[35]

In summary, when preparing to counsel a patient regarding return to sports or other activity after shoulder arthroplasty, it is important to understand the specific ROM and strength requirements for that particular activity as well as the patient's desired level and frequency of participation. Recommendations can then be made on an individual basis.

References

1. McCluskey GI, Uhl T: Total shoulder replacement. *In* Donatelli R (ed): Physical Therapy of the Shoulder, 3rd ed. New York, Churchill Livingstone, 1997, pp 459–476.
2. Brems J: Rehabilitation following total shoulder arthroplasty. Clin Orthop 307:70–85, 1994.
3. Melzak R, Wall P: Pain mechanisms: A new theory. Science 150:971–979, 1965.
4. Muller E: Influence of training and of inactivity on muscle strength. Arch Phys Med Rehabil 51:449–462, 1970.
5. Aren A, Madden J: Effects of stress on healing wounds. J Surg Res 20:93–97, 1976.
6. Hawkins R, Bell R, Jallay B: Total shoulder arthroplasty. Clin Orthop 242:188–94, 1989.
7. Fenlin JJ, Ramsey M, Alardyce T, et al: Modular total shoulder replacement: Design, rationale, indications, and results. Clin Orthop 307:37–46, 1994.
8. Wirth M, Rockwood CJ: Complications of shoulder arthroplasty. Clin Orthop 307:47–69, 1994.
9. Noble J, Bell R: Failure of total shoulder arthroplasty: Why does it occur? Semin Arthroplasty 6:280–288, 1995.
10. Moeckel B, Altchek D, Warren R, et al: Instability of the shoulder after arthroplasty. J Bone Joint Surg 75A:792–797, 1993.
11. Mullaji A, Beddow F, Lamb G: CT measurement of glenoid erosion in arthritis. J Bone Joint Surg 76B:384–388, 1994.
12. Cofield R: Degenerative and arthritic problems for the glenohumeral joint. *In* Rockwood CJ, Matsen FI (eds): The Shoulder. Philadelphia, WB Saunders, 1990, pp 735–742.
13. Harryman D, Sidles J, Harris S, et al: The effect of articular conformity and the size of the humeral head component on laxity and motion after glenohumeral arthroplasty. J Bone Joint Surg 77A:555–63, 1995.

14. Post M, Jablon M, Miller H, Singh M: Constrained total shoulder replacement: A critical review. Clin Orthop 144:135–50, 1979.

15. Iannotti J, Gabriel J, Schnek S, et al: The normal glenohumeral relationships: An anatomical study of one hundred and forty shoulders. J Bone Joint Surg 74A:491–500, 1994.

16. Kibler W: The role of the scapula in athletic shoulder function. Am J Sports Med 26:325–37, 1998.

17. McCann P, Wootten M, Kadaba M, Bigliani L: A kinematic and electromyographic study of shoulder rehabilitation exercises. Clin Orthop 288:179–88, 1993.

18. Dockery M, Wright T, LaStayo P: Electromyography of the shoulder: An analysis of passive modes of exercise. Orthopedics 21:1181–4, 1998.

19. Saha AK: Mechanics of elevation of the glenohumeral joint: Its application in rehabilitation of flail shoulder in brachial plexus injuries and poliomyelitis and in replacement of the upper humerus by prosthesis. Acta Orthop Scand 44:668–678, 1983.

20. Saha A: Mechanism of shoulder movements and a plea for recognition of the zero position of the glenohumeral joint. Clin Orthop 173:3–10, 1983.

21. Poppen N, Walker P: Forces at the glenohumeral joint in abduction. Clin Orthop 135:165–172, 1978.

22. Inman V, Saunders M, Abbot L: Observations on the function of the shoulder joint. J Bone Joint Surg 27:1–30, 1944.

23. Maybach A, Schlegel T: Shoulder rehabilitation for the arthritic glenohumeral joint: Preoperative and postoperative considerations. Semin Arthroplasty 6:297–304, 1995.

24. Collins D, Tenscer A, Sidles J, et al: Edge displacement and deformation of glenoid components in response to eccentric loading: The effect of preparation of glenoid bone. J Bone Joint Surg 74A: 501–607, 1992.

25. Franklin J, Barrett W, Jackins S, Matsen FI: Glenoid loosening in total shoulder arthroplasty. J Arthroplasty 3:39–46, 1988.

26. Kibler W: Shoulder rehabilitation: Principles and practice. Med Sci Sports Exerc 30:S40–S50, 1998.

27. Chen S-K, Simonian P, Wickiewicz T, et al: Radiographic evaluation of glenohumeral kinematics: A muscle fatigue model. J Shoulder Elbow Surg 8:49–52, 1999.

28. Neer CI, Watson K, Stanton F: Recent experience in total shoulder replacement. J Bone Joint Surg 64:319–336, 1992.

29. Lieberson W: Brief isometric exercises in therapeutic exercise. In Basmajain J (ed): Therapeutic Exercise, 4th ed. Baltimore, Williams & Wilkins, 1984.

30. Neer C, Welsh R: The shoulder in sports. Orthop Clin North Am 8:583–91, 1977.

31. Kibler W, Livingston B, Bruce R: Current concepts in shoulder rehabilitation. Adv Operative Orthop 3:249–300, 1995.

32. Mosely J, Jobe F, Pink M, et al: EMG analysis of the scapular muscles during a shoulder rehabilitation program. Am J Sports Med 20:128–134, 1992.

33. Decker M, Hintermeister R, Faber K, Hawkins R: Serratus anterior muscle activity during selected rehabilitation exercises. Am J Sports Med 27:784–91, 1999.

34. Dines DM: Activity after shoulder replacement. In D'Ambrosia R (ed): Orthopedics Special Edition. New York, 1996, pp 36–69.

35. Jenson KL, Rockwood CA Jr: Shoulder arthroplasty in recreational golfers. J Shoulder Elbow Surg 7:362–367, 1998.

40

Results of Shoulder Arthroplasty

•JOHN W. SPERLING and ROBERT H. COFIELD

OVERVIEW

The average age of patients who undergo shoulder arthroplasty is the youngest among all major joint replacements.[76] However, there are exceedingly few reports on the long-term results of shoulder arthroplasty. Wirth and Rockwood noted in their review of the literature from 1975 to 1995 that the average length of follow-up in 41 reported series on shoulder arthroplasty was only 3.5 years.[76] Moreover, of the 21 reports with a minimum follow-up of 2 years, only 5 had a mean follow-up of 5 years or more. The purpose of this chapter is to review the results of (1) hemiarthroplasty, (2) constrained total shoulder arthroplasty, and (3) unconstrained total shoulder arthroplasty.

HEMIARTHROPLASTY (HUMERAL HEAD REPLACEMENT)

Hemiarthroplasty of the shoulder has been available for more than 40 years. The results of the Neer type of humeral head replacement are presented by diagnostic category in Table 40–1. In the past few years, the majority of reports concerning humeral head replacement have been based on the results of trauma. The specific results of hemiarthroplasty for trauma are covered in detail in the specific chapter on this topic. However, as one can see from the table, the results of hemiarthroplasty for trauma are quite mixed in regard to pain relief and restoration of motion.

Osteonecrosis, in contrast, is a very favorable indication for the placement of a humeral head prosthesis when symptoms warrant its use and when the glenoid surface remains largely intact. This is due in no small part to the capsule and rotator cuff remaining nearly normal in this condition. As can be seen from the table, pain relief after humeral head replacement for the treatment of osteonecrosis is usually achieved, and return of movement often approaches normal.

A number of investigators have used humeral head replacement for the reconstruction of shoulders afflicted by osteoarthritis or rheumatoid arthritis (Fig. 40–1). The

landmark article by Neer, in 1974, demonstrated that surprisingly good results could be obtained.[49] In osteoarthritis, as in osteonecrosis, the muscles about the shoulder are nearly normal and afford the opportunity for an excellent return of movement and strength when a stable, relatively painless articulation is created. Unfortunately, the rotator cuff and capsular tissues are often significantly involved in rheumatoid arthritis, and, although pain relief is usually satisfactory, return of movement and strength after humeral head replacement for this condition varies greatly depending on the extent to which the disease involves the periarticular structures.

There are various alternative designs of humeral head replacement in use, the results of which are presented in Table 40–2. Plastic materials have been used in Europe but have not found much use in North America. Worldwide, the isoelastic prosthesis is perhaps the most commonly implanted prosthesis of this type. It would seem that the results parallel those seen with the Neer type of implant, although reports have not supported this. Pain relief is somewhat less frequent, and return of movement is less than one ordinarily anticipates after the Neer type of humeral head replacement. Varian introduced a Silastic cup to serve as an interposition between arthritic joints. This concept has not proved to be viable because component failure and instability of the interpositional cup are frequent.

Steffee and Moore[63] in North America and Jonsson and co-workers in Scandinavia[37,38] have employed a metallic cup to resurface the humeral head. The early results reported by Steffee and Moore are quite good, with pain relief very satisfactory and return of movement similar to that achieved with any style of humeral head replacement. The return of active movement in the patients reported by Jonsson and co-workers is strikingly less than that reported by Steffee and Moore. Patient populations differ somewhat by diagnosis, and perhaps the method of reporting also differs. These investigators have reported almost no complications; however, evaluations of these patients were rather short term, and the type and frequency of complications of this particular design of humeral head replacement are not well established.

511

Table 40–1. RESULTS OF NEER HUMERAL HEAD REPLACEMENT

Diagnosis	Study	Shoulders	Pain Relief	Active Abduction	Result Rating
Old trauma	Tanner[67]	28	89	112	
	Pritchett[55]	7	100		5G, 2F
	Hawkins[36]	9	67	140	6G, 3F
Acute trauma	Boss[9]	20	90	90	
	Goldman[30]	16 Neer	73	107	
		10 Cofield			
Osteonecrosis	Neer[47]	3	100		1E, 2G
	Cruess[20]	5	100		5E
	Cruess[21]	7	100		7S
	Rutherford[57]	11	100	161	11E or S
Osteoarthritis	Neer[49]	47			20E, 20S, 6 US
	Zuckerman[78]	36	83	132	
Rheumatoid arthritis	Neer[48]	26			
	Zuckerman[78]	36	89	106	
	Petersson[52, 53]	11	36	74	
	Koorevaar[42]	19	63	65	
RC arthropathy	Arntz[3]	18	83	112	
	Field[24]	16	81	108	
Mixed	Bell[8]	17	58	91	
	Boyd[11]	64	92		
	Sperling[62]	74	85	124	15E, 24S, 32US

RC = radiocarpal.
Data from references 3, 8, 9, 11, 20, 21, 24, 30, 36, 47–49, 52, 53, 55, 57, 62, 67, 78.

Swanson and co-workers have suggested the use of a bipolar humeral head prosthesis associated with extensive tuberosity and rotator cuff reconstruction.[65,66] Worland and colleagues have also reported on the results of bipolar arthroplasty.[4,77] There are a number of theoretical considerations that may tend to favor the use of an implant such as this, and reported pain relief is quite satisfactory. However, in a practical sense, the return of active movement and strength has been compromised to a greater extent than one might anticipate.

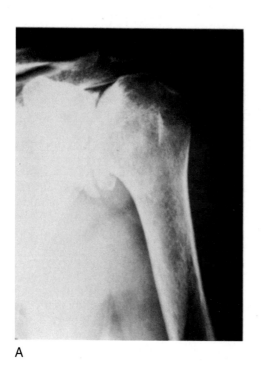
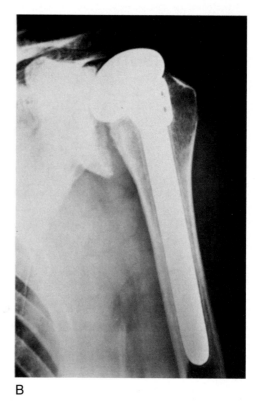

A   B

Figure 40–1. A, Osteoarthritis in the dominant arm of a high-school football coach, 44 years of age, who wished to continue with as many activities as possible. Treatment included use of a Neer-type proximal humeral prosthesis. **B**, This radiograph was taken 3 years after surgery. Pain relief was satisfactory and motion approximated two thirds of normal.

Table 40–2. RESULTS OF VARIOUS DESIGNS OF HUMERAL HEAD REPLACEMENT

Design	Study	Shoulders	Pain Relief	Active Elevation
Metal cup	Steffee[63]	51	82	147
	Jonsson[38]	26	100	57
	Jonsson[37]	5	100	73
Plastic isoelastic	Cockx[16]	25	72	45
	Tonino[69]	14	100	Moderate improvement
	Sait[58]	14		112
Silastic cup	Varian[72]	32	94	Improved in 21
	Spencer[60]	12	42	Little change
Bipolar	Swanson[66]	35	89	71
	Arredondo[4]	48	92	123
	Watson[74]	14	86	
	Worland[77]	108	90	101

Data from references 4, 16, 37, 38, 58, 60, 63, 66, 69, 72, 74, 77.

Mayo Clinic Experience

Over the last 25 years, extensive experience has been gained with the use of humeral head replacement in various diagnostic conditions. This experience is most easily discussed according to the underlying diagnosis.

Fracture

Between 1970 and 1979, 48 patients with 49 shoulders compromised by fractures or fracture-dislocations underwent Neer hemiarthroplasty.[67] Forty-three of the patients were available for follow-up an average of 38 months after surgery; follow-up ranged from 2 to 10 years. Sixteen acute fractures or fracture-dislocations and 28 chronic fracture problems were treated with humeral head replacement. All patients so treated with acute fractures had satisfactory pain relief, and pain relief was satisfactory in 25 of the 28 shoulders with chronic fracture problems. In acute fractures, postoperative average active abduction was 101 degrees; in chronic fracture problems, the postoperative active abduction averaged 112 degrees.

Complications in acute fractures centered on tuberosity and rotator cuff healing. The complications were more common in the chronic fracture and fracture-dislocation situations, and these were usually related to extensive tissue scarring with distortion of anatomy and magnified surgical difficulties.

Based on this experience, we believe that this represents a quite satisfactory treatment option for selected acute and chronic fractures, but, if possible, surgery should be performed early to avoid the problems encountered in the chronic fracture settings.

Primary Arthritis

Zuckerman and Cofield reported on the results of 85 patients who underwent proximal humeral prosthetic replacement for glenohumeral arthritis, specifically osteoarthritis and rheumatoid arthritis.[78] Follow-up greater than 2 years was available in 72 shoulders, with 36 shoulders in each diagnostic category. Satisfactory pain relief was obtained in 83 percent of the shoulders

with osteoarthritis and in 89 percent of the shoulders with rheumatoid arthritis. In osteoarthritis, the return of motion was typically two-thirds to three-fourths normal and in rheumatoid arthritis one-half to two-thirds normal, depending on the severity of involvement of the surrounding soft tissues.

As mentioned earlier, between 80 percent and 90 percent of patients achieved pain relief, but for those who did not, pain often remained quite severe, and at least one half of the unfortunate patients so affected have either seriously considered or have undergone conversion of the humeral head arthroplasty to total shoulder arthroplasty.

Based on this experience, we have come to believe that proximal humeral prosthetic replacement can be a very successful procedure in patients with glenohumeral arthritis; however, the degree and consistency of pain relief is not as great nor as predictable as that achieved by total shoulder arthroplasty. We would continue to consider hemiarthroplasty in patients with rheumatoid arthritis who have severe osteoporosis or glenoid erosion and whose bone would not permit secure glenoid component fixation. We would consider this procedure in a younger osteoarthritis patient or in a patient who wished to be more active and who would accept the possibility of less complete relief in exchange for the benefit of fewer self-imposed restrictions. The operation might also be used in an osteoarthritic patient with compromised glenoid bone volume.

Avascular Necrosis

Osteonecrosis of the shoulder in the nontraumatic setting is almost always associated with the use of steroids. From 1977 to 1983, 31 patients with 42 involved shoulders were treated for osteonecrosis of the proximal humerus.[57] Follow-up evaluation averaged 4.5 years, with a range from 2 to 6.5 years. Of the 19 patients who were treated nonoperatively, 11 patients with 16 affected shoulders were alive and available for review. In 11 of these shoulders there was no collapse or minimal bony collapse. Only 2 of these patients had significant clinical progression; however, in the 5 shoulders with extensive bone collapse, all symptomatically worsened—but not to an extent that required operative treatment. Fourteen patients with 19 affected shoulders with severe pain were selected for surgical treatment.

Thirteen patients with 17 operated shoulders could be evaluated. Seven of these patients with 10 operated shoulders had either no glenoid cartilage changes or minor ones and had a proximal humeral prosthetic replacement. One patient with significant glenoid changes who did not have sufficient glenoid bone to accept a glenoid prosthesis underwent only humeral head replacement. Five patients with 6 affected shoulders and destruction of glenoid cartilage underwent total shoulder arthroplasty. After surgery, pain relief was satisfactory in 16 or the 17 operated shoulders. Average abduction range postoperatively was 150 degrees in patients with total shoulder arthroplasty and 161 degrees in those with a humeral head replacement. External rotation range averaged 67 and 77 degrees, respectively. All the patients with humeral head replacements had excellent or satisfactory results.

Hattrup and Cofield performed a more recent review of 88 shoulders that underwent shoulder arthroplasty for osteonecrosis of the humeral head at our institution by.[34] At an average follow-up of 8.9 years, there was no pain, mild pain, or occasional moderate pain among 77.3 percent of the patients. There were inferior results noted in post-traumatic osteonecrosis, and superior results were noted in steroid-induced osteonecrosis. There was little difference found between humeral head replacement and total shoulder replacement. The most common postoperative complication was rotator cuff tearing, which occurred in 23 of 127 shoulders. The results of this study indicate that the cause of osteonecrosis and previous treatment have important implications for the results of shoulder replacement.

We concluded from our experience that patients with osteonecrosis and minor symptoms should be treated nonoperatively because it is possible that symptom progression may not occur. This is particularly true in those with minor bone deformity. In patients with significant symptoms and bony collapse, either a proximal humeral prosthesis or a total shoulder arthroplasty offers an excellent result. The use of a total shoulder arthroplasty is reserved for those patients with moderate or severe glenoid cartilage changes.

Arthritis with Rotator Cuff Deficiency

In the late 1970s, we recognized a group of patients who had destruction of glenohumeral cartilage and associated severe rotator cuff tearing. This was often linked with instability and some degree of bone loss. Neer and co-workers[50] described a cuff tear arthropathy to better characterize this syndrome, and McCarty and co-workers recognized a similar radiographic appearance in patients who have a pathophysiologic complex that includes crystal deposition.[33]

In 1986, Brownlee and Cofield reported on 20 shoulder replacements performed for cuff tear arthropathy between 1976 and 1982.[15] Fourteen patients with 16 sur-

gically treated shoulders were available for review an average of 4 years after surgery. A proximal humeral replacement used without a glenoid component was performed in 4 shoulders. In these patients, there was a reduction of pain in all shoulders, but there was little change in active movement as a result of surgery. No reoperations were necessary in those who had placement of a proximal humeral prosthesis. However, in the remaining patients who had placement of a glenoid component, revision was needed for glenoid problems in 3 of 12 shoulders.

The results of hemiarthroplasty for rotator cuff arthropathy at the Mayo Clinic in a series of 33 shoulders followed for an average of 5 years was reviewed. Eleven shoulders had undergone between 1 and 4 previous procedures, including an acromioplasty in 8 of them. Hemiarthroplasty was significantly associated with pain relief. However, at the most recent evaluation, 9 patients (27 percent) had moderate pain at rest or pain with activity. Mean active elevation improved from 72 to 91 degrees ($P=0.008$), mean internal rotation improved from L3 to L1 ($P=0.02$), and mean active external rotation improved from 36 to 41 degrees (not significant). Using Neer limited-goal criteria, successful results were achieved in 22 cases (67 percent). However, most patients were satisfied with the outcome of the surgery, and only 4 shoulders were subjectively considered to be the same as or worse than before the operation. Two factors were associated with a less satisfactory outcome: prior subacromial decompression and a significant extent of proximal migration of the humeral head.

A less satisfactory outcome should be expected in patients with prior violation of the coracoacromial arch. The use of either small humeral head sizes in an attempt to facilitate reconstruction of the cuff or large sizes to maximize joint stability does not seem to be justified. Although shoulder hemiarthroplasty is not a perfect answer for patients with rotator cuff arthroplasty, it probably represents the best currently available reconstructive option for this difficult problem.

CONSTRAINED TOTAL SHOULDER ARTHROPLASTY

A strong initial thrust in the design and manufacture of total shoulder prostheses included the development of many constrained or ball-and-socket designs. As orthopedic surgeons became more familiar with the pathology associated with glenohumeral arthritis, it appeared that these designs were seldom needed. The results with the more commonly used constrained designs are tabulated in Table 40–3. Several things should be noted. The first is that pain relief is usually quite satisfactory, the second is that the return of active abduction is typically quite limited, and the third is that the frequency of complications is extraordinarily high. In addition, these complications are often quite serious and include dislocations, component material failure, or component loosening, most of which necessitate major revision surgery.

Table 40–3. RESULTS OF CONSTRAINED TOTAL SHOULDER REPLACEMENT

Study	Prosthesis	Shoulders	F/U (yr)	Pain Relief	Active Abduction
Coughlin[19]	Stanmore	16	2	100	104
Post[54]	Michael Reese	28	1–6	96	
Lettin[44]	Stanmore	40		90	70
Gristina[32]	Trispherical	20	1–3.5	100	58
Kessel[40]	Kessel	33	3.5	85	
Laurence[43]	Glenoid cup	71	6.8	80	76
Brostrom[14]	Kessel	23	7.3	65	35

F/U = follow-up.
Data from references 14, 19, 32, 40, 43, 44, 54.

As an alternative to a completely captive ball-in-socket arrangement, a few hooded or semiconstrained glenoid components have been designed as part of a prosthetic system. The results and complications of these so-called semiconstrained devices are also given in Table 40–4. Unfortunately, the results and complications have not differed dramatically from those seen with the constrained devices. Pain relief is typically satisfactory if a complication does not arise, the return of active abduction is severely limited, and the frequency of complications is extraordinary. Instability can develop adjacent to the overhanging hood. The stresses placed on this hooded component are higher than on a resurfacing component, and loosening is more frequent. Although the concept of a superior glenoid extension to supply additional constraint and stability to a total shoulder arthroplasty is appealing, it has not to date been proved to be a valuable adjunct to patient care problems.

Mayo Clinic Experience

At the Mayo Clinic, we too adhered to contemporary wisdom, and early in our experience with total shoulder arthroplasty, we became involved to a limited extent with the use of constrained total shoulder arthroplasties in patients with various forms of glenohumeral arthritis. One of the early designs of a constrained total shoulder arthroplasty was developed by Dr. William Bickel at the Mayo Clinic (Fig. 40–2). The intent was to incorporate the low-friction concept of Charnley, and for the glenoid component to be entirely encased within the glenoid process of the scapula to maximize the area of bone-cement contact. This design also supplies absolute stability to the shoulder after surgery, which does have some attractive features.

The patient characteristics of those who had a constrained total shoulder replacement at the Mayo Clinic are similar to those of patients who would today receive

an unconstrained device. Unfortunately, this experience was similar to the experience of others (Table 40–5). Significant complications were all too common. These included most notably glenoid loosening and instability. Revision surgery was necessary in 12 of the 27 shoulders (44 percent).

Fifteen shoulders did not have intervening revision surgery and were available for analysis more than 2 years after their initial surgical procedure. As in other series, satisfactory pain relief usually occurred, but

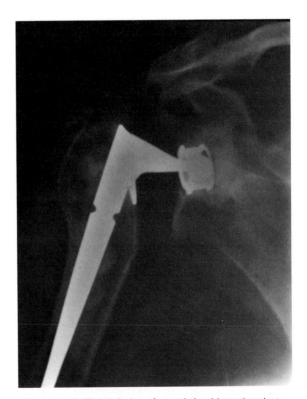

Figure 40–2. Bickel design of a total shoulder arthroplasty.

Table 40–4. RESULTS OF SEMICONSTRAINED TOTAL SHOULDER REPLACEMENT

Study	Prosthesis	Shoulders	F/U (yr)	Pain Relief	Active Abduction
Faludi[22]	English-Macnab	13	3.7		75
McElwain[46]	English-Macnab	13	3.1	85	56
Amstutz[2]	Dana	10	3.5	100	85

F/U = follow-up.
Data from references 2, 22, 46.

Table 40–5. RESULTS OF CONSTRAINED TOTAL SHOULDER REPLACEMENT (MAYO CLINIC EXPERIENCE)

Prosthesis	F/U (Yr)	Shoulders	Active Abduction	Revision
Bickel	12	12	95	8
Stanmore	9	9	93	4
Michael Reese	7	6	73	0

F/U = Follow-up.

return of active abduction was disappointing, averaging between one third and one half of the normal range. Using a rating system similar to Neer's published criteria, there were no excellent results, 5 satisfactory results, and 22 unsatisfactory results.

Based on this experience, it is easy to conclude that the need for a constrained shoulder device is extremely rare. Perhaps it would be considered in an elderly, frail individual with a sedentary lifestyle with bilateral shoulder disease who had failed to improve after an unconstrained arthroplasty and who had severe rotator cuff disease but also had adequate glenoid bone. Such individuals probably exist but likely represent fewer than 1 percent of the entire patient group who would be candidates for prosthetic shoulder arthroplasty.

UNCONSTRAINED TOTAL SHOULDER ARTHROPLASTY

The Neer type of unconstrained total shoulder arthroplasty has become the standard, and, as such, it is the implant against which others must be compared (Fig. 40–3). The results of 1291 Neer total shoulder replace-

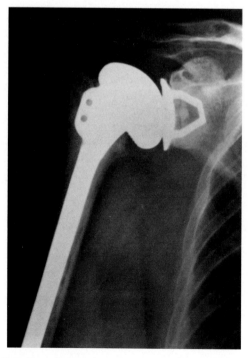

Figure 40–3. Neer design of a total shoulder arthroplasty. Radiograph of the shoulder of a 57-year-old woman with rheumatoid arthritis, now 4 years after surgery.

ments reported by 21 different groups are delineated in Table 40–6. Average follow-up in these studies typically ranges from 2 to 6 years. The diagnostic categories are often mixed but are predominantly osteoarthritis, rheumatoid arthritis, and arthritis secondary to past trauma. As noted, no pain or slight pain is typically present in 90 percent of patients so treated. In some of the series in which the prominent diagnosis is rheumatoid arthritis, the return of active abduction averages about half of the normal range; in other series, the active postoperative abduction range averages approximately two thirds that of the normal range.

It has been clearly shown that patients with osteoarthritis regain approximately three fourths or four fifths of normal movement, whereas patients with rheumatoid disease or those who have arthritis after old trauma are somewhat more compromised in their motion and strength returns after surgery. To address this significant variability in the patient population, Neer has suggested dividing those having this surgery into two groups; one group would participate in a full exercise program and the other would have limited-goals rehabilitation because of muscle or bone deficiencies. This is a novel approach and requires a different mind-set from that typically needed for total knee or total hip arthroplasties. It is, of course, recognized that success in shoulder replacement depends on achieving adequate pain relief and satisfactory stability. Hence, the rationale for a limited or protected rehabilitation program is to maintain stability in patients whose structural integrity is compromised. In this setting, it is not desirable to obtain full movement or strength because of the high probability of catastrophic instability. A method of classifying the result that is predicated on a careful assessment of patient and disease characteristics will probably be used more commonly in the future.

The roentgenographic analysis reveals that a substantial number of changes occur at the glenoid prosthesis-cement and cement-bone interfaces. These are enumerated in Table 40–7. In the series in which the analysis includes a description of the location of the presence of radiolucent zones, it can be seen that at least one third of shoulders have a radiolucent zone at the keel bone-cement interface, but in some series up to two thirds of shoulders exhibit these changes. Some have noted a shift in glenoid component position in certain shoulders that might not otherwise have been seen without sequential radiographs. We have learned from total joint replacement in the hip and the knee that radiolucent zones do not necessarily imply that clinical failure is imminent. Radiolucent zones can be present on the initial postoperative radiograph; they can also develop

Table 40–6. RESULTS OF NEER TOTAL SHOULDER REPLACEMENT

Study	F/U (Yr)	Shoulders	Diagnosis	Pain Relief	Active Abduction	External Rotation
Bade[5]	4.5	38	Mixed	93	118	
Cofield[17]	3.8	73	Mixed	92	120	48
Adams[1]	2.7	33	Mixed	91	96	
Barrett[6]	3.5	50	Mixed	88	100	
Kelly[39]	3.0	40	RA	88	75	40
Frich[27]	2.3	50	Mixed	92	58–78	17–21
Barrett[7]	5.0	140	RA	93	90	40
Brenner[12]	6.4	37	RA, OA	84	115	41
Hawkins[35]	3.3	70	RA, OA	90	131	36
McCoy[45]	3.1	29	RA	93	76	
Vahvanen[71]	1.7	41	RA	98	105	43
Kjaersgaard[41]	2.2	58	Mixed	60	74	16
Friedman[28]	4.5	24	RA	92	81	51
Boyd[10]	4.6	131	Mixed	95	100	33
Bell[8]	1.5	11	Mixed	91	121	
Figgie[25]	5		RA	96	90	
Sneppen[59]	7.5	62	RA	89	74	
Sperling[62]	13.6	34	Mixed	85	104	43
Stewart[64]	9.5	37	RA	89	75	38
Torchia[70]	12.2	89	Mixed	83	117	
Neer[51]	3.1	194	Mixed	Full exercise: 101 E, 28 S, 21 U Limited: 42 S, 1 U		

OA = osteoarthritis; RA = rheumatoid arthritis.
Data from references 1, 5–8, 10, 12, 17, 25, 27, 28, 35, 41, 45, 51, 59, 62, 64, 70, 71.

later during the patient's course and can progress in extent and width. Progressive radiolucency is associated with the development of an increased area of fibrous tissue with or without histiocytic tissue, and, in some patients, revision surgery will be necessary because of pain or pain and bone destruction. At this point, the clinical results with unconstrained total shoulder arthroplasty are very good. The roentgenographic results do cause concern, but, based on available clinical information, only rarely has component revision been necessary because of loosening.

Other types of unconstrained total shoulder arthroplasties, in addition to the Neer design, are available, some of which are listed in Table 40–8. The results of arthroplasty using the Monospherical and Dana systems parallel the results of the Neer total shoulder arthroplasty. Pain relief is typically about 90 percent,

and the return of active abduction approximates two thirds of normal in a mixed patient series. Additionally, the results of newer third-generation implants, such as the Tournier, are reported in the table.[73] These components have modularity of the stem, head, inclination, and offset. The long term results of these new prosthesis have yet to be determined.

Mayo Clinic Experience

For more than 20 years, there has been extensive experience at the Mayo Clinic with the use of the unconstrained total shoulder arthroplasty. In 1984, 73 Neer-type shoulder arthroplasties in 65 patients were evaluated at 2 to 6.5 years after operation.[17] Pain relief was satisfactory in 92 percent of the shoulders. The

Table 40–7. ROENTGENOGRAPHIC ANALYSIS OF GLENOID COMPONENT OF NEER TOTAL SHOULDER REPLACEMENT

Study	Shoulders	Radiolucent Zones		Shift	
		None	Any Area	Keel	Component
Neer[51]	194	70	30		
Bade[5]	38	33	67		
Cofield[17]	73	29	71	33	11
Wilde[75]	38	7	93	68	
Adams[1]	33			36	
Barrett[6]	50	26	74	36	10
Kelly[39]	40	17	83	63	
Frich[27]	50	No Data			
Barrett[7]	140	18	82	55	2
Brenner[12]	37	33	57		2
Hawkins[35]	70	Nearly all			
McCoy[45]	29	14	86		
Vahvanen[71]	41	68	32		
Friedman[28]	24		42		
Torchia[70]	89	12	88		

Data from references 1, 5–7, 12, 17, 27, 28, 35, 39, 45, 51, 70, 71.

Table 40–8. RESULTS OF VARIOUS DESIGNS OF UNCONSTRAINED TOTAL SHOULDER REPLACEMENT

Study	Prosthesis	Shoulders	F/U (Yr)	Pain Relief	Active Abduction
Gristina[31]	Monospherical	100	3.2	90	115
Amstutz[2]	Dana	46	3.5	91	120
Roper[56]	Roper-Day	25	5	100	78
Thomas[68]	Dana	30	2–10		85
Brostrom[13]	Dana St. Georg	26	3.9	76	
Figgie[26]	Custom	27	5		100
Fenlin[23]	Fenlin modular	47	4.5	94	137
Gartsman[29]	Global	27	3		128
Cofield[18]	Cofield	32	4.2	96	145
Sperling[61]	Cofield	87	4.6	87	138
Walch[73]	Tounier	86	2.8		153

F/U = follow-up.
Data from references 2, 13, 18, 23, 26, 29, 31, 56, 61, 68, 73.

return of active abduction averaged 141 degrees in patients with osteoarthritis, 109 degrees in those with traumatic arthritis, and 103 degrees in those with rheumatoid arthritis. The return of active abduction averaged 120 degrees for the entire group. Postoperative external rotation averaged 48 degrees for the 73 shoulders. The amount of postoperative movement obtained was related to the original diagnosis, as noted earlier, and also to the extent of rotator cuff disease.

Complications occurred in 13 patients and included single instances of nerve injury, wound hematoma, and nonfatal pulmonary embolus; 2 patients had reflex dystrophy; recurrent rotator cuff tearing occurred in 5; and, significantly, symptomatic glenoid loosening in 3. Five reoperations were necessary: 1 to treat the wound hematoma, 1 to deal with the nerve injury, and 3 to revise loosened glenoid components. These latter 3 revisions produced satisfactory outcomes for 2 of the patients. From this experience, we concluded that the operation was technically difficult. Particular attention must be paid to repair of the rotator cuff, and the postoperative rehabilitation program must maximize the potential for rotator cuff healing to maximize the potential return of movement and strength; unfortunately, these are somewhat contradictory goals. Also, we learned that clinically significant component loosening was uncommon, but when it did develop, it occurred on the glenoid side and usually rather late. The additional self-evident fact is that the results after unconstrained total shoulder arthroplasty are substantially better than those obtained after the use of semiconstrained or constrained implants.

More recently, the long-term results of 113 total shoulder arthroplasties performed with a Neer prosthesis between 1975 and 1981 were reviewed.[70] The indication for the surgery was moderate or severe pain in association with osteoarthritis, rheumatoid arthritis, and old fractures or dislocations with traumatic arthritis. Analysis included the probability of implant survival, which was 93 percent after 10 years and 87 percent after 15 years. Fourteen shoulders underwent revision surgery. Eighty-nine shoulder arthroplasties were available for follow-up a minimum of 5 years from the time of shoulder arthroplasty (mean, 12.2 years; range, 5 to 17

years). There was relief from moderate or severe pain in 83 percent of shoulders. There was a mean improvement in active abduction of 40 degrees. The amount of abduction that was regained was related to the severity of rotator cuff disease. There was the development of bone-cement radiolucencies in 75 glenoid components, and 39 (44 percent) glenoid components had radiographic evidence of definite loosening. There was a correlation between glenoid loosening and pain. In regard to the humeral component, there was a shift in the humeral component position in 49 percent of the press-fit stems and in none of the cemented stems. There was not an association between humeral component loosening and pain.

We have reviewed the long-term results of shoulder Neer shoulder arthroplasty in patients 50 years of age or younger.[62] There were 74 hemiarthroplasties and 34 total shoulder arthroplasties followed for a minimum of 5 years (mean, 12.3 years) or until revision. There was significant long-term relief of pain as well as improvement in active abduction and external rotation ($P<0.0001$) with Neer shoulder arthroplasty. There was not a significant difference between the two procedures with respect to these variables. A radiolucent line around the humeral component was noted after 24 percent of the hemiarthroplasties and after 53 percent of the total shoulder arthroplasties. A radiolucent line around the glenoid component was seen after 59 percent of the total shoulder arthroplasties. Erosion of the glenoid was found after 68 percent of the hemiarthroplasties. Fifteen hemiarthroplasties had an excellent result; 24 had a satisfactory result; and 35 had an unsatisfactory or unsuccessful result. Four total shoulder arthroplasties had an excellent result; 13 had a satisfactory result; and 17 had an unsatisfactory or unsuccessful result.

Survival estimates for the hemiarthroplasty were 92 percent at 5 years, 83 percent at 10 years, and 73 percent at 15 years. The risk of revision was higher for the 30 shoulders that had undergone hemiarthroplasty for the treatment of the sequelae of trauma than for the 28 that underwent hemiarthroplasty for the treatment of rheumatoid arthritis ($P=0.017$). The estimated survival of the total shoulder prostheses was 97 percent at 5 years, 97 percent at 10 years, and 84 percent at 15 years.

The risk of revision was higher for the 7 shoulders with a rotator cuff tear at the time of the operation than for the 27 that had not had one ($P=0.029$). The data from the study indicated that a shoulder arthroplasty provides marked long-term relief of pain and improvement in motion; however, nearly half of all young patients who have a shoulder arthroplasty have an unsatisfactory result according to a modified Neer result rating system.

In reviewing this experience, we have learned that the clinical results of total shoulder arthroplasty continue to be excellent with this longer follow-up period. The frequency of complications and the need for revision are low. However, when revision surgery is needed, the most common reason is for glenoid loosening. The radiographic analysis suggests that additional revisions may be necessary as the length of follow-up increases. We also believe that care should be exercised when either a hemiarthroplasty or a total shoulder arthroplasty is offered to patients who are 50 years old or younger.

SUMMARY

The humeral head replacement alone is effective in a variety of situations, most notably in certain types of acute fractures and osteonecrosis. It is now generally recognized that if glenoid involvement is moderate or severe, total shoulder arthroplasty of the unconstrained type is usually the better choice. The unconstrained total shoulder arthroplasty has been very effective in relieving pain and typically restoring an ample amount of movement and strength. Thus, the use of constrained or semiconstrained devices seldom, if ever, seems warranted.

References

1. Adams MA, Weiland AJ, Moore JR: Nonconstrained total shoulder arthroplasty: An eight year experience. Orthop Trans 10:232, 1986.
2. Amstutz HC, Thomas BJ, Kabo JM, et al: The Dana total shoulder arthroplasty. J Bone Joint Surg Am 70:1174, 1988.
3. Arntz CT, Jackins S, Matsen FA: Prosthetic replacement of the shoulder for the treatment of defects in the rotator cuff and the surface of the glenohumeral joint [published erratum appears in J Bone Joint Surg Am 75:1112, 1993]. J Bone Joint Surg Am 75:485, 1993.
4. Arredondo J, Worland RL: Bipolar shoulder arthroplasty in patients with osteoarthritis: Short-term clinical results and evaluation of birotational head motion. J Shoulder Elbow Surg 8:425, 1999.
5. Bade HA, Warren RF, Ranawat C, Inglis AE: Long term results of Neer total shoulder arthroplasty. In Bateman JE, Welsh RP (eds): Surgery of the Shoulder. St. Louis, CV Mosby, 1984, p 249.
6. Barrett WP, Franklin JL, Jackins SE, et al: Total shoulder arthroplasty. J Bone Joint Surg Am 69:865, 1987.
7. Barrett WP, Thornhill TS, Thomas WH, et al: Nonconstrained total shoulder arthroplasty in patients with polyarticular rheumatoid arthritis. J Arthroplasty 4:91, 1989.
8. Bell SN, Gschwend N: Clinical experience with total arthroplasty and hemiarthroplasty of the shoulder using the Neer prosthesis. Int Orthop 10:217, 1986.
9. Boss AP, Hintermann B: Primary endoprosthesis in comminuted humeral head fractures in patients over 60 years of age. Int Orthop 23:172, 1999.
10. Boyd AD Jr, Aliabadi P, Thornhill TS: Postoperative proximal migration in total shoulder arthroplasty. Incidence and significance. J Arthroplasty 6:31, 1991.
11. Boyd AD Jr, Thomas WH, Scott RD, et al: Total shoulder arthroplasty versus hemiarthroplasty. Indications for glenoid resurfacing. J Arthroplasty 5:329, 1990.
12. Brenner BC, Ferlic DC, Clayton ML, Dennis DA: Survivorship of unconstrained total shoulder arthroplasty. J Bone Joint Surg Am 71:1289, 1989.
13. Brostrom LA, Kronberg M, Wallensten R: Should the glenoid be replaced in shoulder arthroplasty with an unconstrained Dana or St. Georg prosthesis? Ann Chir Gynaecol 81:54, 1992.
14. Brostrom LA, Wallensten R, Olsson E, Anderson D: The Kessel prosthesis in total shoulder arthroplasty. A five-year experience. Clin Orthop 277:155, 1992.
15. Brownlee RC, Cofield RC: Shoulder replacement in cuff tear arthropathy. Orthop Trans 10:230, 1986.
16. Cockx E, Claes T, Hoogmartens M, Mulier JC: The isoelastic prosthesis for the shoulder joint. Acta Orthop Belg 49:275, 1983
17. Cofield RH: Total shoulder arthroplasty with the Neer prosthesis. J Bone Joint Surg Am 66:899, 1984.
18. Cofield RH, Daly PJ: Total shoulder arthroplasty with a tissue ingrowth glenoid component. J Shoulder Elbow Surg 1:77, 1992.
19. Coughlin MJ, Morris JM, West WF: The semiconstrained total shoulder arthroplasty. J Bone Joint Surg Am 61:574, 1979.
20. Cruess RL: Steroid-induced avascular necrosis of the head of the humerus. Natural history and management. J Bone Joint Surg Br 58:313, 1976.
21. Cruess RL: Corticosteroid-induced osteonecrosis of the humeral head. Orthop Clin North Am 16:789, 1985.
22. Faludi DD, Weiland AJ: Cementless total shoulder arthroplasty: Preliminary experience with thirteen cases. Orthopedics 6:431, 1982.
23. Fenlin JM Jr, Ramsey ML, Allardyce TJ, Frieman BG: Modular total shoulder replacement. Design rationale, indications, and results. Clin Orthop 307:37, 1994.
24. Field LD, Dines DM, Zabinski SJ, Warren RF: Hemiarthroplasty of the shoulder for rotator cuff arthropathy. J Shoulder Elbow Surg 6:18, 1997.
25. Figgie HE, Inglis AE, Goldberg VM, et al: An analysis of factors affecting the long-term results of total shoulder arthroplasty in inflammatory arthritis. J Arthroplasty 3:123, 1988.
26. Figgie MP, Inglis AE, Figgie HE, et al: Custom total shoulder arthroplasty in inflammatory arthritis. Preliminary results. J Arthroplasty 7:1, 1992.
27. Frich LH, Moller BN, Sneppen O: Shoulder arthroplasty with the Neer Mark-II prosthesis. Arch Orthop Trauma Surg 107:110, 1988.
28. Friedman RJ, Thornhill TS, Thomas WH, Sledge CB: Non-constrained total shoulder replacement in patients who have rheumatoid arthritis and class-IV function. J Bone Joint Surg Am 71:494, 1989.
29. Gartsman GM, Roddey TS, Hammerman SM: Shoulder arthroplasty with or without resurfacing of the glenoid in patients who have osteoarthritis. J Bone Joint Surg Am 82:26, 2000.
30. Goldman RT, Koval KJ, Cuomo F, et al: Functional outcome after humeral head replacement for acute three- and four-part proximal humeral fractures. J Shoulder Elbow Surg 4:81, 1995.
31. Gristina AG, Romano RL, Kammire GC, Webb LX: Total shoulder replacement. Orthop Clin North Am 18:445, 1987.
32. Gristina AG, Webb LX. The trispherical total shoulder replacement. In Bayley I, Kessel L (eds): Shoulder Surgery. Berlin, Springer-Verlag, 1982, p 153.
33. Halverson PB, Cheung HS, McCarty DJ, et al: Association of microspheroids containing hydroxyapatite crystals, active collagenase, and neutral protease with rotator cuff defects. II. Synovial fluid studies. Arthritis Rheum 24:474, 1981.
34. Hattrup SJ, Cofield RH: Osteonecrosis of the humeral head: Results of replacement. J Shoulder Elbow Surg 9:177, 2000.
35. Hawkins RJ, Bell RH, Jallay B: Total shoulder arthroplasty. Clin Orthop 242:188, 1989.
36. Hawkins RJ, Neer CS, Pianta RM, Mendoza FX: Locked posterior dislocation of the shoulder. J Bone Joint Surg Am 69:9, 1987.
37. Jonsson E, Brattstrom M, Lidgren L: Evaluation of the rheumatoid shoulder function after hemiarthroplasty and arthrodesis. Scand J Rheumatol 17:17, 1988.
38. Jonsson E, Egund N, Kelly I, et al: Cup arthroplasty of the rheumatoid shoulder. Acta Orthop Scand 57:542, 1986.

39. Kelly IG, Foster RS, Fisher WD: Neer total shoulder replacement in rheumatoid arthritis. J Bone Joint Surg Br 69:723, 1987.
40. Kessel L, Bayley I: The Kessel total shoulder replacement. *In* Bayley I, Kessel L (eds): Shoulder Surgery. Berlin, Springer-Verlag, 1982, p 160.
41. Kjaersgaard-Andersen P, Frich LH, Sojbjerg JO, Sneppen O: Heterotopic bone formation following total shoulder arthroplasty. J Arthroplasty 4:99, 1989.
42. Koorevaar RC, Merkies ND, de Waal Malefijt MC, et al: Shoulder hemiarthroplasty in rheumatoid arthritis. 19 cases reexamined after 1–17 years. Acta Orthop Scand 68:243, 1997.
43. Laurence M: Replacement arthroplasty of the rotator cuff deficient shoulder. J Bone Joint Surg Br 73:916, 1991.
44. Lettin AW, Copeland SA, Scales JT: The Stanmore total shoulder replacement. J Bone Joint Surg Br 64:47, 1982.
45. McCoy SR, Warren RF, Bade HA, et al: Total shoulder arthroplasty in rheumatoid arthritis. J Arthroplasty 4:105, 1989.
46. McElwain JP, English E: The early results of porous-coated total shoulder arthroplasty. Clin Orthop 218:217, 1987.
47. Neer CS: Articular replacement for the humeral head. J Bone Joint Surg 37A:215, 1955.
48. Neer CS: The rheumatoid shoulder. *In* Cruess RR, Mitchell NS (eds): Surgery of Rheumatoid Arthritis. Philadelphia, JB Lippincott, 1971, p 117.
49. Neer CS: Replacement arthroplasty for glenohumeral osteoarthritis. J Bone Joint Surg Am 56:1, 1974.
50. Neer CS, Craig EV, Fukuda H: Cuff-tear arthropathy. J Bone Joint Surg Am 65:1232, 1983.
51. Neer CS, Watson KC, Stanton FJ: Recent experience in total shoulder replacement. J Bone Joint Surg Am 64:319, 1982.
52. Petersson CJ: Painful shoulders in patients with rheumatoid arthritis. Prevalence, clinical and radiological features. Scand J Rheumatol 15:275, 1986.
53. Petersson CJ: Shoulder surgery in rheumatoid arthritis. Acta Orthop Scand 57:222, 1986.
54. Post M, Haskell SS, Jablon M: Total shoulder replacement with a constrained prosthesis. J Bone Joint Surg Am 62:327, 1980.
55. Pritchett JW, Clark JM: Prosthetic replacement for chronic unreduced dislocations of the shoulder. Clin Orthop 216:89, 1987.
56. Roper BA, Paterson JM, Day WH: The Roper-Day total shoulder replacement. J Bone Joint Surg Br 72:694, 1990.
57. Rutherford CS, Cofield RH: Osteonecrosis of the shoulder. Orthop Trans 11:239, 1987.
58. Sait S, Scott WA: Early results of isoelastic hemiarthroplasty in chronic shoulder arthritis. Orthopedics 23:467, 2000.
59. Sneppen O, Fruensgaard S, Johannsen HV, et al: Total shoulder replacement in rheumatoid arthritis: Proximal migration and loosening. J Shoulder Elbow Surg 5:47, 1996.
60. Spencer R, Skirving AP: Silastic interposition arthroplasty of the shoulder. J Bone Joint Surg Br 1986;68:375, 1986.
61. Sperling JW, Cofield RH, O'Driscoll SW, et al: Radiographic assessment of ingrowth total shoulder arthroplasty. J Shoulder Elbow Surg 9:507, 2000.
62. Sperling JW, Cofield RH, Rowland CM: Neer hemiarthroplasty and Neer total shoulder arthroplasty in patients fifty years old or less. Long-term results [see comments]. J Bone Joint Surg Am 80:464, 1998.
63. Steffee AD, Moore RW: Hemi-resurfacing arthroplasty of the shoulder. Contemp Orthop 9:51, 1984.
64. Stewart MP, Kelly IG: Total shoulder replacement in rheumatoid disease: 7- to 13-year follow-up of 37 joints. J Bone Joint Surg Br 79:68, 1997.
65. Swanson AB, de Groot Swanson G, Maupin BK, et al: Bipolar implant shoulder arthroplasty. Orthopedics 9:343, 1986.
66. Swanson AB, de Groot Swanson G, Sattel AB, et al: Bipolar implant shoulder arthroplasty. Long-term results. Clin Orthop 249:227, 1989.
67. Tanner MW, Cofield RH: Prosthetic arthroplasty for fractures and fracture-dislocations of the proximal humerus. Clin Orthop 179:116, 1983.
68. Thomas BJ, Amstutz HC, Cracchiolo A: Shoulder arthroplasty for rheumatoid arthritis. Clin Orthop 265:125, 1991.
69. Tonino AJ, van de Werf GJ: Hemi arthroplasty of the shoulder. Acta Orthop Belg 51:625, 1985.
70. Torchia ME, Cofield RH, Settergren CR: Total shoulder arthroplasty with the Neer prosthesis: Long-term results. J Shoulder Elbow Surg 6:495, 1997.
71. Vahvanen V, Hamalainen M, Paavolainen P: The Neer II replacement for rheumatoid arthritis of the shoulder. Int Orthop 13:57, 1989.
72. Varian JPW: Interposition Silastic cup arthroplasty of the shoulder. J Bone Joint Surg 62B:116, 1980.
73. Walch G, Boileau P: Prosthetic adaptability: A new concept for shoulder arthroplasty. J Shoulder Elbow Surg 8:443, 1999.
74. Watson M: Bipolar salvage shoulder arthroplasty. Follow-up in 14 patients. J Bone Joint Surg Br 78:124, 1996.
75. Wilde AH, Borden LS, Brems JJ: Experience with the Neer total shoulder replacement. *In* Bateman JE, Welsh RP (eds): Surgery of the Shoulder. St. Louis, CV Mosby, 1984.
76. Wirth MA, Rockwood CA Jr: Complications of total shoulder-replacement arthroplasty. J Bone Joint Surg Am 78:603, 1996.
77. Worland RL, Arredondo J: Bipolar shoulder arthroplasty for painful conditions of the shoulder. J Arthroplasty 13:631, 1998.
78. Zuckerman JD, Cofield RH: Proximal humerus prosthetic replacement in glenohumeral arthritis. Orthop Trans 10:231, 1986.

41

Complications in Shoulder Arthroplasty

•STEPHEN J. HATTRUP

In the modern era, Neer introduced shoulder replacement for proximal humeral fractures in the early 1950s and redesigned his prosthesis to allow glenoid resurfacing approximately two decades later.[42,44,45] Over time, the design of shoulder prostheses has evolved in both number and complexity to allow greater adaptation to underlying anatomy and to reduce the frequency of complications. Prostheses are now available that allow bone ingrowth or cement fixation, adjustment of head height, version, offset, diameter, and variable conformity between the glenoid and humeral surfaces. Yet despite these advances, shoulder arthroplasty remains a relatively uncommon and technically challenging procedure for most orthopedic surgeons.[44,58,59] Awareness of the potential complications of this procedure is essential to minimize their occurrence and to ensure proper management.

INCIDENCE

In 1982, Neer published a series of 37 consecutive revision surgeries.[43] The indications for revision surgery perhaps reflected the earlier state of shoulder surgery. These included the presence of a radical acromionectomy or other anterior deltoid deficiency, over-tightened subscapularis, subacromial impingement, loss of humeral length, prominent greater tuberosity, and inadequate rehabilitation. Neer suggested consideration of four conditions to minimize complications, which remain just as valuable today.[45] These are the presence of humeral or glenoid bone deficiency, the possibility of a defective rotator cuff, prior deltoid injury, and chronic instability patterns.

More recently, Cofield has reported two series of reoperations at the Mayo Clinic. The initial series constituted revision surgeries from 1976 through 1988.[17] Indications were glenoid loosening, glenoid arthritis after humeral head replacement, instability, rotator cuff tearing, component failure, humeral loosening, and infection, in order of decreasing frequency. In his second analysis, the Mayo Clinic experience from 1981 through 1991 was reviewed.[13] In 71 revision total

shoulder replacements, indications for reoperation were instability in 47 shoulders, rotator cuff tearing in 42, glenoid loosening in 24, humeral loosening in 20, and component failure in 12, with malposition of 4 components, 3 infections and a single fracture. Some shoulders had more than one indication for revision surgery. Additionally, 32 humeral head replacements were revised. The most common indication for revision surgery was glenoid arthritis, which was present in 26 shoulders. Rotator cuff tearing was found in 7 cases, instability in 5, humeral loosening in 5, component malposition and stiffness in 2 each, and 1 isolated fracture.

Not all complications of surgery require reoperations, and analysis of only revision surgery can distort the true incidence of potential problems with shoulder arthroplasty. To obtain a broad look at this issue, Wirth and Rockwood performed a meta-analysis of complications that occurred in over 1600 shoulder arthroplasties found in 32 peer-reviewed articles.[59] They found that the most common complications in descending order of frequency were component loosening, instability, rotator cuff tearing, periprosthetic fracturing, infection, implant structural failure, and deltoid weakness or dysfunction. However, they were disturbed by the relatively short-term follow-up found in many of the reports they reviewed. Fourteen studies had follow-up of less than 2 years and only 8 reported an average of more than 4 years. The incidence of certain complications, such as loosening, are necessarily underestimated by short-term follow-up (Fig. 41–1). The assessment of complications is a dynamic process as surgical techniques evolve and experience is gained.

INSTABILITY

Postoperative instability patterns can be superior, inferior, posterior, or anterior. Instability can be responsible not only for painful subluxation and dislocation episodes but also for particulate synovitis, osteolysis, and premature loosening of both glenoid and humeral components.[1,22,34,47–49,52,55]

521

Superior. The most frequently recognized pattern is superior instability (Fig. 41–2). Although it is commonly associated with rotator cuff tearing, Boyd has shown that other issues can be responsible as well.[59] He evaluated factors associated with postoperative proximal migration of the humeral component in 131 shoulder replacements at an average follow-up of 55 months. Intra-operatively, 28 of 131 (21 percent) shoulders were discovered to have a torn rotator cuff. Postoperatively, 7 of the 28 shoulders (25 percent) with a documented tear were found to have proximal migration compared with 22 of 103 (21 percent) shoulders with an intact cuff. The

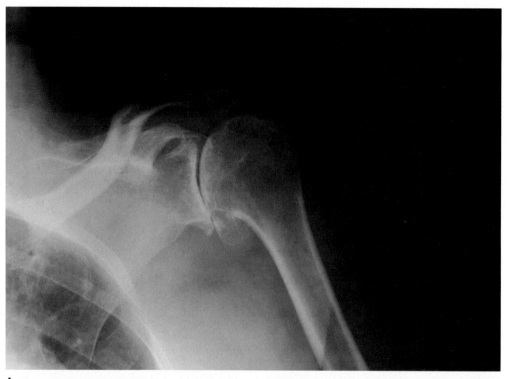

A

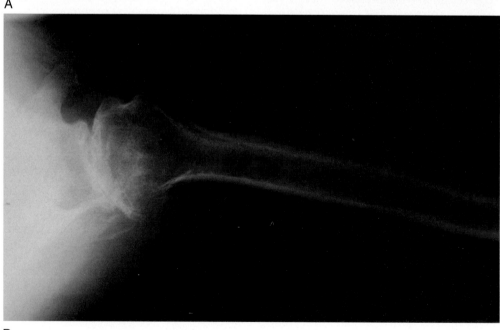

B

Figure 41–1. This patient had symptomatic osteoarthritis of his shoulder, with typical findings of joint space narrowing, osteophyte formation, and posterior erosion of the glenoid present on the radiograph of 9/26/91. **A** and **B**, Total shoulder arthroplasty was performed with an excellent clinical result. Postoperative radiographs on 11/11/91 revealed a reduced shoulder joint. **C** and **D**, Nine years later he presented with 3 months of shoulder pain, which he attributed to a fall. Repeat radiographs of 8/29/00 demonstrated posterior erosion of the polyethylene and metal tray, with subluxation of the joint.

Illustration continued on opposite page

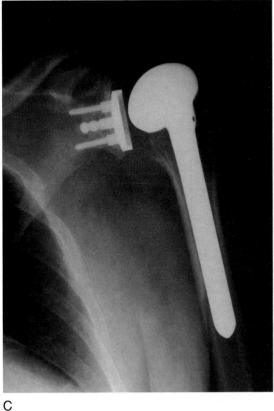

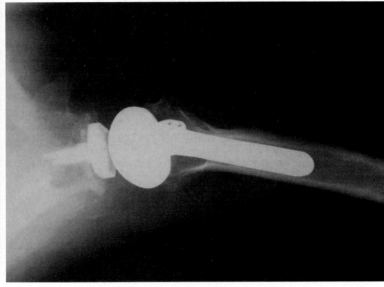

C   D

Figure 41–1. *Continued.*

Illustration continued on following page

lack of correlation between progressive humeral migration and rotator cuff tearing led Boyd to conclude that several factors are relevant to postoperative proximal migration. These include an increased glenoid facing angle, release of the coracoacromial ligament, irreparable rotator cuff tear, proud placement of the humeral component, and dynamic imbalance between a strong deltoid and an attenuated, dysfunctional rotator cuff.

Management. Treatment of patients with superior subluxation or dislocation of the shoulder arthroplasty is dependent on etiology and symptoms. If the displacement is due to an irreparable or incompetent rotator cuff, little may need to be done. Fortunately, the symptoms are often relatively mild.[50,59] If the cause is component malposition or postoperative cuff tearing, revision surgery can be entertained to correct the problem as symptoms indicate. A more challenging issue can be the combination of an absent coracoacromial ligament with cuff disease. These patients can suffer from profound and painful prominence of the humeral head under the anterosuperior shoulder surface as containment within the coracoacromial arch is lost. Reconstruction is difficult and reports sparse. Wiley reported on 4 patients with severe superior dislocation after coracoacromial ligament resection; 3 were associated with cuff repair attempts and 2 with humeral head replacement (HHR).[29] In 2 patients, containment of the humeral head was reestablished with iliac crest bone

graft of the coracoacromial arch in conjunction with capsular release. Both patients had lessening of pain. Alternatively, soft tissue reconstruction can be attempted.

Other surgeons have noted the problem of superior instability from loss of the containment by the coracoacromial arch in a cuff-deficient shoulder. Field reported on 16 cases of HHR for cuff arthropathy.[20] He noted 6 unsuccessful results. Four of the 6 patients had had prior rotator cuff surgery; 3 of these had anterosuperior subluxation and 2 had a deficient deltoid. He concluded that acromioplasty can jeopardize humeral head replacement for cuff arthropathy. Likewise, Gartsman found 3 cases of superomedial instability in 100 consecutive replacements; 2 occurred in instances of cuff tearing with prior coracoacromial ligament resection.[25] Superior instability can also be produced by deltoid injury. Groh described 12 cases of deltoid dysfunction after shoulder replacement.[28] Ten lost function of the anterior and middle deltoid as a result of failed repair and 2 had complete deltoid loss from axillary neuropathy. Average forward flexion was only 33 degrees and anterosuperior dislocation was common with attempted elevation. Function in cases of anterosuperior dislocation is typically extremely poor.

Inferior. Inferior instability is primarily an issue of loss of humeral length after acute fracture reconstruction. Loss of length not only produces painful inferior subluxation or dislocation of the joint but also inefficient

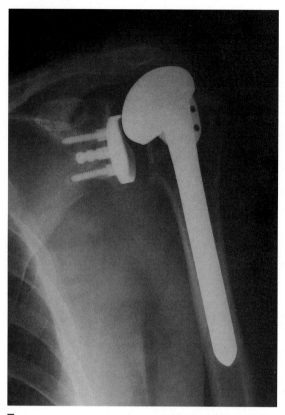

E

deltoid function from inadequate muscle tension. The best treatment is prevention by reconstruction of adequate length in the humeral shaft during prosthetic replacement. Often, proximal humeral fractures involve relatively little bone, and the medial flare of the prosthesis is seated on the calcar in the correct position. On occasion, fracture patterns extend more distally. In these instances, the prosthesis needs to be seated proudly and the interval bone grafted to allow satisfactory healing of the tuberosities to the shaft. The appropriate position of the prosthesis is determined by allowing the humeral head to face the glenoid with the arm in neutral rotation. Gentle traction should be placed across the extremity but sufficient laxity preserved to permit approximately 50 percent translation of the head across the glenoid surface. If the biceps tendon has been preserved, it can be used as an aid in judging soft tissue tensioning. If a replacement is inferiorly positioned, it can only be corrected by revision of the stem to achieve proper tension of the superior capsule and supraspinatus.

Anterior. Anterior instability is generally related to failure of subscapularis repair (Fig. 41–3).[46] Moeckel found 10 cases of revision surgery for instability in 236 shoulder replacements, for an incidence of 4.3 percent.[38] Seven cases were anterior, and all were thought to be secondary to a ruptured subscapularis. Four of these 7 had successful primary repair of the subscapularis, and 3 required calcaneal-Achilles' tendon allograft to reestablish stability. In a series of 11 patients undergoing repeat surgery for instability, Wirth described 3 shoulders with anterior dislocation.[59] All 3 replacements were found to have decreased humeral retroversion, 2 had a

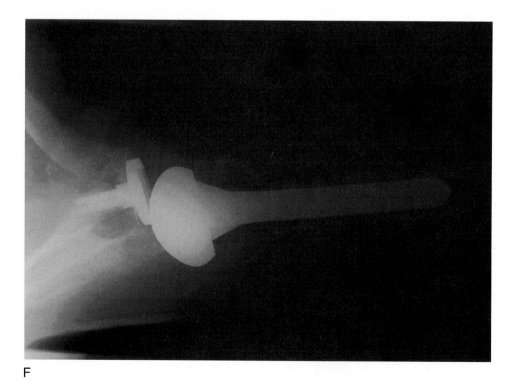

F

Figure 41–1. *Continued.* **E** and **F**, Revision surgery to an all-polyethylene glenoid component with stem exchange was successful.

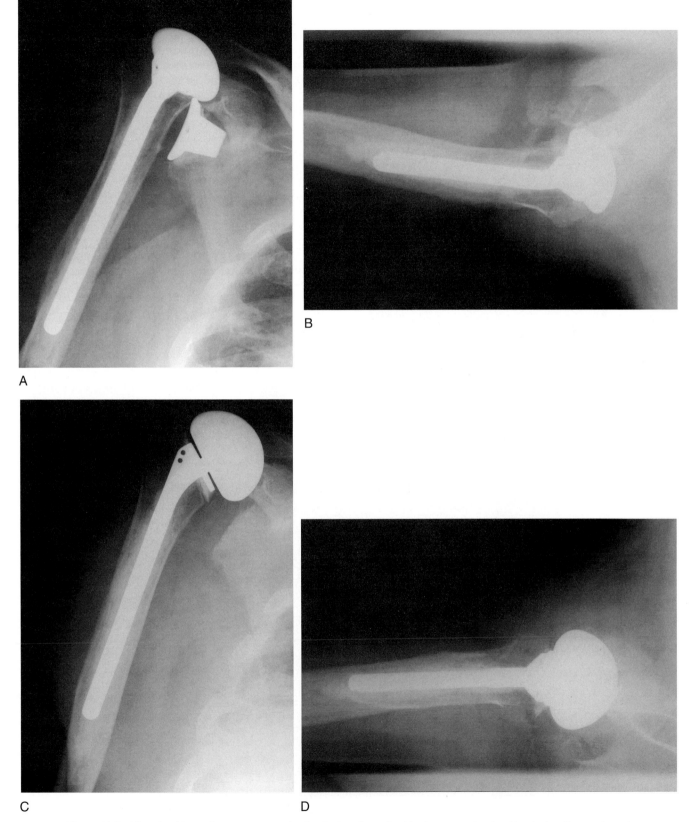

Figure 41–2. After shoulder replacement at another institution, the patient had severe pain, shoulder dysfunction, and crepitus in the shoulder. **A** and **B**, Physical examination and radiographs revealed the humeral prosthesis to be superiorly dislocated and locked onto the top of the glenoid. **C** and **D**, Because the stem was solidly cemented and the rotator cuff was absent, the replacement was revised to a humeral head replacement with an oversized head bridging the interval between the acromion and glenoid for stability.

ruptured subscapularis, and 1 shoulder had anterior glenoid erosion. Factors that were found to have contributed to the failure of the subscapularis were usually poor technique, inadequate tissue, inappropriate physi-

cal therapy, and oversized components that placed excessive tension on the repair.

Management. Treatment of anterior instability involves evaluation of the underlying cause, especially the position of the component and the integrity of the subscapularis. The position of the glenoid component should be checked to ensure that anterior erosion from such problems as rheumatoid arthritis or post-traumatic arthritis has not led to increased glenoid anteversion. Version of the humeral component is likewise assessed. Retroversion as great as 30 to 40 degrees can be accepted, but excessive retroversion needs to be prevented so as not to precipitate posterior instability. Excessive tightness in the posterior capsule can be associated with anterior laxity, and release is frequently necessary to balance the soft tissues. The most important step is restoration or reconstruction of the anterior capsule and subscapularis. Repair of the subscapularis begins with delineation of the tendon edge. The tendon gap is typically filled with thickened bursa and scar tissue, which must be resected to expose the tendon substance. The tendon itself retracts medially, and needs to be mobilized by freeing it not only from the anterior glenoid margin but also circumferencially around to the anterior surface. This procedure cannot be safely performed without identification of the axillary nerve. The objective is to sufficiently mobilize the tendon to allow it to be advanced back to the lesser tuberosity or the cut edge of the humeral neck. Downsizing the humeral head can actually aid in increasing stability by diminishing the volume of the glenohumeral joint and the tension on the repair. If the subscapularis cannot be repaired,

A

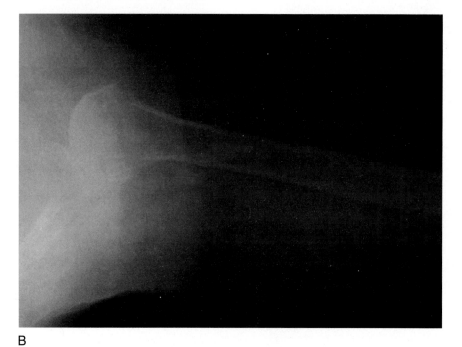

B

Figure 41–3. The diagnosis in this 59-year-old patient was rheumatoid arthritis. **A** and **B**, She underwent total shoulder arthroplasty. Initial physical therapy was unremarkable, but 3 months postoperatively she felt increased pain and developed bruising after a therapy session. Shortly afterward, she began experiencing anterior instability episodes.

Illustration continued on opposite page

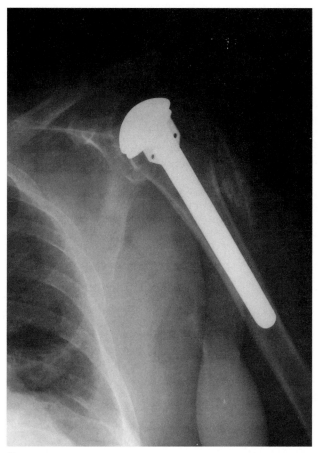

C

reconstruction is necessary. Potential techniques include calcaneal-tendo Achilles allograft or pectoralis major tendon transfer. Both techniques have been successful.[38,59]

Posterior. Posterior instability tends to be multifactorial and associated typically with the osteoarthritic shoulder. The causes include anterior capsular tightness, erosion of the posterior aspect of the glenoid, secondary increased retroversion of the glenoid, posterior subluxation of the humerus, and redundancy of the posterior capsule.[35,58] Moeckel, in his series of 10 revisions for instability, reported 3 shoulders with posterior instability.[23] Contributing problems were found to be excessive retroversion of the glenoid component, capsular redundancy, and humeral malposition (Fig. 41–4). Surgical treatment consisted of 1 case of glenoid revision with posterior glenoid bone grafting, 1 instance of humeral revision to diminish the humeral retroversion, and 1 final procedure of posterior soft tissue repair. Wirth described the surgical pathology in 7 shoulders with posterior instability.[59] Similar issues were reported, including excessive humeral retroversion of greater than 45 degrees in 4 patients, posterior glenoid erosion in 4 shoulders, and 1 instance of nonunion of the greater tuberosity. After revision surgery in a total of 11 cases of instability problems, restoration of stability was accomplished in 10 shoulders and pain relief was uniform. Average postoperative flexion was 100 degrees and external rotation 35 degrees.

The prevention of posterior instability during the primary arthroplasty begins with recognition of these

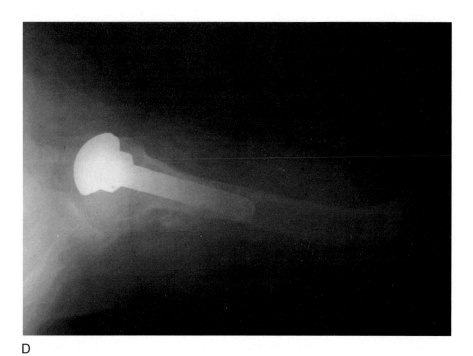

D

Figure 41–3. *Continued.* **C** and **D,** Repeat radiographs revealed anterior subluxation of the shoulder with likely subscapularis failure. She has so far declined repair.

predisposing factors. During the approach to the shoulder, the contracted subscapularis and anterior capsule may need to be lengthened by advancement to the osteotomy edge or Z-plasty.[4,12] More typically, however, the tendon can be adequately mobilized by removal of humeral osteophytes and release from the glenoid margin. If substantial posterior subluxation is noted on the preoperative axillary lateral radiograph, reduction in humeral retroversion offers some benefit in increased posterior capsular tension. Of greater importance is recognition of proper glenoid orientation to avoid inadvertent retroversion. Helpful techniques are utilization of any remaining anterior articular cartilage, which can be curretted down to undisturbed subchondral bone, or palpation of the anterior scapular neck. Use of a larger humeral head can increase stability, but the joint cannot be overstuffed or the subscapularis will either not be reparable or will re-tear. If excessive posterior laxity persists after these steps, posterior capsular imbrication must be carried out. Namba and Thornhill have described a method of posterior capsulorrhaphy whereby heavy nonabsorbable suture was woven through the posterior capsule and posterior cuff tendons and passed through the proximal humerus before stem insertion.[40] Obligatory tightening of the posterior capsule occurs during forward flexion, the position at risk of producing posterior instability. The authors note that the axillary nerve is inferior to the teres minor tendon and the suprascapular nerve medial to the glenoid rim in the region of the capsulorrhaphy. If there is postoperative instability, a similar analysis and correction of the pathology is necessary, with emphasis on the correction of the component position, release of the anterior contracture, and tightening of the posterior soft tissues.

ROTATOR CUFF TEAR

Anterior and Superior. Postoperative rotator cuff tears are most commonly anteriorly through the subscapularis or superiorly through the medial extent of the arthrotomy. Less often, the posterior aspect of the cuff is injured during the humeral neck osteotomy with resulting detachment of the infraspinatus. Although frank tearing can occur, the arthrotomy repair frequently stretches during the rehabilitation. The tendon interval fills with scar tissue, leaving the musculotendinous unit at an ineffective length. A tear manifests itself by instability, as discussed earlier, or by the patient's failure to progress at the expected rate in physical therapy. The diagnosis is relatively easy if dislocation has occurred, and early repair can be planned. In a stable shoulder, the failure of the cuff must be differentiated from other causes of pain and dysfunction, such as stiffness, neurologic injury, deltoid damage, and incomplete patient cooperation. The shoulder with failed healing of the rotator cuff occurring from inappropriate physical therapy or poor tissue can manifest an excessive range of motion, especially in external rotation. Crepitus along the site of the cuff repair is a worrisome finding throughout the healing period. As the patient progresses into active motion exercises, poor motion with disrupted glenohumeral rhythm is indicative of cuff failure. The lift-off and belly press signs are useful to judge subscapularis integrity. Because of the need to protect a potentially intact repair, weakness on manual strength testing is a late finding.

On radiographic examination, proximal humeral migration or anterior subluxation can be evident (Fig. 41–5). Although proximal humeral migration can be associated with other factors, as the acromiohumeral

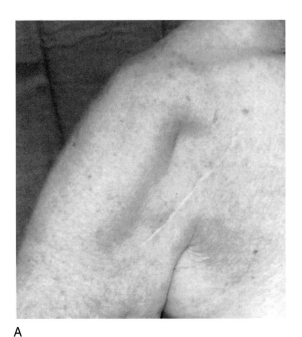

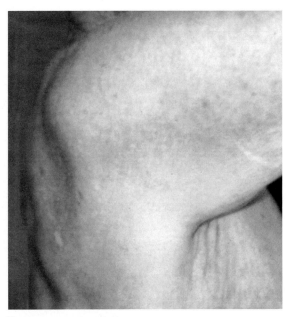

A   B

Figure 41–4. The chief complaint of this 80-year-old patient was that his shoulder was "tricky." He had posterior instability with any forward flexion. **A** and **B**, Physical examination revealed a sunken anterior aspect to the shoulder with posterior prominence on forward flexion. **C** and **D**, Radiographs revealed substantial retroversion of the glenoid component as well as increased retroversion of the humeral component and inferior positioning. Revision surgery was offered but declined to date.

Illustration continued on opposite page

distance narrows, it becomes increasing less likely that any cuff is present superiorly.[5] Arthrographic studies may not be conclusive. Although diagnostic when positive, the tendon gap is often filled with scar tissue obstructing the flow of the contrast material. Magnetic resonance imaging studies are subject to severe artifact distortion. Thus, the diagnosis is often made based on the physical examination and routine radiographs.

Management. Repair is carried out when indicated by instability or dysfunction. Fortunately, many patients have little pain and tolerable function.[2,14] When surgery is attempted, the procedure can be challenging and failures are common.[30,31] The repair is carried out through the original incision for the deltopectoral approach. If there is subscapularis tearing, the deltopectoral incision offers the best exposure, and, in all instances, the deltopectoral access must be available in case humeral head or stem revision is found necessary. The margins of the remaining rotator cuff are then carefully identified. Circumferential mobilization of the tendons from both extra-articular scar tissue and adhesions along the glenoid margin is essential. In the standard manner, the tendons are repaired back to prepared bone beds on the greater and lesser tuberosities, as appropriate. Assessment of the size of the humeral head should be performed as part of the process. An oversized head places excessive tension on the repair; conversely, use of a smaller head relieves stress on the repair and aids in healing. Selective capsulorrhaphy and correction of stem version may be necessary to reestablish stability, especially if stability was originally obtained by choosing an inappropriately large head. As in all cases of shoulder reconstruction, guidance should be given to the physical therapist for establishment of safe motion limits.

PERIPROSTHETIC FRACTURE

Occurrence. Wirth and Rockwood have estimated periprosthetic humeral fractures occur in about 3 percent of shoulder replacements and constitute approximately

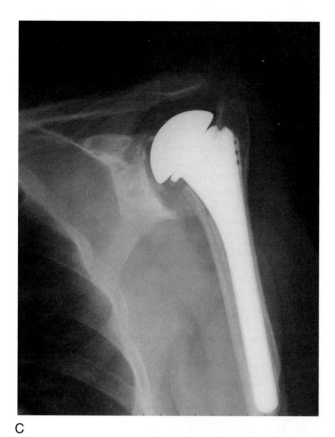

C

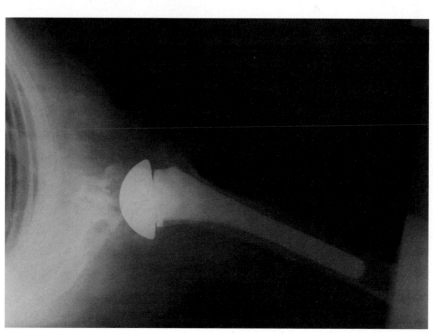

D

Figure 41–4. *Continued.*

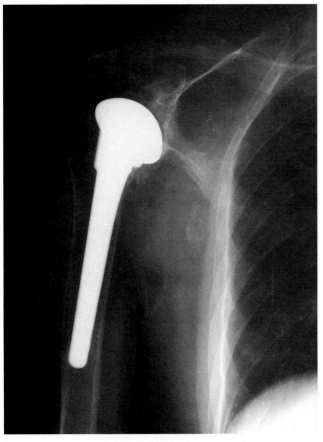

A

20 percent of all complications.[59] The incidence is dependent on technique and length of follow-up, because fractures occur both intraoperatively and postoperatively. Neer reported 4 late fractures in 273 replacements, Brenner encountered 1 fracture in 51 total shoulder arthroplasties (TSAs), Worland found 2 late fractures in 108 bipolar arthroplasties, Walch described 1 intraoperative humeral fracture in 101 prostheses, and Torchia noted 3 humeral fractures in 113 TSAs.[9,45,53,54,60] In these 646 procedures, there were 11 fractures for an incidence of 1.7 percent. These fractures can be difficult to manage. They are often unstable because of increased torsional stresses at the tip of the stem from restriction of motion at the glenohumeral joint, and patients have poor healing from loss of the endosteal blood supply.[8,62]

Classification. Wright and Cofield have classified humeral fractures around a stem as type A, B, or C.[62] Type A fractures were centered at the tip of the prosthesis and extended proximally at least one third the length of the stem. Type B fractures were primarily centered at the tip of the stem, and type C fractures involved the humeral shaft distal to the prosthesis. An alternative but similar classification system was described by Worland.[61] Type A fractures were proximal fractures occurring about the tuberosities. Type B fractures were located about the tip of the prosthesis and were subdivided into three categories. Spiral fractures around a stable prosthesis were B1 fractures, transverse or short oblique fractures with a stable stem were B2, and B3

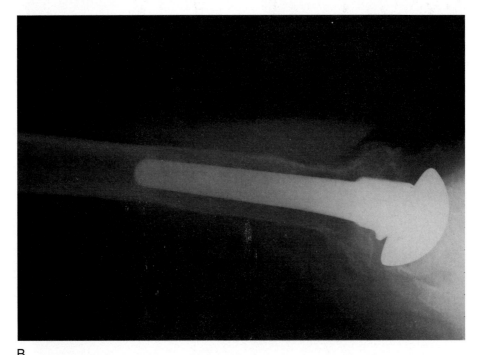

B

Figure 41–5. This 80-year-old man has persistent mechanical pain despite humeral head replacement 2 years earlier. He had subsequently undergone diagnostic arthroscopy and acromioplasty without improvement of symptoms. No substantial inflammation was appreciated at the time of the arthroscopy. Radiographs taken at the time of his examination revealed an undersized but solid humeral component. **A** and **B**, The glenoid showed severe wear and erosion. At surgical exploration, histologic analysis showed significant acute inflammation. **C** and **D**, Resection arthroplasty was performed with insertion of a temporary spacer.

Illustration continued on opposite page

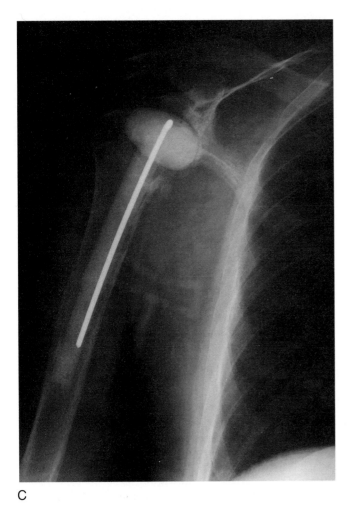

C

fractures had an unstable prosthesis. If the fracture was distal to the stem, it was classified as type C. Both authors believed that their classification systems aided analysis and treatment decision making.

Etiology. These fractures can occur from surgical error intraoperatively or from a traumatic event postoperatively. During surgery, a number of events can lead to a fracture and should be avoided. This begins with exposure in a tight shoulder with osteopenic bone. Excessive torque during dislocation without adequate capsular release can easily produce a fracture. A Darrach retractor or other type of skid device aids in dislocation and reduction by minimizing the forces across the shaft. A second mechanism of injury to the shaft can occur during reaming of the shaft. In the post-traumatic shoulder, distortion of anatomy can lead to eccentric reaming and breakthrough into the cortical canal. Additionally, reaming, if done overzealously, can damage the canal. The humeral cortex is often extremely thin, especially in rheumatoid shoulders. An aggressive approach to the canal produces a fracture. It is safer to stop reaming immediately on cortical contact. Finally, forceful impaction of the stem in an attempt to obtain a tight press-fit in a weak bone is unsafe and can fracture the shaft.

Groh reported on 12 humeral fractures.[27] Eight occurred intraoperatively and 4 postoperatively from an injury. Of the primary fracture cases, 2 resulted from manipulation of the extremity, 1 from reaming, 1 during broaching, and the final 2 after the insertion of the prosthesis. Two additional fractures developed in areas of cortical thinning during revision surgery. Campbell described 21 fractures; 16 were the result of intraoperative

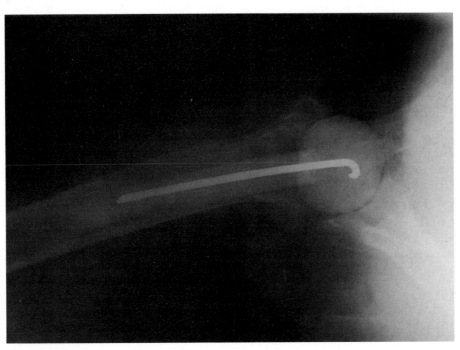

D

Figure 41–5. *Continued.*

Illustration continued on following page

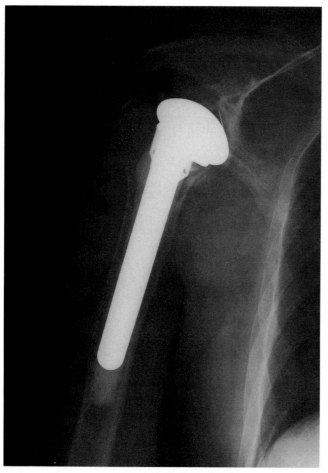

E

complication and 5 happened postoperatively.[11] The most common contributing factor was osteopenia, found in 75 percent of the extremities. In the 7 fractures Boyd discovered after 436 replacements, all occurred late.[8] Six ensued from a fall and 1 from a motor vehicle accident. Five of the patients had rheumatoid arthritis, and this population frequently suffers from osteopenia. Similarly, Wright and Cofield found cofactors of advanced osteopenia in 6 shoulders and an ipsilateral elbow replacement in 2 extremities of 9 late humeral fractures after 499 TSAs.[62] The particular risk that ipsilateral stemmed shoulder and elbow replacements pose to the rheumatoid extremity was delineated. Any vacant segment between the stems or cement columns results in a stress riser. Gill and colleagues recommended use of cemented stems with a continuous cement column to avoid this problem.[26]

Management. Treatment of periprosthetic humeral fractures is complicated by the fact that intraoperative fractures are often not recognized until they are seen on a postoperative radiograph. It may be tempting to treat the fracture nonsurgically, but the outcome is typically poor. Bonutti attempted to treat 4 fractures conservatively; 3 of these were suffered intraoperatively.[4] All failed to heal. He recommended consideration of "vigorous treatment" of these fractures. Boyd treated 7 fractures after arthroplasty without surgery.[8] Six fractures failed to heal and only 1 initially went on to union. One patient refused further treatment; 5 went to union after surgical fixation. In addition, the 1 fracture that did heal initially had a painful nonunion that required revision surgery. Boyd's conclusion was that the technique of

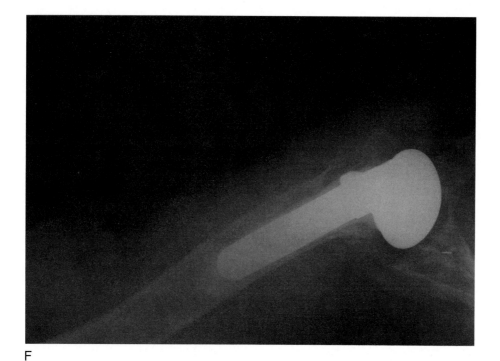

F

Figure 41–5. *Continued.* **E** and **F**, Intravenous antibiotics were administered for 6 weeks, when second-stage reconstruction was carried out.

open reduction and fixation was preferable. Kligman described 5 fractures associated with HHR; 3 of the 5 did heal without surgery.[33] However, time to union was 7 months, and only 1 had a satisfactory result. The 2 treated surgically healed in 2 months. Wright and Cofield reported only marginally better outcome with nonsurgical treatment in their series of 9 fractures.[62] Four did heal without surgery, but 3 others went onto nonunion. Two of these 3 healed with revision surgery and bone grafting, and the 2 treated primarily with internal fixation also healed. They therefore felt that although long oblique and spiral fractures could be managed conservatively, it was better to internally stabilize transverse and short oblique fractures at the tip of the stem or those associated with a loose prosthesis. Distal fractures could be managed conservatively.[27]

The value of aggressive treatment of these fractures was outlined by Campbell and associates.[11] They found improved healing with anatomic reduction and stable fixation. There was significantly less time to union, less influence on rehabilitation, and a trend toward fewer complications. Similarly, anatomic reduction to within 2 mm of displacement was statistically associated with diminished healing time. There is, therefore, a fairly uniform agreement on the value of operative treatment for the majority of these injuries.[8,11,26,27,61,62] Fractures discovered intraoperatively should be stabilized with cerclage wires and a long-stem component as needed to create a stable construct that allows early range of motion postoperatively. The tip of the prosthesis should extend 2 to 3 cortical diameters beyond the fracture. Postoperatively discovered fractures that are proximal to the tip of the stem, especially those with long oblique or spiral patterns, may be stable enough to treat nonoperatively (Wright type A, Worland types A and B1). However, transverse and short oblique fractures require internal stabilization with cerclage cables and a long-stem prosthesis if the fracture extends to within 2 to 3 cortical diameters of the stem tip (Wright type B, Worland type B2 patterns). Similarly, injuries involving an unstable implant are best revised to a long-stem construct (Worland type B3). The more distal fractures, classified as type C by both Wright and Worland, can be treated on their own merits with either internal fixation or bracing, as the fracture pattern and potential elbow involvement dictate.

GLENOID FRACTURES

Glenoid fractures are less common and less troublesome. There are isolated reports but no large series of these injuries.[12,29,32] The glenoid rim is vulnerable anteriorly from the torque applied by reaming, especially when done under power in weak bone. As long as the vault of the glenoid is left intact, resurfacing can still be carried out. Downsizing the choice of the glenoid may be necessary to ensure adequate bone support of the component. If fracture into the glenoid neck occurs, stable fixation with either peg or keeled designs cannot be achieved. The only option in this case is to pack the gle-

noid defect with bone graft from the humeral head and convert to HHR with contouring of the remaining glenoid surface to conform to the humeral head.

INFECTION

Although infection is an uncommon problem, it can be a challenge to diagnose and should be considered whenever there is unexplained pain or premature loosening in a replacement. Neer reported 1 infection in 273 TSAs, Gartsman none in 51 shoulders, Barrett none in 140 TSAs, Walch 2 in 101 prostheses, and Torchia 3 cases of infection in 113 replacements.[2,33,45,53,54] Kozak has reported the Mayo Clinic experience.[35] In 1484 primary cases of arthroplasty, there were 18 infections (1.2 percent). In the 157 revision procedures, infection was subsequently diagnosed in 6 (4.5 percent). An additional 7 primary and 2 revision cases seen after referrals were included. Not surprisingly, pain was the most common symptom and was found in 73 percent of involved shoulders. Other signs and symptoms were drainage in 52 percent, effusion in 36 percent, erythema and stiffness in 33 percent each, and fever in only 21 percent. Laboratory studies of value included an elevated erythrocyte sedimentation rate in 70 percent of patients. An Indium-11 scan was positive in 10 of the 14 shoulders in which it was performed. Cultures revealed the most common organisms to be staphylococci, with Staphylococcus aureus present in 12 shoulders and Staphylococcus coagulase-negative results in 9 patients. Risk factors associated with a higher incidence of infection were systemic immune disorders and multiple prior surgeries.

Management. A number of treatment procedures have been reported. The most successful treatment is a two-stage exchange arthroplasty. This was uniformly successful in 3 shoulders in the Mayo experience, all of which were free of infection at most recent follow-up. Function was also superior in shoulders with retained prostheses. All had no pain or slight pain with active elevation of 98 degrees and external rotation of 26 degrees. The most common treatment was resection arthroplasty. This was performed in 22 patients, who required an average of a little more than two débridements each and who suffered from frequent complications. There were 3 fractures of the humeral shaft, and 5 patients had evidence of recurrent infection. This consisted of 3 superficial infections and 2 recurrent sinus tract formations. Function was also poor in these patients. Fully one half had moderate pain, and average active elevation was limited to 40 degrees. The majority had poor strength.

Other initial treatment programs included 1 of 2 successful arthroscopic débridements. Open débridement with retention of the components was carried out in 3 patients, two of whom later underwent removal of the prostheses. Isolated excision of the sinus tract as the only surgical treatment was tried in 2 patients, with 1 ultimately needing resection arthroplasty. Finally single-stage exchange arthroplasty was successful in 1 of 2 cases. Resection alone was associated with poor function and a relatively high rate of residual infection, with 18 percent showing evidence of ongoing or recurrent infection. Patients with a retained prosthesis had superior pain relief and improved function.

The current treatment of choice is therefore delayed exchange arthroplasty (Fig. 41–6). If the diagnosis is in doubt, the most straightforward evaluation can be frozen section examination of operative tissue by a pathologist who is comfortable with the evaluation of the painful prosthesis. Kozak et al. found that of the 27 patients in whom histologic analysis was carried out, acute inflammation was present in 19, chronic inflammation in 9, and gross purulence in 8.[35] If there is no evidence of substantial inflammation on pathologic evaluation, immediate reconstruction is appropriate. Conversely, if there is evidence of acute inflammation, resection arthroplasty is performed. As second-stage reconstruction is anticipated because of the superior results, it is important to preserve whatever portion of the rotator cuff that remains. In addition, soft tissue management is improved and antibiotic delivery is enhanced with use of an antibiotic-impregnated cement spacer. A Palacos cement spacer is fabricated, combining 4.8 g of tobramycin, 4.0 g of vancomycin, and 2.0 g of cefazolin, which are mixed with each pack of methylmethacrylate. Plastic 5-ml and 12-ml syringes are clamped together as a mold for the spacer, because this provides a tapered shape that typically fits easily down the canal. A "head" is contoured over the top to tension the cuff, and a Rush rod inserted down the construct to add strength. The plastic syringes are cut off after the cement has set, and the spacer is gently inserted down the canal. The remaining rotator cuff is repaired with absorbable sutures around the spacer, and intravenous

antibiotics are administered based on the results of intraoperative cultures. Typically, antibiotics are given for 6 weeks. If the wound has matured with resolution of swelling and erythema, repeat exploration and histologic analysis are undertaken. If persistent acute inflammation is present, repeat cultures are submitted and reimplantation deferred. Otherwise, the prosthesis is implanted. After the multiple violations of the canal, press-fit options are limited and use of cement allows use of further antibiotics, although in lower doses than in the spacer. Usually, only 1.0 g of vancomycin or 1.2 g of tobramycin per pack of methylmethacrylate are used in the final reconstruction, with the choice dependent on the initial cultures. In the 6 reconstructions that I have carried out with this method, there have been no recurrences of infection and uniform relief of pain. Function remains dependent on the integrity of the rotator cuff, as is typical in shoulder arthroplasty.

NEUROLOGIC DEFICIT

Although a problem rarely needing surgery, postoperative neurologic problems can provoke considerable distress for both patient and physician. Lynch found 18 cases of postoperative neurologic deficit after 417 shoulder replacements in 368 patients (4 percent) at the Mayo Clinic.[37] Thirteen of the lesions were brachial plexopathies, primarily upper and middle trunk lesions; in addition, there were 3 instances of idiopathic brachial plexopathy that were considered to be secondary to brachial neuritis, and 1 patient had persistence of a preexisting plexopathy. One patient developed carpal tunnel syndrome. Patients at higher risk for these problems were those who were taking methotrexate, those who had an extended deltopectoral approach for exposure, and those who had shorter operative times. Many factors were found to have no relationship to neurologic complications. These included age of patient, sex, diagnostic category, height, weight, range of motion, prior surgery, rotator cuff tearing, and the presence of diabetes or rheumatoid arthritis. The outcome of the deficits was fairly positive, with 11 of the patients followed at 1 year having a good result and 5 a fair recovery. Only in 4 of the patients was the rehabilitative program disturbed by the nerve injury.

The etiology of the neurologic deficits was thought to be primarily traction.[37] The performance of shoulder arthroplasty involves placing the extremity into various positions of extension and rotation to expose the humeral canal. This manipulation places stress across the brachial plexus, and this stress can be increased through poor positioning of the head. Early in our experience with shoulder replacement, a standard operative table was utilized. Access to the shoulder involved rotation and tilting the cervical spine away from the operative site. This can place addition forces across the plexus and potentially lead to an injury. More recently, use of a table modification allows placement of the head in a neutral position. The typical choice is the utilization of a Mayfield head frame. This permits the top of the table to

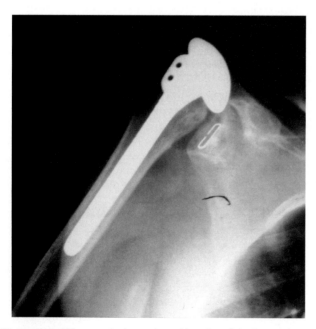

Figure 41–6. When marked superior subluxation of the humeral component is present, the diagnosis of rotator cuff tearing is obvious.

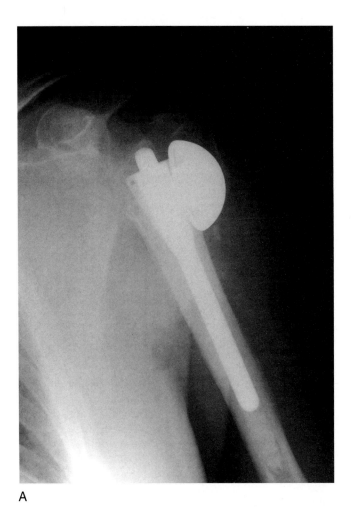

A

be removed, and, in conjunction with lateralization of the patient, eases access to the humeral canal. Alternatively, special table attachments are available for shoulder surgery, which entail removal of the upper quadrant of the table. Access to the posterior aspect of the shoulder is particularly improved, but support of the thorax is diminished, and obese patients are often unstable in these setups. It is up to the surgeons to decide which arrangement works best in their hands. Either situation offers the potential for diminishing the forces across the plexus and reducing the incidence of neurologic injuries.

COMPONENT FAILURE

The design of shoulder prostheses has evolved to include metal backing of the glenoid component, modular and ingrowth glenoid components, modular humeral heads, and bipolar humeral heads. The increased complexity of these designs has introduced new potential methods of failure for shoulder arthroplasty (Fig. 41–7). Blevins has reported occurrences of dissociation of a modular titanium head from the stem through failure of the Morse taper.[3] He identified 13 cases of this complication and calculated an incidence of approximately 1:1000 for that prosthesis. Two important points were emphasized. Investigation revealed that as little as 0.4 ml of fluid contamination of the Morse taper interfered with solid fixation. Additionally, 12 in 13 cases of disassembly occurred within the first 6 weeks after surgery. This suggested problems with the taper lock or possibly in manufacturing and emphasizes the need to that ensure a secure lock is established at surgery.

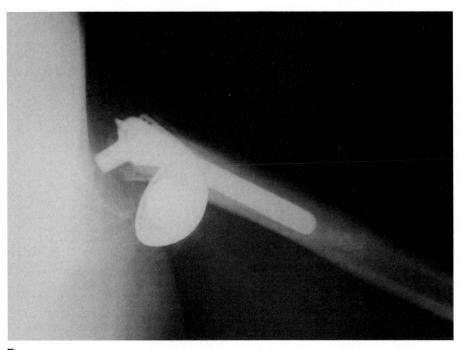

B

Figure 41–7. **A** and **B**, Humeral head replacement was performed outside the United States for an acute fracture of the shoulder in this patient. Failure occurred through disassembly at the Morse taper and disruption of the tuberosity repair.

Problems have also developed with newer glenoid designs. In an attempt to improve glenoid fixation and decrease potential loosening complications, an uncemented bone ingrowth component was developed by Cofield.[16] The design utilized a chromium-cobalt metal tray, two titanium alloy cortical screws, and an ultra-high-molecular-weight polyethylene insert. Although early clinical results were encouraging, episodes of component failure have been noted.[15,16,55,56] In his initial series of 32 shoulder replacements, Cofield found 2 instances of polyethylene dissociation from the metal backing.[16] Glenohumeral instability was thought to be related to these episodes, but the glenoid component was subsequently redesigned to improve the mechanical interlock between the polyethylene insert and the base plate. In a larger series of 180 ingrowth glenoid components, 5 were complicated by polyethylene separation.[15] Three of these occurred in association with substantial polyethylene wear. Similarly, Wallace, in 1999, reported 2 cases of dissociation with use of the same component in a series of 39 uncemented glenoid components.[55] Both episodes occurred late, one at 2 years after surgery and the other after 50 months.[49] Considerable polyethylene wear was associated with the latter case. A metal-backed component is susceptible to catastrophic failure because of the potential for metal-on-metal wear along the glenoid edge in addition to the possibility of polyethylene separation (see Fig. 41–1).

Particulate debris from polyethylene or metal wear can stimulate synovitis and osteolysis as well. Wallace noted that the uncemented glenoid could be associated with eccentric wear of the posterior metal rim and osteolysis, but this process is not unique to one prosthetic design.[55] Sperling described 1 case of particulate synovitis associated with instability in a series of 18 revision arthroplasties.[49] Gartsman found 1 instance of titanium synovitis in 100 consecutive replacements with a Biomet prosthesis.[25] Klimkiewicz described a case report of humeral loosening associated with osteolysis.[34] His analysis suggested that late subsidence of the humeral component resulted in a degree of mechanical instability in the reconstruction. The instability resulted in accelerated polyethylene wear, with osteolysis and, ultimately, loosening of the component as the final outcome.

It seems clear then that the increased complexity of prosthetic designs, which were chosen to reduce previously recognized complications and to restore anatomy more accurately, have introduced additional potential problems. The risk of these problems appears to be increased with any degree of instability in the reconstruction that can cause accelerated wear of the polyethylene surface even with a nonmodular glenoid component.

GLENOID ARTHROSIS

Although HHR has been suggested as an appropriate solution for the shoulder with osteoarthritis or rheumatoid arthritis, these reconstructions can be troubled by persistent pain from the unresurfaced glenoid[6,7,10,51] (Fig. 41–8). In a study of 35 HHRs for osteoarthritis and 32 hemiarthroplasties for rheumatoid arthritis, Cofield found that pain caused 9 of the 35 to be converted to a TSA at average follow-up of 72 months.[53] Two were performed within 2 years of surgery, 2 between 2 and 4 years, and 5 at 4 or more years from the primary reconstruction. Three of the 32 HHRs for rheumatoid arthritis were converted to TSAs. In a review of replacements in patients younger than 50 years old at the time of initial surgery, Sperling reported that of the 15 revisions in 74 HHRs, 11 were necessary for glenoid arthritis.[51] Risk factors included a diagnosis of traumatic arthritis and a history of prior surgery.

In a randomized comparison, Gartsman found poorer pain relief after HHR than after TSA.[24] Three of the 24 HHRs were revised to TSAs. Levine studied the influence of the glenoid contour on the results of HHR.[18] Overall, 23 of 31 (74 percent) of HHRs were considered to have a satisfactory result. If the glenoid wear was concentric, 13 of 15 were satisfactory compared with only 10 of 16 with nonconcentric wear. The pain relief was found to be similar in both groups, but less range of motion was present in the latter group.

The presentation is often worrisome for occult infection, which must be carefully excluded. Pain is associated with any motion, which is typically substantially restricted. The pain may never have been relieved by the HHR, or it may have developed in a delayed manner. Radiographs usually show complete loss of the glenohumeral joint space and frequent evidence of glenoid erosion as well. If concerns are present for substantial glenoid wear, then a computed tomography scan should be obtained to ensure that sufficient bone stock remains for glenoid resurfacing. In theory, revision of a modular HHR to a TSA is a relatively straightforward process, with head removal and insertion of the glenoid component. In practice, however, exposure can be difficult, and extensive capsular releases are necessary. The position of the stem needs to be assessed and may need to be revised for exposure, for malposition, or for soft tissue balancing. Nevertheless, pain relief in these patients can be marked, and they are frequently the most grateful of revision patients.

STIFFNESS

Failure to achieve a degree of motion appropriate to the diagnosis is a complication of surgery. The ultimate range of motion after shoulder arthroplasty can be related to factors beyond the surgeon's control, such as the diagnostic group, the status of the rotator cuff, and the overall condition of the patient.[14,21] Other factors, however, are under the physician's influence and include degree of capsular release, component positioning, and head selection.[21,29] The evaluation of inadequate motion includes review of the preoperative radiograph, the operative report, the initial range of motion, and current radiographs. Superior subluxation of the humeral head can evidence an incompetent rotator cuff; posterior subluxation indicates an instability pattern perhaps compensated for with an oversized humeral head or associated with anterior contracture; and post-traumatic changes suggest circumferential scarring. Physical examination is performed to evaluate the specific directions of restricted motion and the function of the rotator cuff. The areas of stiffness give direction to the releases necessary, although the final decisions are made intraoperatively with the trial prostheses in place. Finally, the

current radiographic films are reviewed for evidence of component malposition and overstuffing of the joint.

Humeral head position should be at or slightly superior to the tip of the greater tuberosity, with the humeral osteotomy typically made just inside the rotator cuff insertion. A high cut can lead to a proud component producing overtensioning of the supraspinatus or superior impingement. A low cut can threaten the cuff insertion. In addition, the uncovered calcar can abut the glenoid

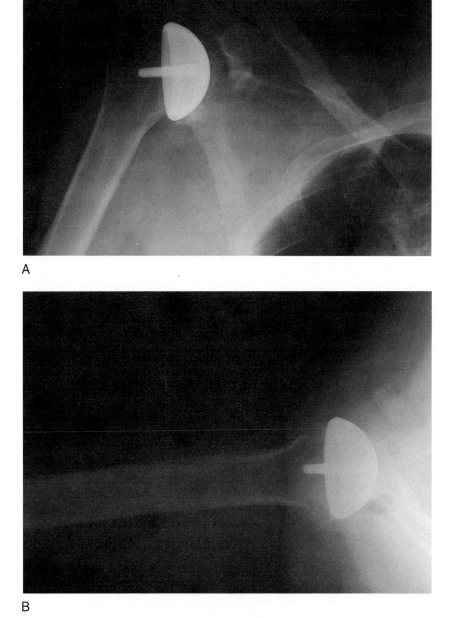

A

B

Figure 41–8. **A** and **B**, This humeral head replacement was unable to relieve the patient's stiffness and pain. Severe glenoid wear and large humeral osteophytes were present on radiographs taken at the time of his examination.

Illustration continued on following page

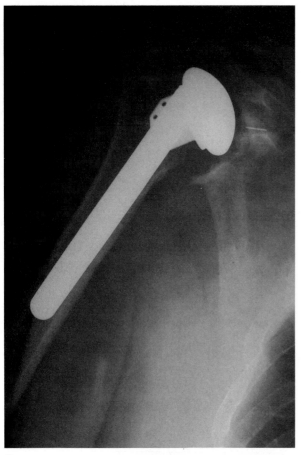

C

and block adduction. Inappropriate version may be related to instability, again compensated by a larger head size. A large head size places abnormal stress on the cuff and limits motion. In 8 cadaveric shoulders, Harryman[29] found that use of a 5-mm oversized head was associated with a marked decrease in motion, ranging from 23 percent to 30 percent in elevation, flexion, and rotation. He also demonstrated the increased tension on soft tissues by seating an anatomic head in a proud position. Figgie similarly noted that use of an enlarged head was related to diminished results, and, conversely, observed restoration of normal glenoid and humeral anatomy with improved results.[21]

At incision, only the head size may need to be changed, or just soft tissue work may be necessary. When there is loss of external rotation to less than a minimum of 30 to 40 degrees, the anterior capsule and subscapularis need to be lengthened. This can be accomplished by mobilization from circumferential adhesions including the glenoid margin, by advancement of the subscapularis to the edge of the humeral osteotomy, or by performance of a Z-plasty lengthening[12] (Figs. 41–9 and 41–10). If internal rotation to 120 degrees is not obtainable, release of the posterior capsule along the glenoid margin should be considered[12,21] (Fig. 41–11). Additional sources of stiffness include impingement of a retained humeral neck, excessive lateral offset from a large humeral head, or malposition of the head in increased retroversion. Blockage of abduction less than 160 degrees is most common from constricted inferior and posterior capsule. Release of the inferior capsule along the humeral neck can be safely carried out to the 6 o'clock position, but if further release is

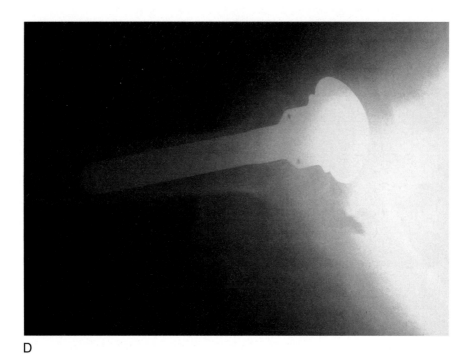

D

Figure 41–8. *Continued.* **C** and **D**, Revision surgery was successful in eliminating the patient's pain.

necessary, it is wise to identify and protect the axillary nerve as the release is directed toward the posterior inferior aspect of the glenoid[12] (Fig. 41–12). Less commonly, superior release is necessary when there is circumferential scarring around the joint (Fig. 41–13).

IMPINGEMENT SYNDROME

In the presence of an intact rotator cuff, the replaced shoulder is subject to the same impingement-related pain as the non-reconstructed shoulder. Freedman

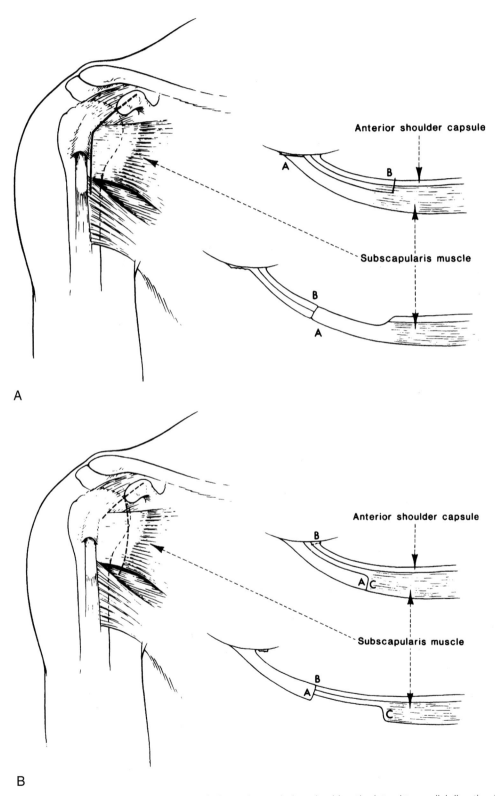

Figure 41–9. Z-plasty lengthening of the subscapularis can be carried out in either the lateral to medial direction (**A**) or the medial to lateral direction (**B**). The choice is up to the surgeon's preference.

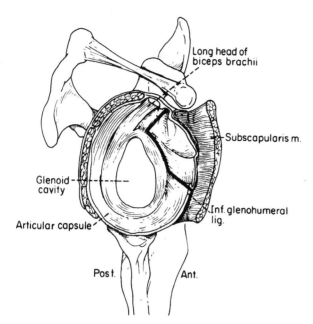

Figure 41–10. The anterior capsule frequently needs to be released along the glenoid margin to allow flexibility of the anterior capsule and the subscapularis; this is the most common means of reestablishing effective external rotation.

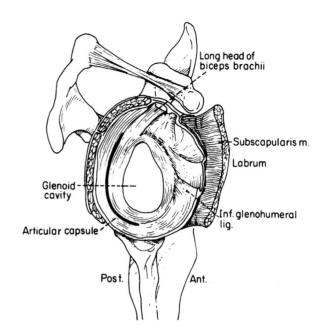

Figure 41–12. Inferior release is carried from the anterior and lateral direction to the posterior and medial direction.

found an incidence of 3 percent in shoulder arthroplasty at his institution.[23] Four patients had pain after TSA and 2 after HHR. All 6 patients were treated with arthroscopic acromioplasty, with a successful outcome in 5 of the 6 shoulders.

Because impingement syndrome does occur in the replaced shoulder, it is prudent during the primary reconstruction to inspect the subacromial space. If an acromial enthesophyte is seen on the preoperative radiograph or palpated during the procedure, it should be

removed. This can be performed through the standard incision, but, if necessary, an accessory approach through the deltoid can be used for the acromioplasty. In a late presentation, it is necessary to differentiate pain caused by impingement tendinitis from other causes of pain. Loosening of the components, rotator cuff tearing, occult infection, component malposition, or instability should be considered. Anteriorly localized shoulder pain with activity, reproduction of the pain with the Neer and Hawkins impingement signs, and relief of

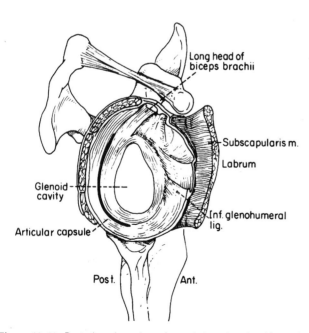

Figure 41–11. Posterior release is performed along the glenoid margin.

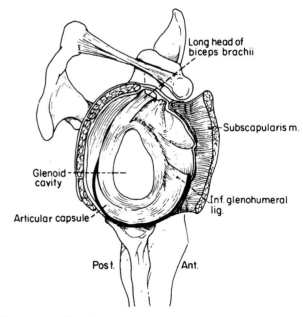

Figure 41–13. Superior release is frequently needed for rotator cuff mobilization during a repair, but, if there is severe capsular scarring, this procedure must also be done to increase glenohumeral volume.

the pain and provocative maneuvers with a subacromial lidocaine injection allow the diagnosis to be reliably established. Initial treatment should be nonsurgical with nonsteroidal anti-inflammatory medication, a limited number of subacromial steroid injections, and, potentially, physical therapy. However if symptoms are persistent, acromioplasty is a reasonable alternative.

HETEROTOPIC OSSIFICATION

Heterotopic ossification (HO) is a frequent finding on postoperative radiographs, although it can be easily overlooked.[19,32,39,50] Fortunately it usually is of limited consequence. Sperling has outlined a grading system that allows that extent of the ectopic bone to be described.[50] In grade 0, there is no bone evident. In grade I the excess bone bridges less than 50 percent of the distance between the lateral aspect of the glenoid and the medial cortex of the humeral shaft or the acromion. If more than 50 percent is ossified, it is classified as grade II disease. Finally, in grade III, there is an osseous bridge. In a study of 58 primary ingrowth TSAs, heterotopic bone was found in 14 cases (24.1 percent).[50] Twelve were grade I and 2 were grade II. The process is usually low grade, appears within 1 to 2 months on radiography, does not progress, and does not affect the result.[50] Similarly, others have confirmed that HO is a frequent finding on postoperative radiographs, but, in almost all cases, little note needs to be taken of the process, and indications for removal of the bone are rare.[32,39]

References

1. Neer CS II, Watson KC, Stanton FJ: Recent experience in total shoulder replacement. J Bone Joint Surg 64A:319–337, 1982.
2. Neer CS II, Brown TH Jr, McLaughlin HL: Fractures of the neck of the humerus with dislocation of the head fragment. Am J Surg 85:252–258, 1953.
3. Neer CS II, Morrison DS: Glenoid bone grafting in total shoulder arthroplasty. J Bone Joint Surg 70A:1154–1162, 1988.
4. Wirth MA, Rockwood CA: Complications of total shoulder arthroplasty. Clin Orthop 307:47–69, 1994.
5. Wirth MA, Rockwood CA: Complications of total shoulder-replacement arthroplasty. J Bone Joint Surg 78A:603–616, 1996.
6. Neer CS II, Kirby RM: Revision of humeral head and total shoulder arthroplasties. Clin Orthop 170:189–195, 1982.
7. Cofield RH, Edgerton BC: Total shoulder arthroplasty: Complications and revision surgery. In Instructional Course Lectures, the American Academy of Orthopedic Surgeons, vol 39. Park Ridge, Ill, American Academy of Orthopedic Surgeons, 1990, p 449.
8. Cofield RH: Revision procedures for shoulder arthroplasty. In Morrey BF (ed): Reconstructive Surgery of the Joints, vol 1. New York, Churchill Livingstone, 1996, p 789.
9. Barrett WP, Franklin JL, Jackins S, et al: Total shoulder arthroplasty. J Bone Joint Surg 69A:865–872, 1987.
10. Franklin JL, Barrett WP, Jackins SE, Matsen FA III: Glenoid loosening in total shoulder arthroplasty: Association with rotator cuff deficiency. J Arthroplasty 3:39–46, 1988.
11. Klimkiewicz JJ, Iannotti JP, Rubash HE, Shanbag AS: Aseptic loosening of the humeral component in total shoulder arthroplasty. J Shoulder Elbow Surg 7:422–426, 1999.
12. Stewart MPM, Kelly IG: Total shoulder replacement in rheumatoid disease. J Bone Joint Surg 79B:68–72, 1997.
13. Søjbjerg JO, Frich LH, Johannsen HV, Sneppen O: Late results of total shoulder replacement in patients with rheumatoid arthritis. Clin Orthop 366:39–45, 1999.
14. Sperling JW, Cofield RH: Revision total shoulder arthroplasty for the treatment of glenoid arthrosis. J Bone Joint Surg 80A:860–867, 1998.
15. Rodosky MW, Bigliani LU: Indications for glenoid resurfacing in shoulder arthroplasty. J Shoulder Elbow Surg 5:231–248, 1996.
16. Wallace AL, Phillips RL, MacDougal GA, et al: Resurfacing of the glenoid in total shoulder arthroplasty. J Bone Joint Surg 81A:510–518, 1999.
17. Boyd AD Jr, Aliabadi P, Thornhill TS: Postoperative proximal migration in total shoulder arthroplasty. Incidence and significance. J Arthroplasty 6:31–37, 1991.
18. Wiley AM: Superior humeral dislocation. A complication following decompression and débridement for rotator cuff tears. Clin Orthop 263:135–141, 1991.
19. Field LD, Dines DM, Zabinski SJ, Warren RF: Hemiarthroplasty of the shoulder for rotator cuff arthropathy. J Shoulder Elbow Surg 6:18–23, 1997.
20. Gartsman GM, Russell JA, Gaenslen E: Modular shoulder arthroplasty. J Shoulder Elbow Surg 6:333–339, 1997.
21. Groh GI, Simoni M, Rolla P, Rockwood CA Jr: Loss of the deltoid after shoulder operations: An operative disaster. J Shoulder Elbow Surg 3:243–253, 1994.
22. Norris TR, Lipson SR: Management of the unstable prosthetic shoulder. In Instructional Course Lectures, the American Academy of Orthopedic Surgeons, vol 47. Park Ridge, Ill, American Academy of Orthopedic Surgeons, 1998, p 141.
23. Moeckel BH, Altcheck DW, Warren RF, et al: Instability of the shoulder after arthroplasty. J Bone Joint Surg 75A:492–497, 1993.
24. Neer CS II: Replacement arthroplasty for glenohumeral osteoarthritis. J Bone Joint Surg 56A:1–13, 1974.
25. Cofield RH: Integral surgical maneuvers in prosthetic shoulder arthroplasty. Semin Arthroplasty 1:112–123, 1990.
26. Namba RS, Thornhill TS: Posterior capsulorrhaphy in total shoulder arthroplasty. Clin Orthop 313:135–139, 1995.
27. Barrett WP, Thornhill TS, Thomas WH, et al: Nonconstrained total shoulder arthroplasty in patients with polyarticular rheumatoid arthritis. J Arthroplasty 4:91–96, 1989.
28. Cofield RH: Total shoulder arthroplasty with the Neer prosthesis. J Bone Joint Surg 66A:899–906, 1984.
29. Hawkins RJ, Bell RH, Jallay B: Total shoulder arthroplasty. Clin Orthop 242:188–194, 1989.
30. Hawkins RJ, Greis PE, Bonutti PM: Treatment of symptomatic glenoid loosening following unconstrained shoulder arthroplasty. Orthopedics 22:229–234, 1999.
31. Brenner BC, Ferlic DC, Clayton ML, Dennis DA: Survivorship of unconstrained total shoulder arthroplasty. J Bone Joint Surg 71A:1289–1296, 1989.
32. Torchia ME, Cofield RH, Settergren CR: Total shoulder arthroplasty with the Neer prosthesis: Long-term results. J Shoulder Elbow Surg 6:495–505, 1997.
33. Walch G, Boileau P: Prosthetic adaptability: A new concept for shoulder arthroplasty. J Shoulder Elbow Surg 8:443–451, 1999.
34. Worland RL, Arredondo J: Bipolar shoulder arthroplasty for painful conditions of the shoulder. J Arthroplasty 13:631–637, 1998.
35. Wright TW, Cofield RH: Humeral fractures after shoulder arthroplasty. J Bone Joint Surg 77A:1340–1346, 1995.
36. Boyd RL, Thornhill TS, Barnes CL: Fractures adjacent to humeral prostheses. J Bone Joint Surg 74A:1498–1504, 1992.
37. Worland RL, Kim DY, Arredondo J: Periprosthetic humeral fractures: Management and classification. J Shoulder Elbow Surg 8:590–594, 1999.
38. Groh GI, Heckman MM, Curtis RJ, Rockwood CA Jr: Treatment of fractures adjacent to humeral prosthesis [abstract]. Orthop Trans 18:1072, 1994–1995.
39. Campbell JT, Moore RS, Ianotti JP, et al: Periprosthetic humeral fractures: Mechanism of fracture and treatment options [abstract]. J Shoulder Elbow Surg 6:176, 1997.
40. Gill DRJ, Cofield RH, Morrey BF: Ipsilateral total shoulder and elbow arthroplasties in patients who have rheumatoid arthritis. J Bone Joint Surg 81A:1128–1137, 1999.
41. Bonutti PM, Hawkins RJ: Fracture of the humeral shaft associated with total replacement arthroplasty of the shoulder. J Bone Joint Surg 74A:617–618, 1992.
42. Kligman M, Roffman M: Humeral fracture following shoulder arthroplasty. Orthopedics 22:511–513, 1999.

43. Gartsman GM, Roddey TS, Hammerman SM: Shoulder arthroplasty with or without resurfacing of the glenoid in patients who have osteoarthritis. J Bone Joint Surg 82A:26–34, 2000.

44. Kozak TKW, Hanssen AD, Cofield RH: Infected shoulder arthroplasty. J Shoulder Elbow Surg 6:177, 1997.

45. Lynch NM, Cofield RH, Silbert PL, Hermann RC: Neurologic complications after total shoulder arthroplasty. J Shoulder Elbow Surg 5:53–61,1996.

46. Blevins FT, Deng X, Torzilli PA, et al: Dissociation of modular humeral head components: A biomechanical and implant retrieval study. J Shoulder Elbow Surg 6:113–124, 1997.

47. Cofield RH, Daly PJ: Total shoulder arthroplasty with a tissue-ingrowth glenoid component. J Shoulder Elbow Surg 1:77–85, 1992.

48. Cofield RH: Uncemented total shoulder arthroplasty. Clin Orthop 307:86–93, 1994.

49. Wallace AL, Walsh WR, Sonnabend DH: Dissociation of the glenoid component in cementless total shoulder arthroplasty. J Shoulder Elbow Surg 8:81–84, 1999.

50. Boyd AD, Thomas WH, Scott RD, et al: Total shoulder arthroplasty versus hemiarthroplasty. Indications for glenoid resurfacing. J Arthroplasty 5:329–336, 1990.

51. Broström L-Å, Kronberg M, Wallensten R: Should the glenoid be replaced in shoulder arthroplasty with an unconstrained Dana or St. Georg Prosthesis? Ann Chir Gyn 81:54–57, 1992.

52. Boyd AD, Thomas WH, Sledge CB, Thornhill TS: Failed shoulder arthroplasty [abstract]. Orthop Trans 14:255, 1990.

53. Cofield RH, Frankle MA, Zuckerman JD: Humeral head replacement for glenohumeral arthritis. Semin Arthroplasty 6:214–221, 1995.

54. Sperling JW, Cofield RH, Rowland CM: Neer hemiarthroplasty and Neer total shoulder arthroplasty in patients fifty years old or less. J Bone Joint Surg 80A:464–473, 1998.

55. Levine WN, Djurasovic M, Glasson J, et al: Hemiarthroplasty for glenohumeral osteoarthritis: Results correlated to degree of glenoid wear. J Shoulder Elbow Surg 6:449–454, 1997.

56. Figgie HE III, Inglis AE, Goldberg VM, et al: An analysis of factors affecting the long-term results of total shoulder arthroplasty in inflammatory arthritis. J Arthroplasty 3:123–130, 1988.

57. Harryman DT, Sidles JA, Harris SL, et al: The effect of articular conformity and the size of the humeral head component on laxity and motion after glenohumeral arthroplasty. J Bone Joint Surg 77A:555–563, 1995.

58. Freedman KB, Williams GR, Iannotti JP: Impingement syndrome following total shoulder arthroplasty and humeral hemiarthroplasty: Treatment with arthroscopic acromioplasty. Arthroscopy 14:665–670, 1998.

59. Sperling JW, Cofield RH, Rowland CM: Heterotopic ossification after total shoulder arthroplasty. J Arthroplasty 15:179–182, 2000.

60. Dines DM, Warren RF, Altchek DW, Moeckel B: Posttraumatic changes of the proximal humerus: Malunion, nonunion, and osteonecrosis. Treatment with modular hemiarthroplasty or total shoulder arthroplasty. J Shoulder Elbow Surg 2:11–21, 1993.

61. Moeckel BH, Dines DM, Warren RF, Altchek DW: Modular hemiarthroplasty for fractures of the proximal part of the humerus. J Bone Joint Surg 74A:884–889, 1992.

62. Kjaersgaard-Anderson P, Frich LH, Søjbjerg JO, Sneppen O: Heterotopic bone formation following total shoulder arthroplasty. J Arthroplasty 4:99–104, 1989.

42

Revision Shoulder Arthroplasty

•JOHN W. SPERLING and ROBERT H. COFIELD

Prosthetic arthroplasty of the shoulder in the form of humeral head replacement began in the United States about 50 years ago. The contemporary style of total shoulder arthroplasty has been used for approximately 25 years. Early experience with total shoulder arthroplasty included rather constrained designs that have been all but abandoned. Therefore, the large majority of experience with patients is with unconstrained shoulder arthroplasty, such as that designed by Neer or some similar variation. As one would expect, most patients with unconstrained total shoulder arthroplasty, as those with the usual types of hip and knee arthroplasty, generally do quite well. However, over time, the need for revision surgery has increased so that now, on a percentage basis, it is not much different from the need for revision in other major joints, such as hip or knee replacements. Although there have been numerous reports concerning the results of primary shoulder arthroplasty, there is little information on revision shoulder arthroplasty. The scientific literature does not reflect the slowly increasing demand for revision total shoulder arthroplasty. Very little material has been published outlining the problems encountered, the techniques for revision, or the outcomes of revision shoulder arthroplasty.

To effectively treat the patient who requires revision shoulder arthroplasty, the surgeon must have information in seven areas. This includes (1) an understanding of the pathoanatomy of the disease that led to the original shoulder arthroplasty; (2) information about the original operative procedure and postoperative care; (3) detailed knowledge of the current situation in the shoulder; (4) the patient's needs, cooperative capacity, and general health; (5) treatment options to solve the problem; (6) technical details of the operative procedure; and (7) recognition of the benefits and limitations of the procedure.

Addressing the last six of the aforementioned areas includes providing data from total shoulder arthroplasty series that outlines the problems identified and their frequency, reviewing the experience with revision surgery, and presenting information from the few articles and book chapters that directly address various aspects of revision surgery. This is then followed by recommendations for diagnostic evaluation, treatment planning, sur-

gical indications, specific technical options, and the complications and limitations of revision shoulder surgery.

REOPERATIONS ON SHOULDER ARTHROPLASTIES (LITERATURE REVIEW)

To collect information about the frequency of reoperation on shoulder arthroplasties, the specific complications encountered, and the treatments used, we reviewed 63 reported patient series. Thirty-four of these series, with 581 operated shoulders, related information on humeral head replacement. Information about these shoulders is displayed in Table 42–1. The majority of revisions were for glenoid arthritis associated with pain, and treatment usually included placing a glenoid component. All other complications were quite infrequent.

Similarly, there were 9 reported series with 307 operated shoulders of reoperations after constrained total shoulder replacements (Table 42–2). The problems leading to reoperation were much more varied than those seen with humeral head replacement alone and were also much more frequent. Because this type of total shoulder replacement is no longer used, which means that few patients are currently seen who need revision of this type of shoulder arthroplasty, additional information about this type of implant and revision techniques are not presented.

Six of the reported patient series of 145 operated shoulders contained information on reoperation for unconstrained total shoulder replacements that was different enough from the design parameters of the Neer type of implants that it was useful to present separate information about them (Table 42–3). Revision surgery was done on 12 shoulders for four well-defined reasons. Finally, 14 reported series with 841 operated shoulders were studied, which defined the reoperations on Neer or Neer-like unconstrained total shoulder replacements. There were 841 reported shoulders; 26 needed revision for 8 different problems; the three most common complications that led to revision surgery were glenoid loosening, rotator cuff tearing, and periprosthetic humeral fracture (Table 42–4).

Table 42–1. REOPERATIONS ON HUMERAL HEAD REPLACEMENTS

Complications	Treatment	No.
Glenoid arthritis	Glenoid component	19
	Revision of humeral head replacement	2
Instability	Revision to total shoulder arthroplasty	2
	Soft tissue repair	1
Rotator cuff tear	Tendon repair	2
Impingement	Acromioplasty	1
	Tuberosity repair	1
Infection	Component removal	1
Nerve injury	Muscle transfer	1
Fractured acromion	Open reduction and internal fixation	1
Not stated		2
		Total 33 (5.7 percent)

ETIOLOGY OF ARTHROPLASTY FAILURE (MAYO CLINIC EXPERIENCE)

Suspicion is triggered by the fact that there are a number of revision shoulder arthroplasties being performed, but the frequency of revision surgery is not reflected in the literature. There is a substantial need for revision shoulder surgery that has been encountered in our practice, including both our own patients who had their initial surgery at our institution and those who were referred for consideration of revision surgery. Tables 42–5 and 42–6 outline the etiologies of failure of humeral head replacement and total shoulder arthroplasty seen in patients treated with revision surgery at our institution. As is reflected in the literature, the major reason for revision of humeral head replacement was painful glenoid arthritis, although in these patients we also encountered a substantial number of rotator cuff or tuberosity problems and glenohumeral instability. Of those 54 shoulders with failure of a humeral head replacement, 28 had only one pathologic abnormality (usually glenoid arthritis), 18 had two pathologic abnormalities, and eight had three pathologic abnormalities needing treatment. Thus, usually, revision surgery for failure of humeral head replacement was not unduly complex (Fig. 42–1).

Failure of total shoulder arthroplasty is somewhat different. The etiologies for failure in 117 shoulders requiring revision are outlined in Table 42–6. It is easy to recognize that many factors are involved with failure of total shoulder arthroplasty and to appreciate that multiple factors may well be present in a single shoulder. In defining this further, we found that 37 shoulders had only one patho-

Table 42–2. REOPERATIONS ON CONSTRAINED TOTAL SHOULDER REPLACEMENTS

Complication	Treatment	No.
Glenoid loosening	Revision	11
	Removal	5
Instability	Revision	10
	Removal	2
Prosthesis bent/fractured	Revision	9
Infection	Removal	5
Fracture	Revision	2
	Removal	1
	Internal fixation	1
Humeral loosening	Revision	2
Humeral and glenoid loosening	Revision	1
Dehiscence	Closure	1
Ankylosis	Clearance	1
Allergy to components	Removal	1
		Total 52 (16.9 percent)

Table 42–3. REOPERATIONS ON UNCONSTRAINED TOTAL SHOULDER REPLACEMENTS OTHER THAN NEER

Complication	Treatment	No.
Instability	Revision	4
Glenoid loosening	Remove component	2
	Component revision	1
Infection	Removal	2
	Revision	1
Rotator cuff tear	Tendon repair	2
		Total 12 (8.3 percent)

Table 42–4. REOPERATIONS ON NEER, UNCONSTRAINED TOTAL SHOULDER REPLACEMENTS

Complication	Treatment	No.
Glenoid loosening	Component revision	6
	Remove component	5
Rotator cuff tear	Tendon repair	5
Fracture	Internal fixation	3
	Component revision	1
Impingement	Acromioplasty	2
Acromioclavicular arthritis	Distal clavicle excision	1
Infection	Remove components	1
Instability	Arthrodesis	1
Nerve injury	Muscle transfer	1
		Total 26 (3.1 percent)

Table 42–5. FAILURE OF HUMERAL HEAD REPLACEMENT (NO. = 54)

Etiologies	No.
Glenoid arthritis	46
Rotator cuff tear, tuberosity problems	18
Instability	10
Component malposition	2
Fracture	2
Heterotopic ossification	1

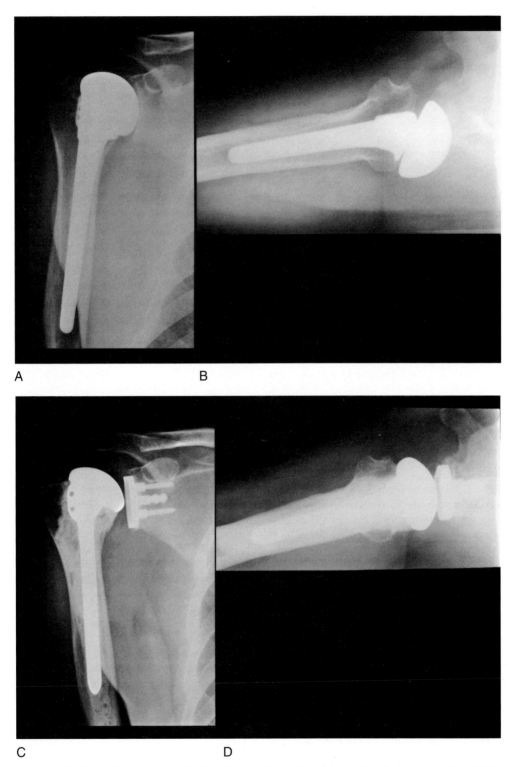

Figure 42–1. **A** and **B**, Example of glenoid arthritis with posterior subluxation after hemiarthroplasty. **C** and **D**, The patient underwent revision to total shoulder arthroplasty with the use of an ingrowth glenoid component.

logic abnormality needing correction, 53 had two, 24 had three, and 3 had four types of etiologic pathologic abnormalities needing correction. The implications of these data lend themselves to rather straightforward recognition. The current shoulder situation requires careful analysis, and detailed preoperative planning is necessary to address all potential etiologies of failure.

PATIENT SERIES ON REVISION PROCEDURES

In 1982, Neer and Kirby reported on revision of humeral head and total shoulder arthroplasties.[8] In their article, they presented a detailed evaluation method, including preoperative, surgical considerations, and postoperative

Table 42–6. FAILURE OF TOTAL SHOULDER REPLACEMENT (NO. = 117)

Etiologies	No.
Instability	73
Rotator cuff tear	54
Glenoid loosening	36
Component material failure	28
Humeral loosening	23
Component malposition	10
Infection	3
Fracture	1

considerations. More than one factor causing failure was present in almost every case. Predominant causes of failure in these patients included deltoid scarring and detachment, tightness of the subscapularis and anterior shoulder capsule, adhesions in the subacromial bursa and impingement of the rotator cuff, prominence of the greater tuberosity or retraction of the tuberosity, loss of humeral bone length, and eccentric glenoid wear or central wear of the glenoid. Finally, the lack of a supervised rehabilitation program contributed to failure in almost all of the arthroplasties that required revision surgery. Thirty-four of the shoulders so evaluated were revised to a total shoulder arthroplasty of the unconstrained type. A full rehabilitation program and return to nearly normal function was obtained in 10 patients, but, overall, the results were not as good as other diagnostic categories for patients undergoing total shoulder arthroplasty. Usually, satisfactory pain relief was achieved, and function for many of the activities of daily living was obtained. Revision was considered a most technically difficult procedure due to a combination of bone loss, scarring, muscle weakness, and infection.

Caldwell and co-authors reported on 18 shoulders requiring revision of prosthetic components, including 10 with previous humeral head replacement and 8 with previous total shoulder arthroplasty.[3] Nine of the humeral head replacements were revised to total shoulder replacements because of glenoid arthropathy. Revision for total shoulder replacements included revision of the glenoid components for loosening or for glenoid malposition in 3, removal of a loosened glenoid component in 2, and revision for instability in 3. Thirteen of the revision arthroplasties were available for follow-up at a minimum of 2 years. The preoperative Hospital for Special Surgery (HSS) shoulder score was 38 and the postoperative score was 70. Five shoulders required further revision surgery. These authors concluded that the outcome of revision arthroplasty did not approach the results of primary arthroplasty, and that some patients need to be rehabilitated with limited goals because of soft tissue or bony defects.

Wirth and Rockwood reviewed data concerning 38 failed, unconstrained shoulder arthroplasties.[12] They also recognized that failure was often multifactorial. The most common complication that led to revision in their patients was symptomatic glenohumeral instability. Other causes of failure included detachment of the anterior deltoid, glenoid component loosening, glenoid bone erosion after hemiarthroplasty, humeral component loosening, greater tuberosity malunion or retraction, fibrous or osseous ankylosis, infection, and dissociation of a modular humeral component.

Moeckel identified 10 of 236 shoulders having replacement arthroplasty that developed symptomatic instability of the shoulder requiring revision arthroplasty.[7] The instability was anterior in 7 and posterior in 3. The anterior instability was caused by rupture of the repaired subscapularis tendon. Operative treatment included mobilization and repair of the tendon, but 3 of the 7 operated shoulders continued to have instability. They underwent reoperation, including anterior tissue reinforcement with a tendo-achilles allograft. This second procedure achieved stability. The posterior instability was caused by many factors, and treatment consisted of correction of any soft tissue imbalance and revision of the implants when needed. After revision surgery for the instability, all patients lost some motion, but pain relief was achieved and the patients were much improved compared with their preoperative situation.

Antuna et al. reviewed the results of 48 shoulders that underwent glenoid component revision surgery at a mean follow-up of 4.9 years (range, 2 to 12 years).[1] The indications for surgery were glenoid component loosening in 29 shoulders, glenoid implant failure in 14 shoulders, and glenoid component malposition or wear leading to instability in 5 shoulders. Thirty shoulders underwent implantation of a new glenoid component and 18 shoulders underwent removal of the component and bone grafting owing to bone deficiencies. There was significant pain relief, improvement in active elevation, external rotation, and satisfaction with revision glenoid surgery ($P<0.05$). Patients without a glenoid component were significantly less satisfied with the procedure than those who underwent reimplantation of a glenoid component ($P=0.01$). Seven shoulders that underwent placement of a new glenoid component and 5 shoulders that underwent removal without reimplantation required revision surgery.

Rodosky and Bigliani[9] reported on surgical treatment of failed glenoid components in nonconstrained shoulder arthroplasty. Twenty-five patients were treated. Eighteen components failed because of loosening, 6 all-polyethylene components fractured at the base of the prosthetic keel, and 1 glenoid had severely worn polyethylene exposing the metal backing. At surgery, 2 of these patients were recognized to have infection. In these patients, both the glenoid and humeral components were removed. The glenoid component was removed in an additional 9 patients, and the component was revised in 14 patients. At an average 5-year follow-up in 24 patients, pain relief was achieved in 19 and there was little or no improvement in pain in 5 patients. Both replacement of the glenoid component and glenoid component removal led to satisfactory results in most patients; however, the results in the replacement group were slightly better overall, both in respect to pain relief and function.

Sperling and Cofield reviewed the results of 18 patients who underwent revision of hemiarthroplasties to total shoulder arthroplasty for glenoid arthritis.[10] The indications for the hemiarthroplasty were trauma (10 shoulders), osteoarthrosis (4), rheumatoid arthritis (2), and osteonecrosis secondary to the use of steroids (2). The mean interval between the hemiarthroplasty and the total shoulder replacement was 4.4 years (range, 0.8 to 12.7 years). The mean score for pain in the shoulder decreased from 4.3 points before the revision to 2.2 points after it ($P = 0.0001$). The mean active abduction increased from 94 degrees before the revision to 124 degrees after revision ($P=0.01$), and the mean external rotation increased from 32 to 58 degrees ($P=0.007$). Two shoulders needed another operation after the revision, 1 because of a late infection and 1 because of particulate synovitis associated with instability. There have been reports about humeral fractures after shoulder arthroplasty. Wright and Cofield identified 9 such fractures after 499 shoulder arthroplasties.[13] The arthroplasties were performed either for rheumatoid arthritis or for the sequelae of trauma. Six fractures were centered at the tip of the prosthesis and 1 fracture was extended proximally. Three other fractures involved the humeral shaft distal to the implant and extended into the distal humeral metaphysis. Two fractures that had unacceptable initial alignment were treated successfully with acute operative intervention. Four other fractures healed with nonoperative treatment. Three others treated with initial nonoperative treatment failed to heal; 2 eventually united after revision of the prosthesis and bone grafting were performed.

Boyd reported that humeral fracture after arthroplasty failed to heal with nonoperative methods in 5 of 7 patients.[2] All 5 ultimately healed after operative treatment. Among the patients in that series, mobility became more restricted compared with the pre-injury status in 5 of the 6 patients in whom the fracture healed. In the series by Wright, 6 of the 8 patients in whom the fracture united had approximately the same range of motion of the shoulder as before the fracture.

Krakauer and Cofield recommended a trial of closed treatment if satisfactory reduction could be obtained and maintained, but, if acceptable alignment could not be achieved, or in the event of a delayed union or nonunion, surgery should be undertaken.[6] This would include internal fixation with a plate, screws, cerclage if the prosthesis were well fixed or revision with a long-stemmed prosthesis if the prosthesis were loose. Autogenous bone grafting should be used in conjunction with surgical intervention.

DIAGNOSTIC EVALUATION

It is clear from the discussion of materials that the major problems encountered have been defined. It is also clear that several problems can coexist in the same shoulder. Information should be collected to define the etiology of difficulty or difficulties in the shoulder, including prior surgical records and radiographs. The surgeon needs to obtain a careful history of the shoulder, of other joint symptoms, and of the patient's general health. Physical examination of the shoulder, the extremity, and the cer-

vical spine should be performed. Plain radiographs of the shoulder include a 40-degree posterior oblique view in internal and external rotation plus an axillary view supplemented with a fluoroscopically positioned spot view of the glenoid when necessary. There should be consideration of adjunctive tests such as a white blood cell count with differential, C-reactive protein, and erythrocyte sedimentation rate for almost all patients with painful arthroplasties. If there is a low suspicion of infection, paired bone and indium-labeled white cell radioisotope scans might be considered to further exclude the possibility of a low-grade infection. If suspicion of infection is moderate or higher, the hematologic studies are combined with a shoulder arthrogram and aspiration. This provides the opportunity to obtain a culture and outline any fistulous tracts that might exist; it also aids in the recognition of rotator cuff tearing or in the identification of substantial synovitis associated with particulate wear. Occasionally, dye is seen tracking between the implant and the cement or the bone. Additionally, if there is substantial muscle weakness present, electromyographic testing may be considered, particularly if the etiology of the initial shoulder problem is trauma.

With the aid of the aforementioned basic information and tests, supplemented by adjunctive tests as necessary, the etiology of the pain and limitation of function leading to implant failure can almost always be defined. Once this is resolved, treatment planning can proceed.

TREATMENT PLANNING

Because there are multiple factors that can lead to failure, it is useful to develop a revision treatment plan or a problem list. The diagnostic evaluation pinpoints the problems, and the problems are then enumerated on the list. There are several possible solutions to these problems. Nonstandard implants may be needed, or a variety of component sizes may be required, which are not usually available and must be requested. Also, it is possible that additional tissue may be required, perhaps bone bank bone graft for small bone deficiencies or autogenous bone graft if the bone defect is more critical to the structural integrity of the composite. If a small amount of autogenous bone graft is needed, bone graft from the anterior iliac crest is adequate; if a larger amount of bone graft is necessary, posterior iliac crest graft is needed, which necessitates changing the position of the patient during the operative intervention. If soft tissue grafting is needed, consideration may be given to supplementation with autogenous fascia lata or a soft tissue allograft, such as a tendo-achilles allograft.

SURGICAL INDICATIONS

The indications for surgery are similar to those of other reconstructive orthopedic procedures, but the margin for error is smaller, and, thus, the indications for surgery must be clearly defined and understood. First, the patient must be experiencing sufficiently serious symptoms, including pain and limitation of function, to warrant the major surgical procedure. Second, clear-cut structural deficiencies must be defined by virtue of the diagnostic evaluation and treatment planning. Third, the surgeon must have a good understanding of the procedure and be able to communicate to the patient the potential benefits and limitations of the surgery. In many situations, patients have soft tissue and bone deficiencies that preclude a high likelihood of obtaining stability, improving movement, and gaining strength. These limitations should be defined. The decision to undertake surgery often hinges on the seriousness (i.e., the intensity) of the pain and the amount of limitation of upper extremity function. In some situations, these limitations are so extensive that it is even to the patient's benefit to consider a surgical procedure with only a fair chance of treatment success, because nonsurgical treatment offers no hope for improvement over time. Alternatively, some elderly patients with lower demands and a reasonable pain situation may well elect to defer any further surgical treatment when the probability of gain in function is so uncertain. Integrating the level of patient symptoms, the extent of structural abnormalities, and the information concerning outcome all lead to an informed judgment.

SURGICAL TECHNIQUE

Operative Exposure

Almost always, the approach is made through the deltopectoral interval. As such, the skin incision is typically vertical on the anterior aspect of the shoulder, slightly lateral to the deltopectoral interval. In revision procedures, there have, of course, been one or more preceding surgical incisions. Every effort is made either to use the old incision or to incorporate it into a longer incision that offers an approach to the deltopectoral interval and retracts the deltoid laterally. If the old scar on the skin has spread, the widened area is excised. The deltopectoral interval is most easily developed just distal to the clavicle, where there is a natural infraclavicular triangle separating the deltoid and pectoralis major muscles. Progresses continues distally. When the cephalic vein is encountered, the deltoid is retracted laterally, leaving the cephalic vein on the medial aspect of the exposure. In revision work, the cephalic vein may have already been ligated or may have been incorporated in scar in such a way that preservation of the vein is not possible. Otherwise, the vein is preserved and allowed to rest medially on the pectoralis major. The anterior border of the deltoid is then mobilized from the clavicle to its insertion on the humerus, and, often, the anterior portion of the insertion is elevated slightly, in continuity with the more distal periosteum of the humerus. Scarring may be less intense inferiorly, and, therefore, the plane between the deltoid and the humerus can be identified in this area. Scarring is often most intense over the midportion of the anterior deltoid. This is a

very dangerous area because the branches of the axillary nerve lie on the undersurface of the deltoid muscle, and the dissection must be meticulous. After the plane is identified distally, it may be wise to discontinue the distal to proximal elevation of the deltoid and to return to the upper portion of the deltoid, elevating this portion and exposing the undersurface of the acromion. The tissue adherent to the undersurface of the acromion can then be incised and the interval between the acromion and humeral head can be developed. Typically, this plane can be extended posteriorly, where scarring is less, and then advanced laterally and anteriorly, completing the elevation of the deltoid off the upper humerus. Occasionally, the scar is so dense and the tissue planes so obscure that this technique does not suffice. Also, the deltoid may be quite thin and frail. In these circumstances (perhaps 5 percent to 10 percent of revision cases), the deltoid origin is incised from the clavicle, acromioclavicular joint, and anterior aspect of the acromion and carefully reflected laterally, to be repaired at the end of the procedure. If the deltopectoral exposure can be accomplished, the deltoid is held laterally with either a Richardson retractor or a Brown-like deltoid retractor.

The next step in developing this plane is to identify the conjoined tendon group and to develop the plane between the subscapularis muscle and this group. The arm is placed in as much external rotation as possible. Usually, scarring is less just distal to the coracoid, and dissection can then progress from superior to inferior and from lateral to medial directions to develop this interval. If there is excellent external rotation, extensive development of this interval is not necessary; unfortunately, external rotation is often limited, and freeing the subscapularis from scar is an important part of the procedure. Dissection in this area must be done very carefully because of the neurovascular group, the axillary nerve, and the musculocutaneous nerve. Therefore, dissection in this area may take a few minutes, or it may take a considerable amount of time to accomplish what needs to be done to free the subscapularis. Scar is then released from around the base of the coracoid, and the shoulder is examined for range of motion.

If motion in abduction is limited to less than 130 or 140 degrees, the need for release of the inferior shoulder capsule can be anticipated. If external rotation is less than 30 degrees, it is probably prudent to incise the subscapularis from the upper humerus rather than incise it through its tendinous substance. Internal rotation is noted. The lower portion of the rotator interval between the subscapularis and supraspinatus is then incised with great care to avoid injury to the long head of the biceps tendon. The subscapularis and anterior shoulder capsule are then elevated from the humerus if there is substantially limited external rotation, or the incision is made through the tendinous substance of the subscapularis, just medial to the humeral capsule insertion if external rotation is ample. This incision is then continued inferiorly when abduction is limited; thus, the inferior shoulder capsule can be carefully incised from the neck of the humerus. This is accomplished by proceeding from an anterior to a posterior direction, with progressive external rotation of the humerus and by careful use of electrocautery so that inadvertent encounter with the axillary nerve can be avoided. When there is limitation of abduction, the inferior shoulder capsule is typically released to the area of the teres minor.

After removal or retraction of the prosthetic humeral head (which is addressed later), the upper humerus is retracted laterally and the joint is inspected. Hypertrophic synovium is débrided. This aids measurably in defining the shoulder capsule. Typically, the anterior-superior shoulder capsule is released from the noon position and relocated to approximately the 3 o'clock position on a right shoulder, with the incision then extending laterally along the superior border of the superior band of the inferior glenohumeral ligament. An elevator can then be placed beneath this portion of the anterior shoulder capsule and the subscapularis, partially freeing these structures from the anterior aspect of the scapula and allowing greater mobility of the anterior soft tissue sleeve; hence, improved external rotation is achieved. It is seldom necessary to release the posterior shoulder capsule. However, in certain very tight shoulders, or, occasionally, in shoulders in which the humeral head implant cannot be removed easily, the posterior shoulder capsule is incised along the glenoid rim. The humerus is then retracted posteriorly and held there either with a Fukuda-like ring retractor, a modified Hohmann-humeral neck retractor, or a large, broad elevator. To facilitate exposure to the glenoid, the arm is typically placed in 70 to 80 degrees of abduction, with neutral flexion-extension, and rotated to the best position for the remaining humeral head and neck behind the retractor. With careful, gentle but persistent pressure, the humerus can almost always be retracted posteriorly enough to expose the glenoid.

The Humeral Component

After completion of the arthrotomy and release of the inferior capsule that is usually required, the humerus is subluxated forward by placement of an elevator along the posterior-inferior aspect of the humeral head. The arm is positioned in slight extension, in adduction, and then progressively externally rotated. Care must be taken to ensure that the proper amount of torque is placed on the humeral shaft to avoid humeral shaft fractures. The rotator cuff attachment is then defined superiorly and posteriorly. The surface of the humeral component is assessed for any wear or other material imperfections, and position is determined. Typically, the height of the prosthetic humeral head is slightly above that of the greater tuberosity. The varus-valgus position of the humeral head is noted relative to the tuberosities and the humeral shaft. The size of the humeral head is evaluated relative to the anticipated size of the patient's usual humeral head, with recognition of the flexibility of the soft tissue envelope determined during exposure. Rotation of the implant is then assessed in relation to the flexed forearm. By evaluating all these things—humeral

surface characteristics, height, varus-valgus positioning (also anterior-posterior positioning), head size, and rotation—one can have a good sense about whether or not the humerus needs to be changed. Attention is then directed to the fixation within the humeral shaft, with an eye toward the need for glenoid work. If there is a one-piece, uncemented humeral implant, the implant is usually removed. If there is a modular humeral head, this is disarticulated. If there is a one-piece humeral prosthesis, it is cemented in a good position; quite typically, this is left in place and retracted posteriorly in the best way possible. If there is a one-piece humeral prosthesis that is cemented in place in poor position, the implant must be removed. Occasionally, it is possible to crack the cement surrounding the upper portion of the implant and then to extract the implant, either by impaction or by use of a humeral component extractor. Many times, however, the stem is so securely cemented in the humerus that this is not possible. The large size of the humeral head usually precludes effective cement removal from the diaphyseal area of the humerus via the upper portion of the humeral canal. It is necessary to make a window in the humerus on its anterolateral aspect, usually about 1 cm in diameter and extending from approximately 3 cm below the cut in the humeral neck to near the end of the cement surrounding the humeral implant. This long, narrow, cortical window is then elevated, cement is removed from within the humeral canal and around the humeral component, and the component is then impacted from the humerus. Additional cement removal then ensues, and the remaining humeral bone is prepared, often with careful use of a high-speed, low-torque bur. When a new component is placed, it must be long enough to bypass the window by 2 to 3 cm, and the window is held in place with cerclage, cables, or heavy sutures. Additional bone graft can be placed surrounding the window if that is thought to be necessary.

Some modular systems allow the creation of a slight offset of the humeral head or placement of a slightly eccentric humeral head on the stem to accommodate some variation in varus, valgus, or anteroposterior placement, or aberrant rotational placement of the implant system. If correction in position of a modular system cannot be accomplished, it is necessary to remove the stem of the modular humeral component. Unfortunately, a number of these components have rather aggressive texturing or tissue-ingrowth capabilities extending down the stem of the component, either to the metaphyseal area or, unfortunately, to the diaphyseal area. These components are extremely difficult to remove, quite likely requiring a humeral window and also very careful use of a high-speed bur to try to cut the interval between the implant and the bone. It is indeed an accomplishment to change such a component without creating any fractures of the humerus. In line with this, after removing a humeral component, it is wise to place a humeral stem trial prosthesis within the humerus before retracting the humerus posteriorly, to guard against inadvertent humeral fracturing.

After completion of work on the glenoid, a humeral component is then repositioned. If a modular system is used and the stem is fixed in good position, adjustment in head size is easily made. If a new stem needs to be secured, it is unlikely that enough metaphyseal and diaphyseal bone will be present in the amount and quality required to seat a press-fitted or tissue-ingrowth component. There are a variety of theories about how to use bone cement in securing a humeral component in the revision setting. Our personal preference is to plug and lavage the canal, to use a cement gun, and then to use finger pressure. The component is then carefully seated in the new cement bed.

The Glenoid Component

After retraction of the humerus posteriorly, scar tissue is excised from around the glenoid component. The surface is then assessed for any wear or deformity. The position is assessed, from superoinferior, anteroposterior, rotational, and angulatory directions relative to anteversion and retroversion. A lever is carefully applied to the edge of the glenoid component, and the integrity of the glenoid fixation is assessed. If the glenoid is grossly loose, it is of course, removed; if there is a moderate amount of loosening, additional tissue is removed from the interface, and the glenoid is carefully levered away from the underlying bone. If the component is loose but is not easily disengaged from the bone of the glenoid, it may be necessary to divide the polyethylene surface of the glenoid component and to then fracture the underlying, interlocking bone cement. If there is metal backing to the polyethylene, the problem is intensified. One often has to work around the edges of the metal to free the component from the underlying bone. Some metal-backed polyethylene components have holes in the center of the metal plate, allowing the polyethylene to be removed and worked through the holes in the metal plate to facilitate component extraction. Fortunately, the majority of tissue-ingrowth glenoid components have—most, if not all, of the tissue-ingrowth surface overlying the face of the glenoid, with very little extending into the glenoid neck. Thus, a narrow, slightly curved osteotome can be used to undermine the metal backing of these types of glenoid components, to remove any screws that are present, and then to extract the component. Needless to say, great care must be taken in removing a slightly loosened glenoid component, because there is only a small amount of glenoid bone, and it is often frail in character. Almost any amount of fracturing of the native glenoid precludes secure replacement of a subsequent glenoid component.

After removal of the old glenoid component, there are typically glenoid rims left intact but with a central cavity of varying size. If the central cavity is large and the walls of the glenoid neck are frail, it is probably a better choice to fill this cavity with bone graft and not to place a new glenoid component for fear that loosening will occur in a very short period of time. On the other hand, if the size of the cavity is small, the bone can be prepared, and a new polyethylene component can be cemented in place. If the cavity is of medium size, consider may be given to

a variation of the Ling technique for the femoral shaft; that is, impacting corticocancellous bone into the defect and then preparing the glenoid for implantation of either a keeled or a column-type device. Our personal preference in this setting has been to prepare the glenoid for a column-type device and to bypass the bone graft with these columns and screws, allowing the surface of the implant to rest on a mixture of native and grafted bone. Usually, bone cement fixation is also used, but, occasionally, it may be omitted.

It is important to recognize that glenoid components now come in a variety of sizes and shapes to aid in correcting special problems that are encountered at the time of revision surgery. Components vary in thickness from 4 to 12 mm, and some components have eccentric configurations to correct for slight abnormalities in glenoid position, and, as mentioned earlier, come in both keel-shaped and column-shaped variants so that a variety of local anatomic changes that are encountered can be addressed. Careful preoperative planning is necessary to ensure that the variety of glenoid components needed to address the spectrum of bone deficiencies are available.

Rarely, in addition to central bone deficiency, there is a peripheral or rim deficiency. Often, scar has filled the area, and the adjacent shoulder capsule adheres densely over this region, precluding the need to place supporting materials to attain shoulder stability. However, if there is a substantial peripheral rim defect and stability cannot be attained by virtue of adaptations in the soft tissues, consideration must given to grafting the defect. Almost always, this requires iliac crest bone grafting with screw fixation into the remaining glenoid neck and the very firm bone at the junction between the glenoid neck and the body of the scapula. After the structural graft is fixed in place, the question of whether or not a glenoid component should be placed on top of this structure can again be addressed.

Soft Tissue Repair

After attending to the glenoid difficulties and repositioning the humeral head, the repair method for the rotator cuff and shoulder capsule can be considered.[4] As a part of the exposure and during the procedure, the coracoacromial arch is inspected and preserved, if possible. Any gross irregularities in the shape of the undersurface of the acromion or distal clavicle are smoothed. The rotator cuff is assessed by observation and palpation, both on its outer and inner aspects. During trial reductions, the stability of the humerus against the glenoid is determined, and adjustments in humeral head size are made. The subscapularis is then repaired. If it was removed from bone, it is sutured to bone through drill holes in the humeral neck. If this type of subscapularis repair is done, it is often helpful to place the sutures before seating the new humeral implant. If the humeral stem was not removed at the time of revision, it is often useful to place bur holes through the humeral cortex on the anterior neck and then to pass sharp, cutting needles through the metaphyseal bone. If the arthrotomy was through tendinous tissue, of course, the tendons are again sutured. It is very important to obtain secure closure of the interval area. It has been our experience that many of the failures of anterior repair occur through this region and do not include substantial disruption of the vertical portion of the subscapularis repair. After closure of the arthrotomy, the shoulder is taken through a range of motion. Translation of the humeral head is assessed anteriorly, posteriorly, and inferiorly, and, if the range in all directions is reasonable, the amount of motion obtained is recorded. This then allows passive motion to occur within these motion limits until tissue healing is moderately firm, usually between 4 and 8 weeks—and often at about 6 weeks. Occasionally, gentle isometric type strengthening can be started before the 6-week period, but often it is prudent to delay strengthening until early soft tissue healing has occurred.

Specific Problems

There can, of course, be *bone deficiencies* underlying both the humeral and the glenoid components.[5] Commonly, the bone deficiency of the upper humerus is in the form of metaphyseal bone loss. It is usually addressed by fixation with bone cement. Occasionally, because of trauma or fracturing, a portion of the upper humerus is absent. This is addressed in three ways. The first is by bone grafting the deficiency. This is usually for small to medium-sized bone deficiencies. The second is by use of an allograft humerus, through which a humeral component has been placed. The third is the use of a custom prosthesis that replaces a portion of the upper humerus and relies on the formation of adjacent scar to attain stability, albeit with substantial weakness. Small amounts of glenoid deficiency can usually be addressed with the use of bone cement. Larger deficiencies require some form of bone grafting. If the area involved is not very important to structure and stability, allograft is probably the most useful choice. If there is an area of structural importance that needs to be replaced or if bone healing is definitely required for maintaining glenoid fixation, autograft bone is preferred.

Instability after total shoulder arthroplasty is a serious problem.[7] Unfortunately, one easily addressed factor is not usually the cause of instability, such as the uncommon situation of anterior instability associated with a subscapularis rupture. The problem is often more complex, involving multiple factors. It is, of course, important to determine the direction or directions and the degree of instability, not only in the office examination but also in the examination under anesthesia. It is important to know whether or not the rotator cuff is intact. If this is not clear during the preoperative evaluation, a shoulder arthrogram may be of some value. The position and size of the components needs to be carefully determined. There is hope that, at the time of revision surgery, soft tissue abnormalities can be corrected to recreate stability, but, all too often, one or both of the components need to be changed. If there is posterior instability and the glenoid is retroverted, which needs to

be corrected. If there is anterior stability and the glenoid is anteverted, which needs to be addressed. If there is posterior instability with the glenoid in a good position the tension across the superior and anterior portions of the rotator cuff as needed but with posterior structures that are too loose, the posterior structures need to be tightened. If there is inferior instability and the humeral component has been placed too low in the humerus, the component needs to be placed more superiorly relative to the humerus, and, quite likely, additional bone graft will need to be added. Instability after shoulder arthroplasty occurs in all directions and is sometimes even multidirectional. It is very important to do detailed preoperative analysis and be prepared to vary the approach to postarthroplasty instability according to the specific abnormalities that can be defined.

Revision surgery needed to correct *rotator cuff tearing* is surprisingly uncommon. There are, of course, individuals with shoulder arthroplasty who subsequently have a dramatic change in shoulder function associated with a rather mild injury. In these settings, it is useful, as in patients who do not have a shoulder arthroplasty, to perform a careful physical examination, which is a deciding factor in whether a substantial rotator cuff tear has occurred, and to consider an early repair if there has been a dramatic change in shoulder function. Usually, however, rotator cuff problems appear in a manner similar to those in patients without a shoulder arthroplasty. That is, the patients have chronic, rather long-term symptoms. Evaluation suggests that tearing of the supraspinatus or supraspinatus and infraspinatus tendons has occurred. There may or may not be substantial pain associated with the presence of these tears, but strength is diminished and active motion may be reduced. In these settings, it is important to identify the magnitude of the tendon tearing and to consider whether or not reconstructive tendon surgery would be of benefit. Often, in this setting, it does not seem as if surgery will help dramatically. The pain is somewhat less than is usually encountered in a patient who has rotator cuff tearing, and the promise of increased function after revision surgery is somewhat less certain. If rotator cuff repair after arthroplasty is undertaken, it is somewhat more difficult than the usual rotator cuff repair. If the shoulder is reasonably stable and the anterior and posterior structures appear to be intact, an anterosuperior approach to the shoulder may be used to address the coracoacromial arch, as is typical for rotator cuff surgery, and a direct repair of the tendon can be performed. If direct tendon repair is not possible, some form of grafting must be done. This repair can make use of either autogenous fascia lata graft or, perhaps, an allograft tendon. Fortunately, this type of surgery is rarely required.

COMPLICATIONS AND LIMITATIONS OF REVISION SURGERY

Unfortunately, there is little scientific information in regard to expected outcomes and the limitations of shoulder arthroplasty revision surgery. Some general guidelines are available. Material to date suggests that should glenoid arthropathy develop in a humeral head replacement, placing a glenoid component usually eliminates pain.[10] If there is a loosened glenoid component that requires revision surgery, somewhere between one half and two thirds of these components can be successfully revised. The remaining one half to one third have such substantial bony deficiencies that only bone grafting the defect is possible.[1] When the humeral component loosens and revision surgery is necessary, revision can typically be successfully performed with use of slightly longer stemmed components and fixation supplemented with bone cement. If there are specific identifiable factors leading to shoulder instability, such as component malposition or disruption of healthy soft tissues, revision surgery to correct instability is quite likely to be successful. If the instability is associated with vague factors, often compounded by inadequate soft tissues, including the rotator cuff tendons, revision surgery is unlikely to be dramatically successful. Certainly, limited-goals rehabilitation is needed, and, therefore, the outcome can be anticipated to be fair at best. When a rotator cuff tear occurs in a rather acute mode, tendon repair is quite likely to be sufficiently helpful to warrant

revision surgery. When chronic attrition ensues, the likelihood of success with larger tears is lessened.

A fracture beneath a humeral prosthesis is usually addressed by immobilization and observation if a satisfactory reduction can be obtained. If the fracture does not progress toward healing, open reduction and fixation with the use of a plate, cerclage, and bone grafting would quite likely be considered in 2 to 4 months. Of course, if the fracture involves a substantial portion of the fixation of the humeral component, revision surgery will be needed that includes revision of the humeral component to a long-stemmed component, possibly additional cerclage fixation, and, quite likely, autogenous bone grafting.

There is not a large amount of information available on the treatment of infection after shoulder arthroplasty.[11] Certainly, classic treatment is removal of the components and any bone cement. The articulation is then treated with rest, as a resection arthroplasty, until stiffening occurs and then gentle stretching and strengthening. It is suggested that about one half to two thirds of patients so treated achieve a satisfactory pain state, and their movement and strength approximate one third of normal capacity. This form of treatment is probably still the first line of treatment for patients with extensive

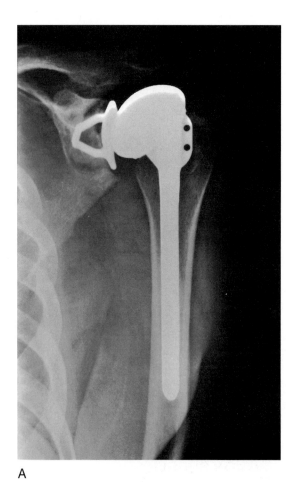

A

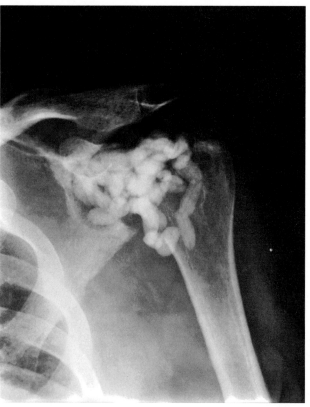

B

Figure 42–2. A, Example of a patient who has an infected total shoulder arthroplasty with a loose glenoid component. **B,** The patient underwent component removal with placement of antibiotic-impregnated cement beads.

Illustration continued on opposite page

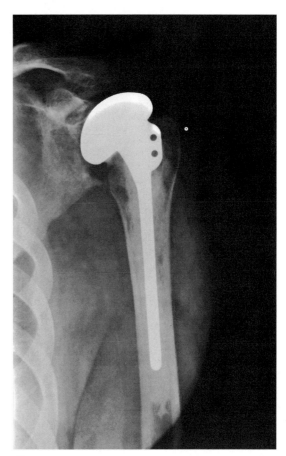

Figure 42–2. *Continued.* **C**, The patient subsequently underwent reimplantation of a hemiarthroplasty 3 months after resection with placement of antibiotics in the cement.

C

infection and osteomyelitis that extends through many areas of the humerus. However, patients with mainly an infectious arthritis picture and only mild changes in the bone can probably benefit from removal of the components, débridement of the tissues, and a delayed reimplantation of either the humerus or the humerus and the glenoid components (Fig. 42–2). There is little information about primary exchange or about treatment of acute joint infections with débridement and antibiotics. The exact guidelines for treatment of the infected shoulder arthroplasty are still unclear, but will likely mirror the guidelines being formulated for the treatment of infections after hip and knee arthroplasty.

SUMMARY

Effective revision total shoulder arthroplasty requires the surgeon to have comprehension of shoulder disease, information about the original operative procedure, detailed knowledge about the current situation in the shoulder, understanding of the patient, ability to define reasonable treatment options, preparation for the technical variations encountered during the operative procedure, and recognition of the limitations of this type of surgery. The literature suggests that revision arthroplasty is indeed uncommon, approximating 3 percent of a large number of shoulder arthroplasties that have been performed and reported. Undoubtedly, though, revision is needed somewhat more commonly than this. The causes of failure are well defined. Unfortunately, they are often multifactorial in a single shoulder. As such, the shoulder must be carefully analyzed, the various problems defined, and the treatment planned meticulously. Surgical indications must take into account the real benefits, but, perhaps more importantly, the real limitations of these procedures. The revision procedure itself is usually technically challenging and often requires adjunctive bone grafting, addresses soft tissue contractures or deficiencies, and involves placement of components that are somewhat unusual in size or ordered specifically for the patient. All these complexities are compounded by the absence of an ample body of scientific information that describes the outcomes of this type of surgery. Only now is this being pieced together. It is quite likely that a decade from now our understanding will be much more complete and our armamentarium for treatment will be increasingly satisfactory.

References

1. Antuna SA, Sperling JW, Cofield RH, Rowland CM: Glenoid revision surgery after total shoulder arthroplasty. Open Meeting of the American Shoulder and Elbow Surgeons. Orlando, FL, 2000.

2. Boyd AD Jr, Thornhill TS, Barnes CL: Fractures adjacent to humeral prostheses. J Bone Joint Surg Am 74:1498, 1992.
3. Caldwell GL: Revision shoulder arthroplasty. Orthop Trans 17:140, 1993–1994.
4. Cofield RH: Integral surgical maneuvers in prosthetic shoulder arthroplasty. Semin Arthroplasty 1:112, 1990.
5. Cofield RH: Total shoulder replacement. Managing bone deficiencies. *In* Craig EV (ed): Shoulder Master Techniques in Orthopaedic Surgery. New York, Raven Press, 1995, p 345.
6. Krakauer JD, Cofield RH: Periprosthetic fractures in total shoulder arthroplasty. Op Tech Orthop 4:243, 1994.
7. Moeckel BH, Altchek DW, Warren RF, et al: Instability of the shoulder after arthroplasty. J Bone Joint Surg Am 75:492, 1993.
8. Neer CS, Kirby RM: Revision of humeral head and total shoulder arthroplasties. Clin Orthop 170:189, 1982.
9. Rodosky MW, Bigliani LU: Surgical treatment of nonconstrained glenoid component failure. Op Tech Orthop 4:226, 1994.
10. Sperling JW, Cofield RH: Revision total shoulder arthroplasty for the treatment of glenoid arthrosis [see comments]. J Bone Joint Surg Am 80:860, 1998.
11. Sperling JW, Kozak TK, Hanssen AD, Cofield RH: Infection after shoulder arthroplasty. Clin Orthop 382:206, 2001.
12. Wirth MA, Rockwood CA Jr: Complications of total shoulder-replacement arthroplasty. J Bone Joint Surg Am 78:603, 1996.
13. Wright TW, Cofield RH: Humeral fractures after shoulder arthroplasty. J Bone Joint Surg Am 77:1340, 1995.

V
The Hip

DAVID G. LEWALLEN • SECTION EDITOR

43

Historical Perspective of Hip Arthroplasty

• MARK B. COVENTRY and BERNARD F. MORREY

No orthopedic procedure of the past century has captured the imagination of both the medical profession and the lay public as has total arthroplasty of the hip. Not only has it been a tremendous boon to the well-being of patients suffering from hip disease, but it has also stimulated the replacement of other joints similarly affected. Total hip arthroplasty is the prototype that led the way.

Deformities of the hip were corrected early in the 19th century (see Chapter 1). Barton[2] of Philadelphia, in 1826, performed osteotomies of the upper femur. Later, Ollier[48] in France published his work on osteotomy in 1885, and Murphy[47] of Chicago combined osteotomy with an interposition of soft tissue between the bone ends. Was this the first hip arthroplasty? Replacing the destroyed joint with an artificial one was long an object of fantasy. Scales[58] credits Gluck, in 1980, with inserting an ivory ball onto the neck of the femur and holding it with screws and a type of "bone glue." Two very important subsequent steps were then taken. They paved the way for total joint replacement.

CUP (MOLD) ARTHROPLASTY

Although arthroplasties using fascia lata, chromicized pig bladder, skin, and other materials were sporadically done, they were rather uniformly unsuccessful. Because of this, the American surgeon, Smith-Petersen,[59] was looking for better interposing material. He and his colleagues observed that a tissue similar to synovium had formed about a piece of glass removed from the thigh of a patient. He reasoned that, if a glass mold could be placed over the head of the femur, synovium would grow as a result, and a successful arthroplasty might eventuate. He did his first glass mold arthroplasty in 1923. Bakelite was then used, and later Pyrex. Both substances tended to break. Venable and Stuck[64] published their work on the alloy of chrome, cobalt, and molybdenum, which had been used by dentists and was uniquely nonreactive in tissue. The trade name for this alloy was Vitallium. Smith-Petersen used Vitallium as an interposing substance in the hip and continued its use

throughout his subsequent vast experience with mold arthroplasty (Fig. 43–1). In retrospect, after clinical evaluation, only about one half of the mold arthroplasties successfully relieved pain. Furthermore, mold arthroplasty could not replace bone deficiencies or correct anatomic abnormalities, such as shortening. However, cup arthroplasty certainly revived the interest in some type of interposing substance to remake the joint, and it was a giant step forward in the concept of total joint replacement.

ENDOPROSTHESIS

A. T. Moore[39] credited Bohlman[7] for the use of a chrome-cobalt ball fitted to a Smith-Petersen triflanged nail to replace the head of the femur. He had inserted such prostheses in 3 patients in 1939. Haboush[29] used a similar device the same year. Moore and Bohlman[40] constructed a special chrome-cobalt endoprosthesis to replace the upper 12 inches of a femur that had been destroyed by a giant cell tumor and reported this in 1943. In 1946, the brothers Judet[30] used an endoprosthesis with a femoral head made of acrylic and with an attached acrylic stem that passed through the intertrochanteric region. Because of severe wear problems, the acrylic prosthesis was replaced by one made of chrome-cobalt alloy (Fig. 43–2). Many modifications of the endoprosthesis were made by McKeever,[36] Valls,[63] Thompson et al.,[61,62] and others, but most failed, as Charnley later wrote, because they had a "defective load-bearing capacity and loosened."[16]

Moore, using his previous experience with Bohlman,[40] reasoned that an intramedullary stem would give more mechanical support to the head than the short stem through the intertrochanteric region. In early 1950 (the exact date is still controversial), he placed his first intramedullary-stemmed Vitallium prosthesis into a patient (Fig. 43–3) (Moore AT: Hip Joint Surgery. Unpublished 1963). In June of the same year, Palmer Eicher of Indianapolis used an intramedullary stainless steel endoprosthesis.[20] The Moore prosthesis was fenestrated to decrease its total weight and perhaps, as Moore

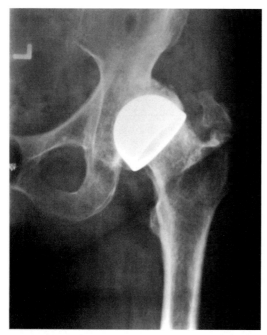

Figure 43–1. Vitallium Smith-Petersen mold (cup) in place for 12 years, with good function. (From Coventry MB: A historical perspective and the present state of total hip arthroplasty. *In* Excerpta Medica International Congress Series. New York, Elsevier, 1983, p 11.)

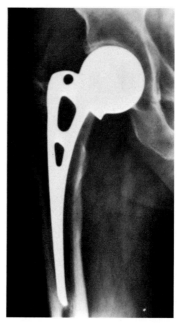

Figure 43–3. Moore's original endoprosthesis. (From Coventry MB: A historical perspective and the present state of total hip arthroplasty. *In* Excerpta Medica International Congress Series. New York, Elsevier, 1983, p 11.)

postulated, to allow some bone growth into the fenestrae. It had a calcar collar. The Moore prosthesis tended to loosen, however, because there was only one basic size to fit all femurs, and the stem was short, thin, and curved. In 1961, Moore designed a straight-stemmed prosthesis with a longer stem of I-beam construction, which allowed three-point contact with the curved medullary canal. Several variations on this prosthesis

were forthcoming. Thompson[61] designed a similar prosthesis but without fenestrations. This meant that later, when methyl methacrylate was available, it could be cemented if desired (Fig. 43–4).

Bipolar Prosthesis

A multiple-bearing endoprosthesis with an interposing, free-riding cup was later designed by Giliberty[26] and by Bateman[3] (Fig. 43–5). The rationale was to lessen friction-

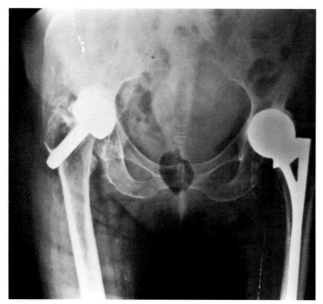

Figure 43–2. Vitallium Judet prosthesis (*left*); Matchett-Brown endoprosthesis (*right*), similar to straight-stemmed Moore endoprosthesis).

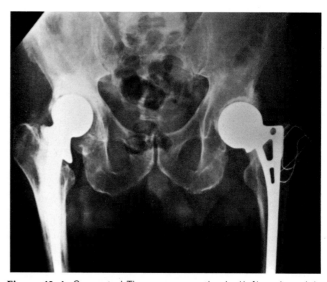

Figure 43–4. Cemented Thompson prosthesis (*left*) and straight-stemmed Moore endoprosthesis (*right*).

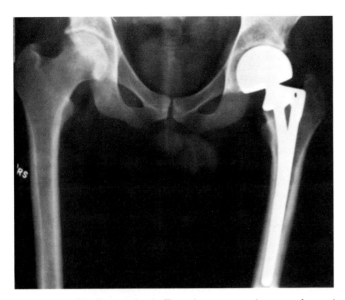

Figure 43–5. Bipolar prosthesis. There is movement between femoral and acetabular units and between acetabular prosthesis and acetabulum. (From Coventry MB: A historical perspective and the present state of total hip arthroplasty. *In* Excerpta Medica International Congress Series. New York, Elsevier, 1983, p 11.)

al forces between the femoral head and the cartilage of the acetabulum. This prosthesis was basically a combination of the cup arthroplasty and the femoral endoprosthesis. The femoral unit could be either secured with cement or press fitted. The acetabular unit was lined with polyethylene so there was no metal-to-metal contact. The bipolar prosthesis, as used today, has rather specific indications. A younger patient with an avascular femoral head has been considered the best candidate.[10] However, an unacceptable failure rate has lessened the enthusiasm for this option. More recently, a report from the Mayo Clinic has demonstrated the value of the bipolar device in refractory instances of instability.[50]

TOTAL HIP ARTHROPLASTY

In 1948, Philip Wiles[67] inserted a ball-and-socket hip prosthesis of stainless steel, but mechanical failure occurred. Three years later, McKee and Watson-Farrar[35] used a stainless steel total hip replacement, modifying McKee's lag screw on the femoral side and utilizing a metal acetabular component. McKee modified this prosthesis in 1956 using a Thompson endoprosthesis and a spherical socket in the acetabulum (Fig. 43–6). Both these units were made of chrome-cobalt. After Charnley had developed methyl methacrylate, the components were cemented.

Methyl Methacrylate

The development of methyl methacrylate as a securing agent for the prosthesis was another tremendous step forward. Although Charnley[15] credited Kiaer and Jansen of Copenhagen and Haboush of New York with first using

methyl methacrylate in 1951, they used only small amounts and did not really create a secure fixation of the components. Wiltse and associates[68] showed that methyl methacrylate was well tolerated in experimental animals (rabbits and monkeys). Cabanela and colleagues[11] later confirmed this in the human from a study of its use to repair cranial defects. Charnley first used methyl methacrylate to "cement" the femoral and acetabular components in 1958. His monumental publication, "Anchorage of the Femoral Head Prosthesis to the Shaft of the Femur,"[13] was a turning point in total hip replacement. Charnley demonstrated that at last firm fixation of the components was possible. Charnley himself stated that his contribution to total hip arthroplasty was "to ream out the marrow cavity and use a large volume of cement into which the tapered stem was introduced." One should review his original writings.[13–16] The basic concept of using methyl methacrylate for fixation of the prosthetic units has remained sound to this day and is owed to Charnley's pioneering effort.

Polyethylene

Charnley's second great contribution to total hip arthroplasty was the use of a plastic material to oppose and articulate with the metal head (see Fig. 43–6).[13,15] He termed this the "low-friction arthroplasty." His first use of Teflon failed because, although the friction was lessened, Teflon wore poorly and its wear particles were reactive. In 1961, he began the use of high-density polyethylene for the acetabular unit. In 1963, Müller[44–46] changed his metal socket to high-molecular-weight polyethylene. In spite of many unsuccessful efforts, the advent of cross-linked polyethylene may truly represent an advance in technology that has a significant effect on decreasing wear debris. The wear advantages of cross-linked polyethylene have been known for years.[6] The advantages to preplacement of the hip are being increasingly investigated.[37]

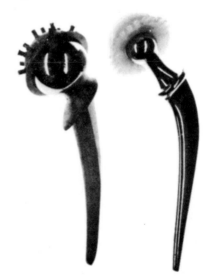

Figure 43–6. McKee (*left*) and Charnley (*right*) total hip prosthesis. (From Charnley J: Evolution of total hip replacement. Ann Chir Gynecol 71:103, 1982.)

Ceramics

Frictional forces were also lessened by Charnley's[13] use of a smaller femoral head than that used by his contemporaries; namely, 22 mm in diameter. Ceramic (alumina, aluminum oxide, porcelain) makes a satisfactory substance to replace the head and, indeed, has been used for both the head and the acetabular component. Boutin[9] published his work on alumina in 1971. Trunnion-bearing principles, pioneered by Weber,[66] were picked up by Mittelmeier and Harms,[38] and they have used the ceramic head on a metal trunnion for the femoral unit, as have others. Fractures of the ceramic head have been reported by Griss and colleagues,[28] by Boutin,[9] and by Salzer.[33,57] Improvements have been made in the manufacture of ceramic, and fracture of the components is alleged to have lessened.

Noncement Fixation

Ring[54,55] devised a unit in which the femoral side was press fitted, basically as was the Moore component, but the acetabular unit was fixed into the pelvis by a stem-and-cup unit placed in considerable valgus (Fig. 43–7). Ring's first design was made in 1960, with a titanium femoral head and a plastic acetabular cup. This failed because of the nature of the plastic, and he then used chrome-cobalt for both units. He modified his prosthesis with a stemmed conical acetabular unit made of polyethylene to avoid metal-on-metal debris that he, McKee, and others found to contribute to synovial reaction and loosening. More recently, further fixation of the acetabular unit with a threaded stem and a Freeman peg was introduced.[19]

The "isoelastic" femoral prosthesis of a polyacetyl resin was introduced in 1973. It is used with a polyethylene cup. Neither unit is secured with methacrylate. Reports on its use were published by Morscher and Dick[43] and by Bombelli et al.[8]

Long-term results of joint replacement are available for a 20-year period and show that loosening continues to be the basic complication. Although loosening is closely related to how fixation by methyl methacrylate is used, other factors contribute to implant failure. Thus, there has emerged the concept of biologic fixation rather than fixation with methyl methacrylate. Historically, press-fit fixation without porous ingrowth has been successful in many cases, but the overall results of press fitting alone were not good enough to consider it as the sole method of fixation. Micromotion is always present. Porous ingrowth, however, allows bone to penetrate the surface of the prosthesis and secure it.

The acetabular side poses a slightly different problem from the femoral side. Anchoring pegs and screws maximize the security of the initial fit of the prosthesis. These are adaptable to metal-backed units, which can be porous coated.

Physiologic fixation may theoretically be either macropore or micropore in nature. Macropore fixation, such as the initial Lord and Judet prostheses,[31,34] and, later, that by Mittelmeier and Harms,[38] did not show intimate contact of bone with the prosthesis. When the prosthesis is microporous coated, bone grows into the micropores and true, complete fixation results. Galante and co-workers[24] were pioneers in this field and published their research work as early as 1971 (Fig. 43–8). Engh's early clinical work was published in 1983.[21] As with all other innovations, however, there are some trade-offs, and the entire issue of porous coating (biologic fixation) is under intensive study.

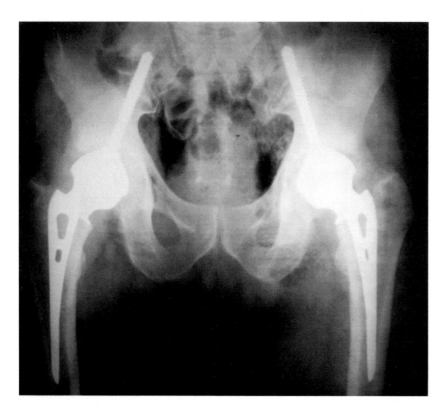

Figure 43–7. Ring prostheses (1966). (From Scales JT: Arthroplasty of the hip using foreign materials: A history. Presented at the Symposium on Lubrication and Wear in Living and Artificial Human Joints, Institution of Mechanical Engineers, Bridgewalk, Westminster, London, 1967.)

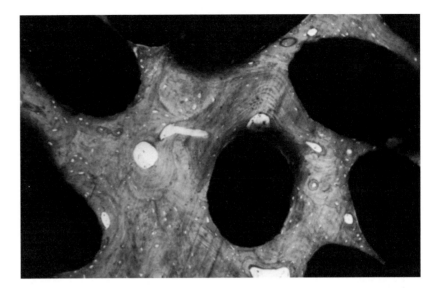

Figure 43–8. Ingrowth of bone into sintered metal covering of femoral endoprosthesis. There is direct contact of bone to metal, with no intervening fibrous cellular layer. (From Coventry MB: A historical perspective and the present state of total hip arthroplasty. *In* Excerpta Medica International Congress Series. New York, Elsevier, 1983, p 11.)

SURFACE REPLACEMENT

So-called surface replacement was developed in an effort to save more bone stock of the upper femur. The femoral head is contoured to accept a metal cap. The acetabulum is treated in a manner similar to that of the usual total hip replacement except that the acetabular component, by necessity, is larger and thus is thinner, with resulting loss of rigidity and resistance to wear. Amstutz and colleagues[1] began work with their THARIES surface replacement in 1973, and other designs were developed about the same time by Wagner,[65] Freeman and colleagues,[23] Gerard and colleagues,[25] Paltrinieri and Trentani,[49] and Capello and Trancik.[12] Younger patients were deemed more appropriate, but the procedure was abandoned because of a high incidence of failure. The concept has, however, been revisited by Amstutz with encouraging early results.[1a]

As the interest in resurfacing replacement has waned, a conservative alternative to resurfacing and medullary stem fixation has been introduced by the so-called medullary fixation devices.[42] The concept has been present for many years and now is growing in interest. The concept of minimal resection implants was an early design feature in the 1920s and has been intermittently revisited ever since (Fig. 43–9).

BIOMECHANICS

Total hip arthroplasty could not have developed to its present state of the art without a change in our understanding of the biomechanical principles of the musculoskeletal system. Knowingly or not, the pioneers in this field used basic biomechanical knowledge, although they had a limited understanding of the specific biomechanics of the hip.[13] Most failures were really mechanical failures. Bioengineering emerged as a specialty in the 1960s, and the bioengineer began playing an essential role in the development of intertrochanteric osteotomy and total hip replace-

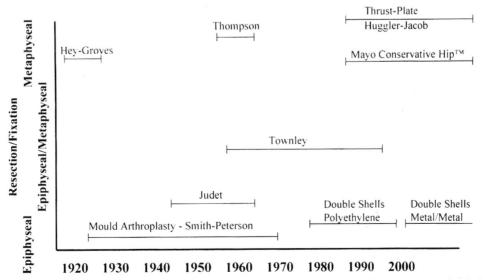

Figure 43–9. Schema of various efforts of hip replacement whereby a minimum amount of bone is removed. (Modified from I. Jacob, personal communication.)

ment. Frederick Pauwels of Aachen, Germany, was the first to describe the basic mechanical principles that apply to the hip.[51,52] He led the way for others to expand on these principles and refine them. Various isolated or combined tensile, compressive shearing and rotational forces on the hip have been analyzed. These analyses can be performed on all present and experimental prosthetic designs. The strength and elasticity of the different available metals have also been evaluated. The designs of both the femoral and acetabular units have been altered to conform to these laboratory tests. The potential for loosening and structural failure has been defined. Methyl methacrylate and polyethylene have also been evaluated as to strength and wear properties. More recently, the metal-on-metal articulation has been the subject of investigation.

BIOLOGIC RESPONSE

Concurrent with biomechanical development has been research into the physiologic response of tissues to the foreign bodies that are part of the total hip arthroplasty. Soft tissue reactions to metal, polyethylene, methyl methacrylate, and, probably, alumina, all occur. The bone itself responds biologically to the stresses on it. Overload may cause pressure necrosis. Increased rigidity may cause stress shielding that in turn may cause bone resorption. These responses are dependent on the design and fixation of the prosthesis. There is also considerable trauma to bone because of reaming, jet lavage, heat generated by polymerization, and other factors.

Many studies have now confirmed Schiller's original implication of the fibrous interface between methacrylate and bone, and metal and bone, as a destructive tissue with properties similar to those of the synovium membrane.[27] This tissue may react similarly to rheumatoid tissue by forming foreign body giant cell and other reactive cell granulomas. These can be destructive, perhaps because of their prostaglandin-forming properties. At present, the extent and possible dangers, including oncogenesis, of this foreign body reaction are still largely undefined. This tissue reaction to foreign material is being extensively studied.[41]

ROLE OF THE MAYO CLINIC

In 1967, the Orthopedic Department at the Mayo Clinic realized that total hip arthroplasty had an important potential for patients with hip disease. After on-site visits to the various centers in Great Britain doing hip replacement, the method of Charnley was selected, and a prospective protocol for its use was established. One type of prosthesis was to be used for a time long enough for surgeons to become familiar with it and to build up enough patient data so that there could be a meaningful statistical analysis. After time, other methods could be used as they developed and seemed to be worthy. All orthopedic department members at Mayo cooperated in this prospective study. Before this study could be undertaken, permission was necessary from the federal Food and Drug Administration to use methyl methacrylate. After the protocols were submitted, the Mayo Clinic was given permission for Investigational New Drug # 1. The first total hip operation at Mayo was done on March 10, 1969 (Fig. 43–10). From this protocol have come considerable data regarding long-term results of total hip arthroplasty (Fig. 43–11).[5]

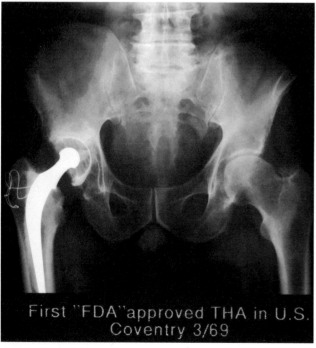

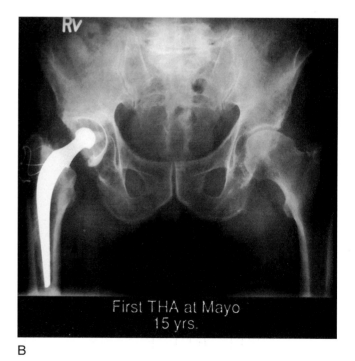

A   B

Figure 43-10. A, The first Food and Drug Administration approval for the use of bone cement occurred at the Mayo Clinic in a patient of Coventry's in March 1969. **B,** An excellent outcome is documented in the Mayo database after 15 years.

CLINICAL ORTHOPAEDICS AND RELATED RESEARCH
Number 344, pp 61–68
© 1997 Lippincott–Raven Publishers

Maintaining a Hip Registry for 25 Years

Mayo Clinic Experience

Daniel J. Berry, MD*; Mary Kessler*; and Bernard F. Morrey, MD*

Figure 43–11. The use of the Mayo Clinic database has been documented in the peer-reviewed literature.

An in-depth study of bacterial flora in the operating room was commenced at the same time.[22] These results likewise had a large part to play in the future development of the operating room environment at the Mayo Clinic. An initial report of our first 2012 total hip arthroplasties[18] was followed by 5-, 10-, 15-, and 20-year studies of the first 333 patients.[4,32,56,60] The 25-year follow-up study is forthcoming.[5a] As of December 31, 1994, 25,500 total hip arthroplasties have been carried out, and data continue to be analyzed regarding them. Currently the Mayo Total Joint Database consists of over 62,000 unique patient entries that comprise Mayo's experience with hip, knee, elbow and shoulder replacements (Table 43–1). The data entry process has developed from a registry to a data base; that is, it possesses the ability to calculate performance scores and to document mode of failure.

ONGOING AND UNSOLVED PROBLEMS

The history of hip replacement may be conceptualized from the perspective of successive problems and their solution[53] (Fig. 43–12). Clearly, there are unsolved and ensuing problems with this technique.

What is the optimal mode of fixation and how can the younger patient best be managed? Will toxic absorption of metallic ions, resulting from the vastly enlarged surface of the ingrowth prostheses, prove harmful? Will a specific design ultimately prove to be better than any other? Will ceramics ultimately find their proper place in the total hip procedure? Clearly, the most challenging questions remain the issue of wear debris and the body's response to it. Will the cross-linked polyethylene be the solution to wear debris that has been so elusive to our specialty? There are many other questions today, still unanswered, that will provide a vast research basis for the future clinically, in the biomechanical laboratory, and for biologic and physiologic investigation. Of particular relevance today is the issue of outcome and cost-effectiveness. These issues are assuming a particularly important role as input in the ongoing issue of research funding, public/political acceptance,control of access, and source and amount of reimbursement.

Table 43–1. MAYO DATABASE FOR MAJOR JOINT REPLACEMENTS 1969–2000

Replacement Anatomic Site	Primary	Revision	Total
Hip	26480	8687	35167
Knee	19223	3485	22708
Shoulder	2590	365	2955
Elbow	978	304	1282
Total	49271	12841	62112

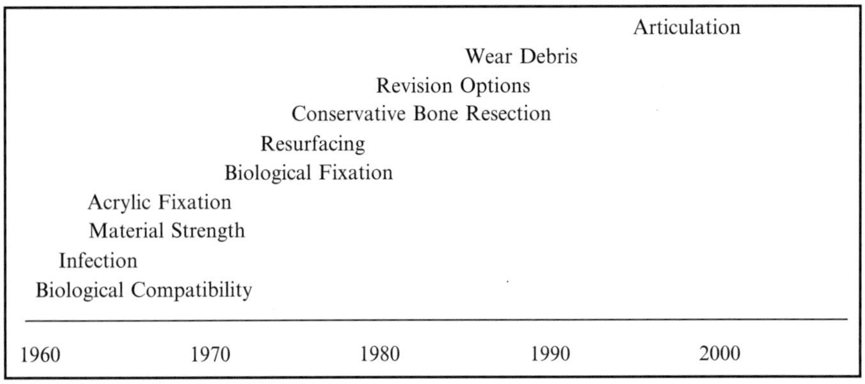

```
                                              Articulation
                                    Wear Debris
                              Revision Options
                        Conservative Bone Resection
                              Resurfacing
                        Biological Fixation

           Acrylic Fixation
           Material Strength
      Infection
      Biological Compatibility

      ──────────────────────────────────────────────────

      1960          1970          1980          1990          2000
```

Figure 43–12. The ebb and flow and problems and solutions have characterized the history of hip replacement. (Modified from Poss R: Natural factors that affect the shape and strength of the aging human femur. Clin Orthop 274:194, 1992.)

References

1. Amstutz HC, Clarke IC, Christie J, Graff-Radford A: Total hip articular replacement by internal eccentric shells. Clin Orthop 128:261, 1977.

1a. Amstutz HC: Arthroplasty options for advanced osteonecrosis. Orthopedics 23:927–928, 2000.

2. Barton JR: On the treatment of ankylosis by the formation of artificial joints. North Am Med J 3:279, 1827.

3. Bateman JE: Experience with a multi-bearing implant in reconstruction for hip deformities [abstract]. Orthop Trans 1:242, 1977.

4. Beckenbaugh RD, Ilstrup DM: Total hip arthroplasty: A review of 333 cases with long follow-up. J Bone Joint Surg 60A:306, 1978.

5. Berry DJ, Kessler M, Morrey BF: Maintaining a hip registry for 25 years. Clin Orthop 344:61, 1997.

5a. Berry DJ, Harmsen WS, Cabanela ME, Morrey BF: Twenty-five-year survivorship of two thousand consecutive primary Charnley total hip replacements: factors affecting survivorship of acetabular and femoral components. J Bone Joint Surg Am 84-A:171–177, 2002.

6. Beveridge C, Sabiston A: Methods and benefits of cross-linking polyolefins for industrial applications. Mater Des 8:263, 1987.

7. Bohlman HR: Replacement reconstruction of the hip. Am J Surg 84:268, 1952.

8. Bombelli R, Gerundini M, Aronson J: Early results of the EM isoelastic cementless total hip prosthesis: 300 consecutive cases with two-year follow-up. In The Hip: Proceedings of the 12th Open Scientific Meeting of the Hip Society. St. Louis, CV Mosby, 1984, p 33.

9. Boutin P: Alumina and its use in hip surgery. Presse Med 79:639, 1971.

10. Cabanela ME: Bipolar endoprosthesis: Mayo Clinic experience with comparison between cemented and uncemented femoral stems. In The Hip, Proceedings of the 12th Open Scientific Meeting of the Hip Society. St. Louis, CV Mosby, 1984, p 68.

11. Cabanela ME, Coventry MB, MacCarty CS, Miller WE: The fate of patients with methyl methacrylate cranioplasty. J Bone Joint Surg 54A:278, 1972.

12. Capello WN, Trancik TM: The Indiana experience. In The Hip, Proceedings of the 10th Open Scientific Meeting of the Hip Society. St. Louis, CV Mosby, 1982, p 167.

13. Charnley J: Anchorage of the femoral head prosthesis to the shaft of the femur. J Bone Joint Surg 42B:28, 1960.

14. Charnley J: Acrylic Cement in Orthopaedic Surgery. Edinburgh, E & S Livingstone, 1970.

15. Charnley J: Total hip replacement by low-friction arthroplasty. Clin Orthop 72:7, 1970.

16. Charnley J: Evolution of total hip replacement. Ann Chir Gynecol 71:103, 1982.

17. Coventry MB: A historical perspective and the present status of total hip arthroplasty. In Excerpta Medica International Congress Series. New York, Elsevier, 1983, p 11.

18. Coventry MB, Beckenbaugh RD, Nolan DR, Ilstrup D: 2,012 total hip arthroplasties: A study of postoperative course and early complications. J Bone Joint Surg 56A:273, 1974.

19. Drabu KJ, Ring PA: Uncemented acetabular cups in dysplastic and protrusio acetabuli. Clin Orthop 210:173, 1986.

20. Eicher P: "Orthopedic Letters Club." Orthop Lett Club August 27, 1951.

21. Engh CA: Hip arthroplasty with a Moore prosthesis with porous coating: A five-year study. Clin Orthop 176:52, 1983.

22. Fitzgerald RH Jr, Nolan D, Ilstrup D, et al: Deep wound sepsis following total hip arthroplasty. J Bone Joint Surg 59A:847, 1977.

23. Freeman MAR, Cameron HU, Brown GC: Cemented double cup arthroplasty of the hip: A five-year experience with the ICLH prosthesis. Clin Orthop 134:41, 1978.

24. Galante JO, Rostoker W, Lueck R, Ray RD: Sintered fiber metal composites as a basis for attachment of implants to bone. J Bone Joint Surg 53A:101, 1971.

25. Gerard Y, Segal PH, Bedoucha JS: Hip arthroplasty by matching cups. Rev Chir Orthop 60(Suppl 2):281, 1984.

26. Giliberty RP: Low-friction bipolar hip endoprosthesis. Int Surg 62:38, 1977.

27. Goldring SR, Schiller AL, Roelke M, et al: The synovial-like membrane at the bone-cement interface in loose total hip replacements and its proposed role in bone lysis. J Bone Joint Surg 65A:575, 1983.

28. Griss P, Silber R, Merkle B, et al: Biomechanically induced tissue reactions after Al_2O_3 ceramic hip joint replacements: experimental and early clinical results. J Biomed Mater Res 7:519, 1976.

29. Haboush EJ: A new operation for arthroplasty of the hip based on biomechanics, photoelasticity, fast-setting dental acrylic, and other considerations. Bull Hosp Joint Dis 14:242, 1953.

30. Judet J, Judet R, LaGrange J, Dunoyer J: Resection Reconstruction of the Hip: Arthroplasty with Acrylic Prosthesis. Edinburgh, E & S Livingstone, 1954.

31. Judet R, Siguier M, Brumpt B, Judet T: Prosthàese totale de hanche en poro-máetal sans ciment. Rev Chir Orthop 64(Suppl 2):14, 1978.

32. Kavanagh BF, DeWitz M, Ilstrup D, et al: Charnley total hip arthroplasty with cement: 15 year results. J Bone Joint Surg 71A:1496, 1989.

33. Knahr K, Salzer M, Plenk H Jr, et al: Experience with bio ceramic implants in orthopedic surgery. Biomaterials 22:98, 1981.

34. Lord GA, Hardy JR, Kummer FJ: An uncemented total hip replacement: Experimental study and review of 300 madreporique arthroplasties. Clin Orthop 141:2, 1979.

35. McKee GK, Watson-Farrar J: Replacement of arthritic hips by the McKee-Farrar prosthesis. J Bone Joint Surg 48B:245, 1966.

36. McKeever DC: Biomechanics of hip prosthesis. Clin Orthop 19:187, 1961.

37. MeKellop H, Shen FW, Lu B, et al: Effect of sterilization method and other modifications on the wear resistance of acetabular cups made of ultra-high molecular weight polyethylene. A hip simulator study. J Bone Joint Surg 82A:1708, 2000.

38. Mittelmeier H, Harms G: Present day state of cement-free anchoring of combined ceramics-metal prostheses. Z Orthopaed 117:478, 1979.
39. Moore AT: Metal hip joint: A new self-locking vitallium prosthesis. South Med J 45:1015, 1952.
40. Moore AT, Bohlman HR: Metal hip joint: A case report. J Bone Joint Surg 25:688, 1943.
41. Morrey BF: The Mechanical, Biological, and Clinical Basis of Joint Replacement Arthroplasty. New York, Raven Press, 1993.
42. Morrey BF, Adams RA, Kessler M: A conservative femoral replacement for total hip arthroplasty. J Bone Joint Surg 82B:952, 2000.
43. Morscher EW, Dick W: Cementless fixation of "isoelastic" hip endoprosthesis manufactured from plastic materials. Clin Orthop 176:77, 1983.
44. Müller ME: Total hop prostheses. Clin Orthop 72:46, 1970.
45. Müller ME: Results 12 years and over [abstract]. Orthop Trans 5:349, 1981.
46. Müller ME: Total hip reconstruction. *In* McCollister EC (ed): Surgery of the Musculoskeletal System. New York, Churchill Livingstone, 1983, p (10):6:223.
47. Murphy JB: Bony lipping of the right acetabular margin and the neck of the femur following a metastatic arthritis; arthroplasty of the hip; cheilotomy. Surg Clin Chicago, Philadelphia, 1915.
48. Ollier LXEK: Traitáe des ráesections et des opáerations conservatrices qu'on pent pratiquáes sur le systáeme osseux. Paris, G. Masson, 1885.
49. Paltrinieri M, Trentani C: A modification of the hip arthroprosthesis. Chir Org 9:85, 1971.
50. Parvizi J, Morrey BF: Bipolar hip arthroplasty as a salvage treatment for instability of the hip. J Bone Joint Surg 82A:1132, 2000.
51. Pauwels F: Der Schenkelhalsbruch ein mechanisches Problem. Stuttgart, Verlage, 1935.
52. Pauwels F: The importance of biomechanics in orthopedics. *In* Ninth Congress of the Sociáetáe Internationale de Chirurgie Orthopáedique et de Traumatologies, Wien, 1963. Wien, Wiener Medizinischen Akademie, 1965.
53. Poss R: Natural factors that affect the shape and strength of the aging human femur. Clin Orthop 274:194, 1992.
54. Ring PA: Replacement of the hip joint. Ann R Coll Surg 48:344, 1971.
55. Ring PA: Ring UPM total hip arthroplasty. Clin Orthop 176:115, 1983.
56. Russotti GM, Coventry MB, Stauffer RN: Cemented total hip arthroplasty with contemporary techniques: A five-year minimum follow-up study. Clin Orthop 235:141, 1988.
57. Salzer M, Knahr K, Locke N, Stark N: Cement-free bioceramic double-cup endoprosthesis of the hip joint. Clin Orthop 134:80, 1978.
58. Scales JT: Arthroplasty of the hip using foreign materials: A history. Presented at the Symposium on Lubrication and Wear in Living and Artificial Human Joints, Institution of Mechanical Engineers, Bridgewalk. London, Westminster, 1967.
59. Smith-Petersen MN: Arthroplasty of the hip. A new method. J Bone Joint Surg 37A:269, 1939.
60. Stauffer RN: Ten-year follow-up study of total hip replacement; with particular reference to component loosening. J Bone Joint Surg 64A:983, 1982.
61. Thompson FR: Two and a half years' experience with a vitallium intramedullary hip prosthesis. J Bone Joint Surg 36A:489, 1954.
62. Thomson JEM, Ferciot CF, Bartels WW, Webster FS: The "light bulb" type of prosthesis for the femoral head. Surg Gynecol Obstet 96:301, 1953.
63. Valls J: A new prosthesis for arthroplasty of the hip. J Bone Joint Surg 34B:308, 1952.
64. Venable CS, Stuck WG: The Internal Fixation of Fractures Springfield, IL, Charles C Thomas, 1947.
65. Wagner H: Surface replacement arthroplasty of the hip. Clin Orthop 134:102, 1978.
66. Weber BG: Total hip replacement with rotation-endoprosthesis. Clin Orthop 72:77, 1970.
67. Wiles P: The surgery of the osteoarthritic hip. Br J Surg 45:488, 1957.
68. Wiltse LL, Hall RH, Stenehjem JC: Experimental studies regarding the possible use of self-curing acrylic in orthopedic surgery. J Bone Joint Surg 39A:961, 1957.

44

Anatomy and Surgical Approaches

• ARLEN D. HANSSEN

Two of the key elements in performing a successful hip arthroplasty are a thorough understanding of the anatomy and knowledge of the various surgical exposures that facilitate the surgical procedure. In general, the vast majority of primary hip arthroplasties can be performed with any of the different surgical exposures; the choice is appropriately influenced by the surgeon's philosophy and personal experience. A large number of revision procedures can be performed with one of the many standard surgical exposures, but the choice may be influenced by the reason for the revision, the surgical exposure used previously, the type of components being revised, the severity of bone deficiency, and the type of implants intended for use at the revision surgery.[10] In complex primary cases with anatomic distortion, or in certain revision cases, several specialized or extensile exposures may be preferable or necessary.

For more than a decade, there has been considerable interest and investigation regarding the anatomic aspects pertinent to hip arthroplasty, particularly with regard to description of new surgical exposures of the hip joint. Because no single surgical approach is appropriate for all situations, the surgeon should be familiar with at least several different approaches by understanding their indications, limitations, and associated complications. The following discussion details some of the anatomic aspects particularly relevant to hip arthroplasty. For a traditional description of the anatomy about the hip joint, the reader is referred to standard anatomy reference books.

ANATOMY

Osteology

Femur. The external geometry of the proximal femur includes the head, neck, lesser and greater trochanters, and proximal femoral diaphysis (Fig. 44–1**A**, **B**). The greater trochanter provides an extensive area for musculotendinous insertion, with the infralateral trochanteric ridge reliably defining the origin of the vastus lateralis muscle. This is a helpful landmark for several surgical approaches that leave the vastus lateralis in continuity with an osteotomized greater trochanter.[39] The lesser trochanter lies posteromedially, provides a site for inser-

tion of the iliopsoas tendon, and is often a helpful intraoperative marker to assess the level of the femoral neck cut.

The hemispheric femoral head diameter averages 46 mm (range, 35 to 58 mm); although it is extremely variable, the adult neck-shaft angle averages 125 degrees (plus or minus 7 degrees).[22,75,94,108] The relative position of the trochanters, the femoral head center, and the femoral shaft are correlated with inclination of the neck-shaft angle.[22,122] Assessment of these relationships provides the surgeon with important intraoperative verification during the hip arthroplasty. For example, in the hip with significant varus inclination of the neck-shaft angle, reaming must be directed more laterally into the greater trochanter to maintain neutral alignment of the reamer, and, ultimately, the prosthesis, within the femoral canal (Fig. 44–2**A**, **B**).

The designers of many of the currently used hip systems have adopted the standard of 135 degrees for the neck-shaft angle of the prosthesis.[75] This angle effectively reduces the femoral offset, which has important implications for hip stability and abductor function.[78] There is no universal shape or size for the proximal femoral canal; thus, there is no single cementless stem design that fits all femurs.[65,94] Approximating the frontal anatomy of 85 percent of femurs with an implant filling the metaphysis requires at least 15 sizes distributed in 3 metaphyseal configurations, each supplied with 2 different neck shaft angles.[75]

Femoral version is determined by the angle between the plane of the femoral condyles and the axis of the femoral neck (see Fig. 44–1). The anteversion angle in adults with a normal hip joint averages 13 degrees (plus or minus 7 degrees), whereas in patients with osteoarthritis, femoral anteversion averages 20 degrees (plus or minus 9 degrees).[107,108] Increased anteversion of the femoral neck likely contributes to the development of osteoarthritis of the hip.[108] In patients with developmental hip dysplasia, the femoral anteversion averages 10 to 14 degrees more than that of control subjects, and this anteversion is independent of the severity of hip subluxation.[123] Extremes of femoral neck version may increase the complexity of hip arthroplasty. If the femoral component is inserted in excessive anteversion or retroversion, the arthroplasty may be unstable. This is particularly true in uncemented arthroplasty, in which

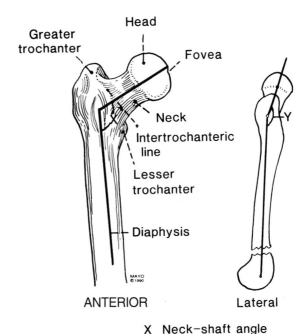

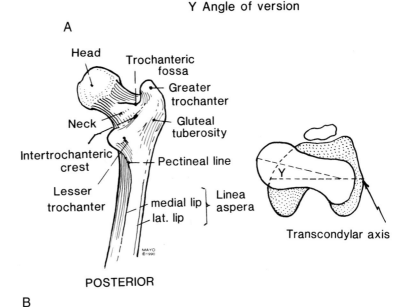

Figure 44–1. Anterior (**A**) and posterior (**B**) views of the external geometry of the proximal femur. X, neck-shaft angle; Y, angle of version.

the anatomic version more rigidly dictates the position of prosthetic insertion.

The proximal femoral metaphyseal region has a complex three-dimensional internal architecture, and most internal dimensions correlate significantly with each other. The neck-shaft angle correlates primarily with external geometry.[94] Canal width, in the vicinity of the lesser trochanter, correlates best with all other proximal internal femoral dimensions.[94] The proximal femoral endosteal geometry is funnel shaped. The canal flare index, a ratio of the intracortical width 2 cm proximal to the lesser trochanter and the width of the canal isthmus, describes the proportionality of the funnel shape.[94] These canal flare index values are age related; values less than 3.0 describe the "stovepipe canal" shape, whereas those greater than 4.7 indicate the "champagne-fluted" shape.[94]

With advancing age, endosteal expansion occurs at a greater rate than periosteal apposition, resulting in cortical thinning, which is most apparent in bones of patients older than 60 years of age.[33,94,105] Prediction of cancellous bone density from these cortical morphology indices is of limited value.[112]

The calcar femorale, a dense vertical plate of bone arising from the posterior medial femoral shaft beneath the lesser trochanter, is formed as a result of traction of the iliopsoas.[131] The calcar femorale extends laterally toward the greater trochanter and contributes to the metaphyseal funnel shape. The calcar femorale and the medial femoral cortex fuse together proximally to form the medial femoral neck, which is often erroneously termed the calcar. With advancing age and ensuing endosteal expansion, the calcar femorale progressively thins or

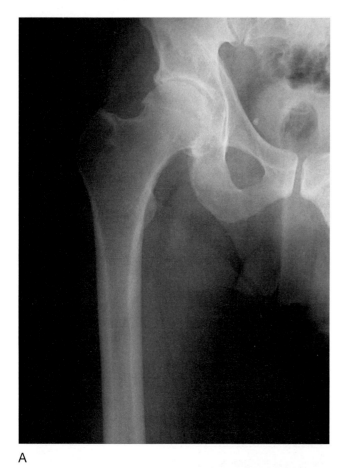

A

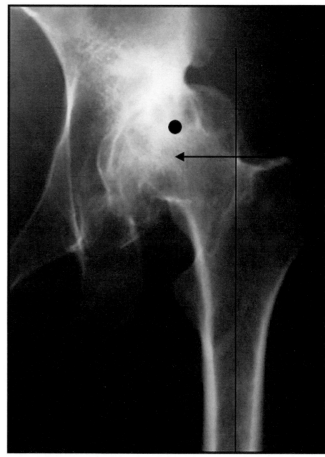

B

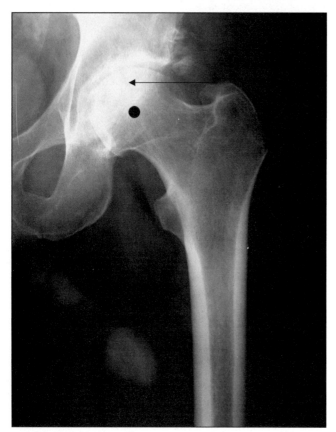

C

Figure 44–2. A, The femoral head center typically lies medial and level with the tip of the greater trochanter with respect to the femoral shaft. **B,** As the neck-shaft angle increases, the head center lies higher than the greater trochanter and closer to the axis of the medullary canal and the greater trochanteric tip is positioned more lateral to the femoral canal. **C,** These relationships change conversely as the neck-shaft angle decreases into varus.

disappears. A centrally placed stem often abuts the calcar femorale, leaving minimal space for the cement mantle.[131] Clearing the calcar region allows space for a cement layer to provide posterior and proximal support of a cemented stem.[131] In contrast, the calcar femorale can provide excellent posterior support for an uncemented implant.

In the lateral projection, the proximal femur has a metaphyseal posterior bow that intersects at the level of the lesser trochanter with the anterior bow of the femoral diaphysis.[94] The posterior bow, created by the anterior cortex and the calcar femorale, averages 10.7 degrees (range, 0 to 24 degrees).[94] It is important for the surgeon to understand these intersecting bows, because it is relatively common for the final placement of the stem to traverse the proximal bow of the femur so that the femoral component is "flexed," particularly if the calcar femorale is robust and the region is not adequately cleared. Variability in the posterior bow of the proximal femur may also change the indication for a straight or anatomically curved uncemented implant. The varus-valgus positioning of femoral components on anteroposterior (AP) radiographs is dependent on limb rotation after total hip arthroplasty.[2] This effect, called pseudoposition, occurs with the posterior positioning of the distal tip of the prosthesis owing to the bow of the femur. External rotation causes pseudovalgus positioning, and internal rotation causes pseudovarus positioning.[2]

Likewise, on the AP projection, significant changes in the measurement of the proximal canal with femoral rotation occur.[30] The distal canal dimensions are not affected significantly by changes in rotation. On the lateral projection, the dimensions of the proximal canal change significantly with internal rotation; however, external rotation has no effect on canal dimensions.[30] Awareness of this phenomenon is important, because excessive reliance on the preoperative template procedure may lead to errors in implant selection if femoral rotation is not obtained in neutral rotation; thus, the presence of this phenomenon emphasizes the need for standardized radiographic technique.

Acetabulum. Fusion of the ischium, ilium, and pubis creates the acetabulum, which provides four functional columns of bony support for the femoral head. The lateral column includes the ilium and superior dome, whereas the pubis and ischium and their associated acetabular walls, respectively, comprise the anterior and posterior columns. The thin medial wall forms the weakest column, and the strongest bone lies superior and posteriorly.[34] The acetabulum faces anteriorly, laterally, and caudally (Fig. 44–3), with the normal anteversion of the acetabulum averaging 17 degrees (plus or minus 6 degrees).[107] Unlike the femoral neck anteversion, acetabular anteversion is similar in patients with osteoarthritis and in normal control subjects.[107]

Radiographically, the true position of the acetabulum (true femoral head center) is based on horizontal and vertical indices measured from the intersection of Kohler's line and a line connecting the radiographic teardrops. Preoperative determination of the true femoral head center has useful clinical application if the acetabulum has been bilaterally destroyed by trauma, by developmental hip dysplasia, or by acetabular bone loss. Most acetabular difficulties encountered are caused by bony deficiencies in one of the four functional columns, which cause lack of structural support or incorrect position of the prosthetic components.

Acetabular bone structure is not the same in all patients and can be defined by a radiolucent triangle superior to the acetabulum.[27] Three different types, or shapes, of the triangle can be defined, and the density of the superior acetabular bone in the triangle can be subdivided as normally radiolucent (stage I); with vertical and transverse trabeculae throughout the triangle (stage II); or filled with bone and cysts (stage III).[27] Type A acetabula, with a thin medial wall, are found more frequently in women, whereas type B acetabula typically occur in men. Type C acetabula are found in patients with subluxation owing to developmental hip dysplasia. These authors emphasize the importance of careful attention to the depth of reaming and press-fitting of the cup at the rim when uncemented hemispherical cup fixation is performed, particularly for type A3 acetabula.[27]

Soft Tissue

Superficial Landmarks. Accurate identification of bony landmarks around the hip joint is difficult because

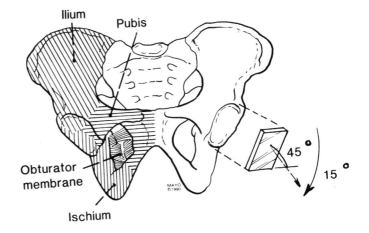

Figure 44–3. The acetabulum faces 45 degrees caudally and 15 degrees anteriorly rather than having a direct lateral opening.

of the large surrounding muscle envelope. The primary landmarks include the anterosuperior iliac spine, the posterosuperior iliac spine, the greater trochanter, and the pubic symphysis. Although a large number of creative descriptions of intersections of these landmarks have been devised, they are not particularly useful during total hip arthroplasty except for the creation of the surgical incision used for the hip replacement.

Capsule and Ligaments. The hip capsule is a strong fibrous tissue that extends down to the intertrochanteric line anteriorly; however, posteriorly, it leaves the femoral neck in an extracapsular position (Fig. 44–4). The capsule becomes less resilient and thickens in patients with degenerative disease processes of the hip joint. Careful posterior capsulorrhaphy or enhancement of the posterior soft-tissue repair may be helpful in preventing posterior dislocation, which can occur in primary total hip arthroplasty performed via a posterior approach.[20,102]

Muscles. There are 21 muscles crossing the hip joint, and, during hip arthroplasty, certain muscles have, of course, major surgical significance (Table 44–1). The tensor fascia lata, the gluteus maximus, and the thick condensation of fascia known as the iliotibial band form the outer layer of the muscular envelope. One of these muscles or the iliotibial tract must be split to gain access to the hip joint. The iliotibial band provides an insertion site for the tensor fascia lata and the majority of the gluteus max-

imus. The iliotibial band has a tendinous connection to the posterior cortex of the femoral shaft that limits the AP excursion of the iliotibial band on the greater trochanter.[58] The tensor fascia lata has the primary function of balancing the weight of the body and the non-weight-bearing leg during walking.[45] The anteromedial fibers of the tensor fascia lata have a greater mechanical advantage for hip flexion than the posterolateral fibers, whereas the posterolateral fibers possess a better mechanical advantage for hip abduction and internal rotation.[100]

Beneath this outer layer, the gluteus medius and minimus muscles and their insertion into the greater trochanter and joint capsule become a focal point of surgical exposure.[23] As detailed later in this chapter, the surgical approaches to the hip joint are designed either to avoid detachment of the gluteus medius or to displace the abductors by mechanisms that facilitate reattachment. The gluteus medius is a three-lobed structure, with each lobe possessing a separate innervation.[45] Electromyographic (EMG) studies have revealed a phasic lobe function rather than a total single muscle action. The gluteus medius and the thick periosteum covering the greater trochanter are in continuity with the fascia of the vastus lateralis and form a functional myofascial unit.[77]

The gluteus minimus inserts into the anterosuperior portion of the hip capsule and the anteroinferior portion of the greater trochanter. The insertion on the greater trochanter shows great variation between an irregular L-shape and a triangular area.[7] As the primary function

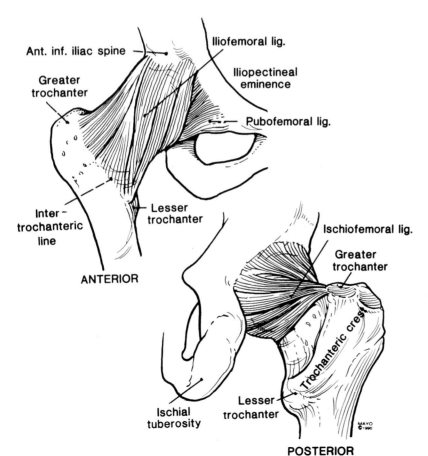

Figure 44–4. The anterior hip capsule is reinforced with the strong iliofemoral ligament and inserts beyond the level of the femoral neck. Posteriorly, the neck is thin and leaves the femoral neck in an extracapsular position.

Table 44–1. MUSCLES OF THE HIP JOINT

Primary Function	Muscle	Nerve	Segmental Innervation	Secondary Function
Extension	Gluteus maximus	Inferior gluteal	L5–S1	External rotation, adduction
	Semimembranosus	Tibial	L5–S1	Internal rotation
	Semitendinosus	Tibial	L5–S1	Internal rotation
	Biceps femoris (longitudinal)	Tibial	L5–S1	
	Adductor magnus (posterior)	Tibial	L4–S1	Internal rotation
Flexion	Iliopsoas	Nn. to iliopsoas	L2–L4	Adduction, external rotation
	Pectineus	Femoral or obturator	L2–L3	Adduction
	Rectus femoris	Femoral	L2–L3	
	Sartorius	Femoral	L2–L3	External rotation
Abduction	Gluteus medius	Superior gluteal	L4–S1	External flexion, external rotation (posterior) Internal rotation (anterior)
	Gluteus minimus	Superior gluteal	L4–S1	Flexion, internal rotation
	Tensor fascia lata	Superior gluteal	L4–L5	Flexion, internal rotation
Adduction	Adductor brevis	Obturator	L3–L4	Flexion
	Adductor longus	Obturator	L2–L3	Flexion
	Adductor magnus (anterior)	Obturator	L3–L5	Flexion
	Gracilis	Obturator	L3–L4	Flexion
	Obturator externus	Obturator	L3–L4	External rotation
External rotation	Piriformis	Nn. to piriformis	S1–S2	
	Obturator internus	Nn. to obturator internus	L5–S2	
	Superior gemellus	Nn. to quadratus femoris	L5–S1	
	Inferior gemellus			
	Quadratus femoris			

of the entire gluteus minimus and the posterior part of gluteus medius is to stabilize the head of the femur in the acetabulum during the gait cycle, extreme care should be taken to restore its insertion with accurate reattachment at closure.[7,45]

The short external rotators include the piriformis, obturator externus, obturator internus, superior gemellus, inferior gemellus, and quadratus femoris. The piriformis provides the key to understanding the neurovascular anatomy of the posterior pelvis. The superior gluteal nerve and superior gluteal artery enter the buttock above the piriformis, whereas all other neurovascular structures enter below. The short external rotators insert into the posterolateral femur and greater trochanter. When encountered during posterior approaches to the hip joint, these muscles can provide additional protection for the sciatic nerve.

Although the vastus lateralis is not a muscle that spans the hip joint, it is often an integral portion of the exposure during hip arthroplasty. Subperiosteal elevation or splitting of the vastus lateralis in association with the gluteus medius is often required for access to the femoral shaft. Maintaining the functional continuity of these muscles allows these muscles to be considered as a digastric muscle. These variations are detailed in the section on surgical exposures.

The remaining muscles are not frequently encountered during exposure for hip arthroplasty unless the anterior approach is used. In this approach, the sartorius and its anatomic relationship to the tensor fascia lata and the relationship of the lateral femoral cutaneous nerve is important. The rectus femoris is also encoun-

tered during the anterior approach, and, occasionally, the reflected head overlying the superior and anterior acetabular rim may need to be released to facilitate surgical exposure.

The iliopsoas tendon inserts into the lesser trochanter posteromedially and functions to flex and externally rotate the hip joint. Release of this insertion is occasionally needed to overcome severe flexion contractures or to increase exposure during difficult revision arthroplasties, particularly when only the acetabular component is revised.[117] Release of the adductors may also be required with severe adduction contractures such as those encountered in patients with Parkinson's disease.

Neurovascular Structures

Vessels. Extensive studies of the arterial anatomy of the hip have primarily emphasized the developmental and adult stages of femoral head vascular supply. This topic is beyond the scope of this description, and the reader is referred to standard anatomic textbooks and the published articles regarding the extensive blood supply to the femoral head. The arterial supply to the remaining structures in the region of the proximal femur and acetabulum has received less attention. Knowledge of the location of these structures is primarily important to the surgeon not only to minimize intraoperative bleeding and vascular complications but also to avoid excessive devascularization of bone. There are primarily seven arteries supplying the region of the hip joint (Fig. 44–5).

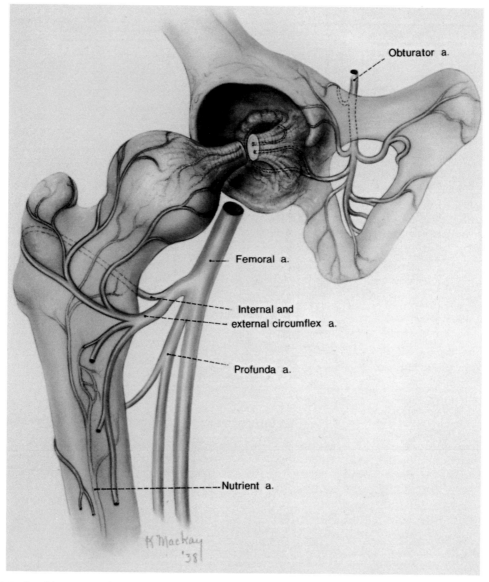

Figure 44–5. Arterial anatomy of the proximal femur showing the contributions of the obturator artery, medial (internal) circumflex artery, lateral (external) circumflex artery, and nutrient artery. The remaining blood supply arises from the superior gluteal artery, inferior gluteal artery, and first perforating artery.

The primary source of the blood supply to the femoral head is the deep branch of the medial femoral circumflex artery.[41] In reconstructive surgery of the hip other than prosthetic replacement, precise knowledge of the extracapsular anatomy of the medial femoral circumflex artery is helpful to prevent iatrogenic avascular necrosis of the femoral head when the posterior approach is used.[41] The medial femoral circumflex artery arises from either the profunda femoris artery or the femoral artery and courses posteriorly between the iliopsoas and the pectineus. It supplies branches to the adductor muscles, gracilis, and obturator externis, and often anastomoses with the obturator artery.

The superior gluteal artery is most at risk at its division at the upper border of the piriformis. This "danger spot" is located three fingerbreadths anterior to the posterosuperior iliac spine and three fingerbreadths caudad to the iliac crest. The deep branch can also be damaged as it traverses with the superior gluteal nerve approximately 4 to 6 cm superior to the acetabular rim. The superior gluteal artery supplies the superior portion of the acetabulum, the posterior rim of the acetabulum, a small portion of the greater trochanter, the gluteus medius, and portions of the gluteus minimus.

The inferior gluteal artery enters the buttock below the piriformis and medial to the sciatic nerve. The transverse branch passes over the posteromedial aspect of the sciatic nerve and supplies a vessel that descends within the substance of this nerve. The transverse branch descends along the posterior acetabulum to the region of the insertion of the short external rotators which it supplies. A deep branch descends anteriorly on the ischium to the external obturator fossa and anastomoses with the obturator artery.

The obturator artery arises from the external iliac artery and sends a branch beneath the transverse ligament into the acetabular fossa. This branch occasionally causes an annoying source of persistent bleeding after the alveolar fat is removed from the acetabular fossa. The lateral femoral circumflex artery originates from the profunda femoris artery or, occasionally, from the femoral artery. It supplies the iliopsoas, vastus lateralis, and vastus intermedius, and sends one branch to the tensor fascia lata. This artery is encountered and requires ligation during the Smith-Petersen approach.[118]

The first perforating artery supplies the posterior aspect of the greater and lesser trochanters. The main vessel traverses the upper adductor magnus and lies beneath the insertion of the gluteus maximus. This branch also supplies the gluteus maximus and adductor magnus. The nutrient artery enters the diaphysis just above the level of the isthmus and contributes to the medullary arterial supply. The anastamoses with the proximal and distal metaphyseal arteries provide a major supply to the entire femoral diaphysis. The diaphysis is also supplied by periosteal arterioles that enter at fascial attachments.

The three major sources of blood supply to the greater trochanter include the gluteus medius and minimus vascularized mainly from the internal iliac artery; the vastus lateralis, vascularized from the descending branches of the lateral circumflex femoral artery; and the transverse branch of the lateral circumflex femoral artery.[91] In a standard trochanteric osteotomy, the supply from the transversing and descending branches of the lateral circumflex artery is lost, suggesting that performance of a digastric trochanteric osteotomy may better preserve the blood supply of the trochanter. In a rabbit model, elevation of the vastus lateralis had little effect on trochanteric blood flow, whereas removal of the gluteus minimus and medius muscles or the abductor slide exposure significantly reduced trochanteric blood flow.[90]

Although injury of major vessels during hip surgery is rare, the incidence has been estimated at 0.25 percent.[89] The mechanisms of severe arterial or nerve injury during surgery of the hip joint have been well outlined.[53,68,89] Orthopedic surgeons have recently developed a new appreciation of the periacetabular neurovascular anatomy and the potential complications associated with transacetabular screw fixation for uncemented acetabular prostheses.[34,59,63,127] An acetabular quadrant system has been described to help avoid neurovascular complications when screws are inserted into the true acetabular region (Fig. 44–6).[127] When screw fixation is used in the true acetabular region, the anterosuperior and anteroinferior quadrants should be avoided to prevent injury to the external iliac artery and vein as wee as the obturator nerve, artery, and vein. Injury can occur during drilling, depth gauging, tapping, or screw insertion. During complex primary or revision hip arthroplasty, when screw fixation is required during insertion of an acetabular cage or with high cup placement, this acetabular quadrant system is not a reliable guide because the intrapelvic neurovascular structures

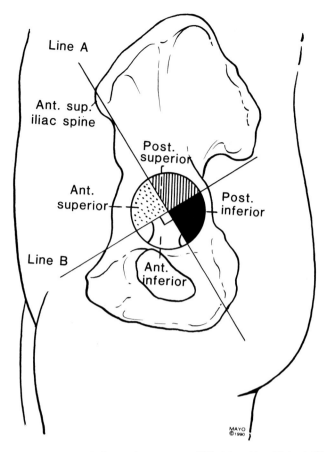

Figure 44–6. Acetabular quadrant system of Wasielewski and Rubash.[127] The anterosuperior and anteroinferior quadrants should be avoided to minimize intrapelvic neurovascular complications associated with drilling, tapping, or screw fixation of an acetabular component.

are also at risk when posteriorly directed screws are employed. Further studies are required to accurately define the periacetabular neurovascular anatomy in the region above the true acetabular region. Accurate knowledge of the anatomy and mechanisms of arterial injury are imperative to avoid these neurovascular vascular complications.

Nerves. The generous supply of sensory innervation to the hip joint capsule has questionable surgical significance. Although retention of the hip capsule may retain hip proprioception, total capsulectomy may also provide more complete pain relief after arthroplasty. Posterior skin flap numbness after primary hip arthroplasty performed via a straight lateral incision was reported in 76 percent of patients; however, none of these patients considered this to be a significant problem.[17]

The nerves of surgical importance during hip arthroplasty include the lateral femoral cutaneous nerve, femoral nerve, superior and inferior gluteal nerves, and sciatic nerve. Clinical assessment alone underestimates the incidence of nerve injury after total hip arthroplasty.[129] It is important to recognize that approximately 48 percent of patients have preoperative electromyographic evidence of chronic injury to the superior gluteal nerve.[61] The lateral femoral cutaneous nerve pierces the deep fascia between the tensor fascia lata and the sartorius approximately 2 to 3 inches below the anterosuperior iliac spine and is most often encountered during anterior approaches to the hip joint. Splitting or transacting the tensor fascia lata to gain access to the hip joint may decrease the incidence of lateral femoral cutaneous nerve damage. The femoral nerve is well out of the field of surgical dissection during hip arthroplasty. Excessive retraction or poorly placed retractors can cause femoral nerve palsy. Femoral artery and nerve compression by bulk allograft used for acetabular reconstruction of the anterior wall have been reported.[12] The Watson-Jones anterolateral approach is associated with a higher prevalence of femoral nerve palsy.[125] In 1000 consecutive hip arthroplasties, there

was an increased prevalence of nerve palsy with revision surgeries compared with primary surgery, regardless of the approach.[92] It has been suggested that the anatomic variations and complexity of the surgical procedure have more causative association with nerve injury than the specific surgical approach.

The sciatic nerve has received great appreciation and respect from hip surgeons (Fig. 44–7). Injuries to this nerve associated with hip arthroplasty are described in Chapter 68. The posterior approach has been associated with a higher prevalence of sciatic nerve injury following the posterior approach; however, a study has been done that refutes this traditional belief.[129] Intraoperative EMG changes of the sciatic nerve occur during lateral retraction of the proximal femur with a transtrochanteric

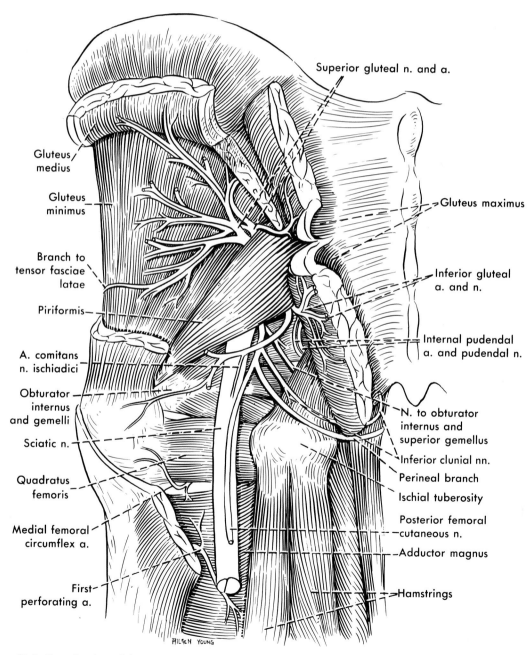

Figure 44–7. Posterior view of the neurovascular structures surrounding the hip joint region. Note the location of the piriformis as the key for locating these structures.

approach, and during anterior retraction of the proximal femur with the posterior approach.[104]

The most reliable way to identify the sciatic nerve during hip arthroplasty is to locate the insertion of the gluteus maximus tendon into the posterolateral aspect of the femur. The nerve can be located two finger-breadths cephalad and two fingerbreadths medial to this insertion and is generally encased in a thick bed of fatty alveolar tissue. When the sciatic nerve requires exposure, it is easiest to identify the nerve here and trace it proximally to dissect it from scar and pseudo-capsule. Additional protection is provided by the short external rotators as they are retracted medially during posterior exposure of the joint. Care must be taken when retractors are inserted behind the posterior wall.

Although injury to the superior gluteal nerve has been primarily associated with the direct lateral or transgluteal approaches, injury occurs subclinically, as documented by EMG, in patients with posterior, lateral, or anterolateral approaches.[1,21] The superior gluteal nerve can be damaged either by direct trauma during muscle splitting or by stretching during muscle retraction. During the transgluteal approach, irritation of the superior gluteal nerve, as measured by intraoperative electromyography, occurs first during gluteus medius splitting, then with increased muscle retraction for acetabular exposure, and, finally, during leg positioning for femoral preparation.[116]

The superior gluteal nerve courses from a posterior to an anterior direction in the interval between the gluteus medius and minimis and separates into 3 branches at the level of the sciatic notch. Entry of the nerve branches on the undersurface of the gluteal muscle bellies is distributed in a splayed pattern with a mean of 7 branches (range, 4 to 10) to the gluteus medius and 1 to 3 separate branches to the gluteus minimus.[57] The most inferior of these branches has been found an average distance of 4.91 cm between the nerve and the superior acetabular rim.[36] In contrast, other investigators have noted the average distance to be 25 mm from the deep inferior branch to the superior edge of the acetabulum.[29]

When reference is made from the midpoint of the superior border of the greater trochanter, it has been suggested that the "safe area" extends 5 cm proximally.[28,57] In another study, the distance measured from the trochanteric tip to the superior gluteal nerve averaged 7.82 cm (range, 6.3 cm to 8.4 cm).[36] In contrast, other authors report that the course of the superior gluteal nerve runs as close as 3 cm from the tip of the greater trochanter.[11,93] The difference in these studies is somewhat resolved by another report that determined the safe area to be 7 cm in the area above and behind the trochanteric tip, 5 cm above the posterior angle of the trochanter and only 3 cm above the anterior angle.[66] It has been demonstrated clinically that proximal gluteal muscle splitting can be successfully limited to less than 5 cm from the trochanteric tip in approximately 95 percent of primary hip arthroplasties when a direct lateral approach is used.[24]

SURGICAL APPROACHES

The basis of designing a good surgical approach is to provide sufficient exposure and facilitate anatomic orientation so that the surgical procedure can be properly and safely performed. Minimizing disruption of important functional structures, providing as close to normal abduction power as possible, and avoiding neurovascular damage are primary considerations. Skin incisions should be created to maximize surgical exposure, and, whenever possible, old surgical scars are incorporated. However, obtaining necessary exposure is given priority and, unlike the knee joint, old scars in the hip region can be crossed or paralleled without concern. Small incisions, especially poorly placed ones, make proper surgical exposure difficult and can be harmful to the tissues. Incisions should be large enough to perform the surgical task, thus preventing excessive retraction and wound edge maceration.

Numerous surgical approaches have been described for hip arthroplasty; however, for more than 10 years, there has been increased interest in development of innovative approaches for complex primary and revision arthroplasties.[14,76] Anatomic distortion caused by the underlying disease process or previous surgery or surgical expertise and personal philosophy often dictate the choice of a given surgical approach. Selection of a specific approach may be influenced by the presence of implants that are potentially difficult to remove or by the need to use implants that require extensile exposure.

McFarland and Osborne categorized existing approaches based on the gluteus medius tendon with anterior and posterior approaches that leave the tendon intact, whereas other approaches have involved detachment of the gluteus medius at its origin or insertion site.[77] Their description of displacement of the gluteus medius in continuity with the vastus lateralis led to the subsequent development of the transgluteal or direct lateral surgical approaches to the hip joint.[6,47] Their method of classification, based on the abductor mechanism and the approach to the joint capsule, does not fully accommodate some of the newly described surgical approaches. The criteria described in the following paragraphs have been used to expand the categories of surgical approaches to the hip joint.

Anterior approaches expose the hip through the sartorius-tensor fascia lata interval with several variations, which include splitting or transecting portions of the tensor fascia lata.[69,118] In general, anterior approaches provide limited exposure unless portions of the gluteus medius insertion are released or trochanteric osteotomy is performed. *Anterolateral* approaches enter the interval between the tensor fascia lata and the gluteus medius. Typically, the anterior portion of the gluteus medius insertion is detached, with or without an underlying bone wafer, to increase exposure.[86,87,119,120,128] The hip is dislocated anteriorly in both anterior and anterolateral approaches. *Posterior* approaches split the gluteus maximus at various levels in line with the muscle fibers. The short external rotator tendons are transected near their insertion or removed along with posterior capsule or a small bone fragment from the posterolateral femur.[42,56,74,83,96,115] The gluteus medius tendon is left undisturbed and the hip is dislocated posteriorly.

Lateral approaches depend on displacement of the abductor mechanism by a variety of methods. Trochanteric osteotomy and division of the fascial continuity between the gluteus medius and vastus lateralis allow superior displacement of the abductor mechanism.[9,16,81] Trochanteric osteotomy and subperiosteal stripping of the vastus lateralis allow anterior displacement of the gluteus medius, greater trochanter, and vastus lateralis in continuity.[70] Splitting the gluteus medius and vastus lateralis longitudinally to maintain fascial continuity allows displacement of the anterior or posterior portions of this functional unit, with or without an underlying trochanteric bone fragment.[6,8,13,18,26,32,36,38,40,43,47-49,52,55,67,73,79,85,88,121] A V-shaped myofascial flap consisting of the proximal part of the vastus lateralis and its fascia with the gluteus medius and minimus, can be reflected off the proximal femur to allow access to the entire capsule of the hip.[80] Dislocation of the hip can be anterior or posterior.

Combined methods incorporate features of several different approaches to provide increased exposure.[64,71] Surgical dissection is increased; therefore, these exposures are usually indicated for revision arthroplasty or complex primary arthroplasties. *Extensile* approaches, often using transfemoral or extended trochanteric osteotomies, allow displacement of the abductor mechanism in continuity with the proximal femur.[3,35,46,62,132] These extensile approaches have become extremely popular in the revision setting, because they allow access anteriorly and posteriorly. *Retroperitoneal* approaches, although rarely required, can be extremely useful for several specific indications.[31,103,111]

Anterior Approaches

Of all the approaches, the anterior exposure is probably the most physiologically based, because the interval is truly "internervous" between the sartorius (femoral nerve) and tensor fascia lata (superior gluteal nerve). Advocates of the anterior approach for hip arthroplasty have declined over the past few years.[69,118]

One anterior approach for hip arthroplasty, described by Light and Keggi (Fig. 44–8), is related in detail in the next paragraph. This anterior approach affords good exposure of the acetabulum and avoids disruption of the abductor mechanism. The principal element of the approach is the incongruency of the skin incision with the plane of the intermuscular interval. Splitting the tensor fascia lata rather than entering the interval between it and the sartorius appears to decrease the incidence of lateral femoral cutaneous nerve damage.

Technique (Light and Keggi)[69]

The patient is positioned supine with a sandbag under the sacrum. A curved transverse incision is made from the anterior superior iliac spine to the tip of the greater trochanter. To expose the hip capsule, the tensor fascia

lata is split longitudinally along the anteromedial aspect in line with the muscle fibers. The tensor fascia lata is retracted posteriorly and the rectus femoris and sartorius are retracted anteriorly. The ascending branch of the lateral femoral circumflex artery is ligated. The anterior capsule is excised and, if required, release of posterior capsule and of the tensor fascia lata origin on the iliac crest increase exposure of the proximal femur. Although rarely needed, anterior to posterior trochanteric osteotomy, can be done easily to

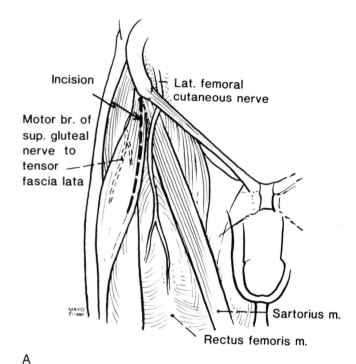

A

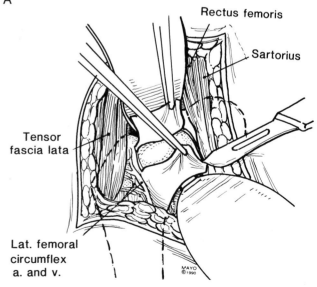

B

Figure 44–8. Anterior approach of Light and Keggi (**A**).[69] The tensor fascia lata is split longitudinally along its anterior border. Note the position of the lateral femoral cutaneous nerve medially (**B**). The rectus femoris and sartorius are retracted anteriorly, the tensor fascia lata is retracted posteriorly, and the ascending branch of the lateral circumflex artery is ligated to expose the hip capsule.

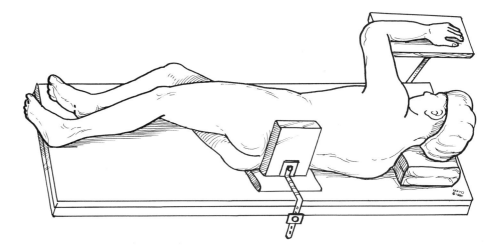

Figure 44–9. The patient is held rigidly between the anterior (*pubic*) and posterior (*sacral*) radiolucent pelvic holders to maintain the lateral decubitus position.

maintain gluteus medius-vastus lateralis continuity.[39] External rotation of the lower extremity facilitates femoral reaming. After insertion of the prosthesis, the tensor fascia lata is reapproximated and the remaining wound is closed in layers.

Anterolateral Approaches

Anterolateral approaches are characterized by the use of the tensor fascia lata-gluteus medius intermuscular interval.[13,87,128] Although early investigators recommended positioning the patient supine, the lateral decubitus position offers better visibility for assistants and allows easier access to the posterior portion of the hip joint. A modification of Müller's anterolateral approach is still used by some of the surgeons at the Mayo Clinic for primary hip arthroplasty.[25,84,87]

Technique (Modified Müller)[25]

The patient is placed in the lateral decubitus position, with the pelvis rigidly supported by padded, radiolucent pelvic holders that compress the pubis and sacrum (Fig. 44–9). The pelvis is accurately positioned and fixed perpendicular to the operating table, which in turn is parallel to the floor, enabling the surgeon to properly orient the prostheses. The skin is prepared and the patient draped so that the limb is freely mobile. A sterile side pocket is created to receive the lower leg after hip dislocation. The incision is centered directly over the midportion of the greater trochanter and courses distally along the line of the femoral shaft. The incision can extend straight proximally or curve posteriorly toward the posterior superior iliac spine, which facilitates exposure for femoral canal preparation (Fig. 44–10).

After incision of the skin and subcutaneous tissues, the iliotibial band is divided longitudinally and held by a self-retaining Charnley-type retractor (Fig. 44–11). The greater trochanteric bursa is excised to expose the gluteus medius insertion into the anterior greater trochanter. The distal and anterior tendinous portions of the gluteus medius insertion are incised to leave a cuff

of tissue, and detachment proceeds posteriorly toward the tip of the greater trochanter. The gluteus medius muscle is split superiorly in line with the muscle fibers approximately 3 cm proximal to the superior acetabular rim. Anterior and cephalad retraction of the gluteus medius exposes the gluteus minimus tendon, and detachment of the gluteus minimus is facilitated by slight flexion and external rotation of the leg. A dull, wide periosteal elevator or sharp dissection can be used to separate the gluteus minimus from the anterior capsule. The glutei are then retracted anterosuperiorly and held by Charnley acetabular pin retractors or a broad, spiked retractor driven into the ilium in the supraacetabular region (Fig. 44–12). The capsule is then incised to expose the femoral head and acetabular rim. The anterior and lateral portions of the capsule may be either excised or preserved for later repair, according to the surgeon's preference.

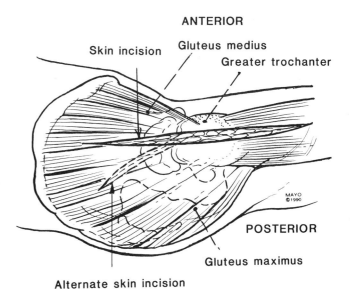

Figure 44–10. The skin incision may either be straight and centered over the femoral shaft or have a gentle proximal posterior curve to facilitate exposure of the femoral canal.

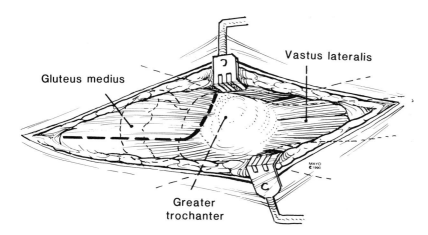

Figure 44–11. The skin, subcutaneous tissue, and fascia are retracted with the Charnley self-retaining retractor. The anterior portion of the gluteus medius is removed from the anterior portion of the greater trochanter and extended proximally through the substance of the muscle approximately 3 cm superior to the superior acetabular rim.

Measurements are taken from the acetabular pins to a point on the femur after the leg is placed in neutral rotation and full extension. A drill bit in the greater trochanter can facilitate accurate localization of this reference point. Dislocation of the hip by adduction, flexion, and external rotation usually is easily performed. If dislocation is difficult, release of remaining capsular attachments, usually anteriorly and inferiorly, and removal of acetabular osteophytes should be performed before dislocation is attempted again. After dislocation, the lower leg is placed into the sterile pocket (Fig. 44–13). The femoral neck is transected at the appropriate level and angle. A large bone hook is placed around the medial femoral cortex above the lesser trochanter to displace the femur posteriorly (Fig. 44–14**A**). Acetabular

exposure is typically improved by positioning the leg so that only the foot remains in the sterile pocket. After acetabular component insertion, the leg is positioned in flexion, external rotation, and adduction so that the lower leg is perpendicular to the floor within the sterile pocket. A large, blunt retractor placed beneath the neck of the femur elevates the femur out of the wound for direct femoral access (see Fig. 44–14**B**). After arthroplasty, secure reattachment of the gluteal muscles can be accomplished by using sutures through drill holes or by passing large bone cutting needles through the greater trochanter. When a drill is used to create trochanteric tunnels, contact with the femoral component should be avoided. The tendinous cuff of gluteus medius tendon is then oversewn with multiple interrupted sutures.

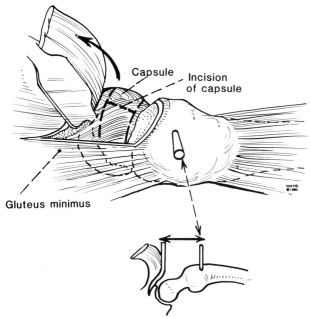

Figure 44–12. The gluteal muscles are retracted superiorly and held with acetabular pin retractors or a broad, spiked (Bickel) retractor driven into the supracetabular region of the ilium. The anterior and lateral portions of the capsule are incised or excised. (*Inset*) Measurements from the acetabular pins to a point on the femur (such as a drill bit) are done with the leg in extension and neutral rotation.

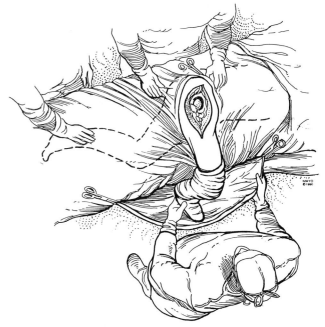

Figure 44–13. After dislocation of the hip by adduction, external rotation, and longitudinal traction, the foot and leg can be placed into the sterile pocket. When the leg is perpendicular to the floor, the surgeon can assess the version of the femoral prosthesis in a clinically reproducible manner.

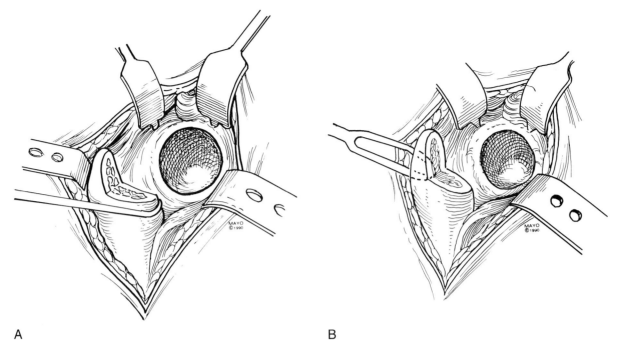

A   B

Figure 44–14. A, A large bone hook placed around the femoral neck assists the posterior retraction of the femur during acetabular exposure and preparation. **B,** A large, spoon-shaped retractor placed beneath the greater trochanter elevated the proximal femur during preparation of the femoral canal and insertion of the femoral prosthesis.

Lateral Approaches

Lateral approaches can be subdivided into transtrochanteric and direct lateral or transgluteal techniques. Both methods displace a portion or all of the entire abductor mechanism. The direct lateral or transgluteal approaches are based on the observation "that the gluteus medius and vastus lateralis can be regarded as being in direct functional continuity through the thick tendinous periosteum covering the greater trochanter."[77] Although this technique was originally described by Bauer et al.,[6] Hardinge has popularized the direct lateral approach to the hip.[47] This approach, performed with the patient in the lateral decubitus position, is currently my own preference and that of several other surgeons at our clinic for both primary surgeries and for many revision procedures.

Technique (Hardinge)[47]

The patient is placed supine, with the greater trochanter at the edge of the table. The skin incision is centered over the greater trochanter and extends 8 cm distally along the anterior border of the femoral shaft (Fig. 44–15**A**). Like the anterolateral approach, proximal extension of the incision can be directed superiorly or posteriorly. After division of the iliotibial band, the gluteus medius tendon is incised and the vastus lateralis is split distally. The gluteus minimus insertion is also partially detached from the greater trochanter. The vastus lateralis and gluteal muscles are then displaced anteriorly in continuity (see Fig. 44–15**B**). After prosthesis implantation, the wound is closed by reattaching the gluteus medius and vastus lateralis by side-to-side repair with multiple interrupted sutures (see Fig. 44–15**C**).

Several technical aspects of this approach are worth noting. The detachment of the gluteus medius should be performed by ensuring that tendinous tissue is left on the greater trochanter for secure reattachment later. Typically, the line of the tendinous incision is along the anterior ridge of the trochanter, and, if the tendon is incised more posteriorly, there is little tendon attachment to allow a secure repair. Sufficient distal splitting of the vastus lateralis is recommended because this minimizes the amount of proximal splitting of the gluteal muscles. Splitting the vastus lateralis with a cautery knife also reduces the amount of heterotopic ossification that develops postoperatively.[113]

Variations of the Direct Lateral Approach

The Dall approach describes elevation of an anterior wafer of bone at the junction of the vastus lateralis and gluteus medius.[26] Repair of this bone wafer and of the attached gluteal tendons into the greater trochanter facilitates a secure repair through bony healing. This technique is often helpful during revision procedures when there is heterotopic bone along the anterior portion of the greater trochanter; otherwise, dissection around the excess bone is through muscle belly, which encumbers a secure repair.

The "Stracathro approach" elevates anterior and posterior bone wafers to provide an extensile exposure.[79]

Transtrochanteric lateral approaches to the hip allow anterior or posterior hip dislocation. These approaches provide excellent acetabular visibility and orientation

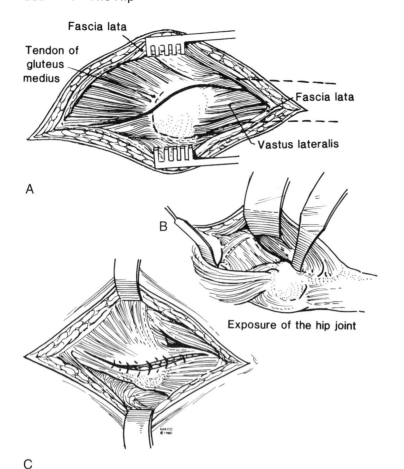

Fascia lata

Tendon of
gluteus
medius

Fascia lata

Vastus lateralis

A

B

Exposure of the hip joint

C

Figure 44–15. The direct lateral approach of Hardinge. **A**, The insertion of the gluteus medius is removed from the anterior portion of the greater trochanter and extended proximally into the substance of the gluteus medius and minimus muscles. The vastus lateralis is split distally. Care is taken to remove the abductors anteriorly so as to leave a tendinous cuff on the trochanter. **B**, The vastus lateralis is subperiosteally elevated, and the entire myofascial unit is retracted anteriorly to expose the hip capsule. **C**, The myofascial unit is repaired in a side-to-side fashion with multiple interrupted sutures that provide a secure reattachment.

and permit trochanteric transfer if desired. Charnley's original concept of total hip arthroplasty emphasized the position of the greater trochanter and the "abductor lever arm." He designed the hip reconstruction to decrease total joint forces by distal and lateral transfer of the greater trochanter, which restored abductor power to the medialized hip joint.[16] Subsequently, the role of trochanteric osteotomy in restoring function and facilitating surgical exposure became a central theme in hip arthroplasty.[37,95] Although the transtrochanteric osteotomy affords excellent exposure, there is a significant incidence of trochanteric complications, which are even more prevalent with revision arthroplasty. Variations of the standard trochanteric osteotomy have been devised to avoid complications and facilitate trochanteric union.[9,39,70,81] The reader is referred to the original articles for a detailed description of classical transtrochanteric approaches. Although trochanteric osteotomy can usually be omitted in primary and revision surgery, the hip surgeon should be prepared to perform a trochanteric osteotomy when necessary.

For approximately a decade, extended trochanteric osteotomies have become popular for a variety of reasons.[3,10,14,18,32,35,48,76,132] These specialized approaches, which include the benefits of trochanteric osteotomy while maintaining the continuity of the gluteus medius and vastus lateralis, are discussed in detail later in this chapter.

Posterior Approaches

The posterior approach is probably the most, or one of the most, commonly used approaches for total hip arthroplasty in the North American continent, primarily because it avoids displacement of the abductor mechanism. It is currently the most popular approach for hip surgery at our clinic. Gibson and Moore popularized the posterior approach.[42,83] Moore's description of the posterior approach is a common posterior approach utilized for hip arthroplasty.[83] There are many variations of the posterior approach, and these differ primarily in the placement of the skin incision and the level of gluteus maximus splitting.

Technique (Moore)[83]

The patient is secured in the lateral decubitus position. The incision is begun just lateral to the sacral prominence and extended anteriorly over the greater trochanteric region and distally in line with the femoral shaft. The iliotibial band is split over the greater trochanter and extended posteriorly in line with the skin incision, splitting the aponeurosis of the gluteus maximus. The gluteus maximus is split bluntly in line with its fibers. The sciatic nerve is identified and protected (Fig. 44–16A). The short external rotators are identified and trisected at their insertion site, leaving a cuff of tendinous insertion for later reattachment. The short rotators are then bluntly dissected from the posterior capsule and retracted medially, providing additional protection for the sciatic nerve. The capsular incision runs obliquely from the acetabular rim to the level of the lesser trochanter (see Fig. 44–16**B**). The femoral head is dislocated posteriorly by adduction and internal rotation (see Fig. 44–16**C**). After completion of the arthroplasty, the capsule is repaired and the short external rotators are reattached to their insertions with multiple interrupted sutures. The remaining wound is closed in layers.

Arthroplasties performed by less experienced surgeons through the posterior approach result in more dislocations.[50,51] Postoperative dislocation may be decreased by proper positioning of the acetabular and femoral prostheses in the appropriate anteversion and by secure reattachment of the capsule and short external rotators. To reduce the incidence of hip dislocation associated with the posterior approach, more attention is being placed on enhanced repair of the posterior soft tissues.[20,56,102] A novel approach describes the use of a posterior trochanteric osteotomy,[115] or posterior bone wafer,[56] devised to facilitate posterior capsule and external rotator repair; this is an attempt to reduce the incidence of postoperative hip dislocation (Fig. 44–17).

Combined Approaches

Certain circumstances may require a combined anterior and posterior approach to the hip joint, which provides a more extensive exposure. Examples include (1) revision surgery requiring acetabular reconstruction with bone graft, (2) prior hip arthrodesis, and (3) severe anatomic distortion requiring extensive exposure. These approaches are characterized by providing simultaneous approaches to the anterior and posterior aspects of the hip joint. Although trochanteric osteotomy can be performed, these approaches are generally designed to avoid a trochanteric osteotomy and are used in situations in which trochanteric osteotomy might usually be preferred for exposure.[64,71]

The combined anteroposterior approach to the hip described by Lusskin et al.[71] essentially approaches the hip joint anteriorly and posteriorly through anterolateral and posterior approaches. If needed, trochanteric osteotomy can be performed. The triradiate exposure[64] requires a triradiate incision centered over the greater trochanter, with two proximal limbs extending anteriorly and posteriorly. This exposure allows anterolateral and posterior capsular exposures and concomitant troch-

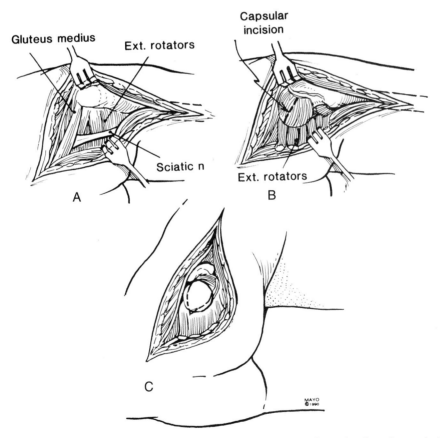

Figure 44–16. The Moore approach to hip arthroplasty. **A,** The iliotibial band is split proximally and posteriorly. The gluteus maximus is split bluntly in line with its fibers. The sciatic nerve is identified and protected. The short external rotators are identified and transected at their insertion. **B,** The external rotators are retracted posteriorly and provide additional protection for the sciatic nerve. The capsular incision runs obliquely from the acetabular rim to the level of the lesser trochanter. **C,** The hip is dislocated posteriorly by adduction and internal rotation.

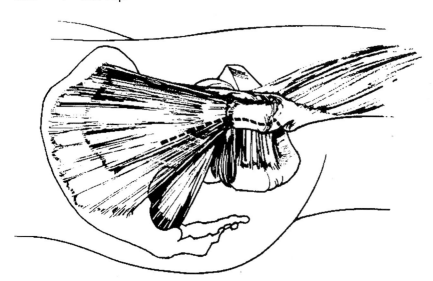

Figure 44–17. The modified posterior approach to the hip joint may be helpful during complex primary or revision procedures. An osteotomy through the posterior third of the greater trochanter is reflected posteriorly in continuity with the short external rotators, joint capsule, and posterior third of the gluteus medius. Closure is accomplished by suture repair of the soft tissues and screw fixation of the trochanteric osteotomy. (From Shaw JA: Experience with a modified posterior approach to the hip joint. A technical note. J Arthroplasty 6:11–18, 1991, with permission of Taylor & Francis Ltd.)

anteric osteotomy if desired. Caution should be exercised using the triradiate incision in older patients, particularly in those with diabetes, multiple previous surgical incisions, or steroid dependency.

Extensile Approaches

Because of the increasing number of complex and difficult revision procedures, the popularity of extensile approaches has been heightened over approximately the past decade.[3,10,14,18,32,35,48,49,76,132] Although these approaches at first may seem disproportionate, familiarity and experience with them reveal that they are more physiologic and friendly to the bone and soft tissues about the hip joint than many of the traditional surgical approaches. The primary indications for the use of an extensile exposure include (1) removal of well-fixed cemented implants; (2) removal of distally well-fixed uncemented implants; (3) removal of a well-fixed endoprosthesis with fenestrations; (4) varus remodeling of the proximal femur associated with a failed implant;

and (5) extraction of an implant associated with acetabular protrusion. Many of these extensile approaches use variations of extended trochanteric or proximal femoral osteotomies.

Vastus Slide (Extensile Exposure)[48,49]

This extensile exposure describes subperiosteal elevation of the entire vastus lateralis anteriorly in continuity with the gluteus medius (Fig. 44–18).[48,49] The majority of the gluteus medius tendon insertion is preserved, and excellent exposure of the entire femoral shaft is easily accomplished.

TECHNIQUE (VASTUS SLIDE)[49]

Through a longitudinal incision centered in line with the femoral shaft, the abductors and vastus lateralis are exposed. A lazy Z-shaped incision through the vastus lateralis and insertion of the gluteus medius is defined by four points, A through D (see Fig. 44–18A). The limbs defined by A to B and A to D are first subperiosteally

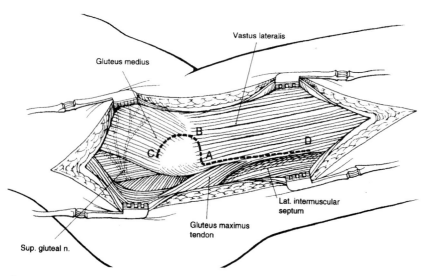

Figure 44–18. In the extensile exposure (vastus slide), the gluteus medius and vastus lateralis are incised with a lazy "Z" incision (**A**). The limbs of the vastus lateralis from A to D and A to B are subperiosteally elevated from a posterior to an anterior direction, which leaves the intermuscular septum and a small fascial cuff attached to the vastus lateralis tubercle.

Illustration continued on opposite page

A

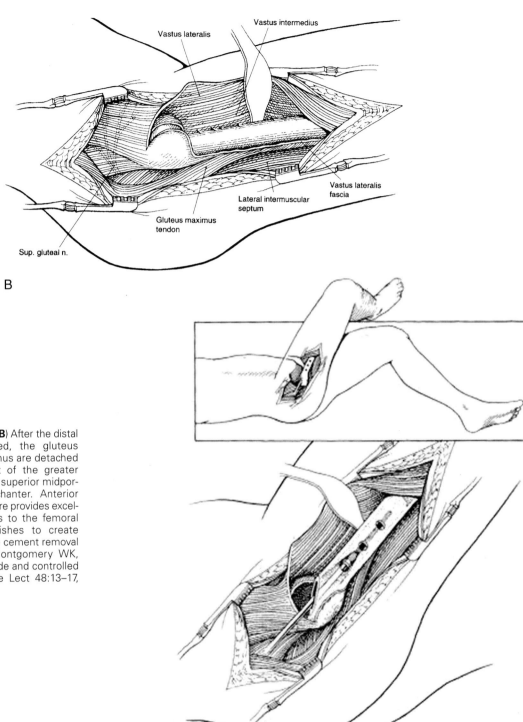

Vastus lateralis

Vastus intermedius

Vastus lateralis fascia

Lateral intermuscular septum

Gluteus maximus tendon

Sup. gluteal n.

B

C

Figure 44–18. *Continued.* (**B**) After the distal exposure is accomplished, the gluteus medius and gluteus minimus are detached from the anterior aspect of the greater trochanter to the proximal superior midportion of the greater trochanter. Anterior retraction of the musculature provides excellent exposure and access to the femoral shaft if the surgeon wishes to create femoral portals to facilitate cement removal (**C**). (From Head WC, Montgomery WK, Emerson RH Jr: Vastus slide and controlled perforations. Instr Course Lect 48:13–17, 1999.)

elevated, with care taken to leave a fascial cuff at the vastus lateralis tubercle for later repair. As the vastus is elevated from the intermuscular septum, perforating vessels are ligated and care is taken to maintain the integrity of the intermuscular septum because this provides a protective barrier for the sciatic nerve. The vastus lateralis can be elevated distally all the way to the knee joint, if necessary, and the extent of distal dissection is determined by the extent of the cement removal

or by the magnitude of femoral reconstruction. Anterior reflection of the vastus lateralis and vastus intermedius is facilitated by placement of retractors around the anterior aspect of the femoral shaft (see Fig. 44–18B).

After distal dissection, the gluteus medius and gluteus minimus tendons are removed from the anterior aspect of the greater trochanter. Again, great care is taken to preserve a tendinous cuff on the greater trochanter for later repair (see Fig. 44–18B). The gluteal detachment proceeds proximally to the superior midportion of the greater trochanter. The substance of the abductor musculature is not violated. The anterior and superior parts of the capsule are excised and the hip joint is dislocated with adduction, external rotation, and longitudinal traction. During acetabular reconstruction, the femur is best positioned in the lateral supine position, whereas intramedullary femoral reconstruction is performed with the foot in a sterile side pocket and with the hip joint in a position of adduction, flexion, and external rotation (see Fig. 44–18C). The exposure of the entire femoral shaft facilitates orientation of the canal during cement removal, placement of femoral portals, and easy application of strut grafts, if necessary. For procedures requiring extensile acetabular exposure, the vastus slide can be extended proximally with incorporation of the Smith-Peterson or the Henry acetabular approach.[49]

Anterior Trochanteric Slide[32,43]

The anterior trochanteric slide technique obviates the need for a standard trochanteric osteotomy by subperiosteal elevation of the vastus lateralis from the anterior and lateral femur and by performance of an osteotomy in the sagittal plane, which includes the origin of the vastus lateralis and the insertion of the gluteus medius and which thereby preserves the continuity of these two structures (Fig. 44–19A). The vastus lateralis is subperiosteally elevated and retracted anteriorly from the intermuscular septum in the same manner as described for the vastus slide exposure (see Fig. 44–19B). The intact musculo-osseous sleeve is displaced anteriorly and provides excellent visibility of the femoral shaft with easy access to the femoral canal.

Extended Trochanteric Osteotomies

Extended trochanteric osteotomies possess the primary advantage of an extremely wide exposure of component fixation surfaces with preservation of soft tissue attachments. The alteration of the proximal femur facilitates accurate and safe distal cement removal and canal machining under direct vision. Furthermore, the proximal femur is allowed to conform to the revision prosthesis and a weakened or damaged trochanter is protected from iatrogenic injury. Soft tissue tension can be adjusted distally, anteriorly, or posteriorly. This approach also reduces operative time. The primary disadvantage of these approaches is that the use of an uncemented, distally fixed femoral component is a requisite portion of the procedure. These osteotomies can be performed in a variety of different ways (Fig. 44–20A–D).

EXTENDED PROXIMAL FEMORAL OSTEOTOMY TECHNIQUE (YOUNGER)[132]

The hip is exposed to the level of the femur by incision of the skin, subcutaneous tissues, and iliotibial band. The extended proximal femoral osteotomy technique involves cutting the anterolateral proximal femur for one third of its circumference with a longitudinal posterior cortical osteotomy procedure (Fig. 44–21A). The osteotomy is extended distally over a variable distance, which is individually determined by the needs of the specific clinical setting. The osteotomy is levered open on an anterolateral hinge of periosteum and muscle to create an intact muscle-osseous sleeve composed of the gluteus medius, greater trochanter, anterolateral femoral diaphysis, and vastus lateralis (see Fig. 44–21B).

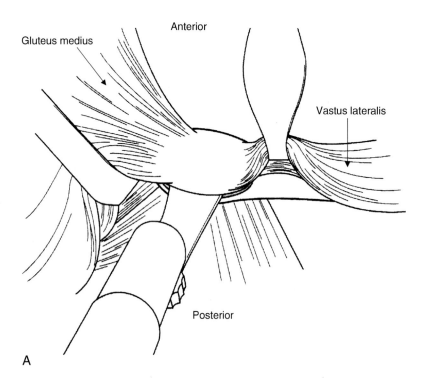

A

Figure 44–19. *See legend on opposite page*

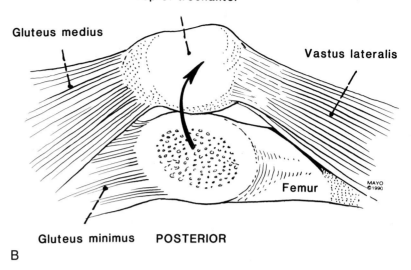

B

Figure 44–19. *Continued.* The anterior trochanteric slide is performed with a sagittal trochanteric osteotomy beneath the level of the gluteus medius insertion and the origin of the vastus lateralis (**A**). The intact musculo-osseous sleeve can be displaced anteriorly after subperiosteal elevation of the vastus lateralis muscle (**B**). (From Engh CA Jr, McAuley JP, Engh C Sr: Surgical approaches for revision total hip replacement surgery: The anterior trochanteric slide and the extended conventional osteotomy. Instr Course Lect 48:3–8, 1999.)

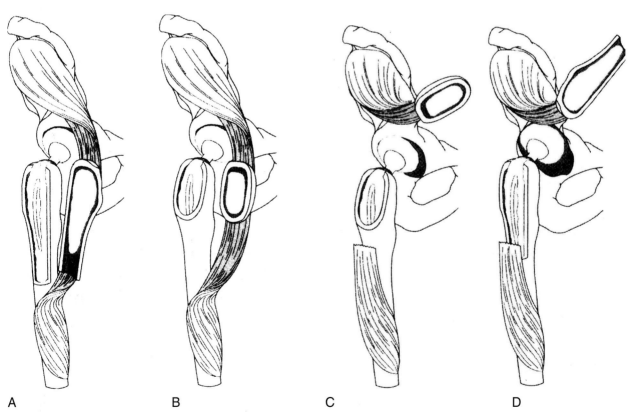

A   B   C   D

Figure 44–20. Four trochanteric osteotomies used for revision total hip arthroplasty: Extended slide (**A**); anterior slide (**B**); conventional (**C**); extended conventional (**D**). (From Engh CA Jr, McAuley JP, Engh C Sr: Surgical approaches for revision total hip replacement surgery: The anterior trochanteric slide and the extended conventional osteotomy. Instr Course Lect 48:3–8, 1999.)

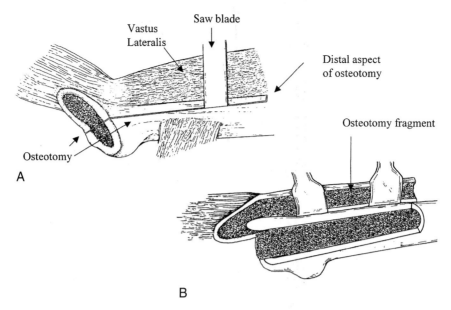

Figure 44–21. In the surgical technique of the extended proximal femoral osteotomy, retracting the vastus lateralis anteriorly exposes the posterolateral aspect of the femur, which creates an osteotomy determined by a preoperative template (**A**). The length of the osteotomy is dependent on the type and length of the prosthesis or the extent and fixation of bone cement. Cross-section of the proximal femur with a pencil bur or drill bit with multiple perforations allows the surgeon to crack the femur from posterior to anterior with several broad osteotomes through the anterior perforations. The osteotomy fragment is hinged anteriorly through the periosteum and carefully preserved attachment of the vastus lateralis to the trochanteric fragment (**B**).

This osteotomy exposes the fixation surface of uncemented implants or distal cement. After implantation of the revision prosthesis, the osteotomy is repaired with cerclage wires or cables. If desirable, the osteotomized fragment can be positioned posteriorly or distally to improve the abductor muscle tensioning.

TRANSFEMORAL APPROACH[46]

This approach is particularly attractive when the proximal femur has deficient bone circumferentially and the surgeon intends to use a proximal femoral allograft or an uncemented femoral component with distal fixation into good host bone. Typically, the vastus lateralis is longitudi-nally split within the muscle substance and a longitudinal femoral osteotomy is performed (Fig. 44–22). This osteoto-my is usually carried proximally, thereby splitting the greater trochanter. This procedure can also be done as a modification of the vastus slide but one must take care to avoid devitalization of the anterior aspect of the femur.

After the osteotomy, perforating drill holes can be placed anteriorly and posteriorly and then the anterior and posterior struts are created by osteoclasis with a broad osteotome. The creation of these struts should leave a medial strut that is continuous with the distal femur. The abductors can be split proximally to increase acetabular exposure, if necessary. If the bone loss requires the use of a proximal femoral allograft, the anterior and

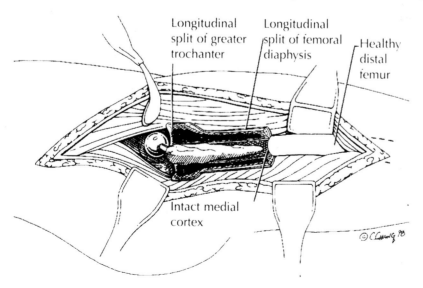

Figure 44–22. In the transfemoral approach, the deficient proximal femur is split longitudinally through the greater trochanter, and the deficient bone is cracked anteriorly and posteriorly to leave an intact medial strut. (From Gross AE: Transfemoral approach to the deficient proximal femur. Instr Course Lect 48:77–78, 1999.)

posterior struts with their attached muscle and blood supply are wrapped around the allograft and secured with circumferential wires during the closure. This often requires lateral translation of these struts around the allograft to obtain a watertight lateral closure of the greater trochanter and vastus lateralis. The resultant anteromedial and posteromedial voids are usually grafted with morcellized cancellous bone before the lateral closure.

Specialized Approaches

Vascularized Scaphoid Window[62]

This technique for creation of a controlled femoral perforation is designed to maintain the viability of the cortical plate by leaving the overlying vastus lateralis carefully attached. Although it may not be important to retain the blood supply when creating femoral portals during many aseptic reconstruction procedures, in the presence of infection, maintenance of bone viability is a requisite. The location of these osteotomy sites is done preoperatively, and these occur typically below the usual extent of surgical dissection and can be done through separate limited incisions. The femur is subperiosteally exposed proximal and distal to the intended osteotomy site (Fig. 44–23A). Narrow retractors are placed at these sites and the vastus lateralis is elevated from the intermuscular septum for only 1 cm at the intended osteotomy site. With an oscillating saw or pencil tip bur, a scaphoid osteotomy is performed from the posterior to the anterior direction through both femoral cortices. The osteotomy is created so as to leave smooth proximal and distal borders, which minimize the stress riser effect. The myo-osseous flap is then elevated anteriorly with the attached overlying muscle. After the procedure, the myo-osseous flap is placed back into its original position and secured with either circumferential wires or large resorbable monofilament sutures.

Retroperitoneal Approach[31,111]

In rare circumstances, revision surgery requires standard or extensile procedures combined with an intrapelvic sur-

gical approach. The most common indication for this approach is the presence of irregularly shaped bone cement that has been extruded into the pelvis through a defect in the acetabular fossa. The risk of life-threatening neurovascular injury during cement removal from the acetabulum requires that surgeons assess this issue during their preoperative planning. The preoperative investigations and consultation with a vascular surgeon are discussed elsewhere in this book. For most surgeons, it is wise to consult with a vascular surgeon who should be available for the surgical procedure.

The extent of intrapelvic exposure can be typically assessed before the procedure. The exposure is similar to approaches used in vascular and renal transplantation surgery. Through an oblique inguinal incision, the external oblique muscle is incised to expose the internal oblique and transverse abdominus muscles (Fig. 44–24A). The hypogastric vessels may need to be ligated if extensive exposure is required. The lateral cutaneous nerve of the thigh is at risk during the exposure and should be protected. The pelvis can be approached medial or lateral to the iliopsoas muscle (see Fig. 44–24B, C). The posterior peritoneum and its contents are retracted medially by blunt dissection to expose the ureter and neurovascular structures (see Fig. 44–24B). In some cases, it is necessary to also detach the iliacus muscle to increase the exposure. The acetabular cement and components can then be removed, and this is often done piecemeal by stabilizing the acetabular contents with intrapelvic retractors and acetabular devices (see Fig. 44–24D).

Clinical Significance

There have been many comparative studies of different surgical approaches with hip arthroplasty.[5,15,44,50,51,54,60, 72,82,84,86,92,97–99,109,110,114,124,126,130] Each surgical approach to the hip joint has certain advantages and disadvantages; however, certain postoperative complications appear more frequently with some approaches. For example, complications of the greater trochanter can be avoided

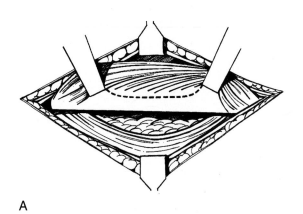

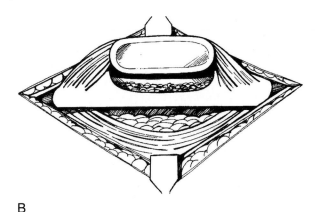

A

B

Figure 44–23. Through a limited exposure of the osteotomy site (**A**), a myo-osseous flap is elevated by careful maintenance of the attachment of the overlying vastus lateralis to the cortical plate in order to maintain viability (**B**). (**A** From Kerry RM, Masri BA, Garbuz DS, Duncan CP: The vascularized scaphoid window for access to the femoral canal in a revision total hip arthroplasty. Instr Course Lect 48:9–11, 1999.)

by using approaches that do not require trochanteric osteotomy. Morrey et al. found more extensive heterotopic ossification with less motion and less patient satisfaction when the transtrochanteric approach was used.[84] Additional reasons for avoiding trochanteric osteotomy include greater blood loss and postoperative hematoma, increased operating time, increased trochanteric bursitis, decreased walking endurance, and slower recovery. In general, trochanteric osteotomy can be avoided in primary hip arthroplasty and used only when absolutely necessary during a difficult primary arthroplasty or revision surgery.

The primary causes of abductor weakness after total hip arthroplasty include failure of abductor reattachment either because of trochanteric nonunion and migration or detachment of the abductor mechanism if it has been removed subperiosteally.[19,95,129] Comparison of the direct lateral approach and a transtrochanteric approach for total hip arthroplasty revealed no difference in the postoperative strength of the hip abductors.[82] Evaluation of the integrity of the abductor repair with the transgluteal (Hardinge) approach was assessed in 97 total hip arthroplasties by sequential measurement of radiographic markers placed in the gluteal-vastus aponeurosis at the time of surgery.[121] Separation of the markers, as a result of displacement of the anterior marker, occurred in the majority of patients. At 1 year, 54 hips had marker separation of more than 1 cm, 21 had marker displacement of more than 2 cm, and 6 hips more than 3 cm. A limp was correlated with separation of more than 2.5 cm; however, pain and function were not affected by any degree of marker displacement. A recent report evaluated the effect of femoral offset on range of motion and abductor muscle strength after total hip arthroplasty.[78] The use of an anterolateral or posterior approach was not a significant variable, and this study points out the need to assess femoral offset when abductor strength is evaluated postoperatively.

Injury to the inferior branch of the superior gluteal nerve may also cause postoperative abductor weakness.[101,106] Comparison of the direct lateral and posterior approaches demonstrated a higher incidence of denervation with the direct lateral approach that was significant at 2 weeks but usually resolved by 3 months.[4] To decrease the incidence of nerve injury, the authors suggest splitting of the vastus lateralis distally to increase exposure rather than proximal splitting of the gluteus medius. In contrast, another study of these same two approaches revealed that most patients had EMG changes postoperatively and the posterior approach had a higher but statistically insignificant incidence of EMG changes.[1] The margin of safety for gluteus medius splitting appears to be 4 cm above the rim of the acetabulum or a band measuring 5 cm from the tip of the greater trochanter.[11,24,36,57,66,93] Superior gluteal nerve injury may also occur by direct injury or traction placed by anterior traction of the gluteal-vastus aponeurosis, particularly when self-retaining retractors are used.

Heterotopic ossification has been reported to be more significant with the transtrochanteric approach com-

pared with an anterolateral and posterior approach.[84] The posterior and transtrochanteric approaches had a threefold higher incidence of heterotopic ossification compared with the anterolateral approach.[126] The Hardinge approach appears to have a higher incidence of heterotopic ossification, and this is particularly true when an anterior bone wafer is elevated with the gluteus-vastus aponeurosis.[36,54] Severe heterotopic bone formation was 5 times more common after the Liverpool approach than after the Hardinge and transtrochanteric surgical approaches.[97,99]

Dislocation after total hip arthroplasty appears to be higher with the posterior approach.[50,51,124,130] Others have demonstrated that, with a careful posterior capsular repair, the incidence of postoperative dislocation can be decreased.[20,102] Removal of an underlying wafer of bone in the posterolateral femur facilitate this repair.[56,115] Positioning of the acetabular and femoral components appears to be more difficult and variable with the posterior approach.[44] This has not been demonstrated to be significant in the available literature.

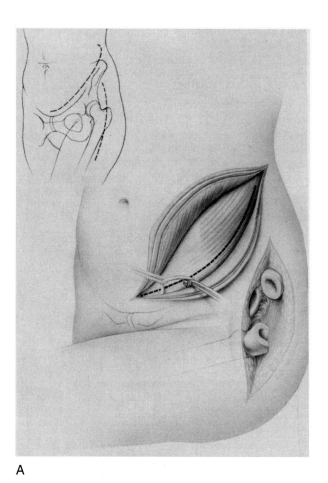

A

Figure 44–24. In the retroperitoneal approach, an inguinal incision (*inset*) is made and the external oblique muscle is incised to expose the internal oblique and transverse abdominis muscles (**A**).

Illustration continued on opposite page

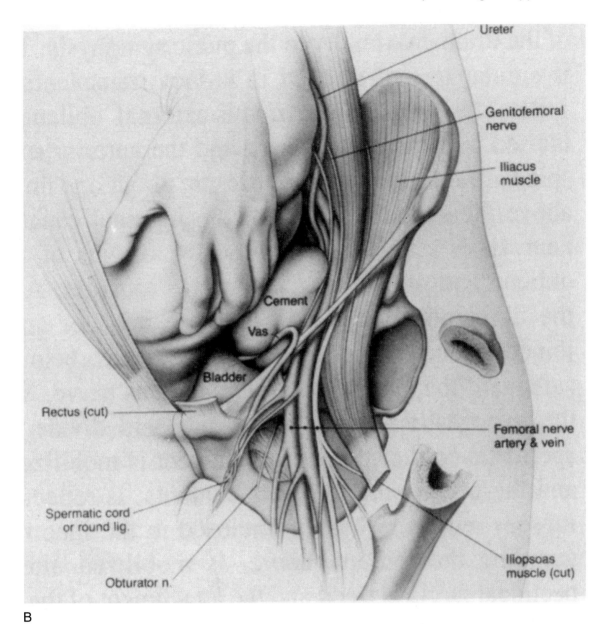

B

Figure 44–24. *Continued.* The hypogastric vessels are divided to expose the intrapelvic structures (**B**). Two access portals are possible by using a medial or lateral approach to the iliopsoas muscle (**C**).

Illustration continued on following page

AUTHOR'S PREFERENCE

Use of a specific approach for hip arthroplasty often depends on personal preference. It is safe to say that the favored approach should be the one in which the surgeon feels most competent. In reality, the hip surgeon needs to be facile with a number of the surgical approaches. For primary total hip arthroplasty and most revision arthroplasties I prefer the transgluteal approach. A secure reattachment of both the gluteus minimus and gluteus medius with nonabsorbable sutures through bone is helpful to maintain good postoperative abductor function. The classic trochanteric osteotomy is rarely used and is reserved for difficult procedures when trochanteric advancement is desirable.

During revision surgery and in the presence of heterotopic ossification, elevating an anterior bone wafer facilitates secure reattachment of the abductor mechanism. The posterior approach is used during revision surgery when the posterior femur is devoid of soft tissue attachment from a prior posterior approach. An extended trochanteric osteotomy is used when a well-fixed porous stem is removed, when femoral components with severe proximal varus remodeling undergo revision, or when an acetabular component with severe intrapelvic protrusion is removed.[35] I prefer to use the transfemoral approach

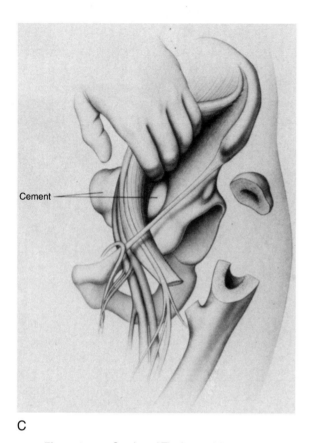

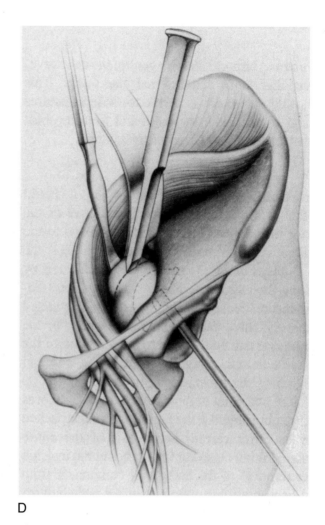

C

D

Figure 44–24. *Continued.* The intrapelvic cement can then be removed piecemeal (**D**). It is best to stabilize the cement mass with retractors in the pelvis and acetabulum during cement fragmentation (**D**). (From Eftekhar NS, Nercessian O: Intrapelvic migration of total hip prostheses. J Bone Joint Surg 71A:1480–1486, 1989.)

for procedures when I anticipate that a proximal femoral allograft will be used; however, the extended trochanteric osteotomy can be used effectively for these large reconstructive procedures.

References

1. Abitbol JJ, Gendron D, Laurin CA, Beaulieu MA: Gluteal nerve damage following total hip arthroplasty. A prospective analysis. J Arthroplasty 5:319–322, 1990.
2. Albert TJ, Sharkey PF, Chao W, et al: Rotation affects apparent radiographic positioning of femoral components in total hip arthroplasty. J Arthroplasty 6(Suppl):S67–S71, 1991.
3. Aribindi R, Paprosky W, Nourbash P, et al: Extended proximal femoral osteotomy. {PRIVATE} Instr Course Lect 48:19–26, 1999.
4. Baker AS, Bitounis VC: Abductor function after total hip replacement: An electromyographic and clinical review. J Bone Joint Surg 7IB:47, 1989.
5. Barber TC, Roger DJ, Goodman SB, Schurman DJ: Early outcome of total hip arthroplasty using the direct lateral vs the posterior surgical approach. Orthopedics 19:873–875, 1996.
6. Bauer H, Kershbaumer F, Poisel S, Oberthalen W: The transgluteal approach to the hip joint. Arch Orthop Trauma Surg 95:47, 1979.
7. Beck M, Sledge JB, Gautier E, et al: The anatomy and function of the gluteus minimus muscle. J Bone Joint Surg 82B:358–863, 2000.
8. Bell SN: Trans-gluteal approach for hemiarthroplasty of the hip. Arch Orthop Trauma Surg 104:109–112, 1985.
9. Berry DJ, Muller ME: Chevron osteotomy and single wire reattachment of the greater trochanter in primary and revision total hip arthroplasty. Clin Orthop 294:155–161, 1993.
10. Blackley HR, Rorabeck CH: Extensile exposures for revision hip arthroplasty. Clin Orthop 381:77–87, 2000.
11. Bos JC, Stoeckart R, Klooswijk AI, et al: The surgical anatomy of the superior gluteal nerve and anatomical radiologic bases of the direct lateral approach to the hip. Surg Radiol Anat 16:253–258, 1994.
12. Bose WJ, Petty W: Femoral artery and nerve compression by bulk allograft used for acetabular reconstruction. An unreported complication. J Arthroplasty 11:348–350, 1996.
13. Burwell HN, Scott D: A lateral intermuscular approach to the hip joint for replacement of the femoral head by a prosthesis. J Bone Joint Surg 36B:104, 1954.
14. Callaghan JJ: Difficult primary total hip arthroplasty: Selected surgical exposures. Instr Course Lect 49:13–21, 2000.
15. Carlson DC, Robinson HJ Jr: Surgical approaches for primary total hip arthroplasty. A prospective comparison of the Marcy modification of the Gibson and Watson-Jones approaches. Clin Orthop 222:161–166, 1987.
16. Charnley J, Ferreira A, De SD: Transplantation of the greater trochanter in arthroplasty of the hip. J Bone Joint Surg 46B:191, 1964.
17. Chatterji U, Fontana A, Villar RN: Posterior skin flap numbness after total hip arthroplasty. J Arthroplasty 11:853–855, 1996.

18. Chen WM, McAuley JP, Engh CA Jr, et al: Extended slide trochanteric osteotomy for revision total hip arthroplasty. J Bone Joint Surg 82A:1215–1219, 2000.

19. Chin KR, Brick GW: Reattachment of the migrated ununited greater trochanter after revision hip arthroplasty: The abductor slide technique. A review of four cases. J Bone Joint Surg 82A:401–408, 2000.

20. Chiu FY, Chen CM, Chung TY, et al: The effect of posterior capsulorrhaphy in primary total hip arthroplasty: A prospective randomized study. J Arthroplasty 15:194–199, 2000.

21. Chomiak J, Slavik M, Stedry V: Electromyographic findings in the gluteal muscles in the Watson-Jones and the Bauer surgical approaches to the hip joint. Acta Chir Orthop Traumatol Cech 57:40–47, 1990.

22. Clark JM, Freeman MAR, Witham D: The relationship of neck orientation to the shape of the proximal femur. J Arthroplasty 2:99, 1987.

23. Clark JM, Haynor DR: Anatomy of the abductor muscles of the hip as studied by computed tomography. J Bone Joint Surg Am 69:1021–1031, 1987.

24. Comstock C, Imrie S, Goodman SB: A clinical and radiographic study of the "safe area" using the direct lateral approach for total hip arthroplasty. J Arthroplasty 9:527–531, 1994.

25. Coventry MB: Hip arthroplasty in older patients with hip dysplasia. In Evarts CM (ed): Surgery of the Musculoskeletal System. New York, Churchill Livingstone, 1983, p 253.

26. Dall D: Exposure of the hip by anterior osteotomy of the greater trochanter. A modified anterolateral approach. J Bone Joint Surg 68B:382–386, 1986.

27. Dorr LD, Bechtol CO, Watkins RG, Wan Z: Radiographic anatomic structure of the arthritic acetabulum and its influence on total hip arthroplasty. J Arthroplasty 15:890–900, 2000.

28. Duparc F, Thomine JM, Dujardin F, et al: Anatomic basis of the transgluteal approach to the hip-joint by anterior hemimyotomy of the gluteus medius. Surg Radiol Anat 19:61–67, 1997.

29. Ebraheim NA, Olexa TA, Xu R, et al: The quantitative anatomy of the superior gluteal artery and its location. Am J Orthop 27:427–431, 1998.

30. Eckrich SG, Noble PC, Tullos HS: Effect of rotation on the radiographic appearance of the femoral canal. J Arthroplasty 9:419–26, 1994.

31. Eftekhar NS, Nercessian O: Intrapelvic migration of total hip prostheses. J Bone Joint Surg 71A:1480–1486, 1989.

32. Engh CA Jr, McAuley JP, Engh C Sr: Surgical approaches for revision total hip replacement surgery: The anterior trochanteric slide and the extended conventional osteotomy. Instr Course Lect 48:3–8, 1999.

33. Fessy MH, Seutin B, Bejui J: Anatomical basis for the choice of the femoral implant in the total hip arthroplasty. Surg Radiol Anat 19:283–286, 1997.

34. Feugier P, Fessy MH, Bejui J, Bouchet A: Acetabular anatomy and the relationship with pelvic vascular structures. Implications in hip surgery. Surg Radiol Anat 19:85–90, 1997.

35. Firestone TP, Hedley AK: Extended proximal femoral osteotomy for severe acetabular protrusion following total hip arthroplasty. A technical note. J Arthroplasty 12:344–345, 1997.

36. Foster DE, Hunter JR: The direct lateral approach to the hip for arthroplasty. Advantages and complications. Orthopedics 10:274, 1987.

37. Free SA, Delp SL: Trochanteric transfer in total hip replacement: Effects on the moment arms and force-generating capacities of the hip abductors. J Orthop Res 14:245–250, 1996.

38. Frndak PA, Mallory TH, Lombardi AV Jr: Translateral surgical approach to the hip. The abductor muscle "split". Clin Orthop 295:135–141, 1993.

39. Fulkerson JP, Crelin ES, Keggi KJ: Anatomy and osteotomy of the greater trochanter. Arch Surg 114:19–21, 1979.

40. Gammer W: A modified lateroanterior approach in operations for hip arthroplasty. Clin Orthop 199:169–172, 1985.

41. Gautier E, Ganz K, Krugel N, et al: Anatomy of the medial femoral circumflex artery and its surgical implications. J Bone Joint Surg 82B:679–683, 2000.

42. Gibson A: Posterior exposure of the hip joint. J Bone Joint Surg 32B:183, 1950.

43. Glassman AH, Engh CA, Bobyn JD: A technique of extensile exposure for total hip arthroplasty. J Arthroplasty 2:11–21, 1987.

44. Gore DR, Murray MP, Sepic SB, Gardner GM: Anterolateral compared to posterior approach in total hip arthroplasty: Differences in component positioning, hip strength, and hip motion. Clin Orthop 165:180, 1982.

45. Gottschalk F, Kourosh S, Leveau B: The functional anatomy of tensor fasciae latae and gluteus medius and minimus. J Anat 166:179–189, 1989.

46. Gross AE: Transfemoral approach to the deficient proximal femur. Instr Course Lect 48:77–78, 1999.

47. Hardinge K: The direct lateral approach to the hip. J Bone Joint Surg 64B:17–19, 1982.

48. Head WC, Mallory TH, Berklacich FM, et al: Extensile exposure of the hip for revision arthroplasty. J Arthroplasty 2:265–273, 1987.

49. Head WC, Montgomery WK, Emerson RH Jr: Vastus slide and controlled perforations. Instr Course Lect 48:13–17, 1999.

50. Hedlundh U, Ahnfelt L, Hybbinette CH: Surgical experience related to dislocations after total hip arthroplasty. J Bone Joint Surg 78B:206–209, 1996.

51. Hedlundh U, Hybbinette CH, Fredin H: Influence of surgical approach on dislocations after Charnley hip arthroplasty. J Arthroplasty 10:609–614, 1995.

52. Heimkes B, Posel P, Bolkart M: The transgluteal approaches to the hip. Arch Orthop Trauma Surg 111:220–223, 1992.

53. Heller KD, Prescher A, Zilkens KW, Forst R: Anatomic study of femoral vein occlusion during simulated hip arthroplasty. Surg Radiol Anat 19:133–137, 1997.

54. Horwitz BR, Rockowitz NL, Goll SR, et al: A prospective randomized comparison of two surgical approaches to total hip arthroplasty. Clin Orthop 291:154–163, 1993.

55. Itokazu M, Ohno T, Itoh Y: Exposure of the hip by anterior osteotomy of the greater trochanter. Bull Hosp Jt Dis 57:159–161, 1998.

56. Iyer KM: A new posterior approach to the hip joint. Injury 13:76–80, 1981.

57. Jacobs LG, Buxton RA: The course of the superior gluteal nerve in the lateral approach to the hip. J Bone Joint Surg 71A:1239–1243, 1989.

58. Kaplan EB: The iliotibial tract. Clinical and morphological significance. J Bone Joint Surg 40A:817, 1958.

59. Keating EM, Ritter MA, Faris PM: Structures at risk from medially placed acetabular screws. J Bone Joint Surg 72A:509–511, 1990.

60. Keene GS, Parker MJ: Hemiarthroplasty of the hip—the anterior or posterior approach? A comparison of surgical approaches. Injury 24:611–613, 1993.

61. Kenny P, O'Brien CP, Synnott K, Walsh MG: Damage to the superior gluteal nerve after two different approaches to the hip. J Bone Joint Surg 81B:979–981, 1999.

62. Kerry RM, Masri BA, Garbuz DS, Duncan CP: The vascularized scaphoid window for access to the femoral canal in revision total hip arthroplasty. Instr Course Lect 48:9–11, 1999.

63. Kirkpatrick JS, Callaghan JJ, Vandemark RM, Goldner RD: The relationship of the intrapelvic vasculature to the acetabulum. Implications in screw-fixation acetabular components. Clin Orthop 258:183–190, 1990.

64. Krackow KA, Steinman H, Cohn BT, Jones LC: Clinical experience with a triradiate exposure of the hip for difficult total hip arthroplasty. J Arthroplasty 3:267–78, 1988

65. Laine HJ, Lehto MU, Moilanen T: Diversity of proximal femoral medullary canal. J Arthroplasty 15:86–92, 2000.

66. Lavigne P, Loriot de Rouvray TH: The superior gluteal nerve. Anatomical study of its extrapelvic portion and surgical resolution by trans-gluteal approach. Rev Chir Orthop Reparatrice Appar Mot 80:188–195, 1994.

67. Learmonth ID, Allen PE: The omega lateral approach to the hip. J Bone Joint Surg 78B:559–561, 1996.

68. Lewallen DG: Neurovascular injury associated with hip arthroplasty. Instr Course Lect 47:275–283, 1998.

69. Light TR, Keggi KJ: Anterior approach to hip arthroplasty. Clin Orthop 152:255–260, 1980.

70. Lindgren U, Svenson O: A new transtrochanteric approach to the hip. Int Orthop 12:37–41, 1988.

71. Lusskin R, Goldman A, Absatz M: Combined anterior and posterior approach to the hip joint in reconstructive and complex arthroplasty. J Arthroplasty 3:313–322, 1988.

72. Macedo CA, Galia CR, Rosito R, et al: Comparation of the anterolateral and posterior approaches in primary total hip arthroplasty. Rev Fac Cien Med Univ Nac Cordoba 56:91–96, 1999.

73. Mallory TH, Lombardi AV Jr, Fada RA, et al: Dislocation after total hip arthroplasty using the anterolateral abductor split approach. Clin Orthop 358:166–172, 1999.

74. Marcy GH, Fletcher RS: Modification of the posterolateral approach to the hip for insertion of the femoral head prosthesis. J Bone Joint Surg 36A:142, 1954.

75. Massin P, Geais L, Astoin E, et al: The anatomic basis for the concept of lateralized femoral stems: A frontal plane radiographic study of the proximal femur. J Arthroplasty 15:93–101, 2000.

76. Masterson EL, Masri BA, Duncan CP: Surgical approaches in revision hip replacement. J Am Acad Orthop Surg 6:84–92, 1998.

77. McFarland B, Osborne G: Approach to the hip. A suggested improvement on Kocher's method. J Bone Joint Surg 36B:364, 1954.

78. McGrory BJ, Morrey BF, Cahalan TD, et al: Effect of femoral offset on range of motion and abductor muscle strength after total hip arthroplasty. J Bone Joint Surg 77B:865–869, 1995.

79. McLauchlan J: The stracathro approach to the hip. J Bone Joint Surg 66B:30–31, 1984.

80. McMinn DJ, Roberts P, Forward GR: A new approach to the hip for revision surgery. J Bone Joint Surg 73B:899–901, 1991.

81. Menon PC, Griffiths WE, Hook WE, Higgins B: Trochanteric osteotomy in total hip arthroplasty: Comparison of 2 techniques. J Arthroplasty 13:92–96, 1998.

82. Minns RJ, Crawford RJ, Porter ML, Hardinge K: Muscle strength following total hip arthroplasty. A comparison of trochanteric osteotomy and the direct lateral approach. J Arthroplasty 8:625–627, 1993.

83. Moore AT: The self-locking metal hip prosthesis. J Bone Joint Surg 39A:811, 1957.

84. Morrey BF, Adams RA, Cabanela ME: Comparison of heterotopic bone after anterolateral, transtrochanteric, and posterior approaches for total hip arthroplasty. Clin Orthop 188:160–167, 1984.

85. Moskal JT, Mann JW III: A modified direct lateral approach for primary and revision total hip arthroplasty. A prospective analysis of 453 cases. J Arthroplasty 11:255–266, 1996.

86. Mostardi RA, Askew MJ, Gradisar IA Jr, et al: Comparison of functional outcome of total hip arthroplasties involving four surgical approaches. J Arthroplasty 3:279–284, 1988.

87. Müller ME: Total hip prostheses. Clin Orthop 72:46, 1970.

88. Mulliken BD, Rorabeck CH, Bourne RB, Nayak N: A modified direct lateral approach in total hip arthroplasty: A comprehensive review. J Arthroplasty 13:737–747, 1998.

89. Nachbur B, Meyer RP, Verkkala K, Zurcher R: The mechanisms of severe arterial injury in surgery of the hip joint. Clin Orthop 141:122–133, 1979.

90. Naito M, Ogata K, Emoto G: The blood supply to the greater trochanter. Clin Orthop 323:294–297, 1996.

91. Najima H, Gagey O, Cottias P, Huten D: Blood supply of the greater trochanter after trochanterotomy. Clin Orthop 349:235–241, 1998.

92. Navarro RA, Schmalzried TP, Amstutz HC, Dorey FJ: Surgical approach and nerve palsy in total hip arthroplasty. J Arthroplasty 10:1–5, 1995.

93. Nazarian S, Tisserand P, Brunet C, Müller ME: Anatomic basis of the transgluteal approach to the hip. Surg Radiol Anat 9:27–35, 1987.

94. Noble PC, Alexander JW, Lindahl LJ, et al: The anatomic basis of femoral component design. Clin Orthop 235:148–165, 1988.

95. Nutton RW, Checketts RG: The effects of trochanteric osteotomy on abductor power. J Bone Joint Surg 66B:180–183, 1984.

96. Osborne RP: The approach to the hip joint: A critical review and a suggested new route. Br J Surg 18:49, 1930.

97. Pai VS: Heterotopic ossification in total hip arthroplasty. The influence of the approach. J Arthroplasty 9:199–202, 1994.

98. Pai VS: Significance of the Trendelenburg test in total hip arthroplasty. Influence of lateral approaches. J Arthroplasty 11:174–749, 1996.

99. Pai VS: A comparison of three lateral approaches in primary total hip replacement. Int Orthop 21:393–8, 1997.

100. Pare EB, Stern JT Jr, Schwartz JM: Functional differentiation within the tensor fasciae latae. A telemetered electromyographic analysis of its locomotor roles. J Bone Joint Surg 63A:1457–1471, 1981.

101. Pascarel X, Dumont D, Nehme B, et al: Total hip arthroplasty using the Hardinge approach. Clinical results in 63 cases. Rev Chir Orthop Reparatrice Appar Mot 75:98–103, 1989.

102. Pellicci PM, Bostrom M, Poss R: Posterior approach to total hip replacement using enhanced posterior soft tissue repair. Clin Orthop 355:224–228, 1998.

103. Petrera P, Trakru S, Mehta S, et al: Revision total hip arthroplasty with a retroperitoneal approach to the iliac vessels. J Arthroplasty 11:704–708, 1996.

104. Pereles TR, Stuchin SA, Kastenbaum DM, et al: Surgical maneuvers placing the sciatic nerve at risk during total hip arthroplasty as assessed by somatosensory evoked potential monitoring. J Arthroplasty 11:438–444, 1996.

105. Poss R, Staehlin P, Larson M: Femoral expansion in total hip arthroplasty. J Arthroplasty 2:259–264, 1987.

106. Ramesh M, O'Byrne JM, McCarthy N, et al: Damage to the superior gluteal nerve after the Hardinge approach to the hip. J Bone Joint Surg 78B:903–906, 1996.

107. Reikeras O, Bjerkreim I, Kolbenstvedt A: Anteversion of the acetabulum and femoral neck in normals and in patients with osteoarthritis of the hip. Acta Orthop Scand 54:18–23, 1983.

108. Reikeras O, Hoiseth A: Femoral neck angles in osteoarthritis of the hip. Acta Orthop Scand 53:781–784, 1982.

109. Roberts JM, Fu FH, McClain EJ, Ferguson AB Jr: A comparison of the posterolateral and anterolateral approaches to total hip arthroplasty. Clin Orthop 187:205–210, 1984.

110. Robinson RP, Robinson HJ Jr, Salvati EA: Comparison of the transtrochanteric and posterior approaches for total hip replacement. Clin Orthop 147:143–7, 1980.

111. Rorabeck CH, Partington PF: Retroperitoneal exposure in revision total hip arthroplasty. {PRIVATE} Instr Course Lect 48:27–36, 1999.

112. Rosson JW, Surowiak J, Schatzker J, Hearn T: Radiographic appearance and structural properties of proximal femoral bone in total hip arthroplasty patients. J Arthroplasty 11:180–183, 1996.

113. Schmidt J, Hackenbroch MH: A new classification for heterotopic ossifications in total hip arthroplasty considering the surgical approach. Arch Orthop Trauma Surg 115:339–343, 1996.

114. Schneeberger AG, Schulz RF, Ganz R: Blood loss in total hip arthroplasty. Lateral position combined with preservation of the capsule versus supine position combined with capsulectomy. Arch Orthop Trauma Surg 117:47–49, 1998.

115. Shaw JA: Experience with a modified posterior approach to the hip joint. A technical note. J Arthroplasty 6:11–18, 1991.

116. Siebenrock KA, Rosler KM, Gonzalez E, Ganz R: Intraoperative electromyography of the superior gluteal nerve during lateral approach to the hip for arthroplasty: A prospective study of 12 patients. J Arthroplasty 15:867–870, 2000.

117. Smith SW, Mankiletow A, Harris WH: Vastus-Psoas release for acetabular exposure in revision hip surgery. J Arthroplasty 12:568–571, 1997.

118. Smith-Petersen MN: Approach to and exposure of the hip joint for mold arthroplasty. J Bone Joint Surg 31A:40, 1949.

119. Soni RK: An anterolateral approach to the hip joint. Acta Orthop Scand 68:490–494, 1997.

120. Stephenson PK, Freeman MA: Exposure of the hip using a modified anterolateral approach. J Arthroplasty 6:137–145, 1991.

121. Svensson O, Skold S, Blomgren G: Integrity of the gluteus medius after the transgluteal approach in total hip arthroplasty. J Arthroplasty 5:57–60, 1990.

122. Sugano N, Noble PC, Kamaric E: Predicting the position of the femoral head center. J Arthroplasty 14:102–107, 1999.

123. Sugano N, Noble PC, Kamaric E, et al: The morphology of the femur in developmental dysplasia of the hip. J Bone Joint Surg 80B:711–719, 1998.

124. Unwin AJ, Thomas M: Dislocation after hemiarthroplasty of the hip: A comparison of the dislocation rate after posterior and lateral approaches to the hip. Ann R Coll Surg Engl 76:327–329, 1994.

125. van der Linde MJ, Tonino AJ: Nerve injury after hip arthroplasty. 5/600 cases after uncemented hip replacement, anterolateral approach versus direct lateral approach. Acta Orthop Scand 68:521–523, 1997.

126. Vicar AJ, Coleman CR: A comparison of the anterolateral, transtrochanteric, and posterior surgical approaches in primary total hip arthroplasty. Clin Orthop 188:152–159, 1984.

127. Wasielewski RC, Cooperstein LA, Kruger MP, Rubash HE: Acetabular anatomy and the transacetabular fixation of screws in total hip arthroplasty. J Bone Joint Surg 72A:501–508, 1990.

128. Watson-Jones R: Fractures of the neck of the femur. Br J Surg 23:787, 1935–1936.

129. Weber M, Berry DJ: Abductor avulsion after primary total hip arthroplasty. Results of repair. J Arthroplasty 12:202–206, 1997.

130. Woo RYG, Morrey BF: Dislocations after total hip arthroplasty. J Bone Joint Surg 64A:1295, 1982.

131. Wroblewski BM, Siney PD, Fleming PA, Bobak P: The calcar femorale in cemented stem fixation in total hip arthroplasty. J Bone Joint Surg 82B:842–845, 2000.

132. Younger TI, Bradford MS, Magnus RE, Paprosky WG: Extended proximal femoral osteotomy. A new technique for femoral revision arthroplasty. J Arthroplasty 10:329–338, 1995.

45
Biomechanics

• BERNARD F. MORREY and ZONG-PING LUO

NORMAL AND POSTREPLACEMENT GAIT

This chapter focuses on some of the biomechanical features of the normal hip and considers them in the context of joint replacement. Because the real goal is to restore function, awareness of the biomedical features of the normal gait are important. In the ideal setting, the replacement can restore this gait cycle to—or approach—"normal" (Fig. 45–1). Measuring physiologic energy expenditure is a valuable method of assessing the penalties caused by gait disabilities. One method to better understand the added physiologic demand caused by a gait disorder is the calculation of the rate of oxygen uptake or energy consumption. Typically, this is done for a normal subject walking at the same speed as the patient with a prosthetic replacement and is determined by subtracting the patient's rate of energy consumption from the normal rate (Fig. 45–2). Severe unilateral osteoarthritis of the hip results in reduced velocity, cadence, stride length, and VO_2, and an increased rate of energy consumption. It has been shown that although there are improvements postoperatively, the average velocity of arthritis patients (55 meters per minute) remains less than the average gait velocity for senior subjects (74 meters per minute).[18]

BASIC BIOMECHANICAL CONSIDERATIONS

For the clinician, as with other joints, it is convenient to discuss the topic of biomechanics according to the three components of function: motion, or kinematics; stability, or constraints; and strength or force transmission.

MOTION—KINEMATICS

The average ranges of normal hip joint motion exhibit a wide variation as a result of differences among individuals of varying physical builds and age groups. Even in nondiseased hips, the arc of motion decreases with increasing age (Table 45–1). Hence, normative data

should serve mainly as guides and not as standards. The patient's opposite extremity is, of course, the best "normal" standard.

Range and Pattern of Hip Motion in Activities of Daily Living

Of importance to the clinician is that adequate motion for daily functions is accomplished by the joint replacement. The mean arcs of hip motion during ambulation of 32 normal subjects are: extension 15; flexion 37 (50-degree arc); abduction 5 and adduction 10; internal rotation 5, and external rotation 9 degrees.[10] The greatest amount of hip flexion occurs when the patient is tying a shoe with the foot resting on the opposite thigh or stooping to pick up something from the floor. The largest amount of hip extension occurs when the patient is walking on sideslopes or engaging in activities such as playing golf. The greatest amount of abduction and internal rotation occurs when the patient is getting into or out of a car, whereas the largest amount of abduction and external rotation occurs during an activity such as golfing (Table 45–2).

PROSTHETIC REPLACEMENT AND MOTION

All hip replacement devices provide for an arc of motion adequate for the performance of daily functions as discussed in the preceding sections. The limiting factors of hip motion in vivo are soft tissue constraints or impingement of the femoral neck on the rim of the prosthetic cup (Fig. 45–3). Exceeding these limits obviously creates an unstable articulation. Increased hand/neck diameter ratios, trapezoidal-shaped prosthetic necks, and asymmetrical and less constrained sockets have been incorporated into various implants to enhance and stabilize prosthetic motion. The newer constrained acetabular implants produce stability at the expense of motion, providing only about 70 to 80 degrees of flexion.

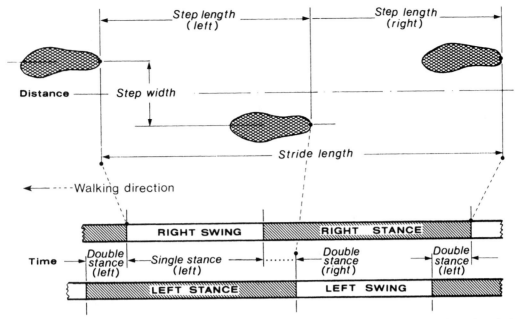

Figure 45–1. A schematic diagram illustrating the typical temporal distance factors in gait analysis. Not shown here is the foot angle, which is the angle between the midline of the foot or shoe and the line of progression. Note that the single-stance period of one leg is the same as the swing phase of the contralateral leg.

CONSTRAINTS—STABILITY

The hip joint is inherently stable because of the congruent ball-and-socket type articulation. The enhanced constraint provided by the ligaments in the normal joint renders this one of the most stable joints in the body. There are few biomechanical considerations in normal hip stability, but this is a major issue with joint replacement (see Chapter 65).

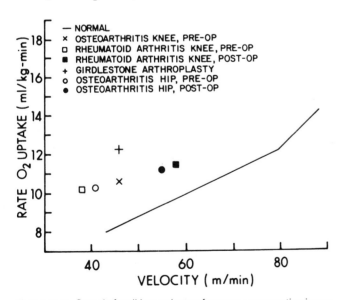

Figure 45–2. Speed of walking and rate of oxygen consumption in normal subjects and in those with gait disorders. Normal baseline data were obtained from normal subjects walking at different speeds. The vertical distance between the data points for the different patient groups and the normal baseline represents the average added energy demand caused by the gait disability.[2,18]

Prosthetic Design and Stability

Hip instability is a complication that rivals or exceeds infection in frequency, morbidity, and financial impact (see Chapter 65). With joint replacement, both articular and ligamentous contributions are altered, and unless a "captive-head" implant is used, the prosthetic joint relies primarily on muscle tone for stability.

On a theoretical basis, a larger prosthetic head is more stable than a smaller one. This is because the greater displacement of the larger head creates increased tissue tension that stabilizes or resists further displacement (Fig. 45–4). The theoretical value of the larger head replacement has not to date been borne out by clinical experience. If the large femoral head implant or enhanced muscle tension are not effective in stabilizing the joint, newer prosthetic designs can provide a stable articulation by means of a captive head within the acetabular component. The implication that

Table 45–1. PASSIVE HIP JOINT RANGE OF MOTION BY AGE

Motion	Age Group (yr)		
	25–39 (No. = 433)	40–59 (No. = 727)	60–74 (No. = 523)
Flexion	122 ± 12	120 ± 14	118 ± 13
Extension	22 ± 8	18 ± 7	17 ± 8
Abduction	44 ± 11	42 ± 11	39 ± 12
Internal rotation	33 ± 7	31 ± 8	30 ± 7
External rotation	34 ± 8	32 ± 8	29 ± 9

Data are mean ± standard deviation.
Data from Roach KE, Miles TP: Normal hip and knee active range of motion: the relationship to age. Phys Ther 71:656, 1991.

this design may increase wear or interface stress has yet to be determined.

Additional variables must also be considered, such as neck impingement and femoral offset.[11] In clinical trials, the amount of femoral offset has been shown to be statistically related to hip stability.[6] By lengthening the distance between origin and insertion, the muscle becomes more efficient. This also results in transmission of less force across the articulation. Trochanteric osteotomy with distal and lateral displacement has been shown to stabilize the unstable hip replacement in selected cases.[6] The concept of offset is important in hip function and for restoration of mechanical "balance" and is discussed later.

FORCE TRANSMISSION

Muscle Strength Potential

The functional strength potential at the hip joint has been estimated for isometric and isokinetic conditions (Table 45–3). The strength is directly correlated with the cross-sectional area of the muscle. The magnitude of this resultant is well known to have been calculated as exceeding times 3 body weight for selected functions such as descending stairs and up to times 8 when tripping and catching one's balance.[17]

As a consequence of these muscle forces, a resultant vector that represents the joint reactive force may be calculated. The orientation of the resultant joint contact force varies over a relatively limited range during the load-bearing portions of normal gait sequences. Generally, the joint contact force on the ball of the hip prosthesis is located in the anterosuperior region. A three-dimensional plot of the resultant joint force during the first cycle of gait with crutches is shown in Figure 45–5. The results of these analytical studies have been confirmed by direct force measurements across the prosthetic head and interface.[1,5,15]

Muscle Moment Arm

The moment arm is defined as the perpendicular distance from the line of action of the muscle force to the point or axis of rotation (Fig. 45-6). Variations in the anatomy of the hip joint change the mechanical advantage of the muscle, which subsequently changes muscle

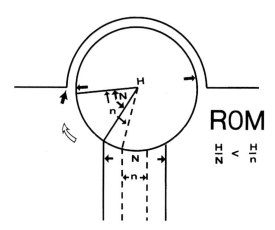

Figure 45–3. The head/neck ratio influences motions before impingement. The motion "n" of the head/neck ratio H/N is less than that "n" of the more narrow neck H/n.

tension and joint contact pressure. An illustration of the moment arm of hip extensor muscles that act in the sagittal plane is shown in Figure 45–7.

During surgical reconstruction of diseased hip joints, the anatomy is altered to achieve the ultimate relationship of the hip joint to the rest of the body and to the muscles acting across the hip joint. These alterations may include the location of the acetabulum and femoral head, thus changing either the origin or the insertion of the muscles as they cross the hip. These biomechanical considerations are currently referred to as offset.

The increasing interest in restoring offset is directed to provide optimal functional efficiency. The efficiency is seen as improving strength, and as the muscle is more efficient, it exerts less force at the joint articulation. In a study of 86 procedures, we have noted a statistically significant relationship between femoral offset, allowing both greater motion and strength.[12] Since the previous edition of this text, the importance of offset is more recognized and some prosthetic systems have been designed with flexibility to adjust the offset of the prosthetic replacement.[11] As noted earlier, prosthetic stability is also enhanced by the proper tensioning of the hip musculature, which is influenced by the design and placement of the implant.

The relationship between neck shaft angle and neck length defines the offset for a specific implant. The value of—and means of—adjusting the offset is being increasingly recognized in femoral prosthetic designs (Fig. 45–8). In fact, it has been estimated that as many as nine discrete femoral size and diminished implants are

Table 45–2. MAXIMUM HIP MOTION IN DAILY ACTIVITIES

	Hip motion (in degrees)					
Function	**Flexion**	**Extension**	**Abduction**	**Adduction**	**Internal Rotation**	**External Rotation**
Walking	65 Stair	10 Slope	14 Stair	5 Slope	5 Stair	9 Ramp
Hygiene	118 Shoe		22 Tub	6 Tub	5 Socks	24 Tub
Household	119 Pick		30 Oven	12 Oven	22 Place	25 Reach
Recreation	108 Car	12 Golf	37 Car	11 Golf	24 Car	33 Golf

From Chao EYS, Rim K, Smidt GL, Johnston RC: The application of 4 × 4 matrix method to the correction of the measurements of hip joint rotations. J Biomech 3:459, 1970.

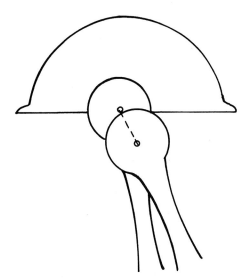

Figure 45–4. Larger femoral head designs require a greater displacement to "escape" the cup.

Table 45–3 HIP FUNCTIONAL STRENGTH POTENTIAL

Function	Isometric (percent)	Isokinetic (percent)
Extension	25	32
Flexion	24	29
Adduction	21	4
Abduction	14	11
Internal rotation	8	14
External rotation	7	10

Data from Fick R: Handbuch der Anatomie des Menschen, vol 2. Berlin, Verlag von Gustav Fisher, 1910, p 175.

necessary to properly fit and "off set" 80 percent of femoral morphologic and size variations.[11]

On the acetabular side, enhanced offset can be gained by a lateral displaced hip center brought about by a special polyethylene insert. The clinical utility of this option has yet to be determined because an increased moment is applied to the polyethylene liner, which could render this unstable. One assessment did show a reasonable difference in the wear rate of a polyethylene acetabular component in a group of patients with "too little" offset.[16]

Bone Remodeling

Major factors in long-term success of joint replacement are stability and component resistance to mechanical failures, which may be expressed as loosening of the prosthesis, lysis of bone, fracture of bone, or fracture of the prosthesis. Thus, understanding the mechanisms of bony response to implantation is the key in achieving a successful joint replacement. Very high stresses act on the bone implant-fixation interface. These tend to be greatest in compression, both proximally and distally, whereas the midportion of the implant is relatively "quiet" (Fig. 45–9). Because the implantation dramatically changes the loading configurations, bone remodeling is an inevitable consequence of the joint replacement. In addition, over time, bony structure remodeling

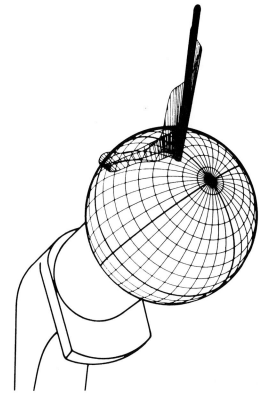

Figure 45–5. Scaled three-dimensional plot of resultant force during the first cycle of gait with crutches. The lengths of the lines indicate the magnitude of force. Radial line segments are drawn at equal increments of time, so the distance between the segments indicates the rate at which the orientation of the force was changing. For higher amplitudes of force during stance phase, line segments in close proximity indicate that the orientation of the force was changing relatively little with the cone angle between 30 and 40 degrees and the polar angle between –25 and –15 degrees. (From Davy DT, Kotzar GM, Brown RH, et al: Telemetric force measurements across the hip after total arthroplasty. J Bone Joint Surg 70A:45, 1989.)

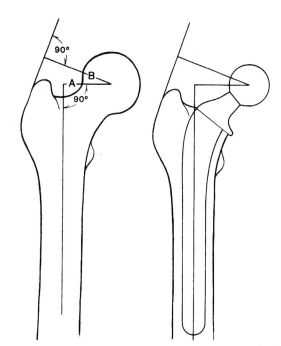

Figure 45–6. The moment arm of a muscle is the perpendicular distance from the line of action to the point or axis of rotation.

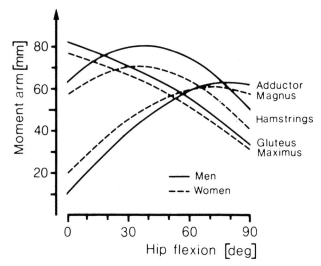

Figure 45–7. Graphic illustration of mean moment arm lengths at different hip angles in 10 men and 10 women.[13]

is continuous and a new equilibrium is continuously established. Otherwise, the prosthesis becomes loose.

The ability of bone to remodel as it adapts structurally to changing loads or signals has been described by what is now known as Wolff's law, first discussed in

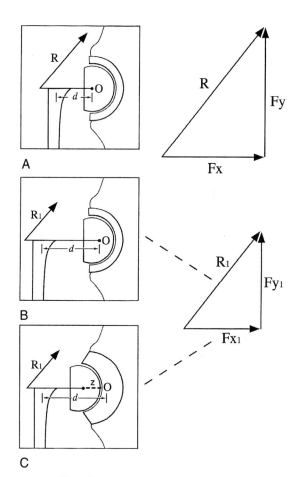

Figure 45–8. The offset of hip replacements is employed to optimize the forces across the prosthetic joint (**A**). The offset can be increased by a laterally placed cup insert (**B**) or by increasing the neck length/angle (**C**).

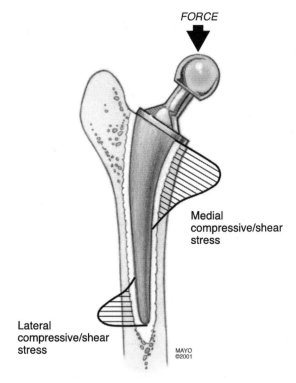

Figure 45–9. The strain distribution of the proximal femur of a cemented stemmed device reveals high compressive stresses proximally, radially, and lateral distally. The mid portion of the stem is "quiet" with low stresses exhibited in this region.

1869.[19] The observation is that the trabecular structure orients in the direction of principal stress.[3]

If the mechanical stress signals exceed an upper or lower discrete threshold described by a "remodeling rule," either bony deposition or resorption occurs. This variation in bony structure in turn alters the stress or strain distribution. The process continues until the remodeling rule is satisfied. In the past, analytic models to predict stress distribution were unable to address the critical issue of these time-dependent changes.

Finite Element Analysis

This type of analytical evaluation, called finite element analysis, is extremely important to estimate long-term

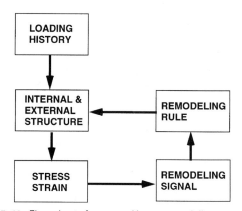

Figure 45–10. Flow chart of proposed bone remodeling process.

femoral changes resulting from implant replacement. The finite element method is a numerical procedure used to determine structural deformation and stress distribution under given loads. The major advantage of the finite element over other mathematical methods is its ability to deal with nonhomogeneous materials and irregular structural geometries, which is ideal for the study of the bone prosthesis composite.

Bone Remodeling Theory

The bone remodeling theory is a mathematical formulation presented in flow chart form in Figure 45–10. Cancellous bone is assumed to be an optimal structure that minimizes an objective function by appropriately distributing the apparent density and trabecular alignment.[8,9]

Practical Application to Uncemented Prosthesis Replacement

An ideal application for the bone remodeling theory is the prediction of the long-term bony response to joint replacement, because of the dramatic changes in the loading configurations. As an example, the predicted bony structure after implantation of the Mayo short-stemmed uncemented femoral replacement component has been evaluated.[13] The purpose of this implant is to provide optimal stress transfer to the metaphysis so that stress shielding can be significantly reduced proximally and stress transfer can be nearly normal distally (Fig. 45–11). The predicted long-term remodeling results after replacement show that the apparent density distribution remains unchanged except for an area of minor resorption at the outside tip of the calcar; this agrees

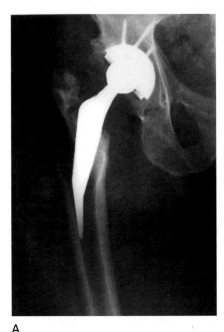

A

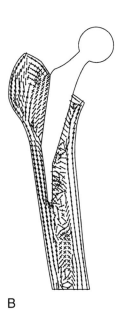

B

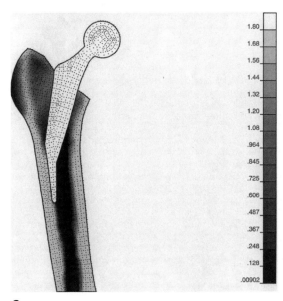

C

Figure 45–11. Bony structure immediately after implantion of Mayo short-stemmed femoral replacement component: **A**, apparent density prediction; **B**, fabric tensor prediction; and **C**, actual bony structure.

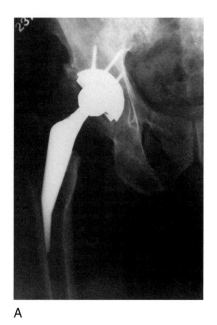

A

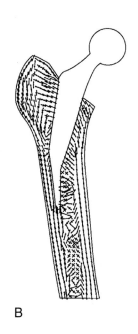

B

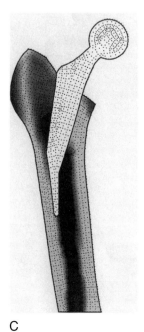

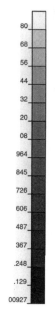

C

Figure 45–12. Bone structure 6 years after implantion of Mayo short-stemmed femoral replacement component: **A,** apparent density prediction; **B,** fabric tensor prediction; and **C,** actual bony structure.

with a 6-year follow-up radiograph (Fig. 45–12). With the increasing use of dual-energy x-ray absorptiometry (DEXA) scans, we can now quantitate the amount of bone present after prosthetic replacement. DEXA scans promise to be of great value in understanding the actual implication of hip replacement on proximal bone remodeling.

References

1. Bergmann G, Graichen F, Rohlmann A: Hip joint loading during walking and running, measured in two patients. J Biomech 16:969, 1993.
2. Brown M, Hislop HJ, Waters RL, Porel L: Walking efficiency before and after total hip replacement. J Am Phys Ther Assoc 60:1259, 1980.
3. Cowin SC: Wolff's law of trabecular architecture at remodeling equilibrium. J Biomech Eng 108:83, 1986.
4. Davy DT, Kotzar GM, Brown RH, et al: Telemetric force measurements across the hip after total arthroplasty. J Bone Joint Surg 70A:45, 1989.
5. English TA, Kilvington M: In vivo records of hip loads using a femoral implant with telemetric output [a preliminary report]. J Biomed Eng 1:111, 1979.
6. Fackler CD, Poss R: Dislocation in total hip arthroplasties. Clin Orthop 151:169, 1980.
7. Fick R: Handbuch der Anatomie des Menschen, vol 2. Berlin, Verlag von Gustav Fisher, 1910, p 175.
8. Fyhrie DP, Carter DR: A unifying principle relating stress to trabecular bone morphology. J Orthop Res 4:304, 1986.
9. Huiskes R, Weinans H, Grootenboer HJ, et al: Adaptic bone-remodeling theory applied to prosthetic-design analysis. J Biomech 20: 1135, 1987.
10. Johnston RC, Smidt GL: Measurement of hip-joint motion during walking. J Bone Joint Surg 61A:1083, 1969.

11. Massin P, Geais L, Astoin E, et al: The anatomic basis for the concept of lateralized femoral stems. A frontal plane radiographic study of the proximal femur. J Arthroplasty 15:93, 2000.

12. McGrory BJ, Morrey BF, Cahalan TD, et al: Effect of femoral offset on range of motion and abductor muscle strength after total hip arthroplasty. J Bone Joint Surg 78B:865, 1995.

13. Morrey BF: Short-stemmed uncemented femoral component for primary hip arthroplasty. Clin Orthop 249:169, 1989.

14. Nemeth G, Ohlsen H: In vivo moment arm lengths for hip extensor muscles at different angles of hip flexion. J Biomech 18:129, 1985.

15. Rydell NW: Forces acting on the femoral-head prosthesis: A study on strain gauge supplied prostheses in living persons. Acta Orthop Scand 88:1 (Suppl 37), 1966.

16. Sakalkale DP, Sharkey PF, Eng K, et al: Effect of femoral component offset on polyethylene wear in total hip arthroplasty. Clin Orthop 388:125, 2001.

17. Walker PS: Design and performance of joint replacements. In Chapman's Orthopedic Surgery, vol 3, 3rd ed. Philadelphia, Lippincott, Williams & Wilkins, 2000, p 2573.

18. Waters RL, Lunsford BR, Perry J, Byrd R: Energy-speed relationship of walking: Standard tables. J Orthop Res 6:215, 1988.

19. Wolff J: Ueber die Bedeutung der Architektur der Spongiosen Substanz. Zent Bl Med Wiss 6:223, 1869.

46

Cemented Acetabular Components

•PANAYIOTIS J. PAPAGELOPOULOS and BERNARD F. MORREY

DESIGN CONSIDERATIONS

Most efforts to improve prosthetic acetabular function and design have been with uncemented devices. The majority of basic and clinical studies are focused on the problem of wear debris. However, additional design features are directed to enhance stability, avoid impingement, optimize motion, preserve bone, and allow for ease of revision.

The concern over acetabular loosening has all but eliminated the use of cemented cups in the United States. This is unfortunate, because an objective assessment of clinical experience does support the continued practice of cementing the cup in the older (more than 70 years of age) patient. Radiographic observation of bone-cement lucency of the ultra-high-molecular-weight-polyethylene (UHMWPE) acetabular cup ranges from 25 percent to 100 percent in various long-term follow-up studies.[1,2,10,13,14,30,32,34] Stauffer reported that the 10-year Mayo Clinic experience with cemented non–metal-backed acetabular components showed some radiographic lucency at a rate approaching 100 percent.[33] Yet one study of 42 Charnley implants followed for 12 to 16 years revealed 2 (5 percent) to be definitely loose by radiographic criteria.[17] I strongly believe that the practice of cementing an all-polyethylene acetabular component should be continued in the older patient and thus has preserved this topic for the third edition of this text.

ANALYTICAL DATA

Cup and Cement Thickness

Finite element studies have shown that, with joint replacement, a reproducible pattern of tendencies results in concentration of stresses (1) in the cancellous bone superior to the cup; (2) in the cement; (3) at the medial wall of the ilium; and (4) in the substance of the acetabulum itself.[7]

Stress levels underlying the subchondral bone increase high-density polyethylene (HDPE) wall thickness decreases,[27] and stress within the polymethylmethacrylate (PMMA) increases as the acetabular component wall thickness decreases. Furthermore, tensile and compressive stresses increase markedly through a spectrum of head sizes. Between the 22- and 44-mm head femoral implants, the maximal tensile stresses increase by 400 percent and maximal compressive stresses by 200 percent.[27] Increasing the thickness of the UHMWPE causes proportionately decreasing microstrain, thus favoring the thicker component (Fig. 46–1). Changes in cement thickness from 1 cm to between 3 and 5 cm not only lessens the torque to failure but also changes the stress distribution of the acetabulum, with a thicker cement mantle resulting in a more uniform and lower stress distribution (Fig. 46–2).

Head Size

The calculated surface contact stress for a simulated 28-mm head system is less than that for the 22-mm head. As the clearance increases from 0.1 to 0.5 mm, the surface stress increases proportionately but not linearly.[3] Hence, head size is not a major determinant of designing the all-polyethylene cup as long as 8-mm thickness is realized by the design.

Metal-Backed Acetabular Implant

Care should be exercised when interpreting and applying such data to the clinical setting.

Theoretical studies of the effect of loading the acetabulum through a prosthetic implant show a tendency for the prosthetic cup to buckle from increased compressive stresses at the apex of the cup and maximum tensile stresses at the periphery[26] (Fig. 46–3). This effect is muted by techniques that enhance the stress distribution of the system such as retaining subchondral bone.[26] Because peak stresses are greater in cancellous than in subchondral bone, cancellous bone is not well suited to withstand stresses imparted through a prosthetic implant. In a normal setting, the posteromedial aspect of the acetabulum is the site of greatest stress. These data from Oonishi[26] indicate that the technique of acetabular preparation should attempt to preserve the subchondral bone and that ideally the position of the resultant vector of force

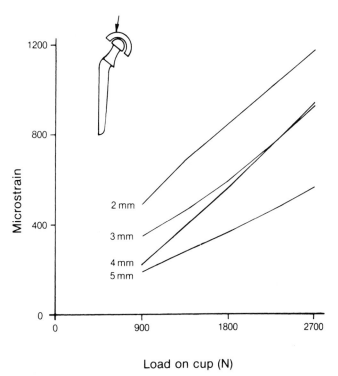

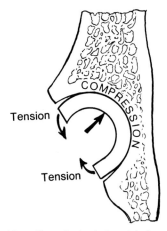

Figure 46–1. Increased strain is observed in the polymethylmethacrylate liner for the thin 2-mm HDPE component compared with those in the thicker 4- and 5-mm models. (From Oh I, Sander TW, Treharne RW: Total hip acetabular cup flange design and its effect on fixation. Clin Orthop 195:304, 1985.)

transmission should be directed posteriorly and superiorly.

The increased stresses in the PMMA that occur after subchondral bone removal are lessened by the use of a metal-backed implant.[4,8,27] In spite of this theoretical value, the clinical experience with cemented metal-backed cups was a disaster. Reviewing their experience from 1980 to 1982, Ritter et al. demonstrated that the likelihood of a

Figure 46–3. Buckling effect of a loaded acetabular component.

loose component with a metal-backed device was statistically greater than that with a polyethylene-cemented implant (P <.001).[28] Other experience supports the poorer clinical results with the metal-backed implant.[22]

The "Ideal Design"

Component design with pod extensions and an undercut groove appear most effective at resisting applied torque. Spacers or pods applied to the surface of the acetabulum ensure a minimal and uniform cement mantle thickness. In addition, experimental studies have demonstrated that, at the time of insertion, a circumferential flange, or lip, provided increased pressurization of the cement into the underlying bone.[24] The conclusion may be drawn that an ideal acetabular component might consist of a series of pods to ensure a uniform cement mantle and a circumferential flange about the lip of the component to enhance cement intrusion into the bone (Fig. 46–4).

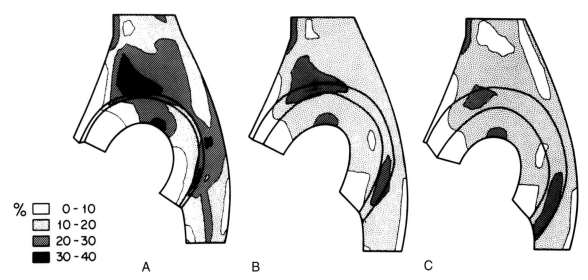

%
- 0 - 10
- 10 - 20
- 20 - 30
- 30 - 40

A   B   C

Figure 46–2. (A) Von Mises' yield contours for total hip replacement with 1 mm of PMMA. (B) Total hip replacement with 3 mm of PMMA. (C) Total hip replacement with 5 mm of PMMA. Note the lessening of the peak stresses with the thicker PMMA preparation. (From Carter DR, Vasu R, Harris WH: Stress distributions in the acetabular region. II. Effects of cement thickness and metal-backing of the total hip acetabular component. J Biomech 15:165, 1982.)

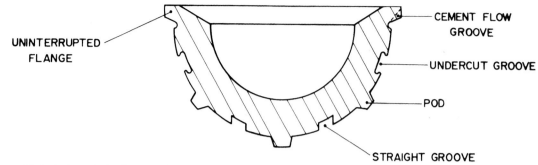

Figure 46–4. Surface design features of the "ideal" UHMWPE acetabular component. (From Oh I, Sander TW, Treharne RW: Total hip acetabular cup flange design and its effect on fixation. Clin Orthop 195:304, 1985.)

INDICATIONS

Most would agree that the indications for cemented HDPE cups are in patients older than 65 or 70 of age or those who have less than 50 percent of host bone available for cement fixation. Current thought also favors the use of HDPE cups for certain revision procedures in the face of cancellous bone graft or to revise well-fixed modular shells.

TECHNIQUE CONSIDERATIONS

Most of the considerable effort directed toward improving the technique has related to (1) preparation of the acetabular bed, (2) attainment of a critical width of a reproducible PMMA layer, and (3) effective use and penetration of PMMA.

Surgical Technique

Serial reaming progresses only to the subchondral bone. A series of satellite defects measuring 3 mm in diameter and 3 mm in depth are placed circumferentially around the rim of the acetabulum, especially in any residual sclerotic areas. Pulsed lavage with 0.05 percent neomycin saline cleanses the interspaces of blood and fat. The acetabulum is dried with sponges, and the cement is inserted at a relatively early (wet) stage.

Cement Mantle

Thumb pressure is used to optimize the intrusion, especially around the superior weight-bearing surface. A silicone plunger is then used to further pressurize the cement. The acetabular component is 2 to 4 mm smaller in diameter than the largest reamer and is placed in 15 degrees of anteversion, with care taken to tilt the component 40 degrees rather than the usual 45 degrees horizontally. Uniform quality bone-cement interfaces are obtained with this technique (Fig. 46–5).

Cement Intrusion

Because PMMA can be the weakest link of fixation, a critical minimal cement thickness has been proposed for optimal fixation. The relationship of PMMA strain according to applied load as a function of different cement layers is shown in Figure 46–1.[8,23] This theoretical observation has been substantiated in the clinical setting as well.[20] To ensure a uniform cement mantle distribution of at least 3 mm in thickness, some cups have been designed with PMMA studs to facilitate reliable attainment of a uniform and adequate mantle thickness. There are no clinical data at this time that demonstrate whether this design feature is only theoretically correct or also of practical value in that it does, in fact, increase the longevity of the interface. Nonetheless, we do over-ream the acetabulum by at least 2 mm to ensure a minimum of 2 to 3 mm of PMMA thickness around the cup.

RESULTS

Radiographic Versus Clinical Results

A major problem confronting the clinician is disparity between radiographic and clinical results, even if the roentgenograms are carefully and systematically

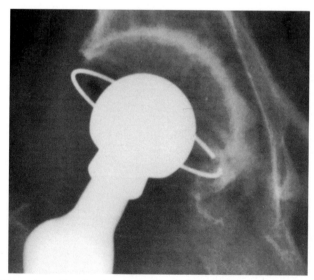

Figure 46–5. Excellent bone-cement interface in all three zones is regularly obtained with the technique described.

measured.[12] In spite of concern about roentgenographic appearances, and in spite of the instruction and preparation of the "younger" orthopedic surgeon, the clinical results of the polyethylene-cemented acetabular components have been surprisingly good (see Fig. 46–5). In an excellent study, Garcia-Cimbrelo and Munuera reported experience with 680 patients followed for an average of almost 13 years.[17] This analysis studied "early" (i.e., less than 10 years after surgery) and "late" (i.e., radiographic or clinical failure more than 10 years after surgery) loosening or failure. Among the 680 patients, loosening occurred early in 29 and late in 32. Clinically, 76 percent of the 29 patients in the early failure group were considered failures, representing 1.5 percent of the overall sample. However, only 28 percent of the 32 patients classified as late failures demonstrated radiographically clinical dissatisfaction. Thus, overall, approximately 2 percent in this patient population were classified as clinical failures. In those showing evidence of lucency in less than 10 years, statistically significant correlations occurred with the underlying diagnosis of congenital hip dysplasia, acetabular fracture, and protrusio acetabuli. In contrast, among those 32 patients demonstrating radiographic lucency more than 10 years after surgery, 56 percent had more than 2 mm of wear (P<.001). The typical radiographic appearance of this sample was a complete radiolucent line around the entire acetabular component.

Further evidence of the effectiveness of cemented HDPE acetabula is reported from Athens by Hartofilakidis and co-workers.[18] After 359 Charnley implants, those patients, who were followed from 1 to 4 years had 98 percent satisfactory results without lucent lines; in those followed from 5 to 9 years, 92 percent demonstrated no significant radiolucent lines. However, in those followed for more than 10 years, a marked dropoff was seen; only 78 percent demonstrated a satisfactory result. Most recently, a Swedish experience averaging 14 years placed the failure rate of the acetabulum at 5 percent.[17]

Cement Failure and Wear Debris

Willert et al. carefully analyzed the histologic findings of loose acetabular components.[35] In this study, samples in which the PMMA had not demonstrated fragmentation showed less loosening than those in which the PMMA had fractured. This implicates the failure of PMMA as a cause of late loosening, but the exact relationship is not clear. It is possible that small fragments of PMMA become lodged between the HDPE and the metal femoral head (three-body abrasion), aggravating and accelerating the wear process.

Consistent with the observation of Willert and Garcia and their colleagues are the findings Wroblewski et al.'s from a study of 59 retrieved acetabular components.[37] In this sample, 19 were demonstrated to have deficient cement between the polyethylene and the bone, indicating that the failure occurred at the bone-cement interface. It was concluded that in possibly as many as 30 percent, loosening of the acetabulum occurred from debris that was generated at the bone-cement interface rather than from the articulation itself.

TECHNIQUE FACTORS

Russotti and colleagues analyzed 251 procedures 5 to 7 years after surgery that employed the so-called contemporary cementing technique for implants inserted at our institution from 1978 through 1980.[29] They identified only 1 patient with definite evidence of radiographic loosening, and no patient underwent cup revision during this period of time. As further support for such clinical results, Cornell and Ranawat reviewed the radiographic appearance of patients who had acetabula prepared with a pulsed lavage.[1] The group whose implants were inserted from 1971 through 1978 without this technique had a significantly greater number of lucent lines than those whose procedures were performed with pulsed lavage between 1979 and 1980.

SELECTION FACTORS

Eftekhar and Nercessian performed a thoughtful analysis of the literature to define the risk factors contributing to radiolucency associated with the acetabular component.[20] One technical factor that was implicated in the presence of radiolucent lines was deepening and widening of the acetabulum, presumably interfering with the strength of the subchondral bone. Further, the extent and frequency of radiolucent lines increased with increased surveillance. In one of the most comprehensive and interesting comparisons, Önsten et al. compared 201 patients with rheumatoid arthritis with 200 who had osteoarthritis.[25] The 10-year survival, free of revision, of the patients with rheumatoid arthritis was 95 percent, compared with 89 percent of those with osteoarthritis. The combined series demonstrates approximately 95 percent likelihood of revision-free survival at 7 years in those who had surgery after 1981 compared with approximately 80 percent of those who had surgery before 1981. These data suggest improved results associated with modified cementing techniques.

Age

Today, our understanding of the indications for, and effectiveness of, the cemented cup is predicated on our own Mayo study of 2000 primary Charnley arthroplasties followed for 25 years.[6] This is the most comprehensive study of its type in the literature. We found that by far, the most dominant factor, correlating to cup survival was the age of the patient at the time of reimplantation. Twenty-five year survivorship free of revision for aseptic loosening was poorer for each decade earlier in life that the procedure was performed and varied from 68.2 percent in patients younger than 40 years of age to 100 percent for patients 80 years of age or older (Fig. 46–6).

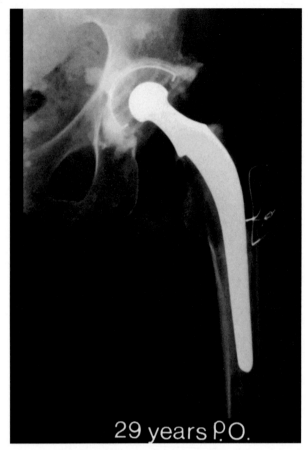

Figure 46–6. Twenty-nine year radiograph of cemented cup in patient 69 years of age at the time of hip replacement.

Male patients had a twofold higher rate of implant revision for aseptic loosening than female patients (25-year survivorship, 95 percent for females versus 81 percent for males, ($P < 0.0001$). The 25-year survivorship rates for acetabular and femoral components free of aseptic loosening were virtually identical (89.6 percent and 89.7 percent, respectively), but acetabular survivorship was worse than femoral survivorship in younger patients (Figs. 46–7 and 46–8).

Previous studies have also demonstrated that, for younger patients, cemented sockets fare worse than cemented femoral implants.[5,31,33] The Mayo Clinic study confirms and extends those findings by providing specific survivorship information for the acetabular and femoral implants for each decade of life. This experience shows that cemented acetabular and femoral component performances are both dependent on age at implantation but that the effect of age is more profound on acetabular component performance.

AUTHOR'S PREFERENCE

Disagreement remains within our institution and within the orthopedic community regarding the indications for using HDPE acetabular components because of the disparity between the radiographic appearance and the clinical performance of the polyethylene acetabulum component. I use cement in all patients who are older than the age of 70 years (Fig. 46–8). I also cement acetabula in those patients for whom I have concern regarding the adequacy of bone to stabilize an uncemented device. The implant I use has a circumferential flange but no pods. The acetabulum is carefully prepared to bleeding subchondral bone, but equal care is taken not to remove the subchondral bone in order to enhance the stability of the underlying substrate. In the superior subchondral bone, 3-mm dimples are also liberally used.

Clinical experience with this technique and selection has been gratifying. Hence, in my opinion, the only two issues remaining are (1) whether there is enhanced stability from the modular implant; and (2) whether techniques for proper cementing are being taught in our residencies now that cemented cups are not being used. I have no solution for the latter issue. However, at the Mayo Clinic, we did compare a 10-year history of cemented and modular cups inserted in patients older than 70 years of age, and we found no statistical difference in the instability rate. Hence, we do believe that the cemented cup should be used for patients older than 70 years of age. The data support this clinical practice.

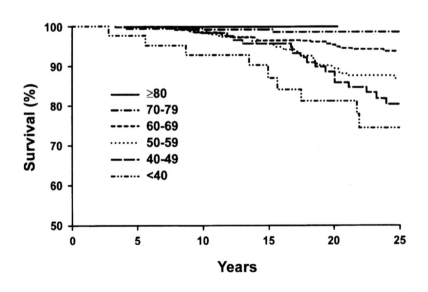

Figure 46–7. Kaplan-Meier survival curve free of revision for acetabular patients stratified by age. Note the excellent 20-year survival rate in patients older than 70 years of age.

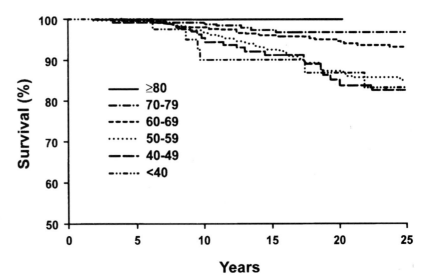

Figure 46–8. Kaplan-Meier survival curve for the femur. The survival rate free of revision is better than that achieved with the cemented cup in patients younger than 60 years of age but no better than in those older than 70 years of age.

References

1. Amstutz HC, Markolf KL, McNiece GM, Gruen TA: Loosening of total hip components: Cause and prevention. *In* The Hip: Proceedings of the 4th Open Scientific Meeting of the Hip Society. St. Louis, CV Mosby, 1976.
2. Andersson GBJ, Freeman MAR, Swanson SAV: Loosening of the cemented acetabular cup in total hip replacement. J Bone Joint Surg 54B:590, 1972.
3. Bartel DL, Bicknele MS, Wright TM: The effect of conformity, thickness, and material on stresses in ultra-high molecular weight components for total joint replacement. J Bone Joint Surg 68A:1041, 1986.
4. Bartel DL, Wright TM, Edwards D: The effect of metal backing on stresses in polyethylene acetabular components. *In* Hungerford DS (ed): The Hip: Proceedings of the 11th Open Scientific Meeting of the Hip Society. St. Louis, CV Mosby, 1983, p 229.
5. Barrack RL, Mulroy RD Jr, Harris WH: Improved cementing techniques and femoral component loosening in young patients with hip arthroplasty. A 12-year radiographic review. J Bone Joint Surg 74B:384, 1992.
6. Berry DJ, Harmsen WS, Cabanela ME, Morrey BF: 25-year survivorship of 2000 consecutive primary Charnley total hip arthroplasties. J Bone Joint Surg 84A:171, 2002.
7. Carter DR: Finite-element analysis of a metal-backed acetabular component. *In* Hungerford DS (ed): The Hip: Proceedings of the 11th Open Scientific Meeting of the Hip Society St. Louis, CV Mosby, 1983, p 216.
8. Carter DR, Vasu R, Harris WH: Stress distributions in the acetabular region. II. Effects of cement thickness and metal-backing of the total hip acetabular component. J Biomech 15:165, 1982.
9. Chandler HP, Reineck FT, Wixson RL, McCarthy JC: Total hip arthroplasty in patients younger than 30 years old: Five year follow-up study. J Bone Joint Surg 63A:1426, 1981.
10. Charnley J, Cupic Z: The nine- and ten-year results of the low friction arthroplasty of the hip. Clin Orthop 95:9, 1973.
11. Cornell CN, Ranawat CS: The impact of modern cement techniques on acetabular fixation in cemented total hip replacement. J Arthroplasty 1:197, 1986.
12. Crowninshield RD, Pedersen DR, Brand RA, Johnston RC: Analytical support for acetabular component metal backing. *In* Hungerford DS (ed): The Hip: Proceedings of the 11th Open Scientific Meeting of the Hip Society. St. Louis, CV Mosby, 1983, p 207.
13. Delee JG, Charnley J: Radiological demarcation of cemented sockets in total hip replacement. Clin Orthop 121:20, 1976.
14. Dorr LD, Cane TJ, Canaty JP: Long-term results of cemented total hip arthroplasty in patients 45 years old or younger. A sixteen year follow-up study. J Arthroplasty 9:453, 1994.
15. Eftekhar NS, Nercessian O: Incidence and mechanism of failure of cemented acetabular component in total hip arthroplasty. Orthop Clin North Am 19:557, 1988.
16. Garcia-Cimbrelo E, Munuera L: Early and late loosening of the acetabular cup after low-friction arthroplasty. J Bone Joint Surg 74:1119, 1992.
17. Garellick G, Herberts P, Strümberg C, Malchau H: Long-term results of Charnley arthroplasty: A 12- to 16-year follow-up study. J Arthroplasty 9:333, 1994.
18. Hartofilakidis G, Stamos K, Ioannidis TT: Fifteen years' experience with Charnley low-friction arthroplasty. Clin Orthop 246:48, 1989.
19. Hozak WJ, Rothman RH, Booth RE, et al: Survivorship analysis of 1,041 Charnley total hip arthroplasties. J Arthroplasty 5:41, 1990.
20. Joshi RP, Eftekhar NS, McMahon DJ, Nercessian O: Osteolysis after Charnley primary low-friction arthroplasty. A comparison of two matched paired groups. J Bone Joint Surg 80B:585, 1998.
21. Kobayashi S, Eftekhar NS, Terayama K, Joshi RP: Comparative study of total hip arthroplasty between younger and older patients. Clin Orthop 339:140, 1997.
22. Mattingley DA, Hopson CN, Kahn A, Geannestras NJ: Aseptic loosening in metal-backed acetabular components for total hip replacement. J Bone Joint Surg 67A:387, 1985.
23. Oh I: A comprehensive analysis of the factors affecting acetabular cup fixation and design in total hip replacement arthroplasty: A series of experimental and clinical studies. *In* Hungerford DS (ed): The Hip: Proceedings of the 11th Open Scientific Meeting of the Hip Society. St. Louis, CV Mosby, 1983, p 129.
24. Oh I, Sander TW, Treharne RW: Total hip acetabular cup flange design and its effect on cement fixation. Clin Orthop 195:304, 1985.
25. Önsten I, Besjakov J, Carlsson AS: Improved radiographic survival of the Charnley prosthesis in rheumatoid arthritis and osteoarthritis: Results of new versus old operative techniques in 402 hips. J Arthroplasty 9:3, 1994.
26. Oonishi H: Mechanical analysis of the human pelvis and its application to the artificial hip joint by means of the three dimensional finite element method. J Biomech 16:427, 1983.
27. Pedersen DR, Crowninshield RD, Brand RA, Johnston RC: An axisymmetric model of acetabular components in total hip arthroplasty. J Biomech 15:305, 1982.
28. Ritter MA, Faris PM, Keating EM, Brugo G: Influential factors in cemented acetabular cup loosening. J Arthroplasty 7(Suppl):365, 1992.
29. Russotti GM, Coventry MB, Stauffer RN: Cemented total hip arthroplasty with contemporary techniques: A five-year minimum follow-up. Clin Orthop 235:141, 1988.
30. Salvati EA, Wright TM, Burnstein AH, Jacobs B: Fracture of polyethylene acetabular cups. J Bone Joint Surg 61A:1239, 1979.
31. Sarmiento A, Ebramzadeh E, Gogan WJ, McKellop HA: Total hip arthroplasty with cement. A long-term radiographic analysis in patients who are older than 50 and younger than 50 years. J Bone Joint Surg 72A:1470, 1990.

32. Stauffer RN: Ten year follow-up study of total hip replacement with particular reference to roentgenographic loosening of the components. J Bone Joint Surg 64A:983, 1982.

33. Sullivan PM, McKenzie JR, Callaghan JJ, Johnston RC: Total hip arthroplasty with cement in patients who are less than 50 years old. A 16 to 22 year follow-up study. J Bone Joint Surg 76A:863, 1994.

34. Sutherland CJ, Wilde AH, Borden LS, Marks KE: A ten-year follow-up of 100 consecutive Müller curved-stem total hip replacement arthroplasties. J Bone Joint Surg 64A:970, 1982.

35. Willert HG, Bertram H, Buchhorn GH: Osteolysis in alloarthroplasty of the hip: the role of bone cement fragmentation. Clin Orthop 258:108, 1990.

36. Wroblewski BM, Lynch M, Atkinson JR, et al: External wear of the polyethylene socket in cement total hip arthroplasty. J Bone Joint Surg 69B:61, 1987.

47

Uncemented Acetabular Components

· ROBERT T. TROUSDALE

Charnley's introduction of methyl methacrylate for prosthetic fixation revolutionized the treatment of patients with arthritic conditions of the hip. Long-term results have proved its efficacy in providing durable, functional improvement in the majority of patients.[20] Although clinical results with cemented techniques remain fairly successful, the long-term radiographic loosening rates of cemented sockets remain high. Up to 48 percent of cemented sockets have been reported to be radiographically loose at 20 years.[1,2,33,45,46,76,80,94] These rates have not been improved with modern cement techniques or metal backing of the cemented sockets.[2,3,60,65] Furthermore, results of cemented revision total hip arthroplasty have been shown to be markedly less durable than the results after primary cemented total hip arthroplasty.

Efforts to improve the fixation of the acetabular components have led to the development of prosthetic designs that obtain more biologic fixation.[18,40,69,73,75,92] Uncemented sockets have many theoretical potential advantages. They are easy to use, and the cup position can be readily changed intraoperatively. The use of modular liners may improve effective cup position, enhancing stability. Ingrowth reliably has been shown to occur in multiple retrieval studies. Since the early 1990s, the use of noncemented sockets has greatly increased and has become the implant of choice in North America for the majority of patients. A matched-pair study comparing cemented acetabular with cementless porous-coated components showed a longer revision rate and lower incidence of radiographic loosening for porous-coated components than for cemented components. It remains to be seen whether the overall clinical and radiographic results in long-term follow-up will be better than those achieved by cemented all-polyethylene designs.

DESIGN

There are basically four design options used to obtain immediate fixation of an uncemented acetabular component: (1) a threaded metal shell, (2) contour of the metal shell, (3) transfixing screws or projections, and (4) a combination of these features.

Threaded Design

Threaded acetabular components were never popular in the United States, and they have fallen further into disfavor for several legitimate reasons: (1) Biologic fixation does not occur predictably and the implants tend to loosen; (2) cups that are loose tend to be painful; (3) removal of an excessive amount of bone may be needed for insertion or removal; (4) orientation can be difficult, and instability can be a problem; and (5) the overall clinical experience in some series has been disappointing.[78,83]

Hemispheric Design

Hemispheric components may be secured by an interference fit or by use of transfixing screws or pegs or both.[18,73,75] Currently, hemispheric cups are most widely used in the United States because they allow great flexibility and proper orientation of the implant and are relatively easy to use. To augment the initial fixation of a hemispheric socket to the acetabulum, lugs, spikes, and screws have been placed in the dome and periphery of the socket. Improvement in acetabular fixation is seen with one, two, and three screws. The fixation that results from three screws, three spikes, or two pegs shows no difference in displacement at 100-kg loads. However, three-screw fixation is associated with the highest load to displacement.[54] Use of more than four screws does not appear to be beneficial in routine case. The placement of the screws also appears to be important. Anterior column screws provide relatively poor fixation and put the iliac vein and obturator artery at risk; for these reasons, they probably should be avoided.[87]

Although screws may reliably provide secondary fixation, there are concerns with their use. These include cold flow and wear of the polyethylene in the screw holes, tracking of polyethylene along the pathway of the screws to the host bone, and fretting at the junction of the screw and the metal-backed cup.[11,12,41,42,56,93] Another method of hemispheric fixation is the addition of a peripheral truncated cone to the shell shape. This cone provides a firm ream fit and obviates the need for axillary screws. Oversizing a hemispheric cup by under-reaming the host bone has been shown to decrease the motion at the implant-bone interface. However, wide gaps in the dome region and decreased contact between the available porous-coated surface and the host bone have been demonstrated in cadaveric studies when the oversizing technique was used. Furthermore, oversizing an implant by 4 mm probably carries an unacceptable rate of acetabular fracture during insertion. Even oversizing a component by 2 mm requires a large force (2000 N) to seat the component.[51]

The noncemented implants currently in use in the United States are made of titanium, cobalt-chrome alloy, or tantalum. The ingrowth of bone has been shown to occur in all three metals. Titanium has the advantages of improved biocompatibility, decreased material stiffness, and the ability to bond chemically to bone.[21,25,36,37] Cobalt-chrome has the theoretical advantages of improved metal hardness, with a subsequent decrease in the amount of wear debris.[55] Cobalt-chrome is also less notch sensitive, making bead application to the substrate more reliable.

BONE INGROWTH

Bone ingrowth into a porous-coated device occurs if the following conditions are met: (1) There must not be excessive motion between the implant and the host bone; (2) there must be intimate contact between the porous surface and the host bone; and (3) pore size must be in the optimal range. If all of these conditions are met, bone ingrowth occurs by a process similar to that of fracture healing—namely, inflammation, repair, and remodeling.[37,43,82,95] Analyses of retrieved acetabular components have demonstrated ingrowth between 0 percent and 100 percent of available porous surfaces.[6,24,26,27,35] The wide reported range of bone growth percentage is explained by varying techniques used for analyzing ingrowth as well as design of implant and time from implantation. Sumner and others[82] evaluated 18 retrieved experimental acetabular components. These components had secondary fixation with screws and a porous titanium fiber mesh ingrowth surface. One implant, removed 1 week after placement, showed no ingrowth. The remaining all demonstrated ingrowth of varying degrees that seemed to correlate with the time after implantation. Those that had been in for a prolonged period of time showed mature bony trabeculae and haversian canals about the implant.

It has become evident that certain surfaces may be more "friendly" to bone ingrowth than others. Certainly, fibermesh and a roughened, "small" beaded surface appear to achieve bony ingrowth easier than a macrobeaded surface. There has been a growing interest in placing bioinductive materials (e.g., hydroxyapatite) onto ingrowth surfaces. Certainly, in the revision setting in which quality is compromised, it is attractive. Whether it is an improvement over other ingrowth surfaces in primary total hip arthroplasty remains to be seen. Since the mid-1990s, tantalum has been used as a bone ingrowth surface, and it appears to achieve bone ingrowth very readily. Tantalum is a very porous metal (80 percent porous by volume) that has high friction characteristics when placed against cancellous bone. It has a modulus of elasticity closer to bone than either cobalt-chrome or titanium. Polyethylene can also be directly molded into the metal, theoretically decreasing the concerns over modularity of the polyethylene (Fig. 47–1A–C).

INITIAL STABILITY

Initial implant stability is a prerequisite for achieving bony ingrowth. Although the exact threshold of relative motion for osseous ingrowth has not been determined, Pilliar and associates have shown that relative motion of less than 28 µm favors bony ingrowth. Motion greater than 150 µm leads to fibrous fixation of the implant.[63] The issue of loading an ingrowth component has been looked at in multiple basic research studies.[30] In a dog titanium fibrous segmental prosthesis, Heck and co-workers found that reduced loading immediately after implantation improved the ultimate shear strength between the bone and the prosthesis.[38] Kim et al. found that immediate weight bearing may be beneficial in a canine acetabular model.[50] Clinically, after primary total hip arthroplasty with a noncemented acetabular component that achieves good initial fixation, weight bearing as tolerated does not seem to compromise fixation. Keeping micromotion to an absolute minimum in order to maximize the chance for bony fixation to occur should be the goal.

INTIMATE CONTACT

Studies from multiple centers have demonstrated that, although bone ingrowth is possible with gaps between the prosthesis and bone interface of up to 3 mm, the process is slower and less consistent than when no gaps are present. Sandborn and associates noted bony ingrowth into gaps of up to 2.0 mm but noted optimal fixation when gaps of less than 0.5 mm were present.[71] Reaming an acetabulum line to line (the last reamer used is the same size as the outer cup diameter) optimizes bony contact but relies on secondary means to obtain fixation. At present, I favor under-reaming a hemispheric cup by 1 to 3 mm, depending on the bone quality, material stiffness, and cup size. One should make sure the cup is not left "proud," leaving large gaps between the dome of the cup and the bone. This can occur with under-reaming by more than 3 to 4 mm in hard, young acetabular bone. Secondary screw fixation may be used to augment the stability obtained by the press-fit cup.

PORE SIZE

A number of authors have addressed the optimal pore size for bony ingrowth, relying primarily on histologic

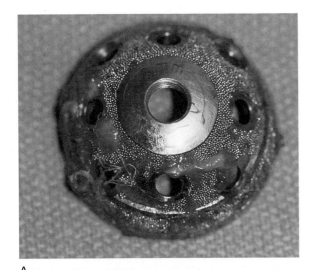

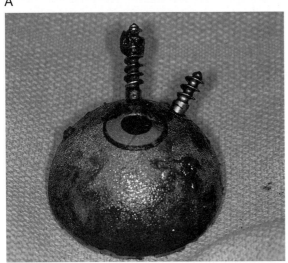

C

Figure 47–1. Examples of three different types of ingrowth surface. **A**, "macrobeaded"; **B**, "microbeaded"; **C**, tantalum. Certainly, each has different potential for ingrowth.

observation and mechanical stability testing. Bobyn and associates, in a canine model with a cobalt-chromium beaded porous surface, noted that implants with pore sizes ranging from 400 to 800 μm had lower fixation strength than those with pore sizes from 50 to 400 μm.[13,14,89] In studies of implants that had pore sizes of less than 100 μm, an increased pore size has been associated with an increased strength of fixation.[69] Other studies using pore sizes in the range of 150 to 400 μm failed to demonstrate a relationship between fixation strength and pore size. Implants of pore size in the 400- to 800-μm range had inferior fixation strength compared with those between 50 and 400 μm.[14,15] From these studies, it can be concluded that the optimal pore size for bone ingrowth is in the range of 100 to 400 μm, but there is certainly conflicting evidence on the relationship between the pore size and the amount of bone ingrowth within this optimal range. Furthermore, as new materials are developed (e.g., tantalum) optimal pore size may vary.

ENHANCING FIXATION

There has been much interest in various methods that may enhance the time-dependent characteristics of bone ingrowth into a metal component. Direct current electrical stimulation has been shown to be effective in enhancing bony ingrowth in porous implants.[23,88] Capacitive coupled field stimulation and pulsed electromagnetic field stimulation have been shown to have no beneficial effects in animal models.[31,44,68]

Autogenous bone grafting possesses osteoconductive and osteoinductive properties and has been shown to enhance bony ingrowth in a porous-coated model in which bone deficiencies were present.[39,48,53,59,70,85] The use of calcium phosphate coatings (hydroxyapatite and tricalcium phosphate) in conjunction with porous materials to enhance fixation has provided inconsistent results.[5,7,10,28,32,66,67,79,89] Controversy remains as to whether a short-acting substance such as tricalcium phosphate or a longer acting substance such as hydroxyapatite is more appropriate for enhancement of bony ingrowth.[57] The optimal surface on which to apply these coatings remains unknown. Certainly, a smooth surface may be less than ideal because when these coatings resorb, fixation may be lost. Whether to put the coatings on a roughened surface or onto an ingrowth surface remains controversial. The fate of these coatings and the exact mechanisms by which they may enhance bony ingrowth have not been fully elucidated.

Any treatment known to adversely affect fracture healing may also inhibit bony ingrowth into a noncemented acetabular component. Inhibition of bony ingrowth can occur when initial prosthesis fixation is not obtained or if there are excessive gaps between the component and the host bone. Treatment of patients with antineoplastic agents, diphosphonates, indomethacin, and low-dose radiation have all been found to decrease the strength of fixation and the amount of bony ingrowth in various animals models.[4,47,49,62,91] These factors should be taken into consideration when these implants are used in this patient population.

The clinical results of the use of porous-coated cementless acetabular components in a 5- to 10-year time frame has been reported from multiple centers. Reliable fixation is obtained in more than 95 percent of cases. Multiple cup designs have been reported to perform well at intermediate surveillance. Clohisy reported on 196 cementless fibermesh acetabular components followed for an average of 122 months.[22] There were no revisions for aseptic loosening and a 5 percent incidence of periacetabular osteolysis. Similar results have been reported with other acetabular cementless designs.[58] In a study of 72 hips followed for 12 years in patients who had had a cobalt-chrome, beaded acetabular component placed, the incidence of both aseptic loosening and acetabular lysis was only 4 percent. The effect of the backside surface finish and the metal type on wear performance of cementless modular acetabular liners was recently evaluated in a laboratory study. The results showed no difference in wear rates between cobalt-chrome and titanium shells.

POTENTIAL DISADVANTAGES OF NONCEMENTED ACETABULAR COMPONENTS

The theoretical advantages of noncemented acetabular components are numerous. They are easy to use. The modular liners may improve effective cup position and diminish dislocation rates. Uncemented cups with modular polyethylene liners are also revision friendly, accommodating to multiple femoral head sizes. Satisfactory ingrowth of bone occurs almost universally.

When assessing clinical results of noncemented acetabular components, one should keep in mind that loosening of cemented sockets has historically not been a problem until at least 5 or 10 years after the operation. Also, although stable implant fixation is achievable with noncemented acetabular components with intermediate follow-up, a variety of other problems not seen with cemented implants have already been reported with noncemented acetabular components with surveillance of less than 10 years. These problems include catastrophic failure of the polyethylene liner, liner-shell dissociation, questionable accelerated polyethylene wear rates, impingement of the iliopsoas tendon on the metal-backed rim, and acetabular osteolysis. Although many authors have stated their enthusiasm for the use of uncemented acetabular components, it may be that we are exchanging the problem of late radiographic loosening seen with cemented cups for a whole host of other problems seen with early designed noncemented acetabular fixation.

Catastrophic failure of the polyethylene liner has occurred in a number of designs of noncemented acetabular components. Berry and colleagues reported on a series of 10 hip inserts of three different designs (PCA, DePuy, and Osteonics) that catastrophically failed at an average of only 4.6 years from index surgery, with a range from 2 to 7.6 years.[9] All of these hips required revision. All acetabular components had a minimal modular polyethylene thickness of less than 5 mm. Half the patients were 40 years of age or younger at the time of primary total hip surgery, and 5 of the hips had vertically oriented acetabular components (50 degrees or more abduction angle). This problem, although well recognized, is poorly understood. It would seem that micromotion of the ultra-high-molecular-weight polyethylene within the shell is a source of wear particles in addition to the wear at the femoral-acetabular interface. Failure is likely to increase in incidence with increased follow-up (Fig. 47–2).

Liner-shell dissociation has also been reported by many authors in multiple cup designs.16,17,19,34,52,61,64,90

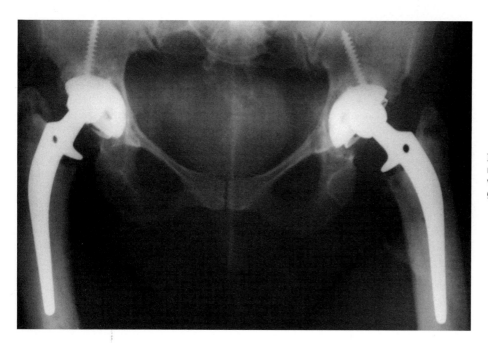

Figure 47–2. Anteroposterior pelvic radiograph showing catastrophic wear in the right hip and progressive gross wear in the left hip.

This may occur early, secondary to a malfunction of the locking mechanism or late secondary to fatigue failure of the polyethylene liner. Revision is required in all instances. Improvement in the locking mechanisms of the modular polyethylene cups, inserting one-piece nonmodular acetabular components, or cementing of a polyethylene liner may decrease the risk of dissociation.

Acetabular fracture can occur during placement of an uncemented acetabular component and may compromise fixation (Fig. 47–3). Sharkey reported on 13 fractures that occurred during insertion of cementless acetabular components.[77] A risk factor was excessive under-reaming of osteoporotic bone in female patients.

A malpositioned uncemented acetabular component may also cause anterior soft tissue impingement.[84] If the component is excessively retroverted, the iliopsoas tendon can become irritated as it extends over the anterior aspect of the acetabulum. This is probably more likely with a noncemented acetabular component than with a cemented one because, with noncemented designs, one attempts to obtain a much tighter interference fit between the implant and the bone than is necessary with the cemented implant. These patients may have activity-related groin pain that is reproduced by external rotation-hyperextension of the hip. This maneuver stretches the iliopsoas over the proud acetabular component. A lateral arthrogram may reveal that the iliopsoas tendon

is tending over the proud acetabular rim. Revision of the component into a more anteverted position may be successful if all other sources of pain are excluded.

As noted earlier, there is strong suspicion of accelerated polyethylene wear rates seen with some noncemented acetabular designs. The DUAL geometry wear rates averaged 0.17 mm per year. Possible causes for this problem may be use of the noncemented acetabular component in younger, higher demand patients. Modularity, polyethylene quality, and use of smaller cups with thin polyethylene liners may all be contributing factors (Fig. 47–4). The modularity and the variable stresses on the surface and within the polyethylene may also be contributing factors.

One of the major concerns with noncemented acetabular components has been the development of pelvic osteolysis, presumably as a result of wear debris, which has been reported in a number of series and again in multiple designs of components (Fig. 47–5).[8,29,72,74] Stulberg, reporting on 199 porous-coated anatomic hip inserts at intermediate follow-up of 5 to 7 years, noted that 30 of 199 had pelvic osteolysis.[81] In our series of HGPI acetabular components, 13 of 116 patients had evidence of radiographic pelvic lysis.[84] The etiology of this lysis is probably multifactorial. Particulate debris from the bearing surface, "backside wear" of the polyethylene metal articulation, and the

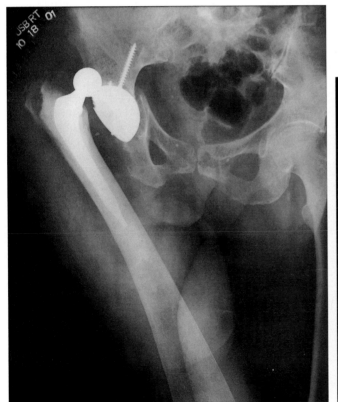

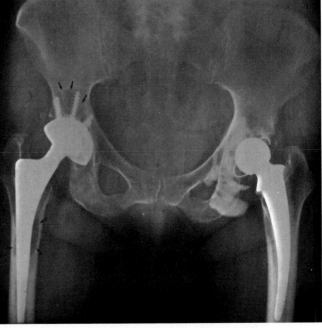

A

B

Figure 47–3. A, Anteroposterior pelvic radiograph 10 days after primary total hip arthroplasty (THA) in which an acetabular fracture occurred during insertion of component. Note displaced component and associated pelvic dissociation. **B,** Anteroposterior pelvic radiograph showing a left cemented THA that has been in place for 21 years. The right THA has marked polyethylene wear, and associated acetabular and femoral lysis has been in place for 8 years.

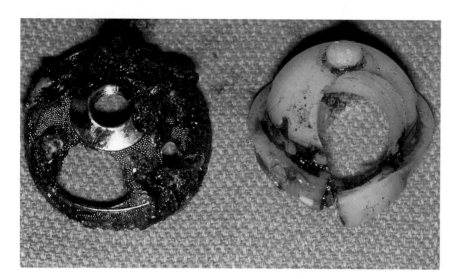

Figure 47–4. Photograph of marked polyethylene wear.

possibility of uncemented socket's providing a conduit for debris access to the pelvis may all be contributing factors.

I currently continue to use noncemented acetabular components, especially in patients who are younger than 70 years of age. However, some surgeons have increased their indications for cemented all-polyethylene components for younger patients. The majority of acetabular components used at present in the Mayo Clinic are hemispherically designed cups made of titanium and either fibermetal or tantalum. Under-reaming of the host acetabulum by 1 to 3 mm is typical, depending on the quality of host bone and the size of the acetabular component being used. Secondary screw augmentation is used according to the surgeon's preference. To date, most uncemented socket designs have relatively low loosening rates. Thin polyethylene should be avoided and, when implanting acetabular components with cup diameters of less than 52 mm, conversion to a 22-mm head on the femoral component may be wise. The rate of highly cross-linked polyethylenes or alternative hard bearing surfaces may also affect the choice of head size and, ultimately, may decide the fate and longevity of uncemented hemispheres (see Chapter 5). Although loosening has not been a problem to date, particulate debris generation, osteolysis, wear rates, and difficulties with the liner-shell mechanism are still of concern.

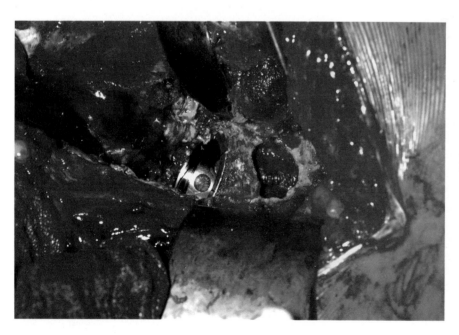

Figure 47–5. Intraoperative photograph of a well-fixed uncemented acetabular shell with marked pelvic osteolysis.

References

1. Andersson GBJ, Freeman MAR, Swanson SAV: Loosening of the cemented acetabular cup in total hip replacement. J Bone Joint Surg 54B:590, 1972.

2. Bartel DL, Bicknele MS, Wright TM: The effect of conformity, thickness, and material on stresses in ultra-high molecular-weight components for total joint replacement. J Bone Joint Surg 68A:1041, 1986.

3. Bartel DL, Wright TM, Edwards D: The effect of metal backing on stresses in polyethylene acetabular components. *In* Hungerford DS (ed): The Hip: Proceedings of the 11th Open Scientific Meeting of the Hip Society. St. Louis, CV Mosby, 1983, p 229.

4. Barth E, Roenningen H, Solheim LF, Saethren B: Influence of cis-platinum on bone ingrowth into porous fiber titanium: Mechanical and biochemical correlations. Trans Soc Biomater 9:170, 1986.

5. Bauer TW, Greesink RCT, Zimmerman R, McMahon JT: Hydroxyapatite-coated femoral stems: Histological analysis of components retrieved at autopsy. J Bone Joint Surg 73A:1439, 1991.

6. Bauer TW, Stulberg BN, Ming J, Geesink RG: Uncemented acetabular components: Histologic analysis of retrieved hydroxyapatite-coated and porous implants. J Arthroplasty 8:167, 1993.

7. Beight J, Radin S, Cuckler J, Ducheyne P: Effect of solubility of calcium phosphate coatings on mechanical fixation of porous ingrowth implants. Trans Orthop Res Soc 14:334, 1989.

8. Berman AT, Avolio A, Delgallo W: Acetabular osteolysis in total hip arthroplasty prevention and treatment. Orthopedics 17:963, 1994.

9. Berry DJ, Barnes CL, Scott RD, et al: Catastrophic failure of the polyethylene liner of uncemented acetabular components. J Bone Joint Surg 76B:575, 1994.

10. Berry JL, Geiger JM, Moran JM, et al: Use of tricalcium phosphate or electrical stimulation to enhance the bone-porous implant interface. J Biomed Mater Res 20:65, 1986.

11. Black J, Sherk H, Bonini J, et al: Metallosis associated with a stable titanium-alloy femoral component in total hip replacement: A case report. J Bone Joint Surg 72A:126, 1990.

12. Black J, Skipor A, Jacobs J, et al: Release of metal ions from titanium-base alloy total hip replacement prostheses. Trans Orthop Res Soc 14:501, 1989.

13. Bobyn JD, Pilliar RM, Binnington AG, Szivek JA: The effect of porous coated, proximally porous coated and fully porous-coated canine hip stem design on bone modeling. J Orthop Res 5:393, 1987.

14. Bobyn JD, Pilliar RM, Cameron HU, Weatherly GC: The optimum pore size for the fixation of porous-surfaced metal implants by the ingrowth of bone. Clin Orthop 150:253, 1980.

15. Bobyn JD, Pilliar RM, Cameron HU, et al: The effect of porous surface configuration on the tensile strength of fixation of implants by bone ingrowth. Clin Orthop 149:291, 1980.

16. Brien WW, Salvati EA, Wright TM, et al: Dissociation of acetabular components after total hip arthroplasty. J Bone Joint Surg 72:1548, 1990.

17. Buecke MJ, Herzenberg JE, Stubbs BT: Dissociation of a metal-backed polyethylene acetabular component: A case report. J Arthroplasty 4:39, 1989.

18. Callaghan JJ, Dysart SH, Savory CG: The uncemented porous-coated anatomic total hip prosthesis: Two-year results of a prospective consecutive series. J Bone Joint Surg 70A:337, 1988.

19. Cameron HU: Disassociation of a polyethylene liner from an acetabular cup. Orthop Rev 22:1160, 1993.

20. Charnley J, Cupic Z: The nine-and ten-year results of the low friction arthroplasty of the hip. Clin Orthop 95:9, 1973.

21. Clemow AJT, Weinstein AM, Klawitter JJ, et al: Interface mechanics of porous titanium implants. J Biomed Mater Res 15:73, 1981.

22. Clohisy JC, Harris WH: The Harris-Galante porous-coated acetabular component with screw fixation: An average ten-year follow-up study. J Bone Joint Surg 81A:66, 1999.

23. Colella SM, Miller AG, Stang RG, et al: Fixation of porous titanium implants in cortical bone enhanced by electrical stimulation. J Biomed Mater Res 15:37, 1981.

24. Cook SD, Barrack RL, Thomas KA, Haddad RJ Jr: Quantitative analysis of tissue growth into human porous total hip components. J Arthroplasty 3:249, 1988.

25. Cook SD, Georgette FS, Skinner HB, Haddad RJ Jr: Fatigue properties of carbon-and porous-coated Ti-6Al-4V alloy. J Biomed Mater Res 18:497, 1984.

26. Cook SD, Thomas KA: Fatigue failure of noncemented porous-coated implants: A retrieval study. J Bone Joint Surg 73B:20, 1991.

27. Cook SD, Thomas KA, Haddad RJ Jr: Histologic analysis of retrieved human porous-coated total joint components. Clin Orthop 234:90, 1988.

28. Cook SD, Thomas KA, Kay JF, Jarcho M: Hydroxyapatite-coated porous titanium for use as an orthopedic biologic attachment system. Clin Orthop 230:303, 1988.

29. Cooper RA, McAllister CM, Borden LS, Bauer TW: Polyethylene debris induced osteolysis and loosening in uncemented total hip arthroplasty: A cause of late failure. J Arthroplasty 7:285, 1992.

30. Curtis MJ, Jinnah RH, Wilson VD, Hungerford DS: The initial stability of uncemented acetabular components. J Bone Joint Surg 74B:372, 1992.

31. Dallant PA, Meunier P, Christel G, et al: Quantitation of bone ingrowth into porous implants submitted to pulsed electromagnetic fields. *In* Lemons JE (ed): Quantitative Characterization and Performance of Porous Implants for Hard Tissue Applications. Special Technical Publication 953. Philadelphia, American Society for Testing Materials, 1987.

32. D'Antonio JA, Capello WN, Crothers OD, et al: Early clinical experience with hydroxyapatite-coated femoral implants. J Bone Joint Surg 74A:995, 1992.

33. DeLee JG, Charnley J: Radiological demarcation of cemented sockets in total hip replacement. Clin Orthop 121:20, 1976.

34. Ferenz CC: Polyethylene insert dislocation in a screw-in acetabular cup. J Arthroplasty 3:201, 1988.

35. Ferro X, Zettl-Schaffer KF, Engh CA, et al: Quantification of bone ingrowth into porous coated acetabular components retrieved postmortem using backscattered SEM techniques. Trans Orthop Res Soc 17:387, 1992.

36. Galante JO, Rivero DP: The biological basis of bone ingrowth in titanium fiber composites. *In* Harris WH (ed): Advanced Concepts in Total Hip Replacement. Thorofare, NJ, Slack, 1985.

37. Haddad RJ Jr, Cook SD, Thomas KA: Current concepts review: Biological fixation of porous-coated implants. J Bone Joint Surg 59A:1459, 1987.

38. Heck DA, Nakajima I, Kelly PJ, Chao EY: The effect of load alteration on the biological and biochemical performance of a titanium fiber-metal segmental prosthesis. J Bone Joint Surg 68A:118, 1986.

39. Hermens KA, Kim WC, O'Carroll PF, et al: Bone morphogenetic protein and cancellous graft use in porous surfaced interface voids. Trans Orthop Res Soc 11:343, 1986.

40. Incavo SJ, DiFazio FA, Howe JG: Cementless hemispheric acetabular components: 2–4 year results. J Arthroplasty 8:573, 1993.

41. Jacobs JJ, Skipor AK, Black J, et al: Metal release and excretion from cementless titanium total knee replacements. Trans Orthop Res Soc 16:558, 1991.

42. Jacobs JJ, Skipor AK, Black J, et al: Release and excretion of metal in patients who have a total hip-replacement component made of titanium-base alloy. J Bone Joint Surg 73A:1475, 1991.

43. Jasty M, Bragdon CR, Maloney WJ, et al: Bone ingrowth into a low-modulus composite plastic porous-coated canine femoral component. J Arthroplasty 7:253, 1992.

44. Jasty M, Schutzer S, Bragdon C, Harris WH: A double blind study of the effects of a capacitively coupled field on bone ingrowth in a canine model [abstract]. Trans Soc Biomater 10:152, 1987.

45. Kavanagh BF, Dewitz MA, Ilstrup DM, et al: Charnley total hip arthroplasty with cement: Fifteen-year results. J Bone Joint Surg 71A:1496, 1989.

46. Kavanagh BF, Wallrichs S, Dewitz M, et al: Charnley low friction arthroplasty of the hip: Twenty year results with cement. J Arthroplasty 9:229, 1994.

47. Keller JC, Trancik TM, St. Mary S, et al: Inhibition of bone ingrowth by Indomethacin. Trans Orthop Res Soc 12:437, 1987.

48. Kienapfel H, Sumner DR, Turner TM, et al: Efficacy of autograft and freeze-dried allograft to enhance fixation of porous coated implants in the presence of interface gaps. J Orthop Res 10:423, 1992.

49. Kim WC, Hermens KW, Rechl H, et al: The effect of irradiation and radiation sheilding on canine porous bone ingrowth hip. Trans Orthop Res Soc 11:341, 1986.

50. Kim WC, Hermens KW, Rechl H, et al: The effect of weightbearing on canine porous hip implants. Trans Orthop Res Soc 11:490, 1986.

51. Kim YS, Callaghan JJ, Ahn PB, Brown TD: Fracture of the acetabulum during insertion of an oversized hemispherical component. J Bone Joint Surg 77A:111, 1995.

52. Kitziger KJ, DeLee JC, Evans JA: Disassembly of a modular acetabular component of a total hip: Replacement arthroplasty. J Bone Joint Surg 72A:621, 1990.

53. Kozin SC, Hedley AK, Urist MR: Augmentation of bone ingrowth. I. Ingrowth into bone morphogenic protein (BMP) impregnated porous implants. Trans Orthop Res Soc 7:181, 1982.

54. Lachiewicz PF, Suh PB, Gilbert JA: In vitro initial fixation of porous-coated acetabular total hip components: A biomechanical comparative study. J Arthroplasty 4:201, 1989.

55. Leland RH, Hofmann AA, Bachus KN, Bloebaum RD: Biocompatibility and bone response of human osteoarthritic cancellous bone to a titanium porous-coated cobalt chromium cylinder. Trans Soc Biomater 14:153, 1991.

56. Lieberman JR, Kay RM, Hamlet N, Kabo JM: Deformation patterns and frictional torque in modular acetabular components. Presented at the annual meeting of the American Academy of Orthopaedic Surgeons, New Orleans, 1994.

57. Manley MT, Capello WN, D'Antonio JA, et al: Fixation of acetabular cups without cement in total hip arthroplasty. A comparison of three different implant surfaces at a minimum duration of follow-up of five years. J Bone Joint Surg 80A:1175, 1998.

58. McAuley JP, Moore KD, Culpepper WJ II, Engh CA: Total hip arthroplasty with porous-coated protheses fixed with cement in patients who are sixty-five years of age or older. J Bone Joint Surg 80A:1648, 1998.

59. McDonald DJ, Fitzgerald RH Jr, Chao EYS: The enhancement of fixation of a porous-coated femoral component by autograft and allograft in the dog. J Bone Joint Surg 70A:729, 1988.

60. Mulroy RD Jr, Harris WH: The effect of improved cementing techniques on component loosening in total hip replacement. J Bone Joint Surg 72B:757, 1990.

61. O'Brien RF, Chess D: Late disassembly of a modular acetabular component: A case report. J Arthroplasty 7S:453, 1992.

62. Pilliar RM, Bobyn JD: The effects of EHDP on the fixation of porous-coated implants by bone growth. Trans Orthop Res Soc 12:438, 1987.

63. Pilliar RM, Lee JM, Maniatopoulos C: Observations on the effect of movement on bone ingrowth into porous-coated implants. Clin Orthop 208:108, 1986.

64. Ries MC, Collis DK, Lynch F: Separation of the polyethylene liner from an acetabular cup metal backing. Clin Orthop 282:164, 1992.

65. Ritter MA, Keating EM, Faris PM, Brugo G: Metal-backed acetabular cups in total hip arthroplasty. J Bone Joint Surg 72A:672, 1990.

66. Rivero DP, Fox J, Skipor AK, et al: Calcium phosphate-coated porous titanium implants for enhanced skeletal fixation. J Biomed Mater Res 22:191, 1988.

67. Rivero DP, Fox J, Skipor AK, et al: Effects of calcium phosphates and bone grafting materials on bone ingrowth in titanium fiber metal. Trans Orthop Res Soc 10:191, 1985.

68. Rivero DP, Landon GC, Skipor AK, et al: Effect of pulsing electromagnetic fields on bone ingrowth in a porous material. Trans Orthop Res Soc 11:492, 1986.

69. Robertson DM, St. Pierre L, Chahal R: Preliminary observation of bone ingrowth into porous materials. J Biomed Mater Res 10:335, 1976.

70. Russotti GM, Okada Y, Fitzgerald RH Jr, et al: Efficacy of using a bone graft substitute to enhance biological fixation of a porous metal femoral component. In Brand RA (ed): The Hip: Proceedings of the 14th Open Scientific Meeting of the Hip Society. St. Louis, CV Mosby, 1987.

71. Sandborn PM, Cook SD, Anderson RC, et al: The effect of surgical fit on bone growth into porous-coated implants. Trans Orthop Res Soc 12:217, 1987.

72. Santavirta S, Konttinen YT, Hoikka V, Eskola A: Immunopathological response to loose cementless acetabular components. J Bone Joint Surg 73B:38, 1991.

73. Schmalzried TP, Harris WH: The Harris-Galante porous-coated acetabular component with screw fixation: Radiographic analysis of 83 primary hip replacements at a minimum of five years. J Bone Joint Surg 74A:1130, 1992.

74. Schmalzried TP, Jasty M, Harris WH: Periprosthetic bone loss in total hip arthroplasty: Polyethylene wear debris and the concept of the effective joint space. J Bone Joint Surg 74A:849, 1992.

75. Schmalzried TP, Wessinger SJ, Hill GE, Harris WH: The Harris-Galante porous acetabular component press-fit without screw fixation: Five year radiographic analysis of primary cases. J Arthroplasty 9:235, 1994.

76. Schulte KR, Callaghan JJ, Kelley SS, Johnston RL: The outcome of Charnley total hip arthroplasty with cement after a minimum twenty year follow-up. J Bone Joint Surg 75A:961, 1993.

77. Sharkey PF, Hozack WJ, Callaghan JJ, et al: Acetabular fracture associated with cementless acetabular component insertion: A report of 13 cases. J Arthroplasty 14:426, 1999.

78. Shaw JA, Bailey JH, Bruno A, Greer RB: Threaded acetabular components for primary and revision total hip arthroplasty. J Arthroplasty 5:201, 1990.

79. Søballe K, Hansen ES, Rasmussen HB, et al: Tissue ingrowth into titanium and hydroxyapatite-coated implants during stable and unstable mechanical conditions. J Orthop Res 10:285, 1992.

80. Stauffer RN: Ten-year follow-up study of total hip replacement with particular reference to roentgenographic loosening of the components. J Bone Joint Surg 64A:983, 1982.

81. Stauffer RN: Contempory current technique—results: Total joint arthroplasty. Presented at the 1991 Hip and Knee Arthroplasty: Current Techniques. Scottsdale, Arizona, 1990.

82. Sumner DR, Turner TM, Urban RM, Galante JO: Remodeling and ingrowth of bone at two years in a canine cementless total hip-arthroplasty model. J Bone Joint Surg 74A:239, 1992.

83. Tallroth K, Slatis P, Ylinen P, et al: Loosening of threaded acetabular components. J Arthroplasty 8:581, 1993.

84. Trousdale RT, Cabanela ME, Berry DJ: Anterior iliopsoas impingement after total hip arthroplasty. J Arthroplasty 10:545, 1995.

85. Turner TM, Sumner DR, Urban RM, et al: A comparative study of porous coatings in a weight-bearing total hip arthroplasty model. J Bone Joint Surg 68A:1396, 1986.

86. Turner TM, Urban RM, Sumner DR, Galante JO: The use of HA/TCP granules in cementless revision of aseptically loosened, cemented THA. Trans Orthop Res Soc 15:208, 1990.

87. Wasielewski RC, Cooperstein LA, Kruger MP, Rubash HE: Acetabular anatomy and transacetabular fixation of screws in total hip arthroplasty. J Bone Joint Surg 72A:501, 1990.

88. Weinstein AM, Klawitter JJ, Cleveland TW, Amoss DC: Electrical stimulation of bone growth into porous Al_2O_3. J Biomed Mater Res 10:231, 1976.

89. Welsh RP, Pilliar RM, McNab I: Surgical implants: The role of surface porosity in fixation to bone and acrylic. J Bone Joint Surg 53A:963, 1971.

90. Wilson AG, Monsees B, Blair VP: Acetabular cup dislocation: A new complication of total joint arthroplasty. Am J Roentgenol 15:133, 1988.

91. Wise MW III, Robertson ID, Lachiewicz PF, et al: The effect of radiation therapy on the fixation strength of an experimental porous-coated implant in dogs. Clin Orthop 261:276, 1990.

92. Wixson RL, Stulberg SD, Mehlhoff M: Total hip replacement with cemented, uncemented, and hybrid prostheses: A comparison of clinical and radiographic results at two to four years. J Bone Joint Surg 73A:257, 1991.

93. Woodman JL, Jacobs JJ, Galante JO, Urban RM: Metal ion release from titanium-based prosthetic segmental replacements of long bones in baboons: A long-term study. J Orthop Res 1:421, 1984.

94. Wroblewski BM: 15–21 year results of the Charnley low friction arthroplasty. Clin Orthop 211:30, 1986.

95. Young FA, Spector M, Kresch CH: Porous titanium endosseous dental implants in rhesus monkeys: Microradiography and histological evaluation. J Biomed Mater Res 13:843, 1979.

48

Cemented Femoral Components

• DANIEL J. BERRY and GAVAN P. DUFFY

Few areas of hip arthroplasty have been the subject of as much controversy, new information, and revisionist thinking since the early 1990s as cemented femoral components. In this time frame, much has been learned about the patients' demographic factors, implant design factors, and surgical technique factors, which have an important influence on femoral component durability. In the early 1990s, a number of studies were published demonstrating good mid- and long-term results with cemented femoral fixation, particularly with the use of modern cementation methods. At the same time, failures of many first-generation uncemented femoral components were published. These studies, in combination with the reliable early clinical results provided by cemented femoral fixation led to a dramatic resurgence of cemented femoral component fixation, even in the young. Unfortunately, in the mid- and late 1990s, a number of authors reported more disappointing results than expected of uncemented femoral fixation used in combination with modern cemented femoral component designs. The problems encountered were mostly related to early failure of grit-blasted stems with a rough (high roughness average [Ra]) surface finish, which led to unacceptable rates of early implant failure associated with component debonding from the cement, abrasion of the cement by the rough stem, particulate debris formation, rapid osteolysis, and clinical failure. These problems led to a re-examination of the interplay among design, component surface finish, cement technique, and patient selection in providing successful long-term results. Several studies also were published showing that even for relatively successful cemented component designs, the failure rate at long term follow-up was not low in young patient populations. Finally, by the end of the 1990s, it became clear that a number of uncemented femoral component designs could provide excellent long-term femoral component fixation and very reliable clinical results in a very high percentage of patients. The consequence of these converging pieces of information has been a decrease in cemented femoral fixation and a gradual increase in uncemented stem use, particularly in younger patients.

DESIGN FEATURES

Many design features must be considered in evaluation of the functional performance of a total hip femoral component. These features may be divided into considerations of femoral head, neck, collar, stem design, and stem surface finish. This chapter focuses on the cemented femoral component; the design concepts and considerations are different (see Chapter 49) when uncemented components are used.

Femoral Head

Important variables in femoral head design include diameter, material, and surface finish. Prostheses are currently available with head diameters of 22, 26, 28, and 32 mm on a routine basis, and even larger femoral heads have been introduced for use with alternative bearing surfaces. Charnley chose 22.225 mm for the head diameter of his original design as a compromise between friction (which varied directly with head size) and wear (which varied inversely with head size).[22,23] Although some investigators have postulated that a larger head size would be more stable, there is no clinical evidence proving a lower rate of dislocation for a larger diameter head up to 32 mm.[38] Theoretically, a 32-mm head allows about 20 percent greater range of motion than a 22-mm head (given the same neck size and acetabular component design), but a difference in hip motion has not been documented in clinical studies.[110] Studies have demonstrated that, although linear wear of a 22-mm femoral head on polyethylene may be greater than that of a 32-mm head, the volume of potentially harmful polyethylene wear debris was considerably larger with a larger head size.[48]

The cemented acetabular component loosening rate is higher for the 32-mm head size.[77] This may be the result of one or both of the following factors: (1) increased head size (increased surface area) increases total friction and increases the torsional stress transmitted to the acetabular component; and (2) increased head size causes increased volumetric polyethylene wear and, therefore, generates more polyethylene debris. This debris formation has been implicated in the formation of a creeping reactive membrane that may lead to loosening of the cemented socket.[103] The 32-mm head size leads to a decreased polyethylene thickness of the acetabular component (assuming the same outside diameter). Especially for metal-backed uncemented sockets, large head sizes matched with small sockets lead to a thin polyethylene liner that may be at risk for accelerated polyethylene wear or catastrophic failure as a result of wear through or fracture.[13] There is no evidence that larger femoral head sizes increase the loosening rate of uncemented cups, but with conventional polyethylene, the osteolysis rate caused by increased volumetric polyethylene wear is greater.

For all the aforementioned reasons, the 32-mm head size in combination with conventional polyethylene has been used much less frequently since the early 1990s. For modular systems, the 28-mm head size provides more options with respect to neck length and head material than the 22-mm-diameter head and, therefore, is used most often. For small acetabular components in which a 28-mm head size compromises satisfactory polyethylene thickness, a 22-mm head size is advocated. With new bearing surfaces such as cross-linked polyethylene and hard-on-hard surfaces that hold the promise of low volumetric wear even with larger femoral head size, there is now an increased interest in exploring larger femoral sizes once again. Larger head sizes increase the range of intra-articular hip motion free of prosthetic impingement and have the theoretical potential to provide better hip stability and lower hip dislocation rates. Whether large head sizes will lead to a reduced rate of dislocation in clinical practice remains to be proved. Likewise, only time will tell if larger head sizes can be used with new bearing surfaces without a high rate of osteolysis.

Femoral head material is an important design variable because different materials have different wear characteristics against polyethylene. Titanium, which is soft and not scratch resistant, has been associated with a higher wear rate in vivo[21] and has been abandoned for the most part. Cobalt-chromium heads have become the standard, and many companies now provide superfinished heads that may further improve the wear characteristics against polyethylene. Ceramic heads, used for some time in Europe, are now more widely available in North America. Ceramics are brittle, and a few ceramic femoral heads have fractured. Ceramics are more wettable and, on wear simulators, appear to have advantageous wear characteristics versus polyethylene. Both alumina and zirconia ceramic heads are now available. Direct comparison of ceramic and cobalt-chromium femoral heads in vivo with respect to polyethylene wear rate and clinical performance on a prospective, randomized basis are not yet available. Several retrospective studies have suggested that ceramic heads may provide a wear-rate advantage, but this remains to be proved.

Femoral Neck

A modular connection between the femoral head and the stem has been incorporated into most modern hip designs. This has many obvious practical clinical advantages in primary and revision settings. The modularity allows easy variation of neck length to optimize tension in the glutei and other muscles of the hip envelope and to optimize leg length, hip stability, and hip biomechanics.

The modular connection does introduce potential problems as well. Wear debris may form at the modular junction, and corrosion at the modular junction may also occur.[26,113] The products of corrosion have been implicated causally, at least in a few cases, in periprosthetic osteolysis. For longer neck lengths, modular systems require a skirt on the femoral head that increases the diameter of the femoral neck and increases the risk of neck impingement on the socket. Neck-socket impingement can lead to instability, polyethylene debris formation, or component loosening.

The neck offset is an important design feature that should be optimized because it profoundly affects the mechanical function of the hip.[55] Offset is determined by the neck-stem angle, the neck length, and the location at which the neck joins the stem (Fig. 48–1). Too large an offset is undesirable and can potentially lead to an increased bending moment or excessive rotational forces on the femoral component, with subsequent stem fracture or loosening. Too small an offset decreases the moment arm of the hip abductors and may cause a persistent abductor limp as well as decrease the moment efficiency, thereby causing an increased resultant compression load across the joint and the potential for component loosening. Insufficient offset may also decrease hip stability because the abductors are under less tension, and thus may increase the risk of dislocation.

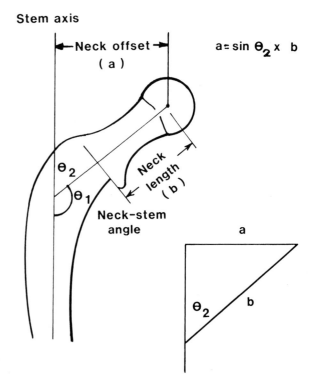

Figure 48–1. Diagrammatic representation of design features of the neck of the femoral component. The neck offset is a function of the neck-stem angle and the neck length.

Collar

The value of having a collar at the base of the femoral neck has been the subject of much debate in recent years.[30,31,34,69,85] When bone cement is used for fixation, the femoral collar functions as an insertion stop, limiting distal insertion of the femoral component into the cement mantle. Initially, it was proposed that a collar might provide some cement pressurization during component insertion; however, the collar has been shown to be ineffective in achieving this purpose. The primary rationale for a collar on a cemented device is to provide a better load transfer environment in the proximal bone and cement. Several experimental and computer modeling studies have indicated a higher (more nearly normal) transmission of compressive stress from the prosthesis into the medial femoral neck bone with a collar (Figs. 48–2 and 48–3).[4,28,62,68,72,111] This effect is beneficial in that it may reduce adaptive bone resorption in the proximal femur (stress shielding), reduce the bending stress in the component stem, and reduce stress in the distal cement (Fig. 48–4).

One of the effects of axial loading of a tapered-stem femoral component is to produce very high hoop stresses (circumferential tensile stresses) in the proximal bone and cement. These hoop stresses may approach the ultimate tensile strength of cement but are theoretically reduced to much safer levels in the presence of a functioning collar.[28] The concerns are that (1) it is technically difficult to fashion an intimate fit between the underside of a component collar and the bone; and (2) any collar-bone contact achieved

at surgery may not be maintained. Even the slightest bone resorption eliminates effective stress transfer, and the beneficial effects of the collar are lost. Mathematical models have indicated that stress can be transferred from a collar through a cement layer to femoral neck bone.[28] In contrast, experimental laboratory studies have shown that, with

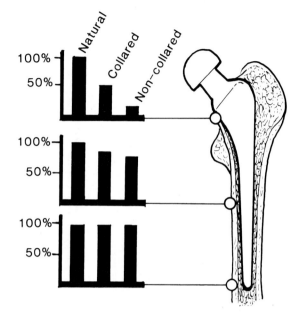

Figure 48–2. Schematic representation of load transferred to the proximal femur in intact and prosthetic hips with and without collars.

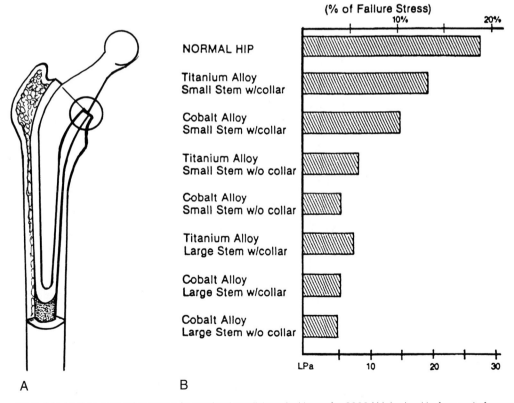

Figure 48–3. Maximal compressive stress in proximal-medial cortical bone for 2000-N joint load before and after prosthetic replacement of the femoral head and neck. (**A** Modified from and **B** from Tarr RR, Lewis JL, Jaycox P, et al: Effect of materials, stem geometry, and collar-calcar contact on stress distribution in the proximal femur with total hip. Trans Orthop Res Soc 4:34, 1979.)

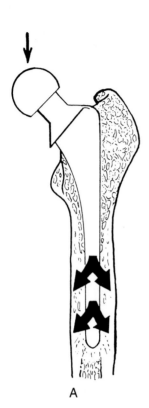

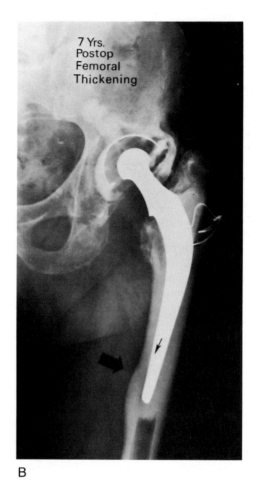

Figure 48–4. A, Schematic representation of maldistribution of load with stress transfer to bone in distal stem region of prosthesis. **B,** Roentgenographic illustration of distal stress transfer with reactive hypertrophy of the femoral shaft at the distal stem of a cemented prosthesis 7 years postoperatively.

axial loading, a layer of cement beneath the collar rapidly fragments. Collarless component designs have been most popular with smooth or polished femoral components that are designed to be able to debond from the cement mantle and function in a taper-slip arrangement. Advocates of these designs suggest that the lack of a collar allows the polished stem to subside slightly to a stable position in a viscoelastic cement mantle, thereby producing positive adaptive bone remodeling. The ability of collarless tapered polished stems to subside into the cement mantle may also provide a self-sealing function that prevents particulate debris from the joint from traveling along the implant stem interface and causing distal osteolysis. Clinical series of cemented stem designs, with or without collars, have both demonstrated very good clinical results. It may turn out that collars are useful for certain stem designs and deleterious for others.

Femoral Stem

Design features of the femoral component stem can be considered under the subheadings of geometric properties (length, shape, cross section), material properties, and surface finish.

Some early devices incorporated a curved stem design. Aside from some other design problems (e.g., a diamond-shaped cross section), these curved stems were abandoned because of the recognized difficulty of maintaining a uniform cement mantle when a curved stem is inserted into a relatively straight (in the frontal plane) femoral medullary canal. A thin cement mantle adjacent to the proximal-lateral and distal-medial aspects of a curved stem is more vulnerable to fatigue failure, with subsequent prosthesis loosening. A straight, slightly tapered stem allows some pressurization of cement on insertion and maintenance of a more uniform layer of cement.[70]

Stem length has been a matter of considerable controversy. Some purely technical factors must be considered, such as ease of insertion and difficulty of removal should that ever become necessary. Mathematical modeling studies have shown that either very short or very long stems produce stress concentrations at some point in the composite.[28] For example, very long stems produce increased stress in the stem and distal stress transfer with shielding of proximal bone. Very short stems produce very high stresses proximally, which may exceed the ultimate strength of cement or bone.

The cross-sectional geometry of a femoral component is a description of the volume and distribution of material along the stem and, at least partially (combined with physical properties of the material), defines the stem's structural features, such as strength and stiffness. Certain section shapes produce a more favorable mechanical environment than others. Sharp corners on the stem should be avoided because they produce marked stress concentrations and may cause cement or bone failure. Stems with a larger volume of material along the lateral border are more resistant to bending and produce less tensile stress in the cement mantle. Those stems that have a relatively thick medial side also produce less compressive stress in the cement. Because bone cement is about three times stronger in compression than in tension, compression loading may be the only safe mode (i.e., the less tensile stress, the less likely that cement will fracture, resulting in component loosening). Figure 48–5 represents the work of Crowninshield et al., indicating the cross-sectional shape that is optimal for use with cement.[29] This analysis was based on the assumption that load passing through the hip would produce bending mainly in the frontal plane. In reality, sagittal plane bending is equally significant, especially during stair and walking activities.

Particularly, since the latter 1990s, it has been recognized that the torsional stability of a stem within the cement mantle is a critically defining feature of its clinical performance. Poor torsional stability owing to excessively rounded implant shapes and small cross-sectional areas have led to early implant debonding from the cement, probably because of the high rotational stresses placed on a stem during daily activities such as stair climbing and arising from chairs. To be successful, implants appear to need a cross-sectional geometry that provides good torsional stability within the cement mantle while avoiding excessively sharp corners in areas that can cause cement fractures.

Stainless steel was used to manufacture many of the early prosthetic femoral devices. Stainless steel is a relatively stiff (i.e., high elastic modulus) material with low fatigue and yield strength characteristics.[111,112] More recent modifications of the metallurgy have, however, produced for prosthetic application stainless steel with excellent fatigue characteristics. Cobalt-chromium alloys have excellent fatigue and yield strengths but have a slightly greater elastic modulus than stainless steel. Titanium alloys have an elastic modulus about one half that of stainless steel or cobalt-chromium (Fig. 48–6).[27,62,68,111] More flexible stems carry less internal stress and transmit more compressive stress to the proximal bone and cement, whereas large, stiff stems reduce the thickness of the cement mantle and produce high tensile stress in the cement distally.[29] Either situation may produce cement failure and component loosening. For cemented devices, the vulnerability of the bone cement appears to make the use of titanium alloys a disadvantageous choice.[98] Titanium is also a soft metal that is easily scratched. Debonding of a titanium stem from cement can lead to rapid particle formation and osteolysis.

Surface finish now is recognized to be a very important design feature and also one that has generated considerable discussion and controversy.[1,5,59] Many of the earliest stem designs had a smooth or polished surface finish. It became recognized that one failure mode of cemented stems was debonding of the stem from the cement mantle. Thus, some cemented prostheses designed in the 1980s and 1990s were manufactured with surfaces that were roughened, porous, or precoated with methyl methacrylate. These surface treatments provide increased adhesion of cement to the stem and thus resist micromotion of the stem within the cement. By maintaining a bond between the prosthesis and the surrounding cement, the surface treatments may reduce cement stresses. However, it is now understood that if such a stem "debonds" from the surrounding cement, the abrasion of the surface on the component with the cement can lead to particulate debris formation (Fig. 48–7).[42,65] Some femoral stems now are polished to reduce the likelihood of debris formation if debonding occurs. Data suggest that certain polished as well as certain surface-"enhanced" femoral designs can work well clinically,[42,87] and data are not yet available to demonstrate a clear clinical advantage of one design type over the other.

Surface roughness is measured with calibrated profilometers. The Ra is the arithmetic average of all departures from the center line of the roughness profile. The mean roughness depth (Rz) is the mean of the depths (highest peak to lowest valley) of the successive sample lengths within the roughness profile. Crowninshield introduced six descriptive terms for implant surface textures: (1) shiny; (2) smooth; (3) stain; (4) matte; (5) rough; and (6) textured.[5] A selection of scanning electron microscopic images of typical implant surfaces is shown in Figure 48–8.

When surface finish is under consideration, there are two important characteristics to assess: (1) push-out strength, which measures the bond between cement and metal and (2) abrasive qualities, which measure the abrasion caused by metal against cement when that cement-metal bond is broken and motion occurs. The cement-metal interface strength is dominated by the mechanical interlock of bone cement into the surface roughness. In abrasion testing, the quantity of cement worn away by various surface finishes is proportional to surface roughness.

One of the concerns regarding the effect of surface finish is how a loose component behaves if motion develops between the metal of a stem and the cement mantle. For a rough stem, debonding often is followed by progressive loosening at the cement-prosthesis interface as a result of cement abrasion by the stem (with maintenance of the bone-cement interface) followed by extensive osteolysis[76] (Fig. 48–9). Smooth surface finish stems appear to behave differently when debonded from the cement. Berry et al. analyzed the effect that debonding, or subsidence, had on the long-term success of the smooth-surface Charnley stem.[14] They found that when the maximal thickness of the radiolucent line between the superolateral border of

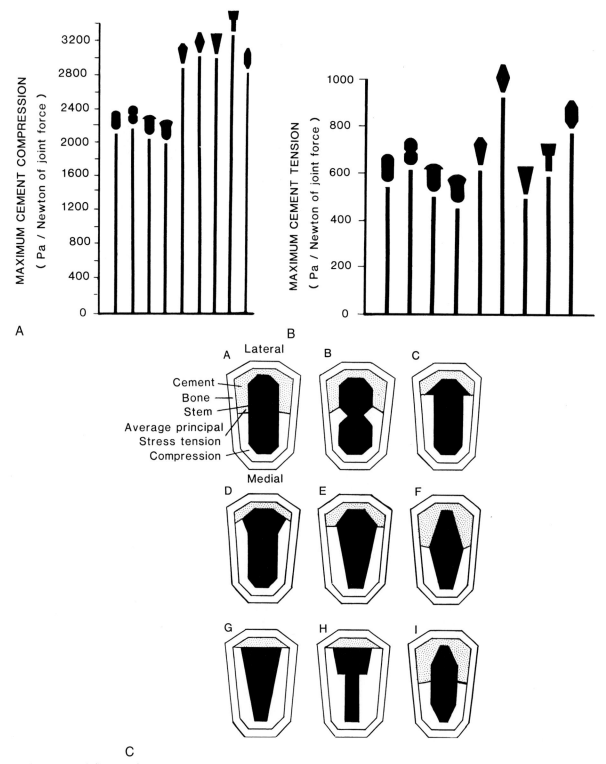

Figure 48–5. Influence of cross-sectional geometry of the femoral stem on the maximal cement compression (**A**) and fusion (**B**). Cross-sectional D shape represents the optimal configuration for use with cement fixation because it generates the least tensile and compression stresses in the cement and exposes the least portion of the cement mantle to tension (**C**). (From Crowninshield RD, Brand RA, Johnston RC, Milroy JC: The effect of femoral stem cross-sectional geometry on cement stresses in total hip reonstruction. Clin Orthop 146:71, 1980.)

the prosthesis and the cement was 2 mm or more, an early appearance of debonding was associated with a significantly poorer (*P*<0.0001) probability of survival of Charnley stem free of revision for aseptic loosening. However, if the thickness of the radiolucent line was less than 2 mm, it had no effect on survivorship. Thus, pronounced early subsidence of the component within the cement mantle had a strong negative impact on the long-term performance of the implant, but debonding associated with mechanical stability of a smooth stem

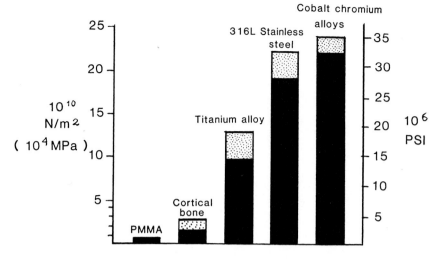

Figure 48–6. Graphic representation of the elastic modulus of implant alloys, bone, and bone cement. (From Tarr RR, Lewis JL, Jaycox P, et al: Effect of materials, stem geometry, and collar-calcar contact on stress distribution in the proximal femur with total hip. Trans Orthop Res Soc 4:345, 1979.)

did not have an adverse effect on long-term implant survivorship. From these data have emerged a more coherent understanding of the effect of stem surface finish on performance. Rough surface stems debond less frequently from the cement, but if they do debond, osteolysis and clinical failure are frequently the consequence. Smooth or polished stems frequently debond from the cement, but if the geometry of the stem and the features of the cement mantle provide mechanical stem stability in the cement, clinical performance is not compromised. Ling and co-workers believe that a further advantage of a polished tapered cemented stem design is its potential to apply favorable loads to the proximal femur as hoop stresses are transferred through the cement mantle. They have produced evidence that cement at body temperature has some viscoelastic characteristics that allow a polished tapered stem to stay stable in the cement and transfer load through the cement to surrounding bone.

POLYMETHYLMETHACRYLATE

Charnley demonstrated the technical utility and biologic compatibility of bone cement many years ago.[22] Even with unsophisticated cementing techniques, polymethylmethacrylate (PMMA) often proves to be a successful and durable substance in prosthetic replacement. However, it has been recognized that bone cement is the weak link in the prosthetic composite. Unfavorable physical properties (e.g., poor fracture toughness, low tensile or fatigue strength, an elastic modulus one third lower than cortical bone) make mechanical failure of the cement a cause of femoral component loosening.[44] Efforts to improve the longevity of cemented total hip arthroplasty (THA) have focused on improving the mechanical characteristics of PMMA itself, optimizing the design of the stem to interact favorably with the cement mantle, and developing techniques to achieve a durable bone-cement interface.[7,8,24,33,63,75]

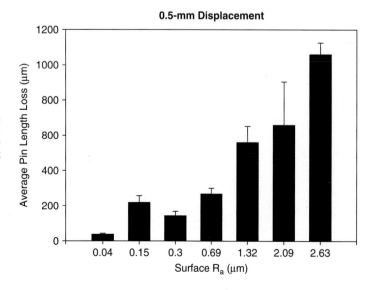

Figure 48–7. Mean abrasion after 250,000 cycles for 0.5 mm cement/metal displacement with different surface roughness. (From Crowninshield RD, Brand RA, Johnston RC, Milroy JC: The effect of femoral stem cross-sectional geometry on cement stresses in total hip reconstruction. Clin Orthop 146:71, 1980.)

A

B

Figure 48–8. Scanning electronic micro-scopic views of implant surfaces. (**A**) Rz = 0.05 μm; (**B**) Ra = 1.22 μm; (**C**) Ra = 2.2 μm. (From Crowninshield RD, Brand RA, Johnston RC, Milroy JC: The effect of femoral stem cross-sectional geometry on cement stresses in total hip recon-struction. Clin Orthop 146:71, 1980.)

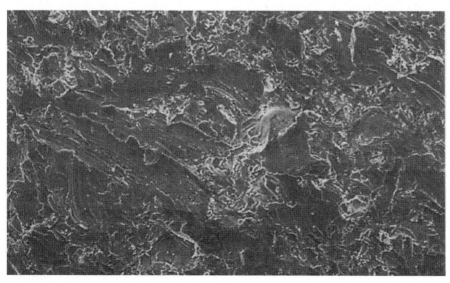

C

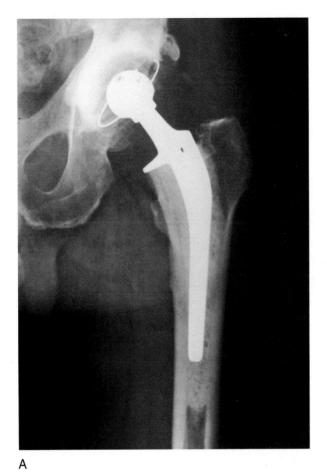

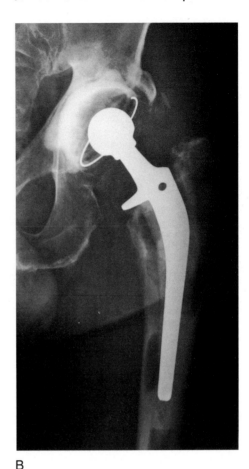

A   B

Figure 48–9. A, Immediate postoperative film of cemented cobalt-chromium femoral component with roughened surface. **B,** Two years later, the stem has debonded and rapid femoral osteolysis is present. The patient was not infected but required revision.

Mechanical Properties

Several brands of PMMA are available to the surgeon. Although the characteristics of tensile strength, compressive strength, and modulus of elasticity are similar among these brands, the fatigue characteristics of different brands under repetitive physiologic loads may be clinically relevant. There are currently no long-term clinical data to validate these concerns.

Clinical proof that all bone cements are not equal, however, has been provided by the European experience with a low-viscosity cement known as Boneloc. In a study of 8579 Charnley prostheses in the Norwegian Joint Registry, the survival rate at 5.5 years was markedly worse (94.1 percent for Boneloc cement versus 98.1 percent for high-viscosity cement; $P<0.0001$).[50]

Because PMMA performs best under compressive loads and poorly in tension, efforts were made to reinforce bone cement with graphite, carbon, or aramide fibers.[61,92,118] Although these composites exhibit improved mechanical characteristics, their application in the clinical setting has proved to be impractical because of handling characteristics and the poor intrusion of these fibers into the cancellous interstices of bone.

Most efforts to improve PMMA have centered around porosity reduction. Burke et al. proposed centrifugation as a method of improving the fatigue properties of PMMA by reducing the number and size of air porosities in cured PMMA.[18] Vacuum mixing has been found by some to reduce porosity better than centrifugation (Fig. 48–10).[2,55] Centrifugation, however, produces more consistent samples, and the standard deviation of fatigue data using vacuum mixing is greater than that for centrifuged specimens.[47] Simplex-P outperforms other brands under fatigue testing regardless of mixing technique.[47,64] Monomer chilling has a deleterious effect on the fatigue life of PMMA; however, this is offset by porosity reduction techniques.[47]

Rimnac et al. have questioned the efficacy of porosity reduction techniques.[96] Their data, supported by those of other investigators, suggest a possible detrimental effect with centrifugation because of significant shrinkage of Simplex-P during curing after porosity reduction.[45] They also questioned the effect of centrifugation on PMMA in the presence of surface irregularities that occur in the clinical setting.[96] Davies et al. subsequently have demonstrated a beneficial effect with centrifugation, even in the presence of surface irregularities.[32]

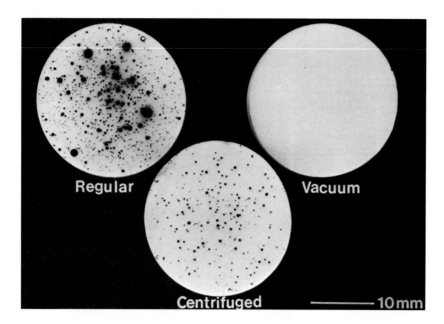

Figure 48–10. Porosities resulting in Simplex-P acrylic bone cement from three different mixing techniques. (From Wixson RL, Stulberg SD, Mehlhoff M: Total hip replacement with cemented, uncemented, and hybrid prostheses. J Bone Joint Surg 73A:257, 1991.)

Results verifying clinical benefits of porosity reduction are not available.

Cement Delivery

Miller and colleagues popularized the concepts of macrointerlock and microinterlock in cemented arthroplasty.[74] Macrointerlock describes the shape assumed by the cement mass within the bone envelope and microinterlock refers to the bone-cement interface after PMMA penetration into the cancellous bone interstices. Improved cementing techniques incorporating careful bone preparation, lavage, hemostasis, cement delivery, and pressurization improve the microinterlock achieved at the bone-cement interface. These techniques also reduce the number of laminations and limit the debris inclusion within the PMMA mantle. The adverse effects of laminations and debris inclusion on the mechanical properties of PMMA have been described.[41,43] Bone preparation, implant geometry, and implant size affect the macrointerlock achieved during arthroplasty.

Intrusion of cement into cancellous bone interstices is dependent on cement viscosity, cement brand, magnitude of pressurization, technique of cement preparation, and quality of preparation and cleansing of the femoral canal. Some investigators have demonstrated the superior penetration of low-viscosity cement compared with regular-viscosity cement.[71,82] Rey et al. demonstrated that cement intrusion depth was proportional to injection pressure for all three brands of cement tested; low-viscosity cement penetrated better than Simplex-P, which in turn was better than Palacos.[94] Chilling of the monomer increased Simplex-P intrusion almost threefold, with the lowest intrusion depth measuring 5.8 mm under 20 psi of pressurization.

In the clinical setting, there is not usually more than 5 or 6 mm of cancellous bone remaining after preparation of the femoral canal; therefore, low-viscosity cement may not provide a significant advantage in the clinical setting, and clinical results of at least the low-viscosity cement, as noted earlier, have been inferior. Concern also has been raised about the effects of pressurization of low-viscosity cement. Bean demonstrated 50 percent to 80 percent penetration of the cortical region with low-viscosity cement at pressures of 60 to 80 psi.[9] In his model, there was no difference in the shear strength at the bone-cement interface between low-viscosity cement and Simplex-P.

Askew et al. have shown PMMA penetration to be a decreasing function of the bone strength, with the ultimate failure load capacity being a balance between the cement penetration allowed by bone porosity and the actual strength of the cancellous bone.[6] Although stronger, denser bone may limit cement penetration, the strength of the composite may be greater than that provided by higher cement penetration into weak cancellous bone. They suggested an optimal penetration depth of 4 mm because only weak bone specimens consistently yielded greater than 4 mm without increasing failure loads.

The strength of the other prosthetic interfaces, which is between the cement and the stem, also has been understood to be affected by the characteristics of the cement. Cement used at an earlier stage in the setting process (i.e., while it has a lower viscosity), adheres more firmly to a rough surface stem than cement used later in the setting process (i.e., while it is more viscous).[106] On the other hand, stem insertion into the cement mantle at a later stage leads to greater cement pressurization, which may improve the quality of bone-cement interface.

Cement Mantle

Satisfactory circumferential thickness of the cement mantle surrounding the femoral component appears to be valuable for two reasons. First, when the mantle becomes very thin, it becomes weak and is at risk of fracture.[54,68] Cement fracture in turn can lead to symptomatic loosening and failure of the arthroplasty. Second, total absence of a cement mantle can give bony access to particulate debris tracking along the implant-cement interface, thereby leading to femoral osteolysis. It should be noted, however, that some surgeons do not believe in the value of a continuous, relatively thick cement mantle. Some have reported good long-term clinical success with a Charnley-style implant inserted with nearly line-to-line broaching and cement. Cement mantle thickness is determined by several factors. The size and dimensions of the femoral canal after preparation in relationship to the size of the component implanted are critical: If the implant system does not "downsize" the femoral component sufficiently compared with the broach (for a given size), an inadequate mantle is provided. Alignment of the femoral component can cause locally thin cement mantles; for example, a component placed in marked varus alignment has a thin cement mantle proximally-medially and distal-laterally. Finally, a component that is not centered well in the prepared canal can be surrounded by areas of locally thin cement or even have areas of complete cement mantle deficiency. Most current prosthesis designs provide means of optimizing component centralization. These include modular or factory-assembled methyl methacrylate spacers that fit on the proximal and distal areas of the component, and, in some cases, proximal component geometries that force the prosthesis into a central position in the prepared femur during implantation.

INDICATIONS

Excellent clinical results combined with a relatively low rate of long-term aseptic loosening and osteolysis make cemented femoral component fixation the standard against which all other means of femoral fixation must be compared (Fig. 48–11).

A good case can be made for using either cemented or uncemented femoral components in the great majority of hip arthroplasties. Cemented femoral fixation probably is not as dependent on femoral bone quality, geometry, or the biology of bone healing as is uncemented fixation; therefore, cemented femoral fixation is versatile and applicable to most clinical situations. Nevertheless, certain femoral canal geometries favor the use of cemented implants, whereas in others uncemented implants are more suitable.

Undoubtedly, cemented femoral component loosening is more frequent in younger, heavier, more active patients. This has led many to advocate the use of uncemented femoral components in young, active patients with good bone quality and suitable geometry for uncemented components (see Chapters 49, 51, and 76).

At the present time, most favor use of a cemented femoral component for older, less active patients. In the very young, active patient with excellent bone, many

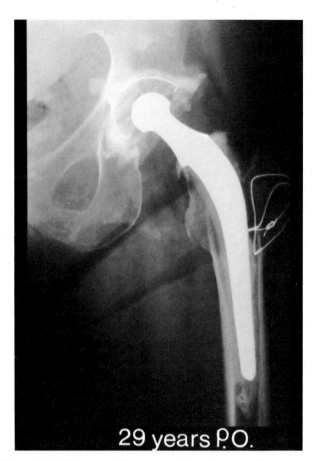

Figure 48–11. Cemented Charnley total hip arthroplasty 29 years after surgery. The femoral component is well fixed.

favor uncemented femoral fixation. For patients between these extremes, the discretion of the surgeon is necessary. For patients younger than age 65, we strongly consider use of uncemented stems if bone quality is satisfactory, whereas for patients older than age 65 we strongly consider use of a cemented stem. However, age is by no means the sole factor used at our institution to determine which type of femoral component fixation to use.

High activity, heavy weight, and male gender all are factors that make us consider uncemented stem fixation more strongly, whereas lower activity and lower life expectancy make cemented fixation attractive. Finally, we emphasize bone geometry and quality in decisions concerning femoral implant fixation. Excellent bone quality with strong cancellous bone and thick cortices is a positive attribute for uncemented fixation, whereas poor bone quality makes cemented fixation more appealing. A thin diaphysis, particularly in the patient with a relatively large femoral neck length and offset, limits the surgeon's ability to choose. It is very difficult to select an implant of adequate size to meet the patient's biomechanical need of matching proximal femoral geometry and yet not implant a stem so large that excessive cancellous bone is removed from the femur. This problem arises as a consequence of proportionality between neck length and base offset and stem size in most implant systems. To achieve success in cemented stem fixation, it is important to maintain cancellous bone in the femoral canal; the presence of cancellous bone makes possible the microinterlock between cement and bone discussed earlier. Thus, in patients with predominantly Dorr type A bone ("champagne-flute"-shaped) femur, we tend to use uncemented implants. On the other hand, for patients with poor bone and a very strong Door type C bone ("stove-pipe"-shaped) femur, we tend to use cemented fixation. Kobayashi has shown that cemented Charnley femoral components exhibit a lower survival rate in stove-pipe-shaped femurs with a low metaphyseal flare index,[60a] but we are concerned that this canal shape may be even more adverse for uncemented stem fixation.

RESULTS

Improvements in prosthesis design and technique logically should lead to improved results. Clinical data are now available that verify the usefulness of some of these changes. However, since the early 1990s, we have learned that not all changes represent steps forward. To determine whether, in fact, a change is truly an advance, each innovation in technique and implant design should be scrutinized and evaluated carefully before it is widely implemented.

The results of cemented THA femoral components vary considerably in different series. Factors affecting reported results may include (1) the makeup of the patient population, (2) the type of prosthesis implanted, (3) the surgical and cementation technique used, (4) the surgeon or group of surgeons performing the surgery, (5) the definitions used to report results, and (6) the length of follow-up.[10,16,39,48–50,57,58,67,73,78,79,89,91,93,94,97,99,101,108,114,117,119]

Demographic factors clearly have a significant impact on the likelihood of prosthesis survivorship. Younger age has been shown in many studies to have an adverse affect on cemented femoral fixation.[52,94,102,105] Likewise, higher weight and higher activity level have been shown to be associated with a higher rate of cemented femoral component failure.[52,105] Male gender also appears to be associated with a higher risk of cemented femoral component loosening.[52,58] The diagnosis also affects the likelihood of failure: Avascular necrosis and post-traumatic arthrosis have both been associated with a higher risk, whereas polyarticular rheumatoid arthritis has been associated with lower risk of cemented femoral failure.[56]

Technical factors, including prosthesis size and position, as well as quality of cement mantle, all appear to play a role in the likelihood of cemented femoral component failure. Prostheses that are too large, as well as prostheses that are too small in proportion to the patient's femoral canal, are at increased risk of failure.[53] Oversized prostheses lead to a thin cement mantle, high cement stresses, and a higher risk of cement failure. Grossly undersized components lead to a thick cement mantle and an overly flexible stem, which may cause higher cement stresses. Significantly undersized stems also are less torsionally stable in the cement mantle. The optimal cement mantle thickness appears to be 2 to 3 mm.[40] Most prostheses are now available in multiple sizes to permit matching of the prosthesis size to the individual femur.[80]

The effect of prosthesis position on survivorship of femoral components is controversial. Most believe that neutral component alignment is desirable.[39] Data suggest an adverse effect from varus femoral component position.[37,93,108] Valgus positioning was once thought to be advantageous, but there are now data suggesting that it may also have adverse consequences.[90] The detrimental effects of alignment other than neutral on prosthesis survivorship probably occur for several reasons, including adverse alterations in hip mechanics and production of locally thin cement mantles.

The quality of the cement mantle and the quality of cement fixation to the surrounding bone can have dramatic effects on the likelihood of long-term success of the procedure. The important contributions of Harris and his co-workers have demonstrated the value of optimizing the manner in which cement is used. They have categorized the quality of the initial cement mantle obtained after THA (Table 48–1). Using this classification scheme, they have shown that the quality of the initial cement mantle has prognostic significance. In a review of 102 hips that were followed for a mean of 15.2 years after cemented THA, they found that 72 patients with grade A, B, or C-1 cement technique had a 4 percent rate of femoral loosening, whereas 21 patients with grade C-2 technique had a 29 percent rate of femoral aseptic loosening.[17] This suggests that steps taken to optimize the quality of the cement mantle at surgery may lead to an improvement in long-term cemented femoral component performance.

The results of cemented THA have been subdivided according to the "generation" of the hip replacement. First-generation THA includes use of stems not made of super alloys and some designs with sharp, narrow

Table 48–1. SURVIVORSHIP OF 2000 HIPS BY TIME FROM SURGERY

Time After Total Hip Arthroplasty (yr)	Survivorship Free of Any Reoperation (percent)	Survivorship Free of Component Removal or Revision for Any Reason (percent)	Survivorship Free of Revision for Aseptic Loosening (percent)
5	96.1	98.0	99.6
10	91.8	94.0	97.1
15	87.1	89.8	93.8
20	81.3	84.1	89.4
25	77.5	80.9	86.5

medial borders. Cement is hand-packed into the femoral canal, and no canal plug is used. Second-generation techniques use super-alloy stems with broad medial borders. The canal is plugged and cement is introduced in a retrograde fashion with a cement gun. Third-generation techniques add surface treatments to femoral prostheses to enhance the stem-cement bond, and cement vacuum mixing or centrifugation is added to reduce cement porosity. In many newer stem designs, proximal and distal spacers have been added to centralize the prosthesis and to help create an even cement mantle.

Further discussion of results is subdivided according to cement generation. However, it should be recognized that not all series from one generation are equivalent because there are significant design variations among prostheses of the same generation.

First-Generation Results: Charnley Total Hip Arthroplasty

The total hip arthroplasty design and technique introduced by Sir John Charnley remains the gold standard to which all others are compared. Berry and co-authors reviewed the Mayo Clinic's 25-year results with this prosthesis.[14] Two thousand consecutive primary Charnley arthroplasties were performed between March 1969 and September 1971. The femoral component used was a smooth-surface stainless steel monoblock, the so-called flat-back Charnley component, with a 22.25-mm head. The mean patient age was 63.5 years. The diagnosis leading to total hip arthroplasty was osteoarthritis in 82 percent. Of the 2000, 97 percent were followed for at least 25 years or until revision operation, component removal, or death. The longest follow-up period was 28.4 years. The survivorship free of component removal for any reason was 80.9 percent (Fig. 48–12). The femoral component survivorship free of revision for aseptic loosening at 25 years was 89.8 percent (see Table 48–3). The 25-year rates of acetabular and femoral component survivorship free of aseptic loosening were similar. There were more femoral than acetabu-lar revisions for aseptic loosening in the first 15 years of the study, but fewer femoral than acetabular revisions in the last 10 years. Age at arthroplasty was the single most important factor affecting durability (Table 48–2), and for each decade earlier in life that the arthroplasty was performed, the revision rate for aseptic loosening increased. Men experienced almost a twofold higher aseptic loosening rate than women. Similarly, Neuman et al. reported a 20-year probability of survival of 88.3 percent in patients younger than 55 years, and 89.3 percent in patients older than 55 years.[78]

Callaghan et al. also reported a 25-year experience with 330 Charnley THA done by a single surgeon.[19] The prevalence of revision because of aseptic loosening of the femoral component was 3 percent, and the prevalance of revision in the 59 hips in the patients still living at the end of the study was 7 percent. Of the 62 hips in patients who lived for at least 25 years after the surgery, 48 (77 percent) had retained the original prosthesis. Schulte et al.[103] reported in more detail the 20-year results of the same group of 330 THAs. Twenty-year survivorship free of revision for aseptic femoral loosening in that series was 95 percent, and 20-year survivorship free of definite radiographic femoral loosening or revision for aseptic femoral loosening was 83 percent. Older, from England, has also reported 20-year results of Charnley THA.[87,88] He found a 3 percent rate of femoral revision for aseptic loosening in 370 Charnley THAs followed for at least 20 years or until death.

One of the reasons for success of the original smooth Charnley stem may be that it is well tolerated by the patient, even if it is debonded from the cement mantle (because of the smooth surface finish that produces little particulate debris when it debonds from the cement). Other factors contributing to its success include: (1) The flat-backed design was rotationally stable in the cement and (2) the 22.225-mm femoral head produced relatively little volumetric polyethylene wear. Finally, it should be noted that results of Charnley THAs done more than 25 years ago were derived from a different type patient population than the present THA group. Thus, in the younger, more demanding patient population now being treated with THA, the Charnley prosthesis may be less durable.

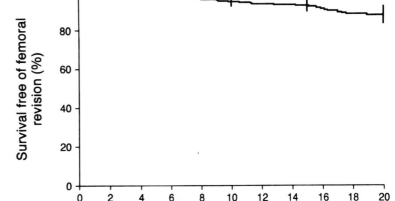

Figure 48–12. Survivorship of Charnley femoral component free of revision or removal for aseptic loosening, by age.

Table 48–2. SURVIVORSHIP[†] BY AGE AT INITIAL ARTHROPLASTY

Age at Total Hip Arthroplasty (yr)[*]	25-Year Survivorship Free of Revision for any Reason	25-Year Survivorship Free of Revision for Aseptic Femoral Loosening	25-Year Survivorship Free of Revision for Aseptic Loosening	25-Year Survivorship Free of Revision for Aseptic Acetabular Loosening
<40	63.7	68.7	82.4	73.7
40–49	62.0	72.7	82.6	80.7
50–59	75.9	81.0	84.6	86.1
60–69	86.9	92.2	92.9	93.6
70–79	92.6	95.9	96.8	98.6
>80	100	100	100	100

*For each column age (P <0.0001 in each case) was a statistically significant determinant of survivorship to the given endpoint.
†Survivorship estimate censored at 20 years because of decreasing number of patients at risk.

The long-term Charnley THA results are better than those reported for other first-generation cemented stems.[37,90] Pavlov reported the 15-year results of 512 Charnley-Müller hip arthroplasties and found a 40-percent rate of failure requiring revision.[90] Dunn and Hamilton reported a 40-percent incidence of loosening of the same stem in 185 hips 10 to 14 years after surgery.[37] Adverse design features of first-generation stems (other than the Charnley) included narrow, sharp medial borders that caused high cement stresses and geometries that caused locally thin cement mantles. Table 48–2 summarizes the results of several long-term studies of cemented femoral component performance.

Second-Generation Results

Several series with 10 or more years of clinical and radiographic follow-up have demonstrated the efficacy of second-generation femoral implants and surgical technique (see Table 48–2). Mulroy and Harris[77] reported 10- to 12.7-year (mean, 11.2 years) results of 105 cemented primary femoral components of several designs implanted with second-generation techniques. At last follow-up, two femoral components had been revised for loosening, and 1 was definitely loose, for an overall aseptic loosening rate of 3 percent. Localized endosteal osteolysis was seen in 6.8 percent of hips.

Stauffer reported 8.8- to 11.5-year[107] (mean, 9.6 years) year results of 222 hip arthroplasties also performed with second-generation techniques and the HD-2 stem. He found a 3.2 percent rate of femoral revision for aseptic loosening and a 4.9 percent rate of definite radiographic femoral loosening. Survivorship free of aseptic femoral loosening at 10 years was 95 percent.

Sanchez-Sotelo et al. reviewed the long-term Mayo Clinic experience with 256 consecutive of HD-2 design THAs performed between 1980 and 1983 with second generation cementing technique.[99] The mean patient age at operation was 66 years and the underlying diagnosis was osteoarthrosis in 71%. At a 15 year median follow-up 7% had been revised for aseptic femoral loosening. Survival free for aseptic loosening at 15 years for the femoral component was 92.2%. When the group was stratified by age the result was significantly worse in patients younger than 50 years of age in whom the survivorship free of mechanical femoral component failure at 15 years was only 72.3 percent.[100] Bourne et al. also reported outcomes of the same Harris Design-2 (HD-2) femoral stem.[15] At a mean of 12 years 97 percent of 191 HD-2 implants were in situ or had been in situ at the time of the patient's death. They did not, however, stratify patients by age. Smith et al. reviewed their 20-year experience with second generation cementing techniques in patients aged 50 years or younger.[106] They found a troublesome loosening rate in the young patients. Four femoral components (8 percent) were revised for osteolysis without loosening and 6 percent were revised for aseptic loosening.

A recent report from Iowa[59] compared the Charnley THA inserted with a second-generation cement technique with the Charnley THA inserted with a first-generation technique. At a minimum of 20 years of follow-up, the failure rate from femoral loosening was lower in the second-generation group, but the difference was not statistically different. The authors could show, however, that adequate filling of the femoral canal was associated with improved stem survival.

Data from the Swedish Joint Registry, which follows all joint arthroplasties performed in Sweden, have demonstrated an improved stem survival rate when second-generation cement techniques were used.[51] Taken together, the bulk of these data[66] support the idea that use of a canal plug and retrograde filling of the canal with a cement gun improve cemented stem survival.

Third-Generation Results

Oishi et al.[86] reported 6- to 8-year (mean, 7 years) results in 100 hybrid THAs (uncemented socket and cemented femur) with third-generation cement technique and a Harris Precoat prosthesis on the femoral side. Only one patient developed femoral loosening requiring revision and none had definite radiographic femoral loosening. Six percent had localized femoral osteolysis. The mean Harris Hip Score was 91 at last follow-up.

Longer term results of third-generation techniques have just started to be reported (Fig. 48–13). Only time

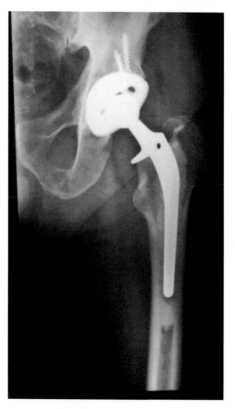

Figure 48–13. Hybrid hip replacement with cemented femoral stem implanted with third-generation technique and centralization.

will tell whether these techniques and implant changes can equal or surpass the high standard set by older designs such as the Charnley THA. The Mayo Clinic experience using third-generation cement techniques with Precoat Stem was reviewed by Duffy et al.[36] Ninety consecutive primary total hip arthroplasties performed for osteoarthritis with Precoat Plus stem were followed for a mean of 12 years. There were 4 revisions (5 percent) for aseptic loosening, debonding, and osteolysis. All 4 aseptic revisions initially had a poor cement grade. Overall survival free of aseptic loosening at 12 years was 95 percent. However, the authors expressed concern that stems with poor cement technique might subsequently debond and fail.[36] Previous reports in the literature have documented failures of this design related to poor cementing technique.[35] Clohisy and Harris reported better results in 121 primary total hips using the Precoat stem.[25] At an average 10-year follow-up, only one femoral component had to be revised for aseptic loosening. Three other femoral components were radiographically loose.

A comparison of two different prosthetic designs implanted by a common third-generation technique also has been studied.[12,20] One hundred fifty Precoat stems had a survivorship rate free of revision or radiographic loosening at 10 years of 98.6 percent, whereas the survivorship of the Iowa hip at 7 years free of aseptic loosening was 90.6 percent. Mohler et al. also reported a high failure rate caused by debonding and osteolysis with the rough surface, round geometry Iowa stem.[75] That stem was thought to have failed at a higher rate for several reasons: (1) It was difficult to achieve a good cement mantle; (2) the round stem geometry provided less torsional stability in the cement mantle (especially in combination with its high offset); (3) the rough surface finish led to a rapid clinical failure because of symptomatic loosening and osteolysis if debonding occurred. Overall, the jury is out on the value of the third-generation technique. Evaluation of the technique has been complicated by the fact that many of the designs placed with third-generation methods have had high failure rates, perhaps more owing to specific features of implant design than to cementation method. Efforts to enhance the stem-cement bond with a rough or precoated surface finish are generally thought to have been a step backward, but cement porosity reduction and stem centralization in the canal probably will prove to have been advantageous.

TECHNIQUE

Several steps in the process of cemented femoral component implantation merit special consideration.

Bone Preparation

Accurate sizing, reaming, and rasping of the proximal femur have contributed to improved implant matching in the wide range of femoral canal geometries encountered in the normal population. Instrument systems that remove almost all of the cancellous bone, although perhaps appropriate to prepare the canal for an uncemented femoral component, are not desirable when preparation is underway for cemented femoral fixation. A good mantle of strong cancellous endosteal bone should be left behind for cement intrusion.

After the endosteal cavity has been prepared to accept the femoral stem, fixation can be improved by removing any loose cancellous bone and debris present. Weber has suggested the use of special brushes, but this can also be accomplished by simply scrubbing the prepared surface with a surgical sponge passed up and down the cavity or by gentle use of a uterine curette.[114] Pulsatile lavage also helps to remove fat debris and blood from the interstices of the bone. This improves cement instrusion and implant fixation, which results in lower rates of femoral component demarcation and loosening.[48,49,81,99] Plugging of the femoral canal before pulsatile lavage allows removal in a retrograde fashion of a significant portion of the debris from the endosteal cavity of the femur.

After the bone has been prepared, it is helpful to achieve as dry a bone surface as possible to avoid the documented adverse affects on cement strength of included fat or blood.[41,43] Methods to reduce bleeding from the endosteal surface of the femur include hypotensive general anesthesia, spinal anesthesia, and topical application of epinephrine or thrombin. Simple packing of the femoral canal with absorbent surgical sponges just before introduction of the cement has also proved effective.

Cement Preparation and Delivery

Significant changes in the preparation of PMMA and its introduction into the femur have occurred since Charnley's original technique was described. The concept of canal plugging, originally introduced by Amstutz, can be accomplished with a separate bolus of PMMA, which can be introduced by a special medullary plug syringe.[3,84] Other options include bone plugs fashioned from the osteotomized femoral head or plastic plugs (available in a variety of sizes and designs). Although the convenience of using commercially available plastic plugs for intramedullary plugging is attractive, work by Beim et al. has documented the superiority of PMMA to bone and two different plastic plug designs with respect to both the level of medullary pressure achieved and subsequent ability of the plug to withstand canal pressurization without cement leakage or distal plug migration.[11]

Oh and Harris reported on the technique of retrograde canal filling using a cement gun after distal plugging. The authors emphasized the potential value of pressurization of the cement mass after its introduction into the canal (Fig. 48–14).[85] A femoral cement compactor was designed by this group to further facilitate the already improved cement intrusion into bone

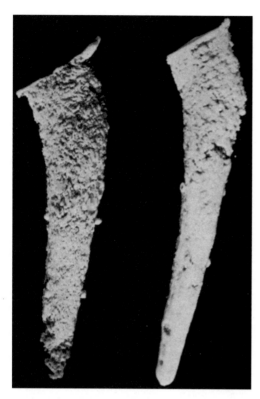

Figure 48–14. Two methacrylate casts of the femoral canals after dissolving the bone with nitric acid: one from a femur with a plug (*left*) and one from a femur without a plug (*right*). The cast from the plugged femur showed fine projections and indentations reflecting the greater penetration of the cement into the cancellous bone. (From Oh I, Harris WH: Proximal strain distribution in the loaded femur: An in vivo comparison of the distribution in the intact femur and after insertion of different hip replacement femoral components. J Bone Joint Surg 60A:75, 1978.)

achieved with simple distal plugging of the canal.[83] Modifications of the cement gun for retrograde canal filling include the addition of a retractable umbrella tip designed to help avoid mixing air, fat, or blood into the cement at the time of cement introduction into the canal. Many systems now allow cement introduction and pressurization by providing various attachments for the same cement gun.

AUTHORS' PREFERENCE

Preoperative planning is an essential ingredient of success. Acetabular component templates are used to determine the desired acetabular component position and the anticipated center of hip rotation. Femoral templates are then used to determine proper femoral component design and size. The femoral component design chosen is based on the surgeon's preferences and on the geometry of the patient's proximal femur. The femoral component size is chosen to match the canal and to provide sufficient room for an adequate cement mantle (at least 2 to 3 mm). The femoral neck osteotomy level is chosen based on the level needed to equalize (when possible) the patient's leg lengths and reproduce the patient's

native hip "offset." Exposure for routine cases may be by anterolateral or posterolateral routes at the surgeon's preference. At the Mayo Clinic, the two are used with about equal frequency. In complex cases, the transtrochanteric approach may be employed.

Before the femoral neck osteotomy is performed, external or internal landmarks are measured to gauge the patient's starting leg length. The femoral neck is osteotomized according to the preoperative plan, using the lesser trochanter and greater trochanter as landmarks. It is wise to make the osteotomy a little higher than the final planned femoral neck resection level.

After the insertion of the socket, the femoral canal is prepared. We prefer instruments that are designed to leave behind good-quality cancellous bone for cement interdigitation. Most systems allow minimal reaming followed by canal preparation with broaches. The goal should be canal preparation to provide neutral prosthesis alignment in the coronal and sagittal planes. When the anterior approach is chosen, there is a tendency— which should be avoided—to flex the component, leading to a locally thin cement mantle proximally (anteriorly) and distally (posteriorly). Component anteversion of approximately 10 to 15 degrees on the femoral side is usually desirable, and, except in cases of distorted anatomy, following the patient's own femoral neck anatomy reproduces appropriate anteversion.

With the final broach in place, trial reduction is performed. Leg length is checked and hip stability is tested. An appropriate neck length is chosen. The femoral neck osteotomy may be revised to optimize leg length, if necessary. If a collared prosthesis is introduced, a calcar planer is used to smooth the femoral neck osteotomy. The broach position is noted to serve as a landmark for positioning of the real femoral component.

A uterine curette, canal brush, or both are then used to gently remove loose fat and very weak cancellous bone from the canal. All good cancellous bone is left behind to optimize conditions for cement interdigitation. The best bone for this is usually within 2 to 3 mm of the endosteum. A canal plug is placed. A well-designed plastic plug or acrylic cement plug may be used. The plug should be placed to provide about a 2-cm cement column distal to the prosthesis tip. The canal is then prepared with a Water Pic. Removal of loose canal contents and fat improves the cement-bone bond. The canal is packed with dilute epinephrine-soaked sponges and then dried meticulously with suction and dry sponges.

Methyl methacrylate cement is mixed under vacuum conditions or mixed and then centrifuged for 1 minute. Usually two and a half batches of cement are satisfactory for smaller femurs; three batches of cement are necessary for larger femurs. Cement is introduced into the canal in a retrograde fashion using a cement gun. Cement is pressurized by the cement gun with an attachment to occlude the top of the canal. Pressurization is most effective if applied for a period of time as opposed to very briefly.

The prosthesis is inserted with the cement in a doughy state. All efforts are made to insert the prosthesis in neutral alignment. At the present time, we prefer a collared stem with a low surface roughness or a tapered collarless stem that is polished. While the cement is hardening, care is taken to avoid moving the leg and the prosthesis. Excess cement is removed as it hardens. Prosthesis systems with proximal and distal centralizers to help ensure good prosthesis alignment and an even, satisfactory, circumferential cement mantle are helpful.

After the methyl methacrylate cement has completely hardened, the hip is reduced and stability retested. Care should be taken to ensure that no debris remains in the socket at the time of reduction, because this can lead to third-body abrasive wear of the polyethylene. Closure in layers is routine. Suction drains are used at the discretion of the surgeon.

The postoperative rehabilitation protocol varies according to the surgeon's discretion and is based on the type of approach and the type of acetabular component fixation.

References

1. Ahmed AM, Raab S, Miller JE: Metal cement interface strength in cemented stem fixation. J Orthop Res 2:105, 1984.
2. Alkire MJ, Dabezies EJ, Hastings PR: High vacuum as a method of reducing porosity of methylmethacrylate. Orthopedics 10:1533, 1987.
3. Amstutz HC, Markolf KL, McNeice GM, Gruen TA: Loosening of total hip components: Cause and prevention. In Evarts CM (ed): The Hip: Proceedings of the Fourth Open Scientific Meeting of the Hip Society. St. Louis, CV Mosby, 1976, p 102.
4. Andriacchi TP, Galnte JO, Belytschko TB, Hamptom S: A stress analysis of the femoral stem in total hip prosthesis. J Bone Joint Surg 58A:618, 1976.
5. Anthony PP, Gie GA, Howie CR, Ling RSM: Localized endosteal bone lysis in relation to the femoral components of cemented total hip arthroplasties. J Bone Joint Surg 72B:971, 1990.
6. Askew MJ, Steege IW, Lewis JL: Effect of cement pressure and bone strength on polymethylmethacrylate fixation. J Orthop Res 1:412, 1984.
7. Bargar WL, Brown SA, Paul HA, et al: In vivo versus in vitro polymerization of acrylic bone cement: Effect on mechanical properties. J Orthop Res 4:86, 1986.
8. Bargar WL, Heiple KG, Weber S, et al: Contrast bone cement. J Orthop Res 1:92, 1983.
9. Bean DJ: Regional variations in bone-cement interface shear strength in the human femur. Orthop Trans 10:73, 1986.
10. Beckenbaugh RD, Ilstrup D: Total hip arthroplasty: A review of 333 cases with long follow-up. J Bone Joint Surg 60A:306, 1978.
11. Beim GM, Lavernia C, Conbery FR: Intramedullary plugs in cement hip arthroplasty. J Arthroplasty 4:139, 1989.
12. Berger RA, Kull LR, Rosenberg AG, Galante JO: Hybrid total hip arthroplasty: 7–10 years results. Clin Orthop 333:134, 1996.
13. Berry DJ, Barnes CL, Scott RD, et al: Catastrophic failure of the polyethylene liner of uncemented acetabular components. J Bone Joint Surg 76B:575, 1994.
14. Berry DJ, Harmsen WS, Cabanela ME, Morrey BF: 25 Year survivorship of 2000 consecutive primary Charnley total hip arthroplasties: Factors governing acetabular and femoral component survivorship. J Bone Joint Surg 84A:171, 2002.
15. Bourne RB, Rorabeck CH, Skutek M, et al: The Haris Design-2 total hip replacement fixed with so-called second-generation cementing techniques. A 10–15 year follow-up. J Bone Joint Surg 80A:1775, 1998.
16. Brady LP, McCutchen JW: A ten-year follow-up study of 170 Charnley total hip arthroplasties. Clin Orthop 211:51, 1986.
17. Bragdon CR, Biggs S, Mulroy WF, et al: Defects in the cement mantle: A fatal flaw in cemented femoral stems for THR. Presented at the 24th Annual Hip Course, Boston, September 29, 1994.
18. Burke DW, Gates EI, Harris WH: Centrifugation as a method of improving tensile and fatigue properties of acrylic bone cement. J Bone Joint Surg 66A:1265, 1984.
19. Callaghan JJ, Johnston RC, Pedersen DR, et al: Why did we leave Charnley total hip arthroplasty? 1994 [submitted for Kappa Delta Award].
20. Cannestra VP, Berger RA, Quigley LR, et al: Hybrid total hip arthroplasty with a precoated offset stem. Four to nine-year results. J Bone Joint Surg 82A:1291, 2000.
21. Cates HE, Faris PM, Keating EM, Ritter MA: Polyethylene wear in cemented metal-backed acetabular cups. J Bone Joint Surg 75B:249, 1993.
22. Charnley J: Arthroplasty of the hip: A new operation. Lancet 1:1129, 1961.
23. Charnley J: Low Friction Arthroplasty of the Hip: Theory and Practice. New York, Springer-Verlag, 1979, p 1.
24. Chin HC, Stauffer RN, Chao EYS: Effect of centrifugation on cement property in an in vitro total hip arthroplasty model. J Bone Joint Surg 72A:363, 1990.
25. Clohisy JC, Harris WH: Primary hybrid total hip replacement, performed with insertion of the acetabular component without cement and precoat femoral component with cement. An average 10-year follow-up study. J Bone Joint Surg 81A:247, 1999.
26. Collier JP, Surprenant VA, Jensen RE, et al: Corrosion between the components of mudlar femoral hip prostheses. J Bone Joint Surg 74B:511, 1992.
27. Crowninshield RD, Brand RA, Johnston RC: A comparison of steel and titanium as femoral component implant materials. Clin Orthop 235:173, 1988.
28. Crowinshield RD, Brand RA, Johnston RC, Milroy JC: An analysis of femoral component stem design in total hip arthroplasty. J Bone Joint Surg 62A:68, 1980.
29. Crowninshield RD, Brand RA, Johnston RC, Milroy JC: The effect of femoral stem cross-sectional geometry on cement stresses in total hip reconstruction. Clin Orthop 146:71, 1980.
30. Crowninshield RD, Brand RA, Johnston RC, Pedersen DR: An analysis of collar function and the use of titanium in femoral prostheses. Clin Orthop 158:270, 1981.
31. Crowninshield RD, Brand RA, Johnston RC, Pedersen DR: An analysis of femoral prosthesis design: The effects on proximal femur loading. Ninth Open Scientific Meeting of The Hip Society. St. Louis, CV Mosby, 1981, p 111.
32. Davies JP, Burke DW, O'Connor DO, Harris WH: Comparison of the fatigue characteristics of centrifuged and uncentrifuged Simplex-P bone cement. J Orthop Res 5:366, 1987.
33. Davies JP, Jasty M, O'Connor DO, et al: The effect of centrifuging bone cement. J Bone Joint Surg 71B:39, 1989.
34. Djerf K, Gilchrist J: Calcar unloading after hip replacement: A cadaver study of femoral stem designs. Acta Orthop Scand 58:97, 1987.
35. Dowd JE, Cha CW, Trakru S, et al: Failure of total hip arthroplasty with a precoated prosthesis. 4–11 year results. Clin Orthop 123, 1998.
36. Duffy G, Lewallen DG: Long-term results of a precoated proximally Macrotextured femoral component. Poster for AAOS, Dallas, 2002.
37. Dunn AW, Hamilton LR: Müller curved-stem total hip arthroplasty: Long-term follow-up of 185 consecutive cases. South Med J 79:698, 1986.
38. Eftekar NS: Dislocation and instability complicating low friction arthroplasty of the hip joint. Clin Orthop 121:120, 1976.
39. Eftekhar NS: Long-term results of cemented total hip arthroplasty. Clin Orthop 225:207, 1987.
40. Estak OM: Strains occurring within the cement mantle. Presented at the 24th Annual Hip Course, Boston, September 29, 1994.
41. Ferracane JL, Wixson RL, Lautenschlager EP: Effects of fat admixture on the strengths of conventional and low-viscosity bone cements. J Orthop Res 1:450, 1984.
42. Fowler JL, Gie GA, Lee AJC, Ling RSM: Experience with the Exeter total hip replacement since 1970. Orthop Clin North Am 19:477, 1988.

43. Gruen TA, Markolf KL, Amstutz HC: Effect of laminations and blood entrapment on the strength of acrylic bone cement. Clin Orthop 119:250, 1976.

44. Gruen TA, McNeice GM, Amstutz HC: Modes of failure of cemented stem-type femoral components: A radiographic analysis of loosening. Clin Orthop 141:17, 1979.

45. Hamilton WH, Cooper DF: Centrifuged cement shrinkage. Orthop Trans 11:212, 1987.

46. Harris WH: The case for cementing all femoral components in total hip replacement. Can J Surg 38:555, 1995.

47. Harris WH, Davies JP: Modern use of modern cement for total hip replacement. Orthop Clin North Am 19:581, 1988.

48. Harris WH, McCarthy JC Jr, O'Neil DA: Femoral component loosening using contemporary techniques of femoral cement fixation. J Bone Joint Surg 64A:1063, 1982.

49. Harris WH, McGann WA: Loosening of the femoral component after use of the medullary plug cementing technique. J Bone Joint Surg 68A:1064, 1986.

50. Havelin LI, Espehaug B, Vollset SE, Engesaeter LB: The effect of the type of cement on early revision of Charnley total hip prostheses. A review of eight thousand five hundred and seventy-nine primary arthroplasties form the Norwegian Arthroplasty Register. J Bone Joint Surg 77A:1543, 1995.

51. Herberts P, Malchau H: How outcome studies have changed total hip arthroplasty practices in Sweden. Clin Orthop 344:44, 1997.

51a. Hozack WJ, Rothman RH, Booth RE Jr, et al: Survivorship analysis of 1,041 Charnley total hip arthroplasties. J Arthroplasty 5:41, 1990.

52. Jaffe W: An eight to twelve year clinical experience with a normalized, proportional cemented hip system. Presented at "State-of-the-Art in Hip and Knee Replacement 1993: Technological Developments to Reduce Wear and Enhance Longevity," Breckenridge, CO, March 1993.

53. Jasty M, Estok D, Harris WH: The mechanisms involved in the failure of fixation of components in total hip arthroplasty. Semin Arthroplasty 4:238, 1993.

54. Johnston RC, Brand RA, Crowninshield RD: Reconstruction of the hip: A mathematical approach to determine optimum geometric relationships. J Bone Joint Surg 61A:639, 1979.

55. Joshi AB, Porter ML, Trail IA, et al: Long-term results of Charnley low-friction arthroplasty in young patients. J Bone Joint Surg 75B:616, 1993.

56. Kavanagh BF, Dewitz MA, Ilstrup DM, et al: Charnley total hip arthroplasty with cement: Fifteen year results. J Bone Joint Surg 71A:1496, 1989.

57. Kavanagh BF, Wallrichs S, Dewitz M, et al: Charnley low-friction arthroplasty of the hip: Twenty-year results with cement. J Arthroplasty 9:229, 1994.

58. Keller JC, Lautenschlager EP, Marshall GW, Mayer PR Jr: Factors affecting surgical alloy/bone cement interface adhesion. J Biomed Mater Res 14:639, 1980.

59. Klapach AS, Callaghan JJ, Goetz DD, Olejniczak JP, Johnston RC: Charnley total hip arthroplasty with use of improved cementing techniques. J Bone Joint Surg 83A:1840, 2001.

60. Knoell A, Maxwell H, Bechtol C: Graphite fiber reinforced bone cement. Ann Biomed Eng 3:255, 1975.

60a. Kobayashi S, Eftekhar NS, Terayama K, Joshi RP: Comparative study of total hip arthroplasty between younger and older patients. Clin Orthop 339:140–151, 1997.

61. Lewis JL, Askew MJ, Wixson RL, et al: The influence of prosthetic stem stiffness and a calcar collar on stresses in the proximal end of the femur with a cemented femoral component. J Bone Joint Surg 66A:280, 1984.

62. Lidgren L, Bodelind B, Moller J: Bone cement improved by vacuum mixing and chilling. Acta Orthop Scand 57:27, 1987.

63. Linden U: Fatigue properties of bone cement: Comparison of mixing techniques. Acta Orthop Scand 60:431, 1989.

64. Ling RSM: Prevention of loosening of total hip components. In Riley LH (ed): The Hip: Proceedings of the Eighth Open Scientific Meeting of the Hip Society. St. Louis, CV Mosby, 1980, p 292.

65. Madey SM, Callaghan JJ, Olejniczak JP, et al: Charnley total hip arthroplasty with use of improved techniques of cementing. The results after a minimum of 15 years of follow-up. J Bone Joint Surg 79:53, 1997.

66. Malchau H, Herberts P, Ahnfelt L, Johnell O: Prognosis of total hip replacement: Results from the national register of revised failures, 1979–1990 in Sweden: A ten year follow-up of 92, 675 THR. Scientific exhibition presented at the 61st annual meeting of the American Academy of Orthopaedic Surgeons, San Francisco, February 18–23, 1993.

67. Manley MT, Stern LS, Gurtowski J, Dee R: Comparison of proximal femoral biomechanics after implantation of titanium and cobalt-chromium femoral components. Trans Orthop Res Soc 8:239, 1983.

68. Manley MT, Stearn LS, Kotzar G, Stulberg BN: Femoral component loosening in hip arthroplasty: A cadaver study of subsidence and hip strain. Acta Orthop Scand 58:485, 1987.

69. Markolf KL, Amstutz HC: In vitro measurement of bone acrylic interface pressure during femoral component insertion. Clin Orthop 121:60, 1976.

70. Markolf KL, Amstutz HC: Penetration and flow of acrylic bone cement. Clin Orthop 121:99, 1976.

71. Markolf KL, Amstutz HC, Hirscholwitz DL: The effect of calcar contact on femoral component micromotion. J Bone Joint Surg 62A:1315, 1980.

72. McCoy TH, Salvati EA, Ranawat CS, Wilson PD Jr: A 15-year follow-up study of 100 Charnley low-friction arthroplasties. Orthop Clin North Am 19:467, 1988.

73. Miller J, Burke DL, Stachiewicz JW, et al: Pathophysiology of loosening of femoral components in total hip arthroplasty: Clinical and experimental study of cement fracture and loosening of the cement-bone interface. In The Hip: Proceedings of the Sixth Open Scientific Meeting of the Hip Society. St. Louis, CV Mosby, 1978, p 64.

74. Miller JE, Stephenson PK: Improved fixation in total hip arthroplasty using pressurized low viscosity cement: A radiological analysis. Orthop Trans 11:489, 1987.

75. Mohler CG, Callaghan JJ, Collis DK, et al: Early loosening of the femoral component at the cement prosthesis interface after total hip replacement. J Bone Joint Surg 77A:1315, 1995.

76. Morrey BF, Ilstrup D: Size of the femoral head and acetabular revision in total hip replacement-arthroplasty. J Bone Joint Surg 71A:50, 1989.

77. Mulroy RD Jr, Harris WH: The effect of improved cementing techniques on component loosening in total hip replacement: An 11 year radiographic review. J Bone Joint Surg 72B:757, 1990.

78. Neumann L, Freund KG, Sørenson KH: Long-term results of Charnley total hip replacement: Review of 92 patients at 15 to 20 years. J Bone Joint Surg 76B:245, 1994.

79. Noble PC, Alexander JW, Lindahl LJ, et al: The anatomic basis of femoral component design. Clin Orthop 235:148, 1988.

80. Noble PC, Jay JL, Cameron BM, et al: Innovations in acrylic bone cement. Scientific exhibit presented at the 53rd Annual Meeting of the American Academy of Orthopaedic Surgeons, New Orleans, February 20–25, 1986.

81. Noble PC, Swarts E: Penetration of acrylic cement into cancellous bone. Acta Orthop Scand 54:566, 1983.

82. Oh I, Bourne RB, Harris WH: The femoral cement compactor: An improvement in cementing technique in total hip replacement. J Bone Joint Surg 65A:1335, 1983.

83. Oh I, Carlson CE, Thomford WW, Harris WH: Improved fixation of the femoral component after total hip replacement using methylmethacrylate intramedullary plug. J Bone Joint Surg 60A:608, 1978.

84. Oh I, Harris WH: Proximal strain distribution in the loaded femur: An in vivo comparison of the distribution in the intact femur and after insertion of different hip replacement femoral components. J Bone Joint Surg 60A:75, 1978.

85. Oh I, Harris WH: A cement fixation system for total hip arthroplasty. Clin Orthop 164:221, 1982.

86. Oishi CS, Walker RH, Colwell CW Jr: The femoral component in total hip arthroplasty: Six to eight-year follow-up of 100 consecutive patients after use of a third-generation cementing technique. J Bone Joint Surg 76A:1130, 1994.

87. Older J: Charnley's by Charnley: A minimum follow-up of 20 years. Presented at the 23rd Open Meeting of the Hip Society, Orlando, FL, February 15, 1995.

88. Older J, Butorac R: Charnley low friction arthroplasty (LFA), a 17–21 year follow-up study. J Bone Joint Surg 74B(Suppl III):251, 1992

89. Pacheco V, Shelley P, Wroblewski BM: Mechanical loosening of the stem in Charnley arthroplasties: identification of the "at risk" factors. J Bone Joint Surg 70B:596, 1988.

90. Pavlov PW: A 15-year follow-up study of 512 consecutive Charnley-Müller total hip replacements. J Arthroplasty 2:151, 1987.
91. Pilliar RM, Bratina WJ, Blackwell R: Mechanical properties of carbon fiber reinforced polymethylmethacrylate for surgical implant applications. In Reifsnider KL, Lauraitis KN: Fatigue of Elementary Composite Material. Special Technical Publication 636. Philadelphia, American Society for Testing Materials, 1977, p 206.
92. Poss R, Brick GW, Wright RJ, et al: The effects of modern cementing techniques on the longevity of total hip arthroplasty. Orthop Clin North Am 19:591, 1988.
93. Ranawat CS, Atkinson RE, Salvati EA, Wilson PD Jr: Conventional total hip arthroplasty for degenerative joint disease in patients between the ages of 40 to 60 years. J Bone Joint Surg 66A:745, 1984.
94. Rey RM, Paiement GD, McGann WM, et al: A study of intrusion characteristics of low viscosity cement, Simplex-P and Palacos cements in a bovine cancellous bone model. Clin Orthop 215:272, 1987.
95. Rimnac CM, Wright TM, McGill DL: The effect of centrifugation on the fracture properties of acrylic bone cements. J Bone Joint Surg 68A:281, 1986.
96. Roberts DW, Poss R, Kelley KK: Radiographic comparison of cementing techniques in total hip arthroplasty. J Arthroplasty 1:241, 1986.
97. Robinson RP, Lovell TP, Green TM, Bailey GA: Early femoral component loosening in DF-80 total hip arthroplasty. J Arthroplasty 4:55, 1989.
98. Russotti GM, Coventry MN, Stauffer RN: Cemented total hip arthroplasty with contemporary techniques: A five-year minimum follow-up study. Clin Orthop 235:141, 1988.
99. Sanchez-Sotelo J, Berry DJ, Harmsen WS: Long-term results of a collared matte-finished femoral component fixed with modern cementing techniques. A fifteen-year-median follow-up study. J Bone Joint Surgery 84A:1636, 2002.
100. Sarmiento A, Ebramzadeh E, Gogan WJ, McKellop HA: Total hip arthroplasty with cement: A long-term radiographic analysis in patients who are older than 50 and younger than 50 years. J Bone Joint Surg 72A:1470, 1990.
101. Schmalzried TP, Harris WH: Hybrid total hip replacement: A 6.5 year follow-up study. J Bone Joint Surg 75B:608, 1993.
102. Schmalzried TP, Kwong LM, Jasty M, et al: The mechanism of loosening of cemented acetabular components in total hip arthroplasty: Analysis of specimens retrieved at autopsy. Clin Orthop 274:60, 1992.
103. Schulte KR, Callaghan JJ, Kelley SS, Johnston RC: The outcome of Charnley total hip arthroplasty with cement after a minimum 20-year follow-up. J Bone Joint Surg 75A:961, 1993.
104. Schurman DJ, Bloch DA, Segal MR, Tanner CM: Conventional cemented total hip arthroplasty: Assessment of clinical factors associated with revision for mechanical failure. Clin Orthop 240:173, 1989.
105. Shepard MF, Kabo JM, Lieberman JR: Influence of cement technique on the interface strength of femoral components. Clin Orthop 381:26, 2000.
106. Smith SE, Estok DM, Harris WH: 20-year experience with cemented primary and conversion total hip arthroplasty using so-called second-generation cementing techniques in patients aged 50 years or younger. J Arthroplasty 15:263, 2000.
107. Stauffer RN: Ten-year follow-up study of total hip replacement: With particular reference to roentgenographic loosening of the components. J Bone Joint Surg 64A:983, 1982.
108. Stauffer RN: Contemporary cement technique results: Total joint arthroplasty. Presented at the 1991 Hip and Knee Arthroplasty Current Techniques Meeting, Scottsdale, AZ, April 5, 1990.
109. Sutherland CJ, Wilde AH, Borden LS, Marks KE: A ten-year follow-up of 100 consecutive Müller curved-stem total hip replacement arthroplasties. J Bone Joint Surg 64A:970, 1982.
110. Tarr RR, Clarke IC, Gruen TA, et al: Total hip femoral component design. Orthop Rev 9:23, 1982.
111. Tarr RR, Lewis JL, Jaycox P, et al: Effect of materials, stem geometry, and collar-calcar contact on stress distribution in the proximal femur with total hip. Trans Orthop Res Soc 4:34, 1979.
112. Urban RM, Jacobs JJ, Gilbert JL, Galante JO: Migration of corrosion products from modular hip prostheses. J Bone Joint Surg 76A:1345, 1994.
113. Van der Schaaf DB, Deutman R, Mulder TJ: Stanmore total hip replacement: A nine to ten year follow-up. J Bone Joint Surg 70B:45, 1988.
114. Weber BG: Pressurized cement fixation in total hip arthroplasty. Clin Orthop 232:87, 1988.
115. Wixson RL, Lautenschlager EP, Novak MA: Vacuum mixing of acrylic bone cement. J Arthroplasty 2:141, 1987.
116. Wixson RL, Stulberg SD, Mehlhoff M: Total hip replacement with cemented, uncemented, and hybrid prostheses. J Bone Joint Surg 73A:257, 1991.
117. Wright TM, Treat PS: Mechanical properties of aramid fiber reinforced acrylic cement. J Mater Sci 14:503, 1979.
118. Wroblewski BM: 15–21 year results of the Charnley low-friction arthroplasty. Clin Orthop 211:30, 1986.
119. Wroblewski BM, Siney PD: Charnley low-friction arthroplasty of the hip. Clin Orthop 292:191, 1993.

49

Uncemented Femoral Components

• DANIEL J. BERRY, BERNARD F. MORREY, and MIGUEL E. CABANELA

Today, implant systems that do not require fixation by acrylic cement are well recognized and accepted. Unlike the knee, where enthusiasm for uncemented implants has waned, uncemented replacement of the hip has rebounded after a short decrease in use caused by failures of early uncemented designs. In this chapter, we review the design rationale and characteristics of uncemented femoral implants, discuss the indications and patient selection, review the technique for implantation, discuss published results and complications, and finally review the Mayo Clinic experience with reoperation for failure of these devices.

DESIGN

Consideration of the material properties from which the device is fashioned, the geometric properties that relate to its shape and function, and the surface characteristics is important for any implant design. These features are discussed in detail in Chapter 3. Here we summarize the design considerations we believe to be most important to the clinician when selecting an implant. However, it is important to note that there is a lack of uniformity of understanding and acceptance of design related to uncemented total hip arthroplasty principles. This point is emphasized by the fact that a survey of 260 hospitals in England found that there were over 30 designs of uncemented femoral components being used,[77] and, in a recent study in Norway, 398 different size and design options were available for uncemented total hip arthroplasty.[53]

Material Properties

Cobalt-chromium and titanium alloys have been most frequently employed for the fabrication of uncemented femoral components. Titanium alloys may have greater affinity for biologic incorporation, but both metals have been found to provide clinically satisfactory osteointegration.[49] Because stress transmission is a major factor in the long-term effectiveness of a device, the modulus of elasticity of the material is of critical importance. In this respect, titanium is the more attractive material because its elastic modulus more closely approximates that of

bone and is about one half that of cobalt-chromium (Fig. 49–1).[40]

One disadvantageous characteristic of titanium is that its strength is markedly reduced if the surface is flawed or notched. The recognized reduction in strength occurring from "notch sensitivity" of this material poses significant design and manufacturing constraints, particularly for surface treatment of the substrate.

The potential toxicity of the material is an additional consideration. Cobalt and chromium are detected in lower concentrations within the body, but, even in smaller concentrations, they tend to be more toxic to cells. In contrast, titanium is associated with greater debris and ionic release but seems to be better tolerated on a cellular level. When titanium prostheses loosen, the soft metal is easily abraded and large amounts of particulate debris may be released. The issue of material proprieties is discussed in detail in Chapters 2 through 7.

Composite materials have been employed to decrease wear and to more closely approximate the modulus of elasticity of bone. Most worldwide experience with composite femoral components has been with the uncemented Isoelastic stem, which, despite being an innovative design, has had a high rate of loosening and clinical failure. However, newer composite materials are at this time being tried in North America, and the preliminary reports appear promising. Given previous experiences, clinical trials are progressing cautiously.

Implant Design

Conceptually, an uncemented implant must (1) attain immediate stability, (2) attain long-term biologic fixation, and (3) provide for favorable biologic compatibility and long-term bony remodeling. To attain these goals, two design philosophies have been adopted: (1) press-fit smooth with a macrolock, and (2) press-fit textured with a microlock.

Stem

An assumption of macro- and microlock concepts for fixation is that a stem shape that closely resembles the anatomy of the proximal and distal femur can achieve stability and thus approximate the stress and strain

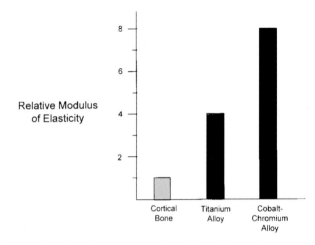

Figure 49–1. Relative modules of elasticity of bone, titanium, and cobalt-chromium.

patterns of the normal femur. Unfortunately, the normal strain pattern in the femur is based on an intact head and neck and is dramatically altered with any intramedullary-loaded system.

The effectiveness of press-fit designs is based on assumptions of bone geometry, the manner of the intramedullary loading, and interface conditions. Factors of major importance to the implantation of all uncemented implants are the considerable variation in the shape of the femur as well as variation of osseous strength. Because of the variation in proximal geometry of the femur, some have concluded that the greatest likelihood of obtaining consistently rigid fixation is in the cortical bone of the medullary canal rather than in the more proximal femur, with its irregular geometry.[48]

In order to obtain rigid fixation without cement, uncemented stems are typically much larger than cemented implants. This results in a significant increase in stiffness, thus predisposing to proximal stress shielding. To avoid this, flutes, slots, and other design features have been employed to allow "fill" without adverse stem stiffness.

A tightly fitting medullary stem is known to be effective in providing initial stability, but the rigidity of implant fixation may lessen after several months as a result of remodeling.[46] Studies in the dog indicate that the tightness of the fit distally does increase strain at the point of contact (thereby relieving strain proximally); however, this does not correlate with changes in long-term bone density.[76] Furthermore, as little as a 0.5-mm oversize difference in the diameter of an implant causes a 100 percent change in microstrain at the time of insertion. This has important implications with regard to hoop stresses and osseous failure, which is known to be associated with press-fit implants.[45] It has been documented in the laboratory that as small as a 1-mm oversized–diameter implant can regularly cause fractures in a dog femur at the time of insertion.[43]

The issue of appropriate fit, whether proximal or distal, continues to be the source of considerable discus-

sion, and great efforts have been made to measure "fill" of the proximal aspect of the femur (Fig. 49–2). Whereas the early designs tended to rely on distal fixation at the isthmus of the canal for rigid fixation, recent concepts favor proximal loading from total surface contact in both the anteroposterior and lateral planes. As can be seen in the Results section of this chapter, both approaches have enjoyed reasonable clinical success.

DESIGN, LOAD, AND SUBSIDENCE

The percentage of fill of the medullary canal with the implant accurately predicts the likelihood of subsidence of a specific design.[71] Yet the force of impaction or implantation is an even greater correlate of subsidence than is the so-called fit-and-fill measurement.[71] Interestingly, early subsidence up to 2 to 3 mm in the axial plane correlates very poorly with pain, but rotational instability of the femoral component does correlate with clinical symptoms of pain, which usually occurs with rising or stair climbing.[64] Studies of the implant geometry reveal that curved stems are better able to withstand out-of-plane torque than are straight stems, even though the stability to axial loading is not dramatically different ($P < 0.0114$). The efficacy of a proximal bow, however, has yet to be demonstrated clinically.

Studies of the change in position of the implant suggest that small amounts of very early longitudinal subsidence may be tolerated and still allow ultimate osteointegration, whereas rotational instability correlates with poor clinical results. As implied above,

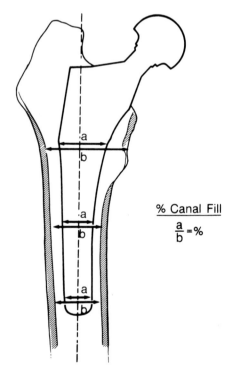

Figure 49–2. Formula for calculation of percentage of canal fill at the three regions of implant contact and fixations. (From Wixson RL, Stulberg D, Mehlhoff M: Total hip replacement with cemented, uncemented, and hybrid prostheses. J Bone Joint Surg Am 73:257, 1991, with permission.)

studies of stability suggest that the manner in which the implant is loaded can be important in demonstrating differences between the various implants and presumably surface treatments. Further investigations have demonstrated that less micromotion is present with cemented implants (average 75 μm) than uncemented devices (approximately 280 μm).[44] Compared to uncemented devices, cemented implants show less stability with an axial load than is shown in rotational stability, as seen with stair climbing.[33]

DESIGN AND REMODELING

Predicting an effective remodeling response is a complex issue, with current designs attempting to impart a load to the proximal metaphyseal portion of the femur. The effectiveness of stress transfer is based on the modulus of elasticity, shape and size of the component, presence of a collar, distribution of the porous coating, and surgical technique.[48,72,82] The difference in the elastic modulus between the titanium and the cobalt-chromium implant results in approximately 30 percent less stress shielding proximally and about 30 percent less shear stress distally with the titanium devices.[40] Remodeling in the experimental animal does not correlate well with the radiographic evidence of fit.[70] Significantly less resorption is predicted with cemented implants compared to uncemented devices.[83]

Collar

Most proximally porous-coated, metaphyseal-filling, uncemented implants are collarless, and this is based on the assumption that the depth of insertion should not be limited by the presence of a collar. Furthermore, the presence of a collar with a tapered stem design might be disadvantageous because a collar would limit the ability of the component to subside slightly early on to a stable position in the medullary canal. There are relatively few scientific or clinical data to suggest the value or the disadvantage of a collar with uncemented femoral devices. It has been demonstrated that the presence of a well-seated collar does increase stability of the uncemented device by as much as a factor of 4. This has been calculated in one-legged stance, but the difference is most demonstrable in stair climbing.[25] Long-stemmed press-fit implants have been shown to cause proximal compressive strains that were approximately 15 percent of normal without a collar, increasing to 50 percent of normal with a collar.[36] Some manufacturers, attempting not to prejudice the choice, have offered their implants with or without a collar as a modular option to be used according to surgeon preference. It is generally considered that, lacking convincing basic studies or clinical material, the collar appears neither to promote proximal bone remodeling nor to prevent stem subsidence.

Extensively coated devices gain most of their rotational stability by a "scratch-fit" in the diaphysis. These devices often do not fill the metaphysis completely, and therefore a collar is helpful to prevent early component subsidence.

Head and Neck

As discussed in Chapter 48, modular heads and necks of mismatched metals are routinely used for uncemented application because many uncemented stems are manufactured of titanium, whereas most femoral heads are cobalt-chromium (considered a superior bearing material). It has been demonstrated that the potential for galvanic corrosion exists between these two dissimilar metal surfaces. Corrosion at this modular junction has been seen in as many as 34 percent of retrieved components with different materials comprising the head and neck, compared to 9 percent when the head and neck are made of the same materials. Crevice and fretting corrosion also appear to play an important role at the modular head-neck junction, and the relative contributions of each type of corrosion at this juncture are still debated.[82]

Surface Treatment

There are two potential design philosophies for uncemented fixation of the femoral component: smooth macrolock and surface-textured microlock. Theoretically, the smooth-stemmed implant causes less proximal stress shielding.[40] However, these projected changes have not been observed clinically or experimentally. It is generally well accepted today that the so-called macrolock implants have less chance of providing long-term pain-free service than does one that is biologically incorporated. Hence, the smooth-stemmed, uncemented femoral component is not in general use at this time.[20]

Optimum surface characteristics known to be consistent with osseous ingrowth are well accepted to include a pore size in the range of 150 to 400 μm in diameter.[49,69] The surface texture allowing osseous incorporation into or onto the implant has taken one of three forms: sintered beads, wire mesh, or plasma spray. Specific density, bonding strength, and porosity characteristics are associated with each of these processes (Fig. 49–3). Review of the literature clearly indicates that ingrowth and remodeling characteristics are less a function of the surface treatment than of the overall component design.

When selecting a device, three aspects of the application of the surface treatment should be considered: (1) patch or circumferential distribution of the porous surface; (2) partial, proximal, or complete extent of the surface coverage; and (3) whether or not the surface is further "enhanced" by the application of a ceramic such as hydroxyapatite or tricalcium phosphate or by growth factors.

Circumferential Surface Treatment

Although not necessary for osseous incorporation, today a circumferential treatment is recommended to lessen the tendency for debris to track distally along the smooth surface of the stem between porous pads (Fig. 49–4). Although the basic science supporting this perception is limited, there is near-universal clinical acceptance of the concept of circumferential surface preparation by most surgeons today.[31,54]

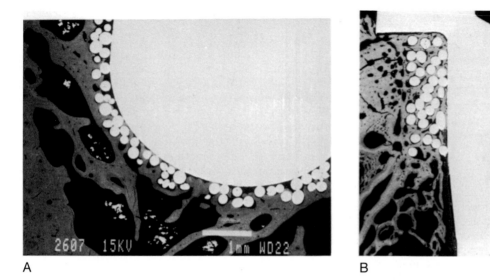

Figure 49–3. A, Electron micrographs of a cobalt-chromium porous-coated stem showing osseous integration. **B,** Same preparation of a titanium alloy wire mesh implant showing osseous integration at 6 weeks.

Extent of Surface Treatment

For primary total hip arthroplasty, most surgeons favor only a proximally, partially coated device because it is thought that this provides a more favorable stress transfer mechanism and a more favorable remodeling environment than does a fully coated device. However, inconsistent clinical performance and concern over inadequate initial fixation have prompted some schools of thought to continue to favor the more fully coated stems even though there is a theoretical and clinically observed tendency for proximal stress shielding.

Certainly the most consistent and reliable results have been experienced with the fully coated anatomic medullary locking (AML) implant, as reported by Engh et al. and discussed below.[23]

Surface Enhancement (Hydroxyapatite Enhancement)

To improve the rapidity and completeness of osseous incorporation and to lessen the likelihood of loosening, hydroxyapatite or tricalcium phosphate has been used

Figure 49–4. A, Wire mesh pad; smooth edges between pads are believed to be a route of particle access to femoral shaft. **B,** Circumferential coating of proximal implant theoretically "seals" proximal femur from wear debris.

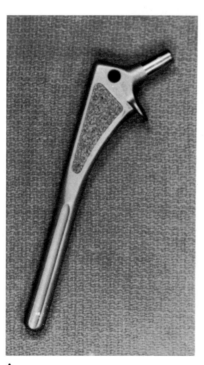

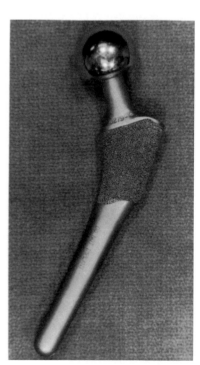

to cover both smooth and treated surfaces. Tricalcium phosphate compounds are biocompatible, with a low potential for systemic toxicity,[37,65] but are resorbed rapidly in vivo, causing unpredictable long-term integrity of the system.[55,75] Hydroxyapatite has the advantage of promoting bone ongrowth but being very slowly resorbed.

One early, well-known manufacturing problem was the production of a nonuniform, thick, irregular hydroxyapatite coating on the substrate. This has been resolved by advances in technology producing a uniform thin application layer. These devices now have much less tendency for cracking, or delamination, which had been implicated as causing or aggravating third-body wear.[3,25] The longevity of hydroxyapatite on the substrate has been questioned, but it has been shown to persist in the experimental animal for up to 10 years.[31] Based on clinical studies with up to 2 years of follow-up, it is clear that the thin application of high-purity hydroxyapatite coatings is particularly effective in resisting delamination.[3,30]

Surface treatments with calcium phosphate and hydroxyapatite consistently reveal radiographic appearances suggesting early osseous incorporation. Although in experimental models these coatings provide more rapid osteointegration than do porous surfaces alone, bone growth into the two types of surfaces is virtually identical at 12 weeks.[15,47] Retrieval studies of the hydroxyapatite-coated implants show a lack of fibrous membrane between the implant and bone at varying sacrifice periods from 2 to 3 weeks up to 2 years after implantation.[29] With thousands of implants inserted, Furlong and Osborn concluded that the only biomaterial capable of creating an intimate bone interface without an intervening membrane is hydroxyapatite ceramic.[27] Whereas some have found that these special coatings do not allow osseous incorporation across gaps,[47] others reported on the enhancement of bone apposition in hydroxyapatite-coated implants that occurs in the presence of implant-bone gaps, with micromotion, or in osteoporotic bone.[16,28,77,81]

The use of hydroxyapatite coating appears to reduce migration of uncemented femoral components when compared to porous coatings.[34] Using sophisticated measuring techniques (approximately 0.2 mm of migration is measurable), Soballe et al. found that implants coated with hydroxyapatite showed less migration than porous components. Furthermore, the hydroxyapatite-coated devices showed no further migration after 12 months, whereas implants without the hydroxyapatite continued to show micromigration ($P <0.05$).[78]

DISADVANTAGES

There are some potential disadvantages to hydroxyapatite coating, as noted above. If the coating is liberated from its point of application on the stem, it may migrate to the articulating joint surface, causing third-body wear and an increase in polyethylene wear debris.[3,6,39] The long-term impact of a biologically active coating is subject to speculation. It is not yet known how bone will remodel around these implants in the long term. At this time, however, with clinical experience of more than 10 years, the early advantage of these coatings, namely the ability to provide faster osteointegration, is accompanied by durable clinical results.

Modular Systems

Emphasis on the need for a precise fit of the prosthesis against endosteal cortical bone in the setting of wide anatomic variation as occurs at the proximal femur prompted the development of modular systems (Fig. 49–5). Variably sized and shaped proximal and distal elements can be attached to a substrate material by interference fit. However, because other techniques exist to assure adequate fit in most primary total hip replacements, concerns about wear debris production at the modular interface have dampened enthusiasm for this design concept.

INDICATIONS

The indication for uncemented implants in general has been the younger, active individual. At the Mayo Clinic, we have typically reserved this procedure for those under the age of 70 with bone stock that was of

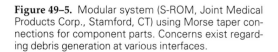

Figure 49–5. Modular system (S-ROM, Joint Medical Products Corp., Stamford, CT) using Morse taper connections for component parts. Concerns exist regarding debris generation at various interfaces.

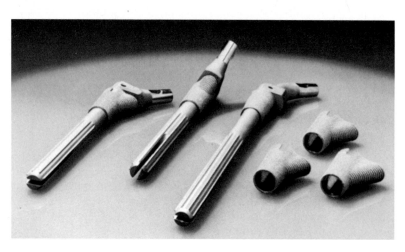

sufficient quality to allow rigid fixation. In most circumstances, we have avoided uncemented implants in patients on chronic steroid therapy or those with chronic debilitating disease, such as rheumatoid arthritis. The uncemented porous-coated implant is also not used in the elderly population sustaining a fracture of the hip. A traditional unipolar, nonbiologically fixed, smooth-surfaced device, such as the Austin-Moore prostheses, is, however, still appropriate in very-low-demand patients.

CONTRAINDICATIONS

Patients with metabolic bone disease and those with poor bone quality, osteoporosis, or limited life expectancy all offer contraindications to uncemented replacement. Typically patients over the age of 70 are not considered candidates for these devices unless they are very active. Patients over the age of 70 are considered best treated with a cemented femoral implant regardless of their level of activity.

TECHNIQUE

Preoperative Planning

The first and basic step for implanting all uncemented devices is that of preoperative planning to assess the optimum fit in the metaphysis and diaphysis of the femur. Because of the significant variation in the relationship of the proximal and distal femur geometry, measurement should be done on both anteroposterior and lateral radiographs. The relative size of the proximal and distal femur indicates the selection of the implant. Thus, canals with very large, trumpet-shaped proximal geometry (type A) may be deemed acceptable only for a total-contact isthmus-filling device. Femurs with relatively normal proximal-distal geometry (type B) might be considered more acceptable for proximal-fitting implant designs. Femurs with a large "stovepipe"-shaped femoral canal (type C) are often better treated with a cemented implant. Some contemporary designs provide various combinations of "mismatched" proximal and distal geometry. The use of templates helps to assure that magnification factors have been considered. This assessment before surgery also allows the operating team to have the appropriate range of sizes available at the time of surgery. The final determination of size can only occur, however, at the time of implantation.

Surgical Technique

Neck Resection

All systems use some form of template to allow accurate estimation of the depth, orientation, and line of femoral neck resection (Fig. 49–6). The level of resection is the most important consideration during removal of the femoral head. Precise orientation of the initial cut is not

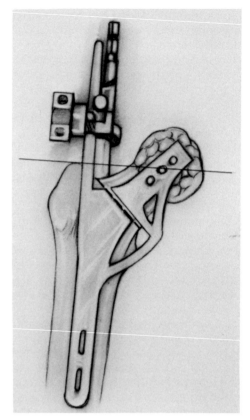

Figure 49–6. Neck resection guide in place.

critical, however, because many uncemented devices are collarless and do not rest on the neck, whereas collared implant systems make use of calcar reamers to assure optimum contact between the collar and the femoral neck.

Canal Preparation

The first step is that of serial reaming of the medullary canal, the initial stages of which are directed by information gathered from the preoperative planning exercise. The central goal of rigid fixation is realized either by proximal metaphyseal or total-contact diaphyseal fixation. In the former instance, the medullary canal may be reamed with a conical reamer (Fig. 49–7). If a total-contact system is being used, some form of cylindrical or straight reaming of the medullary canal will ultimately be necessary (Fig. 49–8). For curved-stemmed design implants, a flexible reamer is used. Straight-stemmed devices use rigid straight reamers. The depth of the reaming process is dictated by the specific design of the implant. The basic rationale of this step is to fashion or customize femora of various sizes to receive a specific-shaped implant with a limited selection of dimensions. The anticipated proximal size of the implant dictates the extent to which the medullary canal is reamed for metaphyseal-filling implants. In contrast, for diaphyseal-filling, extensively coated implants, the size of the prosthesis necessary to obtain intimate diaphyseal fit determines the proximal size to which the metaphysis must be prepared.

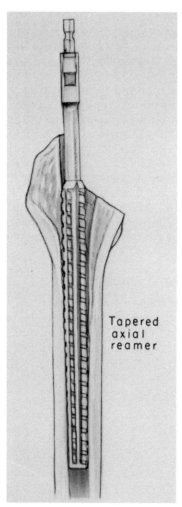

Figure 49–7. Tapered axial reamer.

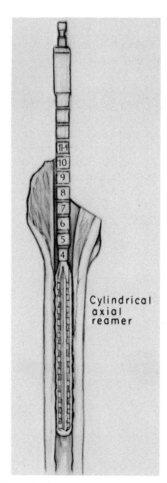

Figure 49–8. Cylindrical axial reamer.

Preparation of the canal by robotics has been suggested and tried on a limited basis. The likelihood of widespread use is limited by the uncertainty of its cost effectiveness and the lack of improvement of clinical results shown in early usage.

After the canal has been reamed, the proximal femur is prepared by serial rasping. The rasp is directed down the canal with the appropriate anteversion for the implant design. In some instances, the rasp is inserted in a neutral position because anteversion is incorporated in the femoral design; otherwise anteversion is dictated by the rasping process. In all instances, the proximal femoral rasping should be conducted in such a way as to provide a very tight fit of the rasp in the proximal femur. Some surgeons recommend verifying the tightness of the fit by the use of a torque wrench to achieve 100 to 125 psi of torque with the rasp in place (Fig. 49–9). No motion of the rasp in the medullary canal indicates adequate fixation with the implant. It has been shown experimentally that the femoral strain associated with the rasp of a precise-fit implant in the experimental animal is approximately 100 microstrain. This increased to 300 microstrain with implant insertion, indicating that the rasp may correlate to but is not an absolute reflection of the stability obtained by the implant itself.[45]

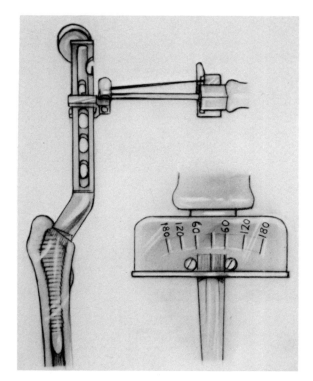

Figure 49–9. Rasp and handle in place, torque wrench applied. When 60 to 80 pounds of torque is applied to rasp, no motion of rasp should occur if it is correctly sized to the femur.

Trial Reduction

Once a rasp of adequate size to obtain rigid fixation of the implant has been seated, a trial reduction with the modular head and neck is prudent. The stability of the hip is assessed by extension and external rotation to assure that there is not excessive anteversion of the stem or acetabular implant and that no impingement between the neck of the implant and the posterior aspect of the acetabular polyethylene occurs. Flexion and internal rotation (the so-called 90-90 test) assures that adequate stability has been obtained, and this should be complemented by testing of stability in mid-position (45 degrees of flexion, adduction, and internal rotation) (Fig. 49–10).

Insertion

Unlike with canal preparation prior to insertion of cement, it has also been shown that irrigation and cleaning of the canal may be harmful rather than of value. It is suggested that blood, bone fragments, and marrow elements enhance osseous incorporation and should not be lavaged and removed from the canal for uncemented devices. Gentle irrigation to remove larger loose cancellous bone debris seems sensible, however.

As the implant is inserted into the femur, it is essential that the proper desired orientation and anteversion are followed. The depth of insertion is dictated by the implant design; most do not use a collar, and therefore the depth of insertion can increase until rigid fixation is obtained. The modular head and neck lengths allow some flexibility to the depth of insertion. It has been shown that the force of impaction does directly correlate with subsequent subsidence.[71] The precise technique to insert the implant consists of a series of firm blows of moderate force. This is in contrast to sharp singular blows to the proximal femur, which may have a tendency to cause proximal femoral fracture. In those instances in which the implant has not been adequately seated, we wait 1 to 2 minutes for strain relaxation and then cautiously attempt further impaction of the device.

Intraoperative Fracture

Intraoperative fracture has been reported in 5 to 20 percent of primary uncemented devices and is discussed in detail in Chapter 67 and subsequently in this chapter. It has been demonstrated in the experimental animal that oversizing the stem by as little as 1 mm regularly causes a diaphyseal fracture that directly correlates with fixation

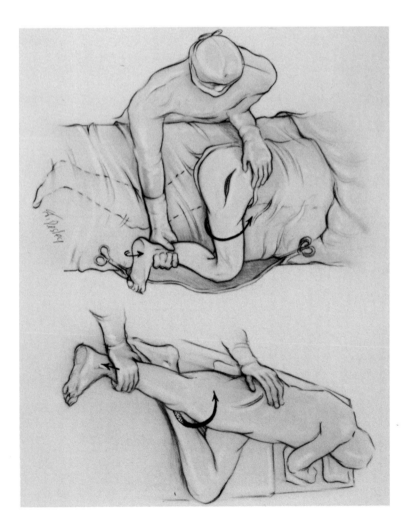

Figure 49–10. The two instability modes are checked after trial reduction. These consist of flexion and internal rotation, to evaluate adequacy of anteversion of the components; and extension and external rotation, to evaluate for excess anteversion of components.

failure.[38] Should a fracture occur in the proximal femur, circumferential wires are placed around the femoral neck.[1,80] This usually provides adequate stability, and, unless the fracture is severely displaced, adverse consequences are infrequent. If a fracture is undisplaced and the femoral component is stable, treatment by protected weight bearing may be adequate; however, circumferential wiring adds a margin of safety and is considered to be the most prudent course. Fractures distal to the neck, involving the femoral shaft, may go unrecognized. To further evaluate the possibility of fracture, intraoperative radiographs in two planes at 90 degrees to each other are often useful and essential when in doubt. Undisplaced fractures, however, may not be evident even by radiographic assessment in two planes, but an argument can be made that a fracture that is not visualized in this manner is seldom of clinical consequence.

Postsurgical Management

Although marked individual variation exists, most current implants appear to be unaffected by early weight bearing. Personal experience should guide one's postoperative plan. We prefer a more conservative approach allowing up to 25 percent weight bearing for 6 weeks, then progressing to full weight bearing over the ensuing 2 to 4 weeks, although patient compliance with this plan is highly variable.

RESULTS

Uncemented porous-coated total hip arthroplasty femoral components have been used in the United States since 1977. Over 10-year results of extensively coated components are now available, whereas few clinical studies of proximally coated devices published to date have a mean follow-up of 10 years. Experience with hydroxyapatite-coated stems also has reached 10 years in a significant number of patients. Although the results may be discussed along several lines, because fundamental differences exist between extensively coated stems, proximally coated stems, and hydroxyapatite-coated stems, each is discussed separately below.

Proximally Porous-Coated Implants

The large number of prosthesis designs and relatively short clinical experience with each makes definitive generalizable conclusions concerning proximally porous-coated stems difficult. As discussed previously in this chapter, components have been made of both cobalt-chromium and titanium; have been coated with beads, wire mesh, and plasma spray; have had patch as well as circumferential porous coatings; have had straight as well as anatomic geometries; have had collared as well as collarless designs; and have been designed to fill and not to fill the diaphyseal portion of the femur (Fig. 49–11). Furthermore, uncemented prostheses have been used in markedly different patient populations depending on each surgeon's indications for use of uncemented femoral components. Finally, some reports are of a surgeon's early experience with a prosthesis and technique, whereas other reports represent the experience of surgeons already expert at implantation of a particular device.

Fixation

The results of a number of series of proximally porous-coated femoral implants are summarized in Table 49–1. The multiple variables involved in obtaining stable femoral fixation make direct comparison between different series and designs impossible. However, from the summarized data, one can conclude that stable bony fixation can be obtained in primary total hip arthroplasties using proximally porous-coated devices of many designs. The rate of mechanical failure (revision for aseptic femoral loosening or radiographic femoral loosening) varies from 2 to 10 percent in most series at 2 to 9 years (Table 49–1). The most favorable series reported fixation as good as any series of cemented femoral stems with a similar follow-up period, whereas less favorable series showed considerably poorer results than those reported with cemented femoral components implanted with modern cement technique. The reasons for these varied results relate to many factors, such as host considerations, technique, and implant design. Although all play a role, we believe implant design may be of paramount importance in determining the final outcome.

Pilliar et al.[69] have shown that initial stem stability is required for bone ingrowth to occur. Logically, then, greater surgical experience and improved surgical technique should increase the likelihood of good component-canal "fit and fill" and consequently also improve the likelihood of femoral bone ingrowth. Callaghan et al. reviewed their first 50 and second 50 consecutive uncemented porous-coated anatomic (PCA) hip implants.[9] They found the second 50 hips had better canal filling with the prosthesis, but they could not demonstrate an improvement in clinical outcome. Kim and Kim reported on 108 PCA hip implants followed a minimum of 6 years.[51] They found that all patients with loose femoral implants or severe thigh pain had undersized femoral components, whereas no patient in their series with a good prosthesis-canal fit in both the coronal and sagittal planes had either femoral component loosening or disabling thigh pain. Hungerford and Jones evaluated their first, second, and third 100 consecutive uncemented PCA stems a minimum of 5 years after surgery.[41] Three of the first 100, one of the second 100, and none of the third 100 stems required revision, leading them to conclude that greater experience with an implant led to better results. Thus, although it is difficult to prove,[38] optimal sizing of proximally coated implants should provide a higher likelihood of initial component stability and a better chance of optimal outcome. Evidence of improved results in recent series (only 2 of 77 PCA stems loose after 10 years of follow-up) probably represents improved rates of femoral

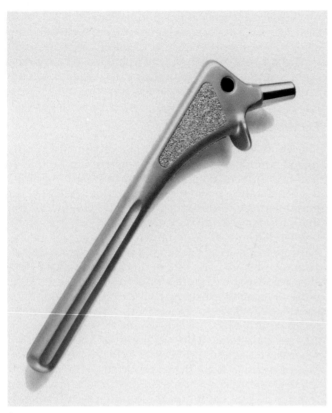

A

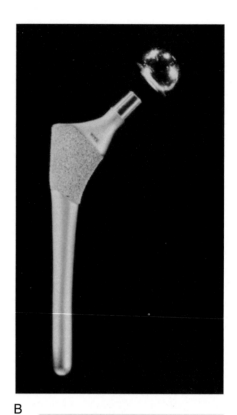

B

Figure 49–11. **A**, Example of a titanium, collared, straight femoral component with proximal titanium mesh patch porous coating (Harris-Galante prosthesis). **B**, Example of a cobalt-chromium collarless, anatomic femoral component with proximal circumferential beaded porous coating (PCA E series). **C**, Example of a titanium, collarless, non–diaphysis-filling femoral component with proximal circumferential plasma sprayed porous coating (Mallory-Head prosthesis).

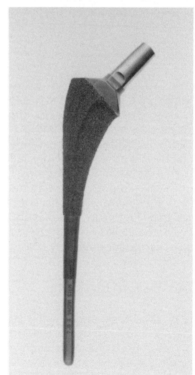

C

Table 49–1. RESULTS WITH PROXIMALLY AND EXTENSIVELY POROUS-COATED FEMORAL IMPLANTS

Reference (Year)	Prosthesis Type	No. of Hips	Mean Patient Age (yr)	Follow-Up (yr)	Femoral Revision for Aseptic Loosening (%)	Definite Femoral Radiographic Loosening (%)	Mechanical Aseptic Femoral Failure Rate (%)
Proximally Coated							
Kim and Kim[51] (1992)	Harris-Galante	82	52	5.0–5.5	5	5	10
Martel et al.[60] (1993)	Harris-Galante	121	49	4.5–6.6	3	6	9
Heekin et al.[35] (1993)	Porous-coated anatomic	100	58	5–7	0	5	5
Owen et al.[66] (1994)	Porous-coated anatomic	226	47	2–9 (mean 5.0)	2.7	4.3	7
Extensively Coated							
Pellegrini et al.[67] (1992)	Trilock (5/8th coated)	57	49	5–8 (mean 6.5)	2	0	2
Engh et al.[23] (1994)	Anatomic medullary locking	227	N/A	Mean 8.4	0.5	1.3	1.8

N/A, not available.

647

fixation resulting from evolution of component design as well as improved surgical techniques.

Thigh Pain

The etiology of thigh pain associated with uncemented femoral components is controversial. Several authors have concluded that component instability is the most common reason for significant thigh pain.[8,11,52] In a minority of patients, significant thigh pain can also occur in the presence of a well-fixed uncemented femoral component. Although the etiology of this phenomenon is not completely understood, mismatch between the stiffness of the implant and the surrounding femoral bone has been suggested as a possible source. A more thorough discussion of thigh pain in association with uncemented components is presented in Chapter 61.

The rate of thigh pain identified in each series of uncemented femoral components varies from 1 to 50 percent (Table 49–2). Reported rates of thigh pain undoubtedly differ for a number of reasons, including how carefully the presence of thigh pain is investigated, how it is defined, and, importantly, the type and stability of the femoral component. In the most favorable reports, the frequency of thigh pain with uncemented stems is similar to that with cemented stems, but most series of proximally coated stems have higher rates of thigh pain than do series of cemented femoral components.[84]

In an effort to reduce the frequency of thigh pain associated with well-fixed uncemented stems, manufacturers have made efforts to reduce the modulus of elasticity of the distal femoral component with slots, flutes, and slimmer midshaft and distal stem geometries (with or without modular distal tips).[10,14] Perhaps testifying to the results of these efforts, Bourne et al., in a study of 105 Mallory-Head prostheses (a titanium, proximally plasma-sprayed implant that does not completely fill the femoral diaphysis), reported mild thigh pain in only 2 percent of hips and moderate thigh pain in only 1 percent of hips 2 years after surgery.[7] These tapered stems, very popular in Europe, performed very well in long-term follow-up studies; in a recent series of 100 hips followed for an average of 10.2 years, results showed no femoral loosening. Reduced rates

of thigh pain are being reported, but it is not clear whether the improved results are due to stem design changes or more reliable bony femoral component fixation.

Osteolysis

Osteolysis may occur around all types of femoral components and is most commonly caused by particulate debris. Rates of localized femoral endosteal osteolysis vary considerably according to prosthesis design and duration of clinical follow-up. Prostheses that are circumferentially porous-coated proximally appear to have less risk of distal lysis than those that are "patch" porous coated. Theoretically "patch" coating provides access channels by which particulate debris can reach distal endosteal bone surfaces, whereas circumferential coating seems to more effectively seal the canal from particulate debris (by forming a so-called gasket seal). Klassen and Cabanela studied the Mayo Clinic's experience with 57 Osteonics Omnifit and 51 Osteonics Omniflex components a mean of 7 and 4 years from surgery, respectively. The rate of distal femoral osteolysis in the "patch" porous-coated implant (Omniflex) was 10 percent, whereas the rate in the circumferentially porous-coated implant (Omnifit) was only 2 percent, despite the fact that the follow-up in the Omniflex group was 3 years less than that in the Omnifit group (see Fig. 49–15 below).[54]

Kim and Kim found a 12 percent rate of osteolysis in 82 primary Harris-Galante total hip arthroplasties (a patch porous-coated titanium stem) in patients 24 to 86 years of age (mean 52 years) followed 5 to 5.5 years.[51] Goetz and colleagues also reported a high rate of osteolysis with the Harris-Galante stem: They found significant distal femoral osteolysis in 29 percent of 41 hips a mean of 4 years after surgery.[31] Although distal osteolysis appears to be more common around patch-coated designs, this relationship is not yet definitely proven, and it is clear that distal osteolysis can occur around any uncemented (or cemented) femoral component, particularly if loosening occurs. Severe osteolysis around well-fixed proximally circumferentially coated designs more often occurs around the proximal femur (Fig. 49–12), although it can occur more distally as well on occasion. When severe, proximal osteolysis can lead to sufficient

Table 49–2. THIGH PAIN ASSOCIATED WITH UNCEMENTED TOTAL HIP ARTHROPLASTY

Reference	Year	Prosthesis Type	No. of Hips	Follow-up (yr)	Thigh Pain (Prevalence)
Haddad et al.[32]	1990	AML (proximally coated and extensively coated)	64	2–4	22%
Kim and Kim[51]	1992	Harris-Galante	82	5–5.5	11% mild activity related 28% moderate-severe activity related 11% moderate-severe (associated with loosening)
Heekin et al.[35]	1993	Porous-coated anatomic	100	5–7	15% activity related
Kim and Kim[53]	1993	Porous-coated anatomic	116	6–7	8% disabling (most were loose)
Capello et al.[14]	1994	Omnifit hydroxyapatite	436	3–5+	1.3%
Bourne et al.[7]	1994	Mallory-Head	105	2	2% mild 1% moderate
Engh et al.[23]	1994	AML (extensively coated)	166	6–13	1.2% activity related
Pellegrini et al.[67]	1992	Trilock (5/8th coated)	57	5–8	3.4% mild

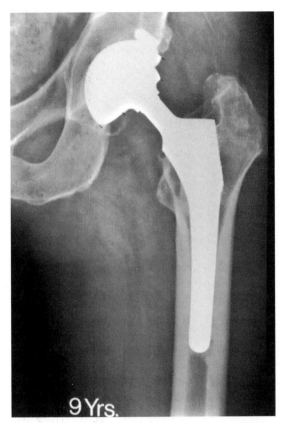

Figure 49–12. Well-fixed PCA implant is asymptomatic at 8 years. Note, however, wear of the cup and early proximal osteolysis.

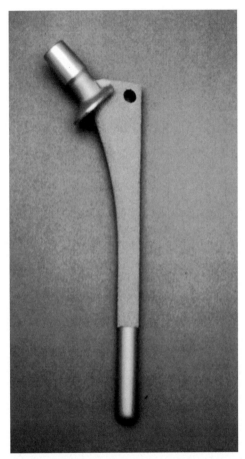

Figure 49–13. Example of an extensively porous-coated cobalt-chromium femoral component (Anatomic Medullary Locking).

bone weakening to cause fracture of the greater or lesser trochanter. In a recent review of 135 patients who received Omnifit microstructured proximally porous-coated stems followed for 13.2 years, we found that the majority of the 28 necessary reoperations were caused by proximal femoral osteolysis.[79]

Extensively Porous-Coated Femoral Implants

Engh and his co-workers have the longest and largest experience with extensively porous-coated femoral implants (Fig. 49–13) for primary total hip arthroplasty in this country. In a preliminary study of the AML prosthesis, they reported the results of 307 hips with a limited inventory of stem sizes followed for 2 to 5 years.[22] In the 195 stems with complete filling of the canal by the prosthesis, they reported that stable fixation occurred in 100 percent (93 percent with bone ingrowth, 7 percent with stable fibrous ingrowth). In contrast, of 112 stems that incompletely filled the canal, only 93 percent were stable and only 69 percent were fixed by bone. Thigh pain was found in 14 percent and limp in 21 percent of patients; both limp and thigh pain were more common in patients with undersized stems.[22] The same group has subsequently published results a mean of 8.4 years after implantation of 227 extensively coated AML stems performed after a full inventory of prosthesis sizes became available.[23] In this group of patients, the revision rate for

aseptic femoral loosening was only 0.4 percent, and only 1.3 percent of unrevised hips had radiographic evidence of femoral component loosening. The thigh pain rate had diminished to 1.2 percent. Pellegrini et al. have also reported favorable results in people 65 years of age and older with an extensively porous-coated femoral component in a series of 196 hips followed for 5 to 14 years (mean of 8.5 years) (see Table 49–1).[67] A review of Table 49–1 suggests that extensively coated stems, at least in series reported thus far, provide stable femoral fixation in a marginally higher percentage of patients than do proximally coated stems. More recent reports have shown 97% stem survival at 12 years.

Stress shielding has been an area of particular concern with extensively porous-coated implants. In a series of 411 AML stems, Engh and co-workers identified severe stress shielding in 4.1 percent and moderate stress shielding in 14.1 percent. Positive correlations were made between stress shielding and (1) distal bone ingrowth into the prosthesis, (2) larger diameter stems, and (3) osteopenic bone prior to surgery.[21,24] Although stress shielding remains a concern, particularly with large stem diameters and in patients with osteoporotic bone, it does not appear to progress radiologically after 2 years. Furthermore, no revision has been reported where stress shielding was the primary cause (Fig. 49–14).

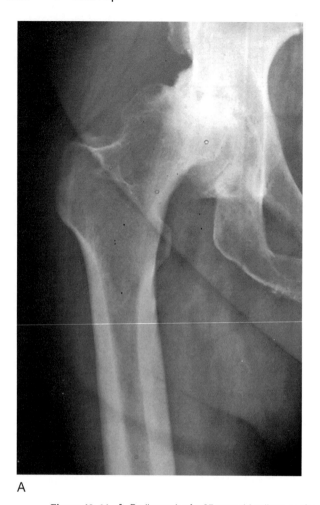

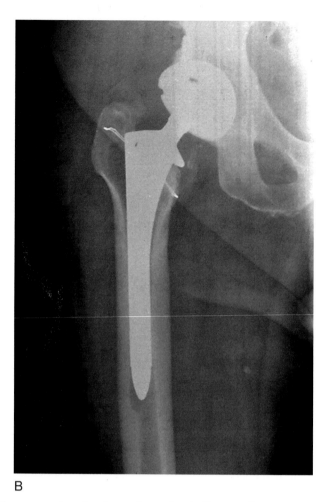

A

B

Figure 49–14. A, Radiograph of a 65-year-old college professor with very symptomatic advanced coxarthrosis. Note excellent bone quality. Patient's weight was 310 pounds. **B**, Radiograph of the same patient 6 years after total hip arthroplasty with an uncemented fully porous-coated stem. Patient has had complete relief of his hip symptoms.

Hydroxyapatite-Coated Stems

Clinical experience with hydroxyapatite-coated femoral implants in North America is limited to several stem designs with modest clinical follow-up periods[2] (Fig. 49–15). McPherson et al. reported on 269 APR hip implants with proximal hydroxyapatite coating over a nonporous surface. At 2.5 to 4 years, they reported a 4.8 percent rate of revision for aseptic loosening or radiographic aseptic loosening.[62] Geesink, from the Netherlands, reported results with 125 Osteonics Omnifit-HA stems (a proximally hydroxyapatite-coated device with underlying macrotexturing of a titanium surface) a minimum of 4 years (mean 5 years) after surgery.[30] In a middle-aged patient population (mean age 53 years), he reported a 0 percent rate of revision for aseptic loosening and a 0 percent rate of radiographic loosening. D'Antonio and associates have reported on a multicenter study of 314 primary total hip arthroplasties performed in the United States and followed 11.1 years after implantation of the same Osteonics Omnifit-HA stem.[12,18] They reported a mean postoperative Harris Hip Score of 95 and significant thigh pain in only 1.6 percent of hips. The mechanical failure rate (revision for

loosening plus radiographic loosening) was 0.5 percent, and all nonrevised stems were considered radiographically stable. Distal femoral osteolysis was seen in only one hip.[18]

The recorded results of hydroxyapatite femoral components are encouraging and parallel those reported in Europe.[27] The long-term impact of osseous incorporation and ultimate hydroxyapatite replacement may provide a fixation environment not fully appreciated at this time.

"Press-Fit" Non–Porous-Coated Uncemented Femoral Components

The most common types of uncemented femoral fixation used in North America have been discussed above. The results of uncemented uncoated, smooth, or macrotextured stems have not matched, for the most part, the results of porous-coated, hydroxyapatite-coated, or cemented femoral components.[68] DuPark and Massin reported on 203 smooth-stemmed, anatomically shaped titanium femoral components.[20] By 2 to 6 years after surgery, 32 hips had already been revised for symptomatic femoral component loosening. Of the 145 cases with

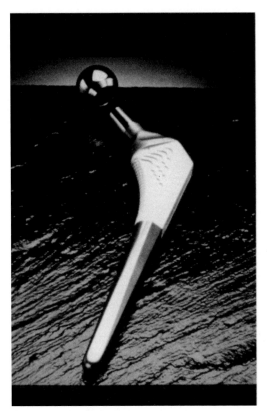

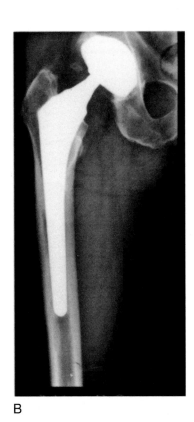

Figure 49–15. A, Example of a titanium proximally hydroxyapatite-coated femoral component (Osteonics Omnifit-HA). **B**, Radiograph of a 48-year-old patient with well-fixed hydroxyapatite-coated femoral component (Omnifit-HA) 2 years after primary total hip arthroplasty.

A   B

satisfactory radiographic follow-up, 59 had extensive radiolucencies and 22 were definitely loose. The femoral survivorship free of revision for aseptic loosening was only 77 percent at 5 years.

In contrast, non–porous-coated, rough-blasted titanium stems, although not widely used in North America, have been reported to provide much better clinical results. Blaha and co-workers reported on 300 total hip arthroplasties performed in Italy using the CLS stem (a titanium, wedge-shaped, tapered, rough-blasted, non–porous-coated implant).[5] At 5 to 8 (mean 7) years, only 0.8 percent had been revised for aseptic loosening and 0.8 percent had radiographic loosening (an aseptic mechanical failure rate of 1.6 percent). This stem continues to be very popular in Europe.

Results in Specific Patient Populations

The majority of uncemented femoral components are utilized in patients with osteoarthritis and good bone quality. Results of uncemented femoral fixation in other patient populations require special consideration.

Young Patients

Young patients are known to be at higher risk than middle-aged or older patients for femoral component loosening with cemented femoral implants. This has led many to advocate the use of uncemented femoral components in young active patients with good bone quality. The results of cemented and uncemented component performance in young patients are discussed in detail in Chapter 53.

Rheumatoid Arthritis Patients

Limited information about the results of uncemented femoral component fixation in patients with inflammatory arthritis is available. Cracchiolo et al. reported on 40 uncemented primary total hip arthroplasties performed in patients with inflammatory arthritis.[17] At 2 to 6 years (mean 3.7 years), no patient had required revision and no stem was definitely loose, but two had subsided. Lachiewicz reported 3- to 6.1-year results in 35 uncemented total hip arthroplasties performed for rheumatoid arthritis; at that time interval, no components had been removed for loosening but three femoral components had subsided.[56] Although these short-term results are not unfavorable, cemented femoral fixation is preferred for most patients with inflammatory arthritis. This preference is based on the excellent reported results of cemented femoral fixation even in young patients with polyarticular inflammatory disease (see Chapter 53). Furthermore, most patients with inflammatory disease are not ideal candidates for uncemented femoral fixation based on poor bone quality, abnormal femoral canal geometry, or use of immunosuppressive agents that may hinder bone ingrowth to uncemented prostheses.

Patients with Avascular Necrosis

Cemented total hip arthroplasty for avascular necrosis of the hip has been associated with poorer long-term results than many other diagnoses, perhaps in part because osteonecrosis often occurs in young, active patients. This finding has prompted enthusiasm for use of uncemented total hip arthroplasty designs for treatment of this problem, but, thus far, limited information on the efficacy of this approach is available. Lins et al. reported on the use of 37 uncemented PCA total hip arthroplasties for osteonecrosis of the femoral head.[57] At 4 to 6 years after surgery, no implant had been revised for femoral loosening, but femoral subsidence was present in 14 percent of hips and femoral bead shedding was present 30 percent of hips. The best reports of an uncemented prosthesis for avascular necrosis have been those of Piston et al., who reported on 35 AML prostheses on young patients followed for 7.5 years (2.9 percent stem failure),[70] and Capello et al., who reported on 53 hydroxyapatite-coated Omnifit stems followed for 6 years with no stem failures.[13] Xenakis and colleagues reported no difference in the clinical results of uncemented PCA prosthesis implants performed in patients with avascular necrosis when compared with patients with osteoarthritis.[85]

COMPLICATIONS

Many of the complications of total hip arthroplasty, such as soft tissue problems, neurovascular problems, and hip instability, are similar in cemented and uncemented total hip replacement. This section focuses on those problems particularly pertinent to implantation of uncemented femoral components: intraoperative fracture, component loosening, osteolysis, stress shielding, and heterotopic ossification.

Intraoperative Femoral Fractures

This topic is discussed in detail in Chapter 67; for completeness, some points pertaining specifically to uncemented total hip arthroplasty implantation are reviewed here. Intraoperative femoral fracture during implantation of cemented femoral components is uncommon. During implantation of uncemented femoral components, the likelihood of fracture is considerably higher, undoubtedly because success of the procedure is predicated on achieving a tight fit of the component in the femoral canal. At the Mayo Clinic, the rate of intraoperative fracture in 2078 primary uncemented components was 3.9 percent, whereas in 17,579 cemented cases the intraoperative fracture rate was only 0.1 percent (see Chapter 67).

Several authors have reported on intraoperative fractures associated with proximally porous-coated devices. Fitzgerald et al. discussed 40 fractures associated with proximally coated devices in 23 revisions and 17 primary hip replacements.[26] Cerclage wires were used in 37 of the 40 cases after the fracture occurred. Loosening or failure occurred in only 3 of the 40 hips but was believed to be associated with the fracture in each case. Martel et

al. reported 10 proximal femoral fractures among 121 primary Harris-Galante total hip arthroplasties.[60] Despite cerclage fixation, 2 of the 10 femoral components loosened. Mont et al. identified 18 cases of intraoperative femur fracture in 730 hips during preparation for an uncemented proximally porous-coated total hip arthroplasty.[63] Management was by cerclage in 14 cases, further impaction of the prostheses in 2 cases, and conversion to cemented femoral fixation in 2 cases. Only 1 of the 16 patients with an uncemented stem had radiographic evidence of loosening, and the authors concluded that properly managed intraoperative femoral fractures did not detract from the results of uncemented proximally porous-coated total hip arthroplasty.

When a fracture occurs during insertion of a proximally porous-coated stem, it usually is a small crack in the proximal femur and can be treated with cerclage fixation. Recognition and treatment of the problem are important to avoid postoperative fracture propagation. In most cases, a proximally porous-coated stem can still be used if a small undisplaced fracture occurs intraoperatively. The decision to switch to a cemented device or an extensively porous-coated distally fixed device is usually made only if satisfactory stability of the proximally porous-coated implant is not present after cerclage fixation of the crack.

Fractures associated with extensively coated diaphyseal-filling stems frequently follow a different pattern than those associated with proximally coated stems and are more often longitudinal diaphyseal split fractures. Schwartz et al. noted a 3 percent rate of fracture associated with placement of the AML prosthesis (which was extensively coated in most of their cases).[74] When the fracture extended distal to the stem tip and was complete, they recommended internal fixation be performed at the time of surgery. Proximal fractures were treated with cerclage and a distally fixed, extensively coated stem. Using this protocol, they found no adverse effects of intraoperative femur fractures 1 to 10 (mean 3) years after surgery.

Component Loosening

Loosening of uncemented stems probably can occur by several mechanisms. Clearly, the most common reason is failure of bone ingrowth to the porous coating in the first several months after implantation. In some cases sufficient fibrous ingrowth may occur to provide a stable, well-functioning prosthesis, but more often the prosthesis becomes loose and clinical failure occurs. The most effective means of avoiding this complication include (1) proper selection of the patient for uncemented femoral component fixation (see Indications earlier in this chapter); (2) proper implant selection; and (3) careful surgical technique emphasizing proper component sizing and rigid component fixation at the time of surgery. Loosening of uncemented stems may also occur by other mechanisms. Severe osteolysis may lead to component loosening in some cases (Fig. 49–16). Jasty et al. have reported that fracture between the bone and interface

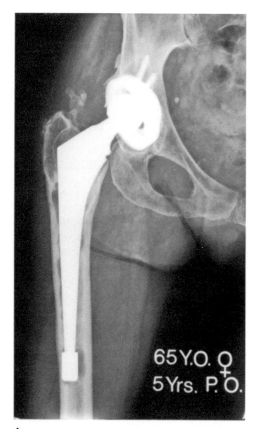

Figure 49–16. **A**, A titanium proximally patch porous-coated stem (Osteonics Omniflex) with marked distal osteolysis 5 years after implantation. **B**, At revision, the channels in the proximal femur by which particulate debris may pass between the porous-coated patches are evident.

A

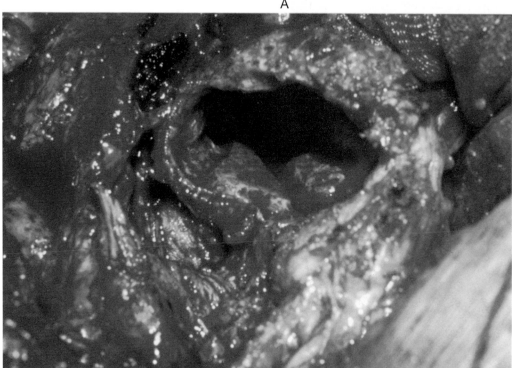

B

of the porous implant may lead to component loosening in some instances.[42]

Evaluation of the painful total hip arthroplasty and diagnosis of uncemented femoral component loosening are discussed extensively in Chapter 61. When the sur-

geon determines that a symptomatically loose femoral component should be revised, there are few data to guide the choice of subsequent implant fixation at the time of revision. We evaluated 51 failed uncemented femoral components revised at the Mayo Clinic to either a cemented stem (31 hips) or an uncemented proximally porous-coated stem (20 hips).[4] At 2 to 6 years after revision, there was a high rate of symptomatic aseptic loosening (50 percent) in the group revised to a proximally porous-coated stem, and we concluded that this option could not be advocated. In the group revised with a cemented stem, the rate of failure was significantly less (re-revision rate 13 percent, symptomatic aseptic loosening rate 19 percent). In the subset of patients with failed uncemented femoral components, the rate of success of cemented femoral revision is less than that typically reported for revision of a failed cemented femoral component. After a failed uncemented femoral component is removed, frequently there is little cancellous bone left for cement interdigitation at the time of revision. When revising a failed uncemented stem for aseptic loosening, we tend to use cement if good cancellous bone is present after removal of the neocortex surrounding the failed implant. If good cancellous bone is not present, we are more likely to use an alternative femoral fixation technique, such as a cemented stem with impacted cancellous allograft or an uncemented extensively porous-coated stem.

Osteolysis

Osteolysis can occur around cemented or uncemented femoral implants, and in both instances particulate debris is the main cause.[58,73] The relationship of proximal patch coating to distal femoral osteolysis is discussed in the earlier section, Proximally Porous-Coated Implants. When osteolysis occurs around a well-fixed, circumferentially coated stem, it is more likely to involve the proximal femur, probably because the "gasket seal" formed by the circumferential coating tends to exclude particulate debris from reaching more distally. Severe proximal bone loss may be found in the calcar region, anteriorly or posteriorly about the proximal femoral component, or in the region of the greater trochanter. Fractures of the greater trochanter associated with osteolysis have been observed, but are an uncommon cause of reoperation.[79]

Treatment of osteolysis around a total hip arthroplasty remains controversial. When significant progressive bone loss resulting from distal lysis is identified, strong consideration should be given to surgical treatment to avoid severe bone loss or periprosthetic fracture (see Fig. 49–16). Most hips with marked, progressive proximal osteolysis will also require surgical intervention. If surgery is embarked upon, lesional treatment (débridement and bone grafting of the lytic areas) is recommended if the component is well fixed. If the femoral component is loose, it is revised. An essential element of surgical treatment of this problem is an attempt to reduce production of the particulate debris causing the osteolysis. The decision about whether to remove a well-fixed femoral component is based on several factors, including the anticipated difficulty of prosthesis removal and the ability of the surgeon to gain access to the areas of osteolysis without component removal.

Stress Shielding

Stress shielding of bone may be associated with any orthopedic implant because of the changes in local bone stresses caused by that implant. For femoral components, marked stress shielding of the proximal femur is most commonly associated with extensively porous-coated stems with distal bone ingrowth. Stiffer, larger diameter prostheses appear to be more likely to cause severe stress shielding than narrower, more flexible implants. Haddad and his co-workers have shown that the quality of a patient's bone also has a significant impact on the likelihood of severe stress shielding. Using dual-energy x-ray absorptiometry (DEXA), they showed that patients with significant osteopenia of the opposite femur were at significantly greater risk for significant stress shielding about a fully porous-coated uncemented hip arthroplasty.[32] Engh and Bobyn suggested that proximal stress shielding, when it occurs, is usually most progressive for the first 1 to 2 years and then stabilizes.[21] Kilgus et al., using DEXA analysis of the AML stem, found some progressive bone loss from 2 to 6 years after implantation as well.[50]

Because there is no good treatment for severe stress shielding associated with a well-fixed implant, at this time most surgeons agree that observation is the best course to follow.

Heterotopic Ossification

Maloney et al. examined the likelihood of heterotopic ossification as a function of femoral fixation and found that the likelihood of symptomatic severe heterotopic ossification formation was somewhat higher in a group of patients treated with uncemented total hip arthroplasty compared to a matched group treated with cemented total hip arthroplasty.[59] In contrast, Duck and Mylod, in a study of 66 hips, did not find a statistically significant difference in risk for heterotopic ossification formation between total hip arthroplasties performed with cemented and those performed with uncemented fixation.[19] The etiology of heterotopic ossification after total hip arthroplasty is multifactorial and is probably related to host factors, surgical technique, and surgical approach, but independent of the type of fixation (see Chapter 66).

AUTHORS' PREFERENCE

The authors and the entire department at the Mayo Clinic favor both extensively coated stems and metaphyseal fit with proximally coated devices without collars. The choice of diaphyseal versus metaphyseal fit and proximal versus full coating is made depending on the bone geometry and quality. In patients with very large metaphyseal areas, tight canals, and excellent cortices, a diaphyseally fitted fully coated stem is preferred. In patient with more normal proximal femoral morphology, a metaphyseally fitted proximally coated stem is the rule; in these instances, proximal circumferential coating is generally used, and hydroxyapatite coating is favored by the majority, but not by all.

References

1. Alikahn MA, O'Driscoll M: Fractures of the femur during total hip replacement and their management. J Bone Joint Surg Br 59:36, 1977.
2. Bauer TW, Geesink RCT, Zimmerman R, McMahon JT: Hydroxyapatite-coated femoral stems. J Bone Joint Surg Am 73:1439, 1991.
3. Bauer TW, Taylor SK, Jiang M, Medendorp SV: An indirect comparison of third-body wear in retrieved hydroxyapatite-coated, porous, and cemented femoral components. Clin Orthop 298:11, 1994.
4. Berry DJ, Cabanela MC, Morrey BF: Revision failed uncemented total hip arthroplasty. Presented at the Annual Meeting of the American Academy of Orthopaedic Surgeons, New Orleans, February 26, 1994.
5. Blaha JD, Grappiolio G, Gruen T, et al: Five to eight year follow-up of a cementless press-fit, non-bone ingrowth total hip stem. Orthop Trans 17:941, 1993-1994.
6. Bloebaum RD, Beeks D, Dorr LD, et al: Complications with hydroxyapatite particulate separation in total hip arthroplasty. Clin Orthop 298:19-26, 1994.
7. Bourne RB, Rorabeck CH, Burkart BC, Kirk PG: Ingrowth surfaces: plasma spray coating to titanium alloy hip replacements. Clin Orthop 298:37, 1994.
8. Burkart BC, Bourne RB, Rorabeck CH, Kirk PG: Thigh pain in cementless total hip arthroplasty. Orthop Clin North Am 24:645, 1993.
9. Callaghan JJ, Heekin RD, Savory CG, et al: Evaluation of the learning curve associated with uncemented primary porous-coated anatomic total hip arthroplasty. Clin Orthop 282:132, 1992.
10. Cameron HU: The two- to six-year results with a proximally modular uncemented total hip replacement used in hip revisions. Clin Orthop 298:47, 1994.
11. Campbell ACL, Rorabeck CH, Bourne RB, et al: Thigh pain after cementless hip arthroplasty: annoyance or ill omen? J Bone Joint Surg Br 74:63, 1992.
12. Capello WN: Outcomes with special devices. Presented at the NIH Consensus Development Conference on Total Hip Replacement, September 12–14, 1994.
13. Capello WN, Colyer RA, Gemlick BF, Feinberg JR: The use of cemented stems in the treatment of osteonecrosis. In Osteonecrosis—Etiology, Diagnosis and Treatment. Rosemont, IL, American Academy of Orthopaedic Surgeons, 1997, pp 397–403.
14. Capello WN, Sallay PI, Feinberg JR: Omniflex modular femoral component: two to five year results. Clin Orthop 298:54, 1994.
15. Cook SD, Enis J, Armstrong D, Lisecki E: Early clinical results with the hydroxyapatite-coated porous LSF total hip system. Dent Clin North Am 36:247, 1992.
16. Cook SD, Thomas KA, Kay JF, Jarcho M: Hydroxyapatite-coated titanium for orthopedic implant applications. Clin Orthop 232:225–243, 1988.
17. Cracchiolo A, Severt R, Moreland J: Uncemented total hip arthroplasty in rheumatoid arthritis diseases: a two to six year follow-up study. Clin Orthop 277:166, 1992.
18. D'Antonio JA, Capello WN, Manley MT, Geesink R: Hydroxyapatite femoral stems for total hip arthroplasty: 10- to-13 years results. Clin Orthop 393:101–111, 2001.
19. Duck HJ, Mylod AG Jr: Heterotopic bone in hip arthroplasties. Clin Orthop 282:145, 1992.
20. Duparc J, Massin P: Results of 203 total hip replacements using a smooth, cementless femoral component. J Bone Joint Surg Br 74:251, 1992.
21. Engh CA, Bobyn DJ: The influence of stem size and extent of porous coating on femoral bone resorption after primary cementless hip arthroplasty. Clin Orthop 231:7, 1988.
22. Engh CA, Bobyn DJ, Glassman AH: Porous-coated hip replacement: the factors governing bone ingrowth, stress shielding and clinical results. J Bone Joint Surg Br 69:45, 1987.
23. Engh CA, Hooten JP Jr, Zettl-Schaffer KF, et al: Porous-coated total hip replacement. Clin Orthop 298:89, 1994.
24. Engh CA, McGovern TF, Bobyn JD, Harris WH: A quantitative evaluation of periprosthetic bone-remodeling after cementless total hip arthroplasty. J Bone Joint Surg Am 74:1009, 1992.
25. Fischer KJ, Carter DR, Maloney WJ: In vitro study of initial stability of a conical collared femoral component. J Arthroplasty 7(Suppl): 389, 1992.
26. Fitzgerald RH Jr, Brindley GW, Kavanagh BF: The uncemented total hip arthroplasty. Clin Orthop Rel Res 235:61, 1988.
27. Furlong RJ, Osborn JF: Fixation of hip prosthesis by hydroxyapatite ceramic coatings. J Bone Joint Surg Br 73:741–745, 1991.
28. Geesink RG, de Groot K, Klein CP: Bonding of bone to apatite-coated implants. J Bone Joint Surg Br 70:17–22, 1988.
29. Geesink RGT: Experimental and clinical experience with hydroxyapatite-coated hip implants. Orthopedics 12:1239, 1989.
30. Geesink RGT: Hydroxylapatite-coated total hip replacement: five year clinical and radiographic results. In Geesink RGT, Manley MT (eds): Hydroxylapatite Coating in Orthopaedic Surgery. New York, Raven Press, 1993, p 117.
31. Goetz DD, Smith EJ, Harris WH: The prevalence of femoral osteolysis associated with components inserted with or without cement in total hip replacements. J Bone Joint Surg Am 76:1121, 1994.
32. Haddad RJ, Cook SD, Brinker MR: A comparison of three varieties of noncemented porous-coated hip replacement. J Bone Joint Surg Br 72:2, 1990.
33. Hagevold HE, Lyberg T, Kierulf P, Reikeras O: Micromotion of cemented and uncemented femoral components. J Bone Joint Surg Br 73:33, 1991.
34. Hamadouche M, Witvoet J, Porcher R, et al: Hydroxyapatite-coated versus grit-blasted femoral stems. A prospective, randomised study using EBRA-FCA. J Bone Joint Surg Br 83:979–987, 2001.
35. Heekin RD, Callaghan JJ, Hopkinson WJ, et al: The porous-coated anatomic total hip prosthesis inserted without cement: results after five to seven years in a prospective study. J Bone Joint Surg Am 75:77, 1993.
36. Holmberg PD, Bechtold J, Sun B, et al: Strain analysis of a femur with long stem press-fit prosthesis. Presented at the 32nd Annual Meeting of the Orthopaedic Research Society, New Orleans, 1986.
37. Hoogendorn HA, Renooij W, Akkermans GMA: Long-term study of large ceramic implants in dog femora. Clin Orthop 187:281, 1984.
38. Horne G: Fit and fill: fashionable fact or fantasy? J Bone Joint Surg Br 74:4, 1992.
39. Howie DW, Haynes DR, Rogers SD, et al: The response to particulate debris [review]. Orthop Clin North Am 24:571, 1993.
40. Huiskes R, Weinans H, Dalstra M: Adaptive bone remodeling in biomechanical design considerations for noncemented total hip arthroplasty. Orthopedics 12:1255, 1989.
41. Hungerford DS, Jones LC: Clinical experience and current status of proximally coated cementless femoral stems. Presented at the NIH Consensus Development Conference on Total Hip Replacement, September 12–14, 1994.
42. Jasty M, Bragdon CR, Maloney WJ, et al: Ingrowth of bone in failed fixation of porous-coated femoral components. J Bone Joint Surg Am 73:1331, 1991.
43. Jasty M, Bragdon CR, Rubash H, et al: Unrecognized femoral fractures during cementless total hip arthroplasty in the dog and their effect on bone ingrowth. J Arthroplasty 7:501, 1992.
44. Jasty M, Burke D, Harris WH: Biomechanics of cemented and cementless prostheses. Chir Organi Mov 77:349, 1992.
45. Jasty M, Henshaw RM, O'Connor DO, Harris WH: High assembly strains and femoral fractures produced during insertion of uncemented femoral components: a cadaver study. J Arthroplasty 8:479, 1993.
46. Jasty M, Krushell R, Zalenski E, et al: The contribution of the nonporous distal stem to the stability of proximally porous-coated canine femoral components. J Arthroplasty 8:33, 1993.
47. Jasty M, Rubash HE, Paiement GD, et al: Porous-coated uncemented components in experimental total hip arthroplasty in dogs: effect of plasma-sprayed calcium phosphate coatings on bone ingrowth. Clin Orthop 280:300, 1992.
48. Kabo JM, Clarke IC: Conventional total hip replacement design including custom considerations. In Amstutz HC (ed): Hip Arthroplasty. New York, Churchill Livingstone, 1991, p 37.

49. Kang JD, McKernan DJ, Kruger M, et al: Ingrowth and formation of bone in defects in an uncemented fiber-metal total hip-replacement model in dogs [review]. J Bone Joint Surg Am 73:93, 1991.

50. Kilgus DJ, Shimaoka EE, Tipton JS, Eberle RW: Dual-energy x-ray absorptiometry measurement of bone mineral density around porous-coated cementless femoral implants. J Bone Joint Surg Br 75:279, 1993.

51. Kim Y-H, Kim VEM: Results of the Harris-Galante cementless hip prosthesis. J Bone Joint Surg Br 74:83, 1992.

52. Kim Y-H, Kim VEM: Early migration of uncemented porous coated anatomic femoral component related to aseptic loosening. Clin Orthop 295:146, 1993.

53. Kim Y-H, Kim VEM: Uncemented porous-coated anatomic total hip replacement: results at six years in a consecutive series. J Bone Joint Surg Br 75:6, 1993.

54. Klassen J, Cabanela MEC: Influence of femoral component design changes on the clinical and radiographic results of uncemented total hip arthroplasty. Presented at the Mid America Orthopedic Association Meeting, West Palm Beach, FL, April 22, 1995.

55. Klein CP, Driessen AA, DeGroot K, Van Der Hooff A: Biodegradation behavior of various calcium phosphate materials in bone tissue. J Biomed Mater Res 17:769, 1983.

56. Lachiewicz PF: Porous-coated total hip arthroplasty in rheumatoid arthritis. J Arthroplasty 9:9, 1994.

57. Lins RE, Barnes BC, Callaghan JJ, et al: Evaluation of uncemented total hip arthroplasty in patients with avascular necrosis of the femoral head. Clin Orthop 297:168, 1993.

58. Maloney WJ, Jasty M, Harris WH, et al: Endosteal erosion in association with stable cementless femoral components. J Bone Joint Surg Am 72:1025, 1990.

59. Maloney WJ, Krushell RJ, Jasty M, Harris WH: Incidence of heterotopic ossification after total hip replacement: effect of the type of fixation of the femoral component. J Bone Joint Surg Am 73:191, 1991.

60. Martel JM, Pierson RH III, Jacobs JJ, et al: Primary total hip reconstruction with a titanium fiber-coated prosthesis inserted without cement. J Bone Joint Surg Am 75:554, 1993.

61. McAuley JP, Moore KD, Culpepper WJ, Engh CA: Total hip arthroplasty with porous-coated prosthesis fixed without cement in patients who are 65 years of age or older. J Bone Joint Surg Am 80:1648, 1998.

62. McPherson EJ, Friedman RJ, Dorr LD: The APR-I experience with hydroxyapatite. In Geesink RGT, Manley MT (eds): Hydroxylapatite Coating in Orthopaedic Surgery. New York, Raven Press, 1993, p 248.

63. Mont MA, Maar DC, Krackow KA, Hungerford DS: Hoop-stress fractures of the proximal femur during hip arthroplasty. J Bone Joint Surg Br 74:257, 1992.

64. Nister L, Blaha JD, Kjellstrom U, Selvik G: In vivo measurements of relative motion between an uncemented femoral total hip component and the femur by roentgen stereophotogrammetric analysis. Clin Orthop 269:220, 1991.

65. Oonishi H, Yamamoto M, Ishimaru H, et al: The effect of hydroxyapatite on bone growth into porous titanium alloy implants. J Bone Joint Surg Br 71:213, 1989.

66. Owen TD, Moran CG, Smith SR, Pinder IM: Results of uncemented porous-coated anatomic total hip replacement. J Bone Joint Surgery Br 76:258, 1994.

67. Pellegrini VD Jr, Hughes SS, Evarts CM: A collarless cobalt-chrome femoral component in uncemented total hip arthroplasty. J Bone Joint Surg Br 74:814, 1992.

68. Phillips TW, Messieh SS: Cementless hip replacement for arthritis: problems with a smooth surface Moore stem. J Bone Joint Surg Br 70:750, 1988.

69. Pilliar RM, Cameron HU, Macnab I: Porous surface layered prosthetic devices. Biomed Eng 10:126, 1975.

70. Piston RW, Engh CA, De Carvalho PI, Suthers K: Cementless total hip arthroplasty in patients with avascular necrosis of the hip. J Bone Joint Surg Am 76:202–214, 1994.

71. Rashmir-Raven AM, DeYoung DJ, Abrams CF Jr, et al: Subsidence of an uncemented canine femoral stem. Vet Surg 21:327, 1992.

72. Rothman RH, Izant TH: Uncemented total hip arthroplasty. In Bolderson RA, et al (eds): The Hip. Philadelphia, Lea & Febiger, 1992, Ch 23.

73. Santavirta S, Hoikka V, Eskola A, Konttinen YT: Aggressive granulomatous lesions in cementless total hip arthroplasty. J Bone Joint Surg Br 72:980, 1990.

74. Schwartz JT Jr, Mayer JG, Engh CA: Femoral fracture during noncemented total hip arthroplasty. J Bone Joint Surg Am 71:1135, 1989.

75. Shimazoki K, Mooney V: Comparative study of porous phosphate as bone substitute. J Orthop Res 3:301, 1985.

76. Skinner HB, Kilgus DJ, Keyak J, et al: Correlation of computed finite element stresses to bone density after remodeling around cementless femoral implants. Clin Orthop 305:178, 1994.

77. Soballe K, Hansen ES, Brockstedt-Rasmussen H, Bunger C: Hydroxyapatite coating converts fibrous tissue to bone around loaded implants. J Bone Joint Surg Br 75:270–278, 1993.

78. Soballe K, Toksvig-Larsen S, Gelineck J, et al: Migration of hydroxyapatite coated femoral prostheses: a roentgen stereophotogrammetric study. J Bone Joint Surg Br 75:681, 1993.

79. Swanson KC, Cabanela ME: Omnifit uncemented total hip arthroplasty: a long term follow-up study. (In preparation).

80. Taylor MM, Myers MH, Harve JP: Intraoperative femur fractures during total hip arthroplasty. Clin Orthop 137:96, 1978.

81. Tisdel CL, Goldberg VM, Parr JA, et al: The influence of a hydroxyapatite and tricalcium-phosphate coating on bone growth into titanium fiber-metal implants. J Bone Joint Surg Am 76:159–171, 1994.

82. Walker PS, Robertson DD: Design and fabrication of cementless hip stems. Clin Orthop Rel Res 235:25, 1988.

83. Weinans H, Huiskes R, Grootenboer HJ: Effects of material properties of femoral hip components on bone remodeling. J Orthop Res 10:845, 1992.

84. Wixson RL, Stulberg D, Mehlhoff M: Total hip replacement with cemented, uncemented, and hybrid prostheses. J Bone Joint Surg Am 73:257, 1991.

85. Xenakis TA, Beris AE, Malizos KK, et al: Total hip arthroplasty for avascular necrosis and degenerative osteoarthritis of the hip. Clin Orthop 341:62–68, 1997.

50

Resurfacing Hip Arthroplasty

•JAVAD PARVIZI and ROBERT T. TROUSDALE

The role of resurfacing hip arthroplasty remains controversial. Although there was early enthusiasm for the use of a surface replacement as an alternative to total hip arthroplasty (THA), an unacceptable number of failures in the early years has led to a decline in the use of resurfacing arthroplasty.[16,21,28,34] With the resurgence of metal-on-metal bearing surfaces and highly cross-linked polyethylenes, some surgeons are returning to the use of resurfacing arthroplasty.

There have been a multitude of resurfacing and conservative replacements described in the past (Fig. 50–1). One advantage of the resurfacing arthroplasty is the conservation of femoral neck bone stock. Unlike hemiarthroplasty and THA that lead to sacrifice of the femoral head and part of the femoral neck, as well as violation of the intramedullary canal for insertion of femoral stem, resurfacing conserves most of the femoral neck bone, allowing for insertion of a conventional stemmed femoral component during hip arthroplasty if or when revision is necessary.

History

One of the earliest reported uses of a foreign material placed between articulating surfaces in the United States was in 1840, when Carnochan used a block of wood as an interposition between the surfaces of the temporomandibular joint. Since that date, surgeons have applied this general principle to the hip and used various types of tissues and materials for interposition. In 1902, Murphy reported on the use of muscle and fascia as an interposing material in diseased joints.[27] In 1918, Baer used chromicized pig's bladder as an interposing material.[3] Smith-Petersen is the first to be credited with resurfacing replacement arthroplasty, or so-called double cup arthroplasty, which can also be thought of as a variation of interposition arthroplasty.[33] He reported a pseudomembrane similar to the synovium of a normal joint, which had developed around a piece of glass that was lodged in the back of his patient. This led him to design a cup made of glass that was placed between the femoral head and the acetabulum for treatment of arthritis. The glass cups were found to be too brittle to withstand the joint forces in the hip, and they frequently fractured. In 1938, he replaced the glass with Vitallium

and implanted over 500 of these cups over the ensuing decade.

During the 1950s, various modifications of cup arthroplasty were developed. Haboush reported on two cases of double cup arthroplasties in which two metallic cups were fixed with acrylic cement, one onto the femoral head and one into the acetabulum. This was perhaps one of the first uses of methacrylate in the performance of hip arthroplasty.[19] Soon after, Townley developed a hemiarthroplasty using a metal cup mounted on a short, curved intramedullary stem.[35] In 1960, Townley introduced an acetabular cup made of polyurethane and, later, polyethylene, which could be used in combination with the femoral stem when THA rather than hemiarthroplasty was desired. The components were fixed with cement. The device was referred to as total articular replacement arthroplasty (TARA). Although Townley initially reported excellent results, loosening of the acetabular component was a serious problem. After 1969, when conventional hip arthroplasty became more widespread, resurfacing arthroplasty fell out of favor.

Resurfacing arthroplasty with various modifications continued to be used in the 1970s and was advocated as an alternative to conventional THA for the young, active patient. This included designs such as the uncemented Müller double-cup arthroplasty in 1968 (Müller), the Luck cup in 1970, Paltrinieri-Trentani in 1970, the evolving Furuya prosthesis in 1971, and the ICLH (Freeman) in 1972.[17,18,36] In 1973, Eicher began to use a device later referred to as the Indiana conservative hip. Capello and associates continued this work.[5,9,10] Amstutz et al. designed the THARIES resurfacing system in early 1980s and have continued to advocate the use of resurfacing arthroplasty.[1,2,4] At present, there are various numbers of resurfacing systems available that differ with respect to materials, component size, profile, instrumentation, and recommended surgical technique.

Rationale

Osteonecrosis of the hip accounts for approximately 10 percent of approximately 250,000 THAs performed yearly in the United States. Many of the patients with osteonecrosis are young, and about 50 percent have bilateral disease. Many joint-conserving procedures, including core

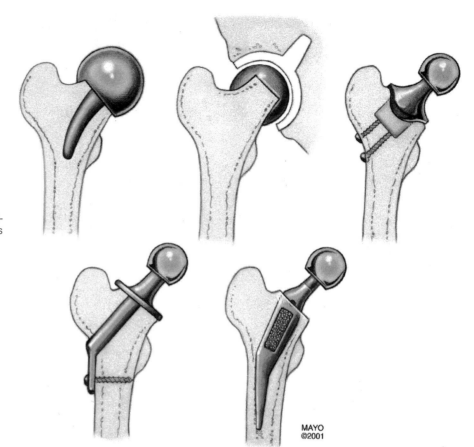

Figure 50–1. Diagram of some of the various resurfacing/conservative hip procedures that have been previously described.

MAYO
©2001

decompression, vascularized and nonvascularized bone grafts, muscle pedicle grafts, osteochondral grafts, and several different types of upper femoral osteotomies have been used, all with varying success.[26,37] However, when the lesion is large (a combined necrotic angle of 200 degrees or involvement of more than 30 percent of the femoral head) and there is also significant subchondral collapse, these more conservative measures are not so successful, and prosthetic replacement of the femoral head is probably the surgical procedure of choice.[14]

The options available in such circumstances include surface replacement arthroplasty, hemiarthroplasty with the use of femoral endoprosthesis, bipolar hemiarthroplasty, and THA. Bipolar hemiarthroplasty has had relatively high failure rates when used for the treatment of osteonecrosis of the femoral head.[7,22,24,25] Although, THA is an effective and predictable option for hip arthritis, the mechanical failure rate after total hip replacement in young patients with osteonecrosis is relatively high.[12,13,29,30] A matched study from our institution observed a failure rate of 79 percent at 17.8 years for patients with osteonecrosis compared with 39 percent for patients with other etiologies.[29] Another comparative study confirmed that patients with osteonecrosis who were younger than 50 years had a significantly higher failure and dislocation rate compared with patients who had osteoarthritis.[30] Because of the limitations of nonarthroplasty surgical procedures and the suboptimal outcome of THA for treatment of osteonecrosis in the young, resurfacing arthroplasty has re-emerged as a

time-buying procedure that provides pain relief and improvement in function without sacrificing the femoral bone stock, which can be used for revision surgery when these young patients outlive their implanted prostheses (Figs. 50–2 and 50–3).

There are three basic types of resurfacing arthroplasty:

1. Partial femoral head replacement
2. Femoral head replacement or so-called hemiresurfacing
3. Total resurfacing arthroplasty, which includes resurfacing of the femoral and acetabular articular surfaces.

Results

Partial Femoral Head Replacement

The results of partial resurfacing replacement for osteonecrosis of the femoral head, although initially encouraging, have, over time, been complicated by relatively high failure rates and osteonecrosis.[32] Based on available reports in the literature, it would be difficult to justify the use of these devices at present.[23,32]

Hemiresurfacing Arthroplasty

Replacement of the femoral side of the joint, or so-called surface replacement hemiarthroplasty has been advo-

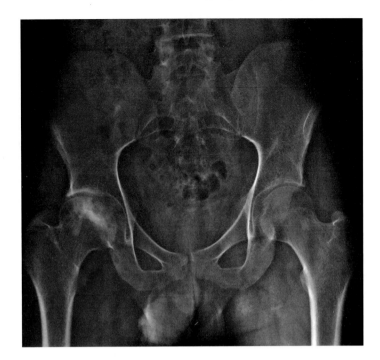

Figure 50–2. Anteroposterior pelvic film of a 22-year-old man with a large collapsed necrotic lesion in the femoral head. The necrotic arc angles on two views added to 195 degrees.

cated as a prudent surgical choice for young patients with osteonecrosis of the femoral head because it has provided reasonable pain relief and improvement in function with greater than 80 percent survivorship at intermediate follow-up.[20] Hungerford et al. reported that when hemiresurfacing arthroplasty was performed for Ficat stage III or early stage IV disease, 30 (91 percent) of 33 hips survived a minimum of 5 years; and at a mean of 10.5 years, 16 (62 percent) of the 26 hips with stage III disease had a good or excellent Harris Hip Score.[20] Krackow et al. reported a good or excellent result in 16 (84 percent) of 19 hips at a mean of 3 years.[23] In another study, Amstutz et al. reported on the results

of hemiresurfacing for osteonecrosis in 31 patients (37 hips), with a mean age of 30 years.[4] There was a significant improvement in function and pain relief after the resurfacing. Eleven cases (30 percent) required conversion at a mean of 7.5 years because of acetabular wear in 10 hips and femoral loosening in 1 hip. Eight hips were converted to THA and 3 hips were converted to metal-on-metal surfacing arthroplasty. The overall survivorship in their series was 79 percent at 5 years, 59 percent at 10 years, and 45 percent at 14 years.[4] In light of these results, we have used this technique for more than 6 years in young patients with large collapsed lesions for whom no other option was reasonable (see Figs. 50–2 and 50–3).

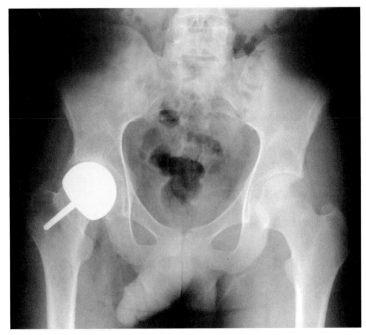

Figure 50–3. Anteroposterior pelvic film one year after hemiresurfacing. The patient has had marked relief of his pain and his functional status is near normal.

Total Resurfacing Arthroplasty

The reports documenting longer follow-up of total articular resurfacing have revealed a substantial number of failures with several designs of resurfacing arthroplasty. Capello et al. reported 6 failures in their first group of 16 replacements with Indiana hip prosthesis, the causes being divided evenly between femoral neck fracture and component loosening.[10] Ritter et al. conducted a prospective, comparative study in 50 patients undergoing concomitant bilateral hip arthroplasty with conventional hip arthroplasty on one side and an articular resurfacing component (Indiana Conservative Hip) on the other side.[31] They reported a significantly higher incidence of radiographic acetabular lucency at the bone-cement interface of the resurfacing arthroplasty, and a higher number of resurfacing components required revision compared with those used in conventional hip arthroplasty.[31] Amstutz et al., in their comparative study between conventional and resurfacing arthroplasty, also reported a higher incidence of acetabular radiolucencies in the surface-replacement group of patients.[2] They did, however, attribute this higher incidence to the younger age of the patients who underwent resurfacing. All the aforementioned series used a resurfacing prosthesis with a polyethylene acetabular component.

In the past few years, the concept of resurfacing the hip with an extremely hard, durable, and wear-resistant bearing surface to provide low friction and wear has been explored. This has included introduction of alternative bearing surfaces such as ceramic, metal-on-metal (CoCr), alumina-on-alumina, and highly cross-linked polyethylene. Beuchel reported the early results of a cementless, titanium nitride ceramic resurfacing hip replacement.[6] The hips were resurfaced with the use of Buechel-Pappas design (Endotec, Inc, South Orange, NJ), which includes a femoral onlay component with an uncoated, short, central, tapered stem mated to a metal-backed, porous-coated, hemispherically shaped UHMW-PE acetabular cup fixed in place by screws. Of the 60 hips in the study, 57 had excellent or good results, with 6-year survivorship of 91.8 percent. This was a significant improvement over the cobalt-chrome components, which had a 67-percent survivorship at the same time interval. However, there were still a number of major complications in that series, including bearing dislocation in 1 case and osteonecrosis of the femoral head in 2 cases.

The most recent important development has been the introduction of modern metal-on-metal bearing surfaces such as the one by Wagner (Sulzer Medica, Wintertur, Switzerland), one by McMinn (Corin, Leicestershire, England), and another by Amstutz (Conserve plus, Wright Medical, Arlington, TX) (Fig. 50–4).[38] Although some of these devices are not presently approved by the Food and Drug Administration (FDA) for use in the United States, they are being implanted as part of multicenter studies. Amstutz et al. reported the results of their initial experience with metal-on-metal resurfacing in 1998. These authors had succeeded in reducing the short-term failure of resurfacing arthroplasty to less than one percent at two years for the metal-on-metal surfaces compared with the 13 to 33 percent for total resurfacing devices containing a polyethylene cup at a similar follow-up (Fig. 50–5).[4] Although results of resurfacing arthroplasty with metal-on-metal bearing surfaces has been encouraging, concerns regarding systemic and tissue toxicity, carcinogenic potential, and other unknown and potentially hazardous effects of metal wear particles hinders some surgeons from implanting these devices in young, active patients.

Mode of Failure

Charnley predicted before 1979 that acetabular loosening would be the primary mode of failure with resurfacing arthroplasty because of transmission of massive forces by the large femoral head to a thin and flexible acetabular component.[11] Femoral failure has also occurred in some reported series. The cause of femoral component failure includes fracture of the femoral

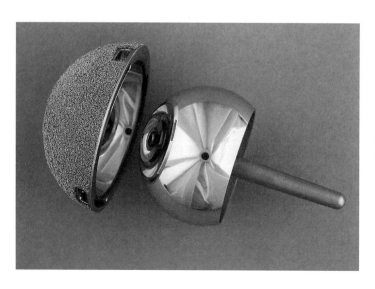

Figure 50–4. Photograph of one design of metal-metal total resurfacing.

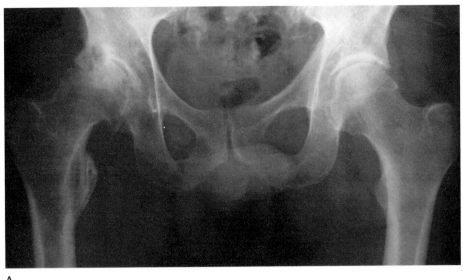

A

B

Figure 50–5. A, Preoperative anteroposterior pelvic film of a severely symptomatic man with right hip arthritis. **B**, Postoperative pelvic film after successful resurfacing performed via trochanteric osteotomy. (Courtesy of Paul Beaule, M.D.)

neck, loosening of the femoral component with or without underlying bone resorption, and component settling.[8,15,18]

The status of the vascular supply and the viability of the femoral head remnant is debated, and remains an important concern. Freeman et al. believe that the femoral head remnant retains its vascularity and does not undergo necrosis. They examined 5 retrieved femoral heads in 2 different series and found the femoral head to be viable.[15,16] Wagner also made similar observations in the few cases that required removal of the femoral head.[38] Other authors, on the other hand, have observed osteonecrosis of the femoral head in patients undergoing revision of the femoral component. Gerard histologically confirmed massive necrosis of the femoral head in 12 patients, with bone resorp-

tion and settling of the uncemented femoral components.[18] Two separate studies, specifically designed to address the vascular status and viability of the femoral head remnant, made conflicting observations. Bogoch et al., in a study of 6 cases, detected evidence of osteonecrosis in three out of the four cases that were being revised for femoral component failure resulting from femoral neck fracture.[5] The femoral head was viable in the other 2 patients who were undergoing revision because of acetabular component failure. They felt that osteonecrosis might have occurred at the time of resurfacing because there was no evidence of foreign body response to methylmethacrylate. Furthermore, they observed areas of bony remodeling at the site of fracture concluding that fracture may have occurred through a weakened zone at the junction of viable and necrotic bone. In a histologic study of 25 retrieved femoral head remnants osteonecrosis was observed in 3 (12 percent) of the femoral heads, all in patients with femoral neck fracture.[8] The conclusion that can be distilled from available literature suggests that osteonecrosis of the femoral head after resurfacing arthroplasty is dependent on the surgical technique, particularly the exposure and reaming of the femoral head, the design of the prosthesis, and the reason for failure of the retrieved femoral heads with osteonecrosis commonly observed after fracture of the underlying femoral neck. It is not known whether the femoral neck fracture is the cause or consequence of osteonecrosis of the remaining femoral head.

Indications

The indications for resurfacing arthroplasty have evolved over the years. Although this procedure used to be carried out for primary and secondary degenerative joint disease such as in cases of slipped capital femoral epiphysis, Perthes disease, developmental dysplasia of the hip and others, the main indication for this procedure in our clinic is still Ficat stage III and early stage IV osteonecrosis of the femoral head in young, active patients who are not good candidates for treatment by conservative measures and other biologic bone-conserving procedures (see Fig. 50-2).

Contraindications

Resurfacing arthroplasty is contraindicated in patients with active infection, malignant disease of the proximal femur or acetabulum, and open physeal plates. It is also relatively contraindicated for patients with severe distortion of the upper end of the femur secondary to congenital or traumatic causes and also for the older patient population. There is no clear-cut age limit for the resurfacing arthroplasty, but in our institution patients older than 50 to 60 years of age are usually considered better candidates for standard THA.

Preoperative Planning

History

It is important to accurately assess the degree, character, and anatomic location of the patient's pain. It is equally important to determine the functional disability from which the patient suffers. A detailed history of all treatments should also be recorded, because patients should exhaust all conservative treatments, such as activity modifications, nonsteroidal anti-inflammatory drugs, and, perhaps, intra-articular steroids. The latter may be useful also to rule out pain that may arise from a different origin.

Examination

The patient's gait should be observed and leg lengths measured and recorded. Resurfacing arthroplasty cannot correct true leg length inequality, but, through the release of contractual deformities, apparent leg length inequality can be overcome in select patients. The location of pain, the function of muscle groups with or without resistance, and the presence of scars should be noted. The hip range of motion should be accurately recorded and an objective hip score determined.

Investigations

Standard anteroposterior and true cross-table lateral view radiographs should be taken to assess the acetabular joint space and the anatomy of the upper end of the femur. The radiographs are also used for creating templates.

Cross-sectional studies such as computeed tomography or magnetic resonance imaging may also be useful in some cases to determine the topography of the proximal femur and assess the severity of femoral head involvement in avascular necrosis.

In patients with suspected occult infection, hip aspiration under radiographic imaging should be performed to rule out deep infection.

Technical Considerations

Surgical preparation of the patient is identical to that used in conventional hip arthroplasty as far as patient positioning, incision placement, and surgical exposure. Hemiresurfacing can be performed easily via a posterior or anterior exposure to the hip joint. The senior author prefers the posterolateral exposure in these young patients to avoid violation of the abductor mechanism. Care should be taken to avoid disruption of the vascular supply to the femoral head (Fig. 50-6).

The proper size hemiresurfacing component is based on intraoperative assessment of the size of the acetabulum using appropriate trials. Once that size is determined, a guide pin is placed into the center of the femoral head (Figs. 50-7 and 50-8). Placement of the guide pin in both planes is confirmed by use of intraoperative fluoroscopy. Once the guide is placed, the femoral head is reamed in line with the calcar axis to the proper dimension (Fig. 50-9). Varus tilting of the femoral component and notching of the superior femoral neck cortex should be avoided (Fig. 50-10). A tapered reamer opens the drill hole dimension with one motion, and the femoral component is impacted onto the prepared surface place (Fig. 50-10). The accurate size of the hemiresurfacing is confirmed with fluoroscopy (Fig. 50-11). It is critical not to undersize or oversize the component (Fig. 50-12). A meticulous closure of the posterior capsule and short rotators is carried out, and the remainder of the closure is according to routine procedure. Patients are allowed to bear

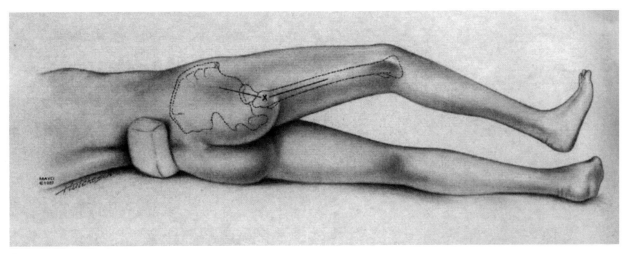

A

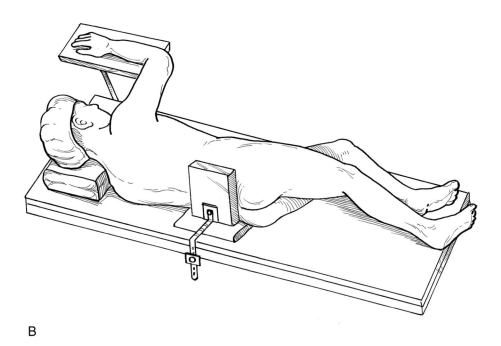

B

Figure 50–6. **A** and **B**, Diagrams showing positioning the patient prior to hemiresurfacing.

weight as tolerated and are typically weaned from ambulatory aids 4 to 6 weeks postoperatively.

CONCLUSIONS

We currently recommend the use of femoral hemiresurfacing arthroplasty for young patients with Ficat stage III and early stage IV osteonecrosis of the femoral head. The results of resurfacing of the femoral head can be a successful interim surgical procedure for treatment of young, active patients with a large osteonecrosis lesion that is not suitable for other treatment options, with the exception of total hip arthroplasty.

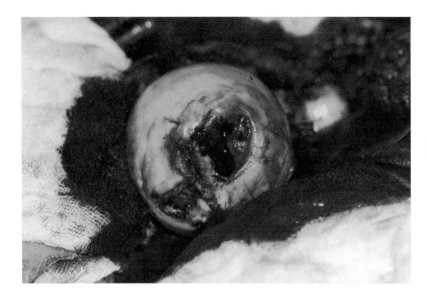

Figure 50–7. Intraoperative photograph of a necrotic femoral head in an active 18-year-old male.

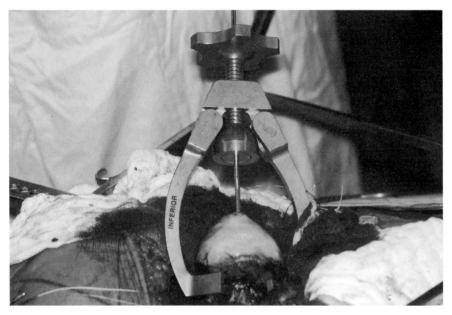

A

Figure 50–8. A, Intraoperative photograph showing placement of guidewire into center of femoral neck. Pin placement can be confirmed with intraoperative fluoroscopy. **B**, Diagram showing placement of pin centrally into the femoral neck.

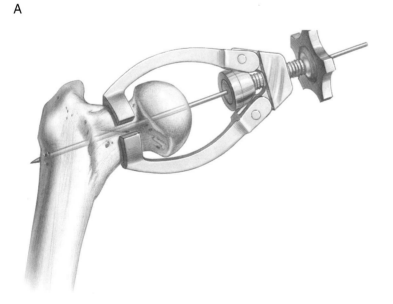

B

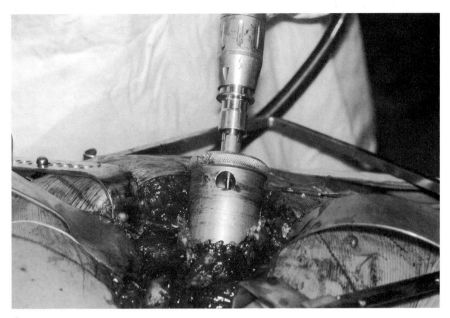

A

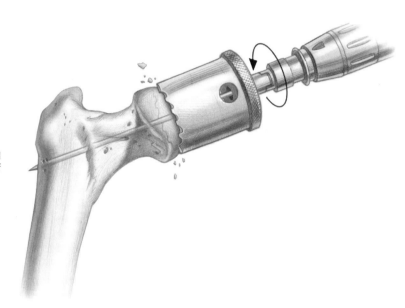

Figure 50–9. A, Photograph showing reaming of femoral head over a guidewire. **B**, Diagram showing reaming of femoral head over guidewire.

B

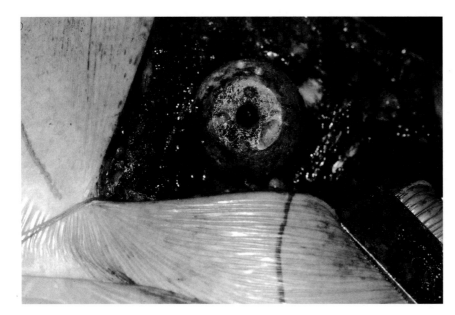

Figure 50–10. Photograph showing prepared proximal femur. Sizing has been done to match acetabulum.

Figure 50–11. Photograph showing trial in place. Hip can be reduced and proper size assessed with fluoroscopy.

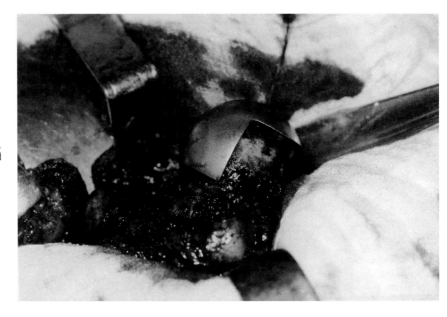

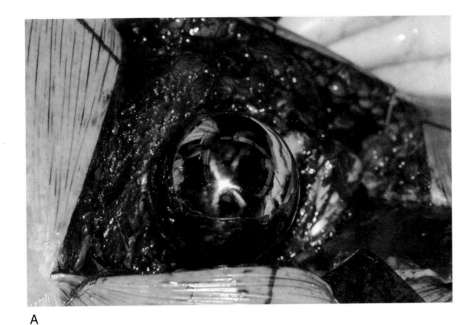
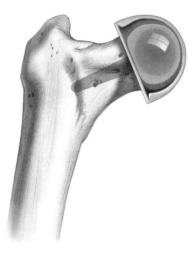

A   B

Figure 50–12. **A**, Photograph with real implant cemented into place. **B**, Diagram showing real implant cemented into place.

References

1. Amustutz HC: The THARIES hip resurfacing technique. Orthop Clin North Am 13:813–832, 1982.
2. Amstutz HC, Thomas BJ, Jinnah R, et al: Treatment of primary osteoarthritis of the hip. A comparison of total joint and surface replacement arthroplasty. J Bone Joint Surg 66A:228–241, 1984.
3. Baer WS: Arthroplasty with the aid of animal membrane. Am J Orthop Surg 16:1–29, 1918.
4. Beaule P, Amstutz H: Hemiresurfacing arthroplasty for osteonecrosis of the hip. Op Tech Orthop 10:123–132, 2000.
5. Bogoch ER, Fornasier VL, Capello WN: The femoral head remnant in resurfacing arthroplasty. Clin Orthop 167:92–105, 1982.
6. Buechel FF: Hip resurfacing revisited. Orthopedics 19:753–756, 1996.
7. Cabanela ME: Bipolar versus total hip arthroplasty for osteonecrosis of the femoral head. A comparison. Clin Orthop 261:59–62, 1990.
8. Campbell P, Mirra J, Amstutz HC: Viability of femoral heads treated with resurfacing arthroplasty. J Arthroplasty 15:120–122, 2000.
9. Capello WN, Ireland PH, Trammell TR, Eicher P: Conservative total hip arthroplasty. A procedure to conserve bone stock. Part I. Analysis of sixty-six patients. Part II. Analysis of failures. Clin Orthop 134:59–74, 1978.
10. Capello WN, Misamore GW, Trancik TM: Conservative total hip arthroplasty. Orthop Clin North Am 13:833–842, 1982.
11. Charnley J: Low friction arthroplasty. Berlin, Springer-Verlag, 1979.
12. Cornell CN, Salvati EA, Pellici PM: Long-term follow-up of total hip replacement in patients with osteonecrosis. Orthop Clin North Am 16:757–769, 1985.
13. Dorr LD, Takei GK, Conaty JP: Total hip arthroplasties in patients less than thirty-five years old. J Bone Joint Surg 65A:474–479, 1983.
14. Ficat RP, Arlet J: Functional investigation of bone under normal conditions. *In* Hungerford D (ed): Ischemia and Necrosis of Bone. Baltimore, Williams and Wilkins, 1980, pp 29–52.
15. Freeman MAR: Some anatomical and mechanical considerations relevant to the surface replacement of the femoral head. Clin Orthop 134:19–24, 1978.
16. Freeman MAR, Cameron HU, Brown GC: Cemented double cup arthroplasty of the hip: A 5-year experience with the ICLH prosthesis. Clin Orthop 134:45–52, 1978.
17. Furuya K, Tsuchiya M, Kawachi S: Socket-cup arthroplasty. Clin Orthop 134:41–44, 1978.
18. Gerard Y: Hip arthroplasty in matching cups. Clin Orthop 134:25–35, 1978.
19. Haboush EJ: A new operation for arthroplasty of the hip based on biomechanics, photoelasticity, setting dental acrylic and other considerations. Bull Hosp Joint Dis 13:242–277, 1953.
20. Hungerford MW, Mont MA, Scott R: Surface replacement hemiarthoplasty for the treatment of osteonecrosis of the femoral head. J Bone Joint Surg 80A:1656–1664, 1998.
21. Jolley MN, Salvati EA, Brown GC: Early results and complications of surface replacement of the hip. J Bone Joint Surg 64A:366–377, 1982.
22. Kim KJ, Rubash HE: Large amounts of polyethylene debris in the interface tissue surrounding bipolar endoprostheses. Comparison to total hip prostheses. J Arthroplasty 12:32–39, 1997.
23. Krackow KA, Mont MA, Maar DC: Limited femoral endoprosthesis for avascular necrosis of the femoral head. Orthop Rev 12:457–463, 1993.
24. Kwok DC, Cruess RL: A retrospective study of Moore and Thompson hemiarthroplasty. A review of 599 surgical cases and analysis of the technical complications. Clin Orthop 169:179–185, 1982.
25. Lachiewicz PF, Desman SM: The bipolar endoprosthesis in avascular necrosis of the femoral head. J Arthroplasty 3:131–138, 1988.
26. Meyers MH: The treatment of osteonecrosis of the hip with fresh osteochondral allografts and muscle pedicle graft technique. Clin Orthop 130:202–209, 1978.
27. Murphy JB: Ankylosis: Clinical and experimental. JAMA 44:1573–1582, 1905.
28. Nelson CL, Walz BH, Gruenwald JM: Resurfacing of only the femoral head for osteonecrosis. J Arthroplasty 12:736–740, 1997.
29. Ortiguera C, Pulliam I, Cabanela ME: Total hip arthroplasty for osteonecrosis. Matched-pair analysis of 188 hips with long-term follow-up. J Arthroplasty 14:21–28, 1999.
30. Parvizi J, Morrey MA, Breen CJ, Cabanela ME: The outcome of uncemented total hip arthroplasty for avascular necrosis in patients under 50 years of age. Transactions of Mid-America Orthopaedic Association, 18th Annual Meeting, Scottsdale AZ, April 26–29, 2000.
31. Ritter MA, Gioe TJ: Conventional versus resurfacing total hip arthroplasty. A long-term prospective study of concomitant bilateral implantation of prostheses. J Bone Joint Surg 68A:216–225, 1986.

32. Siguier T, Siguier M, Judet T, et al: Partial resurfacing arthroplasty of the femoral head in avascular necrosis. Clin Orthop 386:85–92, 2001.

33. Smith-Petersen MN: Evolution of mould arthroplasty of the hip joint. J Bone Joint Surg 30B:59–73, 1948.

34. Steinberg ME: Summary and conclusions. Symposium on surface replacement arthroplasty of the hip. Orthop Clin North Am 13:895–902, 1982.

35. Townley CO: Hemi and total articular replacement arthroplasty of the hip with the fixed femoral cup. Orthop Clin North Am 13:869–894, 1982.

36. Trentani C, Vaccarino F: The Paltrinieri-Trentani hip resurface arthroplasty. Clin Orthop 134:36–40, 1978.

37. Vail TP, Urbaniak JR: Donor-site morbidity with use of vascularized autogenous fibular grafts. J Bone Joint Surg 78:204–211, 1996.

38. Wagner H: Hip arthroplasty by the resurfacing procedure. J Bone Joint Surg 61B:235, 1979.

51

Conservative Replacement Designs: Metaphyseal Fixed Implants

• BERNARD F. MORREY

Although the design and techniques of hip replacement have improved over time, reliable long-term effectiveness in young patients remains problematic. The central problem today is well recognized to be that of the articulation and the generation of wear debris. However, the desire to violate less of the native bone of the proximal femur, allowing a less complicated and more reliable revision procedure, has continued to foster interest in resurfacing and metaphyseal fixed femoral implants. In fact, this was the design philosophy of the earliest of hip replacement designs (Fig. 51–1).

RATIONALE

The goal of any joint replacement is relief of pain that occurs with immediate rigid fixation. The additional goals of "conservative" replacement include: (1) a minimized bone resection, (2) favorable remodeling characteristics, and (3) allowance for ready revision should the implant fail.[35] If these goals can be achieved with nonstemmed devices, this is an attractive option in the opinion of many surgeons.[25,49] The topic of resurfacing hip replacement is discussed in Chapter 50. In this chapter, we deal with metaphyseal fixation of the femoral implant.

Pain Relief

Because pain relief is directly related to rigid fixation,[8,19] any implant not secured with polymethylmethacrylate (PMMA) must attain this goal from either the shape or the surface design or both.[13,40,48] Nonstemmed devices may be fixed directly to the femoral head, to the head and neck, through the neck with a supplemental side plate, or in the proximal metaphyseal portion of the femur. Rigid fixation can be achieved with PMMA or by virtue of the design. Designs that are limited to the head and neck are easily revised, even if cemented, because failure will result in removal of the entire portion of the head replacement so as not to compromise a subsequent

revision. On the other hand, it is logical to conclude that a metaphyseal implant with a wedge-shaped contour in the anterior, posterior, and lateral planes will develop point-contact stabilization in the proximal aspect of the femur, with stability being further enhanced by increased depth of implantation. The validity of this concept has been demonstrated experimentally[24] and is further explored in this chapter.

Conservative Intervention

Any joint replacement device implanted with relatively little bone removed or little violation of the normal anatomy may be viewed as a "conservative" device. This implant should be complemented by conservative intervention of the acetabulum as well. My personal concern with resurfacing the femoral head is the tendency to remove excessive acetabular bone if this is to be replaced as well.

In all instances, minimizing the duration of the procedure and the extent to which the medullary canal of the femur is exposed and refashioned should also lessen the amount of blood loss.

An additional feature of a conservative replacement is the ease of conversion to another device or system should failure occur. An effective and reliable revision is enhanced if the initial implant violates as little bone as possible, specifically leaving intact those elements of fixation needed for traditional implant fixation.

Final considerations are those of cost and inventory. A device that could be used to replace either the left or right side with minimal adjunctive modular features would also be of great value.

Design Options

Resurfacing Implants

The concept of resurfacing arthroplasty dates from the beginning of arthroplasty in the form of cup or mold arthroplasty. Interest has waxed and waned as new concepts emerge.[1,22,44] Unfortunately, new problems

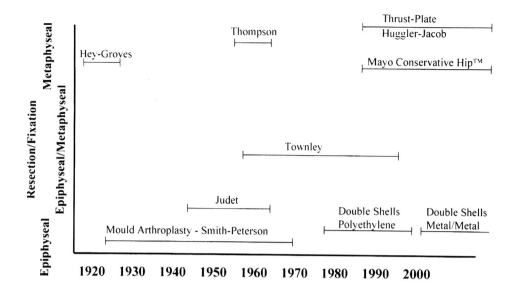

Figure 51–1. Historical perspective of "conservative" fixation in the epiphyseal or metaphyseal aspect of the femur. (Concept modified from I. Jacob, Zurich, Switzerland.)

have arisen with each new effort to reintroduce the resurfacing design. Although the topic is covered in Chapter 50, a few comments help to place this option in the context of the present chapter.

One of the factors that has compromised the effectiveness of femoral resurfacing in the past was avascular necrosis of the femoral head associated with the surgical exposure. It is questionable whether this problem can be completely overcome. The need to remove excessive bone from the acetabulum to ensure sufficient thickness of metal and polyethylene may be addressed by a metal-on-metal articulation or as a bipolar hemireplacement.[36] The improvement in implant fixation may eliminate the need for cement. However, in the final analysis, any femoral resurfacing implant must start with the limiting factor of the neck diameter. The neck diameter determines the minimal effective femoral head diameter, which in turn dictates the minimal cup diameter.

Hence, to date, I continue to be concerned about this issue in total resurfacing replacement. However, as a hemireplacement, this concept is attractive and has been used in carefully selected cases, especially in very young patients (Fig. 51–2).

Metaphyseal Fixation

The alternative to resurfacing is to attain fixation in the metaphyseal portion of the femur but to avoid intramedullary fixation. The two most important design considerations for such implants are the mode of fixation and the sensitivity of the design to the technique of proper placement. In resurfacing implants, the orientation is based on the contour of the head and neck. Most traditional stemmed devices are oriented based on the position of the stem down the canal.[4,30] The absence of stem fixation of metaphyseal fixed prostheses thus introduces additional design and technique considerations.

Nonstemmed-nonresurfacing Devices

The basic concept of metaphyseal fixation of the femoral replacement device is not new. The design philosophies have varied considerably over time, from a head neck replacement with a side plate such as the Thrust Plate device to the double taper Mayo Conservative Hip designed in 1982. The rationale for these designs is briefly discussed.

Remodeling of Metaphyseal Fixed Devices

Given that pain relief is achieved by immediate as well as sustained rigid fixation, favorable long-term remodeling is a desirable characteristic of any conservative device. This implies that the proximal femur should be loaded but not shielded by the device. Studies show that the normal stress pattern of the femur is dramatically altered with any intramedullary system of any material, whether long- or short stemmed, whether cemented or not (Fig. 51–3).[9,10,32,38,48] Systems that replace only the head, or those limited to the head and neck, should have no impact or minimal impact on bone remodeling. Little is known of the optimal stress pattern to ensure long-term compatibility with stemmed implants after head and neck removal. There is no guarantee that a so-called anatomic stem does or can provide an optimal stress distribution pattern for an intramedullary loaded system.[3,5] Furthermore, if adequate immediate fixation is obtained entirely in the proximal femur without a stem, stress shielding would seem to be impossible (Fig. 51–4). Such an approach also has the attractive feature of potentially decreasing or eliminating thigh pain, which continues to exist in a percent of uncemented intramedullary fixed-stem devices.

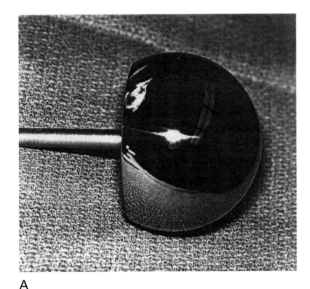

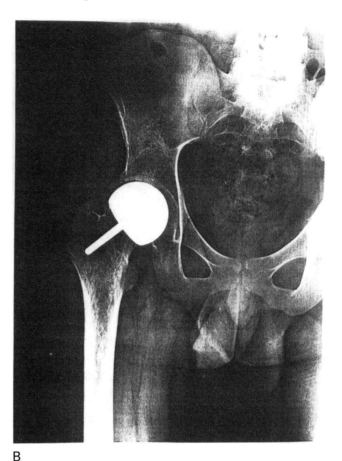

Figure 51–2. A hemiresurfacing implant is useful in a 21-year-old patient with leukemia and steroid-induced osteonecrosis (**A**). Leaving the acetabulum intact adds an additional element of conservative intervention (**B**).

The weight-bearing loads tend to cause a varus moment to be imparted to the replacement device. It has been demonstrated that a narrow medial and wide lateral cross-section geometry creates stresses in the proximal femur that are favorable to bone remodeling[26] and effectively resist the varus moment. As understanding of the loads in the proximal femur has increased, marked rotational stresses, particularly during stair climbing, have been recognized. This load imparts a twisting moment to the prosthetic implant that is proportional to the distance from the femoral head to the center of the femur, hence correlating to femoral offset. The cross-section taper has been shown to be effective in resisting these forces as well.[26]

The Mayo Conservative Hip™

One approach intended to satisfy the aforementioned goals and considerations was that of a double-tapered metaphyseal fixed (60-mm) femoral replacement implant that was designed at the Mayo Clinic in 1982 and modified to provide a circumferential seal in 1998 (Fig. 51–5). Because the design is a radical departure from accepted thinking, several investigations were conducted before it was used in patients.

Fatigue Studies

Fixation

For the Mayo Conservative Hip, a careful study of embalmed cadaver femurs was conducted to better understand the three-dimensional intramedullary anatomy of the proximal femur.[11] The variation of anteversion of the femoral neck and bowing of the proximal femur are important considerations in the design, as confirmed by documenting consecutive patterns of stability attained by several points of fixation. The results of this study indicated that much of the rotatory stability occurs from the favorable multipoint contact geometry between the implant and the proximal femur that has been noted in both the anteroposterior and lateral planes (Fig. 51–6).

To better predict the remodeling behavior of an uncemented implant with a design philosophy that departs from the norm, a two-dimensional finite element analysis was conducted by Huiskes et al.[21] The results demonstrated that the hoop stresses in the simulated model containing this implant were consistent with bone remodeling and were not excessive as subsequently demonstrated in our laboratory (see Fig. 51–5). Rotational forces slightly shifted the maximum stress region posteriorly, but these magnitudes were also not excessive. As

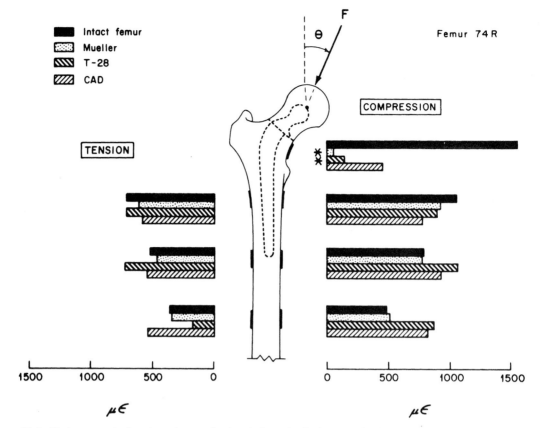

Figure 51–3. Strain gauge studies show that proximal strain is markedly decreased with intramedullary loaded systems. (From Oh D, Harris WH: Proximal strain distributions in the loaded femur. J Bone Joint Surg 60A:75, 1978.)

anticipated, the greatest stresses occurred medially in the frontal plane with a varus-producing force. Subsequent studies to elucidate the effect of varying positions of varus/valgus also revealed little change in the stress distribution of the proximal femur, with slight variations in the varus/valgus orientation in the frontal plane.

Indications

Age is a relative consideration, and metaphyseal devices are used in younger patients and in those with adequate bone quality. Metaphyseal devices may be useful for proximal femoral deformity and when the canal is obstructed by screws or offset from fracture or osteotomy.

Contraindications

The metaphyseal device should not be used if the bone quality is poor, as in patients with extensive osteoporosis. Proximal femoral distortion that does not allow restoration of proper mechanics by these devices is also a contraindication.

Preoperative Planning

Templates, if available, should be used as part of the preoperative planning. Both the anteroposterior and lateral projections should be considered with the templates. For the Mayo Conservative Hip, the dimensions and

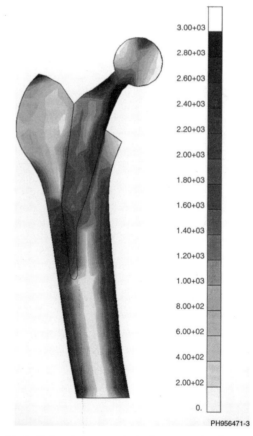

Figure 51–4. Finite element analysis demonstrating favorable stress distribution in the metaphyseal fixed Mayo Conservative Hip.

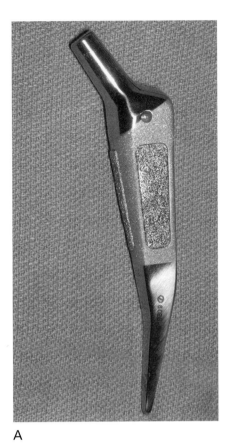

A

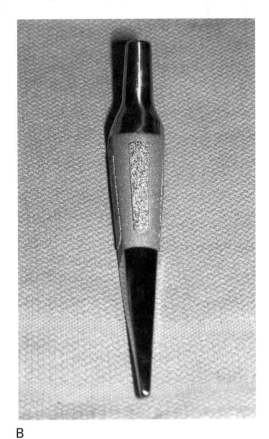

B

Figure 51–5. Mayo Conservative Hip is unchanged from the 1984 design except for the corundumization treatment of the surface added in 1998.

configuration demonstrated by the lateral view are of particular importance when the proper size of the implant is estimated (see Fig. 51–7). The effect of femoral anteversion is also noted because it is also a major determinant of the size of implant to be used (see Fig. 51–6). The final decision on the appropriate size of implant is made at the time of surgery, with use of the rasp as the femoral trial.

SURGICAL TECHNIQUE: MAYO CONSERVATIVE HIP

The lateral decubitus position is used and the anterior approach is preferred, but a posterior approach is also acceptable.

Because the device has no collar, the exact line of resection is not critical, and by the use of a template, the level

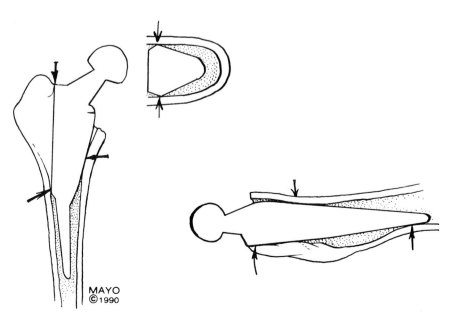

Figure 51–6. Fixation by point contact because of asymmetric geometry of the proximal femur. Note the anteroposterior contact of the prosthesis and femoral neck.

MAYO
©1990

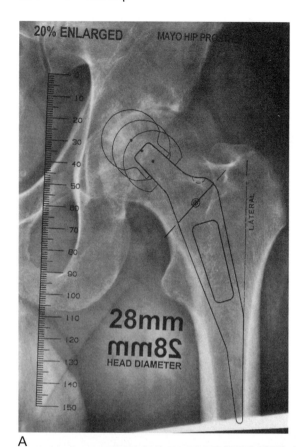

A

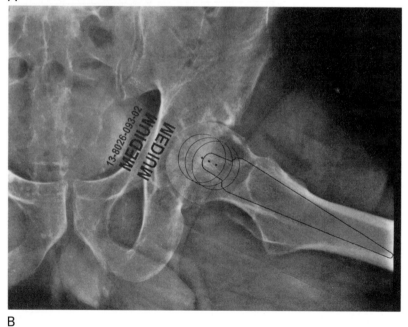

B

Figure 51–7. **A**, Both the anterior, posterior and the lateral projections are studied to estimate the appropriate implant size. **B**, On the lateral view, the depth of insertion is estimated by placing the center of the template over the center of the head.

and orientation of the cut are defined. As with other designs, the usual level of resection is approximately a fingerbreadth above the lesser trochanter. Of particular note and unlike other designs, the neck is left intact. There is no need to violate the trochanter to align with the shaft (Fig. 51–8). By leaving the neck intact, a circumferential seal with the corundumized implant is attained. If the line of osteotomy has been correctly placed, the angle

of the femoral neck cut correlates to the orientation of the rasp, which properly aligns the device.

Femoral Preparation

An awl is placed down the lateral aspect of the neck and medullary canal to locate the lateral cortex of the femur.

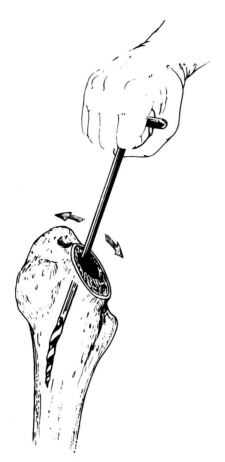

Figure 51–8. The lateral aspect of the femoral neck is left intact, allowing a circumferential seal that lessens the likelihood of wear debris being introduced distally at the prostheses/femur interface. The curved awl identifies the proximal femoral canal.

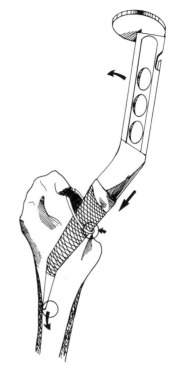

Figure 51–9. Optimal orientation of the implant occurs when the tail of the rasp is parallel to the lateral femoral cortex. The rasp is advanced until stable.

This becomes the landmark for rasp insertion. I remove bone from the femoral neck to assist the initial insertion of the rasp.

The smallest size of femoral rasp is first employed, with the tail of the rasp placed parallel to the lateral cortex of the femur (Fig. 51–9). Modest force exerted by the mallet drives the rasp down the canal. When the rasp no longer advances, the proper size of implant and depth of insertion has been defined.

Component Insertion

The implant is inserted so that the dimple, which is present on the proximal portion of the device, attains the same level as the rasp. Fractures from excessive hoop stresses are rare if the implant is not forced more distally than dictated by the rasp. Trial reduction is again carried out. If there is uncertainty about neck length, the shorter length is invariably the correct decision.

Anteversion of the implant is dictated by the orientation of the femoral neck. If anteversion is excessive, additional neck resection is carried out to allow the implant to fit adequately down the canal at an appropriate depth and rotatory orientation.

Stability is checked in all planes with extension-external rotation and flexion-internal rotation. Closure is of choice after the abductors have been secured with No. 5 nonabsorbable sutures through bone.

Postoperative Management: Mayo Conservative Hip

We continue to use a continuous postoperative rehabilitation program. Thus, the load is increased by 10 to 15 pounds per week. In the second month, load bearing progresses to full body weight, and the patient is weaned off crutches. In the third month, full weight bearing is allowed with use of a cane.

CLINICAL RESULTS

Results

Literature Review

Because the philosophy of conservative replacement favors the younger patient, the relevant frame of reference is a patient population averaging about 50 years of age. Underlying diagnoses and age are important prognostic variables. Studies of younger patients often select avascular necrosis or dysplasia as the underlying diagnosis. One large series of 123 replacements for osteonecrosis of the femoral head revealed a 4 percent revision rate with a mean surveillance of 4.5 years.[18] Most (6) of the failures were of the cup. On the other hand, assessment of

98 replacements for osteonecrosis, with an average patient age of 41 years; followed for a mean of 7 years (range, 2 to 10 years) revealed a 21 percent revision rate in one study.[46] The majority of failures were due to cup wear, and only 4 femoral component failures were documented.[47] Experience with 72 Mittelmeier uncemented femoral replacements for osteonecrosis that were followed for 3 years revealed a mechanical failure of 6 percent for the stem and 8 percent for cups.[17]

Patients with dysplastic hips require replacement at an early age. One study included 41 hips that were followed for 10 years, with a revision rate of 30 percent. Problems with the cup were three times more frequent than with the stem.[39] However, an additional study revealed no loosening among 45 cases of dysplasia an average of 4 years after surgery.[2] In yet another experience using cementless implants in patients younger than 50 years of age, a 5-year mean follow-up revealed that 18 percent had severe wear and lysis. The most extensive problem was with 32-mm head diameters and 6-mm-thick polyethyelene.[12]

In patients with rheumatoid arthritis, the outcome is better than for those with osteonecrosis. A study of 1553 Charnley prostheses in a patient population averaging 53 years of age revealed survival free of revision in 90 percent at 10 years and 83 percent at 15 years. Cup and stem survival was comparable.[28] In a group who primarily had osteoarthritis, experience with an uncemented device in 74 procedures, with a mean patient age of 62 years, revealed a 95 percent success rate of the femoral component.[6] The Wrightington experience with 226 replacements in patients averaging 32 years of age with a 20-year mean follow-up is the most definitive study to date. The 25-year survival rate was 89 percent for those with hip dysplasia; 85 percent in those with rheumatoid arthritis and 74 percent in those with osteoarthritis. Overall, the 25-year survival rate of the femoral component was 81 percent.[45]

The outcomes of precoated implants is very design specific. This is dramatically underscored by noting that when a PMMA precoated implant was used in 45 hips in patients younger than 50 years of age, an 18 percent incidence of stem fixation failure was observed between 5 and 10 years of follow-up.[46]

Metaphyseal Fixation

Metaphyseal femoral fixation,[15] with or without cement, lessens the resorption of proximal bone from stress shielding.[7,9,13,24] Uncemented fixation is attained by osseous incorporation into the implant surface or with a "macrolock" interference fit.[40] The Mayo design features both elements; the multipoint contact in both planes results in an immediate macrolock and metal fiber pads give osseous integration with rigid fixation.[3,8] The value of a tapered device in optimizing bone remodeling in the lateral plane has been demonstrated by Kuiper and Huiskes.[25] The relative lack of thigh pain and proximal resorption that have been reported in other biologically fixed systems are encouraging observations with use of metaphyseal fixed devices.[7,27,31,37,50]

Femoral head and neck replacement with a metaphyseal side plate to stabilize the component has been used in Europe for more than two decades. A series of 52 uncemented Thrust-plate replacements, a mean of 3.5 years after surgery in patients with osteonecrosis, has been reported[15] (Fig. 51–10). A failure rate of 10 percent was observed. These authors emphasize that the outcome for those with osteonecrosis is largely dependent on etiology, and that those who are taking immunosuppressive medication and those with sickle cell disease have the greatest risk of infection and failure.

Mayo Clinic Experience

Of 161 consecutive procedures, 2 patients have died and 2 were lost to follow-up, leaving experience with 159 procedures, with a mean patient age of 51 years.[33] The underlying diagnosis was degenerative arthritis in 63 percent, avascular necrosis in 14 percent, failed previous surgery in 5 percent, post-traumatic arthrosis in 5 percent, rheumatoid arthritis in 7 percent, and congenital dislocation of the hip in 5 percent. A mean surveillance of 6.2 years (range 2 to 13 years) was documented.

Function. The mean arc of motion was typical of most prosthetic replacements, with flexion of 0 to 93, abduction/adduction of 38 to 20, and internal/external rotation of 19 to 34 degrees. After 3 months, 57 percent of patients had a positive Trendelenburg test, and, after 1 year, 5 percent had a clinically detectable limp.

Pain. Moderate pain was present in 4.5 percent at 1 year. One patient eventually required revision for pain. This experience is quite comparable with those data reported for cemented Mayo replacements and other uncemented implant designs.[27,42,50]

Transfusion Requirements. Significantly less blood was required after the Mayo conservative implant compared with that required after an uncemented control implant ($P<.001$). Currently, only 15 percent of patients require transfusion after the Mayo Conservative Hip implant.

Radiographic Changes. These changes are summarized in Table 51–1. Of 159 hips, 127 showed no evidence of a neocortex or lucent line. In the remaining 32, most changes occurred in zones 1 and 2. Evidence of femoral remodeling was considered when there was an increase in bone density in at least one of the seven zones. This occurred in 55 implants, mostly in zone 6 but also in zone 3.[26]

Both the neocortex and increased cortical density are considered favorable because they indicate proximal femoral remodeling rather than stress shielding (Fig. 51–11).

Proximal femoral osteolysis was observed in 11 of the 159 hips (6 percent) and was circumferential in 2 more than 7 years after surgery (Table 51–2). Both required revision. Eight of the 11 had osteolysis in zone 1 or 2 and

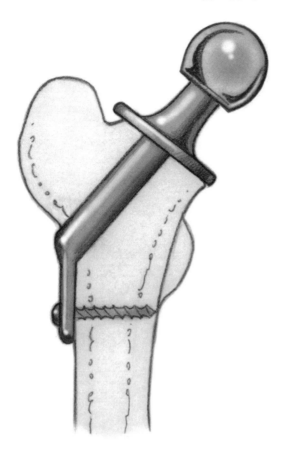

Figure 51–10. The Thrust Plate concept has been employed for a decade in Europe.

6 in zones 6 and 7. Distal osteolysis was uncommon, occurring in only 3 patients, all of whom had extensive acetabular wear.

We estimated wear by using the technique of Livermore and Morrey.[29] In 120 hips (75 percent), no wear could be measured; in 30 (19 percent), 1 mm of wear was observed; in 5, 2 mm (3 percent), and in 4 (2 percent), more than 2 mm. In 37 of the 39 with meas-

urable wear, this was first observed after 5 or more years.

Harris Hip Score. The mean preoperative Harris hip score was 66.3, and at follow-up, 90.4. The Kaplan-Meier rate of probability of survival without revision for mechanical loosening was 98.2 percent, at both 5 and 10 years (Fig. 51–12).

Complications. There were 3 complications not requiring further surgery, 1 hematoma and 2 pulmonary emboli.

There were 12 (7 percent) intraoperative complications. In 10 (6 percent) an undisplaced, type-IA[34] proximal femoral fracture occurred, which did not compromise the result and was not associated with subsidence or reoperation. Each was treated by means of cerclage wire.

The stem alone was revised in 6 cases (3.8 percent), 2 for femoral fracture, 1 as a result of a traffic accident, and 1 because of a fall. Three cases of mechanical loosening occurred because of inadequate fixation (1.8 percent). In 2, the device subsided in the first 3 months after operation, and in 1 an initially stable implant at 6 months became loose when the patient jumped 3 feet from a step and landed on the operated limb. All 3 required revision. In 9 (5.6 percent), delayed femoral osteolysis occurred in association with cup wear, and revision was

Table 51–1. COMPLICATIONS OF 161 CONSECUTIVE HIP REPLACEMENT PROCEDURES USING THE DOUBLE-TAPERED FEMORAL STEM

Complication	No.
Proximal femoral fracture	
Surgery (I, a)*	9
Trauma	2
Instability	
Early	4
Late	3
Loose femoral implants†	1
Loose acetabular implants	2
Sciatic palsy	1
Ectopic bone	1
Late deep infection (tooth abscess)	1
Total	24 (14.6%)

*Ia, undisplaced, proximal to lesser trochanter.
†Radiographic criteria, subsidence greater than 4 mm.

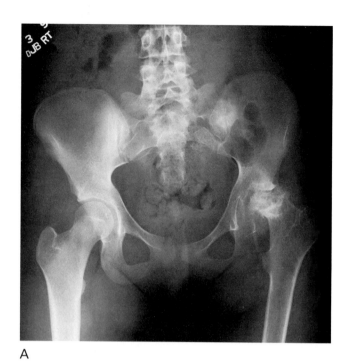

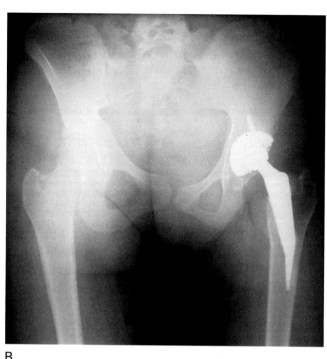

A

B

Figure 51–11. A 61-year-old man with severe coxarthrosis (**A**) is asymptomatic 15 years after replacement with the Mayo Conservative Hip (**B**). Note the remodeling characteristics of proximal femur.

required of both components. The mean time to revision was 7 years (range, 4 to 11 years).

These data compare favorably with those from a multicenter Swedish study reporting migration greater than 5 mm in 22 percent of 539 PCA implants (Howmedica, Rutherford, NJ) requiring 41 femoral revisions (8 percent).[29] Furthermore, Mallory et al.[31] reported stress shielding in 6 percent of 150 patients with a mean follow-up of 6.3 years, and thigh pain in 8 percent.[31]

The incidence of femoral fracture is also comparable with those that occurred in other series with uncemented implants,[16,43] particularly during the time that these prostheses were being introduced. Although fracture may not be as innocuous as once supposed,[23] no patient in the Mayo Clinic series had measurable subsidence or loosening associated with an intraoperative undisplaced fracture of the femoral neck.

Current Design and Outcome Update

Approval from the Food and Drug Administration was granted in December 1997. Since then, the experience has included more than 350 implants. The average patient age at surgery remains at 51 years; and the overall outcome has not substantially changed from that reported earlier. A circumferential treatment by corundumization is currently being used to "seal" the proximal femur and shield the implant/femur interface from wear debris (see Fig. 51–5). This technique of

surface finish for titanium alloy surfaces has been shown to be highly effective in allowing bone ongrowth.[3,14,41]

SUMMARY

Interest in a conservative approach to femoral replacement remains strong. The rationale of resurfacing and metaphyseal fixation is similar in purpose but different in execution. Although the value of the concept appears to be well established, the utility of a given design will be defined in time by careful analysis of long-term outcomes.

Table 51–2. DELAYED COMPLICATIONS REQUIRING REVISION (159 PROCEDURES)

Complication	Number (percent)
Cup	
Loose	1 (0.6)
Unstable	1 (0.6)
Wear	2 (1.2)
Total	4 (2.5)
Stem	
Mechanically loose	3 (1.8)
Pain	1 (0.6)
Trauma/fx femur	2 (1.2)
Total	6 (3.7)
Cup and stem	
Wear/lysis	9 (5.6)

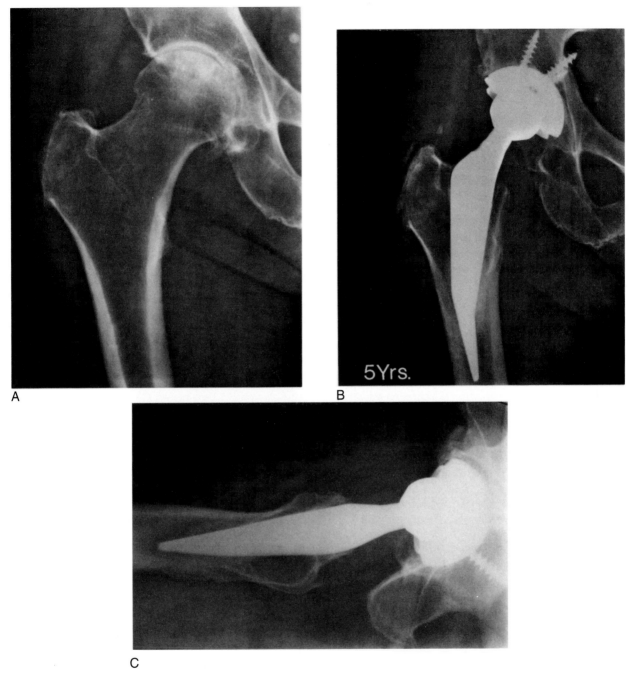

Figure 51–12. A, Preoperative radiographs show significant degenerative arthrosis of the hip. **B**, Five years after implantation, osseous condensation has occurred distal to the greater trochanter and at the level of the lesser trochanter. The femoral neck resection is rounded off. **C**, Lateral view demonstrates the proper orientation of the implant. Note that the femoral component has the same anteversion as does the normal femur. This obviates the need for right and left implants in the inventory.

References

1. Amstutz HC, Grigoris P, Dorey FJ: Evolution and future of surface replacement of the hip. J Orthop Sci 3:169, 1998.
2. Bobak P, Wroblewski BM, Siney PD, et al: Charnley low-friction arthroplasty with an autograft of the femoral head for developmental dysplasia of the hip. The 10- to 15-year results. J Bone Joint Surg 82B:508, 2000.
3. Bobyn JD, Pilliar RM, Cameron HU, Weatherly GC: Osteogenic phenomenon across endosteal bone-implant spaces with porous surfaced intramedullary implants. Acta Orthop Scand 52:145, 1981.
4. Bourne RB, Rorabeck CH: A critical look at cementless stems. Taper designs and when to use alternatives. Clin Orthop 355:212, 1998.
5. Brown JW, Ring PA: Osteolytic changes in the upper femoral shaft following porous coated hip replacement. J Bone Joint Surg 67B:218, 1985.
6. Burt CF, Garvin KL, Otterbreg ET, Jardon OM: A femoral component inserted without cement in total hip arthroplasty. A study of the Tri-Lock component with an average ten-year duration of follow-up. J Bone Joint Surg 80:952, 1998.
7. Callaghan JJ, Dysart SH, Savory CG: The uncemented porous-coated anatomic total hip prosthesis. Two year results of a prospective consecutive series. J Bone Joint Surg 70A:337, 1988.

8. Cameron HU, Pilliar RM, MacNab I: The effect of movement on the bonding of porous metal to bone. J Biomed Mater Res 7:301, 1973.

9. Cook SD, Klawitter JJ, Weinstein AM: The influence of design parameters on calcar stresses following femoral head arthroplasty. J Biomed Mater Res 14:133, 1980.

10. Crowninshield RD, Brand RA, Johnston RC, Milroy JC: An analysis of femoral component stem design in total hip arthroplasty. J Bone Joint Surg 62A:68, 1980.

11. Dai KR, An KN, Hein T, et al: Geometric and biomechanical analysis of the human femur. Orthop Trans 9:256, 1985.

12. Dunkley AB, Eldridge JD, Lee MB, et al: Cementless acetabular replacement in the young. A 5- to 10-year prospective study. Clin Orthop 376:149, 2000.

13. Engh CA, Bobyn JD, Glassman AH: Porous-coated hip replacement. The factors governing bone ingrowth, stress shielding and clinical results. J Bone Joint Surg 69B:45, 1987.

14. Feighan JE, Goldberg VM, Davy D, et al: The influence of surface-blasting on the incorporation of tiatanium-alloy implants in a rabbit intramedullary model. J Bone Joint Surg 77A:1380, 1995.

15. Fink B, Ruther W: Partial and total joint replacement in femur head necrosis. Orthopade 29:449, 2000.

16. Fitzgerald RH Jr, Brindley GW, Kavanagh BF: Fracture and the uncemented total hip arthroplasty. Clin Orthop 235:61, 1988.

17. Fye MA, Huo MHJ, Zatorski LE, Keggi KJ: Total hip arthroplasty performed without cement in patients with femoral head osteonecrosis who are less than 50 years old. J Arthroplasty 13:876, 1998.

18. Garino JP, Steinberg ME: Total hip arthroplasty in patients with avascular necrosis of the femoral head: A 2- to 10-year follow-up. Clin Orthop 334:108, 1997.

19. Haddad RJ Jr, Cook SD, Thomas KA: Biological fixation of porous coated implants. J Bone Joint Surg 69A:1459, 1987.

20. Huggler AH, Jacob HA, Bereiter H, et al: Long-term results with the uncemented thrust plate prosthesis (TPP). Acta Orthop Belg 1(Suppl 59):215, 1993.

21. Huiskes R, Snijders H, Vroemen W, et al: Fixation stability of a short cementless hip prosthesis. Trans Orthop Res Soc 11:466, 1986.

22. Hungerford MW, Mont MA, Scott R, et al: Surface replacement hemiarthroplasty for the treatment of osteonecrosis of the femoral head. J Bone Joint Surg 80A:1656, 1998.

23. Jasty M, Bragdon CR, Rubash H, et al: Unrecognized femoral fractures during cementless total hip arthroplasty in the dog and their effect on bone ingrowth. J Arthroplasty 7:501, 1992.

24. Jasty M, Krushell R, Zalenski AS, et al: The contribution of the nonporous distal stem to the stability of proximally porous-coated canine femoral components. J Arthroplasty 8:33, 1993.

25. Kelsey D, Goodman SB: Design of the femoral component for cementless hip replacement: The surgeon's perspective. Am J Orthop 26:407, 1997.

26. Kuiper JH, Huiskes R: Friction and stem stiffness affect dynamic interface motion in total hip replacement. J Orthop Res 14:36, 1996.

27. Lachiewicz PF, Anspach WE III, DeMasi R: A prospective study of 100 consecutive Harris-Galante porous total hip arthroplasties: 2–5 year results. J Arthroplasty 7:519, 1992.

28. Lehtimaki MY, Kautiainen H, Lehto UK, Hamalainen MM: Charnley low-friction arthroplasty in rheumatoid patients. A survival study up to 20 years. J Arthroplasty 14:657, 1999.

29. Livermore J, Ilstrup D, Morrey B: Effect of femoral head size on wear of the polyethylene acetabular component. J Bone Joint Surg 72A:518, 1990.

30. Malchau H, Wang YX, Karrholm J, Herberts P: Scandivavian multicenter porous coated anatomic total hip arthroplasty study: Clinical and radiographic results with 7 to 10 year follow-up evaluation. J Arthroplasty 12:133, 1997.

31. Mallory TH, Head WC, Lombardi AV, et al: Clinical and radiographic outcome of a cementless, titanium, plasma spray-coated total hip arthroplasty femoral component: Justification for continuance of use. J Arthroplasty 11:653, 1996.

32. Martini F, Kremling E, Schmidt B, et al: Bone mineral density of the proximal femur after unilateral cementless total hip replacement. International Orthopaedics 23:104, 1999.

33. Morrey BF, Adams RA, Kessler M: A conservative femoral replacement for total hip arthroplasty. A prospective study. J Bone Joint Surg 82B:952, 2000.

34. Morrey BF, Kavanagh BF: Complications with revision of the femoral component of total hip arthroplasty. Comparison between cemented and uncemented techniques. J Arthroplasty 7:71, 1992.

35. Morrey BF: Short stemmed uncemented femoral component for primary hip arthroplasty. Clin Orthop 249:169, 1989.

36. Nelson CL, Walz BH, Gruenwald JM: Resurfacing of only the femoral head for osteonecrosis. Long-term follow-up study. J Arthroplasty 12:736, 1997.

37. Nourbash PS, Paprosky WG: Cementless femoral design concerns: Rationale for extensive porous coating. Clin Orthop 355:189, 1998.

38. Oh D, Harris WH: Proximal strain distributions in the loaded femur. J Bone Joint Surg 60A:75, 1978.

39. Porsch M, Siegel A: Artificial hip replacement in young patients with hip dysplasia—long-term outcome after 10 years. Zeitschr Orthop Ihre Grenzg 136:548, 1998.

40. Poss R, Walker P, Specter M, et al: Strategies for improving fixation of the femoral components in total hip arthroplasty. Clin Orthop 235:181, 1988.

41. Robinson RP, Deysine GR, Green TM: Uncemented total hip arthroplasty using the CLS stem: A titanium alloy implant with a corundum blast finish: Results at a mean of 6 years in a prospective study. J Arthroplasty 11:286, 1996.

42. Russotti GM, Coventry MB, Stauffer RN: Cemented total hip arthroplasty with contemporary techniques: A five year minimum follow-up study. Clin Orthop 235:141, 1988.

43. Schwartz JT Jr, Mayer JG, Engh CA: Femoral fracture during noncemented total hip arthroplasty. J Bone Joint Surg 71A:1135, 1989.

44. Siguier M, Judet T, Siguier T, et al: Preliminary results of partial surface replacement of the femoral head in osteonecrosis. J Arthroplasty 14:45, 1999.

45. Sochart DH, Porter ML: The long-term results of Charnley low-friction arthroplasty in young patients who have congenital dislocation, degenerative osteoarthritis, or rheumatoid arthritis. J Bone Joint Surg 79:1599, 1997.

46. Sporer SM, Callaghan JJ, Olejniczak JP, et al: Hybrid total hip arthroplasty in patients under the age of fifty: A five-to ten-year follow-up. J Arthroplasty 13:485, 1998.

47. Stulberg BN, Singer R, Goldner J, Stulberg J: Uncemented total hip arthroplasty in osteonecrosis. Clin Orthop 334:116, 1997.

48. Tarr RR, Lewis JL, Jaycox D, et al: Effect of materials, stem geometry, and collar calcar contact on stress distribution in the proximal femur with total hip. Trans Orthop Res Soc 4:34, 1979.

49. Tennent TD, Goddard NJ: Current attitudes to total hip replacement in the younger patient: Results of a national survey. Ann R Coll Surg Engl 82:33, 2000.

50. Woolson ST, Maloney WJ: Cementless total hip arthroplasty using a porous-coated prosthesis for bone ingrowth fixation: 3 and one-half-year follow-up. J Arthroplasty 7(Suppl):381, 1992.

52

Arthroplasty for Developmental Hip Dysplasia

• ARLEN D. HANSSEN and MARK W. PAGNANO

Developmental hip dysplasia is among the most common diagnoses leading to reconstructive hip surgery in the young adult. Numerous technologic advances have been introduced for both osteotomy and arthroplasty to treat the pain and arthritis associated with this disorder. In general, the indications for total hip arthroplasty include pain with advanced arthritis, older age, and anatomy not suitable for osteotomy. In patients who are not candidates for osteotomy, total hip arthroplasty often is the definitive treatment, even though these patients may be only in the third or fourth decade of life.

The anatomic distortion associated with developmental hip dysplasia varies considerably, from mild subluxation to complete dislocation of the femoral head with no contact with the true acetabulum.[7,9,10] Although mildly dysplastic hips pose no real or additional difficulty to performance of total hip arthroplasty, the completely dislocated hip represents one of the most formidable procedures for the reconstructive surgeon. Charnley and Feagin believed that total hip arthroplasty should be avoided for patients with congenital hip dislocation.[7] Clearly, total hip arthroplasty in these patients is associated with an increased incidence of complications.[7,9,10,14,16,20,34,49]

CLASSIFICATION

Use of a classification system helps to direct surgical strategies and to compare clinical outcomes within subgroups. Although there is no universally accepted classification system, the most commonly used systems are based on the degree of femoral head subluxation out of the true acetabulum.[10,14,23] Hartofilakidis describes three distinct types. In type 1, or dysplasia, the femoral head remains contained within the true acetabulum.[23,24] In type 2, or low dislocation, the femoral head articulates with the false acetabulum, whose inferior lip contacts or overlaps the superior lip of the true acetabulum. Type 3, or high dislocation, describes a femoral head that has migrated superoposteriorly and has no contact with the true or false acetabulum. Eftekhar defined a four-stage system. In stage A, the acetabulum is slightly dysplastic, with mild femoral head deformity; in stage B, there is an intermediate acetabulum[14]; in stage C, there is a high, false acetabulum; and, in stage D, the femoral head has no contact with the ilium.

The Crowe method of classification appears to be the most commonly used system and is the one we prefer. This system is helpful for purposes of preoperative planning and predicts perioperative complications.[6,39] The severity of dysplasia is determined by measuring the vertical perpendicular distance from a horizontal line drawn through the teardrops to a line drawn at the junction of the femoral head and neck (Fig. 52–1A, **B**). The ratio of this measured distance with the measured pelvic height describes the four distinct types of subluxation out of the acetabular region. In patients with type I subluxation, the femoral head has migrated proximally out of the true acetabular region less than 50 percent; in type II, 50 percent to 74 percent; in type III, 75 percent to 100 percent; and, in type IV, there is complete dislocation (Fig. 52–2).

Although many early reports of total hip arthroplasty for developmental hip dysplasia did not characterize the outcome based on different degrees of dysplasia, more current literature has demonstrated that this delineation is meaningful. The following discussion of surgical approaches, surgical techniques, and results of arthroplasty is based on the Crowe classification.

NATURAL HISTORY

The natural history of developmental hip dysplasia has been outlined well previously.[47,48] Patients with complete dislocation (Crowe IV) often have satisfactory function with good range of motion and surprisingly little pain; this is particularly true with bilateral dislocations.[48] The

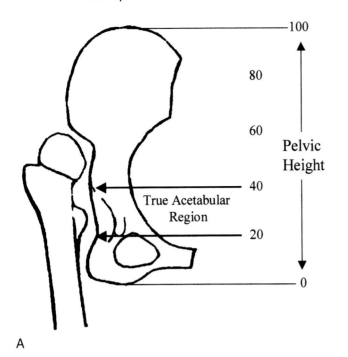

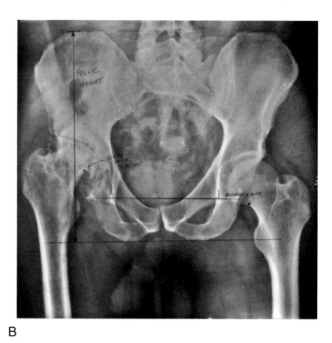

A

B

Figure 52–1. A, The Crowe classification is based on the degree of femoral head subluxation out of the true acetabulum. The vertical height of the true acetabulum is defined as 20 percent of the pelvic height measured from the top of the iliac crest to the ischial tuberosity. The vertical subluxation is measured as the vertical height from the reference line (through the radiographic teardrops) to the femoral head-neck junction. The "degree of subluxation" is then calculated as percent of subluxation = [(amount of vertical subluxation) / (vertical height of the true acetabulum)] ¥ 100. **B,** Anteroposterior pelvic radiograph of a patient with Crowe III developmental hip dysplasia, demonstrating the method of measurement used to determine the severity of the dysplasia.

onset of pain is often delayed until the middle of the fifth decade, and disabling pain is often not present until the seventh decade. The presence of a false acetabulum has predictive value because it portends a poorer prognosis, with earlier onset of clinical symptoms.[48] Patients with unilateral complete dislocation may develop secondary problems such as scoliosis or ipsilateral knee deformity because of limb-length inequality.

Patients with moderate (Crowe II) or severe (Crowe III) dysplasia develop arthritis and clinical disability earlier in life, typically in the third or fourth decade. Once arthritis appears, it tends to progress rapidly, owing to the incongruous contact between the femoral head and the false acetabulum.[9] Patients with mild (Crowe I) dysplasia develop symptoms somewhat later, typically in the fifth or sixth decade (Fig. 52–3).

ANATOMY

A thorough knowledge of the anatomic distortion associated with the different degrees of dysplasia is crucial for planning and performance of the reconstruction (Table 52–1). For a complete description of the anatomic changes of the dysplastic hip, the reader is referred to important early contributions.[7,9,21] Although anatomic variation correlates with dysplasia severity, prior surgical procedures such as pelvic or femoral osteotomy may also cause distortion.

In milder forms of dysplasia, there is bony deficiency of the anterior and posterior segments of the acetabulum as well as a narrow opening and a shallow, sloped socket with deficiency of the superior acetabular segment.[23] In completely dislocated hips, the true acetabulum has a segmental deficiency of the entire acetabular rim, which is hypoplastic, with a soft rhomboid-shaped fossa filled with fibrofatty tissue that is positioned in excessive anteversion. The false acetabulum is formed on the thin bone of the ilium by a thickened joint capsule, and the abductor musculature serves as a roof for the femoral head.

The most commonly acknowledged changes in femoral morphology include a small, deformed femoral head with a short, valgus femoral neck that may be positioned in marked anteversion. The greater trochanter is typically located posteriorly. The femoral canal is straight, with coronal narrowing of the intramedullary canal (so-called femoral stenosis). Anteversion appears to be highly variable and not directly correlated with the severity of the dysplasia.[45] Mildly dysplastic femurs (Crowe I) have anteversion of 12 degrees more than controls, but anteversion of individual cases may exceed 60 degrees. Crowe II, III, and IV femurs have an average anteversion of only 10 to 14 degrees more than normal but with instances of anteversion up to 90 degrees. The increased torsion within the femur occurs in the diaphysis between the lesser trochanter and the isthmus.[45]

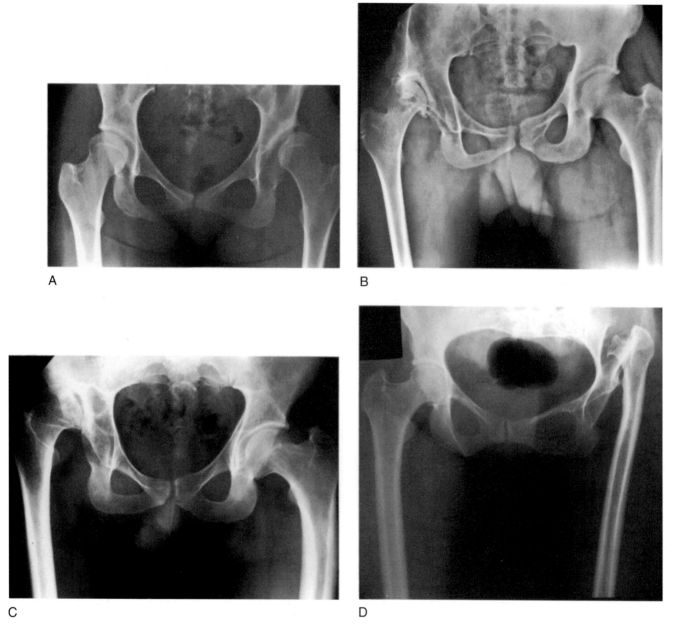

Figure 52–2. Characteristic radiographic findings with dysplasia. **A**, Crowe II hip demonstrating moderate uncovering of the femoral head laterally with well-preserved bone in the true acetabular region and nearly normal proximal femoral anatomy. **B**, Crowe III hip demonstrating significant superolateral bone loss on the acetabular side. Mild changes in the proximal femur can be seen. **C**, Crowe IV hip that has been fashioned with a false acetabulum just above the true acetabular region. The bone in the TAR is well preserved. Narrowing of the proximal femur, particularly in the isthmic portion, is present. **D**, Crowe IV hip demonstrating many of the characteristic changes seen with complete dislocation. A false acetabulum is present high on the ilium; the true acetabulum is shallow and sloping; the femoral head is a shrunken remnant; and there is marked narrowing of the proximal femur.

The soft tissue structures, such as the hip capsule, hamstrings, adductor, and quadriceps muscles, are functionally shortened and make exposure difficult. The abductor muscle mass lies in a horizontal orientation and can be damaged easily. The neurovascular structures are vulnerable to direct and indirect injury during exposure and during limb lengthening. The profunda femoris artery rests at the inferior rim of the acetabulum and is at risk of direct injury. The femoral nerve is vulnerable to traction injury when medial structures are retracted, whereas the sciatic nerve is susceptible when excessive limb lengthening is attempted.

OPERATIVE INDICATIONS

Pain and dysfunction that interfere with the patient's livelihood and ability to sleep and perform activities of daily living have been long-standing indications for total hip arthroplasty in the patient with hip dysplasia.

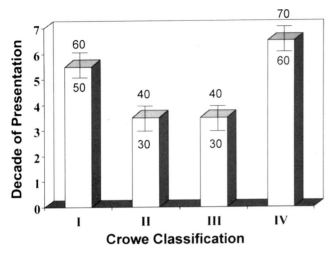

Figure 52–3. The typical ages at which intervention is required as a function of Crowe classification.

Coventry specifically noted that the wish to walk without a waddling gait, the wish to discard a cane or crutches, and the desire to correct limb-length discrepancy were in themselves insufficient indications for total hip arthroplasty.[9] These patients, who are often young with lofty expectations, need to understand that arthroplasty for developmental hip dysplasia has greater association with higher morbidity and inferior outcomes than hip arthroplasties performed for osteoarthritis.

PREOPERATIVE PLANNING

Careful preoperative planning is possibly the most important aspect of total hip arthroplasty for developmental hip dysplasia. Anteroposterior views of the pelvis and hip as well as lateral views of the hip can be supplemented with Judet views to assess acetabular bone stock. In selected situations, a computed tomography scan may be helpful to assess acetabular bone stock and femoral anteversion.[49,51] A vast array of prosthetic options and surgical approaches is required to adequately address the variety of deformities presented at reconstruction. Pelvic tilt, lumbar deformity, hip joint contracture, and limb-length discrepancy should be assessed collectively to determine the desired limb length correction. Assessment should also include the options for a safe and potentially extensile exposure. Previous operations should be appraised as to whether soft tissue dissection will be affected, which will thereby influence the surgical approach or the choice of prosthesis.

In general, it seems logical to address the acetabulum and femur separately based on what type of dysplasia the patient has (Table 52–2). On the acetabular side, preoperative analysis should focus on whether sufficient bone is present to allow placement of the cup in the true acetabulum. The plan should estimate the component size and the need for a bone graft. If more than 30 percent of the cup remains uncovered, consideration must be given to either supplemental bulk acetabular bone graft or to more proximal placement of a smaller acetabular cup. Because small acetabular components are often required, it is also necessary to have 22-mm heads available to ensure that adequate polyetheylene thickness is used.

On the femoral side, the primary problems are anteversion, femoral stenosis, and limb shortening. Radiographs with magnification markers are used to assess the size of the intramedullary canal and the need for shortening with or without rotational osteotomy of the femur. Use of cemented or uncemented fixation is chosen along the usual guidelines of personal preference, bone quality, age, and activity of the patient. A subtrochanteric osteotomy is best performed with an uncemented femoral component. In addition to standard components, the options for prosthesis selection include small straight CDH stems and modular implants that allow intraoperative adjustment of femoral anteversion. Templates are very helpful for determining whether special implants will be required. The use of intraoperative electromyography monitoring has been suggested to monitor sciatic nerve function.[37] All of these considerations are required preoperatively to ensure that the proper equipment is available at the surgical procedure.

SURGICAL APPROACHES

Any standard hip approach may be used in patients who have Crowe I, II, or III dysplasia; however, with Crowe IV hips, a more extensile surgical approach is advisable. The transtrochanteric approach affords excellent acetabular exposure, and trochanteric reattachment facilitates adjustment of abductor tension. The technique of Dunn and Hess[13] facilitates trochanteric reattachment by including a portion of the femoral neck with the trochanteric fragment (Fig. 52–4). Trochanteric reattachment problems can be minimized with use of careful reattachment techniques. The trochanteric slide allows excellent exposure and permits adjustment of abductor tension, and the maintenance of abductor and

Table 52–1. ANATOMIC CHANGES WITH DEVELOPMENTAL HIP DYSPLASIA

Acetabular changes
  Shallow
  Sloping (high acetabular angle)
  Narrow anterior to posterior
  Bone deficiency superolateral and anterior
  Increased acetabular anteversion
Femoral changes
  Proximal femoral hypoplasia (femoral stenosis)
  Posterior attachment of the greater trochanter
  Increased femoral anteversion
  Small, aspherical femoral head
Soft tissue changes
  Elongated, thickened joint capsule
  Abductors "tented" over femoral head
  Iliopsoas, adductors, and rectus femoris contracted
  Sciatic and femoral nerves, femoral and profunda
    vessels shortened

Table 52–2. SURGICAL STRATEGIES FOR DEVELOPMENTAL HIP DYSPLASIA

Acetabulum	Problem	Options	Tips
Crowe I	Anterolateral wall deficiency	Reconstruction at anatomic hip center	Avoid anterior cup overhang (iliopsoas impingement)
Crowe II	Anterolateral wall deficiency Mild superolateral deficiency	Reconstruction at or slightly above anatomic hip center attempting to optimize coverage of socket with native bone	Slight elevation of hip center quite common Bone graft rare
Crowe III	Anterolateral wall deficiency Moderate to severe superolateral deficiency	High hip center with small uncemented cup Anatomic hip center reconstruction beneath large bone graft (less desirable) Custom cups (Oblong) Acetabular reinforcement rings	Slight elevation of hip center quite common Bone graft more common
Crowe IV	Small acetabular fossa with triangular superior shape Osteoporosis	Reconstruction at anatomic hip center with extra small uncemented socket Place cup in psuedoacetabulum (undesirable)	Reverse reaming 22-mm head to increase polyethylene thickness
Femur			
Crowe I	Femoral anteversion Valgus medial femur	Uncemented versus cemented CDH cemented stems Diaphyseal fixation Modular prostheses	Avoid excessive anteversion of uncemented stem
Crowe II	Femoral anteversion Valgus medial femur Increasing femoral stenosis	Uncemented versus cemented CDH cemented stems Diaphyseal fixation Modular prostheses	Avoid excessive anteversion of uncemented stem
Crowe III	Femoral anteversion Valgus medial femur Increased femoral stenosis	Uncemented versus cemented CDH cemented stems Diaphyseal fixation Modular prostheses	Avoid excessive anteversion of uncemented stem Be careful with femoral offset
Crowe IV	Femoral anteversion Femoral stenosis Placement of cup in true acetabulum	Subtrochanteric osteotomy (derotation/shortening) Trochanteric osteotomy Extensile approaches	Careful trochanteric reattachment technique Intraoperative assessment of soft tissue tension with limb lengthening

CDH-congenital dysplasia of the hip.

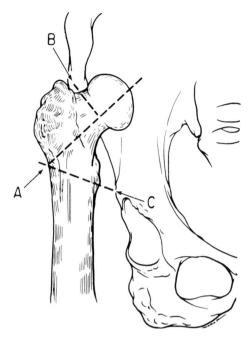

Figure 52–4. Osteotomy of the greater trochanter. Osteotomy along lines A and B allows increased width when the abductor lever arm is re-established. (From Dunn HK, Hess WE: Total hip reconstruction in chronically dislocated hips. J Bone Joint Surg 58A:838–845, 1976.)

vastus lateralis continuity largely prevents trochanteric complications. This approach also allows distal exposure if the decision is made to proceed with a subtrochanteric shortening or derotational osteotomy.

Acetabular Operative Techniques

This portion of the reconstruction is arguably the most important part of the arthroplasty because the ultimate position of the acetabular component often determines many aspects of the femoral reconstruction. The primary objective is to obtain adequate acetabular coverage, and although controversial, placement of the acetabular component within the true acetabular area is ideal because this region frequently has the best available bone stock. Advocates of cemented cups have demonstrated improved durability with modern cementing techniques if the cup is placed within the true acetabular region.[36] Direct placement of a cemented cup in the psuedoacetabulum is associated with a high failure rate.[30] The intermediate results of an uncemented hemispheric cup in either the true acetabular region or in a high hip center position have been excellent.[1,11]

In most patients, careful reaming, with emphasis on medialization into the acetabular fossa, allows placement of a small hemispheric component with adequate cup coverage. Most of these acetabular components are less than 50 mm in diameter. The use of uncemented cups has reduced the need for superolateral structural bone grafting.[1] Several strategies to facilitate placement within the true acetabular region include medialization by perforation of the medial wall, use of a superior

acetabular augmentation such as cement filling or structural bone grafting, or use of reinforcement rings.

Medial Wall Perforation

Deliberate perforation of the medial wall to optimize superior coverage of the acetabular component was originally proposed by Dunn and Hess.[13] This procedure is based on the premise that, biomechanically, medialization is better than superior displacement of the femoral head. This concept has been further popularized by others who have described placement of autogenous graft into the medial defect before cementing a small acetabular component.[23,46] The so-called cotyloplasty procedure has also been reported with the use of an uncemented acetabular component.[37]

The technique of protruding the medial aspect acetabular component beyond the medial wall by controlled reaming has been termed the medial protrusio technique (Fig. 52–5).[12] In general, the amount of medialization required tends to increase as the type of dysplasia worsens.[12] The acetabular reaming remnants used as bone graft in the medial acetabular defect eventually heal and form a new medial wall that can be identified on radiographs. The advantage of this procedure is that the portion of cup covered by the acetabular rim is sufficient to provide intrinsic cup stability and a superior structural graft can be avoided.[12] The theoretical disadvantage of these medialization procedures is that the intentional perforation and associated removal of host bone stock may compromise later revision procedures.

Acetabular Augmentation

Superolateral augmentation needed to provide acceptable acetabular coverage can be done by either filling the defect with cement or with a superolateral structural bone graft. Cement filling of the superior acetabular defect has not produced satisfactory long-term results, and there is a trend toward increased loosening with larger amounts of bulk cement.[33]

Superolateral structural bone grafting can be done with allograft but is done preferably with the patient's own femoral head. These bulk grafts heal reliably to the pelvis. The long-term results achieved with the use of structural bone graft have been variable.[4,5,16,19,22,25,28,31,40–42,44,49] Most of these reported long-term results have been in conjunction with cemented acetabular components (Fig. 52–6). It has not been definitively established that eventual loosening correlates with the amount of initial graft coverage of the acetabular component. Theoretically, uncemented cups may have a better outcome than cemented cups because of better transmission of forces through the graft to the ilium (Fig. 52–7). It is likely that the success of these structural grafts is owed in part to the quality of the initial fixation and the accurate apposition of the graft to the pelvis. The technique described by Barrack and Neumann has been useful in our experience (Fig. 52–8).[3]

Finally, an additional reason for using these structural grafts is to facilitate subsequent revision surgery by

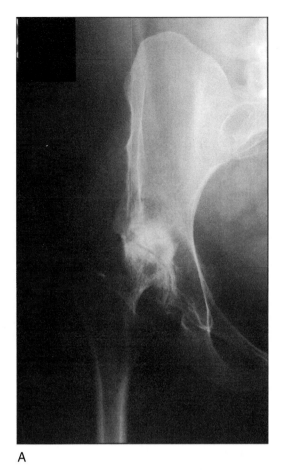

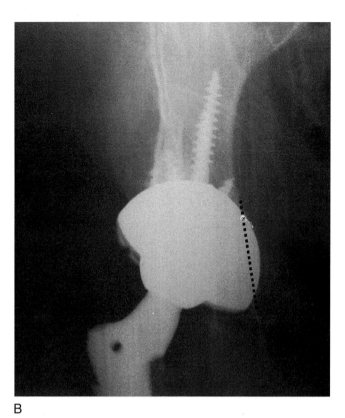

A   B

Figure 52–5. A, Anteroposterior hip radiograph of end-stage arthritis in a patient with Crowe III dysplasia. **B**, Anteroposterior hip radiograph of an uncemented hemispheric cup fixed with multiple screws. The medial protrusio technique facilitated good cup coverage, and the use of superolateral acetabular augmentation with structural bone graft was avoided.

providing additional bone stock.[31] In a small series of patients (who underwent acetabular revision after failure of the cemented components that had been used with superior structural bone graft), the healed bulk graft provided valuable additional bone stock for the support of a revision uncemented acetabular component.[2]

Acetabular Reinforcement Rings

Several reports have emerged concerning the use of acetabular roof-reinforcement rings for developmental hip dysplasia.[17,18] These devices were originally designed to facilitate cup coverage for deficient acetabular bone stock during revision total hip arthroplasty, to restore the anatomic hip center, and to provide adequate fixation for a cemented cup. This technique has been employed especially for Crowe III hips, and the long-term results obtained with these reinforcement rings have been excellent.[17,18] Use of these rings minimizes iatrogenic bone loss and, because the ring and polyethylene cup are inserted independently, the ring can be positioned to maximize host bone contact without regard for version. The polyethylene cup is then cemented in the appropriate position of anteversion. The only

role of cement is in fixation of the cup to the ring, because a risk factor for acetabular component loosening was cement filling of osseous defects.[18] Supplemental bone grafting is indicated when more than 25 percent of the reinforcement ring remains uncovered.

High Hip Center

When it is not feasible to place the acetabular component in the true acetabular region, it is often possible to obtain good apposition of the acetabular component against native bone by superior placement of the cup in a position that is called the high hip center.[1,29] Although the effect of a high hip center on the durability of the arthroplasty remains controversial, there is good evidence for increased rates of femoral and acetabular loosening with initial acetabular cup position outside of the true acetabular region.[38,44] Other authors have argued that isolated superior placement of the cup, without concomitant lateral displacement, is not detrimental to prosthetic component longevity.[33] Most of these poor long-term results are based primarily on the results achieved with cemented cups.[38,44] The use of an uncemented cup with a high hip center has

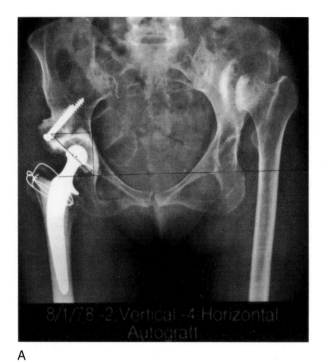

A

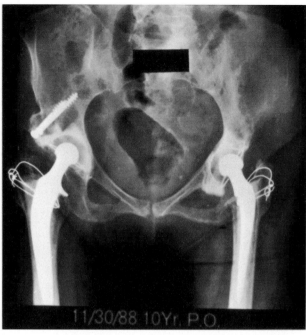

B

Figure 52–6. Total hip arthroplasty with initial cup position within the TAR. **A**, Immediate postoperative radiograph of this 50-year-old woman with Crowe III dysplasia reveals the femoral head center to be within the triangular TAR. **B**, Ten-year follow-up radiographs reveal no evidence of loosening on either the femoral or acetabular sides. We recommend that efforts be made to position the prosthetic femoral head center within the TAR to promote the long-term durability of both the acetabular and femoral components.

been associated with good results as long as there is 75 percent coverage of the cup with native bone and the displacement is superior and not lateral from the true hip center.[1]

In summary, there is still considerable controversy regarding the proper method of acetabular reconstruction. Our current practice is to initially attempt insertion into the true acetabular region of a small, uncemented hemispheric component by means of screw fixation. When more than 30 percent of the cup is uncovered, consideration is given to the use of structural autogenous graft or allograft. Medial protrusion of the cup is occasionally used. A high hip center is considered when elevation of the center of hip rotation will be less than several centimeters. Alternative techniques such as reinforcement rings and the cotyloplasty technique have not been used in our practice.

Femoral Operative Techniques

As previously mentioned, the primary femoral problems are anteversion, stenosis, and limb shortening; also, in many cases, the femoral anatomy requires use of a small, short, straight component. This is particularly true of Crowe IV hips. In most Crowe I and many Crowe II or III hips, the use of small, standard femoral components is sufficient. The decision to use cemented or cementless fixation is primarily based on the usual criteria of personal preference, bone quality, bone geometry,

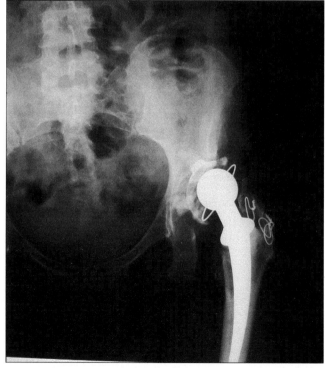

A

Figure 52–7. A, At 10-year follow-up, aseptic loosening of polyethylene cup cemented into the psuedoacetabulum of a Crowe III hip.

Illustration continued on opposite page

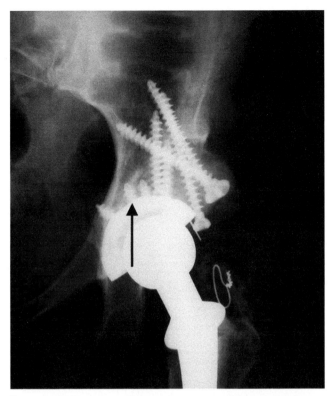

B

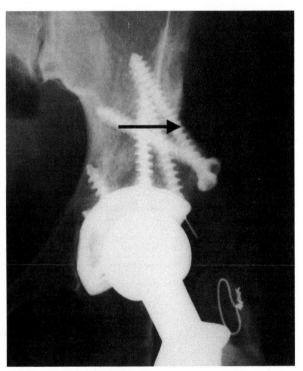

C

Figure 52–7. *Continued.* **B**, Immediate postoperative radiograph of a revision uncemented hemispheric cup with a superolateral structural allograft fixed with screws. The line indicates the junction of host and allograft bone that resulted in approximately 60 percent coverage of the cup with allograft. The femur was not revised, and the small cup and large femoral head required use of a thin polyethylene liner. **C**, Ten-year follow-up radiograph demonstrating excellent incorporation of the bone graft. The lateral aspect of the bone graft has resorbed to the edge of the cup.

and patient age and activity, as well as the need to perform adjunctive procedures such as subtrochanteric osteotomy.

The use of cemented, narrow, straight stem (CDH stems) or custom-made femoral components is much less common than in the past.[50] These implants were most useful in a transtrochanteric approach combined with progressive resection of the proximal femur, which often left a cylindrical femoral tube for placement of the femoral component.[24] The emergence of subtrochanteric osteotomy techniques has decreased the use of this approach. Uncemented femoral fixation can be particularly problematic in the presence of extreme femoral anteversion. A derotational subtrochanteric osteotomy preserves the proximal metaphyseal bone of the femur, and, once anteversion has been corrected, typical monoblock prostheses with proximal fit and fill can be used (Fig. 52–9). Modular proximal fixation prostheses that allow intraoperative adjustment of anteversion are particularly useful (Fig. 52–10**A–C**).[6] A cementless femoral prosthesis with distal fixation allows bypass of the proximal deformity.[43] Cementless femoral components have demonstrated excellent results at intermediate follow-up.[6,26,43]

Subtrochanteric Osteotomy

Particularly when the acetabular component is placed in the true acetabular region, femoral shortening may need to be considered to reduce the risk of sciatic nerve injury. The generally accepted limit of limb lengthening is approximately 4 cm.[20] In addition to progressive resection of the proximal femur, reported techniques of femoral shortening have included transverse, step-cut (Fig. 52–11), double-chevron,[8] and oblique subtrochanteric osteotomies. Femoral osteotomy has become popular because of the dual advantages of shortening as well as femoral derotation. Femoral derotation facilitates preservation and proper orientation of the proximal metaphyseal segment.[52]

The appropriate amount of shortening is determined by careful preoperative planning and then by intraoperatively tailoring. Intraoperative electromyography monitoring should be considered for those cases in which significant lengthening of the limb is necessary. A transverse osteotomy can be used initially. The femur is then derotated and the appropriate orientation and length marked. The rotational stability of the osteotomy site can be significantly enhanced by the use of a step-cut configuration. When a cemented prosthesis is chosen in conjunction with a subtrochanteric osteotomy, it is critical to avoid cement extrusion into the osteotomy site.

Familiarity with a large assortment of femoral prosthetic options is indispensable in dealing with the variety of potential situations that arise when total hip arthroplasty is performed for hip dysplasia. The various facets of femoral reconstruction are not only determined by the variations in femoral anatomy but also by the method of acetabular reconstruction. For example, placement of the acetabular prosthesis in the true

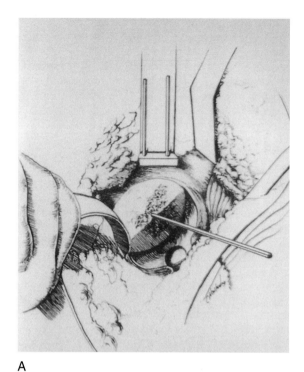

A

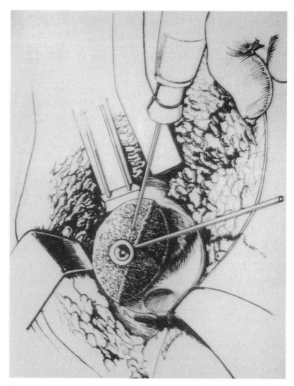

B

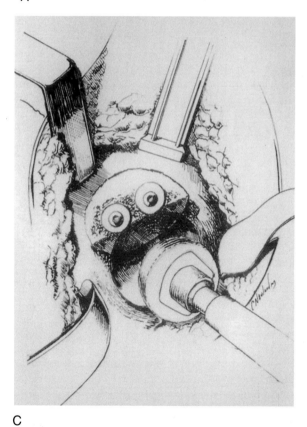

C

Figure 52–8. Bulk femoral head autograft technique. **A,** After initial congruent contouring of the psuedoacetabulum and the femoral head graft, provisional fixation is obtained with Steinmann pins. **B,** Two 6.5-mm AO cancellous screws are placed through the graft in lag screw fashion. **C,** Preparation of the acetabulum proceeds, with simultaneous reverse reaming of the graft and host bone. (From Barrack RL, Newland CC: Uncemented total hip arthroplasty with superior acetabular deficiency. Femoral head autograft technique and early clinical results. J Arthroplasty 5:159, 1990.)

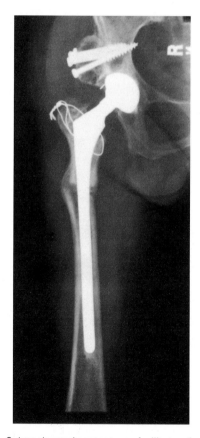

Figure 52–9. Subtrochanteric osteotomy facilitates the use of standard-sized femoral components by preserving the proximal metaphyseal bone. We favor a step-cut osteotomy to improve the rotational stability of the construct.

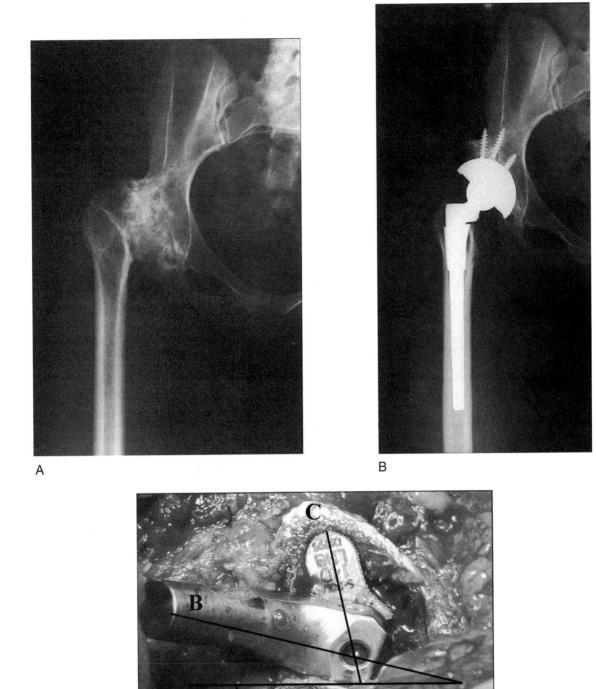

Figure 52–10. **A**, Anteroposterior hip radiograph of end-stage arthritis in a patient with Crowe II dysplasia. **B**, Anteroposterior hip radiograph of an uncemented hip arthroplasty with a modular femoral prosthesis that allows intraoperative adjustment of anteversion. **C**, Intraoperative photograph of femoral component inserted into the proximal femur through a direct lateral approach. Line A represents neutral version, Line B shows the prosthetic neck in 15 degrees of anteversion, and Line C demonstrates that the native femur has 75 degrees of anteversion.

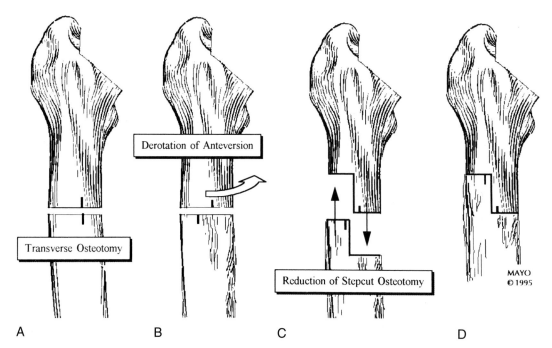

Figure 52–11. Subtrochanteric osteotomy technique. **A,** The initial osteotomy is perpendicular to the long axis of the femur at the subtrochanteric level. **B,** The femur is then derotated to correct the anteversion and the position is marked with an osteotome. **C,** A simultaneous shortening and step-cut osteotomy is then performed. **D,** The femur is reduced in the derotated position and preparation of the femoral canal is then carried out in the standard fashion.

acetabular region may dictate the need for femoral shortening. Likewise, medialization of the cup necessitates increased offset of the femoral component to avoid impingement and to optimize abductor function.

Complications

The usual complications associated with total hip arthroplasty for osteoarthritis are increased in the patient with developmental hip dysplasia.[10,38,44] This is particularly true for patients with complete dislocation.[6] The complications particularly associated with arthroplasty in these patients include nerve palsy,[6,9,16,18,38,44] dislocation,[16,33] and a higher rate of failure.[16,32,38,44] Other complications that are likely to be increased include infection,[36] trochanteric nonunion,[44] and femoral perforation or intraoperative femoral fracture (Table 52–3).[13]

The risk of nerve palsy associated with hip arthroplasty is increased in patients with developmental hip dysplasia.[6,10,15,16,33] The increased incidence of postoperative dislocations is likely owing to trochanteric nonunion or escape, difficulties with acetabular and femoral component position, inadequate femoral offset with a medialized cup, femoral impingement against a pelvis with a high hip center, and the increased surgical dissection required for exposure.

RESULTS

The long-term reported results of total hip arthroplasty for dysplasia are extremely variable owing to a multi-

tude of variables, which include the severity of dysplasia, the wide range of patient age, the method of prosthesis fixation, location of initial cup placement, surgical approach, and length of follow-up. The definitions of failure in most reports vary widely, and most series report survival rates using revision as the endpoint; however, failure rates are significantly higher if failure is defined as definite radiographic loosening or revision.[38] Most of the current surgical techniques with uncemented implants have only short or intermediate follow-up. Patients with Crowe IV dysplasia have a higher incidence of complications and an increased failure rate.[6,35] The reader is referred to the original reports as detailed in Table 52–3, which categorizes some of the variables, such as surgical approach and method of prosthesis fixation. This information enables the reader to evaluate the long-term results in those reports.

AUTHORS' PREFERRED METHOD

Patients with Crowe I dysplasia are treated according to the usual principles of total hip arthroplasty based on assessment of bone quality, patient age, and expected activity levels. Standard anterolateral, direct lateral, or posterior surgical approaches are used for Crowe I, II, and III hips. In Crowe IV hips, transtrochanteric osteotomy still is used occasionally; however, the use of subtrochanteric osteotomy has become more frequent. We prefer an uncemented hemispheric cup placed in the true acetabular region whenever possible but we accept slight elevation of the hip center in Crowe II and III hips if host bone is better maximized in that position. To

Table 52–3. SELECTED SERIES OF TOTAL FOR DEVELOPMENTAL HIP DYSPLASIA

Author	Year	No. of Hips	Prosthesis Fixation	Dysplasia	Approach/Technique	High Hip Center (percent)	FU (yr)	Nerve Palsy (percent)	Dislocation (percent)	Femoral Perforation (percent)	Infection (percent)	Trochanteric Nonunion (percent)	Revisions (percent)
Anderson	1999	24	unc-A both-F	Eftekhar B and C	Transtrochanteric osteotomy; some posterior	38	6.9	4.2	4.2	0	0	5.9	4.2
Cameron	1996	71	unc-A unc-F	Crowe I, II, III, IV	Anterolateral	24	3.5	5.6	1.4		1.4		2.8
Dorr	1999	24	unc-A unc-F	Crowe I, II, III, IV	Anterior Posterolateral Medial Protrusio	0	7						13
Gill	1998	87	Ring-A cem-F	Crowe II, III, IV	Transtrochanteric osteotomy	0	9.4	1.2	2.4	1.2	6.9	3	10
Hartofilakidis	1998	84	cem-A cem-F	Hartofilakidis 2 and 3	Transtrochanteric osteotomy; progressive femoral resection	0	7.1	2.4	5.6	3.6	3.6	1.2	14
Iida	2000	133	cem-A cem-F		Transtrochanteric osteotomy		12.3	0.8	0.8			18.8	7.5
MacKenzie	1996	66	cem-A cem-F	Crowe II, III, IV	Transtrochanteric osteotomy	0	16				3.4		14
Numair	1997	141	cem-A cem-F	Crowe I, II, III, IV	Transtrochanteric osteotomy; some direct lateral			2.1	2.8	0.7			10
Pagnano	1996	145	cem-A cem-F	Crowe II	Transtrochanteric osteotomy, posterior and anterolateral	12.4	14	4.1	0.7	2.1	0.7	1.4	19.3
Stans	1998	90	cem-A cem-F	Crowe III	Transtrochanteric osteotomy, posterior and anterolateral	26	16.6	2.2	2.2	2.2	4.4	8.8	21

cem-cemented; FU-follow-up; unc-uncemented.
Data from references 1, 6, 12, 18, 24, 27, 33, 35, 38, 44.

maximize polyethylene thickness, 22-mm heads are used for cups less than 50 mm in diameter. We try to avoid the use of structural bone grafts if possible and attempt to use medialized cups to achieve this end. A large variety of femoral implants is used currently and includes standard cemented femoral prostheses, proximal cementless modular implants, and cementless implants with diaphyseal fixation.

References

1. Anderson MJ, Harris WH: Total hip arthroplasty with insertion of the acetabular component without cement in hips with total congenital dislocation or marked congenital dysplasia. J Bone Joint Surg Am 81:347–354, 1999.
2. Bal BS, Maurer T, Harris WH: Revision of the acetabular component without cement after a previous acetabular reconstruction with use of a bulk femoral head graft in patients who had congenital dislocation or dysplasia. A follow-up note. J Bone Joint Surg Am 81:1703–1706, 1999.
3. Barrack RL, Newland CC: Uncemented total hip arthroplasty with superior acetabular deficiency. Femoral head autograft technique and early clinical results. J Arthroplasty 5:159, 1990.
4. Becker R, Urbach D, Grasshoff H, Neumann HW: Structural bone grafting in arthroplasty for congenital hip dysplasia: 35 hips followed for 5–10 years. Acta Orthop Scand 70:430–434, 1999.
5. Bobak P, Wroblewski BM, Siney PD, et al: Charnley low-friction arthroplasty with an autograft of the femoral head for developmental dysplasia of the hip. The 10- to 15-year results. J Bone Joint Surg Br 82:508–511, 2000.
6. Cameron HU, Botsford DJ, Park YS: Influence of the Crowe rating on the outcome of total hip arthroplasty in congenital hip dysplasia. J Arthroplasty 11:582–587, 1996.
7. Charnley J, Feagin JA: Low friction arthroplasty in congenital subluxation of the hip. Clin Orthop 91:98–113, 1973.
8. Chareancholvanich K, Becker DA, Gustilo RB: Treatment of congenital dislocated hip by arthroplasty with femoral shortening. Clin Orthop 360:127, 1999.
9. Coventry MB: Total hip arthroplasty in the adult with complete congenital dislocation. In The Hip Society: The Proceedings of the Fourth Open Scientific Meeting of the Hip Society. St. Louis, Mosby, 1976.
10. Crowe JF, Mani VJ, Ranawat CS: Total hip replacement in congenital dislocation and dysplasia of the hip. J Bone Joint Surg 61A:15–23, 1979.
11. Dearborn JT, Harris WH: Acetabular revision after failed total hip arthroplasty in patients with congenital hip dislocation and dysplasia. Results after a mean of 8.6 years. J Bone Joint Surg Am 82:1146–1153, 2000.
12. Dorr LD, Tawakkol S, Moorthy M, et al: Medial protrusio technique for placement of a porous-coated, hemispherical acetabular component without cement in a total hip arthroplasty in patients who have acetabular dysplasia. J Bone Joint Surg Am 81:83–92, 1999.
13. Dunn HK, Hess WE: Total hip reconstruction in chronically dislocated hips. J Bone Joint Surg 58A:838–845, 1976.
14. Eftekhar NS: Principles of Total Hip Arthroplasty. St Louis, CV Mosby, 1978, pp 437–455.
15. Eggli S, Hankemayer S, Müller ME: Nerve palsy after leg lengthening in total replacement arthroplasty for developmental dysplasia of the hip. J Bone Joint Surg Br 81:843–845, 1999.
16. Garvin KL, Bowen MK, Salvati EA, Ranawat CS: Long term results of total hip arthroplasty in congenital dislocation and dysplasia of the hip. A followup note. J Bone Joint Surg 73A:1348–1354, 1991.
17. Gill TJ, Siebenrock K, Oberholzer R, Ganz R: Acetabular reconstruction in developmental dysplasia of the hip: Results of the acetabular reinforcement ring with hook. J Arthroplasty 14:131–137, 1999.
18. Gill TJ, Sledge JB, Müller ME: Total hip arthroplasty with use of an acetabular reinforcement ring in patients who have congenital

19. Gross AE, Catre MG: The use of femoral head autograft shelf reconstruction and cemented acetabular components in the dysplastic hip. Clin Orthop 298:60, 1994.
20. Haddad FS, Masi BA, Garbuz DS, Duncan CP: Primary total hip replacement of the dysplastic hip. J Bone Joint Surg 81A:1462–1482, 1999.
21. Harris WH: Total hip replacement for osteoarthritis secondary to congenital dysplasia or congenital dislocation of the hip. Int Orthop 2:217, 1978.
22. Harris WH, Crothers O, Indong O: Total hip replacement and femoral head bone grafting for severe acetabular deficiency in adults. J Bone Joint Surg 59A:752–759, 1977.
23. Hartofilakidis G, Stamos K, Karachalios T: Congenital hip disease in adults. Classification of acetabular deficiencies and operative treatment with acetabuloplasty combined with total hip arthroplasty. J Bone Joint Surg Am 78:683–692, 1996.
24. Hartofilakidis G, Stamos K, Karachalios T: Treatment of high dislocation of the hip in adults with total hip arthroplasty. Operative technique and long-term clinical results. J Bone Joint Surg Am 80:510–517, 1998.
25. Hasegawa Y, Iwata H, Iwase T, et al: Cementless total hip arthroplasty with autologous bone grafting for hip dysplasia. Clin Orthop 324:179–186, 1996.
26. Huo MH, Zurauskas A, Zatorska LE, Keggi KJ: Cementless total hip replacement in patients with developmental dysplasia of the hip. J South Orthop Assoc 7:171–179, 1998.
27. Iida H, Matsusue Y, Kawanabe K, et al: Cemented total hip arthroplasty with acetabular bone graft for developmental dysplasia. Long-term results and survivorship analysis. J Bone Joint Surg Br 82:176–184, 2000.
28. Inao S, Matsuno T: Cemented total hip arthroplasty with autogenous acetabular bone grafting for hips with developmental dysplasia in adults: The results at a minimum of ten years. J Bone Joint Surg Br 82:375–377, 2000.
29. Jasty M, Anderson MJ, Harris WH: Total hip replacement for developmental dysplasia of the hip. Clin Orthop 311:40–5, 1995.
30. Jensen JS, Retpen JB, Arnoldi CC: Arthroplasty for congenital hip dislocation and dysplasia. Techniques for acetabular reconstruction. Acta Orthop Scand 60:86, 1989.
31. Lee BP, Cabanela ME, Wallrichs SL, Ilstrup DM: Bone-graft augmentation for acetabular deficiencies in total hip arthroplasty. Results of long-term follow-up evaluation. J Arthroplasty 12:503–510, 1997.
32. Linde F, Jensen J, Pilgaard S: Charnley arthroplasty in osteoarthritis secondary to congenital dislocation or subluxation of the hip. Clin Orthop 227:164–171, 1988.
33. MacKenzie JR, Kelly SS, Johnston RC: Total hip replacement for coxarthrosis secondary to congenital dysplasia and dislocation of the hip. Long-term results. J Bone Joint Surg 78A:55–62, 1996.
34. Mulroy RD, Harris WH: Failure of acetabular autogenous grafts in total hip arthroplasty. J Bone Joint Surg 72A:1536–1540, 1990.
35. Numair J, Joshi AB, Murphy JC, et al: Total hip arthroplasty for congenital dysplasia or dislocation of the hip. Survivorship analysis and long-term results. J Bone Joint Surg Am 79:1352–1360, 1997.
36. Okamoto T, Inao S, Gotoh E, Ando M: Primary Charnley total hip arthroplasty for congenital dysplasia: Effect of improved techniques of cementing. J Bone Joint Surg Br 79:83–86, 1997.
37. Paavilainen T, Hoikka V, Solonen KA: Cementless total replacement for severely dysplastic or dislocated hips. J Bone Joint Surg 72B:205, 1990.
38. Pagnano W, Hanssen AD, Lewallen DG, Shaughnessy WJ: The effect of superior placement of the acetabular component on the rate of loosening after total hip arthroplasty. J Bone Joint Surg Am 78:1004–1014, 1996.
39. Ranawat CS, Dorr LD, Inglis AE: Total hip arthroplasty in protrusio acetabuli of rheumatoid arthritis. J Bone Joint Surg 62A:1059–1065, 1980.
40. Ritter MA, Trancik TM: Lateral acetabular bone graft in total hip arthroplasty: A three to eight year followup study without internal fixation. Clin Orthop 193:156, 1985.
41. Rodriguez JA, Huk OL, Pellicci PM, Wilson PD Jr: Autogenous bone grafts from the femoral head for the treatment of acetabular defi-

ciency in primary total hip arthroplasty with cement. Long-term results. J Bone Joint Surg Am 77:1227–1233, 1995.

42. Shinar AA, Harris WH: Bulk structural autogenous grafts and allografts for reconstruction of the acetabulum in total hip arthroplasty. Sixteen-year-average follow-up. J Bone Joint Surg Am 79:159–168, 1997.

43. Silber DA, Engh CA: Cementless total hip arthroplasty with femoral head bone grafting for hip dysplasia. J Arthroplasty 5:231, 1990.

44. Stans AA, Pagnano MW, Shaughnessy WJ, Hanssen AD: Results of total hip arthroplasty for Crowe Type III developmental hip dysplasia. Clin Orthop 348:149–157, 1998.

45. Sugano N, Noble PC, Kamaric E, et al: The morphology of the femur in developmental dysplasia of the hip. J Bone Joint Surg Br 80:711–719, 1998.

46. Symeonides PP, Pournaras J, Petsatodes G, et al: Total hip arthroplasty in neglected congenital dislocation of the hip. Clin Orthop 341:55–61, 1997.

47. Wedge JH, Wasylenko MJ: The natural history of congenital disease of the hip. J Bone Joint Surg 61B:334, 1979.

48. Weinstein SL: Natural history of congenital hip dislocation (CDH) and hip dysplasia. Clin Orthop 225:62, 1987.

49. Wolfgang GL: Femoral head autografting with total hip arthroplasty for lateral acetabular dysplasia: A 12 year experience. Clin Orthop 225:173–185, 1990.

50. Woolson ST, Harris WH: Complex total hip replacement for dysplastic or hypoplastic hips using miniature or microminiature components. J Bone Joint Surg 65A:1099–1108, 1983.

51. Xenakis TA, Gelalis ID, Koukoubis TD, et al: Neglected congenital dislocation of the hip. Role of computed tomography and computer-aided design for total hip arthroplasty. J Arthroplasty 11:893–898, 1996.

52. Zadeh HG, Hua J, Walker PS: Muirhead-Allwood SK Uncemented total hip arthroplasty with subtrochanteric derotational osteotomy for severe femoral anteversion. J Arthroplasty 14:682–688, 1999.

53

The Young Patient: Indications and Results

• GEORGE C. BABIS, BERNARD F. MORREY, and DANIEL J. BERRY

Total hip arthroplasty (THA) has been a remarkably successful operation for treating advanced arthritis of the hip in older patients.[39,56] The high likelihood of pain relief and the excellent restoration of function afforded by this procedure has led this operation to be extended to younger patients, and the short-term clinical results have paralleled the success achieved in older patients. However, as longer term results become available, enthusiasm for the procedure in young patients has been tempered by problems of prosthetic loosening and especially polyethylene wear, and periprosthetic bone loss resulting from osteolysis.

THA failure can be anticipated earlier and more frequently in young patients.[8,15,18,19,21,23,32–34,39,66] Although modern THA serves most older patients well for their lifetime, the increasing expectancy of young patients, now stretching into the eighth and ninth decades, places increased demands on implants. Even in the best-case scenario, many patients younger than 50 years of age may require one or two revision operations in their lifetime. This recognition has led orthopedists to reconsider the alternatives to prosthetic replacement in young patients, including nonoperative treatment, osteotomy, and arthrodesis. Unfortunately, not all patients are candidates, not all are willing to accept any of these alternative treatment methods, and some patients ultimately require prosthetic joint replacement at a young age.

DESIGN OPTIONS

Since the first edition of this book was published, two major changes have occurred that influence the issue of replacement in the young patient: cementless fixation and alternate bearing surfaces.

As reflected by later discussion in this chapter and by information in Chapter 49, a broader selection of increasingly more reliable components designed to be inserted without cement has emerged since the early 1990s. These innovations have provided a more reliable and apparently longer lasting implant, especially in the young patient. This option appears to be further enhanced by hydroxyapatite coating of the stem.[14]

Wear debris, which is particularly problematic in the young patient, may be favorably affected by several material options: cross-linked polyethylene (see Chapter 4), ceramic bearing, and metal-on-metal implants (see Chapter 5).

These innovations have prompted a cautious optimism regarding hip replacement in the patient younger than 60 years of age. However, a reliable solution in those younger than 40 to 50 years of age remains elusive.[37,64]

INDICATIONS

The indications for THA in younger patients are similar to those in older patients: disabling pain and functional deficit caused by advanced arthritis of the hip or advanced hip joint destruction. However, the problems of THA durability in younger patients suggests that criteria for joint replacement should be at least as rigorous as if not more rigorous than those for older patients. Because pain perception and tolerance are not the same for all patients, pain severity should be carefully assessed and always linked to activity. If by modification of activity or other nonoperative means (e.g., ambulatory devices, nonsteroidal anti-inflammatory drugs, weight loss, physiotherapy) pain becomes tolerable, THA can be postponed. Although it is now perhaps less applicable to the older patient population, the "pseudarthrosis test" proposed by Charnley more than 25 years ago[32] continues to be a useful means of determining whether a young patient is a candidate for total hip replacement. The rationale of this test is that even if the patient were to undergo THA and subsequently suffer arthroplasty failure(s) that would preclude further revision and prosthetic reimplantation, would Girdlestone resection arthroplasty cause no worsening of the original preoperative condition?

Three factors—age, anticipated activity level, and availability of acceptable alternatives—are paramount in determining a patient's candidacy for THA. In general, the younger the patient, the more reluctant the orthopedist should be to recommend THA. The surgeon who considers THA when dealing with young patients should at least be familiar with the indications of alternative salvage operations that may alleviate the symptoms and "buy time" for the diseased hip. Postoperative activity level correlates roughly with the number of joints involved by the patient's disease process. Multiple joint involvement is more likely to be an indication for joint arthroplasty at a young age than a single hip joint disease. Patients with bilateral hip disease or co-existent spine, knee, or other lower extremity problems may be less likely to have a satisfactory clinical response to treatment alternatives other than THA.[31] The most frequently encountered diagnoses in young patients that lead to advanced hip joint arthrosis include juvenile rheumatoid arthritis and other polyarticular inflammatory arthritides, developmental dysplasia of the hip, osteonecrosis of the hip, the sequelae of slipped capital femoral epiphysis, Legg-Calvé-Perthes disease, hip trauma, and previous septic arthritis.

PATIENT SELECTION

Even today, there are no ideal candidates for total joint arthroplasty at a young age. However, risk factors for prosthetic failure have been demonstrated that allow classification of patients into two groups with differing postoperative prognoses for prosthetic durability. Patients with a more favorable prognosis include those with multiple joint involvement that limits activity level, patients with bilateral hip disease, patients who are relatively sedentary, and those who are relatively lightweight.[18,19,21,38,46,66] After all, patients with systemic diseases have a shorter life expectancy and their prostheses may sustain for their entire lifetime. Chmell et al.[17] reported a notable mortality rate of 18 percent at an average age of 27.6 years among 39 patients (66 hips) who had undergone because of THA juvenile rheumatoid arthritis. By no means should THA be suggested lightly in this category of patients unless the severity of the symptoms and quality of life demands it.[46] Not surprisingly, unfavorable prognoses are associated with patients who are likely to place high demands on the arthroplasty. Patients with unilateral hip disease without other musculoskeletal problems that limit activity level, patients who must perform heavy labor on a regular basis, and patients who are heavy may also be considered at higher risk for problems with prosthetic durability.[18,19,21,66] Patients who lack the insight to avoid repetitive impact-loading activities or lack the maturity or judgment to understand and abide by the necessary postoperative activity restrictions should also be considered poor candidates for total hip replacement. Patients with severely compromised acetabular or femoral bone stock or compromised abductor muscle function as a result of previous surgery or other disease processes are also less satisfactory candidates for hip arthroplasty. Patients in these groups should be informed frankly that after having a THA they will need to drastically modify their activities. Otherwise they should understand that most likely they will need one or more operations during their life span including the possibility for resection arthroplasty. In the final analysis, the age of the patient remains the most significant factor after long-term survival, with continued difficulty in those younger than 30 to 40 years of age.[26,37] Hence, the decision for THA should be made by a very well-informed patient and not only by the surgeon based on the radiographic appearance of the hip.

TECHNICAL CONSIDERATIONS

The increased demands placed on prostheses in young patients increase the importance of optimizing the technical features of hip arthroplasty in this group of patients. Errors in surgical technique are more likely to manifest themselves as prosthetic failure over the course of time in these patients. Implant selection is also important because high demands magnify the likelihood of prosthetic failure resulting from component loosening, fatigue, or wear.

Careful preoperative planning of the hip arthroplasty is essential. Many of the patients in the younger age group treated with hip arthroplasty have abnormal anatomy of the acetabular or femoral bone. Acetabular bony abnormalities may arise from developmental dysplasia, previous trauma, or previous pelvic osteotomy (Fig. 53–1). On the femoral side, abnormal bone structure may be present as a result of previous surgery (proximal hip osteotomy), previous trauma, or developmental abnormalities.[28,40,48,57,59,63] Patients with juvenile rheumatoid arthritis and patients with developmental dysplasia of the hip may have markedly diminished bone size, requiring special components (Fig. 53–2).[17,36,49,69] By careful preoperative creation of a template, the surgeon can often predict patients who need special prosthetic requirements. Acetabular preoperative templating can frequently identify patients who will require special (such as extra small) prostheses[69] or acetabular bone grafting at the time of surgery.[55] On the femoral side, attention to the size and shape of the femoral canal may identify patients who will need special components. Furthermore, sometimes abnormalities in the femoral canal caused by previous surgery or previous trauma become obvious at the time of templating and allow the surgeon to modify the surgical technique, thereby minimizing the chance of complications when the femoral canal is prepared.

The best method of prosthetic fixation has been debated for both younger and older patients. Since the 1980s, there has been a trend toward the use of uncemented prosthetic components in younger patients.[5,25,39,51] This trend has accelerated as successes have been reported. Long-term information concerning the outcome of cemented component fixation and midterm data concerning the outcome of first-generation uncemented components are now becoming available in this patient population. This information is discussed in more detail later in this chapter. Suffice it to say that high rates of cemented acetabular component failure in young patients have led most

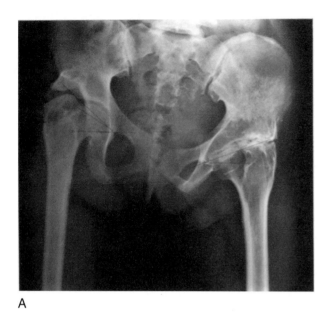
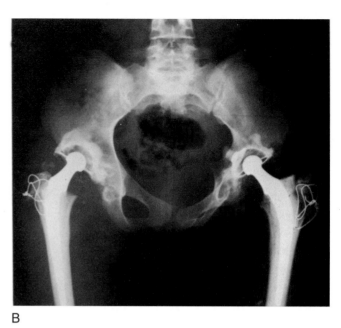

A

B

Figure 53–1. **A**, Failed shelf procedure for bilateral developmental dysplastic hip. **B**, Adequate bone was present for noncustom acetabular and femoral replacement with a good result at 7 years.

surgeons to use uncemented acetabular components in most young patients at the present time.[3,58,63,66] Component fixation with cement has been more successful on the femoral than on the acetabular side, particularly for patients with inflammatory arthritis and multiple joint involvement.[1,8,38,44,47,49,66,68] Good midterm results

have also been reported in selected patients with uncemented femoral implants of specific designs.[45,51] At the present time, justification can be found for using either cemented or uncemented femoral components in young patients. Patients with distorted femoral anatomy, patients with poor bone quality, and patients with

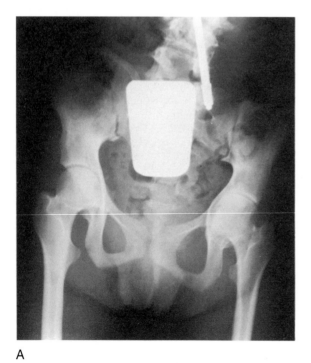
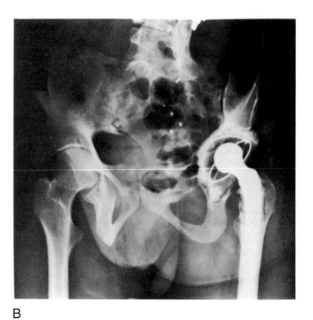

A

B

Figure 53–2. **A**, A 16-year-old dwarf with severe skeletal anomalies, including small femoral canals, valgus coxa magna, and protrusio acetabuli. **B** and **C**, Replacement with a special straight-stemmed implant fit well in the anteroposterior plane (**B**) but violated the posterior cortex on the lateral projection (**C**).

Illustration continued on opposite page

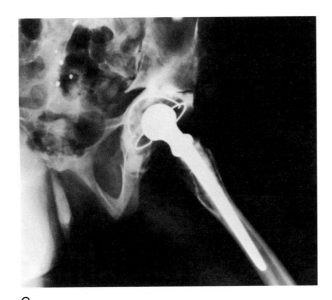

C

Figure 53–2. *Continued.*

systemic diseases that make them less likely to have normally healing bone may have more reliable results from cemented than from uncemented femoral fixation. Patients with excellent bone quality and bony anatomy suitable for good fixation with an uncemented femoral component may be considered for uncemented femoral component fixation. Comparison of the long-term results of modern cement techniques and of more recent uncemented femoral component designs will help guide the choice of femoral prosthetic fixation in the future.

Problems attributable to wear of the bearing surface and formation of particulate debris are particularly troublesome in the young patient population.[4,5,39] If conventional polyethylene is used, efforts should be made to optimize the thickness of the acetabular polyethylene. This provides optimal wear characteristics and reduces the likelihood of catastrophic failure caused by wear-through or polyethylene fracture.[6] For many younger patients, particularly those with smaller sockets and dysplastic hips, a 22-mm head size may be necessary to achieve satisfactory polyethylene thickness.[9] Acetabular components designed to minimize the likelihood of particulate debris formation between the shell and the liner may reduce the amount of polyethylene debris generated.[35] The advantages of using uncemented sockets with screw holes and fixation screws need to be weighed against the potential for providing an avenue for migration of polyethylene debris into the bone of the pelvis. If uncemented femoral components are used, selection of devices with circumferential coating to help provide a "gasket" seal may reduce the risk of distal osteolysis caused by particulate debris produced at the joint-bearing surface.

Advances in polyethylene wear characteristics are promised by the new generation of cross-linked polyethylene acetabular bearings, but their clinical endurance remains to be proved.[53] In addition, alterna-

tives to the routine metal-polyethylene bearing surface are used by some surgeons. Ceramic femoral heads may have improved wear characteristics against polyethylene in vitro, but these potential advantages remain unproved in the clinical setting.[65] Hard-on-hard surfaces, including ceramic-on-ceramic and metal-on-metal articulations, are currently being used in certain centers with promising results.[24,37]

RESULTS

Cemented Total Hip Arthroplasty

Although the short-term clinical results of cemented THA parallel the success achieved in older patients, long-term results have revealed problems with implant durability and fixation. Rates of component loosening and revision for many of the published series of cemented arthroplasty in young patients are summarized chronologically in Table 53–1. Examination of these data allow the following conclusions to be made:

1. Rates of loosening and revision increase with longer follow-up. This is most clearly demonstrated when serial reports of a single series have been published. The short, intermediate, and long-term experience of the Wexham Park Hospital in Slough, England, shows the revision rate increased from 0 percent in an initial report to 25 percent after 11.5 years.[1,67] The consecutive studies of Dorr,[21–23] Collis,[18,19] Halley,[32,33] Klassen,[41,42,66] Johnston,[13,59] and Smith,[58] demonstrate similar increased rates of loosening and revision over time.

2. The younger the patient at the time of THA, the lower the likelihood of long-term prosthetic survival. Studies that incorporate more patients in the 40- to 50-year-old age group report considerably better results than studies limited teenage to patients and those in their 20s, and 30s.[15,17–23] At the Mayo Clinic, Berry et al. assessed the 25-year survival of 2000 patients with primary Charnley THAs, clearly demonstrating the preeminent features of age in survival of both femoral and acetabular components (Figs. 53–3 and 53–4).

3. Implant survival in patients with inflammatory arthritis and multiple joint involvement is better than in patients with other conditions. This finding has been shown by comparing outcomes of THA performed for various diagnoses in individual patient series.[21–23,29,66] It appears that reduced postoperative activity levels outweigh the negative effect of poor bone quality on long-term implant fixation in this group of patients.

4. With longer follow-up, cemented component loosening is definitely more common on the acetabular side than the femoral side of the arthroplasty[12,13, 17,21,43,54,58,64,66] (Fig. 53–5). This finding is more pronounced in series with longer follow-up. Callaghan's[13] review of Johnston's series reported

Table 53-1. PUBLISHED SERIES OF TOTAL HIP ARTHROPLASTY IN YOUNG PATIENTS[a]

Reference (yr)	Cement	No. of Hips	Mean Follow-up yr (range)	Mean Age yr (range)	% Hips w/ Inflammatory Arthritis	Loosening Rate (one or both components)	Acetabular Component Loosening Rate	Femoral Component Loosening Rate	Revision Rate	Acetabular Component Revision Rate	Femoral Component Revision Rate
Halley and Wroblewski[33] (1986)	Y	49	5–15.5	26	17–30	74	16.3	14.3	4	20	18.4	10.2
Witt et al.[68] (1991)	Y	96	11.5	5.3–18.3	16.7	11–26	100	NR	29	21.5	25	22	20
Barrack et al.[3] (1992)	Y	50	12	10–14.8	40.9	18–50	4	46	44	2	22	22	6
Solomon et al.[61] (1992)	Y	130	7.3	3–16	38	10–50	37	19.2	9.2	11.5	10.8	4.6	8.5
Williams and McCullough[67] (1993)	Y	57	4.7	1.7–9	16.4	13.4–24	100	24.6	24.6	7	4	2	2
Sullivan et al.[64] (1994)	Y	89	18	16–22	42	18–49	9	58	50	8	20	13	2
Neumann et al.[54] (1996)	Y	52	17*	15–20.6	51*	34–55	0	6	29	9	10	–	–
Torchia et al.[66] (1996)	Y	63	11	0.3–18.6	17	11–19	32	69.2[†]	67.3[†]	19.2[†]	42.8	38.1	25.4
Chmell et al.[17] (1997)	Y	55	12.8	4–21	19.9	11–29	100 (JRA)	9	9	0	NR	35	18
Sochart and Porter[60] (1997)	Y	43	22.7	0.1–30.3	28.8	19–39	100 (AS)	9.3	9.3	2.3	27.9	25.6	11.3
Sochart and Porter[59] (1997)	Y	226	19.7	2–30	31.7	17–39	44.2 RA, JRA	NR	25	15	NR	27	16
Callaghan et al.[12] (1997)	Y	93	20	1–25	42	18–49	11.8	NR	34	13	22	19	5
Callaghan et al.[12] (1997)	H	45	8.2	5–10	41	26–49	8.9	NR	0	24	18	0	18
Hartofilakidis et al.[34] (1997)	Y	84	16.4	12–24	46	24–55	0	27.4	30.77	20.25	22.6	17.85	21.4
Kobayashi et al.[43] (1997)	CL	66[‡]	14	10–20	37.1	18–50	47.27	32.7	29.1	3.8	20	20	0
Kronick et al.[44] (1997)	H	174	8.3	2–13	37.6	14–50	8	NR	1.4	0.6	8.1	7.5	1.1
Sporrer et al.[62] (1998)	H	45	8.2	5–11	41	25–49	8.9	24.6	0	8.1	18	0	18
Callaghan et al.[13] (1998)	Y	93	23.3	20–25	42	18–49	8.6	23	34.4	12.9	29	15	7.52
Smith et al.[58] (2000)	Y*	47	15.9	0.3–20	41	21–50	NR	NR	55	6	NR	38	19

[a]Series having fewer than 30 hips or less than 5-year mean follow-up were excluded.
[b]Methods used to calculate follow-up intervals were according to the authors and were variable.
[c]Inflammatory arthritis includes juvenile rheumatoid arthritis (JRA), systemic lupus erythematosus, ankylosing spondylitis (AS), dermatomyositis, arthritis of inflammatory bowel disease, and other collagen vascular diseases.
[d]Definitions of loosening were according to the authors and were variable. Rate includes all hips that were considered loose regardless of revision status.
[e]Rate = number of hips revised during follow-up interval/number of hips in series (rates not based on Kaplan-Meier survivorship analysis, except for the series authored by Joshi et al.[32]). Revision defined as removal of one or both components.
[f]NR = information not reported in paper.
Y = both components cemented; H = hybrid, CL = cementless.
*Median.
[†]These percentages are based on the subgroup of 52 hips that had adequate radiographic follow-up.
[‡]Results reported for 55 cups and 53 stems available for 10 to 20 years' follow-up study.
[§]Second-generation cementing technique includes both metal-backed and all-polyethylene cups.

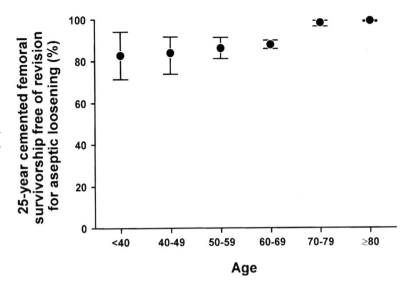

Figure 53–3. Twenty-five year survival free of acetabular revision for aseptic loosening by patient age. (With permission, Mayo Foundation.)

on 93 Charnley THAs performed in young patients. After a mean of 23.3 years of follow-up, there was a 34.4 percent rate of loosening of the acetabular component in 15 percent of those revised compared with 12.9 percent loosening (7.5 percent revised) of the femoral components. Series employing the so-called second-generation cement technique have shown still further improvement in cemented femoral component fixation without a marked improvement in acetabular component performance. Ballard et al.[2] reported on 42 hips in patients younger than 50 years of age followed for a minimum of 10 years. Only 2 femoral components (5 percent) had been revised, but 10 acetabular components (24 percent) had been revised for aseptic loosening. Barrack et al.[3] found similar results in 44 patients younger than 50 years of age who were followed for a mean of 12 years after surgery: No femoral component had been revised for aseptic

loosening and only 1 femoral component was loose; in contrast, 11 hips had been revised for acetabular loosening and 11 more had radiographically loose sockets. Smith et al.[58] reported that over a 20-year span, in 47 cemented THAs performed with use of the second-generation cementing technique, the femoral aseptic loosening was 6 percent, whereas the acetabular component had a loosening rate of 55 percent!

Uncemented Total Hip Arthroplasty

Midterm and long-term results of uncemented prostheses performed in young patients have emerged. Mont et al.[51] reported on 45 hips treated with uncemented porous-coated anatomic (PCA) THAs for noninflammatory arthritis of the hip. Patients were followed for 3 to 7 (mean 4.5) years. The mean preoperative Harris Hip

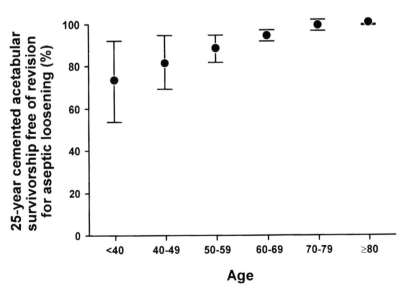

Figure 53–4. Twenty-five year survival free of femur revision for aseptic loosening by patient age. (With permission, Mayo Foundation.)

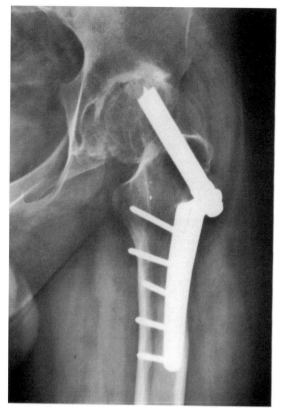

A

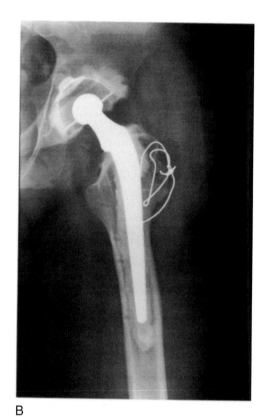

B

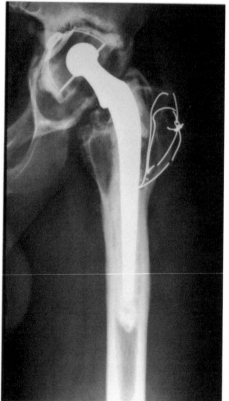

C

Figure 53–5. A, An 18-year-old with degenerative arthritis after treatment of slipped capital femoral epiphysis. **B**, Radiograph immediately after hardware removal and cemented total hip arthroplasty. **C**, Twelve years later, note polyethylene wear and migration of the acetabular component.

Score was 43 points, and the mean postoperative Harris Hip Score was 92 points. Two hips (5 percent) underwent revision, 1 for acetabular loosening and 1 for femoral component loosening.

Radiographically, 2 hips (5 percent) had femoral component loosening and none had definite acetabular loosening. This article did not report on osteolysis, nor did it report on polyethylene wear in this patient population. Kronick et al.[44] reviewed the series of Paprosky and reported on 174 hips in 154 patients younger than 50 years of age (mean 37.6 years) who underwent THA with a cementless acetabular component and an extensive porous-coated femoral stem. Follow-up averaged 8.3 years. Of the 144 porous-coated cups, 5 (3.4 percent) were revised: 3 for wear, 1 for dislocation, and 1 for late loosening as a consequence of osteolysis. Two more cups were found with wear and loosening. Two (1.1 percent) femoral stems were revised, but no other stem was found loose. Fye et al.[29] reported on 72 cementless THAs performed for AVN by a single surgeon. The mean follow-up time was 84 months. Revision rate was 1.5 percent each for the cups and the stems. Femoral osteolysis was observed in 1.5 percent of the hips. Unfortunately, the results of the noncemented THA suffer from the mixture of types of implants used. Conflicting results appear in the literature (i.e., series with no failures in the femoral prosthesis and considerable rates of failure of the acetabular component and vice versa).[50] The Mayo Clinic results with first-generation uncemented devices in young patients also revealed a number of problems and are discussed in the next section. Experience with the short-stemmed device, considered ideal for the younger patient by Morrey, is documented in Chapter 51.

Hybrid Total Hip Arthroplasty

Currently, cemented femoral components have shown good long-term results in young patients, especially with the use of modern cement techniques in young patients.[13,54,58,59] On the other hand, good mid-term results have been accomplished with the use of bony ingrown acetabular components.[62] The hybrid model of fixation seems today to be a reasonable solution.[58] Polyethylene wear and consequent osteolysis remains a considerable risk for all fixation modalities and is a major determining factor for the longevity of THA in the young.[27]

MAYO CLINIC EXPERIENCE

Twenty-five Year Study

A detailed study of 2000 cemented Charnley replacements followed for 25 years allowed Kaplan-Meier survival curves to be calculated for survival of both the femoral and acetabular components in 461 patients. The graphs are self-explanatory in demonstrating the impact of age and survival of the implant (see Figs. 53–3 and 53–4). It is noteworthy that the cemented cup performed much worse than the femoral component in young patients but were equally reliably in the older group.

Adolescent Patients

The frequency of THA performed in adolescent patients at the Mayo Clinic has declined dramatically since 1972. Early enthusiasm for this procedure in very young patients has faded with recognition of increasing failure rates over time. We reviewed 63 cemented THAs placed in 57 patients between 1972 and 1980. Mean age at the time of THA was 17 (range 11 to 19) years. Preoperative diagnoses included juvenile rheumatoid arthritis in 16, developmental dysplasia in 10, slipped capital femoral epiphysis in 8, trauma in 7, tumor in 7, avascular necrosis in 4, spondyloepiphyseal dysplasia in 3, and other miscellaneous diagnoses in 12. So-called first-generation cement technique was used in all patients. Mean follow-up time was 12.6 (range 10 to 18.6) years.

Twenty-seven of the 63 hips had required revision and 2 other hips had symptomatic acetabular component loosening. The probability of prosthetic survival free of revision or symptomatic loosening was 73 percent at 10 years and 55 percent at 15 years. In contrast, the survivorship at 15 years of cemented THA at the Mayo Clinic performed during the same time period in adult patients (mean age 64 years) was significantly better (see Fig. 53–3).

Symptomatic acetabular component loosening was responsible for the majority of failures (76 percent) in our series. The probability of acetabular loosening was three times higher than the probability of femoral loosening after 15 years (see Fig. 53–4). Forty of 52 hips with satisfactory radiographic follow-up had no radiographic signs indicative of any femoral component loosening. Results on the femoral side would have been even better if we had not included 5 cases of stem breakage in the total of 8 hips revised for femoral component aseptic loosening (stem breakage in this group of patients was likely due to the early design, stainless steel femoral components employed).[11,16]

Multivariate survivorship analysis revealed two independent factors associated with a higher probability of THA failure: unilateral arthroplasty ($P = .02$) and history of more than 1 previous hip operation ($P = .0001$). Among the major diagnostic groups, the probability of failure after 10 years was lowest in patients with inflammatory arthritis (11 percent) and highest in patients with previous hip trauma (47 percent) ($P < .05$).

First-Generation Uncemented Total Hip Arthroplasty in Patients Younger than 40 Years of Age

We reviewed all uncemented total hip arthroplasties performed at the Mayo Clinic before 1987 in patients younger than 40 years of age. From 1984 to 1986, a total of 82 uncemented THAs were performed in 72 patients (39 men, 33 women; mean age 32 years; range 17 to 39

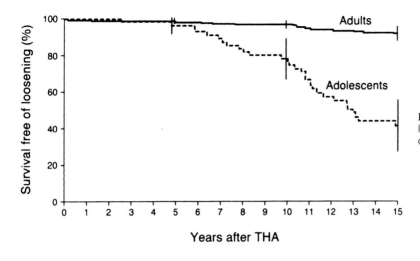

Figure 53–6. Survival free of revision or symptomatic loosening in adolescents versus adults who underwent cemented total hip arthroplasty at the Mayo Clinic.

years). The median follow-up was 10.3 (range 10 to 14) years after arthroplasty. Diagnoses leading to THA were developmental dysplasia in 26, inflammatory arthritis in 15, osteonecrosis in 16, post-traumatic osteoarthritis in 13, and other in 2. The acetabular implant placed was PCA in 39, Harris-Galante HGPI in 22, and Osteonics Dual Geometry in 21. The femoral implant placed was PCA in 39, HGP in 21, Osteonics 19.

Aseptic failure requiring component revision occurred in 24 of the 82 hips (29.3 percent). Twenty-two revisions were for aseptic failure: either aseptic loosening or osteolysis. A total of 17 acetabular components were revised for aseptic failure, 11 for loosening and 6 for osteolysis (Fig. 53–6). Femoral revision was done for loosening in 8 patients, severe osteolysis in 2 patients, and thigh pain without loosening in 10 patients: 10 for aseptic loosening and 3 for osteolysis.

Among patients with surviving prostheses, the Harris Hip Score improved from a mean of 51 preoperatively to 92 postoperatively.

Radiographs demonstrated 13 unrevised hips also had failed. There were 7 failed acetabular components and 7 failed femoral components. Five acetabular components failed radiographically due to marked osteolysis and 2 due to loosening. Four of the femoral components failed due to loosening and 3 due to lysis.

We concluded from this study that uncemented THA provided dramatic pain relief and improvement in function in the majority of our patients (Fig. 53–7). There were, however, major problems with implant durability. The most common reasons for failure were implant loosening and osteolysis. However, the rate of failure—mostly resulting from the related problems of polyethylene liner wear and osteolysis and the problem of femoral component loosening—were of significant concern. These results represent the early experience of a number of surgeons with first-generation implants. Improved techniques, implants, and materials will probably lead to better long-term results in the future than we found in this series of patients.[50] Uncemented THA, like cemented THA, should not yet be considered a complete long-term solution to advanced arthritis of the hip in young active patients. When possible, alternatives to THA in this patient population should still be explored.[7,10,30]

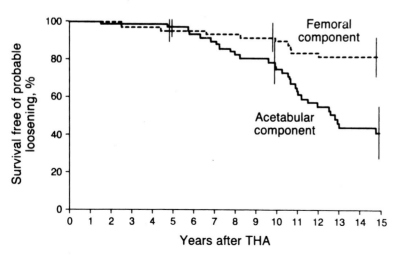

Figure 53–7. Survival free of radiographic component loosening in adolescents who underwent cemented total hip arthroplasty at the Mayo Clinic.

AUTHORS' PREFERENCE

Total hip arthroplasty is recommended reluctantly to young patients only after nonoperative treatment has failed and management with femoral or pelvic osteotomy is not possible. A few patients are candidates for—and willing to accept—hip arthrodesis (see Chapters 51 and 53). Patients with high activity demands, heavy weight, and very young age are poor candidates for THA, whereas patients with multiple joint problems and low activity demands are considered better but still not ideal candidates. Before surgery, the long-term implications of a THA at a young age and the probable need for revision(s) in the future are discussed carefully and candidly with the patient, who is thoroughly informed and then asked to make the final decision.

When THA is performed in young patients, uncemented porous-coated sockets are used in almost all cases (Fig. 53–8). On the femoral side, the type of component fixation is individualized. Patients with good bone quality, bone geometry favorable for use of uncemented components, no biologic factors to retard bone healing, and a long life expectancy are usually treated with uncemented components. In most cases, proximally porous-coated or proximally hydroxyapatite-coated components are currently used at our institution. In some patients with abnormal anatomy, extensively porous-coated stems are used because of their high likelihood of bone ingrowth. The major disadvantage of extensively coated stems is the long-term risks of stress-shielding. A conservative femoral replacement that was designed mainly to avoid stress-shielding, to provide constructive proximal femoral remodeling, and to ensure ease at revision has shown favorable results.[52] Cemented stems are selected for patients with poor bone quality, significant femoral deformity, adverse biologic circumstances for osteointegration, or reduced life expectancy. The best possible cement technique is used, which includes placement of a restriction plug, meticulous canal preparation, cement porosity reduction, retrograde cement filling, and cement pressurization.

Yet, because polyethylene wear is inversely related to age, we have no solution for the acetabular component in this patient group (Fig. 53–8). Specific efforts are made on both sides of the arthroplasty to reduce the likelihood of significant polyethylene wear. Femoral head size is chosen to provide a minimum thickness of 6 to 8 mm (more, if possible) for the polyethylene socket liner. Highly polished cobalt-chromium heads or ceramic femoral heads are used in the hope that they may reduce polyethylene wear (Fig. 53–9). Newer cross-linked polyethylene as well as metal-on-metal or ceramic-on-ceramic bearings should be clinically explored and, if they are successful, they should be used to minimize wear and subsequent osteolysis. Careful instruction regarding appropriate activity after hip arthroplasty is given to all patients. Regularly scheduled clinical follow-up and radiographic follow-up are essential to identify the problems of polyethylene wear, osteolysis, component loosening, and periprosthetic bone loss.

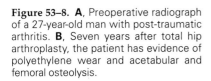

Figure 53–8. A, Preoperative radiograph of a 27-year-old man with post-traumatic arthritis. **B,** Seven years after total hip arthroplasty, the patient has evidence of polyethylene wear and acetabular and femoral osteolysis.

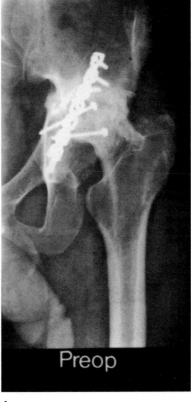

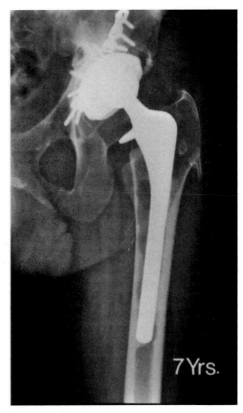

A   B

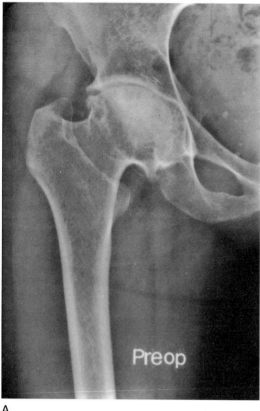

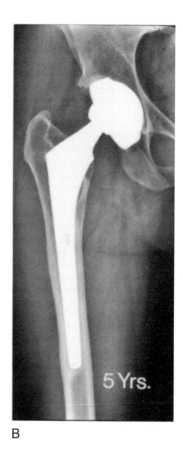

Figure 53–9. **A**, Preoperative radiograph of a 36-year-old woman with hip arthritis. **B**, Five years after total hip arthroplasty, a good clinical and radiographic result.

A

B

References

1. Arden GP, Ansell BM, Hunter MJ: Total hip replacement in juvenile chronic polyarthritis and ankylosing spondylitis. Clin Orthop 84:130, 1972.
2. Ballard WT, Callaghan JJ, Sullivan PM, Johnston RC: The results of improved cementing techniques for total hip arthroplasty in patients less than fifty years old. J Bone Joint Surg 76A:959, 1994.
3. Barrack RL, Mulroy RD Jr, Harris WH: Improved cementing techniques and femoral component loosening in young patients with hip arthroplasty: A 12-year radiographic review. J Bone Joint Surg 74B:385, 1992.
4. Berger RA, Jacobs JJ, Quigley LR, et al: Primary cementless acetabular reconstruction in patients younger than 50 years old. Clin Orthop 344:216, 1997.
5. Berry DJ, Harmsen WS, Cabanela ME, Morrey BF: 25 year survivorship of 2000 consecutive primary Charnley total hip arthroplasties. Factors affecting acetabular and femoral component survivorship. J Bone Joint Surg 84A:171, 2002.
6. Berry DJ, Scott R, Cabanela ME, et al: Catastrophic acetabular component polyethylene failure in total hip arthroplasty. J Bone Joint Surg 76B:575, 1994.
7. Cabanela ME: The painful young adult hip: Surgical alternatives. Perspect Orthop Surg 1:1, 1990.
8. Cage DJN, Granberry WM, Tullos HS: Long-term results of total arthroplasty in adolescents with debilitating polyarthropathy. Clin Orthop 283:156, 1992.
9. Callaghan JJ: Results of primary total hip arthroplasty in young patients. J Bone Joint Surg 75A:1728, 1993.
10. Callaghan JJ, Brand RA, Pedersen DR: Hip arthrodesis: A long-term follow-up. J Bone Joint Surg 67A:1328, 1985.
11. Callaghan JJ, Pellicci PM, Salvati EA, et al: Fracture of the femoral component: Analysis of failure and long-term follow-up of revision. Orthop Clin North Am 19:637, 1988.
12. Callaghan JJ, Forest EE, Sporer SM, et al: Total hip arthroplasty in the young adult. Clin Orthop 344:257, 1997.
13. Callaghan JJ, Forest EE, Olejniczak JP, et al: Charnley total hip arthroplasty in patients less than fifty years old. A twenty to twenty-five-year follow-up note. J Bone Joint Surg 80A:704, 1998.
14. Capello WN, D'Antonio JA, Feinberg JR, Manley MT: Hydroxyapatite-coated total hip femoral components in patients less than fifty years old. Clinical and radiographic results after five to eight years of follow-up. J Bone Joint Surg 79A:1023, 1997.
15. Chandler HP, Reineck FT, Wixson RL, McCarthy JC: Total hip replacement in patients younger than thirty years old. J Bone Joint Surg 63A:1426, 1981.
16. Chao EYS, Coventry MB: Fracture of the femoral component after total hip replacement. J Bone Joint Surg 63A:1078, 1981.
17. Chmell MJ, Scott RD, Thomas WH, Sledge CB: Total hip arthroplasty with cement for juvenile rheumatoid arthritis. Results at a minimum of ten years in patients less than thirty years old. J Bone Joint Surg 79A:44, 1997.
18. Collis DK: Cemented total hip arthroplasty in patients who are less than fifty years old. J Bone Joint Surg 66A:353, 1984.
19. Collis DK: Long-term (twelve to eighteen year) follow-up of cemented total hip in patients who were less than fifty years old: A follow-up note. J Bone Joint Surg 73A:593, 1991.
20. Cornell CN, Ranawat CS: Survivorship analysis of total hip replacements: Results in a series of active patients who were less than fifty-five years old. J Bone Joint Surg 68A:1430, 1986.
21. Dorr LD, Kane TJ III, Conaty JP: Long-term results of cemented total hip arthroplasty in patients 45 years old or younger. J Arthroplasty 9:453, 1994.
22. Dorr LD, Luckett M, Contay JP: Total hip arthroplasties in patients younger than 45 years: A nine-to ten-year follow-up study. Clin Orthop 260:215, 1990.
23. Dorr LD, Takei GK, Conaty JP: Total hip arthroplasties in patients less than forty-five years old. J Bone Joint Surg 65A:474, 1983.
24. Dorr LD, Wan Z, Longjohn DB, et al: Total hip arthroplasty with use of the Metasul metal-on-metal articulation. Four to seven-year results. J Bone Joint Surg 82A:789, 2000.
25. Dowdy PA, Rorabeck CH, Bourne RB: Uncemented total hip arthroplasty in patients 50 years of age or younger. J Arthroplasty 12:853, 1997.
26. Duffy GP, Berry DJ, Rowland C, Cabanela ME: Primary uncemented total hip arthroplasty in patients younger than 40 years old: 10–14 year results using first generation proximally porous coated implants. J Arthroplasty 16(Suppl1):140, 2001.

27. Dunkley AB, Eldridge JD, Lee MB, et al: Cementless acetabular replacement in the young. A 5-to 10-year prospective study. Clin Orthop 376:149, 2000.

28. Ferguson GM, Cabanela ME, Ilstrup DM: Total hip arthroplasty after failed intertrochanteric osteotomy. J Bone Joint Surg 76B:252, 1994.

29. Fye MA, Huo MH, Zatorski LE, Keggi KJ: Total hip arthroplasty performed without cement in patients with femoral head osteonecrosis who are less than 50 years old. J Arthroplasty 13:876, 1998.

30. Ganz RH, Klaue K, Vinh TS, Mast JW: A new periacetabular osteotomy for the treatment of hip dysplasias: Technique and preliminary results. Clin Orthop 232:26, 1988.

31. Greiss ME, Thomas RJ, Freeman MAR: Sequelae of arthrodesis of the hip. J R Soc Med 73:497, 1980.

32. Halley DK, Charnley J: Results of low-friction arthroplasty in patients thirty years of age or younger. Clin Orthop 112:180, 1975.

33. Halley DK, Wroblewski BM: Long-term results of low-friction arthroplasty in patients thirty years of age or younger. Clin Orthop 211:43, 1986.

34. Hartofilakidis G, Karachalios T, Zacharakis N: Charnley low friction arthroplasty in young patients with osteoarthritis. A 12- to 24-year clinical and radiographic study of 84 cases. Clin Orthop 341:51, 1997.

35. Huk OL, Bansal M, Betts F, et al: Polyethylene and metal debris generated by non-articulating surfaces of modular acetabular components. J Bone Joint Surg 76B:568-574, 1994.

36. Huo MH, Salvati EA, Lieberman JR, et al: Custom-designed femoral prostheses in total hip arthroplasty done with cement for severe dysplasia of the hip. J Bone Joint Surg 75A:1497, 1993.

37. Hyder N, Nevelos AB, Barabas TG: Cementless ceramic hip arthroplasties in patients less than 30 years old. J Arthroplasty 11:679, 1996.

38. Joshi AB, Porter ML, Trail IA, et al: Long-term results of Charnley low-friction arthroplasty in young patients. J Bone Joint Surg 75B:616, 1993.

39. Kavanaugh BF, DeWitz MA, Currier BL, et al: Charnley low friction arthroplasty of the hip: Twenty year results with cement. J Arthroplasty 9:229, 1994.

40. Kilgus DJ, Amstutz HC, Wolgin MA, Dorey FJ: Joint replacement for ankylosed hips. J Bone Joint Surg 72A:45, 1990.

41. Klassen RA, Bianco AJ: The young patient. In Morrey BF (ed): Joint Replacement Arthroplasty. New York, Churchill Livingstone, 1991, p 673.

42. Klassen RA, Parlasca RJ, Bianco AJ: Total joint arthroplasty: Applications in children and adolescents. Mayo Clin Proc 54:579, 1979.

43. Kobayashi S, Eftekhar NS, Terayama K, Joshi RP: Comparative study of total hip arthroplasty between younger and older patients. Clin Orthop 339:140, 1997.

44. Kronick JL, Barba ML, Paprosky WG: Extensively coated femoral components in young patients. Clin Orthop 344:263, 1997.

45. Kumar MN, Swann M: Uncemented total hip arthroplasty in young patients with juvenile chronic arthritis. Ann R Coll Surg Engl 80:203, 1998.

46. Lachiewicz PF, McCaskill B, Inglis A, et al: Total hip arthroplasty in juvenile rheumatoid arthritis. J Bone Joint Surg 68A:502, 1986.

47. Lehtimaki MY, Lehto MU, Kautiainen H, et al: Survivorship of the Charnley total hip arthroplasty in juvenile chronic arthritis. A follow-up of 186 cases for 22 years. J Bone Joint Surg 79B:792, 1997.

48. Lubahn JD, Evarts CM, Feltner JB: Conversion of ankylosed hips to total hip arthroplasty. Clin Orthop 153:146, 1980.

49. Maric Z, Haynes RJ: Total hip arthroplasty in juvenile rheumatoid arthritis. Clin Orthop 290:197, 1993.

50. McLaughlin JR, Lee KR: Total hip arthroplasty in young patients. 8- to 13-year results using an uncemented stem. Clin Orthop 373:153, 2000.

51. Mont MA, Maar DC, Krackow KA, et al: Total hip replacement without cement for non-inflammatory osteoarthrosis in patients who are less than forty-five years old. J Bone Joint Surg 75A:740, 1993.

52. Morrey BF, Adams RA, Kessler M: A conservative femoral replacement for total hip arthroplasty. A prospective study. J Bone Joint Surg 82B:952, 2000.

53. Muratoglu OK, Bragdon CR, O'Connor DO, et al: Unified wear model for highly crosslinked ultra-high molecular weight polyethylenes (UHMWPE). Biomaterials 20:1463, 1999.

54. Neumann L, Freund KG, Sørensen KH: Total hip arthroplasty with the Charnley prosthesis in patients fifty-five years old and less. Fifteen to twenty-one year results. J Bone Joint Surg 78A:73, 1996.

55. Ranawat CS, Dorr LD, Inglis AE: Total hip arthroplasty in protrusio acetabuli of rheumatoid arthritis. J Bone Joint Surg 62A:1059, 1980.

56. Schulte KR, Callaghan JJ, Kelley SS, Johnston RC: The outcome of Charnley total hip arthroplasty with cement after a minimum twenty-year follow-up. J Bone Joint Surg 75A:961, 1993.

57. Shinar AA, Harris WH: Cemented total hip arthroplasty following previous femoral osteotomy: An average 16-year follow-up study. J Arthroplasty 13:243, 1998.

58. Smith SE, Estok DM, Harris WH: 20-year experience with cemented primary and conversion total hip arthroplasty using so-called second-generation cementing techniques in patients aged 50 years or younger. J Arthroplasty 15:263, 2000.

59. Sochart DH, Porter ML: The long-term results of Charnley low-friction arthroplasty in young patients who have congenital dislocation, degenerative osteoarthrosis, or rheumatoid arthritis. J Bone Joint Surg 79A:1599, 1997.

60. Sochart DH, Porter ML: Long-term results of total hip replacement in young patients who had ankylosing spondylitis. J Bone Joint Surg 79A:1181, 1997.

61. Solomon MI, Dall DM, Learmonth ID, Davenport JM: Survivorship of cemented total hip arthroplasty in patients 50 years of age or younger. J Arthroplasty 7(Suppl):347, 1992.

62. Sporer SM, Callaghan JJ, Olejniczak JP, et al: Hybrid total hip arthroplasty in patients under the age of fifty: A five- to ten-year follow-up. J Arthroplasty 13:485, 1998.

63. Strathy GM, Fitzgerald RH Jr: Total hip arthroplasty in the ankylosed hip. J Bone Joint Surg 70A:963, 1988.

64. Sullivan PM, MacKenzie JR, Callaghan JJ, Johnston RC: Total hip arthroplasty with cement in patients who are less than fifty years old. A sixteen to twenty-two year follow-up study. J Bone Joint Surg 76A:863, 1994.

65. Sychterz CJ, Engh CA Jr, Young AM, et al: Comparison of in vivo wear between polyethylene liners articulating with ceramic and cobalt-chrome femoral heads. J Bone Joint Surg 82B:948, 2000.

66. Torchia ME, Klassen RA, Bianco AJ: Total hip arthroplasty with cement in patients younger than twenty years: Long-term results. J Bone Joint Surg 78A:995, 1996.

67. Williams WW, McCullough CJ: Results of cemented total hip replacement in juvenile chronic arthritis: A radiological review. J Bone Joint Surg 75B:872, 1993.

68. Witt JD, Swann M, Ansell B: Total hip replacement for juvenile chronic arthritis. J Bone Joint Surg 73B:770, 1991.

69. Woolson ST, Harris WH: Complex total hip replacement for dysplastic or hypoplastic hips using miniature or microminiature components. J Bone Joint Surg 65A:1099, 1983.

54

Proximal Femoral Deformity

•PANAYIOTIS J. PAPAGELOPOULOS and MIGUEL E. CABANELA

Proximal femoral anatomy may be distorted as a result of developmental problems (e.g., developmental hip dysplasia, congenital coxa vara), or secondary, after previous surgical intervention, (e.g., intertrochanteric or subtrochanteric osteotomy or failed total hip arthroplasty). Other, less common situations producing deformity of the proximal femur include cases of malunion or nonunion of proximal femoral fractures, Paget's disease of the femur, and femoral fibrous dysplasia.[23] Each circumstance creates technical difficulties in the performance of a primary or revision total hip arthroplasty.

In addition to the etiologic classification of deformity, Berry[2a] proposes an anatomic classification based on the deformity site: greater trochanter, femoral neck, metaphyseal level, and diaphyseal level. Further categorization can be established by the geometry of the deformity: angular, rotational or translational, abnormal bone size, or a combination of these.

When hip replacement in a patient with proximal femoral deformity is planned, three surgical choices are possible: (1) If the deformity is very proximal, it can simply be *eliminated*; (2) if the deformity is not very severe, the surgeon may be able to *adapt* the procedure to the altered anatomy by modifying the technique or the implant; (3) if the deformity is so significant that the surgeon needs to *correct* it, either simultaneously with the arthroplasty (the most common event) or as a preliminary step before arthroplasty (seldom advisable). Careful preoperative planning helps predict which of these choices may be best suited to situation. Access to a wide range of implants helps the surgeon treat unique femoral geometries. Implants fixed in the diaphysis allow some proximal femoral deformities to be bypassed. Modular or custom implants simplify treatment of certain deformities. If concomitant osteotomy to effect deformity correction is necessary, the requisites of maintaining the blood supply of the bony fragments, achieving satisfactory fixation of the osteotomy (using the implant and/or adjunctive fixation), and obtaining implant stability must be met.

In this chapter, the most frequent causes of proximal femoral deformity are addressed, and the specific needs and techniques applicable to each situation are presented.

DEVELOPMENTAL DISEASE OF THE HIP (DDH)

As far as the proximal femur is concerned, two possibilities exist, depending on whether there has been previous surgery in this area or not.

DDH Without Previous Surgery

There are two main technical problems associated with hip joint replacement in severely dysplastic or dislocated hips. The first involves the proximal femur, which typically shows anteversion exceeding 20 to 30 degrees. If cemented replacement is chosen, a small femoral component is used to reduce the anteversion to a more physiologic level. The void left in the anterior metaphyseal area is filled with cement. However, cement fixation of the femoral component carries a significant incidence of symptomatic mechanical failure in dysplastic hips of young persons with a high level of physical activity.[13,18] This has led most surgeons to use cementless femoral components in these young patients.[5,11,28] However, using a cementless metaphyseal-filling femoral component may result in the insertion of an implant with an unacceptable degree of anteversion that could compromise joint stability; if a smaller cementless metaphyseal-filling component is used to counter the increased anteversion, prosthetic fixation may be compromised. Often distally fixed cementless components with a modified narrower proximal geometry or modular components allow the surgeon to "cheat" the anatomy and provide reliable uncemented fixation.

An additional problem is the positioning of the acetabular component, which must be seated near the anatomic center of rotation of the hip to obtain reliable fixation and to achieve the abductor strength necessary to balance the pelvis.[15] Especially in hips with high dislocation, shortening procedures of the femur are valuable to bring the prosthesis head low enough for reduction.[14,15,20,21] In these complex cases, a reasonable alternative is the use of a proximal femoral subtrochanteric osteotomy combined with distal advancement of the greater trochanter or segmental metaphyseal shortening osteoplasty,[20,21,23] as described in the next section.

DDH with Previous Femoral Osteotomy

Technical problems outlined in the preceding section are significantly worse if the proximal femoral anatomy has been altered by previous osteotomy, the most common being the subtrochanteric Schanz osteotomy.

Mayo Clinic Experience

In a group of 84 patients with DDH and a previous femoral subtrochanteric osteotomy who were operated on between 1969 and 1982, clinical follow-up and radiologic follow-up were obtained in 73 (83 percent) after a mean follow-up of 8.8 years. The operative time, blood loss, and mean hospital stay were somewhat elevated by comparison with these factors in routine total hip arthroplasty. Technical difficulties occurred at the time of exposure of the hip in 63 percent and during preparation of the femoral canal in 60 percent. Osteotomy hardware was removed before surgery in 33.3 percent and at the time of total hip arthroplasty in 62.2 percent; this was difficult in 23.3 percent and hardware breakage occurred during removal in 14.4 percent. Special femoral implants, such as the Charnley straight stem or double-curved stem, were necessary more than half the time. Improvement was generally quite satisfactory (hip score[19] improved from 35 in 80 preoperatively to 77 in 100 at follow-up); however, 39.7 percent of the patients either had revision surgery or experienced disabling pain in the follow-up interval. There were 20 revisions, 5 hips with definite radiographic loosening, and 4 patients with unexplained pain. Stem and socket failure occurred with similar frequency. Of specific interest was the finding that, if the hardware was removed at the time of total hip arthroplasty, the radiographic appearance of the stem was much worse. The revision rate in this study was larger than that reported by Stans et al.[29] in 100 total hip arthroplasties performed in patients with DDH without previous osteotomy. It was thought that this difference was related to the previous femoral osteotomy, particularly if the osteotomy hardware was not removed until the time of total hip arthroplasty. The conclusion from this study was that subtrochanteric femoral osteotomy should be used cautiously, if at all, in the management of arthritis secondary to DDH.

Authors' Preference

If the proximal femoral anatomy is significantly altered by a previous osteotomy, a canal realignment procedure, accompanied, if necessary, by shortening should be done concomitantly with the replacement. This tech-

nique is described later and provides predictable results when combined with the use of cementless femoral stems (Fig. 54–1). Because the diameter of the femoral canal is frequently very narrow in patients with DDH, special stems may sometimes be necessary.

PREVIOUS INTERTROCHANTERIC OSTEOTOMY

Intertrochanteric femoral osteotomy can cause significant deformity in the metaphyseal area of the femur. It is logical to expect that conversion to hip replacement may be more difficult and, therefore, one should expect more perioperative complications and also an effect on the quality of long-term results. Whether cortical defects occasioned by screw removal cause prosthetic loosening is uncertain, but seem these defects to be implicated in some cases.[10] The presence of cortical holes can decrease the quality of cement-bone interdigitation, and the small penetrations of cement through the screw holes may act as stress risers in the mantle and facilitate loosening. Also, in cases of uncemented stem implantation, the presence of screw holes may increase the possibility of intraoperative femoral fracture.

Dupont and Charnley[9] first reported on 121 femoral osteotomies converted to total hip arthroplasty and followed for 1 year. Results from this short follow-up were satisfactory, with 87 percent of patients having no pain and significantly improved range of motion. No data were given for complications, long-term loosening, or revision rates.

In 1982, Benke et al.[2] reviewed 105 femoral osteotomies converted to cemented total hip arthroplasty and followed for a mean of 4.7 years. Eighty-two percent of patients had little or no pain, and 75 percent could walk long distances. The infection rate was 8.6 percent, and technical difficulties, including broken screws and femoral shaft fractures, occurred in 17.1 percent. Long-term revision or radiographic loosening rates were not provided.

More recently, 74 patients who had total hip arthroplasties after femoral osteotomy were compared with a diagnosis-matched control group of 74 patients who had primary procedures performed during the same period[3] and results were assessed between 5 and 10 years. No significant difference was found in the rate of perioperative complications (11 percent each) or in the septic (8 percent versus 3 percent) and aseptic (4 percent each) revision rates. Improved survival was observed in the group without previous osteotomy (90 percent versus 82 percent). The only significant differences were a higher rate of trochanteric osteotomy (88 percent versus 14 percent) and a longer operating time in the osteotomy group. The authors concluded that total hip arthroplasty after previous osteotomy is technically more demanding but not necessarily associated with a higher rate of complications.

In 1998, Shinar and Harris[27] reviewed 22 primary cemented total hip arthroplasties performed by a single surgeon after failed proximal femoral osteotomies and

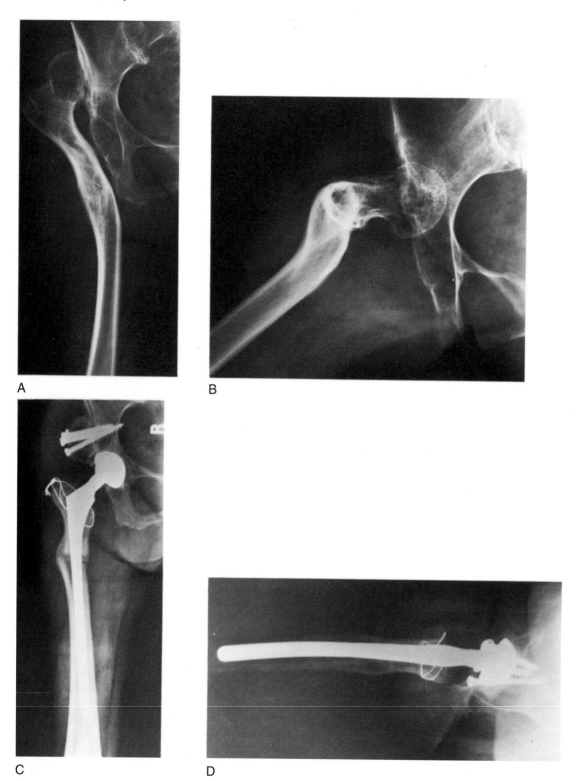

A

B

C

D

Figure 54–1. A, Anteroposterior roentgenograph of the right hip of a 64-year-old woman with painful developmental dysplasia previously treated with a subtrochanteric osteotomy. **B,** Oblique roentgenogram of the same patient. Note the significant femoral deformity. **C,** Anteroposterior roentgenogram at 2-year postoperative follow-up. A step-cut shortening osteotomy of the femur has been carried out. An uncemented femoral component was used. The clinical result was excellent. **D,** Lateral roentgenogram of the same patient.

followed for an average of 15.8 years. Eight reconstructions required custom miniature or calcar replacement components. Two of 19 femoral components (10.5 percent) were revised for aseptic loosening and 2 additional femoral components were loose. Intertrochanteric osteotomy in general did not adversely affect the expected excellent results of the femoral components that were attached with modern cementing techniques. Severe deformity that developed after subtrochanteric osteotomy, however, did adversely affect the outcome.

Mayo Clinic Experience

In a review of 305 total hip arthroplasties in 290 patients who had a previous failed intertrochanteric osteotomy, 215 hips were followed for a minimum of 5 years. Most (91.1 percent) were done for primary or secondary osteoarthritis, and the mean interval between osteotomy and arthroplasty was 7.3 years. All were performed through the intertrochanteric region.

Operative time was longer and blood loss was somewhat greater than for primary total hip arthroplasty, and technical difficulties were encountered in 34.1 percent. Hardware caused problems in about 23 percent. The femoral component was always cemented without a concomitant femoral osteotomy, although this sometimes necessitated the use of a straight or especially curved component. There was a complication rate of 24.9 percent, including intraoperative shaft perforation or fracture, wound infection, nonunion of the greater trochanter, dislocation, and peroneal palsies.

Results were recorded at an average of 10.1 years after replacement, at which time 19.5 percent of stems and 12.6 percent of sockets were probably loose. Of these, 12.1 percent of stems and 7.9 percent of sockets had required revision. The total revision rate was 18.1 percent, of which 3.2 percent were septic.

If time of failure was defined as that of onset of moderate or severe pain or revision, the cumulative probability of failure by pain or revision (Kaplan-Meier method) was 20.6 percent at 10 years, and projected to be 33 percent at 15 years. After a varus osteotomy, the 10-year cumulative failure rate was 29.7 percent and 15.8 percent after valgus osteotomy.

The incidence of positive tissue cultures from the osteotomy site (9 percent), broken plates or screws (20.7 percent), and difficult removal of metal implants (24.3 percent), at the time of total hip arthroplasty all argue in favor of routine removal of such implants after osteotomy healing. This practice would allow reconstitution of the cortices, thereby facilitating subsequent arthroplasty. The incidence of operative technical problems (23 percent), complication rate (24.9 percent), and aseptic revision rate (14.9 percent) are of enough significance to influence the surgical decision toward one or the other procedure—osteotomy or arthroplasty—in certain circumstances.

Authors' Preference

The indications for osteotomy[26] should be strictly followed and the procedure carefully executed so that the mechanical axis of the limb is maintained and the anatomy of the proximal femur is not distorted. Routine hardware removal after oseotomy healing is simple and sensible. When conversion to hip replacement becomes necessary, proper preoperative planning helps determine whether a two-stage procedure is advisable (Fig. 54–2), whether the altered anatomy can be accommodated by the prosthesis or whether an osteotomy to undo the previous osteotomy is necessary. In cases of previous varus intertrochanteric osteotomy, the greater trochanter is often located directly over the femoral canal, and a trochanteric osteotomy or slide is necessary to avoid damage to the abductors during the operation and to restore the hip joint mechanics.

FEMORAL DEFORMITY IN ASSOCIATION WITH FAILED TOTAL HIP ARTHROPLASTY

Revision total hip arthroplasty in the presence of femoral deformity can be particularly challenging when there is proximal bone loss resulting from aseptic loosening and a deformity in the diaphysis of the femur. Proper prosthetic fitting can be very difficult in this circumstance. Femoral deformity can result from: (1) bone remodeling that causes an angular deformity after a short-stemmed prosthesis loosens and migrates into varus; (2) a malunion of an intraoperative or postoperative fracture; or (3) a femoral deformity distal to the loosened prosthesis anteceding prosthetic implantation. In these situations, the use of a femoral corrective osteotomy at the time of revision arthroplasty is currently the procedure of choice.

FEMORAL OSTEOTOMY DURING HIP ARTHROPLASTY

In cases with severe proximal femoral deformity, a corrective femoral osteotomy carried out at the time of arthroplasty can be a very useful strategy.[7,12,16,20–22,24,29] Typically, a femoral prosthesis with a long enough stem is necessary. Clinical situations in which this surgical approach may be advisable include DDH with previous subtrochanteric osteotomy, malunion or nonunion of proximal femoral fractures, pagetoid deformity of the femur, proximal femoral fibrous dysplasia, or previous total hip arthroplasty with secondary deformity as discussed earlier. Generally, uncemented fixation is preferred, and, almost always, all surgical objectives can be met with a single-stage procedure. In our experience, the only indication for a two-stage procedure has occurred in the presence of old fixation hardware, specifically when removal of

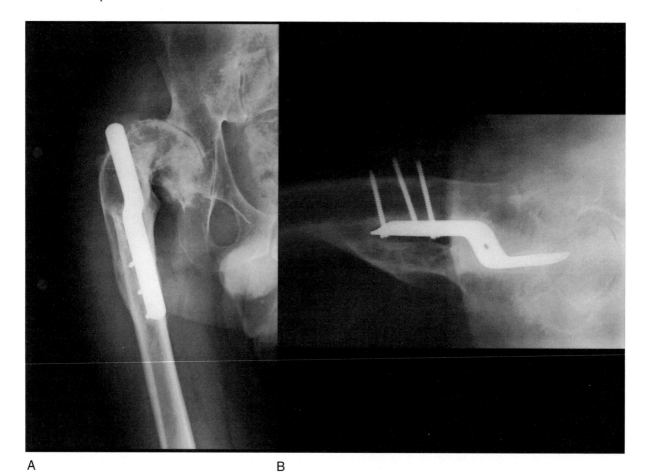

A   B

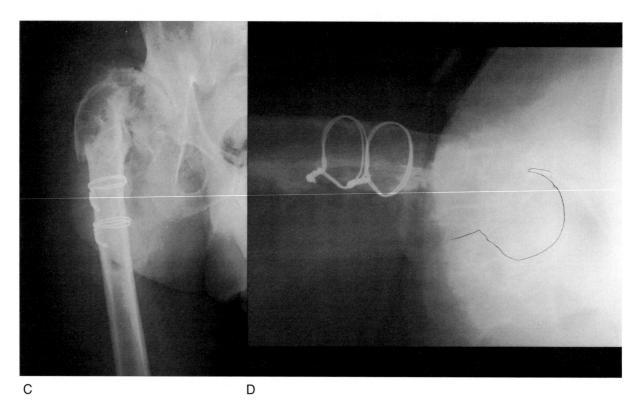

C   D

Figure 54–2. *See legend on opposite page*

this hardware proves to be very time consuming or produces significant bone loss. In these instances, removing the hardware and bone grafting (if necessary) the defect produced at that time, can be followed after a prudent interval (3 to 6 months) by a less risky hip arthroplasty.

Technique

Although each case must be treated individually, proper preoperative planning is essential. Templates made from anteroposterior and lateral radiographs of the entire femur help determine the need for osteotomy, the angle of correction necessary, and whether the correction must be biplanar (a common occurrence).

In general, the osteotomy should be located at the apex of the deformity (Fig. 54–3). Implant size can also be determined at this time, and its length must be such that it extends beyond the osteotomy site for a distance of at least two bone diameters. In cases of DDH, the degree of femoral neck anteversion is estimated, and a derotational osteotomy is planned, when indicated. Careful tracing of the proximal femur and its medullary canal is performed, and the elected femoral prosthesis is templated. The optimal site of the required osteotomy is decided so that the prosthesis can be accommodated in both the metaphysis and the diaphysis of the femur.

The osteotomy itself requires a refined technique. In cases of uniplanar correction, the osteotomy should be incomplete and the wedge of bone should be removed before the deformity is gently corrected by a greenstick fracture of the wedge apex around which, it is hoped, the periosteum and soft tissue attachments have been preserved. In most cases, the proximal and distal fragments can be held in position with bone clamps, and the

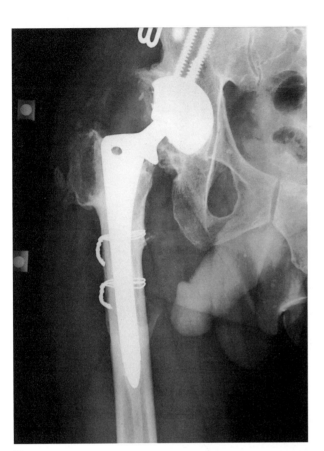

E

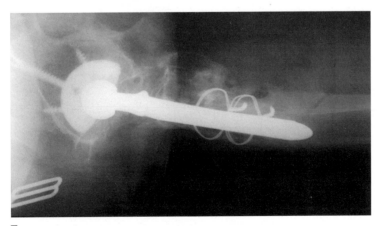

F

Figure 54–2. **A** and **B**, Anteroposterior and lateral roentgenogram of the right hip of a 46-year-old man with severe arthrosis and a significant proximofemoral deformity and a retained plate. Note the intramedullary location of the plate in the lateral view. **C** and **D**, It was deemed advisable to do the reconstruction in two stages. In the first procedure, removal of the hardware required the creation of a cortical window to extract the intramedullary portion of the plate; this window was replaced with wires. Three months later, a total hip arthroplasty was carried out with an uncemented prosthesis. **E** and **F**, Anteroposterior and lateral roentgenogram of the hip of the same patient 3.5 years after surgery. The patient has had an excellent clinical result. Note how it was possible to adapt the prosthesis to the altered proximal femoral anatomy without the need for a corrective osteotomy.

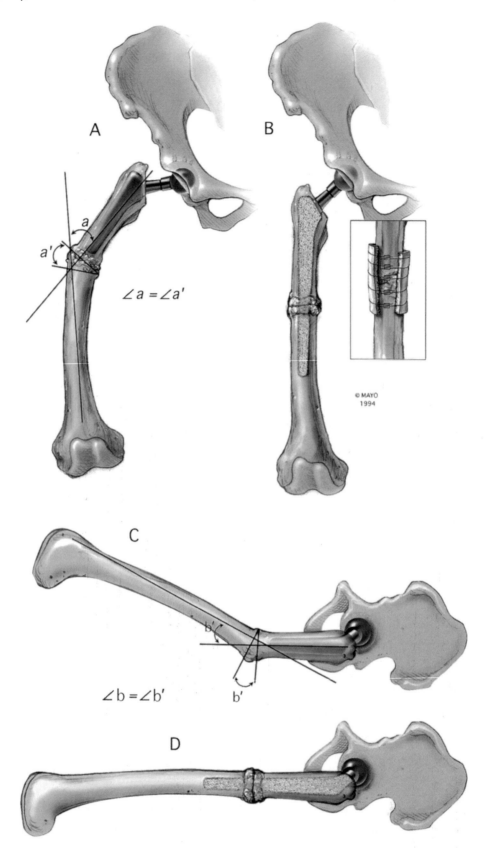

Figure 54–3. Technique of using femoral osteotomy for correction of angular femoral deformity during revision total hip arthroplasty for failed total hip arthroplasty. The corrective osteotomy is located at the apex of the deformity.

femur is then prepared in the usual fashion to receive a cemented or cementless prosthesis. Our experience with cemented fixation has been mixed, and, in general, uncemented fixation is currently preferred. Because achievement of initial stability is essential both for a satisfactory prosthetic result and for osteotomy healing, rigid fixation of the osteotomy is very important.[23] Intramedullary osteotomy fixation is achieved by the implant; rotational stability may be achieved, when needed, with a plate and unicortical screws. An alternative could be to plan the osteotomy with a step-cut configuration, which gives inherent stability and requires only circumferential wires or cables for additional support. Cables combined with allogenic or autogenic cortical struts can be also helpful and are often used. The addition of autologous cancellous bone graft at the osteotomy site is advisable. In cases of DDH with high dislocation, shortening of the femur is necessary. This can be done at the metaphysis, where shortening can be combined with distal advancement of the greater trochanter, or by subtrochanteric diaphyseal shortening, as described later. This then combines maintenance of the proximal femoral anatomy with shortening, which maintains the rotational stability of the femur once the femoral component is in place (Fig. 54–4).

Postoperative protection with a hip spica cast or, at least, a hip guide brace is advisable until early osteotomy union is observed radiographically.

Results of Primary Total Hip Arthroplasty

There are several short reports of osteotomy in combination with primary hip arthroplasty. Satisfactory results with DDH were reported in 1993 by Paavilainen et al., and a good outcome was achieved via previous Schanz osteotomy treated by cementless total hip arthroplasty with femoral shortening and advancement of the greater trochanter.[20,21] The incidence of complications is greater than in primary total hip arthroplasties, however.

In cases of diastrophic dysplasia, osteogenesis imperfecta,[22] or fibrous dysplasia with a significant femoral deformity, osteotomy at one or more levels may be needed to realign the femoral canal and allow insertion of a femoral prosthesis. In 1992, Peltonen et al.[24] described 3 cases of diastrophic dysplasia in which a one-level shortening femoral osteotomy combined with a greater trochanter transfer and tenotomies gave good results. A two-level osteotomy of the proximal and distal femur was required to restore the distorted femoral canal anatomy in 1 of our patients with fibrous dysplasia who had undergone a previous proximal femoral osteotomy.[23]

In 1989, DeCoster et al.[7] reported 3 cases in which a biplanar re-osteotomy at the level of the lesser trochanter was needed to correct the angular deformity from previous surgery. With an average of 3 years of follow-up, all patients had union of the osteotomy and a successful clinical result.[7] All patients were doing well at 10-year follow-up.

In cases of angular femoral deformity (Paget's disease) that cannot be bypassed with a long-stemmed femoral component, a corrective osteotomy may be applicable (see Fig. 54–4). The apex of the deformity is usually recommended as the osteotomy site, and a biplanar osteotomy is most often used.[23]

Total hip arthroplasty in combination with a subtrochanteric double-chevron derotation osteotomy has shown promising short to midterm results in the treatment of complete congenital dislocation of the hip in adults.[1] Chareancholvanich et al.[6] reported, in 1999, on 15 hips in 11 patients with complete congenital dislocation treated by total hip arthroplasty and femoral shortening with a subtrochanteric double-chevron derotation osteotomy at 5.5 years. Excellent results in 5 cases and good results in 7 were recorded (80 percent success rate). The location of the hip center was lowered by a mean of 8.3 cm (range, 5.7 to 10.4 cm). Leg length discrepancy in 7 patients with unilateral involvement was reduced from a mean of 3.9 cm (range, 1.7 to 8.2 cm) before surgery to a mean of 1.4 cm at the latest follow-up (range, 0 to 4 cm). The Trendelenburg sign was corrected from a positive preoperative status to a negative postoperative status in 8 of 10 hips. The only complications were a supracondylar fracture below the femoral component and loosening of the cemented titanium metal-backed acetabular component 1.5 years after surgery.

Yasgur et al., in 1997, reported the results of a transverse osteotomy for subtrochanteric femoral shortening and derotation.[30] Eight patients were followed for an average of 43 months with good to excellent results in 7 of the 8. Eight of 9 osteotomies (89 percent) demonstrated radiographic evidence of healing at an average of 5 months.

Uncemented femoral fixation in conjunction with a subtrochanteric derotational osteotomy has been described in a small series of patients by Zadeh et al.[31] In 7 patients with a mean age of 49 years, an uncemented femoral prosthesis in conjunction with subtrochanteric derotational osteotomy allowed the restoration of the normal proximal femoral anatomy, including the abductor muscle level arm, without the necessity of a greater trochanteric transfer. Correction of the excessive femoral anteversion avoided the tendency for postoperative anterior instability. A CAD/CAM (computer-assisted design/computer-assisted manufacturer) design included a close intramedullary proximal fit with collar, lateral flare, and hydroxyapatite coating to achieve early proximal fixation, and longitudinally cutting fluted stem to provide immediate rotational stability across the osteotomy site. With a mean follow-up period of 31 months, all cases had a satisfactory outcome with evidence of union at the osteotomy site.

More recently, a new technique of subtrochanteric shortening with the prosthesis in situ has been described.[4] The technique minimized complications, allowed correction of severe femoral neck anteversion, and gave excellent rotational stability, while preserving the proximal femur for better press-fitted uncemented fixation. Significant pain relief and functional improvement were reported in 9 cases, and all osteotomies appeared to be healed on radiographs by 12 weeks.[4]

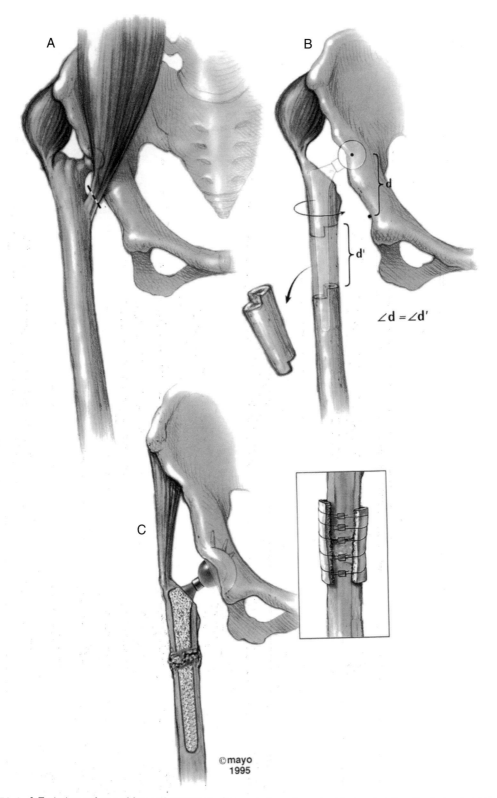

Figure 54–4. A, Technique of use of femoral osteotomy for correction of proximal femoral deformity during total hip arthroplasty in a patient with developmental hip dysplasia. **B**, Subtrochanteric derotational osteotomy can be done in combination with shortening by means of a step-cut osteotomy that maintains the rotational stability of the femur once the femoral component is in place. **C**, A fully coated, uncemented femoral component is preferred. More rotational stability may be achieved when needed with cables, or cables can be combined with allogenic or autogenic cortical struts. Use of autologous cancellous bone graft at the osteotomy site is advisable.

Perka et al.[25] described, in 2000, the implantation of an uncemented straight stem in 15 patients with use of a simultaneous, derotating, and shortening osteotomy. Advantages included a shorter duration of surgery, a lower complication rate, and a more rapid consolidation of the osteotomy. Femur fractures, pseudoarthroses, stem loosening, paresis, and deep infections were not present at 4-year follow-up.

Results in Revision Total Hip Arthroplasty

Revision total hip arthroplasty combined with a corrective femoral osteotomy was reported by Glassman et al.[12] for cases of signicant femoral deformity. A trochanteric osteotomy or slide was done in all cases. All trochanteric and femoral osteotomies healed uneventfully, and the clinical results were excellent. Postoperative immobilization with a hip spica cast was performed in all patients. Holtgrewe and Hungerford[16] reported on 6 similar cases in patients whose average time to radiographic union was 27 months. All of these patients were immobilized postoperatively with a hip spica cast for 5 to 16 weeks. With a follow-up of 46.3 months, clinical results were excellent in 3 patients.

In 1995, Huo et al.[17] reported on a prospective study that was using a technique of oblique femoral osteotomy to correct proximal femoral deformity and to facilitate difficult revision surgery in selected cases. In 25 consecutive patients, 26 osteotomies were performed with a minimum follow-up period of 3 years. The median follow-up period was 50 months, and 81 percent were rated excellent or good. Three stems were revised for aseptic loosening. One additional femoral revision was necessary for nonunion of the osteotomy. Although oblique femoral osteotomy serves as a useful adjunct surgical technique in difficult femoral reconstructions, nearly 25 percent of the hips in this study either failed or were loose at the medium-term follow-up examination.

Mayo Clinic Experience

In 1996, we[23] reported 31 total hip arthroplasties, 20 primary procedures and 11 revisions, performed in 28 patients with concurrent femoral osteotomy. The type of femoral osteotomy used was a uniplanar wedge in 19 cases, a biplanar tool in 4, and a step-cut device in 8. In 4 cases with high hip dislocation, shortening was also performed. Uncemented femoral components were used in 22 cases and cemented in 9 cases. Bone grafting at the osteotomy site was performed in 29 cases.

At 4.5 years, the Harris Hip Score improved from an average of 51 to 77 points in primary cases and from 35 to 73 points in revision cases. The average time until union of the osteotomy was 30 weeks for primary cases and 40 weeks for revision cases. Complications included intraoperative femoral fracture in 7 cases, dislocation in 4, aseptic femoral loosening in 4, osteolysis in 1, deep infection in 1, heterotopic ossification in 6, and osteotomy nonunion in 4. Eight patients (26 percent) had one or more reoperations. Four primary femoral components were revised, and in 2 of the revision cases, the main reasons for revision were aseptic loosening, nonunion, and deep infection. No significant difference was identified in the nonunion rate comparing type of osteotomy, type of fixation of the femoral component (cemented or uncemented), or distance of osteotomy from the lesser trochanter. Because of the high complication rate and the increased technical demands of the procedure, osteotomy is recommended only in complex cases when other techniques are not applicable.

Authors' Preference

In cases of subtrochanteric deformities secondary to Schanz osteotomy, the procedure of subtrochanteric shortening combined with an uncemented long-stemmed femoral component gives the most predictable result. The site of the deformity is identified and circumferentially exposed. A transverse osteotomy is carried out, and the proximal fragment is translated anteriorly to expose the acetabulum, much as in a routine posterior approach to the hip. It is important to try to preserve as many soft tissue attachments as possible on the proximal fragment, including the psoas tendon and the fibers of the vastus lateralis, if this is feasible. If this fragment is flipped up to gain access to the acetabulum, as previously suggested, there is a significant risk of partially devascularization of the proximal femoral diaphysis, which in turn increases the risk of osteotomy nonunion. The section of the femoral neck and head is done in a routine manner, although orientation can be a problem and demands careful attention. This exposure facilitates performance of the acetabular preparation and component fixation. Reaming and rasping of the proximal femoral fragment is then carried out, although many times this preparation is best done with a bur; the distal fragment is typically reamed with cylindrical flexible or stiff reamers. The trial prosthesis of the size to be implanted is introduced into the proximal fragment, the hip is reduced, and the distal femoral diaphysis is placed side by side with the proximal fragment. Manual traction is applied to the distal fragment and a straight transverse osteotomy is made with a sharp, thin blade at the level deemed appropriate and with the goal of preserving as much bone as possible. Attempts to step-cut are not necessary; they complicate the procedure and increase the chances of technical error. Final implantation of the prosthesis can be tricky, and carefully holding the proximal and distal fragments temporarily together with Lowman clamps and a plate may be advisable. Today we prefer to use a fully coated, uncemented prosthesis, which enhances rotational stability. Once

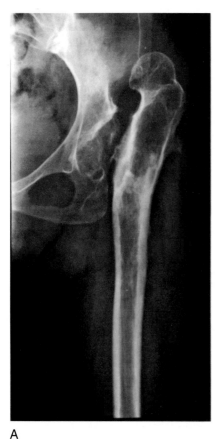

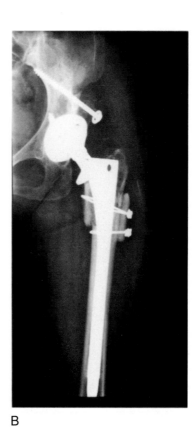

A   B

Figure 54–5. A, Preoperative anteroposterior roentgenograph of the left hip of a 44-year-old nurse who had had a subtrochanteric osteotomy as an adolescent. She has significant instability and moderate pain with activity. B, Six-month postoperative anteroposterior roentgenograph of her hip. She has no pain and her hip is stable.

the prosthesis is inserted and the hip is reduced, the small bone cylinder left from the shortening can be divided longitudinally into two fragments and used as strut grafts fixed with cables or 16-gauge wires to reinforce the osteotomy site (Fig. 54–5). Autologous cancellous bone graft can be used at the osteotomy site, and, if the cortical bone is thinned or if there are segmental cortical deficiencies, employment of strut allografts may be advisable. The size of the prosthetic femoral head is chosen depending on the outer diameter of the socket used, but frequently a 22-mm head is necessary (see Fig. 54–1).

When the procedure is done for revision with a coexistent proximal deformity, modifications of this procedure might be necessary (Fig. 54–6). In fact, the use of the shortening osteotomy is not necessary in this instance (Fig. 54–7).

CONCLUSION

Total hip arthroplasty in the presence of proximal femoral deformity is a complicated proposition. Careful preoperative planning helps determine whether the deformity can be eliminated, whether the procedure can be adapted to the altered anatomy, or whether the deformity has to be corrected by osteotomy. If the latter is necessary, planning includes the accurate location of the site, identification of the type of osteotomy to be carried out, and the type of implant to be used. At this time, our preference is a distally fixed implant, which provides stable fixation of the implant and the osteotomy, essential requirements to avoid nonunion, and secondary failure. Autologous bone graft is helpful and, at times, if cortical bone is lost or weak, strut allograft can help reconstitute bone stock.

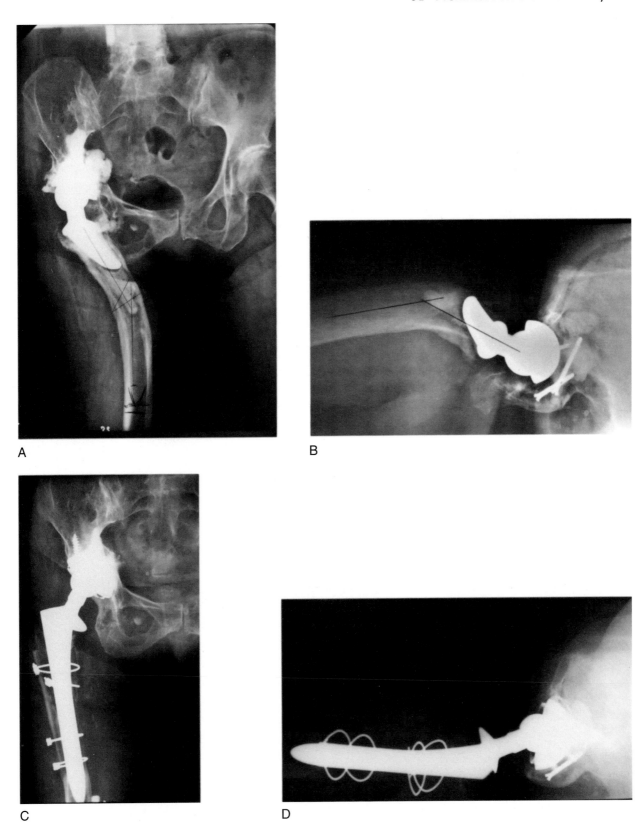

Figure 54–6. A and **B**, Anteroposterior and lateral roentgenograph of right hip and femur of a 60-year-old woman with failed revision of the right hip that used a custom-made prosthesis. Note severe proximal femoral deformity. **C** and **D**, Postoperative anteroposterior roentgenograph of right hip after cementless revision of the femoral component with associated femoral osteotomy and bone grafting. Note the use of homologous cortical struts for supplementary fixation of the osteotomy.

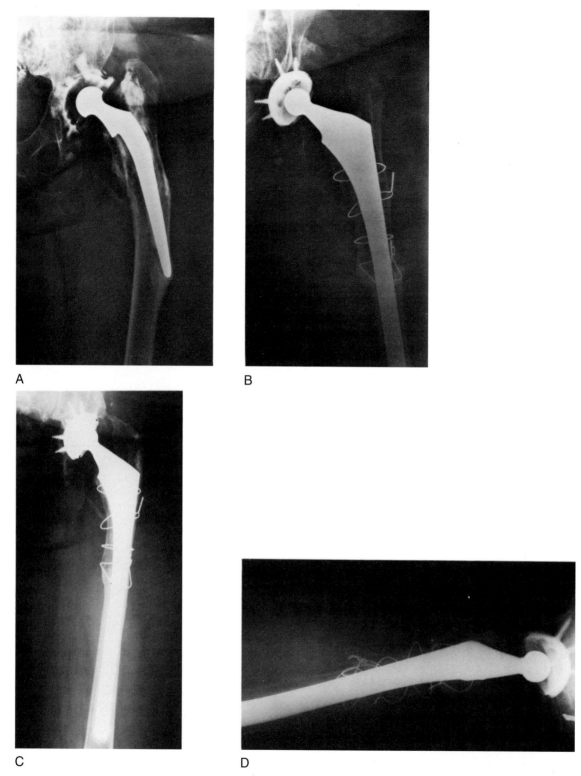

A

B

C

D

Figure 54–7. A, Roentgenogram of the left hip of a 37-year-old woman with loosening of a 7-year-old total hip arthroplasty and significant varus femoral deformity. **B**, Roentgenogram of the same patient immediately after revision surgery. An intraoperative proximal fracture had occurred, necessitating use of circumferential wire. A V-shaped osteotomy at the apex of the femoral deformity was carried out. The osteotomy was fixed with a large, long-stemmed, uncemented prosthesis. The patient was immobilized postoperatively for 6 weeks with a spica mini-cast. **C**, Anteroposterior view of same patient 2 years postoperatively. Note the complete union of the osteotomy. A satisfactory result has been achieved. **D**, Lateral view.

References

1. Becker DA, Gustilo RB: Double-chevron subtrochanteric shortening derotational femoral osteotomy combined with total hip arthroplasty for the treatment of complete congenital dislocation of the hip in the adult. Preliminary report and description of a new surgical technique. J Arthroplasty 10:313, 1995.
2. Benke GJ, Baker AS, Dounis E: Total hip replacement after upper femoral osteotomy: A clinical review. J Bone Joint Surg 64B:570, 1982.
2a. Berry DJ: Total hip arthroplasty in patients with proximal femoral deformity. Clin Orthop 369:262, 1999.
3. Boos N, Kroshell R, Ganz R, Muller ME: Total hip arthroplasty after previous proximal femoral osteotomy. J Bone Joint Surg Br 79:247, 1997.
4. Bruce WJ, Rizkallah SM, Kwon YM, et al: A new technique of subtrochanteric shortening in total hip arthroplasty: Surgical technique and results of 9 cases. J Arthroplasty 15:617, 2000.
5. Callaghan JJ, Dysart SH, Savory CG: The uncemented porous-coated anatomic hip prosthesis: Two-year results of a prospective consecutive series. J Bone Joint Surg 70A:337, 1988.
6. Chareancholvanich K, Becker DA, Gustilo RB: Treatment of congenital dislocated hip by arthroplasty with femoral shortening. Clin Orthop 360:127, 1999.
7. DeCoster TA, Incavo S, Frymoyer JW, Howe J: Hip arthroplasty after biplanar femoral osteotomy. J Arthroplasty 4:79, 1989.
8. DeCoster T, Incavo S, Swenson D, Frymoyer JW: Hip osteotomy arthroplasty: Ten-year follow-up. Iowa Orthop J 19:78, 1999.
9. Dupont JA, Charnley J: Low-friction arthroplasty of the hip for the failures of previous operations. J Bone Joint Surg 54B:77, 1972.
10. Ferguson GM, Cabanela ME, Ilstrup DM: Total hip arthroplasty following failed femoral intertrochanteric osteotomy. J Bone Joint Surg 76B:252, 1994.
11. Fredin H, Sanzin L: Total hip arthroplasty in high congenital dislocation. 21 hips with a minimum five-year follow-up. J Bone Joint Surg Br 73:430, 1991.
12. Glassman AH, Engh CA, Bobyn JD: Proximal femoral osteotomy as an adjunct in cementless revision total hip arthroplasty. J Arthroplasty 2:47, 1987.
13. Halley DK, Wroblewski BM: Long-term results of low-friction arthroplasty in patients 30 years of age or younger. Clin Orthop 211:43, 1986.
14. Harley JM, Wilkinson J: Hip replacement for adults with unreduced congenital dislocation. J Bone Joint Surg 69B:752, 1987.
15. Hartofylakidis G, Stamos C, Ioannidis T: Low friction arthroplasty for old untreated congenital dislocation of the hip. J Bone Joint Surg 70B:182, 1988.
16. Holtgrewe JL, Hungerford DS: Primary and revision total hip replacement without cement and with associated femoral osteotomy. J Bone Joint Surg 71A:1487, 1989.
17. Huo MH, Zatorski LE, Keggi KJ, et al: Oblique femoral osteotomy in cementless total hip arthroplasty. Prospective consecutive series with a 3-year minimum follow-up period. J Arthroplasty 10:319, 1995.
18. Jones LC, Hungerford DS: Cement disease. Clin Orthop 225:192, 1987.
19. Kavanagh BF, Fitzgerald RH Jr: Clinical and roentgenographic assessment of total hip arthroplasty: A new hip score. Clin Orthop 193:133, 1985.
20. Paavilainen T, Hoikka V, Paavolainen P: Cementless total hip arthroplasty for congenitally dislocated or dysplastic hips. Clin Orthop 297:71, 1993.
21. Paavilainen T, Hoikka V, Solonen KA: Cementless total replacement for severely dysplastic or dislocated hips. J Bone Joint Surg 72B:205, 1990.
22. Papagelopoulos PJ, Morrey BF: Hip and knee replacement in osteogenesis imperfecta. J Bone Joint Surg 75A:572, 1993.
23. Papagelopoulos PJ, Trousdale RT, Lewallen DG: Total hip arthroplasty with femoral osteotomy for proximal femoral deformity. Clin Orthop 332:151, 1996.
24. Peltonen JI, Hoikka V, Poussa M, et al: Cementless hip arthroplasty in diastrophic dysplasia. J Arthroplasty 7(Suppl):369, 1992.
25. Perka C, Thomas R, Zippel H: Subtrochanteric corrective osteotomy for the endoprosthetic treatment of high hip dislocation. Treatment and mid-term results with a cementless straight stem. Arch Orthop Trauma Surg 120:144, 2000.
26. Poss R: The role of osteotomy in the treatment of osteoarthritis of the hip. J Bone Joint Surg 66A:144, 1984.
27. Shinar AA, Harris WH: Cemented total hip arthroplasty following previous femoral osteotomy: An average 16-year follow-up study. J Arthroplasty 13:243, 1998.
28. Silber DA, Engh CA: Cementless total hip arthroplasty with femoral head bone grafting for hip dysplasia. J Arthroplasty 5:231, 1990.
29. Stans AA, Pagnano MW, Shaughnessy WJ: Results of total hip arthroplasty for Crowe Type III developmental hip dysplasia. Clin Orthop 348:149-157, 1998.
30. Yasgur DJ, Stuchin SA, Adler EM, DiCesare PE: Subtrochanteric femoral shortening osteotomy in total hip arthroplasty for high-riding developmental dislocation of the hip. J Arthroplasty 12:880, 1997.
31. Zadeh HG, Hua J, Walker PS, et al: Uncemented total hip arthroplasty with subtrochanteric derotational osteotomy for severe femoral anteversion. J Arthroplasty 14:682, 1999.

55A

Proximal Femoral Fracture
Femoral Neck Fracture

• PANAYIOTIS J. PAPAGELOPOULOS and FRANKLIN H. SIM

Femoral neck fractures continue to increase in incidence with the aging of the population, despite better understanding of the epidemiology and prevention of osteoporosis.

Advances in internal fixation have lowered the morbidity from prolonged bed rest and shortened the time to mobilization; however, the incidence of complications after internal fixation of femoral neck fractures, such as nonunion and avascular necrosis, remains high. Likewise, advances in hip arthroplasty techniques, including total hip arthroplasty (THA), bipolar arthroplasty, and modular unipolar arthroplasty have improved the longevity of good results; however, dislocation, infection, and late loosening remain real concerns. The choice of whether hip replacement or internal fixation is the correct surgical operation remains the true challenge.

All would agree that bone union with a viable head is the preferred goal. Fracture pattern and patient profile, however, may doom internal fixation to failure, making arthroplasty the procedure of choice. The physician must then decide whether unipolar, bipolar, or THA is the best option. The choice depends on the surgeon's experience, the needs of the patient, and the fracture characteristics.

INDICATIONS

The indications for hip arthroplasty versus open reduction and internal fixation depend on multiple factors, including type of fracture, comminution, patient age, patient status, bone quality, quality of reduction obtained, and associated disorders.[9,10,27,57] The key is to identify the patient for whom replacement arthroplasty is the best option.

Patient Age and Status

The patient's age is a highly significant and relative factor. Barnes et al.[2] found that only 5 percent of their patients older than 70 years of age showed union by 3 months. However, in the series of Fielding et al.,[21] the incidence of nonunion was highest in the fifth decade. The patient's mental status plays an important role in postoperative management. Patients who are senile and unable to cooperate in limited weight bearing do best with an arthroplasty. Likewise, more active patients have an increased chance of fracture union and may benefit from internal fixation.

Comorbidity

Associated diseases affecting the hip joint or the overall health of the patient, such as inflammatory arthritis or Paget's disease, are best managed by a THA. Patients who are senile and those who have Parkinson's disease are both have a significantly increased risk of dislocation. Controversy exists as to whether these patients are best treated with arthroplasty or internal fixation. Lunceford[47] has found that persistent tremor and inability to use crutches for protected weight bearing leads to a high percentage of fracture complications after open reduction and internal fixation. In 1980, Coughlin and Templeton reported that 37 percent of patients with Parkinson's disease who were treated with a hemiarthroplasty had had a dislocation.[13] They concluded that the low activity level and high rate of dislocation with a hemiarthroplasty make these patients more suited for internal fixation.

A Mayo Clinic retrospective study of 49 patients (50 fractures of the femoral neck) who had Parkinson's disease demonstrated that prosthetic replacement of the femoral head was a satisfactory method of treatment, with only one dislocation. At the time of the report, 19 (80 percent) of the surviving patients could walk. The study showed that particular attention must be addressed to the presence of hip contractures, and that adductor tenotomy may be needed.[62]

Femoral neck fractures occur in up to 10 percent of patients with hemiplegia.[60] Arthroplasty is recommended for patients with marked hemiplegia and limited ambulatory potential.[28] However, attention to treatment of contractures is essential to prevent dislocation.[60]

Hypertonicity and contractures make reduction of displaced fractures difficult and predispose the patient to dislocation after arthroplasty.[11,67,68]

Type of Fracture

The type of fracture is extremely important in determining treatment choice. Although Garden's femoral neck fracture classification is commonly in use (Garden I to IV), these fractures are best classified as either undisplaced or displaced. Garden type I and type II (undisplaced) fractures have reported nonunion rates of 0.5 percent and 5 percent,[2] respectively, whereas nonunion rates of 33 percent have been reported in Garden type III and type IV fractures.[2] Likewise, these investigators have reported an increased incidence of late segmental collapse as high as 27 percent in patients with Garden type III or type IV fractures.

Quality of Reduction and Posterior Comminution

The quality of reduction affects the union rate and must be assessed intraoperatively by satisfactory roentgenographic and fluoroscopic techniques. Banks[1] has shown an increased nonunion rate of 70 percent in Garden type III and type IV fractures with an inadequate reduction. Only 18 percent of those adequately reduced fractures went on to nonunion. Sixty-two percent of his patients with posterior comminution went on to nonunion,[1] but this is a particular problem in those with severe osteoporosis.

TYPE OF ARTHROPLASTY

Our experience indicates that if the patient with an acute femoral neck fracture is a candidate for replacement surgery, the type of replacement arthroplasty should be tailored to the needs of the patient. The choice lies among unipolar, bipolar, and THA.[57]

Unipolar Arthroplasty

Historically, the concept of unipolar arthroplasty for femoral neck fractures was popularized in the 1940s by Judet, who used a unipolar femoral head replacement. With the addition of Vitallium to the armamentarium of orthopedic implants, the Moore and Thompson prostheses soon followed. In the 1960s and 1970s, the addition of methyl methacrylate allowed more secure fixation and less dependence on press fit. In 1958, Reynolds' preliminary report from the Committee on Fractures and Traumatic Surgery on the use of prostheses in the treatment of acute fractures of the femoral neck, indicated that in selected patients, the prosthesis allows more rapid ambulation and a shorter period of hospitalization and postoperative disability. In a classic article in 1964, Hinchey and Day[28] reviewed 294 consecutive cases of fixed endoprosthesis for acute femoral neck fractures, with an excellent discussion of the indications for this procedure.

Subsequent studies have shown that the short-term results are satisfactory with these fixed endoprostheses, with excellent or good results in 60 percent to 80 percent of cases.[19,28,35,39,70] In 1977, Beckenbaugh et al.[4] reported the early Mayo Clinic experience with cemented unipolar arthroplasties. Of 51 patients, 75 percent were older than 76 years of age, and 85 percent had little or no pain after 3 years. However, half of these were not ambulating patients in nursing homes.

A comparative study in 1979 randomized internal fixation versus primary prosthetic replacement in acute femoral neck fractures.[61] The conclusion was that primary prosthetic replacement was associated with earlier postoperative mobilization and was a more definitive treatment with better results at 1 year. The most common complication with all prosthetic replacements is instability.

Acetabular protrusio in uni- or bipolar replacement has been reported to range from 4 percent to 26 percent and stem loosening from 3 percent to 37 percent.[42] D'Arcy and Devas[14] revealed high rates of acetabular erosion and pain in their younger, more active patients. Twenty-six percent of their patients younger than 70 years old had pain and acetabular erosion compared with 14 percent of their patients aged 70 to 79 years and only 1.7 percent of their patients aged 80 to 89 years. Revision rates were also reported to be as high as 37 percent within 2 years of implantation.[38]

In 1996, Jadhav et al. reported the results of the Austin Moore replacement for transcervical fractures of the femur in 40 cases. The patients were reviewed after a period of 12 to 48 months postoperatively. In 30 cases (75 percent), there was mild to severe pain of noninfective origin, starting as early as 6 months postoperatively. This was irrespective of the make, size, or position (varus or valgus) of the prosthesis. Although clinical results were satisfactory in 65 percent of cases, radiologic evidence of complications such as sinking, protrusion, and so forth were seen in the majority of cases. Calcar resorption was seen in 34 cases (85 percent) as early as 4 months postoperatively. They concluded that the Austin Moore replacement should be reserved for elderly, less active, or debilitated patients because of increased acetabular wear over time in the younger individual.[33]

In 1999, Faraj and Branfoot reviewed 101 patients with a mean age of 83.5 years, who were treated for intracapsular femoral neck fracture by Thompson's prosthesis in order to evaluate the use of cement. The prosthesis was fixed in the femoral shaft by means of Palacos cement in 23 percent and was inserted uncemented in 77 percent. They compared the following pre- and postoperative variables in each group: mobility, activity, walking aids, and postoperative thigh pain, and pre- and postoperative hip radiographs. They concluded that that there was no statistically significant difference between the variables in the two groups. Thompson's prosthesis can be inserted uncemented, and patients with radiologic loosening of the prosthesis were not necessarily symptomatic.[20]

In summary, unipolar arthroplasty is indicated in elderly and minimally household-ambulatory patients. Early postoperative recovery and lower complication rates can be expected in this group compared with those who have undergone internal fixation. In previously active community ambulators, the outcome is less predictable, and acetabular erosion is a common complication that requires conversion to THA (Fig. 55A–1).

Bipolar Implant

The bipolar or universal endoprosthesis was developed in an attempt to obviate the problems described in the preceding section. The basic principle of the bipolar prosthetic design is to reduce motion, stress, and wear or erosion of the acetabulum by providing motion between the prosthetic head and the inner bearing insert.

The original bipolar designs used in 1974 were those of Bateman and Giliberty. This design class had the theoretical advantage of increased range of motion and relatively easier conversion to a total arthroplasty than the fixed endoprosthesis. Although the early clinical results were favorable, the longer term complications of femoral stem loosening, acetabular erosion, decreased joint motion, pain, and decreased hip function prompted a re-evaluation of the clinical performance of bipolar hemiarthroplasties.

The early clinical results of bipolar endoprostheses appeared to be significantly better than those achieved with conventional fixed endoprostheses.[3,6,23,41,45,59,65,70] In 1979, Suman,[63] in a comparative study of prosthetic replacement of the femoral head for acute fractures, found that the bipolar replacement gave more complete relief of pain. Drinker and Murray,[17] in a short-term comparison with conventional hemiarthroplasty, suggested that bipolar replacement was the treatment of choice if the patient were younger than 70 years of age.

Bochner et al.[7] observed 90 patients for more than 2 years after bipolar arthroplasties. The mean age in their population was 77 years. Forty-nine percent of these patients retained their preoperative function, and 29 percent required a cane. Only 11 percent needed a walker and 4 percent needed a wheelchair. Ninety-one percent had no pain or mild pain, and 92 percent had satisfactory motion and muscle power. Four percent of the Bateman prostheses dislocated, but this occurred in none of the 46 that had a self-centering design. Only two components were radiologically loose, and there was no evidence of any acetabular erosion.

In 1990, LaBelle and colleagues[40] reported on 79 patients with displaced femoral neck fractures who were followed for an average of more than 7 years. Of 49 surviving patients, 5 had moderate pain with unusual activities, but no patient developed acetabular protrusio. Others have subsequently reported similar outcomes.[24]

In 1996, Goretti et al.[25] presented 98 hips with femoral neck fracture in elderly patients (mean age, 80.5 years) treated by SEM-type bipolar prosthesis. A total of 93 patients (28.3 percent) were followed up for a total of 98 hips submitted to surgery (5 bilateral) after a mean period of 42 months (12 to 96 months). Pain was present in 49 percent of the cases, although it did not significantly invalidate movement; in 60 percent of the cases, there were problems with walking, mostly owing to the general condition of these patients. Wear phenomena in the acetabulum were present in 32 hips (32.6 percent), but there was no correlation with clinical data. Dynamic radiographs showed that only 31 percent of the implants maintained intraprosthetic movement. The authors emphasized the importance of adequate measurement of the prosthetic cup to improve acetabular fit.[25]

Several reports[5,49,54] have further assessed the outcome of bipolar devices, with particular emphasis on function, pain, and acetabular erosion and protrusion. After more than 500 procedures, satisfactory outcomes approached 90 percent, with absence of acetabular problems noted in all three reports.[5,49,54]

Many comparison studies have been performed to compare unipolar fixed-head prostheses with bipolar prostheses, bipolar with modular unipolar bipolar replacement, and cemented with uncemented bipolar arthroplasty. In 1984, a Mayo Clinic comparison study showed better results with the cemented bipolar prostheses than with cemented fixed-head prostheses.[9] Over a 5-year period, 58 patients with displaced femoral neck fractures underwent 59 bipolar replacements with the Bateman prosthesis with cemented femoral stems; these patients were followed for up to 4 years. Forty patients (69 percent) had excellent or good results. However, among the satisfactory results, 11 patients were included who needed a walker for ambulation because of associated medical conditions. These patients, however, had no pain or minimal hip pain, and, excluding them, the results obtained with the bipolar device were comparable with those obtained after conventional total hip replacement.

In 1987, a more comprehensive study by Yamagata et al. at the Mayo Clinic compared a retrospective review of bipolar versus unipolar prostheses.[73] Six hundred eighty-two fixed-head prostheses and 319 bipolar prostheses revealed that the bipolar prostheses provided better hip function as indicated by the Harris Hip Score. The acetabular erosion rate was significantly higher ($P > .05$) in the fixed-head type (Fig. 55A–2), but this finding was thought to be related to length of follow-up, porosity of bone, and fit of the prosthesis-acetabulum. The reoperation rate (Fig. 55A–3), including revision to THA, was higher in the fixed-head group (12.5 percent) than in the bipolar group (7.2 percent). Based on Kaplan-Meier survivorship analysis (see Fig. 55A–3), 13.7 percent of the bipolar hip endoprostheses and 22.9 percent of the fixed-head type were expected to be reoperated 8 years after implantation. Roentgenographic loosening of the femoral component was noted in 25.4 percent of cases but was significantly higher ($P > .05$) in the bipolar groups for follow-up duration of less than 2 years, regardless of the method of fixation used. Cemented fixation of the femoral component led to a higher prosthesis survival rate regardless of type (Fig. 55A–4).

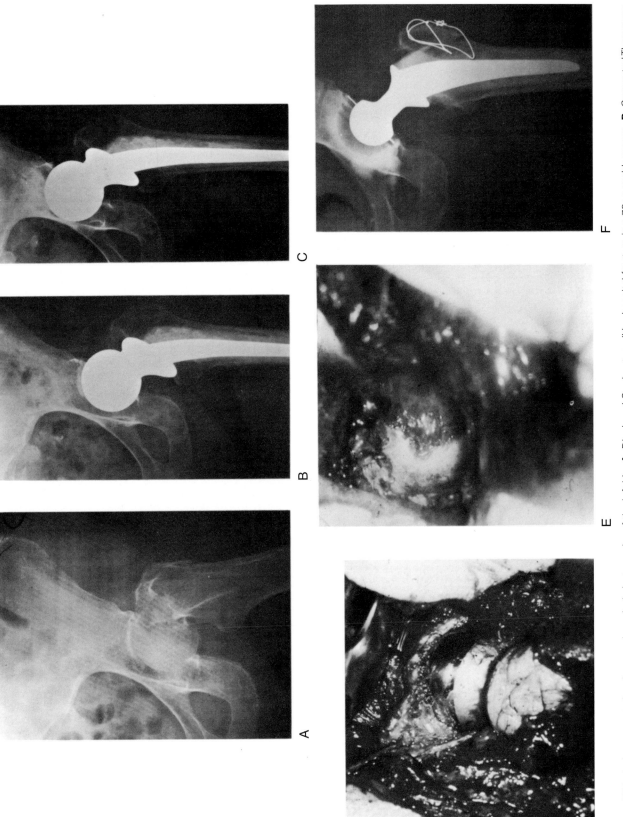

Figure 55A–1. Anteroposterior views and surgical photographs of the left hip. **A,** Displaced Garden type IV subcapital fracture in a 78-year-old woman. **B,** Cemented Thompson prosthesis 3 months after operation. **C,** Joint narrowing and erosion of acetabulum 26 months after operation. **D** and **E,** Revision to total hip replacement. **F,** Extensive erosion of acetabulum is apparent after revision to total hip arthroplasty.

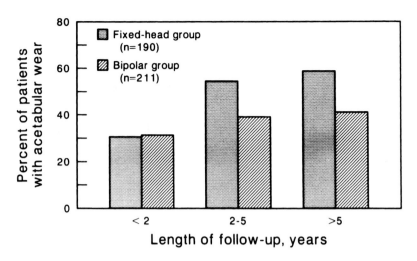

Figure 55A–2. Acetabular erosion (wear greater than 1 mm) of the two groups at different follow-up times. The frequency of acetabular erosion for the fixed-head group was significantly higher (P<.01) than for the bipolar group for follow-up periods longer than 2 years. (From Yamagata M, Chao EY, Ilstrup DM, et al: Fixed head and bipolar hip endoprosthesis. J Arthroplasty 2:327, 1987.)

In 1990, Nottage and McMaster[50] compared bipolar implants with fixed-neck prostheses in femoral neck fractures and found that the mean score for the bipolar group was 85 compared with a mean score of 77 for the fixed-neck group after an average follow-up of 3 years. However, they had a tendency to use the bipolar prosthesis in the younger, more active patient population.

In the period from 1995 to 1998, four comparative studies that assessed bipolar and fixed head implants were reported.[12,48,66,71] In these studies, approximately 600 fixed head and 500 bipolar implants were analyzed. Two of the four assessments found superior function with the cemented bipolar replacement.[48,71] In the other two, the differences were less obvious.[12,66] This led to the recommendation by Cornell et al. to consider the less expensive unipolar implant in elderly patients who were already compromised in their local mobility.[12]

Although the bipolar prosthesis has been recommended in a younger, more active patient, Long and Knight[46] also suggested that there was no advantage in using it in an elderly or inactive patient. Winter[72] also alluded to the significant increase in cost when the bipolar prosthesis was compared with a unipolar model. Without doubt, the most intensely analyzed functional characteristic of the bipolar device is related to the site of insertion, as studied in situ. Several authors have also

shown that the movement of the cup decreases significantly with time.[18,41,51] In several studies, little or no persistent motion has been observed between the two bearings of the prosthesis, possibly causing it to behave in a manner similar to unipolar prostheses. Other studies have shown some persistent movement of the interprosthetic bearing. This may be caused in part by differences in prosthetic design or disease involvement in the acetabulum. Greater intrabearing movement has been demonstrated with the 22-mm head design than with the 32-mm femoral head design.[8] Others have shown that bipolar replacements in patients with osteoarthritis or rheumatoid arthritis, as well as those who have undergone revision have 80 percent motion at the intrabearing articulation. On the other hand, regarding bipolar replacements for fractures, patients with avascular necrosis have exhibited a 50/50 pattern between the intrabearing and outshell/acetabulum articulations.[33]

The impact of stem cement fixation has also been studied.[37,44] With a combined study population of over 600 patients, the cemented implant gave superior results regardless of the implant type and design. These results support the conclusion that the femoral stem should be rigidly stabilized with cement.

Finally, the tribological condition of acetabular tissue before and after bipolar hip surgery was investigated by

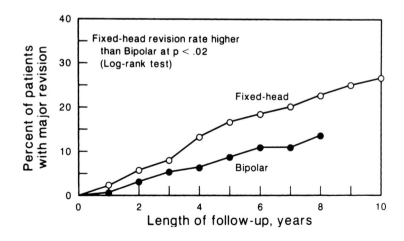

Figure 55A–3. Cumulative incidence of reoperation (Kaplan-Meier survivorship analysis). The bipolar group had a significantly lower (P<.02) incidence of reoperation than the fixed-head group. (From Yamagata M, Chao EY, Ilstrup DM, et al: Fixed head and bipolar hip endoprosthesis. J Arthroplasty 2:327, 1987.)

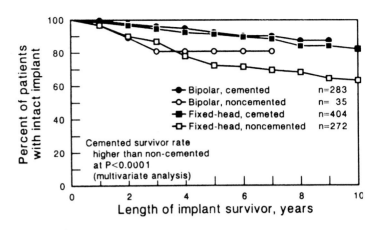

Figure 55A–4. Prosthetic survival rate by method of implant fixation. The cemented group, regardless of type of prosthesis, had a significantly higher survival rate (*P*<.05, multivariate analysis) than the noncemented group. (From Yamagata M, Chao EY, Ilstrup DM, et al: Fixed head and bipolar hip endoprosthesis. J Arthroplasty 2:327, 1987.)

Pickard et al. in 2000. Articular cartilage was taken from the femoral head of patients who were undergoing primary joint replacement as a control. Histology showed major differences between the control cartilage and the bipolar tissue. The control cartilage showed a healthy collagen structure with a good distribution of proteoglycan, whereas the majority of the bipolar tissue had lost tissue architecture and had a sparse fibrous structure. The high friction coefficients with the bipolar tissue imply that the frictional torque at the outer head of the bipolar prosthesis would be large compared with the inner bearing frictional torque. It was, therefore, predicted that the motion of the bipolar prosthesis should occur at the inner bearing.[52]

In summary, bipolar arthroplasties are indicated in a more active and younger patient. The short-term results appear to be significantly better than those seen with the fixed head endoprosthesis.[3,6,41,45,59,65,69] The results do not appear to significantly deteriorate after 7 to 8 years of follow-up. Cement fixation appears to be the preferred method (Fig. 55A–5). There does not appear to be any advantage in using the bipolar endoprosthesis for the treatment of femoral neck fractures in the elderly patient. Moreover, the fact that modular unipolar prostheses cost less than bipolar prostheses provides additional support for their use.[66]

Total Hip Arthroplasty

The improved functional capacity and greater predictability of total joint replacement[4] have broadened the indications for replacement surgery in patients with acute femoral neck fractures. This technique is invaluable in the salvage of complications of femoral neck fractures treated by internal fixation (avascular necrosis, delayed union, and nonunion), particularly if there is loss of articular cartilage in the acetabulum (Fig. 55A–6).[29-31]

In an effort to better define the indications for THA in management of acute femoral neck fractures at the Mayo Clinic, Sim and Stauffer,[58] in 1980, reported early results in 112 patients who had undergone THA after a femoral neck fracture.[15] Eighty-eight percent of these patients had a Garden type III or type IV fracture and

more than 50 percent of the patients also had severe comminution or a high subcapital fracture (Fig. 55A–7). Despite the early satisfactory results, they reported a high dislocation rate (11 percent).

In a more recent study, Lee et al.[43] reported the long-term results of 126 consecutive total hip arthroplasties performed with cement in 18 men and 108 women who had an acute fracture of the femoral neck. The median duration of follow-up was 8.8 years for all patients and 15.7 years for the 22 patients who were alive at the end of the study period. Six hips (5 percent) were revised because of aseptic loosening. Survivorship analysis revealed that the probability of survival of the prosthesis without revision was 95 percent at 5 years, 94 percent at 10 years, 89 percent at 15 years, and 84 percent at 20 years (Fig. 55A–8). Of the 118 patients who were alive at the 1-year postoperative examination, 117 (99 percent) had no pain or mild pain, and 81 (69 percent) had either regained their former level of function or had experienced an improvement over the preoperative level of function. The authors concluded that THA performed in elderly patients for the treatment of acute fracture of the femoral neck was associated with a higher rate of complications than is usually reported for hemiarthroplasty in such patients.

The results of others appear to be similar.[56,57] In 1985, Taine and Armour[64] reviewed 163 total hip arthroplasties that were followed up for 4 years. Sixty-three percent achieved excellent or good results, with an 8 percent dislocation rate. Twelve percent of cases were revised.

In 1987, Delamarter and Moreland[15] reviewed 27 patients treated with total hip replacement for acute fractures, with an average age of 72 years and followed up for an average of 3.8 years. Fifteen of 27 patients had preexisting hip disease. Their results resembled those of patients who had undergone primary total hip replacements for osteoarthritis.

Grenough and Jones[26] reviewed 55 patients younger than 70 years of age, who underwent THA for femoral neck fractures. Thirty-seven patients were followed for an average of 56 months after surgery, and the results contrasted markedly from initial short-term follow-up reports. Twelve patients had already been revised and 6 more were awaiting a revision. The operative technique

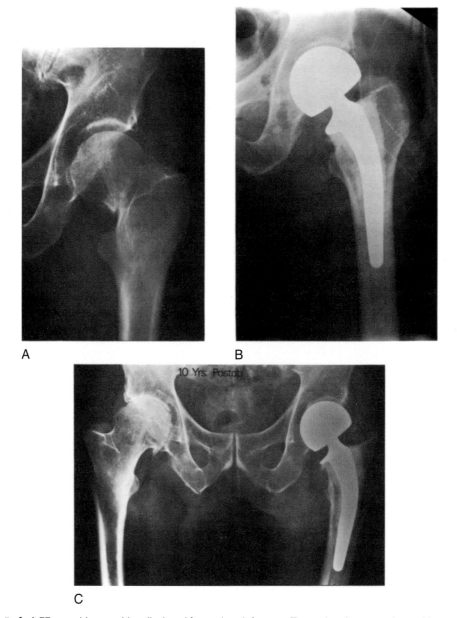

A

B

10 Yrs. Postop

C

Figure 55A–5. A, A 77-year-old man with a displaced femoral neck fracture. The patient is very active and has no preexisting disease. **B,** Two months after bipolar replacement with a Bateman prosthesis, the patient has had a satisfactory recovery. **C,** Ten years postoperatively, the patient has essentially normal motion of the hip and an excellent result with no pain. He remains very active at age 87.

used at the time of arthroplasty included first-generation cementing techniques.

Many comparison studies have been performed to compare THA with internal fixation and either unipolar or bipolar arthroplasty for femoral neck fractures. Gebhard et al.,[22] in 1992, compared the results of THA and unipolar arthroplasties at an average follow-up of 4.5 years. Forty-four patients had uncemented unipolar arthroplasties, 77 had cemented unipolar arthroplasties, and 44 had cemented total hip arthroplasties. Pain, walking, and function scores were higher with THA than with uncemented or cemented hemiarthroplasty. Revision rates were 2.2 percent for THA versus 7.9 percent for cemented hemiarthroplasty and 13 percent for uncemented hemiarthroplasty. The dislocation rates

were 2.3 percent for THA versus 4.9 percent for the hemiarthroplasty groups. Gebhard et al.[22] recommended hemiarthroplasty for older patients who are occasionally active outside the household and THA for more active and healthy patients.

The final consideration is the comparison of the bipolar procedure with a total replacement. In one comparative study, markedly better results were observed after 32 total replacements compared with 42 bipolar replacements.[55] There were no revisions in the total replacement group compared with 28 percent in the bipolar population.

In 2000, Johansson et al.[36] showed that THA should be considered for a displaced femoral neck fracture in elderly patients with normal mental function and high functional demands. In the study, 100 patients 75 years

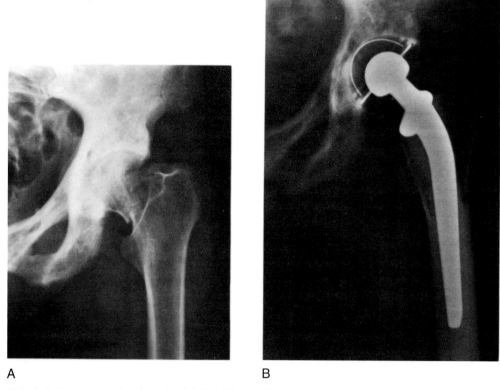

A   B

Figure 55A–6. **A**, Anteroposterior view of pelvis in a 57-year-old patient with associated rheumatoid arthritis. **B**, Sixteen months after total hip arthroplasty. (From Sim FH, Stauffer RN: Management of hip fractures by total hip arthroplasty. Clin Orthop 152:191, 1980.)

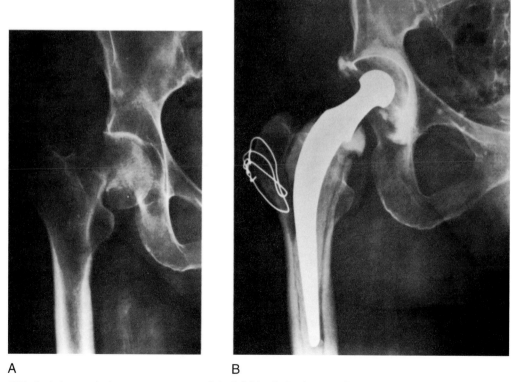

A   B

Figure 55A–7. Anteroposterior roentgenograms of the left hip. **A**, Garden type III midcervical fracture is apparent. There is also Paget's disease involving the innominate bone, with associated narrowing of the joint space. **B**, Two years after total hip arthroplasty.

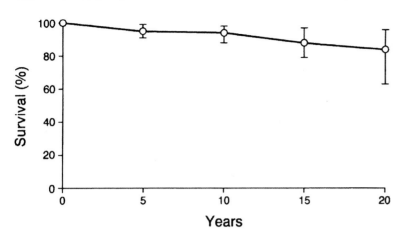

Figure 55A–8. Graph showing the survival of the prosthesis without revision of either component. The I-bars indicate the 95-percent confidence intervals. (From Lee BP, Berry DJ, Harmsen WS, Sim FH: Total hip arthroplasty for the treatment of an acute fracture of the femoral neck: Long-term results. J Bone Joint Surg 80A:70, 1998.)

of age or older, with displaced femoral neck fractures, were randomly assigned to osteosynthesis with two parallel and percutaneously inserted screws (Olmed) or THA (Lubinus IP). Mean age was 84 (range, 75 to 101) years; 74 percent were women and 45 percent had mental dysfunction. General complications were commoner in the arthroplasty group, but the mortality rates did not differ. In the osteosynthesis group, fracture complications were seen in 27 of 50 hips. In the arthroplasty group, dislocation was the main complication and occurred in 11 of 50 cases. After 3 months and after 1 year, the Harris Hip Scores were significantly better in the arthroplasty group. When mental dysfunction was present, the dislocation rate after arthroplasty was 32 percent, whereas the reoperation rate after osteosynthesis was 5 percent. The opposite pattern of complications was found in patients with normal mental function; namely, 12 percent versus 60 percent. The 2-year mortality rate among those with mental dysfunction was 26 of 45, compared with 7 of 55 of those with normal function (P<0.001).[36]

In a comparison study, Ravikumar et al.[53] performed a prospective randomized study with 290 patients older than age 65 years who underwent closed reduction and internal fixation with a sliding compression screw plate, an uncemented Austin Moore hemiarthroplasty, or a cemented Howse II THA. The 13-year results show that there was no statistical difference in the mortality among the three groups (81 percent, 85 percent, and 91 percent, respectively). Internal fixation and hemiarthroplasty groups fared poorly with a revision rate of 33 percent and 24 percent, respectively, compared with 6.75 percent in the THA group. The dislocation rate was 13 percent after hemiarthroplasty and 20 percent after THA. Average Harris Hip Scores were 62, 55, and 80, respectively, for the internal fixation, hemiarthroplasty, and THA groups. In the long term, both internal fixation and hemiarthroplasty resulted in poor outcomes with respect to pain and mobility. Despite high early complications, THA resulted in the least pain and the most mobility in both the short and longterm and showed an encouraging revision rate of only 6.25 percent.[53]

Finally, Iorio et al., in 2001, compared internal fixation, unipolar hemiarthroplasty, bipolar hemiarthroplasty, and THA for treatment of femoral neck fractures.[32] Cost-effectiveness analysis of these four surgical treatment options showed that arthroplasty is the most cost-effective treatment when complication rate, mortality, reoperation rate, and function were evaluated during a 2-year postoperative period. These data were strongly supported by a two-way sensitivity analysis that varied the effectiveness of the interventions and the costs. Literature-derived outcome studies showed that elderly patients with displaced femoral neck fractures achieved the best functional results with a well-healed femoral neck, without osteonecrosis after reduction and internal fixation. Achieving this result may be difficult, and it is not as cost-effective as arthroplasty.

SUMMARY AND AUTHORS' PREFERENCE

Although both THA and bipolar arthroplasty produce satisfactory short-term functional results for displaced femoral neck fractures, THA is associated with a greater morbidity and dislocation rate. However, some studies suggest that THA function continues to improve for up to 2 years, whereas bipolar function levels off.[16] Pain and functional results in THA may also be more predictable. Studies suggest that increased activity and young age of patients lead to a high incidence of early failure in cemented total hip arthroplasties for femoral neck fractures.[26] Newer generations of designs and more refined techniques may reduce these complications.

In our practice, joint replacement arthroplasty is reserved for selected patients with acute femoral neck fractures. Indications for arthroplasty include elderly patients, those with associated disease, and those with unfavorable fracture characteristics. Unipolar arthroplasty is indicated in elderly ambulatory patients. Bipolar arthroplasty is recommended for younger and more active patients.

At this time, the main indication for THA after an acute femoral neck fracture is for a patient with preexisting hip joint disease. In other younger or more active patients, lessening of pain and improvement in functional results in may be more predictable for patients who have undergone THA than for those who have had bipolar arthroplasty. However, THA is associated with a higher morbidity and dislocation rate. Again, newer generation designs and surgical techniques may lessen these problems. Cement fixation is preferred in all unipolar, bipolar, and THAs. Cement fixation is also used for acetabular components because many patients with these components are not ideally suited for ingrowth fixation, and cemented cups in the elderly do not come loose very often. Further studies in the long-term outcome of THA in femoral neck fractures are warranted.

References

1. Banks HH: Factors influencing the result in fractures of the femoral neck. J Bone Joint Surg 44A:931, 1962.
2. Barnes R, Brown JT, Garden RS, Nicoll EA: Subcapital fractures of the femur. J Bone Joint Surg 58B:2, 1976.
3. Bateman JE: Experience with a multi-bearing implant in reconstruction for hip deformities. Orthop Transplant 1:242, 1977.
4. Beckenbaugh RD, Tressler HA, Johnson EW: Results after hemiarthroplasty of the hip using a cement femoral prosthesis. Mayo Clin Proc 52:349, 1977.
5. Bednarek A, Gagala J, Blacha J: Biomechanical principles, indications and early results of bipolar hip arthroplasty. Chir Narzadow Ruchu Ortop Pol 63:133, 1998.
6. Bhuller GS: Use of Giliberty bipolar endoprosthesis in femoral neck fractures. Clin Orthop 162:165, 1982.
7. Bochner RB, Pellici PM, Lyden JP: Bipolar hemiarthroplasty for fracture of the femoral neck. J Bone Joint Surg 70A:1001, 1988.
8. Brueton RN, Craig JS, Hinves BL, Heatley FW: Effect of femoral component head size on movement of the two-component hemiarthroplasty. Injury 24:231, 1993.
9. Cabanela ME: Femoral neck fractures: To pin or not. Orthopedics. 22:833, 1999.
10. Cabanela ME, VanDemark RE Jr: Bipolar endoprosthesis. Hip 68, 1984.
11. Cabanela ME, Weber M: Total hip arthroplasty in patients with neuromuscular disease [Review]. Instr Course Lect 49:163, 2000.
12. Cornell C, Levine D, O'Doherty J, Lyden J: Unipolar versus bipolar hemiarthroplasty for the treatment of femoral neck fractures in the elderly. Clin Orthop 348:67, 1998.
13. Coughlin L, Templeton J: Hip fractures in patients with Parkinson's disease. Clin Orthop 148:192, 1980.
14. D'Arcy J, Devas M: Treatment of fractures of the femoral neck by replacement with the Thompson prosthesis. J Bone Joint Surg 58B:279, 1976.
15. Delamarter R, Moreland JR: Treatment of acute femoral neck fractures with total hip arthroplasty. Clin Orthop 218:68, 1987.
16. Dorr LD, Glousman R, Hoy AL, et al: Treatment of femoral neck fractures with total hip replacement versus cemented and noncemented hemiarthroplasty. J Arthroplasty 1:21, 1986.
17. Drinker H, Murray WR: The universal proximal femoral endoprosthesis: A short-term comparison with conventional hemiarthroplasty. J Bone Joint Surg 61A:1167, 1979.
18. Eiskjer S, Gelinek F, Soballe K: Fracture of the femoral neck treated with cemented bipolar hemiarthroplasty. Orthopedics 12:1545, 1989.
19. Evarts CM: Endoprosthesis as the primary treatment of femoral neck fractures. Clin Orthop 92:69, 1973.
20. Faraj AA, Branfoot T: Cemented versus uncemented Thompson's prostheses: A functional outcome study. Injury 30:671, 1999.
21. Fielding JW, Wilson SA, Ratzan S: A continuing end-result study of displaced intracapsular fractures of the neck of the femur treated with the Pugh nail. J Bone Joint Surg 56:1464, 1974.
22. Gebhard JS, Amstutz HC, Zinar DM, Dorey FJ: A comparison of total hip arthroplasty and hemiarthroplasty for treatment of acute fracture of the femoral neck. Clin Orthop 282:123, 1992.
23. Giliberty RP: Low friction bipolar hip endoprosthesis. Int Surg 62:38, 1977.
24. Goldhill VB, Lyden JP, Cornell CN, Bochner RM: Bipolar hemiarthroplasty for fracture of the femoral neck. J Orthop Trauma 5:318, 1991.
25. Goretti C, Cirilli M, Soldati D, et al: Medial fractures of the femoral neck in the elderly treated by SEM bipolar prosthesis. Chir Organi Mov 81:173–187, 1996.
26. Greenough CG, Jones JR: Primary total hip replacement for displaced subcapital fracture of the femur. J Bone Joint Surg 70B:639, 1988.
27. Gustke KA: Hemiarthroplasty and total arthroplasty in the treatment of intracapsular hip fractures. Instr Course Lect 33:191, 1984.
28. Hinchey JJ, Day PH: Primary prosthetic replacement in fresh femoral neck fractures. J Bone Joint Surg 46A:223, 1964.
29. Hunter GA: A comparison of the use of internal fixation and prosthetic replacement for fresh fractures of the neck of the femur. Br J Surg 56:229, 1969.
30. Hunter GA: A further comparison of the use of internal fixation and prosthetic replacement for fresh fractures of the neck of the femur. Br J Surg 61:382, 1974.
31. Hunter G: Treatment of fractures of the neck of the femur. Can Med Assoc J 117:60, 1977.
32. Iorio R, Healy WL, Lemos DW, et al: Displaced femoral neck fractures in the elderly: Outcomes and cost effectiveness. Clin Orthop 383:229, 2001.
33. Izumi H, Torisu T, Itonaga I, Masumi S: Joint motion of bipolar femoral prostheses. J Arthroplasty 10:237, 1995.
34. Jadhav AP, Kulkarni SS, Vaidya SV, et al: Results of Austin Moore replacement. J Postgrad Med 42:33, 1996.
35. Jensen JS, Holstein P: A long term follow-up of Moore arthroplasty in femoral neck fractures. Acta Orthop Scand 46:764, 1975.
36. Johansson T, Jacobsson SA, Ivarsson I, et al: Internal fixation versus total hip arthroplasty in the treatment of displaced femoral neck fractures: A prospective randomized study of 100 hips. Acta Orthop Scand 71:597, 2000.
37. Kenzora JE, Magaziner J, Hudson J, et al: Outcome after hemiarthroplasty for femoral neck fractures in the elderly. Clin Orthop 348:51, 1998.
38. Kofoed H, Kofoed J: Moore prosthesis in treatment of fresh femoral neck fractures. Injury 14:531, 1983.
39. Kwok DC, Cruess RL: A retrospective study of Moore and Thompson hemiarthroplasty. Clin Orthop 169:179, 1982.
40. LaBelle LW, Colwill JC, Swanson AB: Bateman bipolar hip arthroplasty for femoral neck fractures: A five to ten year follow-up study. Clin Orthop 251:20, 1990.
41. Langen P: The Giliberty bipolar prosthesis: A clinical and radiographical review. Clin Orthop 141:169, 1979.
42. Lausten GS, Vedelo P, Nielsen P: Fractures of the femoral neck treated with a bipolar endoprosthesis. Clin Orthop 218:63, 1987.
43. Lee BP, Berry DJ, Harmsen WS, Sim FH: Total hip arthroplasty for the treatment of an acute fracture of the femoral neck: Long-term results. J Bone Joint Surg Am 80:70, 1998.
44. Lestrange NR: Bipolar arthroplasty for 496 hip fractures. Clin Orthop 251:7, 1990.
45. Lo WH, Chen WM, Huang CK, et al: Bateman bipolar hemiarthroplasty for displaced intracapsular femoral neck fractures. Uncemented versus cemented. Clin Orthop 302:75, 1994.
46. Long JW, Knight W: Bateman UPF prosthesis in fractures of the femoral neck. Clin Orthop 152:198, 1980.
47. Lunceford EM: Use of the Moore self-locking Vitallium prosthesis in acute fractures of the femoral neck. J Bone Joint Surg 47A:832, 1965.
48. Malhotra R, Ayra R, Bhan S: Bipolar hemiarthroplasty in femoral neck fractures. Arch Orthop Trauma Surg 114:79, 1995.
49. Maricevic A, Erceg M, Gekic K: Treatment of femoral neck fractures with bipolar hemiarthroplasty. Lijec Vjesn 120:121, 1998.
50. Nottage NM, McMaster WC: Comparison of bipolar implants with fixed-neck prosthesis in femoral neck fractures. Clin Orthop 251:38, 1990.
51. Poses RM, Berlin JA, Noveck H, et al: How you look determines what you find: severity of illness and variation in blood transfusion for hip fracture. Am J Med 105:198–206, 1998.
52. Phillips JW: The Bateman bipolar femoral head replacement. A fluoroscopic study of movement over a four year period. J Bone Joint Surg 69B:761, 1987.

53. Pickard J, Fisher J, Ingham E, et al: Investigation into the tribological condition of acetabular tissue after bipolar joint replacement hip surgery. Proc Inst Mech Eng [H] 214:361, 2000.

54. Ravikumar KJ, Marsh G: Internal fixation versus hemiarthroplasty versus total hip arthroplasty for displaced subcapital fractures of femur–13 year results of a prospective randomised study. Injury 31:793, 2000.

55. Schatzler A, Mollers M, Stedtfeld HW: Outcome of management of femoral neck fractures with cemented bipolar endoprostheses. Zentralbl Chir 122:1028, 1997.

56. Sim FH, Sigmond ER: Acute fractures of the femoral neck managed by total hip replacement. Orthopedics 9:35, 1986.

57. Sim FH, Stauffer RN: Management of hip fractures by total hip arthroplasty. Clin Orthop 152:191, 1980.

58. Sim FH: Displaced femoral neck fracture: The rationale for primary total hip replacement. In Hungerford DS (ed): The Hip: Proceedings of the 11th Open Scientific Meeting of the Hip Society. St. Louis, CV Mosby, 1983.

59. Simon SR: New concepts in femoral head replacement: The place of the Bateman prosthesis in hip surgery. Bull Hosp Joint Dis 38:59, 1977.

60. Solo-Hall RR: Treatment of transcervical fractures complicated by certain common neurological conditions. Instr Course Lect 17:117, 1960.

61. Soreide O, Molster A, Raugstad TS: Internal fixation versus primary prosthetic replacement in acute femoral neck fractures: A prospective, randomized clinical study. Br J Surg 66:56, 1979.

62. Squires B, Bannister G: Displaced intracapsular neck of femur fractures in mobile independent patients: Total hip replacement or hemiarthroplasty? Injury 30:345, 1999.

63. Staeheli JW, Frassica FJ, Sim FH: Prosthetic replacement of the femoral head for fracture of the femoral neck in patients who have Parkinson disease. J Bone Joint Surg 70A:565, 1988.

64. Suman RK: Prosthetic replacement of the femoral head for fractures of the neck of the femur: A comparative study. Injury 11:309, 1979.

65. Taine WH, Armour PC: Primary total hip replacement for displaced subcapital fractures of the femur. J Bone Joint Surg 67B:214, 1985.

66. VanDemark RE Jr, Cabanela ME, Henderson ED: The Bateman endoprosthesis: 104 arthroplasties. Orthop Transplant 4:356, 1980.

67. Wathne RA, Koval KJ, Aharonoff GB, et al: Modular unipolar versus bipolar prosthesis: A prospective evaluation of functional outcome after femoral neck fracture. J Orthop Trauma 9:298, 1995.

68. Weber M, Cabanela ME: Total hip arthroplasty in patients with low-lumbar-level myelomeningocele [discussion]. Orthopedics 21:709, 1998.

69. Weber M, Cabanela ME: Total hip arthroplasty in patients with cerebral palsy. Orthopedics 22:425-427,1999.

70. West WF, Mann RA: Evaluation of the Bateman self-articulating femoral prosthesis. Orthop Trans 3:17, 1979.

71. Whittaker RP, Abeshaus MM, Scholl HW, Chung SMK: Fifteen years' experience with metallic endoprosthetic replacement of the femoral head for femoral neck fractures. J Trauma 12:799, 1972.

72. Winter WG: Update of fractures of the hip. Clin Orthop 216:1, 1987.

73. Wolfel R, Wagner W, Walther M, Beck H: Hemiprosthesis in femoral neck fracture. Zentralbl Chir 120:721, 1995.

74. Yamagata M, Chao EY, Ilstrup DM, et al: Fixed head and bipolar hip endoprosthesis. J Arthroplasty 2:327, 1987.

55B

Prosthetic Replacement for Intertrochanteric Fracture and Intertrochanteric Nonunion

• GEORGE J. HAIDUKEWYCH

PRIMARY ARTHROPLASTY

Improvements in contemporary sliding screw devices have tempered interest in prosthetic replacement for acute fractures. Early weight bearing and mobilization and rapid return of patients to their prefracture status, however, especially for elderly patients constitute a logical basis for consideration of this option.

Experimental data have shown that the stability of the cemented prosthesis-fracture complex was significantly greater than any nail-reduction complex that was tested.[31] Other potential advantages include fewer reoperations, decreased hospitalization, improved nursing care, and improved function. Potential disadvantages include increased operative time and blood loss, loss of bone stock, prosthetic dislocation, infection, medical complications, and implant loosening. In fact, both early literature from the 1970s and the most current studies do confirm the value of the immediate prosthetic replacement, especially in the unstable fracture.

Tronzo first reported satisfactory results with a Matchett-Brown endoprosthesis in the primary treatment of unstable intertrochanteric fractures in 4 patients who were thought to be senile and unreliable.[38] Their medical conditions were quite severe, and all died within 6 months. Since then, numerous assessments have confirmed the value of acute replacement in these patients.

Rosenfeld et al.[26] reported that 33 of 37 survivors had 64 percent good results with the Lienbach prosthesis. Stern and Goldstein[35] reported 22 fresh and 7 failed internally fixed unstable intertrochanteric fractures that were repaired with Leinbach head and neck prostheses. Eighty-six percent of patients were ambulating 2 to 4 days postoperatively. Reviewing the subsequent literature reveals a great diversity in patient selection, prosthesis, and method. Yet, a number of factors are consistent in most studies. Pho and colleagues[24] reported 8 cases treated with Thompson prostheses. Ambulation without aids was accomplished in 50 percent. Stern and Goldstein's second report[36] of 43 patients treated primarily with the Leinbach prosthesis revealed 88 percent ambulation within the first week, with only 2 percent prosthetic subsidence and pain. Stern and Angerman[34] treated 105 unstable fractures with a Leinbach prosthesis and reported 94 percent return to prefracture ambulatory status. Pinder et al.[25] reported 180 patients with complex intertrochanteric fractures, all of whom returned to prefracture status. Green et al.[8] described 20 patients treated with a head and neck prosthesis; 75 percent were discharged to full weight bearing. Heiman,[15] who has experienced no reoperations or dislocations in more than 100 cases of high-risk elderly osteopenic patients, believes that prosthetic replacement is a better choice than internal fixation in this group. Harwin et al.[14] reported 58 fractures; 88 percent of the patients were ambulatory within the first week and 91 percent were discharged with ambulatory capability. In this series, nearly all patients returned to their prefracture status.

In addition to these specific experiences, several have performed prospective randomized studies. Claes et al.[5] compared a series of unstable intertrochanteric fractures treated with Ender's nails, blade plates, and prosthetic replacement. Return to ambulatory function was by far the best in those patients treated with endoprostheses. Mechanical complications were noted in 4.3 percent of the endoprosthesis group, 28 percent of those with Ender's nails, and 11.3 percent of those with blade plates. Initial postoperative mortality was slightly higher, but at 1 year, mortality was not significantly greater.

Broos[3] reported 388 fractures classified as unstable that were repaired by Ender's nails, angled blade plates, dynamic hip screws, and the Belgian VDP prosthesis. No increase in operative time, blood loss, or mortality occurred with a prosthetic replacement, and final results were worse with use of blade plates or Ender's nails. Of those who were independent before their injury, 64 percent of patients who received dynamic hip screws (DHS) and 65 percent of patients who received prostheses remained independent. However, when the fractures were subdivided, it was concluded that very complex intertrochanteric fractures may do better with endoprosthetic replacement.

No significant difference was noted in a prospective group of 37 patients treated with bipolar prostheses compared with a retrospective group of 42 patients treated with internal fixation, (blade plate) referable to preexisting medical complications, operative time, blood loss, hospital stay, mortality rate, or postoperative complications. Good to excellent results were seen in 75 to 84 percent of patients with prostheses and 60 percent of patients with internal fixation, and rehabilitation was noted to be easier in the prosthesis group. However, meta-analysis of the literature offers few well-controlled studies on which scientific conclusions can be based.[22] Most of the newer reports are found in the European literature and indicate similar satisfactory results, with equal or reduced mortality and morbidity for prosthetic use compared with internal fixation[6,17,19,27,29] (Table 55B–1).

The characteristic features of these experiences are that the implants are reserved for the very elderly; the mean age is commonly greater than 80 years[4,30,40] with unstable fractures. The ideal candidate is one for whom early ambulation is desirable or even essential.[33] The frequency of comorbidity is dramatic in most series, occurring in over half of the patients. Of the numerous coexisting diseases, diabetes mellitus[30] and central neurologic compromise, which cause confusion and falls have been particularly relevant.[4,39] The best outcome occurs with careful medical preparation, brief duration of surgery, and immediate mobilization.[30] In addition, all reports document extremely high complication rates and a comparably high 1-year mortality rate, sometimes as high as 25 percent in 3 months after fixation or replacement (Table 55B–2).[40]

These inordinately difficult features are, of course, inherent in all reports of this fracture, whether treated by fixation or replacement.

TECHNIQUE: ACUTE FRACTURE

Exposure

The patient is placed in the lateral decubitus position, and the pelvis is stabilized with well-padded posts. After sterile preparation and draping, with the involved leg draped free, a lateral incision is made. This is developed through the subcutaneous tissue and the fascia lata. The trochanteric bursa and hematoma are excised. At this point, the fracture is assessed. In many cases, the greater trochanteric fragment is still held in reasonable position with fascial investments. Efforts should be made to leave this intact. If it is intact, a posterior approach is made by dissecting the external rotators off the greater trochanter. If the greater trochanter is displaced, it may be retracted superiorly, thereby diminishing dissection to the external rotators. A T-shaped capsulotomy is made, and the distal femur and greater trochanter are gently retracted anteriorly with a Hohmann retractor and internally rotated. This exposes the head and neck fragment, which is removed with a corkscrew and a hip skid, with care taken not to damage the acetabular articular cartilage. A blunt, curved cobra retractor placed anteriorly aids in the exposure.

Acetabulum

If significant degenerative disease is present, the acetabulum is replaced with a fixed acetabular component; this may be uncemented, but, in the elderly, a cemented polyethylene component may be considered. If the acetabular cartilage is satisfactory, sizing the bipolar component is accomplished based on the sizing of the femoral head and the "suction fit" of the trail heads.

Femur Preparation

Attention is now returned to the femur. The lesser trochanteric fragment is identified and, if large, reduced and fixed with cerclage wires. This may or may not serve to aid in assessing leg length. The femur is then delivered into the wound so that the surgeon may inspect and prepare the medullary canal. Flexible or rigid axial reaming is accomplished carefully. Broaching to the appropriate size then follows. The femoral trial component is then inserted, and the distal fragment is fashioned to provide a broad base of support for the medial calcar flange of the head and neck prosthesis. Anteversion of 10 to 15 degrees is carefully assessed with the knee at a right angle. The height of the body portion of the prothesis is then estimated, and the trial reduction is accomplished.

The greater trochanteric fragment, if in place, has already been prepared during broaching. If the fragment is loose, it is now contoured to fit over the lateral aspect of the prosthesis and reduced. This aids in estimating the length of the prosthetic body. Usually, the center of the head is level with the tip of the trochanter, and the prosthesis should reconstruct this vital relationship. Soft tissue tension is assessed. There should be no visible redundancy or wrinkling of the gluteus medius or vastus lateralis. Tension is manually tested by applying longitudinal traction. The appropriate body section should make contact with the medical calcar and extend to within 1 cm of the tip of the greater trochanter. Stability is assessed in rotational positions, both in extension and flexion. The greater trochanter is now prepared for reattachment. While it is held in a reduced position, holes for cerclage wires are drilled. It is necessary to ensure that the greater trochanter can be reduced and that bone-to-bone contact with the shaft fragment can be obtained. The hip is then dislocated and the trial components removed.

Implant Insertion

Preparation of the canal proceeds with pulsatile lavage and bottle brushing, distal plugging, removal of unstable cancellous bone, and drying of the canal. Vacuum mixing of the cement and retrograde injection with a

Table 55B–1. COMPLICATIONS OF ENDOPROSTHESES

Reference (yr)	No. Patients	Average age (yr)	1-Mo Mortality	1-Yr Mortality	Painful Prosthesis (percent)	Dislocation (percent)	Loosening (percent)	Deep Infection (percent)	Pulmonary Embolus (percent)
Pho et al. (1981)[24]	8	75	0	12	0	12		0	
Staeheli et al. (1986)[32]	64		14	30					
Stern and Angerman (1987)[34]	105	80.4	0	15	2	0	0	2.8	1
Green et al. (1987)[8]	20		5	20	20	0	1	0	
Haentjens et al. (1989)[9]	37	82		35		5		3	
Harwin et al. (1990)[14]	58	78	5		0	0	0	0	
Broos et al. (1991)[3]	145		14	32	27	0.7	0	0	
van Loon et al. (1994)[40]	15	86	4	–	–	1			
Chan et al. (2000)[4]	55	84	10	30	4	0	0	0	1

Table 55B–2. EXPERIENCE WITH ACUTE PROSTHETIC REPLACEMENT FOR EXTRACAPSULAR FEMORAL FRACTURES

Author	Yr	Country	Patients	Study	Age (yr)	Implant	FU	Success	Comment
Stappaerts[33]	1995	Belgium	90	Random	>70	Endoprosthesis (ORIF)	>3 mo	ORIF 60 ENDO 90	Prosthesis recommended
Vahl[39]	1994	Netherlands	22	Selected Unstable	–	Endoprosthesis	–	77	Prosthesis recommended
Schwenk[30]	1994	Germany	136	Selection Criteria	81	Endoprosthesis	–	–	Identified risk factor
Van Loon[40]	1994	Netherlands	15	Unstable	86	Endoprosthesis	–	80	Adjunct wiring of fragments
Haentjens[11]	1994	Belgium	100	Unstable	>75	Bipolar	–	78	
Chan[4]	2000	Texas	55	Consecutive	84	Endoprosthesis	13	–	Confusion: Poor prognosis

ENDO = endoprosthesis; FU = follow-up; ORIF = open reduction and internal fixation.

cement gun is performed. Pressurization of the cement is not recommended in osteoporotic patients with pre-existing cardiac conditions. The prosthesis is inserted at the previously determined degree of anteversion and held until complete polymerization of the methyl-methacrylate occurs. The appropriate modular head and bipolar component are applied and reduction is accomplished. The greater trochanter is applied and fixed with cerclage wires through the prosthesis. Adequate fixation must be obtained to prevent proximal migration of the fragment. Bone graft from the head may be applied about the trochanteric fragments to help ensure fracture healing. The wound is irrigated, the capsule is closed, external rotators are reattached to the greater trochanter, and the wound is closed in layers over suction drainage.

POSTOPERATIVE CARE

The patient is treated like a patient who has had a routine total hip arthroplasty. Postoperatively, the patient is placed in an abduction pillow. Routine prophylactic broad-spectrum intravenous antibiotics are used postoperatively for 24 to 48 hours. Thromboembolic prophylaxis consists of warfarin sodium adjusted by prothrombin time or low molecular weight heparain during hospitalization, and patients are discharged on low-dose aspirin. Sequential gradient hose are worn for 6 weeks postoperatively. Mobilization begins the day after surgery. The patient is started with a bed-to-chair transfer in the morning. Physical therapy is started that afternoon, tilt table and weight bearing are introduced as tolerated with the use of a walker or crutches. Partial weight bearing is recommended if fixation of the greater trochanter was questionable at surgery. Gentle active assisted range of motion and isometric strengthening is begun. Active abduction is avoided until greater trochanteric healing is noted at 6 to 8 weeks. Transfer training is started. When stability is achieved and basic transfers and gait patterns have been learned, the patient is discharged to home or to a rehabilitation center.

THE MAYO CLINIC EXPERIENCE

In 1986, Stahaeli and colleagues[32] reported the Mayo Clinic experience in treating intertrochanteric fractures with endoprostheses; this experience differs somewhat from what has been reported before and after.

Fifty-two patients with unstable fractures had mortality rates at 3, 6, and 12 months of 19, 22, and 30 percent, respectively. At discharge, 18 percent had attained independent ambulation, 39 percent could ambulate with external aids, 36 percent required assistance in walking, and 7 percent were nonambulators. In a carefully matched group of patients who underwent internal fixation of unstable intertrochanteric fractures the failure rate of the devices was 18 percent and reoperations occurred in 13 percent. It was concluded that endopros-

thetic replacement did not favorably influence the results of treatment, largely as a result of an increased mortality. The bulk of the more current literature, however, does justify immediate replacement in selected cases (Fig. 55B–1).

AUTHOR'S PREFERRED TREATMENT

My interpretation of the current and past literature does rather strongly support the use of a cemented endoprosthetic replacement for the unstable fracture; a head/neck implant should be used. On admission, a careful medical assessment is carried out, and we attempt to operate within 24 hours. At the Mayo Clinic, the vast majority of patients with intertrochanteric fractures, however, are treated with encouraging results by sliding screw devices or intramedullary hip screws. Extremely elderly, senile patients with severe osteopenia, unstable fractures, and painful preexisting arthritis are potential candidates for prosthetic replacement. In general, I prefer to reserve arthroplasty for failures of internal fixation discussed later in the chapter. After replacement, we begin ambulation on the first postoperative day. The single most important medical/anesthesia factor that dictates survival outcome is the presence of cardiovascular disease, which is distinct from a functional orthopedic outcome perspective.

ARTHROPLASTY FOR FAILED FIXATION

Unstable intertrochanteric fractures remain a challenge to orthopedic surgeons. Hardware failure with screw cutout and nonunion have all been reported complications when these injuries are encountered in a patient population often plagued by medical comorbidities, dementia, and osteoporotic bone.[1,13,18] Once acute cutout or nonunion has developed, there are several options available for salvage. Some authors have recommended repeat internal fixation, with or without methacrylate augmentation, and bone grafting,[2,13,20,28,37] whereas others have recommended prosthetic replacement.[10,16,20,21,41] Age, activity level, and quality of remaining bone stock influence decision making. Young patients with good remaining bone stock are candidates for repeat internal fixation, whereas older patients with poor bone quality or implant cutout are good candidates for prosthetic replacement.

THE MAYO CLINIC EXPERIENCE

Between 1985 and 1997, 60 patients (49 women and 11 men) with a mean age of 77 years (range, 54 to 96 years) were treated at our institution with hip arthroplasty for salvage of failed internal fixation of an intertrochanteric hip fracture.

Total hip arthroplasty was performed in 32 patients (cemented cups in 24 and uncemented cups in 8), and bipolar hemiarthroplasties were performed in 28.

Cemented stems were used in 57 hips and uncemented stems in 3. A calcar-replacing design was used in 39 of 60 cases (65 percent), an extended neck prosthesis was used in 4 of 60 cases (7 percent), and a long stemmed prosthesis without calcar buildup was used in 12 of 60 cases (20 percent).

The decision of whether to perform a hemiarthroplasty or a total hip arthroplasty was at the discretion of the treating surgeon and was based on the condition of the acetabular cartilage at the time of surgery. There were 4 acute hardware failures (in fewer than 90 days), 21 nonunions with head cutout, and 34 nonunions without cutout.

RESULTS

At last follow-up, 21 patients were alive and 39 were dead. Ten died within the first 2 years (all with implants intact),

and 6 were lost to follow-up. The remaining 44 patients were followed for a mean of 64 months (range, 25 to 185 months). Thirty-one patients of 44 (71 percent) had survived for 2 years and had a minimum of 2 years of radiographic follow-up, with a mean radiographic follow-up of 51 months (range, 25 to 185 months) and a mean clinical follow-up of 65 months (range, 25 to 185 months).

Survivorship

The survivorship free of revision for aseptic loosening was 100 percent at 7 years and 87.5 percent at 10 years (95 percent confidence interval, 67.3 to 100 percent). There were no revisions for sepsis, acetabular wear, or dislocation.

Reoperations

A total of 5 reoperations (8 percent) were performed. One patient underwent revision at 8 years for aseptic loosening

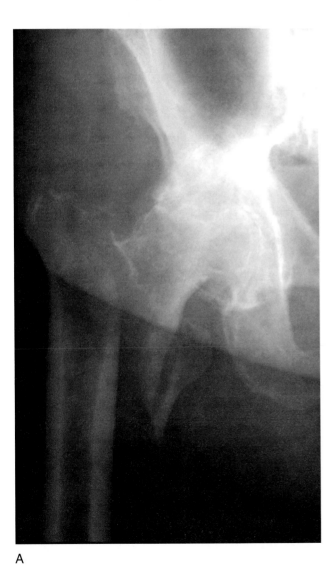

A

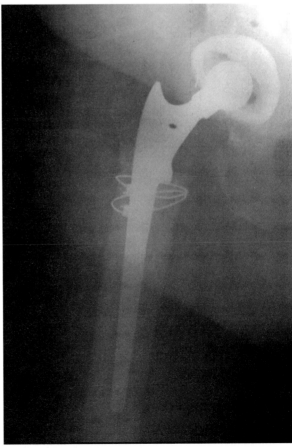

B

Figure 55B–1. A, A 75-year-old woman with three-part intertrochanteric fracture and degenerative arthritis. **B,** She was effectively treated with a cemented implant designed for such fractures.

of both components, and 1 patient had a femoral revision at 10 years for massive osteolysis. There was 1 trochanteric rewiring at 1 year, 1 symptomatic trochanteric hardware removal at 3 years, and 1 débridement of a wound hematoma and fat necrosis (culture negative).

Function

At last follow-up, 39 of 44 (89 percent) had no pain or mild pain and 5 of 44 (11 percent) had moderate to severe pain (all pain was related to the greater trochanter). Forty of 44 patients were ambulatory (91 percent); 26 of the 44 (59 percent) could ambulate with one-arm support or less.

Radiographic Data

At last review, 1 patient of 31 (3 percent) had probable femoral loosening and 1 of 31 (3 percent) had protrusio of her bipolar component. Both had minimal discomfort and had not undergone revision.

Of the 23 patients who had preoperative trochanteric avulsion or transtrochanteric approaches, 21 had adequate follow-up. Twelve healed with obvious bony union (57 percent), 4 healed with fibrous union with no or minimal proximal migration (less than 1 cm), and 5 healed with trochanteric proximal migration greater than 1 cm. Overall, 9 of 21 (43 percent) attempts at achieving bony trochanteric union were unsuccessful.

Discussion

Failed internal fixation of an intertrochanteric fracture presents several challenges to the orthopedic surgeon. Often, the failure is a result of poor bone quality or less than ideal implant placement.[1,13,18] Several studies have documented increased fixation failure rates with poor centering of implants in the femoral head or with certain unstable fracture types.[1,13,18] This patient population often has multiple comorbidites, dementia, and poor postoperative compliance. Options for salvage include repeat internal fixation or prosthetic replacement. Patient age and activity, as well as the status of the articular cartilage and remaining bone stock influence decision making.[20,41] Younger patients with good bone stock may be candidates for repeat internal fixation and bone grafting, whereas older, low-demand patients are often offered prosthetic replacement.

Mariani and Rand[20] reported on 20 patients with intertrochanteric nonunions who were treated between 1961 and 1981. Nine underwent subsequent arthroplasty and 11 underwent repeat internal fixation and bone grafting. Ten of 11 (91 percent) achieved union with repeat internal fixation. Hip scores improved for all patients who were treated with arthroplasty. Repeat internal fixation was used for younger patients (average age, 53 years) and arthroplasty was used in older patients (average age, 73 years). Trochanteric problems were frequent. Stoffelen et al.[37] reported on 7 patients with nonunions after intertrochanteric fractures treated with subsequent arthroplasty. Seventy-two percent reported good to excellent results. Wu et al.[41] reported on fourteen patients treated with repeat internal fixation with methacrylate augmentation of proximal fixation and valgus subtrochanteric osteotomy. All achieved union at an average of five months. Mehlhoff et al.[21] reported on thirteen cases of arthroplasty for failed fixation of intertrochanteric fractures with a mean follow-up of thirty-four months. Two patients required reoperation for instability. One additional patient dislocated and was successfully managed with closed reduction. Average Harris Hip Score at last follow-up was 78. Distortion of the proximal femur caused by medialization of the distal fragment was problematic and resulted in intraoperative fracture with broaching. Only 37 percent of patients reported good to excellent results.

There were several challenges in performing hip arthroplasty after failure of fixation of intertrochanteric hip fractures. The greater trochanter was often ununited and was commonly wired or cabled, and the interface was grafted with autograft from the femoral head. Despite such measures, bony union was achieved in only 57 percent of cases. Additionally, all patients who reported postoperative pain localized it to the greater trochanter. One patient required rewiring of a trochanteric avulsion and 1 required later hardware removal. Patients should be counseled that trochanteric complaints are frequent after such reconstructions.

The femoral side also presented some unique challenges. Proximal anatomy can be distorted by translation of fracture fragments or callus.[13,20] Previous hardware often leaves large lateral cortical defects and distal empty screw holes. Calcar replacement, long stemmed, or extended-neck designs were used frequently in this series to bypass distal stress risers and replace loss of proximal bone stock. I currently favor bypassing cortical stress risers by at least two cortical diameters when selecting stem length.[7] Often, standard reamers and broaches cannot be used owing to proximal deformity and sclerotic bone. A bur may be useful to open the femur proximally to allow access for subsequent canal preparation. In the Mayo Clinic series, there were 2 cases of intraoperative fracture of the femur, with broaching likely caused by distortion of the proximal femoral anatomy; both of these patients successfully treated with cerclage. Patterson et al.[23] have recommended use of unicortical screws in the lateral cortex to prevent cement extravasation during cementation. No late fracture through previous cortical defects were noted in this series. The use of uncemented ingrowth stems in canals with multiple cortical perforations and osteoporotic bone has the theoretical risk of fracture and potential for thigh pain owing to the large diameters often needed for adequate press-fit in elderly patients. I favor cemented stems for those reasons. Additionally, antibiotics can be added to the cement and postoperative weight bearing does not need to be restricted if the greater trochanter has not been disturbed.

Acetabular decision-making was based on the surgeon's assessment of the quality of the remaining cartilage. More recent series[12] have documented excellent survival rates of bipolar hemiarthroplasties, with very low rates of revision for acetabular wear and low dislocation rate. No revisions were necessary in the Mayo Clinic series because of acetabular wear in patients treated with bipolar components; however, 1 patient who underwent a reamed bipolar procedure at index surgery subsequently had protrusio but did not undergo revision because discomfort was minimal. Often, even if the prior implant used to fix the fracture has cut out of the femoral head, the resulting damage to the acetabular cartilage is minimal. Bipolar hemiarthroplasty in this situation may afford better stability and less surgery for these patients who often have multiple comorbidities and low functional demands.

AUTHOR'S PREFERRED TECHNIQUE

Preoperative Evaluation

A thorough history and physical examination should be performed, specifically directed to prolonged wound drainage or other potential clues to underlying infection. A routine laboratory workup should include complete blood count, sedimentation rate, and a C-reactive protein level. Radiographs should be carefully scrutinized for femoral head penetration, remaining bone stock and acetabular joint space, broken screws, and the status of the greater trochanter. A template of the femoral side should be made to ensure that stems are available for adequate bypass of distal stress risers by at least two cortical diameters.

Surgical Technique

The patient is placed in the lateral decubitus position, and intravenous antibiotics are given. Previous incisions are typically used and deepened through the fascia. All previous hardware is removed, and an intraoperative frozen section is performed. If there is any evidence of infection, a resection arthroplasty is performed, an antibiotic-loaded methacrylate spacer is placed, and a delayed arthroplasty is planned after a course of organism-specific intravenous antibiotics. Cultures are routinely sent from the nonunion site and soft tissues around the previous hardware. If there is no evidence of infection, dissection continues. If the trochanter is ununited and proximally displaced, a trans-trochanteric approach is chosen. If the trochanter is united or not fractured, either anterolateral or posterolateral approaches may be used (Fig. 55B–2). The hip is dislocated and the nonunion site exposed. A femoral neck cut is made, usually

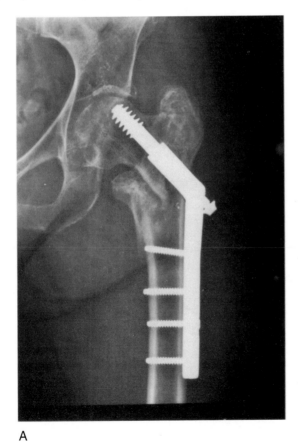
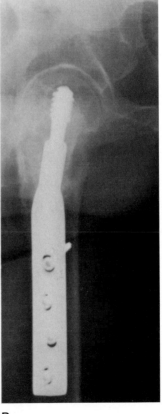

A
B

Figure 55B–2. A 76-year-old woman with intertrochanteric nonunion and a united greater trochanter. She was treated with a cemented calcar, to replace the long-stemmed femoral component and the ingrowth acetabular component.

Illustration continued on following page

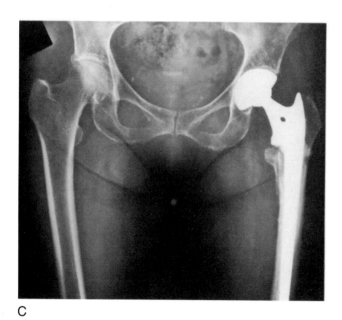

C

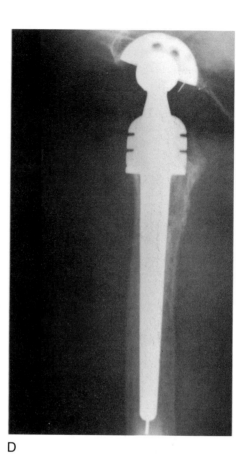

D

Figure 55B–2. *Continued.*

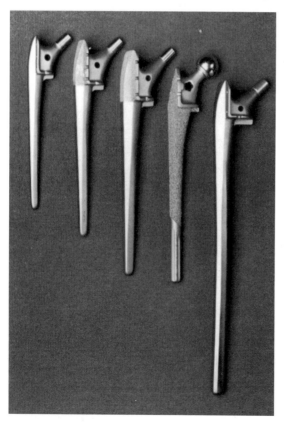

Figure 55B–3. Various designs of modular and nonmodular calcar-replacing prostheses are usually but not always used with cement fixation.

freshening the nonunion site, and the acetabulum is exposed. The quality of the remaining acetabular cartilage is evaluated. If it is unsatisfactory, an acetabular component is implanted in the usual fashion. If the acetabular cartilage is satisfactory, bipolar trial prostheses are inserted until an adequate suction fit of the hemiarthroplasty is achieved. Measuring the diameter of the resected femoral head guides the surgeon to the appropriate size. The femoral canal is opened with a canal finder. Great care is taken in preparation of the proximal femur because previously used hardware can cause sclerotic areas of bone in the metaphysis, which can deflect broaches and reamers and cause intraoperative fractures. I prefer to use a large bur to shape the medullary flare of the proximal femur before broaching. Femoral sizing is performed with trial prostheses, with a goal of adequate distal bypass and replacement of medial bone loss. Often long-stemmed calcar replacement designs are required (Fig. 55B–3). Stems are typically cemented with antibiotics added to the cement. Finger pressure is used over lateral cortical defects during the cementing process. After the hip is reduced, an intraoperative radiograph is performed to evaluate the component's position and size and the presence of extramedullary cement.

If the trochanter was osteotomized or ununited, its undersurface is cleaned of soft tissue until healthy bleeding bone remains. The leg is abducted, and the trochanter is reduced and secured with wires or a cable claw device (Fig. 55B–4). The interface should be

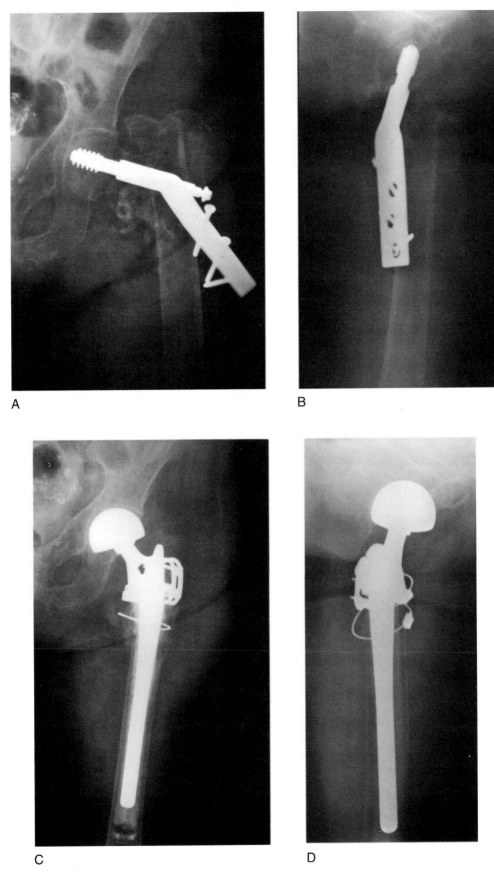

Figure 55B–4. An 80-year-old woman with intertrochanteric nonunion, hardware failure, and greater trochanteric nonunion. She was treated with a cemented calcar replacement femoral component and cerclage and cable fixation of the greater trochanter. A bipolar component was used because of her well-preserved acetabular cartilage at the time of surgery.

autografted with bone taken from the femoral head, if possible. The wound is closed over deep drains in the usual fashion. An abduction pillow is placed.

Postoperative Management

Prophylactic antibiotics are administered for 48 hours. Mechanical and pharmacologic deep vein thrombosis prophylaxis is recommended. If the trochanter was repaired, an abduction orthosis is used to protect the repair until union takes place. Weight bearing is partial for transtrochanteric approaches and as tolerated for cemented arthroplasties. Early mobilization is encouraged.

CONCLUSION

Hip arthroplasty is an effective treatment to salvage failed internal fixation of intertrochanteric hip fractures in elderly patients. The majority of patients have good pain relief and functional improvement. Hip pain is typically related to trochanteric discomfort. Head and neck and long-stemmed implants are often required.

References

1. Baumgaertner MR, Solberg BD: Awareness of tip-apex distance reduces failure of fixation of trochanteric fractures of the hip. J Bone Joint Surg 79B:969, 1997.
2. Blasser KE: Intertrochanteric fracture. In Morrey BF (ed): Reconstructive Surgery of the Joints. Philadelphia, Churchill Livingstone, 1996, pp 1062–1076.
3. Broos PLO: Pertrochanteric fractures in the elderly: Is the Belgian VDP prosthesis the best treatment for unstable fractures with severe comminution? Acta Chir Belg 91:242, 1991.
4. Chan KC, Gill GS: Cemented hemiarthroplasties for elderly patients with intertrochanteric fractures. Clin Orthop 371:206, 2000.
5. Claes H, Broos P, Stappaert SK: Pertrochanteric fractures in elderly patients: Treatment with Ender's nails, blade plate or endoprosthesis. Injury 16:261, 1985.
6. Elberg JF, Peze W: La prothèse dia-céphalique: une nouvelle approche des fractures de la région cervico-trochantérienne chez le vielliard. Acta Orthop Belg 48:823, 1982.
7. Eschenroeder HC Jr, Krackow KA: Late onset femoral stress fracture associated with extruded cement following hip arthroplasty. Clin Orthop 236:210, 1988.
8. Green S, Moore T, Proano F: Bipolar prosthetic replacement for the management of unstable intertrochanteric hip fractures in the elderly. Clin Orthop 224:169, 1987.
9. Haentjens P, Cateleyn PP, De Boeck H, et al: Treatment of unstable intertrochanteric and subtrochanteric fractures in elderly patients: Primary bipolar arthroplasty compared with internal fixation. J Bone Joint Surg 71A:1214, 1989.
10. Haentjens P, Casteleyn PP, Opdecam P: Hip arthroplasty for failed internal fixation of intertrochanteric and subtrochanteric fractures in the elderly patient. Arch Orthop Trauma Surg 113:222, 1994.
11. Haentjens P, Casteleyn PP, Opdecam P: Primary bipolar arthroplasty or total hip arthroplasty for the treatment of unstable intertrochanteric and subtrochanteric fractures in elderly patients. Acta Orthop Belg 60(Suppl 1):124, 1994.
12. Haidukewych GJ, Israel TA, Berry DJ: Long term survivorship of bipolar hemiarthroplasty for fracture of the femoral neck in elderly

13. Haidukewych GJ, Israel TA, Berry DJ: Reverse obliquity of fractures of the intertrochanteric region of the femur. J Bone Joint Surg 83A:643, 2001.
14. Harwin SF, Stern RE, Kulick RG: Primary Bateman-Lienbach bipolar prosthetic replacement of the hip in the treatment of unstable intertrochanteric fractures in the elderly. Orthopedics 13:1131, 1990.
15. Heiman ML: Unstable fractures of the hip. Orthop Rev 17:1047, 1988.
16. Kim Y-H, Oh J-H, Koh Y-G: Salvage of neglected unstable intertrochanteric fractures with cementless porous-coated hemiarthroplasty. Clin Orthop 277:182, 1992.
17. Kipfer M: Traitement des fractures pertrochantériennes du sujet agé par prothèse cervico-céphalique: technique et résultats. Nouvêlle Presse Med 10:2025, 1981.
18. Kyle RF, Gustilo RB, Premer RF: Analysis of 622 intertrochanteric hip fractures. J Bone Joint Surg 61A:216, 1979.
19. Leconte D: La prothèse cervico-céphalique de Merle d'Aubigné-Leinbach dans le traitement des fractures trochantériennes du vieillard. Ann Chir 40:253, 1986.
20. Mariani EM, Rand JA: Nonunion of intertrochanteric fractures of the femur following open reduction and internal fixation. Results of second attempts to gain union. Clin Orthop 218:81, 1987.
21. Mehlhoff T, Landon GC, Tullos HS: Total hip arthroplasty following failed internal fixation of hip fractures. Clin Orthop 269:32, 1991.
22. Parker MJ, Handoll HH: Replacement arthroplasty versus internal fixation for extracapsular hip fractures. Cochrane Database Syst Rev 2:CD000086, 2000.
23. Patterson BM, Salvati EA, Huo MH: Total hip arthroplasty for complications of intertrochanteric fracture. A technical note. J Bone Joint Surg 72A:776, 1990.
24. Pho RWH, Nather A, Tong GO, Korku CT: Endoprosthetic replacement for unstable comminuted intertrochanteric fracture of the femur in the elderly, osteoporotic patient. J Trauma 21:792, 1981.
25. Pinder RC, Durnin CW, Cook PA: Leinbach prosthesis for complex intertrochanteric fractures: 180 cases. Convention Rep 3:1, 1979.
26. Rosenfeld RT, Schwartz DR, Alter AH: Prosthetic replacement for trochanteric fractures of the femur. J Bone Joint Surg 55A:420, 1973.
27. Saraglia D, Carpentier E, Gorfdeeff A, et al: Place des prothèses intermédiaires scellées dans le traitement des fractures du massif trochant rien du vieillard: propos d'une série continue de 110 prothèses. J Chir (Paris) 122:255, 1985
28. Sarathy, MP, Madhavan P, Ravichandran KM: Nonunion of intertrochanteric fractures of the femur. J Bone Joint Surg 77B:90, 1994.
29. Schuckmann P, Schuckmann W: Indikationen zur endoprotetischen Versorgung pertrochantere frakturen. Beitr Orthop Traumatol 36:279, 1989.
30. Schwenk W, Eyssel M, Badke A, et al: Risk analysis of primary endoprosthetic management of proximal femur fractures. Unfallchirurg 20:216, 1994.
31. Sonstegard DA, Kaufer H, Matthews LS: A biomechanical evaluation of implant, reduction and prosthesis in the treatment of intertrochanteric hip fractures. Orthop Clin North Am 5:551, 1974.
32. Staeheli JW, Frassica FJ, Fitzgerald RH: Camparison study of primary endoprosthetic replacement vs. CLAS for unstable intertrochanteric fractures. Orthop Trans 10:481, 1986.
33. Stappaerts KH, Deldycke J, Broos PL, et al: Treatment of unstable peritrochanteric fractures in elderly patients with a compression hip screw or with the Vandeputte (VDP) endoprosthesis: A prospective randomized study. J Orthop Trauma 9:292, 1995.
34. Stern MB, Angerman A: Comminuted intertrochanteric fractures treated with a Leinbach prosthesis. Clin Orthop 218:75, 1987.
35. Stern MB, Goldstein TB: The use of the Leinbach prosthesis in intertrochanteric fractures of the hip. Clin Orthop 128:325, 1977.
36. Stern MB, Goldstein TB: Primary treatment of comminuted intertrochanteric fractures of the hip with a Leinbach prosthesis. Int Orthop 3:67, 1979.
37. Stoffelen D, Haentjens P, Reynders P: Hip arthroplasty for failed internal fixation of intertrochanteric and subtrochanteric fractures in the elderly patient. Acta Orthop Belg 60:135, 1994.

patients. Presented at the Annual Meeting of the Orthopedic Trauma Association, Vancouver, BC, 1998.

38. Tronzo RG: The use of an endoprosthesis for severely comminuted trochanteric fractures. Orthop Clin North Am 5:679, 1974.

39. Vahl AC, Dunki Jacobs PB, Patka P, Haarman HJ: Hemiarthroplasty in elderly, debilitated patients with an unstable femoral fracture in the trochanteric region. Acta Orthop Belg 60:274, 1994.

40. van Loon CJ, de Wall Malefijt MC, Veth RP: Primary treatment of unstable pertrochanteric femoral fractures using a head-neck prosthesis in elderly patients. Ned Tijdschr Geneeskd 138:1810, 1994.

41. Wu CC, Shih CH, Chen WJ, Tai CL: Treatment of cutout of a lag screw of a dynamic hip screw in an intertrochanteric fracture. Arch Orthop Trauma Surg 117:193, 1998.

56

Total Hip Arthroplasty After Acetabular Fracture

• DAVID G. LEWALLEN

Fracture of the acetabulum is usually caused by a severe, high-energy injury that places the long-term function of the hip joint in jeopardy.[5,12,16,23,27,31,33,35] The goals of initial treatment, as in most intra-articular fractures, include restoration of major anatomic relationships, if disrupted, and perfect reduction of the joint surfaces, if significant displacement has occurred.[14,17,23] However, even when these goals are achieved, acetabular fractures carry a high rate of late post-traumatic degenerative changes, ranging up to 57 percent of fractures in some reports.[13,14,16,17,23] In addition, avascular necrosis of the femoral head is a common complication, ranging from 2 to 40 percent in reported series,[5,12–14,16,27,35] which can negate the benefits of the most perfect reduction or skilled osteosynthesis. Total hip arthroplasty is a reasonable consideration if reconstruction is required, whether for failed osteosynthesis, symptomatic joint changes, or because a particular acute fracture is not deemed reconstructable.

INDICATIONS

Established post-traumatic osteoarthritis is a well-accepted indication for joint replacement.[1–3,9,26,37] Other indications for hip arthroplasty include certain pathologic fractures, acute fractures in patients with preexistent significant symptomatic joint changes who were already candidates for hip arthroplasty before injury, and fractures in osteoporotic elderly patients with severe injuries in whom osteosynthesis is unlikely to be successful. In addition, there are rare instances with associated femoral side injuries, such as head-splitting fractures, that preclude a satisfactory result from osteosynthesis of the acetabulum.[8,18,19]

Although other procedures, such as arthrodesis, may be preferred in selected patients (e.g., the young, obese, or individuals who perform heavy manual labor), total hip arthroplasty has a definite role in the treatment of most patients who are disabled by their symptoms, particularly if they are older, more sedentary, or unwilling to accept arthrodesis.

Ipsilateral knee or lumbar spine pathology presents a relative contraindication to hip arthrodesis; hence, total hip arthroplasty may be the best surgical option in these circumstances.[7,20] Coventry reported a staged approach in which the fracture is initially reduced and fixed. If severe arthrosis was anticipated, hip replacement was performed 4 to 6 weeks later. This interval is obviously too short for healing, and one of the first reported cases failed as a result of acetabular component displacement.[6] Although more recent implant fixation methods have been used to allow acute single-stage hip arthroplasty in such cases,[19] total hip arthroplasty should generally be reserved for the late salvage of hips in which the initial treatment of acetabular fracture has failed to prevent significant joint changes and symptoms (Fig. 56–1). Total hip arthroplasty after acute acetabular fracture is rare but is occasionally indicated.[9]

TECHNIQUE

The technique for hip arthroplasty after acetabular fracture usually proceeds in a standard fashion, in many cases according to the surgeon's preference. Often, the surgical approach is complicated by prior surgical procedures and scars. When a previous posterior approach to the hip, such as the Kocher-Lagenbeck, has been employed, a choice must be made whether to formally explore and protect the sciatic nerve, which is often encased in scar, or to use an alternative approach to avoid it altogether. If a posterior approach is used for the hip arthroplasty, nerve exploration or, at least, palpation for identification is recommended. Alternatively, one can elect to avoid repeat exposure through this area of scarring in view of the difficulties encountered in formal identification and protection of the sciatic nerve and the often tedious nature of this surgical exercise. The anterolateral approach may be of great utility in this setting and may actually reduce the risk of neurologic complications in some cases (see Chapter 44). If removal of previous hardware such as plates and screws is required from the posterior column, this is more difficult from an anterolateral approach. Therefore, planned hardware

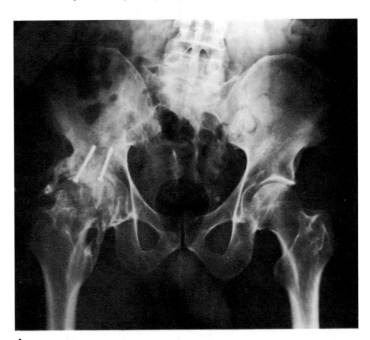

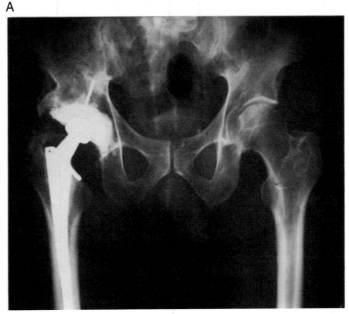

Figure 56–1. Preoperative (**A**) and 2-year postoperative (**B**) radiographs after total hip arthroplasty for post-traumatic changes caused by prior acetabular fracture. Progressive degenerative changes developed despite attempted internal fixation at the time of initial fracture.

A

B

removal may be a reason to select a posterior approach or, alternatively, a more extensile exposure such as trochanteric osteotomy.

When more extensive exposure on the acetabular side is required, conventional trochanteric osteotomy or a trochanteric slide may facilitate reconstruction of acetabular bone loss (see Chapter 44). Osteotomy of tendinous origins from the pelvis can be employed in those rare circumstances in which even wider exposure of the acetabular side is required.[14,25]

Special techniques originally developed for the management of acetabular bone deficiency encountered at revision total hip arthroplasty are often helpful when hip arthroplasty is performed after prior acetabular fracture. A variety of strategies are available depending on the specific defect encountered (see Chapter 62). Two-column support for the acetabular component and restoration of the dome and medial wall should be the goals. Morcellized cancellous graft is recommended for residual cavitary-contained defects on the acetabular side, and structural grafts are reserved for large segmental defects that are not reconstructable without restoration of mechanical support. Internal fixation is routinely employed for structural graft fixation and can range from simple lag screws to multiple pelvic reconstruction plates or antiprotrusio cages, depending on the extent and location of the bony deficiency encountered (see Chapter 62). Rigid internal fixation plus bone grafting are essential when nonunion or major bony discontinuities are encountered at arthroplasty.

Conventional primary arthroplasty methods are entirely sufficient in patients with minimal residual deformity or bone loss. The vast majority of these patients are currently treated with an uncemented porous ingrowth cup after bony reconstruction of the acetabulum.[1] Every effort is made to maximize support for the porous cup on intact patient bone to increase the potential surface area available for bone ingrowth. This is critically important because rates of cup migration, loosening, and revision have been shown to increase significantly when the surface area behind the cup in contact with bone graft increases beyond 50 percent.[22] Adjunctive screw fixation of the porous-coated acetabular cup is frequently employed but is not necessary if excellent cup support and contact are achieved in cases with minimal deformity (Fig. 56–2).

A cemented polyethylene cup remains a viable choice when acetabular bone stock is osteoporotic but relatively intact. In the elderly patient, the use of methyl methacrylate as a "filler" for large bone defects, however, is to be avoided, particularly in critical weight-bearing locations such as the acetabular dome (Fig. 56–3).

POSTOPERATIVE MANAGEMENT

Depending on the stability of the construct, modification of the standard postoperative regimen may be required. In some cases, delays in full weight bearing for 3 months or longer are necessary if healing of an inter-

nally fixed nonunion or incorporation of large areas of bone grafting is required. Heterotopic ossification may complicate the postoperative course, particularly if it is present before arthroplasty as a result of the original fracture or a previous osteosynthesis. Heterotopic bone present at the time of arthroplasty should be excised and postoperative prophylaxis against ectopic bone formation considered. My routine prophylaxis involves low-dose radiation treatment with shielding of uncemented components, fracture lines, or bone graft. Use of certain nonsteroidal anti-inflammatory drugs, such as indomethacin, for prophylaxis is the alternative, particularly in younger patients, for whom there is a wish to avoid even low-dose radiation treatment (see Chapter 66).[4,28,29] However, in general, an attempt is made to avoid the use of radiation treatment or indomethacin when significant bone grafting has been carried out in order to prevent possible adverse effects on graft incorporation and bone healing.

RESULTS

Acute Fracture

The most definitive experience with acute fracture has been reported by Mears et al.[20] Over a 13-year period, 57 procedures were performed, with a mean surveillance of 8 years, in a group averaging 69 years of age. A mean Harris Hip Score of 89 was documented, and 79 percent

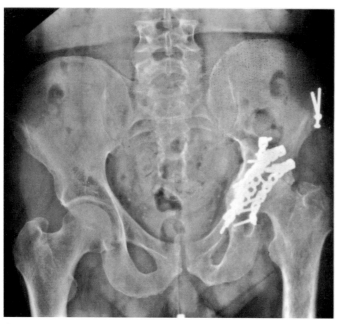

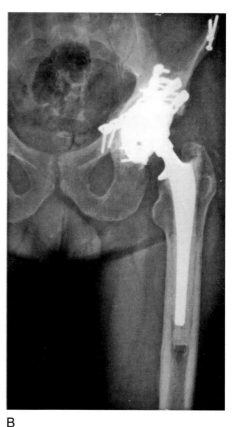

A   B

Figure 56–2. A, Post-traumatic changes after prior internal fixation of a T-fracture. **B**, Use of hybrid fixation allows acetabular morcellized bone grafting, with excellent result at 2 years.

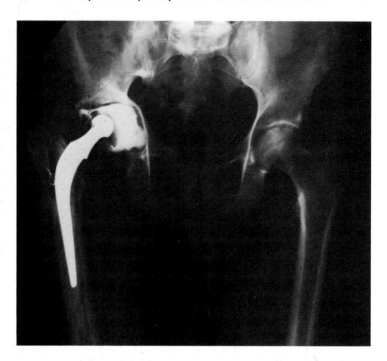

Figure 56–3. Reconstruction of acetabular deficiency resulting from previous acetabular fracture deformity with a large bolus of cement and a relatively undersized, all-polyethylene cup. Note the radiolucent zone at the cement-bone interface, which is the radiographic evidence of acetabular loosening.

had a satisfactory outcome (Fig. 56–4). Subsidence averaging 2 to 3 mm was noted with subsequent stabilization of the cup.

Established Arthrosis: Cemented Acetabular Fixation

Using cemented acetabular fixation, Boardman and Charnley found acceptable results in 66 patients with short term follow-up (mean, 3.5 years).[3,15] Little information was provided by these investigators regarding radiographic loosening rates or appearance, and there were no revisions performed. Their study does suggest that initial results after cemented total hip arthroplasty do not seem to be adversely affected by a prior history of acetabular fracture.[3] Malkin and Tauber reported satisfactory results in using the femoral head as bone graft on the acetabular side in 2 patients so treated.[15]

Mayo Experience

In a review of the Mayo experience with cemented hip arthroplasty in patients with previous acetabular fracture. Romness and Lewallen studied 55 primary total hip arthroplasties in 53 patients[26] with a history of previous acetabular fracture operated between 1970 and 1984. These patients were reviewed retrospectively, at a mean follow-up of 7.5 years, and results were compared and contrasted with 10-year results of cemented total hip arthroplasty, as reported by Stauffer from the same institution.[30] Follow-up ranged from 7 days to 16.6 years, and the average age at fracture was 48.7 years (range, 15 to 83 years). The average age at arthroplasty, 56.2 years (range, 19 to 91 years), was younger than that

usually seen in hip arthroplasty series. Average time from fracture to arthroplasty was 7.8 years (range, 2 months to 45 years). Degenerative changes were present to a significant degree in all hips preoperatively, with 11 percent showing radiographic changes sufficient to allow the diagnosis of avascular necrosis of the femoral head, in an era before magnetic resonance imaging was available.

The original fractures were categorized according to Tile's modification of Letournel and Judet's classification,[14,33] with the majority involving the posterior column, posterior wall, or a combination of the two. Eighty-nine percent of the original fractures were displaced. However, only 22 percent underwent open reduction and internal fixation, a reflection of treatment philosophy during the era in which many of these fractures occurred. Two hips underwent separate bone grafting procedures before the arthroplasty, and only 3 hips underwent bone grafting at the time of the hip arthroplasty.

Criteria for radiographic loosening were identical to those described by Stauffer[29] to allow comparison of results between the two series. Results on the femoral side were remarkably similar to those reported by Stauffer although in a younger patient population and reported at a shorter mean follow-up (7.5 years versus 10 years). Stauffer found a femoral loosening rate of 29.9 percent by radiography, with 12.2 percent symptomatic and 6.1 percent revised. Romness found femoral loosening in 29.4 percent, with 15.7 percent symptomatic and 7.8 percent revised. Results on the acetabular side were not similar, however.

Stauffer found radiographic loosening of the acetabulum in 11.3 percent at 10 years, symptomatic loosening in 5.2 percent, and revision in 3.0 percent. With a history of prior acetabular fracture at arthroplasty, acetabular loosening by radiography occurred in 54.4 percent, sympto-

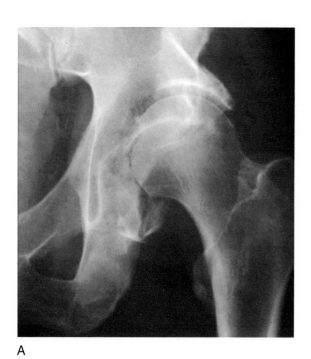

A

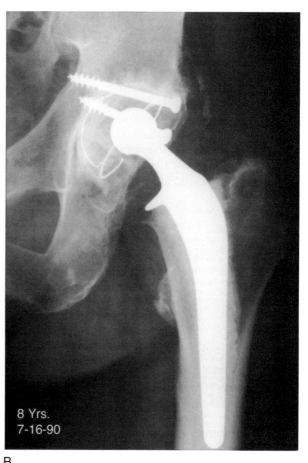

B

Figure 56–4. Preoperative radiograph (**A**) and satisfactory 8-year postoperative radiograph (**B**) of a cemented total hip arthroplasty performed acutely after acetabular fracture. Poor bone quality, fracture comminution, and articular damage had combined to make a successful result from osteosynthesis of the fracture unlikely.

matic loosening occurred in 31.6 percent, and revision had been carried out in 15.7 percent. This demonstrates that the rates of acetabular component loosening and subsequent revision in patients undergoing cemented total hip arthroplasty after prior acetabular fracture are five to six times higher than the rates seen in conventional cemented total hip arthroplasty (Fig. 56–5). One conclusion of this study was that compromised acetabular bone stock from the prior fracture might be contributing to the higher acetabular failure rates.

No failures occurred in 5 cases in which acetabular bone grafting was performed either before or during the total hip arthroplasty, even though this grafting was presumably done in instances of severe bony compromise. These results suggest that reconstruction of bony anatomy after acetabular fractures with significant displacement may have late benefits by facilitating subsequent hip arthroplasty, should this be required, even if the reconstruction has been unsuccessful in preventing post-traumatic degenerative changes. This remains a controversial point, however. A reported study by Karpos et al. compared patients undergoing total hip arthroplasty who had previously had an open reduction and internal fixation for their acetabular fracture with another group in whom treatment of the acetabular frac-

ture had originally been nonoperative.[11] A higher incidence of problems with heterotopic bone removal, excision of extensive scarring or neurolysis, and increased need for structural bone grafting was observed in those patients with prior open reduction and internal fixation. Although this study involved uncemented acetabular components, the problems encountered would be expected to be independent of the type of cup fixation selected.

Uncemented Acetabular Fixation

The advent of biologically fixed acetabular components with adjunctive screw fixation brought about interest in the use of these implants in arthroplasty patients with prior acetabular fracture (see Fig. 56–2). Beginning in the early 1990s, variable results from small series and case reports began to appear.[10,11,24,36] Excellent functional results were reported by Karpos et al. in both patients with a history of prior internal fixation and those originally treated closed.[11] Pritchett and Bortel reported on 19 patients with prior acetabular fracture who required total hip arthroplasty that used a cementless acetabular component and either a cemented or cementless femoral

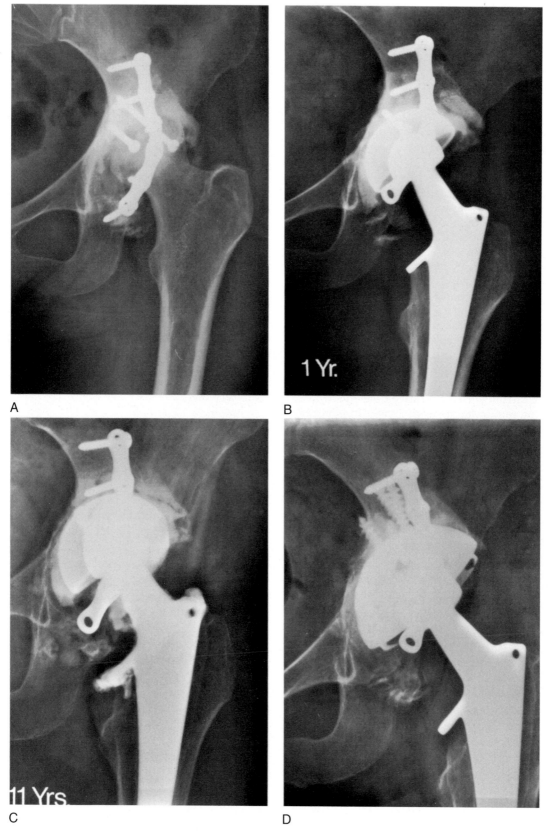

A

B

C

D

Figure 56–5. A 38-year-old woman developed severe arthrosis after a posterior acetabular wall fracture (**A**) 1 year after replacement with cemented metal-backed cup (**B**). At 11 years, gross loosening and pain (**C**) required reoperation. Her hip was readily revised with a biologically fixed cup. The femoral component was solid (**D**).

stem.[24] All patients were followed for a minimum of 2 years, and the mean Harris Hip Score for the series was 84, with no revisions or radiographically loose implants apparent over the period of initial follow-up. Waddell reported on 34 patients with 3-year average follow-up results and also noted initial good results and no loosening or revisions.[36]

Bellabarba et al. reported on 30 hip arthroplasties performed for prior acetabular fracture, all treated with the same porous fiber metal acetabular component.[1] In these 30 cases, 15 had originally received open and 15 closed fracture treatment. Results were compared between the two fracture treatment groups and then with a control group of routine primary arthroplasties without a fracture history. In the groups with prior acetabular fracture, the time from fracture to arthroplasty ranged from 8 months to 37 years, but averaged just over 3 years. Age at arthroplasty averaged 51 years; therefore, similar to previous studies, these patients were younger than the usual arthroplasty population. At an average follow-up postarthroplasty of more than 5 years, implant survivorship with revision or radiographic loosening as the endpoint was 97 percent, and good or excellent results were seen in 90 percent of patients. These results were similar and not statistically different from those seen in the nonfractured cohort. These authors did show that operative time, blood loss, and transfusion requirements were greater in postfracture patients than in the routine arthroplasty group. Also, patients with prior open reduction and internal fixation required longer operative time, more blood, and more frequent need of elevated cup liners to improve hip stability intraoperatively. The closed treatment patients, however, were more likely to require bone grafting of an acetabular defect than were those with previous open reduction and internal fixation. This study shows that the fixation problems encountered with cemented acetabular components in patients with a prior acetabular fracture should be much reduced by the use of uncemented porous ingrowth components and more current methods of bone defect management. Technical difficulties in these patients may include prior surgical scarring, presence of heterotopic bone, residual bone defects or deformity, and the possibility of low-grade infection around hardware used for prior open reduction and internal fixation.

Joly and co-workers documented the potential for problems in arthroplasty cases in which prior internal fixation was performed for severe or displaced fracture patterns.[10] Patients in this series were younger than those reported on in prior studies, averaging 38 years of age and ranging from 12 to 71 years of age. At follow-up, 12 of 30 had failed at an average of only 23 months. Causes of failure included massive heterotopic ossification, implant loosening, and deep infection.[10] Clearly, patients with prior major acetabular injury, and particularly those with residual bone deficits or deformity, will continue to present significant challenges at the time of hip arthroplasty.

SUMMARY

Acetabular fracture places the long-term performance of the hip in jeopardy. If nonreconstructable damage occurs to the joint at the time of injury, primary total hip arthroplasty acutely may be reasonable, especially in the older patient. If fracture treatment is undertaken but is unsuccessful because of failure to achieve fracture union, development of post-traumatic degenerative changes, or avascular necrosis, total hip arthroplasty offers the best subsequent reconstructive option. When disabling symptoms result from joint changes from a prior acetabular fracture, hip arthroplasty using an uncemented acetabular component is the recommended procedure. Despite the successful record of uncemented component fixation combined with cancellous bone grafting, a history of prior fracture can still significantly lengthen and complicate the reconstructive procedures needed during arthroplasty and may exert an adverse effect on long-term performance in some patients. Significant bone deficiency, residual deformity, nonunion, soft tissue scarring, or prior infection can all exert adverse effects on the function and durability of these arthroplasties. Continuing advances in implant design and methods for management of bone deficiency may allow further improvement in the results achieved for these patients.

References

1. Bellabarba C, Berger RA, Bentley CD, et al: Cementless acetabular reconstruction after acetabular fracture. J Bone Joint Surg 83A:868, 2001.
2. Berry DJ: Total hip arthroplasty following acetabular fracture. Orthop 22:837, 1999.
3. Boardman KP, Charnley J: Low-friction arthroplasty after fracture-dislocations of the hip. J Bone Joint Surg 60B:495, 1978.
4. Busse JM, Poka A, Reinert CM, et al: Heterotopic ossification as a complication of acetabular fracture: Prophylaxis with low-dose irradiation. J Bone Joint Surg 70A:1231, 1988.
5. Carnesale PG, Stewart MJ, Barnes SN: Acetabular disruption and central fracture-dislocation of the hip: A long-term study. J Bone Joint Surg 57A:1054, 1975.
6. Coventry MB: Treatment of fracture-dislocation of the hip. J Bone Joint Surg 56A:1128, 1974.
7. Greiss ME, Thomas RJ, Freeman MAR: Sequelae of arthrodesis of the hip. J R Soc Med 73:497, 1980.
8. Hamer AJ, Stockley I: Acetabular fracture treated by primary hip arthroplasty. Injury 25:399, 1994.
9. Jimenez ML, Tile M, Schenk RS: Total hip replacement after acetabular fracture. Orthop Clin North Am 28:435, 1997.
10. Joly JM, Mears DC, Skura DS: Total hip arthroplasty following failed acetabular fracture open reduction/internal fixation. Orthop Trans 17:109, 1993.
11. Karpos PAG, Christie MJ, Chenger JD: Total hip arthroplasty following acetabular fracture: The effect of prior ORIF. Mid Am Trans 52, 1993.
12. Larson CB: Fracture dislocations of the hip. Clin Orthop 151:81, 1980.
13. Letournel E: Acetabular fractures. Clin Orthop 151:81, 1980.
14. Letournel E, Judet R: Fracture of the Acetabulum. Berlin, Springer-Verlag, 1981.
15. Malkin C, Tauber C: Total hip arthroplasty and acetabular bone grafting for unreduced fracture-dislocation of the hip. Clin Orthop 201:5759, 1985.

16. Matta JM, Anderson LM, Epstein HC, et al: Fractures of the acetabulum: A retrospective analysis. Clin Orthop 205:230, 1986.

17. Matta J, Mernt P: Displaced acetabular fractures. Clin Orthop 230:83, 1988.

18. Mears DC: Total hip replacement for acute management of acetabular fractures. Orthop Trans 16:88, 1992

19. Mears DC: Surgical treatment of acetabular fractures in elderly patients with osteoporotic bone. J AAOS 7:128, 1999.

20. Mears D, Velyvis J: Acute total hip arthroplasty for selected displaced acetabular fractures. J Bone Joint Surg 84A:1, 2002.

21. Missiuua PC, Dewar RD: Long-term sequelae of hip fusion surgery. Orthop Trans 12:672, 1988.

22. Patch DA, Lewallen DG: Reconstruction of deficient acetabular using bone graft and a fixed porous ingrowth cup: A 5 year roentgenographic survey. Orthop Trans 17:151, 1993.

23. Pennal GF, Davidson J, Garside H, Plewes J: Results of treatment of acetabular fractures. Clin Orthop 151:115, 1980.

24. Pritchett JW, Bortel DT: Total hip replacement after central fracture dislocation of the acetabulum. Orthop Rev 20:607, 1991.

25. Reinert CM, Busse MJ, Poka A, et al: A modified extensile exposure for the treatment of complex or malunited acetabular fractures. J Bone Joint Surg 70A:329, 1988.

26. Romness DW, Lewallen DG: Long-term results of total hip arthroplasty after prior fracture of the acetabulum. J Bone Joint Surg 72B:761, 1990.

27. Rowe CR, Lowell JD: Prognosis of fractures of the acetabulum. J Bone Joint Surg 43A:30, 1961.

28. Schmidt SA, Kjaersgaard-Anderson P, Pederson NW, et al: The use of indomethacin to prevent the formation of heterotopic bone after total hip replacement: A randomized, double-blind clinical trial. J Bone Joint Surg 70A:834, 1988.

29. Sodemann B, Persson PE, Nilsson OS: Prevention of heterotopic ossification by nonsteroidal anti-inflammatory drugs after total hip arthroplasty. Clin Orthop 237:158, 1988.

30. Stauffer RN: Ten-year follow-up study of total hip replacement. J Bone Joint Surg 64A:983, 1982.

31. Stewart MJ, Mildort LW: Fracture dislocation of the hip: An end result study. J Bone Joint Surg 36A:315, 1954.

32. Tew M, Waugh W: Estimating the survival time of knee replacements. J Bone Joint Surg 65B:579, 1982.

33. Tile M: Fractures of acetabulum. Orthop Clin North Am 11:481, 1980.

34. Tile M: Fractures of the Pelvis and Acetabulum. Baltimore, Williams & Wilkins, 1984, p 177.

35. Urist MR: Fracture dislocation of the hip joint, the nature of the traumatic lesion, treatment, late complication and late results. J Bone Joint Surg 30A:699, 1948.

36. Waddell JP, Morton RN: Total hip arthroplasty following acetabular fracture. Transactions of the 1994 Annual Meeting, Los Angeles. Los Angeles, Orthop Trauma Assoc Trans 88, 1994.

37. Weber M, Berry DJ, Harmsen WS: Total hip arthroplasty after operative treatment of an acetabular fracture. J Bone Joint Surg 80A:1294, 1998.

57

Avascular Necrosis

• FRANK J. FRASSICA, DANIEL J. BERRY, and BERNARD F. MORREY

In the young patient, avascular necrosis (AVN) of the femoral head is a common indication for hip replacement. New cases are diagnosed at a rate of 10,000 to 20,000 per year, with approximately 500,000 individuals having the disease at any given time.[58] The many etiologies of AVN may arise from different pathophysiology but, possibly, a common final pathway. Treatment of AVN of the femoral head remains controversial and varies, depending on the stage of disease, degree of head involvement, age and expectations of the patient, and perceived effectiveness of the intervention.

Hence, we briefly discuss the etiologies, clinical features, staging, radiographic features, and natural history of the femoral head in the adult patient. The classical treatise by Glimcher and Kenzora is an exhaustive analysis of the etiology and pathologic sequelae and remains relevant to all those interested in these features of the disease.[31] The effectiveness of hip replacement is placed in the context of other options.

ETIOLOGIES

Increasing evidence is being accumulated to better define the nature of the AVN and reparative process associated with the vascular insult. The magnitude and effect of the reparative process are dependent on both the extent of the insult and the activity of the local reparative cells. This reparative process weakens the subchondral bone resulting in collapse, after which there is little hope that the hip joint can continue to function as a painless, weight-bearing structure or that it can be reliably salvaged short of joint replacement. For a detailed current review of the various theories causing this problem, the reader is referred to the 2000 instructional course lecture by Mont et al.[58]

Alcoholism, corticosteroid usage, and trauma are the most commonly identified etiologies. Organ transplantation is associated with a high incidence because of the requirement of steroid therapy. Idiopathic AVN (i.e., that for which there is no known etiology) completes the list of the most common etiologies. There are many other precipitating conditions that are uncommon but not necessarily rare, including hemoglobinopathies, Gaucher's disease, Caisson's disease, hematologic neoplasia, systemic lupus erythematosus, pancreatitis, irra-

diation, hyperuricemia, and pregnancy (Table 57–1). Bilateral involvement has been reported in 50 percent to 80 percent of cases.[60]

CLINICAL FEATURES

Patients between 20 and 60 years of age have severe pain over the anterior aspect of the hip, which is worsened with weight bearing and motion of the hip. The pain may be of acute or insidious onset, often with steady progression. Symptoms in the early stages are from effusion and synovitis and from mechanical catching of the separated cartilage in the latter stages.

On examination, an antalgic gait and a positive Trendelenburg sign are common. The hip may be irritable, and gentle range of motion is intensely uncomfortable. Active motion of the hip often causes such intense pain that the patient may be unwilling or unable to flex the hip while supine, especially against resistance. In our experience, these intense symptoms are caused by an initial synovitis that accompanies the acute process.

DIAGNOSIS

There is no single test that is 100 percent reliable to make this diagnosis. However, several studies have shown with some degree of consistency that magnetic resonance imaging (MRI) is approximately 95 percent sensitive and approximately 70 percent specific, leading to an overall accuracy of about 90 percent.[29,36] The bone scan, in contrast, is about 85 percent sensitive and 80 percent specific, with an overall accuracy of about 85 percent.[80,83] The MRI can become positive within 24 hours of insult and one study has used MRI to document the insult a mean of 3.6 months after initiation of steroid use.[22,71] Although it is recognized that occasionally the technetium bone scan may become positive even with a negative MRI,[80] most investigators who have compared these various modalities indicate that MRI is the most reliable mode of diagnosis.[51,70] Because the MRI also provides all-important information about the extent and location of involvement,[58] it is encouraging to see techniques emerging to reduce the cost and increase the effectiveness of the MRI.[48]

Table 57–1. POSSIBLE ETIOLOGIES OF
AVASCULAR NECROSIS

Traumatic
Osseous compartment dysfunction
   Dysbaric (Caisson's disease)
   Gaucher's disease
   Sickle cell disease
   Pancreatitis
   Steroids
   Alcohol
Vascular insult
   Subacute bacterial endocarditis
   Disseminated intravascular coagulation
   Polycythemia rubra vera
   Systemic lupus erythematosus
   Polyarteritis nodosa
   Rheumatoid arthritis
   Giant cell arteritis
   Sarcoid
Metabolic
   Diabetes
   Hyperuricemia
   Blood lipid disorders
Idiopathic

Table 57–2. STAGING SYSTEM OF FICAT AND
ARLET

Stage	0	Preclinical, normal radiograph
Stage	I	Painful hip with normal radiographs
Stage	II	Painful hip with normal femoral head contour with mixed lysis and sclerosis
Stage	III	Painful hip with subchondral collapse and sequestrum formation
Stage	IV	Painful hip with a narrowed joint space and collapse of the femoral head

Hence, when plain radiographs, including oblique views of the hip, are normal and the history and physical examination are consistent with AVN, MRI is a logical next step.

STAGING

Accurate staging of disease progression is most important because options and outcomes of nonreplacement treatment are predicated on these data. In addition to planning treatment, staging helps provide a basis for counseling the patient and comparing the results of surgical intervention. Traditional staging systems are based on anteroposterior, lateral, and frog-leg radiographs of the hip. Although the system described by Marcus et al. is rather detailed,[56] the classification of Ficat and Arlet, which has been modified and updated by Steinberg,[81] continues to be the one most widely used (Table 57–2).[24] The classic radiographic finding of a so-called crescent sign is best demonstrated on the frog-leg lateral projection (see Fig. 57–1). This sign represents subchondral fracture and is pathognomonic for a stage of involvement that cannot be reversed by any current modalities of surgical intervention.

There is no accepted MRI classification system to describe the stages of AVN. However, Mitchell and co-workers have proposed a system based on the MRI signal (Table 57–3).[57] Using this system, a reasonable correlation was found, with the MRI intensity classes A and B being roughly equivalent to stages 1 and 2, and MRI classes C and D roughly equivalent to stage 3 and greater by the radiographic staging systems. That the duration, extent, and distribution of the process is much more accurately defined than has before been possible (Fig. 57–2) has significant treatment implications. As a matter of fact, Sugano et al. have documented the important observation that if the MRI reveals that the contralateral hip is disease free, the likelihood is that this hip will not become involved.[85]

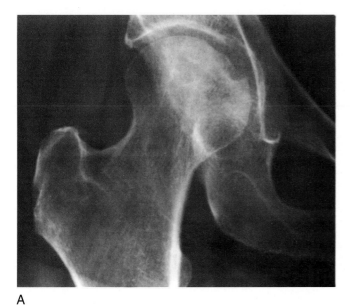

A

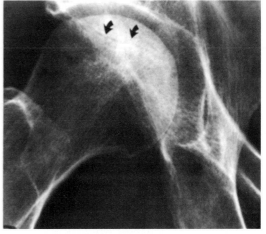

B

Figure 57–1. The frog-leg lateral is the plain view that best demonstrates the crescent sign, which is indicative of subchondral collapse precluding intervention to alter the natural history.

Table 57–3. CORRELATION OF MAGNETIC RESONANCE IMAGING INTENSITY CLASS AND RADIOGRAPHIC STAGE*

MRI Intensity Class	Radiographic Stage	
	I, II[†] (n = 28)	III, IV, V[‡] (n = 28)
A (n = 24)	20 (83)	4 (17)
B (n = 6)	4 (67)	2 (33)
C (n = 14)	4 (29)	10 (71)
D (n = 12)	0	12 (100)

*Data show numbers of hips. Numbers in parentheses indicate percentage of magnetic resonance imaging (MRI) intensity class.
[†]No fracture.
[‡]Fracture.
From Mitchell DG, Rao VM, Dalinka MK, et al: Femoral head avascular necrosis: Correlation of MR imaging, radiographic staging, radionuclide imaging, and clinical findings. Radiology 162:705; 1987.

We have observed with our prospective study that, although traditional MRI is very sensitive to the early stages of the disease, it is a poor modality for following the progression or healing of the process.[7] However, advances use "dynamic" MRI with Gd-DTPA enhancement, a signal representing bone vitality, vascularization, and perfusion after intervention was obtained.[78]

NATURAL HISTORY

The most effective approach to treating AVN of the hip is based on a knowledge of the natural history of the untreated disease for a given etiology and stage of presentation.[17] The natural history of this process is becoming increasingly clear. It has been demonstrated that the lesion can, in fact, heal. Ohzono et al. followed a group of 115 hips with nontraumatic AVN with an average follow-up of more than 5 years.[60] The less involved heads showed up to 91 percent without progression or collapse. With more extensive involvement, even in the early stages, 88 percent of patients advanced from stage II to stage III. Collapse occurred most often when the focus of bone necrosis occupied the weight bearing surface and involved more than 50 percent of the articular surface.[60]

To address the issue of untreated early (Ficat stage I or II) disease, we followed a group of 24 hips with total hip arthroplasty (THA) on one side and an uninvolved (Ficat II or less) contralateral joint.[10] Eight in 24 hips (33 percent) had progressed to collapse by 1 year, and 20 in 24 (83 percent) had collapsed by 3 years (Fig. 57–3). All 24 stage Ficat II hips or those with an earlier stage of disease eventually showed collapse at a mean of 23 months (range, 6 to 63 months). It is important to recognize that these hips were in patients who had rapidly progressed on the opposite side to THA, and who may have been a group with disease features predisposing them to rapid disease progression. Others report that stages I and II of Ficat disease have an estimated timeframe of 9 months before collapse, as predicted by the Kaplan-Meier method. Pavlovcic et al. and Ito et al., on the other hand, reported that 64 percent of patients were asymptomatic 6 years after the diagnoses, especially if the lesion was small.[41,63] In one study, only one of 24 normal hips in patients with AVN in the contralateral joint had progressed at 5 years.[43,85] Clearly, there is much variability in the rate and severity of disease progression in different patient groups. We hope that in the future, stratification for age, diagnosis, etiology of osteonecrosis, stage, lesion size, and lesion location will allow more accurate prediction of prognosis.

Until a better understanding of the natural history of the untreated disease process becomes available, it is

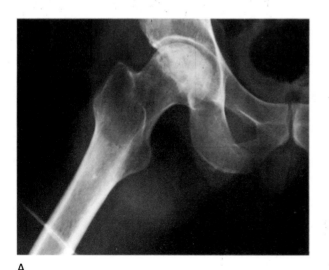

A

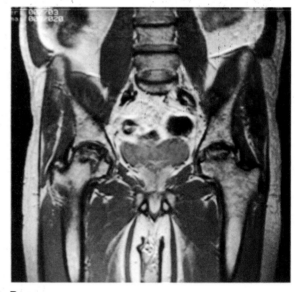

B

Figure 57–2. The extensive process shown in the oblique radiograph (**A**) is more clearly defined by the magnetic resonance imaging study (**B**).

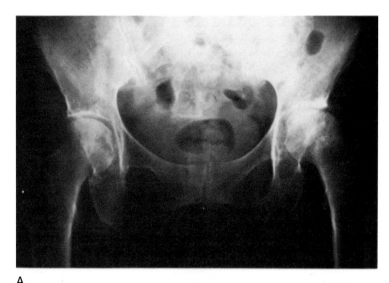

A

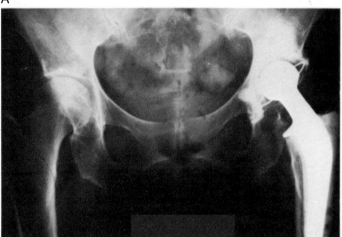

B

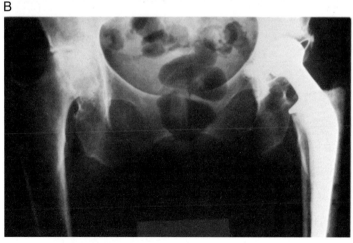

C

Figure 57–3. Patient with stage IV avascular necrosis on the left with a Ficat I hip replacement on the right (**A**). Three years after hip replacement on the left, the opposite hip had not progressed (**B**), but it then progressed to collapse 2 years later (**C**).

difficult to clearly define the indications for observation versus intervention. However, the results of surgical intervention are also obscured by the varied stages in which these treatment modalities have been introduced, adding additional complexity to the accurate analysis of the literature.

TREATMENTS

Treating early stages of AVN of the hip is controversial. Because no treatment modality to date has been shown to be entirely effective in preventing the natural history of the disease process, observation continues to be an acceptable strategy for the asymptomatic hip.[43] We discuss nonreplacement treatment because it is important to place arthroplasty in the proper perspective as a treatment modality.

Nonsurgical Intervention

Pulsed Electromagnetic Field

This technique has been reported to delay the progression and occurrence of subchondral collapse. Thirty-two percent of patients treated with the pulsed electromagnetic field technique were considered failures compared with 56 percent treated with core decompression.[1] Results are better when employed in the early stages of the process; however, the data are incomplete and recommendations regarding the use of this modality cannot be made at this time.

Surgical Options

No Subchondral Collapse

When the sphericity of the femoral head has not been compromised by subchondral fracture or collapse (stage I or II), core decompression continues to be considered as an acceptable form of treatment.

CLINICAL RESULTS

In 1985, Ficat reported 94 percent good results in 82 patients with stage I disease and 82 percent good results in 51 patients with stage II disease[26] (Fig. 57–4). Subsequent investigators, however, have reported quite

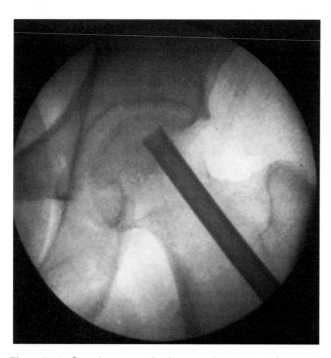

Figure 57–4. Core decompression in a precollapse stage of avascular necrosis.

different results.[94,96] With stage I or II disease, Camp and Colwell demonstrated that 60 percent of patients had a radiographic progression and clinical radiographic failure within 18 months after core decompression.[13] In addition, post- or intraoperative fracture occurred in 4 patients. The latest follow-up revealed further progression in 17 percent with type I disease, 58 percent in those with type IIA disease, and 100 percent in all patients with type IIB disease.[13] In South Africa, Learmonth and colleagues also reported disappointing results after decompression in 41 hips with stage I or II osteonecrosis, with a mean follow-up of 31 months.[53] Clinical or radiographic deterioration occurred in 75 percent of those with stage I disease and 86 percent of those with stage II osteonecrosis. Similarly poor results have been described by others.[38] Yet, Stulberg et al. recommend the procedure based on 70 percent of patients achieving "radiographic and clinical success."[82] A series of recent studies has offered compelling data of more than 90 percent success if decompression is done early, especially in patients with stage I disease.

At the Mayo Clinic, 100 patients with stage I or II disease have been prospectively followed in over 5 years. Approximately half were treated with core decompression and half were treated by observation alone. Although the analysis is not complete, we have not been able to demonstrate any alteration in the rate of progression of the disease process between these two patient populations. The core decompression did, however, relieve pain in approximately 75 percent of this sample.[7]

Subchondral Collapse

CORE AND BONE GRAFTING RESULTS

Currently, the vascularized graft continues to be a popular bone graft technique.[30,76,91] Since the technique was popularized by Bonfigilo and Voke,[9] there have been relatively few reports on the value of stabilizing the avascular section with bone graft.[77]

Daley et al. updated the experience of Bonfigilo and reported that 57 percent of 31 procedures in patients with stage I and stage II disease had satisfactory results, with follow-up ranging from 4 to 27 years.[18] Buckley et al. reviewed 18 of 20 patients and found no progression of the necrosis or collapse after autogenous tibial graft for stage I or stage II atraumatic osteonecrosis.[11] In 2 patients (10 percent), collapse did occur, requiring hip joint replacement.

Urbaniak believes that even more extensive involvement is a suitable indication for vascularized fibula grafting. With follow-up ranging from 8 months to 6 years, only 3 of 50 patients had progressed to the point of requiring hip joint replacement. Femoral head collapse did occur in 3, and a fourth patient had mild or moderate pain.[91] A similar experience was reported by Kane et al. with an 80 percent success rate.[45] Louie et al. report no further surgery at 4 years in 73 percent of 55 patients with vascularized grafts.[54] The procedure is not without risk, however, with an incidence of 2.5 percent intertrochanteric fractures.[2]

Femoral Head Collapse (stages III and IV)

Treatment after subchondral fracture and collapse of the femoral head has occurred (Ficat stages III and IV) is difficult. Interventions have included osteotomy,[27,86] osteochondral allograft, muscle pedicle grafts, vascularized fibular grafts,[91] and prosthetic arthroplasty.[87] Intertrochanteric osteotomy is usually reserved for patients with a limited amount of femoral head involvement, thereby allowing satisfactory delivery or containment of the lesion within the constraints of correction allowed by the osteotomy.

Osteotomy. The amount of femoral head involvement that can be treated by intertrochanteric osteotomy depends to some extent on the location of the lesion. Nevertheless, most agree that lesions encompassing a combined arc of more than 200 degrees (a number obtained by combining the angle subtended by the lesion on the anteroposterior radiograph with the angle subtended on the frog lateral radiographs) are usually not amenable to successful treatment with osteotomy. The limitations to realignment relate to the need to avoid creating a proximal femoral deformity that would make a subsequent hip arthroplasty much more difficult.

Results. Reports on the success of osteotomy have appeared from around the world. After 45 osteotomies, 87 percent had grade III or IV collapse at an average follow-up of 5 years; 60 percent were pain free and 40 percent had satisfactory function. However, it was noted that these patients continued to deteriorate, indicating that osteotomy did not appear to be a long-term solution, particularly in those with more extensive involvement.[59] Maistrelli and co-workers[55] reported an Italian experience with 106 procedures in patients with stage II or greater disease. At follow-up, averaging 8 years, 44 percent of the varus-producing and 41 percent of the valgus-producing osteotomies were considered successful (Fig. 57–5). A report from South Africa on 45 hips, all with type III disease, were followed for an average of 5.5 years.[78] After a valgus flexion osteotomy, 80 percent were considered acceptable without additional procedures at 5 years of follow-up. Patients at risk were those older than 45 years of age with systemic disease, taking certain medications, such as steroids, and those with more extensive involvement. In this country, Jacobs et al. reported on 22 varus-flexion osteotomies with an average follow-up of 5 years.[42] Initially, 73 percent were considered satisfactory; however, at 5 years, less than 50 percent of the sample had a satisfactory outcome. Once again, the best results were achieved with removal of small lesions in a young patient with early-stage disease.

Rotational osteotomy. Rotational osteotomy, popularized by Sugioka in 1983, has been the source of considerable interest, if not controversy, ever since.[86]

Results. Reporting on 158 cases with follow-up averaging approximately 7 years and ranging from 2 to 11 years, Sugioka noted success in 86 percent of patients with stage I and II disease. Furthermore, if one third of the surface was preserved, 95 percent of patients were considered to have a successful outcome.[86] Emphasis was placed on the surgical technique and on obtaining adequate rotation. The complication rate was only 4 percent.[86]

In the United States, two series have reported a 60-percent failure rate among 17 patients at 3 years.[89] From the Mayo Clinic, 18 patients who were followed an average of 5 years[20] revealed radiographic and clinical progression in 15 (87 percent). Twelve had undergone total hip replacement at the time of the report.

In what is a classic study, Ohzono et al. reviewed the results of 4 procedures designed to preserve the joint space and compared these with results from a group of patients without treatment.[60] Although core decompression was performed in patients at earlier stages, clinical and radiographic success was present in only approximately 50 percent. Bone grafting seemed to improve the outcome slightly in patients with stage II disease. Rotational osteotomy was successful in more than 60 percent of cases by both clinical and roentgenographic criteria, and a limited number of varus-producing osteotomies were all successful at the time of the follow-up. These investigators indicated that joint preservation operations were not successful in altering the natural history of the disease compared with the status of hips for which no treatment was offered. The investigators were particularly concerned that core decompression weakened the neck and might have hastened collapse. Regardless, all agreed that further collapse was primarily a function of the size of the lesion.[42,55,60,75]

Joint Replacement Arthroplasty

Four broad categories of joint replacement can be classified for the treatment of avascular necrosis: resurfacing arthroplasty, metaphyseal "conservative" replacement, bipolar replacement, and stemmed total hip arthroplasty. For all options, fixation with or without cement is available.

RESURFACING ARTHROPLASTY

Resurfacing arthroplasty and metaphyseal fixation options are discussed in Chapters 50 and 51. In spite of attractive theoretical value, the disappointing short- and long-term results have reported a high early failure rate of 16 percent to 43 percent within 2 to 8 years of surgery (Fig. 57–6).[3,14,21,26,37,44]

In addition, although surface replacement is a bone-preserving procedure at the proximal femur, a substantial portion of the acetabular bone stock is removed to accommodate the large femoral surface replacement prosthesis. The thickness of the high-density polyethylene of the acetabular cups is limited by the relatively large femoral head and the removal of normal acetabular bone stock. A thin acetabular cup is a disadvantage when the potential of polyethylene

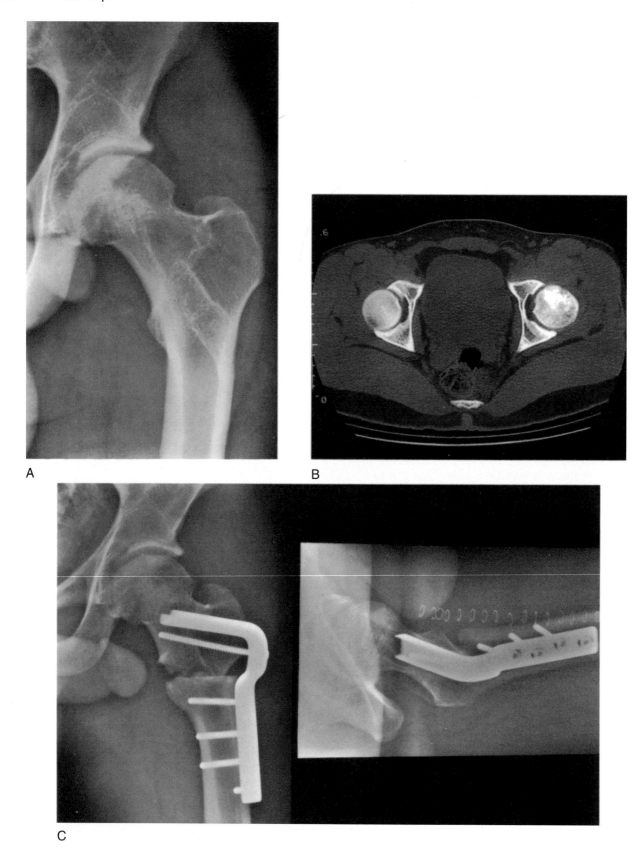

Figure 57–5. Painful collapse after core decompression (**A**) involving 60 percent of the femoral head (**B**). A valgus flexion osteotomy was done (**C**).

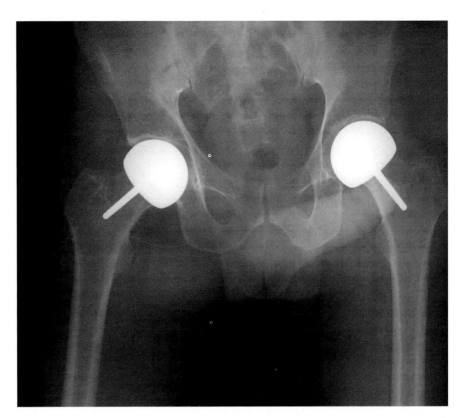

Figure 57–6. Bilateral avascular necrosis (AVN) treated with a "conservative" resurfacing implant that has not loosened at 5 years.

wear is considered in a young population. The concept of biologic fixation and a metal-on-metal articulation has rejuvenated this concept for some, as discussed in Chapter 50.

HEMIARTHROPLASTY

Resurfacing Hemiarthroplasty. Resurfacing hemiarthroplasty is an attractive method for managing avascular necrosis with collapse of the femoral head when the articular cartilage of the acetabulum is well preserved. Like any hemiarthroplasty, the procedure provides less predictable results than THA,[40] but it also is more bone sparing than conventional bipolar or monopolar hemiarthroplasty and burns few bridges for the future. The procedure is discussed in detail in Chapter 50.

Unipolar Replacement. When the acetabular cartilage has not been severely affected, hemisurface arthroplasty and conventional hemiarthroplasty can be employed. Unfortunately, the results of hemiarthroplasty have not been highly predictable, because it is difficult to judge the viability of the acetabular cartilage, and the metal-on-cartilage articulation of a hemiarthroplasty may result in deterioration of the cartilage in the young, active patient.

Unipolar endoprosthetic replacement of the femoral head has not been successful in the young, active patient. Beckenbaugh and co-workers[5] reported an 83 percent failure rate at 40 months of follow-up in 16 patients with AVN treated with a Thompson unipolar endoprosthesis. Seven patients required revision to a total hip arthroplasty and 7 of the remaining hips had significant pain.

Bipolar Replacement. This option has received acceptance for the treatment of fractures, but concern about cartilage integrity and poor outcomes from previous reports have limited its use for AVN.[61] The outcome of a group of 23 fixed-head and 51 bipolar implants inserted without cement revealed satisfactory results in 70 percent of patients with fixed-head devices and 96 percent of those with bipolar devices.[88] Radiographic loosening was observed in 48 percent of the former group but in only 6 percent of the latter group. Furthermore, proximal migration was present in only 9 percent of the bipolar implants and in approximately 60 percent of the fixed-head implants.

For AVN, although the results of bipolar endoprosthetic replacement are significantly better than those of unipolar endoprosthetic replacement, there is still a high failure rate. Cabanela and Vandemark reported failures in 23 percent of 28 bipolar hemiarthroplasties performed at the Mayo Clinic in the mid-1970s. An updated series in 1982 showed better results; however, the failure rate was still significantly higher than for conventional total hip arthroplasty (Fig. 57–7).

Cabanela attempted to resolve the treatment options by comparing various modes of replacement at the Mayo Clinic for the 15-year period from 1971 through 1986.[12] Cemented bipolar implants demonstrated 60 percent satisfactory results at a mean of 9 years after surgery compared with a group of cemented total hip arthroplasty patients assessed from 1982 to 1984. Those with bipolar implants had more complications. All 14 of the total hip

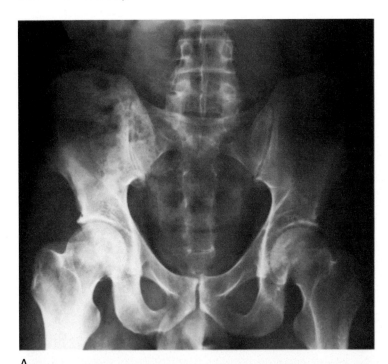

A

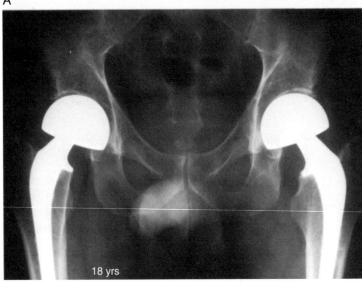

B

Figure 57–7. A, Patient with lupus erythematosus taking high-dose steroids with bilateral significant AVN. **B**, Bilateral press-fit bipolar implants are functioning satisfactorily after 18 years.

replacements were functioning satisfactorily. Total hip arthroplasty provided inferior results in patients with AVN compared with those with degenerative arthrosis. Lachiewicz and Desman[49] noted similar disappointing results, with an overall satisfactory rate of only 48 percent in 31 patients with 38 bipolar endoprostheses.

Yet, hemiarthroplasty is an attractive alternative to total hip arthroplasty. Unfortunately, in the young, active patient, the acetabular cartilage may not be capable of withstanding the stresses of a metal-on-cartilage articulation. This observation was confirmed by a study of 48 procedures followed for a mean of 11 years. Because of a 42 percent radiologic failure rate, these authors, once again, recommend against bipolar replacement for AVN.[40] Steinberg has offered evidence

that acetabular articular cartilage is abnormal in hips with AVN, even when radiographs are normal.[79] Steinberg further reviewed the literature, comparing endoprostheses and total hip replacement for AVN. The results were considered excellent or good in 81 percent of the total hip replacements but in only 58 percent of the endoprostheses. The revision rate for the total hip replacement was 13 percent, compared with 47 percent for the endoprosthetic devices.[85] Interestingly, Fink et al. have also documented an avascular process involving the acetabulum concurrent with avascular involvement of the head in 10 percent of cases of nontraumatic AVN.[25]

In general, the use of the bipolar prosthesis as a treatment for AVN is being abandoned for good reason; the

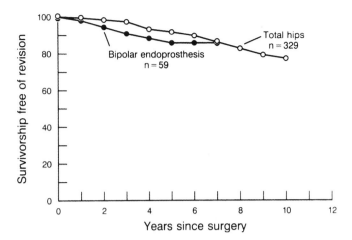

Figure 57–8. Kaplan-Meier survival curves demonstrating the prognosis for patients with avascular necrosis treated with cemented bipolar and cemented total hip arthroplasties.

data are compelling. The Mayo Clinic experience with cemented bipolar and cemented total hip arthroplasty is shown by the Kaplan-Meier survival analysis in Figure 57–8.

TOTAL HIP ARTHROPLASTY

Total hip arthroplasty provides the most reliable pain relief and good early clinical results for patients with advanced stages of AVN. Unfortunately, the excellent short-term results appear to deteriorate at a more rapid rate than in those patients with other diagnoses.[33] Failure of total hip arthroplasty in the treatment of AVN is related to three major variables: age, activity level, and effect of the predisposing condition.[16,28,39,52,66,74] The long-term results deteriorate because of failure of both the acetabular and femoral components.

Many, but not all, series have reported poorer durability of total hip arthroplasty in patients with AVN than in patients with osteoarthritis or rheumatoid arthritis. Whether this is because of the demographic features and underlying condition of patients with AVN or because of something different about the bone of patients with AVN or tissue response to implants in patients with AVN has been debated and remains unknown.

Salvati and Cornell assessed 28 patients undergoing total hip replacement at the Hospital for Special Surgery.[73] Eleven of the 28 arthroplasties failed during the follow-up period, which averaged 8 years: 5 with acetabular loosening, 2 with femoral stem fracture, and 2 with deep infection. Ranawat et al.,[67] in a study from the same institution, noted that 11 of 12 patients were frank failures or had radiographic evidence of a poor prognosis. Saito et al.,[72] in a study of 41 total hip arthroplasties performed in Osaka, Japan, noted a failure rate of 48 percent with a 28 percent revision rate at an average follow-up of 5.5 years. These results support the conclusion that patients with AVN have a poorer prognosis with long-term follow-up compared with patients who have other diagnoses and who receive total hip arthroplasty. Ortiguera and Cabanela from the

Mayo Clinic compared 178 patients with a diagnosis of AVN treated with Charnley total hip arthroplasty to a matched cohort with osteoarthritis.[60a] There was no statistically significant difference in failure rates at a mean of 17.8 years in patients older than 50 years of age who received total hip arthroplasty, but patients younger than 50 years of age with AVN had a higher failure rate than those with osteoarthritis.

On the other hand, these disappointing outcomes are not universally reported. Ritter and Meding[68] compared patients who had idiopathic osteonecrosis with those who had osteoarthritis comparable by age, sex, and complications. Between the 64 osteonecrosis patients and the 615 osteoarthritis patients there was no substantive difference in the complication rate except that those with osteoarthritis had more ectopic bone. Pain was present in 9 percent of the osteonecrotic group and in 6 percent of the osteoarthritic group. Revisions were performed in 1.5 percent of the osteonecrotic patients and in 3.5 percent of the osteoarthritic patients. Xenakis et al. also found no significant difference in clinical outcome or revision rate in two small groups of patients, one with osteoarthritis and one with AVN, at 7 to 8 years of follow-up.[93]

In one of the most definitive studies of this issue, Sarmiento et al. analyzed AVN, rheumatoid arthritis, and osteoarthritis in patients older and younger than 50 years of age.[74] Age-adjusted patients with AVN had more negative radiographic features than patients with other diagnoses. This relationship is shown in Figure 57–9.

Because of the high failure rate of cemented arthroplasties and because of the age of these patients, biologically fixed implants have become more popular (Fig. 57–10).[23,47] There is general agreement that improved cementation techniques have improved the durability of cemented femoral components in patients with AVN. Two studies[28,46,81] have demonstrated lower failure rates with modern cement methods than had been reported in earlier series. Ritter et al. reported on 115 hips with AVN treated with total hip arthroplasty using modern cement techniques.[69] This study confirmed the difference in the diagnosis of AVN and osteoarthritis, but no differences among etiologies of AVN was documented.[69] Because of the high failure rate of cemented total hip arthroplasty in patients with AVN, biologically fixed implants have become popular in this patient population. Several studies have demonstrated a high rate of success with uncemented femoral implants in AVN patients when uncemented femoral components with a favorable track record in the general patient population are used. Piston et al.[65] reported that 94 percent of 35 porous-coated stems in AVN patients were bone ingrown at 5 to 10 years; D'Antonio et al.[19] found that 100 percent of 53 hydroxyapatite-coated stems were stable at 5 years or more; and Xenakis et al.[93] found that 28 of 29 uncemented stems were functioning well at a mean of 7 years in AVN patients. Although it is difficult to compare different series from different eras with different patient populations, all of these reports are more favorable than the great majority of reports of cemented

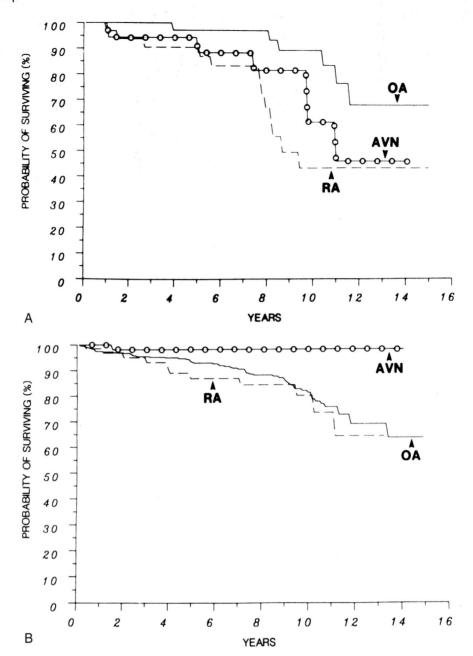

Figure 57–9. A, Survival curves for patients with osteoarthritis are better than those for avascular necrosis (AVN) in a younger age group. **B,** In older patients, the survival curve for AVN is superior to that for both rheumatoid arthritis and osteoarthritis. (From Sarmiento A, Ebramzadeh E, Gogan WJ, McKellop HA: Total hip arthroplasty with cement: A long-term radiographic analysis in patients who are older than fifty and younger than fifty years. J Bone Joint Surg 72A:1740, 1990.)

femoral stems for AVN. For the younger patient with AVN and reasonably good bone quality, uncemented femoral fixation appears to be an attractive option. Unlike cemented sockets, uncemented sockets have enjoyed good fixation in AVN patients, just as in other patient populations. However, as in other young patient groups, the related problems of polyethylene wear and periprosthetic osteolysis have been reported to be frequent in patients with AVN and early uncemented socket designs.[64,65,84] The combination of the good fixation achieved with uncemented sockets and newer bearing surfaces has the potential to markedly improve the

durability of acetabular component durability in the AVN population, just as in other demanding patient groups.

Acetabular Involvement. Avascular necrosis of the acetabulum is quite uncommon. The most common etiology is osteoradionecrosis. In this instance, we recommend a reinforcement ring to avoid reliance on the nonviable bone of the acetabulum (Fig. 57–11).

Complications of Total Hip Arthroplasty in AVN Patients. Although AVN patients are known to be at

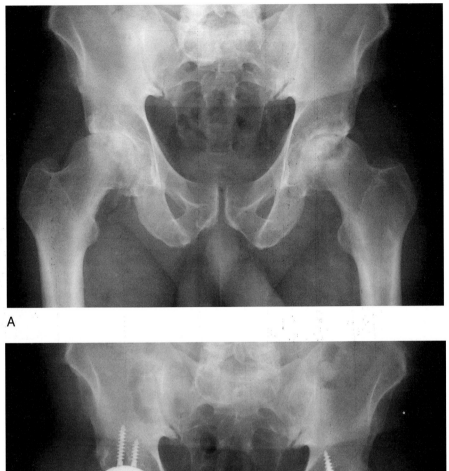

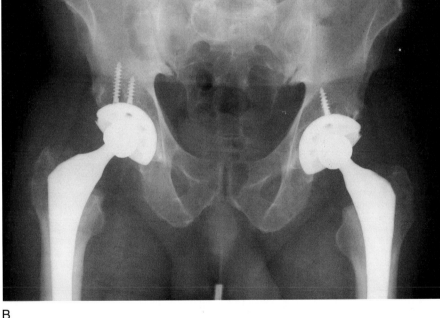

Figure 57–10. Preoperative radiographs of young patient with advanced osteonecrosis of the femoral head and good remaining bone stock (**A**). Radiograph of same patient after uncemented total hip arthroplasty (**B**).

risk for durability problems with THA owing to loosening or osteolysis, it is not always recognized that they may also be at risk for certain other complications. Several authors have suggested that the rate of dislocation may be higher in AVN patients than other patient populations. A Mayo Clinic study of the long-term risk of dislocation after a Charnley total hip arthroplasty demonstrated that AVN patients had more than a twofold higher long-term rate of dislocation than patients with osteoarthritis.[6] Higher dislocations rates in these patients may be related to factors associated with

diagnoses that lead to AVN such as ethanol use, or to structural factors such as less capsular hypertrophy in AVN patients compared with other diagnoses.[6] Patients with AVN on immunosuppressive agents, such as transplant patients or patients with lupus erythematosus, and patients with immunosuppression related to their underlying disease, such as patients with sickle cell disease, probably are at higher risk for prosthetic infection.

Revision. Only a single report of the outcome of a comparison of 19 revisions for AVN and 35 from

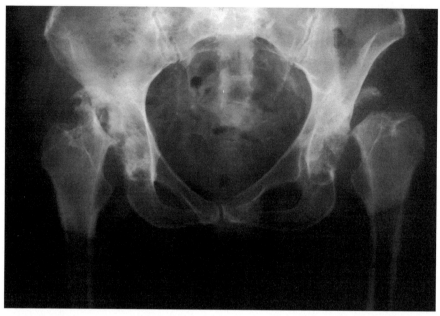

A

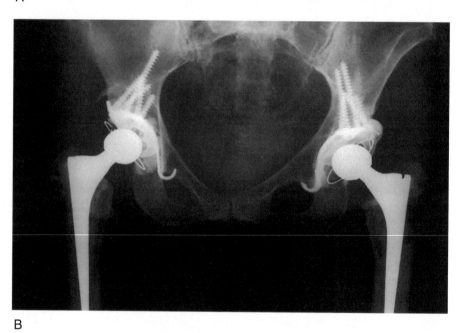

B

Figure 57–11. Hip radiographs of patient with previous radiation treatment of the pelvis and extensive bilateral osteonecrosis of the femoral head (**A**). Patient was treated with cemented total hip replacements with acetabular reinforcement (**B**).

osteoarthritis has been published. The mean age of those with AVN was 54 and for those with osteoarthritis, 67 years. Contrary to the data from primary procedures, the outcome from the revision at 2 years showed no difference by complication, radiographic appearance or need for further revision.[92]

Special Circumstances. Because prognostic and treatment implications are based on etiology, several specific diseases should be reviewed.

Systemic Lupus. Hanssen et al.[35] noted a revision rate of 36 percent in 14 patients with AVN and systemic

lupus erythematosus who had undergone bipolar endoprosthetic replacement. None of the patients in that series who had undergone total hip arthroplasty required revision surgery.

A comparable study by Zangger et al. documented the results of 26 patients with AVN from their disease. A central group was defined. The mean age was 46 years and the mean length of follow-up was 4.5 years. In short-term and mid-term follow-up, results were similar between the two groups.[94]

Gaucher's Disease. Gaucher's disease is a lipid storage disease in which glucocerebroside accumulates in the reticuloendothelial cells secondary to lysosomal acid hydrolase deficiency. Patients may develop AVN and collapse of the femoral head. Most who develop AVN and require orthopedic treatment have type I chronic, nonneuronopathic (adult form) Gaucher's disease.

The results of total hip arthroplasty have been disappointing in these patients, with failure rates approaching 50 percent, most commonly because of loosening of the components.[52] The accumulation of glucocerebroside leads to expansion, thinning, and scalloping of the femoral cortex. Progression of the disease after arthroplasty appears to erode the bone-cement interface, leading to early failure. In addition, there is an unusually high incidence of bleeding diathesis in these patients, and excessive bleeding has been reported in several studies.[4,50] Lachiewicz et al.[50] noted an average blood loss of over 2500 ml in 3 patients. An increased risk of sciatic and peroneal nerve palsies has also been reported, probably secondary to the bleeding diathesis. An alarming 29 percent infection rate has also been noted.[4] Goldblatt et al.[32] observed satisfactory results in 73 percent of 15 arthroplasties in 8 patients, with a mean follow-up of 7.3 years. Four revisions were required for aseptic loosening (2 patients), femoral stem fracture, and protrusion of the acetabular component. The authors cautioned against performing arthroplasties during "Gaucher's bone crises."

When total hip arthroplasty is considered in the patient with Gaucher's disease, several precautions should be taken. Hemostasis should be meticulous, and drainage of the hip is mandatory. The anterolateral approach may be preferable to avoid pressure and irritation of the sciatic nerve if postoperative hemorrhage does occur. Adequate blood components must be available at the time of arthroplasty, and careful technique and postsurgical surveillance are mandatory.

Sickle Cell Disease. Approximately 20 percent of patients with sickle cell hemoglobinopathy[54] develop AVN of the femoral head. Yet, only a relatively small number of these patients develop collapse and sufficient disability to warrant total hip arthroplasty (Fig. 57–12**A**). Hip replacement in these patients is technically difficult, and the incidence of postoperative complications is high. The quality of the bone in the proximal femur may be poor or sclerotic from reported bleeds or infection and severe deformity may be present.[15,34] This makes femoral preparation difficult. Sequestra within the marrow cavity may reduce the cortical thickness to a periosteal rim in some areas. In difficult cases, reaming over a guidewire and radiographic confirmation of broach position is recommended. An uncemented implant may be of value in this setting (Fig. 57–12**B**).

Overall, results have been disappointing. Clarke et al.[15] noted a 59-percent component loosening rate over a 5.5-year period, and 10 of 17 patients had revision surgery at an average of only 43 months after the index arthroplasty. Others have reported a high complication rate, with 5 failures in 8 patients.[3] Bishop and coworkers[7] reported an alarmingly high infection rate of 23 percent.

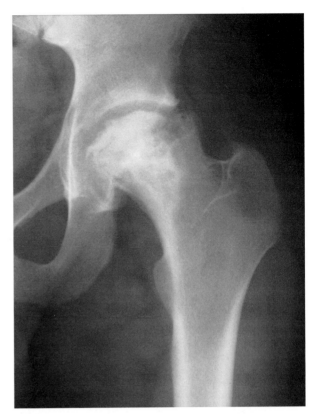

A

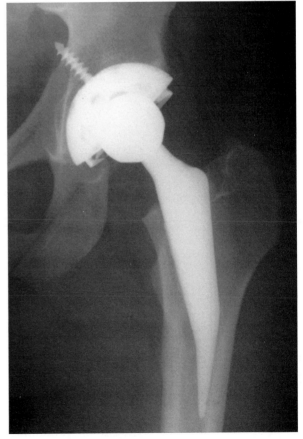

B

Figure 57–12. Sickle cell disease in a 38-year-old male (**A**). Satisfactory result at 2 years with Mayo conservative hip replacement (**B**).

There are numerous perioperative complications after arthroplasty in this group of patients. Several authors have observed vaso-occlusive crises secondary to the stress of surgery.[8,34] This can usually be reduced if exchange transfusion is performed before arthroplasty.[15] Intraoperative bleeding is significant, with an average blood loss of 1390 ml in primary and 2850 ml in revision cases.[8,34] Two of 11 patients in the University of California at Los Angeles (UCLA) experience developed aplastic anemia in the perioperative period. Furthermore, a high reoperation rate in the UCLA experience, with 3 of 11 patients suffering a sciatic neurapraxia and 5 patients having prolonged serious drainage from the wound, underscores the difficult nature of this surgery.[34]

Several principles to reduce the perioperative complication rate have been suggested[15]:

1. Perform exchange transfusion before arthroplasty.
2. Maintain the hematocrit below 40 percent and ideally between 28 percent and 34 percent.
3. Maintain the proportion of sickle cells below 50 percent.
4. Maintain oxygenation level at about 97 percent.
5. In cemented arthroplasties, add gentamicin to the powder.
6. Use epidural anesthesia to improve blood flow to the extremity.
7. Avoid respiratory depression.
8. Maintain a comfortable body temperature.
9. Warm irrigation fluids before use.

Organ Transplant Patients. Successful renal or cardiac transplantation is associated with a risk for AVN of the femoral head and at other sites as well. The vascular insult is probably the result of prolonged immunosuppressive therapy. Most immunosuppressive programs include combinations of both intravenous and oral corticosteroids, azathioprine, and cyclosporine. Radford et al.[66] estimated the risk of femoral head AVN to be 3 percent in 715 patients treated at Addenbrooke Hospital in Cambridge, England. Isono and co-workers[39] found the risk in cardiac transplant patients to be 10 percent at 2 years and 18 percent 5 years after transplant. The Mayo Clinic experience with renal and liver transplant patients revealed excellent long-term results with a complication rate (especially infection) comparable with that of the control group.[62]

Transplant patient would seem to have several risk factors, making them poor candidates for arthroplasty: chronic immunosuppression, young age, and osteoporosis, especially from dialysis. Toomey et al. have correlated a high rate of early radiographic loosening with dialysis therapy.[90] The low demand and reduced life expenctancy lessen the impact of these problems. To date, the results in transplant patients have been excellent, with low infection and aseptic loosening rates. Most surgeons recommend cemented arthroplasties for these patients because they have osteopenia and need chronic immunosuppression.

Isono and co-workers[39] describe a detailed postoperative protocol, including cardiac postoperative intensive care unit monitoring, intravenous perioperative corticosteroid coverage, and reverse isolation. Interestingly, although none of the patients developed wound infections, all had prolonged drainage, which attested to the wound-healing inhibition caused by systemic corticosteroids.

As transplant surgery becomes more successful, there will be greater numbers of transplant patients with symptomatic AVN of the femur. With careful medical support, arthroplasty can be a safe and effective procedure in the transplant patient.

AUTHORS' PREFERENCE

Our approach for the treatment of patients with avascular necrosis is outlined in Figures 57–13 and 57–14.

We use MRI to define the extent of the disease.

Stages 0, I, and II Disease

Patients who have been diagnosed as having stage 0, I, or II and who have no significant pain are often observed, although a discussion of other treatment options, based on etiology and lesion size, is undertaken. If pain limits activity, a period of nonsteroidal anti-inflammatory medication and crutches is prescribed. The patient is reassessed after 3 months. If pain no longer limits activity, the patient is assessed every 6 months clinically and radiographically. If pain limits activity, then a frog-leg radiograph and an anteroposterior pelvis radiograph are obtained. If these do not indicate femoral head collapse, we discuss the three possible options: intra-articular injection, observation and core decompression, and decompression with bone graft.

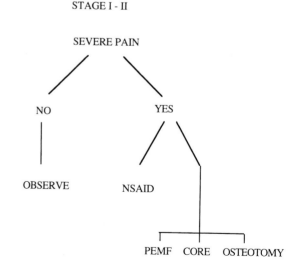

Figure 57–13. Treatment rationale for stages I and II involvement with avascular necrosis.

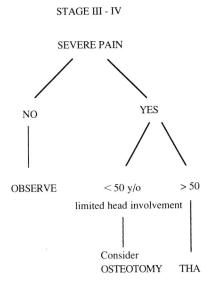

STAGE III - IV

SEVERE PAIN

NO   YES

OBSERVE   < 50 y/o   > 50
           limited head involvement

           Consider
           OSTEOTOMY   THA

Figure 57–14. Treatment rationale for stages III and IV of avascular necrosis.

Our prospective experience with 100 patients treated by core decompression versus observation demonstrates that the former does provide relief from pain, although there is little evidence that it alters the natural history of the disease process. If a patient becomes asymptomatic, activity as tolerated is allowed. However, if patients continue to be symptomatic, if collapse has not occurred in the face of persistent pain, if patients are younger than 55 years of age, and if they have a small osteonecrotic lesion (few patients fulfill these criteria), we discuss osteotomy. If patients are older than age 55, we may consider total hip replacement.

If, at any time during the assessment just described, a crescent sign is noted on the frog-leg lateral radiograph, stage III or IV disease is diagnosed. In this setting, if pain does not limit activity, we simply observe. If pain does limit activity in patients younger than 50 years of age, and if the extent of involvement as recorded by MRI is limited (200 degrees), an appropriate osteotomy is performed if it is determined that this will successfully contain or deliver the osteonecrotic segment. The patient is re-evaluated in 12 months. If symptoms do not limit activity, the patient is allowed to resume functional activity.

If the patient is older than 50 years of age and is symptomatic, with a type III or IV lesion or if the extent of involvement is greater than 200 degrees, we proceed directly to total hip arthroplasty. The preference of the authors varies, although the uncemented acetabular and cemented femoral components are most commonly used. The favorable results reported regarding uncemented femoral fixation in this patient population have led to an increasing tendency to use uncemented femoral fixation for younger patients with adequate bone quality. The senior author employs the short-stemmed Mayo uncemented component if there is no significant osteopenia and if it is determined that there is adequate bone quality present at the time of surgery to rigidly fix the short-stemmed device (see Fig. 57–12).

References

1. Aaron RK, Lennox D, Bunce GE, Ebert T: The conservative treatment of osteonecrosis of the femoral head: A comparison of core decompression and pulsing electromagnetic fields. Clin Orthop 249:209, 1989.
2. Alvuisio FV, Urbaniak JR: Proximal femur fractures after free vascularized fibular grafting to the hip. Clin Orthop 356:192, 1998.
3. Amstutz HC: Surface replacement of the hip with the THARIES system: Two to five year results. J Bone Joint Surg 63A:1069, 1981.
4. Amstutz HC, Carey EJ: Skeletal manifestations and treatment of Gaucher's disease: A review of twenty patients. J Bone Joint Surg 48A:670, 1966.
5. Beckenbaugh RD, Tressler HA, Johnson EW: Results after hemi-arthroplasty of the hip using a cemented femoral prosthesis. Mayo Clin Proc 52:349, 1977.
6. Berry DJ, Harmsen WS: Long-term risk of dislocation after Charnley total hip arthroplasty. American Association of Orthopedic Surgeons, 2002.
7. Berry DJ, Morrey BF, Lewallen DG, Cabanela ME: Core decompression versus observation for early stage osteonecrosis of the femoral head. A prospective study of 87 hips. Orthop Trans. 19:302, 1996.
8. Bishop AR, Roberson JR, Eckman JR, Fleming LL: Total hip arthroplasty in patients who have sickle cell hemoglobinopathy. J Bone Joint Surg 70A:853, 1988.
9. Bonfiglio M, Voke EM: Aseptic necrosis of the femoral head and nonunion of the femoral neck: Effect of treatment by drilling and bone grafting (Phemister technique). J Bone Joint Surg 50A:48, 1968.
10. Bradway JK, Morrey BF: The natural history of atraumatic ischemic necrosis of the femoral head. Clin Orthop Trans 13:518, 1989.
11. Buckley PD, Gearen PF, Petty RW: Structural bone grafting for early atraumatic avascular necrosis of the femoral head. J Bone Joint Surg 73A:1357, 1991.
12. Cabanela ME: Bipolar versus total hip arthroplasty for avascular necrosis of the femoral head: A comparison. Clin Orthop 261:59, 1990.
13. Camp JF, Colwell CW: Core decompression of the femoral head for osteonecrosis. J Bone Joint Surg 68A:1313, 1986.
14. Capello WN, Trancik TM: Indiana conservative hip results: Two to four and one-half year follow-up. Orthop Trans 5:375, 1981.
15. Clarke HJ, Jinnah RH, Brooker AF, Michaelson JD: Total replacement of the hip for avascular necrosis in sickle cell disease. J Bone Joint Surg 71B:465, 1989.
16. Cornell CN, Salvati EA, Pellicci PM: Long-term follow-up of total hip replacement in patients with osteonecrosis. Orthop Clin North Am 16:757, 1985.
17. Cruess RL: Cortisone induced avascular necrosis of the femoral head. J Bone Joint Surg 59B:308, 1977.
18. Daley BJ, Bonfiglio M, Brand RA, Boyer DW: Aseptic necrosis of the femoral head with a forty-year follow-up. J Bone Joint Surg 73A:134, 1991.
19. D'Antonio JA, Capello WN, Manley MT, Feinberg J: Hydroxyapatite coated implants. Total hip arthroplasty in the young patient and patients with avascular necrosis. Clin Orthop 344:124, 1997.
20. Dutton RO, Amstutz HC, Thomas BJ, Hedley AK: THARIES surface replacement in osteonecrosis of the hip. J Bone Joint Surg 64A:1225, 1982.
21. Ensign MF: Magnetic resonance imaging of hip disorders. Semin Ultrasound, CT, MR 11:288, 1990.
22. Fehrle MJ, Callaghan JJ, Clark CR, Peterson KK: Uncemented total hip arthroplasty in patients with aseptic necrosis of the femoral head and previous bone grafting. J Arthroplasty 8:1, 1993.
23. Ficat RP: Idiopathic bone necrosis of the femoral head: Early diagnosis and treatment. J Bone Joint Surg 67B:3, 1985.
24. Fink B, Assheuer J, Enderle A, et al: Avascular osteonecrosis of the acetabulum. Skeletal Radiol 26:509, 1997.
25. Freeman MAR, Cameron HU, Brown GC: Cemented double cup arthroplasty of the hip: A five year experience with the ICLH prosthesis. Clin Orthop 134:45, 1978.

26. Fye MA, Huo MH, Zatorski LE, Keggi KJ: Total hip arthroplasty performed without cement in patients with femoral head osteonecrosis who are less than 50 years old. J Arthroplasty 13:876, 1998.

27. Ganz R, Buchler V: Overview to attempt to neutralize the dead head in aseptic necrosis of the femoral head: Osteotomy and revascularization. In Hungerford DS (ed): The Hip: Proceedings of the Eleventh Open Scientific Meeting of the Hip Society. St. Louis, CV Mosby, 1983, p 296.

28. Garino JP, Steinberg ME: Total hip arthroplasty in patients with avascular necrosis of the femoral head. A 2-to 10-year follow-up. Clin Orthop 334:108, 1997.

29. Genez BM, Wilson MR, Houk RW, et al: Early osteonecrosis of the femoral head: Detection in high-risk patients with MR: imaging. Radiology 168:521, 1988.

30. Gilbert A, Judet H, Judet J, Ayatti A: Microvascular transfer of the fibula for necrosis of the femoral head. Orthopedics 9:885, 1986.

31. Glimcher MJ, Kenzora JE: The biology of osteonecrosis of the human femoral head and its clinical implications. III. Discussion of the etiology and genesis of the pathological sequelae: Comments on treatment. Clin Orthop 140:273, 1979.

32. Goldblatt J, Sacks S, Dall D, Beighton P: Total hip arthroplasty in Gaucher's disease: Long-term prognosis. Clin Orthop 228:94, 1988.

33. Garino JP, Steinberg ME: Total hip arthroplasty in patients with avascular necrosis of the femoral head: A 2- to 10-year follow-up. Clin Orthop 334:108, 1997.

34. Hanker GJ, Amstutz HC: Osteonecrosis of the hip in the sickle cell diseases: Treatment and complications. J Bone Joint Surg 70A:499, 1988.

35. Hanssen AD, Cabanela ME, Michet CJ: Hip arthroplasty in patients with systemic lupus erythematosus. J Bone Joint Surg 69A:807, 1987.

36. Hauzeur JP, Pasteels JL, Schoutens A, et al: The diagnostic value of magnetic resonance imaging in non-traumatic osteonecrosis of the femoral head. J Bone Joint Surg 71A:641, 1989.

37. Head WC: Total articular resurfacing arthroplasty: Analysis of component failure in sixty-seven hips. J Bone Joint Surg 66A:28, 1984.

38. Hopson CN, Siverhus SW: Ischemic necrosis of the femoral head: Treatment by core decompression. J Bone Joint Surg 70A:1048, 1988.

39. Isono SS, Woolson ST, Schurman DJ: Total joint arthroplasty for steroid-induced osteonecrosis in cardiac transplant patients. Clin Orthop 217:201, 1987.

40. Ito H, Matsuno T, Kaneda K: Bipolar hemiarthroplasty for osteonecrosis of the femoral head. A 7- to 18-year follow-up. Clin Orthop 374:201, 2000.

41. Ito H, Matsuno T, Kaneda K: Prognosis of early stage avascular necrosis of the femoral head. Clin Orthop 358:149, 1999.

42. Jacobs MA, Hungerford DS, Krackow KA: Intertrochanteric osteotomy for avascular necrosis of the femoral head. J Bone Joint Surg 71B:200, 1989.

43. Jergesen HE, Khan AS: The natural history of untreated asymptomatic hips in patients who have non-traumatic osteonecrosis. J Bone Joint Surg 79(3):359–363, 1997.

44. Jolley MN, Salvati EA, Brown GC: Early results and complications of surface replacement of the hip. J Bone Joint Surg 64A:366, 1982.

45. Kane SM, Ward WA, Jordan LC, et al: Vascularized fibular grafting compared with core decompression in the treatment of femoral head osteonecrosis. Orthopedics 19:869, 1996.

46. Kantor SG, Huo MH, Huk OK, Salvati EA: Cemented total hip arthroplasty in patients with osteonecrosis. A 6-year minimum follow-up study of second generation cement techniques. J Arthroplasty 11:267, 1996.

47. Katz RL, Bourne RB, Rorabeck CH, McGee H: Total hip arthroplasty in patients with avascular necrosis of the hip: Follow-up observations on cementless and cemented operations. Clin Orthop 281:145, 1992.

48. Khanna AJ, Yoon TR, Mont MA, et al: Femoral head osteonecrosis: Detection and grading by using a rapid MR imaging protocol. Radiology 217:188, 2000.

49. Lachiewicz PF, Desman SM: The bipolar endoprosthesis in avascular necrosis of the femoral head. J Arthroplasty 3:131, 1988.

50. Lachiewicz PF, Lane JM, Wilson PD: Total hip replacement in Gaucher's disease. J Bone Joint Surg 63A:602, 1981.

51. Lang P, Genant HK, Jergesen HE, Murray WPR: Imaging of the hip joint: Computed tomography versus magnetic resonance imaging. Clin Orthop Rel Res 274:135, 1992.

52. Lau MM, Lichtman DM, Hamati YI, Bierbaum BE: Hip arthroplasties in Gaucher's disease. J Bone Joint Surg 63A:591, 1981.

53. Learmonth ID, Maloon S, Dall G: Core decompression for early atraumatic osteonecrosis of the femoral head. J Bone Joint Surg 72B:387, 1990.

54. Louie BE, McKee MD, Richards RR, et al: Treatment of osteonecrosis of the femoral head by free vascularized fibular grafting: An analysis of surgical outcome and patient health status. Can J Surg 42:274, 1999.

55. Maistrelli G, Fusco U, Avai A, Bombelli R: Osteonecrosis of the hip treated by intertrochanteric osteotomy: A four to 15 year follow-up. J Bone Joint Surg 70B:761, 1988.

56. Marcus ND, Enneking WF, Massam RA: The silent hip in idiopathic aseptic necrosis. J Bone Joint Surg 55A:1351, 1973.

57. Mitchell DG, Rao VM, Dalinka MK, et al: Femoral head avascular necrosis: Correlation of MR imaging, radiographic staging, radionuclide imaging, and clinical findings. Radiology 162:705, 1987.

58. Mont MA, Jones LC, Sotereanos DG, et al: Understanding and treating osteonecrosis of the femoral head. AAOS Instructional Course Lect 49:169, 2000.

59. Muller ME: Part I: Intertrochanteric osteotomy in the treatment of the arthritic hip joint. In Tronzo RG (ed): Surgery of the Hip Joint. Philadelphia, Lea & Febiger, 1973.

60. Ohzono K, Saito M, Takaoka K, et al: Natural history of nontraumatic avascular necrosis of the femoral head. J Bone Joint Surg 73B:68, 1991.

60a. Ortiguera CJ: Total hip arthroplasty for osteonecrosis: matched-pair analysis of 188 hips with long-term follow-up. J Arthroplasty 14:21–28,1999.

61. Orwin JF, Fisher RC, Wiedel JD: Use of the uncemented bipolar endoprosthesis for the treatment of steroid induced osteonecrosis of the hip in renal transplantation patients. J Arthroplasty 6:1, 1991.

62. Papagelopoulos PJ, Hay JE, Galanis E, Morrey BF: Infection around joint replacements in patients who have a renal or liver transplantation (79A:36–43, Jan. 1997), Tannenbaum et al (letter; comment). J Bone Joint Surg 80A:607, 1998.

63. Pavlovcic V, Dolinar D, Arnez Z: Femoral head necrosis treated with vascularized iliac crest graft. Int Orthop 23:150, 1999.

64. Phillips FM, Pottenger LA, Finn HA, Vandermolen J: Cementless total hip arthroplasty in patients with steroid-induced avascular necrosis of the hip. A 62-month follow-up study. Clin Orthop 303:147, 1994.

65. Piston RW, Engh CA, DeCarvalho PI, Suthers K: Osteonecrosis of the femoral head treated with total hip arthroplasty without cement. J Bone Joint Surg 76A:202, 1994.

66. Radford PJ, Doran A, Greatorex RA, Rushton N: Total hip replacement in the renal transplant recipient. J Bone Joint Surg 71B:456, 1989.

67. Ranawat CS, Atkinson RE, Salvati EA, Wilson PD: Conventional total hip arthroplasty for degenerative joint disease in patients between the ages of forty and sixty years. J Bone Joint Surg 66A:745, 1984.

68. Ritter MA, Meding JB: A comparison of osteonecrosis and osteoarthritis patients following total hip arthroplasty. Clin Orthop 206:139, 1986.

69. Ritter MA, Helphinstine J, Keating EM, et al: Total hip arthroplasty in patients with osteonecrosis. The effect of cement techniques. Clin Orthop 338:94, 1997.

70. Robinson HJ, Hartleben PD, Lund G, Schreiman J: Evaluation of magnetic resonance imaging in the diagnosis of osteonecrosis of the femoral head: Accuracy compared with radiographs, core biopsy, and intraosseous pressure measurements. J Bone Joint Surg 71A:650, 1989.

71. Sakamoto M, Shimizu K, Iida S, et al: Osteonecrosis of the femoral head: A prospective study with MRI. J Bone Joint Surg 79B2:213, 1997.

72. Saito S, Saito M, Nishina T, et al: Long term results of total hip arthroplasty for osteonecrosis of the femoral head. Clin Orthop 244:198, 1989.

73. Salvati EA, Cornell CN: Long term follow-up of total hip replacement in patients with avascular necrosis. Instruct Course Lect 37:67, 1988.
74. Sarmiento A, Ebramzadeh E, Gogan WJ, McKellop HA: Total hip arthroplasty with cement: A long term radiographic analysis in patients who are older than fifty and younger than fifty years. J Bone Joint Surg 72A:1470, 1990.
75. Scher MA, Jakin I: Intertrochanteric osteotomy and autogenous bone grafting for avascular necrosis of the femoral head. J Bone Joint Surg 75A:1119, 1993.
76. Scully SP, Aaron RK, Urbaniak JR: Survival analysis of hips treated with core decompression or vascularized fibular grafting because of avascular necrosis. J Bone Joint Surg 80A:1270, 1998.
77. Smith KR, Bonfiglio M, Montgomery WJ: Nontraumatic necrosis of the femoral head treated with tibial bone grafting: A follow-up note. J Bone Joint Surg 62A:845, 1980.
78. Solomon L: Idiopathic necrosis of the femoral head: Pathogenesis and treatment. Can J Surg 24:573, 1981.
79. Steinberg ME, Corces A, Fallon M: Acetabular involvement of the femoral head. J Bone Joint Surg 81A:60, 1999.
80. Steinberg ME: Early diagnosis of avascular necrosis of the femoral head. Am Acad Orthop Surg Instruct Course Lect 37:51, 1988.
81. Steinberg ME, Hosick WB, Hartman K: Abstract 300 cases of core decompression with bone grafting for avascular necrosis of the femoral head. Assoc Res Circ Oss News 4:120, 1992.
82. Stulberg BN, Bauer TW, Belhobek GH: Making core decompression work. Clin Orthop 261:186, 1990.
83. Stulberg BN, Bauer TW, Belhobek GH, et al: A diagnostic algorithm for osteonecrosis of the femoral head. Clin Orthop 249:176, 1989.
84. Stulberg BN, Singer R, Goldner J, Stulberg J: Uncemented total hip arthroplasty in osteonecrosis: A 2- to 10-year evaluation. Clin Orthop 334:116, 1997.
85. Sugano N, Nishii T, Shibuya T, et al: Contralateral hip in patients with unilateral nontraumatic osteonecrosis of the femoral head. Clin Orthop 334:85, 1997.
86. Sugioka Y: Transtrochanteric rotational osteotomy in the treatment of idiopathic and steroid induced femoral head necrosis, Perthes disease, slipped capital femoral epiphysis and osteoarthritis of the hip: Indications and results. Clin Orthop 184:12, 1985.
87. Suominen S, Antti-Poika I, Santavirta S, et al: Total hip replacement after intertrochanteric osteotomy. Orthopedics 14:253, 1991.
88. Takaoka K, Nishina T, Ohzono K, et al: Bipolar prosthetic replacement for the treatment of avascular necrosis of the femoral head. Clin Orthop 177:121, 1992.
89. Tooke SM, Amstutz HC, Delaunay C: Hemiresurfacing for femoral head osteonecrosis. J Arthroplasty 2:125, 1987.
90. Toomey HE, Toomey SP: Hip arthroplasty in chronic dialysis patients. J Arthroplasty 13:657, 1998.
91. Urbaniak J, Nunley JA, Goldner RD: Treatment of aseptic necrosis of the femoral head by vascularized fibular graft. Presented at the Eighth Combined Meeting of the Orthopaedic Associations of the English Speaking World. Washington, DC, May 3–8, 1987.
92. Wei SY, Klimkiewicz JJ, Lai M, et al: Revision total hip arthroplasty in patients with avascular necrosis. Orthopedics 22:747, 1999.
93. Xenakis A, Beris AE, Malizos KK, et al: Total hip arthroplasty for avascular necrosis and degenerative osteoarthritis of the hip. Clin Orthop 341:62, 1997.
94. Zangger P, Gladman DD, Urowitz MB, Bogoch ER: Outcome of total hip replacement for avascular necrosis in systemic lupus erythematosus. J Rheumatol 27:919, 2000.

58

Parkinson's Disease

• FRANK J. FRASSICA, JAMES F. WENZ, and FRANKLIN H. SIM

arkinson's disease (paralysis agitans) is a neurologic disorder of the basal ganglia of the brainstem that results in the core syndrome of an expressionless face, rigidity, paucity, slowness of voluntary movement, "resting tremor," stooped posture, and shuffling gait (Fig. 58–1).[11] The peak age of onset of the disease is in the sixth decade of life. The disease may be progressive, resulting in a gait reduced to a shuffle and severe equilibrium problems (Table 58–1). Approximately 1 percent of the United States population older than 50 years of age has Parkinson's disease.

Joint position sense and proprioception are impaired in patients with Parkinson's disease. Zia et al.[28] postulated that the impairment of discrimination of bilateral joint position sense might contribute to the postural abnormalities characteristic of the disease. Patients with Parkinson's disease have a high incidence of hip fractures and reduced bone density.[25] Taggart and Crawford[25] followed 55 patients with Parkinson's disease for 14 to 17 months, noting the incidence of fractures and recording bone mineral density (BMD) values. Interestingly, in both male and female patients, there was a differential reduction in hip BMD compared with spine BMD. They also noted a 10 percent lower BMD for total hip ($P = 0.014$) and 12 percent lower BMD for the neck of the femur ($P < 0.004$) in parkinsonian patients compared with controls. In addition, they reported that during the 14-month follow-up period 11 of the women (38 percent) sustained fractures: hip, 6; distal radius, 4; pelvis, 2; ankle, 2; and nose, 1.

Several studies have shown an increased incidence of hip fractures in patients with Parkinson's disease.[9,14,15] Johnell et al.[14] studied 138 patients who had been newly diagnosed with Parkinson's disease. By 10 years after diagnosis, an estimated 27 percent of the parkinsonian cohort had experienced a new hip fracture. When fractures were considered at eight different skeletal locations (e.g., proximal femur, lumbar vertebra, distal radius), 52 percent of men and 64% percent of women with Parkinson's disease had experienced one or more fractures. When compared with a control population, both male and female parkinsonian patients had especially high risks of proximal femur fractures ($P < 0.001$). The cumulative incidence of new proximal femur fracture was 27 percent (29 percent in men and 26 percent in women) compared with 9 percent in controls.

The increased risk of hip fractures in patients with Parkinson's disease may be due to the propensity to fall and to decreased BMD. Sato and colleagues[22] found a decrease in BMD and a high prevalence of vitamin D deficiency in patients with Parkinson's disease. In addition, many patients had compensatory hyperparathyroidism.

Arthroplasty of the hip in patients with Parkinson's disease is difficult, and several investigators[5,21,26] have reported a subsequent high dislocation rate. Although there are few reports in the literature that specifically discuss hip arthroplasty for arthritis in patients with Parkinson's disease, other studies[6,7,10,24] have indicated that hip arthroplasty is a safe and effective treatment method for displaced femoral neck fractures.

ROLE OF ARTHROPLASTY IN THE TREATMENT OF HIP FRACTURE

Hip fractures are common in the parkinsonian patient. Unfortunately, the systemic medications (e.g., levodopa) used to treat parkinsonism may have the side effect of postural hypotension. The combination of postural hypotension and the dysequilibirum caused by the disease predispose the parkinsonian patient to low-energy accidents.

Hip fractures in the parkinsonian patient should be treated with the standard indications for internal fixation or arthroplasty. We treat Garden[8] stage I and stage II femoral neck fractures with rigid internal fixation and Garden stage III and stage IV fractures with endoprosthetic replacement. Londos et al.[18] reported good results after internal fixation in parkinsonian patients with nondisplaced fractures. In patients with displaced fractures who underwent reduction and internal fixation, only 10 of 19 healed uneventfully. Of the other 9 patients, 6 developed nonunion and 3 had segmental femoral head collapse. Although Soto-Hall[23] believed that the osteosynthesis site was destined to break down in patients with severe parkinsonism, it has been our experience, as well as that of others,[26] that fractures in such patients heal despite their tremors, involuntary movements, and rigidity. The goal of internal fixation should be rigid fixation, because these patients may not be able to maintain a partial weight-bearing or non-weight-

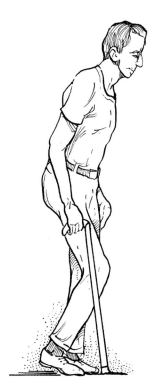

Figure 58–1. Typical patient with Parkinson's disease.

bearing status during their rehabilitation. Unfortunately, the trauma of a fall, hip fracture, or surgery often worsens a patient's deterioration. The primary goal of treatment in such patients is to return them to their prefracture status as quickly as possible. If rigid fixation is not possible because of poor bone stock or comminution after intertrochanteric hip or femoral neck fractures, consideration should be given to prosthetic replacement.

TECHNICAL CONSIDERATIONS

Although several authors[12,13,19] have condemned endoprosthetic replacement in the treatment of femoral neck fractures, more recent reports have shown that hip arthroplasty is safe and effective in the parkinsonian patient.[7,24] The controversy over the merits of endoprosthetic replacement centers around the stability of the prosthetic component (Table 58–2) and the mortality rate after arthroplasty.[2,27] Rothermel and Garcia[21] reported on a series of 23 patients in whom there were 2 dislocations (8.7 percent), and Whittaker et al.[27] reported 2 dislocations (16 percent) in a series of 12 patients. Eventov et al.[7] reported only 1 dislocation in 31 patients who were treated with endoprostheses. Hunter[12,13] strongly advised against prosthetic replacement in patients who have parkinsonism because of what he considered to be an unacceptably high rate of prosthetic dislocation. This opinion was based on the study by Coughlin and Templeton,[5] who reported a 37 percent rate of dislocation and a 75 percent rate of mortality within 6 months postoperatively. Each patient who sustained a dislocation died within 6 months. The authors concluded that internal fixation is the preferred method of treatment and that prosthetic replacement should be avoided. Although Coughlin and Templeton[5] attributed the high rate of dislocation in their series to the use of a posterior (Gibson) approach, Eventov et al.[7] also used a posterior approach but reported only 1 dislocation (1 of 31, 3 percent). Enhanced soft tissue repair has been used to augment the posterior approach.[4,17,20]

RESULTS

The overall treatment and results of hip arthroplasty in the parkinsonian patient are satisfactory, although this group of patients often have more postoperative complications than are found in the general population. Staeheli et al.[24] reported excellent results with the treatment of displaced femoral neck fractures, indicating a dislocation rate of only 2 percent. The mortality rate in that series of 50 patients was 20 percent at 6 months. Although the 20-percent mortality rate was more favorable than those in previous reports of hip fractures in the parkinsonian patient, the rate is somewhat higher than the 13.4 percent 1-year mortality rate reported by Kenzora et al.[16] in the general hip fracture population. The functional status after hip fracture was also better than had been previously reported. Eighty percent of the patients who had been able to walk without an assistive device before the fracture remained able to do so. Before fracture, 50 percent of the patients were nursing home residents; after fracture, 70 percent required nursing home placement. Guyton,[10] DeLee,[6] and others[3,19] also supported the role of endoprosthetic replacement in the treatment of displaced femoral neck fractures.

ELECTIVE TOTAL HIP ARTHROPLASTY IN THE PARKINSONIAN PATIENT

There are no reports in the literature concerned solely with total hip arthroplasty in the parkinsonian patient. Because of the paucity of data on elective total hip arthroplasty, the risks and benefits of arthroplasty can only be extrapolated from reports on arthroplasty for femoral neck fractures.

Table 58–1. COLUMBIA CLASSIFICATION OF THE SEVERITY OF PARKINSON'S DISEASE

Stage	Characteristics	No. Patients
I	Unilateral involvement, little or no functional involvement	10
II	Bilateral or midline involvement, balance not affected	14
III	Early loss of equilibrium, mild or moderate functional disability	16
IV	Severe disability, barely able to stand and walk unaided	7
V	Confined to a wheelchair	0

Table 58–2. INCIDENCE OF PROSTHETIC DISLOCATION AFTER ENDOPROSTHETIC REPLACEMENT OF DISPLACED FEMORAL NECK FRACTURES IN PATIENTS WITH PARKINSON'S DISEASE

Year	Study	No. Patients	No. Dislocations	Rate (percent)
1972	Rothermel et al.[21]	23	8	34.8
1972	Whittaker et al.[27]	12	2	16.7
1980	Coughlin et al.[5]	16	6	37.5
1983	Eventov et al.[7]	31	3	9.6
1988	Staeheli et al.[24]	52	1	1.9

Because there had been no series in the literature, Frassica et al. (unpublished data) reviewed the Mayo Clinic experience with total hip arthroplasty in the parkinsonian patient. Over a 20-year period, 56 arthroplasties were performed in 52 patients (average age, 71 years; range, 60 to 82 years). The preoperative diagnosis was osteoarthritis (26), failed endoprosthesis (7), aseptic loosening after total hip arthroplasty (7), acute femoral neck fracture (4), and 1 each of the following: ancien septic arthritis, degenerative arthritis secondary to Legg-Calvé-Perthes disease, and previous resection arthroplasty. Twenty-seven patents had undergone previous hip surgery, and 40 patients had been taking antiparkinsonism medications preoperatively. Overall, the early functional results after arthroplasty were good. All 6 patients who were nonambulatory preoperatively were able to ambulate independently (3) or with canes or walkers (3) postoperatively. Three patients (5.7 percent) died within 6 months after arthroplasty.

Unfortunately, the long-term results of hip arthroplasty in the parkinsonian patient are related to progression of the neurologic disability. In the series by Frassica et al. (unpublished data), 70 percent of the patients had moderate to severe Parkinson's disease on long-term follow-up. Although only 11 percent of the patients had severe parkinsonism (severe disability, barely able to walk or stand alone) preoperatively, 42 percent had severe parkinsonism 2 to 7 years after arthroplasty.

The prosthesis was successfully implanted in 6 hips (10.7 percent; 6 patients) dislocated. Four of those patients had been taking antiparkinsonism medications; 2 had not. Two of the dislocations occurred in patients who had undergone total hip arthroplasty after an acute femoral neck fracture. Three patients had had previous surgery and 3 had not. The operative approach was transtrochanteric in 4, posterior in 1, and anterolateral in 1. Of the 6 patients who sustained dislocations, 3 experienced dislocation of the prosthesis more than once and 2 required additional surgery. The dislocation rate was 11 percent (4 of 36) for the transtrochanteric approach, 7 percent (1 of 14) for the anterolateral approach, and 16 percent (1 of 6) for the posterior approach.

One patient developed a deep infection that required removal of the prosthetic components.

TECHNICAL FACTORS IN HIP SURGERY IN THE PARKINSONIAN PATIENT

Both Soto-Hall[23] and Rothermel and Garcia[21] alluded to the difficulty in operating on parkinsonian patients because of the presence of a flexion or adduction contracture (or both) of the hip. In another study, 5 of 49 patients who underwent endoprosthetic replacement for femoral neck fractures at the Mayo Clinic had contractures that, when tested intraoperatively, were thought to be severe enough to preclude a stable reduction.[24] Those 5 patients required adductor tenotomies to ensure stable range of motion. Another report indicated that 3 patients who underwent elective total hip arthroplasty also required adductor tenotomies to make stable intraoperative range of motion possible.[3] Adductor tenotomy is a useful and essential adjunct for improving hip motion and reducing the incidence of postoperative dislocation in such patients. When arthroplasty is performed for a femoral neck fracture, it is difficult to discern an adduction contracture perioperatively because of the pain and spasm related to the fracture. If such contractures are not actively sought during the operation, they may be overlooked.

We prefer the anterolateral approach when performing hip surgery on patients with Parkinson's disease because it reduces the risk of dislocation postoperatively and facilitates addressing the problem of hip flexion and adduction contractures. If the contracture is mild, the adductors can be released from the femur. The psoas muscle tendon can also be released if necessary. If abduction of the hip is still limited, the adductors can be released from the pubis (Fig. 58–2).

PREOPERATIVE AND POSTOPERATIVE CARE OF THE PARKINSONIAN PATIENT

Patients with Parkinson's disease should undergo a thorough neurologic evaluation before surgery to ensure that their medical management is optimal. Such patients also require careful medical and neurologic follow-up during the perioperative period.

After elective hip surgery or arthroplasty for a femoral neck fracture, the parkinsonian patient must be treated aggressively with regard to skin care, pulmonary toilet, and genitourinary tract management. Such patients often have skin decubiti (especially over the sacrum or calcaneus) because of extensive time spent in bed. Vigorous pulmonary toilet and early mobilization from bed are necessary to prevent pneumonia and other respiratory complications. Because there is a high incidence of urinary tract infection (approximately 20 percent in the unpublished series by Frassica et al.), antibiotic coverage to prevent sepsis or seeding of the tissues about the implant is necessary.

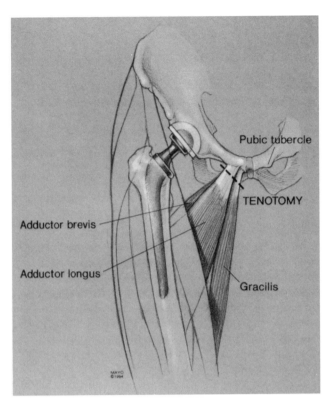

Figure 58–2. Artist's depiction of release of the adductor tendon from the pubis.

During the postoperative period, it is sometimes necessary to brace or cast the parkinsonian patient's hip, maintaining the limb in abduction if it is apparent that the adduction contracture is developing in the early postoperative period. In addition, the caregiver should remember that the severity of the symptoms of Parkinson's disease is often increased by the stress or trauma of fracture or elective surgery.

SUMMARY

Arthroplasty of the hip is generally a safe and effective procedure in the parkinsonian patient. The anterolateral approach to the hip is commonly used, and adductor tenotomy may be necessary to ensure a stable range of motion. During the postoperative period, the surgeon should carefully monitor the patient and initiate appropriate treatment to minimize complications such as skin ulcers, pneumonia, and urinary tract infections. The long-term result of elective total hip arthroplasty often depends on the progression of the neurologic disease.

References

1. Adams RD, Victor M, Ropper AH: Degenerative diseases of the nervous system. Principles of Neurology, 6th ed. New York, McGraw-Hill, 1997, pp 1046–1107.
2. Ali Khan MA, Brakenbury PH, Reynolds IS: Dislocation following total hip replacement. J Bone Joint Surg 63B:214–218, 1981.
3. Bisla RS, Ranawat CS, Inglis AE: Total hip replacement in patients with ankylosing spondylitis with involvement of the hip. J Bone Joint Surg 58A:233–238, 1976.
4. Chiu FY, Chen CM, Chung TY, et al: The effect of posterior capsuolorrhaphy in primary total hip arthroplasty. A prospective randomized study. J Arthroplasty 15:194–199, 2000.
5. Coughlin L, Templeton J: Hip fractures in patients with Parkinson's disease. Clin Orthop 148:192–195, 1980.
6. DeLee JC: Fractures and dislocations of the hip. In Rockwood CA Jr, Green DP, Bucholz RW (eds): Rockwood and Green's Fractures in Adults, 4th ed. Philadelphia, Lippincott-Raven, 1996, pp 1659–1825.
7. Eventov I, Moreno M, Geller E, et al: Hip fractures in patients with Parkinson's syndrome. J Trauma 23:98–101, 1983.
8. Garden RS: Reduction and fixation of subcapital fractures of the femur. Orthop Clin North Am 5:683–712, 1974.
9. Grisso JA, Kelsey JL, Strom BL, et al: Risk factors for falls as a cause of hip fracture in women. The Northeast Hip Fracture Study Group. N Engl J Med 324:1326–1331, 1991.
10. Guyton JL: Fractures of the hip, acetabulum, and pelvis. In Canale ST (ed): Campbell's Operative Orthopaedics, 9th ed. St. Louis, Mosby-Year Book, 1998, pp 2181–2279.
11. Hoehn MM, Yahr MD: Parkinsonism: Onset, progression, and mortality. Neurology 17:427–442, 1967.
12. Hunter GA: Fractures of the neck of the femur. Part I. Displaced fractures of the femoral neck—internal fixation or hemiarthroplasty? Instr Course Lect 29:1–4, 1980.
13. Hunter GA: The rationale for internal fixation and against hemiarthroplasty. In Hungerford DS (ed): The Hip. Proceedings of the Eleventh Open Scientific meeting of the Hip Society. St. Louis, CV Mosby, 1983, pp 34–41.
14. Johnell O, Melton LJ III, Atkinson EJ, et al: Fracture risk in patients with Parkinsonism: A population-based study in Olmsted County, Minnesota. Age Ageing 21:32–38, 1992.
15. Johnell O, Sernbo I: Health and social status in patients with hip fractures and controls. Age Ageing 15:285–291, 1986.
16. Kenzora JE, McCarthy RE, Lowell JD, Sledge CB: Hip fracture mortality. Relation to age, treatment, preoperative illness, time of surgery and complications. Clin Orthop 186:45–56, 1984.
17. Ko CK, Law SW, Chiu KH: Enhanced soft tissue repair using locking loop stitch after posterior approach for hip hemiarthroplasty. J Arthroplasty 16:207–211, 2001.
18. Londos E, Nilsson LT, Stromqvist B: Internal fixation of femoral neck fractures in Parkinson's disease. 32 patients followed for 2 years. Acta Orthop Scand 60:682–685, 1989.
19. Niemann KMW, Mankin HJ: Fractures about the hip in an institutionalized patient population. II. Survival and ability to walk again. J Bone Joint Surg 50A:1327–1340, 1968.
20. Pellicci PM, Bostrom M, Poss R: Posterior approach to total hip replacement using enhanced posterior soft tissue repair. Clin Orthop 355:224–228, 1998.
21. Rothermel JE, Garcia A: Treatment of hip fractures in patients with Parkinson's syndrome on levodopa therapy. J Bone Joint Surg 54A:1251–1254, 1972.
22. Sato Y, Kikuyama M, Oizumi K: High prevalence of vitamin D deficiency and reduced bone mass in Parkinson's disease. Neurology 49:1273–1278, 1997.
23. Soto-Hall R: Treatment of transcervical fractures complicated by certain common neurological conditions. Instr Course Lect 17:117–120, 1960.
24. Staeheli JW, Frassica FJ, Sim FH: Prosthetic replacement of the femoral head for fracture of the femoral neck in patients who have Parkinson disease. J Bone Joint Surg 70A:565–568, 1988.
25. Taggart H, Crawford V: Reduced bone density of the hip in elderly patients with Parkinson's disease. Age Ageing 24:326–328, 1995.
26. Turcotte R, Godin C, Duchesne R, Jodoin A: Hip fractures and Parkinson's disease. A clinical review of 94 fractures treated surgically. Clin Orthop 256:132–136, 1990.
27. Whittaker RP, Abeshaus MM, Scholl HW, Chung SM: Fifteen years' experience with metallic endoprosthetic replacement of the femoral head for femoral neck fractures. J Trauma 12:799–806, 1972.
28. Zia S, Cody F, O'Boyle D: Joint position sense is impaired by Parkinson's disease. Ann Neurol 47:218–228, 2000.

Hip Arthroplasty in Paget's Disease

• JAVAD PARVIZI and FRANKLIN H. SIM

First recognized and described by Sir James Paget in 1877,[31] Paget's disease is a localized disorder marked by increased bone resorption, bone formation, and remodeling, which may lead to substantial osseous deformity with subsequent alteration of joint biomechanics. Because of the associated deformities, the alteration in the quality of the affected bone, and the older age of these patients, a frequent association with disabling hip disease and subsequent need for hip arthroplasty has been reported.[14,28,35] It is imperative to recognize some of the unique problems inherent to this condition in (1) differentiating the source of hip pain preoperatively, (2) determining the technical challenges that may be encountered intraoperatively in the management of osseous deformity and potential bleeding, and (3) identifying measures that may optimize the long-term results and reduce the risk of complications.

PATHOPHYSIOLOGY

Although its incidence may be declining,[6] Paget's disease may affect up to 3.5 percent of persons older than 45 years.[9,11,34] The pelvis and the femur are the most commonly involved bony sites, with radiographic changes reported in 20 to 80 percent of patients with Paget's disease.[15,27,44] It is interesting that symptoms, usually in the form of pain, arise in less than 10 percent of those affected.[43] In symptomatic patients, hip pain either from coxarthrosis or directly from active bone disease occurs in approximately 30 percent of patients and represents one of the most common sites of pain.[43]

Although the exact etiology of Paget's disease remains unknown, a slow viral infection, particularly occurring in individuals with a genetic predisposition, has been implicated.[4,13,29,35,39] The primary abnormality is believed to be an intense focal resorption of normal bone by abnormal osteoclasts.[10] However, because stromal and osteoblastic cells direct osteoclast formation, evidence suggests that osteoblasts may initiate the disease process.[36] Paget's disease evolves through three distinct phases: (1) an initial burst of osteoclastic activity with bone resorption, (2) a mixed phase of both osteoclastic and osteoblastic activity with increased level of bone turnover leading to deposition of structurally

abnormal bone, and (3) a final sclerotic phase during which bone formation outweighs bone resorption.

Depending on the activity of the disease and anatomic site of involvement, different clinical, biochemical, and radiographic pictures may be present. In the active osteoclastic phase, a hypervascular state exists as normal bone is resorbed and the medullary cavity is replaced with fibrovascular connective tissue. The resorption of bone and the hypervascularity may be associated with pain and can lead to increased bleeding during surgery.[17,30,33] Disease activity may be monitored by measuring the serum alkaline phosphatase level, which can be elevated as a result of bone resorption, and urinary hydroxyproline excretion, which reflects breakdown of type I collagen. The increased hydroxyproline level correlates well with the degree of radiographic disease activity and with elevated serum alkaline phosphatase level.[11,20] Radiographically, an advancing V-shaped lytic lesion and a halo of supra-acetabular osteoporosis are indications of osteoclastic activity and bone resorption.[24,37] As compensatory new bone is formed, the characteristic thickened, coarse trabeculae appear radiographically, which correspond histologically to a mosaic pattern of poorly organized lamellar bone. Structurally inferior to normal bone, the new bone deforms under weight bearing and muscle tension forces, leading to bone structure widening, bowing of long bones, coxa vara deformity of the femoral neck, and acetabular protrusio with pelvic involvement (Fig. 59–1).

It is not known if the incidence of osteoarthritis is higher in patients with Paget's disease than in age-matched controls. Some authors have speculated that the pagetic process predisposes patients to degenerative arthritis.[2,17] Altman believed that juxta-articular bony enlargement resulting in articular incongruity, altered biodynamics secondary to bowing and deformity, and altered subchondral support influenced joint function.[2] Guyer and Dewbury, however, found that the actual incidence of hip degenerative changes in patients with Paget's involvement around the hip was the same as that of an age-matched group of patients without Paget's disease.[16] Even if the incidence of osteoarthritis may not be increased in patients with Paget's disease, the pattern of joint disease and bony deformity is clearly influenced by Paget's process. Whereas superior joint space narrowing is commonly associated with idiopathic osteoarthritis, primarily medial or concentric narrowing is seen more frequently in patients with Paget's disease. In a review of 88 patients with hip pain and Paget's involvement, superior joint narrowing was noted in only 3 patients while 78 patients had evidence of medial narrowing and concentric narrowing was seen in 57 patients.[2] In addition, coxa vara deformity of the femoral neck and acetabular protrusio are rare in osteoarthritis yet are a frequent finding in patients with severe Paget's disease. Winfield and Stamp, in reviewing 50 patients with symptomatic Paget's disease, detected acetabular protrusio in 33 percent of patients with pelvic and femoral involvement.[43] In addition, prominent medial joint space narrowing, associated with coxa vara deformity of the femur, was noted in 67 percent of patients in their series.[43]

PREOPERATIVE PLANNING

Source of Hip Pain

Potential sources of hip pain in patients with Paget's disease include bone pain caused by disease activity, osteoarthritis, impending or actual stress fracture (Fig. 59–1), radiculopathy caused by spinal involvement, and Paget's sarcoma. Differentiating the bone pain of Paget's process from the pain secondary to coxarthrosis may be difficult. Both can give a dull, aching pain that may worsen with weight bearing. Relief of discomfort with hip joint injection with local anesthetic would suggest coxarthrosis as the source of pain.[7] Bone pain, however, generally correlates with the activity of the disease. Alkaline phosphatase levels and urinary hydroxyproline excretion are often markedly elevated, and bone scans show intense skeletal uptake. Appropriate therapeutic trial of anti-Paget's medications, such as bisphosphonates and calcitonin, may be beneficial because pain secondary to Paget's disease is improved with treatment.[3,17,26,27] Preoperative consultation with an endocrinologist can be helpful in obtaining disease control and preparing the patient for surgery. Some authors routinely pretreat all potential surgical candidates with calcitonin, diphosphonates, or both.[3,27]

Preoperative Radiographs

In addition to standard hip radiographs, all patients should have a full-length radiographs of the femur obtained prior to arthroplasty, to assess the degree of femoral deformity and the extent of involvement. Based on the radiographs, the need for and the type of femoral osteotomy for correction of the deformity can be determined.

Radiographs should be scrutinized for the presence of complete or stress fractures, which could account for the hip pain. The fractures may be in the region of the femoral neck, intertrochanteric area, or femoral shaft.

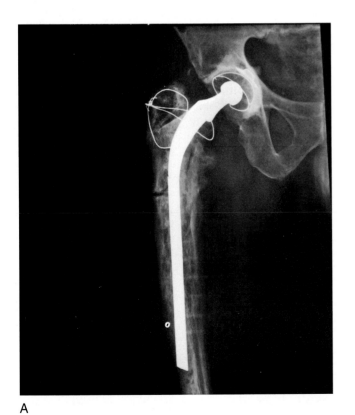

A

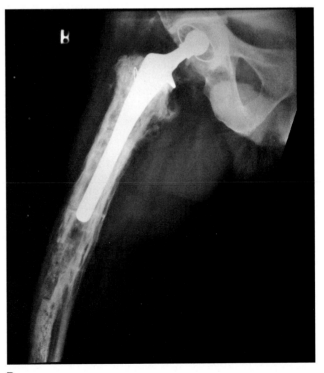

B

Figure 59–1. A, Anteroposterior radiograph of a 69-year-old male who had undergone two prior total hip arthroplasties and presented with severe pain of sudden onset. The patient had sustained fracture of the femur and the femoral component. The femoral component was revised to an uncemented component. **B**, The femur fracture healed uneventfully, and the patient was pain free with ingrown femoral component at 2 years' follow-up.

They are generally associated with skeletal deformity and can present as incomplete or fissure fractures on the tension side of the bone. In our series of 80 Paget's patients who underwent hip arthroplasty, 10 had a previous femoral neck fracture, 2 had femoral shaft fractures, and 1 had a previous intertrochanteric fracture.[26]

Unrelenting pain and radiographic bone destruction inconsistent with Paget's disease alone, particularly if associated with a soft tissue mass, should raise the suspicion of sarcomatous change.[12,18,42] When suspected, adjunctive axial imaging studies such as magnetic resonance imaging or computed tomography scans are indicated to exclude sarcomatous change. Paget's sarcoma represents less than 5 percent of all sarcomas but contributes a much greater percentage of sarcomas in patients over 40 years of age.[8,19,42] Common sites of involvement include the pelvic bones, femur, and humerus, which corresponds to the anatomic distribution of Paget's disease.[18,19,38] When located in the femur, approximately one half of these sarcomas are in the proximal portion and the other half are at the distal level.

TECHNICAL CONSIDERATIONS

Hip arthroplasty in patients with Paget's disease may present special technical challenges.

Hypervascularity

The potential for increased intraoperative bleeding, particularly in patients with active disease, should be anticipated and prepared for preoperatively. Treatment with anti-Paget's medications, prior to surgery, has been shown to be effective in reducing intraoperative blood loss.[28] If hypervascularity is encountered, postoperative treatment with bisphosphonates and calcitonin should be considered because rapid postoperative osteolysis can be concerning.[25] Increased blood loss was observed in patients with Paget's disease undergoing total hip arthroplasty at our institution.[26,33] These patients required greater than usual fluid and blood replacements. Use of an intraoperative blood salvage system should be considered in these patients, particularly those with active disease, when undergoing joint replacement. It is also important to minimize intraoperative bleeding because inability to obtain a dry bed may compromise the interdigitation of cement with bone on the femoral and acetabular side, which may in turn affect the long-term survival of the prosthesis.

Osseous Deformity

Deformities on the femoral side should be recognized and addressed appropriately because proper positioning of the femoral component may be jeopardized otherwise. Coxa vara is a common femoral deformity in patients with Paget's disease that may lead to varus positioning of the femoral component.[28] In our experience, of 22 patients with preoperative coxa vara, 10 had varus positioning of

the component ranging from 2 to 20 degrees.[26] Fortunately, in most patients the degree of varus positioning was mild (average 5.7 degrees), and only the patient with 20 degrees of malposition eventually required revision of the femoral component for aseptic loosening. Occasionally trochanteric or femoral realignment osteotomy may be required to address coxa vara deformity of the femur (Fig. 59–2). If osteotomy of the femur is required at one or more levels, a one-stage approach may be useful in reducing the total period of disability.[32]

On the pelvic side, acetabular protrusio may present difficulties during the total hip arthroplasty in Paget's disease patients (Fig. 59–3). Medial acetabular bone grafting or use of an oversized hemispherical cup may be helpful in restoring the hip center to an anatomic position[22] (Fig. 59–4). The availability of offset acetabular liners for uncemented cup designs provides another option for compensating for medial cup placement in patients with protrusio deformity, depending on its degree. In our series, of the 32 patients with protrusio, 23 had only mild medial displacement and did not require any special reconstructive procedures.[26] Overall, the presence of protrusio was not associated with a poor clinical result. If very poor bone quality is encountered, cement fixation with or without an antiprotrusio cage may be favored.[22] If an uncemented implant is to be used, good peripheral support against an intact rim of the acetabulum and use of multiple screws to supplement fixation may reduce the potential for cup migration.

Implant Choice

Altered bone quality and morphologic features may influence implant choice and fixation methods in patients with Paget's disease. The basic principle of hip arthroplasty in achieving optimal component positioning and adequate fixation should be observed in these patients also. Overall the choice of implant and fixation method is at the discretion of the surgeon and his or her familiarity with specific designs. There are, however, circumstances when special consideration should be given in selecting the type of implant and fixation method. In instances where realignment femoral osteotomy is carried out, a long uncemented femoral stem may be preferred to a cemented stem because cement extravasation into osteotomy gaps may impair bony union. Successful one-stage osteotomy in combination with an uncemented, extensively coated femoral component has been reported.[1]

Conversely, bone quality changes proximally, coupled with deformity from bone enlargement or angulation, make achievement of fit and fill by an extensively porous-coated implant very difficult. Cement fixation or use of a porous-coated implant engaging normal diaphyseal bone may be a better choice in such cases. Occasionally very hard sclerotic bone may be encountered in the pagetoid bone, which precludes the use of standard rasps and instrumentation and may necessitate availability of high-speed burs for bone preparation. It is plausible that cement interdigitation with the hard scle-

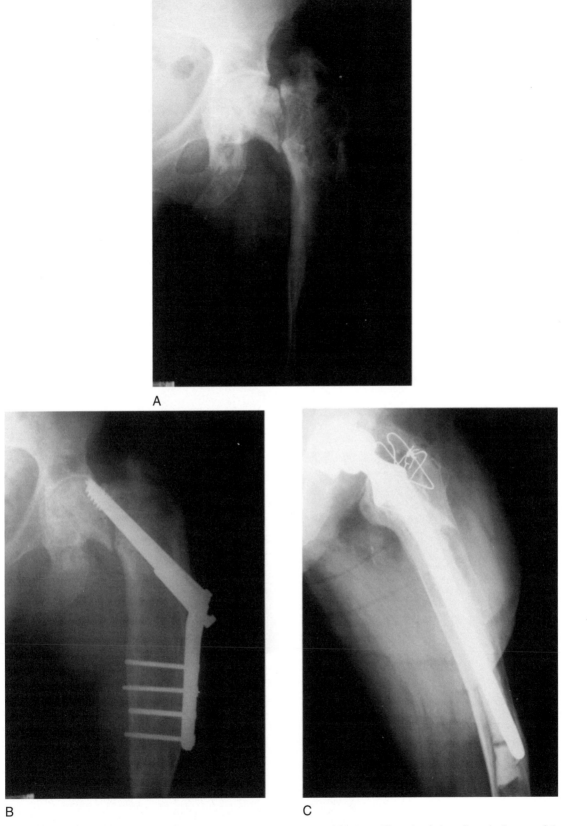

A

B   C

Figure 59–2. A, Anteroposterior radiograph of the left hip in a 73-year-old woman. There is obvious Paget's disease of the proximal femur, with an associated vertical shear-type fracture of the femoral neck. **B**, The patient was treated with open reduction and internal fixation using a compression screw and side plate. Suboptimal fixation of the fracture was achieved, and the screws were cut out of the superior portion of the femoral neck. **C**, The repair was converted to a total hip arthroplasty utilizing a cemented long-stemmed femoral component. Because of the bowing of the femur secondary to the Paget's disease, the tip of the stem was protruding anteriorly and laterally and eventually failed.

Illustration continued on following page

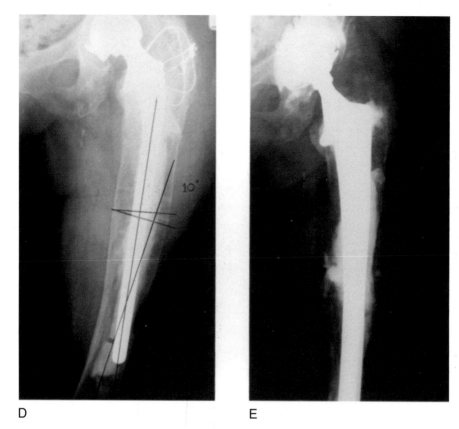

D

E

Figure 59–2. *Continued.* **D**, Preoperative anteroposterior radiograph illustrated the planned osteotomy of the proximal femur in order to correct the deformity at the time of revision arthroplasty. **E**, Postoperative radiograph showing a long cemented femoral stem in the osteotomy site (*arrows*).

Figure 59–3. Severe Paget's disease of the femur and pelvis causing coxa vara and acetabular protrusion. (From McDonald DJ, Sim FH: Total hip arthroplasty in Paget's disease: a follow-up note. J Bone Joint Surg Am 69:766, 1987, with permission.)

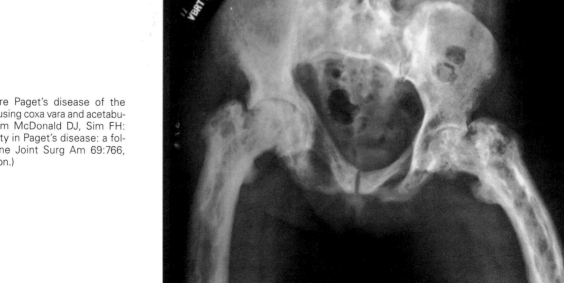

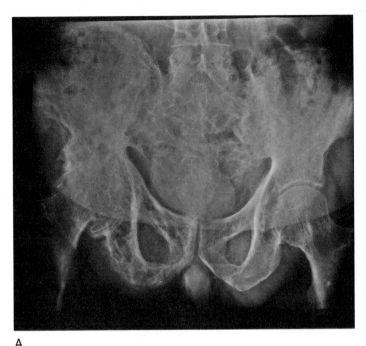

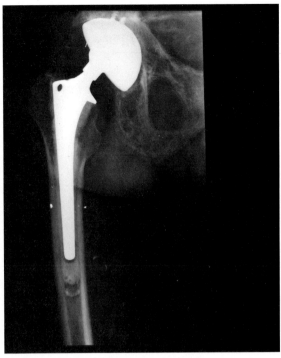

A   B

Figure 59–4. Preoperative anteroposterior radiograph (**A**) of a 72-year-old man with coxa magna and moderate protrusio acetabuli who underwent hybrid hip arthroplasty with the use of a "jumbo" acetabular cup (**B**).

rotic bone may be suboptimal, and in these cases an uncemented component may be more appropriate (Fig. 59–5). The outcome of hip arthroplasty with uncemented components positioned against pagetoid bone at our institution has been very encouraging, with no component loosening in the first decade following joint replacement.[33] In that series, the presence of hard sclerotic bone was the reason for altering the choice of implant and using an uncemented component.

POSTOPERATIVE CARE

Because of the complex nature of arthroplasty in some Paget's disease patients, postoperative care of these individuals may need to be altered. There is theoretical concern that the mechanical effect of prolonged postoperative immobilization or protected weight bearing combined with the metabolic influence of an active disease, may predispose these patients to marked bone resorption. Postoperative treatment with calcitonin and bisphosphonates should help reduce the likelihood of this problem. Early follow-up in the postoperative period is recommended if there is sudden change in status with increasing pain. This may indicate a developing stress fracture or rapid bone resorption. When an associated osteotomy has been performed, it is reasonable to delay full weight bearing until radiographic union has occurred.

RESULTS

There have been several reports on the outcome of total hip arthroplasty in patients with Paget's

disease.[23,26,28,40,41] Ludkowski and Wilson-McDonald reported the results of 37 arthroplasties in 30 patients.[23] At a mean follow-up of 7.8 years (range, 1 to 18.4 years) there were no revisions, and 70 percent of their patients had good to excellent clinical results.[23] They found that the clinical results were influenced by preoperative osseous deformities in the form of coxa vara, protrusio acetabuli, and femoral bowing, with only 34 percent of the patients having a good or excellent result if two or more of the three mentioned deformities were present.[23] Intraoperative technical problems caused by exposure difficulties, excessive bleeding, and hard bone were encountered in 25 percent of their patients.

An earlier report from our institution by Stauffer and Sim[41] also noted technical difficulties but emphasized the excellent early clinical results of 35 cemented hip arthroplasties in 32 patients with Paget's disease. No patients required revision at 2.1 years, and there was a significant improvement in hip scores ($P<0.001$).[41] Merkow et al. confirmed the effectiveness of arthroplasty at relieving symptoms in patients with Paget's disease of the hip, but noted a 9.5 percent incidence of mechanical failure requiring reoperation at a mean follow-up of 5.2 years.[28] In our updated experience, we reported the result of 91 arthroplasties in 80 patients and additionally analyzed 52 arthroplasties in 46 of the 80 patients who underwent surgery before 1975 and in whom minimum 10-year follow-up was available.[26] Comparison was made with 7222 total hip arthroplasties performed between 1969 and 1975 at the Mayo Clinic. In that series, a higher revision rate, radiographic loosening, and significant decline in results were observed in patients with Paget's disease.[26] Fourteen hips (15.4 percent) required revision of one or

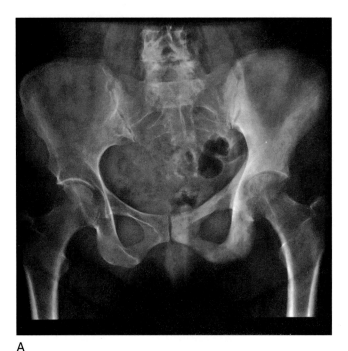

A

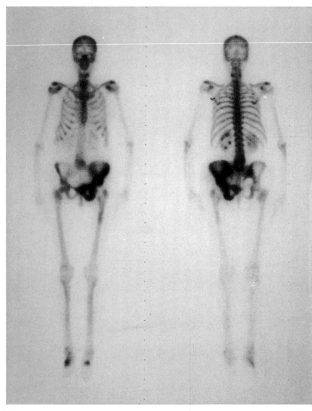

B

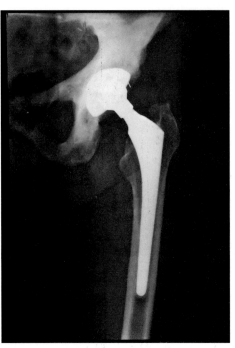

C

Figure 59–5. Preoperative anteroposterior radiograph (**A**) and bone scan (**B**) demonstrating disease activity in a 54-year-old female with Paget's disease affecting the pelvis who underwent uncemented total hip arthroplasty with the acetabular cup being positioned against the active pagetoid bone. **C,** Patient was pain free with stable and ingrown femoral and acetabular components at 7 years.

both components. Twelve revisions (13 percent) were for aseptic loosening and occurred at an average of 7.3 years postoperatively. Overall, 74 percent of patients were considered to have a good or excellent result based on a Mayo Hip Score[21] of 80 or more. In those patients with a minimum 10-year follow-up, aseptic loosening was evident in 30 percent of femoral components and 14 percent of acetabular components (Fig. 59–6). However, actuarial analysis of the survival to aseptic loosening in the 52 patients with 10-year follow-up as a group, compared to our overall experience of 7222 hip arthroplasties performed during the same time period, did show a significant difference in the probability of aseptic loosening at 10 years (Fig. 59–7).

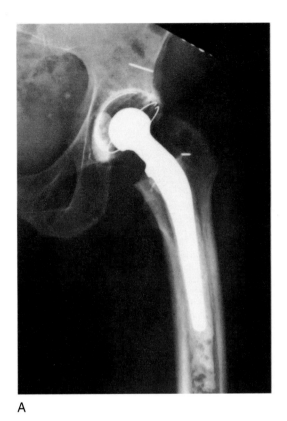

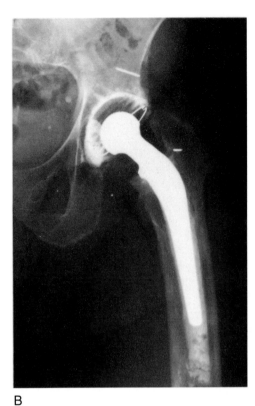

A   B

Figure 59–6. Early femoral loosening. **A,** Initial postoperative radiograph of a 63-year-old patient who had pagetoid involvement of the proximal end of the femur. **B,** One year after surgery, there is a complete radiolucent line at the bone-cement interface. Four millimeters of femoral subsidence has occurred, and a crack is present in the distal mantle of cement. The radiographic score for the femur is zero. At 2.5 years, the patient had only mild symptoms. (From McDonald DJ, Sim FH: Total hip arthroplasty in Paget's disease: a follow-up note. J Bone Joint Surg Am 69:766, 1987, with permission.)

The exact relationship between component loosening and disease activity is not clear. We have not identified a correlation between disease activity, as measured by alkaline phosphatase and urinary hydroxyproline excretion, at the time of arthroplasty and the need for later revision or long-term incidence of aseptic loosening. Other authors have been unable to confirm the effect of disease activity on outcome either. Ludkowski and Wilson-McDonald, after combining their series with six other reported studies to yield a total of 150 patients with Paget's disease receiving cemented total hip arthroplasty, were unable to show a correlation between the results of total hip arthroplasty and disease activity.[23]

The incidence of heterotrophic bone formation in patients with Paget's disease undergoing cemented and uncemented hip arthroplasty at our institution has been higher overall.[26,33] Although the majority of the patients developed mild (Brooker class 1 or 2)[5] heterotrophic ossification, two patients, one in each series, required reoperation for excision of functionally disabling heterotrophic bone. Other studies have also observed a higher incidence of heterotrophic ossification.[23,28]

Figure 59–7. Actuarial analysis of the probability of revision for aseptic loosening in patients who did and did not have Paget's disease. The probability of not having had a revision at 10 years was slightly greater for the patients who did not have Paget's disease. (From McDonald DJ, Sim FH: Total hip arthroplasty in Paget's disease: a follow-up note. J Bone Joint Surg Am 69:766, 1987, with permission.)

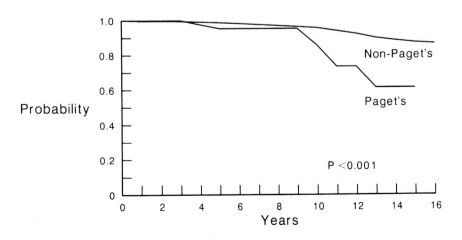

CONCLUSION

Total hip arthroplasty is highly successful in treatment of patients with Paget's disease. Because the results of arthroplasty are similar to or slightly less durable than those seen in patients with osteoarthritis, this information is shared with the patient. The higher risk for heterotrophic bone formation and increased perioperative blood loss due to hypervascularity of the bone is also discussed before surgery. Although in the past cemented devices were preferred, uncemented arthroplasty has shown promising results and is also discussed before surgery in patients with Paget's disease when possible.

References

1. Alexakis PG, Brown BA, Hohl WM: Porous hip replacement in Paget's disease. Clin Orthop 350:138–142, 1998.
2. Altman RD: Musculoskeletal manifestations of Paget's disease of bone. Arthritis Rheum 23:1121, 1980.
3. Avioli LV: Paget's disease: state of the art. Clin Ther 9:567, 1987.
4. Basla MF, Rebel A, Fournier JG, et al: On the trail of paramyxoviruses in Paget's disease of bone. Clin Orthop 217:9, 1987.
5. Brooker AF, Bowerman JW, Robinson RA, Riley LH Jr: Ectopic ossification following total hip replacement: incidence and a method of classification. J Bone Joint Surg Am 55:1629, 1973.
6. Cooper C, Schafheutle K, Kellingray S, et al: The epidemiology of Paget's disease in Britain: is the prevalence decreasing? J Bone Miner Res 14:192–197, 1999.
7. Crawford RW, Gie GA, Ling RS, Murray DW: Diagnostic value of intra-articular anaesthetic in primary osteoarthritis of the hip. J Bone Joint Surg Br 80:279, 1998.
8. Dahlin DC, Unni KK: Bone Tumors: General Aspects and Data on 8542 Cases, 4th ed. Springfield, IL: Charles C Thomas, 1986.
9. Dalinka MK, Aronchick JM, Haddad JG Jr: Paget's disease. Orthop Clin North Am 14:3, 1983.
10. Demulder A, Takahashi S, Singer FR, et al. Abnormalities in osteoclast precursors and marrow accessory cells in Paget's disease. Endocrinology 133:1978–1982, 1993.
11. Franck WA, Bress NM, Singer FR, Krane SM: Rheumatic manifestations of Paget's disease of bone. Am J Med 56:592, 1974.
12. Frassica FJ, Sim FH, Frassica DA, et al: Survival and management considerations in postirradiation osteosarcoma and Paget's osteosarcoma. Clin Orthop 270:120–127, 1991.
13. Gordon MT, Anderson DC, Sharpe PT: Canine distemper virus localized in bone cells of patients with Paget's disease. Bone 12:195–201, 1991.
14. Graham J, Harris WH: Paget's disease involving the hip joint. J Bone Joint Surg Br 53:650, 1971.
15. Guyer PB, Chamberlain AT, Ackery DM, Rolfe EB: The anatomic distribution of osteitis deformans. Clin Orthop 156:141, 1981.
16. Guyer PB, Dewbury KC: The hip joint in Paget's disease (Paget's coxopathy). Br J Radiol 51:574, 1978.
17. Hadjipavlou A, Lander P, Srolovitz H: Pagetic arthritis: pathophysiology and management. Clin Orthop 208:15, 1986.
18. Haibach H, Farrell C, Dittrich FJ: Neoplasms arising in Paget's disease of bone: a study of 82 cases. Am J Clin Pathol 83:594, 1985.
19. Huvos AG, Butler A, Bretsky SS: Osteogenic sarcoma associated with Paget's disease of bone: a clinicopathologic study of 65 patients. Cancer 52:1489, 1983.
20. Kanis JA, Gray RE: Long-term follow-up observations on treatment in Paget's disease of bone. Clin Orthop 217:99, 1987.
21. Kavanagh BF, Fitzgerald RH Jr: Clinical and roentgenographic assessment of total hip arthroplasty: a new hip score. Clin Orthop 193:133, 1985.
22. Lewallen DG: Hip arthroplasty in patients with Paget's disease. Clin Orthop 369:243–250, 1999.
23. Ludkowski P, Wilson-McDonald J: Total arthroplasty in Paget's disease of the hip: a clinical review and review of the literature. Clin Orthop 255:160, 1990.
24. Maldague B, Malghem J: Dynamic radiologic patterns of Paget's disease of bone. Clin Orthop 217:126, 1987.
25. Marr DS, Rosenthal DJ, Cohen GL, et al: Rapid postoperative osteolysis in Paget's disease: a case report. J Bone Joint Surg Am 66:274–277, 1994.
26. McDonald DJ, Sim FH: Total hip arthroplasty in Paget's disease: a follow-up note. J Bone Joint Surg Am 69:766, 1987.
27. Merkow RL, Lane JM: Paget's disease of bone. Orthop Clin North Am 21:171, 1990.
28. Merkow RL, Pellicci PM, Hely DP, Salvati EA: Total hip replacement for Paget's disease of the hip. J Bone Joint Surg Am 66:752, 1984.
29. Mirra JM: Pathogenesis of Paget's disease based on viral etiology. Clin Orthop 217:162, 1987.
30. Namba RS, Brick GW, Murray WR: Revision total hip arthroplasty with correctional femoral osteotomy in Paget's disease. J Arthroplasty 12:591–595, 1997.
31. Paget J: On a form of chronic inflammation of bones. Med Chir Tr 60:37, 1877.
32. Papagelopoulos PJ, Trousdale RT, Lewallen DG: Total hip arthroplasty with femoral osteotomy for proximal femoral deformity. Clin Orthop 332:151–162, 1996.
33. Parvizi J, Schall DM, Sim FH, Lewallen DG: Uncemented total hip arthroplasty in patients with Paget's disease. Paper presented at the 67th Annual Meeting of the American Academy of Orthopaedic Surgeons, Orlando, FL, March 15–19, 2000.
34. Pygott F: Paget's disease of bone: the radiological incidence. Lancet 1:1170–1171, 1957.
35. Renier JC, Fanello S, Bos C, et al: An etiologic study of Paget's disease. Rev Rheum Engl Ed 63:606–611, 1996.
36. Robey PG, Bianco P: The role of osteogenic cells in pathophysiology of Paget's disease. J Bone Min Res 14(2):9–16, 1999.
37. Roper BA: Paget's disease involving the hip joint: a classification. Clin Orthop 80:33, 1971.
38. Schajowicz F, Santini-Araujo E, Berenstein M: Sarcoma complicating Paget's disease of bone: a clinicopathological study of 62 cases. J Bone Joint Surg Br 65:299, 1983.
39. Siris ES: Epidemiological aspects of Paget's disease: family history and relationship to other medical conditions. Semin Arthritis Rheum 23:222–225, 1994.
40. Stauffer RN: Ten-year follow-up study of total hip replacement: with particular reference to roentgenographic loosening of the components. J Bone Joint Surg Am 64:983, 1982.
41. Stauffer RN, Sim FH: Total hip arthroplasty in Paget's disease of the hip. J Bone Joint Surg Am 58:476, 1976.
42. Wick MR, Siegal GP, Unni KK, et al: Sarcomas of the bone complicating osteitis deformans (Paget's disease): fifty years experience. Am J Surg Pathol 5:47–59, 1981.
43. Winfield J, Stamp TC: Bone and joint symptoms in Paget's disease. Ann Rheum Dis 43:769, 1984.
44. Ziegler R, Holz G, Rotzler B, et al: Paget's disease of the bone in West Germany: prevalence and distribution. Clin Orthop 194:199–204, 1985.

60A

Neoplasms: Primary Pathologic Conditions

• THOMAS C. SHIVES and DOUGLAS J. PRITCHARD

A wide variety of primary benign and malignant bone or soft tissue lesions arise in the vicinity of the hip joint.[7] Some of these conditions, obviously, are best treated by alternative methods, but, in some cases, it is appropriate to resect the lesion, sacrificing the hip joint, and then, subsequently, to reconstruct with a total hip device. Some relatively small lesions may require only an endoprosthesis or a conventional total hip device, whereas other, more extensive lesions may require a custom type of total hip arthroplasty. Over the past few years, there have been a number of new developments that have expanded the indications for such procedures. Most recently, there has been interest in the use of composite allografts with conventional total hip devices for the reconstruction of major defects.

Certain pathologic conditions are more commonly treated with resection followed by prosthetic replacement. These may be broadly classified into four distinct groups: primary bone or soft tissue tumors, metastatic cancer, Paget's disease, and other pathologic conditions.

In this portion of the chapter, we discuss the first two topics; the second portion covers the management of metastatic disease, and Paget's disease is discussed in Chapter 59. Other pathologic conditions are discussed elsewhere.

PRIMARY BONE TUMORS

Benign Bone Tumors

Although any benign bone tumor may arise in the region of the hip, certain tumors occur more commonly than others at this site; these include osteoid osteoma, giant cell tumor, and osteochondroma. Usually, these benign conditions can be treated with local excision or excision by curettage (intralesional lesion). However, in some instances, the size, location, and aggressiveness of the tumor may necessitate resection of the proximal femur or a portion of the acetabulum or both. In such a situation, it may be necessary to reconstruct the hip with either an endoprosthesis or a total hip device.[6]

An example of this is a large giant cell tumor in the region of the femoral neck, which recurs after initial treatment by curettage and grafting. In this situation, it may be necessary to resect the upper portion of the femur and reconstruct with an appropriately sized proximal femoral replacement, either an endoprosthesis or a bipolar type of device (Fig. 60A–1).

Nontumors that simulate neoplastic processes include infectious and inflammatory conditions. These are managed in a manner similar to that described in the preceeding paragraphs (Fig. 60A–2).

Malignant Bone Tumors

Chondrosarcoma

One of the most common malignant bone tumors affecting the hip is chondrosarcoma. In Dahlin and Unni's series of 895 chondrosarcomas, 99 arose in the proximal femur and 191 in the periacetabular region or adjacent pelvic bones.[5,12] Many chondrosarcomas arise in the region of the triradiate cartilage, which is the junction of the innominate bone, the pubis, and the ischium. Tumors that arise in this region may be difficult to detect. Indeed, they may be present for several years before they are finally discovered. Because many of these tumors are too large for local excision, more drastic measures, such as a hemipelvectomy, may be necessary. However, there are a number of such chondrosarcomas that do lend themselves to local resection and reconstruction with a prosthetic device.

Chondrosarcoma tends to be one of the most implantable of all tumors. That is, it is easy to seed or spread the tumor into the surrounding soft tissues, with subsequent tumor recurrence. Hence, great care must be taken during the surgical procedure to avoid any spilling of the tumor. Careful planning and execution of the biopsy procedure is necessary so that, once the diagnosis is established, the biopsy wound can be included in the subsequent resection. If it is not, the tumor is likely to recur in the biopsy wound scar.

Careful judgment is required to assess the feasibility and desirability of performing a resection as opposed to

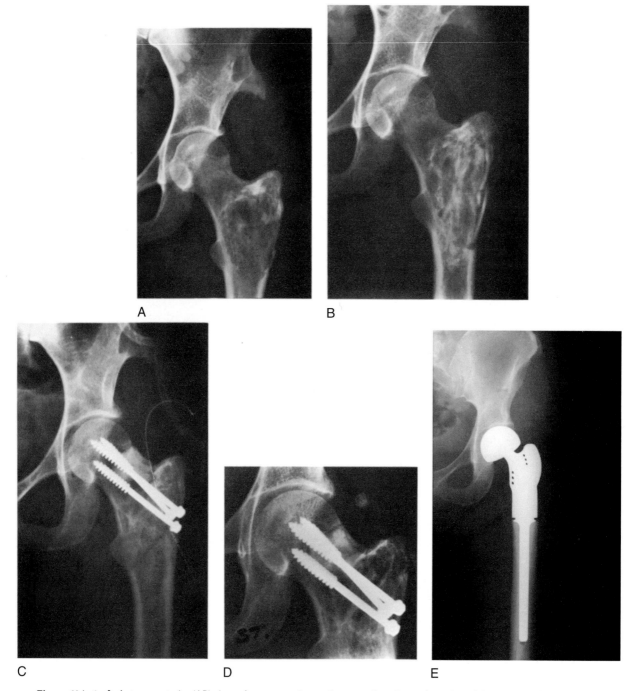

Figure 60A–1. **A**, Anteroposterior (AP) view of recurrent giant cell tumor of trochanteric region of the proximal femur of a 22-year-old woman. **B**, AP view after curettage and bone grafting with autogenous iliac bone. **C**, Further recurrence led to additional resection and reconstruction using methyl methacrylate and internal fixation pins. **D**, Radiographic evidence of further tumor recurrence. **E**, AP view after resection of proximal femur and reconstruction performed with a custom segmental proximal femoral device with a bipolar acetabular component.

a hemipelvectomy. In general, smaller tumors lend themselves more readily to resection, whereas larger tumors generally require hemipelvectomy, either an internal limb-sparing hemipelvectomy or a conventional hemipelvectomy amputation. The type of chondrosarcoma may also influence the decision. For example, clear cell chondrosarcoma, which is rare, tends to involve the femoral head and neck and is relatively indolent. In fact, this lesion may even mimic a

chondroblastoma radiographically. Because this tumor is usually small, resection and reconstruction of the hip joint may be considered. In contrast, another variety of chondrosarcoma, the so-called dedifferentiated chondrosarcoma, tends to be highly malignant. It can be rather large and has considerable soft tissue extension in most cases. Such a tumor is more likely to require more extensive resection or even amputation.

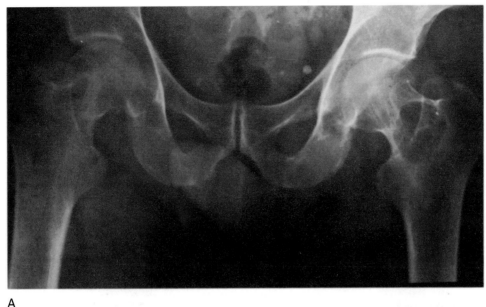

A

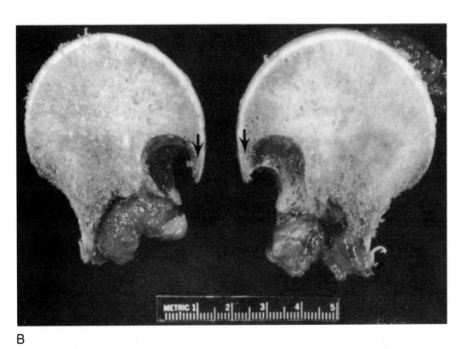

B

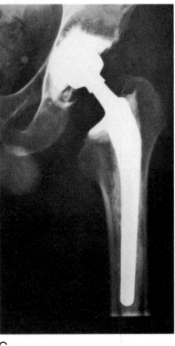

C

Figure 60A–2. A, This 66-year-old man with rheumatoid arthritis had a large osteolytic defect of the base of the femoral neck. **B,** A twisting move caused a spontaneous fracture that required resection. **C,** Because a diagnosis of rheumatoid cyst was confirmed, a hip replacement was carried out.

Osteosarcoma

In Unni's series of 1649 osteosarcomas, 88 occurred in the femoral head and neck and an additional 18 occurred in the region of the acetabulum. One hundred twenty-seven osteosarcomas were located in other parts of the pelvis.[1] As with most tumors in the hip region, pain or a mass was the symptom at onset. Osteosarcoma rarely appears as a pathologic fracture of the hip.

The majority of patients who develop osteosarcoma are younger than 20 years of age. Thus, there is a real dilemma regarding the use of total hip implants in such young patients. However, there is no completely satisfactory method of reconstruction for the young patient who has a hip joint sacrificed to gain tumor control. Osteosarcoma does sometimes arise in the region of the hip joint in the older patient.

For the older patient who has known Paget's disease and then develops a change in symptoms or a change in the radiographic appearance of the lesion, malignant transformation should be suspected. Older patients should also be suspected of having osteosarcoma if they have a prior history of radiation for carcinoma of the pelvic organs or any preexisting condition in the same general region. Radiation sarcoma may arise many years after the radiation treatment.

Because most osteosarcomas that arise in the region of the hip joint are relatively unresectable when initially seen, patients are usually treated with preoperative chemotherapy. Patients should be observed carefully during preoperative treatment; if the tumor responds favorably, it may subsequently prove amenable to resection. In these cases, it is important to resect the tumor together with adjacent muscles and soft tissues (wide excision). Reconstruction usually requires a customized total hip implant. Alternatively, a composite allograft with a conventional total hip may be used for the reconstruction (Fig. 60A–3).

Ewing's Sarcoma

Although Ewing's sarcoma is less common than osteosarcoma, approximately 25 percent of all Ewing's sarcomas arise in the region of the hip.[4]

There is general consensus today that patients with Ewing's sarcoma should be treated with chemotherapy at the outset. After initial chemotherapy, a decision can be made regarding treatment of the primary lesion with surgery or radiation therapy or some combination of the two. The patient will then continue receiving chemotherapy after management of the local lesion.

The decision to use surgery or radiation therapy or both in the region of the hip joint is particularly difficult. If radiation therapy alone is employed, there is a moderate risk of the subsequent development of a local recurrence. In addition, there is considerable morbidity associated with radiation in the region of the hip joint, particularly joint contracture, induration of the soft tissues, and pathologic fracture of the proximal femur. Furthermore, there is some risk of inducing a second malignant tumor at the site of the primary lesion. Resection of the proximal femur and reconstruction with a total hip arthroplasty minimize some of these risks. However, performing total joint replacements on young people, who most commonly have Ewing's sarcoma, may not be orthopedically sound. There is considerable risk that the orthopedic implant will not last indefinitely. There is no unanimity of opinion as to how to proceed with Ewing's sarcoma in this location. Our policy, in general, is to use total hip devices for patients who are somewhat older and to use radiation treatment for younger patients.

SYNOVIAL TUMORS

There are several relatively rare conditions that appear to arise in the synovium of the hip joint. These are nearly always benign. Malignant tumors of the synovium are extremely rare. What is called synovial sarcoma actually seldom arises within a joint. Rather, it arises from the mesenchyma of the adjacent soft tissues and not from preexistent synovial tissue.

In the differential diagnosis of synovial tumors in the region of the hip, consideration must be given to rheumatoid or degenerative cysts and adventitious or bursal enlargements, particularly about the greater trochanter and the iliopectineal region (see Fig. 60A–2).

Pigmented Villonodular Synovitis

Pigmented villonodular synovitis (PVNS) was first described by Jaffe and associates in 1941.[2] This rare condition is more common in the knee joint. In our experience, we have managed 75 patients with PVNS of the knee joint and, during the same period, only 20 patients with this condition involving the hip joint.[9] Patients with PVNS frequently are in the fourth and fifth decades of life. They usually have unilateral hip pain, which is increased by activity and relieved by rest. Roentgenographic findings include multiple cystlike areas in the acetabulum and femoral head and, occasionally, in the femoral neck. These so-called cysts are actually areas of tumor that erode into the subjacent bone and cartilage. There usually are no findings to suggest degenerative arthritis; however, there may be narrowing of the joint space as this disease progresses (Fig. 60A–4).

Most of our patients were symptomatic for an average of 5 years before the diagnosis was established. The condition may be misdiagnosed as osteoarthritis. At the time of surgery, the gross findings are quite characteristic. There is thick, swollen, frondlike synovium and brown discoloration resulting from intra-articular hemorrhage. Microscopically, the synovium is proliferative, with synovial lining cells and stromal cells that fill the interstices and infiltrate the subsynovial fat. The fibroid components are histiocytic, with multinucleated giant cells containing lipoids and hemosiderin. Inflammatory cells may also be present.

Synovectomy is indicated; to achieve this in the hip joint, it is necessary to dislocate the femoral head. When the tumor has invaded the femoral head and/or neck, it is probably advisable to proceed directly to resection of the femoral head and neck and reconstruction with either an endoprosthesis or a total hip device. Sixteen of the 20 diseased hips in our series showed radiographic evidence of bone involvement. Surgical procedures that do not remove all the diseased synovium are more likely to be followed by recurrence of the lesion. However, local recurrence in the hip joint occurs significantly less often than in the knee joint. In fact, none of our hip patients had local recurrences. All were treated by synovectomies accompanied by resection of the femoral head and reconstruction with a prosthetic replacement.

Osteochondromatosis of the Synovium

The term "osteochondromatosis" implies that there may be bone present among the discrete cartilaginous tumors found in the synovium. This is not always the case, however, and sometimes the term "chondromatosis" may be more appropriate.[3] Chondromatosis is a benign chondromatous or a chondro-osseous metaplastic proliferation involving the subsynovial connective tissue of joints, tendon sheaths, or bursa. In the Mayo

Clinic experience, the hip was involved in 16 percent of cases. The average age of these patients was about 40 years, and men were more commonly affected than women. Patient complaints were of pain and limited motion of the hip. The diagnosis may be difficult because the lesion may not be suspected and the roentgenogram may not reveal specific bodies, even when they are grossly present. However, multiple views of the hip may reveal calcified osteochondromatous bodies that become loose and fall into the recesses of the

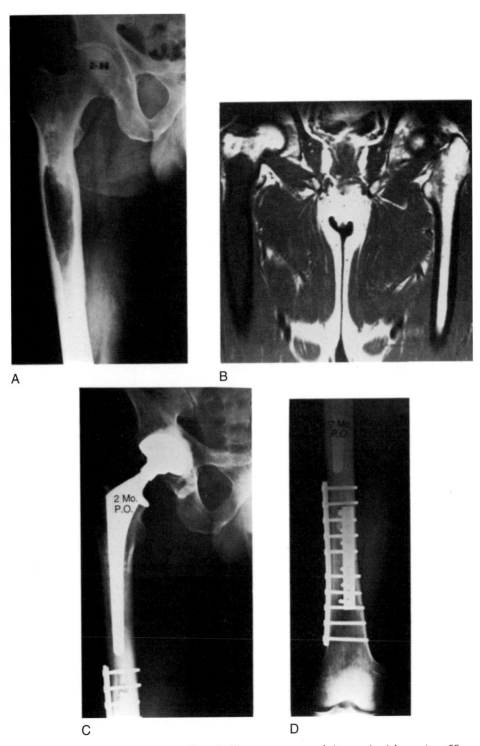

Figure 60A–3. A, Anteroposterior (AP) views of grade III osteosarcoma of the proximal femur in a 65-year-old man. **B**, Magnetic resonance imaging scan clearly delineates the extent of marrow involvement and absence of soft tissue extension. **C**, AP view of the hip after prosthesis-allograft reconstruction. **D**, AP view showing osteotomy site between the allograft and the distal femur.

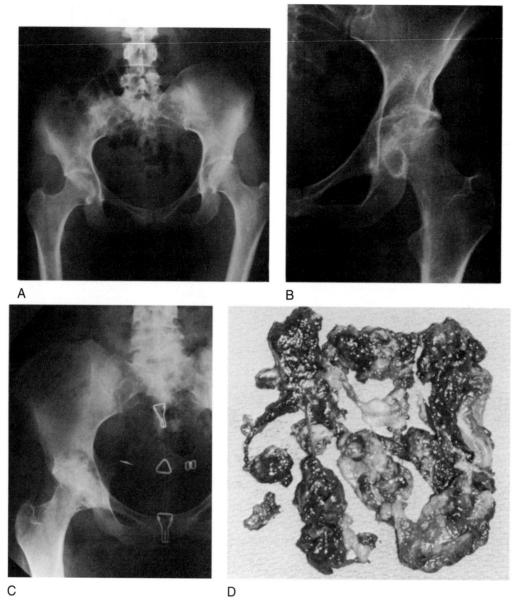

A

B

C

D

Figure 60A–4. Pigmented villonodular synovitis. **A**, Involved right hip of a 32-year-old woman. Note the early changes, chiefly osteoporosis. **B**, More advanced changes are seen in this 30-year-old woman, including cyst formation; the joint space is still fairly normal. **C**, Note the far-advanced changes in this 19-year-old woman, with loss of joint space. This is difficult to differentiate roentgenographically from degenerative arthritis, but the age of the patient makes the diagnosis of osteoarthritis unlikely. **D**, Gross appearance of the synovium of the patient in panel **A**. The pigmented synovium is evident. (From Pritchard DJ, Lunke RJ, Taylor WF, et al: Chondrosarcoma: A clinicopathologic and statistical analysis. Cancer 45:149, 1980.)

joint. The lateral projection is often the most helpful (Fig. 60A–5).

When this condition is suspected or symptoms demand surgical treatment, a diagnostic arthrotomy may be indicated. Once the diagnosis is established by the gross appearance and confirmed by histologic evidence, a synovectomy is indicated. The disease may be quite focal, however, and it is not always necessary to excise the entire synovium, but it is necessary to at least examine the entire synovium grossly. To achieve this, it is usually necessary to dislocate the femoral head from the acetabulum. Of course, this carries the risk of induc-

ing avascular necrosis. This event, however, appears to be minimal if the tissues are handled gently, and the duration that the femoral head is left out of the acetabulum is relatively short. Even with complete excision of all grossly involved tissue, there may be a local recurrence.

Chondromatosis may be accompanied by degenerative changes with narrowing of the hip joint and evident osteoarthritis.

Primary arthroplasty may be advisable when extensive chondromatosis is encountered or when the situation is compounded by the presence of degenerative arthritis.

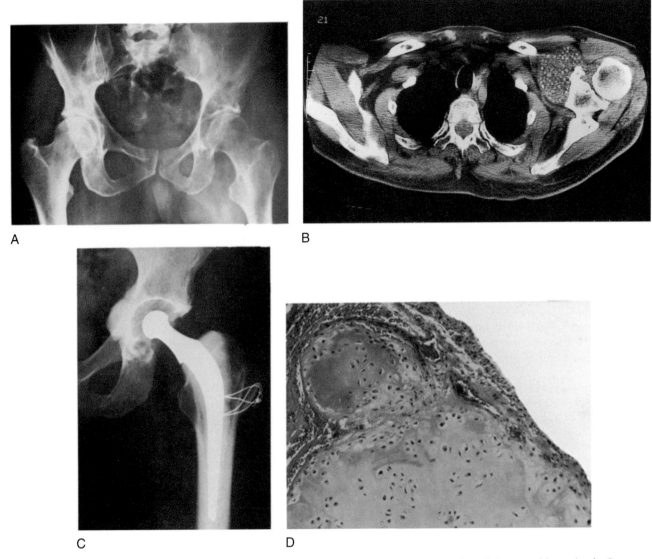

Figure 60A–5. Chondromatosis of the synovium. **A**, A 55-year-old man had had severe pain and almost no hip motion for 3 years. The roentgenogram showed only osteoporosis, but biopsy of the synovium revealed multiple diffuse chondromatosis. **B**, By contrast, there is marked, diffuse osteochondromatosis of the shoulder in this 48-year-old man. **C**, The same case as in panel **A**. The acetabulum was extensively invaded by chondromatosis and was partly excised to remove tumor from the fovea. Reconstruction was possible by total hip arthroplasty after complete synovectomy. This is the appearance 8 weeks after removal and total hip arthroplasty. **D**, The same case as in panels **A** and **C**. Proliferated cartilaginous masses are seen below the synovial layer. (Hematoxylin and eosin; H 175) (From Pritchard DJ, Lunke RJ, Taylor WF, et al: Chondrosarcoma: A clinico-pathologic and statistical analysis. Cancer 45:149, 1980.)

BENIGN AND MALIGNANT SOFT TISSUE TUMORS

There are a variety of benign and malignant soft tissue tumors that may arise in the region of the hip joint. Lipoma is probably the most common benign soft tissue tumor, and it does occur occasionally in the region of the hip joint. When it is located near the surface, the diagnosis may be suspected by the mobility of the tumor and its characteristic soft feel to palpation. However, if it is located deep within the muscle tissue, the clinical examination may not be diagnostic.

Roentgenograms are helpful in that the tumor tends to have the same density as subcutaneous fat. Computed tomography (CT) and magnetic resonance imaging (MRI) are even more helpful in that they show a homogeneous mass of fat density.

If the tumor is symptomatic or enlarging, treatment is by surgical excision. This rarely requires any sort of reconstructive procedure for the hip itself. The same can be said for practically all the benign soft tissue tumors that occur in the region of the hip. For malignant tumors, however, the situation may be entirely different.

Liposarcoma, Fibrosarcoma, and Malignant Fibrous Histiocytoma

As with any soft tissue malignancy, the tumor usually manifests as a mass or an unexplained pain. There may not be any characteristic findings on physical examination. Both CT and MRI are very helpful in characterizing these lesions. For example, a tumor that appears to have a fat density but that is not homogeneous is probably a liposarcoma rather than a lipoma. Indeed, the majority of liposarcomas are not characteristically fatty on CT scan, but rather show multiloculated, inhomogeneous invasive characteristics. Malignant fibrous histiocytoma is the most commonly encountered soft tissue malignant tumor. It is now diagnosed much more commonly than liposarcoma or fibrosarcoma. From a practical standpoint, however, all three of these tumors have characteristics that are similar, and the clinical management is similar. Grade and surgical staging of these tumors are directly related to prognosis and hence dictate the extent of treatment necessary to achieve a good prognosis. In other words, a tumor that is histologically grade I will probably behave in a similar fashion whether it is called a fibrosarcoma or a malignant fibrous histiocytoma. A tumor that is a high-grade extracompartmental lesion (Enneking stage IIB), for example, will behave similarly whether it is a liposarcoma or a fibrosarcoma. Hence, it is vitally important to get accurate staging information. This is best achieved with the use of MRI supplemented with other tests as indicated. Plain radiographs may demonstrate whether there is any bony involvement. Technetium and gallium scans may be helpful in defining the extent of the tumor. Tumors that occur in the anterior part of the hip joint may threaten the neurovascular structures. CT or MRI scans with contrast may be helpful or, alternatively, arteriography may be of benefit in some situations. The more information that is available to the surgeon and the radiation therapist, the more likely it is that goals of tumor management can be achieved; that is, eradication of the tumor with preservation of as much function as possible. Although many of these soft tissue tumors can be treated by soft tissue surgery only, in some cases, the proximity of the proximal femur may dictate the need for resection of the proximal femur and subsequent reconstruction with a hip replacement device. For example, a tumor that appears to arise in the substance of the vastus lateralis muscle may show invasion of the lateral cortex of the proximal femur. This may necessitate sacrifice of the proximal femur.

There are many studies underway that appear to demonstrate the efficacy of preoperative treatment that uses either radiation treatment or some combination of radiation and chemotherapy.[1,8,11] This approach may achieve the same results with less radical surgery. However, if there is actual bony invasion by the soft tissue tumor, sacrifice of that portion of the bone that is involved will almost certainly be necessary.

SURGICAL CONSIDERATIONS

Because these various pathologic conditions appear in different ways, each one must be analyzed individually. No one surgical approach is applicable to every situation. Even routine approaches to the hip joint must be modified on occasion, depending on the specific problem at hand.

Our most frequently used approach to the hip joint, however, is to place the patient in the straight lateral position and to use a straight lateral incision. Almost all regions of the hip are accessible by this approach. Indeed, even tumors in the lesser trochanter are readily approached in this manner, and, in fact, this technique may be far easier to execute than the medial (Ludlof) approach to the hip joint. This lateral approach is particularly useful if a biopsy is planned and followed by immediate resection of the femoral head and neck and whatever soft tissues are to be included in the procedure.

Some tumors involving the hip require resection and reconstruction with a custom type of total hip arthroplasty.[10] This is simply a device that is somewhat longer than the conventional total hip arthroplasty and that is designed to replace whatever segment of femur is sacrificed. Alternatively, if a large segment of the proximal femur is to be resected, the reconstruction may include a combination of an allograft to replace the sacrificed portion of the bone, coupled with a conventional total hip device. The latter procedure may allow reattachment of soft tissues to the allografted bone, which may not be achievable with a customized prosthetic device. However, whichever reconstructive method is to be employed, the technique for resection is the same. The standard lateral approach can be extended distally as far as necessary. The muscles surrounding the proximal femur can be transected at the intended level of bone resection and as much muscle as necessary can be sacrificed to achieve satisfactory tumor margins. An attempt should always be made to achieve at least several centimeters of normal tissue in all planes, including the marrow. All these transections can be verified with frozen sections at the time of the surgical procedure to ensure that the surgeon is cutting through normal tissue rather than tumor.

Once the resection is completed and hemostasis is achieved, reconstruction is relatively easy. If the acetabulum is uninvolved, has not been sacrificed, and looks otherwise healthy, the customized device or composite allograft-femoral component can be coupled with a bipolar acetabular implant. If the acetabulum must be resected or if it is involved with degenerative changes necessitating replacement, a conventional type of acetabular reconstruction can be used.

Perhaps the most important consideration in placing the device, whether it is an endoprosthetic device or a full total hip arthroplasty, is to achieve tension adequate to ensure stability, because, in most of these cases, the muscle is sacrificed, and the only stabilizing factor is the length of the prosthesis, which controls the tension. Thus, as a general rule, it is best to make the prosthetic device as long as possible, so that there is some difficulty in reducing the device into the acetabulum. In some cases, this results in lengthening of the involved side. The patient should be made aware that this is a distinct and even a desirable possibility. Of course, one needs to guard against too much stretching for fear of compromise of the sciatic nerve.

The other major problem is how to achieve abduction in these cases, because the attachments of the abductor muscles are lost. For a number of years, we have used a technique in which the abductor muscles are sutured into the tensor fascia lata (Fig. 60A–6). This method affords surprisingly adequate abductor power in some but not all patients. The more recent use of a composite allograft and total hip device may allow us to achieve better results in this regard, because it is usually possible to attach the abductor muscles directly to the allograft. Of course, with some tumors, it may be necessary to sacrifice all the abductor muscles, and, in this situation, the patient will undoubtedly have a marked Trendelenburg gait and will probably need to use a cane on a permanent basis.

In the past several years, we have increasingly used so-called composites in the reconstruction after resection of the proximal femur. A portion of allograft proximal femur is selected for size and cut to fit. Some prefer to utilize a "step-cut" at the junction of the allograft and the host bone to help control rotation. It is somewhat difficult to achieve precise cuts, however, so some avoid this technique. There are a number of alternative ways to achieve fixation of the prosthetic device and the allograft bone to the host's own bone. One acceptable method involves cementing (with or without antibiotic impregnation of the cement) the femoral prosthesis in the medullary canal of the allograft on the back table and subsequently fixing the composite to the host bone with one or two plates and screws or bands by means of Ogden plates (Fig. 60A–7). Another method is to use a long-stemmed femoral prosthesis to bridge the junction (Fig. 60A–8). No one method appears clearly superior at this time. If the abductor muscles are intact, they can be attached to the trochanteric region of the allograft.

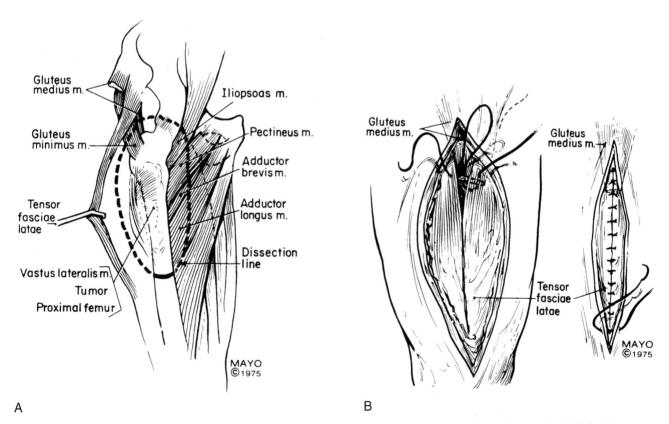

Figure 60A–6. A, Envelopes of muscle mass removed at the time of radical en bloc resection of the proximal third of the femur. **B**, Technique for attachment of the remnant of the gluteus medius to the tensor fasciae latae muscle to provide lateral stability.

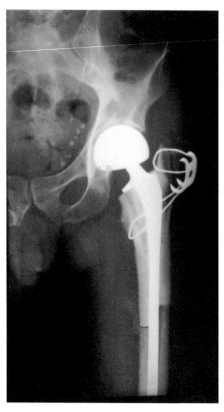

Figure 60A–7. This patient underwent resection of the proximal femur for a chondrosarcoma. A composite allograft/prosthesis was used. Note the "step-cut" at the junction. Iliac bone grafts were also applied at the junction.

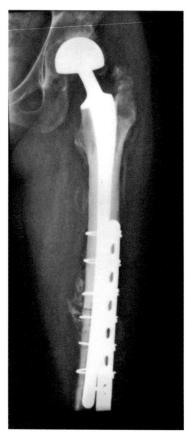

Figure 60A–8. Allograft/prosthesis composite using a long-stemmed device and Dall-Miles plate and cables for fixation.

References

1. Frustia S, Gherlinzoni F, DePaoli A, et al: Adjuvant chemotherapy for adult soft tissue sarcomas of extremities and girdles: Results of the Italian Randomized Cooperative Trial. J Clin Oncol 19:1238, 2001.
2. Jaffe JL, Lichtenstein L, Sutro CJ: Pigmented villonodular synovitis, bursitis and tenosynovitis: A discussion of the synovial and bursal equivalents of the tenosynovial lesion commonly denoted as xanthoma, xanthogranuloma, giant cell tumor or myeloplaxsoma of the tendon sheath, with some consideration of this tendon sheath lesion itself. Arch Pathol 31:731, 1941.
3. Murphy FP, Dahlin DC, Sullivan CR: Articular synovial chondromatosis. J Bone Joint Surg 44A:77, 1962.
4. Pritchard DJ, Dahlin C, Dauphine RT, et al: Ewing's sarcoma: A clinicopathological and statistical analysis of patients surviving five years or longer. J Bone Joint Surg 57A:10, 1975.
5. Pritchard DJ, Lunke RJ, Taylor WF, et al: Chondrosarcoma: A clinicopathologic and statistical analysis. Cancer 45:149, 1980.
6. Pritchard DJ: The surgical management of giant cell tumors of bone. Orthop Surg Wkly Update 1:2, 1980.
7. Pritchard DJ: Tumors. In Tronzo RG (ed): Tumors in Surgery of the Hip Joint, 2nd ed. New York, Springer-Verlag, 1987, p 31.
8. Schray MF, Gunderson LL, Sim FH, et al: Soft tissue sarcoma: Integration of brachytherapy resection and external irradiation. Cancer 66:451, 1990.
9. Schwartz H, Unni KK, Pritchard DJ: Pigmented villonodular synovitis. Clin Orthop 247:243, 1989.
10. Sim FH, Chao EYS: Hip salvage by proximal femoral replacement. J Bone Joint Surg 63A:1228, 1981.
11. Suit HD, Mankin HJ, Wood WC, Proppe KH: Preoperative, intraoperative and postoperative radiation in the treatment of primary soft tissue sarcoma. Cancer 55:2659, 1985.
12. Unni KK: Dahlin's Bone Tumors: General Aspects and Data on 11,087 Cases. Springfield, IL, Charles C Thomas, 1996, p 227.

60B

Neoplasms: Metastatic Disease

• MICHAEL G. ROCK

Metastatic involvement of the hip with compromise of the proximal femur, acetabulum, or both is a common phenomenon. The pelvis is the third most common area of skeletal involvement after the vertebral column and ribs. Additionally, the femur accounts for 61 percent of long bone pathologic fractures, with the majority of these occurring in the proximal third.[23,33] Unlike the upper extremity, impending or actual pathologic fractures in the hip area severely compromises the patient's ambulation. Although greatly impacting a patient's functional capacity, skeletal metastases limited to the upper extremity continue to allow ambulation, thereby avoiding the attendant complications of pressure sores, pneumonia, hypercalcemia, and, with some tumors, disseminated intravascular coagulopathies.

Continued success in the management of primary carcinomas has allowed an increase in clinically significant metastatic disease that may not cause the demise of the patient but that directly affects the quality of life. Of autopsies performed on cancer patients, 60 percent are found to have osseous involvement; specifically, 84 percent in primary tumors of the breast, 84 percent in the prostate, 50 percent in the thyroid, 44 percent in the lung, and 37 percent in the kidney.[5,13] With continued improvement in local control of carcinomas, the management of skeletal metastasis assumes greater significance for the orthopedic surgeon.

Patients with skeletal metastasis generally have wide dissemination, with 50 percent survival at 6 months and 25 percent at 1 year. However, some of the patients most commonly afflicted with skeletal metastasis are those with breast cancer, lymphoma, and myeloma, who collectively have a 75 percent survival at 1 year and an average survival of 21 months.[12,18,19,33,40] Therefore, to perceive skeletal metastasis as representing a preterminal event is not appropriate, and efforts allowing restoration of function and mobility should be sought. The proposed reconstruction should allow for early ambulation and restoration of normal activity, with a negligible possibility of mechanical failure.

NONOPERATIVE OR CONSERVATIVE MANAGEMENT

Historically, skeletal metastasis was considered a preterminal event, and, unless isolated, no surgical attempts at stabilization were performed. Patients were subjected to skin or skeletal traction,[1,9] or possibly even body casts. Because of the attendant risks of maintaining these patients recumbent, their ultimate demise was often expedited by such management. Pathologic fractures were found not to heal in such an environment because of the presence of tumor at the fracture site, the general catabolic condition of the patient, and, possibly, the effect of radiation therapy.[4,6] In excess of 80 percent of pathologic fractures in the proximal femur failed to heal with such conservative measures, thereby inflicting a state of recumbency on these patients until they died of their disease. Pathologic fractures that do unite do so in a delayed fashion, usually exceeding 6 months.[15] Given the patient survival statistics noted above, the vast majority of patients will have died before bone union takes place. Therefore, it becomes mandatory in the lower extremity to achieve appropriate fixation so as to allow restoration of ambulation and function. With the introduction of implants for the management of trauma and arthritic conditions of joints, safe reconstruction or replacement of metastatic deposits are now technically possible, and the goals of pain relief and restoration of function can be achieved.

Conservative, nonoperative management, however, does have a place in the management of extensive skeletal metastasis. In the lower extremity, this principally applies to severely afflicted patients whose life expectancy is less than 1 to 2 months, and whose diffuse involvement may necessitate extensive replacement and numerous operative procedures to achieve ambulation.

The clinical course of metastatic disease includes bone pain, fractures, hypercalcemia, and spinal cord compression, all of which profoundly impair a patient's quality of life. The principal pathogenesis of bone destruction is a stimulation of osteoclastic bone resorption by factors produced by the cancer cells. Evolving and compelling evidence suggests that bisphosphanates and, in particular, pamidronate reduce both the symptoms

793

and complications of bone involvement. In a recent study, the long-term effect of oral pamidronate in the prevention and treatment of skeletal metastasis in patients with breast cancer was reviewed by the Comprehensive Cancer Center in The Netherlands.[45] This study confirmed that the oral administration of pamidronate reduced skeletal morbidity and had a very favorable effect on quality of life. The treatment apparently did not alter the radiographic course of the disease or the overall survival of the patients. The indications for pamidronate are being expanded beyond the experience with breast cancer and myeloma, and ongoing research is evolving in identifying the optimal route, dose, scheduling, and even type of bisphosphanates.[11]

OPERATIVE TREATMENT

The evolution of surgical management of skeletal metastasis in the lower extremity is parallel to that of trauma management and joint replacement surgery. With the advent of new reconstructive alternatives, the management of difficult skeletal metastatic involvement has become possible. The most significant advance in the management of skeletal metastatic disease are those of prophylactic fixation and incorporation of methyl metacrylate to augment existing internal fixation devices and to replace bony architecture destroyed by tumor.

The concept of prophylactic fixation was fostered by studies that showed a reproduceable and predictable effect on bone strength, taking into consideration such factors as cortical destruction of various sizes, shape, and anatomic distribution.[27,29] Defects involving 50 percent of the cortex and those exceeding 2.5 cm in weight-bearing bone had a 50 percent chance of fracture without stabilization. It was also noted that radiation, often used in the management of these conditions, does not effectively allow maturation of these lesions for at least 6, and often 12, weeks after its cessation. During that time frame, the defect may increase in size, further compromising the integrity of the bone. It is, therefore, not uncommon for patients to continue to experience pain, even in the presence of appropriate radiation dose and application.

The indications for prophylactic fixation have evolved from basic biomechanical research and retrospective analysis of clinical data. The radiographic parameters associated with at least a 50 percent chance of fracture are mentioned earlier. Additionally, pain after therapeutic radiation to the lesion has also represented a time-honored indication for prophylactic fixation. More recently, Mirels[30] has refined the indications for surgical stabilization by combining pertinent radiographic and clinical information at the outset. These include four parameters: size, radiographic features, anatomic site, and pain. To each of these four parameters he has ascribed a score of 1 to 3, contingent on the degree of severity or involvement. The collated score, with a minimum of 4 and a maximum of 12, correlates with the fracture probability. The single largest increase in fracture tendency is seen a score between 9 and 10, with 72 per-

cent probability of fracture occurring with the latter. Therefore, prophylactic fixation is recommended for any metastatic deposit for which a collected score of 10 or greater is assigned. High-risk anatomic sites include the weight-bearing lower limb and the peritrochanteric area of the proximal femur, given the high concentration of stresses in these regions[46] (Table 60B–1).

The management of skeletal defects resulting from metastasis in weight-bearing bone, and, in particular, the proximal femur and hip, mandates early surgical stabilization in an effort to avoid pathologic fractures. Prophylactic fixation of metastatic deposits in the hip area is associated with decreased morbidity, operative time, and complications. Futhermore, prophylactic fixation facilitates the administration of radiotherapy and maintenance of patient independence. Therefore, prophylactic fixation should be performed on all patients at risk for impending pathologic fractures. The benefit of prophylactic fixation of femoral fractures has been reinforced by a study that assessed the average length of stay time of and discharge home for patients who had prophylactic fixation versus fixation for actual pathologic fracture. Fixation before fracture resulted in predictably better results than those achieved by fixation after fracture, with decreased length of stay and increased tendency toward being discharged home in an independent and autonomous fashion.[46]

The use of methyl methacrylate in the fixation of joint replacement surgery had already been well established when it was introduced to structurally support a cortical defect by Harrington et al. in 1968.[20] Before its use in metastatic disease, less than half of patients who were subjected to an operative procedure to stabilize metastatic disease in the weight-bearing structures actually regained ambulatory status.[20] The incidence of mechanical failure of the implant, loosening, or both was excessively high. When methyl methacrylate is used to fill a cortical defect, it has been shown to increase actual strength by 50 percent and torsional strength by 69 percent.[37] Although strong in compression, it is less able to resist tension and shear stresses and, therefore, should not be used in isolation for large defects, particularly in weight-bearing structures. However, in conjunction with a nail and plate apparatus, or, possibly, even an intramedullary device, use of methyl methacrylate markedly increases the inherent stability afforded by these implants. The principal application of methyl methacrylate in the hip area is to reconstruct the compromised, possibly missing, calcar, or medial buttress,

Table 60B–1. RISK OF PATHOLOGIC FRACTURE

Score Variable	1	2	3
Site	Upper limb	Lower limb	Peritrochanteric
Pain	Mild	Moderate	Functional
Radiographic appearance	Plastic	Mixed	Lytic
Size: shaft diameter	<1/3	1/3–2/3	>2/3

From Mirels H: Metastatic disease in long bones. Clin Orthop 249:256, 1989.

of the femur. Conventional implants, whether of nail and plate or intramedullary design, fail to achieve compression because of lack of support in this area. The use of adjucant methyl methacrylate made possible a much more successful reconstruction. With the use of methyl methacrylate as an adjunct, mechanical failures have become rare, affording ambulatory status to the vast majority of patients who are reconstructed in this fashion, with pain relief exceeding 85 percent.[16,19]

All patients who have been stabilized for impending or actual pathologic fractures need postoperative radiation therapy to ensure tumor control. The benefits of postoperative radiation therapy were reaffirmed in a study of 64 stabilization procedures in 60 consecutive patients with metastatic diseases to previously unradiated weight-bearing bones with pathologic or impending pathologic fractures. Patients were stratified according to prognostic variables, and endpoint was the functional status as assessed by the patient and the medical provider. On multivariate analysis, only postoperative radiation therapy was significant for the patients' attainment of normal function. The increased functionality of patients who received surgery plus radiation therapy as opposed to those who received surgery alone persisted longer than 1 year after the operation. Additionally, the actuarial median survival of patients in the surgery alone group was 3.3 months compared with 12.4 months for patients with surgery plus radiation therapy, thereby confirming the beneficial association with survival shown by multivariate Cox progression analysis. Although assumed to be an effective adjunct to surgery, the true benefits of postoperative radiation therapy were not fully recognized before this study.[42]

Postoperative radiation therapy may also minimize the possibility of local recurrent disease. In a study in which perioperative radiation therapy was not given, local recurrence was seen in 15 percent of patients, which compromised the reconstructive procedure. All of these patients experienced an actual pathologic fracture, with likely dissemination of tumor cells into the surrounding tissues. This problem is addressed effectively by surgical stabilization, further emphasizing the benefits of prophylactic fixation and perioperative radiation therapy. When this multimodality treatment is given, local recurrence is rare.[6]

MANAGEMENT OF PATHOLOGIC FRACTURES IN THE HIP

Preoperative Assessment

As mentioned previously, every effort should be made to prophylactically stabilize hip lesions. If a fracture has occurred, stabilization should be attained quickly after the diagnosis of metastatic disease has been made. It is not an uncommon event to have a patient who has had no known primary disease suffer a fracture in this region. Given the age of the patient and the radiographic appearance of the pathologic process, metastatic disease may be the most likely possibility. In general, most multifocal lesions are more consistent with metastatic disease or bone tumor simulators.[25] Similarly, unifocal lesions are much more likely to be primary benign or malignant disease. Included are entities that simulate bone tumors, such as intra-osseous ganglions, brown tumors of hyperparathyroidism, infection, cysts attended with degenerative arthritis of the hip joint occurring on either side of the articulation,[14] and rheumatoid pseudocyst (geode of the femoral neck) (Fig. 60B–1).[31] However, a unifocal lesion in patients older than 40 years of age is more likely to represent metastatic than primary disease. One must, however, remember that up to 11 percent of patients who have experienced malignancy will have yet another malignant process diagnosed in their remaining lifetime. Therefore, a known history of cancer

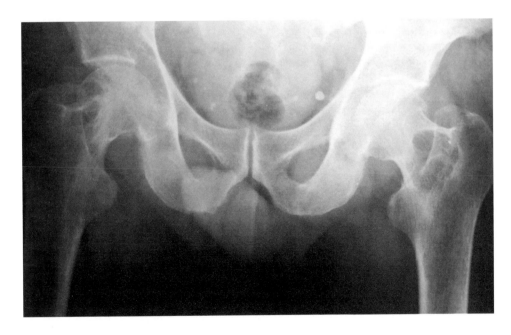

Figure 60B–1. A 58-year-old man with known rheumatoid arthritis has a large rheumatoid pseudocyst of the femoral neck (geode).

with a monostotic lesion to bone is likely but not always consistent with the known primary malignant tumor. Therefore, these lesions may need further investigation to define the nature of the process in bone more effectively and to rule out disease elsewhere, such as in the lung and in the liver, before a formal biopsy is attempted.

Unifocal bone metastasis is seen in approximately 2.5 percent of patients who experience metastasis to bone. Many of these patients will not have a known primary tumor and, therefore, the possible association with an underlying undiagnosed malignancy may seem unlikely.[32,36] An investigative strategy for the older patient with a unifocal lesion in the bone who has had no previously detected primary tumor includes physical examination with emphasis on breast, prostate, and thyroid; laboratory tests that include prostate-specific antigen, serum protein electrophoresis, urinalysis, guaiac test for occult colonic malignancy, a complete blood count and differential test, including sedimentation rate and alkaline phosphatase; and chest and abdominal CT. This strategy detects 85 percent of primary tumors with unifocal bone metastasis. The majority of these tumors are in the lung (63 percent) and kidney (10 percent). If these studies are negative if the history is suggestive, or both, mammography may need to be performed and/or open biopsy of the solitary lytic lesion, although biopsy in and of itself can only identify the histogenesis effectively in approximately 35 percent of cases.

A definitive diagnosis can usually be obtained by either needle biopsy or minimal open biopsy. However, once the diagnosis is confirmed, stabilization or reconstruction should commence immediately. Expedient return to activities and ambulation minimize the complications previously addressed.

Metastatic disease often is present at sites remote from the area principally in question. Therefore, planning reconstructive efforts are planned, it is prudent to obtain sufficient radiographic analysis of the entire bone and contiguous joint. At a minimum, dual-plane radiography should be performed of the entire femur, and anteroposterior plus oblique films of the acetabulum should be obtained. To assist in the detection of tumor that is not noticeable on plain radiographs, scintigraphic scanning may be of value. To document other areas of involvement in the same bone is extremely important because fractures through these areas of additional involvement may negate an otherwise successful reconstruction. Although they are not the primary source of symptoms, these ancillary lesions may have to be addressed at the time of the reconstruction.

One of the distinct advantages of prophylactic fixation of impending fractures is the opportunity to perform an adequate medical evaluation and to reverse clinical parameters that have been rendered abnormal by the underlying systemic nature of the disease. This includes correcting the blood indices to a monocyte count of at least 30 percent, a platelet count exceeding $50,000/cm^3$, and a neutrophil count exceeding $500/cm^3$. Additionally, hypercalcemia, not an uncommon systemic finding, can be corrected with appropriate hydra-

tion, saline diuresis, or the use of mithramycin. Such optimization of medical status before surgery minimizes perioperative morbidity and mortality.

Fractures of the Femoral Neck

Ten percent of patients with disseminated breast cancer and 1.4 percent of all breast cancer patients ultimately sustain a pathologic fracture of the hip, many of which occur within the femoral head and neck.[5] Conventional fixation techniques used for femoral neck fractures should be avoided. Pathologic fractures in this area differ markedly from osteoporotic or traumatic femoral neck fractures. Tumor involvement is often extensive, further compromising the attenuated blood supply associated with fracture. Augmentation with methyl methacrylate is difficult and inadequate. Furthermore, pathologic femoral neck fractures have a high propensity for nonunion.[17]

Therefore, the only viable alternatives in the management of these cases are conversion to a Girdlestone procedure or replacement with a prosthetic device. Girdlestone arthroplasty has been recommended in patients with poor overall general health who require an expedient procedure, or in those whose acetabular involvement is so extensive as to preclude an effective reconstruction (Fig. 60B–2).[38] Furthermore, the goal of managing pathologic fractures in this area is to return the patient to an ambulatory status, or at least obtain pain-free transfer status as rapidly as possible. With the Girdlestone procedure, there has been some discrepancy regarding successful pain management as well as return to function. Continued pain from the Girdlestone procedure often is due to residual bony prominences impinging on the acetabular rim. Performance of the operation through the intertrochanteric line can prevent this complication. If any portion of the femoral neck remains, with or without osteophytes left on the acetabular rim, impingement and pain can be expected. A review of Girdlestone procedures reveals good results, with control of pain and ambulatory status dependent on an external aid, usually a walker.[24] The advantage of the operation is that it can be performed quickly, with minimal blood loss and dissection. The functional results after Girdlestone resection are not nearly as impressive as those achieved with endoprosthetic replacement. However, under isolated circumstances, Girdlestone resection may be indicated.

The vast majority of patients who sustain pathologic fractures of the femoral neck and head can successfully be managed with endoprosthetic replacement.[39] This can take the form of unipolar, bipolar, or total hip replacement contingent on the surgeon's preference and periacetabular involvement. Regardless of the method of proximal articulation selected, the femoral component should be of the long-stemmed variety to stabilize the full length of the femur. It should be recognized that other metastatic foci in the bone are common and, if not stabilized at the same operative procedure, these foci may cause further pathologic fracture distal to the

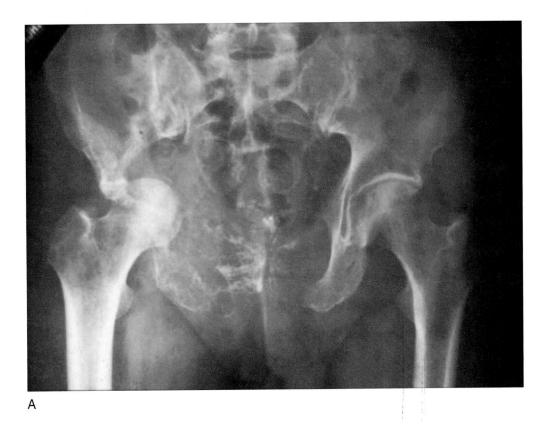

A

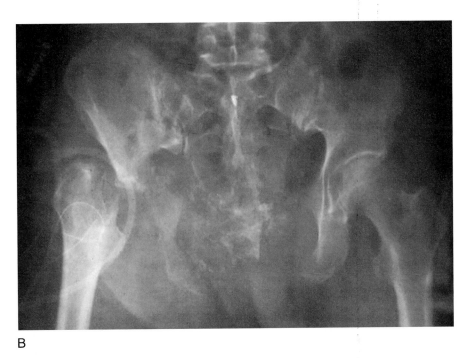

B

Figure 60B–2. A and **B**, Massive destruction of the hemipelvis in this 73-year-old woman with lung metastases. Given the anticipated short life span and the inability to reconstruct, a Girdlestone procedure was performed.

implant (Fig. 60B–3). Given the relatively short life span of most of these patients, use of methyl methacrylate for implant stabilization is routine. Therefore, long-stemmed (142-mm) femoral components should be used with cement extending the full length of the femur.

Because of the compromised medical status of most patients with metastatic disease, including an increased tendency for coagulopathy, attempts should be made to minimize intraoperative and perioperative embolization. In an effort to minimize intraoperative showering

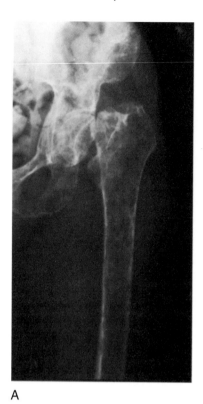

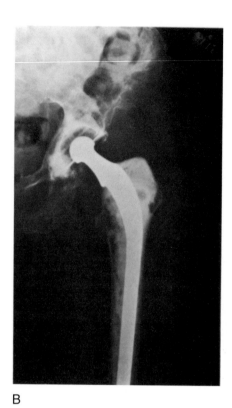

Figure 60B–3. **A,** Extensive skeletal metastasis in a 67-year-old man known to have lung carcinoma. Displaced femoral neck fracture occurred with a minimal twisting injury. **B,** A long-stemmed cemented femoral component was used to bypass additional areas of involvement. A cemented acetabular component was used because of central acetabular involvement by the tumor.

A

B

of fat or tumor emboli, the femur should be vented approximately 4 to 6 cm proximal to the anticipated intramedullary site of the tip of the implant. This venting allows egress of medullary contents during reaming and controlled pressurization of cement at implantation of the component.

Tumor involvement in the acetabulum is not necessarily associated with symptoms. In a study by Haberman et al.[19] of 23 women with breast metastasis involving the femoral head and neck who were to undergo resection or replacement, 19 showed evidence of acetabular metastasis in biopsy specimens without radiographic abnormality. Therefore, Haberman et al. have recommended that total joint replacement be performed on all pathologic femoral neck fractures. However, of 52 patients with femoral neck pathologic fractures treated by hemiarthroplasty who were observed by Harrington,[22] only 3 were found subsequently to experience protrusio or central migration. It is Haberman's recommendation that the additional risks, complications, and operative time associated with acetabular reconstruction are not necessary.

I prefer to use a bipolar articulating endoprosthesis, thereby minimizing the chance of central migration and the operative time needed to deal with the acetabular side of the reconstruction. By appropriately sizing the acetabular component of the bipolar construct and by the inherent mobility between the couplings, the stresses applied through the medial wall are reduced. With significant deficiency of the medial wall or acetabular pillars, it may be necessary to use an acetabular ring and cemented acetabular component to minimize the

chance of migration (Fig. 60B–4). However, the majority of patients can be managed with a bipolar articulation, which allows immediate relief of pain and restoration of ambulation.

The success of endoprosthetic replacement in pathologic fractures is gratifying in the reviews of Harrington[22] and Lane et al.[26] Pain relief was universal, with the patients exhibiting increased independence and with the majority returning to ambulatory status. Of those patients who were capable of ambulation before their pathologic fractures, 72 percent were independent or ambulatory with assisted walkers after a prosthetic replacement, whereas 46 percent of those who were nonambulatory before their fracture management were returned to independent or assisted walking. The average survival in the series of Lane et al.[26] was 5.6 months, whereas in the Harrington[22] series, survival time was 9.8 months. The rapid pain relief and return to functional status associated with endoprosthetic replacement argues favorably for its use with pathologic fractures in this area. Recognizing that metastatic involvement may not be purely isolated to the femoral head and neck and may involve the greater trochanteric region, researchers have developed implants that allow contact between implant and bone, which are capable of transmitting loads rather than relying on a mantle of methyl methacrylate. A wide range of prosthetic implants are now available to address the issue of bone loss in the proximal femur and to afford secure contact. This is particularly important in patients with metastatic renal, thyroid, breast cancer and for those with lymphoma and myeloma, whose average survival may approximate 2 years and in whom tumor

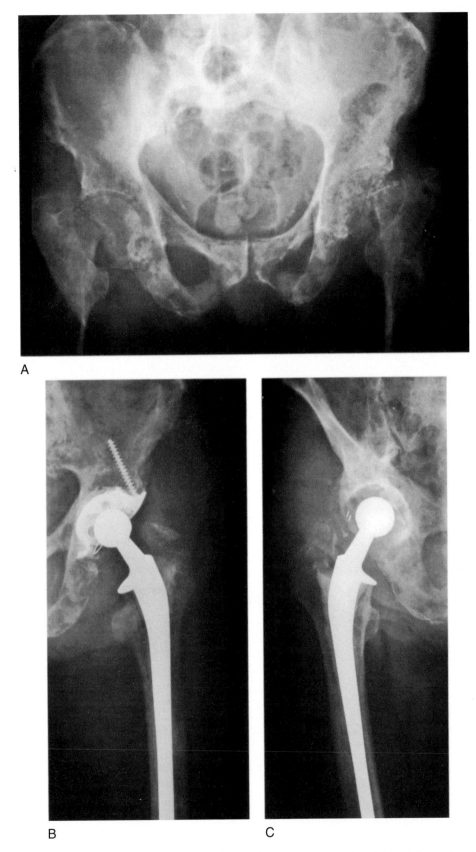

A

B   C

Figure 60B–4. An 87-year-old man known to have metastatic prostate cancer has bilateral femoral neck fractures. Intraoperative assessment of the acetabulum confirms tumor involvement that was suggested on radiographs. To bypass the periacetabular involvement, an antiprotrusio device was employed.

progression may occur in spite of postoperative radiation treatment.

Intertrochanteric Fractures

Pathologic fractures in this area pose a difficult therapeutic management problem. Destruction of bone by tumor, which leads to an intertrochanteric fracture, is often extensive, with failure occurring as a result of marked bone loss on the medial or compressive side of the proximal femur. With weight bearing, displaced and often comminuted fractures are inevitable. Local tumor extent may include the femoral head, neck, and proximal femur, as well as the intertrochanteric region. Therefore, conventional fixation devices, such as sliding nail and plate apparatus for non-neoplastic intertrochanteric fractures are not, by themselves, adequate. The same preoperative planning that was applicable for femoral head and neck fractures is just as significant with intertrochanteric fractures. Preoperative radiographic assessment of the entire femur and acetabular region is necessary before reconstructive considerations. Extensive involvement of the femur below the proposed inferior extent of the side plate warrants alternative reconstructive procedures, such as proximal femoral replacement (Fig. 60B–5).

When the lesion is localized to the intertrochanteric area, screw and plate fixation can be considered if the bone deficiency can be replaced and reinforced with the extensive use of methyl methacrylate (Fig. 60B–6). Anatomic reconstruction is often difficult because of the comminuted aspect of these fractures. Exposure can be gained through a standard lateral incision, and, by reflecting the vastus lateralis both anteriorly and posteriorly, the defects in the intertrochanteric area can be identified; if needed, an additional window can be created anteriorly to allow complete removal of tumor and visualization of the defect. The nail can be advanced into the femoral head and neck in standard fashion by means of appropriate attachment of the angled side plate. At this point, with the defect clearly visible, methyl methacrylate is packed around the nail and areas afflicted by tumor. With the methyl methacrylate still soft and curing, the screws are applied through the plate, lateral cortex, and methyl methacrylate to gain purchase in the medial femoral cortex. With a blunt retractor, the methyl methacrylate can be contoured to reconstruct cortical deficiencies in the proximal femur and avoid extravasation into the medial thigh. Some are of the opinion that additional fixation can be achieved by incorporating methyl methacrylate in the tract used for the femoral nail.[2] This theoretically reinforces the purchase of the nail in the femoral head and neck. This reinforcement, however is gained at the expense of potential complications and difficulties associated with incorporating methyl methacrylate in an area that is not directly seen. Also, the thermal necrosis associated with methyl methacrylate use can potentially induce osteonecrosis. Unless there is evidence of tumor extending

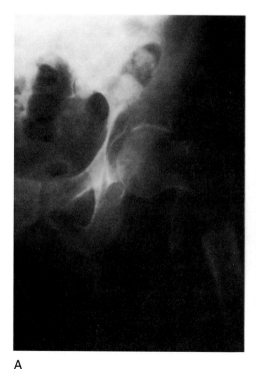

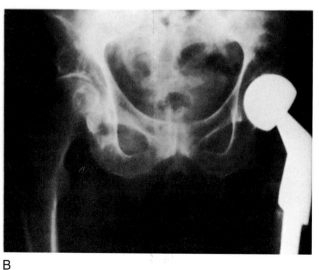

A   B

Figure 60B–5. A, Pathologic intertrochanteric fracture with subtrochanteric extension. Bone loss was too extensive to consider nail/plate fixation even with methyl methacrylate augmentation. **B,** A proximal femoral bipolar prosthesis was used to replace the proximal femur destroyed by the tumor.

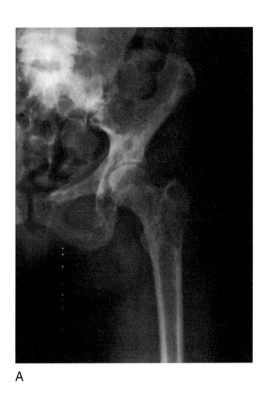

A

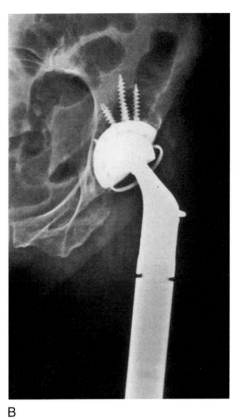

B

Figure 60B–6. A, Intertrochanteric lytic breast metastases in a 75-year-old individual with a fracture. **B**, Cementation plus intramedullary fixation was used for impending fracture.

into the femoral neck and head, the routine use of methyl methacrylate in this area does not seem necessary. Microscopic involvement of the femoral head and neck by tumor can be appropriately controlled by postoperative radiation therapy.

Concomitant involvement of the femoral head and neck, the femoral shaft, or both may not be effectively stabilized by the use of a sliding nail and a side plate. In circumstances in which proximal femoral involvement is too extensive or would necessitate excessive replacement of bone with methyl methacrylate, or if the involvement extends distally, some form of intramedullary device is warranted. A custom proximal femoral prosthesis is the procedure of choice. In this situation, the involved area of the proximal femur is entirely removed, and any involvement in the distal two thirds of the femur is adequately controlled by cementing the intramedullary portion of the implant. The futility of advancing soft tissue into these implants has become apparent with their use. Without soft tissue support, stability is compromised, and, in most large series, dislocation rates approximate 15 percent (Fig. 60B–7).[8,39] This has led to the suggestion of maintaining the acetabular cup more horizontally, between 20 and 30 degrees, with little or no anteversion. Further reduction in dislocations was seen with the introduction of the bipolar articulating endoprosthesis and with attempts at preserving the hip capsule for advancement around the acetabular cup.[34] Abductor power can be partially

retrieved by advancing the tendinous portion of the gluteus medius into the tensor fasciae latae and iliotibial band with the leg maintained in abduction. At maximum, antigravity power can be retained and, although a Trendelenburg gait and stance are inevitable, patients are often sufficiently happy with the result.

The use of proximal femoral replacements does mandate a selection of lengths and intramedullary stem diameters to compensate for patient variability.

Although such megaprostheses are expensive, their use may be appropriate in patients with less virulent metastatic disease, affording rapid pain relief and immediate ambulation.[8,39] Some surgeons have resorted to an abduction splint or some form of abduction harness for 4 to 6 weeks to allow some consolidation of abductor advancement into the iliotibial band.

Intramedullary fixation in the form of Ender nails is mentioned only for the sake of completeness. The main advantages of using Ender nails were decreased morbidity, shorter time, and lack of significant bleeding, because the tumor was never actually exposed. Although theoretically attractive, these implants have uniformly failed in patients with pathologic fractures because of the inevitable collapse, rotation, and backing out of the nails. One of the greatest advancements in management of pathologic conditions is the use of methyl methacrylate, which is not possible if the fracture sit is not actively exposed and made visible. Fracture stabilization is not guaranteed, whereas patients continue to complain of

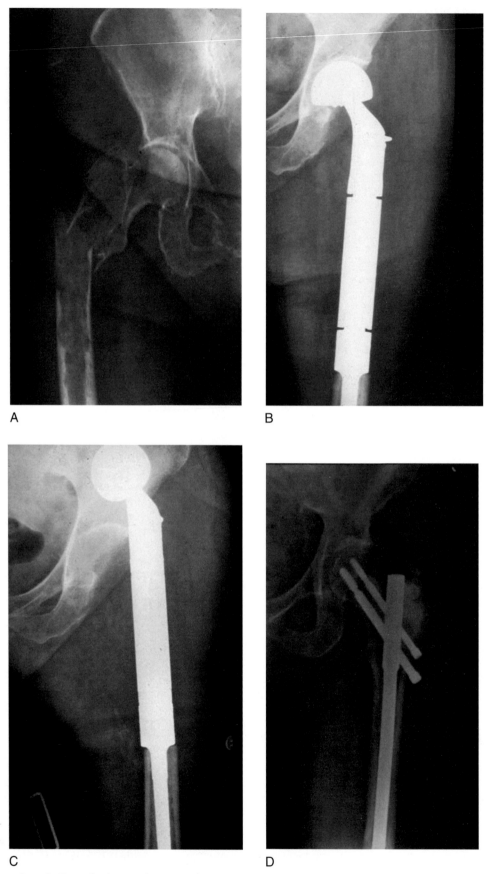

A

B

C

D

Figure 60B–7. A, Extensive intertrochanteric/subtrochanteric metastatic renal cell carcinoma. **B,** Bipolar custom proximal femoral replacement. **C,** Dislocation of bipolar component. **D,** Open reduction and stabilization with constrained acetabular component.

significant pain. Therefore, Ender nail use in the management of pathologic intertrochanteric fracture is severely limited if applicable at all.

Subtrochanteric Fractures

The management of non-neoplastic subtrochanteric fractures of the femur often represents a difficult technical problem for orthopedic surgeons. In neoplastic conditions, loss of bone, possible involvement proximal and distal to the subtrochanteric fracture site, and the general osteoporotic nature of the bone and comminution create an even more difficult reconstructive problem. The use of sliding nail and plate fixation in intertrochanteric fractures may be rationalized because of the augmentation of the nail-collar interface with methyl methacrylate (Fig. 60B–8). However, in subtrochanteric fractures, the bone loss occurs in the vicinity of the proximal portion of the plate, creating tremendous stresses on the implant. Even in the presence of methyl methacrylate, compressive stresses exceed what the implant can safely sustain. The advent of the Zickel nail addressed the need for intramedullary stem fixation combined with proximal fixation into the head and neck. Any osseous defects caused by tumor destruction are reconstructed with methyl methacrylate as has been previously described for intertrochanteric

fractures. There have been isolated reports of difficulties encountered on removal of the Zickel nail. The most notable problem, refracture at the subtrochanteric area, occurs as a result of the lateral and anterior bow of the nail, which impinges on the medial cortex on removal, causing an inframedial to supralateral spiral fracture.[47] The Zickel nail device used for pathologic fracture is not removed under normal circumstances. Therefore, this complication is of greater potential concern in the non-neoplastic indications for the Zickel nail.

The same problems encountered with removal of the Zickel nail often precipitate a pathologic fracture on entry and advancement of the implant into an impending subtrochanteric fracture. Modifications to the technique of Zickel application have been made, which minimize this complication.[3] If the device is introduced, as recommended, through the tip of the greater trochanter, the curve of the component abuts onto the medial aspect of the proximal femur, creating either a fracture in the subtrochanteric area or displacing the implant proximally, precipitating a fracture through the greater trochanter or, possibly, even through the base of the neck. Modifying the entry site from the tip of the trochanter to the posteromedial aspect of the neck at the piriformis tendon insertion, and extending this defect anteriorly and laterally, prevents such a complication from occurring. In the past, an additional problem with the Zickel apparatus was its length, which has now been

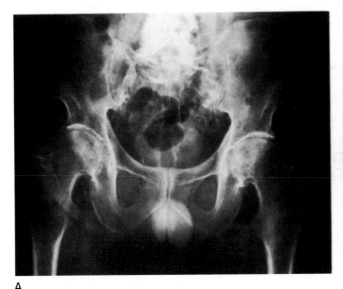

A

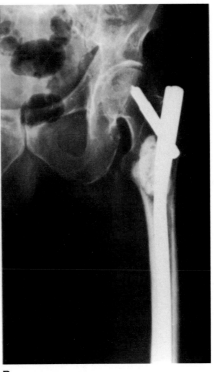

B

Figure 60B–8. **A,** Metastatic hypernephroma in the proximal femur at risk of pathologic fracture. **B,** Prophylactic fixation was achieved by means of a Zickel nail and use of methyl methacrylate.

modified to allow more distal intramedullary fixation in the femur, minimizing periprosthetic fractures in the supracondylar area of the femur.

Recognizing these difficulties with the Zickel nail, researchers have made various modifications to conventional femoral intramedullary rods, which accommodate proximal fixation in the femoral head and neck. Conventional intramedullary rods without provision for proximal locking are associated with subsequent femoral neck fractures in 16 percent of cases.[3,43,44] More recently, the reconstruction nail devised by Russell Taylor has addressed this issue by incorporating two proximal locking screws.[10] This innovation has the added advantage over most intramedullary femoral rods of being nonfluted and, thus, more rigid. If the decision is made to place the patient on a fracture table for an actual pathologic subtrochanteric fracture, it may be difficult to determine the proximal entry hole for the rod and/or to control the proximal segment very effectively because of the unopposed action of the external rotators and, possibly, the iliopsoas on the proximal segment. Under these circumstances, a Steinmann pin can be placed in the anterior aspect of the greater trochanter. This placement allows reduction of the proximal fragment to the distal fragment in an effort to minimize medializing the entry site as well as possibly creating a flexion deformity at the fracture site. Similarly, the proximal fragment tends to be pulled into abduction, which can be corrected by the anteriorly placed Steinmann pin. In an effort to place both proximal locking screws into the femoral head and neck segment, the inferior 8-mm screw should be placed just above the inferior aspect of the femoral neck. In an effort to ensure central positioning of the screw on the lateral radiograph, it may be necessary to obtain oblique films to negate the effect of the bolt and applicator for the proximal aspect of the rod. Radiolucent applicators are becoming available, and they will facilitate imaging. An additional advantage of the reconstruction nail is its ability to lock distally, increasing rotational control (Fig. 60B–9). In treatment of patients with metastatic disease; the success of intramedullary nailing of actual or impending pathologic fractures in the proximal femur has been very gratifying. Pain relief has been reported in 70 to 92 percent of patients, with ambulatory status restored in 84 to 90 percent.[43] The results clearly demonstrate the beneficial effect of intramedullary nailing, particularly as performed prophylactically for metastatic lesions in the proximal femur.

PATHOLOGIC FRACTURES OF THE ACETABULUM AND PELVIS

The pelvis is the second most common site of metastatic deposits to bone.[3] Excluding the sacrum, the pelvis can be considered to have three distinct areas. These are the anterior (ischiopubic), posterior (iliosacral), and periacetabular regions. Involvement of the anterior and poste-

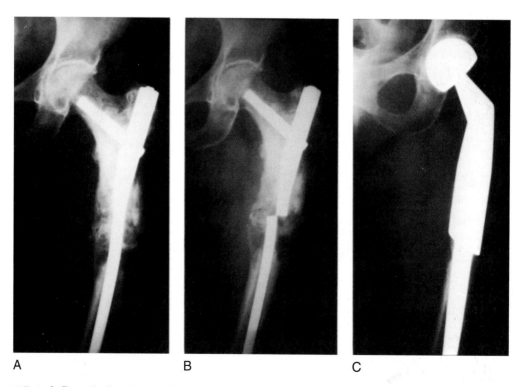

A   B   C

Figure 60B–9. A, Extensive involvement of the proximal third of the left femur by metastatic breast carcinoma; reconstruction was accomplished with a Zickel nail. **B,** Postoperative radiation was not given. Local tumor progression contributed to the mechanical failure of the implant. **C,** With such extensive bone loss, fixation was not possible and a proximal femoral bipolar replacement was performed.

rior segments of the hemipelvis rarely necessitates surgical management. Involvement can be extensive, with pain caused by impending pathologic fracture or by lack of mechanical integrity of the hemipelvic ring. The vast majority of these metastases are amenable to radiation therapy and protected weight bearing until such time as bone maturation and reformation of the involved area occurs. Rarely, with extensive sacral involvement and soft tissue extension, there is lumbosacral plexus irritation, necessitating surgical decompression.

More commonly, the orthopedic surgeon is called to evaluate periacetabular involvement and to stabilize this area in an effort to avoid medial migration of the proximal femur. It has been previously noted by Habermann et al.[17] and Harrington[22] that acetabular involvement can occur in the presence of what appear to be normal radiographs. Anticipating acetabular involvement as the source of continued pain, additional investigations in the form of bone scanning, tomography, or even CT may be necessary to delineate the full extent of disease. As Harrington[22] has pointed out, all patients with acetabular involvement are not necessarily sufficiently symptomatic to warrant any surgical intervention. Conversely, Habermann et al.[19] found sufficient involvement on the acetabular side when reconstructing the proximal femur to recommend total hip replacement in all patients being treated for pathologic femoral neck fractures.

Surgical reconstruction of the compromised acetabulum represents a formidable operative procedure, requiring more time and blood loss and causing more morbidity than conventional joint replacement. Therefore, if acetabular reconstruction is a serious consideration, the patient should be capable of tolerating the procedure and should have an anticipated life span exceeding several months. Ideal patients are those with disseminated renal, thyroid, and breast cancer and cases of myeloma. If the lesion is found to be small, is not directly compromising the weight-bearing surface, and is creating minimal symptoms, serious consideration could be made to irradiating of the area. It must be recognized, however, that with the increased vascularity associated with radiation comes a decrease in the mechanical support of the acetabulum, with the possibility of central or superior migration. Therefore, during radiation and for 6 to 12 weeks afterward, protected weight bearing should be instituted and the patient should be carefully observed with serial radiographs.

In patients with extensive periacetabular disease with impending or actual femoral migration, who are medically debilitated and/or whose life expectancy is short, a Girdlestone resection may be considered. In these isolated patients, the Girdlestone resection may represent the most rational approach.

All other situations demanding some form of acetabular reconstruction have been well addressed in the studies of Levy et al.[28] and Harrington.[21] The degree of periacetabular involvement is categorized as being minor, major, or massive, dictating varied reconstructive alternatives. With minor involvement of the acetabulum not involving the weight-bearing surface, a conventional acetabular cup with medial mesh reinforcement to prevent intrapelvic methyl methacrylate extravasation is recommended. The patient can be ambulatory within several days of the operation, with minimal if any restraints. With larger defects but intact pillars, in which conventional cup replacement carries the risk of migration, an acetabular ring is recommended, reinforced with mesh on the medial wall for the same purpose as stated earlier (Fig. 60B–10). The acetabular ring serves to transmit the stress to the intact columns, avoiding stress on the involved medial and superior aspects of the acetabulum. The acetabular component can be seated in conventional fashion within the ring. Use of a long-neck femoral component avoids the possibility of impingement and lessens the likelihood of dislocation. For massive defects involving the superior, medial, anterior, and posterior columns of the acetabulum, specialized reconstructive methods devised by Harrington[21] need to be employed, including the use of flexible threaded Steinmann pins coursing through the iliac wing into the sacrum to act as a rim onto which the protusio ring can be applied, with support medial from the mesh and superior insertion of methyl methacrylate into the deficiency (Figs. 60B–11 and 60B–12). Universal improvement in the status of patients with minor or major involvement have been recorded by Levy et al.,[28] Harrington,[21] and Sim et al.[41] from the Mayo Clinic. The reconstruction necessary for massive periacetabular bone loss should be reserved for patients who have a favorable prognosis. Apart from relieving pain and attempting to restore realistic function, it is also imperative that an attempt be made to incorporate these patients back into the familiar surroundings of family and friends. Major reconstructions, although technically challenging and gratifying, may not be in the best interest of these patients, given their restricted life span.

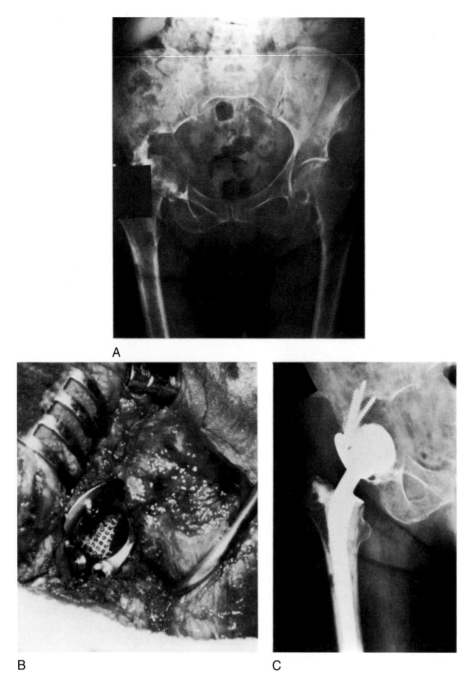

A

B   C

Figure 60B–10. **A**, Diffuse metastatic breast carcinoma involving both sides of the hip joint, allowing medial migration. **B**, Because of massive central acetabular involvement, an acetabular ring was used to gain purchase into the intact interior and posterior pillars. **C**, With a long-stemmed cemented femoral component, the patient was allowed to be ambulatory with protected weight bearing.

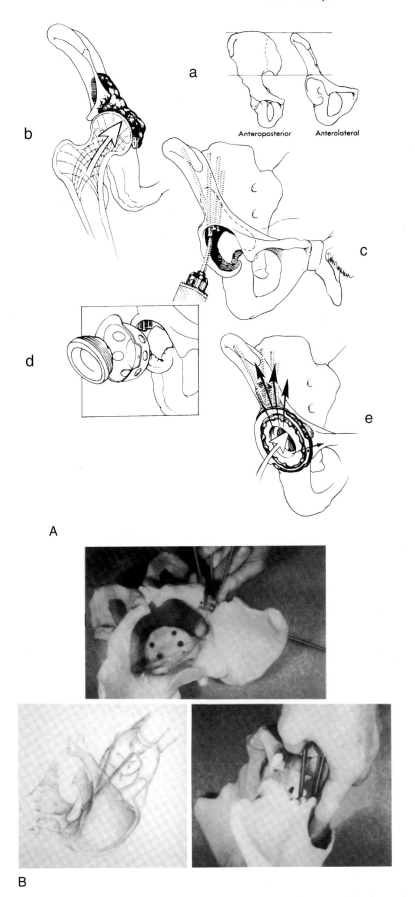

Figure 60B–11. Type III deficiency with proposed reconstruction. **A**, Introduction of threaded Kirschner wires to support the dome and central deficiency of the acetabulum (steps a through e). **B**, Wires guided by the surgeon's finger were introduced through the sciatic notch into the true pelvis. (From Harrington KD: Orthopaedic Management of Metastatic Bone Disease. St. Louis, CV Mosby, 1988.)

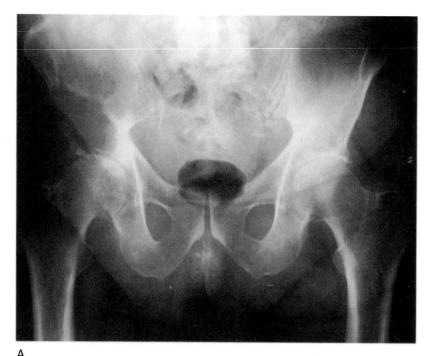

A

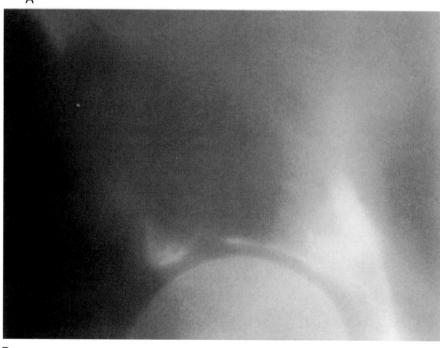

B

Figure 60B–12. A, Radiograph of a 73-year-old man with unifocal renal cell metastases to the right periacetabular region. The patient could not walk and regularly used narcotic analgesics. **B,** Anteroposterior tomogram suggests the lack of dome support.

Illustration continued on opposite page

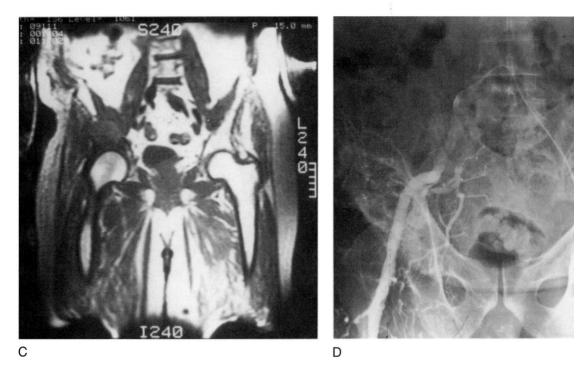

C

D

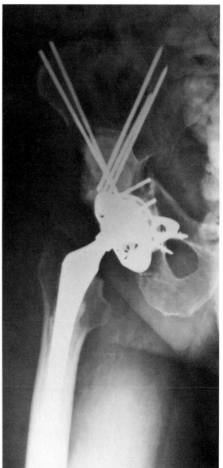

E

Figure 60B–12. *Continued.* **C,** Magnetic resonance imaging reveals expansive lesion involving the weight-bearing dome and pillars, with intrapelvic or extrapelvic soft tissue expansion. **D,** Preoperative arteriography suggests the extensive vascularity of the lesion, prompting embolization before surgery. **E,** Radiograph taken 6 months after reconstruction with threaded Steinmann pins, protrusio ring, mesh, and long-stemmed femoral component. (From Rock MG, Harrington KD: Metastatic bone disease: Pathologic Fractures of the acetabulum and the pelvis. Orthopedics 15:569, 1992.)

References

1. Aufranc OE, Jones WN, Turner RH: Severely comminuted intertrochanteric hip fractures. Surg Gynecol Obstet 112:633, 1961.
2. Bartucci EJ, Gonzalez MH, Cooperman DR, et al: The effect of adjunctive methyl methacrylate on failures of fixation and function in patients with intertrochanteric fractures and osteoporosis. J Bone Joint Surg 67A:1094, 1985.
3. Behr JT, Dobozi WR, Badrinath K: The treatment of pathologic and impending pathologic fractures of the proximal femur in the elderly. Clin Orthop 198:173, 1985.
4. Bonarigo BC, Rubin P: Nonunion of pathologic fractures after radiation therapy. Radiology 88:889, 1967.
5. Cadman E, Bentino JR: Chemotherapy in skeletal metastases. Int Radiat Oncol Biol Phys 1:1211, 1976.
6. Camnasio F, Ravasi F: Modular prostheses in metastatic bone disease of the proximal femur. Bull Hosp Joint Dis 54:211, 1996.
7. Cangeorian BJ, Ryan JR, Salciccioli GG: Prophylactic femoral stabilization with the Zickel nail by closed technique. J Bone Joint Surg 68A:991, 1986.
8. Capanna R, Rock MG, Campanacci M, et al: Femoral megaprosthesis in the management of bone tumor, a study of 49 cases. J West Pacific Orthop 22:33, 1984.
9. Coleman RE: Management of bone metastases. Oncologist 5:463, 2000.
10. Cleveland M, Bosworth DM, Thompson FR: Management of the trochanteric fracture of the femur. JAMA 137:1186, 1948.
11. Coleman MP, Greenough CG, Warren PJ, et al: Technical aspects of the use of the Russell-Taylor reconstruction nail. Br J Accident Surg 22:89, 1991.
12. Douglass HO, Sikekia SK, Mindell E: Treatment of pathological fractures of long bones excluding those due to breast cancer. J Bone Joint Surg 58A:1055, 1976.
13. Drew M, Dickson RB: Osseous complications of malignancy. In Lokich JJ (ed): Clinical Cancer Medicine: Treatment Tactics. Boston, GK Hall, 1988.
14. Eggers GWN, Evans EB, Blumel J, et al: Cystic change in the iliac acetabulum. J Bone Joint Surg 45A:669, 1963.
15. Gainor BJ, Buchert P: Fracture healing in metastatic bone disease. Clin Orthop 178:297, 1983.
16. Gitelis S, Sheinkop MB, Hammerberg K: The treatment of metastatic foci of the proximal femur: A retrospective review. Orthop Trans 5:428, 1961.
17. Graham WD: Pathological fractures secondary to metastatic cancer. J Bone Joint Surg 45B:617, 1963.
18. Gristina AC, Adair DM, Spurr CL: Intraosseous metastatic breast cancer treatment with internal fixation and study of survival. Ann Surg 197:128, 1983.
19. Haberman ET, Sachs R, Stern RE, et al: The pathology and treatment of metastatic disease of the femur. Clin Orthop 169T:70, 1982.
20. Harrington KD, Johnson JO, Turner RH, et al: The use of methyl methacrylate as an adjunct in the internal fixation of malignant neoplastic fractures. J Bone Joint Surg 54A:1665, 1972.
21. Harrington KD: The management of acetabular insufficiency secondary to metastatic malignant disease. J Bone Joint Surg 63:653, 1981.
22. Harrington KD: New tends in the management of lower extremity metastases. Clin Orthop 169:53, 1982.
23. Harrington KD: Orthopaedic Management of Metastatic Bone Disease. St. Louis, CV Mosby, 1988.
24. Hunter GA, Krajbich IJ: The results of medial displacement osteotomy for unstable intertrochanteric fractures of the femur. Clin Orthop 137:140, 1978.
25. Kirschner PT, Simon MA: Current concepts review: Radioisotope evaluation of skeletal disease. J Bone Joint Surg 63A:673, 1981.
26. Lane JM, Sculco TP, Zolan S: Treatment of pathological fractures of the hip by endoprosthetic replacement. J Bone Joint Surg 62A:954, 1980.
27. Leggon RE, Lindsey R, Panjabi M: Strength reduction and the effects of treatment of long bones with defects involving 50% of the cortex. J Orthop Res 6:540, 1988.
28. Levy RN, Sherry HS, Siffert RS: Surgical management of metastatic disease of bone at the hip. Clin Orthop 169:62, 1982.
29. McBroom RJ, Hayes WC: Strength reduction and fracture risk of cortical defects in the diaphysis of long bones. Orthop Trans 9:320, 1984.
30. Mirels H: Metastatic disease in long bones. Clin Orthop 249:256, 1989.
31. Morrey BF: Rheumatoid pseudocyst (geode) of the femoral neck without apparent joint involvement: Case report. Mayo Clin Proc 62:407, 1987.
32. Osteen RT, Kopf G, Wilson RE: In pursuit of the unknown primary. Am J Surg 135:494, 1978.
33. Parrish FF, Murray JA: Surgical treatment for secondary neoplastic fractures. J Bone Joint Surg 52A:665, 1970.
34. Rock MG: The use of the Bateman bipolar proximal femoral replacement for metastatic disease. Presented at the Fourth International Symposium on Limb Salvage, Kyoto, Japan, 1987.
35. Rock MG, Harrington KD: Metastatic bone disease: Pathologic fractures of the acetabulum and the pelvis. Orthopedics 15:569, 1992.
36. Rograff BT, Kaneisl JS, Simon MA: Skeletal metastasis of unknown origin: Prospective evaluation of diagnostic strategy. J Bone Joint Surg 75A:1276, 1993.
37. Ryan JR, Begeman PC: The effects of filling experimental large cortical defects with methyl methacrylate. Clin Orthop 185:306, 1984.
38. Sherry HS, Levy RN, Siffert RS: Metastatic disease of bone in orthopedic surgery. Clin Orthop 169:44, 1982.
39. Sim FH: Diagnosis and Management of Metastatic Disease of Bone: A Multidisciplinary Approach. New York, Raven Press, 1988.
40. Sim FH, Daugherty TW, Ivins JC: The adjunctive use of methyl methacrylate in fixation of pathological fractures. J Bone Joint Surg 65A:40, 1974.
41. Sim FH, Hartz CR, Chao EYS: Total hip arthroplasty for tumor of the hip. In Evarts CM (ed): The Hip: Proceedings of the Fourth Open Scientific Meeting of the Hip Society. St. Louis, CV Mosby, 1976, p 246.
42. Townsend PW, Smalley SR, Cozad SC, et al: Role of postoperative radiation therapy after stabilization of fractures causing metastatic disease. J Clin Oncol 13:2140, 1995.
43. Vanderhulst RRWJ, Vanden Wildenberg FAJM, Vroemen JPAM, Greve JWM: Intramedullary nail with impending pathologic fractures. J Trauma 36:211, 1994.
44. Van Doorn R, van der Hulst RR, van den Wildenberg FA: Intramedullary fixation in impending femoral fractures caused by tumor metastasis. Ned Tijdschr Geneesk 138:2101, 1994.
45. Van Holten-Verzantvoort AT, Papapoulos SE: Oral pamidronate in the prevention and treatment of skeletal metastases in patients with breast cancer. Medicina 1(Suppl 57):109, 1997.
46. Ward WG, Spang J, Howe D, Gordan S. Femoral reconstruction nails for metastatic disease: Indications, technique and results. Am J Orthop 29(Suppl 9):34, 2000.
47. Yelton C, Low W: Iatrogenic subtrochanteric fracture: A complication of Zickel nails. J Bone Joint Surg 68A:1237, 1986.

61

Evaluation of the Painful Total Hip Arthroplasty

• DANIEL J. BERRY

Although total hip arthroplasty is remarkably successful in providing consistent relief of hip pain, a small percentage of patients have pain that requires further evaluation after hip replacement. Accurate identification of the source of the pain is essential for successful treatment management. The symptoms may originate from other anatomic sites, but they more frequently arise from the hip itself.[1] Soft tissue problems, mechanical problems with the arthroplasty, infection, and other, less frequent diagnoses are all potential sources. A systematic approach to the evaluation, with attention directed to key points of the patient's history, physical examination, laboratory test results, and radiographic studies, is necessary to reach a correct diagnosis effectively and efficiently. Since the early 1990s, the diagnostic tests available to the physician have become increasingly sophisticated. At the same time, for uncemented components, the process of distinguishing patients with loose implants from those who have pain for other reasons has grown more difficult. Nevertheless, increased experience has made the diagnosis of loose uncemented implants more accurate. This chapter provides an approach to evaluation of the painful hip arthroplasty and reviews the efficacy of the various diagnostic tests as aids in arriving at the correct diagnosis and treatment.

MANIFESTATION

History

A careful review of the general medical history may suggest diagnoses that would otherwise be overlooked. Prior malignancy or night pain may suggest neoplastic disease (Fig. 61–1). Recent bacterial infection or possible bacteremia should heighten concern that there may be an underlying infection. A history of back problems may suggest the spine as a source of referred pain.[5,29] Metabolic bone problems or a history of severe osteoporosis may alert the orthopedist to the patient at risk for stress fracture. The sudden onset of marked pain in patients with periprosthetic osteolysis suggests the possibility of an acute fracture through an area of bone weakness. Peripheral vascular disease occasionally may appear as discomfort in the hip or thigh area.[10,16,45] Multiple somatic complaints or multiple surgical procedures introduce pain threshold and perception as possible sources of the pain.

Temporal Features

We find it helpful to divide hip pain into that which persists from the procedure, that which occurs in the first few months after surgery, and that which occurs later. In the early postoperative period, pain out of proportion to that expected should lead to consideration of acute infection, heterotopic bone formation, or even component instability. Pain initially felt a few months after the initial procedure suggests other sources: component loosening, chronic infection, soft tissue problems (such as tendinitis or bursitis), or stress fracture (Fig. 61–2).[14,38,43,48,51] Localized osteolysis results from particulate debris, occurs late, and is usually painless. Yet, as it progresses, osteolysis may also be associated with pain caused by particulate debris synovitis or particulate debris reaction along the psoas sheath, an expanded pseudocapsule, or even instability (Fig. 61–3).[41,42]

Location

Problems with the cup are more likely to be felt in the buttock, whereas femoral problems usually are felt in the thigh or knee. Pain in the groin can occur from either cup of femoral problems and is considered the watershed area for pain. Acetabular loosening frequently appears as buttock pain, whereas pain from unipolar or bipolar prostheses often is felt in the groin. Femoral loosening usually is manifested by thigh pain, but femoral component failures, especially of long-stemmed components, also may be felt as pain in the knee in certain patients. Stable uncemented femoral components may also cause persistent thigh pain.

Soft tissue inflammation typically is felt in the anatomic location of the inflammation (Fig. 61–4). Thus,

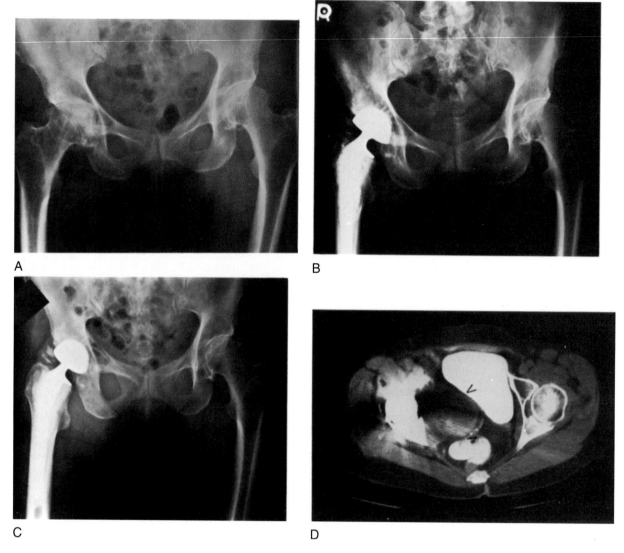

A

B

C

D

Figure 61–1. A, Anteroposterior roentgenogram of patient with painful right hip. **B,** Anteroposterior roentgenogram of total hip replacement. Groin pain persists. **C,** Six months postsurgery, pain is increased with abduction of hip. Lytic area with pathologic fracture noted medial to acetabular component. Same lytic area was present in panels **A** and **B** but is now more evident. **D,** Computed tomographic scan shows mass in pelvis, displacing bladder (*arrow*). Biopsy revealed a chondrosarcoma.

iliopsoas tendonitis usually causes groin pain,[66] whereas trochanteric bursitis mostly causes pain localized over the greater trochanter, sometimes with radiation to the knee along the iliotibial band. Nonunion of the osteotomized trochanter often is not painful, but when symptomatic, it is directly referable to the greater trochanteric region.[59,69]

When the pain occurs almost exclusively in the buttocks or posterior pelvis, there can be a manifestation of referred pain from the back or sacroiliac joints, especially when associated with back discomfort.

Characteristics

Possibly the most important feature is the relationship of pain to activity. Pain with sudden change of position, such as standing from a sitting position or during the

first few steps of ambulation (start-up pain), is typical of a loose component. A triphasic pattern is classic. Pain is sharp with the first few steps of ambulation, is reduced after the patient has walked a moderate distance, and gradually increases after the patient has walked a still greater distance.

Symptoms from instability (subluxation) usually occur in at-risk positions of the hip, and, often, the patient can feel the hip subluxate. Activity-related thigh pain may be design specific and has been associated with uncemented femoral components. Although still not fully understood, activity-related thigh pain seems to represent either loosening of the component or mismatch in the modulus of elasticity between the component and the bone. Pain that occurs at rest or at night should raise concern of infection or tumor problems unless the patient lies on the affected hip, which is characteristic of trochanteric bursitis. Pain that is the same

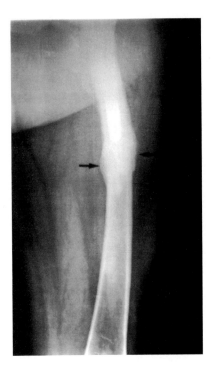

Figure 61–2. Stress fracture of femur in a 37-year-old woman 2 years after revision total hip arthroplasty. An unrecognized perforation had been made at the time of revision total hip arthroplasty. The patient's stress fracture healed with conservative management.

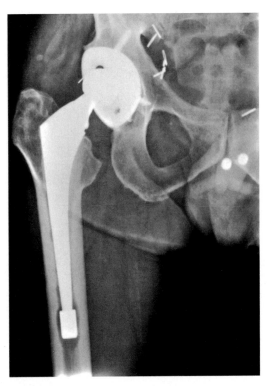

Figure 61–3. Osteolysis around a well-fixed uncemented femoral component. The patient had thigh pain and required revision surgery.

after surgery as before should lead to consideration of an extra-articular source of discomfort.

PHYSICAL EXAMINATION

Simple observation of the patient's gait is extremely helpful. A Duchenne sign (patient leans to the side of the affected hip during stance to compensate for abductor weakness or inhibition) or a Trendelenburg sign suggests hip pathology.

Asking the patient to point to the source of greatest pain and carefully palpating the site may localize the source of the problem. Tenderness over the spine or over the sacroiliac joints may point to pathology in these regions. Pain on palpation of the greater trochanter, the hamstring origins on the ischium, the gluteus maximus insertion, and the piriformis regions can be caused by the soft tissue inflammation of bursitis or tendonitis in these areas. Tenderness over the public rami is common with stress fractures in osteoporosis patients or as an expression of osteitis pubis in younger individuals.

Active or passive pain with motion is a very helpful diagnostic symptom. Exquisite pain with any hip range of motion suggests active synovitis and raises the concern of infection. Pain that occurs at the extremes of hip motion, particularly with maximal hip internal rotation, is commonly associated with loose components. This pain is often felt in the groin or thigh owing to a loose socket or stem, respectively.

I believe that the Stinchfield test (Fig. 61–5) is very effective in distinguishing pain in the hip joint from spine pain. It is positive for both loose cups and stems.

DIAGNOSIS OF INFECTION

The possibility of an infection is of paramount importance, discussed in detail in Chapters 10 and 64, is an essential first step in the assessment process.

IMAGING STUDIES

Despite the proliferation of sophisticated arthrographic studies, nuclear medicine studies, and computed imaging studies, the most helpful radiographic studies for detection of cemented and uncemented prosthetic failure are still good-quality serial plain radiographs of the hip.[3] Plain films may detect infection, osteolysis, tumors, acute fractures, and stress fractures, in addition to prosthetic loosening. Radiostereometry, a sophisticated method based on plain radiographs, is probably the most sensitive test of all for implant loosening but requires multiple intraoperatively placed marker beads and sophisticated biplanar radiographic facilities that are not routinely available.[32] Arthrography is more helpful in detecting loose cemented than loose uncemented components. One study found digital subtraction arthrography to be the most accurate test for predicting implant loosening compared with plain radiographs and scintigraphy.[18,27]

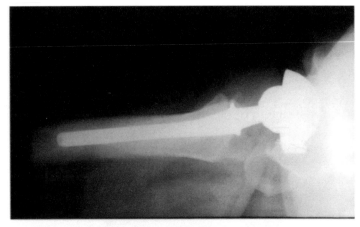

A

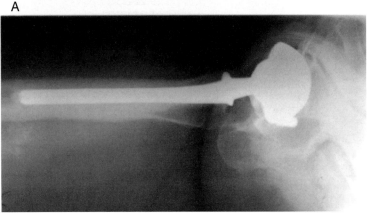

B

Figure 61–4. **A**, Patient with iliopsoas tendinitis caused by tenting of the iliopsoas tendon over the prominent rim of an uncemented acetabular component. **B**, Patient was revised to a less anteverted component with a recessed rim and pain symptoms were relieved.

The role of nuclear medicine scans continues to be debated, but most authors agree they should be considered as a secondary rather than a primary means of looking for loosening.[57] Nuclear arthrography appears to be more sensitive in detecting loosening than standard arthrography,[54] but it is not widely available. Sensitivity, specificity, and accuracy, as well as the criteria for a positive result of each study, are different for cemented and uncemented total hip arthroplasties.[6]

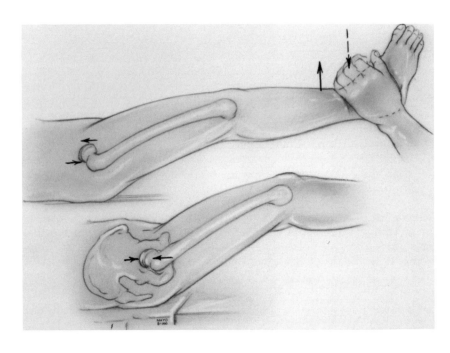

Figure 61–5. The "Stinchfield test" is performed by asking the patient to perform a resisted straight leg raise. The hip joint is loaded, and hip pathology frequently causes pain.

More Recent Tests

One study reported the results of using metabolites of bone turnover to detect implant loosening. Fifty patients with implant loosening proved by surgery were compared with a matched cohort without radiographic evidence of implant loosening.[62] Significantly increased urine levels of several metabolites of bone resorption were identified in patients with loose prostheses compared with controls. The sensitivity and specificity of each metabolite as a predictor of loosening varied, and none were perfect. The role, accuracy, limitations, and practical value of these tests remains to be delineated.

To simplify the discussion, the following sections of the chapter divide patients into those with cemented and those with uncemented components.

Cemented Total Hip Arthroplasty

Plain Radiographs

Regardless of the variations in interpretation and a degree of subjectivity, most authors now agree that certain radiographic findings are highly correlated with prosthetic loosening. As a caveat, one should remember that there remains marked inter- and intraobserver variability in the interpretation of these radiographic findings.[47]

On the acetabular side, loosening is almost certain if serial films show cement fracture, migration, or change of component position.[52] Nevertheless, the predictive value of a complete radiolucent line at the acetabular bone-cement interface has varied in different studies, perhaps reflecting differences of defining subtle acetabular component loosening at surgery. Hodgkinson and colleagues, using a sophisticated means to intraoperatively test cemented acetabular stability at revision, showed that 100 percent of sockets with migration were loose, and 94 percent of sockets with a complete radiolucent line of any width at the bone-cement interface were loose. On the other hand, 79 percent of hips with a radiolucent line in both zones 1 and 2 were loose, and only 5 percent with no migration or a radiolucent line alone in zone 1 were loose.[28]

Yet, O'Neill and Harris (using migration or a 2-mm complete radiolucent line as a criterion) found that plain films identified only 37 percent of loose acetabula.[52] Using similar criteria, others have reported plain films with 81-percent sensitivity and 86-percent specificity[50] and 63-percent sensitivity and 89-percent specificity.[39]

Plain radiographs are more sensitive in identifying cemented femoral component failure.[52,65] Most authors, using migration and a complete radiolucent line of 2 mm or more as criteria, have agreed that cement fracture, gross migration of the component and cement, and a complete radiolucent line at the bone-cement interface predict femoral loosening. Plain films were reported to be 89 percent sensitive and 92 percent specific for femoral loosening.[52] Using similar criteria, Miniaci et al. reported 86 percent sensitivity[50]; on the other hand, partial radiolucent lines at the bone-cement interface may represent adaptive bone remodeling and do not necessarily correlate with prosthetic loosening.[29,40]

In the past, the significance of a radiolucent line at the lateral shoulder of the prosthesis-cement interface, which is frequently called femoral component debonding, was debated. Some authors considered this to be a reliable sign of femoral loosening in as high as 94 percent of patients. Others, including Sir John Charnley himself,[31,55] did not consider this finding to necessarily correlate with symptomatic femoral loosening. In a 20-year follow-up study of 299 Charnley total hip arthroplasties at the Mayo Clinic, femoral debonding associated with a radiolucent line of less than 2 mm at the prosthetic bone-cement interface was not associated with a markedly poorer long-term survival rate for the femoral prosthesis and, in the absence of other signs of loosening, did not correlate statistically with hip pain. It is well known that the smooth, collarless, wedge-shaped Exeter stem has a significant rate of femoral debonding without associated clinical femoral component failure.[17,37] It is also now well recognized that the significance of femoral debonding is specific to component design and component surface finish. Some designs are able to subside slightly to a stable position within the cement mantle but others are not. Implants with a smooth surface and certain wedge like geometry features seem to tolerate debonding well and can function well clinically as a taper-slip arrangement. On the other hand, rough surface or collared implants precoated with polymethylmethacrylate usually produce particulate debris, inflammation, and osteolysis when they debond. Pain with clinical arthroplasty failure, even with minimal implant subsidence within the cement, is common with these implants. When debonding is seen in association with significant thigh pain or other radiographic signs of femoral failure, symptomatic femoral component loosening should be considered likely.

Arthrography

Detection of loose, cemented acetabular components appears to be enhanced by arthrography compared with plain films. Some have found that arthrography improved the sensitivity from 37 percent for plain films to 89 percent,[52] and others reported a 97 percent sensitivity and 68 percent specificity for acetabular arthrography.[46] However, Miniaci et al. found that arthrograms identified only 68 percent of loose sockets.[50]

Less improvement in the detection of loose femoral components is provided by arthrography. Both Minaci et al.[50] and O'Neill and Harris[52] showed that arthrography did not markedly improve the accuracy of predicting the fixation status of the femoral component. However, in O'Neill and Harris' series, one of nine femoral components thought to be well fixed from plain films was correctly proved by arthrography to be loose.[52] Lyons et al. showed that subtraction arthrograms did improve the sensitivity of detecting femoral loosening from 84 percent by plain films to 96 percent.[39] Thus, although most loose femoral components can be detected by plain film, arthrograms to occasionally identify loose components that would not otherwise be detected (Fig. 61–6). Arthrography with postexercise films,[21,26] subtraction arthrography,[61] and radionuclide arthrography[8,58,64] have all been reported to have some advantages over routine contrast arthrography, but this equipment is not available at all institutions. Hence, the addition of the arthrogram at the time of aspiration would seem a logical adjunct to the evaluation of the potentially loose, painful hip arthroplasty.

Technetium Bone Scans

A most helpful means of screening for bony pathology around the hip is the technetium bone scan. Increased uptake can identify tumors and pelvic or femoral stress fractures. The value of bone scans for detecting component loosening has been more controversial and has undergone some revision with time.[27,49,56,60] Early studies showed that technetium bone scans are sensitive but not specific in detecting pathology.[70] Up to 10 percent of patients exhibit abnormal isotope uptake 1 year after total hip arthroplasty.[67] In 35 painful hips, Jensen and Madsen found that sensitivity in detecting loose components was only 77 percent compared with 97 percent

sensitivity for plain films. The specificity was only 46 percent compared with 70 percent for plain films. Their rate of false-positive scans for loosening was 23 percent. Importantly, they identified several instances of unjustified operative exploration based on the positive scan.[30] Lieberman et al. also found that in 54 patients, technetium scans did not provide additional information to plain films. They suggested that the scan be used only when the clinical suspicion for loosening persisted despite negative plain films.[35]

From these studies, the conclusion can be drawn that bone scans, although occasionally helpful, are frequently misleading a specifical is sought for component loosening. The high rate of accuracy of plain films and arthrography makes bone scans of limited clinical value in detecting a loose component.

Uncemented Total Hip Arthroplasty

The increasing popularity of uncemented components has made more difficult the task of determining the source of pain around hip replacements. Radiographic criteria used to detect component loosening in cemented total hip arthroplasty are often not applicable to uncemented total hip arthroplasty. Furthermore, pain without demonstrable component loosening occurs more frequently around uncemented than around cemented total hip arthroplasties. Rates of persistent thigh discomfort in uncemented total hip arthroplasty

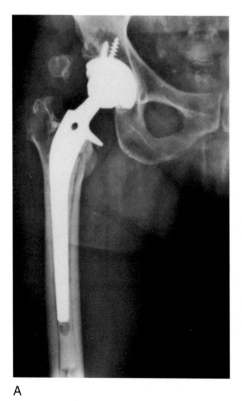
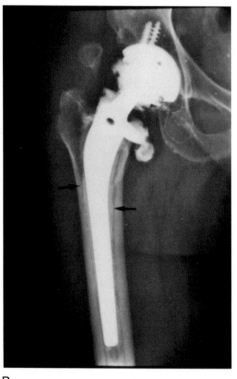

A   B

Figure 61–6. A, Plain films showing a cemented femoral component without definite loosening. **B**, Arthrogram demonstrating femoral component loosening in the same hip.

vary in different series,[12,24,63] but they were as high as 30 percent[20] 2 to 4 years after surgery in some early series. Others have reported a rate of 15 percent to 26 percent up to 7 years after porous-coated anatomic (PCA) replacement.[25]

Thigh pain is the most common complaint after uncemented arthroplasty. In some cases, this is associated with a loose prosthesis, but, in others, it occurs with a stable implant. Campbell et al., in a study of 148 uncemented PCA total hip replacements, found that thigh pain was associated with stem subsidence, bead shedding, and distal periosteal reaction. They concluded that stem instability was the likely cause of pain in most patients.[7] Others have found a positive correlation with thigh pain, suggesting that a mismatch in modulus of elasticity between the prosthesis and the surrounding bone might be a source of pain in some patients.[69] It is also clear that thigh pain does occur in some patients with well-fixed ingrown bone as well as in those with loose femoral components.

Based on the preceding data, it is important from the clinician's standpoint to recognize that there are probably several sources of thigh pain after uncemented total hip arthroplasty. Patients with pain and no loosening are generally selected for observation. Although some eventually require hip exploration or revision, a number (the proportion is debated) improve with time and conservative management. The goal should be identification of patients with pain resulting from loosening, because they are probably less likely to have spontaneous improvement in pain and are thus better candidates for revision.

Plain Films

The Socket

The rate of acetabular loosening in most series of uncemented hemispheric sockets has been low. Although no strict radiographic criteria for uncemented socket loosening are available, most would agree that progressive migration or change in socket position with time indicates acetabular loosening.[44] Fracture of acetabular fixation screws also implies loosening. Heekin et al. have shown that progressive bead shedding from the porous surface more than 2 years after surgery also correlates with migration and, presumably, loosening.[25] Uncemented cup loosening is suggested by the appearance of new radiolucent lines around a socket. Partial radiolucent lines are of uncertain significance, but a complete radiolucent line causes more concern. A new, expanding radiolucent line at the inferior medial bone-implant interface, especially in combination with bony sclerosis at the superior lateral bone implant interface, suggests early tilt of the cup due to loosening.

Because thigh pain is a more frequent problem than acetabular loosening, a body of information is available correlating radiographic findings with uncemented femoral component stability. The classic criteria for categorizing the stability status of the femoral component were established by Engh and co-workers, mostly from studies of the extensively porous-coated anatomic medullary locking stem.[12] Signs suggesting bone ingrowth and stability include (1) no subsidence and (2) lack of a radiodense or radiolucent line at the interface between the bone and the porous coating of the prosthesis. Stable fibrous fixation was suggested by (1) no progressive migration and (2) extensive radiopaque line formation parallel to the porous-coated surface of the stem at the prosthesis-bone interface. Unstable implants were characterized by (1) progressive subsidence of the prosthesis and (2) divergent radiodense lines about the stem. However, a radiolucent or radiodense parallel line around a non–porous-coated region of a femoral implant is a normal response to an uncemented implant and does not indicate loosening. Hence, Engh's criteria should be considered design specific.

Engh and co-workers have subsequently refined the radiographic criteria for assessment of the femoral component into major and minor signs for bone ingrowth and stability.[13] Major signs have an extremely high correlation with implant stability, whereas minor signs have a significant but less conclusive correlation with stability. Major signs of osteointegration include (1) absence of reactive lines at the porous surface of the implant and (2) new bone bridging between the porous surface of the implant and the endosteum (Figs. 61–7 and 61–8). These may be seen as "spot welds" from the endosteum to the porous surface and are more likely to be visible in osteointegrated, extensively coated implants than in osteointegrated proximally porous-coated implants. The major sign of implant instability is progressive implant subsidence or migration. Minor signs suggesting component instability include progressive bead shedding, calcar hypertrophy beneath a collar, and evidence of motion between the smooth portion of the stem and the bone. Minor signs suggesting stability include calcar atrophy and lack of the aforementioned signs of instability.

Pedestal formation (i.e., growth of sclerotic bone at the tip of the component) has been of controversial significance. Some believe it suggests loosening, whereas others do not. Engh et al. observed that pedestal formation with intimate contact between the pedestal and the prosthesis tip suggests distal femoral component stability, whereas pedestal formation associated with a radiolucent line between the pedestal and the prosthesis tip often correlates with distal component instability.[13] Yet, once again, this finding should probably be viewed as design specific.

Over time, the radiographic appearance of uncemented hydroxyapatite-coated implants differs somewhat from that of porous-coated implants. The classical pattern is one of progressive cancellous bone condensation and cortical hypertrophy around the hydroxyapatite-coated portion of the femoral component.[9] Loose hydroxyapatite-coated implants have radiographic findings similar to those of other loose uncemented implants.

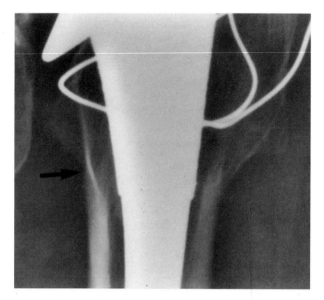

Figure 61–7. A well-fixed proximally porous-coated femoral component showing streaming trabeculae from the porous-coated surface to the endosteum.

The best means of diagnosing uncemented femoral component loosening remains the careful evaluation of good-quality sequential radiographs to look for progressive component change in position or subsidence. In this context, care must be taken not to overinterpret films centered at different points on the femur or on taken in different positions of rotation or with different exposure techniques[19] (Fig. 61–9).

Arthrography

Arthrography for the diagnosis of uncemented component loosening has not been studied well. Barrack et al. reported that in 16 uncemented sockets, arthrography was 29 percent sensitive, 89 percent specific, and 63 percent accurate.[2] On the femoral side, they found a significant rate of false-positives and false-negative results; sensitivity, specificity, and accuracy rates were all 67 percent. The Mayo Clinic experience with a large number of arthrograms used to assess uncemented components has been that the sensitivity rate is low and the study often fails to identify loose components (Fig. 61–10). Fibrous tissue between the bone and the porous coating of components may prevent migration of contrast dye, even around loose and symptomatic components.

Technetium Bone Scan

Radioisotope scans may seem a particularly attractive diagnostic alternative because of the difficulty in assessing the stability of uncemented components by plain radiography and arthrography. The presence of thigh pain is associated with a higher incidence of positive technetium bone scans.[27] Unfortunately, the process of bone remodeling around uncemented stems

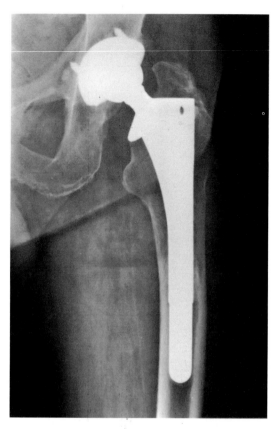

Figure 61–8. A well-fixed extensively porous-coated femoral component showing streaming trabeculae between the porous coating and the endosteum. Note that there is some proximal stress shielding, also consistent with distal bone ingrowth.

is a gradual and prolonged one[33,36,67] and probably varies with implant design. This prolonged remodeling would be expected to manifest itself on bone scan, and, in fact, Oswald et al. found abnormal technetium isotope uptake at the prosthesis tip in 72 percent of uncemented hips 2 years after surgery.[53] Thus, although clinical studies comparing bone scans with component stability at revision are lacking in uncemented total hips, it appears that definitive interpretation of bone scans after uncemented total hip arthroplasty is problematic.

Diagnostic Injection of the Hip Joint with Local Anesthetic

Injection of local anesthetic may be useful after a complete evaluation if the source of the patient's pain is still uncertain. Marcaine may be injected into the hip joint under fluoroscopic guidance. Good pain relief for a period commensurate with the activity of the local anesthetic suggests an intra-articular source of the patient's pain. The contrary is probably not true; if no pain relief occurs, one cannot conclude that the pain source is necessarily extra-articular, because failure of the local anesthetic to reach all parts of the arthroplasty is probably not uncommon (just as contrast does not always reach

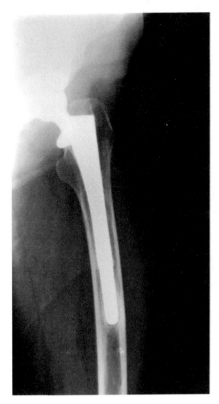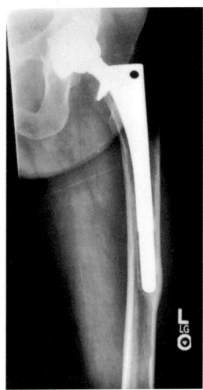

Figure 61–9. Anteroposterior radiographs of the same patient's femur taken on the same day. Note that slight differences in hip rotation give the false appearance that the component is in a different position on the two films.

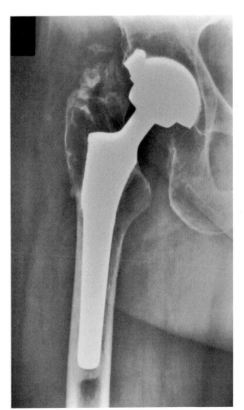

Figure 61–10. A, Plain film showing loose uncemented femoral component (note nonparallel complete radiolucent line at interface between porous coating and bone, bead shedding, and distal pedastal). **B,** A false-negative arthrogram shows no contrast around the femoral component. At revision, the femoral component was proved to be loose.

A

B

portions of a loose arthroplasty during arthrography). The surgeon using injection to evaluate pain around a prosthesis also must be mindful of the fact that injection can have a placebo effect. Yet again, this is a useful adjunct, especially if an aspiration is being done to exclude an infection.

Dynamic Computed Tomography

Little is known of the value of this test. Donaldson et al. first reported the results of using dynamic computed tomography to assess rotational instability of uncemented femoral components.[11] Because most loose femoral components manifest motion in response to rotational testing, forced internal and external rotation of the hip causes the femur to move with respect to the loose femoral component. Instability may then be visible on computed tomogram cuts taken with the hip in maximal internal and external rotation. In a series of 10 patients, 100 percent sensitivity with this technique was reported.[11] Subsequent confirming reports have not appeared to date in the literature.

CONCLUSION

When pain occurs around the total hip arthroplasty, its source usually can be identified by obtaining a careful description of the pain, performing a thorough yet focused physical examination, and scrutinizing good-quality serial plain radiographs of the arthroplasty. When the source of pain remains elusive despite these investigations, other, more sophisticated tests, including arthrography and nuclear medicine scans, may be helpful. The usefulness of the studies is different for cemented and uncemented components.[34]

I have found this logic to be amenable to an algorithmic approach (Figs. 61–11 and 61–12).[15,22,23] Still, evaluation of the painful total hip arthroplasty requires clinical judgment and varies, based on the patient's individual circumstances and the accuracy of specific diagnostic tests available to individual surgeons at each institution. Finally, the individual surgical experience and judgment are the ultimate arbitrators in the most difficult cases.

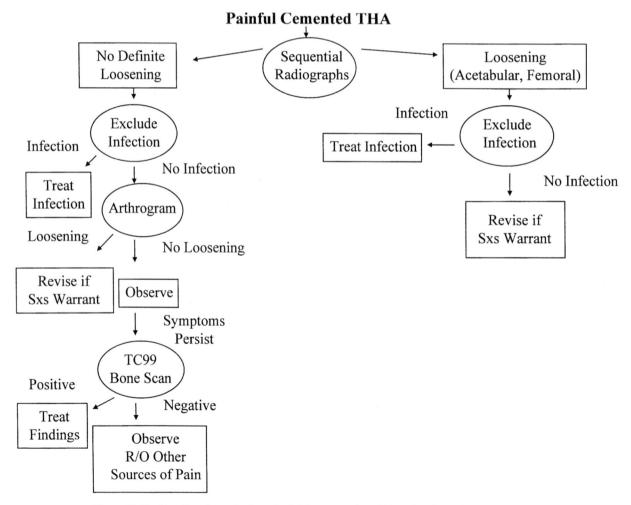

Figure 61–11. Algorithm for evaluation of painful cemented total hip arthroplasty. Sxs = symptoms.

Painful Uncemented THA

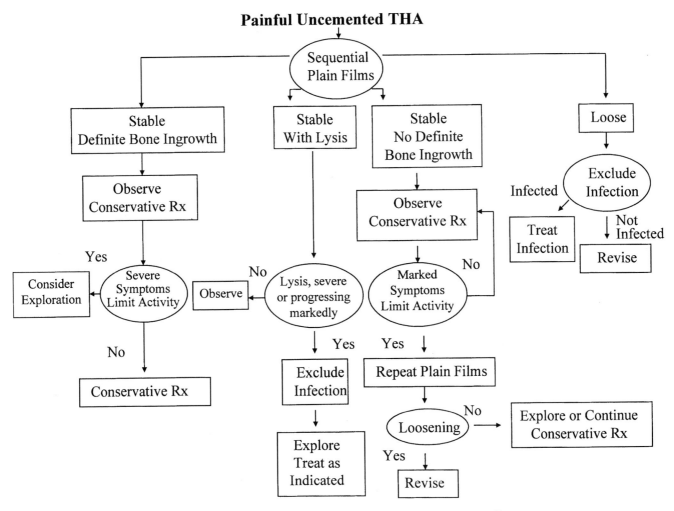

Figure 61–12. Algorithm for evaluation of painful uncemented total hip arthroplasty. Rx = treatment.

References

1. Barrack RL: Assessment of the symptomatic total hip. Orthopedics 17:793, 1994.
2. Barrack RL, Tanzer M, Kattapuram SV, Harris WH: The value of contrast arthrography in assessing loosening of symptomatic uncemented total hip components. Presented at the 58th Annual Meeting of the American Academy of Orthopaedic Surgeons, Washington, DC, February 20–22, 1992.
3. Barrack RL: Assessment of the symptomatic total hip. Orthopedics 17:793, 1994.
4. Berry DJ, Wallriches BL, Ilstrup DM: The natural history of femoral component debonding and its impact on long-term survivorship of Charnley total hip arthroplasty. Orthop Trans 19:302, 1995–1996.
5. Bohl WR, Steffee AD: Lumbar spinal stenosis: A cause of continued pain and disability in patients after total hip arthroplasty. Spine 4:168, 1979.
6. Boubaker A, Delaloye AB, Blanc CH, et al: Immunoscintigraphy with antigranulocyte monoclonal antibodies for the diagnosis of septic loosening of hip prostheses. Eur J Nucl Med 22:139, 1995.
7. Campbell ACL, Rorabeck CH, Bourne RB, et al: Thigh pain after cementless hip arthroplasty. J Bone Joint Surg 74B:63, 1992.
8. Capello WN, Vri BG, Wellman HN, et al: Comparison of radiographic and radionuclide hip arthrography in determination of

9. femoral component loosening of hip arthroplasty. *In* The Hip: Proceedings of the 13th Open Scientific Meeting of the Hip Society. St. Louis, CV Mosby, 1985, p 157.
9. D'Antonio JA, Capello WN, Manley MT: Remodeling of bone around hydroxyapatite-coated femoral stems. J Bone Joint Surg 78A:1226, 1996.
10. DeWolfe VG: Intermittent claudication of the hip and the syndrome of chronic aortoiliac thrombosis. Circulation 9:1, 1954.
11. Donaldson TK, Wasilewski RL, Rubash HE: A dynamic test for the diagnosis of loosened uncemented femoral components. Presented at the 58th Annual Meeting of the American Academy of Orthopaedic Surgeons, Washington, DC, 1992.
12. Engh CA, Bobyn JD, Glassman AH: Porous-coated hip replacement. J Bone Joint Surg 69B:45, 1987.
13. Engh CA, Massin PM, Suthers KE: Roentgenographic assessment of the biologic fixation of porous-surfaced femoral components. Clin Orthop 257:107, 1990.
14. Eschenroeder HC Jr, Krackow KA: Late onset femoral stress fracture associated with extruded cement following hip arthroplasty. A case report. Clin Orthop 236:210, 1988.
15. Fisher DA: Evaluation of the painful total hip arthroplasty. Semin Arthroplasty 3:229, 1992.
16. Floman Y, Bernini PM, Marvel JPJ, Rothman RH: Low-back pain and sciatica following total hip replacement: A report of two cases. Spine 5:292, 1980.

17. Gie GA, Flowler JL, Lee AJC, Ling RSM: The long-term behavior of a totally collarless, polished femoral component in cemented total hip arthroplasty. J Bone Joint Surg 72B:935, 1990.

18. Ginai AZ, van Biezen FC, Kint PA, et al: Digital subtraction arthrography in preoperative evaluation of painful total hip arthroplasty. Skeletal Radiol 25:357, 1996.

19. Goodman S, Rubenstein J, Schatzker J, et al: Apparent changes in the alignment of the femoral component in hip arthroplasties associated with limb positioning. Clin Orthop 221:242, 1987.

20. Haddad RJJ, Skalley TC, Cook SD, et al: Clinical and roentgeno-graphic evaluation of noncemented porous-coated anatomic medullary locking (AML) and porous-coated anatomic (PCA) total hip arthroplasty. Clin Orthop 258:176, 1990.

21. Hardy DC, Reinus WR, Totty WG, Keyser CK: Arthrography after total hip arthroplasty: Utility of postambulation radiographs. Skeletal Radiol 17:20, 1988.

22. Harris WH, Barrack RL: Contemporary algorithms for evaluation of the painful total hip replacement. Orthrop Rev 22:531, 1993.

23. Harris WH, Barrack RL: Developments in diagnosis of the painful total hip replacement. Orthop Rev 22:439, 1993.

24. Hedley AK, Gruen TA, Borden LS, et al: Two-year follow-up of the PCA noncemented total hip replacement. In The Hip: Proceedings of the 14th Open Scientific Meeting of the Hip Society. St. Louis, CV Mosby, 1987.

25. Heekin RD, Callaghan JJ, Hopkinson WJ, et al: The porous-coated anatomic total hip prosthesis, inserted without cement. J Bone Joint Surg 75A:77, 1993.

26. Hendrix RW, Wixson RL, Rana NA, Rogers LF: Arthrography after total hip arthroplasty: A modified technique used in the diagnosis of pain. Radiology 148:647, 1983.

27. Herzwurm PJ, Simpson SL, Duffin S, et al: Thigh pain and total hip arthroplasty: Scintigraphy with 2.5 year follow-up. Clin Orthop 336:156, 1997.

28. Hodgkinson JP, Shelley P, Wroblewski BM: The correlation between the roentgenographic appearance and operative findings at the bone-cement junction of the socket in Charnley low friction arthroplasties. Clin Orthop 228:105, 1988.

29. Jasty M, Maloney WJ, Bragdon CR, et al: Histomorphological studies of the long-term skeletal responses to well fixed cemented femoral components. J Bone Joint Surg 72A:1220, 1990.

30. Jensen JS, Madsen JL: Tc-99m-MDP scintigraphy noninformative in painful total hip arthroplasty. J Arthroplasty 5:11, 1990.

31. Johnston RC, Crowninshield RD: Roentgenologic results of total hip arthroplasty: A ten year follow-up study. Clin Orthop 181:92, 1983.

32. Karrholm J, Herberts P, Hultmark P, et al: Radiostereometry of hip prostheses. Review of methodology and clinical results. Clin Orthop 344:94, 1997.

33. Kim HS, Suh JS, Han CD, et al: Sequential Tc-99m MDP bone scans after cementless total hip arthroplasty in asymptomatic patients. Clin Nucl Med 22:6, 1997.

34. Levitsky KA, Hozack WJ, Balderston RA, et al: Evaluation of the painful prosthetic joint. Relative value of bone scan, sedimentation rate, and joint aspiration. J Arthroplasty 6:237, 1991.

35. Lieberman JR, Huo MH, Schneider R, et al: Evaluation of painful hip arthroplasties. J Bone Joint Surg 75B:475, 1993.

36. Lifeso RM, Abdel-Nabi M, Meinking C: Triphasic bone scanning following porous-coated hip arthroplasty. Clin Orthop 269:38, 1991.

37. Ling RSM: The use of a collar and precoating on cemented femoral stems is unnecessary and detrimental. Clin Orthop 285:73, 1992.

38. Lotke PA, Wong RY, Ecker ML: Stress fracture as a cause of chronic pain following revision total hip arthroplasty. Clin Orthop 206:147, 1986.

39. Lyons CW, Berquist TH, Lyons JC, et al: Evaluation of radiographic findings in painful hip arthroplasties. Clin Orthop 195:239, 1985.

40. Maloney WJ, Jasty M, Burke DW, et al: Biomechanical and histologic investigation of cemented total hip arthroplasties: A study of autopsy-retrieved femurs after in vivo cycling. Clin Orthop 249:129, 1989.

41. Maloney WJ, Jasty M, Harris WH, et al: Endosteal erosion in association with stable uncemented femoral components. J Bone Joint Surg 72A:1025, 1990.

42. Maloney WJ, Jasty M, Rosenberg A, Harris WH: Bone lysis in well-fixed cemented femoral components. J Bone Joint Surg 72B:966, 1990.

43. Marmor L: Stress fracture of the pubic ramus simulating a loose total hip replacement. Clin Orthop 121:103, 1976.

44. Massin P, Schmidt L, Engh CE: Evaluation of cementless acetabular component migration. J Arthroplasty 4:245, 1989.

45. Matos MH, Amstutz HC, Machleder HI: Ischemia of the lower extremity after total hip replacement. J Bone Joint Surg 61A:24, 1979.

46. Maus TP, Berquist TH, Bender CE, Rand JA: Arthrographic study of painful total hip arthroplasty: Refined criteria. Radiology 162:721, 1987.

47. McCaskie AW, Brown AR, Thompson JR, Gregg PJ: Radiological evaluation of the interfaces after cemented total hip replacement. Interobserver and intraobserver agreement. J Bone Joint Surg 78B:191, 1996.

48. McElfresh EC, Coventry MB: Femoral and pelvic fractures after total hip arthroplasty. J Bone Joint Surg 56A:483, 1974.

49. McInerney DP, Hyde ID: Technetium 99Tcm pyrophosphate scanning in the assessment of the painful hip prosthesis. Clin Radiol 29:513, 1978.

50. Miniaci A, Bailey WH, Bourne RB, et al: Analysis of radionuclide arthrograms, radiographic arthrograms, and sequential plain radiographs in the assessment of painful hip arthroplasty. J Arthroplasty 5:143, 1990.

51. Oh I, Hardacre JA: Fatigue fracture of the inferior pubic ramus following total hip replacement for congenital hip dislocation. Clin Orthop 147:154, 1980.

52. O'Neill DA, Harris WH: Failed total hip replacement: Assessment by plain radiographs, arthrograms, and aspiration of the hip joint. J Bone Joint Surg 66A:540, 1984.

53. Oswald SG, Van Nostrand D, Savory CG, et al: Three-phase bone scan and indium white blood cell scintigraphy following porous coated hip arthroplasty: A prospective study of the prosthetic hip. J Nucl Med 30:1321, 1989.

54. Oyen WJ, Lemmens JA, Claessens RA, van Horn JR, et al Nuclear arthrography: Combined scintigraphic and radiographic procedure for diagnosis of total hip prosthesis loosening. J Nuclear Med 37:62, 1996.

55. Pacheco V, Shelley P, Wroblewski BM: Mechanical loosening of the stem in Charnley arthroplasties. Identification of the "at risk" factors. J Bone Joint Surg 70B:596, 1988.

56. Pearlman AW: The painful hip prosthesis: Value of nuclear imaging in the diagnosis of late complications. Clin Nucl Med 5:133, 1980.

57. Pfahler M, Schidlo C, Refior HJ: Evaluation of imaging in loosening of hip arthroplasty in 326 consecutive cases. Arch Orthop Trauma Surg 117:205, 1998.

58. Resnik CS, Fratkin MJ, Cardea JA: Arthroscintigraphic evaluation of the painful total hip prosthesis. Clin Nucl Med 11:242, 1990.

59. Ritter MA, Gioe TJ, Stringer EA: Functional significance of nonunion of the greater trochanter. Clin Orthop 159:177, 1981.

60. Rushton N, Coakley AJ, Tudor J, Wraight EP: The value of technetium and gallium scanning in assessing pain after total hip replacement. J Bone Joint Surg 64B:313, 1982.

61. Salvati EA, Ghelman B, McLaren T, Wilson PDJ: Subtraction technique in arthrography for loosening of total hip replacement fixed with radiopaque cement. Clin Orthop 101:105, 1974.

62. Schneider U, Breusch SJ, Termath S, et al: Increased urinary crosslink levels in aseptic loosening of total hip arthroplasty. J Arthroplasty 13:687, 1998.

63. Shaw JA, Bruno A, Paul EM: The influence of age, sex, and initial fit on bony ingrowth stabilization with the AML femoral component in primary total hip arthroplasty. Orthopedics 15:687, 1992.

64. Swan JS, Braunstein EM, Wellman HN, Capello W: Contrast and nuclear arthrography in loosening of the uncemented hip prosthesis. Skeletal Radiol 20:15, 1991.

65. Tehranzadeh J, Schneider R, Freiberger RH: Radiological evaluation of painful total hip replacement. Radiology 141:355, 1981.

66. Trousdale RT, Cabanela ME, Berry DJ: Anterior iliopsoas impingement after total hip arthroplasty. J Arthroplasty 10:546, 1995.

67. Utz JA, Lull RJ, Galvin EG: Asymptomatic total hip prosthesis: Natural history determined using Tc-99m MDP bone scans. Radiology 161:509, 1986.

68. Volz RG, Brown FW: The painful migrated ununited greater trochanter in total hip replacement. J Bone Joint Surg 59A:1091, 1977.

69. Vresilovic EJ, Hozack WJ, Rothman RH: Incidence of thigh pain after uncemented femoral prosthesis as a function of stem size. Presented at the Annual Meeting of the American Academy of Orthopaedic Surgeons, Washington, DC, February 22, 1992.

70. Weiss PE, Mall JC, Hoffer PB, et al: 99m Tc-methylene diphosphonate bone imaging in the evaluation of total hip prostheses. Radiology 133:727, 1979.

62

Acetabular Revision: Techniques and Results

• DAVID G. LEWALLEN and DANIEL J. BERRY

Revision of the acetabulum will be required in 5 to 10 percent of patients within the first 20 years after cemented total hip arthroplasty[40] (also see Chapter 46). When cemented total hip arthroplasty is performed in younger patients, the acetabular revision rate is considerably higher.[10,23,25,27] Uncemented components still fail in some cases as a result of prosthesis loosening, component malposition, infection, or polyethylene wear and osteolysis.[3] Similar techniques may be utilized for either cemented or uncemented acetabular reconstruction. However, recently the need to revise the failed polyethylene liner of well-fixed uncemented acetabular components has given rise to a new form of acetabular revision: polyethylene liner exchange, shell retention, and bone grafting.

Early experience with revision using cement has been disappointing. Kavanagh et al.[42] found a 25 percent rate of "probable" acetabular component failure at 4.5 years after cemented acetabular revision in a Mayo Clinic study, and series by multiple other authors have reported similar results.[11,61,62] The inadequacy of cemented acetabular fixation in the revision setting led to widespread use of uncemented porous-coated acetabular components when they became routinely available in the mid-1980s. Ten-year results for these uncemented components are now available and show a considerable improvement over cemented sockets in the revision setting.[46] The predictable results of uncemented porous-coated sockets, in combination with their versatility and ease of insertion, have led to their routine use in most revision situations. Just as the value of uncemented sockets in most acetabular revisions is being established, their limitations in hips with extreme pelvic bone loss are also becoming apparent. Alternative methods of managing severe acetabular bone deficiencies are developing. Longer term results of structural and particulate bone grafting of acetabular defects are now available, and the role of bone allografts for acetabular reconstruction is evolving. Use of anti-protrusio cages and reinforcement rings for protection of grafts and spanning of major defects has become accepted in

certain complex cases, and oblong or bilobed implants and modular acetabular systems have been introduced in order to attempt to allow for maximal host bone support of the reconstruction during management of major bone deficiency problems, helping to maximize the likelihood of a satisfactory and durable result.

A successful revision is predicated on several key steps: removal of the failed component without causing excessive damage to the remaining native bone stock; assessment of the acetabular bone loss; treatment of the osseous deficiency; selection of an implant that can provide maximal support on host bone; and, finally, implantation of a mechanically stable prosthesis in appropriate orientation. Achieving these goals is facilitated by a systematic means of classifying acetabular bone deficiencies, a familiarity with the techniques available for acetabular reconstruction, ability to judge the quality and location of bone remaining in the acetabulum, and knowledge of the results of available methods for acetabular reconstruction. After assessing these factors, the final step is proper application of the appropriate technique to the specific acetabular reconstruction problem.

CLASSIFICATION OF ACETABULAR BONE DEFICIENCIES

A classification system for acetabular bone deficiencies is necessary, both because it provides a common language to discuss the problem of acetabular reconstruction and because it gives the surgeon a framework within which to organize the available methods of treating acetabular bone deficiency problems. The system most commonly utilized in the United States is the American Academy of Orthopaedic Surgeons classification (Fig. 62–1).[14] This system subdivides deficiencies into type I (segmental), type II (cavitary), type III (combined segmental and cavitary), type IV (pelvic discontinuity), and type V (previous arthrodesis). These deficiencies may be subdivided by their superior, posterior, anterior, or medial location.

824

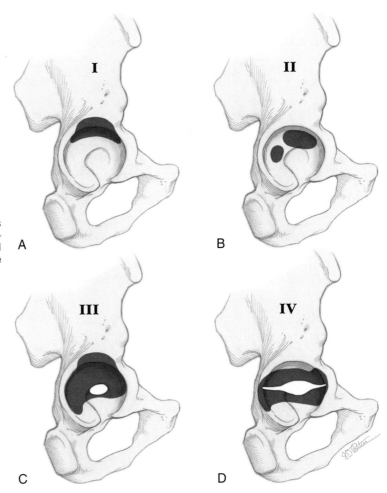

Figure 62–1. American Academy of Orthopaedic Surgeons classification of acetabular bone deficiencies. **A**, Type I segmental deficiency. **B**, Type II cavitary deficiency. **C**, Type III combined segmental and cavitary deficiency. **D**, Type IV bone deficiency (pelvic discontinuity).

TREATMENT OPTIONS: EFFECTIVENESS OF SPECIFIC TECHNIQUES

Bone Cement for Prosthesis Fixation and Treatment of Acetabular Deficiency

Cement provides immediate fixation, fills residual defects, and is simple technically. Unfortunately, a number of series have shown relatively high failure rates with this technique at mid- to long-term follow-up.[1,11,38,41,42,61,62] The probable reason for a high reported rate of failure is the poor ability of cement to gain satisfactory fixation in the sclerotic attenuated bone remaining after removal of a failed acetabular component. Jasty and Harris have reported that, for larger bone defects, particularly those with a large medial deficiency, the results of this technique are especially poor. In 28 hips followed for a mean of 6.3 years after revision, a 14 percent aseptic failure rate of type II (cavitary) deficiencies and a 75 percent aseptic failure rate for patients with large medial segmental deficiencies was recorded.[38]

Cement Fixation and Structural Bone Graft for Acetabular Deficiencies

This technique provides immediate cup fixation with cement and uses bone grafting to make up for bone deficiencies and to provide restoration of a normal center of hip rotation. Several authors have reported high graft union rates in this setting.[21,22,25,26,30,37,39,54,80] With longer term follow-up, however, bulk allograft collapse may be seen to occur, particularly when the graft is relied on to provide structural support for a large portion of the socket.[28,53,87]

Using this technique, Jasty and Harris found a 33 percent acetabular failure rate in 38 hips followed for a mean of 5.9 years. When the bulk graft covered less than one third of the socket, the failure rate was zero, but when it covered more than two thirds of the socket, the failure rate was 58 percent.[39] In a longer term follow-up report of the same patients, Kwong et al. found that acetabular component failure caused by loosening occurred in 11 of 22 hips a mean of 10 years after revision.[44]

The Mayo Clinic experience with acetabular bone graft augmentation in both primary and revision arthroplasty was recorded in 54 hips evaluated at an average follow-up of 10.2 years.[45] After 5 years, the mechanical failure rate (radiographic loosening plus revision for loosening) was 16 percent, and at 10 years it had increased to 30 percent. The survivorship free of acetabular revision at 5 years was 85 percent, at 10 years 70 percent, and at 12 years 54 percent. However, it was noted that, even among those implants that failed, in many instances the presence of a well-healed graft facilitated the subsequent revisions by increasing the amount of bone stock available for support of the new implant.

Cement Fixation and Impacted Morselized Bone Grafting for the Acetabulum

Sloof and co-workers have reported successful results of densely packed cancellous bone used to completely fill the deficient acetabular cavity combined with a socket cemented into the cancellous graft within the reconstructed acetabulum.[74,77] Despite variable amounts of socket migration as studied by stereoradiographic methods, the majority of the patients so treated predictably experienced significant symptomatic relief.[56] Recent bone biopsy results presented in a series of patients reoperated after a prior impaction graft in the acetabulum have documented gradual restoration of viable living bone by resorption and replacement of the necrotic graft, even in those patients with unstable, loose cemented sockets requiring repeat revision.[5,7] Although this method has been used in a wide range of acetabular revision problems, it may deserve consideration in selected circumstances where results using other methods described here have proven suboptimal. The originators of this technique have combined wire mesh with the graft so as to allow containment of the graft and dense impaction of the graft bed prior to cementation of the socket, which may allow extension of the technique to some of the more challenging segmental deficiencies encountered.[74] Experience with this technique in North America has been limited to this point.

Bipolar Prosthesis and Bone Graft

This technique is simple and tends to resist dislocation, and was originally considered to be the first stage of a two-stage procedure.[58] Despite favorable short-term results,[76] longer term results have shown an unacceptably high rate of failure, primarily as a result of graft resorption, prosthetic migration, and pain.[6,57,84] Brien et al. reported a 61 percent failure rate in 18 hips followed for 2.9 years after this method of reconstruction.[6] Papagelopoulos et al. reported the Mayo Clinic experience of 81 hips treated with bipolar prosthesis and bone graft during revision total hip arthroplasty. Survivorship free of acetabular re-revision was only 47 percent at 6.5 years, and a large number of patients had pain (37 percent) or significant bipolar migration (85 percent) (Fig. 62–2).[58]

Anti-Protrusio Devices

These devices provide immediate secure fixation of the prosthesis to the pelvis and bridge bone defects, providing a foundation for prosthetic support on native bone.[8,24,33,47,51,52,55,59,65,66,70,71,73,86,88] They facilitate grafting of bone deficiencies while providing an environment in which the graft is protected from excessive mechanical forces that may lead to graft failure.[5] In recent years, improved implants and techniques have led to more favorable results (Fig. 62–3). Fuchs et al. reported on 68 hips revised at the Hospital for Special Surgery with acetabular reinforcement rings or metallic shells.[20] Two to 5 years after revision, no components had been re-revised and only 3 percent were considered to have radiographic evidence of loosening. Rosson and Schatzker found only a 7.5 percent incidence of acetabular re-revision in 66 hips revised with either a Müller reinforcement ring or a Burch-Schneider cage.[67] The best long-term results reported for the anti-protrusio cage in revision surgery have been reported by Wachtl et al., who used this implant in 38 revisions followed up at a mean of 12 years postsurgery but up to 21 years postrevision. These authors noted one case of cage loosening and overall survivorship of 92%.[82]

Results can be expected to be less durable when the technique is limited to cases of extreme bone deficiency. Using the Burch-Schneider cage selectively for revision of 42 hips with severe acetabular bone deficiencies (combined type III deficiencies), Berry and Müller reported a failure rate at a mean of 5 years of 12 percent as a result of aseptic loosening.[2] Schatzker and Wong have reported on 57 patients treated with an acetabular roof ring and compared these to 38 subsequent cases treated with the larger anti-protrusio cage and showed a failure rate of 12.5 percent for the roof rings at a mean of 8.3 years postoperatively and a failure rate of 5.4 percent for the cages at a slightly shorter mean follow-up of 6.6 years postsurgery. These authors concluded that the anti-protrusio cage was a reasonable choice for major combined segmental cavitary defects requiring extensive grafting and suggested that roof rings be reserved for more limited isolated cavitary or segmental defects where very good bone support remains.[72]

A key technical point that has emerged recently is that successful use of anti-protrusio devices is enhanced by placement of the implant so that it is well supported by native bone, especially in the area superiorly in the region of the weight-bearing dome. When large structural grafts are needed, anti-protrusio rings may protect the graft from collapse caused by revascularization and mechanical overload. Efforts to avoid any gaps in this area between implant and host bone are critical to long-term implant stability.[2,9,67,88] Bone graft healing and incorporation behind these devices is predictable.[2,63,67,81,88] These devices provide a foundation for the socket and thereby allow more frequent use of particulate graft, which has been shown to incorporate more quickly and completely than structural bone grafts.[34]

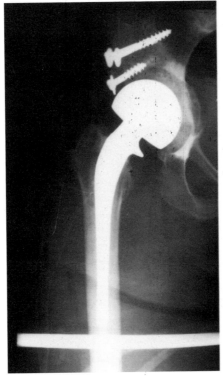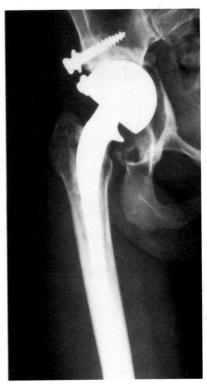

Figure 62–2. Immediate postoperative (**A**) and 4-year follow-up (**B**) radiographs of a patient treated with bipolar component and bone graft for acetabular reconstruction. Note the resorption of bone graft and marked migration of the bipolar component. The patient required another revision surgery.

A   B

It is important to realize that cages are not porous-coated implants and do not have the potential for biologic fixation. For this reason, their use would seem best restricted to the selected few cases in which there is inadequate host bone to provide initial mechanical stability or a reasonable likelihood of long-term biologic fixation with an uncemented cup.

Uncemented Porous-Coated Hemispherical Acetabular Component

Uncemented porous-coated sockets are presently the implant of choice for the great majority of acetabular

component revisions (Fig. 62–4). These components are straightforward to use and are versatile.[23,31,32,35] Several large series reporting the results of these components over the first decade postimplantation are now available, and it is clear that they work very well for the vast majority of acetabular revision circumstances.[46,50] Of 140 hips revised with the Harris-Galante prosthesis, the aseptic loosening rate was only 1 percent 2 to 6 years (mean 3.4 years) after revision.[79] Padgett et al. reported on 129 hips followed for 3 to 7.5 years after revision with the same prosthesis and found no failures caused by aseptic loosening.[57] Paprosky and colleagues reported on 147 uncemented hemispherical sockets followed for

Figure 62–3. **A**, Anteroposterior radiograph of patient with polyethylene wear and severe acetabular osteolysis. **B**, Two-year postoperative radiograph following reconstruction of acetabulum with Ganz anti-protrusio ring and particulate allograft. Note good incorporation of the allograft bone and stable acetabular component.

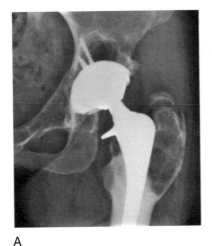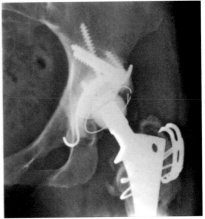

A   B

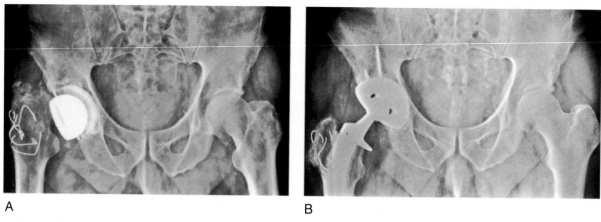

A   B

Figure 62–4. A, Preoperative radiograph showing failed acetabular component with cavitary (type II) bone deficiency. **B,** Postoperative radiograph showing successful reconstruction with particulate bone graft and uncemented porous-coated hemispherical acetabular component fixed with screws.

3 to 9 years (mean 5.7 years) and found that only 6 sockets (4 percent) required revision for aseptic loosening or had radiographic evidence of aseptic loosening.[59]

Uncemented hemispherical sockets also appear to work well in combination with limited acetabular bone grafting. In the series of Tanzer et al., 127 of the sockets required bone grafts (particulate graft only in 115, bulk and particulate in 12).[79] None of the grafts provided major structural support. All grafts showed radiographic evidence of osseous union. In Padgett et al.'s series, 107 of the 129 hips required bone grafting.[57] Only two non-contained structural grafts were used; the remainder were grafts placed in cavitary defects or medial segmental defects. No graft failures were identified.

In a recent update of the Rush-Presbyterian experience, Leopold et al. reported 138 consecutive cementless revisions followed for a mean of 10.5 years and demonstrated 84 percent survivorship at 11.5 years using the Kaplan-Meier method. Only two components (1.8 percent) were radiographically loose, but 17 percent of cases demonstrated osteolysis around the cup, and this problem was noted to be more common with increasing follow-up.[46] Even those patients with very significant initial bone deficiency from underlying dysplasia, if revised because of loosening of the original socket, experience a high rate of success when good contact on host bone is achieved at the time of revision using an uncemented acetabular component, even when this requires some elevation of the hip center.[15]

There are, however, infrequent but select circumstances in which uncemented porous-coated sockets have a high failure rate. Such can occur when (1) acetabular bone quality is so poor that an uncemented socket cannot be rigidly fixed at the time of revision, (2) acetabular bone loss is so massive that satisfactory contact between the porous-coated socket and native bone cannot be achieved, or (3) high-dose radiation has been administered previously. When stable fixation cannot be achieved in revision surgery, early failure of an uncemented socket is likely. Several authors have shown that uncemented sockets will fail when they are placed against a bed largely consisting of allograft bone. In

Paprosky et al.'s series, the overall failure rate was only 4 percent, but the rate was 100 percent (six of six hips) in patients with severe combined (type III) bone deficiencies in which the socket rested primarily on bone graft.[59] McAllister and Borden reported that 97 percent of 187 porous sockets used in revisions with a good acetabular rim remaining were stable, but only 48 percent of 31 hips in which less satisfactory native bone contact was achieved were stable at follow-up.[48] Pollock and Whiteside reviewed 23 uncemented sockets placed against large allografts and followed them for more than 2 years. They found a 30 percent rate of socket re-revision, and only 35 percent of sockets were well fixed without radiographic signs of loosening at last follow-up.[64]

MAYO EXPERIENCE

The Mayo Clinic experience includes 60 hips followed for at least 5 years with first-generation uncemented hemispherical socket designs.[60] A 12 percent rate of acetabular failure was found in those hips with less than 25 percent graft socket coverage, and a remarkable 78 percent radiographic or clinical failure rate was found in 27 hips with greater than 50 percent coverage (Fig. 62–5).[60]

In a review of all uncemented acetabular components inserted at the Mayo Clinic over a 15-year period from 1984 to 1998, a steady and increasing rate of acetabular failure and re-revision beyond the first decade post-surgery was documented, clearly showing that further improvements in initial fixation and subsequent durability are needed (Fig. 62–6). Largely fibrous fixed sockets, even if initially clinically successful, can be expected to be much less resistant to the effects of any particulate debris generated than those implants that are fixed by solid bone ingrowth. Whether improvements in materials available for bone ingrowth and the advantages of improved bearing surfaces and reduced wear will result in significant improvements in the long-term results of these revision procedures remains to be shown.

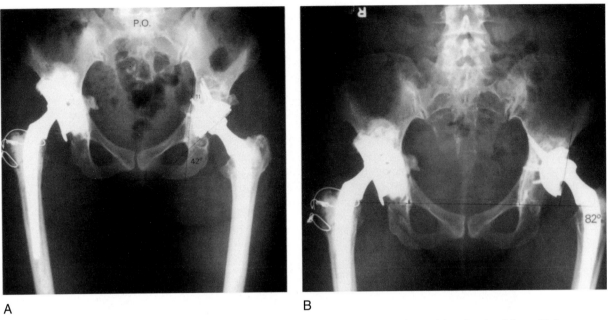

A   B

Figure 62–5. Radiographs taken immediately postoperatively (**A**) and at 6.5 years after revision showing failure of left uncemented socket placed on large amount of allograft bone (**B**).

Conclusion. When native bone contact with porous coating falls below a certain threshold, there is an increased risk of failure. The minimum acceptable amount of contact with native bone is not yet clear, but is probably at least 50 percent. It is probable that native bone strength, location of contact between the bone and the socket, and the biologic activity of remaining acetabular bone also affect the amount of contact compatible with a durable result. Ultimately, judgment is required when deciding the amount of contact required for a successful procedure.

SPECIAL TECHNIQUES USING UNCEMENTED POROUS-COATED HEMISPHERICAL SOCKETS

Two techniques have been developed to increase the reliability of this strategy: the use of extra-large sockets and the use of small sockets placed in a "high" position. Extra-large sockets (Fig. 62–7) are useful because they allow maintenance of a relatively normal hip center of rotation and yet maximize contact between the cup and native bone.[19] During preparation small, segmental, and cavitary defects are often obliterated or made small enough to be dealt with easily using limited particulate

Figure 62–6. Overall survivorship curves for all 7814 cemented acetabular components performed at Mayo Clinic over a 15-year period from 1984 through 1998. For both primary and revision cases, a disturbing progressive and nonlinear increase in uncemented acetabular component failure is seen, especially as these populations enter the second decade postsurgery.

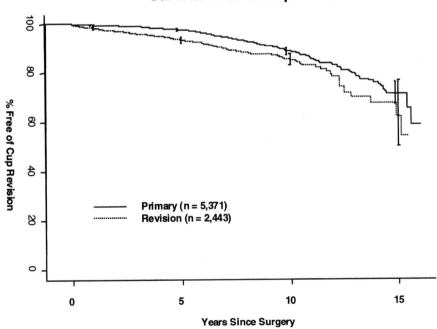

Survival Free of Cup Revision

% Free of Cup Revision

Primary (n = 5,371)
Revision (n = 2,443)

Years Since Surgery

bone grafts. Extra-large sockets often optimize the contact of the component with the remaining rim of acetabular bone, thereby providing a better press fit of the component and enhanced initial cup stability. Dearborn and Harris reported a single surgeon's series of 24 cases in which an oversized or so-called jumbo hemispherical ingrowth cup of 66 mm or larger was used and no radiographic loosening or revision for loosening was observed.[16]

During acetabular revision, the anterior-to-posterior dimension of the acetabulum between the anterior and posterior columns limits the maximum size of the reamer and uncemented cup that can be used. Excessive ream-

ing can severely compromise remaining support of the socket. Large, oblong-shaped defects cannot always be filled with a hemispherical cup because of anterior-to-posterior size constraints, unless one column, usually the anterior, is sacrificed.

Restoring the hip center to its normal location has many advantages,[85] but in revision surgery, where compromises and trade-offs must of necessity be made, some elevation of the hip center can be accepted if the benefit is much improved socket contact with native bone not achievable by reaming to a larger size at the level of the original hip center (Fig. 62–8).[29,36] Most authors agree that placement of the socket in a high, but

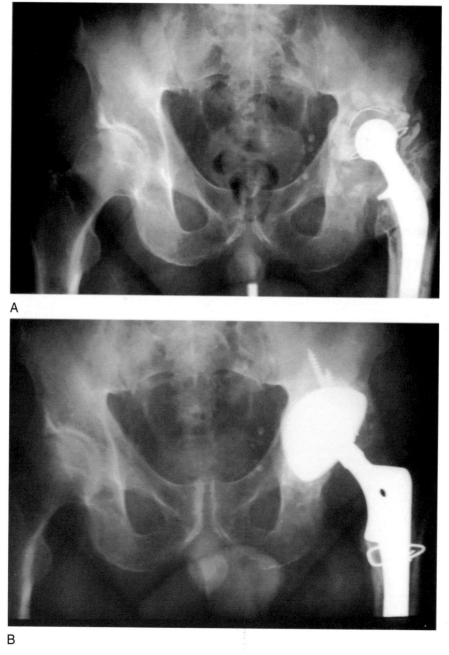

A

B

Figure 62–7. **A,** Radiograph of failed acetabular component with combined (type III combined segmental and cavitary) bone deficiency. **B,** Reconstruction with extra-large uncemented porous-coated hemispherical acetabular component.

not markedly lateralized, position does not have significant adverse biomechanical effects on the socket itself,[44,68,75] although there is some concern that a very high socket position can have negative effects on the performance of the femoral component.[43,85] Because the ilium narrows above the normal acetabulum, smaller sockets are often needed when a high hip center is used. Schutzer and Harris have reported the results of using uncemented sockets placed in a high hip center position in 49 hip revisions. At a mean of 40 months after surgery, no socket was revised for loosening and no socket showed definite radiographic loosening.[75] Dearborn and Harris updated and extended this report on the senior author's experience with a consecutive series of 61 hips with dysplasia requiring revision of a failed previously placed socket. At a mean follow-up of 8 years, a 3 percent mechanical loosening rate was observed in this series where 64 percent of the patients required a high hip center to achieve good contact on host bone.[15]

Mayo Experience. In a review of the Mayo experience with jumbo cups, Whaley and Berry reviewed 89 porous titanium wire mesh acetabular components used for revision where cups of over 62 mm were used in the women and cups 66 mm or larger were used in the men in order to fill the large acetabular defects encountered during those revisions.[83] At an average follow-up of about 7 years, only 2 of 89 had required repeat revision for aseptic loosening, and only two other cups had definite radiographic evidence of loosening.

In spite of these advantages, the technique also has some negative practical consequences. Significant leg length discrepancy may result, and greater trochanteric advancement may be necessary to provide satisfactory soft tissue tension and abductor function. Instability resulting from femoral impingement against the pelvis can be a problem. Finally, for very large superior bone

defects, the markedly reduced width of the ilium may be unsatisfactory to support even the smallest sockets.

CONCLUSION

Most acetabular deficiencies can be managed successfully with uncemented porous-coated hemispherical sockets. Use of extra-large cups and willingness to accept some elevation of the hip center when necessary can expand the circumstances in which good native bone support for the cup is achieved, and this is the essential element for long-term success with these components. In rare circumstances in which severe bone loss requires such extensive bone grafting that little native bone contact with the uncemented cup would be present, alternative forms of reconstruction should be considered (see below).

Oblong Acetabular Components

Bilobed or oblong acetabular components have become available for use in revision with a range of sizes and some options with regard to cup version and inclination of the face of the acetabular opening. These devices have been specifically developed to address cases with large oval or oblong acetabular bone defects, where alternatives would be superolateral structural graft, elevation of the hip center, or excessive over-reaming of the acetabulum beyond that allowed by patient dimensions (Fig. 62–9). DeBoer and Christie have reported on 18 cases, of which 15 were revisions, at a mean of 6.5 years' follow-up, with only one implant unstable and having required revision at last follow-up—a case of massive bone loss and grafting.[17] Berry et al. have reported results in 38 cases followed for a mean of 3 years, with

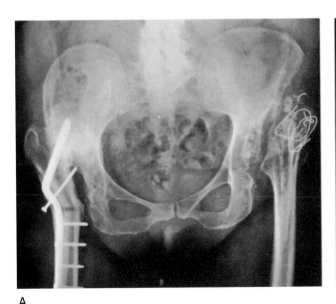

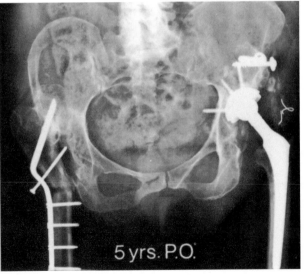

A   B

Figure 62–8. A, Radiograph of failed acetabular component with large superior (type I) segmental bone deficiency. **B**, Radiograph 5 years after operation showing reconstruction with hemispherical socket placed mostly on native bone at a high hip center.

one cup requiring revision in a case where a structural graft was used as the main support for the majority of the implant.[4]

In a review of the use of bilobed cups in 37 hips by Chen et al., the long-term performance of these implants in cases of severe bone loss was called into question. These cases represented a selected subgroup out of a total of 414 acetabular revision cases performed by the authors during the same time frame. At a mean of 41 months, probable or definite loosening was present in 24 percent, with most of the failures in those cases with disruption of the medial wall or upward migration of the previous failed implant of 2 cm or more. These authors concluded that routine use of these devices could not be recommended in the face of more severe bone defects.[12] Our experience with bilobed cups suggests that these implants fit only a limited number of patients well. In other patients, the seating of the implant will require excessive bone removal or the implant gains poor primary stability in the complex-shaped acetabular defect. Presently we limit the use of these implants to the few patients with a superolateral

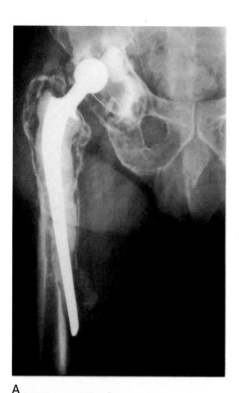

A

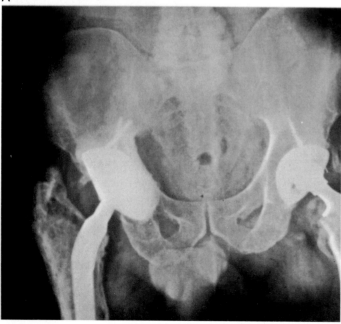

B

Figure 62–9. **A**, Radiograph of patient with a combined (type III) acetabular bone deficiency with a large superior segmental deficiency. **B**, Two years after successful reconstruction with oblong off-the-shelf porous-coated uncemented acetabular component.

acetabular deficiency, in whom the prosthesis appears to provide an excellent fit without excessive bone reaming.

Custom Acetabular Components

Interest has developed over the past decade in the use of custom acetabular components fabricated from computed tomography—generated models of the acetabular bone defect present. Use of these implants has been focused on cases where massive bone defects exist that would not be easily addressed by traditional off-the-shelf implants and methods. This technique is limited by difficulties in achieving accurate modeling of the bone defect when significant metal artifact is present, difficulties in predicting the quality of the bone that remains for support of the new implant, the delay needed for fabrication, and the very significant expense of these implants. However, a report by Christie et al. on a triflanged custom acetabular component offers encouraging results, with adjunctive support achieved by the addition of three flanges from the periphery of the implant similar, to those used in cage devices, for support on intact host bone on the ilium and ischium around the periphery of the acetabular defect.[13] In 67 hips available for follow-up at an average of 53 months, no uncemented custom triflange cup had required removal despite major bone defects in all cases and pelvic discontinuity in half the cases at the time of the original revision. This concept of an uncemented cage and cup combination may have a role in the management of massive bone loss cases not reconstructible with stable support on host bone using traditional methods.

AUTHORS PREFERRED TECHNIQUE

Acetabular revision involves a stepwise progression, designed to maximize the chances of success, with key components as follows: (1) careful preoperative planning; (2) adequate surgical exposure; (3) acetabular component removal; and (4) acetabular reconstruction specific to the bone defect present and the location and quality of acetabular bone remaining. Each of these important areas is discussed in turn.

Preoperative Planning

Good-quality anteroposterior and lateral pelvic films are essential. An effort should be made to delineate the severity and location of any bone deficiency present and to identify the specific technical challenges likely to be encountered during surgery. It is helpful to consider anticipated problems of (1) exposure, (2) failed prosthesis removal, (3) bone deficiency reconstruction, (4) implant placement, and (5) hip stability. If pelvic discontinuity is suspected, Judet views of the pelvis may be useful. In cases of gross intrapelvic protrusion of the acetabular component, further study of the course of intrapelvic arteriovenous structures or the ureter may

be helpful.[18,69] Preoperative templating should be carried out to help plan the optimal acetabular reconstruction. Arrangements are made for unusual prosthetic needs and procurement of anticipated bone grafts. If it is anticipated that either the acetabular shell or femoral component may be kept and revision limited to the other single component of the previous arthroplasty, actual records from the prior procedure can be invaluable in assuring that proper replacement components, such as modular heads and polyethylene inserts, are available. Self-sticking manufacturers' labels on the components from the original procedure are more likely to be accurate than dictated surgical notes, which can contain errors.

Exposure

The exposure for acetabular component revision is determined partly by the surgeon's preference and partly by the demands imposed by the specific circumstances encountered. For most routine acetabular revisions in which the femoral component is also being revised, a posterolateral, anterolateral, or direct lateral approach can be utilized successfully. For more complex revisions, trochanteric osteotomy or an extensile approach to the hip may be necessary[78] (see Chapter 44). When it is anticipated that the femoral component will be retained, a more extensile approach may be useful to facilitate acetabular exposure.[50] When problems with soft tissue tension or hip stability after acetabular revision are anticipated, a transtrochanteric approach may be preferable to allow trochanteric advancement and tightening of the abductor mechanism.

Acetabular Component Removal

Removal of the loose acetabular component, either cemented or uncemented, is usually not terribly difficult once good acetabular exposure has been established. Curved osteotomes are helpful for component removal. If necessary, all-polyethylene components may be quartered using a high-speed burr or osteotome to facilitate their removal. Especially when the remaining bone is poor, gentle handling of the instruments is important to reduce bone loss during prosthesis removal.

When a well-fixed acetabular component must be removed (for reasons such as infection, malposition, or osteolysis), component removal may be considerably more difficult. Removal can usually be effected by gently passing a curved osteotome around the entire periphery of the well-fixed component before attempting removal. The area of maximum danger is medial, and hand-held osteotome instruments must be kept as close to the socket as possible to avoid injuring intrapelvic structures or causing severe medial bone loss. Well-fixed all-polyethylene components can be reamed away until a thin layer remains, which usually separates from the underlying cement mantle quite easily. For well-fixed uncemented components, a recently introduced curved osteotome system attached to a central femoral head that rests inside the original polyethylene insert or a trial insert greatly facilitates removal of these implants. A curved blade available in two lengths and in a range of sizes corresponding to the cup diameter is passed down the developing interface between the well-fixed cup and the bone around the periphery of the acetabular component. This system facilitates removal of extremely well-fixed implants with minimal host bone damage (Fig. 62–10).

It is important preoperatively to recognize circumstances in which the component or cement has protruded medially in an intrapelvic position and may impinge on or be adherent to intrapelvic structures. When this situation is encountered, imaging of vascular anatomy with angiography and preoperative consultation with a vascular surgeon may be advisable, particularly if assistance with an intrapelvic approach for component removal is needed. Controlled exposure and retraction

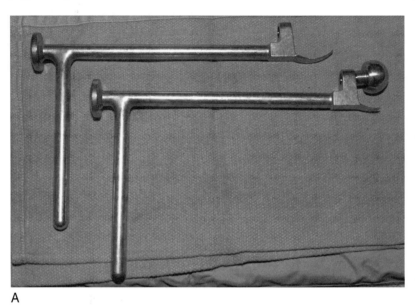

A

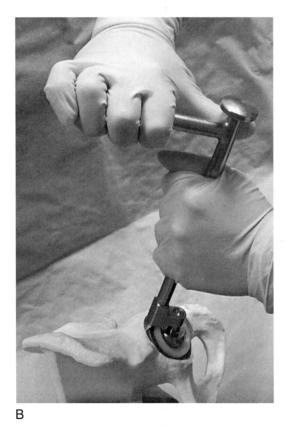

B

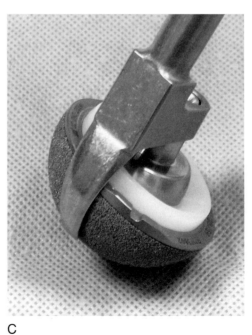

C

Figure 62–10. **A**, System of curved blades for division of implant-bone interface and removal of a well-fixed uncemented bone ingrown acetabular component. **B** and **C**, Availability of different sizes in 2-mm increments and a centering head in 22-, 28-, and 32-mm sizes allows division of the interface with controlled positioning of the blade and minimal bone loss.

of intrapelvic vessels is preferred to emergent efforts at control of sudden potentially life-threatening and massive bleeding from a retroacetabular intrapelvic source.

After the failed acetabular component and any remaining cement have been removed, all of the fibrous membrane that had been surrounding the component is meticulously removed from the acetabulum. The acetabular bone deficiency is classified and reconstruction undertaken.

Acetabular Reconstruction

The majority of acetabular component revisions can be managed successfully with an uncemented hemispherical porous-coated acetabular component and cancellous bone grafting or residual defects. After exposure of the socket, it is reamed until a good hemisphere of native bleeding bone is present. Usually, further medialization is not necessary and will compromise already deficient medial bone stock. Care is taken to avoid reaming the socket to an excessive size that could compromise the remaining acetabular rim or anterior and posterior columns. Remaining defects are grafted, usually using particulate allograft. The graft can be packed into the defects by hand and shaped to fit the hemisphere precisely by using the hemispherical reamers in "reverse." Before choosing the socket size, trial components are used to ensure that the chosen socket will be neither too large nor too small for the prepared socket. A hemispherical uncemented porous-coated socket, usually 2 to 3 mm larger than the reamer size, is then press-fit into the bone. In most circumstances for revision cases, socket fixation into the pelvis is augmented with multiple screws placed through the socket into the pelvic bone. If the host bone is soft and screw purchase is inadequate, the screws may be cemented in place. This is done by injecting the soft cement into the drill holes with a 10-ml syringe and a 14-gauge soft needle and advancing the screw into final position before the cement hardens. The screw is tightened in a serial fashion as the cement hardens.

Type I: Segmental Deficiencies

Most small to moderate segmental bone deficiencies can be treated with hemispherical uncemented porous-coated sockets. Frequently preparation of the socket by reaming will obliterate small segmental deficiencies. Medial segmental deficiencies may be grafted with morselized cancellous bone, and small peripheral segmental deficiencies frequently can be ignored. Moderate-sized peripheral segmental defects may be treated with bone grafting, not for cup support, but to restore bone stock for the future. Small to moderate superior deficiencies can sometimes be managed successfully by accepting a slightly elevated hip center for the socket, thereby allowing placement of an uncemented socket with good mechanical support on a bed of viable host bone. Large defects in a critical superolateral location may require a bulk structural graft for mechanical support of the cup. Use of an uncemented socket alone resting on such a graft markedly increases the risks of cup migration. An alternative method, such as use

of an anti-protrusio cage, should be considered in such circumstances.

Type II: Cavitary Deficiencies

Most cavitary deficiencies can be treated satisfactorily with hemispherical uncemented sockets. After preparation of the socket, small cavitary deficiencies can be filled with particulate cancellous bone graft. For large cavitary deficiencies, extra-large sockets and larger quantities of particulate bone graft may be needed. Massive irregular or oblong cavitary defects may require an alternative method as discussed below.

Type III: Combined Segmental and Cavitary Deficiencies

Most combined defects can also be treated successfully with extra-large uncemented porous-coated hemispherical sockets. The principles and techniques described above for treating segmental and cavitary deficiencies should be followed. An effort should be made to place the socket against the maximum surface of native bone possible. Cancellous grafts may be used to fill small remaining bone deficiencies. Extra-large sockets will almost always be necessary to optimize contact of the socket with native bone in these circumstances. Slight elevation of the hip center may be accepted when it facilitates placement of the socket on better native bone. Offset acetabular inserts available for use with many implant systems can greatly facilitate correction of a medialized or elevated hip center, and thereby improve mechanics of the hip and reduce the risk of hip instability.

Special Cases

Three specific bone deficiencies are difficult to manage successfully with hemispherical sockets alone: (1) large oblong-shaped deficiencies, (2) large medial deficiencies in which the native bone provides no medial support for a hemispherical socket, and (3) huge global acetabular deficiencies. The authors' preferred treatment options for each of these specific circumstances are described below.

LARGE SUPERIOR SEGMENTAL BONE DEFICIENCIES

Large oblong acetabular deficiencies are not uncommon and result from superior migration of the socket with resultant segmental and cavitary loss of the superior acetabular bone. When the defect is quite large, a large hemispherical uncemented socket cannot be placed without extensive compromise of anterior and posterior columns. Alternative treatment options available for this problem include: (1) a high hip center, (2) a large superior structural segmental bone graft, (3) impaction grafting in combination with a cemented cup, and (4) special oblong uncemented acetabular components. The pros and cons of the high hip center technique have been discussed above. A large superior structural graft can also be used to fill the defect. Rigid fixation of the graft to the pelvis with internal fixation is necessary. As a general rule, if more than 50 percent of the socket is supported by structural graft, and especially when this involves the superior weight-bearing portion of the acetabulum, we prefer a cemented socket. However, the high rates of graft collapse and failure when cemented sockets are used alone with bulk grafts has led us to the use of an anti-protrusio device in combination with the cemented socket in order to protect the allograft from long-term overload and collapse in most of these cases. Use of impaction grafting and placement of a cemented socket as recommended by Sloof et al.[77] might be reasonable for these difficult cases, although creation of very massive volumes of cancellous graft may slow or prevent incorporation, and thus this technique may have some limitations with the most massive of defects. We have very limited experience with this method.

Another means of treating large oblong defects is via an oblong uncemented porous-coated off-the-shelf acetabular component designed to fill the bone deficiency with metal (see Fig. 62–10). Theoretical advantages of this technique are (1) the normal hip center is restored, (2) increased contact area between the porous prosthesis and native bone can in theory be achieved, and (3) the need for a large superior structural bone graft is obviated. The usual dilemma with this method involves difficulty in achieving good contact without gaps or irregularities between the implant and bone, the potential need for excessive reaming in an already deficient acetabular cavity to achieve optimal bone contact, and difficulty in assessing how much contact has actually been achieved behind the cup. These problems have made it difficult for us to employ these implants except in the very occasional instance where the defect very closely matches the available size and shape of the off-the-shelf oblong implants. Even in those circumstances where excellent fit and contact against the host is achieved, there may be problems in terms of implant version or inclination that can increase the potential for hip instability. These problems in combination have limited the use of these implants in our hands and have stimulated the development of a system of modular acetabular augments designed to be used with a hemispherical shell (Fig. 62–11). The goal is to maximize contact against host bone by creation of an implant at surgery that matches the patient's defects, while facilitating placement of the acetabular cup and insert in proper version and as near to the anatomic level as possible (Fig. 62–12). This modular approach to filling in these large irregular and segmental deficiencies is experimental, and long-term results will be needed to validate this concept before it can be recommended for general use.

MASSIVE COMBINED DEFICIENCIES

Huge global deficiencies of the socket, especially when coupled with medial acetabular bone so deficient that it provides no resistance to medial socket migration, represents another situation that is very difficult to treat successfully with uncemented hemispherical components alone. In such circumstances, satisfactory support from native bone is unlikely to be achieved, and the likelihood of stable long-term biologic fixation is reduced. In these circumstances, we have utilized extensive bone grafting to restore pelvic bone stock and have protected these bone grafts with anti-protrusio devices (Fig. 62–13). Secure screw fixation of these devices to the pelvis is necessary, and the devices must be placed and oriented so that they rest on a secure foundation of native bone while allowing appropriate orientation of the acetabular cup. Bone deficiencies are filled with cancellous bone graft in most cases, but occasionally structural graft is used when this is deemed necessary for initial stability of the construct or to span large defects and serve as a strut from the ilium to the ischium when the volume of cancellous graft needed would be excessive and unlikely to ever revascularize and incorporate. An all-polyethylene socket or constrained acetabular insert, if needed, is then cemented into the reinforcement device in appropriate orientation. The addition of porous or hydroxyapatite surfaces to the backside of such anti-protrusio devices or cage-like additions to traditional hemispherical cups in order to achieve biologic fixation and supplement the mechanical fixation initially provided by interference, fit, and screws may help improve the long-term durability of these devices, especially in higher demand younger patients.

Type IV: Pelvic Discontinuity

Patients with pelvic discontinuity present some of the most challenging problems in acetabular reconstruction. Preoperative radiographs may demonstrate the presence of a discontinuity, but frequently this problem is not clearly visible on preoperative radiographs (even if Judet views are obtained). Thus the surgeon must be attentive during the reconstruction to check for pelvic discontinuity and to treat it appropriately if identified. Failure to address pelvic discontinuity at the time of revision surgery carries with it a high likelihood of failure of the reconstruction.

Successful treatment of pelvic discontinuity requires stabilization of the discontinuity (which generally represents a transverse acetabular fracture nonunion). Stabilization of the pelvis may be achieved with anterior and posterior column plating or, in some cases, posterior column plating alone (Fig. 62–14). The 3.5-mm pelvic reconstruction plates used for acetabular fractures work well for this purpose. The anti-protrusio cages with both iliac and ischial flanges allow screw fixation to the ilium and, on the ischial side, either screw placement or, more often in our hands, insertion of the flange into the ischium, where it can act as a blade plate. Such a device may be used alone to attempt to stabilize the discontinuity associated with severe bone loss, but it is usually employed wherever possible in combination with a separate posterior column plate when adequate room and bone stock exist for both implants. Treatment of any remaining acetabular bone deficiency and placement of an appropriate acetabular component are based on the tenets outlined in the above sections.

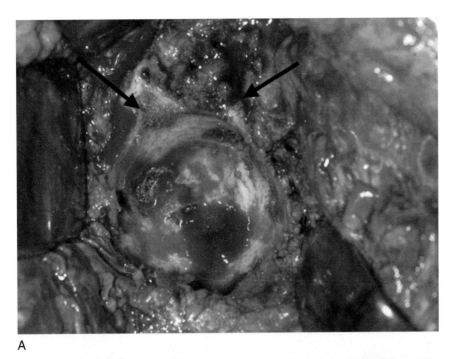

A

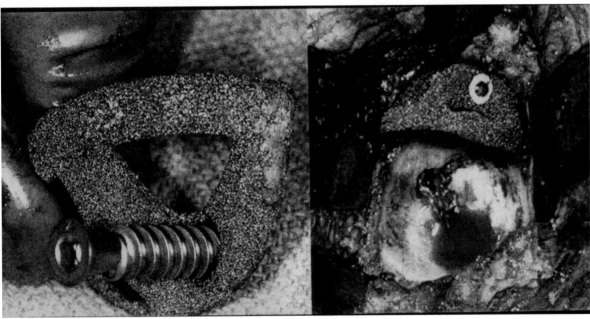

B1   B2

Figure 62–11. A, Acetabular defect present after removal of loose cup and failed resorbed superior structural bone graft (*arrows*). **B,** Porous tantalum acetabular augment fixed into place on rim of acetabulum.

Illustration continued on following page

CONCLUSIONS

Reconstructive challenges faced during acetabular revision surgery may range from trivial problems similar to those encountered during primary surgery all the way to massive defects that do not seem readily reconstructible with any method. The size of the challenge posed by certain failed arthroplasties seems to be increasing as time goes by, perhaps related to a larger population at risk and the effects of osteolysis in what are more and more active patient populations receiving hip arthroplasties. Acetabular component revision is now far more successful than in the early years of revision total hip replacement. A systematic approach to the problem of acetabular revision provides the surgeon with the highest likelihood of success. Revision of each failed acetabular component is based on the type of bone deficiency present, the location and quality of the bone remaining, the individual circumstances of the patient, and the surgeon's own preferences and available resources.

Text continued on page 841

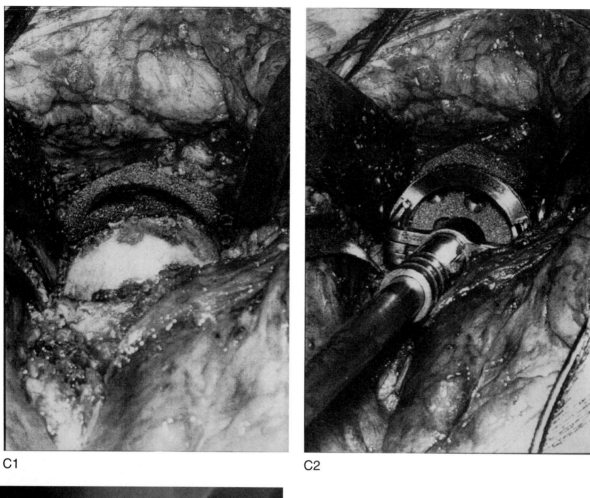

C1

C2

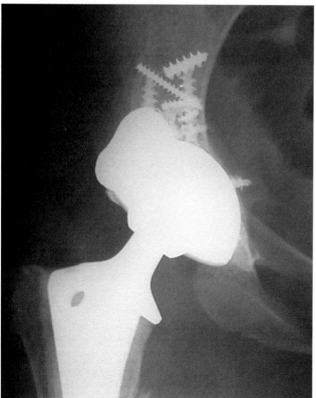

D

Figure 62–11. *Continued.* **C,** Cup placement into acetabulum and against augment. Cement fixation is used between augment and cup but with porous implant and bone graft in contact with host. **D,** Radiograph of cup and augment construct fixed with screws to acetabulum.

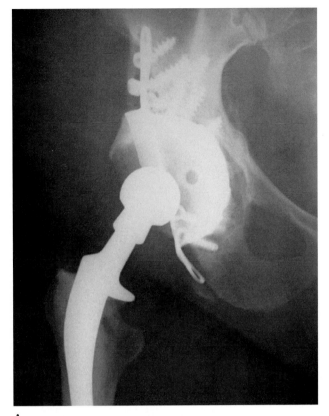

A

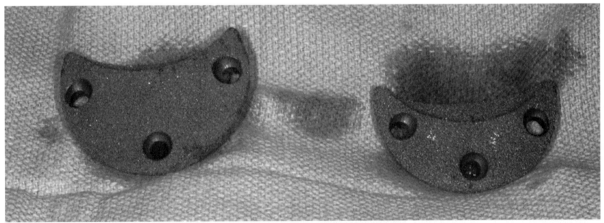

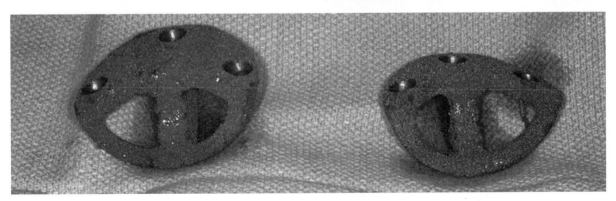

B

Figure 62–12. A, Pre-revision radiograph showing a failed anti-protrusio cage that has migrated in a large associated bone defect with failed prior structural grafting. **B**, Example of a porous tantalum acetabular augment with fenestrations for use with a hemispherical cup and cancellous bone graft in the fenestrations.

Illustration continued on following page

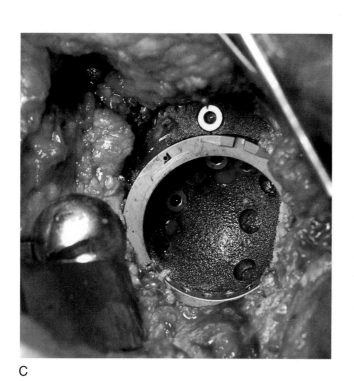

C

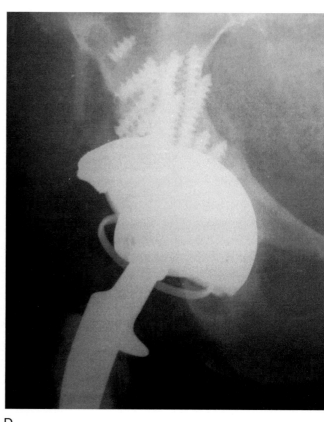

D

Figure 62–12. *Continued.* **C**, Acetabular augment in place cemented to the hemispherical porous cup, providing maximal host bone contact and restoration of the anatomic hip center. **D**, Postoperative radiograph.

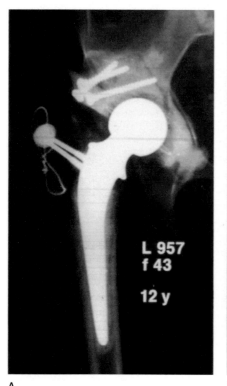

A

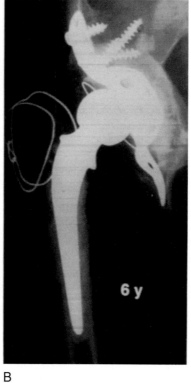

B

Figure 62–13. A, Radiograph showing massive acetabular bone deficiency (type III). **B**, Reconstruction with Burch-Schneider anti-protrusio cage and particulate allograft at 6 years showing excellent graft incorporation.

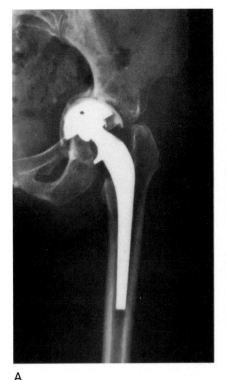
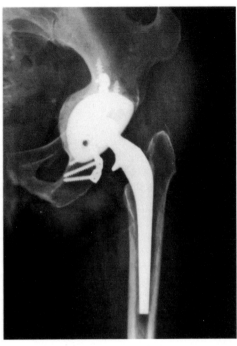

A   B

Figure 62–14. A, Radiograph showing failed acetabular component with associated pelvic discontinuity. **B,** Two years after reconstruction with uncemented porous-coated acetabular component, plating of the posterior column, autogenous grafting of the discontinuity, and particulate allograft bone grafting of the cavitary deficiencies. Radiograph shows healing of the discontinuity and stable acetabular component.

The majority of acetabular revisions can and should be managed with uncemented hemispherical sockets. These implants have emerged as the workhorse of acetabular revision surgery but do have limitations, and will fail if satisfactory initial stability and good contact on viable host bone are not achieved. In such circumstances, knowledge of other treatment options is mandatory, and these alternative treatment choices must be available and used when appropriate. The full extent of the acetabular defects and relative quality and location of host bone remaining is not always apparent preoperatively and may not be completely clear until during the procedure. In particular, some portions of the procedure, such as acetabular component removal, can change the characteristics and extent of the bone defect present. Availability of a variety of implants and graft materials greatly facilitates the successful reconstruction of these always unique and frequently challenging problems.

References

1. Amstutz HC, Ma SM, Jinnah RH, Mai L: Revision of loose total hip arthroplasties. Clin Orthop 170:21, 1982.
2. Berry DJ, Müller ME: Revision arthroplasty using an anti-protrusio cage for massive acetabular bone deficiency. J Bone Joint Surg Br 74:711, 1992.
3. Berry DJ, Scott R, Cabanela ME, et al: Catastrophic acetabular component polyethylene failure in total hip arthroplasty. J Bone Joint Surg Br 76:575, 1994.
4. Berry DJ, Sutherland CJ, Trousdale RT, et al: Bilobed oblong porous coated acetabular components in revision total hip arthroplasty. Clin Orthop 371:154, 2000.
5. Bohm P, Banzhaf S: Acetabular revision with allograft bone: 103 revisions with three reconstruction alternatives followed for 0.3–13 years. Acta Orthop Scand 70:240–249, 1999.
6. Brien WW, Bruce WJ, Salvati EA, et al: Acetabular reconstruction with bipolar prosthesis and morselized bone grafts. J Bone Joint Surg Am 72:1230, 1990.
7. Buma P, Lamerigts N, Schreurs BW, et al: Impacted graft incorporation after cemented acetabular revision: histological evaluation in eight patients. Acta Orthop Scand 67:536–540, 1996.
8. Burch H: La Chirurgie Orthopédique. [Die orthopädische Chirurgie.] Berne: Hans Huber, 1978.
9. Cabanela ME: Reconstruction rings and bone graft in total hip revision surgery. Orthop Clin North Am 29:255–262, 1998.
10. Callaghan JJ: Results of primary total hip arthroplasty in young patients. J Bone Joint Surg Am 75:1728, 1993.
11. Callaghan JJ, Salvati EA, Pellicci PM, et al: Results of revision for mechanical failure after cemented total hip replacement, 1979 to 1982: a two to five year follow-up. J Bone Joint Surg Am 67:1074, 1985.
12. Chen WM, Engh CA Jr, Hopper RH Jr, et al: Acetabular revision with use of a bilobed component inserted without cement in patients who have acetabular bone stock deficiency. J Bone Joint Surg Am 82:197–206, 2000.
13. Christie MJ, Barrington SA, Brinson MF, et al: Bridging massive acetabular defects with the triflange cup: 2–9 year results. Clin Orthop 393:216–227, 2001.
14. D'Antonio JA, Capello WN, Borden LS, et al: Classification and management of acetabular abnormalities in total hip arthroplasty. Clin Orthop 243:126, 1989.
15. Dearborn JT, Harris WH: Acetabular revision after failed total hip arthroplasty in patients with congenital hip dislocation and dysplasia: results after a mean of 8.6 years. J Bone Joint Surg Am 82:1146–1153, 2000.
16. Dearborn JT, Harris WH: Acetabular revision arthroplasty using so-called jumbo cementless components: an average 7 year follow-up study. J Arthroplasty 15:8–15, 2000.
17. DeBoer DK, Christie MJ: Reconstruction of the deficient acetabulum with an oblong prosthesis: three to seven year results. J Arthroplasty 13:674, 1998.

18. Eftakhar NS, Ohanner N: Intrapelvic migration of total hip prostheses. J Bone Joint Surg Am 71:1480, 1989.

19. Emerson RH Jr, Head WC: Dealing with the deficient acetabulum in revision hip arthroplasty: the importance of implant migration and use of the jumbo cup. Semin Arthroplasty 4:2, 1993.

20. Fuchs MD, Salvati EA, Wilson PD, et al: Results of acetabular revisions with newer cement techniques. Orthop Clin North Am 19:649, 1988.

21. Gordon SL, Binkert BL, Rashkoff ES, et al: Assessment of bone grafts used for acetabular augmentation in total hip arthroplasty. Clin Orthop Rel Res 201:18, 1985.

22. Gross AE, Lavoie MV, McDermott P, Marks P: The use of allograft bone in revision of total hip arthroplasty. Clin Orthop 197:115, 1985.

23. Gustke KA, Grossman RM: Acetabular reconstruction in primary and revision total hip arthroplasty. Tech Orthop 2:65, 1987.

24. Haentjens P, Handelberg F, Casteleyn PP, Opdecam P: The Müller acetabular support ring. Int Orthop (SICOT) 10:223, 1986.

25. Harris WH: Allografting in total hip arthroplasty: in adults with severe acetabular deficiency including surgical technique for bolting graft to the ilium. Clin Orthop 162:150, 1982.

26. Harris WH: Bone grafting for acetabular deficiency in association with total hip replacement. In The Hip: Proceedings of the 14th Open Scientific Meeting of the Hip Society. St. Louis, CV Mosby, 1987, p 39.

27. Harris WH: The first 32 years of total hip arthroplasty: one surgeon's perspective. Clin Orthop 274:6, 1992.

28. Harris WH: Bulk versus morselized bone graft in acetabular revision total hip replacement. Semin Arthroplasty 4:68, 1993.

29. Harris WH: Reconstruction at a high hip center in acetabular revision surgery using a cementless acetabular component. Orthopedics 21:991–992, 1998.

30. Harris WH, Crothers O, Oh I: Total hip replacement and femoral-head bone-grafting for severe acetabular deficiency in adults. J Bone Joint Surg Am 59:752, 1977.

31. Harris WH, Krushell RJ, Galante JO: Results of cementless revisions of total hip arthroplasties using the Harris-Gallante prosthesis. Clin Orthop 235:120, 1988.

32. Hedde C, Postel M, Kerboul M, Courpied JP: La réparation du cotyle par homogreffe osseuse conservée au cours des révisions de prothèse totale de hanche. Rev Chir Orthop Reparatrice Appar Mot 72:267, 1986.

33. Hedley AK, Gruen TA, Ruoff DP: Revision of failed total hip arthroplasties with uncemented porous-coated anatomic components. Clin Orthop 235:75, 1988.

34. Hirose I, Kawauchi K, Kondo S, et al: Histological evaluation of allograft bone after acetabular revision arthroplasty: report of two cases. J Orthop Sci 5:515–519, 2000.

35. Hozack WJ: Techniques of acetabular reconstruction. Semin Arthroplasty 4:72, 1993.

36. Jasty M: Jumbo cups and morcellized graft. Orthop Clin North Am 29:249–254, 1998.

37. Jasty M, Harris WH: Total hip reconstruction using frozen femoral head allografts in patients with acetabular bone loss. Orthop Clin North Am 18:291, 1987.

38. Jasty M, Harris WH: Results of total hip reconstruction using acetabular mesh in patients with central acetabular deficiency. Clin Orthop 237:142, 1988.

39. Jasty M, Harris WH: Salvage total hip reconstruction in patients with major acetabular bone deficiency using structural femoral head allografts. J Bone Joint Surg Br 72:63, 1990.

40. Kavanaugh BF, DeWitz MA, Currier BL, et al: Charnley low friction arthroplasty of the hip: twenty year results with cement. J Arthroplasty 9:229, 1994.

41. Kavanagh BF, Fitzgerald RH: Multiple revisions for failed total hip arthroplasty not associated with infection. J Bone Joint Surg Am 69:1144, 1987.

42. Kavanagh BF, Ilstrup D, Fitzgerald RH: Revision total hip arthroplasty. J Bone Joint Surg Am 67:517, 1985.

43. Kelley SS: High hip center in revision arthroplasty. J Arthroplasty 9:503, 1994.

44. Kwong LM, Jasty M, Harris WH: High failure rate of bulk femoral head allografts in total hip acetabular reconstructions at 10 years. J Arthroplasty 8:341, 1993.

45. Lee BP, Cabanela ME, Wallrichs BS, Ilstrup DM: Bone graft augmentation for acetabular deficiencies in total hip arthroplasty: results of long-term follow-up. J Arthroplasty 12:503–510, 1997.

46. Leopold SS, Rosenberg AG, Bhatt RD, et al: Cementless acetabular revision: evaluation at an average of 10.5 years. Clin Orthop 369:179–186, 1999.

47. Mayer G, Hartseil K: Acetabular reinforcement in total hip replacement. Arch Orthop Trauma Surg 105:227, 1986.

48. McAllister CM, Borden LS: Allograft reconstruction of the acetabulum in revision hip surgery. Semin Arthroplasty 4:80, 1993.

49. Morsi E, Garbuz D, Gross AE: Revision total hip arthroplasty with shelf bulk allografts: a long-term follow-up study. J Arthroplasty 11:86–90, 1996.

50. Moskal JT, Danisa OA, Shaffrey CI: Isolated revision acetabuloplasty using a porous-coated cementless acetabular component without removal of a well-fixed femoral component: a 3 to 9 year follow-up study. J Arthroplasty 12:719–727, 1997.

51. Müller ME: Acetabular revision. In The Hip: Proceedings of the Ninth Open Scientific Meeting of the Hip Society. St. Louis, CV Mosby, 1981, p 46.

52. Müller ME, Jaberg H: Total hip reconstruction. In Evarts CM (ed): Surgery of the Musculoskeletal System, 2nd ed, vol 3. New York, Churchill Livingstone, 1990, p 2879.

53. Mulroy RD Jr, Harris WH: Failure of acetabular autogenous grafts in total hip arthroplasty. J Bone Joint Surg Am 72:1536, 1990.

54. Oakeshott RD, Morgan DAF, Zukor DJ, et al: Revision total hip arthroplasty with osseous allograft reconstruction: a clinical and roentgenographic analysis. Clin Orthop 225:37, 1987.

55. Oh I, Harris WH: Design concepts, indications, and surgical technique for use of the protrusio shell. Clin Orthop 162:175, 1982.

56. Ornstein E, Franzen H, Johnsson R, et al: Migration of the acetabular component after revision with impacted morcellized allografts: a radiostereometric two year follow-up analysis of 21 cases. Acta Orthop Scand 70:338–342, 1999.

57. Padgett DE, Kull L, Rosenberg A, et al: Revision of the acetabular component without cement after total hip arthroplasty. J Bone Joint Surg Am 75:663, 1993.

58. Papagelopoulos PJ, Lewallen DG, Cabanela ME, et al: Acetabular reconstruction using bipolar endoprosthesis and bone grafting in patients with severe bone deficiency. Clin Orthop 314:170, 1995.

59. Paprosky WG, Perona PG, Lawrence JM: Acetabular defect classification and surgical reconstruction in revision arthroplasty: a 6 year follow-up evaluation. J Arthroplasty 9:33, 1994.

60. Patch DA, Lewallen DG: Reconstruction of deficient acetabula using bone graft and a fixed porous ingrowth cup: a 5 year roentgenographic study. Orthop Trans 17:151, 1993.

61. Pellicci PM, Wilson PD, Sledge CB, et al: Revision total hip arthroplasty. Clin Orthop 170:34, 1982.

62. Pellici PM, Wilson PD, Sledge CB, et al: Long-term results of revision total hip replacement: a follow-up report. J Bone Joint Surg Am 67:513, 1985.

63. Peters CL, Curtain M, Samuelson KM: Acetabular revision with the Burch Schneider antiprotrusio cage and cancellous allograft bone. J Arthroplasty 10:307–312, 1995.

64. Pollock FH, Whiteside LA: The fate of massive allografts in total hip acetabular revision surgery. J Arthroplasty 7:271, 1992.

65. Postel M: Prothesenwechsel an der Hüfte. Orthopade 18:382, 1989.

66. Postel M, Courpied JP: Le remplacement d'une prothese totale de hanche defaillante. Rev Rhum 53:133, 1986.

67. Rosson J, Schatzker J: The use of reinforcement rings to reconstruct deficient acetabula. J Bone Joint Surg Br 74:716, 1992.

68. Russotti GM, Harris WH: Proximal placement of the acetabular component in total hip arthroplasty. J Bone Joint Surg Am 73:587, 1991.

69. Salvati EA, Bullough P, Wilson PD: Intrapelvic protrusion of the acetabular component following total hip replacement. Clin Orthop 111:212, 1975.

70. Samuelson KM, Freeman MAR, Levak B, et al: Homograft bone in revision acetabular arthroplasty: a clinical and radiographic study. J Bone Joint Surg Br 70:367, 1988.

71. Schatzker J, Glynn MK, Ritter D: A preliminary review of the Müller acetabular and Burch-Schneider anti-protrusio support rings. Arch Orthop Trauma Surg 103:5, 1984.

72. Schatzker J, Wong MK: Acetabular revision: the role of rings and cages. Clin Orthop 369:187–197, 1999.
73. Schneider R: Total Prosthetic Replacement of the Hip: A Biomechanical Concept and Its Consequences. Toronto: Hans Huber, 1989.
74. Schreurs BW, Slooff TJJH, Gardeniers JWM, Buma P: Acetabular reconstruction with bone impaction grafting and a cemented cup: 20 year's experience. Clin Orthop 393:202–215, 2001.
75. Schutzer SF, Harris WH: High placement of porous-coated acetabular components in complex total hip arthroplasty. J Arthroplasty 9:359, 1994.
76. Scott RD, Pomerov D, Oser E, et al: The results and technique of bipolar revision hip arthroplasty combined with acetabular grafting. Orthop Trans 11:450, 1987.
77. Sloof TJJH, Huiskes R, Van Horn J, Lemmens AJ: Bone grafting in total hip replacement for acetabular protrusion. Acta Orthop Scand 55:593–596, 1984.
78. Stiehl JB: Acetabular allograft reconstruction in total hip arthroplasty: surgical approach and aftercare. Orthop Rev 20:425, 1991.
79. Tanzer M, Drucker D, Jasty M, et al: Revision of the acetabular component with an uncemented Harris-Galante porous coated prosthesis. J Bone Joint Surg Am 74:987, 1992.
80. Trancik TM, Stuhlberg BN, Wilde AH, Feiglin DH: Allograft reconstruction of the acetabulum during revision total hip arthroplasty: clinical, radiographic, and scintigraphic assessment of the results. J Bone Joint Surg Am 68:527, 1986.
81. van der Linde M, Tonino A: Acetabular revision with impacted grafting in a reinforcement ring: 42 patients followed for a mean of 10 years. Acta Orthop Scand 72:221–227, 2001.
82. Wachtl SW, Jumg M, Jakob RP, Gautier E: Burch Schneider anti-protrusio cage in acetabular revision surgery: a mean follow-up of 12 years. J Arthroplasty 15:959–963, 2000.
83. Whaley AL, Berry DJ, Harmsen WS: Extra-large uncemented hemispherical acetabular components for revision total hip arthroplasty. J Bone Joint Surg Am 83:1352–1357, 2001.
84. Wilson MG, Nikpoor N, Aliabadi P, et al: The fate of acetabular allografts after bipolar revision arthroplasty of the hip. J Bone Joint Surg Am 71:1469, 1989.
85. Yoder SA, Brand RA, Pedersen DR, O'Gorman TW: Total hip acetabular component position affects component loosening rates. Clin Orthop Rel Res 228:79, 1988.
86. Young C, Hastings DE, Schatzker J: Acetabular reinforcement in total hip replacement. J Bone Joint Surg Br 67:311, 1985.
87. Young SK, Dorr LD, Kaufman RL, Gruen TAW: Factors related to failure of structural bone grafts in acetabular reconstruction of total hip arthroplasty. J Arthroplasty 6(Suppl): S73, 1991.
88. Zehtner MK, Ganz R: Midterm results (5.5–10 years) of acetabular allograft reconstruction with the acetabular reinforcement ring during total hip revision. J Arthroplasty 9:469, 1994.

63

Femoral Revision Without Structural Augmentation

• MIGUEL E. CABANELA

About 200,000 total hip replacements are performed annually in the United States. It is estimated that revision is necessary at a rate of approximately 1 percent per year in this group of patients. This translates to about 10,000 to 15,000 revisions being done yearly in the United States. At my own institution, revisions have increased slightly and slowly since the early 1990s, to encompass about one third of the total number of approximately 1000 hip arthroplasties performed annually. It has also been noted that the complexity of revision procedures continues to increase, making comparison with historical studies very difficult. However, our ability to deal with more complex problems has also improved, and with it the quality of the revision results.

Reasons for femoral revision include infection, stem fracture, dislocation, stem loosening, and, more recently, femoral osteolysis. Infection and dislocation are discussed elsewhere (see Chapters 64 and 65). With the advent of the superalloys, stem fracture has practically disappeared. Thus, the most common indications of revision surgery today are loosening of the stem, osteolysis, or a combination of both.

REMOVAL OF OLD PROSTHESIS

The first step in any femoral revision procedure is the removal of the old prosthesis, followed by the preparation of the femoral canal for insertion of the new device. Removal of the old prosthesis can be very time consuming and requires different techniques and instruments, depending on the type of prosthesis to be removed.

Cemented Prosthesis

In general, the removal of the prosthesis itself is simple. The removal of the cement, however, can be extremely difficult and time consuming, particularly if the primary mode of loosening was at the cement-prosthesis interface (mechanical loosening, debonding). Conversely, if loosening has occurred at the cement-bone interface, cement

removal is not a problem, but removal of the intervening membrane must be very complete so that the medullary canal of the femur is left as clean as possible for the surgeon to proceed with the revision technique elected.

Accidents occurring cement removal include cortex penetration, additional loss of cortical bone stock, and femoral fracture. After trying different methods, my colleagues and I have settled on removal of the proximal cement by means of hand tools. Osteotomes with different types of heads—straight, curved, chisel-type, and T-head—are available, which split the cement and allow piecemeal removal. It is essential to have long rongeurs as well as a headlight or a fiberoptic type of light for canal visualization. Removal of distal, well-fixed cement can be very taxing. Image intensification often helps to avoid cortical penetration. Power burs can be used but the risk of cortical penetration is high. The use of the ultrasonographic cement extractor, with its aural warning of cortex penetration, has proved to be valuable, safe, and quick for removal of long, distal, well-fixed cement plugs. Patience, repeated irrigation, careful observation, and repetition of the same moves can make the job of cement removal safer, but it remains a somewhat tedious part of the procedure. The need for complete cement removal cannot be overemphasized, particularly if a long-stemmed prosthesis is to be used for revision. In this instance, leaving cement remnants on one side of the endosteal canal can force the long stem into an unnecessary and dangerous penetration of the cortex. That is why, in instances of failure by debonding, when the cement remains very well fixed to the bone, we more frequently use an extended femoral osteotomy for the approach, as proposed by Paprosky,[43] particularly when we plan to use a fully porous-coated stem for the revision. This approach facilitates both cement and membrane removal.

Proximally Coated Stems

Usually, removal of proximally coated uncemented stems is not a problem if loosening is the cause of the revision. In cases of well-fixed, proximally coated stems that are revised for thigh pain, one must break proximal bone bonds by using flexible osteotomes or a pencil-tipped power bur. Even in cases of very firm osseous integration, judicious use of the aforementioned instruments allows fairly quick removal of these components, with minimal destruction of the metaphysis of the femur.

Fully Porous-Coated Femoral Stems

Removal of a well-fixed, fully porous-coated femoral stem can be an extremely time consuming and even disastrous affair. Of all the described methods of removal, perhaps the extended proximal femoral osteotomy proposed by Paprosky, although somewhat radical, is the safest.[34,35] This procedure is performed through an extended posterolateral approach and consists of removing a portion of bone about one third of the circumference of the femur, involving the greater trochanter and hinging the window anteriorly. This facilitates visualization of the component, which can then be cut with a metal cutting bur; the proximal metaphyseal portion of the prosthesis can then be freed with use of a pencil-tipped power bur, flexible osteotomes, and, sometimes, a Gigli saw. The distal cylindrical portion of the prosthesis can be removed by means of dedicated trephines. Usually this procedure is combined with use of a fully porous-coated, long-stemmed, straight, or curved prosthesis for revision. At the termination of the procedure, the osteotomy is closed and fixed with circumferential wires or cables, occasionally with additional strut grafts for reinforcement of the lateral cortex, if it is very weakened.

ASSESSMENT OF FEMORAL DEFICIENCY

Once the prosthesis, or cement, or both are removed and the entire proximal femur is clean and free of membrane and soft tissue, the next step is evaluation of the femoral defect. The Committee of the Hip of the American Academy of Orthopaedic Surgeons has popularized a classification[7] of femoral defects that divides them into segmental, cavitary, combined, malaligned, stenotic, and discontinuous; they are further subdivided by geographical location as well as by size (see Table 63–1). The assessment of the type, size, and location of the defect must precede the decision of which type of reconstruction to use.

Table 63–1. AMERICAN ACADEMY OF ORTHOPAEDIC SURGEONS CLASSIFICATION OF FEMORAL DEFECTS

1. Segmental, proximal, partial, complete, intercalary greater trochanter
2. Cavitary, cancellous, cortical, ectasia
3. Combined segmentary and cavitary
4. Malalignment, rotational angular
5. Stenosis
6. Discontinuity

RECONSTRUCTION ALTERNATIVES

Many factors should be considered during the decision-making process in selecting the reconstruction alternative. The patient's age and activity level, the type of bone deficiency, the quality of the remaining bone, the previous procedure, and the conditions responsible for the revision are all factors that must be considered.

Cemented Revision

Logically, the use of cement in revision surgery is the alternative with which we have the longest experience and the greatest amount of follow-up information.

Cement fixation for revision has been used in elderly patients with reasonably good femoral bone stock. This group includes (1) patients who have preservation of proximal cancellous bone (previously uncemented Moore prosthesis or previous cemented prosthesis that has left proximal cancellous bone in the femur); (2) patients with lesser bone quality but limited life expectancy who are good candidates for cement use; (3) patients with a failed porous-coated uncemented prosthesis and good proximal bone stock; and (4) patients in whom reimplantation for previous infection is undertaken, especially if rigid prosthetic fixation can be obtained, because this facilitates the use of antibiotic-impregnated bone cement. In addition, cement is necessary when a proximal femoral allograft-prosthetic composite is used.

In contrast, cement is contraindicated if the metaphysis of the femur contains defects or if the bone is thin and very fragile. Young, active patients may not be good candidates for a cemented prosthesis. Also, if the proximal endosteal surface of the femur is very sclerotic and poor bone pressurization is anticipated, cement is not the best choice.

All the published results of cemented femoral revision using so-called first-generation cementing technique[6,10,23,24,34,46,47,56,57] demonstrated very high re-revision rates (4 percent to 29 percent), with follow-ups of 4 to 8 years. In addition, radiographic loosening was present in 18 percent to 24 percent of the implants.

Improvements in cement technique (second-generation technique) and, perhaps, better implant designs have lowered the re-revision rate, but the numbers quoted are 10 percent re-revision and an additional 10 percent of radiographic loosening with 12 years of follow-up.[13,51] These figures are not quite so good in patients younger than 55 years of age.[54,55]

The use of a long-stemmed cemented prosthesis provides a larger cement fixation surface that reduces the unit load on the cement and the prosthesis, allows bypass of bone deficiencies present, and permits distal cement interdigitation into, perhaps, better bone (Fig. 63–1). However, disadvantages include increased difficulty with prosthesis extraction if revision becomes necessary and the possibility of stress shielding in an already deficient proximal femur. Intermediate results have been satisfactory.[56] A calcar replacement cemented

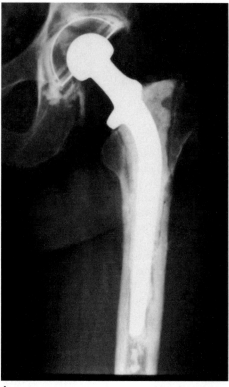

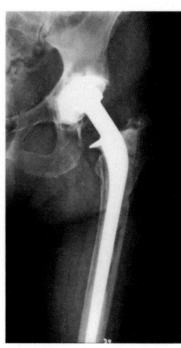

A   B

Figure 63–1. A, Radiograph of an 80-year-old woman with a painful, loose prosthesis. The bone quality after removal of the prosthesis and cement was acceptable. **B**, Same patient, 10 years after implantation of a long-stemmed cemented component. She has had an excellent result and, at age 90, she is unlikely to need another revision.

prosthesis can be utilized in situations in which bone loss below the lesser trochanter is present.

Technical Aspects of Cemented Revision

When cement is considered for revision, four aspects must be precise. First, preparation of the receiving bone surface must include, as previously mentioned, complete removal of the cement membrane and, if it is present, the neoendocortex. This preparation exposes as much of the underlying cancellous bone as possible in order to ameliorate cement interdigitation. If the proximal femur is sclerotic, microtexturing it with a small pencil-tipped bur can improve the receiving cortex. Adequate fixation is a balance between cement penetration allowed by bone porosity and the inherent strength of the bone; thus, if the bone is very weak, it cannot provide strong fixation, even with adequate cement penetration.[1] In this instance, the cemented femoral revision has a higher and more rapid failure rate than is found with cemented revisions performed in minimally compromised or normal bone. Because of this fact, if the cement-bone interface in the original prosthesis is excellent and if there is no evidence of membrane on the interface, the technique of cementing within the cement mantle can provide a stronger construct than that achieved by removing the cement and leaving behind the weakened bone. Excellent results have been reported[16] with the technique of cement within cement, and we have been pleased with its performance in a few selected instances (Fig. 63–2), including a broken stem with an intact distal cement mantle; removal of a femoral component for revision of a loose cup to obtain

better exposure, with or without changed leg length or increased offset; and debonding of a femoral component with an intact cement mantle. The old cement surface must be dry and roughened to increase surface area, and the new cement must be injected during the fluid phase to prevent lamination.

Second, a proper implant design must be selected. Today, the ideal implant is made of cobalt-chromium and has smooth edges, a polished surface finish, a tapered geometry, and a surrounding proper cement mantle (i.e., a mantle 2 to 3 mm thick and extending at least 2 cm beyond the tip of the prosthesis).

Third, cement preparation includes porosity reduction methods such as vacuum mixing or centrifugation.

Fourth, cement delivery includes not only the preparation of a "bone-dry" surface obtained by using adrenaline-impregnated sponges as well as proper suction, but also by filling the retrograde canal via a cement gun to avoid admixture of the cement with blood or fat. The filling is followed by pressurization of the cement into the canal. The long-term effects of pressurization remain unknown, however. Proper alignment of the stem within the canal, particularly if the canals are patulous, is important. However, minor deviations into the varus or valgus have not proved deleterious to the long-term results.

Uncemented Proximally Porous-Coated Femoral Stems

The first reports of cemented femoral revisions in the mid-1980s coincided with the advent of proximally porous-coated uncemented femoral stems. This discovery

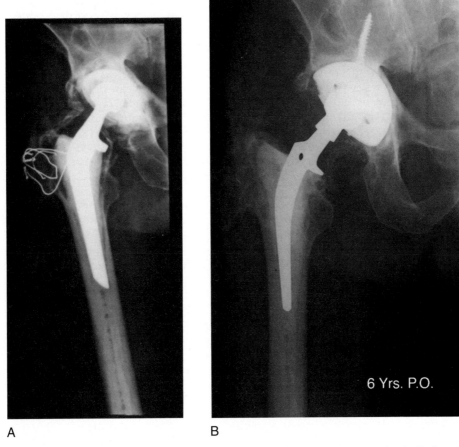

Figure 63–2. **A**, A 68-year-old man seen 10 years after a revision procedure. He has groin and buttock pain. Radiographs show loosening of the acetabulum. The femoral component is not loose. However, this is a monoblock titanium component. At surgery, there was significant titanium metallosis. The femoral component was removed, but the cement was very firmly embedded. Note the long cement distal plug. Therefore, a cement-within-cement technique was used. **B**, Six years postoperatively, the patient is asymptomatic.

naturally led to the use of these components for revisions, because they provided the potential for biologic implant fixation. Thus, in the second half of the 1980s, a very large number of these prostheses were used for revision. Initial reports were encouraging.[18,41] However, it soon became apparent that these prostheses had failed to provide the improvements expected over the cemented femoral results. Galante[15] found a 37-percent survivorship to the point of revision or progressive femoral subsidence in 54 hips, with an average of 5 years follow-up after revision with a BIAS prosthesis. Hussamy and Lachiewicz[20] reported favorable clinical results in 41 hips in which the same prosthesis was used, but they also found a significant rate of prosthetic subsidence at a mean of 5 years after surgery. Trousdale and Morrey reported similar results with the same prosthesis (Personal communication between Trousdale RT and Morrey BF). Woolson[61] reported a re-revision rate of 20 percent and a subsidence rate of 45 percent in 28 hips revised with use of the Harris-Galante prosthesis and followed for a mean of 5.5 years. Malkani et al.[33] reported on 69 femoral component revisions that used an uncemented, long-stemmed, metaphyseal-filling, proximally coated cobalt-chromium curved prosthesis (Omnifit long stem). With a mean follow-up of 3 years,

re-revision had occurred in 9 percent of patients. Intraoperative fractures were a frequent complication (46 percent). Survivorship free of revision or moderate pain at 5 years was 82 percent for the entire group but only 58 percent at 4 years for those with intraoperative femoral fracture.

The most complete report on the use of proximally porous-coated femoral components in revision was that of Berry and co-workers[2] in 1995. They reviewed 375 consecutive revisions performed at the Mayo Clinic between 1985 and 1989, which used six different but similar stem designs: the Harris-Galante prosthesis, the BIAS, the Omnifit, the Omnifit long stem, the porous-coated anatomic (PCA), and the PCA long stem.

The mean patient age was 60 years, and the group consisted of 152 men and 223 women. The diagnosis was failed total hip arthroplasty with aseptic loosening in 80 percent, instability in 4 percent, fracture in 3 percent, and a two-stage procedure for infected total hip replacement in 13 percent. The types of prostheses used were as follows: 51 Harris-Galante, 94 BIAS, 72 Omnifit, 52 Omnifit long stem, 49 PCA, and 57 PCA long stem. The removed prostheses were cemented in 76 percent, uncemented in 7 percent, cemented long stem in 14 percent, and uncemented long stem in 3 percent. The bone loss was graded as minimal in 13 percent, level 1 in 16 percent, level 2 in 58 percent, level 3 in 10 percent, and as periprosthetic fractures in 3 percent.

With an average of 4.7 years of clinical follow-up and 4.3 years of radiographic follow-up, the revision rate revealed that 20 percent and 24 percent of patients, respectively, had moderate or severe pain, and 29 percent had mild pain. Forty percent of the prostheses were radiographically loose, and an additional 17 percent were possibly loose. The 8-year survivorship rate free of revision for aseptic failure was 58 percent, but the survivorship free of aseptic loosening (radiographic loosening or revision for loosening) was only 20 percent, and the survivorship rate free of symptomatic loosening was 46 percent. Although there were statistically significant differences among prosthetic types with respect to survivorship, these were probably due to selection criteria among patients. All prostheses had a significant failure rate. Both increased subsidence and poorer survivorship were associated with severe bone loss.

Intraoperative fracture, a common fact of revision surgery, occurred in 26 percent of the revisions, and it appeared to portend a poor survivorship, although it was not statistically significant.

This work has probably written the last chapter on the use of proximally porous-coated prostheses in femoral revision surgery. The reason for the failure of these devices is related to several factors, listed as follows:

1. The proximal femur is often weakened and is sclerotic in revision.
2. These prostheses rely on fixation in the metaphysis.
3. The quality of the initial fixation is often compromised, particularly if an intraoperative fracture has occurred.
4. The geometry of the prosthesis and the geometry of the proximal femur may not be congruent, and because of this, the contact of bone with the porous-coated metaphysis of the prosthesis may be very limited.
5. The combination of poorly vascularized weakened proximal bone in limited contact with a less than optimally stable prosthesis provides a poor environment for biologic fixation.

At my institution, the use of porous-coated implants in revision femoral surgery has practically been discontinued.

Extensively Porous-Coated Femoral Stems

Despite improvements with modern cement techniques, the results of cemented femoral revisions with certain patients or with certain types of bone are poor. Femurs with sclerotic or weakened proximal canals and little remaining cancellous bone are not well suited for fixation with cement. Likewise, the results of cement fixation for revision in younger patients have shown an increased number of re-revisions and loosening.[28,29] Extensively porous-coated devices were designed to bypass the proximal deficient femur and obtain fixation in the well-preserved diaphyseal cortical bone.[18] This bone is better suited to provide rotational stability and late biologic fixation (Fig. 63–3). The results reported so far are largely satisfactory. Engh and colleagues[12,27] reported 174 femoral revisions that used a fully porous-coated stem. With a follow-up of 5 years or more, the re-revision rate was 4.6 percent for aseptic loosening, with an additional 1.7 percent of the remaining hips being radiographically loose. Survivorship of 10 years was calculated at 90.5 percent. Paprosky[44] reported 297 uncemented femoral revisions with a mean follow-up of 5.1 years. The failure caused by aseptic loosening was 2 percent (5 patients) and there were an additional 2 patients who had radiographic loosening but who had not been revised. All patients who failed had poor canal filling by the prosthesis. More recently, Paprosky[43,63] reported on 170 femoral revisions done with extensively coated stems and followed for a mean of 13.2 years (range, 10 to 16 years). A prosthetic survivorship greater than 95 percent was reported, with 82 percent showing radiologic evidence of bony ingrowth and 13.9 percent exhibiting stable fibrous fixation. The overall mechanical failure rate was 4.1 percent, and only 9 percent of the patients had thigh pain. Moreland,[39] at the Annual Meeting of the Hip Society in 1995, reported on 185 hip revisions that had used either an anatomic medullary locking stem or a Solution stem; both of these are fully coated prostheses. A re-revision rate of 2.4 percent for aseptic failure was reported. In addition, 83.4 percent of femoral components had bony ingrowth, and an additional 15 percent had stable fibrous ingrowth. Severe stress shielding occurred in 7 percent of the bone-ingrown cases. More recently, the same author[40] reported on 137 hips treated with extensively porous-coated stems and followed for 9.3 years (range, 5 to 16 years). Eighty-three percent of the stems achieved bony ingrowth. Significant thigh pain was reported in 7 percent of the bone-ingrown stems, 16 percent of the stable fibrous-fixated stems, and 75 percent of the unstable stems.

Technical Aspects of Fully Porous-Coated Prostheses

The technique of using uncemented fully porous-coated prostheses requires the following:

1. Canal preparation should be similar to that performed for any other prosthesis and requires complete cement removal. Preparing the femur with straight or flexible reamers is the next step. The difference between reamer size and prosthesis size is based on the type of prosthesis as well as the patient's bone quality. In general, under-reaming by 0.5 cm is advisable with straight stems, but with curved stems, line-to-line reaming is often necessary.
2. A prosthetic system that includes stems of different lengths and geometries (straight as well as bowed stems) and the potential to make up for deficient proximal femoral bone (calcar replacement) is helpful.
3. A diaphyseal fit with intimate prosthesis-bone contact of at least 5 cm is recommended. Most canals

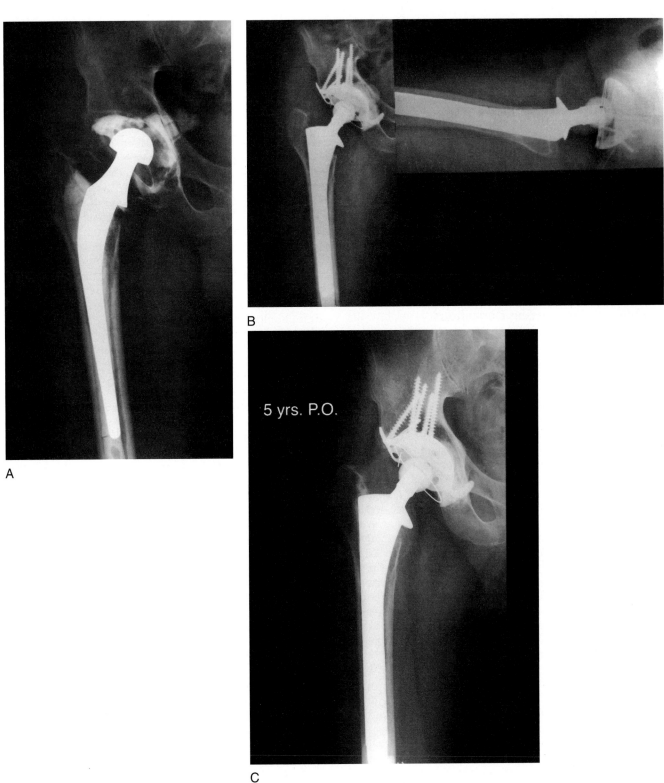

Figure 63–3. A, Radiograph of the hip of a 57-year-old man taken 8 years after implantation. Patient has significant weight-bearing groin and thigh pain. **B,** Anteroposterior and lateral radiograph of the same patient after revision of both components, the femur with a fully porous-coated stem. **C,** Anteroposterior radiograph 5 years after surgery. The patient has no pain and is doing very well. Note the distal osteointegration of the stem.

have larger anteroposterior than medial-lateral diameter; thus, some excess reaming in the medial-lateral diameter is usually advisable.

4. As with other types of reconstructions, bone deficiencies must be treated with cortical struct

grafts in the manner described elsewhere in this chapter.

Potential problems with these types of devices occur. In the first place, not all femurs are suited for this type of fixation. Femurs with very large canal diameters require excessively large femoral components, and components with diameters greater than 18 mm are associated with a higher risk of thigh pain even when osseous integration occurs, as well as a high risk of proximal femoral bone loss as a result of stress shielding. Paprosky[43] observed that stress shielding was greatest in patients with stems larger than 16.5 mm and in those with osteoporotic bone. The long-term effect of these stems in the proximal femurs of young patients remains unknown but is a reason for some concern. Finally, removal of an osseously integrated, extensively coated stem (e.g., in cases of infection or poor position of the stem) is very difficult and may lead even to destruction of the femur.

Extensively coated femoral components remain a very important tool in the armamentarium of the revision hip surgeon.

Intrafemoral Impaction Cancellous Allograft and Cement (Ling Technique)

This method of femoral component revision, which was first used by Ling and reported by Gie et al.,[16] was based on a method of acetabular reconstruction first reported by Slooff et al.[53] The method employs compressed morcellized cancellous allograft to rebuild bone stock in the endosteal aspect of the femur, combining this with a cemented, collarless, polished type of stem. This method has acquired some popularity in the United States since the early 1990s. Initially, as often happens with new methods, it was applied somewhat indiscriminately for all types of revision surgeries. It is my opinion, based on 8 years of experience, that this method should be reserved for cavitary deficiencies (metaphyseal and diaphyseal) with an intact periosteal envelope. Small segmental (wall) deficiencies are not a contraindication to the method because they can be reconstructed with wire mesh, reconstruction plates, or strut allografts. Over the last few years, prostheses of different lengths have become available, and these have somewhat extended the applicability of this method.

In 1993, Gie and colleagues[16] reported the results of this technique in 68 hips followed for a mean of 30 months. Of 56 hips reviewed, the scores for function and movement improved and appeared to maintain with time. The incidence of lucent lines was low and subsidence of the stem within the cement occurred in over one half the hips within the first 6 months, but subsidence of the cement within the bone mantle occurred much less commonly. Complications included a 4.4-percent dislocation rate and a similar incidence of intra- and postoperative femoral fractures. There were no revisions done and no infections developed. In 1997, Gie reported on the same group of patients. Twenty-one were dead and 42 had been followed for a minimum of 6 years. After this time, there were no reoperations and only 1 progressive radiological failure.

Since the mid-1990s, there has been a plethora of reports from Europe[8,14,19,35,38,45,58] and North America[9,25,28,36] of femoral revisions done with this technique. Although the overall initial assessments are favorable, problems that began appearing included intraoperative fractures resulting from the impaction, postoperative fractures and dislocations, and early subsidence.[22,25,36,45] It appears that some of these problems are related to the technique, which has a somewhat steep learning curve. Although some reports have appeared of the use of this technique with precoated prostheses,[28] the method rests on the concept that a polished, tapered prosthesis will have the ability to subside slightly within the cement mantle (taking advantage of the ductility of the methylmethacrylate) and in that manner provide circumferential hoop stresses beneficial to incorporation of the impacted graft.

My colleagues and I have elected to reserve impaction grafting for selected indications, typically metaphyseal or diaphyseal cavitary deficiencies (Fig. 63–4), although we have accepted small segmental deficiencies and reconstructed them with cobalt-chromium, Vicryl mesh, or strut allografts. Between 1993 and 1997, we performed 55 revisions with this technique, using a CPT prosthesis and fresh frozen cancellous allograft chips. This represented 14 percent of our revision practice. All cases had severe cavitary or combined deficiencies. Thirty-two were men and the mean age was 62.7 years (range, 36 to 79 years). Strut allografts were used for shaft reinforcement in 40 hips. The mean follow-up was 4 years and no patient was lost. Forty-six patiens had moderate or severe pain preoperatively, but only 3 had moderate pain at follow-up. Aside from 1 patient who became infected 2 years postoperatively and whose implant was removed, there was no instance of loosening, and in only 1 hip did we observe subsidence greater than 3 mm. Besides the 1 infection, there were 4 intraoperative fractures treated with strut reinforcement and cerclage wires or cables, 2 dislocations treated by closed reductions without recurrence, and 1 partial sciatic palsy that resolved. Our worst problem was the 5 postoperative fractures that commonly occurred quite late, often years after the surgery. All were treated successfully with plate osteosynthesis and strut grafting, and in no instance was the prosthesis fixation compromised. Thus, with the exception of the infected prosthesis that was removed, no other prosthesis was revised in our first 8 years of using this technique.

This is the reason we continue to use this technique for the selected indications mentioned: cavitary meta-diaphyseal deficiencies with an intact or almost intact cortical envelope.

The histology of the grafted bone was studied in the experimental animal by Schreurs et al.,[52] who performed a series of femoral impaction grafts in goats. They showed how an initial necrosis of the inner third of the cortex was repaired by a remodeling process that reached the graft by 6 weeks and continued to replace the graft by a process of graft lysis combined with simultaneous new host bone deposition. Similarly, the histology of the grafted bone was studied in biopsy specimens as well as

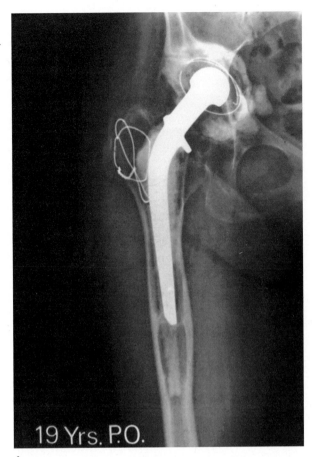

A

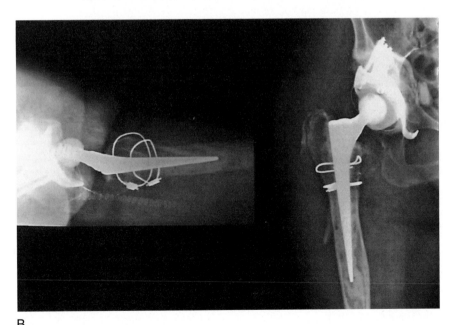

B

Figure 63–4. A, Radiograph of the right hip of a 62-year-old woman 19 years after implantation of a total cemented total hip arthroplasty for degenerative disease secondary to dissociated double hypertropia. Note the significant metaphyseal and diaphyseal cavitary osteolysis. **B,** Anteroposterior and lateral radiograph of the same hip after revision with intrafemoral impaction allograft and cement.

Illustration continued on following page

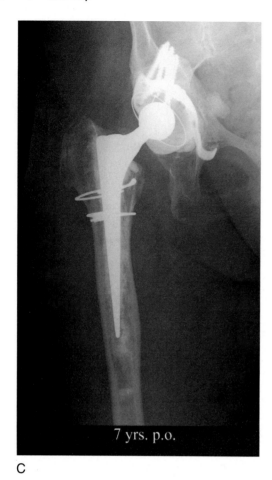

7 yrs. p.o.

C

Figure 63–4. *Continued.* **C**, Radiograph of the same hip 7 years after surgery. Note the lack of subsidence and what appears to be radiologic incorporation of the graft.

in postmortem femurs of patients who succumbed at different times after impaction grafting revision to problems other than the arthroplasty.[30,31,37,42] In all instances, there was a viable cortical shell, and the cancellous grafts were partially remodeled or, at times, surrounded by dense fibrous tissue that appeared capable of carrying load. It is possible that the impact of the graft on a vascularized bed has the potential for substitution and incorporation of this graft. In addition, the hoop stresses on the cement mantle generated by the collarless polished tapered stem may help the graft revascularization. Furthermore, because the graft is well fixed to the composite cement mantle and because the rotational stability is excellent, remodeling of the bony trabeculae may be facilitated.

Technical Aspects of the Procedure

The technique is complex and time consuming, requires great meticulousness, and is very expensive (a large amount of allograft is usually needed). Complete removal of the previous femoral component, as well as cement, fibrous membrane, and debris constitutes the usual first step. The endosteal surface of the femur must be perfectly cleaned. Reconstruction of segmental

defects with some type of screen (cobalt-chromium or Vicryl) or allograft struts is the next step. The femoral canal is then occluded 3 cm below the most distal cavitary deficiency or the most distal tip of the implant to be used (whichever is more distal). Use of a plastic cement restrictor or a cement plug is usually advisable.

Cancellous bone taken from allograft femoral heads, distal femurs, or both is prepared by means of rongeurs and a mechanized bone mill. Small fragments of 4 to 6 mm in size are advisable. Using a centering guide and then successive size packers and oversize tamps, the graft is impacted vigorously into the femoral canal until a new medullary canal is obtained. Emphasis must be placed on the vigor required for the impaction effort. Exquisite attention to the tamp rotation is, of course, essential when the new medullary canal is being prepared to avoid component malrotation. After a trial reduction, the cement is vacuum mixed, injected in retrograde fashion, and pressurized, and the stem is cemented. Postoperative care is routine and ambulation is encouraged, with touch-toe weight bearing for the first 8 weeks, followed by progression as tolerated.

The impaction cancellous allograft appears to be promising, particularly for restoration of bone stock in young patients with severe deficiencies, but longer follow-up of these patients is obviously necessary.

Distal Fixation with Tapered, Fluted, Grit-blasted Stems

In the last few years, a femoral component revision that started in Europe and has gained more adepts in North America is the use of fluted, tapered, grit-blasted titanium stems. These stems achieve longitudinal (axial) stability by their conical geometry and rotational stability by the presence of flutes, whereas a certain amount of ongrowth is obtained by their rough surface and their metallurgy (titanium alloy).

The precursor of these stems was the Wagner "self-locking stem,"[59] a monoblock fluted titanium alloy stem that has been used extensively in Europe but less in North America. Results reported with the use of this stem in revision have been satisfactory, with follow-ups of up to 10 years.[3,4] Birchers et al.[3] reported a 92 percent 10-year survivorship in 99 revisions, and Bohm and Bischel[4] reported only 6 reoperations after 129 revisions with this stem were followed for 4.8 years. Other authors[5,17,21,26,48,50,60] have also reported favorable results with medium-term follow-up. There are, however, two problems with this stem. The first is unacceptable implant subsidence; this is probably related to the monoblock nature of the stem. Moreover, the inherent difficulty in reaching optimal position relative to implant stability and limb length leads to insertional errors. The learning curve with this stem is steep and costly. The second problem, which is in part related to the first and also to the relatively short offset of this stem related to the pronounced valgus direction of the neck-shaft angle, is that there is a relatively high incidence of dislocation. My limited experience with the Wagner stem has confirmed the problems of subsidence and instability.

In an effort to solve the problems of the Wagner stem and keep its advantages, modular stems were developed. These stems allow independent engagement of the distal tapered, fluted stem in the femoral diaphysis, achieving axial and rotational stability and combining these features with a proximal body that allows optimization of leg length, femoral offset, and prosthetic joint stability. The modular junction located at a critical level of the component has been tested at least in one model[49] and found to be able to withstand high stresses and to be capable of long-term endurance. However, no clinical results of use of stems have been reported in the literature.

Indications for this type of stem are in a state of flux. They appear to be useful for certain periprosthetic fractures, because they can be used to bypass the fracture and achieve adequate stability (Fig. 63–5). Likewise, they may offer superior fixation in cases of femoral deformity that require shaft osteotomy at the time of arthroplasty. Moreover, in patients with very large femoral canals, they may produce less stress shielding than comparable sized, fully porous-coated stems.

Technical Aspects of Modular, Tapered, Fluted, Grit-blasted Titanium Stems

Because these stems require the creation of a tapered cone in the femoral canal, enough of the isthmus needs to be present to provide initial axial and rotational stability. Therefore, if there is not enough diaphysis to be milled to a supporting tapered cone, stability may not be reliably achieved. In addition, because the cone is created with straight reamers, if a long stem is needed, the normal anterior femoral bow introduces the risk of femoral perforation. The solution to this problem is to use an anterior extended femoral osteotomy, popularized by Wagner, that allows the surgeon to gain a straight path down the curved femur and avoid anterior perforation.

AUTHORS' PREFERENCE

The selection of a specific revision technique depends on a number of factors, most importantly the amount and quality of the remaining bone stock, the age and functional demands of the patient, the reason for failure

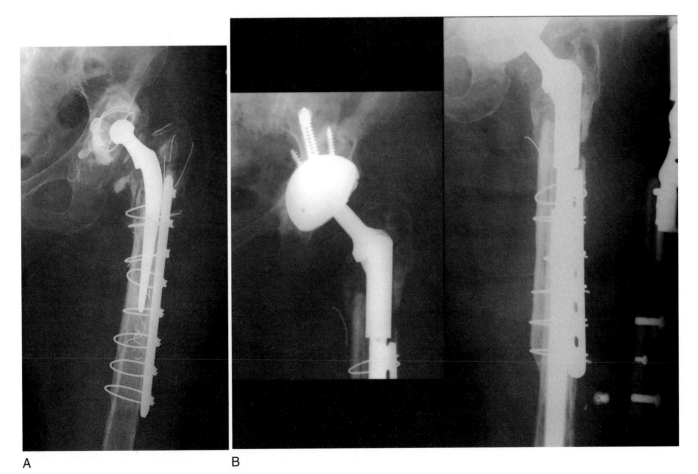

A   B

Figure 63–5. A, Radiograph of the left hip of an 85-year-old woman who had had a cemented total hip arthroplasty 16 years ago and had two additional surgeries in the past year for a periprosthetic fracture. She is unable to walk because of severe thigh pain. **B,** At surgery the fracture was found to be ununited, and a modular, tapered, fluted, grit-blasted titanium prosthesis was used to bypass the fracture. The patient was walking without pain 6 months after surgery.

of the primary procedure, and the judgment and personal preference of the surgeon. Each case must be studied individually, but the current preferences of my colleagues and I are described in the following paragraphs.

When the bone loss is minimal, especially if some of the cancellous bone is preserved, cemented stem fixation is our preference in the elderly patient. If a cemented stem is being revived and the original cement-bone interface remains good, we favor the cement-within-cement technique, which appears to provide excellent results.

In younger patients with minor bone loss and longer expected survival, the current trend is toward uncemented fixation, most commonly using an extensively coated prosthesis.

When moderate bone loss is present, cortical defects should first be repaired with cortical strut allografts before prosthetic reconstruction is performed. Then, if the diaphyseal bone is of good quality and the canal diameter is not in excess of 18 mm, an extensively porous-coated straight or curved stem of the proper length (6, 8, or 10 inches) is the preferred method of revision.

When significant cavitary defects, both metaphyseal and diaphyseal, are present after femoral preparation (rarer circumstances), we favor the use of impaction cancellous allograft and cement for femoral reconstruction, regardless of the patient's age. This is also our choice for very large, patulous femoral canals, although in some instances of signicant proximal bone loss with very large canals, we have more recently favored the use of modular, tapered, fluted, grit-blasted titanium stems. We have had very limited experience with modular stems of the S-ROM type.

Finally, in the very rare instances of major or massive bone loss, replacement of the proximal part of the femur with a prosthesis or, more frequently, with an allograft-prosthetic composite is our procedure of choice.

References

1. Askew MJ, Stege JW, Lewis JL, et al: Effect of cement pressure in bone strength on polymethylmethacrylate fixation. J Orthop Res 1:412, 1984.
2. Berry DJ, Harmsen WS, Ilstrup D, et al: Survivorship of uncemented proximally porous coated femoral components in revision total hip arthroplasty (in press).
3. Bircher HP, Riede U, Luem M, Ochsner PE: The value of the Wagner SL revision prosthesis for bridging large femoral defects. Orthopade 30:294, 2001.
4. Bohm P, Bischel O: Femoral revision with the Wagner SL revision stem: Evaluation of 129 revisions followed for a mean of 4.8 years. J Bone Joint Surg 83A:1023, 2001.
5. Boisgard S, Moreau PE, Tixier H, Levai JP: Bone reconstruction, leg length discrepancy, and dislocation rate in 52 Wagner revision total hip arthroplasties at 44-month follow-up. Rev Chir Orthop Reparatrice Appar Mot 87:147, 2001.
6. Callaghan JJ, Salvati EA, Pellicci PN, et al: Results of revision for mechanical failure after cemented total hip replacement. J Bone Joint Surg 67A:1074, 1985.
7. D'Antonio J, McCarthy JC, Barger WL, et al: Classification of femoral abnormalities in total hip arthroplasty. Clin Orthop 296:133, 1993.
8. De Roeck, Drabu KJ: Impaction bone grafting using freeze-dried allograft in revision hip arthroplasty. J Arthroplasty 16:201, 2001.
9. Duncan LP, Masterson EL, Masri BA: Impaction allografting with cement for the management of femoral bone loss. Orth Clin North 29:297, 1998.
10. Echeverri A, Shelly P, Wroblewski BM: Long-term results of hip arthroplasty for failure of previous surgery. J Bone Joint Surg 70B:49, 1988.
11. Elting JJ, Zycat BA, Mikhail WEN, et al: Impaction grafting: Report of a new method for exchange femoral arthroplasty. Orthopedics 18:107, 1995.
12. Engh CA, Glassman AH, Griffin WL, Meyer JG: Results of cementless revision for failed cemented total hip arthroplasty. Clin Orthop 235:91, 1988.
13. Estok DN, Harris WH: Long-term results of cemented femoral revision surgery using second generation techniques: Average 11.7 years follow-up. Clin Orthop 299:190, 1994.
14. Flugsrud GB, Ovre S, Grogaard B, Nordsletten L: Cemented femoral impaction bone grafting for severe osteolysis in revision hip arthroplasty. Good results at 4-year follow-up of 10 patients. Arch Orthop Trauma Surg 120:386, 2000.
15. Galante JO: Cementless femoral revision: BIAS results. Presented at the 24th Annual Hip Course, Boston, 1994.
16. Gie GA, Linder L, Ling RS, et al: Impacted cancellous allografts and cement for revision total hip arthroplasty. J Bone Joint Surg 75B:14, 1993.
17. Grunig R, Morscher E, Ochsner PE: Three-to-seven year results with the uncemented SL femoral revision prosthesis. Arch Orthop Trauma Surg 116:187, 1997.
18. Gustilo RB, Bechtold JE, Giacchetto J, Kyle RF: Rationale: Experience of long stem femoral prosthesis. Clin Orthop 249:159, 1989.
19. Hostner J, Hultmark P, Karrholm J, et al: Impaction technique and graft treatment in revision of the femoral component: Laboratory studies and clinical validation. J Arthroplasty 16:76, 2001.
20. Hussamy O, Lachiewicz PF: Revision total hip arthroplasty with the BIAS femoral component. J Bone Joint Surg 76A:1137, 1994.
21. Isacson J, Stark A, Wallensten R: The Wagner revision prosthesis consistently restores femoral bone structure. Int Orthop 24:139, 2000.
22. Karrholm J, Hultmark P, Carlsson L, Malchau H: Subsidence of a nonpolished stem in revisions of the hip suing impaction allograft. Evaluation with radiostereometry and dual-energy X-ray absorptiometry. J Bone Joint Surg 81:135, 1999.
23. Kavanagh BF, Fitzgerald RH Jr: Multiple revisions for failed total hip arthroplasty not associated with infection. J Bone Joint Surg 69A:1144, 1987.
24. Kavanagh BF, Ilstrup DN, Fitzgerald RH Jr: Revision total hip arthroplasty. J Bone Joint Surg 67A:517, 1985.
25. Knight JL, Helming C: Collarless polished tapered impaction grafting of the femur during revision total hip arthroplasty: Pitfalls of the surgical technique and follow-up in 31 cases. J Arthroplasty 15:159, 2000.
26. Kolstad K, Adalberth G, Mallmin H, et al: The Wagner revision stem for severe osteolysis. Thirty-one hips followed for 1.5–5 years. Acta Orthop Scand 67:541, 1996.
27. Lawrence JN, Engh CA, Macalino GE, Lauro GR: Outcome of revision hip arthroplasty done without cement. J Bone Joint Surg 76A:965, 1994.
28. Leopold SS, Berger RA, Rosenberg AG, et al: Impaction allografting with cement for revision of a femoral component. A minimum four-year follow-up study with use of a pre-coated femoral stem. J Bone Joint Surg 81:1080, 1999.
29. Lieberman JR, Moeckel BH, Evans BG, et al: Cement-within-cement revision hip arthroplasty. J Bone Joint Surg 75B:869, 1993.
30. Linder L: Cancellous impaction grafting in the human femur: Histological and radiographic observations in six autopsy femurs and eight biopsies. Acta Orthop Scand 71:543, 2000.
31. Ling RSN, Timperley AJ, Linder L: Histology of cancellous impaction grafting in the femur. J Bone Joint Surg 75B:693, 1993.
32. Lord G, Marotte JH, Guillamon JL, Blanchard JP: Cementless revision of failed aseptic cemented and cementless total hip arthroplasties. Clin Orthop 235:67, 1988.
33. Malkani AL, Lewallen DG, Cabanela ME, Wallrichs SL: Femoral component revision using an uncemented, proximally coated, long stem prosthesis (in press).

34. Marti RK, Schuller HM, Besselaar PP, Haasnoot ELV: Results of revision hip arthroplasty with cement: A 5–14 year follow-up study. J Bone Joint Surg 72A:346, 1990.
35. Mazhar Tokgozoglu A, Aydin M, Atilla B, Caner B: Scintigraphic evaluation of impaction grafting for total hip arthroplasty revision. Arch Orthop Trauma Surg 120:416, 2000.
36. Meding JB, Ritter MA, Keating EM, Faris PM: Impaction bone-grafting before insretion of a femoral stem with cement in revision total hip arthroplasty. A minimum two-year follow-up study. J Bone Joint Surg 79:1834, 1997.
37. Mikhail WE, Weidenhielm LR, Wretenberg P, et al: Femoral bone regeneration subsequent to impaction grafting during hip revision: Histologic analysis of a human biopsy specimen. J Arthroplasty 14:849, 1999.
38. Mikhail WE, Wretenberg PF, Weidenhielm LR, Mikhail MN: Complex cemented revision using polished stem and morselized allograft. Minimum 5 years' follow-up. Arch Orthop Trauma Surg 119:288, 1999.
39. Moreland J: Cementless revision arthroplasty. Presented at the Annual Meeting of the Hip Society Orlando, FL, February 1995.
40. Moreland JR, Moreno MD: Cementless femoral revision arthroplasty of the hip: Minimum 5 years follow-up. Clin Orthop 393:194–201, 2001.
41. Morrey BF, Kavanagh BF: Complications with revision of the femoral component of total hip arthroplasty: Comparison between cemented and uncemented techniques. J Arthroplasty 7:71, 1992.
42. Nelissen RG, Bauer TW, Weidenhielm LR, et al: Revision hip arthroplasty with the use of cement and impaction grafting. Histological analysis of four cases. J Bone Joint Surg 77:412, 1995.
43. Paprosky WG, Greidanus NV, Antoniou J: Minimum 10-year results of extensively porous-coated stems in revision hip arthroplasty. Clin Orthop 369:230, 1999.
44. Paprosky WJ: Twenty-fourth annual Hip Course. Harvard Medical School, Boston, September 1994.
45. Pekkarinen J, Alho A, Lepisto J, et al: Impaction bone grafting in revision hip surgery. A high incidence of complications. J Bone Joint Surg 82B:103, 2000.
46. Pellicci PN, Wilson PD, Sledge CB, et al: Long-term results of revision total hip arthroplasty: A follow-up report. J Bone Joint Surg 67A:513, 1985.
47. Pellicci PN, Wilson PD, Sledge CB, et al: Revision total hip arthroplasty. Clin Orthop 170:134, 1982.
48. Ponziani L, Rollo G, Bungaro P, et al: Revision of the femoral prosthetic component according to the Wagner technique. Chir Organi Mov 80:385, 1995.
49. Postak PD, Greenwald AS: The influence of modularity on the endurance performance of the Link® MP™ hip stem. Orthopaedic Research Laboratories. Cleveland, 2001.
50. Rinaldi E, Marenghi P, Vaienti E: The Wagner prosthesis for femoral reconstruction by transfemoral approach. Chir Organi Mov 79:363, 1994.
51. Rubash HE, Harris WH: Revision of non-septic loose cemented femoral components using modern cement techniques. J Arthroplasty 3:241, 1988.
52. Schreurs BW, Huiskes R, Slooff TJJH: The initial stability of cemented and noncemented femoral stems fixated with a bone grafting technique. Clin Mater 16:105, 1994.
53. Slooff TJ, Schimmel JW, Buma P: Cemented fixation with bone grafts. Orthop Clin North Am 24:667, 1993.
54. Stromberg CN: A multicenter 10 year study of cemented revision total hip arthroplasty in patients younger than 55 years old: The follow-up report. J Arthroplasty 9:595, 1994.
55. Stromberg CN, Herberts P, Ahnfelt L: Revision total hip arthroplasty in patients younger than 55 years: Clinical and radiologic results after four years. J Arthroplasty 3:47, 1988.
56. Stromberg CN, Palnertz B: Cemented revision hip arthroplasty: A multicenter 5–9 year study of 204 first revisions for loosening. Acta Orthop Scand 63:111, 1992.
57. Turner RH, Mattingly VA, Scheller A: Femoral revision total hip arthroplasty using a long stem femoral component: A clinical and radiographic analysis. J Arthroplasty 2:247, 1987.
58. van Biezen FC, ten Have BL, Verhaar JA: Impaction bone-grafting of severely defective femora in revision total hip surgery. 21 hips followed for 41–85 months. Acta Orthop Scand 71:135, 2000.
59. Wagner H, Wagner M: Femoral revision prosthesis with severe bone loss. In Kusswetter W(ed): Noncemented Total Hip Replacement: International Symposium. New York, Thieme Medical Publishers, 1990, p 301.
60. Wehrli U: Wagner revision of prosthesis stem. Z Unfallchir Versicherungsmed 84:216, 1991.
61. Woolson ST: Cementless femoral revision: Harris-Galante prosthesis. Presented at the 24th Annual Hip Course, Boston, 1994.
62. Younger TI, Bradford MS, Magnus MD, Paprosky WG: Extended proximal femoral osteotomy: A new technique for revision arthroplasty. J Arthroplasty 10:329, 1995.
63. Younger TI, Bradford MS, Paproski WG: Removal of a well-fixed cementless femoral component with an extended proximal femoral osteotomy. Contemp Orthop 30:375, 1995.

64

Diagnosis and Treatment of the Infected Hip Arthroplasty

• MARK J. SPANGEHL, ARLEN D. HANSSEN, and DOUGLAS R. OSMON

Deep wound infection after hip arthroplasty is one of the most distressing complications affecting this enormously successful surgical procedure. At the Mayo Clinic, for more than 30 years, deep infection has affected approximately 1 percent of 35,000 total hip arthroplasty patients, which is less than that for total knee arthroplasty.[5] Diligence with recognized prevention measures to reduce bacterial contamination, augment the host response, and optimize the wound environment in the preoperative, perioperative, and postoperative time periods are necessary to reduce the incidence of deep infection (see Chapter 10). Despite all precautions, infection occasionally and inevitably occurs after hip arthroplasty, and the subsequent treatment challenges the therapeutic resources of the orthopedic surgeon and infectious disease specialist. Although treatment methods and surgical techniques have improved significantly, rapid diagnosis and expeditious use of established treatment principles are essential to a successful outcome.

CLASSIFICATION

One available classification describes the mechanisms by which the bacteria are presented to the wound environment in four different modes: surgical contamination, hematogenous spread, recurrent infection, and infection from direct inoculation or contiguous spread.[108] This classification was based on 42 infected total hip arthroplasties, diagnosed from a cohort of 3215 hips. Thirteen hip infections were determined to be from surgical contamination, 19 were from a hematogenous source, 13 represented recurrent infection, and 4 were presumed to be from direct inoculation. Although this classification clearly depicts the various mechanisms of bacterial delivery to the wound, it is quite clear that when deep infection occurs, the specific mechanism of bacterial delivery to the wound is often unknown and that retrospective or emperic assignment is often arbitrary. Furthermore, the usefulness of this classification to guide management decisions in a specific clinical situation is quite limited.

Classification schemes are most useful when they provide prognostic information and effectively direct management decisions. Coventry's original classification of deep infection after total hip arthroplasty separated the clinical presentation of symptoms into three stages.[19,35] In this classification, stage I infections include the classic fulminant postoperative infection, the infected hematoma, and the superficial infection that progresses to a deep infection. Stage II infections include the chronic indolent infection that becomes apparent 6 to 24 months postoperatively. Stage III infections develop in a previously asymptomatic total hip arthroplasty 2 or more years postoperatively and are believed to be hematogenous in origin. Analysis of the first 3215 total hip arthroplasties performed at the Mayo Clinic revealed postoperative infection in 42 hips (1.3 percent), and in these hips, the diagnosis of infection was made in the first 3 months in 17 hips, between the 4th and 20th months in 18 hips, and between the 20th and 51st months in 7 hips.[35]

Coventry's three-stage classification system has been refined to more clearly articulate treatment guidelines according to current management concepts (Table 64–1).[117] This system describes 4 categories: (1) positive intraoperative culture (PIOC): diagnosed by two or more intraoperative cultures positive for the same organism and treated with 6 weeks of intravenous antibiotics and no surgical intervention; (2) early postoperative infection (EPOI): infection that develops within 1 month of prosthesis implantation and treated with débridement, exchange of polyethylene liners, retention of components, and intravenous antibiotics for 4 weeks; (3) late chronic infection (LCI): infection that becomes apparent more than 1 month from surgery and is characterized by an insidious clinical onset and treated with débridement, removal of prosthetic components, appropriate antibiotic treatment, and subsequently managed with various treatment options; and (4) acute hematogenous infection (AHI): acute onset of clinical symptoms in a previously well-functioning arthroplasty.

Table 64–1. CLASSIFICATION OF DEEP PERIPROSTHETIC INFECTION

	Type 1	Type 2	Type 3	Type 4
Timing	Positive intraoperative culture (PIOC)	Early postoperative infection (EPI)	Acute hematogenous infection (AHI)	Late (chronic) infection (LCI)
Definition	Two or more positive cultures at surgery	Infection occurs within the first month after surgery	Hematogenous seeding of previously well functioning arthroplasty	Chronic indolent clinical course; infection present for more than 1 month
Treatment	Appropriate antibiotics	Attempt at débridement with prosthesis salvage	Attempt at débridement with prosthesis salvage or prosthesis removal	Prosthesis removal

DIAGNOSIS

The basic fundamentals of diagnosis include a high index of suspicion combined with a thorough history, physical examination, plain radiographs, arthrocentesis, and several simple hematologic studies. Radionucleide studies and evaluation of surgical tissue specimens or the appearance of the hip joint are occasionally necessary to establish the diagnosis.

Clinical Presentation

Pain is the most common symptom in the patient with an infected hip arthroplasty and typically occurs while the patient is at rest. Onset of acute and fulminant infection in the immediate postoperative period is observed only rarely, most likely because of a decreasing incidence of deep infection caused by intraoperative contamination but also as a result of overuse of antibiotics, such as for persistent postoperative wound drainage. The use of antibiotics in this setting modulates the signs and symptoms of infection so that the diagnosis is delayed and is often made much later in the clinical course, when the chance for prosthesis salvage is less likely.

When purulent material drains from a red and swollen wound in a febrile patient, the diagnosis of postoperative infection is easily established. The major challenge encountered during the immediate postoperative period is differentiating between superficial and deep infection because there are no diagnostic, laboratory, roentgenographic, or scintigraphic techniques that establish this differentiation. Formal débridement with culture of deep tissue specimens is often the only way to diagnose the infected hip arthroplasty in the immediate postoperative setting. Spontaneous discharge of hematoma, wound dehiscence, or prolonged postoperative wound drainage are the most common indications for proceeding with open débridement.[35] When the patient is returned to the operating room for débridement of a draining wound, it is very difficult to determine whether the infection emanates from beneath the fascia. In contrast, a patient with a late hematogenous infection in a previously well functioning arthroplasty usually has acute onset of symptoms such as malaise, chills, fever, and an extremely painful hip, which usually facilitates rapid diagnosis.[35]

An entity termed incisional cellulitis has been reported in 16 cases of erythematous eruption on the skin within the flaps of the surgical incision after 2200 primary total hip replacement.[101] The symptoms began within 9 months of operation in 13 hips, and 2 to 3 years after surgery in 3 patients. All the patients had a similar appearance of the skin eruption, which began at the posterior skin flap and spread radially. The cause was unclear; however, compromise of the venous and lymphatic circulation around the skin flaps may have been responsible. All were treated with antibiotics (15 intravenous, 1 oral), with complete resolution of the eruption within 1 to 6 days. The primary difficulty was the determination of incisional cellulitis versus an underlying prosthetic infection.

Infections appearing in the subacute or chronic setting represent the greatest diagnostic challenge. These patients do not typically have systemic signs of infection, and the diagnosis is frequently overlooked. Persistence of a painful total hip arthroplasty should always alert the surgeon to the possibility of infection, and historical factors, such as persistent pain since the arthroplasty, prolonged postoperative wound drainage, and antibiotic treatment for difficulties with primary wound healing, should be specifically assessed in the patient with a painful prosthesis. For these individuals, laboratory tests are often important adjuncts in establishing the presence of deep infection.

Laboratory Parameters

The use of laboratory tests to diagnose an acute postoperative infection is often very confusing because the hemoglobin level, peripheral leukocyte count, and erythrocyte sedimentation rate are usually abnormal during this time period in the uncomplicated total hip arthroplasty. The diagnosis of infection in the immediate postoperative setting is not easily differentiated with laboratory, roentgenographic, or scintigraphic techniques. Diagnosis of the acute hematogenous infection in a previously painless arthroplasty is usually quite obvious and does not require sophisticated laboratory techniques. The patient with a painful prosthesis resulting from a chronic indolent infection represents the primary reason for the use of additional investigative laboratory tests. No test is 100 percent sensitive and 100 percent specific; therefore, the diagnosis of infection relies on the surgeon's judgement of the clinical presentation, the physical examination findings, and the results of previous investigations combined with the results of new laboratory tests.

The white blood cell count is rarely abnormal in patients who have an infection after a total hip arthroplasty, and it is not helpful for ruling infection in or out.[14,79] Some care must be taken in interpreting the erythrocyte sedimentation rate (ESR) or the C-reactive protein (CRP) level, because other factors, such as rheumatoid arthritis, recent surgery, neoplasia, collagen vascular disease, or an inflammatory condition also affect these tests. In the absence of these other variables, an ESR of more than 30 or 35 mm per hour and a CRP level of more than 10 mg per liter should be considered abnormal and should warrant additional investigation to rule out infection.[37,47,104,112] The ability of the CRP level to return to normal much faster than the ESR enables it to be a more sensitive indicator of infection, particularly in the early postoperative period.

In one study, none of the infected hips in which the implants had been in situ for more than 5 years were associated with a normal ESR.[62] We have observed otherwise and have seen patients with nonvirulent organisms and a normal ESR who develop infection more than 5 years after their index arthroplasty. It should be noted that the sensitivity of the ESR and the CRP are markedly diminished in the setting of a nonvirulent organism in the chronic indolent infected hip arthroplasty.[14,79,106] In 23 patients with a bacteriologically proven deep infection with a low virulent organism, the maximum ESR value was a median of 50 (range, 22 to 110 mm) mm and the maximal CRP value was 35 (range, 9 to 95 mg/L) mg/L.[106] When taken in isolation, normal values for CRP and ESR were observed in 26 percent of patients; however, when used in combination, only 1 patient had a normal value for both tests.[106] Based on this information, especially in the chronic setting of evaluation of a painful prosthesis, we believe the ESR or CRP, as isolated laboratory tests, are not suitable screening assays. In contrast, the combination of the ESR and the CRP has been labeled as the most useful screening investigation for the diagnosis of infection after hip arthroplasty and, when elevated, constitute the basis for obtaining additional tests to document the presence of infection.[112]

A newly described exocellular glycolipid antigen produced by coagulase-negative staphylococci produce can be detected with the enzyme-linked immunosorbent assay (ELISA).[95] The ELISA test for this antigen has been reported to have potential for the diagnosis of infection by distinguishing between staphylococcal infection around prostheses and aseptic loosening.[95] There were significant differences between the serum IgG and IgM levels in 15 patients with culture-proven infection of prostheses compared with a control group of 32 patients without infection ($P < 0.0001$).[95] We have no experience with this technique, but it or similar immunologic tests may be of increasing importance in the years ahead.

Plain Radiography

In the immediate postoperative period, and in the patient with late hematogenous infection, plain radiographs are usually normal, but it is extremely impor-

tant to obtain them because the status of prosthesis fixation is an important variable in the management decision process. Plain radiographs are of limited value in establishing the diagnosis of infection because many radiographic findings, such as loosening, osteolysis, and endosteal scalloping, are present in both septic and aseptic failure. Occasionally, findings such as periostitis, rapidly progressive and diffuse osteolysis, or endosteal scalloping strongly suggest infection.[69] Sequential review of all radiographs is necessary to improve the detection of these radiographic signs. Periosteal new-bone formation, with or without loosening of a component, has been considered by some to be pathognomonic of deep infection (Fig. 64–1).[37,47]

Arthrography

Arthrography of the hip can be helpful in the evaluation of the painful hip prosthesis. In 178 painful hip arthroplasties 75 (43 percent) had a pseudobursa demonstrated by arthrography and 12 (16 percent) of these hips with pseudobursa demonstrated a communicating irregular pattern.[6] Nine (75 percent) of the 12 hips with the irregular communicating bursae had a proven deep infection, which suggests that this arthrographic finding is a significant diagnostic clue for the presence of infection. The true value of arthrography is that fluid obtained by aspiration can be cultured.

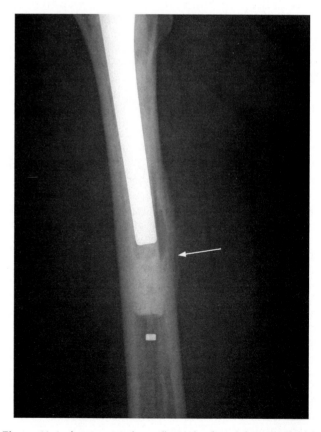

Figure 64–1. Anteroposterior radiograph of an infected total hip arthroplasty demonstrating the pathognomonic radiographic sign of periosteal new bone formation (arrow).

Aspiration of the Hip Joint

Routine use of aspiration in the evaluation of a painful hip arthroplasty is not indicated; rather, aspiration should be used selectively in patients with a history of wound-healing problems, radiographic changes, and elevated laboratory values.[30] When there is any suspicion regarding the presence of infection, aspiration remains one of the best preoperative tools available to document the presence of infection.[38,60,62,65,100,111,117] The reported rates of sensitivity and specificity of aspiration for culture have varied widely, with sensitivity ranging from 0.50 to 0.93 and specificity ranging from 0.82 to 0.97.[111] These results suggest that aspiration is better for ruling infection in than for ruling it out. The variability of results obtained from aspiration in prior series is in part due to the sample type obtained at aspiration, the number of samples obtained, the number of repeat aspirations, the unrecognized or unreported use of antibiotics before aspiration, and the lack of a so-called gold standard for comparison.[112] For example, in a prospective review, 12 patients with an infection had been receiving antibiotics before aspiration and only 6 had a positive result on aspiration.[110] Another reason is probably the technique of aspiration and how the samples are transported or handled after retrieval of fluid or tissue for culture. To improve accuracy, it has been proposed that a standard protocol should be established.[112]

This protocol requires discontinuation of all antibiotics 2 to 3 weeks before the aspiration, adherence to strict aseptic technique, use of local anesthetics only in the skin and not in the joint (because they are bacteriostatic), and verification of the intracapsular position of the needle with arthrography.[112] If sufficient fluid is obtained, the specimen is separated into three samples for culture; when insufficient fluid is obtained, the joint is irrigated with nonbacteriostatic saline solution and reaspirated. A needle biopsy of synovial tissue is also obtained at the time of the aspiration. The diagnosis is established when all three specimens reveal the same organism and these results correlate with the clinical profile. When only one sample is positive, the aspiration is repeated, and any repeat aspiration that reveals the same organism and antibiotic-sensitivity profile, confirms the diagnosis. When two of three samples are positive, the result is interpreted according to other tests. For example, if hematologic parameters are elevated without other apparent cause apart from infection, infection is likely, and the aspiration is not repeated. However, if the results of the laboratory investigations are normal or the parameters are elevated for other reasons, the aspiration is repeated.[112]

Radionuclide Imaging

Interest in scintigraphy continues but is limited by the cost and time required and the persistent unreliability of these scans in many different clinical settings. The technetium-99 scan has been recommended as an initial screening tool because this technique is very sensitive but nonspecific. If the technetium scan is negative, infection is unlikely and if the technetium scan is positive, other methods of scintigraphy can be performed. Gallium-67 citrate scans are also very nonspecific and are not recommended for the investigation of deep periprosthetic infection.[60]

The usefulness of indium-111-labeled white blood cells for the diagnosis of infection after hip arthroplasty remains controversial.[38,60,74,107,115] In one study of 98 patients with possible infection who had surgery within 14 days of the scans, it was determined that indium-111 scanning had an 88 percent sensitivity, 73 percent specificity, and 81 percent accuracy for the diagnosis of infection.[70] Another study that used sequential indium-111-labeled scans and complementary technetium-99-sulfur colloid imaging in suspected infected total hip arthroplasties, reported a 100 percent sensitivity, 97 percent specificity, and 98 percent accuracy.[86] Unlike others,[54] we have been impressed with the improvement in accuracy when we use these sequential scanning techniques; however, the interpretation of these scans still remains subjective. Therefore, although we do not rely solely on these tests, we continue to use them in equivocal cases.

Many new methods, such as 99Tc(m)-polyclonal human IgG (99Tc[m]-HIG) scintigraphy,[23] indium-111-labeled immunoglobulin scintigraphy,[80,82] or 18F-fluorodeoxyglucose (FDG) and positron emission tomography (PET) scanning,[127] are currently being developed and evaluated but require further appraisal before they are universally applied. One distinct disadvantage of many labeled antibody or immunoglobulin techniques is that these tests can be used only once in a given patient because of their antigenic nature and, therefore, sequential monitoring to assess response to therapy is not possible with many of these techniques.

Intraoperative Investigations

The Gram stain has been used as an investigation to confirm the presence or absence of bacteria in tissue specimens obtained from the failed hip arthroplasty. Although the Gram stain may be specific, it lacks any acceptable level of sensitivity.[32,60,111] The Gram stain is extremely unreliable and should not be used as a basis for determining treatment.[22] As such, we do not send tissue samples for Gram stain evaluation.

Intraoperative frozen sections are a valuable tool in the diagnosis of infection and are most useful in equivocal situations when preoperative investigations are confounding. Most investigators have reported favorable results with a sensitivity of 0.80 or more and a specificity of 0.90 or more.[2,32,67,83,84,93,111] As with aspiration, some of the variation is due in part to the low prevalence of infection and the variablility of criteria in some of the series.[87] Some have used an overall histologic picture rather than a specific number of polymorphonuclear cells per high-power field,[31] whereas others have recommended the use of 10 rather than 5 polymorphonuclear cells per high-power field to improve specificity without reducing sensitivity.[67] In this prospective analysis, the specificity improved from 0.96 to 0.99, whereas the sensitivity remained the same when 10 instead of 5 polymorphonuclear leukocytes per high-power field were used.[67] An important observation from that study is that tissue should be obtained from areas that appear to be most inflamed and that the pathologist should be experienced in interpretation of these specimens. We have found a substantial number of interobserver variations among pathologists in the interpretation of tissue obtained from patients with a failed total hip replacement.

Despite normal preoperative investigations, the appearance of some hips may appear infected to the surgeon during the surgical procedure. Frank pus and abscess formation are the most obvious signs of infection, whereas features such as diffuse synovitis, turbid joint fluid, and formation of slime are also suspicious. Sometimes the appearance of the joint is so suspicious for the presence of infection that the surgeon cannot proceed with the intended reconstructive procedure and chooses to wait for the results of cultures from tissue specimens obtained during the surgical procedure. Sometimes, these are false impressions, and, in our experience, when subsequent cultures are negative, we have found that wear debris from severe erosion of the polyethylene liner is potentially responsible for the tissue reaction observed by the surgeon. Unfortunately, the true value of the surgeon's intraoperative opinion may never be known because it is difficult to quantitate these opinions, and preoperative findings also influence these opinions. In one study, the association between the surgeon's intraoperative opinion and the pathologist's interpretation found a sensitivity of 0.70 and a specificity of 0.87.[32] The treatment options for these patients include leaving the prosthesis in place, performing a single-stage exchange, or performing resection arthroplasty and obtaining multiple specimens for culture, with reoperation later when the final results of culture are available.

An additional problem for the surgeon is the determination of whether there is persistent infection at the time of reimplantation after a period of treatment with a resection arthroplasty. In one study, analysis of frozen sections at the time of reimplantation after resection arthroplasty had a sensitivity of 25 percent, a specificity of 98 percent, a positive predictive value of 50 percent, a negative predictive value of 95 percent, and an accuracy of 94 percent.[21] This study suggests that a negative finding on intraoperative analysis of frozen sections has a high predictive value with regard to ruling out the presence of infection; however, the sensitivity of the test for the detection of persistent infection is poor.

Microbiology

The diagnosis of deep infection primarily rests on the isolation of the microorganism(s) from tissue specimens obtained about the hip through aspiration, biopsy, or surgery. Accurate identification of the pathogenic microorganism is critical, and preoperative cultures are helpful to direct intitial postoperative antibiotic therapy. Coagulase-negative staphylococci are the most common microorganisms (28 percent) recovered from an infected total hip arthroplasty at our institution, whereas Staphylococcus aureus (17 percent) is the second most common. This distribution is distinctly different compared with the infected total knee arthroplasty, where S. aureus is most common. In the absence of the isolation of microorganisms from clinical material, histologic examination of the tissue about the hip must demonstrate changes characteristic of infection. Our current definition of prosthetic infection includes a combination of clinical symptoms and signs, histologic analysis of tissue, and results of cultures. The diagnosis of definite infection is made if evaluation of the hip joint establishes at least one of the following criteria: (1) two or more cultures obtained by aspiration or deep tissue specimens obtained at surgery that yield the same organism; (2) histopathologic evaluation of intra-articular tissue reveals changes of acute inflammation; (3) gross purulence is observed at the time of surgery; or (4) there is an actively discharging sinus tract.

There are many potential problems with routine culture and sensitivity testing of specimens, which include appropriate handling, transport, and the technique of plating. Open communication between the physician and the microbiology laboratory is essential so that special culture techniques are performed when there is clinical suspicion of atypical microorganisms or when specific antibiotic sensitivity testing is required. For example, Staphylococcus lugdunensis, a coagulase-negative bacterium, is more virulent than other coagulase-negative staphylococci and, in many clinical situations, behaves like S. aureus and frequently produces a clumping factor resulting in a positive slide (short) coagulase test result.[103] If the microbiology laboratory does not use the tube coagulase (long) test, the organism may be misidentified as S. aureus. Because S. lugdunensis is susceptible to many antibiotics, specific testing of the isolates helps the clinician to choose the appropriate antibiotic. Moreover, correct identification also clarifies the epidemiology, pathogenesis, and correct treatment to combat this organism in prosthetic joint infections.

Another problem is that some bacteria are simply not isolated by routine culture techniques. A technique involving immediate transfer of prostheses to an anaerobic atmosphere was followed by mild ultrasonication to dislodge adherent bacteria. This approach resulted in the culture of quantifiable numbers of bacteria from 26 of the 120 implants, whereas the same bacterial species were cultured by routine techniques in only 5 corresponding tissue samples.[119] Tissue removed from the culture-positive implants showed that inflammatory cells were present in all samples. This suggests that these implants may have been infected by bacteria not isolated by the routine techniques of culture. We are currently investigating this ultrasonication technique in a prospective evaluation of aseptic and septic hip and knee arthroplasties.

TREATMENT

Among the multitude of therapeutic approaches, the common basic treatment objectives have been eradication of infection, alleviation of pain, and restoration of function. Fundamental treatment principles include appropriate use of antibiotics combined with thorough surgical débridement. There are multiple variables and considerations directing the physician and patient to the most appropriate choice of a treatment plan. The six basic management options include: (1) antibiotic suppression, (2) open débridement, (3) resection arthroplasty, (4) arthrodesis, (5) reimplantation of another prosthesis, and (6) amputation (Table 64–2). With the exception of chronic antibiotic suppression, which does not eliminate infection, the cornerstone principles of these treatment options include thorough surgical débridement combined with the appropriate use of antibiotics.

Treatment with Antibiotics Only

Antibiotic Suppression

Occasionally, in elderly or frail individuals, suppressive antibiotic therapy may be selected, with full recognition that the infection will not be eliminated. This method of management should be rarely selected and used only when the following criteria are met: (1) prosthesis removal is not feasible (usually because of a medical condition that precludes an operative procedure), (2) the microorganism has low virulence, (3) the microorganism is susceptible to an oral antibiotic, (4) the antibiotic can be tolerated without serious toxicity, and (5) the prosthesis is not loose.[41,118] Combining limited clinical data reveals that antibiotic suppression was successful, defined only as retention of the prosthesis, in 9 (31 percent) of 29 hips.[37,41,47,118] Despite the fact that most patients fail to meet all of these criteria, this method of treatment is more commonly attempted than the literature suggests, a practice that, unfortunately, prolongs the presence of infection and often complicates subsequent treatment attempts. In particular, this practice in younger, healthy patients is to be condemned because the use of suppressive therapy can convert a relatively localized infectious process with a susceptible organism into an extensive and recalcitrant condition with a much more resident organization, making eradication of the infection a formidable or impossible task.

Treatment with Surgical Intervention

General Principles

Many aspects of the surgical débridement are similar regardless of the selected treatment approach. Old incisions are used to expose the hip unless exposure will be compromised. Many incisions are invaginated, and it is often advisable to excise the scar and any adjacent sinus tracts so that the skin and subcutaneous tissue layers are well vascularized and will heal readily. Antibiotics are withheld until tissue specimens are obtained from the pseudocapsule and the bone-prosthetic interfaces of both components. Thorough débridement is an essential factor, but it is recognized that this variable is difficult to quantify and assess. Retained bone cement is one of the variables related to adequacy of débridement and has been shown to be associated with an increased risk of recurrent infection after a delayed reconstruction technique.[34,73,117] Most surgeons are cognizant of the difficulty in localizing and removing all cement, and, despite the most careful efforts, additional pieces of cement are often accidentally discovered in obscure areas of the wound. The ability to assess the presence of retained cement postoperatively is actually quite limited, and this may be one factor accounting for the differences in success among studies. The use of a 10-mm laparoscope can be extremely helpful in the search for retained cement in the medullary canal.

It is also difficult to know how many sequential procedures should be performed to acheive adequate débridement. Currently, the vast majority of infected hips at our clinic are treated with one surgical débridement unless there is extensive soft-tissue necrosis or other extenuating circumstances. For example, if there is extreme difficulty localizing or removing all bone cement, additional tests, such as tomograms or CT scanning, are occasionally helpful, and additional débridement can be performed in several days.[18] Open wound management should be avoided in the care of the infected hip arthroplasty because wound contracture often leads to a recalcitrant hip wound,[74] and the wound often becomes infected with multi–drug-resistant nosocomial organisms.

Débridement with Prosthesis Retention

Open débridement is occasionally indicated for acute, fulminant infection in the immediate postoperative period or for the late hematogenous infection of a

Table 64–2. TREATMENT OF INFECTED THA

Variables	Options	Goals
• Depth of infection	• Antibiotic suppression	• Eradication of infection
• Time elapse since surgery	• Débridement	• Alleviation of pain
• Soft-tissues	• Resection arthroplasty	• Maintenance of function
• Prosthesis fixation	• Arthrodesis	
• Pathogens	• Amputation	
• Host factors	• Reimplantation	
• Physician capabilities		
• Patient expectations		

securely fixed and previously functional prosthesis. Suggested criteria for use of this management technique include (1) short duration of symptoms (less than 3 to 4 weeks), (2) susceptible gram-positive organisms, (3) no prosthetic loosening, and (4) absence of excessive scar tissue from prior surgical procedures.[10,20,114] There is a relative contraindication for débridement and attempted salvage of the prosthesis for the patient with multiple joint replacements; the rationale of the relative contraindication is to reduce the risk of metachronous infection to these other joints.[76] The available results of débridement are difficult to assess because of variability in the time to treatment, differences in microbiology and susequent antibiotic management, extent and completeness of débridement, status of implant fixation, quality of the surrounding soft tissues, and the criteria for success in each report.

The original Mayo Clinic experience detailed surgical débridement in 18 infected total hip arthroplasties.[35] Fifteen of these débridements were performed in the first month after implantation and were successful in 6 of 8 infected hematomas that were judged to extend beneath the deep fascia. The other 7 débridements were unsuccessful, and factors responsible for failure included excessive scar tissue from multiple prior surgical procedures and onset of deep infection after prolonged postoperative wound drainage, which may have indicated that the infection was present for a long time before the débridement was attempted. Of two patients with acute onset of late hematogenous infection, one was successfully treated with débridement.

In a large series of 41 infected total hip arthroplasties treated with surgical débridement, 35 hips were treated in the first month after arthroplasty (EPOI) and 6 were treated for AHI.[117] Débridement was successful in 26 (74 percent) EPOI hips and 3 (50 percent) AHI hips. In contrast with the results reported in the combined literature, the reports detailed earlier in this chapter suggest that urgent and aggressive surgical débridement is occasionally reasonable and relatively successful if the treatment indications and patient selection criteria outlined earlier are rigidly applied.

Our experience over the past few years details surgical débridement in 42 additional infected total hip arthroplasties, all with well-fixed components.[20] After a mean duration of follow-up of 6.3 years, only 6 patients (14 percent) were successful. Four of 19 who had had an early postoperative infection and 2 of 4 who had had an acute hematogenous infection were managed successfully, whereas all 19 patients who had a late chronic infection were deemed to have had a failure of treatment. Débridement had been performed at a mean of 6 days (range, 2 to 14 days) after the onset of symptoms in the patients who had been managed successfully, and at a mean of 23 days (range, 3 to 93 days) in those for whom treatment had failed. Based on this experience, we believe débridement with retention of the prosthesis is potentially successful for early postoperative infection or acute hematogenous infection, provided that it is performed in the first 2 weeks after the onset of symptoms and that the prosthesis previously had been functioning well. This procedure has not been successful when it has been performed more than 2 weeks after the onset of symptoms. This window of opportunity is much smaller when the offending organism is *S. aureus*, because prostheses that were débrided more than 2 days after onset of symptoms were associated with a higher probability of treatment failure than those that were débrided within 2 days of onset (relative risk, 4.2; 95 confidence interval, 1.6 to 10.3).[10] The important conclusions drawn from this experience are that expeditious treatment is essential, and prosthesis retention in patients who have a chronic infection universally fails.

A report of arthroscopic irrigation and débridement for late, acute periprosthetic infection in 8 hips was successful in all cases at an average of 70 months of follow-up.[50] These authors stressed that effective treatment requires early diagnosis, prompt arthroscopic débridement, well-fixed components, a sensitive microorganism, and the patient's tolerance of and compliance with antibiotic therapy. It is also important to note that these patients were carefully selected, and all were placed on long-term suppressive antibiotic therapy. We have had no experience with this technique in such a clinical setting and prefer open débridement over arthroscopic débridement for the infected hip arthroplasty.

Resection Arthroplasty

Resection arthroplasty of the hip with excision of all foreign material has been the most definitive method of eradicating infection.[14,16,42] Although resection arthroplasty often provides marked relief from pain, most patients require the use of ambulatory aids, fatigue easily, have a Trendelenburg gait, experience hip joint instability, and have a large limb-length discrepancy.[8,42,56,92,109] Implantation of another prosthesis for the failed, infected total hip arthroplasty provides the patient with markedly better functional recovery than a resection arthroplasty.[4,88,109] Some patients are not candidates for reimplantation, and for these patients, a resection arthroplasty is then performed as a definitive procedure (Fig. 64–2). It should also be recognized and conveyed to the patient that choosing resection arthroplasty as the initial treatment option does not "burn any bridges," and if that patient desires implantation of another prosthesis many years later and is an acceptable candidate for reimplantation, an arthroplasty can be performed at that time.

Arthrodesis

Unlike the knee joint, arthrodesis of the hip joint after the treatment of an infected total hip arthroplasty has only rarely been advocated.[59] In a series of 14 patients treated with hip arthrodesis for a failed hip arthroplasty, 7 hips failed because of infection. The average age of patients with an infected arthroplasty was 39 years (range, 24 to 67 years), and many were engaged in high-demand occupations. All hips were successfully fused with a modification of the A-O technique, with use of a laterally placed cobra plate, an anteriorly contoured Dynamic A-O compression plate, and autogenous bone

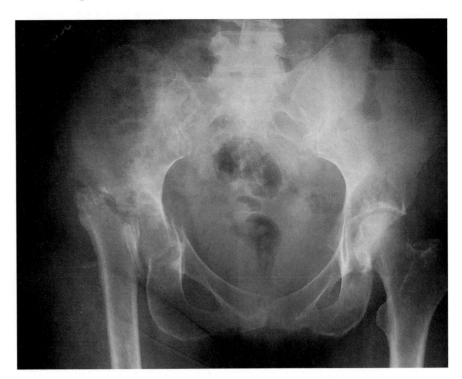

Figure 64–2. Anteroposterior radiograph of a patient treated by resection arthroplasty of the hip for treatment of an infected hip arthroplasty.

graft. Postoperatively the patients were placed in a hip spica cast. These authors strongly recommend this formidable but definitive procedure for the young, active patient with a failed arthroplasty.

Amputation (Disarticulation)

Although hip disarticulation is occasionally required to control life-threatening infection, the need for this procedure for the infected hip joint is exceedingly rare and has been reported from only one center.[12,33] These authors performed hip disarticulation in 11 (1.3 percent) of 857 infected total hip arthroplasties and indicated that this procedure was required for (1) life-threatening infection, (2) severe loss of soft tissue and bone stock, and (3) vascular injury. Combining multiple series, which allow assessment of outcomes for all patients treated for an infected hip arthroplasty in that medical center for the time period of the reported study, indicate that hip disarticulation occurred in 0.7 percent of 1682 infected total hip arthroplasties.[37,47]

Although we also performed several hip disarticulations for the treatment of an infected hip arthroplasty, a new technique termed the tibia-hindfoot osteomusculocutaneous rotationplasty with calcaneopelvic arthrodesis has been developed in an effort to avoid hip disarticulation (Fig. 64–3).[91] This procedure is indicated for the patient who would otherwise require hip disarticulation for severe loss of bone stock but who has a good limb distal to the knee joint. After resection of the remaing distal femur, the lower leg is prepared by removing the skin and subcutaneous tissue and disarticulating the foot distal to the calcaneus. The leg is then "turned up" and placed within the soft tissue envelope of the thigh so that the calcaneus is placed and fused within the acetabular defect. The proximal tibia is thus positioned distally and serves as a weight-bearing stump, whereas the tibiotalar joint allows reasonable motion at the level of the previous hip joint. This procedure has successfully allowed these patients to function at a low thigh amputation level or knee disarticulation level, which is a vast improvement over the function achieved after hip disarticulation.

Insertion of Another Prosthesis

General Principles and Controversies

Reimplantation of another prosthesis has become the desirable method of treatment for most patients with an infected total hip arthroplasty.[37,72] The potential for improved functional outcome with another prosthesis must be balanced against the disadvantage of a higher reinfection rate compared with a definitive resection arthroplasty. Generally accepted contraindications for reimplantation include (1) persistent or recalcitrant infection, (2) medical conditions that prevent multiple reconstructive procedures, and (3) severe local soft tissue damage or systemic conditions that will most likely predispose toward reinfection.

Controversies and questions regarding the reimplantation of another prosthesis include (1) the proper duration and route of antibiotic therapy; (2) the concept of organism "virulence"; (3) the role of local antibiotic delivery systems, such as antibiotic-impregnated bone cement spacers, beads, or antibiotic-loaded prostheses; (4) the efficacy of antibiotic-impregnated bone cement for the revision surgery; (5) the proper time delay from removal of the infected prosthesis to insertion of another prosthesis; (6) the method of fixation of reimplantation prostheses; (7) the role of spacers in promoting ease

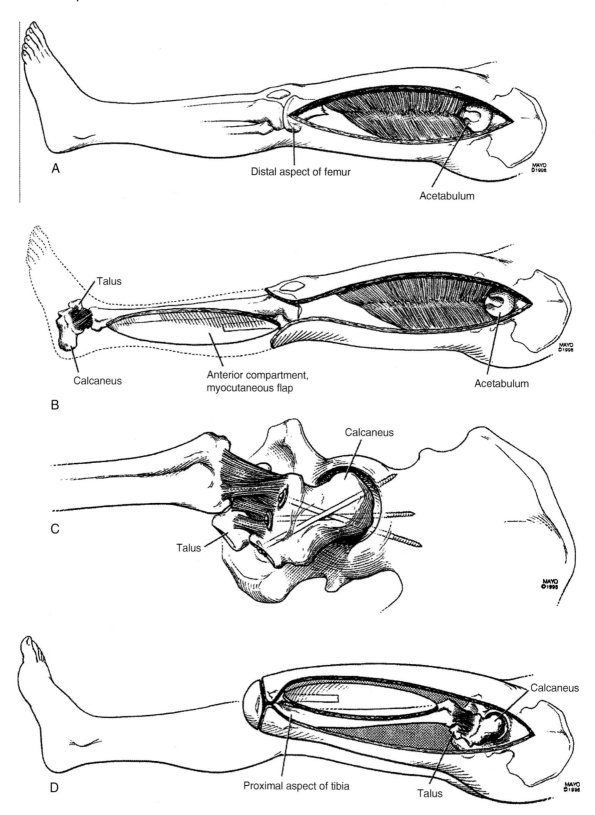

Figure 64–3. **A**, The soft tissue envelope in the thigh is contoured to accept the tibia. **B**, The acetabulum is reamed to expose bleeding cancellous bone approximately the same size as the calcaneal tuberosity. An ovoid musculocutaneous flap, centered over the muscles of the anterior compartment of the leg, is created. **C**, The remaining portion of the distal femur and the proximal tibia are resected. The tibia and musculocutaneous flap are rotated and the calcaneal tuberosity is twisted in the reamed acetabulum. The calcaneus then is fixed into the acetabulum with cancellous-bone screws and supplemented with morcellized cancellous bone graft. **D**, The abductor muscles are sutured to the fascia lata, and the tibial soft tissue envelope is closed. The adductor muscles are sutured through holes in the tibia to facilitate stump control. (From Peterson CA II, Koch LD, Wood MB: Tibia-hindfoot osteomusculocutaneous rotationplasty with calcaneopelvic arthrodesis for extensive loss of bone from the proximal part of the femur. A report of four cases. J Bone Joint Surg 79A:1504–1509, 1997. By permission of Mayo Foundation for Medical Education and Research.)

of surgical technique or final clinical function; and (8) the use of structural allografts for reconstruction.

Many of these variables are codependent and analysis in most reports is hindered by small patient numbers and the effect of historical perspective because there have been many changes and improvements that have evolved simultaneously since the early 1970s. We believe that a staging system that clearly delineates infection type, host, and wound variables is necessary to stratify patients appropriately so that different treatment approaches can be effectively analyzed.[5,94] We are currently involved in a consensus group of the Musculoskeletal Infection Society to develop such a staging system.

Antimicrobial Therapy

The optimal duration of intravenous antibiotics for the treatment of patients with an infected total hip arthroplasty has not been definitively established. Although some have recommended 6 weeks of intravenous antibiotics, others have empirically chosen 4 weeks of intravenous antibiotics, and review of available reports reveals the duration of antibiotic therapy to be extremely variable, ranging from 0 to 9 weeks of intravenous therapy and no oral antibiotics to more than 2 years of oral therapy.[14,40,49,123,128]

Although there are some general guidelines for the use of intravenous antibiotic therapy, there is no consensus on the proper use of oral antibiotics for the treatment of an infected total hip arthroplasty. There has been interest in the safety and efficacy of long-term treatment with oral antibiotics, particularly in combination with rifampin, for the treatment of infected orthopedic implants.[25,26,113,123,128] Some of these regimens have been a combination of initial intravenous therapy followed by oral antibiotics and have been performed with or without initial surgical débridement. In a randomized, placebo-controlled, double-blind trial, 33 patients with culture-proven staphylococcal infection of stable orthopedic implants with a short duration (less than 1 year) of symptoms were treated.[128] Treatment consisted of initial débridement and a 2-week intravenous course of flucloxacillin or vancomycin with rifampin or placebo, followed by either ciprofloxacin-rifampin or ciprofloxacin-placebo. The cure rate was 100 percent in the ciprofloxacin-rifampin group compared with 58 percent in the ciprofloxacin-placebo group (P=.02).[128] Only 24 patients fully completed the trial, with a follow-up of 34 months, because 9 of 33 patients dropped out due to adverse events (No.=6), noncompliance (No.=1), or protocol violation (No.=2). The addition of oral rifampin with intravenous antibiotics also appears to be effective in animal models[51] and in the clinical setting with traditional two-stage treatment protocols.[48,52]

Salvati and co-workers have paid the most attention to the optimal type and duration of antibiotic therapy needed to treat deep periprosthetic joint infection.[66,102] They have recommended a two-stage reimplantation protocol in selected patients consisting of resection arthroplasty and followed by 6 weeks of intravenous antibiotics in doses sufficient to achieve a postpeak serum bactericidal titer (SBT) of at least 1:8, in which the SBT represents the highest serum dilution, killing 99 percent of the infecting organism.[66,102] By definition, the use of this strict protocol prevents any comparative determination about the necessary duration of antibiotic therapy.

In a retrospective study of delayed hip reconstruction at our clinic, 35 patients received less than 4 weeks of intravenous antibiotics, whereas 44 had more than 4 weeks.[73] Antibiotic-impregnated beads or spacers were not used and antibiotic-impregnated cement was not used at reimplantation. Although reinfection occurred in 7 (20 percent) of 35 patients receiving less than 4 weeks of therapy compared with 4 (9 percent) of 44 patients receiving 4 or more weeks of therapy, this difference was not statistically significant (P=0.19).

Organism Virulence

Although many orthopedic surgeons have been of the opinion that gram-negative infections are more difficult to treat and are more susceptible to recurrence,[12,17,35,55] others have demonstrated no difference in the incidence of recurrent infection with either gram-positive or gram-negative organisms.[4,36,66,73,79] It is our current opinion that certain organisms, such as S. aureus, are indeed more virulent and more prone to treatment failure with procedures such as débridement with porsthesis salvage[10] and may have a higher risk of failure with delayed reimplantation protocols.[9] These concerns regarding S. aureus have been previously reported.[40]

It is important to distinguish between the concepts of virulence and resistance. In the current era, a higher proportion of patients have organisms that are considered as multi–drug-resistant.[46,53,58] Infections caused by methicillin-resistant staphylococci are currently the most commonly encountered resistant organisms; however, others such as vancomycin-resistant enterococci are now being encountered. The primary problem with these resistant organisms is that the options for available antibiotics, particularly oral agents, are limited, and thereby the treatment options of débridement with prosthesis retention or single-stage exchange are severely restricted.[46,53,58]

Certain bacteria are capable of forming an exopolysaccharide-glycocalyx or "slime," which was previously considered to be a protective biofilm permitting microbial growth with protection from antibodies and antibiotics. Although tests are available to determine the production of glycocalyx in laboratory cultures, the association between glycocalyx production and recurrence of infection is not available, and, therefore, these tests are not currently clinically relevant.

Subsequent studies suggest that antibiotic resistance is not related to the ability to produce slime but rather is associated with metabolic characteristics associated with surface colonization, and that these changes are dependent on the specific type of biomaterial substrate.[77] This study demonstrated that consistently higher mean inhibitory concentration (MIC) levels were required for adherent bacteria and this was particularly true of bacteria adherent to polymethylmethacrylate compared with bacteria adherent to polyethylene.[77] This concept of changing antibiotic susceptibility, based on a specific organism combined with a specific biomaterial, has significant bearing on many of the treatment concepts already discussed. For example, the serum bactericidal titer and MIC testing methods performed in vitro may not reflect the true antibiotic susceptibility of the infecting organism if retained pieces of bone cement or other foreign objects remain in the wound.

Antibiotic-impregnated Bone Cement

The concept of local antibiotic delivery by incorporation of gentamicin into acrylic bone cement was initially proposed by Buchholz as a prophylactic method and subsequently developed into a therapeutic application.[12] Investigators have evaluated the elution of a wide assortment of antibiotics from a variety of different acrylic bone cements under a variety of different conditions.[24,27,39,57,61,89,90] Antibiotics leach in higher concentrations and over longer time periods from Palacos bone cement than from Simplex-P, C.M.W., and Sulfix acrylic bone cements.[89] The amount of antibiotic elution is highly dependent on the porosity of the bone cement and the concentration of antibiotics present in the cement.[6,14,61] The addition of 25 percent dextran, which increases porosity, greatly facilitates elution of antibiotics.[61] Lincomycin and tetracycline are deactivated by the polymerization process of polymethylmethacrylate, whereas the addition of rifampin prevents the polymerization of the bone cement.[24,47] Combining two antibiotics in bone-cement improves elution of both drugs, and the minimal combination of 2.4 g tobramycin and 1.0 g vancomycin per 40-g packet of bone cement powder has been suggested.[89]

Antibiotic-impregnated cement as a local antibiotic-delivery system can be used in the form of beads or spacers between the time of resection arthroplasty and reimplantation (and also at reimplantation) when incorporated in bone cement used for prosthesis fixation. A distinct disadvantage of using beads about the hip joint is the extreme difficulty of removing these beads after approximately 6 weeks. Large amounts of antibiotic powder (up to 8 or 9 g of antibiotic per 40-g packet of bone cement) can be added to the cement for beads and spacers, but most physicians use only 1 to 2 g of antibiotic powder per batch of cement prepared for prosthesis fixation to avoid significant mechanical weakening of the acrylic mixture.[24] Elson has frequently used up to 4.5 g per batch in the bone cement used for prosthesis fixation, at 12 years of follow-up, with survival analysis in 239 hips, no difference in mechanical loosening was observed when comparison was made using ratios of less than or more than 2.5 g per 40 g of cement.[28] The clinical experience with antibiotic-impregnated cement has been widespread.[11,13,15,36,43–46,48,49,52,53,57,58,66,68,71,78,81,96–99,102,105,117,120–122,125,126] The use of antibiotic-impregnated cement for prosthesis fixation has been almost universal in conjunction with use of a direct-exchange technique but has been controversial among surgeons who have favored delayed reconstruction. The potential efficacy and results obtained with antibiotic-impregnated cement and time delay are discussed later in this chapter (Fig. 64–4).

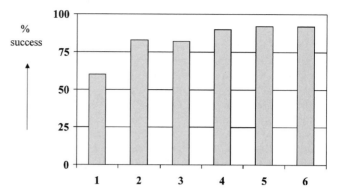

Figure 64–4. Graph demonstrating the independent beneficial effects of delayed reconstruction and the use of antibiotic-loaded bone cement for prosthesis fixation at the time of reimplantation. 1 = Direct exchange without antibiotic-loaded bone cement (60 percent success); 2 = direct exchange with antibiotic-loaded bone cement (83 percent); 3 = delayed reimplantation without antibiotic-loaded bone cement (82 percent success); 4 = delayed reconstruction, no antibiotic-impregnated beads or spacers, and antibiotic-impregnated cement for the reimplantation (90 percent success); 5 = delayed approach with antibiotic-impregnated beads or spacers for local antibiotic delivery in addition to the use of antibiotic-impregnated cement at reimplantation (92 percent success); and 6 = use of antibiotic-loaded beads or spacers and an uncemented femoral component during a delayed reconstruction approach (92 percent).

Direct-Exchange Reconstruction

One of the primary decisions facing the physician treating an infected hip arthroplasty is the selection of a direct-exchange technique or a delayed reconstruction. Advocates of the direct-exchange method cite lower morbidity in their patients who escape from the time period with a resection arthroplasty, lower costs because of the absence of a second hospitalization and surgical procedure, and avoidance of the technical difficulty associated with implanation in delayed reconstructive techniques.[13,15,28,75,96–98,105,120] Disadvantages of this approach include the inability to add antibiotics to the bone cement based on cultures from surgical tissue samples and the distinct possibility that the newly implanted prosthesis may be exposed for days to organisms not covered by the antibiotics in the bone cement or by those provided intravenously until culture results from the surgery have been obtained.

Based on a large literature review, the factors associated with a successful direct exchange included (1) absence of wound complications after the initial total hip replacement; (2) good general health of the patient; (3) methicillin-sensitive *Staphylococcus epidermidis*, S. aureus, and streptococcus species; and (4) an organism that was sensitive to the antibiotic mixed into the bone cement.[53] Factors associated with failure included (1) polymicrobial infection; (2) gram-negative organisms, especially pseudomonas species; and (3) certain gram-positive organisms such as methicillin-resistant *S. epidermidis* and group D *Streptococcus*.[53] These authors noted that methicillin-resistant organisms have become more common, many current revision surgical techniques use cementless implants, fixation without antibiotic-impregnated cement may be a contraindication to direct exchange, and that there essentially are no data on the use of bone graft in association with direct exchange. For these reasons, the authors have changed their view on direct exchange and stated that the current indications for this technique are limited.

We reviewed 37 infected hip arthroplasties treated consecutively to test the feasibility of published patient selection criteria for direct exchange arthroplasty.[46] These criteria include the requirement of a healthy patient with good soft tissue, minimal femoral bone loss, and an organism identified preoperatively as an antibiotic-sensitive gram-positive organism.[120] Only 4 patients (4 hips) (11 percent) were deemed potential candidates for a direct exchange procedure. Infected arthroplasties excluded from a primary exchange included 14 patients (15 hips) with gram-negative or methicillin-resistant gram-positive organisms obtained from preoperative joint aspirations, 10 patients (10 hips) with moderate or severe femoral bone loss, 4 patients (4 hips) who required a proximal femoral osteotomy for component removal, 2 patients (2 hips) with poor health status, and 2 patients (2 hips) with poor soft tissue. We concluded that with the increasing emergence of antibiotic-resistant bacteria and an increased prevalence of revision arthroplasties with associated bone loss, the feasibility of published selection criteria for direct exchange is limited.

Contrary to generally accepted criteria for direct-exchange,[13,120] Raut et al. have detailed in several reports their experience with one-stage revision of infected total hip arthroplasty associated with a draining sinus or in the presence of a gram-negative organism.[96-98] They reported an 86 percent cure rate in 57 hips with draining sinuses at an average follow-up of 7.4 years,[97] and a cure rate of 93.4 percent for patients with gram-negative infections at an average follow-up of 8 years.[96] They attributed their success to meticulous surgical technique and use of preoperative parenteral antibiotics and antibiotic-loaded cement. These results have yet to be reproduced by other investigators.

If the choice is made to perform a direct exchange, the use of antibiotic-impregnated cement for prosthesis fixation appears to be quite important. Direct exchange using plain bone cement not impregnated with antibiotics has been successful in 40 (60 percent) of 67 infected total hip arthroplasties, whereas success was achieved in 1352 (83 percent) of 1630 hips treated with the use of antibiotic-impregnated cement (Fig. 64–4).[47] Although the use of a direct exchange technique is far more common in Europe than in North America, if this approach seems desirable in individual patients, we would suggest careful preoperative selection combined with use of antibiotic-impregnated cement for prosthesis fixation. In our opinion, a philosophy of delayed reconstruction for the treatment of the infected hip arthroplasty seems most appropriate in the current era of patient treatment.

Delayed Reconstruction

Delayed reconstruction techniques allow the physician to observe the patient's response to therapy and to assess the possibility of recurrence after antibiotics are stopped.

Disadvantages of this approach include the hardship experienced by patients with a resection arthroplasty, the need and attendant costs of a second surgical procedure, and the technical difficulties associated with prosthesis implantation on a delayed basis. Advocates of the delayed reconstructive approach have been interested in determining the shortest acceptable delay between resection arthroplasty and reimplantation to minimize patient hardship, improve functional results, and decrease the difficulty of the revision procedure as well as to maintain the lowest possible reinfection rate. This interest has been somewhat diminished with the introduction of the prosthesis of antibiotic-loaded acrylic cement (PROSTALAC).[43,125,126]

The initial Mayo Clinic experience of a two-staged reconstruction technique detailed 82 hips in which prostheses were fixed with plain acrylic bone cement without the admixture of antibiotics; there was a success rate of 87 percent at a mean of 5.5 years of follow-up.[73] Only 7 percent of the 56 hips reconstructed 1 or more years after resection arthroplasty had recurrent infection, but 27 percent of the 26 hips reconstructed less than 1 year following resection arthroplasty developed recurrent infection ($P<0.001$). This study, in the absence of antibiotic-impregnated bone cement, suggests that delayed reconstruction and the length of that time delay are important variables. When multiple series of delayed reconstructions using bone cement without antibiotic admixture are combined, 130 (82 percent) of 159 hips were successful at final follow-up (Fig. 64–4).[47] It is important to note that none of these patients were treated with antibiotic-impregnated beads or spacers between the time of the resection arthroplasty and the reimplantation. This cure rate for infection is remarkably similar to the success achieved with antibiotic-impregnated cement used for a direct exchange and strongly indicates that both variables—delayed reconstruction and antibiotic-impregnated cement for prosthesis fixation—deserve credit when consideration is given to the factors responsible for the successful treatment of an infected total hip arthroplasty.

Accordingly, it seems logical to hypothesize that patients treated with a delayed reconstructive technique that uses antibiotic-impregnated cement for the reimplantation prosthesis would have a higher cure rate for infection. Combining multiple series of patients treated with delayed reconstruction, no antibiotic-impregnated beads or spacers, and antibiotic-impregnated cement for the reimplantation prosthesis reveals a successful outcome in 354 (90 percent) of 382 patients (Fig. 64–4).[47] If patients treated with a delayed approach have had antibiotic-impregnated beads or spacers for local antibiotic delivery in addition to the use of antibiotic-impregnated cement at reimplantation, a successful outcome in a complied series was observed in 174 (92 percent) of 189 hips (Fig. 64–4).[47] These data suggest that antibiotic-impregnated cement has an independent effect as a local antibiotic delivery system before reimplantation as well as at the time of revision surgery when used for prosthesis fixation. Although analysis based on combined series with innumerable variables has significant shortcomings, these results seem to suggest that delayed reconstruction, local antibiotic delivery systems, and antibiotic-impregnated cement for prosthesis fixation are meaningful determinants of treatment that predict a successful outcome of an infected total hip arthroplasty.

Prostalac

The PROSTALAC was developed in an effort to reduce patient morbidity and decrease the technical difficulties associated with a delayed reconstruction.[125,126] This hip prosthesis facsimile has a thin polyethylene acetabulum and modular stainless steel femoral endoskeleton that are coated with antibiotic-loaded cement to act as a local antibiotic delivery system as well to maintain limb length and anatomic relationships. Patients are mobilized rapidly and enjoy a shorter hospitalization and more comfortable existence as they await reimplantation. In 48 patients undergoing a two-stage revision of an infected hip using a PROSTALAC who were followed for an average of 43 months, 3 (7 percent) had a further episode of infection.[126] Two became reinfected with different organisms and 1 with the same organism. Finally, treatment of an infection associated with extensive loss of the proximal part of the femur is a challenging problem that is particularly suited

for the use of a PROSTALAC.[44,125] The prosthesis acts as an internal splint to maintain the length of the femur, allows flexibility for the interval period, facilitates safer and easier exposure at reimplantation, and allows the potential for allograft reconstruction at reimplantation.

We have used the PROSTALAC primarily for patients with severe proximal femoral bone loss, but we have had difficulties with dislocation of the prosthesis. In the presence of good acetabular bone stock, hip instability can be reduced with a snap-fit articulation between the femoral prosthesis and the acetabular polyethylene liner. In patients with poor acetabular bone stock, it is difficult to use these prosthetic designs and hip stability remains a significant issue. In patients with good proximal femoral bone stock, we have discontinued the use of a PROSTALAC because, in these situations, the femoral medullary bone stock becomes very sclerotic during the interval between resection arthroplasty and reimplantation, and this sclerotic bone essentially mandates the use of an uncemented femoral component.

Rather, in the presence of good femoral bone stock we have been using an intramedullary femoral dowel of antibiotic-impregnated cement and a block spacer in

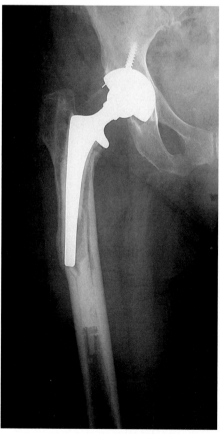
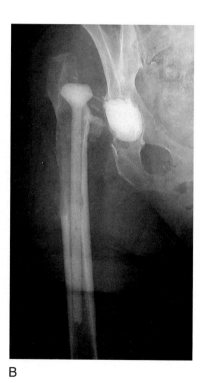
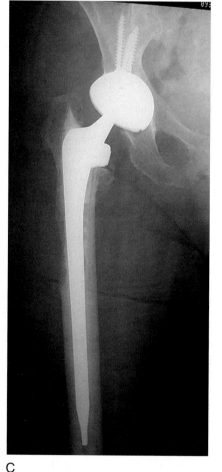

A   B   C

Figure 64–5. A, Anteroposterior radiograph of a total hip arthroplasty chronically infected with methicillin-resistant coagulase-negative *Staphylococcus.* **B,** Anteroposterior radiograph of hip joint after removal of the implant and insertion of an antibiotic-loaded femoral medullary dowel and a block acetabular spacer. **C,** Postoperative radiograph, after an interval of 3 months, of a reimplantation prosthesis with an antibiotic-loaded, cemented femoral component and of a highly porous acetabular component with antibiotic-loaded cement for fixation of the polyethylene liner into the acetabular shell.

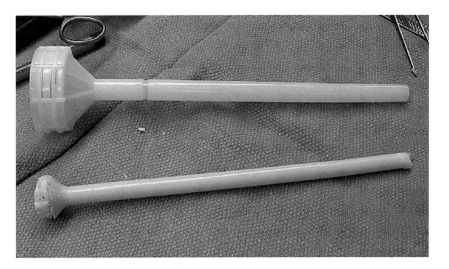

Figure 64–6. The antibiotic-loaded femoral medullary dowel is fabricated by using a readily available cement gun and allowing the antibiotic-loaded cement to fully polymerize within the cement gun spout. The dowel is then removed from the spout in a retrograde fashion. The gently tapered dowel is easily removed at the delayed reconstruction.

the acetabulum and treating the patient as we would with a traditional resection arthroplasty (Fig. 64–5). This dowel is made within the spout of a cement gun that has a gentle taper from its base to tip (Fig. 64–6). When the dowel is used, the femoral canal undergoes cancellization during the time period between resection and reimplantation, which provides an excellent bed for cement intrusion if antibiotic-impregnated cement is chosen for prosthesis fixation (Fig. 64–5). The block spacer within the acetabulum facilitates the ease of acetabular exposure at reimplantation.

Uncemented Prostheses

Many surgeons prefer the use of uncemented femoral fixation, and, in some situations, the femoral bone stock is not favorable for cement fixation.[124] Our initial experience with delayed reconstruction, in which we used uncemented prostheses, detailed 34 patients followed for an average of 4 years. The procedure was successful in 28 hips (82.3 percent).[79] It is important to note that antibiotic-impregnated cement beads or spacers were not used in the time interval between resection and reimplantation. Combining series that used an uncemented femoral component and antibiotic-loaded beads or spacers during a delayed reconstruction approach revealed successful eradication of infection in 160 (92 percent) of 174 patients (see Fig. 64–4).[29,45,63,64,117]

We are unaware of any available data regarding the success associated with acetabular components fixed with antibiotic-loaded cement compared with uncemented acetabular components. Traditionally, we have used uncemented acetabular components and have used bone graft admixed with antibiotics to fill the cavitary bone defects behind the acetabular components. We are currently evaluating the use of highly porous uncemented acetabular components in which the acetabular polyethylene component is cemented within the acetabular shell, and we are investigating the levels of antibiotic that diffuse through the shell to the host bone of the acetabulum when antibiotic-loaded cement is used.

Use of Bone Graft

The use of morcellized cancellous, small structural fragments, or massive structural bone grafts for reconstruction of a previously infected total hip arthroplasty have not been associated with an increased risk of reinfection.[1,7,45,68,79] We have found that the need for these massive femoral allografts for delayed reconstruction in the treatment of patients with infected total hip arthroplasties appears to be increasing, and we remain concerned with their use in the setting of prior infection (Fig. 64–7). When these grafts are used, we prefer to use antibiotic-impregnated cement for fixation of the femoral component through the allograft.

Recurrent Infection Following Reimplantation

In 34 patients treated for an infected total hip arthroplasty with removal of the prosthesis and implantation of another prosthesis, infection recurred an average of 2.2 years after reimplantation.[85] This occurrence was seldom compatible with a good functional outcome. Resection arthroplasty was reliable in eradicating reinfection but led to poor function and was associated with persistent pain. Reimplantation of a third prosthesis allowed 3 patients to achieve an excellent result, but the 8 hips that failed a third reimplantation attempt had the worst functional results. Those patients in whom the same single microorganism could be identified from the failed primary total hip and from the failed first reimplantation, might be reasonable candidates for another attempt at a two-stage reimplantation of a third prosthesis. This is particularly true when a deficiency in prior antibiotic therapy or surgical technique can be identified.

AUTHORS' PREFERRED METHOD

Careful preoperative evaluation of the patient with a painful total hip arthroplasty usually allows the preoperative diagnosis of infection, and aspiration of the hip remains the most important diagnostic technique in our

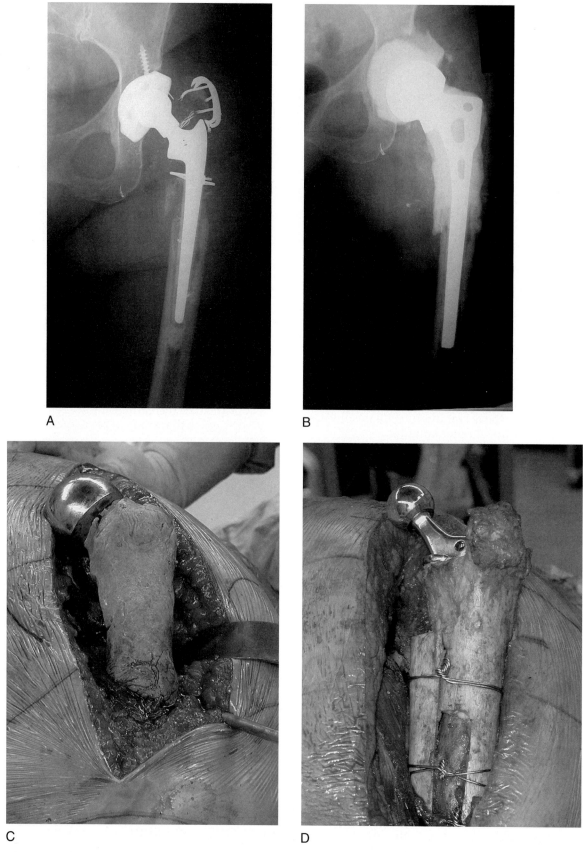

A

B

C

D

Figure 64–7. A, Anteroposterior radiograph of a chronically infected total hip arthroplasty with severe proximal femoral bone loss. **B**, Anteroposterior radiograph of a hand-molded prosthesis surrounded with antibiotic-loaded cement to maintain femoral length and facilitate surgical exposure at reimplantation. **C**, Intraoperative photograph of the hand-molded prosthesis surrounded with antibiotic-loaded cement. **D**, Intraoperative radiograph of a large structural allograft used for the femoral reconstruction. **E**, Anteroposterior radiograph of a reimplantation allograft-prosthetic femoral reconstruction with antibiotic-loaded cement for prosthesis fixation.

Illustration continued on opposite page

hands. In elderly patients with medical problems, suppressive antimicrobial therapy can be attempted, with the understanding that the infectious process can become worse. In the patient with an acute postoperative infection or a late hematogenous infection in an otherwise well functioning arthroplasty, débridement and 4 weeks of intravenous antibiotics can occasionally be effective, and we then individualize the decision to continue prolonged oral antibiotics after intravenous therapy.

Once the decision has been made to perform a resection arthroplasty, the patient can be treated definitively with the resection arthroplasty, a direct exchange technique, or a delayed reconstructive technique. Although in carefully selected situations a one-stage procedure can be effective, we prefer a delayed reconstruction, and most patients are reimplanted 3 months after resection arthroplasty. Selection of the reimplantation prosthesis should be based on the status of host bone stock and the anticipated activity level of the patient. Most of the present reimplantations at the Mayo Clinic use the hybrid concept with an uncemented acetabulum and a femoral component fixed with antibiotic-impregnated bone cement. We limit the use of the PROSTALAC to patients with severe femoral bone loss and prefer the use of a femoral medullary dowel and acetabular block spacer to provide delivery of local antibiotics in the time interval between resection arthroplasty and insertion of the new prosthesis. A global summary of the approach to the infected total hip arthroplasty is shown in a treatment algorithm (Fig. 64–8).

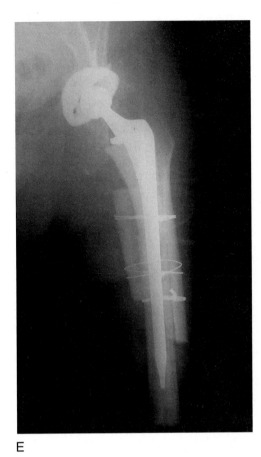

E

Figure 64–7. *Continued.*

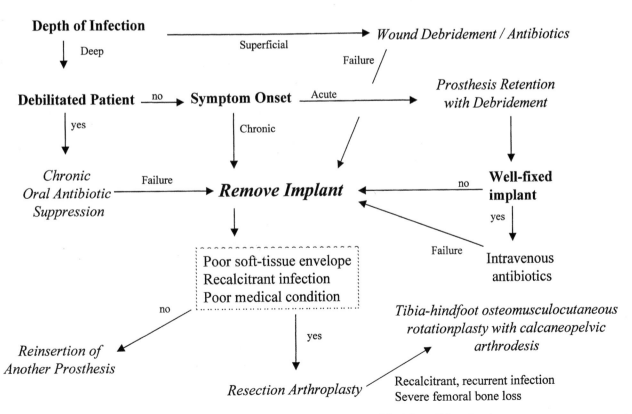

Figure 64–8. A treatment algorithm for the management of the infected hip arthroplasty.

References

1. Alexeeff M, Mahomed N, Morsi E, et al: Structural allograft in two-stage revisions for failed septic hip arthroplasty. J Bone Joint Surg 78B:213–216, 1996.

2. Athanasou NA, Pandey R, de Steiger R, et al: Diagnosis of infection by frozen section during revision arthroplasty. J Bone Joint Surg 77B:28–33, 1995.

3. Baker AS, Greenham LW: Release of gentamicin from acrylic bone cement. Elution and diffusion studies. J Bone Joint Surg 70A:1551–1557, 1988.

4. Balderston RA, Hiller WDB, Iannotti JP, et al: Treatment of the septic hip with total hip arthroplasty. Clin Orthop 221:231–237, 1987.

5. Berbari EF, Hanssen AD, Duffy MC, et al: Risk factors for prosthetic joint infection: Case-control study. Clin Infect Dis 27:1247–1254, 1998.

6. Berquist TH, Bender CE, Maus TP, et al: Pseudobursae: A useful finding in patients with painful hip arthroplasty. Am J Radiol 148:103–106, 1987.

7. Berry DJ, Chandler HP, Reilly DT: The use of bone allografts in two-stage reconstruction after failure of hip replacements due to infection. J Bone Joint Surg 73A:1460–1468, 1991.

8. Bourne RB, Hunter GA, Rorabeck CH, MacNab JJ: A six-year follow-up of infected total hip replacements managed by Girdlestone's arthroplasty. J Bone Joint Surg 66B:340–343, 1984.

9. Brandt CM, Duffy MC, Berbari EF, Hanssen AD, et al: *Staphylococcus aureus* prosthetic joint infection treated with prosthesis removal and delayed reimplantation arthroplasty. Mayo Clin Proc 74:553–558, 1999.

10. Brandt CM, Sistrunk WW, Duffy MC, et al: *Staphylococcus aureus* prosthetic joint infection treated with débridement and prosthesis retention. Clin Infect Dis 24:914–919, 1997.

11. Brien WW, Salvati EA, Klein R, et al: Antibiotic impregnated bone cement in total hip arthroplasty. An in vivo comparison of the elution properties of tobramycin and vancomycin. Clin Orthop 296:242–248, 1993.

12. Buchholz HW, Elson RA, Englebrecht E, et al: Management of deep infection of total hip replacement. J Bone Joint Surg 63B:342–353, 1981.

13. Callaghan JJ, Katz RP, Johnston RC: One-stage revision surgery of the infected hip. A minimum 10-year followup study. Clin Orthop 369:139–143, 1999.

14. Canner GC, Steinberg ME, Heppenstall RB, Balderston R: The infected hip after total hip arthroplasty. J Bone Joint Surg 66A:1393–1399, 1984.

15. Carlsson AS, Josefsson G, Lindberg L: Revision with gentamicin-impregnated cement for deep infections in total hip arthroplasties. J Bone Joint Surg 60A:1059–1064, 1978.

16. Castellanos J, Flores X, Llusa M, et al: The Girdlestone pseudarthrosis in the treatment of infected hip replacements. Int Orthop 22:178–181, 1998.

17. Cherney DL, Amstutz HC: Total hip replacement in the previously septic hip. J Bone Joint Surg 65A:1256–1265, 1983.

18. Colyer RA, Capello WN: Surgical treatment of the infected hip implant. Two-stage reimplantation with a one-month interval. Clin Orthop 298:75–79, 1994.

19. Coventry MB: Treatment of infections occurring in total hip arthroplasty. Orthop Clin North Am 6:991–1003, 1975.

20. Crockarell JR, Hanssen AD, Osmon DR, Morrey BF: Treatment of infection with débridement and retention of the components following hip arthroplasty. J Bone Joint Surg Am 80A:1306–1313, 1998.

21. Della Valle CJ, Bogner E, Desai P, et al: Analysis of frozen sections of intraoperative specimens obtained at the time of reoperation after hip or knee resection arthroplasty for the treatment of infection. J Bone Joint Surg 81A:684–689, 1999.

22. Della Valle CJ, Scher DM, Kim YH, et al: The role of intraoperative Gram stain in revision total joint arthroplasty. J Arthroplasty 14:500–504, 1999.

23. Demirkol MO, Adalet I, Unal SN, et al: 99Tc(m)-polyclonal IgG scintigraphy in the detection of infected hip and knee prostheses. Nucl Med Commun 18:543–548, 1997.

24. De Palma L, Greco F, Ciarpaglini C, Caneva C: The mechanical properties of "cement-antibiotic" mixtures. Ital J Orthop Traumatol 8:461–467, 1982.

25. Drancourt M, Stein A, Argenson JN, et al: Oral treatment of staphylococcus spp. infected orthopaedic implants with fusidic acid or ofloxacin in combination with rifampicin. J Antimicrob Chemother 39:235–240, 1997.

26. Drancourt M, Stein A, Argenson JN, et al: Oral rifampin plus ofloxacin for treatment of *Staphylococcus*-infected orthopedic implants. Antimicrob Agents Chemother 37:1214–1218, 1993.

27. Duncan CP, Masri BA: The role of antibiotic-loaded cement in the treatment of an infection after a hip replacement. J Bone Joint Surg 76A:1742–1751, 1994.

28. Elson RA: One-stage exchange in the treatment of the infected total hip arthroplasty. Semin Arthrop 5:137–141, 1994.

29. Fehring TK, Calton TF, Griffin WL: Cementless fixation in 2-stage reimplantation for periprosthetic sepsis. J Arthroplasty 14:175–181, 1999.

30. Fehring TK, Cohen B: Aspiration as a guide to sepsis in revision total hip arthroplasty. J Arthroplasty 11:543–547, 1996.

31. Fehring TK, McAlister JA Jr: Frozen histologic section as a guide to sepsis in revision joint arthroplasty. Clin Orthop 304:229–237, 1994.

32. Feldman DS, Lonner JH, Desai P, Zuckerman JD: The role of intraoperative frozen sections in revision total joint arthroplasty. J Bone Joint Surg 77A:1807–1813, 1995.

33. Fenelon GC, von Forester G, Engelbrecht E: Disarticulation of the hip as a result of failed arthroplasty. J Bone Joint Surg 62A:441–446, 1980.

34. Fitzgerald RH Jr, Jones DR: Hip implant infection. Treatment with resection arthroplasty and late total hip arthroplasty. Am J Med 78 (Suppl 68):225–228, 1985.

35. Fitzgerald RH Jr, Nolan DR, Ilstrup DM, et al: Deep wound sepsis following total hip arthroplasty. J Bone Joint Surg 59A:847–855, 1977.

36. Garvin KL, Evans BG, Salvati EA, Brause BD: Palacos gentamicin for the treatment of deep periprosthetic hip infections. Clin Orthop 298:97–105, 1994.

37. Garvin KL, Hanssen AD: Infection after total hip arthroplasty. Past, present, and future. J Bone Joint Surg 77A:1576–1588, 1995.

38. Glithero PR, Grigoris P, Harding LK, et al: White cell scans and infected joint replacements. Failure to detect chronic infection. J Bone Joint Surg 75B:371–374, 1993.

39. Gonzalez Della Valle A, Bostrom M, Brause B, et al: Effective bactericidal activity of tobramycin and vancomycin eluted from acrylic bone cement. Acta Orthop Scand 72:237–240, 2001.

40. Goodman SB, Schurman DJ: Outcome of infected total hip arthroplasty. An inclusive, consecutive series. J Arthroplasty 3:97–102, 1988.

41. Goulet JA, Pelicci PM, Brause BD, Salvati EA: Prolonged suppression of infection in total hip arthroplasty. J Arthroplasty 3:109–116, 1988.

42. Grauer JD, Amstutz HC, O'Carroll PF, Dorey FJ: Resection arthroplasty of the hip. J Bone Joint Surg 71A:669–679, 1989.

43. Haddad FS, Masri BA, Campbell D, et al: The PROSTALAC functional spacer in two-stage revision for infected knee replacements. Prosthesis of antibiotic-loaded acrylic cement. J Bone Joint Surg Br 82B:807–812, 2000.

44. Haddad FS, Masri BA, Garbuz DS, Duncan CP: The treatment of the infected hip replacement. The complex case. Clin Orthop 369:144–156, 1999.

45. Haddad FS, Muirhead-Allwood SK, Manktelow AR, Bacarese-Hamilton I: Two-stage uncemented revision hip arthroplasty for infection. J Bone Joint Surg 82B:689–694, 2000.

46. Hanssen AD, Osmon DR: Assessment of patient selection criteria for treatment of the infected hip arthroplasty. Clin Orthop 381:91–100, 2000.

47. Hanssen AD, Rand JA: Evaluation and treatment of infection at the site of a total hip or knee arthroplasty. Instr Course Lect 48:111–122, 1999.

48. Hofmann AA: Two-stage exchange is better than direct exchange in the infected THA. Orthopedics 22:919, 1999.

49. Hope PG, Kristinsson KG, Norman P, Elson RA: Deep infection of cemented total hip arthroplasties caused by coagulase-negative staphylococci. J Bone Joint Surg 71B:851–855, 1989.

50. Hyman JL, Salvati EA, Laurencin CT, et al: The arthroscopic drainage, irrigation, and débridement of late, acute total hip arthroplasty infections: Average 6-year follow-up. J Arthroplasty 14:903–910, 1999.

51. Isiklar ZU, Darouiche RO, Landon GC, Beck T: Efficacy of antibiotics alone for orthopaedic device related infections. Clin Orthop 332:184–189, 1996.
52. Isiklar ZU, Demirors H, Akpinar S, et al: Two-stage treatment of chronic staphylococcal orthopaedic implant-related infections using vancomycin impregnated PMMA spacer and rifampin containing antibiotic protocol. Bull Hosp Jt Dis 58:79–85, 1999.
53. Jackson WO, Schmalzried TP: Limited role of direct exchange arthroplasty in the treatment of infected total hip replacements. Clin Orthop 381:101–105, 2000.
54. Joseph TN, Mujtaba M, Chen AL, et al: Efficacy of combined technetium-99m sulfur colloid/indium-111 leukocyte scans to detect infected total hip and knee arthroplasties. J Arthroplasty 16:753–758, 2001.
55. Jupiter JB, Karchmer AW, Lowell DJ, Harris WH: Total hip arthroplasty in the treatment of adult hips with current or quiescent sepsis. J Bone Joint Surg 63A:194–200, 1981.
56. Kantor GS, Osterkamp JA, Dorr LD, et al: Resection arthroplasty following infected total hip replacement arthroplasty. J Arthroplasty 1:83–89, 1986.
57. Kendall RW, Duncan CP, Smith JA, Ngui-Yen JH: Persistence of bacteria on antibiotic loaded acrylic depots. A reason for caution. Clin Orthop 329:273–280, 1996.
58. Kordelle J, Frommelt L, Kluber D, Seemann K: Results of one-stage endoprosthesis revision in periprosthetic infection cause by methicillin-resistant *Staphylococcus aureus*. Z Orthop Ihre Grenzgeb 138:240–244, 2000.
59. Kostuik J, Alexander D: Arthrodesis for failed arthroplasty of the hip. Clin Orthop 188:173–182, 1984.
60. Kraemer WJ, Saplys R, Waddell JP, Morton J: Bone scan, gallium scan and hip aspiration in the diagnosis of infected total hip arthroplasty. J Arthroplasty 8:611–615, 1993.
61. Kuechle DK, Landon GC, Musher DM, Noble PC: Elution of vancomycin, daptomycin, and amikacin from acrylic bone cement. Clin Orthop 264:302–308, 1991.
62. Lachiewicz PF, Rogers GD, Thomason HC: Aspiration of the hip joint before revision total hip arthroplasty. Clinical and laboratory factors influencing attainment of a positive culture. J Bone Joint Surg 78A:749–754, 1996.
63. Lai KA, Shen WJ, Yang CY, et al: Two-stage cementless revision THR after infection. 5 recurrences in 40 cases followed 2.5–7 years. Acta Orthop Scand 67:325–328, 1996.
64. Lecuire F, Collodel M, Basso M, et al: Revision of infected total hip prostheses by ablation reimplantation of an uncemented prosthesis. 57 case reports. Rev Chir Orthop Reparatrice Appar Mot 85:764, 1999.
65. Levitsky KA, Hozack WJ, Balderston RA, et al: Evaluation of the painful prosthetic joint relative value of bone scan, sedimentation rate, and joint aspiration. J Arthroplasty 6:237–244, 1991.
66. Lieberman JR, Callaway GH, Salvati EA, et al: Treatment of the infected total hip arthroplasty with a two-stage reimplantation protocol. Clin Orthop 301:205–212, 1994.
67. Lonner JH, Desai P, Dicesare PE, et al: The reliability of analysis of intraoperative frozen sections for identifying active infection during revision hip or knee arthroplasty. J Bone Joint Surg 78A:1553–1558, 1996.
68. Loty B, Postel M, Evrard J, et al: One stage revision of infected total hip replacements with replacement of bone loss by allografts. Study of 90 cases of which 46 used bone allografts. Int Orthop 16:330–338, 1992.
69. Lyons CW, Berquist TH, Lyons JC, et al: Evaluation of radiographic findings in painful hip arthroplasties. Clin Orthop 195:239–251, 1985.
70. Magnuson JE, Brown MI, Hauser MF, et al: In-111-labeled leukocyte scintigraphy in suspected orthopedic prosthesis infection: Comparison with other imaging modalities. Radiology 168:235–239, 1988.
71. Masri BA, Duncan CP, Beauchamp CP: Long-term elution of antibiotics from bone-cement: An in vivo study using the prosthesis of antibiotic-loaded acrylic cement (PROSTALAC) system. J Arthroplasty 13:331–338, 1998.
72. Masterson EL, Masri BA, Duncan CP: Treatment of infection at the site of total hip replacement. Instr Course Lect 47:297–306, 1998.
73. McDonald DJ, Fitzgerald RH Jr, Ilstrup DM: Two-stage reconstruction of a total hip arthroplasty because of infection. J Bone Joint Surg 71A:828–834, 1989.

74. Meland NB, Arnold PG, Weiss HC: Management of the recalcitrant total-hip arthroplasty wound. Plast Reconstr Surg 88:681–685, 1991.
75. Mulcahy DM, O'Byrne JM, Fenelon GE: One stage surgical management of deep infection of total hip arthroplasty. Ir J Med Sci 165:17–19, 1996.
76. Murray RP, Bourne MH, Fitzgerald RH Jr: Metachronous infection in patients who have had more than one total joint arthroplasty. J Bone Joint Surg 73A:1469–1474, 1991.
77. Naylor PT, Myrvik QN, Gristina AG: Antibiotic resistance of biomaterial-adherent coagulase-negative and coagulase-positive staphylococci. Clin Orthop 261:126–133, 1990.
78. Nelson CL, Evans RP, Blaha JD, et al: A comparison of gentamicin-impregnated polymethylmethacrylate bead implantation to conventional parenteral antibiotic therapy in infected total hip and knee arthroplasty. Clin Orthop 295:96–101, 1993.
79. Nestor BJ, Hanssen AD, Ferrer-Gonzalez R, Fitzgerald RH Jr: The use of porous prostheses in delayed reconstruction of total hip replacements that have failed because of infection. J Bone Joint Surg 76A:349–359, 1994.
80. Nijhof MW, Oyen WJ, van Kampen A, et al: Hip and knee arthroplasty infection. In-111-IgG scintigraphy in 102 cases. Acta Orthop Scand 68:332–336, 1997.
81. Ochsner PE, Brunazzi MG, Picard CM: Salvage surgery in chronic infection following total hip prosthesis. Orthopade 24:353–359, 1995.
82. Oyen WJ, vanHorn JR, Claessens RA, et al: Diagnosis of bone, joint, and joint prosthesis infections with In-111-labeled nonspecific human immunoglobulin G scintigraphy. Radiology 182:195–199, 1992.
83. Pace TB, Jeray KJ, Latham JT Jr: Synovial tissue examination by frozen section as an indicator of infection in hip and knee arthroplasty in community hospitals. J Arthroplasty 12:64–69, 1997.
84. Padgett DE, Silverman A, Sachjowicz F, et al: Efficacy of intraoperative cultures obtained during revision total hip arthroplasty. J Arthroplasty 10:420–426, 1995.
85. Pagnano MW, Trousdale RT, Hanssen AD: Outcome after reinfection following reimplantation hip arthroplasty. Clin Orthop 338:192–204, 1997.
86. Palestro CJ, Kim CK, Swyer AJ, et al: Total hip arthroplasty: Periprosthetic indium-111-labeled leukocyte activity and complementary technetium-99-sulfur colloid imaging in suspected infection. J Nucl Med 31:1959–1965, 1990.
87. Pandey R, Drakoulakis E, Athanasou NA: An assessment of the histological criteria used to diagnose infection in hip revision arthroplasty tissues. J Clin Pathol 52:118–123, 1999.
88. Pazzaglia UE, Ghisellini F, Ceffa R, et al: Evaluation of reimplant total hip prostheses and resection arthroplasty. Orthopedics 11:1141–1145, 1988.
89. Penner MJ, Duncan CP, Masri BA: The in vitro elution characteristics of antibiotic-loaded CMW and Palacos-R bone cements. J Arthroplasty 14:209–214, 1999.
90. Penner MJ, Masri BA, Duncan CP: Elution characteristics of vancomycin and tobramycin combined in acrylic bone-cement. J Arthroplasty 11:939–944, 1996.
91. Peterson CA II, Koch LD, Wood MB: Tibia-hindfoot osteomusculocutaneous rotationplasty with calcaneopelvic arthrodesis for extensive loss of bone from the proximal part of the femur. A report of two cases. J Bone Joint Surg 79A:1504–1509, 1997.
92. Petty W, Goldsmith S: Resection arthroplasty following infected total hip arthroplasty. J Bone Joint Surg 62A:889–896, 1980.
93. Pons M, Angles F, Sanchez C, et al: Infected total hip arthroplasty—the value of intraoperative histology. Int Orthop 23:34–36, 1999.
94. Poss R, Thornhill TS, Ewald FC, et al: Factors influencing the incidence and outcome of infection following total joint arthroplasty. Clin Orthop 182:117–126, 1984.
95. Rafiq M, Worthington T, Tebbs SE, et al: Serological detection of Gram-positive bacterial infection around prostheses. J Bone Joint Surg 82B:1156–1161, 2000.
96. Raut VV, Orth MS, Orth MC, et al: One stage revision arthroplasty of the hip for deep gram negative infection. Int Orthop 20:12–14, 1996.
97. Raut VV, Siney PD, Wroblewski BM: One-stage revision of infected total hip replacements with discharging sinuses. J Bone Joint Surg 76B:721–724, 1994.

98. Raut VV, Siney PD, Wroblewski BM: One-stage revision of total hip arthroplasty for deep infection. Long-term followup. Clin Orthop 321:202–207, 1995.

99. Robbins GM, Masri BA, Garbuz DS, Duncan CP: Primary total hip arthroplasty after infection. J Bone Joint Surg 83A:602–614, 2001.

100. Roberts P, Walters AJ, McMinn DJW: Diagnosing infection in hip replacements. The use of fine-needle aspiration and radiometric culture. J Bone Joint Surg 74B:265–271, 1992.

101. Rodriguez JA, Ranawat CS, Maniar RN, Umlas ME: Incisional cellulitis after total hip replacement. J Bone Joint Surg 80B:876–878, 1998.

102. Salvati EA, Callaghan JJ, Brause BD, et al: Reimplantation in infection. Elution of gentamicin from cement and beads. Clin Orthop 207:83–93, 1986.

103. Sampathkumar P, Osmon DR, Cockerill FR III: Prosthetic joint infection due to *Staphylococcus lugdunensis*. Mayo Clin Proc 75:511–512, 2000.

104. Sanzen L: The erythrocyte sedimentation rate following exchange of infected total hips. Acta Orthop Scand 59:148–150, 1988.

105. Sanzen L, Carlsson AS, Josefsson G, Lindberg LT: Revision operations on infected total hip arthroplasties. Two to nine year follow-up study. Clin Orthop 229:165–172, 1988.

106. Sanzen L, Sundberg M: Periprosthetic low-grade hip infections. Erythrocyte sedimentation rate and C-reactive protein in 23 cases. Acta Orthop Scand 68:461–465, 1997.

107. Scher DM, Pak K, Lonner JH, et al: The predictive value of indium-111 leukocyte scans in the diagnosis of infected total hip, knee, or resection arthroplasties. J Arthroplasty 15:295–300, 2000.

108. Schmalzried TP, Amstutz HC, Au M-K, Dorey FJ: Etiology of deep sepsis in total hip arthroplasty. The significance of hematogenous and recurrent infection. Clin Orthop 280:200–207, 1992.

109. Schroder J, Saris D, Besselaar PP, Marti RK: Comparison of the results of the Girdlestone pseudarthrosis with reimplantation of a total hip replacement. Int Orthop 22:215–218, 1998.

110. Spangehl MJ, Masri BA, O'Connell JX, Duncan CP: Prospective analysis of preoperative and intraoperative investigations for the diagnosis of infection at the sites of two hundred and two revision total hip arthroplasties. J Bone Joint Surg 81A:672–683, 1999.

111. Spangehl MJ, Masterson E, Masri BA, et al: The role of intraoperative gram stain in the diagnosis of infection during revision total hip arthroplasty. J Arthroplasty 14:952–956, 1999.

112. Spangehl MJ, Younger AS, Masri BA, Duncan CP: Diagnosis of infection following total hip arthroplasty. Instr Course Lect 47:285–295, 1998.

113. Stein A, Bataille JF, Drancourt M, et al: Ambulatory treatment of multidrug-resistant staphylococcus-infected orthopedic implants with high-dose oral co-trimoxazole (trimethoprim-sulfamethoxazole). Antimicrob Agents Chemother 42:3086–3091, 1998.

114. Tattevin P, Cremieux AC, Pottier P, et al: Prosthetic joint infection: When can prosthesis salvage be considered? Clin Infect Dis 29:292–295, 1999.

115. Teller RE, Christie MJ, Martin W, et al: Sequential indium-labeled leukocyte and bone scans to diagnose prosthetic joint infection. Clin Orthop 373:241–247, 2000.

116. Tigges S, Stiles RG, Meli RJ, Roberson JR: Hip aspiration: A cost-effective and accurate method of evaluating the potentially infected hip prosthesis. Radiology 189:485–488, 1993.

117. Tsukayama DT, Estrada R, Gustilo RB: Infection after total hip arthroplasty. A study of the treatment of one hundred and six infections. J Bone Joint Surg Am 78A:512–23, 1996.

118. Tsukayama DT, Wicklund B, Gustilo RB: Suppressive antibiotic therapy in chronic prosthetic joint infections. Orthopedics 14:841–844, 1991.

119. Tunney MM, Patrick S, Gorman SP, et al: Improved detection of infection in hip replacements. A currently underestimated problem. J Bone Joint Surg 80B:568–572, 1998.

120. Ure KJ, Amstutz HC, Nasser S, Schmalzried TP: Direct-exchange arthroplasty for the treatment of infection after total hip replacement. An average ten-year follow-up. J Bone Joint Surg 80A:961–968, 1998.

121. Wang JW, Chen CE: Reimplantation of infected hip arthroplasties using bone allografts. Clin Orthop 335:202–210, 1997.

122. Went P, Krismer M, Frischhut B: Recurrence of infection after revision of infected hip arthroplasties. J Bone Joint Surg 77B:307–309, 1995.

123. Widmer AF, Gaechter A, Ochsner PE, Zimmerli W: Antimicrobial treatment of orthopedic implant-related infections with rifampin combinations. Clin Infect Dis 14:1251–1253, 1992.

124. Wilson MG, Dorr LD: Reimplantation of infected total hip arthroplasties in the absence of antibiotic cement. J Arthroplasty 4:263–269, 1989.

125. Younger AS, Duncan CP, Masri BA: Treatment of infection associated with segmental bone loss in the proximal part of the femur in two stages with use of an antibiotic-loaded interval prosthesis. J Bone Joint Surg 80A:60–69, 1998.

126. Younger AS, Duncan CP, Masri BA, McGraw RW: The outcome of two-stage arthroplasty using a custom-made interval spacer to treat the infected hip. J Arthroplasty 12:615–623, 1997.

127. Zhuang H, Duarte PS, Pourdehnad M, et al: The promising role of 18F-FDG PET in detecting infected lower limb prosthesis implants. J Nucl Med 42:44–48, 2001.

128. Zimmerli W, Widmer AF, Blatter M, et al: Role of rifampin for treatment of orthopedic implant-related staphylococcal infections: A randomized controlled trial. Foreign-Body Infection (FBI) Study Group. JAMA 279:1537–1541, 1998.

65

Dislocation

• BERNARD F. MORREY

Instability is one of the major complications of hip replacement arthroplasty.[6,7,18,24,40,46,51,59,60,62,64] It may necessitate prolonged hospitalization, rehabilitation, and, if recurrent, imply a certain level of functional impairment that requires surgical treatment.[13] The reported incidence of postoperative dislocation has ranged from less than 1 percent to almost 10 percent.[23,66] The cost of managing this complication has been estimated at $70,000,000 annually in the United States.[56] In this chapter, the current understanding of risk factors, strategy, and outcomes of management of the problem are discussed.

INCIDENCE

The true incidence of this problem is not known with certainty. Instability in the form of subluxation may not be noted, and unless long-term follow-up is obtained, many cases may be missed.[17,74] A review of 16 reports from 1973 through 1987 revealed a dislocation rate of 2.23 percent after 35,000 procedures were performed (Table 65–1). Of the several studies that specifically address the issue of prosthetic hip dislocation, Khan et al.[42] reported an incidence of 2.1 percent after 6774 procedures and Kristiansen et al.[43] reported 4.9 percent after 427 operations. At the Mayo Clinic, Woo and Morrey[74] reviewed over 10,500 primary and revision total hip arthroplasties, noting 331 dislocations for a rate of 3.2 percent. The Mayo Clinic experience with 26,480 primary procedures performed from 1969 to 2000 has been updated, revealing instability in 624 for a rate of 2.4 percent There does not appear to be a significant learning curve, at least at our institution, because this complication has occurred with a frequency of 2 percent to 3 percent each year for more than three decades.

MECHANISM

The prosthetic hip is unstable in one of two motions. Hip flexion, adduction, and internal rotation causes a posterior dislocation, typically associated with patients sitting in low chairs and rising from a sitting position.[74]

Extension, adduction, and external rotation results in the less common anterior dislocation. In contrast to the two motions described, the second type of dislocation occurs most frequently after an anterior surgical approach and when excessive anteversion is imparted to one or both components.

RISK FACTORS

Real or perceived factors shown or suspected to be associated with an unstable total hip arthroplasty are considered as preoperative, perioperative, and postoperative variables. A more detailed method of assessment is according to disease features, patient characteristics, technique/design consideration, and postsurgical variables (Table 65–2).

DISEASE FEATURES

Most total joint replacements are performed for five diagnoses: degenerative arthritis, rheumatoid arthritis, avascular necrosis, congenital hip dislocation, and trauma. The frequency of these diagnoses in a controlled series compared with the incidence in populations of unstable hips is shown in Table 65–3. Low-grade sepsis can be a subtle cause of late dislocation.[12,66] The possibility of delayed-onset sepsis specifically must be considered in the patient whose hip dislocation has developed several years after implantation.

PATIENT CHARACTERISTICS

Gender has been consistently proven to be an important risk factor in dislocations because it occurs twice as frequently in females than in males in the early stages after operation.[42,43,54,74] In fact, the incidence in females exceeds that in males by a 3:1 to 4:1 ratio in those with delayed (more than 5 years) dislocation.[17,25,49,71] The risk increases with age, and one series reported the rate of instability in those older than 80 years as 4 percent.[25] The implications of an increased lever arm effect or of increased forces associated with patient height and weight have not proved to be relevant.

Table 65–1. FREQUENCY OF HIP INSTABILITY REPORTED IN THE LITERATURE

Author	Year	Procedures	No.	Dislocations or Subluxations Percent
Bergstrom et al.[7]	1973	283	13	4.6
Charnley and Cupic[14]	1973	185	3	1.6
Lazansky[46]	1973	501	22	1.6
Coventry et al.[18]	1974	2012	60	3.0
Eftekhar[23]	1976	1560	11	0.7
Ritter[66]	1976	502	35	7.0
Carlson and Gentz[11]	1977	351	17	4.8
Etienne et al.[26]	1978	9815	56	0.6
Lewinnek et al.[50]	1978	300	9	3.0
Khan et al.[42]	1981	6774	142	2.1
Chandler et al.[13]	1981	800	43	5.4
Woo and Morrey[74]	1982	10500	331	3.2
Williams et al.[72]	1982	1280	32	2.6
Roberts et al.[67]	1983	506	7	1.4
Kristiansen et al.[43]	1985	427	21	5.0
Dall et al.[19]	1986	98	2	2.0
Total		35,894	804	2.25

Data from references 7, 11, 13, 14, 18, 19, 23, 26, 42, 43, 46, 50, 66, 67, 72, 74.

Table 65–2. RISK FACTORS CONSIDERED TO RELATE TO DISLOCATIONS AFTER TOTAL HIP ARTHROPLASTY

Preoperative	Perioperative	Postdislocation
Age	Approach	Dislocation versus subluxation
Sex	Aftercare	
Side	Component head size	Time to dislocation
Bilaterality	Range of motion	Direction of dislocation
Previous surgery	Leg length discrepancy	Redislocation
Diagnosis	Cup version	Reoperation
Height	Cup obliquity	
Weight	Trochanteric position/avulsion	

Modified from Woo RYG, Morrey BF: Dislocations after total hip arthroplasty. J Bone Joint Surg 64A:1295, 1982.

Table 65–3. RELATIONSHIP OF INSTABILITY AND OPERATIVE DIAGNOSIS AS REPORTED IN THE LITERATURE

Underlying Diagnosis	Control (percent)	Dislocation (percent)	Percent of Total
Degenerative joint disease	2872 (60)	77 (46)	2.6
Rheumatoid arthritis	771 (16)	27 (16)	3.5
Avascular necrosis	223 (4)	8 (5)	3.6
Congenital dislocation of hip	334 (7)	9 (5)	2.7
Fracture	607 (12)	46 (28)	7.6
Total	4807	167	3.5

Alcoholism, Psychological, and Neurologic Factors

There is now clear evidence of a markedly increased incidence, up to a factor of 5, with excessive alcohol consumption.[36,37,61] However, emotional problems were not, in themselves found to be a contributing factor to instability.[37] Cerebral dysfunction associated with increased age has also been shown to be a significant risk factor.[71,73]

Underlying Diagnosis: Prior Surgery

Prior hip surgery has been recognized by every investigator as playing a significant role in subsequent hip instability.[11,21,22,27,42,74] The most dramatic differences were reported by Williams et al.,[72] who noted a 0.6 percent incidence of dislocation after primary procedures and a 20 percent incidence after revision operations. Combining the data in several large series revealed 98

Table 65–4. RELATIONSHIP OF UNDERLYING DIAGNOSIS AND PREVIOUS SURGERY AND HIP INSTABILITY

Underlying Diagnosis	Previous Surgery	Number of Hip Dislocations (percent)		Total
		No. Previous Surgery		
Degenerative joint disease	195 (7.2)	1573 (1.9)		1768 (2.5)
Rheumatoid arthritis	27 (7.4)	278 (3.6)		305 (3.9)
Avascular necrosis	33 (9.1)	117 (2.6)		150 (4.0)
Congenital dislocation of hip	108 (6.5)	126 (0.8)		234 (3.4)
Fracture	376 (5.9)	138 (10.1)		514 (7.0)
	4.8	2.4		3.1

Modified from Woo RYG, Morrey BF: Dislocations after total hip arthroplasty. J Bone Joint Surg 64A:1295, 1982.

dislocations after 4753 primary procedures, for an incidence of 2 percent. This contrasts with 82 dislocations after 1290 revision operations (6.3 percent).[11,27,72,74] In the Mayo Clinic experience of 10,500 procedures, instability developed in 2.4 percent of the 7241 procedures that were performed on patients who did not have previous surgery and in 4.8 percent of the 3259 procedures that were done on patients who had some type of previous hip surgery (P<.001) (Table 65–4).[74] Even more significant is the frequency of instability after prosthetic revision. Alberton's literature review documented a rate of instability of 12 percent after 1856 revision procedures. The Mayo Clinic experience revealed an incidence of 7.5 percent after 1548 revision procedures performed at the Mayo Clinic between 1970 and 1999.[2]

PERIOPERATIVE FACTORS

Surgical Expertise

One study of the relationship of surgical experience and the complications of instability revealed a direct correlation, with the patients of less experienced surgeons having a greater dislocation rate.[36] No difference was present after an experience of more than 30 procedures has been obtained.

Surgical Approach

A documented increase of up to threefold in hip instability has been associated with a posterior surgical approach to the hip (4 percent) compared with the anterior surgical exposure (1.3 percent).[67] Woo and Morrey report that the anterior surgical approach was associated with a 2.3 percent incidence of dislocation compared with 5.8 percent among those with posterior procedures.[74] We have also documented a higher frequency of dislocation after posterior surgical approaches while considering other factors with use of multivariable statistical analysis (Table 65–5 and Fig. 65–1). Considering the surgical approach and femoral head size, the posterior approach was associated with more instability than the anterior or lateral trochanteric approach for 22-mm, 28-mm, and 32-mm femoral head dimensions (P<.01) (Table 65–5). Mallory et al. have performed an exhaustive review of the literature documenting a 4 percent instability rate after 11,000 procedures from 11 authors who used a posterior approach. The anterior approach had a rate of 2.1 percent after 6677 procedures from 10 authors. Mallory described an anterior split technique with an .8 percent rate after 1518 operations.[53] Of interest is a report that shows that if the capsule is left intact[2] or if the posterior capsule is repaired, the posterior exposure appears to be as stable as the anterior approach.[63]

Component Head Size

The assumption and logic of the larger head size is that greater displacement must occur before the hip can dislocate, which therefore imposes increased tension on the soft tissues (Fig. 65–2). Clinical experience, however, has not confirmed the reality of this logic. In fact, when the issue has been specifically addressed, no correlation can be found between head size and prosthetic instability.[27,66,74] Woo and Morrey[74] reviewed the Mayo Clinic experience of over 10,000 procedures. Among 331

Table 65–5. RELATIONSHIP BETWEEN SURGICAL APPROACH, COMPONENT HEAD SIZE, AND HIP INSTABILITY

Surgical Approach	Hip Instability (percent)*			Total
	Head Size (22 mm)	Head Size (28 mm)	Head Size (32 mm)	
Anterior	2.6	1.3	2.1	2.3
Lateral	2.7	4.1	3.4	3.1
Posterior	6.8	6.0	3.5	5.8
All approaches	2.9	4.7	3.3	3.5

*Percentage data are average dislocation rates.

All Head Sizes

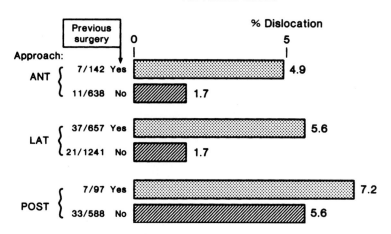

Figure 65–1. Interrelationship of surgical approach, previous surgery, and component head size.

implants, an incidence of 2.9 percent instability was noted in the 22-mm implants compared with 3.3 percent for the 32-mm implants. This difference was not statistically significant. The presently available clinical data clearly demonstrate little or no correlation between 32-mm and 22-mm head size and hip instability (Table 65–5).[27,32,42,58,72,74] However, this issue continues to be assessed and debated.

Range of Motion

The relationship of laxity and stability is not well addressed in the literature. Coventry noted that the range of motion in patients with hip instability had a slight increase in internal and external rotation among those who experienced early dislocation and greater flexion in the group with late dislocation.[17] The total arc of motion, adding all five functions of flexion, abduction, adduction, and internal and external rota-

tion, has shown that the greatest overall arc occurs in individuals with late dislocations. This important observation is presumably related to stretching of the pseudocapsule (Fig. 65–3).[17] Additional studies are warranted to further study this question, particularly with late instability.

Head Neck Ratio: Skirted Neck Implants

The issue of impingement has long been shown to be at the heart of the issue of head/neck/cup, rim interaction. The elevated rim limits motion, and impingement occurs

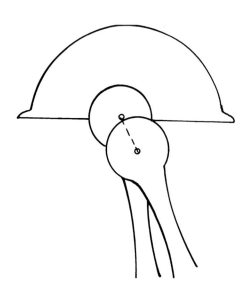

Figure 65–2. The larger femoral head must displace by a greater amount to sublux. Thus, the larger head should theoretically be more stable.

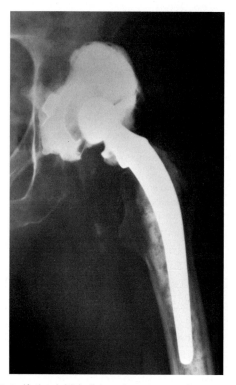

Figure 65–3. If the initial dislocation occurs after several years, stretching of the pseudocapsule is a likely contributing cause, as shown by this arthrogram of an unstable hip.

with a lessened arc of motion, depending on design characteristics. The elongated modular head/neck implant frequently has a "skirt" in the longer dimensions. A review of our experience with this implant reveals a sixfold increased instability rate compared with a nonskirted device,[47] whereas both groups had selection bias inherent in the clinical selection for the long-necked, skirted device. The difference in stability rates is alarming (P<.01). In another study, Kelly et al. made an interesting observation concerning the relationship of head/cup ratio and instability.[41] With a 22-mm femoral head, a 14 percent incidence of dislocation occurred among cups greater than 62 mm in diameter, and in 4 percent of those with a 60-mm or smaller acetabular implant.

Tissue Balance

This is probably the most important variable when expressed as trochanter nonunion. Limb length inequality, abduction weakness, and offset variation are also considered but are less clearly related.

Trochanteric Nonunion

The presence of a migrated, uncemented trochanter is one of the most commonly demonstrated and dominant causes of instability, increasing the risk by a factor of 6![38,70,74] Although trochanteric osteotomy is less commonly performed today, this finding serves to demonstrate the importance of its dynamic contribution to the stability of the implant. Although trochanteric osteotomy is not necessary to properly orient the components, advancement may be associated with enhanced stability, but this is unproved for primary procedures. Nonunion occurs in 5 percent of cases, and, when it is present, more than 15 percent are unstable[5,11,17,68,74] (Fig. 65–4).

Limb Length Inequality

Limb length shortening is a commonly considered factor in hip instability.[11,26,27,43,50,74] Yet, relative leg length as a measure of myofascial tension has not been shown to be associated with instability. In our experience and that of Fackler and Poss,[27] the unstable hip measured 1.5 mm longer than the nonoperated control.[74] Coventry also found that the limb was equal to the preoperative limb in 75 percent of 32 late dislocators and was shorter than the opposite side in only 8 of these 32 (25 percent).[17] On the other hand, Kristiansen et al.[43] compared 21 dislocations with 21 controls and showed that the unstable hip was slightly more proximal than the opposite hip. In contrast, Carlsson and Gentz[11] also showed a statistical correlation (P<.05) between the proximally placed implant and dislocation.

Offset

Fackler and Poss have emphasized the relationship of femoral offset to hip instability after prosthetic replacement.[27] A statistical correlation was found between the hip with decreased offset and instability. This is logical because (1) the decreased offset decreases the arc of motion before impingement occurs, and (2) the myofascial tension of the gluteus musculature is increased by increased offset. My clinical experience supports Fackler and Poss' observation. Fortunately, the amount of offset can be controlled with modular head and neck implants and the eccentric cup liners and should be considered

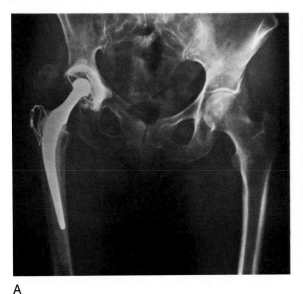

A

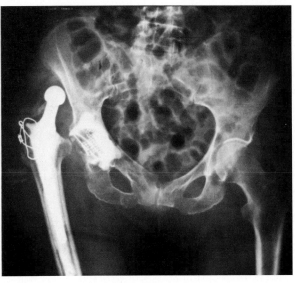

B

Figure 65–4. Trochanteric nonunion and migration (**A**) is clearly documented to be associated with hip instability (**B**). (From Woo RYG, Morrey BF: Dislocations after total hip arthroplasty. J Bone Joint Surg 64A:1295, 1982.)

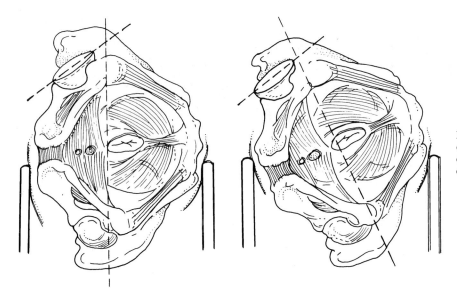

Figure 65–5. If arthroplasty is done in the lateral decubitus position, forward tilt of the pelvis may cause inadvertent retroversion of the acetabular component.

when the femoral and acetabular components for hip replacement are selected.

Abduction Weakness

The direct measurement and correlation of abductor strength has been presented. Although poorly controlled, abductor weakness was considered a constant feature in several categories of instability studied by Door and Wan.[21]

Component Orientation

Component orientation has long been recognized as a critical feature in providing stability to the replaced joint.[11,23,26,27,43,66,74] Acetabular orientation is the most difficult to achieve consistently. Variations in positioning the patient on the operating table lead to inaccurate estimates of cup orientation at the time of surgery. The unnoticed forward rotation of the pelvis in the lateral decubitus position causes an unnoticed retroverted positioning of the cup (Fig. 65–5). Posterior exposure to the capsule is associated with less anteversion of the cup than is observed from the anterior exposure.[43,74]

Cup orientation is difficult to measure on the plain roentgenograms in nonmetalic components. Furthermore, the anteversion angle varies according to the amount of lateral tilt (obliquity) that is present. Several studies have addressed the difficult problem of accurately determining cup orientation from the radiograph,[1,32] but most provide data or formulas that are too difficult or complex to use clinically. Nonetheless, acetabular orientation is probably the most sensitive variable in predisposition to a hip dislocation.[42,66]

Cup obliquity or abduction-adduction has been studied by several investigators, and most have not found a close correlation unless the cup is placed in an extreme position.[43,50] One careful study demonstrated a so-called

safe position of anteversion of 15 to 10 degrees and abduction of 40 to 10 degrees (Fig. 65–6). In the experience of Lewinnek et al.,[50] an instability rate of 1.5 percent occurred in the safe range, compared with a 6 percent average rate for acetabula oriented outside this range. This safe zone was statistically more stable than if one of these parameters was exceeded ($P<.05$).[50]

There has been relatively little attention paid to femoral component anteversion other than recommending that this be oriented to 15 degrees. The rotation of the femoral component is difficult if not impossible to measure accurately by radiography. Nonetheless, Fackler and Poss[27] showed that 44 percent of their 34 dislocation cases had malposition of one or both components, compared with only 6 percent of the control population. Importantly, they demonstrated that the most common orientation error was excessive femoral anteversion, and that this was independent of whether or not a trochanteric osteotomy was used as the surgical approach.

Extended Acetabular Wall

Acetabular design is known to be potentially capable of placing the hip at risk due to impingement.[10] Charnley first suggested and designed an extended posterior wall of the acetabular component to lessen the likelihood of posterior dislocation.[14] With the advent of modular components, more flexibility becomes available to position the implant (Fig. 65–7). Both 10-degree and 20-degree elevations are also now commercially available in virtually all acetabular component designs. Although the theoretical advantage of the design modification is obvious, there are some potential disadvantages with this concept. Increasing the extent of one portion of the socket decreases the arc of motion. This can allow impingement to occur, particularly if the orientation of the elevated wall is improperly placed.[57] In fact, Krushell et al. demonstrated that the arc of motion

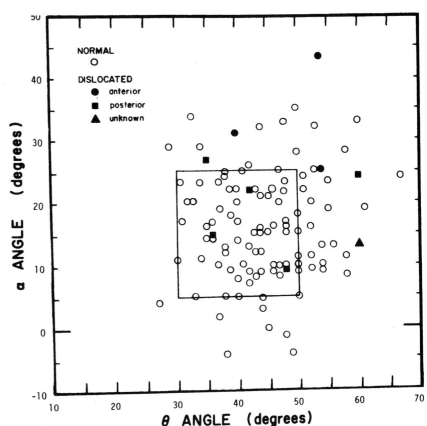

Figure 65–6. The so-called safe zone, 15 degrees plus or minus 10 degrees of anteversion and 40 percent plus or minus 10 percent of valgus or abduction, statistically decreases the chance of instability. (From Lewinnek GE, Lewis JL, Tarr R, et al: Dislocations after total hip replacement arthroplasties. J Bone Joint Surg 60A:217, 1978.)

with this design is not significantly altered but simply reoriented.[45] Nonetheless, concern does exist with regard to impingement and increased torque with the extended wall (Fig. 65–8).[8,31,34,54,57]

An additional concern exists because of the increased surface area exposed to the femoral head. This may result in increased wear debris with resulting osteolysis and eventually could even render the hip more unstable than if the elevated liner were not present (Fig. 65–9). In fact, case reports of femoral loosening have also been associated with impingement on an extended posterior wall acetabular component.[7]

Given these several theoretical advantages and disadvantages of this concept, it is somewhat surprising that

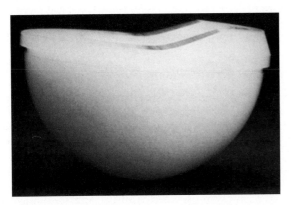

Figure 65–7. Extended acetabular wall can be oriented to resist the unstable position of hip replacement.

there is relatively little clinical material supporting either position.[58] To address this question, we analyzed more than 5000 total hip arthroplasties performed at the Mayo Clinic from 1985 through 1991. In this group, approximately 2500 had an elevated (ELEV) design and approximately 2700 had a traditional (STD) design.[16] The 2-year probability of dislocation was 2.19 percent for the ELEV group and 3.85 percent for the STD group ($P<.001$) (Fig. 65–10). Increased stability was cross-correlated with other variables. The ELEV acetabular component revealed enhanced stability regardless of surgical approach, mode of fixation, gender, and whether the procedure was primary or revision. However, the difference in stability was more noticeable in patients with revision procedures, suggesting that this particular acetabular design might be reserved for the at-risk patient.[16]

Postoperative and Postdislocation Variables

Dislocation Versus Subluxation

Although a distinction is recognized clinically between frank hip dislocation and subluxation, this distinction is not clearly made in the literature. It appears that most reports discuss frank dislocations, but, often, the distinction is not mentioned and what constitutes instability is not defined. When the issue is addressed, subluxation is primarily based on the perception of the patient and

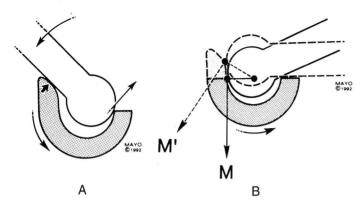

Figure 65–8. An extended portion of the acetabulum causes impingement of the neck (**A**), lessens the arc of motion, and (**B**) increases the torque applied to the component because of the asymmetry.

is characterized by not requiring physician assistance or an anesthetic for reduction. Given this definition, in one study of 35 unstable hips, 7 were frank dislocations and 28 (75 percent) were subluxations.[66] Typically, subluxation is spontaneously reduced and thus is a much less significant clinical entity. At times, however, the functional incapacity from subluxation justifies surgical intervention.[20]

Rehabilitation

One interesting study, published in 1995, found no difference in the rate of instability if the patient was rehabilitated in an acute care facility or in a formal rehabilitation unit.[44]

Time to Dislocation

In the early experience, it was thought that dislocation usually occurred in the first year after surgery. A distinct pattern of late dislocations was noted by Woo and Morrey[74] as well as others[42] (Fig. 65–11). The data of Khan et al.[42] reveal that the greatest risk of dislocation is within the first 5 weeks after surgery, although our data suggest that only 40 percent of the dislocations occur within the first month. The experience of Williams et al.[72] indicates that 70 percent of dislocations occur within the first 30 days. These investigators further made an important distinction between dislocation of primary procedures that occurred with a mean time of

31 days and those that developed recurrence after having sustained the initial dislocation at 106 days.

At the Mayo Clinic, 23 percent of the 311 patients experienced dislocation 1 year after surgery.[74] Coventry,[17] expanding on this study, reported on 32 patients who had developed initial instability 5 to 10 years after surgery. An increased ratio (3:1) of women to men in the late dislocation group was observed, and, of interest, prior surgery was a less important variable in this population. It was also noted that those with delayed instability patterns seemed to have a greater range of motion than the controls, which was thought to be the result of enlarged pseudocapsules that had developed with time (see Fig. 65–3). The findings of von Knoch et al. have updated our experience.[71] Between 1969 and 1995, 616 primary hip replacements were unstable after 25,465 procedures (2.4 percent). Of the 616,165, 27 percent first dislocated 5 or more years after surgery, averaging 11 years, with a range of 5 to 25 years! The increased risk for late dislocation was reaffirmed in females ($P<.02$). Other factors that correlated significantly were neurologic impairment and wear. Also of particular note is that 55 percent late dislocations did require a revision stabilization procedure.[42]

Direction of Dislocation

An accurate statement regarding the causes of recurrence after the initial dislocation is probably not possible because of the numerous variables involved. However, a very important question for the clinician is: If my patient sustains a dislocated hip, what are the chances of its being treated in such a way that it will not recur? The time when the dislocation occurs may be an important prognostic factor.

Instability After Revision Surgery

The high incidence of instability after revision surgery is well recognized. A review of 26 reports in the literature documenting 1856 revisions reveals an instability rate of 11.9 percent.[2] The Mayo experience with 1548 revision procedures, with a mean follow-up of 8.1 years, has been analyzed.[2] This assessment revealed 115 dislocations (7.5 percent). In this experience, the risk factors of dislocation were carefully analyzed and compared with those of a matched control group. It is of interest to note that the risk factors described in the pre-

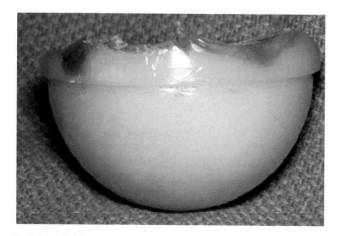

Figure 65–9. The extended wall is also the source of increased wear from impingement as evidenced by this Charnley cemented cup.

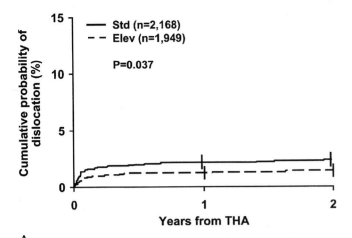

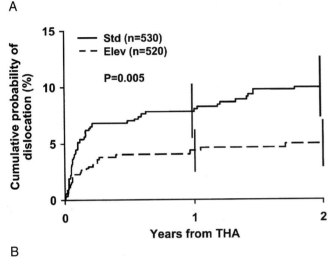

Figure 65–10. The elevated liner is associated with enhanced stability in primary (**A**) and revision (**B**) procedures.

cent) or whether both implants were revised (7.3 percent). There were, however, three variables that were shown to be statistically relevant: size of the femoral head, elevated rim liners, and trochanteric nonunion. The 22-mm head was shown to be statistically significantly more unstable after a revision procedure ($P<.05$). Elevated rim liners also demonstrated a tendency for enhanced stability, with a dislocation rate after revision of 2.4 percent compared with 8.7 percent ($P<.05$). Finally, as has been documented in virtually every other series, whether acute or revision, trochanteric nonunion with migration revealed an instability rate that was significantly associated with residual instability after revision ($P<.001$).

TREATMENT

Nonoperative Treatment

The nonoperative treatment for a patient with a dislocated or unstable primary hip replacement tends to be effective, particularly if the initial event occurred within 3 months of the procedure.[20] Review of the available literature may be simply summarized by observing that using one of several accepted postdislocation modalities to immobilize the hip for 6 to 12 weeks has a two-in-three chance to eliminate or prevent future recurrence.[42,43,74] At the Mayo Clinic, a hip brace that limits flexion and internal rotation for 6 to 8 weeks is the preferred means of treatment for the first-time dislocater. Ritter[66] reports that casting for a 6-week period was successful in 63 percent of cases, and Dorr et al.[22] reported that 10 of 12 patients were successfully treated with a brace for 3 months (83 percent). A detailed study of the nonoperative management for hip dislocations reports that 13 of 32 patients were treated by closed reduction and casting for 3 to 6 weeks. An additional 11 of 32 were treated by open reduction and casting for 3 to 6 weeks with comparable satisfactory results.[72] Rao and Bronstein cleverly demonstrated that 98 patients with a posterior exposure did not have a single incidence of dislocation when they were treated with a knee immobilizer while they were in bed.[65] Hence, this

ceding paragraphs do not necessarily relate to the patient who is at risk after undergoing a revision. Specifically, there was no statistical correlation with age, sex, laterality, and inclination of the acetabular implant. In addition, we could determine no propensity for instability whether the femur alone was revised (7.1 percent), the acetabulum alone was revised (9.0 per-

Figure 65–11. Dislocations that initially occur within the first several weeks or months after surgery are less likely to recur (**A**) than those that initially occur late (**B**). (From Khan MA, Brakenbury PH, Reynolds ISR: Dislocation following total hip replacement. J Bone Joint Surg 63B:214, 1981.)

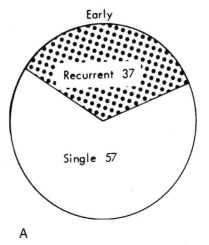

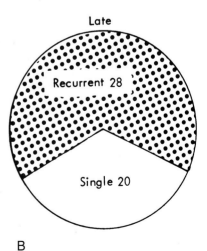

simple technique should prove effective in treating the patient who has sustained a dislocation.

In summary, nonoperative treatment is successful in two thirds of cases of instability after primary replacement.

Surgery for the Unstable Primary Hip

Fortunately, since the first two editions of this book were published, a moderate amount of literature has become available regarding the outcome of managing this condition.

Incidence

According to the Mayo experience, approximately 3 percent of patients develop an unstable hip, and, of those, 2 of 3 will be rendered stable by nonoperative management. Thus, only about 1 of every 100 patients undergoing total hip arthroplasty has required revision surgery directed at hip instability. Similarly, in an extensive survey of more than 97,000 hip replacement procedures performed between 1978 and 1990, approximately 2 percent underwent a surgical procedure for hip instability.[52] In general, when surgical intervention is performed for instability, the cause of the dislocation must be defined clearly before surgery[20,30]; otherwise, there is no obvious explanation for why case salvage may require an inherently constrained implant.[27] Under all circumstances, the success of reoperation for chronic instability is variably reported as between 40 percent and 80 percent.[1,15,18,20,25,42,65,75]

Pathology Defined and Correctable

Based on a Mayo experience of almost 100 reoperations, the defined causes of hip instability are shown in Table 65–6.[20] Of the various explanations for prosthetic instability, retroversion of the cup is probably the most commonly identified and most readily corrected. Yet, no one feature dominates, because malposition of a single component was observed by Ali Kahn et al.[42] in only 40 percent of their cases and in only half of those who underwent revision at the Mayo Clinic.[20]

Repositioning of the cup is a successful strategy in approximately 70 percent of reoperations.[20] A variation of this option is augmentation of the rim of the cup by securing an additional wedge of ultrahigh-molecular-weight-polyethylene to the portion of the cup that exhibits the instability. This procedure was originally described by Olerud and Karlstrom[60] with limited clinical experience, but Bradbury and Milligan have documented 14 of 16 successful procedures[9] (see Fig. 65–4).

Pathology Undefined or Global

As reported in the preceding sections, a specific subset of this group with undefined or global pathology

Table 65–6. DIAGNOSIS AND SUCCESS OF REVISION IN 98 CASES OF HIP INSTABILITY AT THE MAYO CENTER

Type of Revision	No.	Success (percent)
Component revision	48	33 (69)
Trochanteric advance/revision	24	15 (62)
Removal of impingement	6	2 (33)
Multiple treatment modalities	20	10 (50)
Total	98	60 (60)

includes those patients who have late dislocation of their hip and those in whom no obvious cause is present or identified. In the Mayo Clinic experience, intervention was successful only in approximately 50 percent of instances when no definite cause was identified before surgery.[20] The one procedure that was seen to be an exception was trochanteric advancement.

Advancement or reattachment of the trochanter is a highly useful technique. This is performed by carefully leaving the pseudocapsule to be plicated as a separate component of the procedure (Fig. 65–12). The trochanteric segment is small enough to leave an osseous bed but large enough to contain the attachment of the gluteus medius and minimus. This segment is advanced approximately 2 cm and fixed with a cruciate, monofilament wire technique. Fraser and Wroblewski[29] used the technique of trochanteric advancement and reported success in 80 percent of 20 patients. Similarly, Kaplan et al.[39] observed success in 80 percent after 21 patients were treated similarly. Ekelund et al.[25] studied 21 patients with this procedure and reported an identical 80 percent success rate. Hence, in those patients with no observable cause of instability, advancement of the trochanter is an important adjunct or essential treatment strategy (Fig. 65–13). Stabilization by fascia lata also has been reported as successful in up to 80 percent of cases, but this is not a commonly performed procedure.[69]

Captive Articulations

In some circumstances, the instability has been well established but no obvious malalignment of the component is definable, or the osseous and soft tissue integrity has been compromised or eliminated irreparably. Either a captive or a bipolar articulation may be the only option short of a resection arthroplasty in this patient type. Prostheses that are inherently stable—specially designed to provide articular stability to the hip—are becoming increasingly popular (Fig. 65–14). Devices that lock the femoral head into the acetabulum obviously transmit force to the bone-implant interface, thus possibly causing predisposition to acetabular component loosening. Anderson et al.[4] reported experience with 21 constrained acetabular components, documenting a 71 percent success rate with a minimum follow-up of 2 years. They recognized no radiographic evidence of cup loosening in their

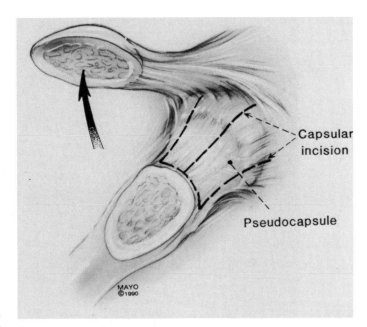

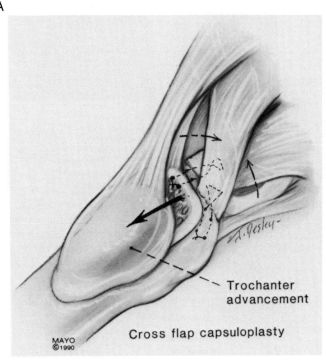

Figure 65–12. A, If there is a large pseudocapsule present, an inverted-T incision is made over the pseudocapsule after the components have been oriented, the impingement has been removed, or the acetabular wall has been lengthened. **B,** Closure of the pseudocapsule is performed in a cruciate fashion, bringing the tissue as close to the femoral neck as possible and attaching the tissue with nonabsorbable suture placed through the proximal femur.

study. The 5 failures were attributable to dissociation of the ultra-high-molecular-weight polyethylene insert from the metal cup rather than from failure at the bone prosthesis interface.

One note did, however, describe 2 mechanical failure of this implant.[28] A considerable experience with 101 captive Omnifit devices with at least 2 years' surveillance was reported by Goetz et al.[33] In this group, 55 percent had evidence of prior instability. Of these, 54 of 56 had no recurrence at a mean of more than 4 years. Of interest, pain persisted in about 50 percent of those in whom pain was part of their initial complaint.

Bipolar Replacement

Parvizi et al.[60a] reviewed the Mayo Clinic experience with 27 patients who had undergone bipolar hip arthroplasty as a salvage procedure for recurrent instability, with a mean surveillance of 5 years (range, 2 to 12 years). No patient was lost to follow-up. Sixty-seven percent in the study had undergone at least two, and, on average, three, stabilizing surgical procedures on the hip before bipolar arthroplasty. In 9, no specific single cause of the instability could be identified. At final follow-up, 25 patients (93 percent) had stable hips

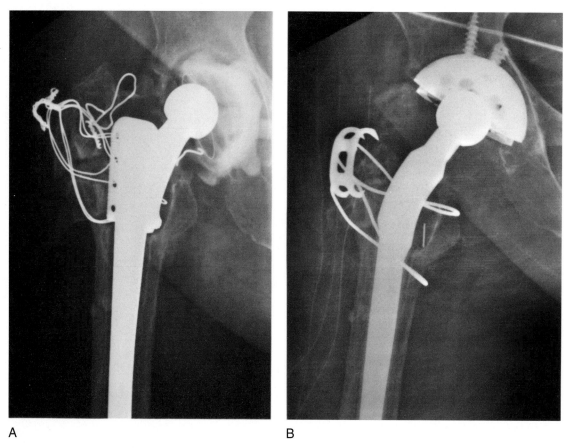

A   B

Figure 65–13. A, Patient with unstable hip who had trochanteric osteotomy and advancement that failed to unite. Revision consisted of reorienting the elevated liner to a more anterior direction because the patient was found to be unstable in extension and external rotation. **B,** The trochanter was reattached with cables. A one-half spica cast was applied for 6 weeks.

(Fig. 65–15). All patients in the study had objective improvement in hip function and mobility as measured by the Harris Hip Score (*P*<0.05). The long-term results of this study indicate that bipolar hip arthroplasty has a valuable role in the salvage management of recurrent instability of the hip in patients, particularly for those in whom other stabilization procedures have failed.

A variation of the bipolar design was also offered for use with unstable prostheses. One French design reported a successful outcome in 12 of 13 patients.[48] A similar concept of a tripolar device was reported to be successful in all 8 patients in whom it was used.[35]

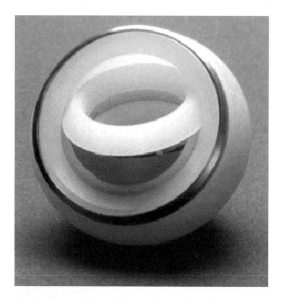

Figure 65–14. One version of the captive head implant consists of two articulating captive articular surfaces.

The Management of the Unstable Hip After Revision Surgery

There is little in the literature regarding this other than the Mayo Clinic experience.[2] A review of 115 dislocations after revision procedures showed that 103 were treated closed; of these, 67 redislocated (65 percent). This is the exact opposite expectation after closed reduction of a primary hip, in which approximately 67 percent are stable without additional surgery. Of the 67 patients who were treated with closed reduction, 38 ultimately underwent an additional re-revision procedure (57 percent). Of these 38 who underwent a surgical procedure to correct instability after revision, only 37 percent were stable at final follow-up, averaging more than 8 years. The specific analysis of these patients is rather complex and is best summarized in a flow diagram as depicted in Figure 65–16.

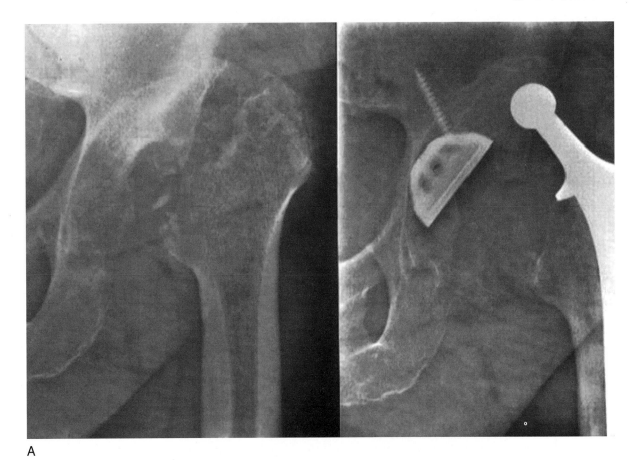

A

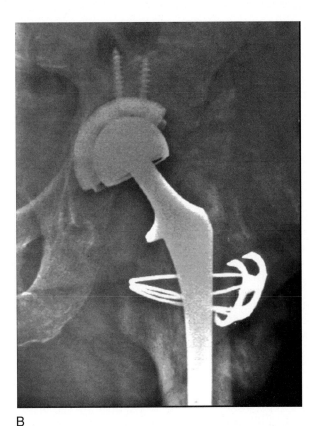

B

Figure 65–15. A bipolar replacement successfully addressed this unstable hip 2 years after surgery (**A**) and salvaged a failed effort to supplement the hip rim in another instance (**B**).

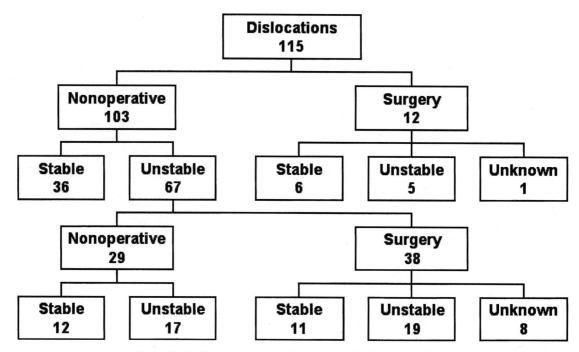

Figure 65–16. Treatment outcome for the unstable hip after revision.

AUTHOR'S PREFERENCE

For an individual with recurrent dislocation and in whom conservative modalities such as a hip guide brace have failed, the workup proceeds as follows:

1. The time of the initial dislocation is determined. Early dislocations imply trochanteric nonunion, problems with myofascial tension, inadequate scarring about the hip, improper component orientation, neuromuscular deficiency, or impingement or cognitive impairment. Late dislocations suggest stretching of the soft tissues and enlarged pseudocapsule, poor myofascial tension, or cognitive deficiency.
2. The precise direction of dislocation is determined by history and by any radiographs that may be available. Extension external rotation tends to cause anterior dislocation, and flexion internal rotation produces a posterior force and dislocation. Straight lateral dislocation is seen in some instances, usually with a vertically oriented acetabular component or nonunion of a trochanter.
3. The physical examination specifically elicits the degree of hip motion. If the patient dislocated early, this is of less value. For patients who have dislocated after several years, a greater than anticipated internal and external rotation and, possibly, hip flexion suggest a stretching of the pseudocapsule. Care is taken not to be too aggressive during examination of the patient in order to avoid a dislocation in the office!
4. Anteroposterior, lateral, and, if necessary, frog-leg radiographs are obtained to measure precisely both the component orientation and the possibility of impingement.

5. A magnetic resonance arthrogram is performed on patients whose cause of instability is not obvious and on those who have sustained the first dislocation several years after the procedure. A large pseudocapsule in a patient with a late dislocation, in my judgment, is a circumstance that requires surgical correction.

Surgical Procedure

If it appears that limb length inequality or myofascial tension is a problem, the trochanter should be osteotomized but the capsule preserved. The pseudocapsule is then incised in an inverted-T fashion in such a way as to allow distal advancement of the femoral attachment (see Fig. 65–12). The orientation of the components is then assessed, and the hip is dislocated to precisely define the direction and mechanism of the instability. If an impingement is found to be a problem, it is removed. The orientation of the component is carefully scrutinized. If a modular implant has been used, the liner is removed and rotated to see whether it provides stability. If the orientation of the acetabulum is grossly abnormal and obviously the cause of the problem, it is changed. The same is true for the femoral component, although the femoral component is rarely revised for instability unless the orientation is grossly abnormal. Usually, an excessive anteversion is found.

The closure of the capsule is important in my judgment. The femoral side of the pseudocapsule is advanced in a cruciate fashion, bringing the anterior pseudocapsule posteriorly and the posterior pseudocapsule together anteriorly, and attaching it through holes placed in the bone as close to the neck as possible. The trochanter is then advanced if it has been removed.

A simple osteotomy of the trochanter and advancement should render approximately 80 percent of such hips stable. Reattachment is performed by circumferential cable, with care taken to obtain good fixation of the trochanter. In those patients whose trochanteric component is small, the Dall-Miles cage[19] is used to capture what remnants of the trochanter (see Fig. 65–4).

In refractory cases or in those who do not have a defined cause, the constrained liner is being used more frequently. The bipolar device may be considered if it uniquely matches the femoral articulation, but the indications for this are roughly equivalent to those of the constrained designs.

Postoperatively, we apply a hip guide brace that is used for 6 to 12 weeks from the time of surgery. The patient is carefully instructed to avoid the mechanism that is thought to be most at risk based on the findings at surgery.

References

1. Ackland MK, Bourne WB, Uhthoff HK: Anteversion of the acetabular cup. J Bone Joint Surg 68B:407, 1986.
2. Alberton GM, High WA, Morrey BF: Dislocation after revision total hip arthroplasty and analysis of risk fractures and treatment outcomes. J Bone Joint Surg 84A:2002.
3. Altchek M: Avoiding dislocation in prosthetic hip replacement. Orthop Rev 22:644, 1993.
4. Anderson MJ, Murray WR, Skinner HB: Constrained acetabular components. J Arthroplasty 9:17, 1994.
5. Amstutz HC, Maki S: Complications of trochanteric osteotomy in total hip replacement. J Bone Joint Surg 60A:214, 1978.
6. Beckenbaugh RD, Ilstrup DM: Total hip arthroplasty: A review of three hundred and thirty-three cases with long follow-up. J Bone Joint Surg 60A:306, 1978.
7. Bergstrom B, Lindberg L, Persson BM, Onnerfalt R: Complications after total hip arthroplasty according to Charnley in a Swedish series of cases. Clin Orthop 95:91, 1973.
8. Bosco JA, Benjamin JB: Loosening of a femoral stem associated with the use of an extended-lip acetabular cup liner: A case report. J Arthroplasty 8:91, 1993.
9. Bradbury N, Milligan GF: Acetabular augmentation for dislocation of the prosthetic hip. A 3 (1–6) year follow-up of 16 patients. Acta Orthop Scand 65:424, 1994.
10. Brien WW, Salvati EA, Wright TM, Burstein AH: Dislocation following THA: Comparison of two acetabular component designs. Orthopedics 16:869, 1993.
11. Carlsson AS, Gentz CF: Postoperative dislocation in the Charnley and Brunswik total hip arthroplasty. Clin Orthop 125:177, 1977.
12. Chan CLH, Norman-Taylor F, Vollar RN: Septic dislocation of a total hip replacement: A forgotten complication. J Orthop Rheum 8:176, 1995.
13. Chandler RW, Dorr LD, Perry J: The functional cost of dislocation following total hip arthroplasty. Clin Orthop 182:168, 1981.
14. Charnley J, Cupic Z: The nine and ten year results of the low-friction arthroplasty of the hip. Clin Orthop 95:9, 1973.
15. Clayton ML, Thirupathi RG: Dislocation following total hip arthroplasty: Management by special brace in selected patients. Clin Orthop 177:154, 1983.
16. Cobb TK, Morrey BF, Ilstrup DM: The stabilizing effect of elevated acetabular rim liners after THA. J Bone Joint Surg 79A:1361, 1977.
17. Coventry MB: Late dislocations in patients with Charnley total hip arthroplasty. J Bone Joint Surg 67A:832, 1985.
18. Coventry MB, Beckenbaugh RD, Nolan DR, Ilstrup DM: 2012 total hip arthroplasties: A study of postoperative course and early complications. J Bone Joint Surg 56A:273, 1974.
19. Dall DM, Grobbelaar CJ, Learmonth ID, Dall G: Charnley low-friction arthroplasty of the hip. Clin Orthop 211:85, 1986.
20. Daly PJ, Morrey BF: Surgical correction of the unstable total hip arthroplasty. J Bone Joint Surg 74A:1334, 1992.
21. Dorr LD, Wan Z: Causes of and treatment protocol for instability of total hip replacement. Clin Orthop 355:144, 1998.
22. Dorr LD, Wolf AW, Chandler RW, Coventy JP: Classification and treatment of dislocation of total hip arthroplasty. Clin Orthop 173:151, 1983.
23. Eftekhar NS: Dislocation and instability complicating low friction arthroplasty of the hip joint. Clin Orthop 121:120, 1976.
24. Ejsted R, Olsen NJ: Revision of failed total hip arthroplasty. J Bone Joint Surg 69B:57, 1987.
25. Ekelund A, Rydell N, Nilsson OS: Total hip arthroplasty in patients 80 years of age and older. Clin Orthop 281:101, 1992.
26. Etienne A, Cupic A, Charnley J: Postoperative dislocation after Charnley low-friction arthroplasty. Clin Orthop 132:19, 1978.
27. Fackler CD, Poss R: Dislocation in total hip arthroplasties. Clin Orthop 151:169, 1980.
28. Fisher DA, Kiley K: Constrained acetabular cup disassembly. J Arthroplasty 9:325, 1994.
29. Fraser GA, Wroblewski BM: Revision of the Charnley low-friction arthroplasty for recurrent or irreducible dislocation. J Bone Joint Surg 63B:552, 1981.
30. Garcia CE, Munueral I: Dislocation in total hip arthroplasties. J Arthroplasty 7:145, 1992.
31. Gie A, Scott T, Ling RSM: Cup augmentation for recurrent hip replacement dislocation. J Bone Joint Surg 71B:338, 1989.
32. Goergen TG, Resnick D: Evaluation of acetabular anteversion following total hip arthroplasty: Necessity of proper centering. Br J Radiol 48:259, 1975.
33. Goetz DD, Capello WN, Callaghan JJ, et al: Salvage of total hip instability with a constrained acetabular component. Clin Orthop 355:171, 1998.
34. Graham GP, Jenkins AIR, Mintowt CZYZW: Recurrent dislocation following hip replacement: Brief report. J Bone Joint Surg 70B:675, 1988.
35. Grigoris P, Grecula MJ, Amstutz HC: Tripolar hip replacement for recurrent prosthetic dislocation. Clin Orthop 304:148, 1994.
36. Hedlundh U, Ahnfelt L, Hybbinette C-H, et al: Surgical experience related to dislocations after total hip arthroplasty. J Bone Joint Surg 78B:206, 1996.
37. Hedlundh U, Sanzen L, Fredin H: The prognosis and treatment of dislocated total hip arthroplasties with a 22 mm head. J Bone Joint Surg 79V:374, 1997.
38. Joshi A, Lee CM, Markovic L, et al: Prognosis of dislocation after total hip arthroplasty. J Arthroplasty 13:17, 1998.
39. Kaplan SJ, Thomas WH, Poss R: Trochanteric advancement for recurrent dislocation after total hip arthroplasty. J Arthroplasty 2:119, 1987.
40. Kay NRM: Some complications of total hip replacement. Clin Orthop 95:73, 1973.
41. Kelley SS, Lachiewicz PF, Hickman JM, Paterno SM: Relationship of femoral head and acetabular size to the prevalence of dislocation. Clin Orthop 355:163, 1998.
42. Khan MA, Brakenbury PH, Reynolds ISR: Dislocation following total hip replacement. J Bone Joint Surg 63B:214, 1981.
43. Kristiansen B, Jorgensen L, Holmich P: Dislocation following total hip arthroplasty. Arch Orthop Trauma Surg 103:375, 1985.
44. Krotenberg R, Stitik T, Johnston MV: Incidence of dislocation following hip arthroplasty for patients in the rehabilitation setting. Am J Phys Med Rehabil 74:444, 1995.
45. Krushell RJ, Burke DW, Harris WH: Elevated-rim acetabular components: Effect on range of motion and stability in total hip arthroplasty. J Arthroplasty 6(Suppl):53, 1991.
46. Lazansky MG: Complications revisited: The debit side of total hip replacement. Clin Orthop 95:96, 1973.
47. Lawton R, Morrey BF: Hip instability associated with long neck skirted femoral head comonents. Orlando, FL, American Academy of Orthopaedic Surgeons, February 2000.
48. Leclercq S, el Blidi S, Aubriot JH: Bousquet's device in the treatment of recurrent dislocation of a total hip prosthesis. Apropos of 13 cases. Rev Chir Orthop Reparatrice Appar Mot 81:389, 1995.
49. Levy RN, Levy CM, Snyder J, Digiovanni J: Outcome and long-term results following replacement in elderly patients. Clin Orthop 316:25, 1995.
50. Lewinnek GE, Lewis JL, Tarr R, et al: Dislocations after total hip replacement arthroplasties. J Bone Joint Surg 60A:217, 1978.
51. Lowell JD: Complications of total hip replacement. Instr Course Lect 23:209, 1974.

52. Malchau H, Herberts P, Ahnfelt L: Prognosis of total hip replacement in Sweden. Follow-up of 92,675 operations performed 1978–1990. Acta Orthop Scand 64:497, 1993.

53. Mallory TH, Lombardi AV Jr, Fada RA, et al: Dislocation after total hip arthroplasty using the anterolateral abductor split approach. Clin Orthop 358:166, 1999.

54. McCollum DE, Gray WJ: Dislocation after total hip arthroplasty: Causes and prevention. Clin Orthop 261:159, 1990.

55. Morgensen B, Arnason H, Jonsson GT: Socket wall addition for dislocating total hip. Acta Orthop Scand 57:373, 1986.

56. Morrey BF: Difficult complications after hip joint replacement. Clin Orthop 344:179, 1997.

57. Murray DW: Impingement and loosening of the long posterior wall acetabular implant. J Bone Joint Surg 74B:377, 1992.

58. Nicholas RM, Orr JF, Mollan RAB, et al: Dislocation of total hip replacements: A comparative study of standard, long posterior wall and augmented acetabular components. J Bone Joint Surg 72B:418, 1990.

59. Nolan DR, Fitzgerald RH, Beckenbaugh RD, Coventry MB: Complications of total hip arthroplasty treated by reoperation. J Bone Joint Surg 57A:977, 1975.

60. Olerud K, Karlstrom G: Recurrent dislocation status post total hip replacement. J Bone Joint Surg 67B:402, 1985.

60a. Parvizi J, Morrey BF: Bipolar hip arthroplasty as a salvage treatment for instability of the hip. J Bone Joint Surg Am 82A:1132-1139,2000.

61. Paterno SA, Lachiewicz PF, Kelley SS: The influence of patient-related factors and the position of the acetabular component on the rate of dislocation after total hip replacement. J Bone Joint Surg 79A:1202, 1997.

62. Patterson FP, Brown CS: Complications of total hip replacement arthroplasty. Orthop Clin North Am 4:503, 1973.

63. Pellicci PM, Bostrom M, Poss R: Posterior approach to total hip replacement using enhanced posterior soft tissue repair. Clin Orthop 355:224, 1998.

64. Pellicci PM, Salvati EA, Robinson HJ: Mechanical failures in total hip replacement requiring reoperation. J Bone Joint Surg 61A:28, 1979.

65. Rao JP, Bronstein R: Dislocations following arthroplasties of the hip: Incidence, prevention and treatment. Orthop Rev 20:261, 1991.

66. Ritter MA: Dislocation and subluxation of the total hip replacement. Clin Orthop 121:92, 1976.

67. Roberts JM, Fu FH, McClain EJ, Ferguson AB: A comparison of the dislocated and anterolateral approach to total hip arthroplasty. Clin Orthop 187:205, 1983.

68. Robinson RP, Robinson HR, Salvati EA: Comparison of transtrochanteric and posterior approaches for total hip replacement. Clin Orthop 147:143, 1980.

69. Stromsoe K, Eikvar K: Fascia lata plasty in recurrent posterior dislocation after total hip arthroplasty. Arch Orthop Trauma Surg 114:292, 1995.

70. Turner RS: Postoperative total hip prosthetic femoral head dislocations. Incidence, etiologic factors, and management. Clin Orthop 301:196, 1994.

71. von Knoch M, Berry DJ, Morrey BF: Late dislocation after total hip arthroplasty. J Bone Joint Surg (in press).

72. Williams JF, Gottesman MJ, Mallory TH: Dislocation after total hip arthroplasty: Treatment with an above-knee hip spica cast. Clin Orthop 171:53, 1982.

73. Woolson ST, Rahimtoola ZO: Risk factors for dislocation during the first three months after primary total hip replacement. J Arthroplasty 14:662, 1999.

74. Woo RYG, Morrey BF: Dislocations after total hip arthroplasty. J Bone Joint Surg 64A:1295, 1982.

75. Wyssa B, Raut VV, Siney PD, Wroblewski BM: Multiple revision for failed Charnley low-friction arthroplasty. J Bone Joint Surg 77B:303, 1995.

66

Ectopic Bone

• FRANK J. FRASSICA, DEBORAH A. FRASSICA, and DANIEL J. BERRY

eterotopic ossification is characterized by normal bone formation at ectopic sites. Many authors use the terms heterotopic ossification and ectopic bone interchangeably in the orthopedic literature. Ectopic bone may form within the musculoskeletal system after trauma or elective surgery, or as a manifestation of genetic disorders. There are no reliable animal models in which to study ectopic bone formation after hip arthroplasty. The most common animal models of ectopic bone formation involve the surgical implantation of bone morphogenic proteins (BMPs). These BMPs induce enchondral bone formation. When this process is studied histologically, there is an early fibroproliferative phase followed by chondrocyte differentiation, vascularization, osteoblast differentiation with bone matrix formation, and subsequent mineralization of the osteiod.[46] The formation of ectopic bone after hip arthroplasty may be secondary to release of BMPs after exposure of the hip and the arthroplasty. To be effective, ectopic bone prevention methods must be initiated during the early fibroproliferative phase of bone formation.

The formation of bone in the soft tissues (heterotopic or ectopic ossification) about the hip can compromise the major goals of total hip arthroplasty. A significant amount of ectopic bone can both limit motion about the hip and result in unexpected postoperative pain.

The development of ectopic bone is common after total hip arthroplasty.[8,10,24,26,39,45] However, only a small number of patients develop it in sufficient amounts to compromise the overall result.[42] The phenomenon of ectopic bone is not unique to modern total hip arthroplasty but was noted after both cup arthroplasty[24,56] and endoprosthetic replacement.[3] Indeed, it may be found with any operation about the hip. Charnley reported that 5 percent of his patients developed significant ectopic bone after total hip arthroplasty.[10]

Although many have speculated on the etiology of ectopic bone about the hip, there is no evidence to incriminate a single cause. Surgical factors such as bone dust, muscle damage, hematoma formation, and disrupted periosteum have all been implicated but were not statistically significant in one study of 224 patients with ectopic bone.[28] The role of the transtrochanteric approach is debated.[15,16] In a study of more than 500 procedures at the Mayo Clinic, the lateral transtrochanteric approach was associated with more ectopic bone than the anterolateral or posterolateral approach, but the differences lack statistical significance (Table 65–1).[42] Spinal cord injured patients often form large amounts of ectopic bone about the hip in the absence of fractures and surgical trauma.[18] The etiology is probably multifactorial and involves an inducing agent, osteogenic precursor cells, and an environment conductive to osteogenesis.[48]

Several researchers have characterized the process of ectopic bone development after arthroplasty as intramembranous ossification.[53,58] Others[64–66] have demonstrated that bone formation in soft tissues in experimental models with bone morphogenic protein follows a cascade, resembling endochondral ossification of the growth plate.

CLASSIFICATION SYSTEMS

There are several classification systems[15,28,42,52,53] that quantitate the amount of ectopic bone in the soft tissues about the hip. Most systems are two dimensional and use the anteroposterior radiograph. The system of Brooker et al.[8] is simple and is most commonly used. This system quantitates the amount of ectopic bone on an incremental scale of 1 to 4 (Fig. 66–1):

Class I: Islands of bone within the soft tissues about the hip
Class II: Bone spurs from the pelvis or proximal end of the femur, leaving at least 1 cm between opposing bone surfaces.
Class III: Bone spurs from the pelvis or proximal end of the femur, reducing the space between opposing bone surfaces to less than 1 cm.
Class IV: Apparent ankylosis of the hip.

An equally simple scheme has been used by Morrey et al.[42] from the Mayo Clinic (Fig. 66–2):

Grade I: Less than 5 mm
Grade II: Less than 50 percent of the distance from trochanter to acetabulum
Grade III: More than 50 percent of the distance from trochanter to acetabulum
Grade IV: Apparent ankylosis on the anteroposterior view

Table 66–1. RELATION OF EXTENT OF HETEROTOPIC BONE TO SURGICAL APPROACH

Surgical Approach (No.)	Extent of Heterotopic Bone (grade)* (percent)				
	None (0)	<5 mm (I)	< 50 percent (II)	> 50 percent (III)	Bridged (IV)
Anterior (145)	19	27	26	23	5
Transtrochanteric (238)	21	24	26	21	8
Posterior (124)	26	21	31	18	4

*Definition in text.
From Morrey BF, Adams RA, Cabanela ME: Compression of heterotopic bone after anterolateral transtrochanteric and posterior approaches for total hip arthroplasty. Clin Orthop 188:160, 1984.

Although practical, these classification systems have limitations that should be understood. Many patients with significant ectopic bone on the anteroposterior radiograph are asymptomatic and have good hip motion. In such patients, lateral views of the hip often show that the bone bridge is not as severe as expected from the anteroposterior radiograph. Cobb et al. showed that ectopic ossification on the anteroposterior film correlated only imperfectly with hip range of motion.[11]

INCIDENCE AND PREDISPOSING CONDITIONS

The incidence of ectopic bone in large series of unselected patients varies between 20 and 80 percent.[15,16,26,42,43,45] Fortunately, this is significant in only 5 to 10 percent of patients who form Brooker class III or IV ectopic bone.[42] In general, ectopic bone is present on the radiographs within 6 weeks after surgery and may be seen as soon as

3 weeks if looked for carefully. If bone has not formed within the soft tissues after 3 months, it is unlikely to form, and although ectopic bone at 3 months is not fully mature, it usually does not increase further in amount.

There are no laboratory studies to predict the patient at risk for significant ectopic bone formation. Serum alkaline phosphatase levels have had no predictive value.[41] There are, however, several clinical groups of patients who are at high risk. Patients with active ankylosing spondylitis, diffuse idiopathic skeletal hyperostosis (DISH syndrome), a history of ectopic bone after previous hip surgery, and limited preoperative hip motion are predisposed to formation of ectopic bone after arthroplasty (Fig. 66–3).

Bisla et al.[5] reported that ectopic bone occurred in 61.7 percent of their patients with ankylosing spondylitis who underwent total hip arthroplasty. Brooker class III or IV involvement was present in 39 percent of the patients in that series. Coventry and Scanlon,[12] however, noted no increase in ectopic bone unless the spondylitis was "active." Those patients with "burned-out"

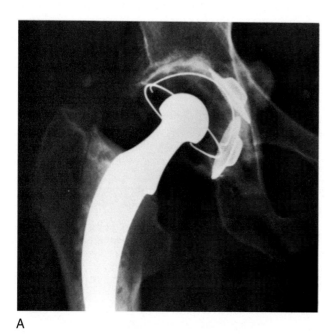

A

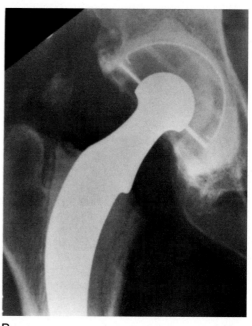

B

Figure 66–1. Radiographs showing Brooker classification of ectopic bone about the hip: class I, bone islands (**A**); class II, greater than 1-cm gap (**B**); class III, less than 1-cm gap (**C**); and class IV, apparent bridge (**D**).

Illustration continued on opposite page

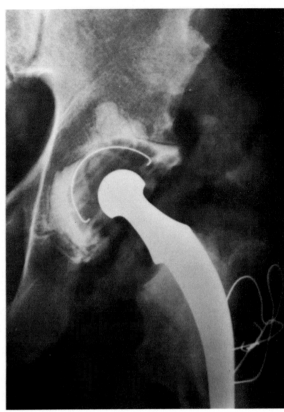

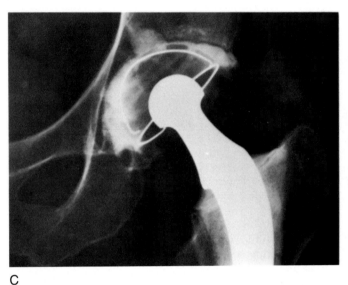

C

D

Figure 66–1. *Continued.*

rheumatoid spondylitis had no increase in incidence of ectopic bone. In a letter to the *Annals of Rheumatologic Diseases* in 1998, Tani et al. reported a significant correlation between elevated serum C reactive protein and the formation of ectopic bone in 20 arthroplasties in 16 patients with ankylosing spondylitis.[61] Kilgus and colleagues,[31] after a study of 53 hip replacements in 31 patients with ankylosing spondylitis, recommended prophylactic treatment when the following criteria were met: (1) a previous arthroplasty resulting in class III or IV heterotopic ossification or a large amount of class I heterotopic ossification (prophylaxis for the ipsilateral or contralateral hip); (2) when a second operation on the hip is performed; and (3) when the hip is ankylosed preoperatively. Sundaram and Murphy[59] noted an overall rate of 40 percent in primary arthroplasties and 55 percent in patients with previous hip surgery. Class II[15] involvement was noted in only 11 percent. Walker and Sledge[70] reported a 77 percent incidence of heterotopic ossification in 26 hips in patients with ankylosing spondylitis who had no prophylactic treatment. Thirty percent had Brooker class III or IV involvement. Three hips (15 percent) in 2 patients suffered complete reankylosis.

Several investigators have noted that men with hypertrophic osteoarthritis are more apt to develop ectopic bone after total hip arthroplasty than women.

Ritter and Gioe,[52] in a study of 507 total hip arthroplasties, reported that men are twice as likely as women to develop ectopic bone (*P*<.005), a finding similar to that reported by Morrey et al.[42] Blasingame et al.[6] further delineated the high-risk male subgroup of patients with skeletal hyperostosis (Forestier disease). Although the strict diagnosis of Forestier disease requires the presence of flowing ossification in at least four contiguous vertebral bodies, they correlated the amount of spinal osteophytes with the risk of ectopic bone after total hip arthroplasty. In their study of 69 arthroplasties, 38 percent of the patients with grade III or IV spinal osteophytosis developed Brooker class III or IV changes. Fifty percent of the patients with Forestier disease (grade IV spinal osteophytosis) developed ectopic bone of class III or IV.

Patients who have developed ectopic bone after previous arthroplasty or hip surgery are prone to develop this complication again. Ritter and Vaughan[52] reported that each of 23 patients with a history of ectopic bone again developed ectopic bone, and in each patient, the quantity of bone was the same as that following the original arthroplasty. Several studies[15,66] have shown the risk of ectopic bone in bilateral arthroplasty to be 60 percent to 90 percent if ectopic bone developed in the contralateral hip.

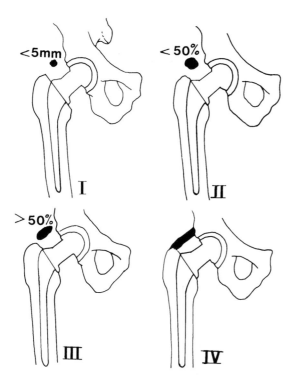

Figure 66–2. Mayo classification of ectopic bone: grade I, less than 5 mm; grade II, less than 50 percent; grade III, greater than 50 percent; grade IV, apparent bridge. (Data from Morrey BF, Adams RA, Cabanela ME: Compression of heterotopic bone after anterolateral transtrochanteric and posterior approaches for total hip arthroplasty. Clin Orthop 188:160, 1984.)

Resection of Established Ectopic Bone

Patients who develop significant ectopic bone after arthroplasty of the hip generally have decreased hip range of motion and may or may not have significant pain. A small percentage of patients have significant pain without a significant loss of hip motion. Most symptomatic patients have Brooker class III or IV ectopic bone. The reverse is not true: Many patients with Brooker class III or IV ectopic bone are pain free and have a functional arc of hip motion.

The results of ectopic bone excision for poor range of motion have been favorable (Fig. 66–4). Warren and Brooker[71] reported that 11 of 12 patients had a successful result after resection of their ectopic bone and treatment with low-dose radiation. The average improvement in hip flexion was 45 degrees and that in abduction 25 degrees. None of the patients developed class III or IV ectopic bone on follow-up. Nollen[44] reported the results of excision followed by ethylhydroxydiphosphonate therapy in 10 patients. Thirty percent had a major recurrence of the ectopic bone and 20 percent had a poor result. An average of 35 degrees of improvement in hip flexion was found. Kjaersgaard-Andersen and Schmidt[35] reported good results after resection and a 6-week course of indomethacin in 8 patients. Stiffness decreased in all patients (average improvement in combined hip motion was 123 degrees), and significant ectopic bone recurred in 2 patients but did not affect the result. van der Werf et al.[68] reported the results of resection and low-dose irradiation (beginning on the fifth postoperative day) in 7 patients. All but 1 patient had a reduction in preoperative pain, and there was an average improvement in combined hip motion of 137 degrees.

Most articles combine informations on patients treated with ectopic bone excision alone and those treated with ectopic bone excision in the course of a revision total hip arthroplasty. Cobb et al. reported on 53 hips treated with ectopic bone excision without implant

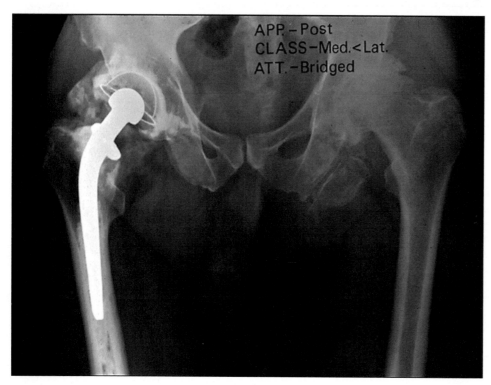

Figure 66–3. The presence of extensive hypertrophic reactive arthritis is a strong predictor of the development of ectopic bone after surgery.

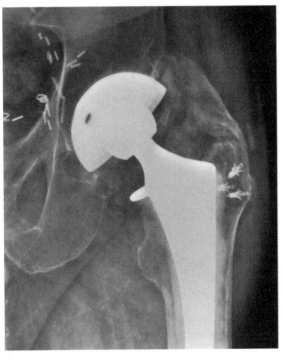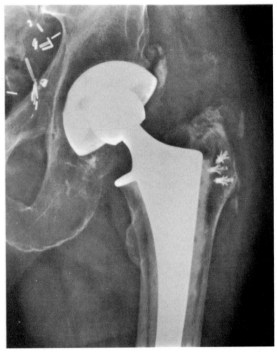

A   B

Figure 66–4. (**A**) Brooker class IV of heterotopic ossification in a 65-year-old man with painful limitation of motion. (**B**) After complete resection. The patient has improved overall motion by 80 degrees and has decreased discomfort by one grade.

revision at the Mayo Clinic. Indications were loss of motion in 60 percent, pain alone in 9 percent, both pain and limited motion in 26 percent, and other in 5 percent. Motion improved (P <.001) in all planes: The mean flexion arc improved by 34 degrees, the mean abduction-adduction arc by 22 degrees, and the mean rotation arc by 21 degrees.[11]

Although hip pain occurs frequently as heterotopic bone is actively forming, most patients do not experience marked pain once the ectopic bone has matured. If pain persists after ectopic bone has matured, careful evaluation must be undertaken to exclude other sources of pain, such as deep infection, loosening of the components, subluxation/dislocation, trochanteric bursitis, or abductor weakness. The results of excision of mature ectopic bone for pain are less predictable than the results of ectopic bone excision for hip stiffness. In the series of van der Werf et al. all but 1 of 7 patients had a reduction in pain postoperatively.[68] In the series by Cobb, the overall group treated with ectopic bone excision experienced a mild reduction in pain (by an average of one class on a pain scale of 1 to 4). It is noteworthy, however, that in the select group of 5 patients in that series treated with ectopic bone excision with pain alone as the indication, no mean improvement in pain was noted for the group.[11]

In summary, most studies have reported a significant increase in hip range of motion, and some have reported a reduction in pain after resection of ectopic bone.[35,71] Prophylaxis against ectopic bone recurrence with low-dose radiation or nonsteroidal anti-inflammatory agents should be used to prevent recurrence. When coun-

seling a patient preoperatively, we generally expect an improvement in hip flexion of 30 to 45 degrees. Some patients have significant pain improvement; however, many continue to have discomfort. Patients with pain and adequate range of motion (90 degrees of hip flexion) generally do not have sufficient improvement postoperatively to warrant exploration and resection.

Resection of ectopic bone can be difficult. Computed tomography scans are useful to identify the location and pattern of ectopic bone. Blood loss may range from 200 to 2000 ml. The mean blood replacement in the series reported by Cobb was 1.5 units with a range of zero to 5 units.[11] Intraoperative radiographs are necessary to verify that the ectopic bone has been excised. Some authors advocate dislocation of the prosthesis to accomplish complete resection of the ectopic bone.[70] At least two suction drains should be used to minimize the risk of hematoma formation. Appropriate postoperative adjuvant therapy to reduce the risk of recurrence of the ectopic bone is essential.

PREVENTION OF ECTOPIC BONE

The prevention or minimization of ectopic bone is the goal of all hip surgeons. This can be best accomplished by preoperative identification of high-risk patients and subsequent treatment of those patients, when possible, with some form of adjuvant prophylactic treatment.

Although there are no studies that correlate surgical technique with the formation of ectopic bone, there are several aspects of good surgical technique that might, logically, lower the risk of ectopic bone. Bone dust and debris should be removed from the soft tissues. Trauma to the abductor and adductor muscle groups of the hip should be minimized, and the supra-acetabular periosteum of the ilium should not be irritated. Drainage of the wound should be adequate to reduce hematoma formation. When a bone graft is added to either the femoral or acetabular component, it should be stable and not free to migrate into the soft tissue.

There are three postoperative adjuvant methods advocated to reduce the risk of ectopic bone: low-dose irradiation, diphosphonates, and nonsteroidal anti-inflammatory agents. Although various reports have supported the efficacy or oral agents, low-dose irradiation remains the most effective form of treatment.

Diphosphonate Therapy

Diphosphonates are pyrophosphate analogues that have been used to inhibit the formation of ectopic bone.[19,20,50] They inhibit the growth of hydroxyapatite crystal in vitro by chemisorption. Etidronate disodium is the most commonly used agent.[50] There is no evidence that diphosphonates inhibit the formation of osteoid matrix, and, when diphosphonates are discontinued, mineralization of the osteoid occurs. Diphosphonates must be given preoperatively and continued for 3 to 4 months. The effect is dose related, and long-term use may produce osteomalacia. Although preliminary reports[17] were favorable, Thomas and Amstutz[62] reported in 1985 that disphosphonates were ineffective in preventing ectopic bone when administered preoperatively for 2 to 4 weeks and postoperatively for 3 months.

Nonsteroidal Anti-inflammatory Agents

Nonsteroidal anti-inflammatory agents (prostaglandin formation inhibitors such as indomethacin, ibuprofen, Naproxen, and diclofenac)[1,9,22,33–36,44,57,63,68–70,72] and aspirin[21,47] have also been employed for the prevention of heterotopic ossification. Because of favorable reports, many authors advocate their use in high-risk patients rather than low-dose irradiation. In addition, some authors[51] recommend that all patients who undergo total hip arthroplasty should have prophylaxis with nonsteroidal anti-inflammatory agents.

It has been reported that ibuprofen (400 mg three times a day) was effective in the prevention of ectopic bone in a small number of patients. In a similar study, Ritter and Gioe found that indomethacin was effective.[52] Other reports have confirmed the efficacy of nonsteroidal anti-inflammatory medications for the control of heterotopic bone.[22,33,40,51,57,63,69,72]

Gebuhr and co-workers,[22] in a prospective randomized study, found that naproxen was effective in reducing the formation of heterotopic bone. Naproxen (500 mg) was given in suppository form twice on the day of operation followed by 4 weeks of oral dosing (250 mg three times a day). In the treatment group, only 1 of 27 patients (3.7 percent) developed significant ectopic bone, whereas, in the placebo group, 8 of 27 (29.6 percent) developed significant ectopic bone. Kjaersgaard-Andersen et al.[33] reported a prospective, double-blind, randomized study of indomethacin prophylaxis (indomethacin 25 mg three times a day for 2 weeks). The incidence of significant ectopic bone was significantly less in the treated group (5 versus 27 percent; P=.002).

The necessary duration of nonsteroidal treatment has not been well established. Many authors recommend 4 to 6 weeks. Whereas Kjaersgaard-Andersen et al.[33] found 2 weeks of indomethacin 25 mg three times a day to be effective, Ahrengart et al.[1] found ibuprofen 500 mg three times a day to be ineffective. Van der Heide noted an overall incidence of ectopic bone formation of 74 percent with Brooker grade III formation of 16 percent in a prospective study of 19 patients treated with a 3-day trial of indomethacin.[67] Several studies have shown that an 8- to 14-day treatment course is effective.[2,13,34,37,40,73] Amstutz[2] found excellent ectopic bone prevention with no cases of Brooker Grade III or IV bone formation in 196 patients who completed a 10-day course of oral indomethacin (25 mg three times daily).

Major disadvantages of nonsteroidal anti-inflammatory medication are noncompliance and side effects such as gastrointestinal distress, fluid retention, and adverse renal effects. Contraindications to nonsteroidal anti-inflammatory treatment include: (1) active gastric ulcer, (2) significant gastritis within 6 months, (3) previous history of allergy or intolerance to the specific agent, and (4) severe renal, cardiac, or hepatic insufficiency.[1,34,72] In properly selected patients, intolerance to nonsteroidal anti-inflammatory medication develops in 10 to 35 percent.[9,22,33,51,57,69]

Amstutz[2] reported significant postoperative bleeding in 4 of 106 patients when a 10-day course of indomethacin was combined with warfarin to prevent deep venous thrombosis.

Low-Dose External Beam Irradiation

Low-dose external beam irradiation has been shown to be an effective and safe method of preventing heterotopic ossification in high-risk patients. Coventry and Scanlon[12] popularized its use in 1981, using 2000 cGy in 10 fractions (1 centiGray [cGy]=1 rad). Numerous studies in the literature have demonstrated efficacy using lower doses of irradiation.[4,14,30,49] Ayers and associates, in 1986, reported the effective use of 1000 cGy in five divided doses. In that study, only a single patient (1.5 percent) developed Brooker class III ectopic bone.[4]

Pellegrini and colleagues,[38,49] in a study of 6222 hips in 55 high-risk patients, found that a single postoperative dose of 800 cGy of external beam irradiation was an effective as 1000 cGy delivered in five fractions. In that study, no patients developed Brooker class IV ectopic bone. In patients receiving the single 800 cGy fraction, only two (6 percent) developed class III ectopic bone. Both patients had previous ectopic bone formation after arthroplasty of the ipsilateral hip, and in only 1 was the class III bone formation progressive from a previous class II. Ectopic bone occurred outside of the radiation portal over the vastus lateralis ridge of the greater trochanter in 31 percent of the hips. Sixteen percent of the hips with extrafield ectopic bone needed more than one cortisone injection secondary to a painful greater trochanter. Healy et al.[25] reported similar results in a series of 34 hips treated with a single 700-cGy fraction on the first postoperative day. A single patient developed class III ectopic bone postoperatively (2.9 percent).

Trochanteric nonunion has been reported to occur in 30 percent of patients after low-dose irradiation.[4,49] Nonunion of the greater trochanter is multifactorial and may not always be specifically related to the irradiation.

Postoperative external beam irradiation can be inconvenient from a logistic point of view (e.g., pain, nursing staff requirements, risk of dislocation). Based on the basic science study (in vivo, pre- and postoperative irradiation of demineralized bone matrix) of Kantorowitz et al.,[29] two centers have conducted randomized studies of preoperative external beam single-fraction irradiation versus single-fraction postoperative irradiation.[23,54,55] Both studies showed no significant difference in efficacy between pre- and postoperative irradiation. In both protocols, the preoperative irradiation is delivered *within 4 hours of the planned operation*. Gregoritch and co-workers reported class III ectopic bone in only 1 (3.7 percent) of 27 patients treated with preoperative irradiation.[23] In the study by Seegenschmiedt et al.,[55] 2 of 9 patients who had their radiation more than 4 hours before surgery developed heterotopic ossification and were considered treatment failures.

AUTHORS' PREFERENCE

At this time, we favor the use of low-dose irradiation as an adjuvant in high-risk patients. There are three groups of patients we consider to be at high risk for the formation of ectopic bone: (1) patients with active ankylosing spondylitis, (2) patients with osteoarthritis of the hip and the DISH syndrome, and (3) patients who have demonstrated a predilection to form heterotopic bone after a previous hip operation. Nonsteroidal anti-inflammatory agents are an effective alternative as a means of prophylaxis. Noncompliance and intolerance may occur in up to one third of patients. In addition, although these agents have been shown to reduce heterotopic ossification significantly, some heterotopic ossification (Brooker class III) occurs in up to 5 percent of patients despite nonsteroidal therapy in unselected hip arthroplasty patients in prospective randomized studies.[22,36] In contrast, single-fraction external beam irradiation in *high-risk patients* results in less than a 2 percent risk of heterotopic ossification.[4,49]

Low-dose irradiation is effective and safe. When the anterolateral or lateral approach to the hip is used, the skin incision is not within the field of irradiation. If the posterior approach is selected, we still believe that irradiation is safe because there has been no evidence of wound breakdown in these patients. The surgical technique is modified slightly, with skin suture being used in lieu of metal staples, because staples may cause scatter of the radiation if they are in the irradiated field. Irradiation is begun on the first postoperative day, when feasible, and always within the first 72 hours postoperatively. Delaying radiation beyond the fourth postoperative day substantially compromises the result. Currently, a single fraction of 700 to 800 cGy is delivered within the first 72 hours postoperatively.

Because low-dose irradiation is very effective in controlling ectopic bone after total hip arthroplasty, we have been concerned that it may inhibit bone ingrowth into porous-coated prosthetic components. It may also compromise incorporation of the bone grafts and healing of the osteotomized trochanter, or of abductors to the trochanter. Accordingly, a custom shielding technique similar to the method of Jasty and colleagues[27] was developed to reduce the irradiation dose to the bone ingrowth areas of the prostheses and to bone-grafted areas. Our early results employing low-dose irradiation to control ectopic bone in porous-coated prostheses were favorable and led to the use of Cerrobend shields, which are particularly helpful after placement of uncemented implants (Fig. 66–5). There have been no early failures of the prosthetic components (Figs. 66–6 and 66–7). Our preliminary results are similar to those of Sylvester et al.[60] They appear to be as effective as the previously proven 2000-cGy administration. In some instances, the value of this technique appears particularly dramatic. Proper shielding of the hip is essential to the outcome of the surgery, and we believe the orthopedic surgeon should provide information regarding the type of prosthesis and location of the porous coating to the radiation oncologist before radiation is given.

The risk of inducing malignant disease with ionizing radiation in the treatment of patients without a malignant disease is always a concern. Both Kim et al.[32] and Brady[7] found that all patients with radiation-induced sarcomas had been treated with more than 3000 rads over a 3-week period. In addition, in a review of 130 postradiation sarcomas treated at the Mayo Clinic, no case of sarcoma has developed after low-dose irradiation for the control of ectopic bone. In women of childbearing age, it is more prudent to use a prostaglandin blocker than risk the potential of scattered radiation to the ovaries.

Irradiation Technique for Cemented Arthroplasty

A total dose of 700 to 800 cGy is delivered as a single fraction through parallel opposed anteroposterior and posteroanterior fields. The field covers both the abductor and adductor muscle groups. The radiation fields are planned on a simulator, and the fields are checked by portal verification radiographs. Areas that have been bone grafted and trochanteric osteotomy sites are shielded via hand-placed blocks, custom cadmium-lead alloy blocks, or via use of the multileaf collimator.

Irradiation Technique for Noncemented Arthroplasties

A single dose of 700 to 800 cGy is delivered through parallel opposed anteroposterior and posteroanterior fields. The radiation fields are planned on a simulator to cover both the abductor and adductor muscle groups (see Fig. 66–5). The porous-coated (bone ingrowth) areas of the prosthesis are identified on the postoperative radiographs and shielded (see Fig. 66–5B). In addition, bone defects that have been grafted and trochanters that have been osteotomized are shielded. After simulation, the area to be irradiated is checked with portal verification radiographs (see Fig. 66–5).

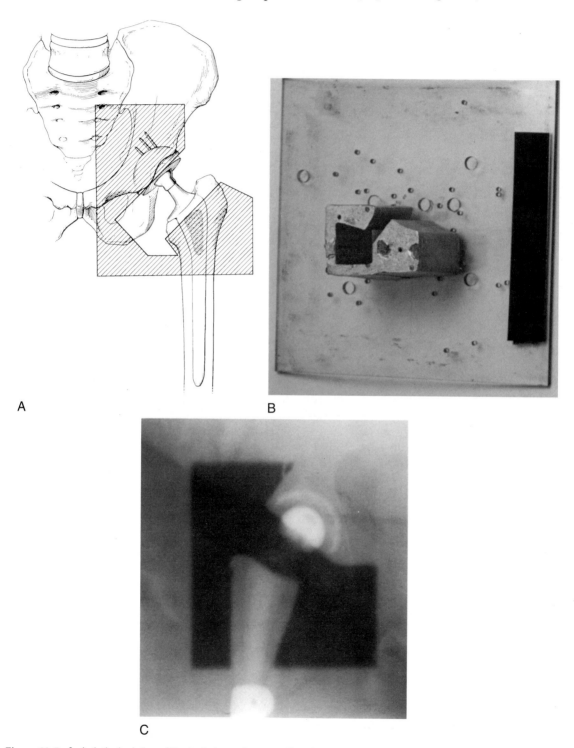

A

B

C

Figure 66–5. A, Artist's depiction of the technique of custom Cerrobend blocks to shield the porous-coated component. **B**, Photograph of the Cerrobend custom block designed to shield the porous-coated areas of both the femoral and acetabular components. **C**, Portal verification radiograph demonstrating excellent shielding of the porous-coated areas of the femoral and acetabular components.

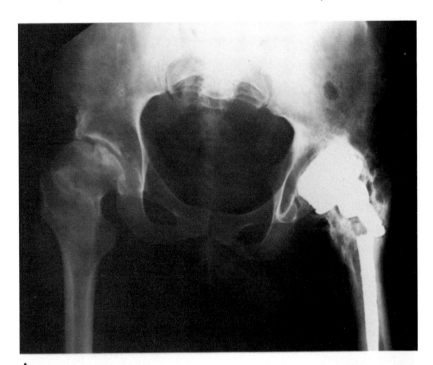

Figure 66–6. **A**, Anteroposterior radiograph of a 26-year-old woman who developed grade IV heterotopic ossification after arthroplasty with the Judet prosthesis. Revision was necessary secondary to fracture of the femoral stem. **B**, Anteroposterior radiograph after revision with adjuvant low-dose external beam irradiation. There is no heterotopic ossification in the abductor muscle group, with only grade II heterotopic ossification in the area of the adductor muscles.

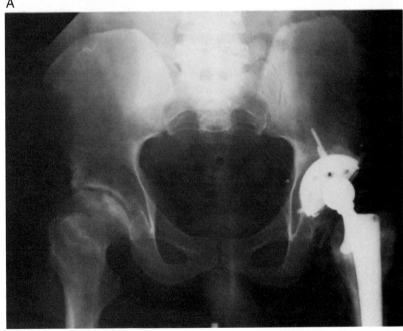

B

SUMMARY

Heterotopic ossification, or development of ectopic bone after total hip arthroplasty may compromise the postoperative result by limiting hip range of motion and causing postoperative pain. Patients at risk for the formation of ectopic bone include those with active ankylosing spondylitis and diffuse idiopathic skeletal hyperostosis (DISH syndrome), as well as those who experienced formation of ectopic bone after a prior arthroplasty or surgical procedure. Low-dose irradiation delivered as a single fraction postoperatively within 3 days of the arthroplasty is a most effective method of controlling ectopic bone. Porous ingrowth prostheses and bone-grafted areas should be shielded. Radiation fields should be planned on a simulator and checked with portal verification radiographs.

ACKNOWLEDGMENT

We wish to express our gratitude to Paula Schomberg, M.D., for her advice during the preparation of this chapter.

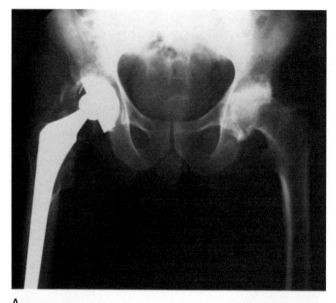

A

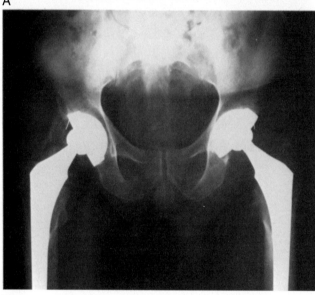

B

Figure 66–7. A, Anteroposterior radiograph of a 61-year-old man who had developed grade III heterotopic ossification after a right total hip arthroplasty. He also had significant osteoarthritis of the spine. **B,** Anteroposterior radiograph after left total hip arthroplasty with adjuvant external beam irradiation. There is essentially no heterotopic bone formation.

References

1. Ahrengart L, Blomgren G, Tornkvist H: Short-term ibuprofen to prevent ossification after total hip arthroplasty: No effects in a prospective randomized study of 47 arthrosis cases. Acta Orthop Scand 65:139, 1994.
2. Amstutz HC, Fowble VA, Schmalzried TP, Dorey FJ: Short-course indomethacin prevents heterotopic ossification in a high risk population following total hip arthroplasty. J Arthroplasty 12:126, 1997.
3. Andersen G, Nielson JM: Results after arthroplasty with Moore's prosthesis. Acta Orthop Scand 43:397, 1972.
4. Ayers DC, Evarts CM, Parkinson JR: The prevention of heterotopic ossification in high-risk patients by low-dose radiation therapy after total hip arthroplasty. J Bone Joint Surg 68A:1423, 1986.

5. Bisla RS, Ranawat CS, Inglis AE: Total hip replacement in patients with ankylosing spondylitis with involvement of the hip. J Bone Joint Surg 58A:233, 1976.
6. Blasingame JP, Resnick D, Coutts RD, Danzig LA: Extensive spinal osteophytosis as a risk factor for heterotopic bone formation after total hip arthroplasty. Clin Orthop 161:191, 1981.
7. Brady LW: Radiation induced sarcomas of bone. Skeletal Radiol 4:72, 1979.
8. Brooker AF, Bowerman JW, Robinson RA, Riley LH: Ectopic ossification following total hip arthroplasty: Incidence and method of classification. J Bone Joint Surg 55A:1629, 1973.
9. Cella JP, Salvati EA, Sculco TP: Indomethacin for the prevention of heterotopic ossification following total hip arthroplasty: Effectiveness, contraindications, and adverse effects. J Arthroplasty 3:229, 1988.
10. Charnley J: The long term results of low-friction arthroplasty of the hip performed as a primary intervention. J Bone Joint Surg 54B:61, 1972.
11. Cobb T, Berry DJ, Morrey BF: Functional outcome of excision of heterotopic ossification after total hip arthroplasty. Clin Orthop 361:131, 1999.
12. Coventry MB, Scanlon PW: The use of irradiation to discourage ectopic bone: A nine-year study in surgery about the hip. J Bone Joint Surg 63A:201, 1981.
13. Dorn U, Grethen C, Effenberger H: Indomethacin for prevention of heterotopic ossification after hip arthroplasty: A randomized comparison between 45 and 8 days of treatment. Acta Orthop Scand 69:107, 1998.
14. DeFlitch CJ, Stryker JA: Postoperative hip irradiation in prevention of heterotopic ossification: Causes of treatment failure. Radiology 188:265, 1993.
15. DeLee J, Ferrari A, Charnley J: Ectopic bone formation following low friction arthroplasty of the hip. Clin Orthop 121:53, 1976.
16. Errico TJ, Fetto JF, Waugh TR: Heterotopic ossification: incidence and relation to trochanteric osteotomy in 100 total hip arthroplasties. Clin Orthop 190:138, 1984.
17. Finerman GAM, Krengel WF Jr, Lowell JD, et al: Role of diphosphonates (EHDP) in the prevention of heterotopic ossification after total hip arthroplasty: A preliminary report. In The Hip: Proceedings of the Fifth Open Scientific Meeting of the Hip Society. St. Louis, CV Mosby, 1977; p 222.
18. Finerman GAM, Stover SL: Heterotopic ossification following hip replacement or spinal cord injury: Two clinical studies with EHDP. Metab Bone Dis 5:337, 1981.
19. Frances MD: The inhibition of calcium hydroxyapatite crystals by polyphosphonates and polyphosphates. Calcif Tissue Res 3:151, 1969.
20. Frances MD, Russell RGG, Fleisch H: Diphosphonates inhibit formation of calcium phosphate crystal in vitro and pathological calcification in vivo. Science 165:1264, 1969.
21. Freiberg AA, Cantor R, Freiberg RA: The use of aspirin to prevent heterotopic ossification after total hip arthroplasty. Clin Orthop 267:93, 1991.
22. Gebuhr P, Soelberg M, Orsnes T, Wilbek H: Naproxen prevention of heterotopic ossification after hip arthroplasty: A prospective control study of 55 patients. Acta Orthop Scand 62:226, 1991.
23. Gregoritch SJ, Chadha M, Pellegrini VD, et al: Randomized trial comparing preoperative versus postoperative irradiation for prevention of heterotopic ossification following prosthetic total hip replacement: Preliminary results. Int J Radiat Oncol Biol Phys 30:55, 1994.
24. Hamblen DL, Harris WH, Rottger J: Myositis ossificans as a complication of hip arthroplasty. J Bone Joint Surg 53B:764, 1971.
25. Healy WL, Lo TCM, Covall DJ, et al: Single-dose radiotherapy for prevention of heterotopic ossification after total hip arthroplasty. J Arthroplasty 5:369, 1990.
26. Ilstrup DM, Nolan DR, Beckenbaugh RD, Conventry MB: Factors influencing the results in 2012 total hip arthroplasties. Clin Orthop 95:250, 1973.
27. Jasty M, Schutzer S, Tepper J, et al: Radiation-blocking shields to localize periarticular radiation precisely for prevention of heterotopic bone formation around uncemented total hip arthroplasties. Clin Orthop 257:138, 1990.
28. Jowsey J, Coventry MB, Robins PR: Heterotopic ossification: Theoretical consideration, possible etiologic factors, and a clinical

review of total hip arthroplasty patients exhibiting this phenomenon. *In* The Hip: Proceedings of the Fifth Open Scientific Meeting of the Hip Society. St. Louis, CV Mosby, 1977, p 210.

29. Kantorowitz DA, Miller GJ, Ferrara JA, et al: Preoperative versus postoperative irradiation in the prophylaxis of heterotopic bone formation in rats. Int J Radiat Oncol Biol Phys 19:1431, 1990.

30. Kennedy WF, Gruen TA, Chessin H, et al: Radiation therapy to prevent heterotopic ossification after cementless total hip arthroplasty. Clin Orthop 262:185, 1991.

31. Kilgus DJ, Namba RS, Gorek JE, et al: Total hip replacement for patients who have ankylosing spondylitis: The importance of the formation of heterotopic bone and of the durability of fixation of cemented components. J Bone Joint Surg 72A:834, 1990.

32. Kim JH, Chu FC, Woodward HQ, et al: Radiation induced soft tissue and bone sarcoma. Radiology 129:501, 1978.

33. Kjaesgaard-Andersen P, Nafei A, Teichert G, et al: Indomethacin for prevention of heterotopic ossification: a randomized controlled study in 41 hip arthroplasties. Acta Orthop Scand 64:639, 1993.

34. Kjaersgaard-Andersen P, Ritter MA: Short-term treatment with nonsteroidal anti-inflammatory medications to prevent heterotopic bone formation after total hip arthroplasty: A preliminary report. Clin Orthop 279:157, 1992.

35. Kjaersgaard-Andersen P, Schmidt SA: Indomethacin for prevention of ectopic ossification after hip arthroplasty. Acta Orthop Scand 57:12, 1986.

36. Kjaersgaard-Andersen P, Schmidt SA: Total hip arthroplasty: The role of anti-inflammatory medications in the prevention of heterotopic ossification. Clin Orthop 263:78, 1991.

37. Kjaersgaard-Andersen P, Nafei A, Teichert G, et al: Indomethacin for prevention of heterotopic ossification. Acta Orthop Scand 64:639, 1993.

38. Konski A, Pellegrini V, Poulter C, et al: Randomized trial comparing single dose versus fractionated irradiation for prevention of heterotopic bone: A preliminary report. Int J Radiat Oncol Biol Phys 18:1139, 1990.

39. Kromann-Andersen C, Sorenson TS, Hougaard K, et al: Ectopic bone formation following Charnley hip arthroplasty. Acta Orthop Scand 51:633, 1980.

40. McMahon JS, Waddell JP, Morton J: Effect of short-course indomethacin or heterotopic bone formation after uncemented total hip arthroplasty. J Arthroplasty 6:259, 1991.

41. Mollan RAB: Serum alkaline phosphatase in heterotopic para-articular ossification after total hip arthroplasty. J Bone Joint Surg 61B:433, 1979.

42. Morrey BF, Adams RA, Cabanela ME: Compression of heterotopic bone after anterolateral transtrochanteric and posterior approaches for total hip arthroplasty. Clin Orthop 188:160, 1984.

43. Nolan DR, Fitzgerald RH, Beckenbaugh RD, Coventry MB: Complications of total hip arthroplasty treated by reoperation. J Bone Joint Surg 57A:977, 1975.

44. Nollen AJG: Effects of ethylhydroxydiphosphonate (EHDP) on heterotopic ossification. Acta Orthop Scand 57:358, 1986.

45. Nollen AJG, Sloof TJJH: Para-articular ossifications after total hip replacements. Acta Orthop Scand 44:230, 1973.

46. O'Connor JP: Animal models of heterotopic ossification. Clin Orth 346:71, 1998.

47. Pagnani MJ, Pellicci PM, Salvati EA: Effect of aspirin on heterotopic ossification after total hip arthroplasty in men who have osteoarthrosis. J Bone Joint Surg 73A:924, 1991.

48. Parkinson JR, Evarts CM, Hubbard LF: Radiation therapy in the prevention of heterotopic ossification after total hip arthroplasty. *In* The Hip: Proceedings of the 10th Open Scientific Meeting of the Hip Society. St. Louis, CV Mosby, 1982, p 211.

49. Pellegrini VD, Konski AA, Gastel JA, et al: Prevention of heterotopic ossification with irradiation after total hip arthroplasty. J Bone Joint Surg 74A:186, 1992.

50. Plasmans CMT, Kuypers W, Sloof TJJH: The effect of ethane-1-hydroxy-1, 1-diphosphonic acid (EHDP) on matrix induced ectopic bone formation. Clin Orthop 132:233, 1978.

51. Reis HJ, Kusswetter W, Schellinger T: The suppression of heterotopic ossification after total hip arthroplasty. Int Orthop 16:140, 1992.

52. Ritter MA, Gioe TJ: The effect of indomethacin on para-articular ectopic ossification following total hip arthroplasty. Clin Orthop 167:113, 1982.

53. Rosendahl S, Christofferson J, Norgaard M: Para-articular ossification following hip replacement. Acta Orthop Scand 48:400, 1977.

54. Seegenschmiedt MH, Goldmann AR, Wolfel R, et al: Prevention of heterotopic ossification (HO) after total hip replacement: Randomized high versus low dose radiotherapy. Radiother Oncol 26:271, 1993.

55. Seegenschmiedt MH, Martus P, Goldmann AR, et al: Preoperative versus postoperative radiotherapy for prevention of heterotopic ossification (HO): First results of a randomized trial in high risk patients. Int J Radiat Oncol Biol Phys 30:63, 1994.

56. Slatis P, Kiviluoto O, Santavirta S: Ectopic ossification after hip arthroplasty. Ann Chir Gynaecol 67:89, 1978.

57. Sodemann B, Persson PE, Nilsson OS: Nonsteroidal anti-inflammatory drugs prevent the recurrence of heterotopic ossification after excision. Arch Orthop Trauma Surg 109:53, 1990.

58. Stover SL, Hataway CJ, Zieglas HE: Heterotopic ossification in spinal cord injured patients. Arch Phys Med Rehabil 56:199, 1975.

59. Sundaram NA, Murphy JCM: Heterotopic bone formation following total hip arthroplasty in ankylosing spondylitis. Clin Orthop 207:223, 1986.

60. Sylvester JE, Greenberg P, Selch MT, et al: The use of postoperative irradiation for the prevention of heterotopic ossification after total hip replacement. Int J Radiat Oncol Biol Phys 14:471, 1988.

61. Tani Y, Nishioka J, Inoue K, Hukuda S: Relation between ectopic ossification after total hip arthroplasty and activity of general inflammation in patients with ankylosing spondylitis. Ann Rheum Dis 5:634, 1998.

62. Thomas BJ, Amstutz HC: Results of administration of diphosphonates for the prevention of heterotopic ossification after total hip arthroplasty. J Bone Joint Surg 67A:400, 1985.

63. Tozun R, Pinar H, Yesiller E, Hamzaoglu A: Indomethacin for prevention of heterotopic ossification after total hip arthroplasty. J Arthroplasty 7:57, 1992.

64. Urist MR: The bone induction principle. Clin Orthop 53:243, 1967.

65. Urist MR, Hay PH, Dubue F: Osteogenic competence. Clin Orthop 64:194, 1969.

66. Urist MR, Strates BS: Bone formation in implants of partially and wholly demineralized bone matrix. Clin Orthop 71:271, 1970.

67. Van der Heide HJL, Koorevaar RT, Schreurs BW, et al: Indomethacin for 3 days is not effective as prophylaxis after primary total hip arthroplasty. J Arthroplasty 14:796, 1999.

68. van der Werf GJIM, Hasselt NGN, Tonimo AJ: Radiotherapy in the prevention of recurrence of para-articular ossification in total hip prostheses. Arch Orthop Trauma Surg 104:85, 1985.

69. Wahlstrom O, Risto O, Djerf K, Hammerby S: Heterotopic bone formation prevented by diclofenac. Acta Orthop Scand 62:419, 1991.

70. Walker LG, Sledge CB: Total hip arthroplasty in ankylosing spondylitis. Clin Orthop 262:198, 1991.

71. Warren SB, Brooker AB: Excision of heterotopic bone followed by irradiation after total hip arthroplasty. J Bone Joint Surg 74A:201, 1992.

72. Wurnig C, Eyb R, Auersperg V: Indomethacin for prevention of ectopic ossification in cementless arthroplasties: A prospective 1-year study of 100 cases. Acta Orthop Scand 63:628, 1992.

73. Wurnig C, Auersperg V, Boehler N, et al: Short-term prophylaxis against heterotopic bone after cementless hip replacement. Clin Orthop 344:175, 1997.

67

Periprosthetic Fractures Associated with Hip Arthroplasty

• DAVID G. LEWALLEN and DANIEL J. BERRY

Fractures of the femur adjacent to the femoral component of the hip arthroplasty can vary from minor, with barely perceptible effects on outcome, to catastrophic and nearly unreconstructable, with a major impact on the final outcome.[1,4,16,26,28,32,45,53] Better algorithms for treatment, improved implants, and better surgical techniques have led to marked advances in management of this challenging problem. The event may occur during surgery, be associated with significant trauma, or occur as a result of routine day-to-day loads about the hip when loosening, osteolysis, or local stress risers are present. The frequency with which periprosthetic fractures are encountered has been increasing, in large part as a result of the growing population at risk after more than 30 years of hip arthroplasty in this country. The causes, the means of prevention, and the postevent management of these fractures is becoming well understood. Since the last edition was published, a clearer picture of the frequency of acetabular fracture and its management has emerged. This is discussed at the end of this chapter.

FEMORAL FRACTURES

Classification

Fractures of the femur are described by when they occur relative to index arthroplasty, etiology, and anatomic location.

A description of when the fracture occurs results in two major categories: (1) intraoperative fractures, which occur during the course of the index arthroplasty or as a result of removal of a prior failed implant; and (2) postoperative fractures, which occur some days, months, or, more typically, years after the original procedure.

The cause of the fracture is not always clear, but, when possible, classification by etiology assists with regard to treatment and prevention of future problems. Thus, management may vary considerably for an acute periprosthetic fracture associated with major trauma versus a fracture through a stress riser such as a screw hole or cortical window after low-level stress. In addi-

tion, both of these problems are considerably different from stress fractures that occasionally occur adjacent to the implant tip.

Although these considerations are important, the majority of classification schemes have dealt with the location and pattern of the fracture lines relative to the femur and the prosthesis. Attention is often given to the relationship of the fracture and the tip of the femoral stem, because this relationship may significantly influence treatment options and outcome.

Whitaker and colleagues used a three-zone system, with fractures proximal to the lesser trochanter designated as type I, fractures below the lesser trochanter

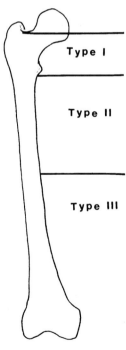

Figure 67–1. Morrey classification of intraoperative fractures related to the anatomy of the femur and subdivided by displacement. (From Morrey BF, Kavanagh BF: Complications with revision of the femoral components of total hip arthroplasty: Comparison between cemented and uncemented techniques. J Arthroplasty 7:71, 1992.)

902

down to the stem tip as type II, those at or below the stem tip as type III.[54] Bethea and associates also suggested classification into three types, with type A distal to the stem tip; type B proximal to the stem tip; and type C comminuted, involving the proximal femur.[4]

Johansson et al. suggested yet another division into three types, with type I proximal to the stem tip; type II both proximal and distal, involving a long spiral fracture; and type III, entirely distal to the stem tip.[26]

With the introduction of uncemented implants and a sharp increase in the incidence of intraoperative cracks and fractures of the femur,[37,43,55] designations of com-

plete versus incomplete and division into distal versus proximal fractures have been suggested.[45]

Morrey et al.[38] categorized intraoperative fractures encountered during uncemented implantation, incorporating some of the features of several of the previous systems discussed, with type IA proximal to the lesser trochanter and undisplaced; type IB, the same but displaced 2 mm or more; type IIA, between the lesser trochanter and the isthmus and undisplaced; type IIB, the same as IIA but with 2 mm or more of displacement; type IIIA, distal to the isthmus; and type IIIB, the same as IIIA but displaced more than 2 mm (Fig. 67–1).[27] The system is effective for uncemented implants and references the anatomy of the femur, because in some cases these cracks are produced during preparation for insertion.

A review of 487 patients from 26 reports (including several of those cited earlier) prompted Mont et al. to propose a six-type classification system: intertrochanteric (type I), proximal femur (type II), spanning the stem tip (type III), distal to the tip (type IV), comminuted (type V), and supracondylar (type VI).[36]

Duncan and Masri have proposed a modified classification system, again consisting of three types designated type A, trochanteric fracture; B, fracture around or just below the stem tip; and C, fracture well below the stem tip (Fig. 67–2). In this classification scheme, type A is subcategorized into fractures involving the lesser (A₁) or greater (A₂) trochanter. Type B fractures are subdivided into those in which the stem is well fixed (B₁), the stem is loose (B₂), or there is extremely poor bone stock in the proximal femur, usually with comminution or significant osteolysis (B₃).[10] This classification system, which fits well with an algorithm suitable to guide contemporary fracture management, is now the most widely used.

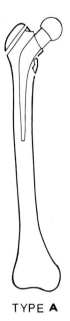

A   TYPE **A**

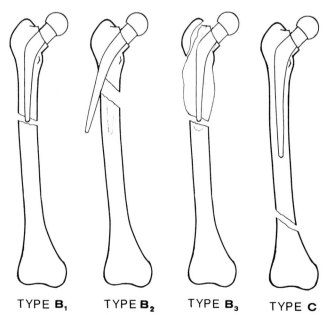

B   TYPE **B₁**   TYPE **B₂**   TYPE **B₃**   TYPE **C**

Figure 67–2. Classification of periprosthetic fractures of the femur associated with total hip arthroplasty as proposed by Duncan and Masri. **A,** Type A₁, at the lesser trochanter (type A₂, at the greater trochanter, is not shown). **B,** Type B₁, around or just below the stem with the stem well fixed. Type B₂, at or just below the stem with the stem loose. Type B₃, at or just below the stem with poor bone stock in the proximal femur. Type C, well below the stem. (From Duncan C, Masri BA: Fractures of the femur after hip replacement. Instr Course Lect 44:293, 1995.)

Table 67–1. INCIDENCE OF INTRAOPERATIVE FEMORAL FRACTURE ASSOCIATED WITH TOTAL HIP ARTHROPLASTY

Reference (yr)	Primary vs. Revision	Cemented vs. Uncemented	Stem Type	Total No. of Hips	Fracture Incidence (percent)
Taylor et al.[52] (1978)	Both	Cemented	Multiple	14,000	1
Federici et al.[13] (1988)	Both	Uncemented	Multiple	122	4.1
		Cemented	Multiple	480	1.7
Fitzgerald et al.[16] (1988)	Primary	Uncemented	Multiple	499	3.5
	Revision	Cemented	Multiple	131	17.6
Christensen et al.[6] (1989)	Revision	Cemented	Not specified	159	6.3
Schwartz et al.[45] (1989)	Primary	Uncemented	AML	1059	3
	Revision	Uncemented	AML	259	3
Stuchin[51] (1990)	Both	Uncemented	Multiple	79	13
Morrey and Kavanagh[38] (1992)	Revision	Uncemented	BIAS*	91	18
		Cemented	Multiple	94	3
Malkani et al.[32] (1993)	Revision	Uncemented	Osteonics long stem	69	46
Trousdale and Morrey[53] (1994)	Revision	Uncemented	BIAS*	96	19

AML = anatomic medullary locking.
*Bias, Zimmer International, Warsaw, IN.
Data from references 6, 13, 16, 32, 38, 45, 51–53.

INCIDENCE

Intraoperative Fractures

The rate of femoral fractures has been estimated to range from 0.1 percent to 3.2 percent with cemented primary total hip arthroplasties, and from 3 percent to 12 percent for cemented revisions (Table 67–1). For uncemented primary and revision total hip arthroplasty, intraoperative fracture rates range from 3 percent to 46 percent. Clearly, the introduction of uncemented implants, with the goal of a tight-fitting implant in the femoral cavity, has produced a significant increase in the incidence of intraoperative fractures.[16,17,32,33,38,45,46,53]

Postoperative Fracture

Postoperative fractures of the femur have been reported to occur anywhere from several days to a decade or more after the index procedure.[1,13,22,24,26,30,31] Many fractures occur in patients who have had a prior arthroplasty or some other type of hip procedure (Table 67–2). Adolphson et al. reviewed 32 fractures of the femur after total hip arthroplasty and found that 62 percent of the patients had had two or more prior procedures.[1] Bethea et al. showed that 18 of 31 perioprosthetic fractures (60 percent) had had at least two prior procedures and that loosening or cortical thinning caused by the failed total hip arthroplasty was present before fracture in 75 percent.[4]

Mayo Clinic Experience

Most reports of postoperative fractures associated with total hip arthroplasty deal with cemented implants, and there are limited data on the rates in uncemented, primary, or revision arthroplasty. To better understand this issue, we assessed the Mayo Hip Replacement Database from 1969 to 1998. There were 30,329 hip arthroplasties performed at the Mayo Clinic. Of these, 6349 were revisions, and uncemented implants were used in approximately one fifth of procedures (Table 67–3).[2]

Table 67–2. INCIDENCE OF POSTOPERATIVE FEMORAL FRACTURE ASSOCIATED WITH TOTAL HIP ARTHROPLASTY

Reference (yr)	Primary vs. Revision	Cemented vs. Uncemented	Stem Type	Total No.	Fracture Incidence (percent)	Follow-up	Mean Time to Fracture (range)
McElfresh and Coventry[33] (1974)	Both	Cemented	Charnley	5400	0.1	—	107 mo (4–20 mo postoperative)
Scott et al.[46] (1975)	Both	Cemented	Multiple	?	0.1	Estimated	1.5–12 mo
Adolphson et al.[1] (1987)	Both	Cemented	Multiple	1539	1.1	3.2 yr	2.5 yr
Fredin et al.[17] (1987)	Primary	Cemented	Not Specified	1961	0.6	54 mo (12–92 mo postfracture)	58 mo (2–142 mo)
Lowenhielm et al.[31] (1989)	Primary	Cemented	Multiple	1442	1*	Up to 15 yr	3.1 yr (3 mo–10 yr)

*Accumulated postoperative risk of fracture by 15 years = 25.3 per 1000.
Data from references 1, 17, 31, 33, 46.

Table 67–3. PERIPROSTHETIC FEMUR FRAC-TURES AROUND TOTAL HIP ARTHROPLASTY

	No.	Fractures	Percent
Intraoperative primary	23980	170	1
Cemented		68	0.3
Uncemented	20859	170	5.4
	3121		
Intraoperative revision	6349	497	7.8
Cemented	4813	175	3.6
Uncemented	1536	322	20.9
Postoperative primary	23980	262	1.1
Postoperative revision	6349	252	1.1
Totals	30329	1249	4.1

Intraoperative. There was an overall 1 percent incidence of femoral fracture intraoperatively for primary total hip arthroplasty and a 7.8 percent incidence at revision (Table 67–4). The incidence varied greatly according to fixation technique and ranged from 0.13 percent for the 20,859 primary cemented total hip arthroplasties to 5.4 percent for the 3121 primary uncemented total hip arthroplasties. These rates compare with an intraoperative fracture rate of 3.6 percent for the 4813 cemented revision procedures and a 20.9 percent fracture rate for the 1536 uncemented revision procedures. Many intraoperative fractures represent small cracks that are of little consequence, but some are major fractures that markedly change the intraoperative management of the femoral reconstruction.

Postoperative. In the Mayo Clinic experience, fractures occurred after surgery in 1.1 percent of 23,980 primary

Table 67–4. INCIDENCE OF FEMORAL FRACTURE ASSOCIATED WITH TOTAL HIP ARTHROPLASTY AT MAYO CLINIC (1969–1990)

Procedure	Intraoperative Fractures (percent)	Postoperative Fractures (percent)
Primary (No. = 19657)		
Cemented	0.1	0.6
Uncemented	3.9	0.4
Total	0.5	0.6
Revision (No. = 4397)		
Cemented	1.9	2.8
Uncemented	14.0	1.5
Total	5.0	2.4

arthroplasties. A fracture was documented in a much higher proportion—4 percent—of the 6349 revisions.

CONTRIBUTING FACTORS

Multiple factors have been implicated alone and in combination with the development of either intraoperative or postoperative femoral fracture. These can be grouped generally into patient-related, surgeon-controlled, and implant design factors (Table 67–5).

Patient-related Factors

Intraoperative fractures of the femur are 12 times more common in cemented revisions than in cemented primary arthroplasties and 4 times more common for uncemented revisions compared with uncemented arthroplasties. This is because failure of the prior implant, generally caused by loosening, frequently produces osteolysis and bone weakness.[18] Osteolysis associated with a failed total hip arthroplasty is the single most common factor producing increased risk of intraoperative fracture (Fig. 67–3). Osteoporosis, from senility or disuse, and other pathologic processes of bone also predispose the patient to periprosthetic fracture. Femoral perforation, which produces a defect in the cortex at or near the tip of the femoral stem, markedly increases the risk of fracture at the time of revision and during the postoperative period (Fig. 67–4).

In patients with a history of prior intertrochanteric osteotomy, Ferguson and colleagues documented intraoperative femoral fracture in 33 percent. These fractures resulted from distortion of the femoral anatomy in the presence of stress risers in the form of screw holes or larger defects.[14] The mechanical effect of a cylindrical defect that constitutes 50 percent of the bone diameter is a reduction in torsional strength of 62 percent and a reduction in energy to failure of 82 percent.[11] This effect is exaggerated when the femoral stem tip ends at the same level as the defect.

Surgeon-controlled Factors

Special note should be taken of variables that are within the control of the surgeon. These are exposure, implant

Table 67–5. FEMORAL FRACTURE ASSOCIATED WITH REVISION TOTAL HIP ARTHROPLASTY: CONTRIBUTING FACTORS

Patient	Surgeon Controlled	Implant
Osteoporosis	Exposure	Number of sizes
Small size	Implant removal	Proximal wedge effect
Deformity	Cement removal	Stem length
Osteolysis/loosening	Bone preparation	Stem bow
Prior surgery (defects)	Implant sizing (mismatch)	Instrumentation
Trauma	Implant insertion	Fixation made
Excessive loads	Postoperative management	Stem stiffness

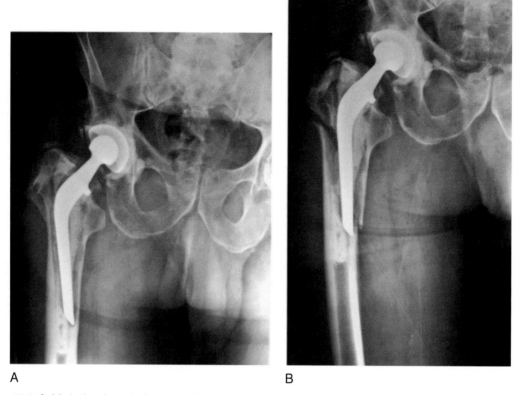

A   B

Figure 67–3. A, Marked periprosthetic osteolysis 7 years after implantation. The recommended revision was deferred by the patient because of mild pain. **B,** Periprosthetic fracture occurred 3 months later, after a fall.

and cement removal, bone preparation, stem insertion, and implant design features.

Exposure

During revision surgery, care must be taken to provide adequate exposure for delivery of the proximal femur. This is necessary both to access the acetabulum and to gain good visibility down the femoral canal. The amount of dissection varies, depending on the amount of scarring and the quality of the soft tissues, but it may need to be extensive in some cases. Good exposure not only helps avoid excessive torsion at dislocation but is essential to clean and prepare the canal adequately for the revision implant. Extended greater trochanteric osteotomy can reduce the fracture risk markedly when applied in the proper setting.

Implant Removal

Removal even of loose implants must be done carefully to avoid trochanteric fracture or avulsion (Fig. 67–5).

Cement Removal

Obvious dangers exist with regard to perforation or fracture of the femur during the use of osteotomes or high-speed burs for cement removal. The introduction

of the extended trochanteric osteotomy has dramatically decreased the risk of inadvertent femoral cortex perforation (Fig. 67–6). Use of ultrasonically driven tools is also of great help.

Bone Preparation

During both primary and revision surgery, bone preparation may be complicated by alterations in femoral anatomy and reduction in bone quality in the proximal femur. To achieve torsional control of uncemented implants, optimal endosteal preparation is obligatory. Areas at particular risk for fracture are the medial or anterior neck and calcar region, particularly with metaphyseal filling implants.

Stem Insertion

Intraoperative fractures most frequently occur during insertion of uncemented press-fit devices. It is important to recognize that some implant systems have the prostheses intentionally oversized relative to the rasp. Insertion of a stem that is larger than the preparing rasp by only 0.5 mm causes very high strains in the proximal femur as well as fractures.[18] The length of the stem also has an effect. During revision surgery, it is necessary to achieve several bone diameters of

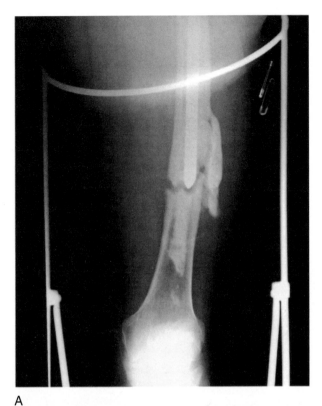

A

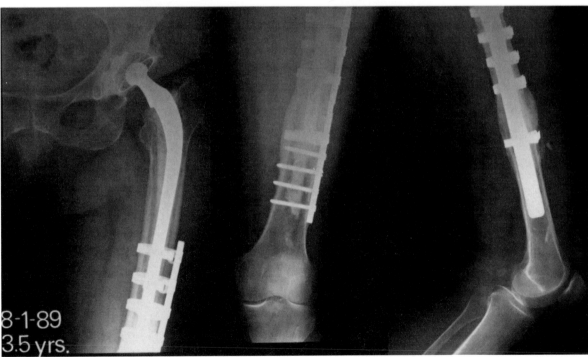

B

Figure 67–4. A, Femoral defect created at the time of revision total hip arthroplasty with extruded cement near the stem tip. **B,** Subsequent fracture at this stress riser was treated successfully with an Ogden-type plate without disturbing the well-fixed stem.

fixation beyond any stress risers caused by cortical defects or scalloping.[30] However, with uncemented stems, this increased length may result in an increased risk of intraoperative fracture or cracking.[25,32,51,53] This risk seems greatest in instances where a large proximal prosthesis cross section or wedge-shaped design in both planes is used in combination with a long stem.[29] This may relate to mismatching between the bow of the prosthesis and the patient's own femur.

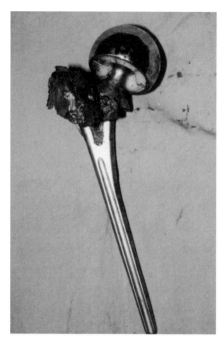

Figure 67–5. Fractures may be produced during otherwise routine revision cases if care is not taken during implant extraction, as evidenced by this trochanteric fracture produced by hasty disimpaction of a grossly loose press-fitted endoprosthesis.

Implant Design Factors

There are several design parameters that can influence the frequency of fractures, especially in uncemented devices. These include stem length, the bow of the stem (match or mismatch to the patient's anterior femoral bow), and proximal stem geometry, with some aggressive proximal wedge shapes more likely to cause femoral splitting. A multitude of sizes and shapes are needed for optimal fit both in primary surgery and (especially) in revision cases. The wide variation in implant systems that are now readily available allows some degree of customization with use of these much more cost-effective alternatives.

Finally, familiarity with the implant system being used is necessary to avoid problems related to under-reaming or under-rasping as the optimal fit is sought.

PREVENTION OF PERIPROSTHETIC FRACTURES

Several considerations are important in preventing femoral fractures, either at the time of primary or revision surgery or subsequent to the index arthroplasty. Prevention is always preferred to treatment. Recommendations include the following:

1. Good-quality multiplanar preoperative radiographs with magnification markers
2. Careful preoperative planning and templating
3. Removal of sufficient bone and scar to avoid trochanteric fracture at the time of device removal
4. Flexibility in use of the implant system, especially for revision, and not forcing one implant system to solve all problems
5. Selected use of extended trochanteric osteotomy for revisions
6. Avoidance of femoral perforation or creation of defects
7. Cerclage before rasping or stem insertion in high-risk patients[22]
8. Avoidance of excessive canal debris
9. Correct alignment of instrumentation during bone preparation
10. Elimination of localized areas of bone impingement or prominence
11. Stem bypass of cortical defects or stress risers
12. Patience (see Fig. 67–5)
13. Intraoperative radiographs at preparation or insertion
14. Regular radiographic follow-up to detect impending fracture from osteolysis

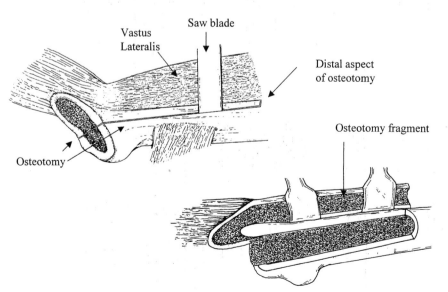

Vastus Lateralis

Saw blade

Distal aspect of osteotomy

Osteotomy fragment

Osteotomy

Figure 67–6. The extended trochanteric osteotomy has markedly decreased inadvertant cortical penetration and fracture during cement removal.

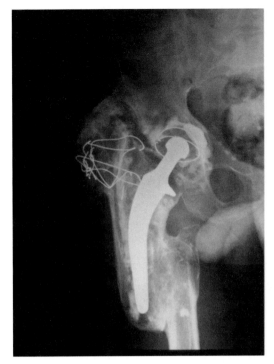
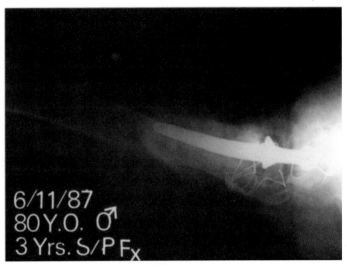

Figure 67–7. Femoral malunion 3 years after closed treatment of a periprosthetic femoral fracture, making revision of the loose, painful stem impossible without simultaneous osteotomy.

TREATMENT METHODS

Nonoperative Treatment

Nonoperative treatments such as casting and protected weightbearing have been effective in certain select cases if the fracture is stable and the device well fixed. Minimally displaced trochanteric fractures are especially amenable to management in this way.[21,42] For displaced shaft fractures, nonoperative management in the past has included traction followed by cast or cast brace immobilization and has been suggested as an alternative to operative intervention. Mixed results have been reported with nonoperative methods, with an increased risk of femoral malunion and nonunion as well as other, more general complications (Fig. 67–7).[4,26,35,54] The increased costs and potential for medical complications associated with prolonged traction and bed rest, combined with the high reported risk of fracture complications, render this option no longer viable except in unusual circumstances.

Cerclage Fixation

The mainstay of treatment for periprosthetic femoral fractures has been cerclage fixation. Cerclage wires and, more recently, cables and nylon bands can be passed around the femur in cases of long oblique or spiral fracture lines.[15,28,47,50] It is desirable for the stem to extend beyond the fracture site and to avoid excessive soft tissue stripping. Supplemental morcellized bone graft should be considered, and adjunctive onlay cortical struts can be added as well (Fig. 67–8).[40] Cerclage is inadequate mechanically

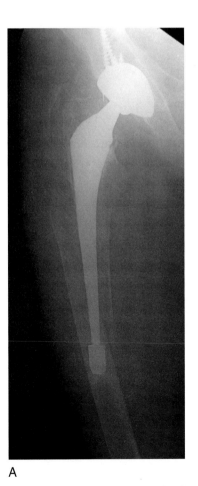

A

Figure 67–8. **A**, Vancouver Type B_2 fracture with a loose stem but good quality bone.

Illustration continued on following page

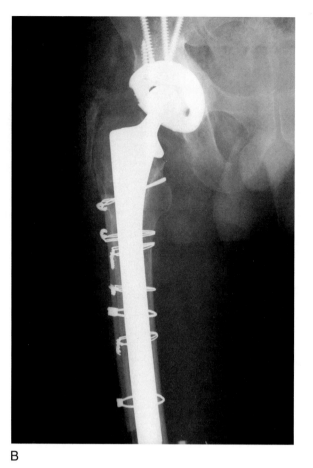

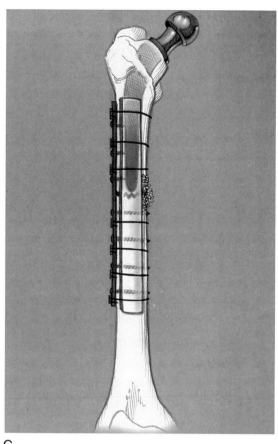

B   C

Figure 67–8. *Continued.* **B,** Revision with a fully coated stem and strut allograft. **C,** If greater stability should be required, a plate may be incorporated at a 90-degree angle to the bone struct.

when used alone without an intramedullary stem for fixation of most unprotected fracture lines.

Prophylactic cerclage can be used to prevent fractures in cases at risk.[13] Cerclage can be of help with long spiral intraoperative fractures that occur during stem insertion.[8,16,23,48]

Femoral Revision

Revision is the treatment of choice when a periprosthetic fracture occurs in association with a loosened stem. Either a cemented or an uncemented stem may be used during the revision surgery. Adjunctive fixation in the form of cerclage, plate fixation, or onlay cortical struts is usually needed (Fig. 67–9). One study has documented the superiority of a cerclage plate to cerclage bone struct fixation.[50] Cemented fixation improves stability and still allows bone union as long as methacrylate is not allowed to extrude into the fracture site.[5,9] This is particularly well suited to fractures occurring in elderly patients whose bone quality is poor.[4] Uncemented femoral stems, especially those with extensive porous coating, can achieve distal diaphyseal fixation, allow reconstruction of the fractured proximal femur, and facilitate local bone grafting efforts. Adjunctive fixation is also often beneficial as circumstances dictate.

Markedly comminuted fractures associated with extensive osteolysis may require replacement of the proximal femur with either a proximal femoral placement prosthesis or allograft-prosthetic composite (Fig. 67–10) or a fracture stem that gains axial and rotational stability distal to the fracture site. Proximal femoral replacement is usually reserved for elderly patients for whom rapid mobilization is sought at the possible expense of function. Allograft-prosthetic composites allow wrapping of the fragmented femur around the allograft to facilitate soft tissue attachment, hip stability, and function (Fig. 67–11). Today, modular designs allow management of even the most severe problems, often without the need for custom implants or bone struts. This level of management has been facilitated by the use of a modified trochanteric osteotomy (Figs. 67–12**A** and 67–13).

Open Reduction and Internal Fixation

Open reduction and internal fixation of periprosthetic fractures usually is limited to Vancouver type B_1 fractures, with a well-fixed, well-functioning stem and fracture at the stem tip. It is uncommon for a conventional compression plate fixation to be of value in these fractures. Fortunately, current plate designs allow for and accommodate cerclage wire fixation.[39] These devices

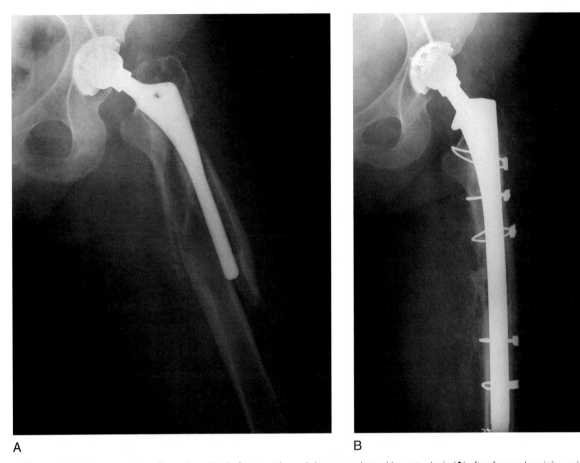

A

B

Figure 67–9. Vancouver Type B$_2$ periprosthetic fracture through bone weakened by osteolysis (**A**) after femoral revision with an extensively coated stem. Vascularity of all bone fragments was maintained and healing occurred without strut grafting (**B**).

allow solid fixation with less soft tissue dissection and can reduce violation of the cement mantle or scoring of the stem proximal to the fracture site (see Fig. 67–12).

Experimental evidence now reveals the cerclage/ plate construct is quite stable, and statistically more rigid than cerclage and bone struts.[8,29,56] A multicenter report demonstrated excellent results when Vancouver type B fractures were salvaged with an internal fixation procedure that used a plate and struct graft or strut graft alone. The strut grafts, when placed so as to minimize excessive periosteal stripping, improve the mechanical stability of these fractured hips and also appear to enhance the potential for healing.[19]

Bone Grafting

The combination of intramedullary and extramedullary disruption of blood supply to the bone during surgery in many of these cases makes delayed or nonunion problems quite possible, even when fixation is excellent (see Fig. 67–11). Cancellous bone graft may help prevent this complication and should be used routinely.

Onlay cortical strut allografting[12] has been proved to be of great value, particularly as an adjunct to the management of periprosthetic femoral fractures. One or more cortical struts may be used alone or in combination with conventional plate fixation to provide mechanical stability and facilitate union (see Fig. 67–8). Wire or cables are used to secure the struts after they have been fashioned with a bur or saw to span the fracture and achieve good cortical contact. Cancellous graft can be placed beneath the strut to fill in the gaps and attempt to speed union to the femoral shaft. High rates of union of cortical struts to the host bone in revision total hip surgery have been reported, with more than 90 percent of the grafts radiographically healed at follow-up.[12] Technically, with osteoporotic bone, two struts may be required to prevent the tightening cable or wire from cutting into the soft osteoporotic host bone.

Results

Considerably greater information about treatment outcome is available since the previous editions of this book were published.

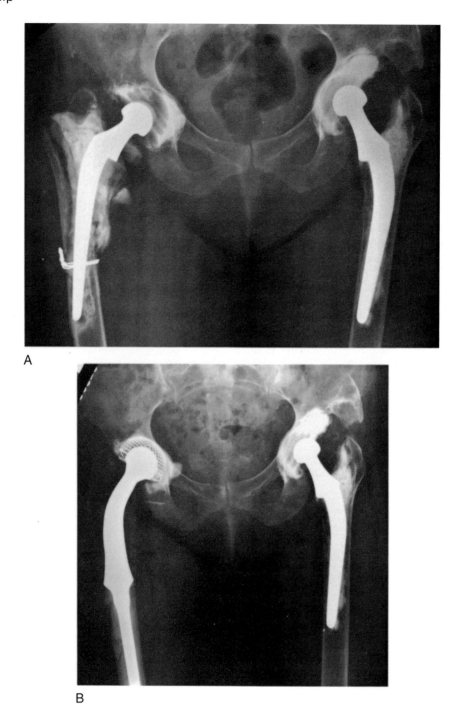

A

B

Figure 67–10. A, Periprosthetic fracture associated with a loose, painful femoral component in an elderly patient with very poor proximal bone stock. **B,** This case was managed with a proximal femoral replacement implant that allowed rapid mobilization of the patient.

Historical Results

As early as 1982, Bethea et al. reported 31 cases in which fractures occurred 4 weeks to 10 years after arthroplasty.[4] Sixty-five percent had loosening or cortex erosion before fracture. Nonoperative treatment yielded poor results. The best results were seen in the group with long-stemmed revisions.[4]

Johansson et al. reported 37 fractures, of which 23 were intraoperative and 14 postoperative fractures. Average follow-up was 3.9 years, with a range of 2 to 9 years. Both operative and nonoperative treatment was used. Operative measures included cerclage, plates, revision with and without long stems, and excisional arthroplasty. Complications occurred in 60 percent of patients, and a satisfactory result was achieved in only

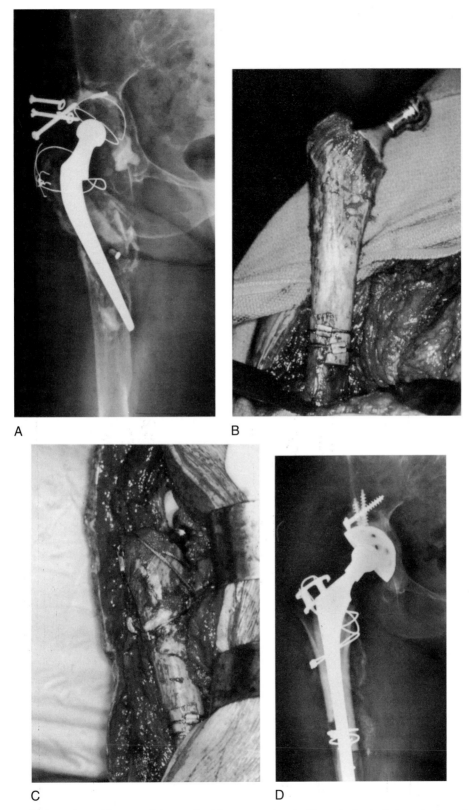

Figure 67–11. A, Comminuted fracture of the proximal femur associated with marked osteolysis and extremely poor quality of residual bone in the proximal femur. **B**, Treatment involved insertion of an allograft-prosthetic composite with cementing of the device to the allograft and step-cut osteotomy at the graft-host junction. **C** and **D**, Note the cerclage fixation of the residual proximal femoral bone around the allograft, which facilitates soft tissue attachment, hip stability, and union of the graft to the host.

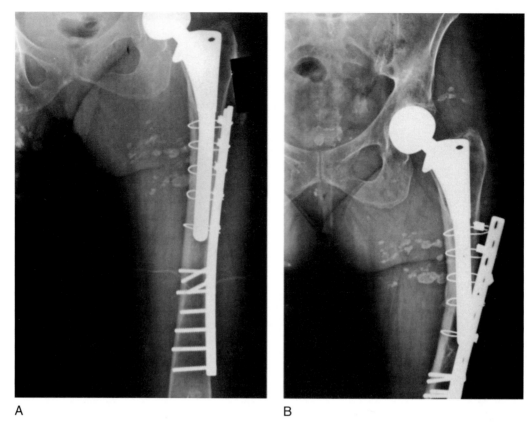

A   B

Figure 67–12. **A**, Use of a specially designed plate with cables proximally and screws distally to allow fixation of a fracture below the tip of a well-fixed, extensively porous-coated stem. **B**, Despite an anatomic reduction originally, nonunion resulted. No adjunctive bone grafting was used at the time of the original procedure. Routine use of bone graft is encouraged because this may facilitate union before failure of the internal fixation.

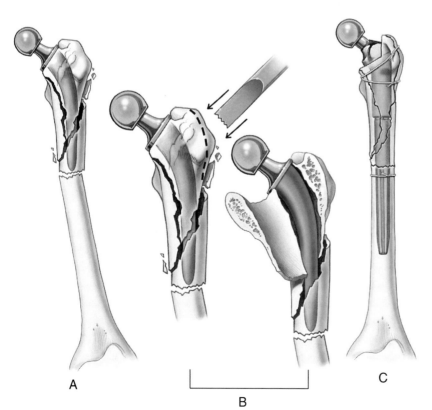

A   B   C

Figure 67–13. **A**, Vancouver Type B$_3$ periprosthetic femur fracture. The proximal bone is very lytic and nonsupportive. **B**, A lateral trochanteric splitting approach preserves osseous generation potential. **C**, Reconstruction with modular, fluted, tapered, grit-blasted titanium stem. The stem bypasses the fracture and obtains axial and rotational stability in the diaphysis. Vascularity of the proximal fracture fragments was maintained and the fracture is healing.

43 percent of intraoperative fractures and 36 percent of postoperative fractures.[26]

Early experience with intraoperative fractures from the Mayo Clinic was documented by Fitzgerald et al.[16] A review of a sample of a certain uncemented design noted that intraoperative fractures occurred in 23 revision and 17 primary total hip arthroplasties, all during uncemented implantations. Eighteen of 23 cases involved fractures proximal to the lesser trochanter. Cerclage was used in 37 of 40 patients. Loosening or failure occurred at final follow-up in 3 of the 40, and all were believed to be fracture related.

Modern Results

INTRAOPERATIVE FRACTURES

Schwartz et al. reviewed 1059 primary and 259 revision arthroplasties performed with an uncemented, porous-coated femoral prosthesis. They found a 3 percent fracture rate in both the revision and primary total hip arthroplasty groups.[45] Cerclage plus fully coated or four-fifths coated stems was used if proximal fractures occurred. Open reduction and internal fixation was performed if the fracture was distal to the stem tip and complete. These authors found no adverse effect related to any of the intraoperative fractures a mean of 37 months after surgery.

POSTOPERATIVE FRACTURES

Haddad et al. reported the results of a multicenter study evaluating the treatment of Vancouver B_1 periprosthetic fractures associated with a well-fixed femoral component and a fracture near the tip of the stem.[19] All the fractures were treated with internal fixation that included the use of a cortical strut bone graft. In 19 of the fractures, two cortical strut grafts were used alone, and in 21, strut grafts were used in combination with a lateral metal plate. Thirty-nine of 40 fractures healed. There were no marked malunions. The authors concluded that use of cortical strut grafts could enhance the mechanical stability as well as the potential for healing of these difficult fractures in a high-stress region.

Springer et al. reported the modern Mayo Clinic experience with revision hip arthroplasty to treat periprosthetic femur fractures.[49] A total of 120 hips were followed for at least 2 years (mean, 5.1 years) after revision. Twenty-two femoral components subsequently were revised or removed; 11 for loosening, 5 for infection, 3 for loosening with nonunion, 2 for recurrent dislocation and 1 for a new periprosthetic femur fracture. Of the 98 patients with surviving implants, 78 had no pain or mild pain and 70 required a one-handed gait aid or less. Failure, defined as revision, component removal, or radiographic prosthesis loosening or nonunion was present in 17 of 42 cemented implants; 19 of 28 uncemented, proximally coated implants; 8 of 32 extensively porous-coated implants; and 7 of 18 allograft prosthetic composites or femur protheses. Although the treatment groups were not identical, the best results were achieved with use of extensively porous-coated implants that gained fixation distal to the fracture site in the well-preserved diaphyseal bone. If bone quality allows reconstruction with an uncemented femoral component that gains mechanical stability and biologic fixation distal to the fracture site, this appears to be a good method for most femoral revisions for periprosthetic femur fracture.

Nonunion of periprosthetic femur fracture represents an uncommon and uniquely challenging problem. Crockarell et al. reported on 23 such cases and concluded that there was a high rate of complications related to treatment and that functional outcomes were relatively poor.[7] The authors noted that prevention of the problem by optimal treatment of the initial periprosthetic fracture was important.

AUTHORS' PREFERENCE

We prefer to categorize periprosthetic fractures according to the system of Duncan and Masri because this system provides an algorithm that, when loosely followed, is very valuable as a guide to treatment. Vancouver Type A fractures—those that occur around the lesser or greater trochanter—are treated nonoperatively if fracture displacement is minimal and if the prosthesis is functioning well. Most of these fractures, however, occur in association with periprosthetic osteolysis. In this setting, marked periprosthetic lysis usually proves to be an indication for operative management. These fractures mostly occur through very thin bone, which is usually not amenable to fixation. We frequently prefer to treat the fracture conservatively for several months, in many cases allowing it to heal, and then operate to manage the associated problems of bearing surface wear and periprosthetic osteolysis. Frequently, the thin shell of trochanteric bone is left in place with an intact soft tissue sleeve. The osteolytic bone defects are grafted with retention of implants if they are well fixed. Measures to reduce particulate debris formulation, such as polyethylene liner exchange and femoral head exchange, usually are performed concomitantly.

The great majority of Vancouver Type B fractures (those occurring around the stem or at the tip of the stem) are treated operatively. For Vancouver type B_1 fractures (those fractures that occur at the stem tip in association with a well-fixed, well-functioning stem) we usually perform internal fixation. Our preferred method is to use a lateral cable plate and anterior cortical strut graft for fixation. The cable plate allows screw fixation distal to the fracture site and cerclage fixation proximal and distal to the fracture site. When possible, in addition to proximal cable fixation, we also try to use unicortical screws, or screws angled through the plate into the posterior cortex, proximal to the fracture site, because these screws enhance stability. It is desirable to avoid excessive periosteal stripping of the bone during the internal fixation procedure. We use autogenous bone graft when possible to augment fracture healing at the fracture site.

For Vancouver type B_2 fractures (those around the stem or stem tip associated with a loose implant), we prefer femoral component revision. We individualize the type of femoral component fixation according to patient demographic features, bone quality, and fracture pattern. For simple fractures that can be anatomically reduced in very old patients with poor bone, long cemented stems can be used successfully. It is important to avoid cement extrusion through the fracture site that may reduce the potential for healing. For most fractures of this pattern, however, we use long uncemented femoral components. The key tenets of treatment are (1) to gain fracture stability, (2) to gain implant stability, and (3) to create favorable biologic conditions for fracture healing. To achieve these goals in most circumstances, we use long uncemented stems that bypass the fracture site and gain fixation of implant and fracture in the isthmus distal to the fracture site. We prefer to use uncemented, extensively porous-coated stems or fluted, tapered, grit-blasted stems for this purpose. Fracture stability can be enhanced if necessary with cortical bone strut grafts. It is desirable to avoid excessive stripping of the fracture site when applying strut grafts.

For Vancouver type B_3 fractures (those around the stem associated with unreconstructable bone), we individualize the treatment according to the quality of the remaining distal bone as well as patient demographic factors. For very old patients, we consider use of a cemented tumor prosthesis. For younger patients, we prefer to use an allograft prosthetic composite or, when bone quality allows, a fluted, tapered, grit-blasted stem, which gains axial and rotational stability in the isthmus of the femur distal to the fracture site. When this technique is used, we try to avoid any stripping of the muscle attached to the comminuted proximal fragments of bone. We gain access to the fracture by simply lifting the fracture fragments away from the failed prosthesis. At closure, we wrap the fragments around the new prosthesis with minimal disruption of the blood supply to the fracture fragments.

We treat Vancouver type C fractures (those that occur well distal to the stem of an implant) as we would any other femur fracture; that is, with internal fixation. Needless to say, antegrade nailing is not possible; therefore, these fractures usually are treated with retrograde supracondylar nails or plate fixation.

In summary, the best approach is based on the following principles, which, in general, are supported by the literature:

1. If the fracture is displaced, fix it as rigidly as possible.
2. If the stem is loose, revise it with a stem long enough to extend well past the fracture site.
3. Use cancellous bone graft routinely along fracture lines.
4. Consider onlay cortical struts as needed as a biologic and mechanical adjunct.
5. When poor bone quality in the proximal femur and associated comminution at the fracture site preclude reconstruction, salvage conducted with either a proximal femoral replacement stem or an allograft prosthesis composite should be considered.

These principles have been summarized in a treatment by Duncan and Masri (Fig. 67–14).[10] We have found this a useful guide to decision-making in the treatment of these problems. It is important to recognize, however, that the final decision regarding optimal implant choice and treatment method may hinge on intraoperative findings. Flexibility is the byword in thought, technique, and implant selection.

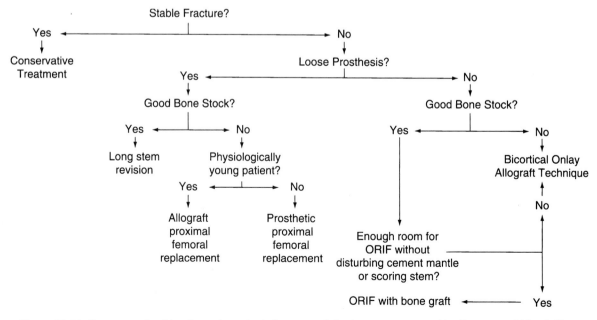

Figure 67–14. Treatment algorithm for periprosthetic fractures of the femur as proposed by Duncan and Masri. (From Duncan C, Masri BA: Fractures of the femur after hip replacement. Instr Course Lect 44:293, 1995.)

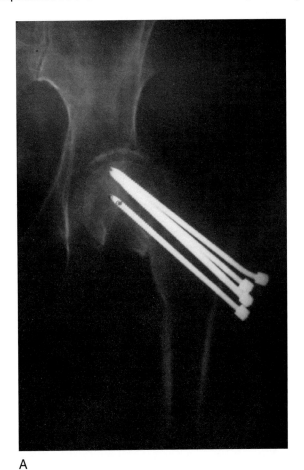

Figure 67–15. A 68-year-old woman demonstrates a nonunion 14 months after femoral neck fracture (**A**). A central fracture occurred through the osteoporotic central wall of the acetabulum (**B**).

A

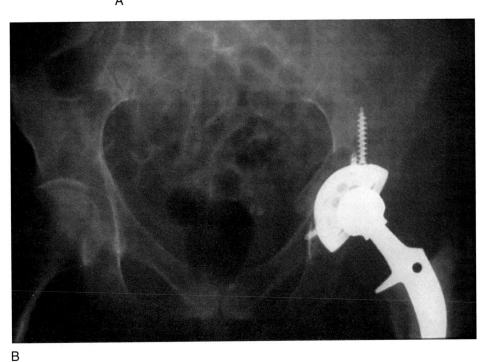

B

Acetabular Fractures

Since the first and second editions of the book were published, additional information has become available about periprosthetic fractures of the acetabulum.

Acetabular fractures can occur both intraoperatively and postoperatively.

Experimental studies have evaluated the occurrence of intraoperative acetabular fractures. This complication is almost exclusively associated with use of uncemented acetabular implants that are press-fitted into the acetabulum. Experimental studies have demonstrated that acetabular fractures occur most commonly when there is marked oversizing of the acetabular component relative to the reamed bone. Assessment of 30 fresh or embalmed cadaveric specimens revealed a fracture in 18 (6 percent) after insertion of a metal-backed acetabular component oversized by 2 to 4 mm. The conclusion of the study was that one caution must be used when a socket is inserted that is markedly oversized relative to the reamed dimensions of the acetabulum. Insertion of a cup more than 2 mm bigger than the reamed size of the acetabulum usually should be avoided.

In a multicenter study that included the Mayo Clinic, Sharkey et al.[47] evaluated fractures that occurred with insertion of uncemented acetabular components. They found that these fractures often were nondisplaced partial fractures of the wall of the acetabulum, which did not compromise implant stability. The key finding of the study, however, was that, on some occasions, unrecognized major fractures of the pelvis occurred with insertion of uncemented implants. Such fractures can lead to early and catastrophic implant failure. The authors concluded that the surgeon should be vigilant about the possibility of a pelvic fracture when uncemented implants are inserted, and if a fracture is identified, appropriate measures should be taken intraoperatively to ensure that the implant and pelvis are stable. In cases of minor fractures, little change in treatment may be needed (augmentation screws may be added to the socket if they are not already used), but in cases of more severe fracture, more involved reconstruction techniques are required intraoperatively.[3]

The Mayo Clinic experience of postoperative acetabular fractures was reported by Peterson and Lewallen who described 11 patients with a postoperative periprosthetic fracture.[41] In 8, the fracture was associated with a stable acetabular component, and in 3, it was not. The fractures associated with a loose cup usually were treated operatively. Six of the 8 fractures associated with a well-fixed cup healed with nonoperative management, although several of the acetabular components loosened later.[3]

Sanchez-Sotelo et al. reported on a new type of periprosthetic fracture of the acetabulum that occurs through osteolytic lesions of the pelvis.[44] Marked osteolysis of the pelvis leads to a risk of periprosthetic fracture. Prevention of this problem by timely reoperation for severe osteolysis is important.

Pelvic discontinuity identified at the time of revision arthroplasty represents another unique type of acetabular periprosthetic fracture. These fractures usually are stress fracture nonunions that occur through areas of weak and deficient bone of the pelvis (Fig. 67–15). Pelvic discontinuity requires complex management techniques. The details of treatment and management of the difficult problem of prior acetabular fracture are discussed further in Chapter 56.

References

1. Adolphson P, Jonsson U, Kalen R: Fractures of the ipsilateral femur after total hip arthroplasty. Arch Orthop Trauma Surg 106:353, 1987.
2. Berry DJ: Epidemiology: Hip and Knee. Orthop Clin North Am 30:183, 1999.
3. Berry DJ, Lewallen DG, Hanssen AD, Cabanela ME: Pelvic discontinuity in revision total hip arthroplasty. J Bone Joint Surg 81A:1692, 1999.
4. Bethea JS, DeAndrade JR, Fleming LL, et al: Alignment: Proximal femoral fractures following total hip arthroplasty. Clin Orthop 170:95, 1982.
5. Charnley J: The healing of human fractures in contact with self-curing acrylic cement. Clin Orthop 47:157, 1966.
6. Christensen CM, Seger BM, Schultz RB: Management of intraoperative femur fractures associated with revision hip arthroplasty. Clin Orthop 248:177, 1989.
7. Crockarell J Jr, Berry DJ, Lewallen DG: Nonunion after periprosthetic femur fracture associated with total hip arthroplasty. J Bone Joint Surg 81A:1073, 1999.
8. Dennis MG, Simon JA, Kummer FJ, et al: Fixation of periprosthetic femoral shaft fractures: A biomechanical comparison of two techniques. J Orthop Trauma 15:177, 2001.
9. Dumez JF, Gayet LE, Avedikian J, Clarac JP: Treatment of femoral fractures on a total hip prosthesis using Charnley's "long stem" prosthesis. Apropos of 18 cases. Rev Chirurgie Orthop Reparatrice Appar Mot 82:225, 1996.
10. Duncan C, Masri BA: Fractures of the femur after hip replacement. Instr Course Lect 44:293, 1995.
11. Edgerton BC, An KN, Morrey BF: Torsional strength reduction due to cortical defects in bone. J Orthop Res 8:851, 1990.
12. Emerson RH Jr, Malinin TI, Cuellar AD, et al: Cortical strut allografts in the reconstruction of the femur in revision total hip arthroplasty: A basic science and clinical study. Clin Orthop 285:35, 1992.
13. Federici A, Carbone M, Sanguineti F: Intraoperative fractures of the femoral diaphysis in hip arthroprosthesis surgery. Ital J Orthop Trauma 14:311, 1988.
14. Ferguson GM, Cabanela ME, Ilstrup DM: Total hip arthroplasty after failed intertrochanteric osteotomy. J Bone Joint Surg 76B:252, 1994.
15. Fishkin Z, Han SM, Ziv I: Cerclage wiring technique after proximal femoral fracture in total hip arthroplasty. J Arthroplasty 14:98, 1999.
16. Fitzgerald RH Jr, Brindley GW, Kavanagh BF: The uncemented total hip arthroplasty: Intraoperative femoral fractures. Clin Orthop 235:61, 1988.
17. Fredin HO, Lindberg H, Carlsson AS: Femoral fracture following hip arthroplasty. Acta Orthop Scand 58:20, 1987.
18. Gill TJ, Sledge JB, Orler R, Ganz R: Lateral insufficiency fractures of the femur caused by osteopenia and varus angulation: A complication of total hip arthroplasty. J Arthroplasty 14:982, 1999.
19. Haddad FS, Duncan CP, Berry DJ, et al: Periprosthetic femoral fractures around well fixed implants: An independent observer multicenter study of the use of cortical onlay allografts or cortical onlay allografts with plates (in press).
20. Hardinge K: The direct lateral approach to the hip. J Bone Joint Surg 64B:17, 1982.
21. Heekin RD, Engh CA, Herzwurm PJ: Fractures through cystic lesions of the greater trochanter. A cause of late pain after cementless total hip arthroplasty. J Arthroplasty 11:757, 1996.
22. Herzwurm PJ, Walsh J, Pettine KA, et al: Prophylactic cerclage: A method of preventing femur fracture in uncemented total hip arthroplasty. Orthopedics 15:143, 1992.
23. Incavo SJ, DiFazio F, Wilder D, et al: Longitudinal crack propagation in bone around femoral prosthesis. Clin Orthop 272:175, 1991.
24. Jasty M, Bragdon CR, Rubash H, et al: Unrecognized femoral fractures during cementless total hip arthroplasty in the dog and their effect on bone ingrowth. J Arthroplasty 7:501, 1992.
25. Jasty M, Henshaw RM, O'Connor DO, Harris WH: High assembly strains and femoral fractures produced during insertion of uncemented femoral components: a cadaver study. J Arthroplasty 8:479, 1993.
26. Johansson JE, McBroom R, Barrington TW, et al: Fracture of the ipsilateral femur in patients with total hip replacement. J Bone Joint Surg 63A:1435, 1981.
27. Kim YS, Callaghan JJ, Ahn PB, Brown TD: Fracture of the acetabulum during insertion of an oversized hemispherical component. J Bone Joint Surg 77A:111, 1995.

28. Kligman M, Otramsky I, Roffman M: Conservative versus surgical treatment for femoral fracture after total or hemiarthroplasty of hip. Arch Orthop Trauma Surg 119:79, 1999.

29. Kligman M, Otramsky I, Roffman M: Mennen plate in hip and shoulder joint replacement. Bull Hosp J Dis 56:84, 1997.

30. Larson JE, Chao EYS, Fitzgerald RH: Bypassing femoral cortical defects with cemented intramedullary stems. J Orthop Res 9:414, 1991.

31. Löwenhielm G, Hansson LI, Kärrholm J: Fracture of the lower extremity after total hip replacement. Arch Orthop Trauma Surg 108:141, 1989.

32. Malkani AL, Cabanela ME, Lewallen DG: Cementless total hip arthroplasty using proximally coated, chrome cobalt, long stem, curved prosthesis: Two to five year results. Orthop Trans 17:586, 1993.

33. McElfresh EC, Coventry MB: Femoral and pelvic fractures after total hip arthroplasty. J Bone Joint Surg 56A:483, 1974.

34. McGrory BJ: Periprosthetic fracture of the acetabulum during total hip arthroplasty in a patient with Paget's disease. Am J Orthop 28:248, 1999.

35. Missakian ML, Rand JA: Fractures of the femoral shaft adjacent to long stem femoral components of total hip arthroplasty: report of seven cases. Orthopedics 16:149, 1993.

36. Mont MA, Maar DC: Fractures of the ipsilateral femur after hip arthroplasty: A statistical analysis of outcome based on 487 patients. J Arthroplasty 9:511, 1994.

37. Moroni A, Faldini C, Piras F, Giannini S: Risk factors for intraoperative femoral fractures during total hp replacement. Ann Chir Gynaecol 89:113, 2000.

38. Morrey BF, Kavanagh BF: Complications with revision of the femoral component of total hip arthroplasty: Comparison between cemented and uncemented techniques. J Arthroplasty 7:71, 1992.

39. Ogden WS, Rendall J: Fractures beneath hip prostheses: A special indication for Parham bands and plating. Orthop Trans 2:70, 1978.

40. Pekkarinen J, Alho A, Lepisto J, et al: Impaction bone grafting in revision hip surgery. A high incidence of complications. J Bone Joint Surg 82B:103, 2000.

41. Peterson CA, Lewallen DG: Periprosthetic fracture of the acetabulum after total hip arthroplasty. Bone Joint Surg 78A:1206, 1996.

42. Probst A, Wetterkamp D, Neuber M: Iatrogenic avulsion of the greater trochanter during prosthetic replacement of the hip. Unfallchirurg 102:497, 1999.

43. Radl R, Aigner C, Hungerford M, et al: Proximal femoral bone loss and increased rate of fracture with a proximally hydroxyapatite-coated femoral component. J Bone Joint Surg 82B:1151, 2000.

44. Sanchez-Sotelo J, McGrory B, Berry DJ: Acute periprosthetic fracture of the acetabulum associated with osteolytic pelvic lesions: A report of three cases. J Arthroplasty 15:126, 2000.

45. Schwartz JT Jr, Mayer JG, Engh CA: Femoral fracture during noncemented total hip arthroplasty. J Bone Joint Surg 71A:1135, 1989.

46. Scott RD, Turner RH, Leitzes SM, et al: Femoral fractures in conjunction with total hip replacement. J Bone Joint Surg 57A:494, 1975.

47. Sharkey PF, Hozack WJ, Booth RE Jr, Rothman RH: Intraoperative femoral fractures in cementless total hip arthroplasty. Orthop Rev 21:337, 1992.

48. Shaw JA, Daubert HB: Compression capability of cerclage fixation systems: A biomechanical study. Orthopedics 11:1169, 1988.

49. Springer BD, Berry DJ, Lewallen DG: Femoral revision to treat periprosthetic hip fractures following total hip arthroplasty (unpublished).

50. Stevens SS, Irish AJ, Vachtsevanos JG, et al: A biomechanical study of three wiring techniques for cerclage-plating. J Orthop Trauma 9:381, 1995.

51. Stuchin SA: Femoral shaft fracture in porous and press-fit total hip arthroplasty. Orthop Rev 19:153, 1990.

52. Taylor MM, Meyers MH, Harvery JP: Intraoperative femur fractures during total hip replacement. Clin Orthop 137:96, 1978.

53. Trousdale RT, Morrey BF: Uncemented femoral revision of total hip arthroplasty with the BIAS prosthesis (in press).

54. Whittaker RP, Sotos LN, Ralston EL: Fractures of the femur about femoral endoprostheses. J Trauma 14:675, 1974.

55. Younger AS, Dunwoody I, Duncan CP: Periprosthetic hip and knee fractures: The scope of the problem. Instr Course Lect 47:251, 1998.

56. Zenni EJ Jr, Pomeroy DL, Caudle RJ: Ogden plate and other fixations of fractures complicating femoral endoprostheses. Clin Orthop 231:83, 1988.

Nerve Palsy After Total Hip Arthroplasty

• BERNARD F. MORREY

Although risk to the sciatic nerve is well recognized with total hip arthroplasty, problems with the femoral, gluteal, and obturator nerves are also possible and increasingly recognized (Fig. 68–1).

INCIDENCE

Overall, neural injury probably occurs in approximately 1 to 2 percent of cases. Clinically detectable injury to the sciatic nerve occurs in approximately 0.6 to 1 percent.[8,21,26,29,34] Because of the infrequency of recognized palsies in the gluteal or obturator nerves, the incidence of injury to these structures has not been well defined. Such injuries must be quite uncommon, with the exception of injury to the gluteal nerve, which is associated with some surgical exposures.[13] The frequency with which nerve injury can be diagnosed by electromyography (EMG) is greater than is clinically recognized.[34]

In a study by Ahlgren et al. that followed 50 consecutive cases with electromyograph (EMG) analysis, 4 had electrical evidence of sciatic nerve involvement but only 1 of the 4 revealed any clinical evidence of damage.[2] Overall, these investigators placed the incidence of clinically significant sciatic palsy at 0.6 percent. One series of 1000 replacements reported an incidence of sciatic palsy of .8 percent.[19]

It is of interest that the occurrence appears to be a function of the learning curve. Johanson et al. reported a 1 percent frequency in the first 7 years of their experience with primary hips, but only 0.3 percent in the second 6 years' experience.[14] Schmalzried and colleagues studied more than 3000 cases of 53 palsies; 48 of the 53 (90 percent) palsies involved the sciatic nerve.[25] Simmons and associates analyzed 440 cases and found 10 with femoral neuropathy, all associated with the Hardinge surgical approach.[28] These investigators implicated the use of anterior retractors as the cause of the symptoms, and all 10 recovered.

Mayo Experience

At the Mayo Clinic, sciatic palsy was diagnosed in 76 patients after 26,480 procedures (.3 percent) over a span of almost 30 years, from 1970 to 1999.

ANATOMY

Sciatic Nerve

The anatomic relationship and proximity of the sciatic nerve to the posterior acetabulum and femur is well known (Fig. 68–2). The nerve variably traverses the piriformis, placing it at risk from retraction, particularly during posterior exposures. In this regard, the peroneal distribution is considered to be at greater risk because of the proximity of this segment of the nerve to retractors. This portion may also be vulnerable because of the relative fixation of the sciatic nerve, both in the notch and at the neck of the fibula. This selectively places the peroneal portion at risk of stretching. Edwards et al. studied the anatomy of the nerve and explained the high EMG incidence of injury to the short head of the biceps femoris, on the basis of stretch to the proximal aspect of the nerve.[9]

Femoral Nerve

The location of the femoral nerve at the level of the acetabulum also places it at risk from anterior retractors (Fig. 68–3). The inferior retractor near or under the iliopsoas tendon, which is used with the Hardinge approach, places the nerve and its branches to the sartorius and rectus femoris at particular risk.[25] Inserting the retraction more proximally allows protection at this level owing to the bulk effect of the muscle.

Gluteus Nerve

The superior gluteal nerve traverses the interval between the gluteus medius and minimus. The vertical muscle component of the Hardinge exposure makes the nerve vulnerable during this surgical approach[1] (Fig. 68–4).

The obturator nerve is at risk of penetration by the medial wall of the acetabulum.[18]

RISK FACTORS

Risk factors have been well documented. For primary procedures, patients with developmental dysplasia of

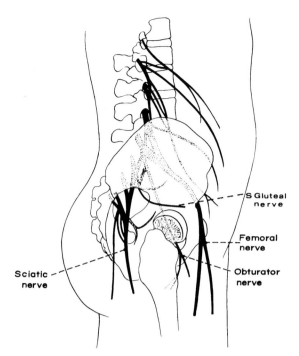

Figure 68–1. The course of the four nerves at risk with hip replacement. (Modified from Weber ER, Daube JR, Coventry MD: Peripheral neuropathies associated with total hip arthroplasty. J Bone Joint Surg 58A:66, 1976.)

the hip (DDH) have an incidence of sciatic lesions as high as 13 percent.[30] The analysis of Schmalzried et al. revealed a 5.2 percent incidence of neural involvement with DDH, which was approximately four times greater than the 1.3 percent occurrence after other primary diagnoses.[25] Others have reported a similar risk with DDH.[21] Revision hip replacement has been shown to increase the risk of nerve injury in virtually every study; 3.2 percent of patients with revision surgery had neural injury in the study by Schmalzreid et al. Johanson and co-workers implicated the increased surgical time and increased blood loss associated with these particular types of procedures as possible causes of nerve injuries.[14] They fur-

ther considered the decreased incidence in more recent years to reflect improved surgical technique and awarenesses of the potential cause of nerve damage.

Surgical Exposure

Sciatic Nerve. The role, if any, of surgical exposure and sciatic nerve injury is not well established. Most believe that the sciatic nerve is injured by retraction rather than being at risk because of the exposure itself. Navarro et al. reported no statistical difference between the .6 percent incidence after a posterior approach and the 1 percent incidence after a lateral trochanteric approach.[19]

In addition to the specific risks mentioned in the preceding paragraphs, it has long been recognized that females have a markedly greater risk of developing palsy than males.[8,9,34] In the series of Edward et al., 74 percent of cases involved women,[9] and in the analysis of Black and co-workers, approximately 80 percent of patients with nerve palsy were women.[5] Twelve of 14 patients with palsy in the Mayo Clinic series were also women (85 percent) compared with 52 percent of the overall population of total hip arthroplasty patients who were women.[30] While possibly related to diagnoses, the exact cause of increased risk of nerve palsies in women is undefined.

CLINICAL PRESENTATION

The onset and recognition of nerve injury may be acute or delayed.

Acute

In most instances, the problem is noted immediately after surgery, usually invading the sciatic nerve. Cohen and colleagues reported two delayed sciatic palsies that

Figure 68–2. Cross-sectional anatomy of the pelvis demonstrating the vulnerability of the femoral and sciatic nerves. (From Weber ER, Daube JR, Coventry MD: Peripheral neuropathies associated with total hip arthroplasties. J Bone Joint Surg 58A:66, 1976.)

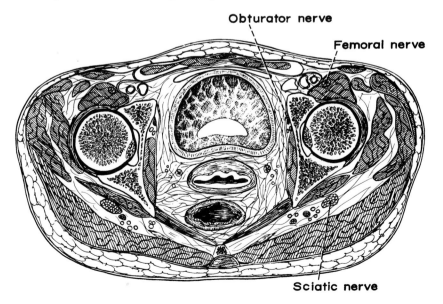

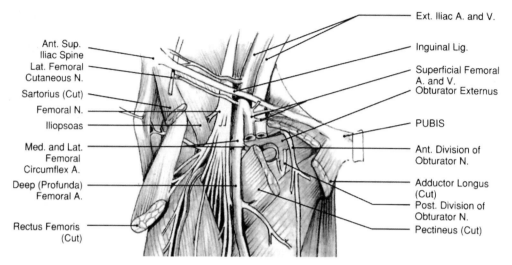

Figure 68–3. The anatomy of the femoral nerve and the femoral triangle. (From Reckling FW, Reckling JB, Mohr MC: Orthopedic Anatomy and Surgical Approaches. St. Louis, Mosby–Year Book, 1990.)

developed 3 days after surgery.[7] Femoral palsies are often not diagnosed until the patient begins physical therapy, although, clearly, these most commonly occur at the time of the procedure.

Delayed

It may be a surprise to learn that not all nerve injuries are identified immediately after surgery.[10] In 1991, Cohen et al. reported a patient with well-documented delay 27 hours after surgery and found four other such instances in the literature.[7]

Hemorrhage

This is a well-known cause of delayed or subacute sciatic nerve palsy, with the use of anticogulation being implicated as the cause.[6,11] Typically, these patients have acute onset of marked pain in the buttock or in the groin. Sciatic and, less commonly, femoral palsy follows. The diagnosis may be difficult because hemorrhage cannot always be appreciated on clinical examination. The sciatic stretch test is positive. Because the condition is reversible by timely decompression of the nerve, the proper diagnosis is imperative.

Late Presentation

There have been occasional reports of patients with significant neural injury that occurred months or even years after surgery.[20] Edwards et al.[10] reported an instance of significant sciatic dysfunction secondary to the sharp edge of polymethylmethacrylate at the margin of the acetabulum, which caused impingement on the sciatic nerve. Symptoms were relieved by removing the prominence. This instance justifies careful radiographic assessment to assure containment of the cement or screws at the acetabulum. A report has also

been made of injury to the sciatic nerve from a fractured trochanteric wire that migrated into the sciatic nerve 6 years after the surgery.[4]

An instance of delayed femoral nerve palsy occurred secondary to penetration of the medial wall of the acetabulum during preparation for arthroplasty. A large hematoma ultimately developed, causing pressure on the femoral nerve.[35] The hematoma resolved with return of neural function.

ETIOLOGY

In less than 50 percent of cases, the exact cause of the neuropathy is identifiable. Johanson et al. reported 47 percent of identifiable causes in 34 patients.[14] Schmalzried was able to define the cause of palsy in 42 percent of the 53 cases among a total of 3126 procedures.[25]

Sciatic Nerve Palsy

The most commonly recognized or unusual cause of sciatic palsy is limb lengthening (Fig. 68–5). Sunderland noted that axial neural stretch of 6 percent of the length of a nerve causes measurable dysfunction.[32] The average length of the sciatic nerve is approximately 75 cm; 6 percent is approximately 4 cm. In careful review by Stans et al. of 100 patients treated at the Mayo Clinic with total hip arthroplasty for congenital dislocation, some measure of sciatic nerve injury was detectable in 13. There were no sciatic palsies in the 54 hips lengthened by less than 4 cm. In contrast, among those hips that had greater than 4 cm of lengthening, the incidence of nerve palsy was 28 percent ($P<.0001$).

Yet, the overall correlation of leg length inequality in primary hip replacement and sciatic nerve injury is not so well established.[3] The use of somatosensory evoked potentials shows little correlation between leg

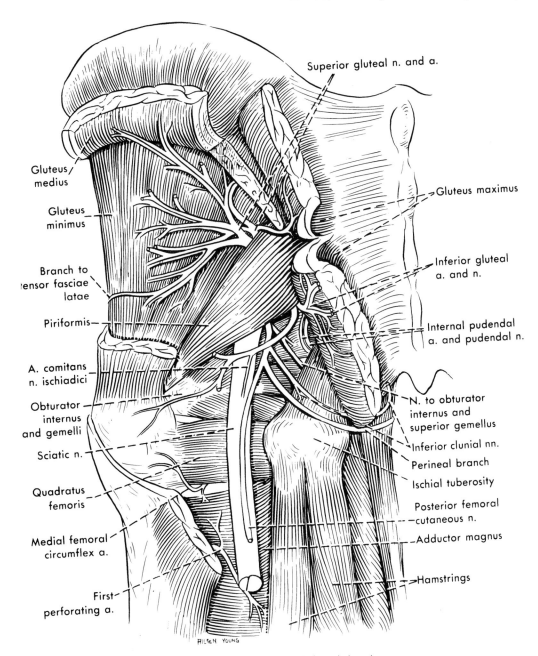

Figure 68–4. The anatomy of the sciatic and gluteal nerves.

length inequality and sciatic nerve injury.[5] Edwards et al., however, noted that, in 10 of 12 patients with palsies involving the sciatic distribution, the average limb lengthening was approximately 2.7 cm, and in 4, the lengthening was greater than 4 cm[9] (Fig. 68–6). Pekkarinen et al. observed no correlation of nerve palsy and leg length after 4339 procedures.[21] Hence, this issue is controversial.

Edwards et al. also implicated direct trauma[9] in 4 of 11 cases of sciatic palsies. Direct trauma occurs from pressure of retraction or from the retractor itself and may be more common after difficult dissections and in patients with tight or stiff hips. In an interesting study performed by Zechmann and Reckling, there was no correlation

between the preoperative range of motion and the development of sciatic palsy.[36] Nonetheless, most authors, including myself, believe that the difficulty of the dissection and stiffness of the hip do predispose patients to nerve palsies (see Fig. 68–6).[2] Moreover, direct injury can occur from pressure caused by a dislocated femoral component and also can be seen at the time of reduction.[31] Uchio et al. have also described entrapment of the sciatic nerve from scarring of the piriformis muscle.[33]

Entrapment

Direct injury to the sciatic nerve caused by securing the trochanter has been reported by several authors.[4,12,16]

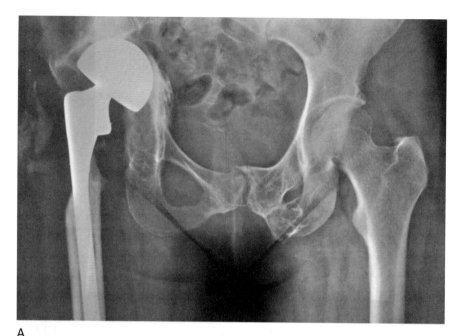

A

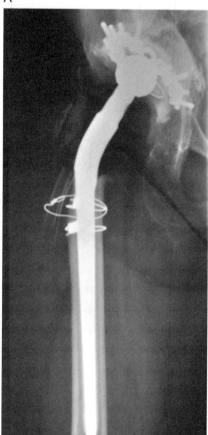

B

Figure 68–5. A, Loss of proximal femoral bone and shortening. **B,** Relative lengthening of the extremity occurred at the time of revision. The patient had sensory and motor dysfunction for 1 year; eventually, nearly total resolution was achieved.

Gudmundson and Pilgaard have offered a technique of trochanteric wiring designed to minimize the chance of injury to the sciatic nerve.[12] I operated on a patient whose sciatic nerve was entrapped at the edge of the acetabulum by the acetabular component. This has also been observed with the use of a protrusio ring.[17]

Femoral Nerve Palsy

The femoral nerve is vulnerable to direct pressure from retraction but is more at risk from a surgical exposure in which the gluteus is split. In Solheim and Hagen's study, the femoral nerve was involved in 2 of 6 patients with neural involvement after 825 hip replacements.[29]

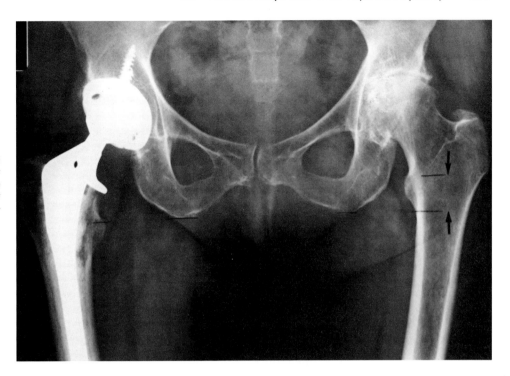

Figure 68–6. A 66-year-old woman developed complete sciatic palsy after lengthening of 2.5 cm after hip replacement. Spontaneous recovery was documented 1 year after surgery.

A femoral palsy was reported in 2.3 percent of patients in whom the anterior Hardinge approach was used, with spontaneous recovery in all 10 patients.[28] Injury to the femoral nerve from hematoma has also been reported.[11,35] EMG studies have demonstrated that the femoral nerve is the second most frequently involved, and subclinical injury seems to occur relatively frequently (unpublished data).

Gluteal Nerve Palsy

It has been estimated that splitting the gluteus medius more than 4 cm places the nerve at risk.[1] One patient was referred to us in whom this nerve appeared to have been severely damaged, with complete denervation of the gluteus medius after a difficult revision procedure in which this exposure was used.

Obturator Nerve Palsy

The obturator nerve is at particular risk with protrusion of methyl methacrylate through defects in the acetabulum.[18,27] This protrusion may cause a delayed manifestation and seems to respond well to late decompression.

PREVENTION

It has been observed that an increased awareness is the most important factor in preventing this complication.[14] In my experience, subtrochanteric femoral resection for the severely dysplastic hip markedly decompresses the sciatic nerve, lessening the likelihood of nerve injury with difficult procedures for congenital dysplasia of the

hip (CDH). Careful preoperative planning that decreases the incidence of leg length inequality to less than 1 to 2 cm is also an important variable (see Chapter 70). Strict avoidance of lengthening more than 4 cm under any circumstances is strongly supported by Sunderland's theoretical observations,[32] by Edwards et al.,[9] and by Stans et al. in their review of the CDH experience at the Mayo Clinic.[30]

Somatosensory Evoked Response

The use of somatosensory evoked response has been applied to total hip replacement in hopes of identifying the at-risk patient. Although the data Kennedy et al. suggest that monitoring the somatosensory evoked potential was of value in 23 consecutive revisions,[15] this has not been substantiated by other investigators.[5,22,23] In an excellent study by Black et al. of 100 consecutive cases, 18 individuals had positive somatosensory evoked potentials during surgery.[5] Of these, 18 had demonstrable clinical symptoms after the procedure. In these instances, an altered potential was observed at the time of closure. These investigators also demonstrated that reaming the femur also evokes potentials, indicating that this may be one period of risk during the technique. They also implicated prior surgery as a risk factor but were not able to correlate leg length inequality with nerve palsy. They concluded that monitoring somatosensory evoked potential did not significantly protect the nerve or allow technique modification to lessen the likelihood of nerve injury. Rasmussen et al.,[23] in a prospective study using somatosensory evoked response, observed no benefit in this monitoring technique. Porter and associates, in contrast, did reveal that extensive somatosensory responses, such as simultaneous decrease of amplitude and increase of latency, were predictive of nerve injury.[22] The problem is that none of these studies offers confidence that this technique actually protects the patient.

TREATMENT

Treatment of nerve palsy after total hip arthroplasty is predicated on etiology. However, in approximately half of these patients, no obvious or subtle cause can be identified.

Patients with femoral neuropathy, particularly thought to be associated with a surgical approach, are clearly managed by expectant observation. In approximately 50 percent of patients in whom an apparent cause is known, intervention may be indicated.

INTERVENTION

Leg Length Inequality

Patients with leg length inequality and sciatic nerve palsy noted immediately after surgery may be treated by shortening the femoral head and neck, if a modular component has been used. Flexing the knee to decompress the personeal portion of the sciatic nerve may also be effective in this setting.

Hematoma

There is strong evidence to support immediate decompression of a hematoma. Fleming et al. demonstrated that 4 of 5 patients treated with decompression improved or completely recovered, whereas the 1 in whom observation was carried out failed to recover.[11] Brantigan and colleagues have also recommended prompt decompression of a hematoma.[6] The major concern, therefore, is missing the diagnosis. Acute onset of pain 1 or 2 days after surgery and a subacute development of the nerve palsy are the hallmarks of this particular clinical presentation, usually in an excessively anticoagulated patient.

Impingement

Delayed development of nerve palsies requires careful assessment to investigate the possibility of impingement, such as from protruded methyl methacrylate or, possibly, from a screw securing the acetabulum. Delayed-onset injuries do tend to respond to removal of the offending cause.[27]

PROGNOSIS FOR RECOVERY

Recovery from nerve injuries after total hip arthroplasty is very much a function of the etiology. The prognosis is generally categorized as being complete, incomplete, or

with severe residual deficiency. In Johanson and colleagues' experience of 28 procedures, 79 percent had incomplete recovery.[14] Edwards et al. thought that patients with lesions of the sciatic nerve with personeal distribution had a better prognosis than those with complete sciatic lesions.[9] In Schmalzried and associates' study, 7 of 53 patients recovered completely, all within 21 months. Thirty-three of the 53 had some residual symptoms, and 13 of 53 had severe residual deficiencies.[25] In Stans' experience with primary surgery for DDH, 12 patients were followed an average of 10 years. Of these, seven (58 percent) had complete recovery and five (42%) were left with some residual motor and sensory deficiency. Schmalzried revisited the patients in his 1991 review and observed favorable prognosis if some residual motor function was present after surgery or within 2 weeks.[26] Delayed-onset nerve compression treated by removal of the compression source is associated with relief of symptoms in the majority of instances.

AUTHOR'S PREFERENCE

In my practice, the focus on treatment of nerve palsies is to prevent their occurrence. This may be brought about by a healthy appreciation of the circumstances in which these occur: more common in (1) females, (2) revision surgery, (3) type III or IV CDH, and (4) the stiff hip. Patients with a history of laminectomy may also be at risk. Although this has not been well documented in the literature, I have made this correlation with nerve palsies after total knee arthroplasty. Spinal anesthesia may also play a role and thus is avoided in patients who are otherwise thought to be at risk for the development of nerve palsy.

The treatment of nerve injuries once they have occurred is based on whether an etiology is definable or not. Observation and reassurance are the treatment modalities for those without known cause.

In those patients in whom the etiology is definable, hematoma, leg lengthening, or impingement are the three most readily recognized causes. A very careful examination for hematoma, including magnetic resonance imaging, is appropriate in the acute stage. Immediate decompression of a hematoma is the most dramatic treatment option and one that is strongly recommended if not absolutely indicated.

Impingement is investigated with internal and external pelvic oblique films, along with a true lateral film of the hip. We specifically observe the status of acetabular screws.

If leg length difference is the apparent cause, and sensory or only mild motor dysfunction is present, I use a split mattress technique in which the knee is flexed approximately 60 to 90 degrees. This relaxes the sciatic nerve. The extension at the knee is gradually increased over the next several days. I particularly use the split mattress technique if the lesion is of the personeal distribution. If a more profound palsy is diagnosed, and if a modular head and neck prosthesis has been used, I shorten the extremity with the shortest neck length available. If stability is a concern, the trochanter may be advanced and a cast may be used or the hip may be protected with a splint.

References

1. Abitbol JJ, Gendron D, Laurin CA, Beaulieu MA: Gluteal nerve damage following total hip arthroplasty: A prospective analysis. J Arthroplasty 5:319, 1990.
2. Ahlgren SA, Elmqvist D, Ljung P: Nerve lesions after total hip replacement. Acta Orthop Scand 55:152, 1984.
3. Amstutz HC, Ma SM, Jinnah RH, Mai L: Revision of aseptic loose total hip arthroplasties. Clin Orthop 170:21, 1982.
4. Asnis SE, Hanley S, Shelton PD: Sciatic neuropathy secondary to migration of trochanteric wire following total hip arthroplasty. Clin Orthop 196:226, 1985.
5. Black DL, Reckling FW, Porter SS: Somatosensory-evoked potential monitored during total hip arthroplasty. Clin Orthop 262:170, 1991.
6. Brantigan JW, Owens ML, Moody FG: Femoral neuropathy complicating anticoagulation therapy. Am J Surg 132:108, 1976.
7. Cohen B, Bhamra M, Ferris BD: Delayed sciatic nerve palsy following total hip arthroplasty. Br J Clin Pract 45:292, 1991.
8. DeHart MM, Riley LH Jr: Nerve injuries in total hip arthroplasty. J AAOS 7:101, 1999.
9. Edwards BN, Tullos HS, Noble PC: Contributory factors and etiology of sciatic nerve palsy in total hip arthroplasty. Clin Orthop 218:136, 1987.
10. Edwards MS, Barbaro NM, Asher SW, Murray WR: Delayed sciatic palsy after total hip replacement: Case report. Neurosurgery 9:61, 1981.
11. Fleming RE, Michelsen CB, Stinchfield FE: Sciatic paralysis: A complication of bleeding following hip surgery. J Bone Joint Surg 61A:37, 1979.
12. Gudmundsson GH, Pilgaard S: Prevention of sciatic nerve entrapment in trochanteric wiring following total hip arthroplasty. Clin Orthop 196:215, 1985.
13. Hagen R: Peripheral nerve injuries. J Norway Med Assoc 90:945, 1970.
14. Johanson NA, Pellicci PM, Tsairis P, Salvati EA: Nerve injury in total hip arthroplasty. Clin Orthop 179:214, 1983.
15. Kennedy WF, Byrne TF, Majid HA, Pavlak LL: Sciatic nerve monitoring during revision total hip arthroplasty. Clin Orthop 264:223, 1991.
16. Mallory TH: Sciatic nerve entrapment secondary to trochanteric wiring following total hip arthroplasty: A case report. Clin Orthop 180:198, 1983.
17. McLean M: Total hip replacement and sciatic nerve trauma. Orthopedics 9:1121, 1986.
18. Melamed NB, Satya-Murti S: Obturator neuropathy after total hip replacement [letter]. Ann Neurol 13:578, 1983.
19. Navarro RA, Schmalzried TP, Amstutz HC, Dorey FJ: Surgical approach and nerve palsy in total hip arthroplasty. J Arthroplasty 10:1, 1995.
20. Oleksak M, Edge AJ: Compression of the sciatic nerve by methylmethacrylate cement after total hip replacement. J Bone Joint Surg 74B:729, 1992.
21. Pekkarinen J, Alho A, Puusa A, Paavilainen T: Recovery of sciatic nerve injuries in association with total hip arthroplasty in 27 patients. J Arthroplasty 14:305, 1999.
22. Porter SS, Black DL, Reckling FW, Mason J: Intraoperative cortical somatosensory evoked potentials for detection of sciatic neuropathy during total hip arthroplasty. J Clin Anesth 1:170, 1989.
23. Rasmussen TJ, Black DL, Bruce RP, Reckling FW: Efficacy of corticosomatosensory evoked potential monitoring in predicting and/or preventing sciatic nerve palsy during total hip arthroplasty. J Arthroplasty 9:53, 1994.
24. Reckling FW, Reckling JB, Mohr MC: Orthopedic Anatomy and Surgical Approaches. St. Louis, Mosby–Year Book, 1990.
25. Schmalzried TP, Amstutz HC, Dorey FJ: Nerve palsy associated with total hip replacement: Risk factors and prognosis. J Bone Joint Surg 73A:1074, 1991.
26. Schmalzried TP, Noordin S, Amstutz HC: Update on nerve palsy associated with total hip replacement. Clin Orthop 344:188, 1997.
27. Siliski JM, Scott RD: Obturator-nerve palsy resulting from intrapelvic extrusion of cement during total hip replacement: Report of four cases. J Bone Joint Surg 67A:1225, 1985.
28. Simmons C Jr, Izant TH, Rothman RH, et al: Femoral neuropathy following total hip arthroplasty: Anatomic study, case reports, and literature review [Review]. J Arthroplasty 6(Suppl):S57, 1991.
29. Solheim LF, Hagen R: Femoral and sciatic neuropathies after total hip arthroplasty. Acta Orthop Scand 51:531, 1980.
30. Stans AA, Pagnano MW, Shaughnessy WJ, Hanssen AD: Results of total hip arthroplasty for Crowe type III developmental hip dysplasia. Clin Orthop 348:149–157, 1998.
31. Stockley I, Bickerstaff D: Sciatic palsy following reduction of a dislocated prosthesis: Brief report. J Bone Joint Surg 70B:329, 1988.
32. Sunderland S: Nerve and Nerve Injuries. Edinburgh, Churchill Livingstone, 1978.
33. Uchio Y, Nishikawa U, Ochi M, et al: Bilateral piriformis syndrome after total hip arthroplasty. Archiv Orthop Trauma Surg 117:177, 1998.
34. Weber ER, Daube JR, Coventry MD: Peripheral neuropathies associated with total hip arthroplasty. J Bone Joint Surg 58A:66, 1976.
35. Wooten SL, McLaughlin RE: Iliacus hematoma and subsequent femoral nerve palsy after penetration of the medial acetabular wall during total hip arthroplasty: Report of a case. Clin Orthop 191:221, 1984.
36. Zechmann JP, Reckling FW: Association of preoperative hip motion and sciatic nerve palsy following total hip arthroplasty. Clin Orthop 241:197, 1989.

69

Vascular Injuries Associated with Hip Arthroplasty

• DAVID G. LEWALLEN

Vascular injuries are rare but potentially devastating complications that have been reported in association with hip arthroplasty. They may appear either with acute hemorrhage during the procedure or with delayed postoperative bleeding problems. Injury may occur to either arterial or venous structures in the neighborhood of the hip. Anatomically, structures at risk include the femoral artery and vein, obturator artery and vein, external iliac artery and vein, common iliac artery and vein, and profunda femoris branches more distally in the thigh. The potential problems resulting from vascular injury include thrombosis of either arterial or venous structures, with emboli that may migrate proximally in the case of the venous system or shower distally in the case of injury to atherosclerotic arterial vessels.[9,11,15,16,24,31] Injury may also result in formation of an arteriovenous fistula or false aneurysm.[9,10] Clinically, symptoms of vascular injury may be noted immediately during the course of the surgery, in the subsequent hours or days after the procedure, or years after the index arthroplasty, when, for example, flow changes resulting from a pseudoaneurysm may become apparent. Ischemia occlusion or embolization and frank bleeding at the time of a subsequent revision procedure may all appear as the initial signs of a much earlier vascular insult.

PREVALENCE

Reports of vascular complications suggest a prevalence between 0.2 percent and 0.3 percent.[21] The most commonly injured arterial structures by report are the external iliac artery and the common femoral artery.[30] In a review by Shoenfield, 68 vascular complications collected from the literature revealed 36 external iliac artery injuries and 17 common femoral artery injuries, with two thirds occurring on the patient's left side.[20] Disruption of normal anatomic relationships, scarring about the hip from prior surgery, component migration, and encroachment by implants or cement on neighboring vascular structures make vascular injury more common during revision hip surgery than during primary hip replacement.[19,30] The true prevalence of vascular injury depends on what threshold is set for the definition of a significant

vascular problem because, obviously, any surgical exercise results in bleeding and damage to minor vascular structures. If "excessive bleeding" is used as the threshold, an incidence of approximately 1 percent (19 of 2012 arthroplasties) was reported by Coventry in an early review of a large arthroplasty experience, with 6 of the 19 patients requiring a reoperation. Clearly, not all these patients were thought to have had an injury to a major named vascular structure.[6] More serious problems tend to be those that make their way into the literature as case reports. Nonetheless, in Shoenfield's review of a collection of 68 arthroplasties requiring reoperation for associated vascular injury, the mortality rate was 7 percent and amputation was ultimately required in 15%, documenting the dread outcomes possible with these injuries.[30] Despite more recent advances in methods of recognition and treatment of vascular injuries, Feugier et al. published a report in 1999, documenting a 37 percent mortality rate associated with vascular injuries seen over a 12-year period.[7]

ETIOLOGY OF VASCULAR INJURY

Vascular injuries may occur directly from sharp instruments such as knives or osteotomes and may also occur indirectly from stretching, tearing, or compression during placement of retractors, manipulation of the limb, or even postoperative dislocation.[16] Although direct injury by sharp instruments usually involves immediately adjacent vascular structures, stretching or tearing can occur to vascular structures at some distance from the operative field. Exact mechanisms of injury can include common iliac vein injury or arterial injury by violation of the medial wall of the acetabulum as a result of excessive acetabular reaming or placement of drills or screws.[12,18,32,33] Sharp-tipped retractors such as a Hohmann type of instrument can produce direct vascular injury when placed anteriorly over the rim of the acetabulum, or, alternatively, when placed medial to the femoral neck, with respective damage to the common femoral artery or to the medial and lateral circumflex femoral vessels. Bleeding, ischemia caused by occlusion, and late formation of pseudoaneurysm requiring operative repair have all been documented from this mechanism.[2,14,21,27] In a report of 6 cases related to the use of the Hohmann retractor, the resulting vascular injury led to amputation in 1 patient.[21]

Vascular injury has also been described during extraction of failed acetabular components at the time of revision surgery. Particularly at risk are those patients who have intrapelvic extrusion of methacrylate cement that occurred at the time of their prior surgery. Depending on the extent or location of the extruded cement, there may be encroachment on—or even complete encirclement of—vascular structures by the methacrylate, with the result that subsequent extraction of the loose implant and attached cement bolus produces inevitable and poten-

tially catastrophic vascular damage.[3,5] Vascular injury has also been reported that has arisen from compression or kinking of atherosclerotic vessels, with resultant arterial thrombosis or atherosclerotic arterial emboli to the more distal extremity.[2,22,31] In a report by Nachbur of 15 cases of vascular complications, 2 were thought to be instances of postoperative ischemia brought on by thrombosis.[21] Postoperative ischemia may also occur in the absence of direct injury because of limb lengthening, particularly when preoperative vascularity is marginal owing to underlying atherosclerosis or prior radiation (Fig. 69–1).[19] One report has even documented aortic thrombosis after acetabular component revision in an elderly man with

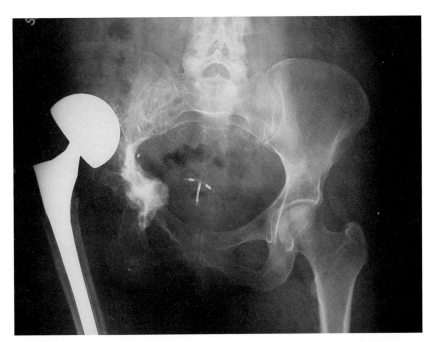

Figure 69–1. A, Multiply operated right hip, with a history of high-dose radiation after desmoid tumor excision from the right hemipelvis and several subsequent failed arthroplasty attempts. **B**, After reconstruction. No excess bleeding was noted intraoperatively or after surgery. There was no change in limb vascularity while the patient was in the hospital.

Illustration continued on following page

A

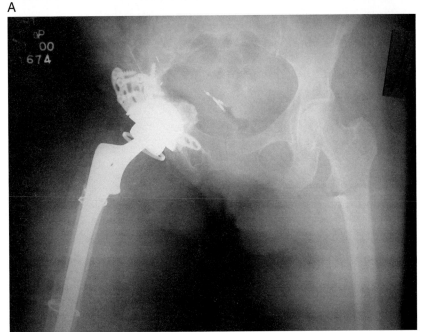

B

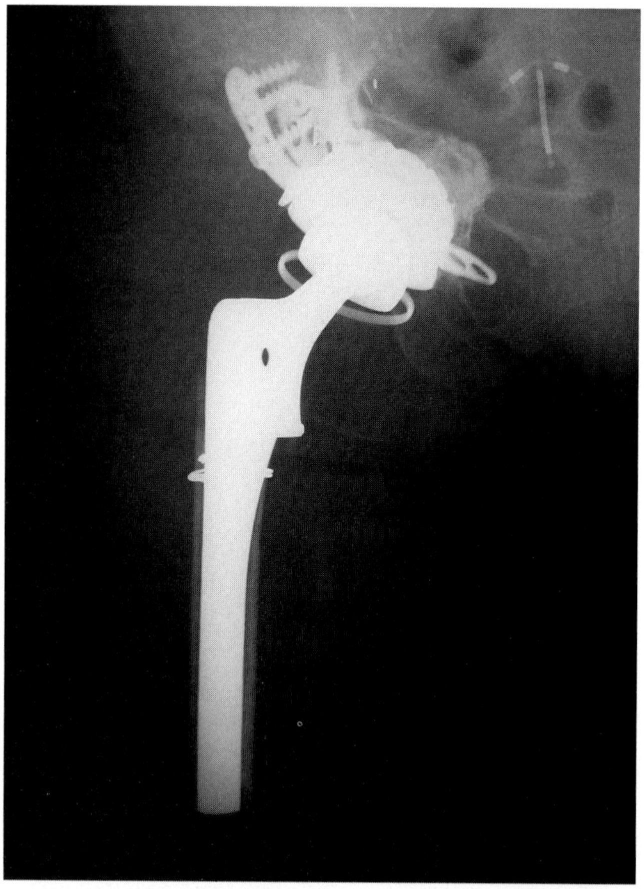

recurrent postoperative episodes of dislocation of the hip.[16]

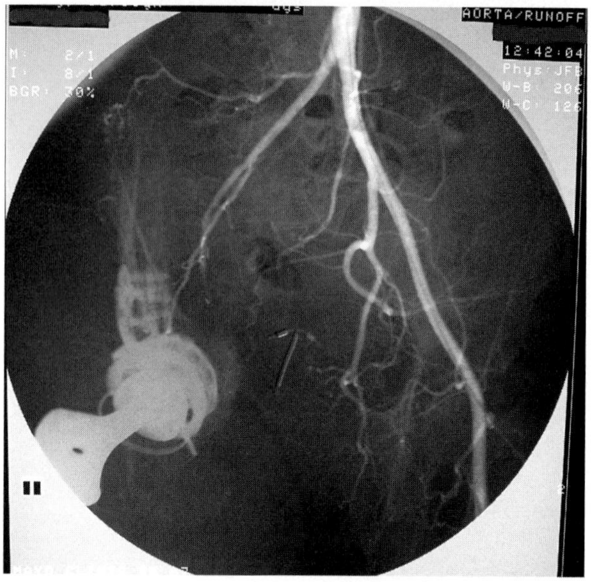

With the advent of widespread use of uncemented, hemispheric, porous ingrowth, acetabular components fixed with adjunctive screws, a new potential risk to vascular structures has been introduced. Drills or screws projecting beyond the bone medial to the acetabulum can cause vascular injury. Beginning in the early 1990s, reports of the potential for major hemorrhage and even death related to screws that were used with an uncemented acetabular component began to appear.[12,13] The proximity of the intrapelvic vessels to the track of various fixation screws placed in a hemispheric cup has been nicely demonstrated in subsequent anatomic studies by Keating et al. and by Wasielewski et al.[12,32] (Fig. 69–2). In particular, the external iliac vessels, obturator nerve and vessels, and superior and inferior vesicular venous plexus on the medial aspect of the acetabulum are at risk. Wasielewski et al. have described a system of quadrants that help guide the surgeon to safe screw placement, with the anterosuperior and anteroinferior portion of the acetabulum representing the at-risk area or so-called zone of death (Fig. 69–3). The mechanical strength and quality of screw fixation is best in the posterosuperior and posteroinferior quadrants anyway, and because there is significant risk with screws placed in the anterior quadrants, where mechanical quality of fixation is poor, there really is no reason to subject the patient to the risk of attempted screw placement into bone in those regions. Even if safe screw placement is accomplished at the time of surgery, the potential risk of screws does not end there, because later intrapelvic migration of the cup stemming from failure of fixation

Figure 69–1. *Continued.* **C,** Sudden change in limb status was noted after a prolonged plane ride to home, with hip flexed, pain, pallor, and pulselessness consistent with acute arterial occlusion. Attempted embolectomy and arterial reconstruction were unsuccessful, leading to subsequent above-knee amputation. **D,** Angiogram showing small or absent arterial branches in the entire right hemipelvis as a result of prior radiation. Femoral artery occlusion was thought to be caused by a combination of stretch from limb lengthening, radiation effects, and prolonged compression from the long plane ride with the hip flexed.

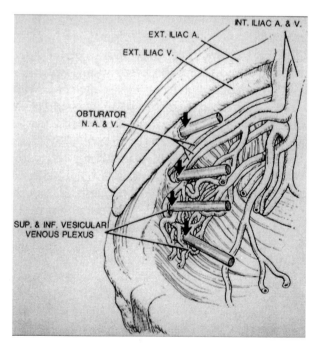

Figure 69–2. Intrapelvic vascular structures with a trajectory of acetabular screws shown by solid rods. (From Keating EM, Ritter MA, Faris PM: Structures at risk from medially placed acetabular screws. J Bone Joint Surg 72A:509–511, 1990.)

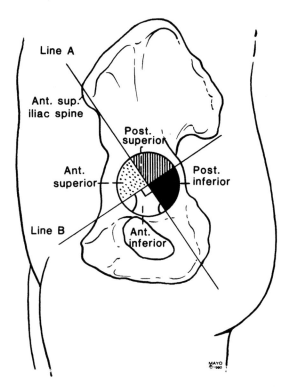

Figure 69–3. Acetabular zones demonstrating anterosuperior and anteroinferior quadrants, which should be avoided during acetabular screw placement to prevent intrapelvic vascular injury. (Adapted from Wasielewski RC, Cooperstein LA, Kruger MP, Rubash HE: Acetabular anatomy and the transacetabular fixation of screws in total hip arthroplasty. J Bone Joint Surg 72A:501–508, 1990.)

gentle retraction of soft tissue structures, can help prevent damage to adjacent vessels. Simple techniques, such as use of scalpels or other sharp instruments away from rather than toward adjacent neurologic or vascular structures, can help reduce the risk of inadvertent direct injury. Careful retractor placement intraoperatively is important, first, careful surgical dissection, and then by placement of the retractor into an already created free space adjacent to bone, the least risky technique. Preoperative vascular assessment and consultation may be reasonable for selected patients with a history of pre-existing severe peripheral vascular disease or an anatomic abnormality that might place vessels in proximity to the required surgical field. Preoperative angiography has been recommended for those circumstances, in which significant intrapelvic migration of failed acetabular components or extravasated cemented may place the intrapelvic vessels at some risk.[1,5,9,10,25,28] In selected cases, planned medial intrapelvic exposure has been used as well as mobilization of the iliac vessels with the assistance of a general or vascular surgeon. These techniques prevent inadvertent vascular injury during removal of markedly displaced intraplevic implants. Thorough knowledge of vascular anatomy in the region of the hip helps the surgeon to avoid risky maneuvers and subsequent vascular injury. In particular, it is essential that acetabular screws not be placed into the hazardous zones as determined by the adjacent vascular anatomy medial to the acetabulum (Fig. 69–5).

Delayed injury to vascular structures can occur with failure of arthroplasties that have been in place for many years. Acetabular component migration or migration of disintegrated portions of the implant, such as the locking ring of a constrained cup, can result in vascular erosion and pseudoaneurysm formation.[8,20,26,29] Implant wear or loosening can produce synovitis and cyst formation, which can sometimes become large and extend intrapelvically, causing vascular compression by the pseudotumor.[17]

and loosening or from periprosthetic acetabular fracture can result in life-threatening bleeding from laceration of intrapelvic vessels (Fig. 69–4).[23] As with most major complications associated with hip arthroplasty, prevention is always preferred over treatment. Careful exposure during surgery and equally careful technique, with

Figure 69–4. Intrapelvic migration of cup and screws after motor vehicle accident and pelvic fracture. The patient died soon after arrival at the hospital, despite efforts at bleeding control and resuscitation, because of laceration of the iliac vessels and massive intrapelvic hemorrhage.

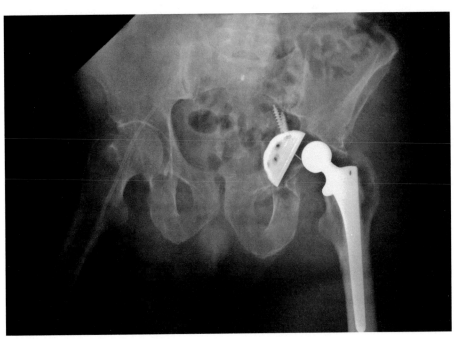

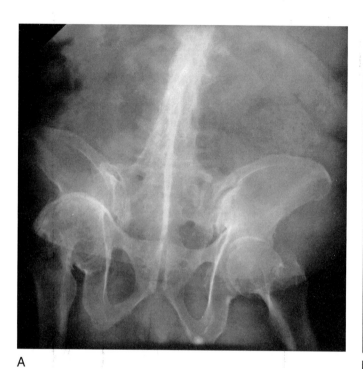

A

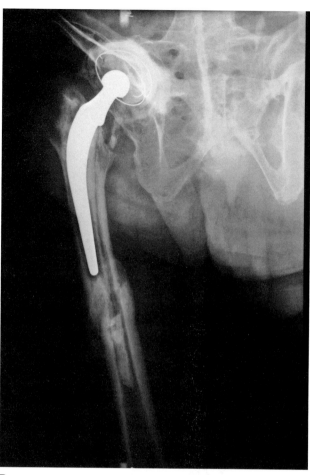

B

Figure 69–5. A, Original preoperative radiograph. **B,** Radiograph of failed, loose total hip arthroplasty in a patient with pelvic deformity from childhood tuberculosis and adult ankylosing spondylitis. Revision surgery was complicated by sudden massive bleeding anteriorly adjacent to the hip, which was subsequently found to be caused by injury to the femoral artery as it coursed over the anterior rim of the acetabular component. Local control and emergent vascular bypass grafting preserved limb vascularity and allowed completion of the revision surgery, but an associated femoral nerve palsy, likely from damage during bleeding control efforts, proved to be permanent.

Large, bulky reconstructions, such as can occur with some structural allografts, can cause compression of adjacent vascular structures during certain limb positions.[4]

MANAGEMENT OF VASCULAR INJURY

Successful management of sudden vascular injury requires knowledge of local anatomy and some degree of contingency planning if the most effective and rapid response is to be mounted. Prompt recognition of vascular injury is important. When such an injury is identified intraoperatively, the initial critical step is, of course, bleeding control. Coagulation or ligation of smaller vessels can be effective, and packing can provide temporary control, or, in some cases, may even achieve hemostasis as a result of thrombosis of the injured vessel, particularly when venous injury has occurred. Injury to major named vessels most often requires operative control and may necessitate repair. The operating orthopedic surgeon should have a thorough knowledge of pertinent regional

vascular anatomy and some familiarity with necessary adjunctive emergent operative approaches, such as the ilioinguinal or McBurney incision for retroperitoneal or intrapelvic exposure. Emergent proximal vascular control can prove to be a life-saving procedure and allow operative repair with the assistance of a vascular surgeon or a surgeon who has comparable expertise. Such assistance can be invaluable in the event of major vascular injury that requires formal vascular repair. Preoperative consultation with a vascular surgeon can greatly facilitate availability of such an individual for intraoperative assistance should vascular injury occur, and, in some cases, will result in the vascular surgeon's recommendation of elective mobilization and protection of the vascular structures at risk. I have found such collaboration particularly helpful in patients with markedly distorted pelvic anatomy or a history of prior vascular injury repair, or in selected cases with marked intrapelvic migration of components and cement (see Fig. 69–5).

Recognition of vascular injury may be delayed and may become apparent because of excessive blood loss or transfusion requirements in the hours after surgery.

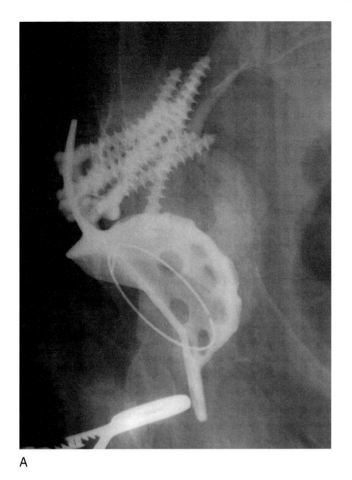

A

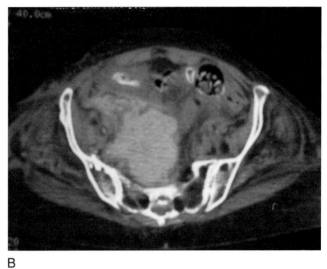

B

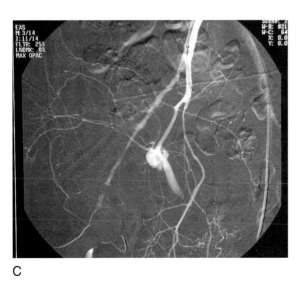

C

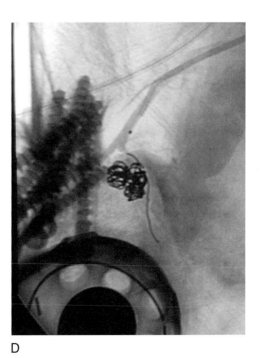

D

Figure 69–6. A, Intraoperative radiograph taken during complex revision total hip arthroplasty performed with an acetabular cage. Note the screw tips protruding beyond the bone medially. **B,** Computed tomography scan of the pelvis obtained post-operatively because of ongoing blood loss reveals large intrapelvic hematoma in the iliac fossa displacing the pelvic contents. **C,** Angiogram showing intrapelvic bleeding. **D,** Radiodense coil used for angiographic embolization of bleeding adjacent to the tip of the screw.

Documentation of the bleeding source with use of axial imaging or radiography and intra-arterial embolization for control can sometimes prevent the need for repeat surgery (Fig. 69–6). Very late symptoms from false aneurysm formation can be nonspecific or confusing but may well require surgical treatment once the diagnosis is confirmed.

SUMMARY

Vascular injuries associated with hip arthroplasty are very uncommon but may be catastrophic and life endangering. Thorough knowledge of local vascular anatomy, care during operative maneuvers that place vascular structures at risk, and thorough knowledge of local vascular anatomy about the hip can reduce the risk of such problems.[16] In addition, collaboration, when appropriate, with an experienced vascular surgeon, both preoperatively and in some cases intraoperatively, can help reduce the risk of inadvertent vascular injury. Should vascular injury occur, prompt recognition is essential to allow appropriate treatment and to reduce the chances of adverse outcomes.

References

1. Al-Salmon M, Taylor DC, Beauchamp CP, Duncan CP: Prevention of vascular injuries in revision total hip replacement. Can J Surg 35:261–264, 1992.
2. Aust JC, Bredenberg CE, Murray DG: Mechanisms of arterial injuries associated with total hip replacement. Arch Surg 116:345–349, 1981.
3. Bergqvist D, Carlsson AS, Ericsson BF: Vascular complications after total hip arthroplasty. Acta Orthop Scand 54:157–163, 1983.
4. Bose WJ, Petty W: Femoral artery and nerve compression by bulk allograft used for acetabular reconstruction. An unreported complication. J Arthroplasty 11:348–350, 1996.
5. Brentlinger A, Hunter JR: Perforation of the external iliac artery and ureter presenting as acute hemorrhagic cystitis after total hip replacement. Report of a case. J Bone Joint Surg 69A:620–622, 1987.
6. Coventry MB, Beckenbaugh RD, Nolan DR, Ilstrup DM: 2,012 total hip arthroplasties: A study of postoperative course and early complications. J Bone Joint Surg 56A:273–284, 1974.
7. Feugier P, Fessy MH, Carret JP, et al: Total hip arthroplasty. Risk factors and prevention of iatrogenic vascular complications. Ann Chir 53:127–135, 1999.
8. Giacchetto J, Gallagher JJ: False aneurysm of the common femoral artery secondary to migration of a threaded acetabular component. A case report and review of the literature. Clin Orthop 231:91–96, 1988.
9. Heyes FLP, Aukland A: Occlusion of the common femoral artery complicating total hip arthroplasty. J Bone Joint Surg 67B:533–535, 1985.
10. Hopkins NFG, Vanhegan JAD, Jamieson CW: Iliac aneurysm after total hip arthroplasty. Surgical management. J Bone Joint Surg 65B:359–361, 1983.
11. Jonsson H, Karlstrom G, Lundqvist B: Intimal rupture and arterial thrombosis in revision hip arthroplasty. Case report. Acta Chir Scand 153:621–622, 1987.
12. Keating EM, Ritter MA, Faris PM: Structures at risk from medially placed acetabular screws. J Bone Joint Surg 72A:509–511, 1990.
13. Kirkpatrick JS, Callaghan JJ, Vandemark RM, Goldner RD: The relationship of the intrapelvic vasculature to the acetabulum. Implications in screw-fixation acetabular components. Clin Orthop 258:183–190, 1990.
14. Kroese A, Molleaud A: Traumatic aneurysm of the common femoral artery after hip endoprostheses. Acta Orthop Scand 46:119, 1975.
15. Lewallen DG: Neurovascular injury associated with hip arthroplasty. J Bone Joint Surg 79A:1870–1880, 1997.
16. Leung AG, Cabanela ME: Aortic thrombosis after acetabular revision of a total hip arthroplasty. J Arthroplasty 13:961–965, 1998.
17. Madan S, Jowett RL, Goodwin MI: Recurrent intrapelvic cyst complicating metal-on-metal cemented total hip arthroplasty. Arch Orthop Trauma Surg 120:508–510, 2000.
18. Mallory TH: Rupture of the common iliac vein from reaming the acetabulum during replacement. J Bone Joint Surg 54A:276–277, 1972.
19. Matos MH, Amstutz HC, Machleder HI: Ischemia of the lower extremity after total hip replacement. J Bone Joint Surg 61A:24–27, 1979.
20. Mody BS: Pseudoaneurysm of external iliac artery and compression of external iliac vein after total hip arthroplasty. Case report. J Arthroplasty 9:95–98, 1994.
21. Nachbur B, Meyer RP, Verkkala K, Zurcher R: Mechanisms of severe arterial injury in surgery of the hip joint. Clin Orthp 141:122, 1979.
22. Parfenchuck TA, Young TR: Intraoperative arterial occlusion in total joint arthroplasty. J Arthroplasty 9:217–220, 1994.
23. Peterson CA II, Lewallen DG: Periprosthetic fracture of the acetabulum after total hip arthroplasty. J Bone Joint Surg 78A:1206–1213, 1996.
24. Ratliff AHC: Arterial injuries after total hip replacement [editorial]. J Bone Joint Surg 67B:517–518, 1985.
25. Reiley MA, Bond D, Branick RI, Wilson EH: Vascular complications following total hip arthroplasty. A review of the literature and a report of two cases. Clin Orthop 186:23–28, 1984.
26. Ryan JA, Johnson ML, Boettcher WG, Kirkpatrick JN: Mycotic aneurysm of the external iliac artery caused by migration of a total hip prosthesis. Clin Orthop 186:57–59, 1984.
27. Salama R, Stavorovsky MM, Iellin A, Weissman SL: Femoral artery injury complicating total hip replacement. Clin Orthop 89:143–144, 1972.
28. Schullin JP, Nelson CL, Beven EG: False aneurysm of the left external iliac artery following total hip arthroplasty. Report of a case. Clin Orthop 113:145–149, 1975.
29. Sethuraman V, Hozack WJ, Sharkey PF, Rothman RH: Pseudoaneurysm of femoral artery after revision total hip arthroplasty with a constrained cup. J Arthroplasty 15:531–534, 2000.
30. Shoenfield NA, Stuchin SA, Pearl R, Haveson S: The management of vascular injuries associated with total hip arthroplasty. J Vascular Surg 11:549–555, 1990.
31. Stubbs DH, Dorner DB, Johnston RC: Thrombosis of the iliofemoral artery during revision of a total hip replacement. A case report. J Bone Joint Surg 68A:454–455, 1986.
32. Wasielewski RC, Cooperstein LA, Kruger MP, Rubash HE: Acetabular anatomy and the transacetabular fixation of screws in total hip arthroplasty. J Bone Joint Surg 72A:501–508, 1990.
33. Wasielewski RC, Crossett LS, Rubash HE: Neural and vascular injury in total hip arthroplasty. Orthop Clin North Am 23:219–235, 1992.

70

Leg Length Inequality

• ROBERT T. TROUSDALE and BERNARD F. MORREY

The well-known problem of limb length inequality after total hip replacement is usually within the control of the surgeon. It is the opinion of some surgeons that the length of the extremity, although important, is a secondary consideration compared with hip stability,[11] but all agree that marked differences (plus or minus 2 cm) do interfere with a favorable clinical result. An otherwise excellent clinical and radiographic result can be perceived as a failure by the patient if a large leg length discrepancy exists.

INCIDENCE

It appears that because of increased awareness and the flexibility of modularity,[9] the problem is less common today than in the past.[12] In 1978, Williamson and Reckling reported that 144 of 150 patients had lengthening of the operated limb averaging 16 mm.[20] Twenty-seven percent required a shoe lift and 3 percent who had lengthening also had a sciatic nerve palsy. Turula et al. noted that 10 of 35 patients with limb length inequality after unilateral hip replacement were subjectively aware of the limb length difference. All had a limp, and all had more than 14 mm of lengthening of the operated leg.[16] Since the early 1990s, several series reported a mean difference of about 1 cm.[1] Woo and Morrey reported an average radiographic leg lengthening in 333 total hip replacements of 10 mm.[20] When attention is focused on this potential problem before surgery, the differences usually can be reduced to within 1 or 2 mm.[21] Woolson and Harris reported more favorable results because only 2.5 percent of patients' limbs were lengthened more than 6 mm in their series of 84 total hip replacements.[22] Today, we estimate that about 5 percent of patients require a shoe lift after primary hip replacement.

Functional Leg Length Inequality

The concept of fixed pelvic tilt or "functional instability" may be even more common but less well recognized[6] (Fig. 70–1). All orthopedic surgeons have had patients who complain of leg length inequality but who radiographically have equal lower limbs by measurement.

The concept introduced by Hoikka et al. was carefully assessed by Ranawat and Rodriguez. Although leg length inequality was demonstrated in 14 of their patients, all but about 1 percent tended to resolve with time, apparently because of adjacent joint/spine accommodation.[15]

SIGNIFICANCE

Abraham and Dimon noted that considerable disparity exists with regard to the significance of leg length inequality. Some authors think that up to 2 cm may be acceptable.[1] It has also been argued that limb lengthening is necessary and common after hip replacement to prevent laxity of the joint and subsequent instability leading to dislocation.[17] Discrepancies of less than 1 cm have, in general, been well tolerated; those greater than this amount can be corrected with appropriate shoe lifts. Limb shortening can also cause functional impairment, with diminished abductor function and the potential for increased instability secondary to soft tissue laxity.[2]

In one of the first such reports, Weber et al. from the Mayo Clinic correlated lengthening to an increased risk of sciatic palsy.[19] Williamson and Reckling reported that 5 of 150 patients undergoing total hip arthroplasty developed partial or complete sciatic palsies.[20] In this group, the mean lengthening of the operated extremity was 17 mm (Fig. 70–2). However, this measurement was not statistically different from the mean 16-mm difference in the overall series. These investigators correlated the risk of sciatic palsy with the female gender and prior surgery. Kennedy et al. recognized that the risk of sciatic palsy increased with prior surgery and the preoperative shortening that may have occurred from the pathologic process. These investigators reported use of intraoperative somatosensory evoked potentials when revision procedures were performed on limbs that had undergone shortening before revision.[10] In this sample, there were no peripheral nerve complications, with an average increase of 18 mm in leg length, ranging from 6 to 43 mm.

Several studies have reported that low back pain occurs with increased frequency in the presence of

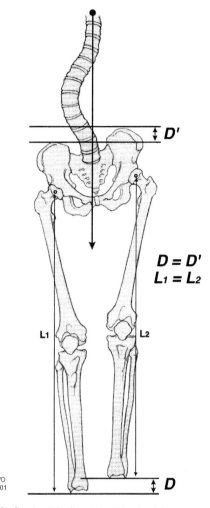

$$D = D'$$
$$L_1 = L_2$$

MAYO
©2001

Figure 70–1. If a fixed pelvic tilt exists, this should be accounted for in the preoperative planning. The leg will be "short" by distance "D" even if the leg to ankle length is equal.

limb inequality.[3,4] Some have also theorized that unequal extremities may produce gait disturbances that cause increased joint forces, which in turn may lead to premature mechanical failure.[5] Turula et al. studied 55 patients with leg length inequality averaging 9 mm in unilateral and 12 mm in bilateral cases after total hip arthroplasty.[17] Their data were interpreted as suggesting that such inequality may also be a source of aseptic loosening and, possibly, unexplained pain in patients after hip replacement surgery. A similar conclusion was revealed by Visuri et al., who noted a 15 percent incidence of loosening after 7 years if 7 to 8 mm of lengthening had occurred.[18] We have not been able to confirm this observation from our experience, but it does observe further analysis.

With the exception of sciatic palsy, which occurs rarely and inconsistently, there have been relatively few well-documented complications directly attributed to leg length inequality other than patient inconvenience. Nonetheless, it is important to inform the patient of this potential problem. This can be a most distressing problem for the patient, and malpractice suits have occurred over this issue.

PREVENTION

Preoperative Planning

Both true and functional leg length inequality should be assessed. A true inequality is a direct reflection of unequal limb length of the femur and the tibia; a functional, or apparent, inequality results from pelvic obliquity caused by spinal deformity and/or adduction, abduction, or flexion contractures. The goal of preoperative assessment should be first to identify whether a leg

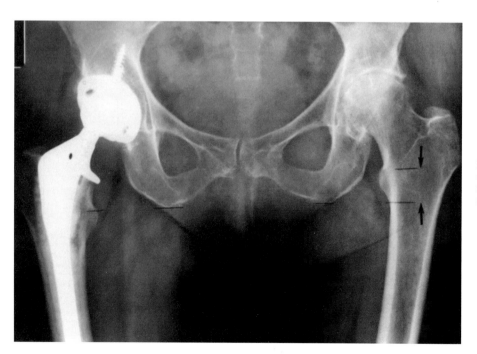

Figure 70–2. Moderate lengthening of the extremity undergoing hip replacement has resulted in sciatic palsy, which resolved over a 2-year period.

length discrepancy exists and second, to plan for correction, noting that the goal is to correct the functional discrepancy and not necessarily the actual leg length difference from hip to ankle.

Abraham and Dimon make the following recommendations: (1) determine by history whether or not the patient perceives limb inequality regardless of the actual measurement; (2) discuss the possibility of leg length inequality before surgery; (3) be aware of apparent leg length inequality such as occurs with fixed adduction or flexion contractures (see later); and (4) provide a consistent pre-, intra-, and postoperative method of assessment. Preoperative planning is necessary for estimation of the proper femoral neck osteotomy level (Fig. 70–3). In addition, the specific issue of offset, as well as axial length, should be considered in the preoperative planning. Finally, some form of direct intraoperative assessment is strongly advised if any question exists, especially in those with preoperative contracture or discrepancies.

Clinical Assessment

Preoperative assessment in the office, although not precise,[3] can be very useful and even necessary to determine the functional significance of leg length differences.[6,15] The patient should also be asked whether the legs feel equal in length before surgery. The following physical measurement techniques are used to further evaluate:

1. *Gait.* The effect of length discrepancy is probably best and most simply detected by observing the patient's gait.
2. *Soft tissue flexibility, joint contracture, and pelvic tilt limit the accuracy of this method. Measure the distance from the anterior superior iliac crest to the medial malleolus.*
3. *Flexion test (patella sight test).* With the patient supine, flexion of the hips to 60 degrees flattens the spine and compensates for hip flexion contracture. Flexing the knee 70 to 90 degrees allows a reasonably accurate estimation of femoral and tibial length differences (Fig. 70–4).
4. *Umbilicus: medial malleolus distance.* This is a reasonable method to estimate apparent and functional inequalities but does not provide an accurate measurement of true extremity length differences.
5. *Pelvic tilt.* This may be the most accurate means of assessing significant real or functional leg length differences. Leveling the pelvic crests with shims placed under the foot compensates for spinal distortion and adaptive changes (Fig. 70–5). This method is easy and is the best to detect either true or functional leg length inequality before or after surgery.

Radiographic Assessment

Of the numerous skeletal landmarks used to evaluate extremity length, Hoikka et al. demonstrated that the

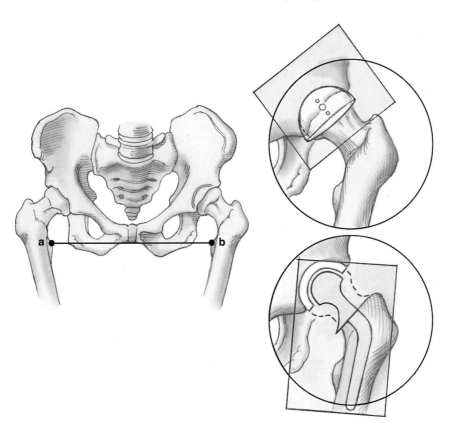

Figure 70–3. Accurate measurement of the anticipated implant size, level of resection, and hip center lessens the likelihood of leg length inequality.

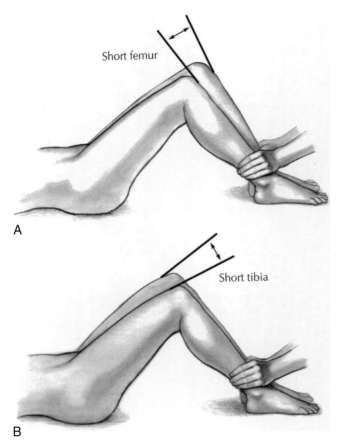

A

B

Figure 70–4. Patella sight test. Tangential view of patellas with hips and knees flexed provide an estimate of femoral length differences (**A**) and tibial length differences (**B**).

ischial tuberosities are more accurate reference points than the vertices of the femoral heads.[6] These investigators further analyzed the clinical and radiographic impact of leg length inequality and pelvic tilt.[8] The data suggest that as part of preoperative planning, consideration should be given to adjustment of leg length during hip replacement, aiming more for correction of the pelvic tilt than for the limb length measured from the apex of the hip to the floor. They introduced the concept of a "functional" leg length, which is a combination of the axial measurement of the extremity along with the position of the hip joint referable to the pelvic wall.[7] At the Mayo Clinic, direct and precise measurement is provided by a "scanogram" (Fig. 70–6). The x-ray source is mounted on a trolley that moves down the extremity, exposing 14 × 17-cm films with a scale that allows direct measurement of femoral, tibial, and overall length (Fig. 70–7).

Careful radiographic and clinical planning is most useful in minimizing occurrence of unequal extremities after replacement. Woolson and Harris studied preoperative templating of both femoral and acetabular components in an effort to plan and properly perform resections to minimize leg length inequality.[23] Using such an approach, an average discrepancy of only 2.8 mm was observed in a series of 84 patients. Only two (2.5 percent) with unilateral replacement had inequalities of more than 6 mm.[21] In the revision setting, preoperative templating can aid in the choice of proper

implants that will aid in gaining appropriate length. It is of interest that the limb is prone to be left short after revision, which may account in part for the high incidence of instability after this procedure (Fig. 70–8). In some instances, intraoperative electromyographic monitoring may be useful when lengthening greater than 3 to 4 cm is anticipated.[14]

Intraoperative Assessment

Several intraoperative methods to assess limb length have been suggested. These have typically included skeletal markers in the pelvis and femur and gross observation or measurement of the position of the knees or ankle before and after hip replacement. Although there are few studies that verify the overall accuracy of any of these methods, the originators have reported that these techniques are effective and reproducible in their hands.[23]

Tension Test

Charnley used an intraoperative stretch test performed by putting traction on the extended limb to determine the pullout tension of the hip (this test is probably still used by most orthopedic surgeons). This simple test depends on the level of anesthesia, axial rotation of the limb, state of muscle relaxation, and pericapsular scar tissue. This is obviously only a very crude estimate of tissue tension, the accuracy of which depends on the

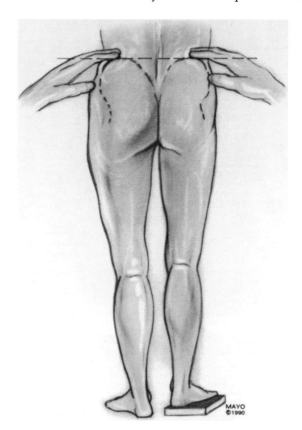

Figure 70–5. Leveling the pelvis with a shim under the foot is an effective clinical means to measure effective leg length differences.

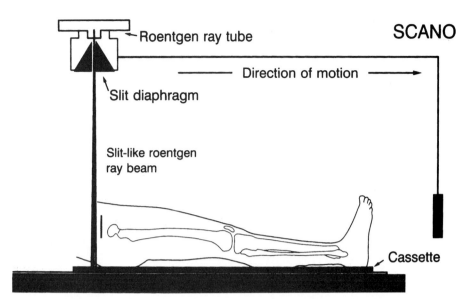

Figure 70–6. The scanogram is made by exposing the cassette from a moving roentgen ray tube that travels down the extremity.

manner in which the test is performed. The limb must be in neutral extension, abduction, adduction, and neutral rotation. The pull is applied longitudinally in the line of the limb, putting a distalward force on the proximal femur. Tension perpendicular to the long axis, such as occurs with an attempt to pull the joint apart, distorts

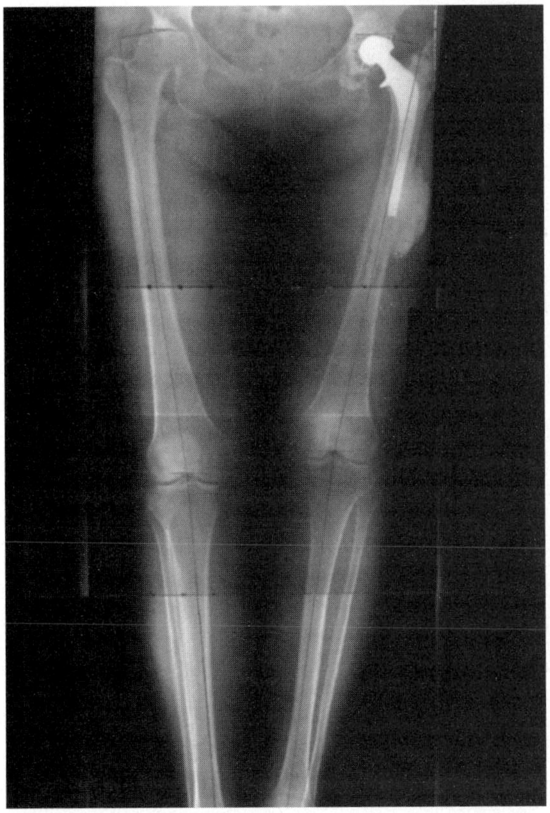

Figure 70–7. Example of hip-to-ankle roentgenogram made with scanogram technique that allows direct and accurate radiographic measurement to within a fraction of a millimeter. In this instance, the operated extremity is shorter than the contralateral extremity, as is common with revision surgery.

the tension on the hip and leads to overtightening and subsequent increased limb length.

Templates

With the advent of accurate templating systems and jigs for cutting the femoral neck, the distance of the femoral neck cut can be measured above the lesser trochanter. Preoperative templating can regularly approximate the proper length of the extremity to, within an error of plus or minus 2 to 3 mm.

The precise level of the femoral neck resection is the key to proper length, and this is determined before surgery by templating. The corollary is that the relationship of the neck cut and neck length system of the implant being used is clear.

Direct Intraoperative Measurement

Direct measurement of pre- and postreplacement pelvic-femoral length has been recommended by several authors.[11,13,23] Most systems employ skeletally fixed devices placed in both the pelvic and proximal femur. The distance before the hip is dislocated and after arthroplasty can then be accurately measured.

Woolson and Harris have described a jig that uses three pins in the iliac crest and a caliper fixed to a discrete point on the femur to measure the length before and after joint replacement.[23] Subsequently, Woolson reported less than 3 mm average discrepancy after 84 procedures. Only 11 percent had more than 6 mm of lengthening using pre- and intraoperative planning and assessment.[22] Hoikka et al. used two Steinmann pins but admitted to a 5- to 10-mm error in their measuring system.[6] McGee and Scott have described a method of determining leg length that uses a pin inserted into the iliac crest, which is bent so that the inferior aspect of the pin rests on the greater trochanter.[13] The pin can be rotated out of the surgical field during the arthroplasty and placed back into position after reduction of the hip to confirm leg length.

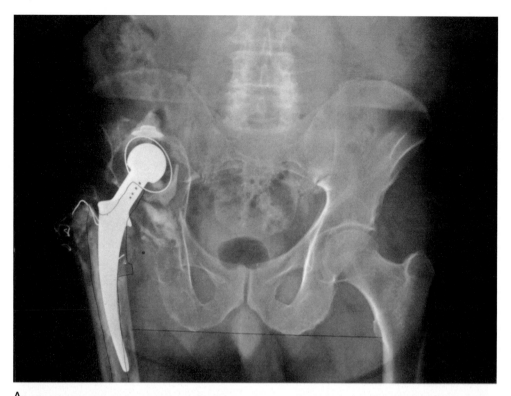

A

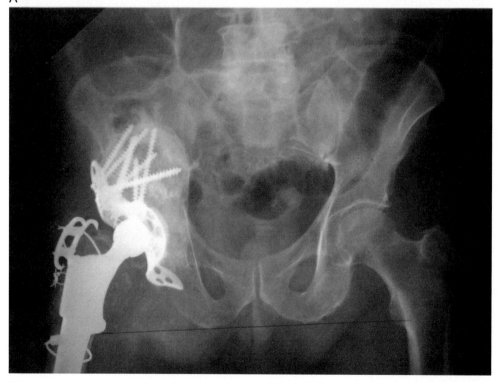

B

Figure 70–8. (A) Preoperative and **(B)** postoperative radiograph of patient who has a large acetabular defect and leg length discrepancy. Revision was performed by intraoperative electromyographic monitoring, with restoration of leg length equality. The patient experienced no sciatic nerve problems postoperatively.

In our department, if intraoperative measurement is to be performed, a spike retractor reflects the abductor mechanism and also may serve as a pelvic reference point, whereas a spike or marker placed in the greater trochanter provides a distal landmark reference. Care should be taken to make these assessments with the hip slightly extended (Fig. 70–9).

AUTHORS' PREFERENCE

Accurate restoration of leg lengths need not be burdensome or time-consuming. Clinically, we observe the gait pattern and use the pelvic tilt test for estimating functional inequalities. We view the patient from the back, with the physician's hands placed on each pelvic

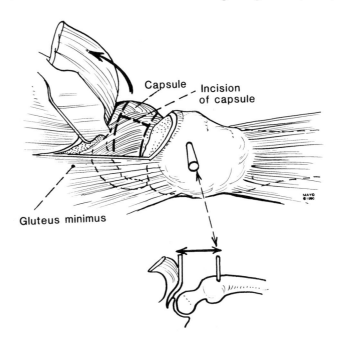

Capsule   Incision
of capsule

Gluteus minimus

Figure 70–9. A, A spike in the ilium and one in the trochanter is the simplest means of measuring leg length before and after surgery. **B,** Intraoperative assessment of leg lengths both pre- and postarthroplasty, measuring the distances with the knees perfectly aligned, can be a helpful gross estimate of the length in surgery.

A

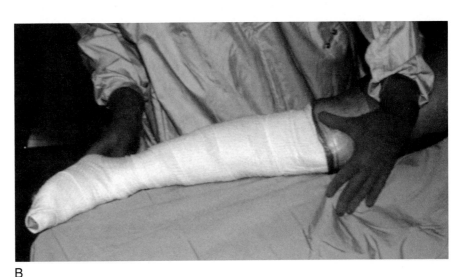

B

crest. The short leg is shimmed by having the patient stand on different thicknesses blocks until the pelvis is judged to be level (see Fig. 70–5). The patella sight tests are used to quickly estimate femoral versus tibial discrepancies (see Fig. 70–4). If needed, an accurate radiographic measurement is obtained by scanogram (see Fig. 70–6).

We personally rely heavily on the preoperative assessment of the level of resection and component position (Fig. 70–10). The line of neck resection is typically 1.5 to 2 cm above the lesser trochanter. Acetabular preparation just to the inner table and a neck length commensurate with this landmark accurately replicates the opposite leg length if this is normal. If a trial reduction is performed, 4 to 7 mm distal translation is to be expected. Gross differences are easily assessed by resting the operated on the unoperated leg.

TREATMENT

Shoe Lift

About 5 percent to 10 percent patients require a lift, but some have reported an incidence of up to 25 percent.[2] The lift is very rarely needed for differences less than 1 cm. Thus, discrepancies of 2.5 cm or more are usually managed with a lift. Typically we prescribe a heel lift that is approximately 5 mm less and a sole lift generally 8 to 10 mm less than the measured leg length inequality.

Surgery

If the difference is extreme or symptomatic, surgical intervention is considered. This may be simply

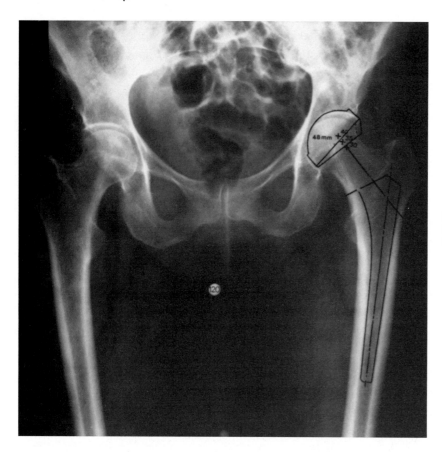

Figure 70–10. Preoperative templating is probably the single most important technique for prevention of gross limb length differences.

accomplished by changing modular neck lengths dependent on the system being used.[7] In some cases, advancement of the greater trochanter can provide excellent stability when improved soft tissue tension is required and there is no plan to further lengthen the limb. Assessment of the soft tissue tension is important to ensure that the hip remains stable.

If the discrepancy exceeds 3 to 4 cm in younger patients who are active, closed femoral shortening of the contralateral femur is discussed.

References

1. Abraham WD, Dimon JH III: Leg length discrepancy in total hip arthroplasty. Orthop Clin North Am 23:201, 1992.
2. Edeen J, Sharkey PF, Alexander AH: Clinical significance of leg-length inequality after total hip arthroplasty. Am J Orthop 24:347, 1995.
3. Friberg O: Clinical symptoms and biomechanics of lumbar spine and hip joint in the leg length inequality. Spine 8:643, 1983.
4. Giles LGF, Taylor JR: Low-back pain associated with leg length inequality. Spine 6:510, 1981.
5. Gore DR, Murray MP, Gardner GM, et al: Roentgenographic measurements after Müller total hip replacement. J Bone Joint Surg 59A:948, 1977.
6. Hoikka V, Paavilainen T, Lindholm TS, et al: Measurement and restoration of equality in length of the lower limbs in total hip replacement. Skeletal Radiol 16:442, 1987.
7. Hoikka V, Santavirta S, Eskola A, et al: Methodology for restoring functional leg length in revision total hip arthroplasty. J Arthroplasty 6:189, 1991.
8. Hoikka V, Vankka E, Tallroth K, et al: Leg length inequality in total hip replacement. Ann Chir Gynaecol 80:396, 1991
9. Hozack WJ, Mesa JJ, Rothman RH: Head-neck modularity for total hip arthroplasty. Is it necessary? J Arthroplasty 11:397, 1996.
10. Kennedy WF, Byrne TF, Majid HA, Pavlak LL: Sciatic nerve monitoring during revision total hip arthroplasty. Clin Orthop 264:223, 1991.
11. Knight WE: Accurate determination of leg lengths during total hip replacement. Clin Orthop 123:22, 1977.
12. Love BRT, Wright K: Leg length discrepancy after total hip joint replacement. J Bone Joint Surg 65B:103, 1983.
13. McGee HM, Scott JH: A simple method of obtaining equal leg length in total hip arthroplasty. Clin Orthop 194:269, 1985.
14. McGrory BJ, Trousdale RT: Sterile electromyographic monitoring during hip and pelvis surgery. Orthop Rev 23:274-276, 1994.
15. Ranawat CS, Rodriguez JA: Functional leg-length inequality following total hip arthroplasty. J Arthroplasty 12:359, 1997.
16. Turula KB, Friberg O, Haajanen J, et al: Weight-bearing radiography in total hip replacement. Skeletal Radiol 14:200, 1985.
17. Turula KB, Friberg O, Lindholm TS, et al: Leg length inequality after total hip replacement. Clin Orthop 202:163, 1986.
18. Visuri T, Lindholm TS, Antti-Poika I, Koskenvuo M: The role of overlength of the leg in aseptic loosening after total hip arthroplasty. Ital J Orthop Trauma 19:107, 1993.
19. Weber ER, Daube JR, Coventry M: Peripheral neuropathies associated with total hip arthroplasty. J Bone Joint Surg 58A:66, 1976.
20. Williamson JA, Reckling FW: Limb length discrepancy and related problems following total hip replacement. Clin Orthop 134:135, 1978.
21. Woo RY, Morrey BF: Dislocation after total hip arthroplasty. J Bone Joint Surg 64A:1295, 1982.
22. Woolson ST: Leg length equalization during total hip replacement. Orthopedics 13:17, 1990.
23. Woolson ST, Harris WH: A method of intraoperative limb measurement in total hip arthroplasty. Clin Orthop 194:207, 1985.

VI
The Knee

MARK W. PAGNANO • SECTION EDITOR

71

Anatomy and Surgical Approaches

• MICHAEL J. STUART

This chapter reviews the anatomy of the knee, with particular reference to surgical approaches and joint replacement arthroplasty. The osteology, neurovascular supply, and soft tissue anatomy of the knee are discussed. The surgical approaches detailed are not exhaustive but reflect the commonly used exposures and those associated with revision and management of complications.

OSTEOLOGY

Tibia

The medial tibial plateau is slightly concave, and the lateral plateau is slightly convex. In the saggital plane, the tibial condyles slope posteriorly approximately 10 degrees. In the frontal plane, the condyles are essentially perpendicular to the longitudinal axis of the tibia.[15] The highest pressure concentrations are located on the uncovered cartilage of the medial compartment and on the menisci as well as on the uncovered cartilage of the lateral compartment.[10] Trabecular bone of the tibial epiphysis and metaphysis is responsible for load transmission. Compressive strength and stiffness depend on bone density and trabecular architecture.[16] The medial tibial plateau is a high-strength area, especially centrally and anteriorly. Strength is reduced at both plateaus toward the periphery. Trabecular bone strength is significantly reduced at a distance greater than 5 mm from the surface.[12] Preservation of tibial bone stock during total knee arthroplasty (TKA) should be considered, because optimal support is achieved by resecting 10 mm or less of the tibial plateau.[18] Excessive bone resection may contribute to prosthetic loosening and alteration of the desired component position.

Femur

The femoral condyles are asymmetric, with the medial condyle being smaller in the anteroposterior and mediolateral dimensions (Fig. 71–1). This accounts for the normal rotation of the tibia during extension. The sagittal curvature of the condyles has a radius that decreases posteriorly. The condyles converge anteriorly to form the trochlea, which articulates with the patella. The highest bone strength is found at the posterior aspects of the condyles, with the central area being relatively weak. In contrast to the tibia, femoral trabecular bone strength is greater with increased distance from the subchondral plate.[16]

Normal bone strength parameters are altered in the presence of axial malalignment.[16] Deviation from the normal mechanical axis of zero degrees or the anatomic axis of 2 to 12 degrees of valgus results in abnormal load sharing between the condyles. High-strength areas are found in the medial tibial plateau in varus knees, and distal tibial weakening is evident. Mechanical testing has shown that the tibias of osteoarthritic knees have significantly altered stiffness patterns compared with those of normal tibias.[9] Unicompartmental osteoarthritis is associated with increased stiffness of the cancellous bone underlying the involved compartment and decreased stiffness of the bone underlying the opposite compartment. Bone strength is less in knees with rheumatoid arthritis compared with those with osteoarthritis. Steroid medication does not seem to influence bone strength in the rheumatoid knee.[16]

Patella

The articular surface of the patella is divided into medial and lateral facets by a major vertical ridge. The medial facet is usually smaller (Wiberg type II) than the lateral. A second vertical ridge near the medial border produces the narrow "odd" facet. The trabecular structure of the patella and the femoral trochlea is aligned normally to the joint surfaces.[15]

NEUROVASCULAR SUPPLY

Vessels

Eight arteries provide the major blood supply to the knee: supreme genicular artery, medial and lateral superior genicular arteries, medial and lateral inferior genicular arteries, middle genicular artery, anterior and posterior tibial recurrent arteries (Fig. 71–2).[28] The supreme genicular artery arises from the femoral artery

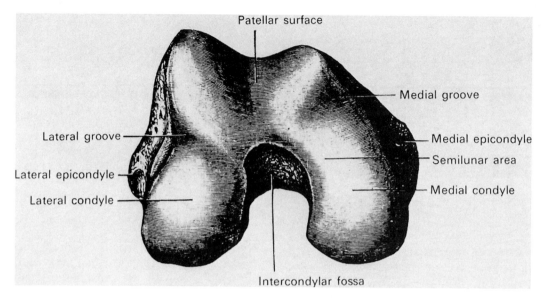

Figure 71–1. Axial view of the distal femur depicting the condyles and trochlear or patellar surface. (From Clemente CD [ed]: Gray's Anatomy: 30th American ed. Philadelphia, Lea & Febiger, 1985, p 280.)

just above the opening of the adductor canal and gives off saphenous, muscular, articular, and deep oblique branches. The medial and lateral superior genicular arteries are branches of the popliteal vessel. Periosteal, muscular, and capsular branches contribute to the epiphyseal circulation and to the anterior anastomosis. The medial and lateral inferior genicular arteries also arise from the popliteal vessel and run toward the front of the knee deep to the collateral ligaments. These vessels are vulnerable to injury during meniscal excision and

exposure of the posterior corners of the knee. The anterior and posterior recurrent branches of the anterior tibial artery supply the anterior aspect of the knee, the superior tibiofibular joint, and the lateral condyle of the tibia.

The popliteal vessels are surprisingly close to the bone at the level of the tibial cut. A magnetic resonance study documented this distance as 3 to 12 mm in extension and 6 to 15 mm in 90-degree flexion.[31]

The patella is supplied by two systems of vessels: the midpatellar vessels penetrating the middle third of the anterior surface and the polar vessels entering the apex behind the patellar ligament. A vascular anastomotic ring surrounds the patella, with oblique branches converging on the anterior surface (see Fig. 71–2).[27] The distal half of the patella has a dual blood supply, but the upper half is supplied only by the midpatellar vessels. The patella is susceptible to ischemia if these vessels are damaged. Excision of the prepatellar fat pad and lateral retinacular release during total knee arthroplasty may result in devascularization. Cadaver knee injection studies showed that vascular filling was absent after a medial arthrotomy incision too close to the patella, radical incision of the fat pad, lateral retinacular release performed too close to the patella, and cauterization of the prepatellar vessels.[20] These data provide some of the basis for the subvastus medialis approach to the knee.[13]

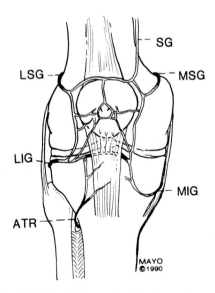

Figure 71–2. Diagram of the major blood supply to the knee. Branches of the anastomotic ring converge on the anterior surface of the patella. SG = supreme genicular artery; MSG = medial superior genicular artery; LSG = lateral superior genicular artery; MIG = medial inferior genicular artery; LIG = lateral inferior genicular artery; ATR = anterior tibial recurrent artery. (Adapted from Scapinelli R: Blood supply of the human patella: Its relation to ischemic necrosis after fracture. J Bone Joint Surg 49B:563, 1967.)

Nerves

Anterior and posterior groups of afferent nerves supply the knee.[12] The anterior group includes branches of the femoral, common peroneal, and saphenous nerves. Articular afferents form the terminal portions of the nerve to the vastus medialis, vastus lateralis, and vastus intermedius. The lateral articular and recurrent peroneal nerves originate from the common peroneal supplying the lateral capsule and collateral ligament. The primary articular afferent branch of the saphenous nerve is the infrapatellar branch, which innervates the inferomedial capsule, the patellar tendon, and the anterior skin (Fig. 71–3). Transection of these branches with a medial skin incision may result in bothersome numbness for the patient. The posterior group is composed of the posterior articular and obturator nerves. The posterior articular nerve is a branch of the posterior tibial nerve, and its fibers penetrate the oblique popliteal ligament and the posterior capsule. These fibers supply the capsule, peripheral menisci, cruciate ligaments, and infrapatellar fat pad.

Fusiform mechanoreceptor structures are located on the surface of the cruciate ligaments beneath the synovial membrane.[29] These receptors resemble Golgi tendon organs, which may function in a proprioceptive reflex arc to protect the knee from excessive displacements. Axons, neural bundles, free nerve endings, and specialized receptors are present within the perimeniscal capsular tissues.[21] Capsular distention from intra-articular fluid inhibits the quadriceps contraction reflex.

SOFT TISSUE ANATOMY

An understanding of the soft tissue anatomy about the knee is essential for surgical exposures to preserve joint stability after total knee arthroplasty.

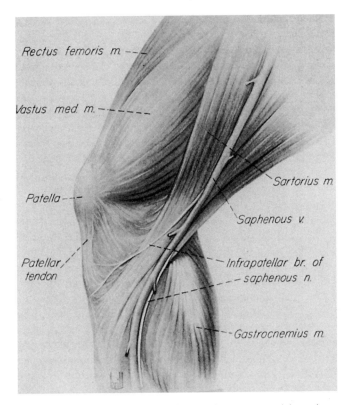

Figure 71–3. Infrapatellar branch of the saphenous nerve lying subcutaneously on the medial aspect of the knee. (From DePalma AF: Disease of the knee. Philadelphia, JB Lippincott, 1954, p 652.)

Anterior Structures and Exposures

The extensor mechanism includes the quadriceps muscle, quadriceps tendon, patella, and patella tendon. The distal quadriceps complex represents an aponeurosis of four muscle bellies at the anterior aspect of the knee.[26] Centrally, the rectus femoris tendon continues over the anterior surface of the patella and is the only quadriceps component with continuity to the infrapatellar ligament. A portion of the vastus medialis fibers (vastus medialis obliquus) are oriented at an angle of approximately 60 degrees to the rectus tendon. The muscle fibers become tendinous for only a few millimeters and insert directly into the patella or contribute to the medial retinaculum. The vastus medialis fibers are routinely disrupted during a medial parapatellar approach for total knee arthroplasty. The vastus lateralis fibers are oriented at an angle of approximately 30 degrees to the rectus tendon. These fibers insert into the superolateral corner of the patella and contribute to the lateral retinaculum. The vastus intermedius lies deep to the other three muscles and inserts directly into the superior border of the patella.

The infrapatellar tendon is composed primarily of rectus femoris fibers that extend distally over the anterior surface of the patella.[26] The tendon ranges in length from 3.5 to 5.5 cm. The infrapatellar tendon inserts over a broad expansion at the tibial tubercle and blends with the fascia on the anterior surface of the tibia. The tendon and its insertion must be carefully protected during exposure of the knee joint. An arthritic knee with an extensor mechanism contracture and limited flexion is especially vulnerable. A safe exposure and improved postoperative flexion may be achieved with a modified V-Y quadricepsplasty for a quadriceps contracture and a tibial tubercle osteotomy for a patellar tendon contracture[30,36] (see later).

Skin Incisions

Routine surgical exposure for total knee arthroplasty involves an anterior skin incision followed by a medial parapatellar arthrotomy in an effort to minimize disruption of the medial lymphatic drainage and saphenous nerve branches.[14]

In general, prior transverse-type skin incisions can be ignored in favor of a straight anteromedial or anterolateral approach to the knee; however, if a previous longitudinal incision exists, care must be taken to avoid a new incision that is within 2 to 3 cm of the prior one, because skin necrosis can occur in the intervening segment. Furthermore, as a general principle, it must be remembered that straight skin lincisions heal quite well and are favored over more curvilinear types of incisions. Finally, because the lymphatic drainage of the knee is oriented from a lateral to a medial direction, lateral incisions are more desirable than longitudinal incisions. Unfortunately, the majority of reconstructive procedures are best performed by translating the patella laterally, thus favoring an anteromedial approach.

EXPOSURES

The Medial Joint

The fascia, ligaments, and capsule of the medial side of the knee are arranged in three distinct layers (Fig. 71–4).[33] The first layer encountered after a medial skin incision is the deep fascia that invests the sartorius muscle and overlies the structures of the popliteal fossa. The second layer is defined by the fibers of the superficial medial collateral ligament. Tendons of the gracilis and semitendinosus (pes anserinus) separate the first and second layers. The third layer represents the true capsule of the knee joint. Thick vertical fibers of this layer form the deep medial ligament or middle capsular ligament, which extends from the femur to the midportion of the peripheral margin of the meniscus and tibia. The posteromedial corner of the knee is formed by the condensation of the middle and deep layers with the semimembranosus tendon sheath (Fig. 71–5). The semimembranosus tendon inserts directly into bone at the posteromedial corner of the tibia and beneath the superficial medial ligament. The semimembranosus tendon sheath extends across the posterior aspect of the knee to the lateral femoral condyle, forming the oblique popliteal ligament. Additional fibrous expansions of the sheath extend to the posterior capsule and superficial medial ligament.

Insall et al.[19] described a medial release during total knee arthroplasty for a knee with a fixed varus deformity. This involved elevating a subperiosteal sleeve of tissue that included the pes anserinus tendons, superficial medial ligament, semimembranosus, and posterior capsule from the tibia. This sleeve preserves medial stability but allows correction of angular deformity. Others recommend semimembranous tendon lengthening if a release is required.[14]

Anteromedial Exposure

INDICATIONS

This is the universal approach to the knee. It is particularly useful for joint replacement arthroplasty in its various forms. Extensor mechanism realignment or release, either proximal or distal, can be conducted through the same incision. Anterior cruciate ligament reconstruction, although commonly performed arthroscopically, can be achieved with an open technique by means of the anteromedial capsular approach. Finally, arthrolysis, synovectomy, and joint débridement are readily performed with lateral subluxation of the extensor mechanism.

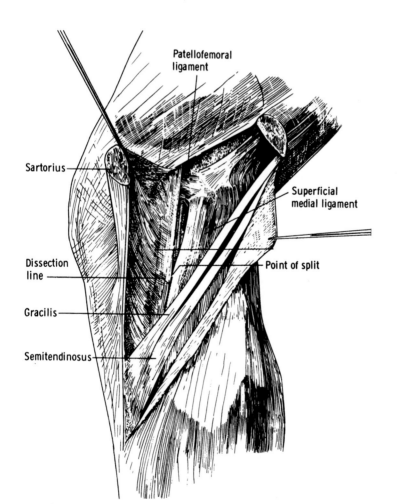

Figure 71–4. First and second layers of the medial side of the knee after reflection of the sartorius. (From Warren LF, Marshall JL: The supporting structures and layers on the medial side of the knee. J Bone Joint Surg 61A:56, 1979.)

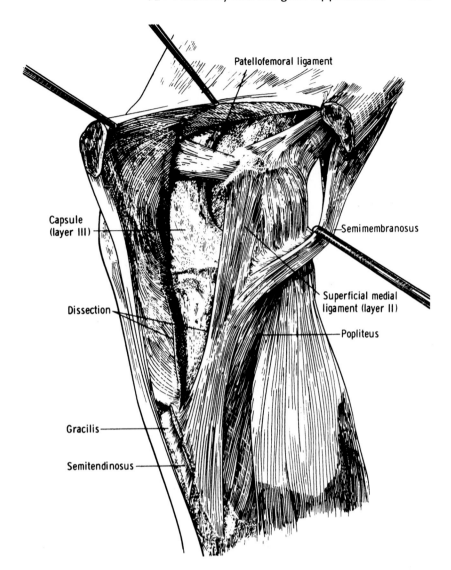

Figure 71–5. Superficial medial ligament and the third layer of the medial side of the knee after removal of the gracilis and semitendinosis. (From Warren LF, Marshall JL: The supporting structure and layers on the medial side of the knee. J Bone Joint Surg 61A:56, 1979.)

CONTRAINDICATIONS

Longitudinal skin incisions lateral to the midline are a contraindication to a subsequent anteromedial skin incision because the narrow skin bridge is at risk for necrosis. Contraction and scarring of the extensor mechanism preclude adequate exposure through a routine anteromedial approach, thus necessitating an extensile technique such as the quadriceps snip, the modified V-Y quadricepsplasty, or tibial tubercle osteotomy, which are described in the following sections.

TECHNIQUE

A straight skin incision just medial to the midline, beginning approximately 7 cm proximal to the patella, is carried distally to the inferior pole of the patella, ending just at the medial aspect of the tibial tubercle (Fig. 71–6). A centimeter of soft tissue medial to the tibial tubercle is preserved to allow repair of the capsule at the time of closure. The dissection carries through the subcutaneous tissue, exposing the quadriceps tendon. The joint is entered just to the medial aspect of the patella and the quadriceps tendon is split longitudinally in line with these fibers. The dissection carries distally, reflecting the anteromedial capsule from

the tibia. The synovium is excised along with any fat pad laterally as necessary to provide adequate visibility of the lateral compartment. Reflection and lateral rotation of the extensor mechanism allow the knee to flex, which exposes the entire knee joint from anterior to posterior.

Should exposure of the proximal femur be desirable, the incision is simply carried proximally through the quadriceps tendon. The rectus femoris muscle is split, exposing the shaft of the femur.

CLOSURE

Closure is with interrupted absorbable sutures in a single layer. The tissues on either side of the capsular incision are almost always of adequate quality to allow secure closure that accommodates virtually normal flexion and extension without interruption of the suture line. Plication at the time of closure may be done to prevent slight lateral subluxation or maltracking of the extensor mechanism. Some have advocated closing the retinaculum in flexion to more easily attain full flexion after surgery. A statistically significant improvement in knee flexion after TKA—118 compared with 113 degrees—has been documented.[8]

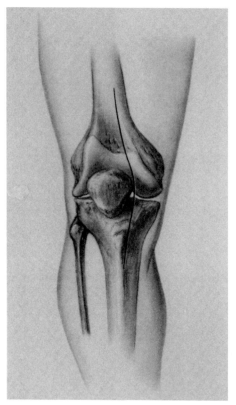

A

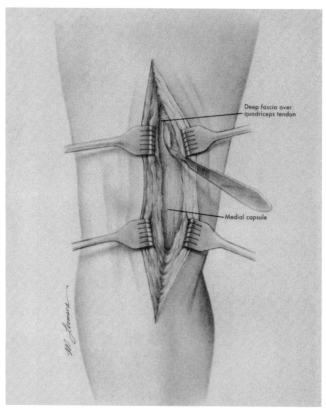

Deep fascia over
quadriceps tendon

Medial capsule

B

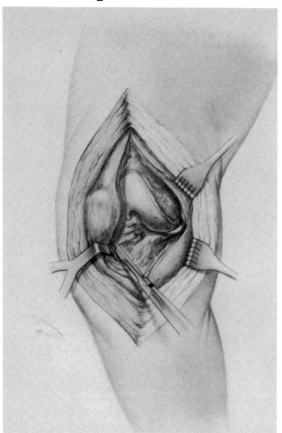

C

Figure 71–6. *See legend on opposite page*

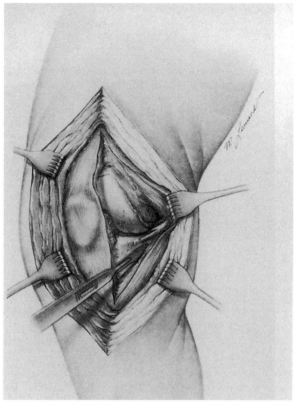
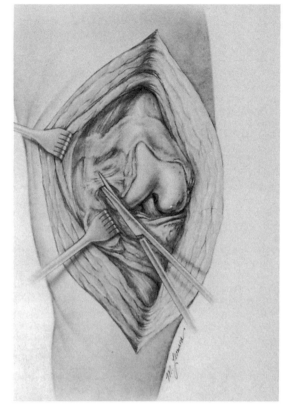

D   E

Figure 71–6. Anteromedial exposure. The skin incision is straight just at the medial margin of the patella (**A**). The dissection carries through the subcutaneous tissue, exposing the medial capsule and deep fascia of the quadriceps tendon (**B**). The capsule is entered and the quadriceps muscle is split proximally. Sharp dissection frees the medial margin of the patella (**C**). The dissection then elevates the capsule from the medial aspect of the tibia. I prefer to release the meniscus from the coronoid ligament at this time, facilitating the subsequent removal of the medial meniscus (**D**). Exposure of the lateral tibia requires a tangential resection of the fat pad and release of the lateral capsule from the tibia. The tendinous attachment of the lateral aspect of the patella is released, allowing the patella to be everted, and the knee is flexed, providing full exposure of the knee joint (**E**). If lateral reflection of the patella and extensor mechanism is difficult, the lateral patella plica and the patellofemoral ligament may be released to allow more extensive reflection of the extensor mechanism. (From Krackow KA: The Techniques of Total Knee Arthroplasty. St. Louis, CV Mosby, 1990.)

Subvastus Approach (Hofmann et al.)

The original description of this approach by Erkes dates to 1929, and is found in the German literature. This exposure has been revisited and has been popularized by Hofmann et al.[13] for knee replacement.

INDICATIONS

The indications for the subvastus approach are similar to those described for the anteromedial approach; however, this has the theoretical advantage of decreasing patellofemoral complications of subluxation, dislocation, and avascular insult.

CONTRAINDICATIONS

Instances in which it is desirable to leave the extensor mechanism intact to facilitate rehabilitation or in circumstances when the patella has been previously operated, raising a question regarding its vascularity, are contraindications to the subvastus approach. Relative contraindications include revision total knee arthroplasty, because prior arthrotomy causes scarring of the

extensor mechanism, making exposure difficult. Prior proximal tibial osteotomy and short patient stature likewise may result in less than adequate exposure.

SURGICAL TECHNIQUE

With the knee flexed 90 degrees, a straight anteromedial skin incision is performed as described in the previous section. The incision continues distally one fingerbreadth distal to the tibial tubercle (Fig. 71–7). Identification of the fascial layers follows. The first fascial layer is incised just medial to the patellar tendon to avoid injury to the plexus of patellar vessels. Blunt dissection is then carried out proximally, and the vastus medialis is lifted from its thin, perimuscular fascia. The inferior edge is identified and the muscle is further released from the femur and intermuscular septum with a periosteal elevator or by blunt dissection distally to the adductor tubercle. With the knee flexed, an attempt to reflect the muscle anteriorly allows definition of the tendinous insertion of the vastus medialis to the medial capsule. This is incised at the level of the midpatella. Efforts are made to avoid intra-articular incision at this point. The extensor mechanism is then elevated

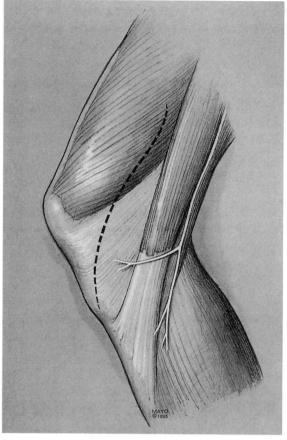

A

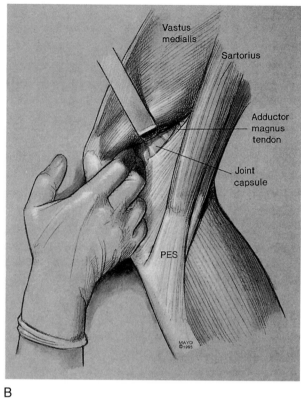

B

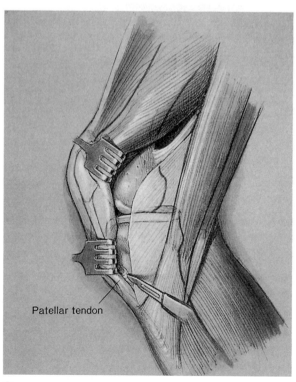

C

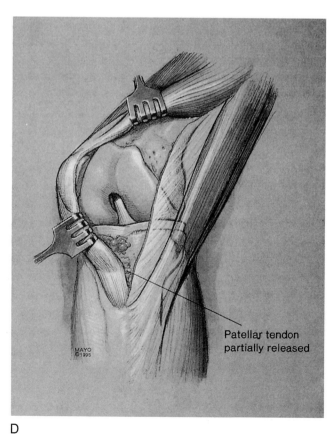

D

Figure 71–7. *See legend on opposite page*

anteriorly and laterally and a curvilinear medial arthrotomy is performed along the medial edge of the fat pad. Sharp dissection of the fat pad from the tibia is carried out and a small portion of the patellar tendon insertion at the tubercle can be released to provide easy lateral translation. The patella is then everted and dislocated laterally while the knee is extended. The knee is then slowly flexed, with further dissection of the vastus medialis muscle from the intermuscular septum being carried out during flexion of the knee, as necessary, to complete the exposure.

At the completion of the procedure, if there is a tendency for lateral subluxation or tracking of the patella, a lateral release is carried out from an intra-articular approach.

Closure is routine, with absorbable sutures. There is no need to reattach the muscle belly to the intermuscular septum because it will spontaneously reattach. Distally, the capsule is closed with interrupted sutures, and the remainder of the closure is routine. Straight leg lift exercises are begun within 24 hours. A compressive dressing is removed at 1 to 2 days, and active and passive exercises and range of motion are begun.

Mid-vastus Splitting Approach

This exposure is suggested as an alternative for TKA. Instead of separating the vastus medialis from the quadriceps tendon (Fig. 71–8), the incision proceeds proximally into muscle. A prospective study by White et al. documented fewer lateral retinacular releases and less pain with this approach compared with the parapatellar tendon splitting approach. Another study documented less blood loss with this muscle-splitting approach, but 43 percent had asymptomatic abnormal electromyography changes in the muscle.[24] More evidence is required before this can be considered a superior exposure.

Anterolateral Approach

INDICATIONS

The anterolateral approach is indicated for lateral intra-articular adhesions, lateral retinacular release, and as an adjunct to quadricepsplasty, particularly when proximal extension is necessary to observe the vastus lateralis and intermedius. It is also the technique preferred by some surgeons for valgus knee arthroplasty.

CONTRAINDICATIONS

A relative contraindication to this approach is joint replacement for a varus knee, because medial displacement of the extensor mechanism is extremely difficult. Medial reflection of the extensor mechanism does not afford an adequate exposure for reconstructive procedures of the knee joint.

TECHNIQUE

A straight longitudinal incision equidistant proximally and distally to the patella is carried out as described by Kocher.[17] The capsule is entered at the lateral aspect of the patella and the exposure extends distally over the anterolateral aspect of the tibia and proximally into the vastus lateralis just lateral to the quadriceps tendon (Fig. 71–9). This allows necessary release of the extensor mechanism and some limited joint visibility.

Techniques to Expose the Difficult Knee

A more extensile approach may be required for a stiff knee resulting from previous surgery, septic arthritis, prior fracture, or radiation treatment. Other challenging exposures may be associated with obesity, rheumatoid arthritis, severe varus or valgus deformities, and flexion or extension contractures.[25] The pathoanatomy includes a contracted extensor mechanism, contracted collateral ligaments, scarred suprapatellar pouch, scarred medial and lateral gutters, tibial tubercle malposition, and thick adipose tissue. These exposures may be essential in order to avoid patellar tendon avulsion. I prefer to start with a posteromedial tibial release and lateral retinacular release, followed by a quadriceps snip if necessary. The modified V-Y quadricepsplasty is reserved for severe quadriceps contracture. The tibial tubercle osteotomy is indicated in the setting of tubercle transfer, severe patella infra, or with difficult tibial component stem extraction.

PROXIMAL PROCEDURES: QUADRICEPS SNIP, MODIFIED V-Y QUADRICEPSPLASTY

Incision into the extensor mechanism allows the patella to be reflected laterally without compromising the patellar tendon attachment. In severe cases, the quadriceps

---

Figure 71–7. Subvastus (southern) approach of Hofmann et al. After the routine preparation and under tourniquet control, the knee is flexed 90 degrees to make the skin incision. A direct anteromedial skin incision is then carried out, beginning approximately four fingerbreadths above the patella and ending about one fingerbreadth distal to and just medial to the tibial tubercle (**A**). Because the knee is flexed, the tissues separate as the skin incision is made, allowing observation of the deep structures. The first fascial layer is identified proximally and is incised in line with the skin incision at the level of, and just medial to, the patella to avoid injury to the vessels. This fascial layer is then elevated off the thinner perimuscular fascia of the vastus medialis and down to its insertion. This allows identification of the inferior margin of the vastus medialis. This is then elevated from the periosteum and the intermuscular septum by blunt dissection about 10 cm proximal to the adductor tubercle (**B**). The descending genicular artery and the saphenous nerve are not endangered by this maneuver. The vastus medialis muscle is then tensed anteriorly and the tendinous insertion of the vastus medialis to the medial capsule, measuring 2 to 3 cm, is identified and transversely incised near the midpatella. Efforts are made not to enter the joint at this time. Lifting the extensor mechanism allows exposure of the joint and, beginning in the superior pouch, an arthrotomy is carried out that ends at the medial aspect of the tibial tubercle (**C**). Placing this incision at the medial margin of the patella and fat pad minimizes bleeding. Sharp dissection is then required to release this extensor mechanism from the proximal anteromedial and lateral portions of the tibia; however, the patellar tendon insertion site is left intact. The patella is everted and dislocated laterally with the knee in full extension. The knee is then slowly flexed while the vastus medialis muscle belly is bluntly dissected off the intermuscular septum proximally, thus allowing free lateral translation and eversion of the extensor mechanism (**D**).

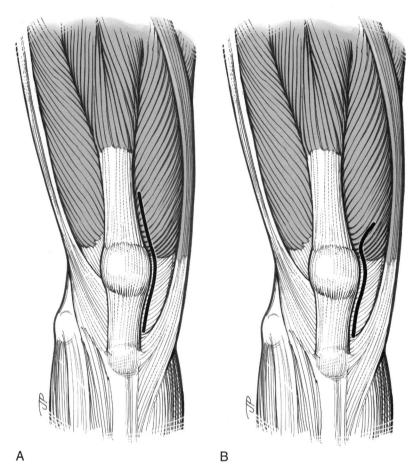

A   B

Figure 71–8. The standard parapatellar incision in the quadriceps tendon (**A**) compared to that of the vastus split approach (**B**). (From Parentis MA, Rumi MN, Deol GS, et al: A comparison of the vastus splitting and median parapatellar approaches in total knee arthroplasty. Clin Orthop 367:107, 1999.)

tendon and patella can be reflected distally to provide access to the anterior aspect of the knee and then lengthen the extensor mechanism. This exposure, originally described by Coonse and Adams,[5] has been modified by Insall.[17] Proximal releases are contraindicated when the quality of soft tissue proximal to the patella is poor and the contractility of the muscle is limited. Distal osteotomy exposures are preferred in such instances or when tibial tubercle malposition requires transposition (Fig. 71–10).

DISTAL PROCEDURES: TIBIAL TUBERCLE OSTEOTOMY

The extensor mechanism may be released by osteotomy of the tibial tubercle.[23] This permits the tubercle to be hinged, advanced proximally or distally, or translated medially or laterally as necessary. The technique of Whiteside[36] appears attractive based on the reported effectiveness, low complication rate, and technical use. Distal osteotomy is contraindicated after previous procedures in which the width or substance of the tibial tubercle is thin, compromising the ability to obtain an osseous union. It is also contraindicated when lengthening of a scarred proximal extensor mechanism is required.

TECHNIQUES

Quadriceps Snip. A standard medial arthrotomy incision is extended at the apex of the rectus tendon in an oblique and lateral direction. The patella is everted and the knee flexed. A routine repair with absorbable or nonabsorbable suture is performed and postoperative rehabilitation is not altered.

Results. Barrack et al.[3] reported on 123 revision arthroplasties, including 94 with a medial approach, 31 with a quadriceps snip, 15 with a tibial tubercle osteotomy, and 14 with a quadriceps turndown. The quadriceps snip group was found to be clinically equivalent to the group who had received the standard arthrotomy exposure. Garvin et al.[11] used the quadriceps snip in 10 revision and 6 primary arthroplasties. Postoperative flexion contracture averaged 7 degrees (range, 5 to 10 degrees). No differences in strength were found when the quadriceps snip group compared with the contralateral TKA group.

Modified V-Y Quadricepsplasty (Insall Modification of Coonse-Adams Turndown). A straight longitudinal skin incision is performed either through the previous incision or, ideally, an anteromedial skin inci-

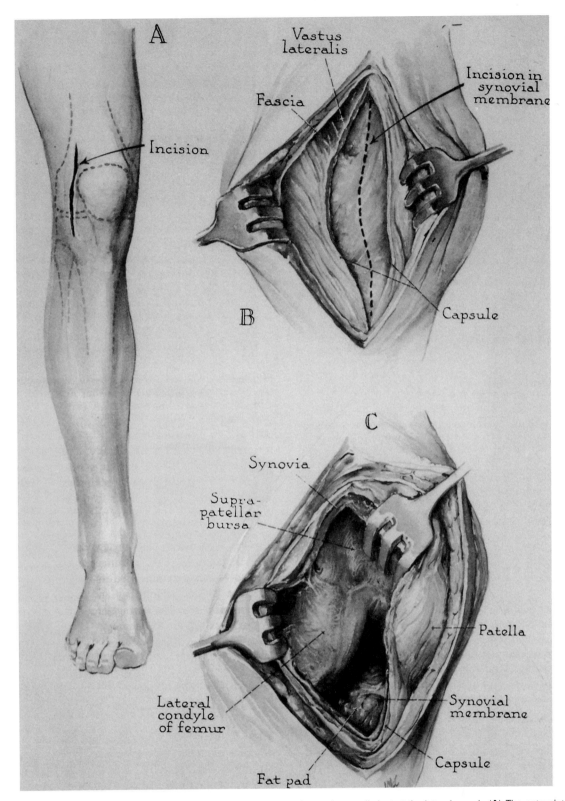

Figure 71–9. Anterolateral exposure. The skin incision is centered over the patella just at the lateral margin (**A**). The anterolateral capsule is identified and is incised in line with the skin incision (**B**). This allows exposure of the lateral aspect of the joint, including the suprapatellar pouch and the extensor mechanism in the region of the patella tendon (**C**). For quadricepsplasty, the incision is extended proximally. The vastus lateralis is elevated off the lateral aspect of the femur. Perforating vessels are ligated and the entire femur may be exposed as necessary by proximal extension of this incision. (From Banks S, Laufman H: An Atlas of Surgical Exposure of the Extremities, 2nd ed. Philadelphia, WB Saunders, 1987.)

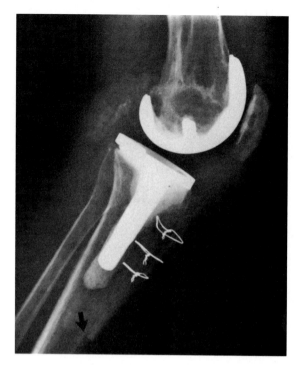

Figure 71–10. Whitesides osteotomy with proximal advancement (*arrow*) at reimplantation in patient with 30 degrees' flexion after antibiotic spacers for infection.

sion just medial to the midline. The capsular and quadriceps release is identical to that described earlier for an anteromedial approach, with the capsule being entered just at its medial aspect and the quadriceps tendon being split along its substance lateral to the vastus medialis (Fig. 71–11). During the procedure, a contracted quadriceps mechanism or scarred anterior extensor mechanism may make lateral reflection of the patella difficult. The rectus femoris incision is extended laterally and distally from the apex, with about a 45-degree angle as an inverted "V." This incision avoids the muscular fibers and transects the lateral retinaculum at an oblique angle, and terminates after incising the anterior fibers of the iliotibial band at the tibia. The extensor flap is then reflected distally and laterally, allowing access to the knee joint. In such circumstances, generalized joint contracture is common. The capsuloligamentous structures are then dissected from the tibia medially, which allows the knee to flex. If lengthening of the extensor mechanism is necessary, a V-Y quadricepsplasty is performed by suturing the rectus tendon together at the apex of the "V." This exposure requires postoperative flexion stops in a rehabilitation brace determined by the intraoperative assessment of the quadriceps repair tension with passive knee motion. Partial weight bearing is allowed with the brace locked in full extension.

Results. Trousdale et al.[32] reviewed the Mayo Clinic experience with a proximal V-Y quadriceps modification of the Coonse-Adams exposure used in 9 instances as an adjunct for revision arthroplasty and in 5 patients

for primary arthroplasty. The average arc of motion after the procedure was 4 to 85 degrees. Biomechanical testing, however, indicated significant weakness in comparison with the normal contralateral knee. This difference was statistically significant ($P<.05$) compared with the normal knee but not statistically significant if the contralateral knee had undergone a routine knee replacement. Aglietti et al.[1] used the modified V-Y quadricepsplasty in 11 primary posterior stabilized total knee arthroplasties. Elimination of the knee extension lag required 2 months, but no permanent extension lag was encountered.

Tibial Tubercle Osteotomy. Tibial tubercle osteotomy is performed in four clinical settings: (1) to realign the extensor mechanism, typically following total knee arthroplasty after the demonstration of patella maltracking; (2) for exposure of the stiff knee undergoing knee replacement; (3) for transfer of a malpositioned tibial tubercle; and (4) for extensor mechanism release after contracture (Fig. 71–12).

Technique (Whitesides). The typical parapatellar incision is extended 8 to 10 cm below the tibial tubercle. A medial arthrotomy extends proximally about 6 cm above the patella and is medial to the quadriceps tendon. A long fixed segment of the anterior crest is elevated along with the tibial tubercle (Fig. 71–13). Whiteside and Ohl[36] prefer the use of an oscillating saw to transect the medial linear component of the tibial crest; separation of the tubercle and crest from the tibia is performed with a curved osteotome. Leaving the soft tissue attachments to the lateral aspect of the pretibial region, the osteotomized segment is rotated laterally. The lateral attachments of the quadriceps expansion are also left to the lateral tibial flair. After the procedure, reattachment occurs with two wires passing through the tibial tubercle and the medial cortex of the tibia. Screws and staples are not used. Postoperative care includes early motion as tolerated, as well as full weight bearing as tolerated during the first week of the recovery period.

Results. Introduced in 1983 by Dolan[7] as an adjunct to expose the stiff knee, this approach is attractive because it provides the opportunity for bone-to-bone healing, which is stronger than the healed proximal turndown procedures. In addition, there is less potential for scarring of the quadriceps mechanism, which will decrease the compliance of the soft tissue and hence decrease the ultimate arc of motion. The osteotomy also allows for lengthening of the extensor mechanism. Finally, as a means of exposing the knee, this provides better visibility than the turndown techniques can offer. However, osteotomy is technically more demanding. Since Dolan's original description was published, several techniques have been described.[36,37] Wolff et al. reported 26 procedures of the tibial tubercle osteotomy for the purpose of exposure.[37] Although several variations of the techniques were used, typically, a relatively small portion of the tibia other than the tubercle itself

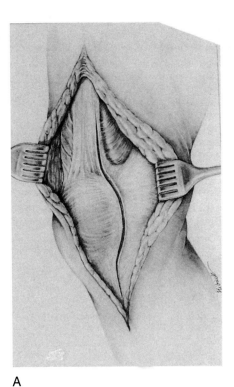

A

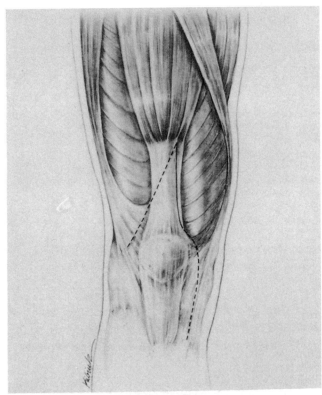

B

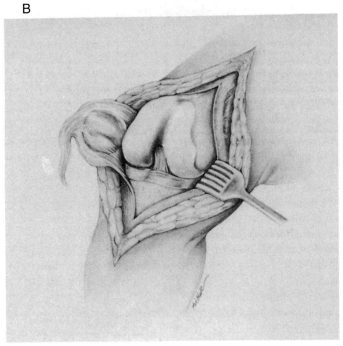

C

Figure 71–11. Coonse-Adams turndown procedure (Insall modification). **A,** The knee joint is exposed through a typical anteromedial skin incision, with the joint entered through the anteromedial retinaculum and capsule. **B,** At the proximal extent of the rectus femoris tendon, an incision is made with approximately a 45-degree angle distally, severing the quadriceps tendon and carrying across the lateral retinaculum to the level of the tibia. **C,** The patella with the quadriceps tendon is then reflected anterolaterally and the knee is flexed, providing full exposure of the knee joint. (From Krackow KA: The Techniques of Total Knee Arthroplasty. St. Louis, CV Mosby, 1990.)

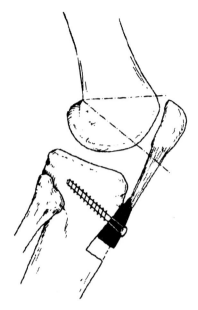

Figure 71–12. The DeLee tubercle osteotomy procedure is designed to release a contracted patellar tendon and improve flexion.

was included in the osteotomy. The range of motion before surgery was 48 degrees and changed to 77 degrees after the procedure. These investigators reported 23 percent complications related to the osteotomy. This was particularly seen in patients with rheumatoid arthritis. Nonunion occurred in 11 percent of their patients and 4 percent had tendon rupture. A more effective method is that described by Whitesides and Ohl.[36] This technique includes the crest of the tibia along with the tibial tubercle. Measuring approximately 8 to 10 cm in length, the osteotomized bone fragment is rotated laterally while the lateral soft tissue hinge is preserved. Experience with 71 patients who underwent a more extensive osteotomy revealed a mean flexion arc of 3 to 97 degrees after surgery. There were no nonunions and no serious complications. Whitesides also reported on 136 total knee arthroplasties exposed with a tibial tubercle osteotomy. The mean postoperative total range of motion was 94 degrees (range, 15 to 140 degrees).[35] Two patients sustained a partial tubercle avulsion, 2 had painful fixation wires, and no nonunions occurred.

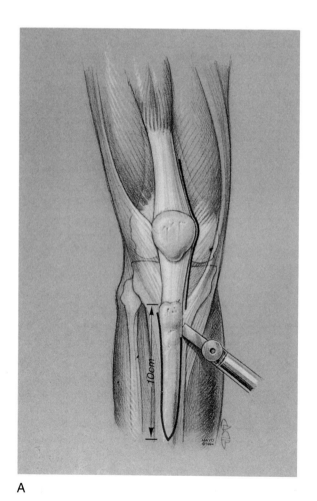

A

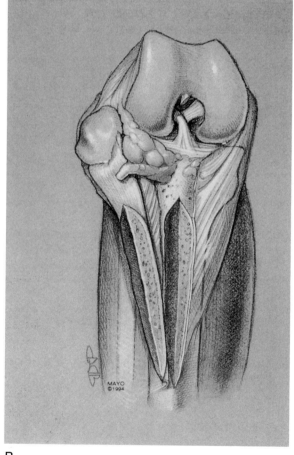

B

Figure 71–13. **A,** The Whitesides tubercle osteotomy technique exposes and osteotomizes approximately 10 cm of the tibial crest distal to the tubercle. **B,** The osteotomized segment is rotated on soft tissue laterally, allowing exposure of the knee. **C,** Repair is by cerclage wire placed through holes in the medial cortex.

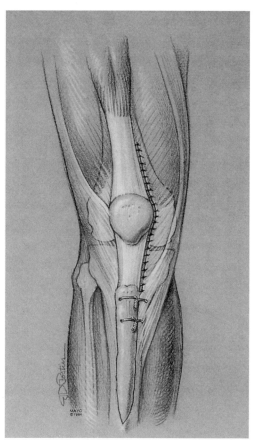

C

Figure 71–13. *Continued.*

References

1. Aglietti P, Windsor RE, Buzzi R, Insall JN: Arthroplasty for the stiff or ankylosed knee. J Arthroplasty 4:1, 1989.
2. Banks S, Laufman H: An Atlas of Surgical Exposure of the Extremities, 2nd ed. Philadelphia, WB Saunders, 1987.
3. Barrack R, et al: The Ranawat Award. Comparison of surgical approaches in total knee arthroplasty. Clin Orthop 356:16, 1988.
4. Clemente CD (ed): Gray's Anatomy: 30th American ed. Philadelphia, Lea & Febiger, 1985, p 280.
5. Coonse K, Adams JD: A new operative approach to the knee joint. Surg Gynecol Obstet 77:344, 1943.
6. DePalma AF: Disease of the Knee. Philadelphia, JB Lippincott, 1954, p 652.
7. Dolan MG: Osteotomy of the tibial tubercle in total knee replacement: A technical note. J Bone Joint Surg 65A:704, 1983.
8. Emerson RH Jr, Ayers C, Higgins LL: Surgical closing in total knee arthroplasty. A series follow-up. Clin Orthop 368:176, 1999.
9. Finlay JB, Bourne RB, Kramer WJ, et al: Stiffness of bone underlying the tibial plateaus of osteoarthritic and normal knees. Clin Orthop 247:193, 1989.
10. Fukubayashi T, Kurosawa H: The contact area and pressure distribution pattern of the knee: A study of normal and osteoarthritic knee joints. Acta Orthop Scand 51:871, 1980.
11. Garvin KL, Scuderi G, Insall JN: Evolution of the quadriceps snip. Clin Orthop 321:131, 1995.
12. Harada Y, Wevers HW, Cooke TD: Distribution of bone strength in the proximal tibia. J Arthroplasty 3:167, 1988.
13. Hofmann AA, Plaster RL, Murdock LE: Subvastus (Southern) approach for primary total knee arthroplasty. Clin Orthop 269:70, 1991.
14. Hungerford DS, Krackow K, Kenna D: Total Knee Arthroplasty: A Comprehensive Approach. New York, Williams & Wilkins, 1984.
15. Hvid I: Mechanical strength of trabecular bone at the knee. Dan Med Bull 35:345, 1988.
16. Hvid I: Trabecular bone strength at the knee. Clin Orthop 227:210, 1988.
17. Insall JN: Surgical approaches to the knee. *In* Surgery of the Knee. New York, Churchill Livingstone, 1984, p 41.
18. Insall JN: Technique of the total knee replacement. *In* Dorr LD (ed): The Knee: Papers of the First Scientific Meeting of the Knee Society. Baltimore, University Park Press, 1985, p 23.
19. Insall JN, Ranawat CS, Scott WN: The total condylar knee prosthesis: A report of 220 cases. J Bone Joint Surg 61A:173, 1979.
20. Kayler DE, Lyttle D: Surgical interruption of patellar blood supply by total knee arthroplasty. Clin Orthop 229:221, 1988.
21. Kennedy JC, Alexander IJ, Hayes KC: Nerve supply of the human knee and its functional importance. Am J Sports Med 10:329, 1982.
22. Krackow KA: The Techniques of Total Knee Arthroplasty. St. Louis, CV Mosby, 1990.
23. Merritt P, Conaty JB, Dorr LD: Effects of soft tissue releases on results of total knee replacement. *In* Total Arthroplasty of the Knee: Proceedings of the Knee Society. Rockville, MD, Aspen Publishers, 1987, p 25.
24. Parentis MA, Rumi MN, Deol GS, et al: A comparison of the vastus splitting and median parapatellar approaches in total knee arthroplasty. Clin Orthop 367:107, 1999.
25. Paulos LE, Wnorowski DC, Greenwald AE: Infrapatellar contracture syndrome: Diagnosis, treatment and long-term follow-up. Am J Sports Med 22:440, 1994.
26. Reider B, Marshall JL, Koslin B, et al: The anterior aspect of the knee joint: An anatomical study. J Bone Joint Surg 63A:351, 1981.
27. Scapinelli R: Blood supply of the human patella: Its relation to ischemic necrosis after fracture. J Bone Joint Surg 49B:563, 1967.
28. Scapinelli R: Studies on the vasculature of the human knee joint. Acta Anat 70:305, 1968.
29. Schultz RA, Miller DC, Kerr CS, Micheli L: Mechanoreceptors in human cruciate ligaments. J Bone Joint Surg 66A:1072, 1984.
30. Scott RD, Siliski IM: The use of a modified V-Y quadricepsplasty during total knee replacement to gain exposure and improve flexion in the ankylosed knee. Orthopedics 8:45, 1985.
31. Smith PN, Gelinas J, Kennedy K, et al: Popliteal vessels in knee surgery: A magnetic resonance imaging study. Clin Orthop 367:158, 1999.
32. Trousdale RT, Hanssen AD, Rand JA, Cahalan TD: VY quadricepsplasty in total knee arthroplasty. Clin Orthop 286:48, 1993.
33. Warren LF, Marshall JL: The supporting structures and layers on the medial side of the knee. J Bone Joint Surg 61A:56, 1979.
34. White RE Jr, Allman JK, Trauger JA, Dales BH: Clinical comparison of the midvastus and medial parapatellar surgical approaches. Clin Orthop 367:117, 1999.
35. Whiteside LA: Exposure in difficult total knee arthroplasty using tibial tubercle osteotomy. Clin Orthop 321:32, 1995.
36. Whitesides LA, Ohl MD: Tibial tubercle osteotomy for exposure of the difficult total knee arthroplasty. Clin Orthop 260:6, 1990.
37. Wolff AM, Hungerford DS, Krackow KA, Jacobs MA: Osteotomy of the tibial tubercle during total knee replacement: A report of 26 cases. J Bone Joint Surg 71A:848, 1989.

72A

Biomechanics of the Knee

• KENTON R. KAUFMAN

An understanding of knee biomechanics is essential for management of various orthopedic problems. This chapter reviews the basic biomechanics of the normal knee joint. The characteristics of the joint articulating surface are discussed, with particular relevance to the active and passive motion of the tibiofemoral joint. The joint contact area is reviewed and constraints and ligamentous stability are outlined. Tibiofemoral and patellofemoral joint kinetic forces and contact pressure distribution are presented. Finally, design considerations of prosthetic replacement are discussed and placed in context.

JOINT ARTICULATING SURFACES

The tibiofemoral joint is a double condyloid joint composed of medial and lateral articular surfaces. There are marked differences in the shape of both the medial and lateral femoral and tibial condyles. The profile of the femoral condyle varies with the condyle examined (Fig. 72A–1; Table 72A–1). The medial condyle projects extensively, both longitudinally and medially, to offset the lateral medial angulation of the femur as the shaft progresses distally. The shaft of the femur is not vertical but is angled in such a way that the femoral condyles do not lie immediately below the femoral head but somewhat medial. Given the obliquity of the shaft of the femur, the lateral condyle lies more directly in line with the shaft than the medial condyle (Fig. 72A–2). The femoral condyles differ in anterior/posterior dimension and configuration, which is important for joint movement. The medial and lateral condyles both decrease their radii from anterior to posterior. This means that the distance from the center of rotation to the condylar surface is greatest toward the anterior portion of the femur and progressively decreases along the distal edge of the bone to the posterior surface.

The medial and lateral compartments of the tibial plateau also have substantial bony differences. The medial condyle of the tibia is concave superiorly (the center of curvature lies above the tibial surface), with a

radius of curvature of 80 mm.[28]* The lateral condyle is convex superiorly (the center of curvature lies below the tibial surface), with a radius of curvature of 70 mm.[28] The tibial plateau widths are greater than the corresponding widths of the femoral condyles (Fig. 72A–3; Table 72A–2). However, the tibial plateau depths are less than those of the femoral condyle distances. The articulating surface of the medial tibial condyle is 50 percent larger than the surface of the lateral condyle that corresponds to the larger medial femoral condyle. When the large articular condyles of the femur are placed on the shallow cavities of the tibial condyles, the incongruence of the knee joint is evident.

The triangular patella is the largest sesamoid bone in the body. The posterior surface of the patella is covered by articular cartilage and divided by a vertical ridge located approximately in the center of the patella, which divides the articular surface into approximately equal medial and lateral patellar facets. The patella-articulating surface of the femur is the intercondylar groove, or femoral sulcus, of the anterior aspect of the distal femur. The femoral surfaces are concave side to side but convex top to bottom.[21] The patellofemoral joint is the least congruent joint of the body.[44] The geometry of the patellofemoral articular surfaces remains relatively constant as the knee flexes. The knee sulcus angle changes only plus or minus 3.4 degrees from 15 degrees to 75 degrees of knee flexion. The mean depth index varies by only plus or minus 4 percent over the same flexion range. Similarly, the medial and lateral patellar facet angles (Fig. 72A–4) change by less than a degree throughout the entire knee flexion range. However, there is a significant difference between the magnitude of the medial and lateral patellar facet angle, probably to control the tendency for lateral displacement of the patella via the pull of the quadriceps muscles.

MOTION

Global Motion

The tibiofemoral joint displays two degrees of freedom. The first degree of freedom allows movements of flexion

---

*For all references cited in this chapter, see the reference section of Chapter 72B.

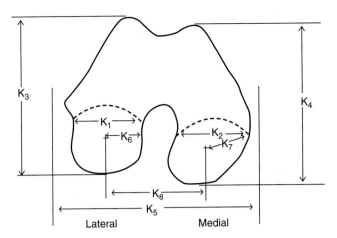

Figure 72A–1. Geometry of the distal femur. The distances are defined in Table 72A–1.

and extension in the sagittal plane. The axis of rotation intersects the femoral condyle at an angle to the mechanical and anatomic axes.[28] Both fixed axes and screw axes

have been calculated (Fig. 72A–5). The optimal axes are fixed, whereas the screw axis is instantaneous. The symmetric optimal axis is constrained in such a way that the axis is the same for both the right and left knees. The screw axis may sometimes but not always coincide with the optimal axis, depending on the motion of the knee joint. The second degree of freedom is axial rotation around the long axis of the tibia. There is an automatic axial rotation that is involuntarily linked to flexion and extension. When the knee is flexed, the tibia internally rotates. Conversely, when the knee is extended, the tibia externally rotates. This coupled motion is called the screw-home mechanism. Several explanations have been given for this rotational movement.[49] It has been suggested that the unequal curvature of the femoral condyles may cause this rotational movement because different degrees of rotation are required for the different bony geometry. Similarly, different anterior/posterior femoral condyle dimensions may be a cause. Soft tissue factors have also been cited. This may involve tightening of either or both the anterior and posterior cruciate ligaments. However, the most likely explanation is that the rotation is a combination of these factors.[18]

Table 72A–1. GEOMETRY OF THE DISTAL FEMUR

| | Condyle | | | | | |
| | Lateral | | Medial | | Overall | |
Parameter	Symbol	Distance (mm)	Symbol	Distance (mm)	Symbol	Distance (mm)
Medial/lateral distance	K1	31 ± 2.3 (male) 28 ± 1.8 (female)	K2	32 ± 31 (male) 27 ± 3.1 (female)		
Anterior/posterior distance	K3	72 ± 4.0 (male) 65 ± 3.7 (female)	K4	70 ± 4.3 (male) 63 ± 4.5 (female)		
Posterior femoral condyle spherical radii	K6	19.2 ± 1.7	K7	20.8 ± 2.4		
Epicondylar width					K5	90 ± 6 (male) 80 ± 6 (female)
Medial/lateral spacing of center of spherical surfaces					K8	45.9 ± 3.4

See Figure 72A–1 for location of measurements.[32,58]

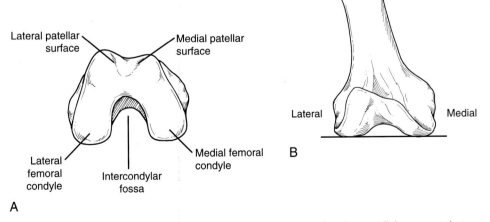

Figure 72A–2. A, The patellar surface is separated from the tibial articular surface by two slight grooves that run obliquely across the condyles. The medial femoral condyle is longer than the lateral femoral condyle. **B,** The lateral femoral condyle lies more directly in line with the shaft than the medial condyle. (From Norkin CC, Levangie PK: Joint Structure and Function: A comprehensive Analysis, 2nd ed. Philadelphia, FA Davis 1992.)

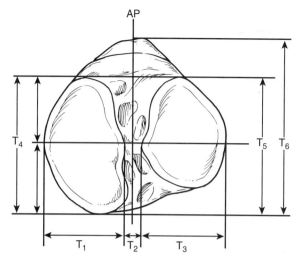

Figure 72A–3. Contour of the tibial plateau (transverse plane). The distances are defined in Table 72A–2. (From Yoshioka Y, Siu D, Scudamore RA, et al: Tibial anatomy in functional axes. J Orthop Res 7:132, 1989. Copyright 1989, by Orthopaedic Research Society.)

Tibiofemoral Joint Articulating Surface Motion

The planar motion of two adjacent body segments can be described by the concept of the instant center of motion. As one body segment rotates about the other, at any instant, there is a point that does not move. This point has zero velocity and acts as a center of rotation. This technique yields a description of motion at one point only and is not applicable if motion of 15 degrees or greater exists in other planes. When the instantaneous center of rotation is at the contact point between the femur and tibia, the instantaneous velocity is zero and the tibia is rolling around the femoral surface. An understanding of the motion between the articulating surfaces of the knee joint is important for understanding causes of wear, instability, and loosening of implants after total knee arthroplasty.

Frankel and colleagues[16] analyzed the surface motion of the tibiofemoral joint from 90 degrees of flexion to full extension in 25 normal knees and thereby determined ·the instant center pathway. They found the pathway to be semicircular and located in the femoral condyle (Fig. 72A–6). The centers fall within a circle with a diameter

of 2.3 cm. They also determined the instant center pathway for the tibiofemoral joint in 30 knees with internal derangement. They found that in all cases the instant center was displaced from its normal position at some point during the knee motion. They were able to correlate wear of the articular cartilage surface with specific abnormalities noted in instant center analysis.

Knee articulating motion is a combination of gliding and rolling between the femoral and tibial surfaces.[28] The ratio of rolling to gliding is not constant throughout the range of flexion and is controlled by both the anatomy of the joint surfaces and the constraints imposed by the anterior and posterior cruciate ligaments. Müller[41] considered the rolling/gliding ratio to be controlled by the basic model of a crossed four-bar linkage. In this model, the tibial and femoral insertions of both cruciate ligaments are fixed to their respective surfaces and can be represented by two crossed bars. The cruciate bars are linked together at their attachments to the tibia and femur, and this link constitutes the two additional bars of the four-bar linkage. The four-bar crossed-link model guides the femoral and tibial surfaces past one another. The tibiofemoral contact point has been shown to move posteriorly as the knee is flexed, reflecting the coupling of anterior/posterior motion with flexion/extension (Fig. 72A–7). During flexion, the weight-bearing surfaces move backward on the tibial plateaus and become progressively smaller (Table 72A–3). It has been shown that in an intact knee at full extension, the center of pressure is approximately 25

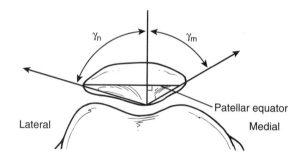

Figure 72A–4. Medial (γ_m) and lateral (γ_n) patellar facet angles. (From Ahmed AM, Burke DL, Hyder A: Force analysis of the patellar mechanism. J Orthop Res 5:69, 1987. Copyright 1987 by Orthopaedic Research Society.)

Table 72A–2. GEOMETRY OF THE PROXIMAL TIBIA

Parameter	Symbols	All Limbs	Male	Female
Tibial plateau widths (mm)				
Medial plateau	T_1	32 ± 3.8	34 ± 3.9	30 ± 22
Lateral plateau	T_3	33 ± 2.6	35 ± 1.9	31 ± 1.7
Overall plateau	$T_1 + T_2 + T_3$	76 ± 6.2	81 ± 4.5	73 ± 4.5
Tibial plateau depths (mm)				
AP depth, medial	T_4	48 ± 5.0	52 ± 3.4	45 ± 4.1
AP depth, lateral	T_5	42 ± 3.7	45 ± 3.1	40 ± 2.3
Interspinous width (mm)	T_2	12 ± 1.7	12 ± 0.9	12 ± 2.2
Intercondylar depth (mm)	T_6	48 ± 5.9	52 ± 5.7	45 ± 3.9

See Figure 72A–3 for location of measurements.[59]

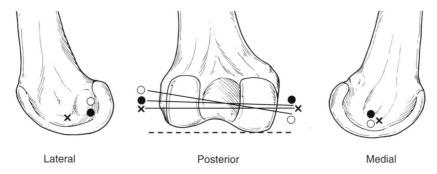

Lateral   Posterior   Medial

Figure 72A–5. Approximate location of the optimal axis (nonsymmetric and symmetric), and the screw axis on the medial and lateral condyles of the femur of a human subject for the range of motion of 0 to 90 degrees of flexion (standing to sitting). (From Lewis JL, Lew WD: A method for locating an optimal "fixed" axis of rotation for the human knee joint. J Biomech Eng 100:187, 1978.)

mm from the anterior edge of the knee joint line.[3] This contact point moves posteriorly with flexion to approximately 38.5 mm from the anterior edge of the knee joint.

Patellofemoral Motion

During knee flexion, the patella makes a rolling/gliding motion along the femoral articulating surface. Throughout the entire flexion range, the gliding motion is clockwise (Fig. 72A–8). The mean amount of patellar gliding for all knees is approximately 6.5 mm per 10 degrees of flexion between zero degrees and 80 degrees and 4.5 mm per 10 degrees of flexion between 80 degrees and 120 degrees.

The patellofemoral contact area is much smaller than the tibiofemoral contact area (Table 72A–4). As the knee joint moves from extension to flexion, a band of contact moves upward over the patellar surface (Fig. 72A–9). As knee flexion increases, the contact area not only moves superiorly but also becomes larger. At 90 degrees of knee flexion, the contact area has reached the upper level of the patella. As the knee continues to flex, the contact area is divided into separate medial and lateral zones.

KNEE JOINT STABILITY

The muscles, ligaments, menisci, osseous geometry, and joint capsule all combine in a complex manner to produce joint stability. If any of these structures malfunction or are disrupted, knee joint instability occurs. These factors are all interdependent and serve the function of both determining normal motions and limiting motion beyond a certain point.

Joint Surface

The constraints provided by the femoral and tibial joint surfaces are not adequate for functional stability. The distal femur is convex, whereas the proximal tibia is partially flat, slightly concave medially, and slightly convex

laterally. However, the tibial intercondylar eminence and the articular geometry do provide some potential for stability. Hsieh and Walker[23] found that geometric conformity of the condyles was the most important criterion for decreasing laxity under load bearing. They stated that in order to perform anterior/posterior, rotary, and medial/lateral movements, the femur must ride upward on the tibial curvature. Similarly, to rotate, the femur "screws out," giving an upward movement. Medial/lateral motion produces this effect to an even greater degree because of the tibial spines. This is called the "uphill principle." These authors concluded that under low loading conditions, the soft structures (ligaments, capsule, meniscus) provided joint stability, and that as loading increases, the condylar surface conformity becomes the most important factor.

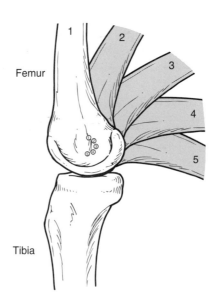

Figure 72A–6. The instant center of rotation for the knee. (From Frankel VH, Burstein AH, Brooks DB: Biomechanics of internal derangement of the knee. Pathomechanics as determined by analysis of the instant centers of motion. J Bone Joint Surg 53A:945, 1971.)

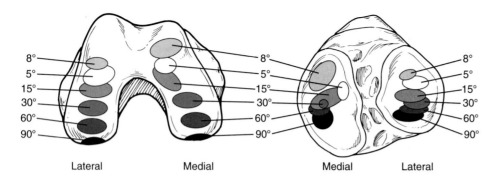

Lateral   Medial   Medial   Lateral

Figure 72A–7. Tibiofemoral contact area as a function of knee flexion angle. (From Iseki F, Tomatsu T: The biomechanics of the knee joint wiht special reference to the contact area. Keio J Med 25:37, 1976.)

Table 72A–3. TIBIOFEMORAL JOINT FORCES: COMPRESSION

Author	Activity	Knee Angle (degrees)	Force (× BW)
Ericson and Nisell, 1986[15]	Cycling	85	1.2
Komistek et al., 1998[31]	Walking	–	1.7–2.3
Taylor et al., 1998[51]	Walking	25	2.4
Morrison, 1970[39]	Walking	15	3.0
Harrington, 1976[22]	Walking	–	3.5
Kuster et al., 1997[33]	Walking	20	3.9
Collins, 1995[13]	Walking	20	4.1–6.0
Morrison, 1969[40]	Downstairs	60	3.8
	Upstairs	45	4.3
Kaufman et al., 1997[30]	Isokinetic extension at 60 degrees/sec	55	4.0
	180 degrees/sec	55	3.8
Ellis et al., 1984[14]	Rising from chair	–	3–7
Kuster et al., 1994[34]	Downhill walking		
	Males	40	7.1
	Females	40	8.5

BW = body weight.
Data from references 13–15, 22, 30, 31, 33, 34, 39, 40, 51.

Ligamentous Stability

The ligament structures are able to resist translational forces and thus prevent translation of their bony attachments if that translation takes place in the direction of the ligament fibers. This principle is particularly relevant for provision of anterior/posterior translational stability. Li et al.[36] have shown that the hamstrings provide an active restraint to anterior displacement in the tibia. This restraint indicates that muscle contraction and co-contraction contribute to the stability of the knee joint by increasing the stiffness of the joint.

The collateral ligaments provide varus/valgus stability of the knee. The rotational forces are not resisted by the ligaments acting alone. Increased compressive force generated at the joint articular surface produces a torque that resists the rotational moment. Burstein and Wright[9] have also indicated the importance of muscle forces contributing to knee joint stability in the frontal plane. At full knee extension the knee may be expected to show a balance of compressive forces between the medial and lateral compartments in response to axial loading. If a medially directed force is applied at the foot in addition to axial loading, rotation occurs about the anatomic center of the joint and causes a varus moment at the knee. This moment cannot be resisted by a single force but rather must be resisted by a couple force. In this case, the varus knee moment is resisted by the forces in the medial and lateral joint compartments. The resisting force on the medial side increase joint compression between the femoral and tibial surfaces, whereas the lateral compartment experiences a decrease of joint compressive load.

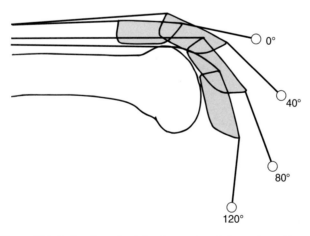

0°
40°
80°
120°

Figure 72A–8. Position of patellar ligament, patella, and quadriceps tendon and location of the contact points as a function of the knee flexion angle. (From van Eijden TM, Kouwenhoven E, Verburg J, Weijs WA: A mathematical model of the patellofemoral joint. J Biomech 19:219, 1986. Copyright 1986, with permission of Elsevier Science.)

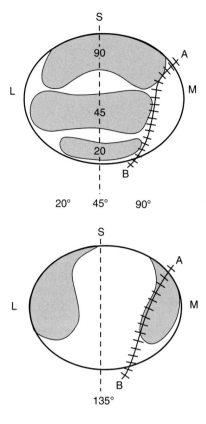

Figure 72A–9. Diagrammatic representation of patellar contact areas for varying degrees of knee flexion. (From Goodfellow J, Hungerford DS, Zindel M: Patello-femoral joint mechnanics and pathology. 1. Functional anatomy of the patello-femoral joint. J Bone Joint Surg 58B:287, 1976.)

The force distribution in the collateral ligaments and on the knee plateaus is a function of lower limb alignment. Key anatomic landmarks were identified (Fig. 72A–10). The tibiofemoral angle ($\theta_2-\theta_1$) was 1.2 degrees plus or minus 2.2 degrees varus. There was no significant gender or age difference. When the femoral anatomic valgus was measured, the section of the anatomic axis of the femur was important because the proximal femoral, distal femoral, and overall femoral anatomic axes were different. Based on the distal anatomic axis, the femoral anatomic valgus for the entire population studied was 4.2 degrees plus or minus 1.7 degrees. When the proximal femoral anatomic axis was used, the femoral anatomic valgus became 5.8 degrees plus or minus 1.9 degrees as opposed to 4.9 degrees plus or minus 0.7 degrees when the overall anatomic axis was used. Gender and age did not cause any significant differences. The patellofemoral

Table 72A–4. PATELLOFEMORAL CONTACT AREA

Knee Flexion (degrees)	Contact Area (cm²)
20	2.6 ± 0.4
30	3.1 ± 0.3
60	3.9 ± 0.6
90	4.1 ± 1.2
120	4.6 ± 0.7

From Hubert HH, HayesWC: Patellofemoral contact pressures:The influence of Q-angle and tendofemoral contact. J Bone Joint Surg 66A:5, 1984.

Q angle was 5.8 degrees plus or minus 6.7 degrees for the entire group, and there were no gender-related differences. However, the patellotibial Q angle was significantly larger in female patients (9.9 degrees plus or minus 4.9 degrees) than in male patients (6.8 degrees plus or minus 5.9 degrees), whereas age did not produce any significant variation. The anatomic Q angle was also significantly greater in the female patients (18.8 degrees plus or minus 4.6 degrees) compared with that of male patients (15.6 degrees plus or minus 3.5 degrees).

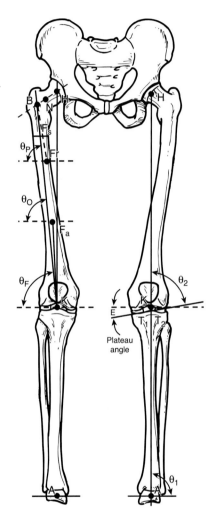

Figure 72A–10. A schematic diagram illustrating the key roentgenographic landmarks used to define the axial alignment parameters. H = femoral head center; N = midpoint of femoral neck base; F_s = midpoint of cortical width at lesser trochanter; F_r = midpoint of cortical width at a proximal third of femoral length; HN = bisector of femoral neck; F_sF_r = anatomic axis of proximal femur; B = intersection of line HN and F_sF_r; F_a = midpoint of distal third of femoral length; K = knee-joint center; HK = mechanical axis of femur; A = ankle joint center; KA = mechanical axis of tibia; F_aK = anatomic axis of distal femur; BK = overall anatomic axis of femur; θ_1 = tibial mechanical axis orientation angle; θ_2 = femoral mechanical axis orientation angle; θ_f = distal femoral axis orientation angle; θ_p = proximal femoral axis orientation angle; θ_0 = overall femoral axis orientation angle. (From Hsu RWW, Himeno S, Coventry MB, Chao EYS: Normal axial alignment of the lower extremity and load-bearing distring distribution at the knee. Clin Orthop 255:215,1990.)

JOINT LOADING

Understanding the loads across the knee joint is important for understanding knee prosthetic design and preference. The knee muscles are relatively inefficient because of small, effective moment arms compared with the externally applied forces and moments. This constraint requires the muscles to contract at high forces to maintain joint equilibrium. Consequently, knee joint contact and shear forces are surprisingly high in magnitude. Joint forces during stair ascent and descent are slightly higher than those used for walking. The forces increase during isokinetic exercise and in rising from a chair, and are greatest during downhill walking (see Table 72A–3). Moreover, the peak forces during stair walking and exercise, either isokinetic or cycling, occur at greater degrees of knee flexion.

Wear or dislocation of the polyethylene element is especially sensitive to shear forces. The tibiofemoral joint anterior shear forces are low for cycling, walking, and stair descent, being .05, .4 and .6, respectively. The anterior shear forces are larger for stair ascent and isokinetic exercise. They are greatest for squatting activities and exceed 3.5 times body weight (BW). The direction of the force imposed on the cruciate ligaments can be defined in terms of the ligaments' attachment relative to the tibia. Of greatest relevance to the design of the prosthetic knee is that the anterior-directed shear forces reflect a load on the posterior cruciate ligament, limiting posterior displacement of the tibia.

The peak posterior shear forces (see Fig. 72A–10) reflect a load on the anterior cruciate ligament, limiting anterior displacement of the tibia relative to the femur. The maximal posterior shear forces are less than $0.2 \times$ BW for activities of daily living and up to $0.4 \times$ BW during exercise. The largest shear forces occur during downhill walking. With the exception of cycling,

the peak posterior shear forces occur at knee flexion angles less than 30 degrees.

The maximum patellofemoral joint compression force is lowest during walking, .5 times BW. It is increased for cycling, rising from a chair, walking up and down stairs, and walking downhill. Isokinetic exercises place five times BW compressive force on the patella.[30] Further, a patellofemoral contact force of $20 \times$ BW has been suggested for athletic activities that involve jumping. More importantly, during weight lifting a patellofemoral joint reaction as high as $25 \times$ BW could occur. Further, the peak patellofemoral joint contact force during walking occurs at nearly full extension, whereas the peak patellofemoral force for other activities occurs at much larger flexion angles. The patellofemoral joint compressive forces are distributed over a limited area in both the normal and replaced joint. Thus, the contact stresses can be very large for either.

KNEE MECHANICS DURING GAIT

The major aim of treating patients is to correct joint deformity and restore normal function. Other than the accepted knee scores, a more detailed means of precisely quantitating structural or functional change is with gait analysis. Gait parameters can be categorized into three basic groups: temporal distance factors, motion, and forces.

Temporal-distance Factors

Temporal-distance factors provide a measure of overall gait function. These factors can be defined on the basis of a footprint diagram (Fig. 72A–11). Walking speed is expressed in meters per minute. Cadence is defined as the number of strides per minute. This has been a useful

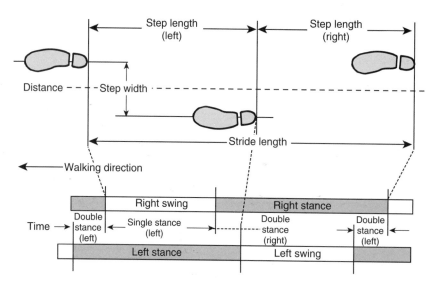

Figure 72A–11. Typical temporal distance factors used in gait analysis. Note that the single stance period of one leg is the same as the swing phase of the contralateral leg. (From Chao EY, Laughman RK, Schneider E, Stauffer RN: Normative data of knee joint motion and ground reaction forces in adult level walking. J Biomech 16:219, 1983. Copyright 1983, with permission of Elsevier Science.)

parameter to discriminate the performance variations after knee replacement.

Knee Motion

Chao et al.[11] reported the three-dimensional motion of the knee during level walking. Ten key parameters were defined from the motion curves. Total ranges of knee joint motion in each plane were very consistent.

Kaufman et al.[29] collected knee kinematics during level walking as well as during stair ascent and stair descent. The knee kinematic patterns were different for each of the walking conditions (Fig. 72A–12). For all walking conditions, the maximum knee flexion occurred during swing phase. The knee flexion angle on stairs was greater than on level ground. Maximal knee flexion angle was 60 degrees during level walking, 87 degrees during stair descent, and 94 degrees during stair ascent.

Knee Kinetics

Kinetics is a branch of mechanics that studies the relationship between the forces acting on a body and the changes they produce in the motion of the body. Forces between the foot and the ground are measured by means of a force plate capable of resolving the time history of the ground reactive forces.

Kaufman et al.[29] measured the knee kinetics during level walking and demonstrated an internal flexor moment initially, followed by an internal extensor moment to provide knee stability. During stair ascent, there was an initial internal knee extensor moment required to initiate the upward displacement of the body. Conversely, during stair descent the initial knee moment was an internal flexor moment that changed to an internal knee extensor moment required for joint stabilization during stair descent. The peak knee extensor moment during stair descent (8.2 percent BW-height [HT]) is greater than four times the knee moment during stair ascent (2.2 percent BW-HT) or level walking (1.9

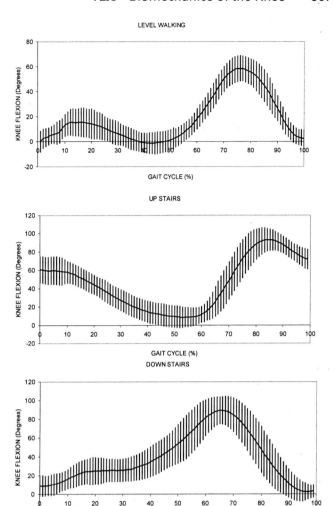

Figure 72A–12. Knee flexion during level walking, stair ascent, and stair descent for normal subjects. Notice that full extension is rarely achieved. Those patients with 5 degrees of flexion contracture demonstrate normal gait under most conditions. (From Kaufman K, Hughes C, Morrey B, et al: Gait characteristics of adults with knee osteoarthritis. J Biomech 34:907, 2001.)

percent BW-HT). This is consistent with the known greater difficulty in descent than ascent for most of the knee replacements.

72B

Biomechanics and Design of Artificial Knee Joints

•KENTON R. KAUFMAN and PETER S. WALKER

DESIGN GOALS

In broad terms, the design goals of any knee replacement are relief of pain, unlimited functional ability, durability for the life of the patient, reproducibility in the operating room, and low cost. Since the 1970s, when condylar metal-plastic total knees were first introduced, clinical experience and biomechanical studies have combined to reach a consensus on many of the design features that are necessary to achieve these goals. Just as importantly, design characteristics that can lead to future problems have also been identified.

Although pain relief is usually achieved, exceptions occur when the patella is not resurfaced or when there is interface micromotion, the latter occurring most often with uncemented components. Unlimited function can be considered to be a range of flexion of 135 degrees and no restriction on the desired activities of the individual. However, in practice, the average maximum flexion angle for different total knee designs is typically 110 degrees, with greater motion being the current expectation.

Since the early 1980s, there have been major improvements in design and technique such that the incidence of loosening and instability has been markedly reduced. This has been the result of a better understanding of the need for accurate alignment to correct ligament tensioning and to improve the design of surface geometry. However, a fatigue wear mechanism of the polyethylene, known as delamination, has emerged as the most serious threat to durability, occurring in some designs less than 10 years postoperatively. This wear of the plastic, together with wear debris from modular parts such as metal trays and screws, has also caused severe bone lysis in many patients.

Although simplicity of surgical technique is ideal, present-day systems show increasing complexity because of the wide range of sizes, design types, and modular options. The variation of inherent stabilities in the different designs of standard condylar replacements, with surfaces ranging from flat to fully dished, indicates the lack of comparative biomechanical data on performance. Other design issues today include the question of whether meniscal bearing designs indeed offer enhanced durability and performance, and whether rotating hinged designs, which offer reliable stability, should take the place of the unlinked constrained condylar type of designs, which are more prone to instability. An inevitable consequence of expanding component options and complexity of instrumentation has been that cost has increased to some extent.

SURFACE GEOMETRY AND CONTACT STRESS

To achieve normal joint mechanics, the surfaces of a joint replacement should be reasonably anatomic and provide normal laxity and stability in combination with the remaining soft tissues.[23] The profiles of the femoral condyles in the sagittal plane have been described in terms of spirals, circular arcs, and polynomials, but, with suitable parameters, any of these methods can provide a close representation.[61] After accounting for size, there are differences in the sagittal contour among different knees, with a standard deviation of about 1 mm.[19]

In the frontal plane, the bearing spacing (BS) defines the lowest points on the condyles on each side (Fig. 72B–1). The inner and outer frontal femoral radii (RFI and RFO) are defined separately, to account for designs with relatively shallow or even flat outer surfaces. The radius of the distal intercondylar groove is defined, although the sections of the patella flange itself can be specified to provide a more anatomic match to the natural patella.

The femoral profile that articulates with the tibial surface in the sagittal plane can be defined by three radii, AB, BC, and CD. An important parameter is the transition point between the distal and posterior radii, called the PDTA angle. For the natural knee, this angle is around 10 to 15 degrees and divides the posterior radius, about 20 mm on average, from the larger distal radius. The lateral distal radius is much larger than that on the medial side, facilitating the internal rotation that occurs in early flexion[46] as a result of the relatively different medial and lateral rolling distances. In like manner, the

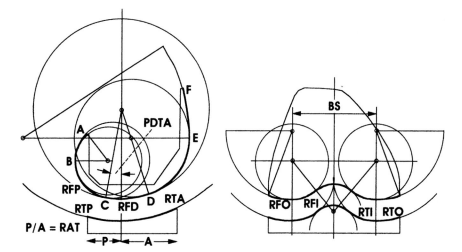

Figure 72B–1. Description of the geometry of the femoral and tibial bearing surfaces using parametrized dimensions. Refer to text for definition of abbreviations.

sagittal profile of the patellar groove can be represented by two additional radii, DE and EF, which are important for correct tracking, providing stability, and preventing excess soft tissue tensions.[2]

The starting point for the surfaces of the tibial component is, again, the bearing spacing, which generally is the same as for the femoral component.[32] In the frontal plane, the inner and outer tibial radii (RTI and RTO) are defined relative to the femoral values, ranging from the same values as the femoral to giving complete conformity to infinite radii or flat surfaces. However, conformity must be distinguished from constraint. The former can be described by the parameter "relative radius of curvature" (R), which is defined in terms of the femoral and tibia radii (RF and RT) as: $1/R = 1/RF + 1/RT$, in which convex is positive and concave is negative. Constraint, in contrast, refers to the effect of a displacement from the neutral position on the increase in relative height and is hence an indicator of stability.[56] The intercondylar radius is less than that of the femoral component to avoid impringement. In the sagittal plane, three parameters are important, the first being the location of the lowest point on the tibial surface, which can be defined by the ratio P : A (see Fig. 72B–1). This is a key parameter because it defines the femoral-tibial contact point at all angles of flexion when only axial compressive forces are acting. The anterior and posterior radii (RTA and RTP) are defined separately to allow for the smaller RTA, which maximizes stability, and the larger RTP, which facilitates rollback of the contact point.

Using the above description of the condylar surfaces, the contact stresses at the contact points can be calculated.[27] The goal is to minimize the stresses on the plastic surface, because this is one of the factors that minimizes the deformation and wear of the material.

This goal implies that the highest possible conformity in both planes is preferable, consistent with other criteria such as adequate laxity and preventing transmission of high shear stresses to the component-bone interface. Because the polyethylene does not behave completely elastically and because the contact dimensions are not

small compared with the radii, the analytical solutions to determine contact stress are not strictly valid. However, an apparent value of 600 MPa was determined experimentally.[51,54]

The lowest stresses occur when the femoral and tibial surfaces conform closely in both the frontal and sagittal planes. Low conformity in both planes produces a point contact situation producing maximal stresses. This applies to designs whose femoral condyles are biconvex, articulating on relatively flat tibial surfaces. An intermediate situation occurs when there is close conformity in the frontal plane but relatively low conformity in the sagittal plane. This configuration has the potential advantage of allowing for adequate anteroposterior (AP) displacement and internal-external rotation.[46] On rotation, the contact points move outward to the peripheries of the plastic.[47] This not only produces elevated contact stresses but can lead to severe deformation and even splitting at the sides of the plastic.[22]

LAXITY, STABILITY, AND MOTION

In the natural joint, laxity and stability depend on the geometry of the articulating surfaces, combined with the tension patterns and elastic properties of the ligaments and soft tissues during the flexion range.[5,17,46] In the natural knee, the dishing of the medial tibial condyle plays an important role under weight bearing,[37] but friction between the joint surfaces is minimal.

Numerous studies have shown the anterior cruciate ligament generally to be more important in early flexion and the posterior cruciate ligament (PCL) in late flexion. The PCL produces a posterior displacement of the femur on the tibia as flexion proceeds, whereas the relatively greater stability on the medial side of the joint, compared with the lateral results in a differential rollback, produces an internal rotation.[46]

As flexion progresses, the center of the femur moves posteriorly relative to the tibia, by a total of 8 mm on average through the 0 to 120 degrees of flexion range.[46]

In parallel with the posterior displacement of the femur, there is a steady internal rotation of the tibia about its own long axis of 10 degrees.

A number of explanations have been put forward for this displacement-rotation behavior. The posterior displacement has been attributed to the tension in the PCL, which was well illustrated in the studies by Rovick et al.[46] The behavior of the PCL in AP displacement has been described in further detail by Zavatsky and O'Connor.[60] At any particular flexion angle, in response to an increasing posterior force on the femur, those fibers that are in tension are highlighted, with more and more fibers being recruited with increasing force.

Explaining the rotation is more difficult. Some authors have attributed it to the greater radius of the distal lateral femoral condyle compared with the medial femoral condyle, the postulation being that rolling occurs during early flexion, resulting in a greater posterior excursion on the lateral side, and thereby producing the internal rotation. The shape of the intercondylar femoral and tibial surfaces has also been shown to contribute to a rotational behavior, although the effect is limited to early flexion.

In the recent past, designs with low inherent stability that preserve the PCL have been widely used, because of the advantages of freedom of motion and allowance of rollback. However, given that flatter geometries tend to have high contact stresses and allow considerable sliding, both of which tendencies are believed to accelerate wear,[7] there has been a tendency for geometries to become more conforming, particularly with more controlled techniques of PCL balancing and release.[4,45] When the surfaces themselves allow little laxity, the role of the existing ligaments can be questioned. Also, at surgery, even though ligament balancing may appear to be satisfactory under lightly loaded conditions, the reduced laxity of the surfaces under weight bearing may still lead to excessive ligament tensions and restriction of motion.

To represent functional conditions, the effect of a compressive force, together with the friction between metal and polyethylene, which is much higher than that between cartilage surfaces, must also be taken into account.[53]

For the normal knees, under non–weight-bearing conditions, the AP displacement has a mean of 8.9 mm.[53] With half body weight, the displacements were reduced by a mean of 29 percent, consistent with the results of Markolf et al.[37] In comparing the values for normals with those of other studies, it is important to recognize whether or not other degrees of freedom were constrained during the test, with reduced values occurring when there is constraint. This important principle has been termed "coupled displacements." When all degrees of freedom were unconstrained during the AP drawer test, the mean displacements under no compressive load were 9.1 mm[37] and 13 mm,[17] whereas under test conditions generally similar to ours, values were 5.5 mm[38] and 4.7 mm.[57]

Using an analytic method to calculate forces (Fig. 72B–2) and displacement with a friction coefficient

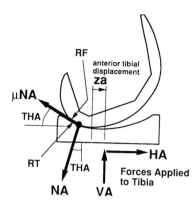

Figure 72B–2. Forces at the femoral-tibial contact points for a combination of a compressive force and a shear force. The frictional force is significant. Refer to text for definition of abbreviations.

of 0.05, the theoretical values for the total AP displacement were found to agree with the data from the patients and from the tests on the prosthetic components themselves. The theory can be extrapolated to predict the AP displacement under conditions of higher load bearing in functional situations in which the compressive forces can reach three times body weight.

Data in the range of level walking with an axial compressive force of 1500 N (approximately two times body weight), an AP shear force of 200 N, and a low flexion angle such that the distal radii of the femoral components are applicable, show that, for both constraints, the AP displacements are less than 3 mm. If the shear force increases to 300 N, the AP values are still only 3 to 5 mm. In the case of load bearing with a flexed knee, as in ascending or descending stairs, with axial compression of 2000 N (approximately three times body weight) and AP shear force of 300 N, and when the posterior radii of the femoral component are applicable, the AP values are 7.4 mm for the designs of moderate constraint and 4.3 mm for the high-constraint design. If the shear force increases to 400 N, the displacements are 11.3 and 6.5 mm.

The effect of the coefficient of friction is substantial. For a range of 0.0 to 0.1, the AP displacements reduce from 4.5 to 1.1 mm for the moderate-constraint design in extension and from 11.9 to 2.9 mm in flexion.

The displacements for level walking when the flexion angle is small show that, for the moderate-constraint design, the maximum total AP laxity is 3 to 7 mm depending on the shear force, whereas for the higher conformity designs, the values are only 2 to 5 mm.

With the knee in flexion, however, the situation is different because the condyles are much less stable as a result of the small posterior femoral radius, and the PCL is likely to be taut. For the moderate-constraint design, the displacements based on the condylar surfaces are in the range of 3 to 11 mm, so that soft tissues may well be required to limit the AP sliding, especially the PCL. With the higher constraint design, which sacrifices the PCL, the surface stability is sufficient in function, even without the intercondylar stabilizing cams. However, the cams would be needed if there were moderate shear forces in combination with low compressive forces.

In conclusion, it appears that higher constraint designs with differences in sagittal femoral and tibial radii in early flexion of around 12 mm provide complete stability to the forces that apply to normal walking, with only a few millimeters of AP sliding. The soft tissues contribute little if anything to stability, and all of the shear forces are carried at the condylar surfaces. In the low-constraint designs with a radii difference averaging 17 mm, the surfaces are capable of providing all of the stability in walking, but the amount of AP laxity is likely to result in some contribution from soft tissues. As the radii difference increases beyond 20 mm, more and more of the shear forces are carried by soft tissues and correspondingly less by the condylar surfaces.

WEAR AND DAMAGE OF THE PLASTIC

From the discussion in the preceding section, it is apparent that in condylar designs, to allow for adequate AP and rotational laxity, and because of the reduced femoral-tibial conformity in flexion, there is a requisite lack of complete conformity, resulting in higher than ideal contact stresses. In this situation, wear is an important concern.

The study by Blunn et al.[6] comprised over 280 retrievals of a range of knee designs obtained from a number of European centers, with the emphasis on long-term follow-up. Over a third of the cases were in the range of 10 to 20 years of follow-up.

There are three types of wear mechanisms in plastic material. The first is *adhesive* wear, occurring at local contact points between the metal and the plastic within the overall contact area. Typically, this generates small particles and shreds in the range 0.1 to 10 μm, as well as thin sheets up to about 10 μm in width. *Abrasive* wear is caused by the cutting of the plastic surface by a harder surface or by particles. In *two-body abrasion*, the roughness is integral with the hard surface, such as a carbide inclusion or a scratch. In *three-body abrasion*, interposed particles of metal, acrylic cement, bone, or other material cause the surface cutting. Finally, there is *delamination* wear, which is a fatigue phenomenon whereby high subsurface stresses lead to propagation of cracks within the plastic, with the cracks eventually coalescing and reaching the surface. This typically results in surface destruction to depths of several millimeters, even down to the metal baseplate.

Surface wear occurs at microscopic adhesive points. When there is sufficient lubrication between the femoral and tibial surfaces, the plastic surface displays fine ripples with spacing from 2 to 10 μm. Thin sections through such surfaces, viewed under polarized light, showed that at these contact points there is a considerable buildup of strain energy. When this energy reaches a critical level, particles are released from the surface. This type of wear results in very small particles and shreds, of approximately 1 μm or less.[48]

However, the most severe type of wear is delamination, which causes destruction of the plastic to a depth of several millimeters. The important characteristic of delamination is that it is time dependent. Up to 8 years, the delamination scores were close to zero, but after 8 years, the scores increased rapidly. Hence, it would be misleading to judge the wear resistance of a particular design in relatively short-term follow-up, because the most severe delamination wear could take place precipitously after a certain elapsed time. The lines of maximum shear stress show that the highest value occurs below the surface. The significance of this is that the initiation and propagation of the cracks depends on the input of strain energy, which is highest in the regions of the highest shear stresses. For direct loading with no sliding, the depth below the surface is 25 percent the width of the contact area, or, typically, 1 to 2 mm.[27]

However, for the subsurface stresses to produce delamination wear, there need to be sites for the initiation of cracks. There is good evidence that these sites are intergranular defects where inadequate bonding has taken place between polyethylene granules during the extrusion or molding processes (Fig. 72B–3).[6,12] Once a crack has initiated in this way, it can propagate as a result of the energy provided at the crack tip by the cyclic stresses. Multiple cracks can occur if there are sufficient numbers of defects in the regions of high shear stress.[57]

A disadvantage of flat plastic surfaces with low constraint is that the contact point locations during activities are both variable and unpredictable. Although the ideal contact region is in the middle third of the plastic surface, small variations of tibial slope or PCL tension can result in abnormal contact locations and excessive sliding motions. The sliding is a result of AP or internal-external rotation. This produces extensive wear over the surface as well as severe wear damage at the anterior or posterior edge of the plastic. Wear studies on specimens have highlighted the increased wear caused by sliding, which is greatly reduced under rolling or when the contact point is in the same location.[7]

At the other end of the spectrum, designs that have high constraint and hence large contact areas and low contact stresses are often thought to produce extremely low wear rates and be free of delamination wear.

From the standpoint of minimizing wear of the plastic, a number of design and materials criteria can be specified. The provision for functional laxity by partial constraint is seen to be compatible with reducing wear because of the adverse consequences of excessive constraint, not only for wear but for fixation also. Although cobalt-chromium surfaces are adequate, to minimize the surface wear in the long term, surfaces such as ceramics, which are harder and more wettable, are preferable. Perhaps the most important variable is the quality of the plastic itself, in terms of complete consolidation with a minimal number of fusion defects or voids, and with the minimal amount of oxidation at the time of implantation. In the next section, the variations in the design configuration are described, including a reference to mobile bearing designs, which are intended to minimize wear of all types.

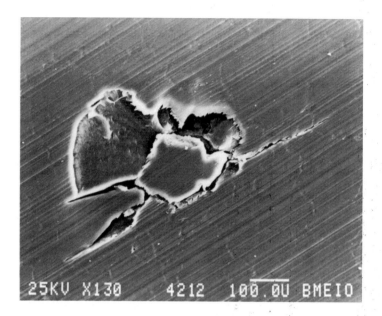

Figure 72B–3. A subsurface intergranular defect in a retrieved tibial component. Cracks can be seen emanating from the corners.

DESIGN CONFIGURATIONS

Most designs can be considered to fall into one of four categories, described in terms of the forces and moments they are capable of transmitting (Fig. 72B–4). The simplest form is the condylar replacement, whose surfaces carry out the same mechanical function as the original joint surfaces and the menisci. Forces in the direction of the tibial long axis are carried at the lateral and medial contact points. AP shear forces are transmitted by a combination of friction and the degree of conformity between the bearing surfaces.[53] If the tibial surfaces are flat in the AP direction, friction provides the only shear force. However, if the total compressive force is 2000 (three times body weight) and the friction coefficient is 0.1, the frictional shear force is 200 N, which is comparable with the shear force calculated for normal activities.[39,40] This means that, in many instances, free sliding within the joint is less than for the normal joint or may not even occur at all. The surfaces transmit axial torque when the lateral and medial shear forces act in opposite directions, again by friction and partial conformity of the surfaces. For flat surfaces, this torque is comparable to the values applied in function as a result of the friction.

One type of design substitutes for the absence of one or both cruciates by an intercondylar stabilizing arrangement. One of the main advantages is that posterior subluxation of the tibia can be prevented. This can be turned to further advantage by arranging the cam actions so that there is some rollback of the femoral contact points. Rollback facilitates a high range of flexion by reducing impingement of the posterior structures. Theoretically, the forces on the tibial component produce less AP rocking compared with the basic condylar type because the result of the posterior contact point force and the force on the peg is in line with the center of the component. However, this may not always apply because of the variety of force combinations that occur

in practice. The intercondylar cam should ideally allow for internal-external rotation laxity by suitable radiusing of the cam surfaces.

If the intercondylar tibial post and box are extended further upward, varus-valgus moments can now be transmitted. Provision for internal-external rotation laxity can be made by suitable rounding off of the intercondylar surfaces, the control preferably being passed to the condylar surfaces. This type of joint design differs from a fixed hinge in that certain laxities and lack of constraints are allowed.

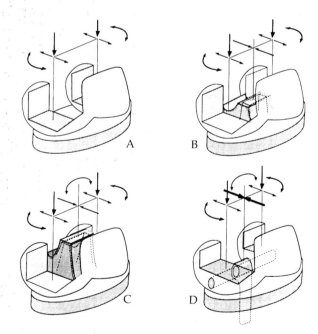

Figure 72B–4. Design configurations of total knees based on the forces and moments carried across the joint. **A,** Partially constrained condylar replacement. **B,** Stabilized condylar replacement. **C,** Superstabilized condylar replacement. **D,** Rotating or fixed linked hinge.

The fixed hinge is the maximally constrained configuration allowing no freedom except flexion-extension. All the forces and moments are directly transmitted by the joint and transferred to the fixation stems. A fixed hinge can be justified in old and infirm patients, in cases of serious instability, or in cases of bone tumor prosthesis in which soft tissue and muscle stabilization are clearly deficient. However, rotational laxity, in which the displacements are more and more restrained by the axial force as the displacement from the neutral position increases, reduces the magnitude of the forces and moments transmitted across the joint components by allowing soft tissues and muscles to absorb some of the energy. Nonetheless, provision for rotational laxity has its price in added mechanical complexity.

Whichever type of joint is used, the tensions and lever arm of the various structures around the knee can significantly affect the function of the joint as a whole. Thus, surgical placement of the components is an important consideration. It can be assumed that in a device preserving the PCL, maximal flexion is reached when the tension in the PCL is at the maximal allowable strain of 15 percent.[10] A posterior tilt of 10 degrees allows an extra 30 degrees of flexion because, as the femur rolls back on the tibial surface in flexion, it is able to do so without distraction. Conversely, an anterior tilt of 10 degrees blocks flexion by 25 degrees. Posterior tilt is compatible with the anatomy of the upper tibia, and a more uniform upper tibial cut can be made at surgery.

A design configuration that was intended not only to optimize function but also to minimize wear is the meniscal bearing, or mobile bearing, concept. In its original form (the Oxford knee), the part of the femoral condyle that articulated with the tibia was replaced with a metal component with a spherical surface. A smooth metal plate was fixed onto the upper tibia. Between these metal parts was a plastic meniscus, in complete conformity with both surfaces but allowing unrestricted freedom of motion. Cruciate ligaments were intended to provide stability and to preserve the "four-bar linkage" mechanism.[8,50] Retrieval studies indicated a low wear rate, although the design has limitations in terms of having no provision for the patella, requiring both cruciates, and needing precise surgery. The design was extended by others, by arranging for the lateral and medial parts to run in tracks and by providing a patella flange. However, in these configurations, the distal profile of the femoral component provides for full conformity only at full extension. As soon as flexion occurs, there is complete contact only on the posterior half of the plastic.

A further development of the mobile bearing concept has been to use a single piece of plastic that articulates on a polished flat metal tibial plate. This concept has a number of advantages, including mechanical strength, simplicity, and comparative ease of surgery. Methods for restricting the motion of the plastic "meniscus" are shown in Figure 72B–5. The central pivot point, used in the New Jersey Rotating Platform design,[43] allows freedom of rotation but no translations. A more anatomic motion can be provided by

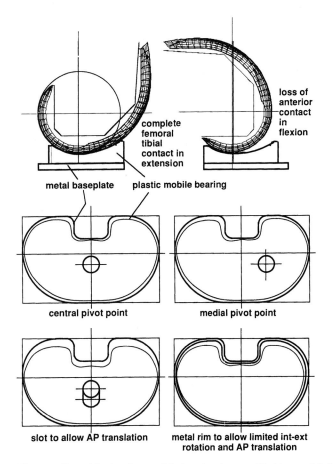

Figure 72B–5. Meniscal or mobile bearing knees. *(Top)* Loss of full contact occurs with flexion. *(Bottom)* Different schemes for limiting the motion of a single piece of plastic on a flat metal tibial tray.

defining a medial pivot point. To allow for translation as well as rotation, a slot can be provided, although a PCL with the correct tension would be required to provide a femoral rollback that was progressive with flexion angle. A scheme that allows both rotation and translation, but within defined amounts, is provided by containing the plastic within a metal rim. "Flip-up" of the plastic can be prevented by a suitable mechanical arrangement. In terms of stability and laxity characteristics, mobile bearing designs need special consideration. Although any required stability can be obtained in a standard condylar replacement by suitable radii of curvature, a mobile bearing knee works effectively as a condylar replacement with flat tibial surfaces. The stability is then provided by soft tissues such as the cruciate ligaments, by an immediate constraint (such as in the rotating platform design), or by limit stops. At this time, there are limited biomechanical data to define the optimal arrangement.[55]

FUTURE DESIGNS

The basic design principles for successful total knee replacements are well established. Today, most designs show similar general characteristics, yet it is likely that relatively small differences in radii and fixation methods could result in significant differences in performance, long-term wear, and long-term fixation, although such differences may not become apparent until after 10 years of follow-up. There is a growing perceived need for a "high-performance" knee that will provide superior performance, especially flexion, and longevity. It was hoped that a design form of the mobile bearing type would be the most likely candidate to fulfill this role. To date, this expectation has not been realized (see Chapter 77). At the same time, the durability of the standard condylar knees is likely to be further improved by an upgrade in the polyethylene quality and, possibly, by a harder material or coating for the femoral component. Performance itself, as well as consistency, is likely to be enhanced by advances in instrumentation, with respect to bone cuts and soft tissue tensions. Most knee problems can be addressed by modern systems, which include several design forms and augmentations, although a customized approach for the more unusual or difficult cases is advisable. A significant reduction in cost of knee components is only likely if there is a radical change of manufacturing methods or materials.

ACKNOWLEDGMENT

Much of the work in this chapter is condensed from studies carried out by many researchers in our biomechanics laboratories; the full references are quoted in the text. Thanks are due to various funding organizations, including the United Kingdom Department of Health, North-East Thames Health Authority, Bristol-Myers, Zimmer, and Howmedica.

References

1. Ahmed AM, Burke DL, Hyder A: Force analysis of the patellar mechanism. J Orthop Res 5:69, 1987.
2. Ahmed AM, Duncan NA, Tanzer M: The medial-lateral shift and spin of the patella are correlated with geometric features of the femoral trochanter. Trans Orthop Res Soc 19:823, 1994.
3. Andriacchi T, Stanwyck TS, Galante JO: Knee biomechanics in total knee replacement. J Arthroplasty 1:211, 1986.
4. Arima J, Martin JW, White SE, et al: Partial posterior cruciate ligament release and knee kinematics after total knee arthroplasty. Proc Orthop Res Soc 19:87, 1994.
5. Blankevoort L, Huiskes R, De Lange A: The envelope of passive knee joint motion. J Biomech 21:705, 1988.
6. Blunn GW, Joshi AB, Lilley PA, et al: Polyethylene wear in unicondylar knee prostheses. Acta Orthop Scand 63:247, 1992.
7. Blunn GW, Walker PS, Joshi A, Hardinge K: The dominance of cyclic sliding in producing wear in total knee replacement. Clin Orthop 273:253, 1991.
8. Bradley J, Goodfellow JW, O'Connor JJ: A radiographic study of bearing movements in unicompartmental Oxford knee replacements. J Bone Joint Surg 69B:598, 1987.
9. Burstein AH, Wright TM: Basic biomechanics. In Insall J, Scott W (eds): Surgery of the Knee. New York, Churchill-Livingstone, 2001, pp 215–231.
10. Butler DL, Kay MD, Stouffer DC: Comparison of material properties in fascicle-bone units from human patella tendon and knee ligaments. J Biomech 19:425, 1986.
11. Chao EY, Laughman RK, Schneider E, Stauffer RN: Normative data of knee joint motion and ground reaction forces in adult level walking. J Biomech 16:219, 1983.
12. Collier JPM, Mayor MB, McNamara JL, et al: Analysis of the failure of 122 polyethylene inserts from uncemented tibial knee components. Clin Orthop 273:232, 1991.
13. Collins JJ: The redundant nature of locomotor optimization laws. J Biomech 28:251, 1995.
14. Ellis MI, Seedhom BB, Amis AA, et al: Forces in the knee joint whilst rising from normal and motorized chairs. J Biomech 8:33, 1979.
15. Ericson M, Nisell R: Tibiofemoral joint forces during ergometer cycling. Am J Sports Med 14:285, 1986.
16. Frankel VH, Burstein AH, Brooks DB: Biomechanics of internal derangement of the knee. Pathomechanics as determined by analysis of the instant centers of motion. J Bone Joint Surg 53A:945, 1971.
17. Fukubayashi T, Torzilli PA, Sherman MF, Warren RF: An in vitro biomechanical evaluation of anterior-posterior motion of the knee: Tibial displacement, rotation and torque. J Bone Joint Surg 64A:258, 1982.
18. Fuss FK: Principles and mechanisms of automatic rotation during terminal extension in the human knee joint. J Anat 180:297, 1992.
19. Garg A, Walker PS: Prediction of total knee motion using a 3-D computer graphics model. J Biomech 23:45, 1990.
20. Goodfellow J, Hungerford DS, Zindel M: Patello-femoral joint mechanics and pathology. 1. Functional anatomy of the patello-femoral joint. J Bone Joint Surg 58B:287, 1976.
21. Gray H: In Williams PL, Warwick R (eds): Gray's Anatomy. Philadelphia, WB Saunders, 1978, pp 183–189.
22. Harrington IJ: A bioengineering analysis of force actions at the knee in normal and pathological gait. Biomed Eng May:167, 1976.
23. Hsieh H, Walker PS: Stabilizing mechanisms of the loaded and unloaded knee joint. J Bone Joint Surg 58A:87, 1976.
24. Hsu RWW, Himeno S, Coventry MB, Chao EYS: Normal axial alignment of the lower extremity and load-bearing distribution at the knee. Clin Orthop 255:215, 1990.
25. Hubert HH, Hayes WC: Patellofemoral contact pressures: The influence of Q-angle and tendofemoral contact. J Bone Joint Surg 66A:5, 1984.
26. Iseki F, Tomatsu T: The biomechanics of the knee joint with special reference to the contact area. Keio J Med 25:37, 1976.
27. Johnson KL: Contact Mechanics. Cambridge, England, Cambridge University Press, 1985.
28. Kapandji IA: The physiology of the joints. In Lower Limb, vol 2. Edinburgh, Churchill-Livingstone, 1987.
29. Kaufman K, Hughes C, Morrey B, et al: Gait characteristics of adults with knee osteoarthritis. J Biomech 34:907, 2001.
30. Kaufman KR, An KN, Litchy WJ, et al: Dynamic joint forces during knee isokinetic exercise. Am J Sports Med 19:305, 1991.
31. Komistek RD, Stiehl JB, Dennis DA, et al: Mathematical model of the lower extremity joint reaction forces using Kane's method of dynamics. J Biomech 31:185, 1998.
32. Kurosawa H, Walker PS, Abe S, et al: Geometry and motion of the knee for implant and orthotic design. J Biomech 18:487, 1985.
33. Kuster M, Wood GA, Sakurai S, Blatter G: Downhill walking: A stressful task for the anterior cruciate ligament? A biomechanics study with clinical implications. Knee Surg Sports Traumatol Arthrosc 2:2, 1994.
34. Kuster MS, Wood GA, Stachowial GW, Gachter A: Joint load considerations in total knee replacements. J Bone Joint Surg 79B:109, 1997.
35. Lewis JL, Lew WD: A method for locating an optimal "fixed" axis of rotation for the human knee joint. J Biomech Eng 100:187, 1978.
36. Li G, Rudy TW, Sakane M, et al: The importance of quadriceps and hamstring muscle loading on knee kinematics and in-situ forces in the ACL. J Biomech 32:395, 1999.
37. Markolf KL, Bargar WL, Shoemaker SC, Amstutz HC: The role of joint load in knee stability. J Bone Joint Surg 63A:570, 1981.
38. Markolf KL, Mensch JS, Amstutz HC: Stiffness and laxity of the knee: The contributions of the supporting structures. J Bone Joint Surg 58A:583, 1976.
39. Morrison JB: Function of the knee joint in various activities. Biomed Eng 4:473, 1969.
40. Morrison JB: The mechanics of the knee joint in relation to normal walking. J Biomech 3:51, 1970.
41. Müller W: The Knee: Form, Function, and Ligament Reconstruction. New York, Springer-Verlag, 1983.
42. Norkin CC, Levangie PK: Joint Structure and Function: A comprehensive Analysis, 2nd ed. Philadelphia, FA Davis, 1992.

43. Pappas MJ, Makris G, Buechel FF: Wear in prosthetic knee joints. Scientific exhibit at the 59th Annual Meeting of the American Academy of Orthopaedic Surgeons, Washington, DC, February 1992.

44. Radin EL: A rational approach to the treatment of patellofemoral pain. Clin Orthop 144:107, 1979.

45. Ritter MA, Faris PM, Keating EM, et al: Posterior cruciate ligament balancing during total knee arthroplasty. J Arthroplasty 3:323, 1988.

46. Rovick JS, Reuben JD, Schrager RJ, Walker PS: Relation between knee motion and ligament length patterns. Clin Biomech 6:213, 1991.

47. Sathasivam S, Walker PS: Optimisation of the bearing surface geometry of total knees. J Biomech 27:255, 1994.

48. Schmalzried TP, Jasty M, Rosenberg A, Harris WH: Polyethylene wear debris and tissue reactions in knee as compared to hip replacement. J Appl Biomater 5:185, 1994.

49. Soderberg JL: Kinesiology: Application to Pathological Motion. Baltimore, Williams & Wilkins, 1997, pp 263–310.

50. Soudry M, Walker PS, Reilly DT, et al: Effects of total knee replacement design on femoral-tibial contact conditions. J Arthroplasty 1:35, 1986.

51. Taylor SJ, Walker PS, Perry JS, et al: The forces in the distal femur and the knee during walking and other activities measured by telemetry. J Arthroplasty 13:428, 1998.

52. van Eijden TM, Kouwenhoven E, Verburg J, Weijs WA: A mathematical model of the patellofemoral joint. J Biomech 19:219, 1986.

53. Walker PS, Amberek MB, Morris JR, et al: Anterior-posterior stability in partially conforming condylar knee replacement. Clin Orthop 310:87, 1995.

54. Walker PS, Blunn GW, Joshi AB, Sathasivam S: Modulation of delamination by surface wear in total knees. Trans Orthop Res Soc 18:499, 1993.

55. Walker PS, Sathasivam S: The design of guide surfaces for fixed-bearing and mobile-bearing knee replacements. J Biomech 32:27, 1999.

56. Walker PS, Wang CJ, Masse Y: Joint laxity as a criterion for the design of condylar knee prostheses. In Proceedings of the Conference on Total Knee Replacement. Institution of Mechanical Engineers, London, 1974.

57. Warren PJ, Olankolun TK, Cobb AG, et al: Laxity and function in knee replacements. Clin Orthop 305:200, 1994.

58. Yoshioka Y, Siu D, Cooke TDV: The anatomy and functional axes of the femur. J Bone Joint Surg 69A:873, 1987.

59. Yoshioka Y, Siu D, Scudamore RA, et al: Tibial anatomy in functional axes. J Orthop Res 7:132, 1989.

60. Zavatsky AB, O'Connor JJ: A model of human knee ligaments in the sagittal plane. Part 1, response to passive flexion. Part 2, fiber recruitment under load. Proc Inst Mech Eng [H] 206:125, 135, 1992.

61. Zoghi M, Hefzy MS, Fu KC, Jackson WT: A three-dimensional morphometrical study of the distal human femur. Proc Inst Mech Eng [H] 206:147, 1992.

73

Posterior Cruciate Ligament Retaining Total Knee Arthroplasty

• MARK W. PAGNANO and JAMES A. RAND

The controversy over retention or substitution of the posterior cruciate ligament (PCL) continues. The excellent long-term results of total knee arthroplasties done with cemented condylar components of cruciate-sacrificing, cruciate-substituting, and cruciate-retaining designs ensures that this debate will continue. The central concept is focused on whether PCL retention can reliably and reproducibly promote femoral rollback as the knee flexes (Fig. 73–1). An assessment of the theoretical issues and clinical results of knee arthroplasty assists in the analysis of this controversy. Important new data from the fields of biomechanics, histology, gait-analysis, radiology, as well as from the operating room have sharpened the PCL debate. The interested reader can find a review article that extensively explores each of those issues.[10] Historically, the potential advantages of PCL preservation are seen as maintenance of the joint line, femoral rollback, proprioception, maintenance of a central contact point of articulation, and low shear stress on the bone-cement interface of the tibial component. The disadvantages of PCL preservation are higher polyethylene stresses, a seesaw effect from femoral glide (Fig. 73–2), difficulty in soft tissue balance, and the fact that PCL retention is not always possible.[1]

INDICATIONS AND CONTRAINDICATIONS

The indications for a PCL-preserving total knee arthroplasty are fixed flexion of less than 30 degrees, varus of less than 20 degrees, and valgus of less than 25 degrees; joint subluxation of no more than 1 cm; structurally intact PCL; and technical ability of the surgeon. For patients with large fixed deformities, soft tissue balance may require sacrifice of the PCL to facilitate proper soft tissue balance. A surgeon's technical ability to balance the PCL is important. A lax PCL is not functional but is preferable to an excessively tight PCL. A tight PCL limits knee motion and may be a source of pain and abnormal polyethylene wear patterns. Contraindications to PCL preservation are severe fixed deformities, technical

inability to balance the PCL, and anatomic abnormality of the PCL, such as severe ligamentous degeneration.

TECHNIQUE

Preservation and balance of the PCL must be combined goals of surgery. The tibial attachment of the PCL is located posterior and distal to the tibial plateau. The tibial attachment of the PCL is vulnerable to injury during the tibial resection for total knee arthroplasty. Excessive bone resection from the proximal tibia (i.e., greater than 1 cm) or a large posteriorly sloped cut may jeopardize the tibial attachment of the PCL. The PCL may be injured during a correct tibial resection by excessive posterior travel of the saw blade. Placing an osteotome anterior to the PCL during tibial resection serves to protect it. Once the tibial plateau bone has been removed, any remaining bone island anterior to the PCL can be trimmed to allow placement of the tibial component.

Balancing the PCL can be difficult. A slightly lax PCL is preferable to one that is excessively tight. Balance of the PCL should be assessed *after* correction of any varus or valgus ligamentous imbalance. Varus or valgus imbalance can affect assessment of PCL tension. Soft tissue balance is always tested in both extension and flexion (Fig. 73–3). The gap or space between the femoral and tibial cut surfaces should be within 1 to 2 mm of each other in both flexion and extension. PCL tension is best assessed with the trial total knee prosthesis in place. An excessively tight PCL results in (1) anterior translation of the tibia from beneath the femur (Fig. 73–4); (2) anterior liftoff of the trial polyethylene from the tibia tray in flexion; and/or (3) displacement of the femoral component in flexion (see Fig. 73–4). A useful test of the relative balance of the PCL is the so-called POLO (pullout, liftoff) test introduced by Dr. Richard Scott. In this test, a trial reduction is done with a stemless tibial trial prosthesis and a curved tibial insert. The Pullout portion of the test is done at 90 degrees of flexion and confirms that the PCL is not too loose if the tibial insert can not be subluxed (pulled out) anteriorly from beneath the femur. The Liftoff portion is done while putting the knee

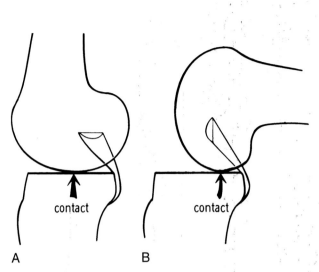

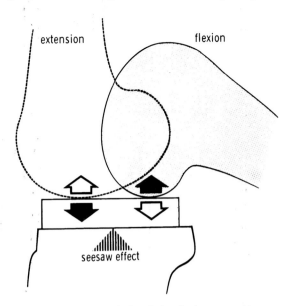

A   B

Figure 73–1. A, With an intact posterior cruciate ligament (PCL) in extension, the tibial femoral contact area is near the mid tibia. **B**, With flexion, the contact area is posteriorly placed because of the rollback effect that occurs with a functional posterior cruciate ligament. (From Insall JN: Historical development, classification, and characteristics of knee prostheses. *In* Insall JN, Windsor RE, Scott WN, et al [eds]: Surgery of the Knee, 2nd ed. New York, Churchill Livingstone, 1993, p 677.)

Figure 73–2. Femoral translation during flexion caused by posterior cruciate ligament retention may cause a see-saw effect on the tibial implant. (From Insall JN: Historical development, classification, and characteristics of knee prostheses. *In* Insall JN, Windsor RE, Scott WN, et al [eds]: Surgery of the Knee, 2nd ed. New York, Churchill Livingstone, 1993, p 677.)

through a range of motion up to 120 degrees and ensuring that the tibial insert does not book open (lift off) in flexion, indicating that the PCL is too tight. Scott postulates that if the PCL is neither too loose nor too tight, it must be just right.

If the PCL is excessively tight, the tension can be decreased by several techniques. Increased tibial bone resection is only appropriate if the knee is tight in both flexion and extension. If the knee is tight only in flexion, increasing tibial bone resection leaves the knee lax in extension, resulting in symptomatic instability. If the knee is tight only in flexion, the posterior slope of the

tibial cut should be assessed. The tibia normally has a 3- to 7-degree posterior slope. The amount of posterior slope cut on the tibia is dependent on the prosthetic design. Some implants have an inherent posterior slope in the articular geometry and require less posterior slope than knees with a flat geometry in the sagittal plane. Increasing posterior slope for the tibial resection relaxes the PCL. Posterior tibial slope should not exceed 10 degrees to avoid risk of injury to the tibial attachment of the PCL. Posterior cruciate recession consists of selective release of the anterior fibers of the PCL from their tibial attachment. Release of the anterior 10 percent to 20

Figure 73–3. Soft tissue tension after correction of varus-valgus and contracture deformity is measured with the knee in full extension. Proper balance of the soft tissue occurs with a flexion gap that is equal to the extension gap.

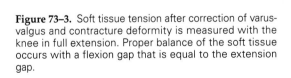

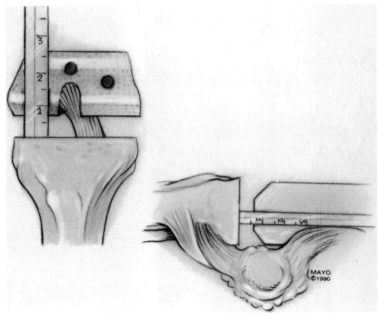

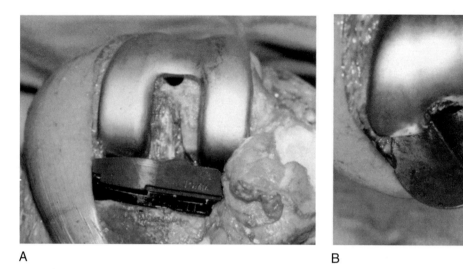

A

B

Figure 73–4. A, In flexion, the tibial tray lifts off if the posterior cruciate ligament (PCL) is too tight. **B**, With a tight PCL, the tibia rotates anteriorly and laterally with flexion.

percent of the PCL results in correct soft tissue balance. If more than 75 percent of the PCL is released, a PCL-substituting prosthesis should be considered. The remaining 25 percent of the PCL fibers may rupture with activity, leading to instability (Fig. 73–5).[11] If the PCL is released or absent, the tibial tray should be more conforming, because rollback does not occur (Fig. 73–6). Hence, the surgeon should match the constraints of the soft tissue with the inherent constraints of the knee system being used.

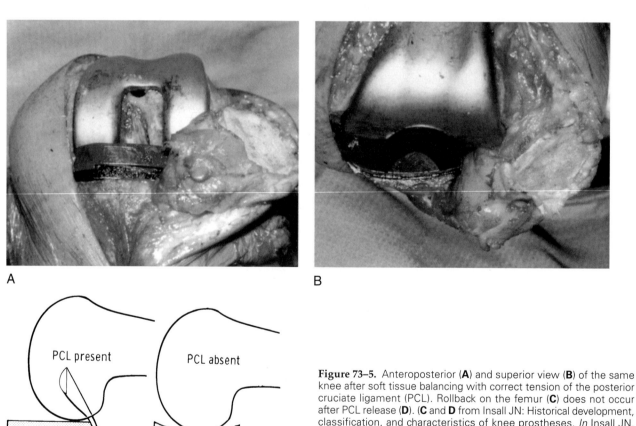

A

B

PCL present

PCL absent

C

D

Figure 73–5. Anteroposterior (**A**) and superior view (**B**) of the same knee after soft tissue balancing with correct tension of the posterior cruciate ligament (PCL). Rollback on the femur (**C**) does not occur after PCL release (**D**). (**C** and **D** from Insall JN: Historical development, classification, and characteristics of knee prostheses. *In* Insall JN, Windsor RE, Scott WN, et al [eds]: Surgery of the Knee, 2nd ed. New York, Churchill Livingstone, 1993, p 677.)

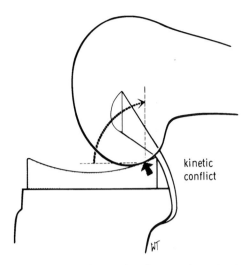

Figure 73–6. If the posterior cruciate ligament is retained, the tibial component should have posterior conformity to allow the femur to roll back. (From Insall JN: Historical development, classification, and characteristics of knee prostheses. *In* Insall JN, Windsor RE, Scott WN, et al [eds]: Surgery of the Knee, 2nd ed. New York, Churchill Livingstone, 1993, p 677.)

RESULTS AND COMPLICATIONS

Early ligament-retaining prostheses, such as the polycentric and geometric designs, were not able to provide predictable results. Prior editions of this textbook provide an extensive discussion of the results obtained with these and other early knee designs.

The Miller-Galante I (MG-I) prosthesis had a relatively flat articular geometry and multiple sizes. The objective was to reproduce normal knee kinematics. A study of 116 cemented prostheses at 3.5 years of follow-up found 88 percent good or excellent results.[16] The range of motion was 105 degrees. Reoperation was required in 9 percent of the knees, with revision in 6 percent. When inserted without cement, the results with the MG-I prosthesis have been termed problematic. Berger et al. reported the 11-year follow-up of 113 consecutive cementless MG-I total knees.[2] Cementless femoral fixation in that study was deemed excellent, whereas tibial components had a 6 percent rate of revision. The cementless metal-backed patella used in that series was poor, with a 30 percent rate of revision. Those authors have now abandoned cementless fixation in total knee arthroplasty.

The posterior cruciate-sparing modification of the total condylar prosthesis was the cruciate condylar prosthesis. The same femoral component was used for both the total and cruciate condylar implants. The tibial component of the cruciate condylar differed from that of the total condylar by having a posterior cruciate recess posteriorly (Fig. 73–7). The objective of the cruciate condylar prosthesis was to encourage femoral rollback and motion.[14] The long-term results of this design have been reported by three separate groups.[4,7,12] A 9-year study of 144 knees found 95 percent good or excellent results.[9] Mean knee motion was 106 degrees. Tibial radiolucent lines were present in 41 percent, of which 12 percent were progressive. Eight of the knees were failures. A review of 78 knees in 63 patients followed for a mean of 10 years at the Mayo Clinic was performed.[12] Good or excellent results were achieved in 93 percent of knees. Mean flexion was 102 degrees. Radiolucent lines were present adjacent to 57 percent of the knees. Using an endpoint of revision, survivorship was 96 percent at 10 years. There were no significant differences in survivorship, radiolucent lines, or knee scores among knees with

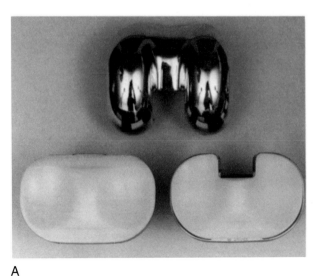

A

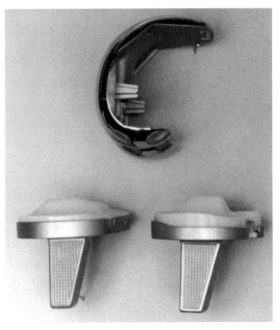

B

Figure 73–7. The total condylar prosthesis with a cruciate-sacrificing and cruciate-sparing tibial implant.

an all-polyethylene or metal-backed tibial component. Complications consisted of deep sepsis in 1 percent, loosening in 1 percent, and supracondylar fracture in 3 percent. In yet another study of 42 knees followed at 11 years, 93 percent good or excellent results were achieved.[4] The range of motion was 104 degrees. Incomplete radiolucent lines were observed in 75 percent. The complication rate was 17 percent and the reoperation rate was 19 percent.

The kinematic condylar prosthesis had metal backing of the tibial component and separate right and left femoral components (Fig. 73–8). The tibial plateau was flattened in the sagittal plane in an attempt to improve motion by encouraging femoral rollback. A study of 192 knees followed for a mean of 6 years found 88 percent good or excellent results.[18] Mean knee motion was 109 degrees. Radiolucent lines were present adjacent to 40 percent of the tibial and 60 percent of the patellar components. Reoperation was performed in 11 knees, of which 4 were for patellar loosening and 1 for patellar fracture. In a study from the Mayo Clinic, 119 knees were evaluated at 10 years.[8] Good or excellent results were achieved in 87 percent. Mean knee motion was 105 degrees. Joint line height was changed by a mean of 1 mm. A 2-mm radiolucent line was identified adjacent to 2 patellar, 1 femoral, and 1 tibial component. Patellar component loosening was identified in 6 knees. Aseptic loosening of the tibial and femoral component occurred in 2 knees. Using an endpoint of revision, survivorship was 96 percent at 10 years.

The press fit condylar (PFC) prosthesis was introduced with a keeled tibial component designed to resist offset loading while preserving tibial bone stock (Fig. 73–9). A survivorship analysis of 1000 consecutive posterior cruciate-retaining PFC knees, reported in 2000, revealed a 10-year survivorship free of mechanical failure of 98.7 percent.[3] The PFC design is available in both cemented and cementless versions. A comparison of 51 cemented and 55 cementless PFC knees was done at 10 years.[5] Survivorship with revision as the endpoint was 96 percent for the cemented knees and 88 percent for the cementless knees. Knee Society scores for pain and function were 92 and 72 for the cemented knees and 88 and 66, respectively, for the cementless knees. Another 10-year follow-up study included 155 knees from an initial study group of 235 knees.[17] Cementless fixation was used in more than half of the femoral components and less than 10 percent of the tibial components. Knee Society pain and function scores were 95 points and 84 points, respectively. Survivorship to revision was reported as 92 percent at 10 years.

The anatomic graduated component (AGC) prosthesis includes a one-piece metal-backed component with direct compression molded polyethylene. A multicenter study of 2001 AGC knees was done.[15] The predominant diagnosis was osteoarthritis (91 percent) and the follow-up was from 3 to 10 years, with 71 knees having 10-year data. Knee Society pain and function scores were 75 and 86, respectively, at last follow-up. A survivorship analysis (that excluded metal-backed patellar failures) predicted a 98 percent 10-year survivorship free of revision. A consecutive series of 387 knees done with the AGC design and using thin (4.4 mm) tibial polyethylene was reported at an average of 10 years of follow-up. Survivorship with revision or loosening as the endpoint was 98.7 percent at 5 years, 95.4 percent at 10 years, and 94.3 percent at 15 years.[9]

The Mayo Clinic experience with 9200 total knee arthroplasties was reviewed.[13] Of 3907 posterior cruciate-

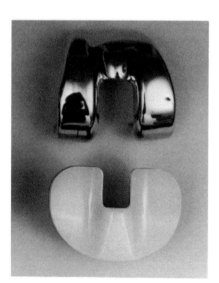
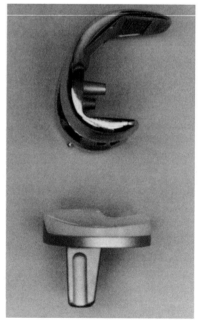

Figure 73–8. The kinematic condylar prosthesis.

A   B

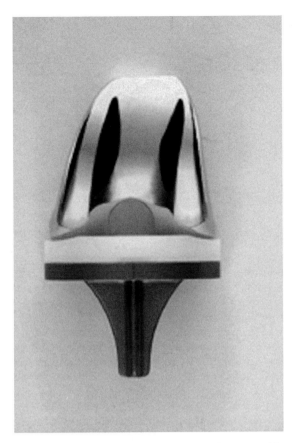

Figure 73–9. The press-fit condylar prosthesis. (Courtesy of Deputy Inc., Warsaw, IN.)

retaining total knee arthroplasties with a metal-backed tibial component, a 91 percent survivorship at 10 years was predicted. Therefore, the results of posterior cruciate-retaining prostheses appear durable. Good or excellent results can be anticipated in 79 to 96 percent. There appears to be little difference between metal-backed and all-polyethylene tibial components or between meniscal and fixed bearing implants. A longer duration of experience will be required to determine whether these design differences affect long-term results.

AUTHOR'S PREFERENCE[3]

One of the authors (MWP) prefers to routinely excise the posterior cruciate and substitute for it with a posterior stabilized knee design. The other author's preference (JAR) is to preserve the posterior cruciate when feasible during total knee arthroplasty. The latter author has found it possible to preserve a posterior cruciate that is present in 90 percent of knees. It is extremely important to be sure that the posterior cruciate is appropriately balanced. It is better to have a slightly lax than an excessively tight posterior cruciate, and it is preferable to sacrifice the posterior cruciate rather than leave a knee unbalanced with residual varus deformity. In approximately 10 percent of knee arthroplasties in which the posterior cruciate is saved,

some of the anterior fibers are released to avoid excessive tension in the posterior cruciate. If the posterior cruciate must be sacrificed to achieve soft tissue balance, the decision regarding posterior cruciate substitution or not is based on the anteroposterior laxity of the knee with a trial prosthesis in place and the extensor mechanism reduced. When the posterior cruciate is sacrificed at surgery, the use of a slightly thicker tibial polyethylene allows adequate stability of the knee in 50 percent of patients. A posterior-stabilized implant is used for those knees that tend to sublux posteriorly during trial reduction.

References

1. Andriacchi TP, Galante JO: Retention of the posterior cruciate in total knee arthroplasty. J Arthroplasty 3:S13, 1988.
2. Berger RA, Jacobs JJ, Rosenberg AG, et al: Problems with cementless total knee arthroplasty at eleven years follow-up. Paper #5 presented at American Association of Hip and Knee Surgeons 10th Annual Meeting, Dallas, TX, November 3–5, 2000.
3. Berry DJ, Whaley A, Harmsen WS: Survivorship of 1000 consecutive cemented cruciate-retaining total knee arthroplasties of a single modern design: Results at a mean of 10 years. Paper #7 presented at American Association of Hip and Knee Surgeons 10th Annual Meeting, Dallas TX, November 3–5, 2000.
4. Dennis DA, Clayton ML, O'Donnell S, et al: Posterior cruciate condylar total knee arthroplasty. Clin Orthop 281:168, 1992.
5. Duffy GP, Berry DJ, Rand JA: Cement versus cementless fixation in total knee arthroplasty: Results at 10 years of a matched group. Clin Orthop 356:66, 1998.
6. Insall JN: Historical development, classification, and characteristics of knee prostheses. In Insall JN, Windsor RE, Scott WN, et al (eds): Surgery of the Knee, 2nd ed. New York, Churchill Livingstone, 1993, p 677.
7. Lee JG, Keating EM, Ritter MA, Faris PM: Review of the all-polyethylene tibial component in total knee arthroplasty. Clin Orthop 260:87, 1990.
8. Malkani AL, Rand JA, Bryan RS, Wallrichs SL: Total knee arthroplasty with the kinematic condylar prosthesis: A ten-year follow-up study. J Bone Joint Surg 77A:423, 1995.
9. Meding JB, Ritter MA, Keating EM, Faris PM: Total knee arthroplasty with 4.4 millimeters of tibial polyethylene: Average ten year follow-up study. Paper #6 presented at American Association of Hip and Knee Surgeons 10th Annual Meeting, Dallas TX, November 3–5, 2000.
10. Pagnano MW, Cushner FD, Scott WN: Whether to preserve the posterior cruciate ligament in total knee arthroplasty. J Am Acad Ortho Surg 6:176,1998.
11. Pagnano MW, Hanssen AD, Lewallen DG, Stuart MJ: Flexion instability after primary posterior cruciate retaining total knee arthroplasty. Clin Orthop 356:39, 1998.
12. Rand JA: A comparison of metal-backed and all polyethylene tibial components in total knee arthroplasty. J Arthroplasty 8:307, 1993.
13. Rand JA, Ilstrup DM: Survivorship of total knee arthroplasty: Cumulative rates of survival of 9,200 total knee arthroplasties. J Bone Joint Surg 73A:397, 1991.
14. Ritter MA, Gioe TJ, Stringer EA, Littrell D: The posterior cruciate condylar total knee prosthesis: A five-year follow-up study. Clin Orthop 184:264, 1984.
15. Ritter MA, Worland R, Saliski J: Flat-on-flat, non-constrained compression molded polyethylene total knee replacement. Clin Orthop 321:79, 1995.
16. Rosenberg AG, Barden RM, Galante JO: Cemented and ingrowth fixation of the Miller-Galante prosthesis. Clin Orthop 260:71, 1990.
17. Schai PA, Thornhill TS, Scott RD: Total knee arthroplasty with the PFC system: Results at a minimum of ten years and survivorship analysis. J Bone Joint Surg Br 80:850, 1998.
18. Wright J, Ewald FC, Walker PS, et al: Total knee arthroplasty with the kinematic prosthesis. J Bone Joint Surg 72A:1003, 1990.

74

Posterior Cruciate-Substituting and -Sacrificing Total Knee Arthroplasty

·CEDRIC J. ORTIGUERA, ARLEN D. HANSSEN, and MICHAEL J. STUART

Total knee arthroplasty designs can be classified into cruciate-retaining, cruciate-sacrificing, cruciate-substituting (posterior-stabilized), constrained condylar, and hinged designs (Fig. 74–1). Cruciate-retaining designs, which rely on the integrity of the collateral and posterior cruciate ligaments, require less conforming articular surfaces to allow proper ligament function during knee range of motion. Cruciate-sacrificing designs compensate for the absence of the posterior cruciate ligament by cupping of the tibial component, which increases articular conformity to reduce translation and rotation during knee flexion.[16] Posterior stabilized designs evolved from cruciate-sacrificing components with the addition of a tibial post and femoral housing mechanism to prevent posterior subluxation. Posterior-stabilized prostheses require the presence of competent collateral ligaments and should not be regarded as a constrained design, which also provides medial-lateral stability. Constrained condylar prostheses, with the added height and conformity of the polyethylene tibial spine and femoral housing, render medial-lateral stability and are used primarily in complex arthroplasties with compromised or absent collateral ligaments. Hinged designs provide the most inherent stability but have an increased incidence of complications, including mechanical loosening. Hinged components are rarely used today except for unique situations such as tumor excision necessitating resection of the collateral ligaments.

DESIGN CONSIDERATIONS

The most widely used posterior cruciate-sacrificing prosthesis has been the total condylar device, which was developed at the Hospital for Special Surgery in 1974. This prosthetic design includes a femoral component with symmetric, anatomic condyles that have a decreasing radius of curvature from anterior to posterior and an all-polyethylene or metal-backed tibial component with biconcave plateaus. Conformity of the articulation increases in extension and decreases in flexion, which allows rotation and gliding motions. Although this

prosthesis proved to be durable, it was found to offer limited knee motion.

The original posterior-stabilized condylar knee design, the Insall-Burstein, introduced in 1978, was specifically developed to improve range of motion and stair climbing while preventing posterior subluxation.[11] The initial posterior-stabilized design introduced a central polyethylene tibial spine that articulated with a transverse femoral cam to prevent posterior tibial subluxation and to produce controlled femoral rollback on a posteriorly inclined tibial surface. This design effected an improved range of motion and a resultant compressive joint force at the prosthesis-bone interface.[11] A metal-backed tibial component was introduced in 1980 in an attempt to improve the load transmission across the interface.

Since the introduction of the first posterior-stabilized design, the use of cruciate-substituting arthroplasties has increased dramatically. Although the substituting prosthesis was developed to address severe angular knee deformity accompanied by contraction of the posterior cruciate ligament (PCL), the use of this design now encompasses the entire spectrum of primary and revision knee arthroplasty. With more than two dozen total knee arthroplasty designs now available on the market, nearly all manufacturers offer a dedicated posterior-stabilized design or posterior-stabilized version in their line.

Although the basic concept of ligament substitution is maintained, it is important to realize that not all posterior-stabilized designs are the same. Most posterior-stabilized designs incorporate an increased articular conformity that results in transfer of the resisted rotational and translational forces to the prosthetic-bone interface.[34] Modifications of posterior-stabilized components incorporate flat tibial surfaces to decrease articular constraint.[3] This reduction of articular conformity decreases the contact surface area, with a resultant increase in the contact stresses measured at the articular surface.[3] The authors compared the results of two posterior-stabilized total knee arthroplasty designs. One group had an anatomic femoral component, a modular cam segment, and a flat-on-flat tibial articular surface,

982

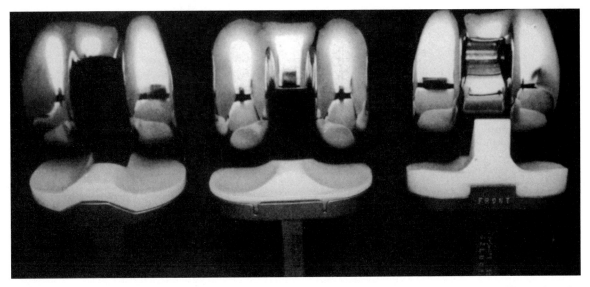

Figure 74–1. (*Left*) The kinematic condylar prosthesis—posterior cruciate ligament-retaining design. (*Middle*) The total condylar prosthesis—posterior cruciate ligament-sacrificing design. (*Right*) The kinematic stabilizer prosthesis—posterior cruciate-substituting design. (From Hanssen AD, Rand JA: A comparison of primary and revision total knee arthroplasty using the kinematic stabilizer prosthesis. J Bone Joint Surg 70A:491, 1988.)

whereas the other had a nonanatomic femoral component with a fixed cam mechanism and high congruency between the tibial articular surface and femoral condyles. At 32 months of follow-up, the group with the flat-on-flat articular surface was found to have significantly higher presence of effusion, synovitis, and aseptic tibial component loosening with associated polyethylene wear (unpublished data). These differences may be attributable to the unconstrained tibial articular congruity and mechanical abrasion of the modular cam against the tibial post.

RETENTION, RESECTION, OR SUBSTITUTION?

In the normal knee, the PCL functions as part of the four-bar linkage, producing femoral rollback and movement of the tibiofemoral contact point posteriorly with knee flexion. This results in an increase in the quadriceps lever arm and improved quadriceps efficiency. In most total knee arthroplasties, the anterior cruciate ligament is deficient or resected, altering the complex interaction of the four-bar linkage. Whether to retain, resect, or substitute for the PCL during total knee arthroplasty is a controversial decision that has persisted for several decades.

Suggested advantages of PCL retention include absorption of anteroposterior and varus-valgus shear or tensile forces by the PCL. These forces are otherwise transferred to the prosthetic-bone interface and the articulating surface of the prosthesis.[2] Additionally, the femoral rollback mechanism of the PCL theoretically facilitates increased range of motion by preventing femoral impingement on the posterior tibia during max-

imal knee flexion.[2] This rollback mechanism requires minimally conforming articular surfaces best achieved with flat tibial plateaus. Patients with an intact PCL after total knee arthroplasty demonstrate a more normal pattern of stair-climbing compared with patients with sacrificing or substituting designs.[1,2] The PCL may also preserve proprioception and provide patients with a more natural feeling in the knee joint, but reports have failed to show any clinical difference in proprioception when comparing cruciate-sparing versus cruciate-sacrificing total knee arthroplasties.[38–40] In studies comparing patient satisfaction with bilateral cruciate-sparing and cruciate-sacrificing knees, no significant differences were found in patient preference.[3,41]

Arguments against cruciate sacrifice include limitation of surgical exposure, restriction of deformity correction, and compromise of soft tissue balancing. Although proponents of cruciate retention argue that more normal kinematics can be maintained, flouroscopic studies have failed to confirm this because cruciate-retaining knees actually exhibit a paradoxical anterior femoral translation with knee flexion, with no appreciable rollback occurring in one study.[46,49]

PCL-sacrificing components have increased articular surface conformity that provides a large contact area, resulting in decreased contact stress and, in theory, decreased polyethylene wear. Soft tissue balancing with equalization of the flexion and extension gaps is made easier at the time of surgery. Advocates of posterior-stabilized designs cite the same possible advantages of lower articular surface point contact stresses owing to better prosthetic conformity and facilitation of deformity correction, along with more reliable knee stability, improved range of motion, and removal of a potential constraining force should the PCL be tensioned too tightly.[29]

Several clinical situations favor the use of a posterior-stabilized prosthesis. Superior clinical results are obtained in the postpatellectomy patient with a posterior-stabilized prosthesis than with cruciate-retaining arthroplasty.[13] Paletta and Laskin reported on 22 patients with osteoarthritis and a prior patellectomy. Nine patients received a posterior-stabilized total knee arthroplasty and 11 had a cruciate-retaining condylar arthroplasty. The mean preoperative knee scores of 45 and 47 points improved postoperatively to 89 points in the stabilized group and 67 points in the cruciate-retaining arthroplasty group ($P<0.001$). Final range of motion was also significantly better (113 degrees versus 105 degrees) in the posterior-stabilized arthroplasty group (<0.01). At an average of 5 years after surgery, 12 of the 13 cruciate-retaining arthroplasties had more than 1 cm of anteroposterior translation at 90 degrees of flexion compared with only 1 of 9 posterior-stabilized arthroplasties. If the PCL is absent, dysfunctional, or requires removal during primary or revision surgery, the use of a posterior-stabilized prosthesis seems advisable.

Beyond these considerations, reasons for retention or substitution of the PCL are theoretical and philosophical. The continuing controversy centers around primary total knee arthroplasty, in which the PCL is present in 99 percent of knees.[23] The vast majority of primary knee arthroplasties, including those with severe angular deformity, permit retention of the PCL.[22,29] In the presence of a severe valgus or varus deformity or a severe flexion contracture, posterior cruciate sacrifice may facilitate appropriate soft tissue balancing and alignment of the limb.[27] Laskin compared the results of a group of patients with a preoperative fixed varus or combined varus and flexion contracture of at least 15 degrees who were undergoing total knee arthroplasty.[41] Compared with patients who had cruciate retention, patients with posterior stabilized arthroplasties had less pain, less incidence of bone cement radiolucencies, and an increased eventual flexion arc (108 degrees versus 86 degrees, $P<0.01$). Ten-year Kaplan-Meier survivorship was 72 percent for the cruciate-retaining group versus 92 percent for the posterior-stabilized group.

The remaining question concerns the actual function of the PCL in a total knee arthroplasty. In the absence of the anterior cruciate ligament and with consequent loss of the normal four-bar linkage mechanism, the PCL does not function normally and acts more as a posterior tether. The ability to insert a prosthesis and restore physiologic PCL tension throughout the full arc of knee motion is extremely difficult. An in vivo study measuring PCL tension after cruciate-retaining arthroplasty revealed wide variation.[16] Thirty percent of knees reached high levels of strain prematurely in early flexion, which caused high contact pressures on the posterior tibial plateau with continued flexion; 60 percent of knees had a lax PCL throughout the range of motion, and only 10 percent had normal ligament tension throughout the range of motion. This study seriously questions the ability to consistently achieve normal PCL tension during total knee arthroplasty.

Arguments against cruciate sacrifice include decreased efficiency during ambulation, alteration of stair-climbing pattern, limited knee flexion, and increased stress at the prosthesis-bone interface. Resection of the PCL without posterior substitution, such as with the total condylar prosthesis, has currently fallen out of favor despite the excellent clinical results achieved with this design.[20,21,26] Substitution for the PCL is also associated with an abnormal pattern of stair climbing and increased stress at the prosthesis-bone interface, but increased distal femoral bone resection is also required to accommodate for the housing of the component. This has led to the concern of bone deficiency at the time of revision arthroplasty. Mintzer et al. have shown that pronounced stress shielding occurs beneath the anterior femoral flange regardless of component design, suggesting that the remaining bone in the notch region is of poor quality. Because most revision arthroplasties are performed with a posterior-stabilized knee, the bone loss is likely inconsequential.

Because of the concern for distal femoral bone loss with posterior-stabilized designs, interest has been increasing regarding the use of more conforming implants as an alternative to the use of a cam and post for sagittal plane stability. Laskin and colleagues reported on the use of a deep-dished congruent ultrahigh-molecular-weight-polyethylene component.[44] Compared with the posterior-stabilized insert, the medial-lateral configurations were identical. In the sagittal plane, the deep-dish implant had a deeper concavity, whereas the posterior-stabilized implant had an intercondylar eminence. At short term follow-up, there were no differences in mean range of motion (116 degrees), ability to ascend and descend stairs in a bipedal manner, pain scores, knee scores, stability, or lack of anterior knee pain. The authors believe that this type of implant obviates the need for intercondylar bone resection, decreasing the potential for fracture and maximizing bone volume for future revision surgery. Longer term follow-up is needed to prove the durability of this design.

Clinical studies, using historical controls, have suggested that cruciate-retaining arthroplasties have an increased range of motion compared with cruciate-sacrificing arthroplasties.[2] Knee flexion is enhanced with posterior cruciate-substituting designs because of increased femoral rollback on the tibia. A prospective study of 242 patients revealed a significantly greater range of motion in the posterior cruciate-substituting group of patients (103 degrees versus 112 degrees; $P<0.001$).[9] Other authors have reported mean arcs of motion as high as 110 degrees to 115 degrees with posterior-stabilized designs.[5,11,42] Careful clinical evaluation has also revealed a significantly greater translation in the anteroposterior plane at 30 degrees and 90 degrees of knee flexion in cruciate-retaining arthroplasties compared with cruciate-substituting designs ($P<0.01$).[12] This increased translation and the corresponding change in point of contact pressures during prosthetic translation raises concern about the possibility of increased polyethylene wear in cruciate-retaining total knee arthroplasty designs.

Delayed onset of spontaneous PCL insufficiency after cruciate-retaining total knee arthroplasty, associated with knee instability and symptoms leading to revision surgery, has been reported.[19] We have also observed patients with the clinical phenomenon of delayed and spontaneous PCL deficiency resulting in "symptomatic flexion instability" and posterior tibial polyethylene wear (Fig. 74–2). PCL insufficiency in cruciate-retaining arthroplasties, caused by a variety of mechanisms, may be a much more frequent cause of painful dysfunction than previously realized.

A cadaver study demonstrated that PCL failure by avulsion occurs after an average of 8.6 mm of tibial bone resection.[19] The level of tibial bone resection during total knee arthroplasty often approaches or surpasses 8 mm, and, despite the appearance of a competent ligament at surgery, the ligament may be compromised enough to eventually fail postoperatively. To avoid compromise of the PCL, tibial bone resection must be kept to a minimum, especially when the osteotomy is performed with a posterior inclination. Minimal bone resection and retention of the PCL mandate the use of thin polyethylene tibial components, which heightens the concern for eventual polyethylene failure. Interestingly, the emerging epidemic of catastrophic polyethylene failure after total knee arthroplasty has been primarily reported in cruciate-retaining designs and is essentially unheard of with cruciate-substituting designs.[31]

SURGICAL TECHNIQUE

The surgical approach for the cruciate-sacrificing knee design is the same as for cruciate-retaining designs except that resection of the PCL often facilitates soft tissue balancing and minimizes the extent of ligamentous release required to achieve appropriate extremity alignment. Tibial plateau exposure improves after resection of the PCL because of the increased ease of anterior tibial subluxation. Although most of the surgical technique is similar to that used for the cruciate-retaining total knee arthroplasty, there are some specific differences.

Careful preoperative templating usually alerts the surgeon to the possibility of femoral-tibial size mismatch in a given patient. Many current posterior-stabilized designs do allow mismatching of the tibial and femoral components, but when a system is used that does not allow this mismatch, it is helpful to cut and size the tibia before the femur. Although this size mismatch is uncommon, it is best to anticipate this difficulty and use a knee system that allows mismatch or preserves the PCL for the total knee arthroplasty in these knees.

Resection of the PCL, beginning with the femoral attachment, is best performed with a cautery knife in an effort to coagulate the multiple small vessels surrounding the posterior cruciate ligament (Fig. 74–3). These vessels can be difficult to address if the tourniquet is deflated after insertion of the tibial component.

A femoral alignment reference system is used in all designs (Fig. 74–4). The femoral housing of the posterior-stabilized prosthesis requires additional removal of bone in the intercondylar notch region by either resection or reaming, depending on the design chosen. During the removal of bone, the medial-lateral location of the intercondylar resection guide must be carefully positioned to avoid excessive excavation of a femoral condyle or excessive prosthesis translation. Use of

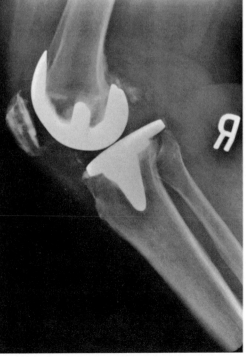
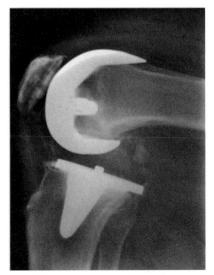

Figure 74–2. Lateral (**A**) and stress view (**B**) radiographs demonstrating posterior tibial subluxation caused by posterior cruciate ligament insufficiency of spontaneous onset 9 months following cruciate-retaining total knee arthroplasty.

A   B

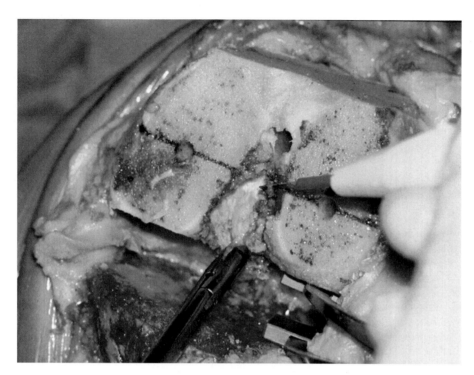

Figure 74–3. To minimize bleeding, both cruciate ligaments are released from the intracondylar notch by cautery knife.

sizing jigs or careful observation of the intercondylar notch sizing with the trial components is important to avoid condylar fracture during the seating of an uncemented femoral component. Osteoporotic bone is prone to fracture if the component is impacted with the bone cement in a viscous or doughy state of polymerization because the femoral housing and cement may act as a wedge against the epicondyle. Finally, the tibial cut does

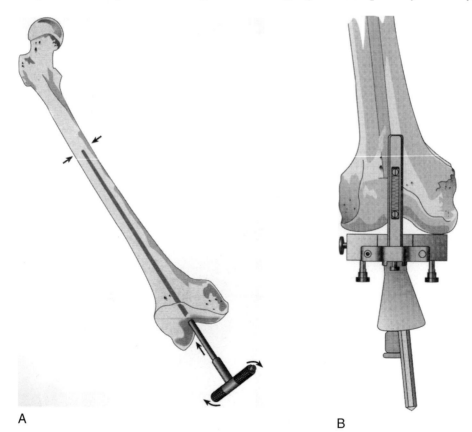

A

B

Figure 74–4. **A**, Posterior cruciate-substituting systems typically employ intramedullary femoral alignment systems. **B**, The femoral valgus orientation may be varied depending on the pathology. This is of value with the design for angular deformity.

Illustration continued on opposite page

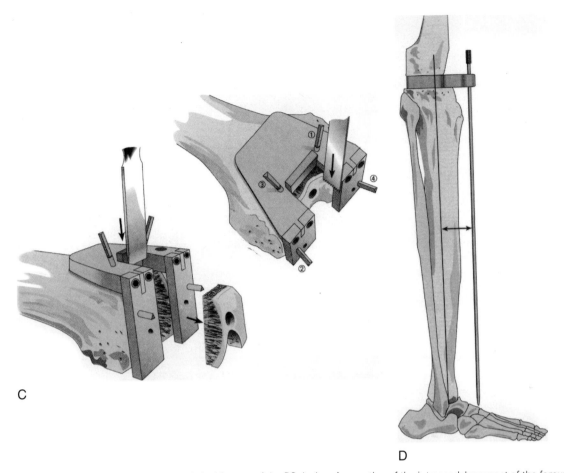

C

D

Figure 74–4. *Continued.* **C**, The unique technical feature of the PS design. A resection of the intracondylar aspect of the femur has been performed to accommodate a femoral component design that articulates with the tibial insert. (**D**) Although all systems align with the long axis of the tibia, the posterior tilt of the tibial cut is eliminated or minimized in most systems.

not employ a posterior slope because this can cause impingement on the tibial condylar eminence at full extension.

For modular metal-backed tibial designs, the tourniquet can be deflated before placement of the polyethylene insert; however, if an all-polyethylene tibial component is chosen, we recommend that hemostasis with tourniquet deflation and reinflation be obtained before the tibial component is cemented.

CLINICAL RESULTS

Numerous retrospective studies of posterior cruciate-sacrificing total knee arthroplasties have demonstrated consistently good clinical results and excellent intermediate-term survival. In 224 total condylar arthroplasties with an all-polyethylene tibial component, the 15-year success rate was 91 percent, with an annual failure rate of 0.65 percent.[25] Ranawat documented clinical survivorship of 91 percent and roentgenographic survivorship of 89 percent at 11 years of follow-up after total condylar arthroplasty.[20] Despite these favorable results, knee function was compromised by limitation of postoperative flexion to less than 100 degrees and an abnormal pattern of stair climbing.

The posterior-stabilized knee design met the initial goals of improved range of knee motion and stair climbing.[11] In the initial report of Insall, the mean range of motion improved from 95 degrees preoperatively to 115 degrees postoperatively. One third of patients achieved greater than 120 degrees of knee flexion. Seventy-six percent of patients were able to navigate stairs without aids, a significant improvement compared with the total condylar design. Other authors have suggested that ultimate range of motion is not dependent on knee design but rather is directly correlated with the preoperative range of motion only.[17] The only prospective randomized study available demonstrates a significantly better range of motion with the posterior-stabilized knee design.[9]

Although stair climbing was significantly improved with the posterior-stabilized design, it has been shown that the gait in these patients is abnormal when ascending stairs.[1,2] This abnormal pattern of stair climbing is characterized by a forward lean of the body and decreased knee flexion, however, the clinical significance of this abnormal gait pattern is unknown.

In a comparative study of 30 patients with paired bilateral total knee arthroplasties, one cruciate retaining and one cruciate substituting, no significant differences in knee scores or patient satisfaction were correlated with knee design at 2 to 5 years after surgery.[3] One third of patients preferred the posterior-stabilized design, one third chose the cruciate-retaining design, and one third indicated no preference. These authors suggested that the final decision regarding the choice of prosthesis design would hinge on the long-term survival of the various implants and not on knee function.

Long-term survival of the posterior-stabilized knee design has been very encouraging.[5,22,24–26,28,38,42,43,48,49] Font-Rodriquez and colleagues[48] reported on survival without revision or recommended revision in 91 percent of 215 PCL-sacrificing arthroplasties at 20 years, 94 percent of 265 PCL-stabilized arthroplasties (all-polyethylene tibia) at 16 years, 98 percent of 2036 PCL-stabilized arthroplasties (metal-backed tibia) at 14 years, and 94 percent of 49 PCL-stabilized arthroplasties (modular components) at 10 years.[47] The trend of improved results in this retrospective cohort analysis may reflect refinement of surgical technique. The 2-year, 5-year, and 10-year survival rates of the cruciate-retaining condylar knee arthroplasty have been reported as high as 99 percent, 98 percent, and 91 percent, respectively, whereas the posterior-stabilized design has 2-year and 5-year survival rates of 99 percent and 97 percent.[22] This analysis included only metal-backed tibial cruciate-retaining components and both all-polyethylene and metal-backed tibial posterior cruciate-substituting components. The posterior stabilized design was selectively used for the more complex arthroplasties.[8,22]

In an original cohort of 289 cemented posterior-stabilized total knee arthroplasties with an all-polyethylene tibial component, the 13-year survivorship was 94 percent for an annual failure rate of 0.4 percent.[28] From the same institution, of 102 consecutive total knee arthroplasties with a cemented posterior-stabilized design using a metal-backed tibial component, there were no instances of tibial loosening, polyethylene failure, or massive osteolysis.[5] The 12-year survivorship in these patients was 96.4 percent, with an annual failure rate of 0.3 percent.

In Laskin's review of total knee arthroplasties in the presence of fixed varus contracture of at least 15 degrees, 10-year Kaplan Meier survivorship was 92 percent, with a posterior-stabilized design (Insall-Burstein), and 72% with a cruciate-retaining design ($P < 0.01$).[42]

Similar outcomes have been obtained with other stabilized designs. Emmerson and colleagues have shown a cumulative survival rate of 95 percent at 10 years and 87 percent at 13 years with the kinematic stabilizer prosthesis.[48] Ranawat and colleagues reviewed the 4- to 6-year results with the press-fit condylar modular posterior-cruciate substituting design.[43] They found the rate of survival to be 97 percent of 125 knees, with nonprogressive radiolucent lines present at the cement-bone interface in 39 percent.

These results are unmatched by any other knee design, and there are no reports of cruciate-retaining knee arthroplasties with this length of follow-up and excellent success of implant survival. Based on the available literature, some believe that the cemented posterior-stabilized knee design represents the gold standard for implant survival.

COMPLICATIONS

Complications have been reported that are specifically related to, or more commonly associated with, the posterior-stabilized knee prosthesis.

The Patella

Patellofemoral complications appear to be more common with the posterior-stabilized design compared with the sacrificing (total condylar) design.[11] Significant patellofemoral complications were noted in 11 percent of patients in retrospective reviews of posterior-stabilized prostheses.[8,11] The overall rate of patellar fracture in posterior-stabilized total knee arthroplasties was 7 percent of 100 Insall-Burstein I total knee prostheses.[45] Patellar fractures in knees with posterior-stabilized components have been correlated with the need for lateral release[33] and the thickness of the patellar button.[11]

There have been no comparative clinical series between the cruciate-retaining and cruciate-substituting designs regarding patellofemoral malfunction and the difficulties observed with metal-backed patellae have further complicated the ability to compare these knee designs.

Patellar clicking at the terminal extension was described in 16 patients with a posterior-stabilized total knee arthroplasty who did not meet specific implant position criteria.[6] These criteria include (1) posterior positioning of the tibial component on the tibial plateau, (2) joint line height alteration of more than 8 mm, and (3) maintenance of patellar height between 10 and 30 mm. Careful preoperative planning to place the tibial components in the optimal position and to maintain the joint line height within the suggested range of implant position offers optimal function and avoidance of terminal patellar clicking with the posterior-stabilized total knee arthroplasty.[6]

Eleven of 635 patients developed symptomatic peripatellar intra-articular fibrous bands, the so-called tethered patella syndrome, characterized by painful popping, catching, grinding, or jumping of the patellar component in the radiographic absence of patellar malalignment.[30] Two of the 11 prostheses were cruciate-retaining designs, whereas the remaining prostheses were posterior stabilized. Three types of fibrous bands were identified at arthroscopy: (1) a transverse band preventing patellar seating in the femoral component sulcus; (2) a band extending from the infrapatellar fat pad to the superolateral patella, which tethers the patella laterally; and (3) a band extending from the inferior pole of the patella to the intercondylar region, which tethers the patella inferiorly. Arthroscopic resection of these bands was successful in all patients.

The patellar clunk syndrome describes a phenomenon observed exclusively in the posterior-stabilized design.[2,4,10,34] Patients experience an audible, painful clunk because of a suprapatellar fibrous nodule that wedges into the intercondylar notch during knee flexion and dislodges during knee extension at approximately 35

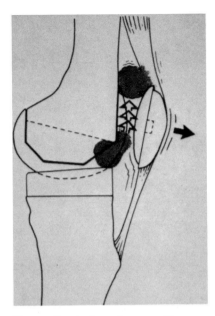

Figure 74–5. The patellar clunk syndrome—a fibrous nodule trapped in the intercondylar notch becomes dislodged with knee extension at 30 to 40 degrees. (From Hozack WJ, Rothman RH, Booth RE Jr, Balderston RA: The patellar clunk syndrome: A complication of posterior stabilized total knee arthroplasty. Clin Orthop 241:203, 1989.)

degrees (Fig. 74–5). Onset of symptoms in 20 patients occurred postoperatively at an average of 10.7 months (range, 2 to 34 months).[2] Unlike patients with the tethered patella syndrome, these patients do not have diminished range of motion. Initial nonoperative management of quadriceps rehabilitation and injection was successful in 4 patients, and duration of nonoperative management averaged 5 months. Arthroscopic resection of the fibrous nodule was successful in 7 of 11 patients, and resection at arthrotomy was successful in 3 others. Although earlier reports had implicated proximal overhang of the polyethylene patellar dome as an etiologic factor,[10] subsequent experience has demonstrated that the sharp edge of the femoral sulcus of the original Insall-Burstein design is the primary underlying factor.[2] After identification of these patellofemoral problems, modification of this femoral component reduced the incidence of patellofemoral complications in this design to 3 percent.[50]

Ranawat's experience with the press-fit condylar prosthesis has shown a low prevalence of patellofemoral complications with this design.[43] Eight percent (10 of 125 knees) had symptoms of pain or effusion at 4.8-year follow-up. There was 1 vertical patella fracture and no knees with patellar clunk or instability. Overall, with modern femoral component designs, patellofemoral complications now appear to be no more common in posterior-stabilized designs than in cruciate-retaining designs.

Fracture

Intercondylar distal femoral fracture is a unique complication of posterior-stabilized total knee arthroplasty, reported in 40 of 898 knees.[15] Nondisplaced fractures in 35 knees and 4 displaced fractures fixed with AO screws caused no adverse effect with the routine postoperative rehabilitation protocol. A sizing block for the intercondylar bone resection has apparently eliminated this complication because no fractures have occurred in the subsequent 532 arthroplasties.[15]

Dislocation

Dislocation of a posterior-stabilized prosthesis has been sporadically reported and associated with revision surgery or extensive lateral release in a patient with severe preoperative valgus limb alignment.[7,8] The largest series, describing 15 cases of dislocation in a group of 3032 posterior-stabilized arthroplasties, correlated dislocation with a change in the prosthetic design.[14] Four dislocations (0.02 percent) occurred with the original Insall-Burstein design (IB-I) compared with 10 (2.5 percent) with the IB-II design, which had diminished the tibial post height by 2 mm and additionally moved the post posteriorly another 2 mm. The IB-II modified design restored the original height and position of the tibial spine, and the incidence of dislocation was reduced to 0.2 percent. Reduction under anesthesia followed by long leg casting for 2 to 3 weeks, quadriceps rehabilitation, and a gradual knee flexion program was successful in 11 of 15 patients. Three of the IB-II designs redislocated and were successfully treated with conversion to an IB-II-modified tibial tray.

Wear, Osteolysis

Although there have been no major series revealing an increased incidence of osteolysis, there have been isolated case reports of this problem. Our interpretation of this experience is that the modular posterior-cruciate-substituting (PS) design is considerably more prone to excessive wear than the monoblock PS design (Fig. 74–6). In fact, modularity is probably of greater relevance in the posterior–cruciate-retention (CR) than in the PS design when wear and osteolysis are considered.

Mayo Clinic Experience

Although the currently published data are encouraging, we are beginning to see a disturbing increase in problems with the tibial component of the design most commonly used at the Mayo Clinic. The reasons for reoperation for tibial component problems, wear and osteolysis, are shown in Table 74–1. These reasons are not dramatically different from problems and lysis

Table 74–1. CAUSES OF 125 CRUCIATE-SUBSTITUTING TIBIAL INSERT REVISIONS

Revision Etiology	No.
"Failed" tibial implant	95
Osteolysis	19
Wear	11
Total	125

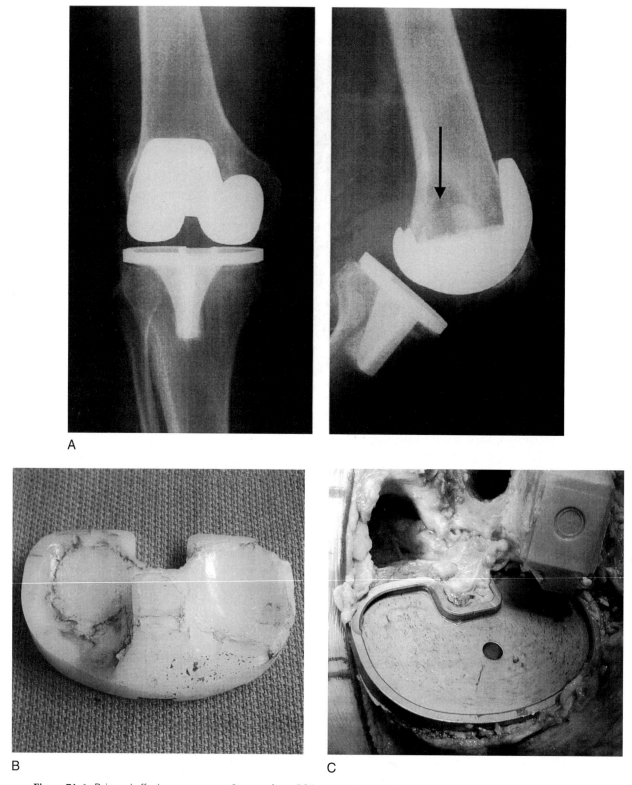

Figure 74–6. Pain and effusion was present 6 years after a PS knee replacement in a 56-year-old man. Osteolysis was present (*arrow*) (**A**). At revision, considerable wear was present at the medial eminence and at both weight-bearing portions of the tray (**B**). The "underside" wear was considerable and the probable cause of most of the lysis (**C**).

associated with cruciate-retaining designs. The problems are principally related to the modular design, regardless of the management of the cruciate ligament. We are currently analyzing these data to better understand the issue, even as this text goes to press.

AUTHOR'S PREFERRED METHOD

Historically, the philosophy at the Mayo Clinic has been to preserve the posterior cruciate ligament whenever possible during total knee arthroplasty; however,

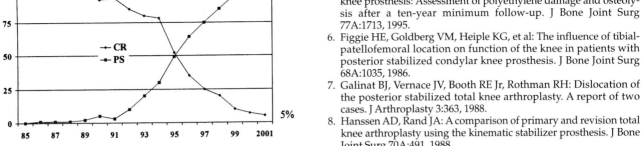

Figure 74–7. Depiction of the trend of Mayo Clinic use of posterior–cruciate-retention (CR) and posterior–cruciate-substituting (PS), designs 1985–June 2001.

this view has changed in the past few years (Fig. 74–7). Currently, 95 percent of our primary total knee arthroplasties use a posterior-stabilized design. Many surgeons have lowered their threshold for the use of a posterior–cruciate-substituting prosthesis in the presence of severe flexion contracture or severe angular malalignment. The best reported survivorship of posterior-stabilized total knee arthroplasty with a metal-backed tibial component is 98 percent at 14 years, and this rate represents the standard by which other knee designs must be judged.[5] However, we must emphasize that this implant was a single-piece, nonmodular design. Although we continue to find the PS design philosophy very attractive, we are currently reassessing our experience and approach, based on data acquired on this design. The hope and expectation is that the problems that do exist with the PS concept are amenable to femoral/tibial design modifications, especially those related to the modular design.

Editor's Note

The topic and issue of osteolysis will emerge as a major consideration over the next several years, just as it has been known to exist with the modular cruciate-retaining implants. Increasing problems with osteolysis are beginning to emerge with the PS designs as well. The extent of these problems appears to be design specific. We recommend continued caution in selection of the CR or PS designs (BFM).

References

1. Andriacchi TP, Galante JO: The influence of total knee-replacement design on walking and stair climbing. J Bone Joint Surg 64A:1328, 1982.
2. Andriacchi TP, Galante JO: Retention of the posterior cruciate in total knee arthroplasty. J Arthroplasty 3(Suppl):S13, 1988.
3. Becker MW, Insall JN, Faris PM: Bilateral total knee arthroplasty: One cruciate retaining and one cruciate substituting. Clin Orthop 271:122, 1991.
4. Beight JL, Yao B, Hozack WJ, et al: The patellar "clunk" syndrome after posterior stabilized total knee arthroplasty. Clin Orthop 299:139, 1994.
5. Colizza WA, Insall JN, Scuderi GR: The posterior stabilized total knee prosthesis: Assessment of polyethylene damage and osteolysis after a ten-year minimum follow-up. J Bone Joint Surg 77A:1713, 1995.
6. Figgie HE, Goldberg VM, Heiple KG, et al: The influence of tibial-patellofemoral location on function of the knee in patients with posterior stabilized condylar knee prosthesis. J Bone Joint Surg 68A:1035, 1986.
7. Galinat BJ, Vernace JV, Booth RE Jr, Rothman RH: Dislocation of the posterior stabilized total knee arthroplasty. A report of two cases. J Arthroplasty 3:363, 1988.
8. Hanssen AD, Rand JA: A comparison of primary and revision total knee arthroplasty using the kinematic stabilizer prosthesis. J Bone Joint Surg 70A:491, 1988.
9. Hirsch HS, Lotke PA, Morrison LD: The posterior cruciate ligament in total knee surgery. Save, sacrifice, or substitute? Clin Orthop 309:64, 1994.
10. Hozack WJ, Rothman RH, Booth RE Jr, Balderston RA: The patellar clunk syndrome. A complication of posterior stabilized total knee arthroplasty. Clin Orthop 241:203, 1989.
11. Insall JN, Lachiewicz PF, Burstein AH: The posterior stabilized condylar prosthesis: A modification of the total condylar design. Two- to four-year clinical experience. J Bone Joint Surg 64A:1317, 1982.
12. Khoury F, Stern SH, Cardin L, Stulberg SD: Anterior posterior translation in total knee arthroplasty: Does the posterior cruciate ligament function in vivo? Presented at the Annual Meeting of the American Academy of Orthopaedic Surgeons. New Orleans, March 1, 1994.
13. Paletta G, Laskin RS: Total knee arthroplasty after a previous patellectomy. J Bone Joint Surg 77A:1708, 1995.
14. Lombardi AV, Mallory TH, Vaughn BK, et al: Dislocation following primary posterior stabilized total knee arthroplasty. J Arthroplasty 8:633, 1993.
15. Lombardi AV, Mallory TH, Waterman RA, Eberle RW: Intercondylar distal femoral fracture: An unreported complication of posterior stabilized total knee arthroplasty. J Arthroplasty 10:643, 1995.
16. Lotke PA, Corces A, Williams JL, Hirsch HS: Strain characteristics of the posterior cruciate ligament after total knee arthroplasty. Am J Knee Surg 6:104, 1993.
17. Maloney WJ, Schurman DJ: The effects of implant design on range of motion after total knee arthroplasty. Total condylar versus posterior stabilized total condylar designs. Clin Orthop 27:147, 1992.
18. McLain RF, Bargar WF: The effect of total knee design on patellar strain. J Arthroplasty 1:91, 1986.
19. Ochsner JL, McFarland G, Baffes GC, Cook SD: Posterior cruciate ligament avulsion in total knee arthroplasty. Orthop Rev 22:1121, 1993.
20. Ranawat CS, Boachie-Adjei O: Suvivorship analysis and results of total condylar knee arthroplasty: Eight-to eleven-year follow-up period. Clin Orthop 266:6, 1991.
21. Ranawat CS, Hansraj KK: Effect of posterior cruciate sacrifice on durability of the cement-bone interface. A nine-year survivorship study of 100 total condylar knee arthroplasties. Orthop Clin North Am 20:63, 1989.
22. Rand JA, Ilstrup DM: Survivorship analysis of total knee arthroplasty. Cumulative rates of survival of 9200 total knee arthroplasties. J Bone Joint Surg 73A:397, 1991.
23. Scott RD, Volatile TB: Twelve years experience with posterior cruciate-retaining total knee arthroplasty. Clin Orthop 206:100, 1986.
24. Scott WN, Rubinstein M: Posterior stabilized knee arthroplasty: Six years' experience. Clin Orthop 205:138, 1986.
25. Scott WN, Rubinstein M, Scuderi G: Results after knee replacement with a posterior cruciate-substituting prosthesis. J Bone Joint Surg 70A:1163, 1988.
26. Scuderi GR, Insall JN, Windsor RE, Moran MC: Survivorship of cemented knee replacements. J Bone Joint Surg 71B:798, 1989.
27. Stern SH, Moeckel BH, Insall JN: Total knee arthroplasty in valgus knees. Clin Orthop 273:5, 1991.
28. Stern SH, Insall JN: Posterior stabilized prosthesis. Results after follow-up of nine to twelve years. J Bone Joint Surg 74A:980, 1992.
29. Teeny SM, Krackow KA, Hungerford DS, Jones M: Primary total knee arthroplasty in patients with severe varus deformity. A comparative study. Clin Orthop 273:19, 1991.

30. Thorpe CD, Bocell JR, Tullos HS: Intra-articular fibrous bands. Patellar complications after total knee replacement. J Bone Joint Surg 72A:811, 1990.

31. Tsao A, Mintz L, McRae CR, et al: Failure of the porous coated anatomic prosthesis in total knee arthroplasty due to severe polyethylene wear. J Bone Joint Surg 75A:19, 1993.

32. Tria AJ, Harwood DA, Alicea JA, Cody RP: Patellar fractures in posterior stabilized knee arthroplasties. Clin Orthop 299:131, 1994.

33. Vernace JV, Rothman RH, Booth RE Jr, Balderston RA: Arthroscopic management of the patellar clunk syndrome following posterior stabilized total knee arthroplasty. J Arthroplasty 4:179, 1989.

34. Walker PS, Hsieh HH: Conformity in condylar replacement knee prostheses. J Bone Joint Surg 59B:222, 1977.

35. Walker PS, Garg A: Range of motion in total knee arthroplasty. A computer analysis. Clin Orthop 262:227, 1991.

36. Whiteside LA, Amador DD: Rotational stability of a posterior stabilized total knee arthroplasty. Clin Orthop 242:241, 1989.

37. Windsor RE, Scuderi GR, Moran MC, Insall JN: Mechanisms of failure of the femoral and tibial components in total knee arthroplasty. Clin Orthop 248:15, 1989.

38. Cash RM, Gonzalez MH, Garst J: Proprioception after arthroplasty. Role of the posterior cruciate ligament. Clin Orthop 331: 172, 1996.

39. Simmons S, Lephart S, Rubash H, et al: Proprioception following total knee arthroplasty with and without the posterior cruciate ligament. J Arthroplasty 11:763, 1996.

40. Lattanzio PJ, Chess DG, MacDermid JC: Effect of the posterior cruciate ligament in knee-joint proprioception in total knee arthroplasty. J Arthroplasty 13:580, 1998.

41. Pereira DS, Jaffe FF, Ortiguera C: Posterior cruciate ligament-sparing versus posterior cruciate ligament-sacrificing arthroplasty. J Arthroplasty 13:138, 1998.

42. Laskin RS: Total knee replacement with posterior cruciate ligament retention in patients with a fixed varus deformity. Clin Orthop 331:29, 1996.

43. Ranawat CS, Luessenhop CP, Rodriguez JA: The press-fit condylar modular total knee system. Four- to six-year results with a posterior-cruciate substituting desing. J Bone Joint Surg 79A, 1997.

44. Laskin RS, Maruyama Y, Villaneuva M, Bourne R: Deep-dish congruent tibial component use in total knee arthroplasty. A randomized prospective study. Clin Orthop 380:36, 2000.

45. Thadani PJ, Vince KG, Ortaaslan SG, et al: Ten- to 12-year followup of the Insall-Burstein I total knee prosthesis. Clin Orthop 380:17, 2000.

46. Stiehl JB, Komistek RD, Dennis DA: Detrimental kinematics of a flat on flat total condylar knee replacement. Clin Orthop 365:139, 1999.

47. Stiehl JB, Komistek RD, Dennis DA, et al: Pluoroscopic analysis of kinematics after posterior-cruciate-retaining knee arthroplasty. J Bone Joint Surg 77B:884, 1995.

48. Font-Rodriguez DE, Scuderi GR, Insall JN: Survivorship of cemented total knee arthroplasty. Clin Orthop 345:79, 1997.

49. Emmerson, KP, Moran CG, Pinder, IM: Survivorship analysis of the kinematic stabilizer total knee replacement. A 10- to 14 year follow-up. J Bone Joint Surg 78-B:441, 1996

50. Scuderi, GR, Insall, JN: Performance of cruciate ligament substituting total knee arthroplasty. In Insall, JN, Scott, WN, Scuderi GR (eds): Current Concepts in Primary and Revision Total Knee Arthroplasty. Philadelphia, Lippincott-Raven, pp 41-45, 1996 .

75

Uncemented Total Knee Arthroplasty

• MARK W. PAGNANO, PANAYIOTIS J. PAPAGELOPOULOS, and JAMES A. RAND

OVERVIEW

The purported benefits of uncemented fixation in total knee arthroplasty (TKA) include more durable long-term fixation than can be achieved with cement. The rationale behind uncemented fixation is that a dynamic biologic interface between prosthesis and bone will hold up better over time than the static interfaces between prosthesis-cement-bone. A review of the available data, however, shows that uncemented TKA is not more durable than cement and has proved less reliable, in most instances, than cemented fixation. For those reasons, uncemented total knee prostheses have not been used at the Mayo Clinic since the early 1990s. Nonetheless, uncemented fixation continues to enjoy some degree of popularity in the United States, particularly as part of a so-called hybrid knee arthroplasty with an uncemented femoral fixation and a cemented tibial component.

The "Hybrid." It is very difficult to determine whether bone grows into the implant. Almost all retrieved implants have been surgical specimens from symptomatic patients. Bone ingrowth has occurred in less than 10 percent of the porous surfaces and has been located most frequently adjacent to porous-coated pegs or screws (Fig. 75–1).[23] Bone ingrowth has been found most consistently adjacent to the femoral component. The frequency of fibrous tissue ingrowth into tibial components has been high. Whether or not fibrous ingrowth will provide long-term satisfactory fixation is unknown. Therefore, some have advocated cement fixation for the tibial implant. Hence, the rationale for the hybrid implant.

INDICATIONS AND CONTRAINDICATIONS

The indications for uncemented TKA remain controversial. Uncemented fixation typically has been suggested for those patients who are (1) physiologically young, (2) of ideal body weight, (3) cooperative and willing to restrict activities after surgery, and (4) who have good bone quality and quantity.

Uncemented TKA is contraindicated in patients who are (1) of markedly advanced age; (2) have metabolic bone disease; (3) have osteopenia; and (4) who are unwilling or unable to cooperate with restricted weight bearing early after surgery.

Hybrid Total Knee Arthroplasty. A cemented tibia coupled with an uncemented femur has come to be considered a compromise between the two forms of fixation (Fig. 75–2). More problems have emerged on the tibial side of uncemented designs as the degree and extent of bone ingrowth have been variable and unpredictable. In contrast, femoral fixation has been reliably obtained with many uncemented designs and loosening has been less problematic. Uncemented knee components do cost more than comparable cemented components and appear to require a greater degree of surgical accuracy in implantation, thus calling into question the usefulness of the hybrid approach. Because isolated femoral component loosening is an uncommon cause of revision after cemented TKA arthroplasty, the hybrid approach probably adds little benefit. The hybrid knee is discussed in detail in the following sections.

Final Determination. The surgeon must make the final decision whether to use uncemented fixation at the time of surgery. Good surgical technique is required to prepare the bony surfaces for an uncemented implant. Implant-to-bone apposition must be ensured, with no gaps of more than 1 mm at all interfaces. The implant must also be inherently stable throughout a range of motion, with no tendency to rock or toggle, particularly in deep flexion. If any of these criteria are not satisfied, the surgeon is obligated to proceed with cemented fixation of the implant.

PROCEDURE

Implant Selection

A wide variety of uncemented implant designs are currently available. The optimal pore size is probably in the range of 200 to 400 mm with a 20- to 30-percent porosity.[10] Fixation pegs and stems should not be

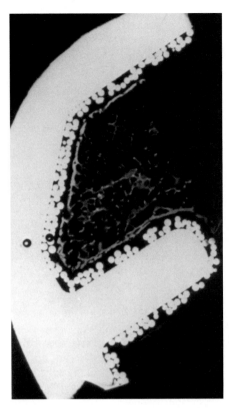

Figure 75–1. Histologic appearance of retrieved porous femoral component, revealing primarily fibrous tissue ingrowth.

porous coated, in order to prevent stress shielding and bone resorption in the metaphysis.[9] Whether porous pegs; long, straight stems; polyethylene pegs; screws; or finned stems should be used for proximal fixation is undetermined. The trend has been to increase the quality of initial tibial fixation. Hence, the optimal amount and type of fixation that will provide initial stability for ingrowth yet prevent long-term problems of stress shielding are unknown. In an in vitro study under eccentric loading of 225 N, sinking on the loaded side occurred with liftoff on the opposite side.[52] An implant with a central stem and peripheral pegs displayed less motion than did designs with short medial and lateral pegs. Another in vitro study that used an axial load of 500 N and an anterior shear force of 750 N, a central stemmed or bladed design provided the best resistance to offset loading.[56] In shear and torque, short pegs close to the periphery or a central stem with blades produced the least interface displacement.[56] In yet another in vitro study, the most rigid implant fixation occurred with use of four peripherally placed, 6.5-mm cancellous screws.[35] A central stem added only stability to the screws in cases of poor-quality bone (Fig. 75–3). In a final in vitro study, four cancellous screws piercing the proximal tibial cortex decreased liftoff and sinking of the tibial component under cyclic loading.[37] The addition of a central sleeve decreased liftoff but not sinking. In 447 cementless tibial components inserted without screws, partial radiolucent lines were present in 24 percent compared with 4 percent of 1442 components fixed with screws.[59] The possibility of press-fit, uncemented, noningrowth fixation has been assessed.[21] A comparison of 26 cemented and 49 uncemented tibial components using a press-fit Kinematic prosthesis found 96 percent good or excellent results in the cemented knees compared with 77 percent in the press-fit knees.[38] Ten of the press-fit tibial components required revision.

The Patella. Patellar fixation with uncemented implants has typically been reliable, but most metal-backed patellar components have suffered because of problems with premature polyethylene wear. A notable exception has been the mobile bearing metal-backed patellar component of the low contact stress design, which has demonstrated a good track record.[11] Nonetheless, strong consideration should be given to the use of a cemented, all-polyethylene patellar component in all TKAs.

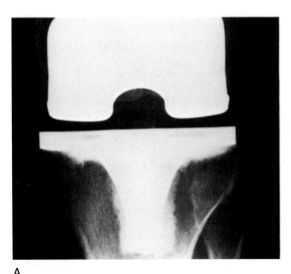

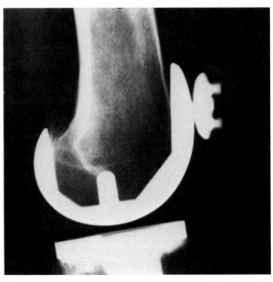

A   B

Figure 75–2. Anteroposterior (**A**) and lateral (**B**) radiographs of hybrid press-fit condylar knee with cemented tibia and uncemented femur and patella.

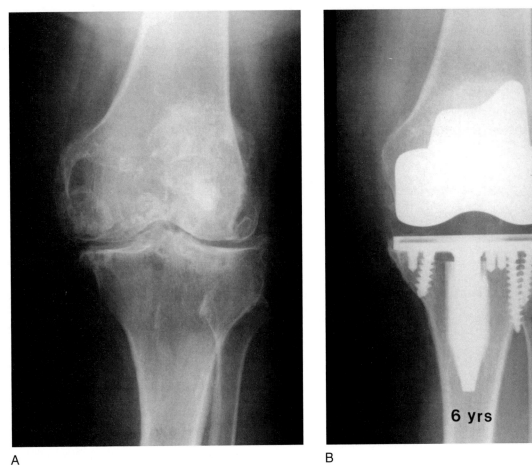

A   B

Figure 75–3. Severe arthritis in an 80-year-old woman (**A**) with a successful clinical and radiographic outcome 6 years after replacement with an uncemented, stemmed implant (Arthroloc) (**B**).

Surgical Technique

The surgical technique for uncemented fixation is similar to that used in cemented arthroplasty. Implant position, alignment, and soft tissue balance must be correct, with good stability and adequate motion. One of the major advances in TKA in the past two decades has been the development of instrumentation systems that produce accurate bone cuts. Regardless of the implant selected, almost all instrumentation systems are accurate and combine intramedullary and extramedullary alignment guides. Soft tissue balance in both flexion and extension remains of great importance and must be thoroughly assessed by the surgeon.

Careful surgical technique is required to achieve bone apposition within 1 mm on all cut surfaces. The saw blade should be allowed to work slowly through the bone. A saw that is forced through the bone with pressure may deviate from the desired path. Each cut surface must be checked to ensure that both the medial and lateral sides are parallel and flat. Because each subsequent bone cut relies on the accuracy of the previous cut, accuracy in the initial bone cuts is essential. Instrument systems that use a milling device instead of a saw blade may improve the precision of bony preparation needed for an uncemented implant.

After the bone cuts have been completed, trial reduction of the components should reveal no bone implant gaps greater than 1 mm. The implants must be stable in both flexion and extension, with balanced soft tissues. A common problem is to have anterior liftoff of the tibial component from the tibia-on-knee flexion. The posterior capsule tightness and the inclination of the tibial cut in the sagittal plane should be checked. A 5- to 7-degree position slope of the tibia usually prevents posterior tibial impingement in flexion. The degree of tibial slope depends on implant type. If the posterior cruciate is too tight, a posterior cruciate recession (selective release of the anterior fibers from the tibia) should be performed.

Once a satisfactory trial reduction has been achieved and the appropriate holes for implant fixation are made, a slurry of bone is placed over the cut tibial bone surface. An acetabular reamer, as used in total hip arthroplasty, is used to obtain bone from the previously removed tibial plateau. The ground bone is mixed with a small amount of saline and crushed in a small basin to a fine slurry. This bone paste is placed on the tibial surface to fill the spaces between bone trabeculae.

The real tibial component is then impacted into position. The real femoral component is placed. If any small gaps are present between implant and bone, some of the bone slurry is placed in the gap. The polyethylene patellar implant should be cemented. Once all components are placed, stability of the implants and knee stability and motion are assessed. If all implants are stable, routine closure is performed. If any implant shows rocking or motion between the implant and bone, it should be removed and fixed with cement.

Rehabilitation

Physical therapy is begun on postoperative day 1 or 2. Active and active-assisted motion exercises and quadriceps strengthening are started. The goal is for the patient to achieve 90 degrees of knee flexion before dismissal from the hospital. Toe-touch weight bearing is enforced for the first 4 to 8 weeks postoperatively. Between 4 and 8 weeks postoperatively, progressive weight bearing then is performed with bilateral support. At 8 to 12 weeks, the patient progresses to a single cane or no aids, as tolerated.

RESULTS

The outcome of uncemented replacement is best discussed according to type of implant design, *hybrid fixation*, and Mayo Clinic experience.

Porous-coated Arthroplasty (PCA)

A comparative study of 100 cemented kinematic knees and 50 uncemented PCA knees at 2 years found higher knee scores for the cemented arthroplasties; the reoperation rate was 4 percent for the cemented knees and 12 percent for the uncemented prostheses.[48] Another study of 55 uncemented PFC TKA was compared retrospectively with a matched group of 51 cemented PFC TKA at a mean follow-up of 10 years.[20] There were 10 revisions in the uncemented group for tibial or femoral loosening or lysis compared with 2 revisions in the cemented group. Survival to revision of the femoral or tibial component or radiographic failure was 94 percent in the cemented group and 72 percent in the uncemented group at 10 years (Fig. 75–4).

In a prospective study of the PCA prosthesis, 26 knees with uncemented fixation were compared with 25 knees with cement fixation at 3 years.[18] Good or excellent results were achieved in 69 percent of the uncemented and 68 percent of the cemented knees (nonsignificant). Blood loss was higher and radiolucent lines, loose beads, and tibial components subsidence were more frequent in the uncemented knees.

The PCA design provided 92 percent to 95 percent good to excellent results with uncemented fixation at 2 years and 93 percent good to excellent results at 5 years with or without cement fixation.[24] An additional comparative study of 110 cemented kinematic knees and 50 uncemented PCA knees at 2 years found higher knee scores for the cemented arthroplasties; the reoperation rate was 4 percent for the cemented knees and 12 percent for the uncemented prostheses.[48]

The Miller-Galante prosthesis has been extensively studied, and in several randomized studies, it has been reported this knee revealed comparable results with cemented and uncemented fixation.[31,39,47,49] The results have declined over time.[5,31,47,49] A comparison of 116 cemented with 123 cementless prostheses was performed at 3 to 6 years after arthroplasty.[49] Failure occurred in 7 cemented and 5 cementless knees. In a prospective randomized study of the Miller-Galante prosthesis, 183 knees with cementless fixation were

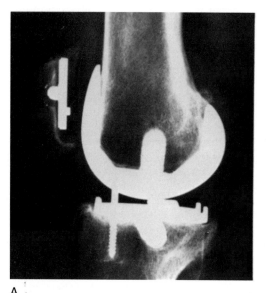
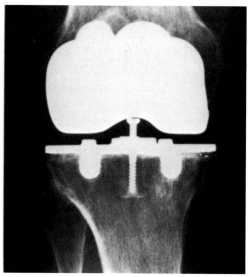

A   B

Figure 75–4. Anteroposterior (**A**) and lateral (**B**) radiographs of porous-coated anatomic knee at 5 years. There are loose beads adjacent to the tibial component, which has subsided anteriorly into the tibia. The patella is loose radiographically.

compared with 209 knees with hybrid fixation.[47] At 3 years after arthroplasty, the Hospital for Special Surgery (HSS) score was 85 in the cemented and 87 in the cementless knees. The reoperation rate was 9 percent for the cemented compared with 8 percent for the cementless knees. One study included 113 consecutive cementless Miller-Galante I knees that were prospectively followed for a mean of 11 years.[5] Five tibial components loosened and were revised, and more than 50 percent of the tibias had clear radiolucent lines beneath the tray. Three large osteolytic lesions developed beneath stable tibial components. No femoral components were revised for loosening, but 12 were revised because of damage induced by wear-through of a metal-backed patellar component. Based on these results, those authors have abandoned cementless fixation in TKA.

Low Contact Stress (LCS)

The results of cementless fixation with the meniscal bearing and rotating platform versions of the low contact stress (LCS) design have been satisfactory (Fig. 75–5). Sorrells et al. reported on 665 cementless rotating platform LCS knees operated between 1984 and 1995 and found an 11-year survivorship of 94.7 percent.[53] Jordan et al. reported on 473 cementless meniscal-bearing LCS knees operated between 1985 and 1991.[28] Seventeen revisions were done in that series, and the cumulative rate of survival with mechanical failure as the endpoint was 94.6 percent at 8 years. Buechel and Pappas followed 25 knees with the cementless bicruciate retaining meniscal bearing LCS knee and had a 6-year survivorship of 100 percent.[12] These same authors reported 98.1 percent 6-year survivorship with the cementless rotating platform LCS knee and 97.9 percent 6-year survivorship with the cementless meniscal bearing LCS design.[12]

OTHER EXPERIENCE

The results of completely uncemented total knee arthroplasty have consistently been less satisfactory than those of cemented designs at short-term follow-up (2 to 5 years) and at mid-term follow-up (5 to 10 years). The early results with the Freeman-Swanson and Freeman-Samuelson designs provided satisfactory results in 81 to 82 percent of cases.[1,2,8]

The results of other experiences with uncemented fixation have varied. Using the Tricon prosthesis with cementless fixation of both components report good or excellent results in all 48 knees at 7 years after arthroplasty.[34] However, tibial component subsidence of 1 to 2 mm occurred in 10 percent, and 3 percent had more than 2 mm of subsidence. With an endpoint of revision, a 92 percent survivorship was predicted at 7 years. Using the Anatomic Graduated Component (AGC) prosthesis with cementless fixation in 72 knees, at 3 years the mean HSS knee score was 92.[29] However, tibial component subsidence occurred in 4 patients. With an endpoint of revision, a survivorship of 88 percent at 3 years was found for the cementless knees compared with 99 percent for a prior series of cemented knees using the same prosthesis design.

An additional survival analysis and radiologic review was performed on a comparative series of cemented (150) and uncemented (201) implants.[15] The incidence of loosening of the femoral component at 6 years was 9.8 percent with uncemented fixation and 0.6 percent with cement (*P*<0.05).[15] Among uncemented prostheses, there was no difference in the survival or radiologic outcome with the use of either a stem or two condylar pegs.

Yet, in another randomized prospective study, the results of 139 prostheses were reported at 5 years. No statistically significant difference was found between cemented and uncemented fixation.[36] Overall, knee motion was similiar in both groups, from 5 to 100 degrees of flexion. On the basis of the knee scoring system of the HSS, 97 percent of the cemented knees and 83 percent of the uncemented knees achieved good to excellent results (*P* <.05). This difference could not be attributed to differences in the preoperative knee scores (similar in both groups).[36]

Using the AGC prosthesis with uncemented fixation in 72 knees, at 3 years the mean HSS knee score was 92.[34] However, tibial component subsidence occurred in 4 patients. With an endpoint of revision, a survivorship of 88 percent at 3 years was found for the uncemented knees compared with 99 percent for a

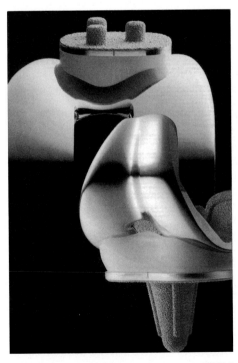

Figure 75–5. The uncemented low contact stress (LCS) knee has a reported survivorship of more than 95 percent at 8 to 11 years of follow-up. In no studies to date, however, has the durability of the cemented Insall-Burstein I knee or the cemented anatomic graduated component knee been met or exceeded by an uncemented design at comparable periods of follow-up.

prior series of cemented knees that used the same prosthesis design.

More recently, 144 knees showed a survival rate at 79 percent at a follow-up period of 10 years. Uncemented fixation of this design with use of macrointerlocking pegs and no other stabilization resulted in poor fixation and a high revision rate.[45]

In a retrospective study of 1000 performance TKAs, 584 were uncemented and 416 were cemented in both femoral and tibial components. The average subjective and functional Knee Society scores were 91.2 and 90.1 for patients with uncemented and 89.6 and 83.5 for those with cemented knee replacements.[4]

Whitesides assessed 184 Ortholock-I uncemented femoral and tibial components employing a tibial stem.[60] One knee loosened during the 15- to 18-year follow-up period and was revised, and 5 knees were revised for infection. Survival rate at 18 years, considering loosening, was 98.6 percent (see Fig. 75–3).

In another prospective randomized study, 96 cemented and 96 noncemented TKAs were performed. The mean duration of the operation was significantly longer (more than 10 minutes) for the cemented prostheses, and the total scores for the two groups were similar (143 and 140, respectively). Although the clinical outcomes were comparable, the quality of the fixation was significantly better with cemented arthroplasty.[22]

Mayo Clinic Experience—Complete Uncemented Fixation

Comparative Study. The Mayo Clinic experience with uncemented fixation began in November 1981, with the PCA prosthesis, as part of a multicenter prospective study; a comparison group of cemented implants of the same design was matched retrospectively to the prospectively studied uncemented design.[44]

Forty-one uncemented knees were compared with 50 cemented knees at 2 years after operation. The patients receiving the uncemented implant were, on average, 10 years younger than the cemented implant group and had had more previous surgery. The uncemented group had a longer recovery time than the cemented group. At 2 months postoperatively, the uncemented group had more pain, limp, need for ambulatory support, and need for support when ascending stairs. However, at 2 years, these differences had largely disappeared.

The press-fit condylar prosthesis, which incorporates a larger, finned stem in the tibia, has been studied by us with cemented and uncemented fixation.[43] A prospective study of 59 uncemented and 59 cemented knees was performed at 2.8 years postoperatively. The groups were not exactly comparable because the patients in the uncemented group were 9 years younger than those in the cemented group. The preoperative knee scores were similar at 56 plus or minus 11 in both groups. At review, the HSS score was 88 plus or minus 7 in the cementless knees compared to 86 plus or minus 10 in the cemented knees (nonsignificant).

HYBRID RESULTS

Midterm results with hybrid TKAs fail to show a clinically significant benefit in regard to implant durability, reliability of fixation, pain relief, or improvement in function for uncemented fixation over cemented fixation. The gold standard in implant durability is the cemented posterior-stabilized Insall-Burstein I implant with a one-piece metal-backed tibial component that has a 14-year survivorship of 98.7 percent.

Mayo Clinic Experience—Hybrid Fixation

Two reports outline our experience with hybrid fixation and with uncemented fixation on both the femoral and tibial sides. Duffy et al. retrospectively matched a group of 55 uncemented press fit condylar (PFC) knees with a group of cemented PFC total knees at a mean of 10 years of follow-up.[20] Survival to revision or radiographic failure was 94 percent in the cemented group and 72 percent in the uncemented group. Campbell et al. reviewed 74 consecutive hybrid PFC total knees at a mean follow-up of 7.4 years and found that 9 knees had been revised and that the femoral component was the source of failure in 8 of those 9 cases.[13] Implant survivorship at 5 years was 85 percent. In contrast, a survivorship analysis done by Whaley et al. of our experience with 1000 consecutive cemented cruciate-retaining PFC total knees showed a 10-year survivorship of 97.3 percent.[58] In light of these results, we remain committed to cemented fixation at this time. We are vigilant for opportunities with new materials or prosthetic designs that one day could make the promise of improved fixation with an uncemented knee implant a reality. Hydroxyapatite has been applied to some knee systems to address the issue of fixation.[45,46] Early results are progressing.

Complications

There are no differences in incidence of thrombophlebitis whether cement is or is not used.[16] Most complications relate to implant fixation.

Implant subsidence into the tibia was a frequent finding in the uncemented PCA knees but not in those with cemented fixation.[18,19] The subsidence was anterior and medial into the tibia and resulted in a medial displacement of the mechanical axis of the limb. Implant subsidence also has been observed with the Freeman-Samuelson,[2] Miller-Galante,[32] and Tricon-M[33] prostheses. Implant subsidence appears to stop once a new subchondral plate forms beneath the tibial component, as evidenced by a sclerotic line on the radiograph.

Radiolucent lines have been observed frequently with cementless fixation. Fluoroscopically positioned radiographs are essential to identify radiolucent lines. In the PCA experience, radiolucent lines were observed adjacent to 26 percent of the cemented knees and 65 percent of the uncemented knees (P <.0001). Radiolucent lines were progressive in 3 percent of the cemented knees and 18 percent of the uncemented PCA knees. Tibial radiolucent lines correlated with more varus positioning of the tibial component, whereas femoral radiolucent lines correlated with a less valgus limb alignment. In the PFC knee, radiolucent lines 1 mm wide or greater were observed adjacent to the tibial component in 86 percent of the uncemented knees compared with 41 percent of the cemented knees. On the femoral side of the PFC knees, radiolucencies were seen in 50 percent of the uncemented knees and 20 percent of the cemented knees.

Loosening of beads from the porous coating was very frequent with the PCA device. Most of the bead shedding occurred either at operation or during the first 2 months postoperatively; it stopped once ingrowth stabilized the implant. In our uncemented PFC experience, 19 percent of tibial components and 8 percent of femoral components had shed beads. The only time progressive bead loosening was observed was when implant fixation was unstable. Rosenqvist et al.[50] found bead loosening in 19 of 32 uncemented PCA components; 73 percent of the loose beads occurred more than 3 months postoperatively. In another study,[14] loose beads were detected in 23 of 40 PCA knees at 13 months. Loosening of a few beads from the porous surface probably is not important in terms of structural integrity of the porous surface.[24] Bead loosening is only of concern if it is a progressive phenomenon, indicating unstable fixation.

Bone Ingrowth

It is very difficult to determine the frequency of fixation of porous implants by bone ingrowth.[42,51,54,57] Almost all retrieved implants have been surgical specimens from symptomatic patients. Bone ingrowth has occurred in less than 10 percent of the porous surfaces and has been located most frequently adjacent to porous-coated pegs or screws (see Fig. 75–1).[23] Bone ingrowth has been found most consistently adjacent to the femoral component. The frequency of fibrous tissue ingrowth into tibial components has been high. Whether or not fibrous ingrowth will provide long-term satisfactory fixation in unknown. The use of hydroxyapatite on the implant has revealed improved fixation characteristics.[46]

Metal Ion Release

A final unanswered question concerning uncemented implants concerns the long-term effects of metal ion release and corrosion. Ion release can be anticipated in view of the increased surface area provided by porous implants compared with nonporous implants. Metabolic, bacteriologic, immunogenic, and oncogenic effects of metals have been reported in experimental animals.[7] A study of ion release adjacent to the PCA knee prosthesis found no difference in levels of cobalt, chromium, and nickel in the urine of patients with cemented and uncemented prostheses.[26] Similar results have been reported from titanium devices.[25]

Polyethylene Wear and Osteolysis

There are few wear/lysis issues unique or characteristic of uncemented implants, and they can be seen around well fixed implants.[6] Catastrophic failure from polyethylene wear has been associated with posterior cruciate-retaining total knee designs with relatively flat articular surface geometries. In a study of 122 retrieved tibial components of cementless total knees, there was significant wear in 62 percent.[17] There was a positive correlation between the extent of wear and the level of contact stress, with noncongruent designs displaying greater wear. The PCA prosthesis has demonstrated a 4.5 percent revision rate in 176 knees at 4 years (Fig. 75–6).[30] Nine additional knees had more than 30 percent thinning of the polyethylene thickness. At revision, 4 of the knees had osteolytic areas in bone filled with particulate polyethylene debris. In another series of PCA prostheses, failure occurred in 19 of 108 cementless knees by 5 years.[27]

Osteolysis has been identified to 16 percent of 174 total knee arthroplasties with cementless fixation.[41] The areas of osteolysis correlated with polyethylene particles. The medial aspect of the tibial metaphysis was the most common location of osteolysis.

Osteolysis adjacent to screw holes was frequent, suggesting a pathway for polyethylene wear debris into the metaphysis.

Osteolysis from so-called backside or nonarticular surface wear of modular tibial inserts has emerged as a concern. Both uncemented and cemented implants can be affected. The cement-bone interface may act as a barrier

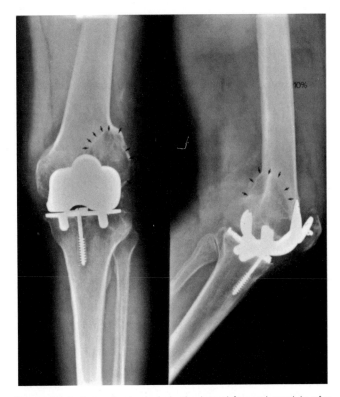

Figure 75–6. Area of osteolysis in the lateral femoral condyle of a 74-year-old man, resulting from polyethylene wear 9 years after insertion of a porous-coated anatomic total knee arthroplasty.

to the underlying metaphyseal bone, which may delay the onset of osteolysis in cemented TKAs. In contrast, the screws associated with some uncemented tibial trays may act as a conduit for wear debris and allow osteolytic lesions to develop more rapidly after uncemented TKAs.

AUTHOR'S PREFERENCE

It is our preference to use cement to fix all three components in TKA. Cemented fixation has proved reliable and durable, and the potential benefits of biologic fixation with an uncemented implant have not materialized. In our analysis, the concept of hybrid fixation is flawed. The surgeon and patient endure the added operative time to let the cement harden on the tibial and patellar sides and incur the added cost of an uncemented implant on the femoral side, but they gain no measurable benefit in regard to implant durability. We remain interested in future progress with implant materials and implant designs that could make uncemented TKA a reliable and durable option.

If an uncemented fixation is selected, surgical technique must be meticulous to avoid gaps between the implant and the host bone as well as to achieve initial stability. All bone cuts should be made with cutting blocks. There should be a gap of no more than 1 mm on any single cut bone surface with stable fixation of the implant. Smaller areas of bone deficiency should be filled with ground bone obtained from the cancellous bone removed at the time of arthroplasty. When an uncemented tibial component is used, ground bone graft is placed over the cancellous surface of the tibia, to fill voids in the cancellous bone followed by placement of the tibial component. Ancillary fixation of the tibial component with screws, pegs, or stems should be considered to improve initial fixation and prevent subsidence. There must be no motion of the tibial component throughout a range of motion or it should be removed and cement fixation used. Uncemented fixation of the patellar component is not used, because of problems of wear of metal-backed patellar components. Once all of the implants have been placed, it is essential to be sure that there is stability through a range of motion and appropriate soft tissue balance.

Rehabilitation after uncemented fixation is delayed compared with cement fixation. It is our preference to place the patient on partial weight bearing for the first 4 weeks to minimize micromotion around the cut surfaces, and then to progress to weight bearing gradually through 8 weeks, at which time crutches are discontinued commensurate with the patient's quadriceps strength after rehabilitation.

References

1. Albrektsson BEJ, Carlson LV, Freeman MAR, et al: Proximally cemented versus uncemented Freeman-Samuelson knee arthroplasty: A prospective randomized study. J Bone Joint Surg 74B:233, 1992.
2. Audell RA, Cracchiolo A III: The use of implants with polyethylene peg fixation in total knee arthroplasty. In Rand JA, Dorr LD (eds): Total Arthroplasty of the Knee: Proceedings of the Knee Society, 1985–1986. Rockville, MD, Aspen Publishers, 1987, p 179.
3. Baldwin JL, El-Saied R, Rubinstein RA Jr: Uncemented total knee arthroplasty: Report of 109 titanium knees with cancellous-structured porous coating. Orthopedics 19:123, 1996.
4. Bassett RW: Results of 1000 performance knees: Cementless versus cemented fixation. J Arthroplasty 13:409, 1998.
5. Berger RA, Jacobs JJ, Rosenberg AG, et al: Problems with cementless total knee arthroplasty at 11 years' follow-up. Presented at American Association of Hip and Knee Surgeons, Dallas, November 3–5, 2000.
6. Berry DJ, Wold LE, Rand JA: Extensive osteolysis around an aseptic, stable, uncemented total replacement. Clin Orthop 293:204, 1993.
7. Black J: Does corrosion matter? J Bone Joint Surg 70B:517, 1988.
8. Blaha JD, Insler HP, Freeman MAR, et al: The fixation of a proximal tibial polyethylene prosthesis without cement. J Bone Joint Surg 64B:326, 1982.
9. Bobyn JD, Cameron HU, Abdulla D, et al: Biologic fixation and bone modeling with an unconstrained canine total knee prosthesis. Clin Orthop 166:301, 1982.
10. Bobyn JD, Pilliar RM, Cameron HU, Weatherly GC: The optimum pore size for the fixation of porous-surfaced metal implants by the ingrowth of bone. Clin Orthop 150:263, 1980.
11. Buechel FF, Rosa RA, Pappas MJ: A metal backed rotating bearing patellar prosthesis to lower contact stress. An 11 year clinical study. Clin Orthop 248:34, 1989.
12. Buechel FF, Pappas MJ: Long term survivorship analysis of cruciate-sparing versus cruciate sacrificing knee prostheses using meniscal bearings. Clin Orthop 260:162, 1990.
13. Campbell MD, Duffy GP, Trousdale RT: Femoral component failure in hybrid total knee arthroplasty. Clin Orthop 356:58, 1998.
14. Cheng CL, Gross AE: Loosening of the porous coating in total knee replacement. J Bone Joint Surg 70B:377, 1988.
15. Chockalingam S, Scott G: The outcome of cemented vs. cementless fixation of a femoral component in total knee replacement (TKR) with the identification of radiological signs for the prediction of failure. Knee 7:233, 2000.
16. Clarke MT, Green JJ, Harper W, Gregg P: Cement as risk factor for deep-vein thrombosis. Comparison of cemented TKR, uncemented TKR and cemented THR. J Bone Joint Surg 80B:611, 1998.
17. Collier J, Mayor MB, McNamara JL, et al: Analysis of the failure of 122 polyethylene inserts from uncemented tibial knee components. Clin Orthop 273:232, 1991.
18. Collins DN, Heim SA, Nelson CL, Smith P: Porous-coated anatomic total knee arthroplasty: A prospective analysis comparing cemented and cementless fixation. Clin Orthop 267:128, 1991.
19. Dodd CAF, Hungerford DS, Krackow KA: Total knee arthroplasty fixation: Comparison of the early results of paired cemented versus uncemented porous-coated anatomic knee prostheses. Clin Orthop 260:66, 1990.
20. Duffy GP, Berry DJ, Rand JA: Cement versus cementless fixation in total knee arthroplasty. Clin Orthop 356:66, 1998.
21. Ewald FC, Walker PS, Poss R, et al: Uncemented, press-fit total knee replacement. In Rand JA, Dorr LD (eds): Total Arthroplasty of the Knee: Proceedings of the Knee Society, 1985–1986. Rockville, MD, Aspen Publishers, 1987, p 173.
22. Guicquel P, Kempf JF: Comparative study of fixation mode in total knee arthroplasty with preservation of the posterior cruciate ligament. Rev Chir Orthop Reparatrice Appar Mot 86:240, 2000.
23. Haddad RJ Jr, Cook SD, Thomas KA: Biological fixation of porous-coated implants. J Bone Joint Surg 69A:1459, 1987.
24. Hungerford DS, Krackow KA, Kenna RV: Two- to five-year experience with a cementless porous-coated total knee prosthesis. In Rand JA, Dorr LD (eds): Total Arthroplasty of the Knee: Proceedings of the Knee Society, 1985–1986. Rockville, MD, Aspen Publishers, 1987, p 215.
25. Jacombs JJ, Silverton C, Hallab NJ, et al: Metal release and excretion from cementless titanium alloy total knee replacements. Clin Orthop 358:173, 1999.
26. Jones L, Hungerford D, Kenna V: Metal ion release from cemented and cementless porous coated knee prosthesis. Orthop Trans 8:267, 1984.

27. Jones SMG, Pinder IM, Moran CG, Malcolm AJ: Polyethylene wear in uncemented knee replacement. J Bone Joint Surg 74B:18, 1992.

28. Jordan LR, Olivo JL, Voorhorst PE: Survivorship analysis of cementless meniscal bearing total knee arthroplasty. Clin Orthop 338:119, 1997.

29. Kavolus CM, Ritter MA, Keating EM, Faris PM: Survivorship of cementless total knee arthroplasty without tibial plateau screw fixation. Clin Orthop 273:170, 1991.

30. Kilgus DJ, Moreland JR, Finerman GAM, et al: Catastrophic wear of tibial polyethylene inserts. Clin Orthop 273:223, 1991.

31. Kobs JK, Lachiewicz PF: Hybrid total knee arthroplasty two to five year results using the Miller-Galante prosthesis. Clin Orthop 286:78, 1993.

32. Landon GC, Galante JO, Maley MM: Noncemented total knee arthroplasty. Clin Orthop 205:49, 1986.

33. Laskin RS: Tricon-M uncemented total knee arthroplasty: A review of 96 knees followed for longer than 2 years. J Arthroplasty 3:27, 1988.

34. Laskin RS: Total knee arthroplasty using an uncemented polyethylene tibial implant. Clin Orthop 288:270, 1993.

35. Lee RW, Volz RG, Sheridan DC: The role of fixation and bone quality on the mechanical stability of tibial knee components. Clin Orthop 273:177, 1991.

36. McCaskie AW, Deehan DJ, Green TP, et al: Randomized, prospective study comparing cemented and cementless total knee replacement: Results of press-fit condylar knee replacement at five years. J Bone Joint Surg 80B:971, 1998.

37. Miura H, Whiteside LA, Easley JC, Amador DD: Effects of screws and a sleeve on initial fixation in uncemented total knee tibial components. Clin Orthop 259:160, 1990.

38. Nafei A, Neilsen S, Kristen O, Hvid I: The press-fit Kinemax knee arthroplasty. J Bone Joint Surg 74B:243, 1992.

39. Nilsson KG, Karrholm, Linder L: Femoral component migration in total knee arthroplasty: Randomized study comparing cemented and uncemented fixation of the Miller-Galante I design. J Orthop Res 13:347, 1995.

40. Parker DA, Rorabeck CH, Bourne RB: Long-term follow-up of cementless versus hybrid fixation for total knee arthroplasty. Clin Orthop 388:68, 2001.

41. Peters PC, Engh GA, Dwyer KA, Vinh JN: Osteolysis after total knee arthroplasty without cement. J Bone Joint Surg 74A:864, 1992.

42. Pilliar RM, Lee JM, Maniatopoulos C: Observations on the effect of movement on bone ingrowth into porous-surfaced implants. Clin Orthop 208:108, 1986.

43. Rand JA: Cement or cementless fixation in total knee arthroplasty? Clin Orthop 273:52, 1991.

44. Rand JA, Bryan RS, Chao EYS, Ilstrup DM: A comparison of cemented versus cementless porous-coated anatomic total knee arthroplasty. In Rand JA, Dorr LD (eds): Total Arthroplasty of the Knee: Proceedings of the Knee Society, 1985–1986. Rockville, MD, Aspen Publishers, 1987, p 195.

45. Regner L, Carlsson L, Kärrholm J, Herberts P: Clinical and radiologic survivorship of cementless tibial components fixed with finned polyethylene pegs. J Arthroplasty 12:751, 1997.

46. Regner L, Carlsson L, Kärrholm J, Herberts P: Tibial component fixation in porosis and hydroxyapatite-coated total knee arthroplasty. A radiostereometric evaluation of migration and inducible displacement after 5 years. J Arthroplasty 15:681, 2000.

47. Rorabeck CM, Bourne RB, Lewis PL, Nott L: The Miller-Galante knee prosthesis for the treatment of osteoarthrosis. J Bone Joint Surg 75A:402, 1993.

48. Rorabeck CH, Bourne RB, Nott L: The cemented Kinematic-II and the non-cemented porous-coated anatomic prostheses for total knee replacement: A prospective evaluation. J Bone Joint Surg 70A:483, 1988.

49. Rosenburg AG, Barden RM, Galante JO: Cemented and ingrowth fixation of the Miller-Galante prosthesis. Clin Orthop 260:71, 1990.

50. Rosenqvist R, Bylander B, Knutson K, et al: Loosening of the porous coating of bicompartmental prostheses in patients with rheumatoid arthritis. J Bone Joint Surg 68A:538, 1986.

51. Samuelson KM: Fixation in total knee arthroplasty: Interference fit. In Rand JA, Dorr LD (eds): Total Arthroplasty of the Knee: Proceedings of the Knee Society, 1985–1986. Rockville, MD, Aspen Publishers, 1987, p 249.

52. Shimagaki H, Bechtold JE, Sherman RE, Gustilo RB: Stability of initial fixation of the tibial component in cementless total knee arthroplasty. J Orthop Res 8:64, 1990.

53. Sorrells RB: The rotating platform mobile bearing TKA. Orthopedics 19:793, 1996.

54. Stulberg SD, Stulberg BN: The biological response to uncemented total knee replacements. In Rand JA, Dorr LD (eds): Total Arthroplasty of the Knee: Proceedings of the Knee Society, 1985–1986. Rockville, MD, Aspen Publishers, 1987, p 143.

55. Summer DR, Turner TM: Effect of pegs and screws on bone ingrowth in cementless total knee arthroplasty. Clin Orthop 309:150, 1994.

56. Walker PS, Hsu HP, Zimmerman RA: A comparative study of uncemented tibial components. J Arthroplasty 5:245, 1990.

57. Walldius B: Arthroplasty of the knee using an endoprosthesis: 8 years' experience. Acta Orthop Scand 30:137, 1960.

58. Whaley D, Berry DJ, Harmsen SS: Survivorship of 1000 consecutive press-fit condylar total knees at an average 10 year follow-up. Presented at American Association of Hip and Knee Surgeons, Dallas, November 3–5, 2000.

59. Whiteside L: Four screws for fixation of the tibial component in cementless total knee arthroplasty. Clin Orthop 299:72, 1994.

60. Whitesides LA: Long-term follow-up of the bone-ingrowth Ortholoc knee system without a metal-backed patella. Clin Orthop 388:77, 2001.

76

Unicompartmental Knee Arthroplasty

• MARK W. PAGNANO and JAMES A. RAND

After three decades of experience with unicompartmental knee replacement, the procedure remains controversial, with conflicting results of success and failure. The conflicting data in the literature reflect differing patient selection criteria, variable surgical techniques, changing implant designs, and varying lengths of study after arthroplasty. In the 1990s, unicompartmental knee replacement was largely abandoned by most academic institutions in the United States. That was certainly the case at the Mayo Clinic; of more than 8500 primary total knee replacements that were done there in the 1990s only 3 unicompartmental knee replacements were performed. Unicompartmental replacement fell out of favor for several different reasons, but their unpopularity was attributable in large part to the remarkable success of total knee replacement. However, there has been a resurgence of interest in unicompartmental knee replacement. That interest has been sparked by the introduction of the so-called minimally invasive surgical technique and by the publication of favorable long-term survivorship data from several centers.

Unicompartmental arthroplasty has been advocated as a conservative surgical procedure. Because only the diseased compartment is resurfaced, the patellofemoral and contralateral compartments remain relatively undisturbed. In a study of 19 osteoarthritic knees, Brocklehurst et al. found that visually normal-appearing articular cartilage from osteoarthritic knees had values of water content, proteoglycan synthesis rates, and cell counts similar to those of normal controls.[7] Therefore, if the unresurfaced compartments appear "normal," resurfacing of the entire knee may be unnecessary. The mechanical durability of the cartilage and the effects of polyethylene and cement debris are unresolved.

The potential advantages of unicompartmental arthroplasty include preservation of bone stock, proprioception by the retained cruciate ligaments, relatively normal knee kinematics, and increased flexion, low infection rate, and little bleeding. A surgical technique that uses a small (3-inch) incision and avoids eversion of the patella and violation of the extensor mechanism has gained notice. Two groups of surgeons have applied this minimally invasive surgical technique to unicompart-

mental knee arthroplasty. The potential disadvantages of unicompartmental replacement are (1) failure to resurface all of the joint, which allows potential disease progression; (2) difficulty in surgical technique; and (3) high polyethylene stresses that may lead to loosening or wear a combination of the two (Table 76–1).

INDICATIONS AND CONTRAINDICATIONS

The ideal patient for unicompartmental total knee arthroplasty must be selected by age, weight, activity level, and extent of deformity. The physiologically older patient should be considered for unicompartmental or tricompartmental total knee arthroplasty, whereas the younger patient should be selected for osteotomy. The obese or high-activity-level patient will place excessive stresses on the arthroplasty, leading to loosening or accelerated polyethylene wear. Patients selected for unicompartmental arthroplasty should be close to their ideal body weight and lead sedentary lifestyles. Symptoms should be localized to the diseased compartment, with minimal symptoms in the patellofemoral joint. Preoperative rest pain should be minimized, with primarily weight-bearing pain.[25]

The range of motion of the knee should be from a flexion contracture of less than 5 degrees to at least 90 degrees of flexion.[25] Other authors have suggested that flexion contractures up to 15 degrees can be corrected with unicompartmental arthroplasty.[48] The extent of varus or valgus deformity should be limited. Varus angular deformity of up to 10 to 20 degrees or valgus angular deformity of up to 15 degrees of valgus has been successfully treated by unicompartmental arthroplasty.[25,48] We select knees with 10 degrees or less of valgus or varus deformity. Knees with more extensive deformity are more likely to have degenerative changes that could progress with time in the unresurfaced compartments. Knees with more extensive deformity may require soft tissue release to balance the ligaments of the knee. Because ligament releases are contraindicated in unicompartmental arthroplasty, severe deformities cannot be corrected adequately.

Table 76–1. UNICOMPARTMENTAL TOTAL KNEE

Advantages	Disadvantages
Preserves bone	Technically difficult
Preserves both cruciates	Strict patient selection
Increased range of motion	Potential increased wear
More normal proprioception	Higher failure rate
More normal kinematics	Disease progression

The contraindications to unicompartmental arthroplasty include inflammatory arthritis and chondrocalcinosis. The underlying disease process in inflammatory arthritis leads to progressive damage in the unresurfaced compartments. Relative contraindications include obesity, high activity level, fixed angular deformity, deficient anterior cruciate ligament, and prior patellectomy.

The ultimate decision of whether to perform unicompartmental or tricompartmental total knee arthroplasty must be made at surgery. There is no substitute for visual inspection of the joint surfaces and cruciate ligaments and assessment of soft tissue balance after joint débridement. If the anterior cruciate ligament is absent, tricompartmental replacement should be selected.[15] If eburnated bone is present in either the patellofemoral joint or the unresurfaced compartment, unicompartmental replacement should not be performed.[25]

It is extremely difficult to provide a meaningful comparison and analysis of the literature to determine the indications and relative value of the several options for treating unicompartmental disease. Nonetheless, what little data are available are shown in Table 76–2. A more comprehensive discussion of each relevant study would seem appropriate.

In a prospective study of 228 knees in 165 patients, each of the compartments of the knee at arthroplasty was graded for arthritic changes.[42] Criteria used for unicompartmental replacement were (1) age older than 60 years, (2) weight less than 82 kg, (3) relatively sedentary lifestyle, (4) flexion contracture no greater than 5 degrees; (5) angular deformity less than 15 degrees, (6) intact anterior cruciate ligament, and (7) no significant cartilage erosion in the opposite compartment. Only 13 knees (6 percent) fulfilled all selection criteria.[42] In contrast, when slightly different criteria were used, 207 of 208 knees prospectively studied were considered to be candidates for unicompartmental total knee arthroplasty.[11]

A comparison of 49 high tibial osteotomies (followed for 7.8 years) and 42 unicompartmental total knee arthroplasties (followed for 5.8 years) was performed.[8] Satisfactory clinical results were achieved in 76 percent of the unicompartmental arthroplasties compared with satisfactory results in 43 percent of the osteotomies. The latter figure is moderately less than what is typically reported in the literature. The revision rate was 7 percent for the unicompartmental arthroplasties compared with 20 percent for the osteotomies. Twenty patients with a unicompartmental arthroplasty in one knee and a total knee arthroplasty in the contralateral knee were evaluated at 3 years.[9] Good knee scores were obtained in 90 percent of the total knee group compared with 80 percent of the unicompartmental knee group at 1 year. The range of motion of the knee was 120 degrees for the unicompartmental group compared with 105 degrees for the total knee group. In another study of 23 patients with a unicompartmental arthroplasty of one knee and a total knee arthroplasty on the contralateral side who were followed for 81 months, 44 percent preferred the unicompartmental procedure, 12 percent preferred the total knee operation, and 44 percent could not tell the difference.[28] The range of motion was 123 degrees for the unicompartmental group compared with 100 degrees for the total knee arthroplasty group. In yet another study of 42 patients followed at 6.5 years, 50 percent preferred the unicompartmental side, 21 percent the total knee side, and 29 percent could not tell the difference.[13] A comparison of 120 unicompartmental arthroplasties and 81 tricompartmental total knee arthroplasties was performed at a mean of 78 and 68 months, respectively.[36] The Knee Society knee score averaged 85 for the tricompartmental arthroplasty group compared with 90 for the unicompartmental arthroplasty group. The reoperation rate was 4 percent for the unicompartmental patients compared with 19 percent for the total knee arthroplasty patients. The high reoperation rate in the total knee group reflected the use of older total knee designs.

Table 76–2. COMPARISON OF UNICOMPARTMENTAL TOTAL KNEE ARTHROPLASTY (UNI-TKA) WITH OSTEOTOMY OR TRICOMPARTMENTAL TOTAL KNEE ARTHROPLASTY

	Uni-TKA vs. Osteotomy					
	Osteotomy			Uni-TKA		
Authors	No. of Knees	Follow-Up (yr)	Good (percent)	No. of Knees	Follow-Up (yr)	Good (percent)
Broughton et al.[8]	49	5–10	43	42	5–10	76
Ivarsson and Gillquist[19]	10	1	40	10	0.5	80
	Uni-TKA vs Tricompartmental TKA					
	Tricompartmental			Uni-TKA		
	No. of Knees	Follow-Up (yr)	Good (percent)	No. of Knees	Follow-Up (yr)	Good (percent)
Cameron and Jung[9]	20	3	90	20	3	80
Laurencin et al.[28]	23	7	83	23	7	96
Newman et al.[34]	51	5	xx	51	5	xx

Newman et al. prospectively randomized 102 knees with unicompartmental disease to either unicompartmental or total knee replacement. Both groups had a preponderance of female patients with a mean age of 69 years. The patients in the unicompartmental group had less perioperative morbidity and an earlier hospital discharge than those in the tricompartmental group. At the 5-year follow-up, 2 unicompartmental knees and 1 total knee had been revised. The unicompartmental group had more excellent results and more knees able to flex beyond 120 degrees.

PROSTHESIS SELECTION

Making a decision regarding prosthesis selection requires that for unicompartmental arthroplasty the following alternatives be considered: prosthetic constraint, fixation mode, use of mobile or nonmobile polyethylene bearing, instrumentation for insertion, and choice of a metal-backed or all-polyethylene tibial component. Inherent in the concept of a unicompartmental prosthesis are design limitations. Because all ligaments are preserved, a minimal-constraint (i.e., flat) geometry for the tibial component must be employed, or a kinematic mismatch will exist between cruciate ligament retention and prosthetic constraint. Hodge and Chandler reported considerably better results after an unconstrained design was used than were achieved after use of a design with a more constrained geometry.[17] However, the low congruity between the femoral and tibial components implies the potential for high polyethylene stresses and polyethylene wear (Fig. 76–1).[17] A unique approach to this design problem is found in the meniscal-bearing Oxford prosthesis (see Fig. 76–9).[6,15] In a radiographic study of 20 knees, the bearings were found to move backward a mean of 4.4 mm in the medial compartment and 6.0 mm in the lateral compartment.[6]

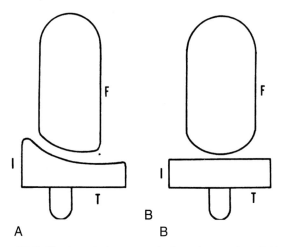

Figure 76–1. The two design concepts for unicompartmental knee replacement: (**A**) Constrained and (**B**) unconstrained. (From Hodge WA, Chandler HP: Unicompartmental knee replacement: A comparison of constrained and unconstrained designs. J Bone Joint Surg 74A:877, 1992, with permission.)

During rotational motion of the knee, the bearings in the medial and lateral compartments move in opposite directions. Bearing movement was confirmed at 5 years after arthroplasty. That prosthesis, however, is not approved for use in the United States.

The issue of bone preservation or sacrifice and the use of metal backing of the tibial component are interrelated. Thin polyethylene tibial components (less than 9 mm) have had a higher incidence of loosening.[32] If a thicker all-polyethylene tibial component is used, loosening decreases but bone is sacrificed. If a metal-backed tibial tray is used, fixation of the tibial component is improved. However, metal backing requires 2 to 3 mm of metal thickness, resulting in a thinner liner of polyethylene and the potential for polyethylene wear. A metal-backed component with a thicker polyethylene liner sacrifices additional bone.

TECHNIQUE

Each design has its own unique features for bone preparation. What is emphasized here are the principles, with no particular technique being favored or illustrated.

The technique of unicompartmental arthroplasty obviously differs from that of total knee arthroplasty. Surgical exposure should be performed through an anteromedial arthrotomy, even if a lateral unicompartmental replacement is performed. Because the decision regarding unicompartmental versus total knee arthroplasty is made at surgery, total knee replacement is more easily performed through an anteromedial than an anterolateral arthrotomy. The articular cartilage of the patella and the unresurfaced compartment must be protected to prevent damage or dessication. The anterior horn of the contralateral meniscus must be protected. A thorough débridement of osteophytes should be performed, which allows passive correction of alignment. The femoral and tibial components should cover the entire weight-bearing surface of the diseased compartment. The anterior edge of the femoral component must not impinge on the patella. The components should be inserted to allow slight opening of the knee in full extension, which avoids excess tension on the implant.[25,48] The mechanical axis of the limb must *not* be overcorrected to avoid overload of the unresurfaced compartment. The ideal location of the mechanical axis is in the midline of the knee or slightly toward the resurfaced compartment (Fig. 76–2).

The minimally invasive approach allows the unicompartmental knee to be operated through a smaller incision (Fig. 76–3). Typically, a 3-inch incision is employed for medical compartment arthroplasty, starting at the superomedial border of the patella and extending to the proximal medial border of the tibia. A vertical medial arthrotomy is made in line with the skin incision. Superiorly, the arthrotomy is extended medially by 1 inch, as in the initial portion of a subvastus approach to the knee. Distally, the medial meniscus and capsular tissue are freed from the anterior border of the tibia.

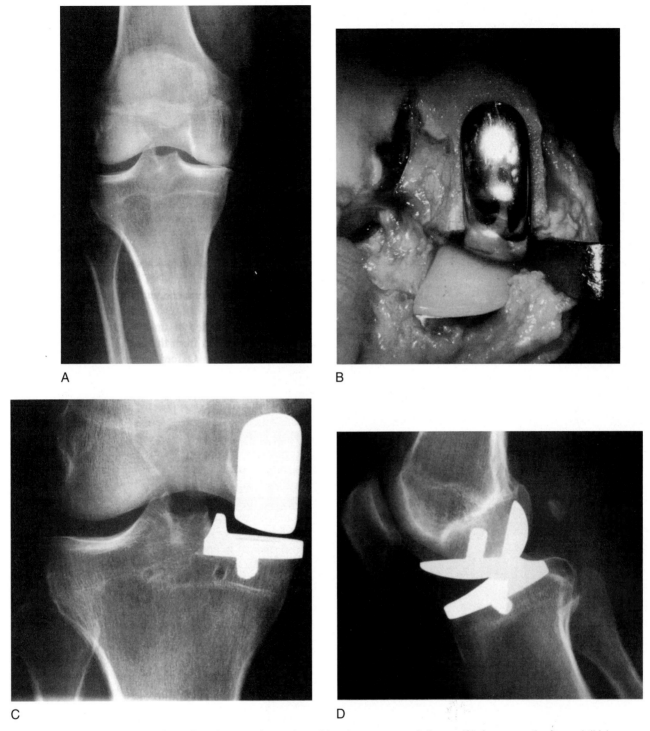

Figure 76–2. A 67-year-old man in 5 degrees of varus but with unicompartmental disease (**A**). At surgery the femoral-tibial alignment is well restored in extension and in flexion (**B**). The radiographs confirm the position and well-covered tibial bone by the implant in both frontal (**C**) and lateral (**D**) projections.

To provide additional exposure of the distal medial femoral condyle, a small portion of the medial facet of the patella can be removed. With combined distraction of the tibia and femur and external rotation of the tibia, reasonable exposure of the medial compartment can be achieved. Special instrumentation for the particular knee system selected is often of substantial benefit if the surgeon elects to try the minimally invasive approach.

RESULTS

Several studies have provided 10-year survivorship data regarding unicompartmental knee replacement.[3,5,23,33,35,37,41,44,46] In nearly all of these studies, the patients were predominantly women in the latter part of the seventh decade of life. Murray et al.[33] used the Oxford meniscal-bearing design in 143 knees with medial compartment disease and an intact anterior cruciate ligament. The clinical follow-up was a mean of 7.6 years. There were 5 revision operations done for a survival rate of 98 percent at 10 years. Squire et al.[41] reviewed a single surgeon's experience with the Marmor knee design, which incorporates an inset, all-polyethylene tibial component. One hundred-forty unicompartmental knees were done in that series, and 14 knees have subsequently been revised. The cumulative rate of survival at 22 years was estimated at 84 percent. Berger et al.[3] reported 62 consecutive unicompartmental knees done with a cemented, metal-backed tibial component in 51 patients with a mean age of 68 years. The mean follow-up was 7.5 years. The 10-year survivorship was reported as 98 percent. Those three studies have helped fuel the resurgence of interest in unicompartmental knee replacement. Nonetheless, the results of unicompartmental arthroplasty often are difficult to interpret because of differing implant designs, variable surgical technique, and different evaluation systems.

A review of results by implant design may provide a better understanding of results than a review of the results of a single surgeon.

The St. George Sled prosthesis was an early unicompartmental prosthesis that used an all-polyethylene, minimally constrained tibial component (Fig. 76–4).[14] A prospective study of 115 knees at 4.5 years revealed good or excellent results in 86 percent.[30] Survivorship using an endpoint of significant pain was 76 percent at 6 years. Seven knees were revised. In another prospective study of 102 knees, followed for 8 years, 78 percent good or excellent results were achieved.[26] The revision rate was 5 percent and the loosening rate 4 percent. In yet another study of 34 knees followed for 8 years, 68 percent satisfactory results were achieved.[21] A study of 575 knees over 9 years found a 1.2 percent revision rate and a 2.4 percent reoperation rate.[12]

The polycentric prosthesis was another early design that was frequently used for unicompartmental arthroplasty (Fig. 76–5). In a series of 207 unicompartmental

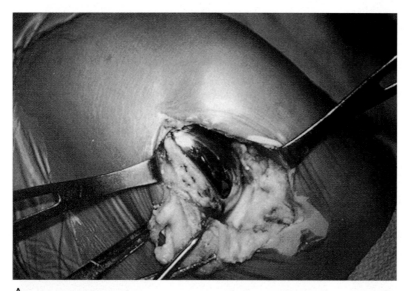

A

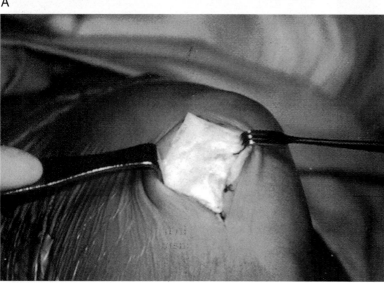

B

Figure 76–3. The so-called minimally invasive approach to unicompartmental knee arthroplasty involves the use of a 3-4 inch incision (**A**). The patella may be subluxed laterally but is not everted. With proper retractors a reasonable view of the medial compartment is afforded with this limited incision (**B**) and excellent results achieved (**C**).
Illustration continued on opposite page

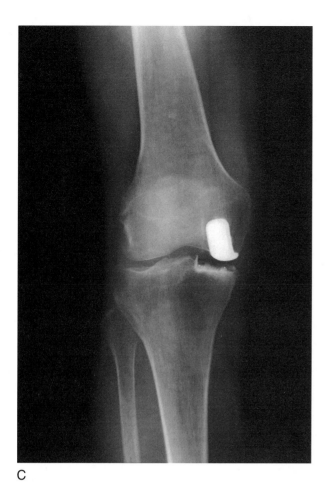

C

Figure 76–3. *Continued.*

arthroplasties followed for 2.6 years, of which 188 were polycentric implants, there was an 11 percent failure rate.[22] Varus limb alignment correlated with prosthetic failure, with 52 percent of the knees aligned in varus failing. Failure was also seen in those with technically well-performed procedures, probably the result of an inadequate early design. The polycentric prosthesis was modified into the Gunston-Hult unicompartmental design with a flat tibial plateau.[2] Of 77 knees followed for 10 years, there were 75 percent good or excellent results, with a 10 percent reoperation rate.[2] When properly balanced, this device was associated with a highly successful functional outcome (Fig. 76–6).

The Marmor modular prosthesis has been one of the most widely used unicompartmental arthroplasties (Fig. 76–7). In a report of 37 knees followed for 2 years, pain relief was achieved in only 65 percent.[27] The reoperation rate was 22 percent. Lateral compartment replacements appeared to have better results than medial compartment replacements. In a 4-year follow-up of 59 knees, 76 percent good or excellent results were achieved, with a 12-percent reoperation rate.[39] In contrast, a study of 72 knees at 4 years revealed 90 percent excellent pain relief, with only 1 reoperation.[1]

Using the second-generation modular prosthesis, 91 percent satisfactory results in 159 arthroplasties occurred at 4 years.[10] The revision rate was 5 percent. Marmor reported the results of 60 knees at a mean of 11 years.[32] Sixty-three percent good or excellent results were achieved. Nine of 21 failures were caused by loosening of 6-mm tibial components. A study of 63 unicompartmental knees at 7.4 years found 90 percent good or excellent results, with an 8 percent revision rate.[43] The results of Squire et al. with the Marmor implant have been noted earlier.

Figure 76–4. St. George Sled prosthesis. (From Engelbrecht E: The "Sled" prosthesis: A partial prosthesis for destructions of the knee joint. Chirurg 11:510, 1971. Copyright 1971, Springer-Verlag, with permission.)

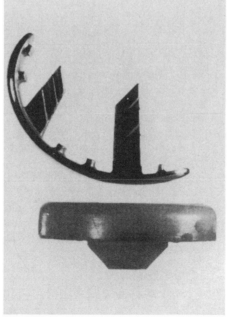
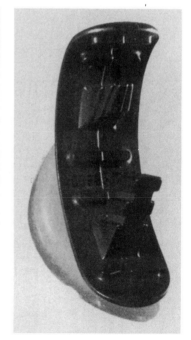

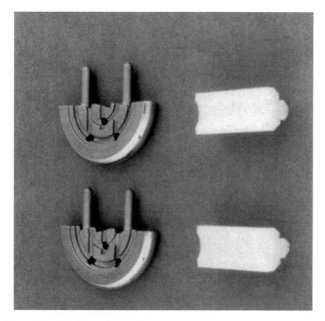

Figure 76–5. Polycentric prosthesis.

The Robert Breck Brigham Hospital prosthesis used a flat, all-polyethylene tibial component with cement fixation (Fig. 76–8).[38] Of 100 knees followed for 3.5 years, 92 percent achieved good pain relief. The average knee flexion was 114 degrees. At 7 years, the revision rate for this series was 7 percent[37] and at 10 years, it was 13 percent.[47] A study of 68 knees followed for 51 months revealed 80 percent good or excellent results, with 6 failures.[40] The prosthesis was modified to include a metal-backed tibial component. A study of 50 knees with the metal-backed tibial component, followed for 5.5 years, had 90 percent good or excellent results with no revision.[24]

The Oxford meniscal-bearing prosthesis was studied in 103 knees that were followed for 36 months (Fig. 76–9).[15] Pain relief was achieved in 96 percent, with a mean of 105 degrees for knee flexion. Nine knees required reoperation. The failure rate was 16 percent if the anterior cruciate ligament was deficient, compared with 4.8 percent if the anterior cruciate ligament was intact. As noted previously, Murray et al. have achieved a 10-year survivorship of 98 percent with use of this implant in selected patients.

Cementless fixation of unicompartmental prostheses has been less satisfactory than cement fixation. Of 28 PCA knees with cementless fixation followed for a minimum of 2 years, 71 percent had good or excellent results (Fig. 76–10).[4] Eleven knees had either been revised or were considered to be potential failures. A study of 41 cemented and 43 cementless PCA knees at 1 to 4 years found that 82 percent had good or excellent results, with 2 failures (1 in each group).[29] A study of 51 PCA knees with cementless fixation found at 2 years 90 percent satisfactory results.[31] A study of 82 cementless arthroplasties at 4 years revealed a 12 percent failure rate.[45] Survivorship was estimated at 81 percent at 8.5 years.

A study of 87 unicompartmental prostheses compared 50 knees with a flat, unconstrained tibial plateau with 26 PCA knees that had a constrained, sloped tibial plateau.[17] At 53 months, 98 percent of the unconstrained knees had good or excellent results compared with 70 percent of the constrained knees. Subsequent revision was required for 27 percent of the constrained prostheses compared with 8 percent of the unconstrained designs. A multicenter study of 294 unicompartmental cemented knees with an all-polyethylene tibial component revealed an 82 percent, 12-year survivorship.[16] There was no difference in survivorship between medial and lateral replacements.

COMPLICATIONS

The complications inherent in unicompartmental arthroplasty include all the problems associated with total knee arthroplasty, with the exception of patellar implant loosening. Sepsis is less frequent in unicompartmental than in total knee arthroplasty, being reported in less than 1 percent of knees.[12,15,17,32,38,43,45] Loosening has been the most frequent complication and is generally associated with thin, all-polyethylene tibial components[18,32] (Fig. 76–11). There are some additional complications unique to unicompartmental arthroplasty that are not seen with total knee arthroplasty. Progressive degeneration of the unresurfaced contralateral compartment of the knee occurs in 1 to 10 percent of knees.[17,32,43,45] Progressive degeneration of the unresurfaced compartment has frequently been related to overcorrection of limb alignment, with placement of excessive load on the unresurfaced compartment. Impingement of the anterior portion of the femoral component against the patella can cause pain in up to 3 percent of knees.[25] Subluxation of the tibia referable to the femur may occur because of poor ligament balance or component malposition.[25,47,48] Meniscal-bearing dislocation can occur with the meniscal-bearing knee in up to 3 percent of knees, more frequently in knees with a deficient anterior cruciate ligament.[15]

AUTHOR'S PREFERENCE

My preference (MWP) is to perform osteotomy about the knee for patients who are young, usually younger than 45 years of age. The ideal candidate for unicompartmental total knee arthroplasty is a lightweight, relatively sedentary person 70 years of age or older. Of course, the ultimate decision regarding unicompartmental or tricompartmental replacement must be made at the time of surgery based on the appearance of the articular surface and the status of the ligaments. Mild chondromalacic changes in the patellofemoral joint or lateral compartment are not considered contraindications to unicompartmental replacement, provided the patient meets the other criteria. A deficient

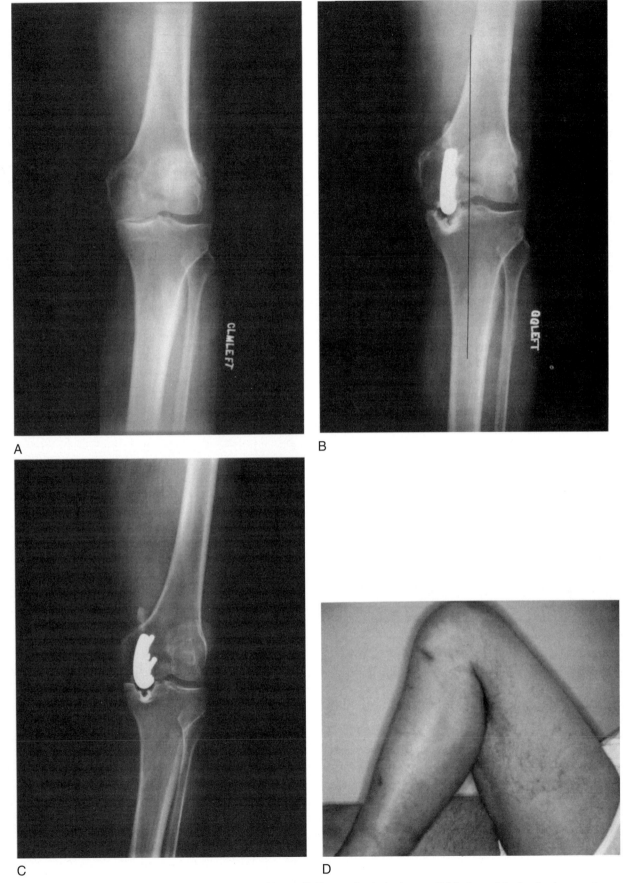

Figure 76–6. A, Medial gonarthrosis in a 64-year-old man. **B**, The mechanical axis was slightly toward the involved compartment after replacement. Nineteen years later, the implant is not loose (**C**) and excellent function persists (**D**).

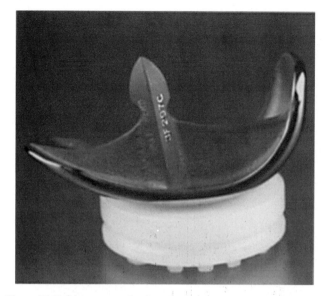

Figure 76–7. Marmor prosthesis.

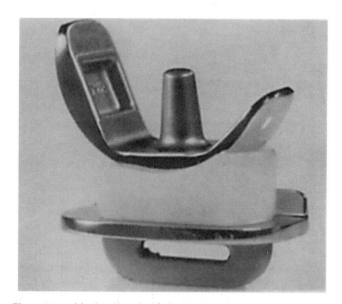

Figure 76–9. Meniscal-bearing Oxford prosthesis.

anterior cruciate ligament would be considered a contraindication to unicompartmental arthroplasty.

It is my (MWP) contention that at the present time, unicompartmental knee replacement represents an intellectually attractive option for the patient with isolated unicompartmental disease. However, several questions should be answered before the indications for unicompartmental arthroplasty are expanded: (1) Will unicompartmental replacement in younger patients be durable enough to supplant upper tibial osteotomy?

(Remember that most of the current long-term data are from elderly female patients.) (2) Can revision of minimally invasive unicompartmental "pre-total knees," in fact, be done without penalty? (Remember earlier reports of substantial bone loss requiring grafting or augmentation during conversion to total knee replacement.) (3) Will patients and surgeons be willing to accept a potentially higher rate of failure for lower morbidity and cost? (Minimally invasive techniques will always have a series of tradeoffs.)

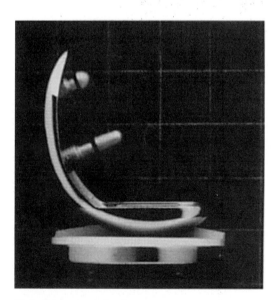

Figure 76–8. Brigham prosthesis.

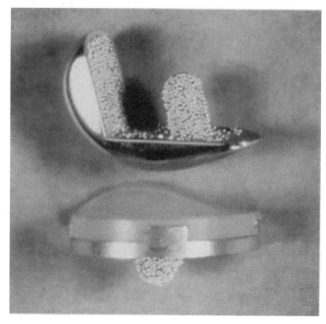

Figure 76–10. Porous-coated arthroplasty prosthesis.

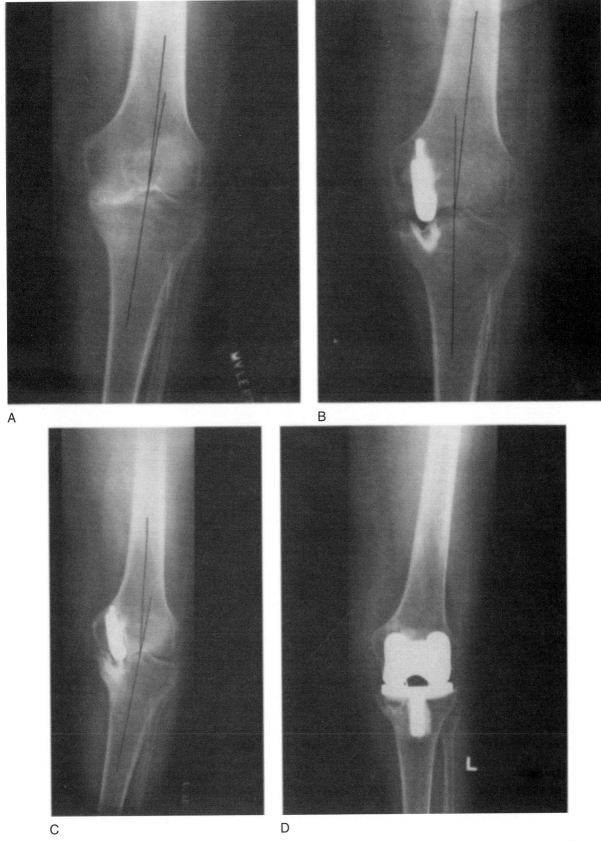

Figure 76–11. Medial gonarthrosis in a 60-year-old man (**A**). A polycentric replacement recreated a 4-degree anterior valgus alignment (**B**). This knee failed in 4 years (**C**), requiring a conversion to a condylar replacement (**D**).

References

1. Bae DK, Guhl JF, Keane SP: Unicompartmental knee arthroplasty for single compartment disease. Clin Orthop 176:233, 1983.
2. Barck AL: 10-year evaluation of compartmental knee arthroplasty. J Arthroplasty 4(Suppl):49, 1989.
3. Berger RA, Nedeff D, Borden R, Sheinkop R: Unicompartmental knee arthroplasty: clinical experience at 6-10 year follow up. Clin Orthop 367:50, 1999.
4. Bernasek TL, Rand JA, Bryan RS: Unicompartmental porous coated anatomic total knee arthroplasty. Clin Orthop 236:52, 1988.
5. Bert JM: 10 year survivorship of metal backed unicompartmental arthroplasty. J Arthroplasty 13:901, 1998.
6. Bradley J, Goodfellow JW, O'Conner JJ: A radiographic study of bearing movement in unicompartmental Oxford knee replacements. J Bone Joint Surg 69B:598, 1987.
7. Brocklehurst R, Bayliss MT, Maroudas A, et al: The composition of normal and osteoarthritic articular cartilage from human knee joints. J Bone Joint Surg 66A:95, 1984.
8. Broughton NS, Newman JH, Baily RAJ: Unicompartmental replacement and high tibial osteotomy for osteoarthritis of the knee. J Bone Joint Surg 68B:447, 1986.
9. Cameron HU, Jung YB: A comparison of unicompartmental knee replacement with total knee replacement. Orthop Rev 17:983, 1988.
10. Cartier P, Cheaib S: Unicondylar knee arthroplasty. J Arthroplasty 2:157, 1987.
11. Chesnut WJ: Preoperative diagnostic protocol to predict candidates for unicompartmental arthroplasty. Clin Orthop 273:146, 1991.
12. Christensen NO: Unicompartmental prosthesis for gonarthrosis: A nine-year series of 575 knees from a Swedish hospital. Clin Orthop 273:165, 1991.
13. Cobb AG, Kozinn SC, Scott RD: Unicondylar or total knee replacement: patient preference. J Bone Joint Surg 72B:166, 1990.
14. Engelbrecht E: The "Sled" prosthesis: A partial prosthesis for destructions of the knee joint. Chirurg 11:510, 1971.
15. Goodfellow JW, Kershaw CJ, Benson MK, O'Connor JJ: The Oxford knee for unicompartmental osteoarthritis. J Bone Joint Surg 70B:692, 1988.
16. Heck DA, Marmor L, Gibson A, Rougraff BT: Unicompartmental knee arthroplasty: A multicenter investigation with long-term follow-up evaluation. Clin Orthop 286:154, 1993.
17. Hodge WA, Chandler HP: Unicompartmental knee replacement: A comparison of constrained and unconstrained designs. J Bone Joint Surg 74A:877, 1992.
18. Insall JN, Aglietti P: A five to seven year follow-up of unicondylar arthroplasty. J Bone Joint Surg 62A:1329, 1980.
19. Ivarsson I, Gillquist J: Rehabilitation after high tibial osteotomy and unicompartmental arthroplasty. Clin Orthop 226:139, 1991.
20. Ivarsson IS, Gillquist J: The strain distribution in the upper tibia after insertion of two different unicompartmental prostheses. Clin Orthop 279:194, 1992.
21. Johnell O, Sernbo I, Gentz CF: Unicompartmental knee replacement in osteoarthritis: An 8 year follow-up. Arch Orthop Trauma Surg 103:371, 1985.
22. Jones WT, Bryan RS, Peterson LFA, Ilstrup DM: Unicompartmental knee arthroplasty using poly centric and geometric hemicomponents. J Bone Joint Surg 63A:946, 1981.
23. Knutson K, Lewold S, Robertsson O: The Swedish knee arthroplasty register: A nationwide study of 30,003 knees. Acta Orthop Scand 65:375, 1994.
24. Kozinn SC, Marx C, Scott RD: Unicompartmental knee arthroplasty: A 4.5 to 6 year follow-up study with a metal backed tibial component. J Arthroplasty 1(Suppl):1, 1985.
25. Kozinn SC, Scott R: Current concepts review: Unicondylar knee arthroplasty. J Bone Joint Surg 71A:145, 1989.
26. Larsson SE, Larsson S, Lundkvist S: Unicompartmental knee arthroplasty: A prospective consecutive series followed for six to eleven years. Clin Orthop 232:174, 1988.
27. Laskin RS: Unicompartmental tibiofemoral resurfacing arthroplasty. J Bone Joint Surg 60A:182, 1978.
28. Laurencin CT, Zelicof SB, Scott RD, Ewald FC: Unicompartmental versus total knee arthroplasty in the same patient. Clin Orthop 273:151, 1991.
29. Lindstrand A, Stenstrom A, Egund N: The PCA unicompartmental knee. Acta Orthop Scand 59:695, 1988.
30. MacKinnon J, Young S, Baily RAJ: The St. George Sled for unicompartmental replacement of the knee. J Bone Joint Surg 70B:217, 1988.
31. Magnussen PA, Bartlett RJ: Cementless PCA unicompartmental joint arthroplasty for osteoarthritis of the knee. J Arthroplasty 5:151, 1990.
32. Marmor L: Unicompartmental arthroplasty of the knee with a minimum ten year follow-up period. Clin Orthop 228:171, 1988.
33. Murray DW, Goodfellow JW, O'Connor JJ: The Oxford medial unicompartmental arthroplasty: A ten-year survival stusy. J Bone Joint Surg 80-B:983, 1998.
34. Newman JH, Akroyd CE, Shah NA: Unicompartmental or total knee replacement? Five-year results of a prospective, randomised trial of 102 osteoarthritic knees with unicompartmental arthritis. J Bone Joint Surg 80B:862, 1998.
35. Robertsson O, Knutson K, Lewold S, Lidgren L: The routine of surgical management reduces failure after unicompartmental knee arthroplasty. J Bone Joint Surg 83B:45, 2001.
36. Rougraff BT, Heck DA, Gibson AE: A comparison of tricompartmental and unicompartmental arthroplasty for the treatment of gonarthrosis. Clin Orthop 273:157, 1991.
37. Schai PA, Jeung-Tak S, Thornhill T, Scott R: Unicompartmental knee arthroplasty in middle aged patients: A 2–6 year followup evaluation. J Arthroplasty 13:365, 1998.
38. Scott RD, Santore RF: Unicondylar unicompartmental replacement for osteoarthritis of the knee. J Bone Joint Surg 63A:536, 1981.
39. Shurley TH, O'Donoghue DH, Smith WD, et al: Unicompartmental arthroplasty of the knee. Clin Orthop 164:236, 1982.
40. Sisto DJ, Blazina ME, Heskicoff D, Hirsh LC: Unicompartmental arthroplasty for osteoarthritis of the knee. Clin Orthop 286:149, 1993.
41. Squire MW, Callaghan J, Goetz D, Sullivan P: Unicompartmental knee replacement: A minimum 15 year followup study. Clin Orthop 367:61, 1999.
42. Stem SH, Becker MW, Insall JN: Unicondy lar knee arthroplasty: An evaluation of selection criteria. Clin Orthop 286:143, 1993.
43. Stockelman RE, Pohl K: The longterm efficacy of unicompartmental arthroplasty of the knee. Clin Orthop 271:88, 1991.
44. Svard UC, Price AJ: Oxford medial unicompartmental knee arthroplasty. A survival analysis of an independent series. J Bone Joint Surg 83B:191, 2001.
45. Swank M, Stuhlberg SD, Jiganti J, Machairas S: The natural history of unicompartmental arthroplasty: An eight year follow-up study with survivorship analysis. Clin Orthop 286:130, 1993.
46. Tabor OB, Tabor OB: Unicompartmental arthroplasty: A long-term followup study. J Arthroplasty 13:373, 1998.
47. Thomhill TS, Scott RD: Unicompartmental total knee arthroplasty. Orthop Clin North Am 20:245, 1989.
48. Thomhill TS: Unicompartmental knee arthroplasty. Clin Orthop 205:121, 1986.
49. Whiteside LA, McCarthy DS: Laboratory evaluation of alignment and kinematics in a unicompartmental knee arthroplasty inserted with intramedullary instrumentation. Clin Orthop 274:238, 1992.

77

Mobile-Bearing Knee

• BERNARD F. MORREY and MARK W. PAGNANO

Despite the excellent results that have been reported with a wide variety of design concepts and fixation strategies, there are continued issues in total knee arthroplasty that have prompted and justified ongoing basic and clinical investigation. Probably the most important recent initiative in this regard is that of the so-called mobile-bearing knee. Generically this may be defined as any knee in which there is an intercalary element that has at least one degree of freedom both at the femoral articulation and at the tibial base plate. The characteristic features relate principally to (1) the degree of congruency between the mobile element and the femoral component; (2) the degrees of freedom with regard to the mobility of the bearing—rotation, confined translation, or unrestricted rotation and translation; (3) the means of posterior stabilization; and (4) the method of fixation.

RATIONALE

There is an ever-increasing expectation from a younger patient population of improved function and increased longevity with prosthetic replacement. The two major goals for improving knee joint design, and hence function, are (1) to decrease the wear characteristics, particularly if the increased activity is expected or allowed; and (2) to increase the amount of motion. Based on these clinical expectations, the design goals of the mobile-bearing knee may be summarized as follows:

1. To decrease wear by replicating normal kinematic motion
2. To increase motion
3. To allow a reproducible surgical technique by a competent orthopedic surgeon
4. To provide a reliable long-term functional outcome
5. To avoid complications, specifically those that are related to the design

NORMAL KNEE KINEMATICS

It is believed that replication of normal knee kinematics will, by decreasing abnormal motion, lessen the likelihood of wear at the articulation or at the mobile-bearing–tibial interface. Hence, the design rationale is predicated on replicating normal kinematics. The available arc of flexion and extension typically averages about 140 degrees. Normal gait occurs with knee flexion between 5 and 20 degrees.[26] It has been demonstrated that the axis of flexion can be simulated or at least approximated by the transepicondylar axis.[17] Studies by Walker et al. have also confirmed that the axial rotation of the tibia on the femur for the most part also is replicated by a line through the base of the medial aspect of the medial tibial spine.[32] Normally with an intact posterior cruciate ligament, posterior excursion of the femur referable to the tibia during flexion is approximately 14 mm (Fig. 77–1). In addition, axial rotation is maximal at 30 degrees of flexion.[20] The average internal and external rotation in flexion and extension in normal subjects is 6 to 9 degrees, ranging up to 14 degrees in some instances.[10] Furthermore, femoral rollback occurs principally at the lateral femoral-tibial articulation, while essentially "pivoting" with a smaller excursion path at the medial articulation. It is for this reason that variable sagittal axes of rotation have been suggested for the knee replacement in order to replicate these kinematic features.

Forces

The forces across the knee joint are particularly important referable to implant design and articular surface stresses. Up to three to four times body weight has been demonstrated to occur during a normal gait cycle.[22] The greatest force is at approximately 20 degrees of flexion, but force is relatively high in the 0 and 45 degree arc of flexion.

KNEE REPLACEMENT DESIGN

Kinematics of Wear

Theoretical and experimental data have demonstrated that surface stresses are significant at the femoral-tibial articulation. These stresses increase dramatically when the femur articulates with a less congruent, that is, the more flat, tibial component. As the congruity increases between the tibial-femoral articulation, the surface area increases and the surface stresses decrease.[2] It has been

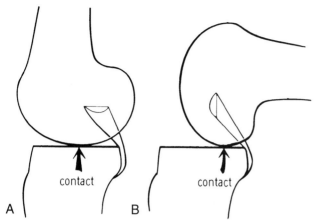

Figure 77–1. A, With an intact posterior cruciate ligament (PCL) in extension, the tibial-femoral contact area is near the midtibia. **B**, With flexion, the contact area is posteriorly placed because of the rollback effect that occurs with a functional PCL. (From Insall JN: Historical development, classification, and characteristics of knee prostheses. *In* Insall JN, Windsor RE, Scott WN, et al. [eds]: Surgery of the Knee, 2nd ed. New York, Churchill Livingstone, 1993, p 677.)

calculated that the difference between a round-on-flat compared to a highly conformed femoral-tibial component changes the surface contact area by a factor of 5. The contact area of a nonconforming round-on-flat type of articulation is approximateliy 200 mm² compared to 1000 mm² on a highly conforming implant.[31] It has also been demonstrated that this change in surface area is directly correlated with the change in surface stress, which decreases by a factor of 5 with the more constrained femoral components. Approximately 25 MPa of surface stress occurs on the nonconforming and only 5 or less MPa on the highly conforming implant surface.[19]

The problem or dilemma is to reconcile the need for the femur to roll posteriorly on the tibia during flexion while still maintaining a high degree of congruence.

Furthermore, because rollback is a function of an intact posterior cruciate ligament, the rationale of the total condylar implant was that, by removing the posterior cruciate ligament, the obligatory rollback would not occur. Thus a more congruent femoral-tibial articulation could be employed. Although this was and still is a viable design option, it causes increased forces at the anterior-posterior articular margins and thus attains a decrease in surface stress at the expense of normal knee kinematics (Fig. 77–2). Hence the interest in the mobile-bearing concept.

The highly congruent femoral-tibial sagittal articulation decreases surface stress but does not allow rollback of the femur on the tibia. This means that a sheering stress at the tibial implant–bone interface is introduced by such designs. The sheering forces first cause stress at the bone-cement interface in monoblock knee and secondarily cause micromotion of the modular knee. In the modular knee, this micromotion is known to cause so-called back-side wear.[23] The logical solution is to allow and even encourage the "backside" motion that occurs with normal rollback at the insert-tray interface by employing a highly polished tibial tray. If the tibial articulation is allowed to move on the tibial base plate, this will limit the forces at the bone-cement interface, and possibly decrease the likelihood of loosening. In addition, if the surface of the tibia and the mobile-bearing implant are highly polished, this should also decrease the likelihood of excessive wear. Although the flat tibial surface allows rollback, it also causes high stresses on the articular surface, and it is these high stresses that tend to cause delamination and wear of the tibial component. If the posterior cruciate ligament is removed, then anterior-posterior translation is eliminated; however, some means of stabilizing the knee must be introduced into the articulation. The resolution of the problem, therefore, is to allow translation while introducing high congruity of the articulation. This is the basis of the mobile-bearing knee concept (Fig. 77–3).

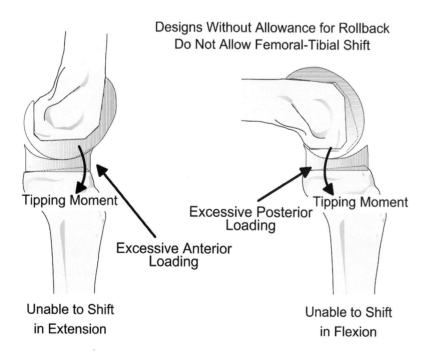

Figure 77–2. A highly constrained articulation with an intact posterior cruciate ligament imposes tilting forces on the articulation in the sagittal plane. (From Pappas MJ, Buechel FE: Biomechanics and design rationale: New Jersey LCS® Knee Replacement System. DePuy Sales Training Seminars, Biomedical Engineering Trust, South Orange, NJ, 1993.)

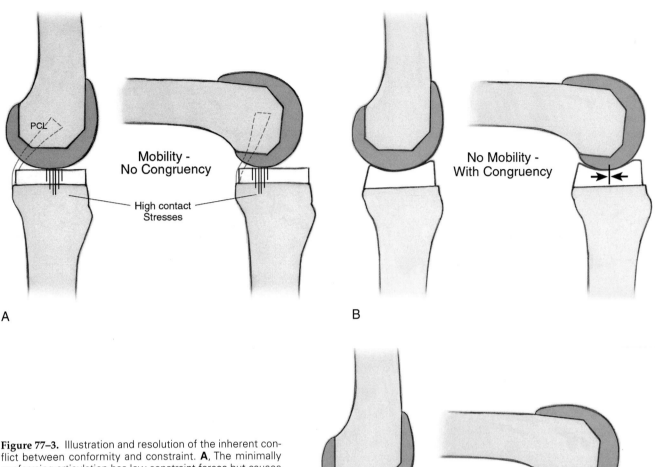

Figure 77–3. Illustration and resolution of the inherent conflict between conformity and constraint. **A,** The minimally conforming articulation has low constraint forces but causes high contact stress in the polyethylene. **B,** The highly conforming articulation has low contact stress but high constraint forces that could lead to implant loosening. **C,** The conflict can be resolved by allowing motion with a highly conforming intercalary tibial acetabular component.

The Ideal Design

The ideal design, therefore, will first enhance the conformity at the femoral-tibial articulation with a more conforming surface geometry that decreases the stresses imparted to the tibial surface and, second, allow the articulating element to rotate or translate at the tibia to accommodate the posterior rollback. If these design parameters are met, it is thought that the likelihood of wear, even with the currently available replacement materials, will be reduced and hopefully knee flexion may also increase, and possibly even approach normal.[12]

If the basic rationale is relatively straightforward and attractive, as with so many other such circumstances, the "devil is in the details." Specifically, how are these goals embodied in a design? How is the posterior cruci-

ate ligament accommodated, or is it preserved? How are the axes of motion defined? Is the goal to "replicate" motion, or is the normal motion "replaced" by allowing degrees of freedom that accommodate but do not actually replicate the more normal kinematics? An additional concern is that an absent posterior cruciate ligament may lead to instability. Hence the so-called hybrid concept was introduced by designing a stabilizing element to help control rollback in the absence of a posterior cruciate ligament.

Design Options

The essential design consideration is to accommodate the femoral rollback. This may be accomplished by a number of design approaches: (1) floating menisci on two independently moving condylar elements; (2) defined motion pattern of the meniscus; (3) rotating platforms; (4) rotating and translating platforms; and (5) freely mobile articulations. Normally[7,8] rollback tends to pivot about the medial femoral condyle and tends to glide on the lateral condyle. Because the femoral rollback occurs more laterally than medially, an axial rotation of the tibia on the femur occurs during this motion. This kinematic feature can be approximated, although not totally replicated, by simple rotation of the tibial articulating element. This therefore provides the basis of the two major design philosophies: a rotating platform or a variable mobile bearing that allows both rotation and translation (Fig. 77–4). A further considera-

tion is whether the posterior cruciate ligament is either retained or substituted. Some of these characteristics are summarized in Table 77–1.

Prosthetic Kinematics: The Function of the Mobile-Bearing Knee

Analytical and bench studies have revealed in general that axial rotation patterns are replicated by meniscal but not rotating platform designs. Most designs allow 4 to 5 degrees' rotation instead of the normal 10 to 12 degrees. In addition, the translation of the mobile-bearing knee has not been demonstrated to obtain the 10 to 15 degrees that is normally seen. A typical tendency observed in

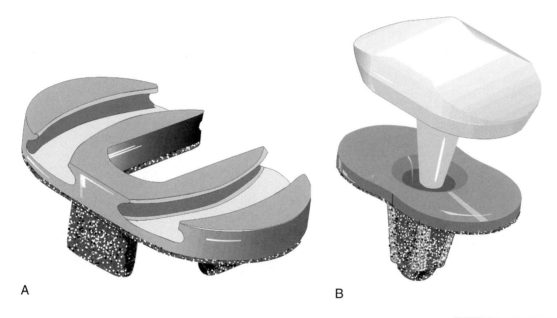

A   B

Figure 77–4. The major philosophies of design in mobile-bearing knees are illustrated. The early design of meniscal-bearing articulation that glides in troughs (**A**) has given way to the rotating platform (**B**), which allows simple rotation around a central axis. **C**, The MBK knee (Zimmer, Warsaw, IN) allows both rotation and translation while favoring medially biased kinematics.

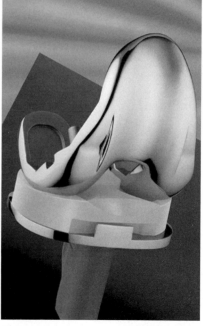

C

Table 77–1. DESIGN CHARACTERISTICS OF SOME OF THE "EARLY" MOBILE-BEARING KNEE IMPLANTS

Name	Company	Introduced	Articulation	Motion	PCL	Fixation
Partially Conforming						
LCS	DePuy (Warsaw, IN)	1970s	Coronal conforming sagittal conforming	RP	Sacrified	Cement, noncement
SAL	Sulzer (Houston, TX)	1987	Coronal nonconforming sagittal conforming	RP	Retained	Cement preferred
Highly Conforming						
Oxford	Biomet (Warsaw, IN)	1976	Coronal conforming sagittal conforming	Sliding	Retained	Cement, noncement

LCS, low contact stress; PCL, posterior cruciate ligament; RP, rotating platform; SAL, self-aligning.

fluoroscopic studies is for the femur to initially roll posteriorly but, with additional flexion, actually roll more anteriorly once again on the tibia.[7] It is of particular interest to note that this same pattern is that which is seen in many of the fixed-bearing knees.[7,11,30] However, it is for these reasons that two mobile-bearing knee with no preferred axis have been designed: the Zimmer Medial Biased Kinematic (MBK) and the Sulzer Orthopedic Self-Aligning (SAL) implants. These designs do not dictate the movement pattern but allow it to be determined by the dynamic and ligamentous constraints. Although this would seem to be an attractive and desirable goal, it may potentially be associated with increased wear, so there is some skepticism about allowing a freely mobile, nondefined pattern of intercalary motion.[14]

Studies have shown that the function of the mobile bearing is discretely defined during gait and with stair walking. In fact, stairs offers the most discriminating activity to determine the replication of more normal motion. It has also been shown that 1 to 2 mm of varus-valgus tilt or lift-off also occurs during gait in up to 75 percent of patients with fixed-bearing[9] and mobile-bearing[29] prosthetic replacements. This appears to be present to some extent in essentially all designs and increases the relevance of the issue of articular conformity in the coronal plane.

SURGICAL TECHNIQUE

There is relatively little discussion of the unique technical issues regarding the implantation of the various mobile-bearing implants. There are three overriding considerations in this regard: (1) the basic principles of knee joint replacement apply for all designs; (2) there are some unique technique considerations that are specifically applicable to mobile-bearing knees; and (3) there are also some specific features of technique based on individual mobile-bearing implant design.

The technical considerations to be considered are summarized below:

1. In general, mobile-bearing knees are, at this time, considered a more challenging technical procedure, not more forgiving. This is in contrast with the posterior-stabilized knee, wherein the removal of the posterior cruciate ligament redefines the kinematics and hence allows correction of contractures and angular deformity.

2. The flexion and extension gap must be equalized in this as with any well-done joint replacement arthroplasty. A loose flexion gap may allow the rare but dramatic and disconcerting problem of bearing spin-out.

3. The anterior-posterior slope of the tibial cut is a design-specific issue. For the most part, it is recommended that a posterior tibial slope be established; however, this can occur either by design at the articulation or with the cut of the tibia. If the posterior slope is introduced from the cut on the tibia, this is generally less than the 5 to 10 degrees recommended with fixed-bearing implants, and in some designs a 0-degree cut is recommended.

4. Most mobile-bearing knees require a slightly increased amount of bone removal. Should the implant fail, although not yet confirmed by data, our impression is that the revisions may be somewhat more challenging because of an increased amount of bone loss.

Sequence of Cuts

Some designs are based on a strategy that starts with the tibial cut and bases the alignment and the remainder of the resection from this frame of reference. The reason for this is that resection of the tibia has the same impact on flexion and extension gaps and, thus, possibly makes the preparation of the femur more easily performed. Regardless of the system used, the senior author has always initiated knee preparation with the tibial cut.

Cementation

Even experienced surgeons often cement the mobile-bearing knee components separately. When this is done, the tibia is secured first, followed by the femoral component, because of the obvious difficulty of inserting the tibia when the femoral component is in place.

Postoperative Care

There is no dramatic difference in the postoperative management between mobile-bearing and fixed-bearing designs.

RESULTS

Although it is possible to report the results that have appeared in the literature, a comparison among various designs and experiences is not readily made because of the differences in reporting technique. Nonetheless, an effort to summarize the literature to date regading the various mobile-bearing knees is shown in Table 77–2. Several different design philosophies are embodied in the reports appearing in the current literature.

Oxford Unicompartmental Meniscal-Bearing Knee

This implant was designed specifically as a unicompartmental replacement. The popularity if not the indications for such an implant, regardless of the design, has waxed and waned somewhat over the years, at least in the United States. Currently there is not universal enthusiasm for the design philosophy of a unicompartmental knee because, at this point in time, the early failure of these implants is still higher than that reported for condylar designs. However, the concept is attractive because it allows preservation of the normal compartment and does allow more normal function when successful. It is in this context that the Oxford mobile-bearing knee was designed. According to the designers, the specific indications for this implant are (1) symptomatic medial unicompartmental involvement; (2) a functional anterior cruciate ligament; (3) absence of fixed varus deformity; (4) less than 15 degrees of fixed flexion contracture; and (5) minimum, if any, patellofemoral disease. In a 10-year report from the designing institution, an implant survival rate of 95 percent was recorded.[21] These investigators have found that 25 percent of the patients they see in their practice are candidates for the mobile-bearing knee. The Swedish registry records almost 700 knees from 19 centers and documents a 90 percent implant survival rate at 5 years.[17] Most surgeons in the United States apply more strict criteria for the unicompartmental replacement. In one prospective study, 228 knees were assessed for eligibility for a hemi-replacement device, revealing only 6 percent of the patients to have met the stated criteria.[28] This topic is discussed in detail in Chapter 76.

Low Contact Stress Knee

The Low Contact Stress (LCS) design was conceived over two decades ago by DePuy Orthopaedics. As is the case with most implants, the greatest clinical experience is that reported by the innovators. This particular design concept has evolved from three variations or philosophies, each available for fixation with or without bone cement (Fig. 77–5). The longest experience of 21 cement-fixed bicruciate retention implants revealed that, at 12 years, the survival rate was 91 percent.[3] A 6-year survival of 25 knees fixed without cement was 100 percent. It is difficult to understand how an otherwise identical implant could have a better short-term survival when cement is not used, and one might question whether or not this difference is statistically or clinically significant. In any event, the posterior cruciate–sparing version was used without cement and revealed a 6-year survival of 98 percent in 57 knees. The rotating platform version of their experience involves 108 procedures fixed both with and without cement. A surveillance period of 8 years reveals 98 percent satisfactory results with no distinction between the cemented and uncemented implants.[12] Others have reported similar surgical results (see Table 77–2). An extensive and independent assessment of this implant was reported by Sorrells. After 665 LCS rotating platform procedures, an 11-year survivorship of 95 percent was reported. The mechanical technical complication rate was only 3 percent.[27] Others have reported a 9 percent dislocation rate of the posterior cruciate–retaining rotating platform version of this knee.[1] Of particular note is the low mechanical failure of the rotating platform thus far reported.

Self-Aligning Mobile-Bearing Knee

The SAL system allows both rotation and translation of the articular surface of the tibial insert. The device can be implanted with or without cement. From a clinical experience of 172 implants, careful analysis of 61 cases revealed a 5.5-year survival rate of 95 percent.[16] Assessment of 115 patients revealed two mechanical failures, one resulting from wear and one from stiffness.[5] Overall the results of this design seem to be comparable to those of other systems, especially when fixed with cement.

P.F.C. Sigma RP

A nonpeer review of 90 implants in patients averaging 64 years has been reported from DePuy Orthopaedics. Both posterior cruciate–retaining (72) and posterior cruciate–substituting (18) implants were available for insertion. With an average follow-up of only 1 year, the mean flexion was 102 degrees. Two percent had moderate pain.[24]

Medial-Biased Kinematics Knee

The design considerations of the MBK include reduced wear, smooth patellar tracking, medial-based kinematics, freedom of rotation of the femur on the tibia, limited translation of the tibial-based plate, stability of the interposed high-density polyethylene bearing, interchangeability of femur and tibial sizes, increased base plate strength, and theoretically physiologic flexion and extension (see Fig. 77–4). Insall identified three groups of patients, representing 69 procedures, with an average age of 67. Surveillance of 61 patients for 1 to 5 years

Table 77–2. RESULTS AFTER ARTHROPLASTY WITH MOBILE-BEARING KNEE DESIGNS

Study	Implant	Design Type	No. of Knees	Patient Age (yr)	Mean Time Follow-up (yr)	Rate of Survival (%)	No. (%) Mechanical Failures
Lewold et al. (1995)[17]	Oxford unicompartmental	Anterior-posterior translation	699		5	90	
Murray et al. (1998)[21]	Oxford unicompartmental	Anterior-posterior translation	144	35–90	10	98	1 (1.5)
Price and Svard (2000)[25]	Oxford unicompartmental	Anterior-posterior translation	378		10	95	3 (1)
Buechel and Pappas (1990)[4]	LCS posterior cruciate–retaining meniscal-bearing	Anterior-posterior translation, rotation	57		6	98	
Jordan et al. (1997)[15]	LCS posterior cruciate–retaining meniscal-bearing	Anterior-posterior translation, rotation	473	29–87	8	95	17 (4)
Sorrells (1996)[27]	LCS rotating platform	Rotation	665	70 mean	11	95	3 (.5)
Callaghan et al. (2000)[6]	LCS rotating platform	Rotation	119		9	100	0
Callaghan et al. (2000)[5]	SAL	Anterior-posterior translation, rotation	115	47–90	5.6	95	3
Buechel (1990)[3]	Rotating platform	Rotation	108	8	98		
Insall et al. (2001)[12]	Rotoglide	R/T	1600		8	99	

LCS, low contact stress; R/T, rotation/translation; SAL, self-aligning.

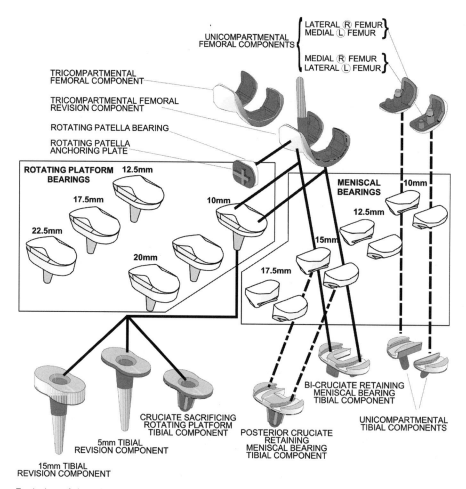

UNICOMPARTMENTAL
FEMORAL COMPONENTS {
LATERAL ®ᴿ FEMUR
MEDIAL ©ᴸ FEMUR
}

{
MEDIAL ®ᴿ FEMUR
LATERAL ©ᴸ FEMUR
}

TRICOMPARTMENTAL
FEMORAL COMPONENT

TRICOMPARTMENTAL FEMORAL
REVISION COMPONENT

ROTATING PATELLA BEARING

ROTATING PATELLA
ANCHORING PLATE

ROTATING PLATFORM
BEARINGS   12.5mm

17.5mm

22.5mm

20mm

10mm

MENISCAL
BEARINGS   10mm

12.5mm

15mm

17.5mm

BI-CRUCIATE RETAINING
MENISCAL BEARING
TIBIAL COMPONENT

POSTERIOR CRUCIATE
RETAINING
MENISCAL BEARING
TIBIAL COMPONENT

UNICOMPARTMENTAL
TIBIAL COMPONENTS

CRUCIATE SACRIFICING
ROTATING PLATFORM
TIBIAL COMPONENT

5mm TIBIAL
REVISION COMPONENT

15mm TIBIAL
REVISION COMPONENT

Figure 77–5. Evolution of thought and design of the LCS system. (DePuy Orthopaedics, Warsaw IN). (From Pappas MJ, Buechel FE: Biomechanics and design rationale: New Jersey LCS® Knee Replacement System. DePuy Sales Training Seminars, Biomedical Engineering Trust, South Orange, NJ, 1993.)

(mean 2.5 years) revealed 57 percent excellent and 38 percent good results, for an overall 95 percent satisfactory result (Fig. 77–6). In a European clinical trial of 249 MBK implants, none had yet been revised, but the follow-up averaged only 1 year.[12]

COMPLICATIONS

Other than those accepted complications of total knee arthroplasty, the major specific complication associated with the mobile-bearing knee is that of dislocation or "spin-out" of the articular element. This was seen particularly in those early meniscal-bearing knees.[1] Most problems currently seem to relate to fixation and patellar tracking. Potential issues regarding ease of revision must await greater clinical experience.

AUTHORS' PREFERENCE

There is great enthusiasm for the mobile-bearing concept within the orthopedic community. The value appears to be largely design and technique sensitive. These implants are more expensive than fixed-bearing knees, and the surgical technique may be more demanding. The authors currently believe that the ideal indication is the young active patient. Increased motion is also desirable, but the available data do not necessarily suggest that this will occur with the devices currently available. Our final opinion is deferred pending more data. This will hopefully be realized from the outcomes of a prospective study of the MBK device and a prospective, randomized study of the rotating platform and fixed-bearing versions of the P.F.C. Sigma implant that are ongoing in our department.

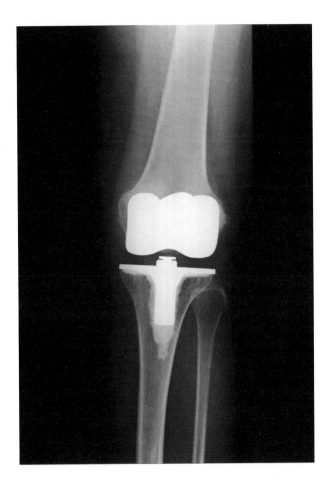
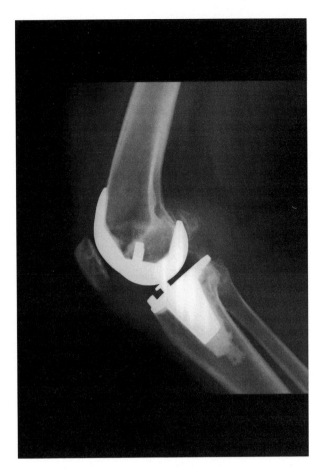

Figure 77–6. Postoperative view of the MBK.

References

1. Bert JM: Dislocation/subluxation of meniscal bearing elements after New Jersey Low-Contact Stress total knee arthroplasty. Clin Orthop 254:211–215, 1990.
2. Blunn GW, Walker PS, Joshi A, Hardinge K: The dominance of cyclic sliding in producing wear in total knee replacements. Clin Orthop 273:253–260, 1991.
3. Buechel FF: Cemented and cementless revision arthroplasty using rotating platform total knee implants: a 12 year experience. Orthop Rev 71(Suppl), 1990.
4. Buechel FF, Pappas MJ: Long-term survivorship analysis of cruciate-sparing versus cruciate-sacrificing knee prostheses using meniscal bearings. Clin Orthop 260:162–169, 1990.
5. Callaghan JJ, Insall JN, Greenwald AS, et al: Mobile-bearing knee replacement. J Bone Joint Surg Am 82:1020–1041, 2000.
6. Callaghan JJ, Squire MW, Goetz DD, et al: Cemented rotating-platform total knee replacement: a nine to 12-year follow-up study. J Bone Joint Surg Am 82:705–711, 2000.
7. Dennis DA, Komistek RD, Hoff WA, Gabriel SM: In vivo knee kinematics derived using an inverse perspective technique. Clin Orthop 331:107–117, 1996.
8. Dennis DA, Komistek RD, Stiehl JB, et al: Range of motion after total knee arthroplasty: the effect of implant design and weight-bearing conditions. J Arthroplasty 13:748–752, 1998.
9. Dennis DA, Komistek RD, Walker SA, et al: Femoral condylar lift-off in vivo in total knee arthroplasty. J Bone Joint Surg Br 83:33–39, 2001.
10. Goodfellow J, O'Connor J: The mechanics of the knee and prosthesis design. J Bone Joint Surg Br 60:358–369, 1978.
11. Hoff WA, Komistek RD, Dennis DA, et al: A three dimensional determination of femorotibial contact positions under in vivo conditions using fluoroscopy. J Clin Biomech 13:455–470, 1998.
12. Insall JN: Historical development, classification, and characteristics of knee prostheses. In Insall JN, Windsor RE, Scott WN, et al. (eds): Surgery of the Knee, 2nd ed. New York, Churchill Livingstone, 1993, p 677.
13. Insall JN, Aglietti P, Baldina A, Easley ME: Meniscal-bearing knee replacement. In Insall S (ed): Surgery of the Knee, 3rd ed. New York, Churchill Livingstone, 2001, pp 1717–1738.
14. Jones VC, Fischer J, Barton DC, et al: An experimental model of tibial counterface polyethylene wear in mobile bearing knees: the influence of design and kinematics. Biomed Mater Eng 9:187–196, 1999.
15. Jordan LR, Olivo JL, Voorhorst PE: Survivorship analysis of cementless meniscal bearing total knee arthroplasty. Clin Orthop 338:119–123, 1997.
16. Kaper BP, Smith PN, Bourne RB, et al: Medium-term results of a mobile bearing total knee replacement. Clin Orthop 367:201–209, 1999.
17. Lewold S, Goodman S, Knutson K, et al: Oxford meniscal bearing knee versus the Marmor knee in unicompartmental arthroplasty for arthrosis: a Swedish multicenter survival study. J Arthroplasty 10:722–731, 1995.
18. Menchetti PPM, Walker PS: Mechanical evaluation of mobile bearing knees. Am J Knee Surg 10:73–82, 1997.
19. Morra EA, Postak PD, Greenwald AS: The influence of mobile bearing knee geometry on the wear of UHMWPE tibial inserts: a finite element study. Orthop Trans 22:148–149, 1998–1999.
20. Morrison JB: The mechanics of the knee joint in relation to normal walking. J Biomech 3:51–61, 1970.

21. Murray DW, Goodfellow JW, O'Connor JJ: The Oxford medial unicompartmental arthroplasty: a ten-year survival study. J Bone Joint Surg Br 80:983–989, 1998.
22. Pappas MJ, Buechel FF: Biomechanics and design rationale: New Jersey LCS® Knee Replacement System. DePuy Sales Training Seminars, Biomedical Engineering Trust, South Orange, NJ, 1993.
23. Parks NL, Engh GA, Topoleski LD, Emperado J: Modular tibial insert micromotion: a concern with contemporary knee implants. Clin Orthop 356:10–15, 1998.
24. Perka C: A prospective single-center study: durability of the P.F.C. SigmaRP. Orthop Today Dec:18–19, 2000.
25. Price A, Svard U: An independent survival analysis of the Oxford unicompartmental meniscal bearing knee replacement. Presented as a Scientific Poster at the annual meeting of the American Academy of Orthopaedic Surgeons, Orlando, FL, March 15–19, 2000.
26. Smidt GL: Biomechanical analysis of the knee. J Biomech 6:79–102, 1973.
27. Sorrells RB: The rotating platform mobile bearing TKA. Orthopedics 19:793–796, 1996.
28. Stern SH, Becker MW, Insall JN: Unicondylar knee arthroplasty: an evaluation of selection criteria. Clin Orthop Rel Res 286:143, 1993.
29. Stiehl JB, Dennis DA, Komistek RD, Crane HS: In vivo determination of condylar lift-off and screw-home in a mobile-bearing total knee arthroplasty. J Arthroplasty 14:293–299, 1999.
30. Stiehl JB, Komistek RD, Dennis DA, et al: Fluoroscopic analysis of kinematics after posterior-cruciate retaining knee arthroplasty. J Bone Joint Surg Br 77:884–889, 1995.
31. Szivek JA, Anderson PL, Benjamin JB: Average and peak contact stress distribution evaluation of total knee arthroplasties. J Arthroplasty 11:952–963, 1996.
32. Walker PS, Sathasivam S: The design of guide surfaces for fixed-bearing and mobile-bearing knee replacements. J Biomech 32:27–34, 1999.

78

Managing Deformity: Total Knee Arthroplasty Techniques

• ROBERT T. TROUSDALE and BERNARD F. MORREY

Restoration of a deformed arthritic knee to proper axial, sagittal, and rotational alignment is one of the principle goals of total knee arthroplasty. Over the past several decades, it has become clear that the perioperative alignment directly influences the postoperative alignment and that the postoperative alignment directly influences long-term implant survivorship.[8,10,12,27,30] In this chapter, we review the current data regarding alignment and techniques of deformity correction and discuss the long-term implications of the proper management of such problems.

TECHNIQUE OF CORRECTION OF FIXED DEFORMITY

Given the importance of proper limb alignment, it seems essential to address the means of soft tissue release and balance to realize correct axial load distribution. Sculco[33] credits Freeman with recognizing the problem of soft tissue balance in 1977. Since then, Insall, Krackow, and others have written extensively on this issue and have provided excellent theoretical[16] and technical[17] insight into the problem. The clinical assessment consists of determining whether the malalignment is fixed or correctable. Overall, the technique for soft tissue release is well known, and the general principles should be followed in incremental steps. It is essential to avoid over-releasing "tight" medial or lateral structures because this can cause ligamentous imbalance (most commonly in flexion) and incompetence leading to knee instability after this arthroplasty.

Basic Concepts

To achieve proper alignment after total knee arthroplasty, proper bony cuts and soft tissue releases need to be performed.[38,40] Proper bony cuts typically involve resecting the distal femur perpendicular to the mechanical axis, which is typically 5 to 7 degrees of valgus alignment from the right femur.[3,7,34] The tibia is cut perpendicular to its mechanical axis.[4,29] This combined with appropriate soft tissue releases will restore normal limb alignment. The need to obtain a long-leg radiograph prior to the arthroplasty has been evaluated by McGrory et al.[24] In a prospective randomized trial, they found that a preoperative long-leg radiograph was not helpful in obtaining a normally aligned limb postoperatively. They recommended not obtaining this film in the routine patient but stated that it may still be helpful in patients with a prior history of hip surgery, femur or tibia fracture, or severe limb deformity.

A clear understanding of two basic concepts is necessary for the proper management of fixed angular deformities. First, it is necessary to define the specific etiology or the cause of the deformity. Several classification systems have been offered to help in this regard. Second, one must recognize the relationship between soft tissue release/balance and implant selection.[32]

A practical guideline used by the senior author to assure an adequate release is the attainment of 1 to 2 mm of separation of the components opposite of the direction of the deformity, measured in 5 degrees of flexion. This assures that there is not an uncorrected soft tissue contracture that causes persistent deformity even if the osseous cuts have been performed in such a way as to provide an optimum osseous mechanical axis. Mild postoperative laxity of the ligaments is not generally considered to be detrimental if the ligaments are balanced and the limb is well aligned. In fact, performance may be enhanced if the ligaments are slightly lax but balanced. Edwards et al. report 63 knee replacements followed from 1 to 7 years, all with competent collateral ligaments and adequate alignment.[6] Those with greater varus-valgus laxity had better results than those that were put in "tight." Among the former group, 9 percent had pain, compared to 38 percent in those whose implants were inserted with a so-called stable technique. It should be emphasized that no patient in the former group had instability and all were well aligned.

Kaufer and Matthews stated that optimal results cannot be obtained with a nonconstrained total knee arthroplasty when there is greater than 30 degrees of fixed flexion or greater than 20 degrees of fixed valgus or varus deformity preoperatively.[13] They recommended the use of constrained prostheses in this group of patients. In our experience, most deformities, even if they are fixed, can be managed properly with nonconstrained condylar knee designs and appropriate soft tissue releases. Laskin and others have shown that, for fixed deformities exceeding 15 degrees, excision of the posterior cruciate ligament (PCL) and use of a PCL-substituting prosthesis obtains the best results.[21]

Fixed Varus Deformity

A fixed varus deformity is the most common deformity encountered because degenerative arthritis of the knee has a predilection for medial compartment involvement.[20] To the extent that the varus malalignment is not excessive (i.e., < 10 degrees of anatomic alignment), varus contracture can be reliably corrected at the time of joint replacement arthroplasty. This is predicted by the ability to correct the deformity at least to a neutral position by valgus stress during the preoperative examination (Fig. 78–1). This simple test is used by the authors to predict the difficulty of attaining optimum alignment and balance.

Technique

Two technical principles are accepted: (1) a varus correction is not corrected by bone resection, and (2) soft tissue releases are performed from the tibia.[22] Preoperative templating determines the anticipated osseous resection from the tibia and the femur. This provides a reliable measure for verifying the intraoperative resection as suggested by the alignment instrumentation.

SOFT TISSUE RELEASE

The component elements are released in the following order:

1. Osteophytes are removed from the femur and tibia. Typically, a large osteophyte develops under the femoral attachment of the medial collateral ligament. The osteophytes must be removed from the entire margin of the medial femoral condyle as well as from the tibia, including the posteromedial margin.
2. The capsule is released. The anteromedial and posteromedial portions of the capsule are reflected subperiosteally by sharp dissection at the time of the exposure. Additional release is performed after the tibial cut and after osteophyte removal if a residual contracture is observed with trial reduction of the components.
3. The semimembranosus is released from the posteromedial aspect of the joint.
4. If the knee remains contracted, the superficial portion of the medial collateral ligament is released from the tibia.

After each of these measures, the varus-valgus stability of the knee is examined. Care should be taken not to "over-release" the tight medial side. If excessive lateral laxity is considered to be present, it can be corrected by the use of a stabilizing implant (Fig. 78–2).[5]

Lateral Collateral Ligament Retensioning (Krackow). An alternative solution to residual lateral instability is lateral collateral ligament (LCL) reconstruction, or retensioning, according to Krackow et al.[19] There are few experiences documenting the effectiveness of either

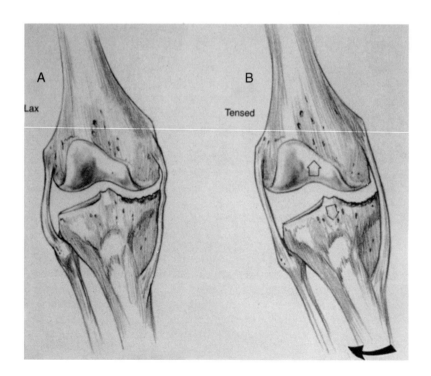

Figure 78–1. Determination of fixed versus correctable deformities is most important. If a varus deformity can be corrected to neutral by valgus stress (**A**), this indicates a significant soft tissue release will not be necessary (**B**). (From Scuderi GR, Insall JN: Fixed varus and valgus deformities. In Lotke P [ed]: Masters Techniques: Knee Arthroplasty. New York, Raven Press, 1995, p 112.)

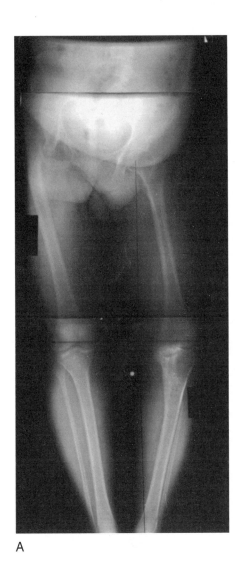

A

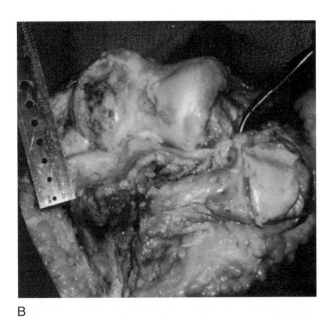

B

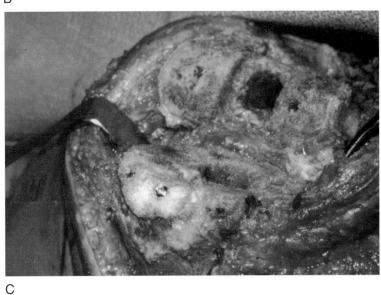

C

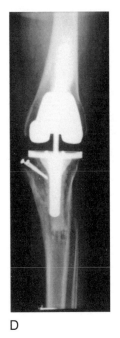

D

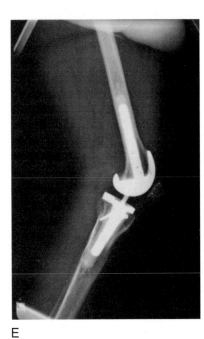

E

Figure 78–2. A, Long-leg standing radiograph of a severe varus deformity with medial compartment bone loss. **B** and **C**, Intraoperative photos showing the extensive medial release from the tibial side and the peripheral bone loss (**B**), treated with autogenous bone grafting and fixation with two screws (**C**). **D** and **E**, Postoperative anteroposterior and lateral radiographs showing restoration of a normal anatomic axis and use of a semiconstrained condylar knee design secondary to excessive lateral laxity.

approach. We have no experience with Krackow's procedure but have had some success with soft tissue ligament reconstruction. An ancillary incision is made 3 cm above and 4 cm distal to the fibular styloid. The peroneal nerve is identified and mobilized (Fig. 78–3). The fibula is predrilled to receive either a 4.5- or 6.5-mm cancellous AO screw. The fibula is osteotomized approximately 2 cm distal to its articular surface with an oscillating saw perpendicular to its long axis. After the fibula is dissected free of its tibiofibular capsular attachments, and with the knee in about 10 degrees of flexion, the fibula is brought distally and overlapped to the extent necessary to provide adequate tension on the fibular collateral ligament. This determines the amount of the bone resection that is necessary. The fibula is then attached with an AO screw placed through the predrilled proximal fragment and into the medullary canal distally. Careful range of motion and varus-valgus stress testing is performed to assure proper tensioning of the advanced ligament.

Results

Teeny and associates have reviewed their experience with 27 knees presenting with more than 20 degrees of varus angulation and compared the results with 40 knees having a preoperative varus angulation of less than 5 degrees.[37] A minimally constrained cruciate-sparing prosthesis was used, and the follow-up averaged approximately 5 years. Although the more complicated procedures took an average of 30 minutes longer than the less complicated ones, the overall Harris Hip Score was quite comparable: 92 in the control and 89 in the group

with the more severe deformity. The mean alignment was 3 degrees of varus in the severe-deformity group and 0 degrees in the control group. The range of motion was also somewhat different, averaging 98 degrees of flexion in those with preoperative deformity and 107 degrees in the control group.[37] Laskin and Schob also reported their experience with 68 knees after a simple medial capsular release followed for an average of approximately 5 years. Seventy-three percent of cases had less than 5 degrees of varus-valgus instability after surgery; however, the authors did report that 2 of 68 cases underwent medial collateral ligament tear. All patients had adequate postoperative alignment.[22]

Valgus Malalignment

Valgus malalignment has received more attention than has varus deformity despite it being much less common.[35] Knowing the amount of valgus correctable by varus stress is again helpful to plan the extent of release and degree of implant constraint that may be needed. In addition to the tight lateral structures, there is often attenuation of the medial collateral ligament. In the elderly and low-demand patient, it may be reasonable to utilize the more constrained implant rather than perform extensive soft tissue release. It is important to recognize that the osseous deficiencies of the valgus knee usually comprise a hypoplastic or defective femoral condyle and tibial plateau laterally. Peters et al. have recently compared two different lateral release sequences and quantified the effects of sequential lateral capsular ligamentous structure release.[28] They found that releasing in a five

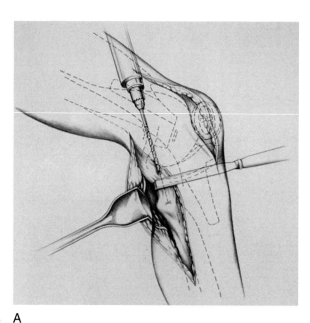

A

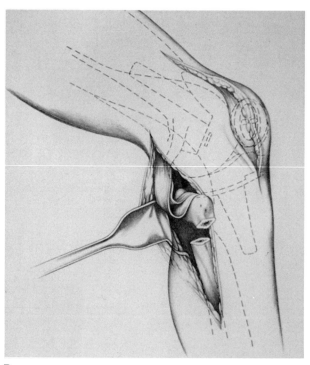

B

Figure 78–3. *See legend on opposite page*

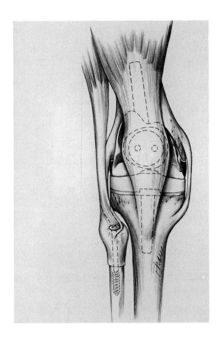

C

Figure 78–3. The approach is through a supplemental posterolateral incision, exposing the fibular head, which is predrilled. **A,** The peroneal nerve is identified and protected. The neck of the fibula is osteotomized, and traction is placed distally, simulating the desired tension on the fibular collateral ligament. **B,** The amount of overlap is resected. **C,** The fibula is then attached with a single AO cancellous screw and placed in the predrilled tract. (From Krackow KA: Deformity. *In* The Technique of Total Knee Arthroplasty. St. Louis, CV Mosby, 1990, p 329.)

step sequence—PCL, posterolateal capsule, iliotibial band, popliteus tendon, and LCL—produced more symmetrical flexion-extension gaps than did releasing in a four step sequent (PCL, iliotibial band, popliteus tendon/LCL complex, biceps).

Technique

ANTEROMEDIAL APPROACH

After the tibia has been cut using an extramedullary alignment system and as predicted by the template constructed preoperatively, the intramedullary alignment system is used to resect the distal femur. A trial reduction, usually with a thin implant, is carried out, and an estimate of the varus-valgus soft tissue tension is noted. In our practice, when modular tibial components are used, at least a 10-mm-thick high-density polyethylene component is employed in all cases. Thus, if the soft tissue is excessively taut (the 2-mm rule), a lateral release is carried out.

The anatomic components that contribute to the lateral contracture are assessed, consisting of the biceps tendon, the popliteus tendon, the iliotibial band, the LCL, and the arcuate complex (Fig. 78–4). In a fixed valgus deformity, particularly in rheumatoid patients, there may also be a fixed external rotation deformity of the tibia secondary to contracture of the iliotibial band.

Additional osseous deformity is typically present at either the femur or tibia as one of the components of deformity (Fig. 78–5).

Soft Tissue Release. Hungerford and Lennox have classified valgus deformities as those in which the medial collateral ligament is competent (type I) versus those in which the medial collateral ligament is deficient (type II).[11] The appropriate management is predicated on this classification system.

Type I Contracture: Competent Medial Collateral Ligament. The sequence of release is generally well accepted. After trial reduction, if excessive tension persists,

1. Any remaining femoral or tibial osteophytes are removed.
2. The capsule is released from the lateral and posterolateral tibial margin.
3. The iliotibial band is released proximal to the joint, aligned with either an oblique Z-plasty or multiple perforations. This is performed through the arthrotomy incision with the patella reflected laterally. The iliotibial band is dissected from the subcutaneous tissue and is well defined so that the appropriate release may be carefully and completely carried out.
4. The LCL is then released with a fleck of bone from its attachment on the femur, along with the popliteus tendon.
5. If the "separation" requirement is still not satisfied, then the biceps tendon must be released. A separate incision is made over the taut biceps tendon. This is dissected free of the peroneal nerve and a Z-lengthening of the structure just proximal to its insertion is carried out.
6. Finally, if the knee remains contracted, failing the separation test, the femoral attachment of the lateral gastrocnemius is released.

For contracture requiring release of the LCLs, or steps 5 and 6 described above, a constrained implant is required.

Type II Contracture: Deficient Medial Collateral Ligament. If the laxity of the medial compartment is mild, capsule and deep collateral ligaments may be reattached or advanced.

Medial Capsule Reefing (Mayo). A simple means we use to advance the capsule is to place nonabsorbable sutures through the medial tibial cortex about 1 cm distal to the surface of resection (Fig. 78–6). With the knee extended to about 10 degrees and with varus stress, the sutures are placed through the capsule and ligament remnant and tied. Assessment of integrity and tension with flexion and extension is confirmed.

After surgery, a knee stabilizing brace is used during gait for 3 weeks.

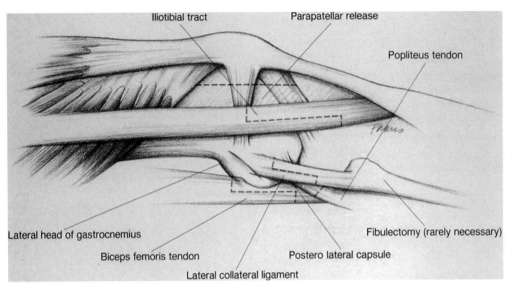

Figure 78–4. The components that contribute to valgus contracture and the manner of release. (From Hungerford DS, Lennox DW: Management of fixed deformity at total knee arthroplasty: fixed valgus deformity. *In* Hungerford DS, Krackow KA, Kenna RV [eds]: Total Knee Arthroplasty. Baltimore, Williams & Wilkins, 1984.)

Medial Advancement Technique (Hungerford). If the valgus deformity is associated with an incompetent medial collateral ligament after adequate release, medial ligamentous complex advance can be achieved. The medial aspect of the arthrotomy incision is extended to expose the pes anserine tendons. With the knee flexed, the pes anserine tissue is relaxed and released subperiosteally and posteriorly as a flap using sharp dissection (Fig. 78–7). This flap of tissue includes a portion of the capsule, the superficial medial collateral ligament, and the pes anserine tendons. The sleeve of tissue is then advanced distally with the knee held in proper alignment and with some varus stress as the knee is flexed 10 degrees. Reattachment is performed with a ligament staple as distally as possible; otherwise the mechanics of the ligament will be altered. Two staples typically are used to assure adequate fixation of the advanced collateral ligament complex.

Collateral Absence with Achilles Tendon Allograft Reconstruction (Mayo). Complete absence of the medial collateral ligament must be managed by either a constrained implant, graft reconstruction, or both. We have limited but encouraging experience with Achilles tendon allograft reconstruction.

The anatomic origin of the medial collateral ligament is located at the medial epicondyle. The tubular portion of the Achilles tendon is "locked" into a tunnel made at this origin and tied with No. 5 nonabsorbable suture securely to the lateral cortex. With the knee extended, the posterior fibers are attached with a No. 5 nonabsorbable suture to the area of attachment of the superficial medial collateral ligament. With the knee flexed to 60 degrees, the anterior fibers are drawn taut and secured with No. 5 nonabsorbable sutures attached to the tibia through bone holes (Fig. 78–8).

Postoperative Care. Postoperative management usually consists of a knee immobilizer full time for at least 3 weeks. This is removed for supervised flexion and extension. The immobilizer may be continued if there is any question about the integrity or the maturity of the healing medial collateral ligament complex. In some instances, a prestressed knee brace may be used to allow earlier motion and still protect the ligament surgery.

LATERAL EXPOSURE AND RELEASE (KEBLISH)

Keblish has reported a surgical approach from the lateral parapatellar exposure that allows direct visualization and release of the various components of the lateral contracture.[14] This procedure is more difficult and time consuming, but it is reported to provide access to the static elements comprising the contracture. We have no experience with this exposure.

A standard linear incision is made just lateral to the midline and extends approximately 2 cm lateral to the patellar tendon, terminating distally over the anterior compartment. The peroneal nerve is identified and protected and the iliotibial band is released with a Z or V-Y technique. The amount of release required is judged according to the severity of the valgus deformity. If this does not allow proper alignment with varus stress, then the posterolateral corner comprising the arcuate complex is released. For more severe deformities, including tibial rotation and valgus that is greater than 40 degrees, the anteromedial fascia is elevated from Gerdy's tubercle along with partial or complete resection of the fibular head in order to decompress the peroneal nerve and minimize the longitudinal stretch that occurs with the correction of such an extensive degree of deformity. The patellar tendon and extensor mechanism is reflected medially along with a portion of the insertion in order to allow adequate release for medial translation. On occasion, complete elevation of the tendon insertion is required, using a periosteal feathering

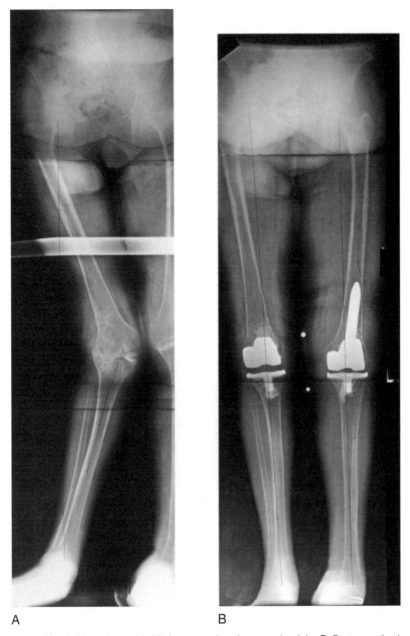

Figure 78–5. A, Rheumatoid arthritis patient with 36-degrees valgus knee on the right. **B**, Postoperative long-leg view showing restoration of a mechanical axis and use of a posterior-stabilized knee design. Patient required lateral iliotibial band, lateral collateral ligaments, and popliteus release to adequately balance the knee.

technique, or the insertion may be released with an osteotome.

Once the knee is flexed and the extensor mechanism is reflected medially, the necessary soft tissue releases, including the posterolateral corner, may be carried out, and the medial compartment is exposed only after the release of the lateral structures. The PCL is almost always sacrificed with such severe contractures. With correction of the alignment, a significant capsular defect is present laterally. Keblish recommended immobilizing the fat pad or a margin of the lateral meniscus so that the void over the implant may be protected. Skin closure is routinely obtained, and drains are recommended. Keblish offered many specific hints

and technical points, and the reader is referred to the original description.[14]

Results

Keblish reported experience with 79 patients using his extensive lateral approach. Fifty-three had over a 2-year follow-up. Scores of excellent or good were recorded in 93 percent of cases. He used a nonconstrained implant and has had no problem with instability.[14]

Whiteside has reported on 135 patients with valgus deformity measuring a mean of 16 degrees before surgery, achieving an average of 7 degrees of valgus alignment after surgery.[39] At 7 years of follow-up, he reported

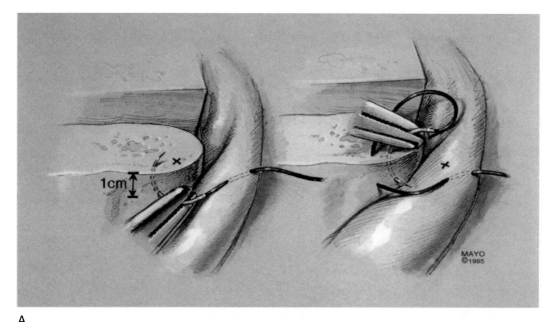

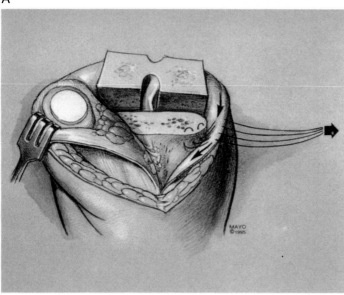

A

B

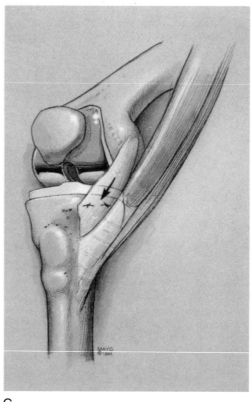

Figure 78–6. A, Two nonabsorbable sutures are placed 1 cm from the cut surface and embedded in the cancellous bone. **B,** The medial collateral ligament and medial capsule are grasped proximally. **C,** Proper tension and placement are confirmed with a trial reduction, and the sutures are tied after the prosthesis has been cemented in place.

C

no functional impairment of this group of patients. He did note, however, that if greater than 25 degrees of valgus exists preoperatively, then postoperative laxity is observed medially. This suggests that a valgus deformity of greater than 20 to 25 degrees may well require medial collateral ligament advancement or capsular reattachment. Whiteside also emphasized the fact that patellar malalignment may occur, although this was observed in only 1 of his 135 patients.

Miyasaka et al. reviewed 108 knees with valgus angulation of 10 degrees or greater in 83 patients undergoing primary total knee arthroplasty with an average surveillance of 14.1 years.[26] They found that 24 percent of the knees had mild to moderate instability.

Krackow et al. reported the results of 99 patients from 2 to 10 years after surgery that included soft tissue release for valgus deformity. In those with bone loss and soft tissue contracture, simple release of the contracture

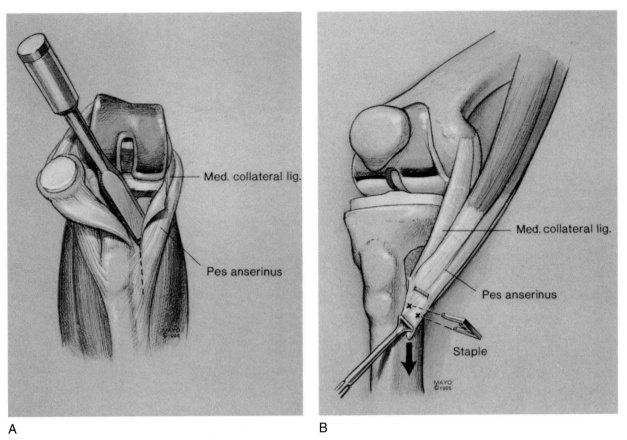

A   B

Figure 78–7. A, The medial collateral ligament and pes anserine tendons are elevated en masse subperiosteally from the anteromedial aspect of the proximal tibia. **B**, With the knee partially flexed, the medial tissues are advanced to attain proper balance and stabilized with two staples.

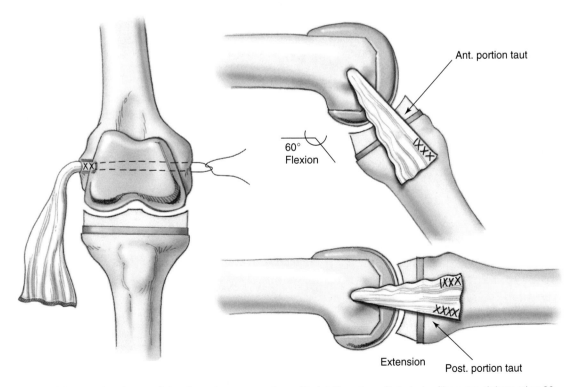

Figure 78–8. Diagram showing medial collateral reconstruction with Achilles allograft. Anterior fibers are tightened at 60 degrees of flexion and posterior fibers tightened in full extension.

was adequate. However, the medial collateral ligament was advanced if severely deficient. They reported a 90 percent excellent or good result with both types of deficiencies. Compared to 40 control patients with less deformity, 98 percent were reported as excellent or good.[19]

Buechel classified valgus deformity as mild, moderate, or severe and recommended using an unconstrained implant with a design different from but mechanics similar to that used by Krackow et al. He reported satisfactory results with a sequence of release similar to that described above.[2]

Furthermore, Krackow and Holtgrewe noted a set of patients in whom valgus deformity was due to a failed proximal tibial osteotomy with osseous malalignment.[18] This type of problem has been described by Wolff et al., who classified this as extra-articular etiology of malalignment.[41] In Krackow and Holtgrewe's opinion, such deformity requires a medial ligament reconstruction, and, in five patients so treated, all had a satisfactory result. A minimally constrained implant was used in this group of patients.[18] Others have also reported postosteotomy or fracture deformity as a cause of malalignment. Roffi and Merritt reported only 8 of 13 patients with fracture deformities having excellent or good results with very short follow-up, averaging only 27 months.[31] Thus it appears as though secondary osseous-induced malalignment (osteotomy and fracture) may have a poorer prognosis than would be expected from that occurring as an integral part of the disease process.

Complications

One of the most devastating complications of correcting a valgus deformity is well recognized to be personeal palsy. Horlocker et al. reported that valgus malalignment of greater than 10 degrees preoperatively may predispose to peroneal nerve palsy, whereas valgus alignment of less than 10 degrees was not associated with postoperative palsy.[9] Careful monitoring during surgery and exposure of the nerve has been suggested, but no studies to date have proven the efficiency of these precautions. Evoked potential monitoring may be of value when greater than 15 degrees of valgus is being corrected.

Flexion Deformity

Relatively little has been written regarding fixed flexion contractures, yet this is one of the most common deformities observed. If greater than 5 to 10 degrees of residual flexion deformity exists following joint replacement arthroplasty, increased work is required of the quadriceps mechanism. Functional leg length discrepancy and secondary back pain can also occur with a persistent postoperative flexion contracture. Krackow has analyzed flexion contracture management in some detail.[15] More aggressive resection of bone from the distal femur does allow the knee to come into full extension; however, tightness is present during flexion becuase the flexion gap is not altered by the excessive distal femoral cut (Fig. 78–9). Further correction of the contracture by bony resection unbalances the collateral ligaments, resulting in kinematic abnormalities. Similarly, excessive removal of the proximal tibia allows the knee to come into full extension. However, this results in an increased flexion gap, making the knee unstable in flexion (Fig. 78–10). Thus a severe flexion contracture cannot be completely solved by osseous resection of either the femur or the tibia. As a general rule, if the amount of bone resected is greater than that which is needed to accommodate the implant, some form of imbalance will be present either in flexion or in extension. However, if the contracture is so great that some additional bone must be resected, this is better tolerated from the femur than the tibia because

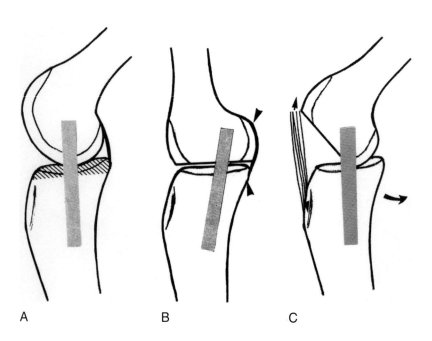

A   B   C

Figure 78–9. A, Fixed flexion contractures consist of contracted collateral ligaments, cruciate ligaments, and posterior capsule. **B,** Correction by resection of bone from the femur results in the ability to bring the leg straight with a tight posterior capsule. **C,** With flexion, however, the tightened structures anteriorly, the taut collateral ligaments, and the presence of the posterior femoral condyle prevent full flexion.

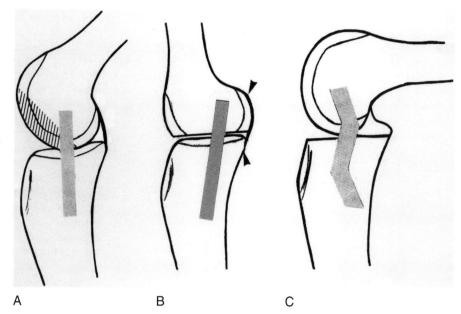

Figure 78–10. **A**, Fixed flexion contracture. **B**, Correction from the tibia allows the leg to come out straight with a tight posterior capsule and collateral ligament. **C**, With flexion, however, a significant gap occurs, the collateral ligament is lax, and the knee is unstable.

A   B   C

excess removal of the femur renders the knee stable in flexion, whereas excessive removal of tibial bone does not.

If greater than 30 to 40 degrees of flexion contracture is present before surgery, some effort should be considered to resolve this soft tissue contracture before the total knee arthroplasty. This has been accomplished either by serial casting or, in the past, by in-hospital use of dynamic splints. If greater than 60 degrees of flexion contracture is present, then consideration of a staged procedure is appropriate. This consists of a posterior capsular release procedure and casting to allow stretching of the posterior structures, followed by total knee arthroplasty. We have observed temporary peroneal palsy with release of flex-

ion contracture greater than 60 degrees, further justifying consideration of the staged procedure. The release is also compromised if the joint is destroyed, and pain does not allow maintenance of the extension gained.

Technique

Intraoperatively, the flexion contracture is managed first by removing the distal femur and proximal tibia in the usual fashion. Residual contracture is then addressed by releasing the posterior capsule from the femur. Following this, the posterior condyles are osteotomized to further release the soft tissue structures (Fig. 78–11). If residual contracture remains, then the

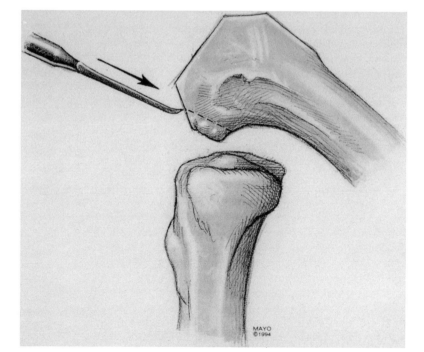

Figure 78–11. Care must be taken to assure that any posterior condylar osteophytes are removed with an osteotome as a further method of decompressing and releasing the posterior capsule.

PCL is released from the tibia and a PCL-substituting implant is employed. In our experience, release of the PCL is the single most important element in resolving moderately severe flexion contractures.

PCL-sacrificing implant designs effectively stabilize the knee after cruciate resection. If the knee is still tight in extension, elevation of the joint line by removing 2 to 6 mm of distal femur may be performed to further increase the extension gap.

Results

There are virtually no results in the literature regarding the management of fixed flexion contracture. It is of interest, however, to note that Tanzer and Miller have demonstrated that residual flexion contracture after replacement does improve with time.[36] They observed 35 knees with a residual flexion contracture averaging 13 degrees at the time of surgery that were decreased to a mean of 3 degrees 55 weeks after surgery. It is emphasized that in none of these 35 knees was there greater than 30 degrees of residual flexion contracture after the procedure. Similarly, Aglietti and co-workers reported on 20 knees with less than 50 degrees of preoperative motion.[1] After surgery, flexion improved from an average of 60 degrees to 85 degrees and extension improved from an average contracture of 28 degrees to 7 degrees' residual contracture at 4 to 5 years. McPherson et al. have just reported similar findings in a series of 28 cases. They note no apparent difference in the natural history of those patients with preoperative contractures of up to 30 degrees.[23] We must emphasize, however, that this experience has not been observed by all and, in general, if the knee does not come out into full extension at the time of surgery, it is not wise to assume significant resolution in the postoperative period.

Hyperextension Deformity

Very rarely patients will present with a preoperative hyperextension knee deformity. Most commonly this is seen in patients with neuromuscular problems (i.e., polio). Very little has been written about the technique and outcome in this patient subgroup. One must be careful with patients who ambulate with a hyperextension gait because ambulation may become difficult if the patient cannot "lock" the knee in extension. Meding and others recently reviewed the results of 58 cruciate-retaining total knee arthroplasties in 53 patients with at least 5 degrees of preoperative hyperextension. No cases of major ligamentous instability, neuromuscular disease, or inflammatory arthropathy were identified before surgery. At an average of 4.5 years, no knee replacement was revised for any reason. Postoperative extension averaged 0 degrees, and only two knees had a hyperextension deformity after surgery.[25]

It makes sense in this patient subgroup to do all one can to "tighten" the extension gap. This can be accomplished by resecting a minimal amount of distal femur with or without the use of distal augments. Using a thick tibial insert will also "tighten" the extension gap but it will also tighten and limit flexion. Recurrence of

the hyperextension deformity postoperatively can occur from soft tissue stretch. Because of this, some surgeons favor proceeding to a hinged implant that will mechanically block hyperextension. Use of this implant should help in decreasing the chance of recurrence of hyperextension but of course puts more stress on the implant-bone-cement interface.

AUTHORS' PREFERENCE

The techniques described above for mild to moderate varus and valgus deformity have been effective in our experience. We would emphasize the following points:

1. Great care is taken to avoid excessive osseous resection that results in seating the implants on weak metaphyseal bone; if concern exists, stemmed implants are used.
2. Release is carried out to the extent that the separation test is satisfied to assure adequate relaxation on the contracted side.
3. We prefer a stabilized implant design over ligament reconstruction in most instances.
4. The Achilles tendon allograft has been an effective adjunct for those patients with severe deficiencies.

References

1. Aglietti P, Windsor RE, Buzzi R, Insall JM: Arthroplasty for the stiff or ankylosed knee. J Arthroplasty 4:1, 1989.
2. Buechel FF: A sequential three-step lateral release for correcting fixed valgus knee deformities during total knee arthroplasty. Clin Orthop 260:170, 1990.
3. Cates HE, Ritter MA, Keating EM, Faris PM: Intramedullary versus extramedullary femoral alignment systems in total knee replacement. Clin Orthop 386:32, 1993.
4. Dennis DA, Channer M, Susman MW, Stringer EA: Intramedullary versus extramedullary tibial alignment systems in total knee arthroplasty. J Arthroplasty 8:43, 1993.
5. Donaldson WF III, Sculco TP, Insall JN, Ranawat CS: Total Condylar III-knee prosthesis: long-term follow-up study. Clin Orthop 226:21, 1988.
6. Edwards E, Miller J, Chan KH: The effect of postoperative collateral ligament laxity in total knee arthroplasty. Clin Orthop 236:44, 1988.
7. Engh GA, Petersen TL: Comparative experience with intramedullary and extramedullary alignment in total knee arthroplasty. J Arthroplasty 5:1, 1990.
8. Faris PM, Herbst SA, Ritter MA, Keeting EM: The effect of preoperative knee deformity on the initial results of cruciate-retaining total knee arthroplasty. J Arthroplasty 7:527, 1992.
9. Horlocker TT, Cabanela ME, Wedel DJ: Does postoperative epidural analgesia increase the risk of peroneal nerve palsy after total knee arthroplasty? Anesth Analg 79:495, 1994.
10. Hsu HP, Garg A, Walker PS, et al: Effect of knee component alignment on tibial load distribution with clinical correlation. Clin Orthop 248:135, 1989.
11. Hungerford DS, Lennox DW: Management of fixed deformity at total knee arthroplasty: fixed valgus deformity. In Hungerford DS, Krackow KA, Kenna RV (eds): Total Knee Arthroplasty. Baltimore, Williams & Wilkins, 1984.
12. Karachalios TH, Sarangi PP, Newma JH: Severe varus and valgus deformities treated by total knee arthroplasty. J Bone Joint Surg Br 76:938, 1994.
13. Kaufer H, Matthews LS: Spherocentric arthroplasty of the knee. J Bone Joint Surg Am 63:545, 1981.

14. Keblish PA: The lateral approach to the valgus knee: surgical technique and analysis of 53 cases with over two-year follow-up evaluation. Clin Orthop 271:52, 1991.
15. Krackow KA: Management of fixed deformity at total knee arthroplasty: fixed flexion contracture. *In* Hungerford DS, Krackow KA, Kenna RV (eds): Total Knee Arthroplasty. Baltimore, Williams & Wilkins, 1984.
16. Krackow KA: Management of fixed deformity at total knee arthroplasty: general principles. *In* Hungerford DS, Krackow KA, Kenna RV (eds): Total Knee Arthroplasty. Baltimore, Williams & Wilkins, 1984.
17. Krackow KA: Deformity. *In* The Technique of Total Knee Arthroplasty. St. Louis, CV Mosby, 1990, p 249.
18. Krackow KA, Holtgrewe JL: Experience with a new technique for managing severely overcorrected valgus high tibial osteotomy at total knee arthroplasty. Clin Orthop 258:213, 1990.
19. Krackow KA, Jones MM, Teeny SM, Hungerford DS: Primary total knee arthroplasty in patients with fixed valgus deformity. Clin Orthop 273:9, 1991.
20. Laskin RS: Management of fixed deformity at total knee arthroplasty: fixed varus deformity. *In* Hungerford DS, Krachow KA, Kenna RV (eds): Total Knee Arthroplasty. Baltimore, Williams & Wilkins, 1984.
21. Laskin RS, Rieger M, Schob C, Turen C: The posterior stabilized total knee prosthesis in the knee with severe fixed deformity. Am J Knee Surg 1:199, 1988.
22. Laskin RS, Schob CJ: Medial capsular recession for severe varus deformities. J Arthroplasty 2:313, 1987.
23. McPherson EJ, Cushner FD, Schiff CF, Friedman RJ: Natural history of uncorrected flexion contractures following total knee arthroplasty. J Arthroplasty 9:499, 1994.
24. McGrory B, Trousdale RT, Pagnano M: Preoperative long leg radiographs in total knee arthroplasty: a randomized prospective trial. Presented at the meeting of the Knee Society, American Academy of Orthopaedic Surgeons, 2002.
25. Meding JB, Keating M, Ritter MA, et al: Total knee replacement in patients with genu recurvatum. Clin Orthop 393:244, 2001.
26. Miyasaka KC, Ranawat CS, Mullaji A: A 10–20 year follow-up of total knee arthroplasty for valgus deformities. Clin Orthop 345:29, 1997.
27. Moreland JR: Intramedullary vs. extramedullary total knee instrumentation. *In* Goldberg VM (ed): Controversies of Total Knee Arthroplasty. New York, Raven Press, 1991.
28. Peters CL, Mohr RA, Bachus KN: Primary total knee arthroplasty in the valgus knee. J Arthroplasty 16:721–729, 2001.
29. Petersen TL, Engh GA: Radiographic assessment of knee alignment after total knee arthroplasty. J Arthroplasty 3:67, 1988.
30. Ritter MA, Faris PM, Keating EM, Meding JB: Postoperative alignment of total knee replacement: its effect on survival. Clin Orthop 299:153, 1994.
31. Roffi RP, Merritt PO: Total knee replacement after fractures about the knee. Orthop Rev 19:614, 1990.
32. Scuderi GR, Insall JN: Fixed varus and valgus deformities. *In* Lotke P (ed): Masters Techniques: Knee Arthroplasty. New York, Raven Press, 1995, p 111.
33. Sculco TP: Soft tissue balancing in total knee arthroplasty. *In* Goldberg VM (ed): Controversies of Total Knee Arthroplasty. New York, Raven Press, 1991.
34. Smith JL Jr, Tullos HS, Davidson JP: Alignment of total knee arthroplasty. J Arthroplasty 4(Suppl):S55, 1989.
35. Stern SH, Moeckel BH, Insall JN: Total arthroplasty in valgus knees. Clin Orthop 273:5, 1991.
36. Tanzer M, Miller J: The natural history of flexion contracture in total knee arthroplasty: a prospective study. Clin Orthop 248:129, 1989.
37. Teeny SM, Krackow KA, Hungerford DS, Jones M: Primary total knee arthroplasty in patients with severe varus deformity: a comparative study. Clin Orthop 273:19, 1991.
38. Tew M, Waugh W: Tibiofemoral alignment and the results of knee replacement. J Bone Joint Surg Br 67:551, 1985.
39. Whiteside LA: Correction of ligament and bone defects in total arthroplasty of the severely valgus knee. Clin Orthop 288:234, 1993.
40. Windsor RE, Scuderi GR, Moran MC, Insall JN: Mechanisms of failure of the femoral and tibial components in total knee arthroplasty. Clin Orthop 248:15, 1989.
41. Wolff AM, Hungerford DS, Pepe CL: The effect of extraarticular varus and valgus deformity on total knee arthroplasty. Clin Orthop 271:35, 1991.

79

Extensor Mechanism Problems Following Total Knee Arthroplasty

• MARK J. SPANGEHL and ARLEN D. HANSSEN

Extensor mechanism complications are the most frequent reason for early reoperation in an aseptic total knee arthroplasty (TKA) using contemporary total condylar prosthetic designs. The prevalence of complications involving the extensor mechanism in large series has ranged from 1.5 to 12 percent.[15,17,38,72,95] Patient selection, operative technique, and implant design all influence the frequency of these complications. This chapter reviews and summarizes causes, surgical considerations, and treatment options pertaining to extensor mechanism problems in TKA.

BIOMECHANICS

The patella serves a number of significant functions (Table 79–1), the most important being its mechanical role.[58] These features have already been discussed in some detail in Chapters 71 and 72. TKA has several biomechanical effects on the patellofemoral joint.[36] The designs of patellar implants may be considered as axisymmetric (dome), one-plane symmetric (anatomically shaped), or two-plane symmetric (modified dome shaped). The more conforming designs boast a larger load-bearing surface area and a reduction in contact stresses, and suggest increased stability.[17,33,60,67,72,75] When seven different designs of TKAs were compared, the total contact area of the patellofemoral joint was only 21 percent of that of the intact knee joint.[60] Contact areas of the axisymmetric design decreased less with malalignment than did contact areas of the one-plane symmetric design. There was a tendency for the prosthetic patella to shift medially on knee flexion, in contrast to the control patella, which shifted laterally.[60] These alterations of knee kinematics and the decrease in patellofemoral contact area after TKA may be responsible for complications such as polyethylene wear, loosening, and subluxation.

OPTIMIZING COMPONENT POSITION

Component position and soft tissue balance are two of the most important ingredients to maximize the mechanical performance of the extensor mechanism in TKA. Modern total knee instrumentations all have generic resemblances with respect to alignment systems and cutting guides, and their evolution has made bone resection and prosthetic positioning more accurate and reproducible.[24,25] Yet numerous studies have cited problems with implant alignment and soft tissue balance as a leading cause of extensor mechanism complications.[6,15,27,33,35,39,68,76,81,82] Additionally, component malrotation, without clinically apparent patellar instability, has been implicated as a cause of anterior knee pain.[7,89] Therefore, it is worthwhile to review the surgical technique of component positioning, emphasizing potential pitfalls, optimizing component position, and thereby minimizing extensor mechanism complications.

Varus/Valgus

Excessive postoperative limb alignment of greater than 10 degrees of valgus has consistently correlated with patellofemoral problems.[38,79,107] This situation accentuates the quadriceps (Q) angle, increasing the lateral force vector on the patella.[79,98] Causes of valgus malalignment include excessive valgus resection of the distal femur or proximal tibia. Incomplete seating of a component on accurate bone preparation can also lead to this end result. Overall limb alignment and mechanical axis should be assessed with trial components.

Translation

The medial-lateral displacement of the femoral and tibial components also influences the extensor mechanism function. Ideally, the femoral component should coincide with the resected margin of the lateral femoral condyle. The epicondyles and the intercondylar notch can be used as references for medial-lateral positioning, and the prosthetic patellar groove should approximate that of the native trochlear groove. Femoral component medialization should be avoided, and slight lateral translation may improve patellar tracking (Fig. 79–1B).[102]

Table 79–1. PATELLAR FUNCTIONS

Increase quadriceps moment arm
Provide cartilage surface with low coefficient of friction
Centralize force of quadriceps
Protect quadriceps and patellar tendons from attritional wear
Shield joint from direct trauma
Cosmesis

Similarly, tibial component medialization adversely affects patellar stability by causing relative lateral displacement of the tibial tubercle, thus increasing the Q angle. Inadequate lateral exposure or a deficiency of the lateral tibial plateau tempts medial translation of the tibial prosthesis. This circumstance may be encountered in a knee with a previous valgus upper tibial osteotomy or lateral tibial plateau trauma with significant bone loss.

Axial Rotation

Femoral

Proper rotational orientation of femoral and tibial components is vital to arthroplasty function, and malrotation has clearly been associated with extensor mechanism complications.[11,22,31,37,51,103,106] Internal rotation of the femoral component has a detrimental effect on patellar tracking by displacing the femoral trochlea medially, resulting in an increased Q angle (Fig. 79–1A). A small amount of external rotation is favorable and has been shown to improve tracking in anatomic studies; however, excessive external rotation should be avoided.[2,102,103] The references for judging femoral component rotation are the epicondylar axis, approximately 3 degrees of external rotation relative to the posterior femoral condylar axis, and a perpendicular axis

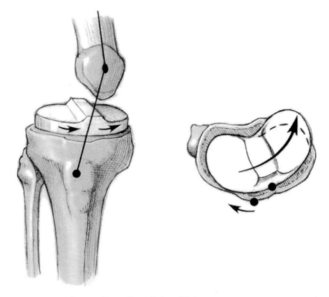

Figure 79–2. Internal rotation of the tibial component accentuates the Q angle by causing a relative lateral displacement of the tibial tubercle, leading to patellar maltracking.

to the femoral trochlear groove or the anterior-posterior axis of the knee.[3,26,93] The epicondylar axis is useful in situations where the posterior condyles are distorted or deficient, as in a rheumatoid knee with erosion and valgus deformity or in the revision arthroplasty setting.[12] Although the posterior femoral condyles are commonly used to judge femoral component rotation, the epicondylar axis has been shown to be most accurate for re-establishing proper femoral component rotation.[26,80,87,93] Finally, resection of the lateral trochlear ridge on the anterior distal femur should be greater than its medial counterpart, and slightly more bone should be removed from the posteromedial femoral condyle than from the posterolateral condyle, when using a femoral component with symmetric posterior condyles. If this does not appear to be the case, one should suspect internal malrotation of the cutting guide, and the position of the cutting guide should be reassessed.

Tibial

Tibial component rotation determines the position of the tibial tubercle. Excessive internal rotation of the tibial prosthesis has been identified as a cause for patellar subluxation and dislocation, by displacing the tibial tubercle laterally and increasing the Q angle (Fig. 79–2).[7,11,16,31,61,79] References for tibial component rotational orientation include the medial to middle third of the tibial tubercle and the tibial crest (although individual variation does exist).[61] Rotational alignment can be assessed with the limb in full extension, allowing the tibial component to be evaluated in relation to the femoral prosthesis, tibial tubercle, and ankle mortise. Maneuvering the knee through a range of motion allows the trial tibial tray to "auto-adjust" its position relative to the femoral component and is helpful prior to determination of its final

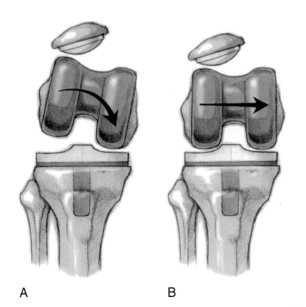

A   B

Figure 79–1. Malpositions of the femoral component adversely affecting patellar tracking. Internal rotation (**A**) and medial displacement (**B**) both cause medialization of the patellar groove and increased lateral retinacular tension.

position. The selected rotational position typically places the medial to middle third of the tibial tubercle in line with the midportion of the tibial prosthesis. Poor exposure is a common cause of malrotation and medial translation of the tibial component.[14]

Patella

Patellar resurfacing principles include re-creating the original thickness with the patella-prosthetic composite, avoiding asymmetry of the residual patella following resection, positioning the implant in the correct location, and obtaining proper soft tissue balance and patellar tracking.[4,89] Whereas over-resection may leave the patella thin and susceptible to fracture, under-resection can result in increased patellofemoral forces, reduced knee flexion, and increased lateral retinacular tension, causing patellar instability.[48,115] The major vertical ridge of the patella is located an average of 4.6 mm medial to the midpatella.[86] Therefore, with simple dome-shaped implant designs, slight medialization is one important ingredient for the restoration of proper patellar tracking.[16,31,37,127]

PATELLAR INSTABILITY

Instability of the patella after TKA may occur with or without resurfacing of the patella. The prevalence of symptomatic patellar instability leading to reoperation is low: 0.5 percent (25 of 5463 cases) to 0.8 percent (24 of 2887 cases) in centers where a large number of arthroplasties are performed.[17,38] The causes of instability can be multiple (Table 79–2), but most involve errors in surgical technique.[5,16,17,38,71,79,96] Component malposition, excessive valgus alignment of the knee, soft tissue imbalance, and trauma are the most common culprits of patellar instability.[16,17,38,79,95]

Recognition of a patient predisposed to patellar instability following TKA is important. Excessive preoperative valgus alignment, especially chronic situations, predisposes to patellofemoral instability postoperatively.[16,55,71,79] A patient with a history of subluxation, recurrent dislocation, or ligamentous laxity may be at higher risk. Preoperative radiographic assessment should include a full-length standing anteroposterior view, a lateral view, and a Merchant image of the knee.[78] Patients with preoperative patellar displacement or tilt

Table 79–2. ETIOLOGIES OF PATELLAR MALTRACKING FOLLOWING TOTAL KNEE ARTHROPLASTY

Component malposition
Residual valgus limb alignment
Static soft tissue imbalance
Dynamic soft tissue imbalance
Trauma/capsular dehiscence
Prosthetic design
Patella alta
Soft tissue impingement
Postoperative hemarthrosis

had a twofold greater likelihood of having these postoperatively, and half as many demonstrated central patellar tracking compared to patients without preoperative tilt or displacement following TKA.[14]

The presentation of patellar maltracking may be one of pain and/or mechanical symptoms, which can include catching, giving way, subluxation, or frank dislocation. Intermittent instability is more of a discomfort than a significant disability, unless persistent or complete dislocation occurs resulting in sudden loss of quadriceps power. The chief morbidity may be the potential for component loosening, patellar fracture, and excessive patellar wear, with the generation of particulate debris.[5,61,98]

Etiology

Identifying the underlying cause(s) of the instability is critical so that the appropriate treatment can be selected. The cause can be difficult to ascertain; thus an accurate chronicle of events, in addition to a thorough clinical and radiographic evaluation, is essential. Gait, limb alignment, muscle mass, and patellar mobility and tracking must be assessed. Radiographs are used to measure mechanical and anatomic axes as well as tibial and femoral component positions relative to their respective bones. However, femoral and tibial component rotation is difficult to judge with plain radiographs. Computed tomography, using the epicondylar axis as a reference for the femoral component and the tibial tubercle for the tibial component, can be used to assess component malrotation.[11]

Contemporary femoral components of TKA essentially factor out significant trochlear groove variation from the instability equation, leaving soft tissue tension and component positions as the only remaining variables. Axial patellofemoral images allow patellar tilt, displacement, and subluxation assessment.[14,37,40,95,96] The patellar implant location and symmetry of the bony resection can also be evaluated.[96]

Conservative Treatment

The treatment of symptomatic patellar maltracking and instability following TKA is directed at the cause(s). Conservative treatment may be undertaken for dynamic subluxation. This dynamic muscle imbalance is due to the vastus lateralis overpowering the vastus medialis, causing lateral subluxation. Terminal extension strengthening exercises may resolve this situation by balancing the muscle dynamics controlling the patella.[5] Other nonoperative treatments attempted have consisted of the use of patellar "cutout" braces, iliotibial band stretching, or taping methods.

Surgical Indications and Technique

In most instances of chronic subluxation or atraumatic dislocation, nonoperative treatment is unsuccessful and surgical intervention is required.[61,120] The surgical indications for symptomatic patellar instability include pain, functional disability, unacceptable weakness or extensor lag, and failed conservative treatment.[17,38]

Soft Tissue Procedures

When operative intervention is necessary, the surgical approach should be methodical. Capsular dehiscence is an uncommon cause of subluxation and instability, but should be considered in those patients with a more sudden onset, usually within the first 3 months following surgery.[17,38] Overly aggressive physiotherapy, excessive extensor mechanism tension, massive hemarthrosis, improper suture material, or inadequate arthrotomy repair can be the basis for the problem. A soft tissue defect is frequently palpable at the superomedial capsulotomy site. An arthrogram may be helpful but often is unnecessary. Direct surgical repair is typically uncomplicated.

A careful intraoperative assessment of patellar tracking is mandatory through the range of motion. The "rule of no thumb" states that the patella should track in the midline without the surgeons' thumb stabilizing the lateral border. Ideally, the medial articular surface of the patellar prosthesis should contact the medial femoral condyle throughout the range of knee motion. However, there are limitations to intraoperative assessment of central patellar tracking. First, this is only a static evaluation at best, while the patient is under anesthesia, eliminating the influence of dynamic muscle balance. Second, the thigh tourniquet alters the normal quadriceps excursion. Knee flexion prior to tourniquet inflation can limit tethering of the quadriceps mechanism, and tourniquet deflation when testing patellar tracking allows more accurate conditions for assessment.[43]

If the limb is well aligned and patellar tilting with medial lift-off, subluxation, or dislocation occurs, a lateral release is recommended.[5,17,52,96,107,114] This maneuver may be adequate for symptomatic subluxation but is usually insufficient treatment when dealing with recurrent or chronic patellar dislocation.

Proximal Alignment

Patellar instability, in the presence of properly placed components, should be treated with a proximal soft tissue realignment procedure if persistent tilt or subluxation exists despite lateral retinacular release.[1,38,52,53,61, 79,96,107] This involves medial imbrication or advancement of the medial quadriceps laterally and distally at the time of arthrotomy closure. Insall's technique is popular, and successful results have been reported (Fig. 79–3).[1,38,79] We ensure proper tracking with closure by placing two or three sutures in the peripatellar region of the medial arthrotomy. This allows extensor mechanism tension and patellar tracking to be visualized and judged throughout the range of motion, and, if satisfactory, closure may proceed with careful, intermittent reassessment of tracking. Rarely, further steps are necessary to achieve proper patellar tracking. In these situations, proximal soft tissue

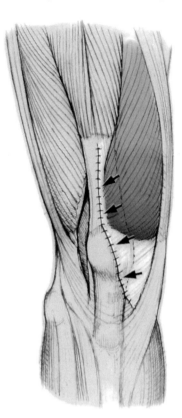

Figure 79–3. Vastus medialis advancement for correcting lateral patellar subluxation if lateral release alone is insufficient.

realignment procedures using modified V-Y quadricepsplasties have been described for the most difficult reconstructive cases, often involving chronic dislocations.[93] Quadricepsplasty in TKA has been shown to cause moderate weakness in extension, yet near-normal active extension is present when objectively tested using a Cybex machine.[118]

Distal Reconstruction

Distal realignment procedures involving tibial tubercle osteotomy have been employed, although their use is debated.[5,16,38,53,61,73,97,123,125] Advocates have used tibial tubercle transfer in combination with lateral retinacular release in knees with patellar instability.[16,61,73,122,123,125] The controversy develops when mild or moderate malrotation exists in the presence of a securely fixed component. The debate focuses on revision of the well-fixed, mildly malpositioned component versus tibial tubercle osteotomy in situations in which proximal soft tissue realignment procedures are inadequate to correct patellar instability.[5,16,38,61,73,79,122] Those opposing osteotomy cite the numerous complications reported, including skin slough and infection, loss of fixation, nonunion, tibial fracture, and compartment syndrome.[38,73,79] Patellar tendon rupture has also been reported and is one of the most dreaded complications of TKA.[28,38,82,100] Additional challenges of osteotomy fixation may be encountered as a result of poor bone quality and prosthetic stem interference. Proponents of osteotomy caution against taking too thin a wafer of bone and, with modifications of previously described techniques, claim improved results, although data are scarce.[16,61] Refinements have included larger and longer bone blocks, retention of soft tissue attachments, preparation of recipient bone beds, and improved understanding of necessary fixation methods.[16,61,73] Kirk et al. reported no recurrent dislocations or ruptures of the patellar ligament in 15 knees in which patellar dislocation following TKA had been treated with distal transfer of the patellar ligament with the use of a modified Trillat procedure.[61]

Authors' Recommendations

Our approach is to perform proximal soft tissue realignment maneuvers or component revision when necessary, avoiding distal realignment procedures. If the implants appear in an appropriate position and a previous soft tissue procedure has not been performed, then proximal realignment is more likely to be successful. However, if the implants are malpositioned, then revision surgery should be undertaken because a soft tissue procedure is unlikely to be successful. It is advisable that the surgeon always be prepared to perform an entire revision arthroplasty in every instance when surgically addressing patellar instability.

Results

Reviewing multiple larger series of surgically treated symptomatic patellar instability after TKA, one can see that the results are reasonable, but not outstanding.[17,38,61,79,122] Of the three series containing knee scores, 80.8 percent (42 of 52 knees) had good or excellent results and 19.2 percent (10 of 52 knees) had fair or poor results. The combined series accumulated a 19.6 percent (20 of 102 knees) complication rate, while 6.8 percent (7 of 102 knees) developed recurrent subluxation or dislocation.

PATELLAR FRACTURES

The prevalence of patellar fractures after TKA has ranged from 0.1 percent (12 of 8249 cases) to 8.5 percent (10 of 118 cases).[17,39,85,104,110] Fractures occur in both resurfaced and unresurfaced patellas. In a study by Grace and Sim, the rate of fracture after TKA was 0.05 percent (3 of 5530 cases) for unresurfaced patellas compared with 0.33 percent (9 of 2719 cases) for resurfaced patellas.[39] The rate of fracture was higher after revision (0.61 percent; 3 of 495 cases) than after primary TKA (0.12 percent; 9 of 7754 cases).

Etiology

Factors implicated in patellar fractures following TKA are numerous (Table 79–3).[120] A patellar fracture may be due to trauma, fatigue, or stress.[124] Fatigue fractures

Table 79–3. FACTORS IMPLICATED IN PATELLAR FRACTURE AFTER TKA

Demand
Weight
General activity
Flexion
Patellofemoral Component Design
Increased thickness
Leg length
Weak bone
Osteopenia
Steroid therapy
Thermal necrosis caused by cement
Surgery
Patellar cut
    Excessive resection
    Inadequate resection
    Removal of lateral subchondral bone
    Removal of peripheral bone
Avascular necrosis caused by lateral release
Lateral shear of patella
Anterior tibial displacement
Component malalignments
Fixation Failure
Patellar implant loosening

Adapted from Vince KG, McPherson EJ: The patella in total knee arthroplasty. Orthop Clin North Am 23:675, 1992.

are more common than traumatic fractures. The etiology of a fatigue fracture may be avascularity, component malalignment, excessive bone resection, or use of a large central fixation peg on the patellar implant.[39,59,76,110,112,121]

The vascular supply to the patella is at risk when an anteromedial arthrotomy is performed in conjunction with a lateral retinacular release.[18] Osteonecrosis of the patella may follow, in part because of violation of the lateral superior genicular vessels.[108,112,1121] If a lateral release is necessary, it is best performed at least 1 cm lateral to the patellar border. There is evidence suggesting less interference with the patellar blood supply using this guideline compared to a lateral release performed closer to the patella.[59] Radical excision of the fat pad, combined with a lateral release, can also potentially compromise patellar blood supply.[59] Osteonecrosis has been identified in some patellas that had fatigue fractures following TKA.[45,110] In an earlier study by Ritter et al., patellar fractures were identified in 4 percent of knees that had not had a lateral release compared to 1 percent of knees that had had such a release; however, in an updated study with a larger sample size, patellar fractures occurred in 4 percent of patients with lateral release and in 0.5 percent of patients without lateral release, suggesting that lateral release and vascularity are important in the etiology of these fractures.[104,105] Preserving the vascularity of the patella, by minimizing the fat pad resection, and preserving the superior lateral genicular vessels when lateral release is necessary, may minimize the occurrence of patellar fractures.

Excessive patellar bone resection, or removal of the strong subchondral cancellous bone or peripheral bone, weakens the remaining patella.[57,95,108] A minimum thickness of 15 mm of residual patellar bone has been recommended.[101] Reproduction of the original thickness of the patella after resurfacing is optimal. Conversely, inadequate bone resection, leaving the patella excessively thick, tenses the extensor mechanism and surrounding retinacula, increasing the strain on the patella.[16,82,104,107] Other technical factors, such as creation of a large central defect or violation of the anterior patellar cortex, may create an area of stress concentration, leaving the patella vulnerable to fracture.[57,108]

Classification

Ortiguera and Berry have described a classification system based on implant stability, integrity of the extensor mechanism, and quality of bone stock[85] (Table 79–4). Type I fractures have an intact extensor mechanism and a stable implant. In type II fractures, the extensor mechanism is disrupted and the implant may be well fixed or loose. Type III fractures are characterized by a loose patellar component and an intact extensor mechanism. Type III fractures are subtyped into A (good bone stock with a loose patellar component) and B (poor bone stock with a loose patellar component) (Fig. 79–4). Treatment (as described below) is guided by the fracture type.

Treatment

Treatment of patellar fractures is individualized and dependent on a number of factors. Variables that influence the treatment are location of the fracture, amount of displacement, integrity of the extensor mechanism, patellar component stability, and the extent of comminution and quality of the bone fragments.[35,37,39,85]

Nonoperative Treatment

Nonoperative treatment is recommended for fractures that are "nondisplaced"; however, the definition of displacement has varied widely.[46,110,124] Nonoperative treatment is recommended for fractures with an intact extensor mechanism and a secure implant (type I) or a loose implant that is asymptomatic (some type III fractures).[85] These fractures typically are nondisplaced or minimally displaced without significant comminution. Acutely diagnosed fractures are treated with a knee immobilizer or cylinder cast with protected weight bearing for 6 weeks, followed by progressive range of motion. However, many type I and III fractures are noted incidentally at follow-up, when fragmentation of the patella is noted on routine radiographs.[85] The large majority of these occur within the first 3 years following surgery. These patients are often asymptomatic and do not require any specific treatment. In the series by Ortiguera and Berry, 44 percent (34 of 77 patients) were asymptomatic or minimally symptomatic when the fracture was discovered, and 82 percent of the fractures were identified within 3 years of surgery.[85]

Surgical Intervention

Operative treatment is necessary for fractures that are associated with disruption of the extensor mechanism (type II) or symptomatic loosening of the patellar implant (some type III fractures). A partial patellectomy with repair of the extensor mechanism provides a better result than attempts at open reduction and internal fixation for a single major fragment with a secure implant. Comminuted fractures with a loose implant are managed by removal of the loose component and all cement. If there are multiple fragments, only those fragments that may cause impingement are resected. Deficient bone stock often precludes prosthetic reimplantation; thus patellar resection arthroplasty (patelloplasty) or patellectomy with extensor mechanism reconstruction is required. Overall, satisfactory results following surgical treatment of patellar fractures have been reported in approximately half of the patients, and complications occurred in almost as many.[17,35,39,46,85]

Results

Reports addressing the results of treatment of patellar fractures after TKA seem to indicate that surgical care is less predictable. However, it must be noted that these results are often not comparable because of differing criteria used to select treatment, either operative or non-

Table 79–4. CLASSIFICATION OF PATELLAR FRACTURES

Fracture Type	Description	Treatment
I	Intact extensor mechanism Stable implant	Immobilization
II	Disrupted extensor mechanism (implant fixed or loose)	Extensor mechanism repair with partial or complete patellectomy vs. open reduction and internal fixation
III	Intact extensor mechanism (implant loose)	Surgery only if symptomatic Component revision
III A	Good bone stock	vs. resection
III B	Poor bone stock	vs. partial patellectomy vs. complete patellectomy

Adapted from Ortiguera CJ, Berry DJ: Patella fracture after total knee arthroplasty: J Bone Joint Surg 84A:532-540,2002.

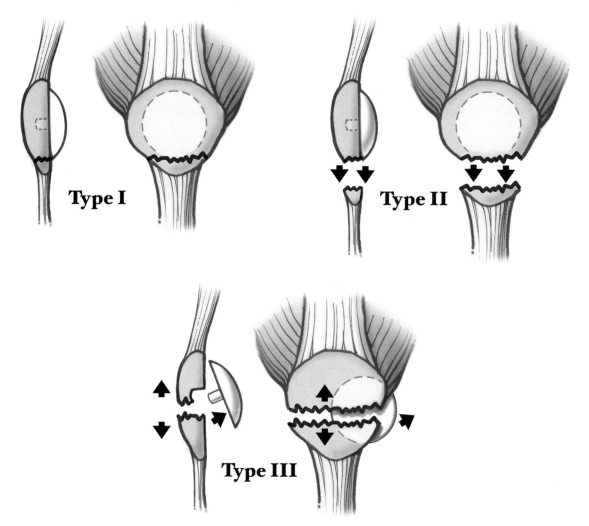

Figure 79–4. Mayo Clinic classification system based on stability and integrity of the extensor mechanism. (Courtesy of the Mayo Foundation.)

operative, for patients with patellar fractures. Generally, the more severe fractures and those with extensor mechanism disruption will be selected for surgery, whereas those fractures that are undisplaced or minimally displaced will be treated nonoperatively, thereby inherently selecting a group with a more difficult problem for surgery. With these limitations in mind, results in patients treated with surgery are generally poorer than in those treated nonoperatively. Combining three series totaling 111 cases, satisfactory results were reported in 91 percent (50 of 55) of the cases treated nonoperatively and only 46 percent (26 of 56) of the cases treated surgically, with a complication rate of roughly 45 percent.[39,46,85] Therefore, the results of the literature suggests that those patients requiring surgery have a high complication rate, but, if the fracture type is at all suitable for nonoperative treatment, this should be recommended.

PROSTHETIC WEAR

Prosthetic wear occurs with both all-polyethylene and metal-backed patellar implants. Metal backing of patellar polyethylene was introduced to reduce strain in the patella and attempt to improve implant fixation to bone.[37] However, failure appears to be a universal problem that affects many different designs.[6,8,32,50,68,69,106,116] The prevalence of failure from wear of a metal-backed implant is dependent on the duration of the evaluation, but also on prosthetic design.[27,63] Although metal-backed patellar implants generally have a higher failure rate than all-polyethylene implants, the failure of metal-backed implants is also design specific.[19,44,63] The rate of failure from clinically symptomatic wear has ranged from 5 percent (7 of 131 cases) to 11 percent (16 of 150 cases) within 2 years after the TKA.[69,106,116]

Mechanisms of metal-backed patellar component failure include wear of the polyethylene, exposing the metal backing; fracture of the polyethylene with separation from the metal backing; and fracture of the fixation pegs from the metal baseplate of the patellar implant.[6,106,116] Design features of the implant that can lead to failure include thin polyethylene over the edge of the metal plate; lack of bonding of the polyethylene to the metal plate; thin polyethylene overall; a sharp, angled transition point between the trochlear surface and the condylar weight-bearing surfaces of the femur; and the use of a titanium femoral component.[6,65,81,116,126]

Various biomechanical factors also affect wear of the polyethylene. These factors include the degree of patellofemoral congruity, shear forces associated with maltracking, and the inherently high patellofemoral joint forces with high flexion angles.[34,49] Laboratory analyses of a variety of all-polyethylene and metal-backed designs have been conducted examining patellofemoral contact stresses, deformation, and wear.[20,34,49,77] The all-polyethylene components experienced local deformation and osseous failure, whereas metal-backed implants failed because polyethylene wear exposed the metal backing.[49] The more highly congruent designs produced less wear and deformation.[75] However, this conformity may yield a more constrained articulation, increasing the risk of osseous patellar fracture and component loosening. Point loading, precipitating accelerated polyethylene wear, may also result if maltracking is present. A metal-backed patellar implant with a polyethylene articular surface that freely rotates with reference to the metal backing has been reported to cause less wear than other designs. Using this design, no wear-related failures were reported in 331 knees that had been followed for 2 to 11 years.[21] Predisposing or associated factors related to failure of patellar components have also been identified and include young age, male sex, increased body weight, high activity level, a diagnosis of osteoarthritis, flexion of more than 115 degrees, increased patella-implant composite thickness, and malalignment of the implant with improper tracking.[44,68,106,116] Additionally, there is evidence that a failed metal-backed patellar component may be a risk factor for the development of periprosthetic infection, possibly related to the metal debris and chronic synovitis.[91]

Diagnosis

Patellar wear has two characteristic clinical presentations. One scenario is a sudden onset of patellar failure, with a sensation of a crack or pop, swelling, and pain, especially with active knee flexion or extension. The other presentation is one of a gradual onset of increasing pain, swelling, synovitis, and crepitus. Audible metallic crepitus at the patellofemoral articulation and synovitis suggest the diagnosis.[84] Auscultation over the patella during active range of motion may generate a distinctive metal-on-metal grating sound. In longstanding cases, aspiration of the knee will reveal metallic debris and skyline radiographs of the patella may demonstrate metal-on-metal contact. Standard radiographic views may display radiodense clouds of metallic synovitis within the surrounding soft tissue or more sizable portions of metallic debris from fracture of the metal baseplate (Fig. 79–5). Arthroscopy has been used in some situations to diagnose early suspected component failures.

Treatment

Treatment of a failed patellar prosthesis consists of component removal, a thorough synovectomy to remove particulate debris, and femoral component revision if metal abrasion is significant. Correction of patellar tilt or

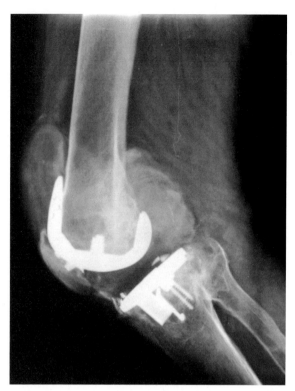

Figure 79–5. Catastrophic metal-backed patellar implant failure with metallic synovitis, wear, and fracture of the metal baseplate 5 years after index total knee replacement.

maltracking should be performed because these factors can contribute to patellar component failure. The alignment of the femoral and tibial components should be assessed, and malposition corrected if present, to prevent tracking problems. Revision of the patella is dependent on the quality and quantity of bone stock remaining (see next section). The best results of treatment occur with early diagnosis and patellar revision before severe synovitis and foreign body reaction ensue.

LOOSENING AND PATELLAR IMPLANT REVISION

Loosening of the patellar implant has been reported in 16 of 2887 (0.6 percent) to 180 of 4287 (4.2 percent) TKAs.[10,15,17] Factors associated with loosening of cemented patellar implants include use of a small central fixation peg, deficient patellar bone stock, malposition of the patellar component, trauma, and lateral release.[10,17] With use of a three-peg patellar component in 577 total knee arthroplasties, Mason and colleagues reported no loosening at an average follow-up of 3 years.[74] However, in another large series, Berend et al. noted 180 loose patellar components out of 4287 patellar implants.[10] Average time to loosening was 2.3 years. Loosening was related to lateral release and was therefore thought to be an avascular process. Other loosening catalysts include asymmetric bone resection, excessive loading by high-activity patients, and patients achieving higher degrees of flexion.

Treatment

Treatment of patellar implant loosening depends on the patient's symptoms and adequacy of the remaining patellar bone stock. If the patient is asymptomatic, a loose all-polyethylene component may not require any treatment. Only 15 of 180 loose patellar components required revision over a 15-year period.[10] Failed metal-backed patellar components generally require revision because of symptoms, or concern about damage to the femoral prosthesis.[27] Additionally, the failed metal-backed patellar component may place the knee at risk for the development of periprosthetic infection.[91]

If sufficient bone is available, with potential for cement interdigitation, reimplantation is performed. Often, a concave central defect remains after removal of the loose implant and cement. In this situation, a biconvex patellar implant satisfactorily fills in for the deficient patellar bone (Fig. 79–6).[98] If patellar bone stock is insufficient to allow resurfacing, patelloplasty (patellar resection arthroplasty) may be performed.[6,88,90] Results with this procedure reveal improved postoperative pain and function scores.[88,90] However, one third to one half of patients still reported pain ranging from mild to severe following this procedure.[88,90] Parvizi et al. also stressed the importance of component position (Fig. 79–7). These authors noted a poorer outcome in patients who underwent isolated patellar component resection versus those in whom patellar resection was performed in conjunction with femoral or tibial revision. The former group had a much higher need (13 of 19 vs. 3 of 16) for lateral release, suggesting that subtle, uncorrected component malposition may be a contributing factor for a poorer result and subsequent need for reoperation.[90]

A new technique of patellar bone grafting as an alternative to patelloplasty has been described.[42] Cancellous bone is inserted into the patellar shell and held in place with a tissue flap. Results at a mean of 37 months suggest that this procedure has the potential to restore patellar bone stock. Patellectomy is reserved as the final

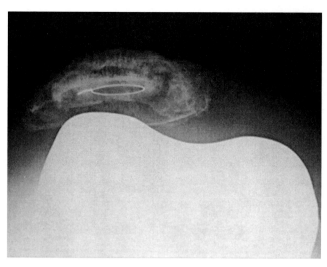

Figure 79–7. The subluxed patella poses a particularly difficult reconstructive problem. Merchant radiograph of failed patellar component with severe bone loss. Note the lateral subluxation of the patellar construct and internal rotation of the femoral component.

alternative, and some extensor weakness should be expected.[64,66,94]

Patellar Bone Grafting Technique

This procedure is indicated in patients in whom severe cavitary patellar bone loss leaves only the anterior cortex and variable amounts of the peripheral patellar rim (a patellar shell) (Fig. 79–8A). A tissue flap, created from peripatellar fibrotic tissue, a free tissue flap obtained from the suprapatellar pouch, or a fascia lata graft is obtained (Fig. 79–8B). The fibrous tissue on the undersurface of the quadriceps tendon is the most common area to elevate a tissue flap (Fig. 79–8C). It is helpful to avoid débridement of the peripatellar fibrosis around the patellar shell because this tissue is necessary for eventual placement of sutures. The tissue flap is sewn to the peripheral patellar rim with multiple sutures to provide a watertight closure. An opening is left in the flap closure to allow introduction of the cancellous bone graft.

Cancellous bone graft, either locally harvested autograft or morselized allograft, is tightly impacted into the patellar defect. The consistency of the bone graft should be similar to that of the graft used for impaction bone grafting techniques such as the Ling procedure, because this provides some structure but allows graft compaction. The graft should be packed so that it appears to be excessive because it will compress in the first year or so after arthroplasty (Fig. 79–8D).

The tissue flap contains the bone graft and serves as an interposition between the femoral trochlea and bone graft. The patellar shell–bone graft construct undergoes remodeling against the trochlea, and the retropatellar surface assumes the shape of the prosthetic trochlear groove (Fig. 79–8E). Postoperative rehabilitation is unchanged from the usual revision knee protocol. It is important to ensure that proper positioning of the femoral and tibial components has been achieved

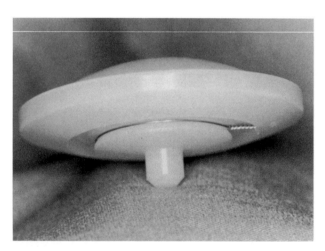

Figure 79–6. Biconvex patella implant.

because excessive shear forces or persistent patellar maltracking will be detrimental for this procedure as for other patellar reconstructive techniques.

Results

Revision of a failed patellar prosthesis is not to be taken lightly. In two large series of isolated patellar component revision after TKA, the authors concluded that this seemingly elementary surgical procedure is associated with a significant complication rate.[13,72] Berry and Rand reported an 83 percent (30 of 36 cases) good or excellent result, but a 34 percent (14 of 41 cases) complication rate was experienced.[13] There were five patellar fractures, three patients with patellar instability, two cases of peroneal palsy, two cases of polyethylene wear, and infection and extensor lag in one patient each. Lynch et al. reported a 24 percent rate of complications (9 of 37 cases) after isolated revision of the patellar component.[72]

Authors' Recommendations

Asymptomatic loose all-polyethylene patellar components do not require surgery unless there are indications of progressive osteolysis. If the patellar component becomes displaced, it may become symptomatic, requiring revision surgery. Failed metal-backed patellar components should be revised to prevent the generation of significant amounts of metal particulate debris and damage to the femoral component. If sufficient bone is present for reimplantation of a new prosthesis, reimplantation is preferable to resection arthroplasty. However, if only a shell of bone remains, attempts at reimplantation of a new prosthesis should be avoided because this may result in fracture of the patella and subsequent loosening of the patellar component. Additionally, femoral and tibial component position should be carefully inspected, and revised if the components are malpositioned. Leaving malpositioned components, which may have contributed to the original failure of the patellar component, is likely to result in ongoing problems.

PATELLAR AND QUADRICEPS TENDON DISRUPTION

Disruption of the extensor mechanism can be a result of patellar or quadriceps tendon disruption, patellar fracture, or tibial tubercle avulsion. The prevalence of patellar tendon rupture following TKA has ranged from 0.22 percent (18 of 8288 cases) to 0.55 percent (5 of 915 cases).[23,100] Etiologies of disruption include inadvertent intraoperative detachment from the tibial tubercle during knee exposure as a result of excessive dissection of the patellar ligament or excessive tension during surgery. The stiff knee with limited motion and patients with previous upper tibial osteotomy are at greater risk

for patellar ligament avulsion. A too-aggressive patellar osteotomy may partially disrupt and weaken both patellar and quadriceps tendon insertion sites to bone. Impingement of the prosthesis on the tendon or ligament, causing attritional wear and extensor mechanism failure, has also been reported.[41] Late atraumatic patellar ligament rupture infrequently occurs in patients with diabetes mellitus, collagen-vascular disease, or prolonged steroid use. Late traumatic rupture has been reported after a fall or a violent contraction of the quadriceps in a slightly flexed knee. Knee manipulation and failure of the fixation of the patellar ligament after realignment of the distal extensor mechanism have also been reported as etiologies of disruption after TKA.[38,99,100]

Prevention

This catastrophic complication presents a challenging reconstructive problem with outcomes that are often less than satisfactory. Therefore, emphasis on prevention is critical to try to avoid this complication. Prevention of patellar ligament rupture by careful surgical technique and recognition of high-risk patients is critical. Host risk factors include an ankylosed or stiff knee, patella infra, and previous surgery.[99] In these situations, the use of a more extensile approach, such as a "rectus snip" or modified Coonse-Adams extensor mechanism turndown, may be beneficial to lessen the tension on the patellar insertion. Another method for exposing the stiff knee involves subperiosteal skeletonization of the posteromedial soft tissue sleeve of the proximal tibia combined with external tibial rotation. This maneuver allows excellent exposure and avoids undue tension on the extensor mechanism and patellar ligament insertion by translating them laterally. A tibial tubercle osteotomy may also be considered to enhance exposure, particularly in cases of patella infra, in which repositioning of the tubercle somewhat more proximally may be desired in order to avoid impingement of the patella on the tibial insert. However, it is our preference to use soft tissue methods to gain exposure if all possible and avoid tibial tubercle osteotomy because of potential associated complications.[38,99,100,109]

Results

The majority of reported results after treatment of patellar ligament rupture are discouraging. One study found no satisfactory results using suture alone and 50 percent satisfactory results after staple fixation in the cases of acute rupture.[56] In a study by Rand et al., only 4 of 16 knees in which a patellar ligament rupture after TKA had been treated operatively had a successful result.[100] After treatment, 11 of the knees had a persistent rupture and infection developed in 4, leading to arthrodesis in 2 and an above-knee amputation in 1. Of the nine patients originally managed with fixation with sutures, the repair failed in six and infection developed in three. Of the four

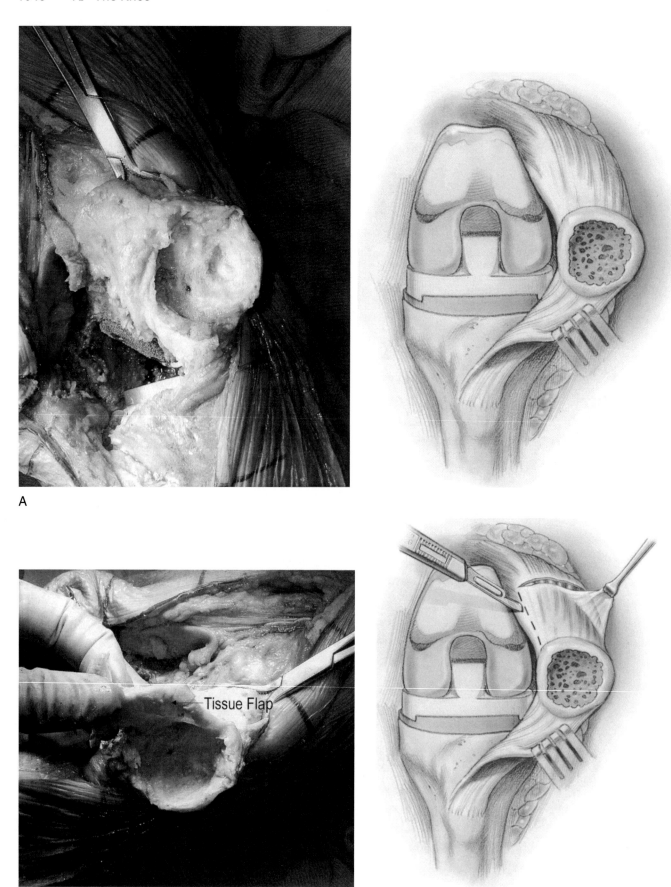

A

B

Tissue Flap

Figure 79–8. *See legend on opposite page*

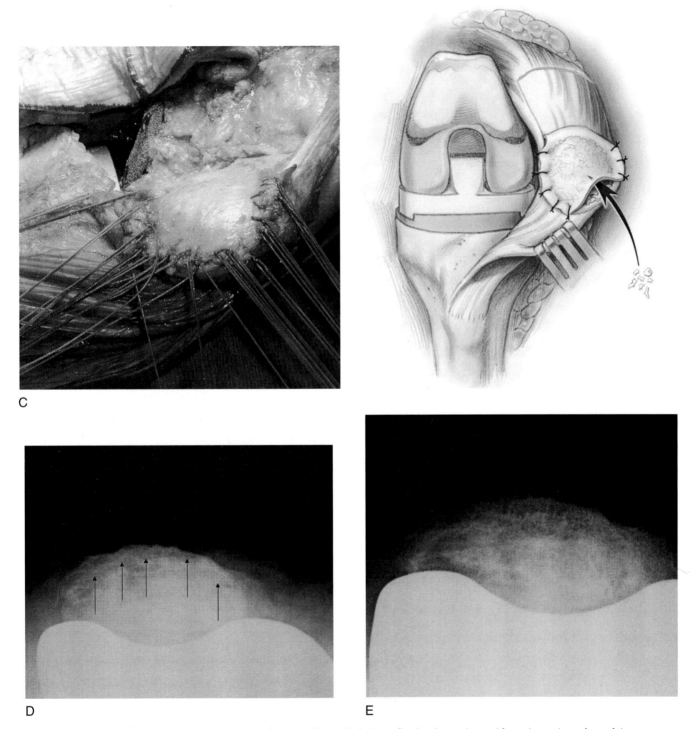

Figure 79–8. A, Intraoperative photograph of the patellar shell. A tissue flap has been elevated from the undersurface of the quadriceps tendon. **B** and **C,** The tissue flap is transposed so that it can be secured to the circumference of the patellar shell with multiple interrupted nonabsorbable sutures. **D,** Postoperative Merchant radiograph of the patellar bone-grafting construct. The *arrows* indicate the junction between the bone graft and the patellar shell. Note the volume of graft used to obtain a thick patellar construct. **E,** Two-year follow-up Merchant radiograph of same patient. Note the consolidation and compression of bone graft, which has molded to the contour of the femoral trochlea.

cases treated with staple fixation, two were successful. The two knees reconstructed with a xenograft (no longer available) had successful results, but the one knee treated with reconstruction using semitendinosus tendon had an unsuccessful result.[99,100] Other reports have varying results. Cadambi and Engh achieved successful results in

all seven knees that had been treated for patellar ligament rupture (after TKA) with an autogenous graft consisting of the semitendinosus tendon followed by 6 weeks of immobilization in a cast, although only three knees achieved more than 90 degrees of flexion (Fig. 79–9).[23] Emerson et al. updated their series and reported on 15

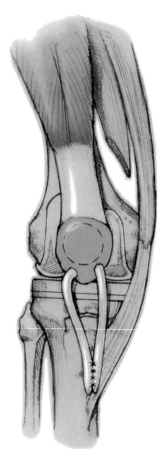

Figure 79–9. Diagram showing the reconstruction (or reinforcement) of the patellar ligament with the use of autogenous semitendinosus tendon.

operatively, potentially sacrificing some knee flexion to protect the repair. Patients may touch weight-bear with a walker provided they are compliant. Patients are changed to a hinged knee brace at 6 weeks, and gradual flexion is allowed over 3 months.

Longstanding ruptures can be complicated by adaptive contracture of the extensor mechanism. In these situations, mobilization of the extensor mechanism well proximal to the joint is required. If the tendon can be reattached to the tibial tubercle without unreasonable tension, acute repair techniques are employed. If the tendon is of poor quality, is absent, or cannot be mobilized distally, allograft reconstruction may be considered. Late reconstruction of a patellar ligament rupture using an allograft consisting of a composite of quadriceps tendon, patella, patellar ligament, and tibial tubercle may be used. We have found the Achilles tendon, with the extensive fascial component, effective for those patients with autogenous tissue deficiency (Fig. 79–10). As discussed above, successful outcome seems to depend on tensioning the graft in full extension, with 6 weeks of

knees of which 9 had more than 2 years of follow-up.[28,29] Two of the allografts reruptured, and three patients had extensor lags of 20 degrees or more. Using the same technique, Leopold et al. reported unsuccessful results in all seven knees, because of a persistent extensor lag greater than 30 degrees in all patients.[67] The largest series, and that with the most successful results, has been reported by Nazarian and Booth.[83] Thirty-four of 36 patients with a minimum 2-year follow-up had a successful outcome; however, 8 patients required repeat allograft reconstruction because of rupture of the original graft. Fifteen patients had an average extensor lag of 13 degrees; the remainder had no lag.

Authors' Recommendations

In some low-demand, elderly patients, functional loss may be inadequate to merit surgical intervention, and a drop-lock knee brace may be an acceptable treatment. Intraoperative or perioperative ruptures should be reattached as soon as possible with No. 5 nonabsorbable suture, synthetic tape, screw, or staple fixation. Autogenous semitendinous tissue, heavy suture, or tape should be used to reinforce and protect an acute repair. Patients should be immobilized in full extension post-

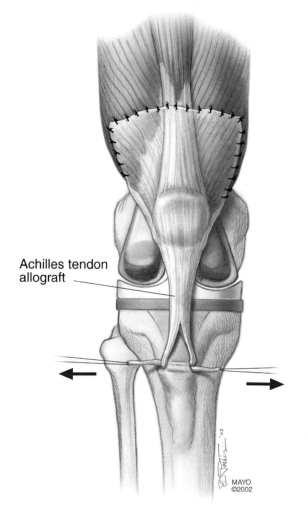

Achilles tendon allograft

Figure 79–10. We (B.F.M.) have had gratifying results using an Achilles tendon allograft to reconstruct the extension mechanism. The tendinous portion is split and attached through drill holes in the anterior tubercle. The fascial component provides strong structural attachment to the quadriceps muscle.

immobilization postoperatively followed by a gradual flexion, with 0 to 90 degrees' flexion not allowed until 3 months postoperatively.

Knee arthrodesis is a salvage procedure in treating extensor mechanism insufficiency when other means of reconstruction have failed and knee stability is preferred over bracing methods.

Quadriceps tendon rupture as a complication after TKA is very rare, as are literature reports.[30,41,71] Suspected risk factors include inflammatory arthritis, prolonged use of steroids, previous surgery, tendon devascularization during surgery, and anterior femoral flange component impingement of an overly flexed prosthesis. Quadriceps tendon rupture with functional extension power loss warrants surgical repair. Surgical repair by direct suturing and a Scuderi type of tenoplasty may be insufficient.[30,41,111] By resection of the rupture zone back to healthy tendon, mobilization of the quadriceps, and preparation of the proximal patellar pole for tendon reattachment, successful results can be maximized. A No. 5 nonabsorbable suture woven through the quadriceps tendon and anchored in patellar bone via drill holes provides a secure repair. Reinforcement of the repair followed by immobilization postoperatively, as for patellar tendon ruptures as outlined above, is recommended.

SOFT TISSUE IMPINGEMENT

Soft tissue impingement can occur following TKA. The patellar clunk syndrome is primarily associated with the use of a posterior-stabilized prosthesis.[9,47] However, it may also occur in cruciate-retaining designs and in patients who have significant knee flexion and has also been described in unresurfaced patellas.[113] A prominent fibrous nodule develops at the junction of the proximal pole of the patella and the quadriceps tendon. During knee flexion, the fibrous nodule enters the intercondylar notch of the femur and catches in this location on extension of the knee (Fig. 79–11). Arthroscopic removal of the nodule has been successful in the relief of symptoms.[47,70,119] Lucas et al. reported successful treatment in all 32 knees that underwent arthroscopic excision, with only one patient reporting persistent anterior knee pain, but no clunk.[70]

During TKA, thickened synovial tissue is often noted at the superior pole of the patella. This tissue may hypertrophy; therefore, excising this tissue may be beneficial. However, it has not been proven whether or not excising this tissue reduces the incidence of clunk.

Hypertrophy of the fat pad with the development of patella infra can be a source of pain after TKA.[19] Excision of the hypertrophic fat pad with freeing of the patellar ligament from scar tissue is recommended.[92] Patella infra after TKA is not always symptomatic. A study of 61 knees that had at least a 10 percent decrease in the Insall-Salvati ratio (patellar ligament length divided by patella length on a lateral radiograph of the knee) after TKA found no association between the range of motion or the strength of the quadriceps and the degree of patella infra.[54,62] Intra-articular fibrous bands that created a tethered patella syndrome were reported after 11 of 635 TKAs.[117] After removal of the fibrous bands, all of the symptoms resolved.

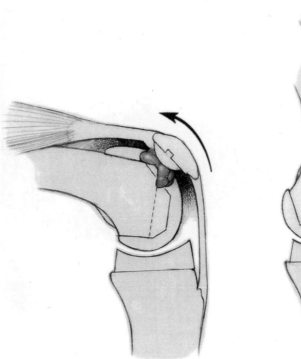
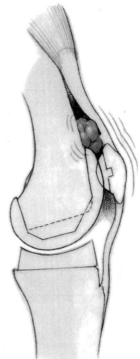

Figure 79–11. The patellar "clunk" syndrome occurs when a suprapatellar mass of fibrous-synovial tissue catches between the femoral and patellar components during knee extension. The "clunk" is created by the nodule disengaging from its intercondylar notch position.

SUMMARY

Treatment of extensor mechanism problems following TKA remains one of the few obstacles plaguing successful results. Complications affecting the extensor mechanism have become the most frequent reason for reoperation following insertion of a total knee replacement. The surgical methods employed to deal with extensor mechanism problems are themselves fraught with significant complication rates and often result in less than optimal outcomes. Complications related to the extensor mechanism after TKA can best be avoided by meticulous operative technique, with specific attention directed at ensuring optimal component position.

REFERENCES

1. Aglietti P, Buzzi R, Insall JN: Disorders of the patellofemoral joint. *In* Insall JN (ed): Surgery of the Knee, 2nd ed. New York, Churchill Livingstone, 1993, p 241.
2. Anouchi YS, Whiteside LA, Kaiser AD, Milliano MT: The effects of axial rotational alignment of the femoral component on knee stability and patellar tracking in total knee arthroplasty demonstrated on autopsy specimens. Clin Orthop 287:170, 1993.
3. Arimi J, Whiteside LA, McCarthy DS, White ES: Femoral rotational alignment, based on the anteroposterior axis in total knee arthroplasty in a valgus knee. J Bone Joint Surg Am 77:1331–334, 1995.
4. Barlett DH, Franzen J: Accurate preparation of the patella during total knee arthroplasty. J Arthroplasty 8:75, 1993.
5. Barnes CL, Scott RD: Patellofemoral complications of total knee replacement. Instr Course Lect 42:303, 1993.
6. Barrack RL, Matzkin E, Ingraham R, et al: Revision knee arthroplasty with patella replacement versus bony shell. Clin Orthop 356:139–43, 1998.
7. Barrack RL, Scharder T, Bertot AJ, et al: Component rotation and anterior knee pain after total knee arthroplasty. Clin Orthop 392:46–55, 2001.
8. Bayley JC, Scott RD: Further observations on metal-backed patellar component failure. Clin Orthop 236:82, 1988.
9. Beight JL, Yao B, Hozack WJ, et al: The patellar "clunk" syndrome after posterior stabilized total knee arthroplasty. Clin Orthop 299:139–42, 1994.
10. Berend ME, Ritter MA, Keating EM, et al: The failure of all-polyethylene patellar components in total knee replacement. Clin Orthop 388:105–11, 2001.
11. Berger RA, Corssett LS, Jacobs JJ, Rubash HE: Malrotation causing patellofemoral complications after total knee arthroplasty. Clin Orthop 356:144–53, 1998.
12. Berger RA, Rubash HE, Seel MJ, et al: Determining the rotational alignment of the femoral component in total knee arthroplasty using the epicondylar axis. Clin Orthop 286:40, 1993.
13. Berry DJ, Rand JA: Isolated patellar component revision of total knee arthroplasty. Clin Orthop 286:110, 1993.
14. Bindelglass DF, Cohen JL, Dorr LD: Patellar tilt and subluxation in total knee arthroplasty: relationship to pain, fixation, and design. Clin Orthop 286:103, 1993.
15. Boyd AD Jr, Ewald FC, Thomas WH, et al: Long-term complications after total knee arthroplasty with or without resurfacing of the patella. J Bone Joint Surg Am 75:674, 1993.
16. Briard JL, Hungerford DS: Patellofemoral instability in total knee arthroplasty. J Arthroplasty 4(Suppl):87, 1989.
17. Brick GW, Scott RD: The patellofemoral component of total knee arthroplasty. Clin Orthop 231:163, 1988.
18. Brick GW, Scott RD: Blood supply to the patella: significance in total knee arthroplasty. J Arthroplasty 4(Suppl):75, 1989.
19. Bryan RS: Patella infra and fat-pad hypertrophy after total knee arthroplasty. Tech Orthop 3:29, 1988.
20. Buechel FF, Pappas MJ, Makris G: Evaluation of contact stress in metal-backed patellar replacements: a predictor of survivorship. Clin Orthop 273:190, 1991.
21. Buechel FF, Rosa RA, Pappas MJ: A metal-backed, rotating-bearing patellar prosthesis to lower contact stress: an 11-year clinical study. Clin Orthop 248:34, 1989.
22. Burr DB, Cook LT, Cilento EV, et al: A method for radiographically measuring true femoral rotation. Clin Orthop 167:139, 1982.
23. Cadambi A, Engh GA: Use of a semitendinosus tendon autogenous graft for rupture of the patellar ligament after total knee arthroplasty: a report of seven cases. J Bone Joint Surg Am 74:974, 1992.
24. Cates HE, Ritter MA, Keating EM, Faris PM: Intramedullary versus extramedullary femoral alignment systems in total knee replacement. Clin Orthop 286:32, 1993.
25. Chew JTH, Steward NJ, Hanssen AD, et al: Differences in patellar tracking and knee kinematics among three different total knee designs. Clin Orthop 345:87–98, 1997.
26. Churchill DL, Incavo SJ, Johnson CC, Beynnon BD: The transepicondylar axis approximates the optimal fixation axis of the knee. Clin Orthop 356:111–18, 1998.
27. Crites BM, Berend ME: Metal-backed patellar components: a brief report on 10-year survival. Clin Orthop 388:103–104, 2001.
28. Emerson RH Jr, Head WC, Malinin TI: Reconstruction of patellar tendon rupture after total knee arthroplasty with an extensor mechanism allograft. Clin Orthop 260:154, 1990.
29. Emerson RH, Head WC, Malinin TI: Extensor mechanism reconstruction with an allograft after total knee arthroplasty. Clin Orthop 303:79–85, 1994.
30. Fernandez-Baillo N, Garay EG, Ordonez JM: Rupture of the quadriceps tendon after total knee arthroplasty: a case report. J Arthroplasty 8:331, 1993.
31. Figgie HE, Goldberg VM, Heiple KG, et al: The influence of tibial-patellofemoral location on function of the knee in patients with the posterior stabilized knee prosthesis. J Bone Joint Surg Am 68:1035, 1986.
32. Francke EI, Lachiewicz PF: Failure of a cemented all-polyethylene patellar component of a press-fit condylar total knee arthroplasty. J Arthroplasty 2:234–237, 2000.
33. Freeman MA, Samuelson KM, Elias SG, et al: The patellofemoral joint in total knee prostheses: design considerations. J Arthroplasty 4(Suppl):69, 1989.
34. Glaser FE, Gorab RS, Lee TQ: Edge loading of patellar components after knee arthroplasty. J Arthroplasty 14:493–499, 1999.
35. Goldberg VM, Figgie HE III, Inglis AE, et al: Patellar fracture type and prognosis in condylar total knee arthroplasty. Clin Orthop 236:115, 1988.
36. Goldstein SA, Coale E, Weiss AP, et al: Patellar surface strain. J Orthop Res 4:372, 1986.
37. Gomes LSM, Bechtold JE, Gustilo RB: Patellar prosthesis positioning in total knee arthroplasty: a roentgenographic study. Clin Orthop 236:72, 1988.
38. Grace JN, Rand JA: Patellar instability after total knee arthroplasty. Clin Orthop 237:184, 1988.
39. Grace JN, Sim FH: Fracture of the patella after total knee arthroplasty. Clin Orthop 230:168, 1988.
40. Grelsamer RP, Bazos AN, Proctor CS: Radiographic analysis of patellar tilt. J Bone Joint Surg Br 75:822, 1993.
41. Gustilo RB, Thompson R: Quadriceps and patellar tendon ruptures following total knee arthroplasty. *In* Rand JA, Dorr LD (eds): Total Arthroplasty of the Knee. Rockville, MD, Aspen Publishers, 1987, p 41.
42. Hanssen AD: Bone-grafting for severe patellar bone loss during revision knee arthroplasty. J Bone Joint Surg Am 83:171–76, 2001.
43. Hanssen AD, Rand JA: Management of the chronically dislocated patella during total knee arthroplasty. Tech Orthop 3:49, 1988.
44. Healy, WL, Wasilewski SA, Takei R, Oberlander M: Patellofemoral complications following total knee arthroplasty. J Arthroplasty 10:197–201, 1995.
45. Holtby RM, Grosso P: Osteonecrosis and resorption of the patella after total knee replacement. Clin Orthop 328:155–58, 1996.
46. Hozack WJ, Goll SR, Lotke PA, et al: The treatment of patellar fractures after total knee arthroplasty. Clin Orthop 236:123, 1988.
47. Hozack WJ, Rothman RH, Booth RE Jr, Balderston RA: The patellar clunk syndrome: a complication of posterior stabilized total knee arthroplasty. Clin Orthop 241:203, 1989.

48. Hsu HC, Luo ZP, Rand JA, An KN: Influence of patellar thickness on patellar tracking and patellofemoral contact characteristics after total knee arthroplasty. J Arthroplasty 11:69–80, 1996.

49. Hsu HP, Walker PS: Wear and deformation of patellar components in total knee arthroplasty. Clin Orthop 246:260, 1989.

50. Huang CH, Lee YM, Lai JH, et al: Failure of the all-polyethylene patellar component after total knee arthroplasty. J Arthroplasty 14:940–944, 1999.

51. Huberti HH, Hayes WC: Patellofemoral contact pressures: the influence of Q-angle and tendofemoral contact. J Bone Joint Surg Am 66:715, 1984.

52. Insall JN: Surgical techniques and instrumentation in total knee arthroplasty. In Insall JN (ed): Surgery of the Knee, 2nd ed. New York, Churchill Livingstone, 1993, p 739.

53. Insall JN, Haas SB: Complications of total knee arthroplasty. In Insall JN (ed): Surgery of the Knee, 2nd ed. New York, Churchill Livingstone, 1993, p 891.

54. Insall J, Salvati E: Patella position in the normal knee joint. Radiology 101:101, 1971.

55. Johnson DP, Eastwood DM: Patellar complications after knee arthroplasty: a prospective study of 56 cases using the kinematic prosthesis. Acta Orthop Scand 63:74, 1992.

56. Jones EC, Insall JN, Inglis AE, Ranawat CS: Guepar knee arthroplasty results and late complications. Clin Orthop 140:145, 1979.

57. Josefchak RG, Finlay JB, Bourne RB, Rorabeck CH: Cancellous bone support for patellar resurfacing. Clin Orthop 220:192, 1987.

58. Kaufer H: Mechanical function of the patella. J Bone Joint Surg Am 53:1551, 1971.

59. Kayler DE, Lyttle D: Surgical interruption of patellar blood supply by total knee arthroplasty. Clin Orthop 229:221, 1988.

60. Kim W, Rand JA, Chao EYS: Biomechanics of the knee. In Rand JA (ed): Total Knee Arthroplasty. New York, Raven Press, 1993, p 9.

61. Kirk P, Rorabeck CH, Bourne RB, et al: Management of recurrent dislocation of the patella following total knee arthroplasty. J Arthroplasty 7:229, 1992.

62. Koshino T, Ejima M, Okamoto R, Morii T: Gradual low riding of the patella during postoperative course after total knee arthroplasty in osteoarthritis and rheumatoid arthritis. J Arthroplasty 5:323, 1990.

63. Kraay MJ, Darr OJ, Salata MJ, Goldberg VM: Outcome of metal-backed cementless patellar components: the effect of implant design. Clin Orthop 392:239–244, 2001.

64. Larson KR, Cracchiolo A III, Dorey FJ, Finerman GAM: Total knee arthroplasty in patients after patellectomy. Clin Orthop 264:243, 1991.

65. Laskin RS, Bucknell A: The use of metal-backed patellar prostheses in total knee arthroplasty. Clin Orthop 260:52, 1990.

66. Lennox DW, Hungerford DS, Krackow KA: Total knee arthroplasty following patellectomy. Clin Orthop 223:220, 1987.

67. Leopold SS, Greidanus N, Paprosky WG, et al: High rate of failure of allograft reconstruction of the extensor mechanism after total knee arthroplasty. J Bone Joint Surg Am 81:1574–579, 1999.

68. Lewellen DG, Rand JA: Failure of metal backed patellae in total knee arthroplasty. Presented at the 57th Annual Meeting of the American Academy of Orthopaedic Surgeons, New Orleans, February 13, 1990.

69. Lombardi AV Jr, Engh GA, Volz RG, et al: Fracture/dissociation of the polyethylene in metal-backed patellar components in total knee arthroplasty. J Bone Joint Surg Am 70:675, 1988.

70. Lucas TS, DeLuca PF, Nazarian DG, et al: Arthroscopic treatment of patellar clunk. Clin Orthop 367:226–229, 1999.

71. Lynch AF, Rorabeck CH, Bourne RB: Extensor mechanism complications following total knee arthroplasty. J Arthroplasty 2:135, 1987.

72. Lynch JA, Baker PL, Lepse PS, et al: Solitary patellar component revision following total knee arthroplasty. Presented at the 60th Annual Meeting of the American Academy of Orthopaedic Surgeons, San Francisco, February 20, 1993.

73. Masini MA, Stulberg SD: A new surgical technique for tibial tubercle transfer in total knee arthroplasty. J Arthroplasty 7:81, 1992.

74. Mason MD, Brick GW, Scott RD, et al: Three pegged all polyethylene patellae: 2 to 6 year results. Orthop Trans 17:991, 1994.

75. McLain RF, Bargar WF: The effect of total knee design on patellar strain. J Arthroplasty 1:91, 1986.

76. McMahon MS, Scuderi GR, Glashow JL, et al: Scintigraphic determination of patellar viability after excision of infrapatellar fat pad and/or lateral retinacular release in total knee arthroplasty. Clin Orthop 260:10, 1990.

77. McNamara JL, Collier JP, Mayor MB, Jensen RE: A comparison of contact pressures in tibial and patellar total knee components before and after service in vivo. Clin Orthop 299:104–13, 1994.

78. Merchant AC, Mercer RL, Jacobsen RH, Cool CR: Roentgenographic analysis of patellofemoral congruence. J Bone Joint Surg Am 56:1391, 1974.

79. Merkow RL, Soudry M, Insall JN: Patellar dislocation following total knee replacement. J Bone Joint Surg Am 67:1321, 1985.

80. Miller MC, Berger RA, Petrella AJ, et al: Optimizing femoral component rotation in total knee arthroplasty. Clin Orthop 392:38–45, 2001.

81. Milliano MT, Whiteside LA, Kaiser AD, Zwirkoski PA: Evaluation of the effect of the femoral articular surface material on the wear of a metal-backed patellar component. Clin Orthop 287:178, 1993.

82. Moreland JR: Mechanisms of failure in total knee arthroplasty. Clin Orthop 226:49, 1988.

83. Nazarian DG, Booth RE Jr: Extensor mechanism allografts in total knee arthroplasty. Clin Orthop 367:123–129, 1999.

84. Nwaneri UR, Manderson EL: Failed metal-backed patella in total knee arthroplasty. Orthopedics 17:179, 1994.

85. Ortiguera CJ, Berry DJ: Patella fracture after total knee arthroplasty. J Bone Joint Surg 84A:532-540,2002.

86. Pace TB, Kennedy EJ, Hofmann AA, Kane KR: Normal patella anatomy: medial eccentricity of the thickest anterior-posterior dimension. Presented at the 61st Annual Meeting of the American Academy of Orthopaedic Surgeons, New Orleans, February 27, 1994.

87. Pagnano MW, Hanssen AD: Varus tibial joint line obliquity: a potential cause of femoral component malrotation. Clin Orthop 392:68–74, 2001.

88. Pagnano MW, Scuderi GR, Insall JN: Patellar component resection in revision and reimplantation total knee arthroplasty. Clin Orthop 356:134–38, 1998.

89. Pagnano MW, Trousdale RT: Asymmetric patella resurfacing in total knee arthroplasty. Am J Knee Surg 13:228–233, 2000.

90. Parvizi J, Seel MJ, Hanssen AD, Morrey BF: Patellar component resection arthroplasty for the severely compromised patella. Clin Orthop 2002 (in press).

91. Petrie RS, Hanssen AD, Osmon DR, Illstrup D: Metal-backed patellar component failure in total knee arthroplasty: a possible risk for late infection. Am J Orthop 27:172–76, 1998.

92. Pettine KA, Bryan RS: A previously unreported cause of pain after total knee arthroplasty. J Arthroplasty 1:29, 1986.

93. Poilvache PL, Insall JN, Scuderi GR, Font-Rodriguez DE: Rotational landmarks and sizing of the distal femur in total knee arthroplasty. Clin Orthop 331:35–46, 1996.

94. Railton GT, Levack B, Freeman MA: Unconstrained knee arthroplasty after patellectomy. J Arthroplasty 5:255, 1990.

95. Ranawat CS: The patellofemoral joint in total condylar knee arthroplasty: pros and cons based on five- to ten-year follow-up observations. Clin Orthop 205:93, 1986.

96. Rand JA: Patellar resurfacing in total knee arthroplasty. Clin Orthop 260:110, 1990.

97. Rand JA, Bryan RS: Results of revision total knee arthroplasties using condylar prostheses: a review of fifty knees. J Bone Joint Surg Am 70:738, 1988.

98. Rand JA, Gustilo RB: Technique of patellar resurfacing in total knee arthroplasty. Tech Orthop 3:57, 1988.

99. Rand JA, Morrey BF, Bryan RS: Patellar tendon rupture following total knee arthroplasty. Tech Orthop 3:45, 1988.

100. Rand JA, Morrey BF, Bryan RS: Patellar tendon rupture after total knee arthroplasty. Clin Orthop 244:233, 1989.

101. Reuben JD, McDonald CL, Woodard PL, Hennington LJ: Effect of patella thickness on patella strain following total knee arthroplasty. J Arthroplasty 6:251, 1991.

102. Rhoads DD, Noble PC, Reuben JD, Tullos HS: The effect of femoral component position on the kinematics of total knee arthroplasty. Clin Orthop 286:122, 1993.

103. Rhoads DD, Noble PC, Reuben JD, et al: The effect of femoral component position on patellar tracking after total knee arthroplasty. Clin Orthop 260:43, 1990.

104. Ritter MA, Campbell ED: Postoperative patellar complications with or without lateral release during total knee arthroplasty. Clin Orthop 219:163, 1987.

105. Ritter MA, Herbst BA, Keating EM, et al: Patellofemoral complications following total knee arthroplasty: effect of a lateral release and sacrifice of the superior lateral geniculate artery. J Arthroplasty 11:368–372, 1996.

106. Rosenberg AG, Andriacchi TP, Barden R, Galante JO: Patellar component failure in cementless total knee arthroplasty. Clin Orthop 236:106, 1988.

107. Scott RD: Treatment of patellar instability associated with total knee replacement. Tech Orthop 3:9, 1988.

108. Scott RD: Duopatellar total knee replacement: the Brigham experience. Orthop Clin North Am 13:89, 1992.

109. Scott RD, Siliski JM: The use of a modified V-Y quadricepsplasty during total knee replacement to gain exposure and improve flexion in the ankylosed knee. Orthopedics 8:45, 1985.

110. Scott RD, Turoff N, Ewald FC: Stress fracture of the patella following duopatellar total knee arthroplasty with patellar resurfacing. Clin Orthop 170:147, 1982.

111. Scuderi C: Ruptures of the quadriceps tendon. Am J Surg 95:626, 1958.

112. Scuderi G, Scharf SC, Meltzer LP, Scott WN: The relationship of lateral releases to patellar viability in total knee arthroplasty. J Arthroplasty 2:209, 1987.

113. Shoji H, Shimozaki E: Patellar clunk syndrome in total knee arthroplasty without patellar resurfacing. J Arthroplasty 11:198–201, 1996.

114. Simmons E, Cameron JC: Patella alta and recurrent dislocation of the patella. Clin Orthop 274:265, 1992.

115. Starr MJ, Kaufman KR, Irby SE, Colwell CW: The effects of patellar thickness on patellofemoral forces after resurfacing. Clin Orthop 322:279–285, 1996.

116. Stulberg SD, Stulberg BN, Hamati Y, Tsao A: Failure mechanisms of metal-backed patellar components. Clin Orthop 236:88, 1988.

117. Thorpe CD, Bocell JR, Tullos HS: Intra-articular fibrous bands: patellar complications after total knee replacement. J Bone Joint Surg Am 72:811, 1990.

118. Trousdale RT, Hanssen AD, Rand JA, Cahalan TD: V-Y quadricepsplasty in total knee arthroplasty. Clin Orthop 286:48, 1993.

119. Vernace JV, Rothman RH, Booth RE, Balderston RA: Arthroscopic management of the patellar clunk syndrome following posterior stabilized total knee arthroplasty. J Arthroplasty 2:281, 1987.

120. Vince KG, McPherson EJ: The patella in total knee arthroplasty. Orthop Clin North Am 23:675, 1992.

121. Wetzner SM, Bezreh JS, Scott RD, et al: Bone scanning in the assessment of patellar viability following knee replacement. Clin Orthop 199:215, 1985.

122. Whiteside LA: Distal realignment of the patellar tendon to correct abnormal patellar tracking. Clin Orthop 344:284–289, 1997.

123. Whiteside LA, Ohl MD: Tibial tubercle osteotomy for exposure of the difficult total knee arthroplasty. Clin Orthop 260:6, 1990.

124. Windsor RE, Scuderi GR, Insall JN: Patellar fractures in total knee arthroplasty. J Arthroplasty 4(Suppl):63, 1989.

125. Wolff AM, Hungerford DS, Krackow KA, Jacobs MA: Osteotomy of the tibial tubercle during total knee replacement: a report of twenty-six cases. J Bone Joint Surg Am 71:848, 1989.

126. Wright TM, Bartel DL: The problem of surface damage in polyethylene total knee components. Clin Orthop 205:67, 1986.

127. Yoshii I, Whiteside LA, Anouchi YS: The effect of patellar button placement and femoral component design on patellar tracking in total knee arthroplasty. Clin Orthop 275:211, 1992.

80

Revision Total Knee Arthroplasty: Techniques and Results

• MARK W. PAGNANO and JAMES A. RAND

Despite improvements in component design, instrumentation, and surgical technique, failures of total knee arthroplasty and the need for revision continue. Aseptic loosening was a dominant mode of failure in the 1970s, while metal-backed patellar failure and catastrophic wear-through of thin tibial inserts dominated the 1980s and early 1990s. The challenge for the new millenium appears to be osteolysis from polyethylene particulate debris. Salvage of the failed total knee arthroplasty presents a challenge for even the most experienced surgeon because of bone loss, soft tissue deficiencies, and patient expectations that are often unrealistic.

CAUSES OF FAILURE

The cause of failure in early designs of total knee arthroplasties was largely loosening at the bone-cement interface. Failure may be considered in terms of (1) poor patient selection, (2) improper implant design, and (3) incorrect surgical technique.

Correct patient selection is mandatory. The markedly obese patient or the patient who wishes to return to impact-loading sports will place stresses that exceed safe levels across the knee. The result will be implant loosening, breakage, or accelerated wear with resultant failure. Although obese patients do experience marked improvements in pain and function after total knee arthroplasty, they likely have higher rates of failure after both primary and revision arthroplasties.[14,48,57]

Minimally conforming or moderately conforming (total condylar type) resurfacing implants will minimize stresses on the bone-cement interface and theoretically decrease loosening. In contrast, highly conforming implants such as the original geometric design place high loads on the bone-cement interface, and predispose to loosening. Implants with long intramedullary stems are not necessary for primary arthroplasty in most patients. The more bone sacrificed at the initial arthroplasty, the more difficult will be any subsequent salvage procedure. The long-accepted approach has been that the surgeon should be conservative at the initial arthro-

plasty and attempt to preserve as much normal anatomy as feasible (i.e., bone stock, collateral ligaments, and the posterior cruciate ligament). In reality, though, the surgeon must strike a balance at the time of the initial arthroplasty: minimal tibial resections must be offset by the need for at least 8-mm polyethylene inserts, and the posterior cruciate ligament should not be retained if it causes difficulty in balancing the knee.

Incorrect surgical technique is the most important cause of failure of arthroplasties. The surgeon has little control over patients or implant design but can control the quality of the surgical technique. The major advances in total knee arthroplasty in the last 10 years have been an awareness of correct implant placement and the development of instrumentation systems to allow reproducible surgical technique. The importance of obtaining a correct mechanical axis of the limb, avoiding varus tibial component placement, and maintaining the joint line are now accepted principles of surgical technique.[12,16,17,24,42] Current instrumentation systems combine intramedullary and extramedullary alignment guides and a series of cutting blocks to aid in correct implant placement. Instrumentation systems, however, are only as good as the person using them. Complex deformities sometimes require deviation from the instrumentation systems. Furthermore, the importance of appropriate ligament balancing in both flexion and extension, a focal point with the early total condylar technique, has not been emphasized adequately over the last decade. Failures continue to occur, even with modern implants placed with current instrumentation, because of surgical errors.

Malalignment of the limb or of the implant will predispose to failure. Limb alignment must be assessed in terms of the mechanical axis of the limb, not the axial alignment (tibiofemoral angle) (Fig. 80–1). The mechanical axis should be within the central one third of the joint to maintain even loading of the prosthesis. Either increased valgus or, especially, increased varus will predispose to failure through loosening or wear caused by excessive compressive loads on the side of the tibial component and tensile loads on the other side. Varus placement of the tibial component greater than 3 degrees in relation to the

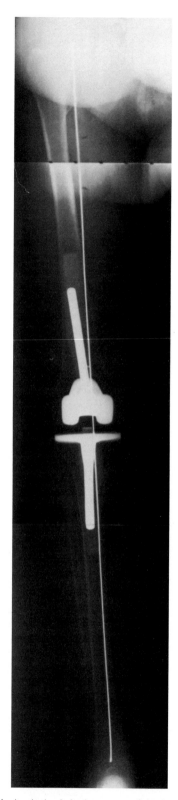

Figure 80–1. Mechanical axis in the center of the knee after revision arthroplasty.

tibia has been associated with failure and radiolucencies with many designs.[12,16,28,44,46]

Ligament imbalance may result in clinical symptoms of functional instability. Ligament balance must be present throughout a range of motion and correlates closely with maintenance of the joint line. Although asymmetric collateral ligament imbalance may result initially in only minimal clinical symptoms, ligament imbalance can affect limb alignment and result in loosening and wear (Fig. 80–2). Similarly, the knee must be stable in the anteroposterior plane in flexion. So-called flexion instability has recently been identified as a cause of failure after cruciate-retaining total knee arthroplasty as well as posterior stabilized total knee arthroplasty.

Extensor mechanism problems of instability, fracture, and wear are the most frequent sources of reoperation after total knee arthroplasty with current designs. Implant breakage, subsidence, component or bone fracture, and limited motion are less frequent causes of failure leading to revision.[48]

The surgeon should beware of the patient who presents with chronic pain after total knee arthroplasty without an apparent cause. The patient who has pain after arthroplasty with an appropriately positioned implant that is not infected, loose, or unstable in flexion or extension is unlikely to benefit from revision surgery.

INDICATIONS AND CONTRAINDICATIONS

The indication for revision total knee arthroplasty is mechanical failure of a previous arthroplasty in a symptomatic patient or marked and progressive bone loss in an asymptomatic patient.[6,7,22,29,31,53,55] Mechanical failures include loosening, instability, severely limited motion, severe malalignment, and significant extensor mechanism dysfunction. Prerequisites for revision are (1) a psychologically stable patient who is motivated and cooperative, (2) adequate remaining bone stock, (3) adequate soft tissues, and (4) generally satisfactory health patient for a potentially prolonged operative procedure.

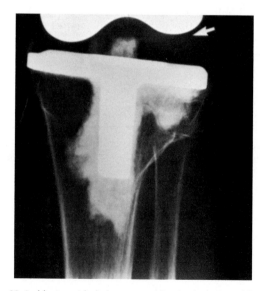

Figure 80–2. Ligament imbalance resulting in alteration of limb alignment.

EVALUATION OF THE FAILED TOTAL KNEE ARTHROPLASTY

All failed arthroplasties should be carefully evaluated for possible deep infection. The evaluation should include erythrocyte sedimentation rate, C-reactive protein, differential technetium-99m/indium-111 bone scans, and knee aspiration. Although results positive for infection are helpful, infection may be present despite normal laboratory findings. A history of problems with wound healing, prolonged drainage, or need for reoperation after arthroplasty should raise suspicion of septic failure. Persistent pain since, or even before, the arthroplasty often is reported by the patient who has a chronic pain behavior problem. In contrast, the patient who initially does well but subsequently experiences gradual development of pain or instability usually has a mechanical cause of failure.

Physical examination should be directed to the entirety of both lower extremities. Ipsilateral hip disease may present as a painful ipsilateral total knee arthroplasty. Contralateral or ipsilateral hip ankylosis or contralateral knee disease may affect gait adversely, resulting in failure of a total knee arthroplasty.

Examination of the knee should begin with an assessment of the location of previous surgical incisions. Previous incisions may have been placed suboptimally (Fig. 80–3). Potential problems with both exposure and wound healing must be anticipated.

The integrity of the extensor mechanism, its mobility, and muscle strength are of paramount importance. A nonfunctioning extensor mechanism because of a longstanding patellar ligament avulsion is an extremely difficult problem to correct. A paralyzed extensor mechanism is a contraindication to revision arthroplasty.

Anteroposterior stability has been underemphasized in the past and should be carefully assessed. A posterior cruciate ligament–retaining knee that presents with diffuse anterior knee pain and recurrent swelling combined with an exam that shows a posterior sag or excessive anteroposterior motion suggests the diagnosis of so-called flexion instability.[36] Collateral ligament integrity, or at least integrity of the joint capsule, should be assessed. In the presence of a loose implant with bone loss, collateral ligament integrity is difficult to determine. Careful palpation of the knee on stress testing will often define an intact capsular structure that will provide adequate stability at revision.

The extent of soft tissue scarring may be inferred from the thickening of the soft tissues and the amount of motion preoperatively. The neurovascular status of the extremity must be carefully assessed. If there are concerns about neurologic (usually peroneal nerve) or vascular status, an electromyogram or vascular flow studies, or both, should be obtained preoperatively.

Radiographic evaluation of the failed arthroplasty includes full-length standing radiographs of the lower extremity, anteroposterior and lateral radiographs of the knee, tangential patellar views, and fluoroscopically positioned views of the bone-cement or implant-bone interface. Use of fluoroscopically positioned radiographs has enabled detection of radiolucencies that

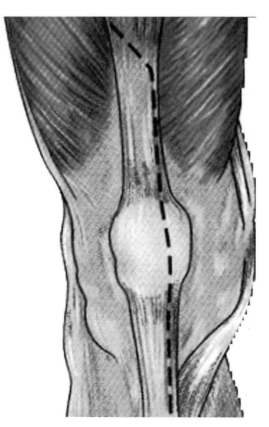

Figure 80–4. The quadriceps snip is a versatile exposure option in the [AU] moderately stiff knee. (From Insall JN, Scott WN: Surgical Exposures. Citation *In* Insall JN [ed]: Surgery of the Knee, 3rd ed. New York, Churchill missing Livingstone, 2001, p 521.)

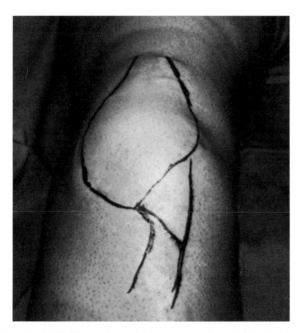

Figure 80–3. Multiple prior incisions complicate the choice of exposure. Usually, the most lateral incision on the anterior aspect of the knee should be utilized.

would not be visualized on routine radiographs.[33] The plain radiographs should be studied for limb alignment, component position, soft tissues, remaining bone stock, and implant loosening. A careful study of the remaining bone stock will allow assessment of the feasibility of revision and the type of implant necessary. Comparison of sequential radiographs at different time intervals is very helpful in determining progression of radiolucencies (i.e., loosening). Periosteal new bone formation or rapidly progressing osteolysis suggests infection. Bone and indium scans are helpful in distinguishing between loosening and infection.

THE REVISION

Preoperative Planning

Surgical exposure, implant design, and type of management of bone deficiency must be chosen carefully. Exposure must be planned in view of previous surgical incisions and the status of the extensor mechanism. Implant choice will depend on the integrity of the posterior cruciate and collateral ligaments as well as the extent of bone deficiency. In most patients a posterior-stabilized implant is used in the revision setting. For moderate collateral ligament insufficiency, a constrained-condylar design that supplements the collateral ligaments is appropriate. For true collateral ligament loss or a grossly marked imbalance between the flexion and extension spaces, a rotating hinge design should be utilized. The interrelationship of anatomic considerations and implant selection is summarized in Table 80–1.

Technique

The principles of revision total knee arthroplasty are the same as those of primary arthroplasty: (1) correct limb alignment, (2) proper component position, (3) soft tissue balance to provide stability throughout a range of motion, and (4) adequate motion for activities of daily living. Although the objectives of revision and primary arthroplasty are the same, it is more difficult to achieve

these goals in revision surgery. The most frequent problems are soft tissues, the previous bone-cement interface, and bone loss.

Exposure

Surgical exposure should utilize pre-existing incisions whenever feasible. In general, the most laterally placed anterior incision should be selected. Dissection between the skin and the extensor mechanism should be minimized to prevent skin ischemia. If soft tissue flaps must be elevated, the flap should be full-thickness skin, subcutaneous fat, and superficial fascia to maintain the blood supply to the skin. A medial parapatellar arthrotomy is utilized for the arthroplasty. Scarring in the extensor mechanism often will prevent eversion of the patella and knee flexion without compromising the patellar ligament attachment to the tibia.

Exposure is gained by freeing all the scar from the suprapatellar pouch and the medial and lateral gutters and excising any hypertrophic fat pad. A subperiosteal elevation of the deep portion of the medial collateral ligament is done along the medial tibia to the posteromedial border of the tibia. Often, external rotation of the tibia combined with flexion of the knee will allow the extensor mechanism to be dislocated laterally. If the extensor mechanism still cannot be dislocated, we perform a quadriceps snip. Most knees can be exposed in this manner without the need for a lateral release or an extended exposure, such as a V-Y quadricepsplasty.[54,60]

An alternative exposure is osteotomy of the tibial tubercle. This appears to have been first described by Dolan in 1983.[11] A detailed analysis by Wolff et al. revealed 13 tubercle osteotomies for revision total knee arthroplasty.[63] Whiteside has described a long tibial tubercle anterior crest osteotomy in which the extensor mechanism is simply rolled laterally (Fig. 80–5).[61,62] After the procedure, the extensor mechanism is reapproximated by its osseous attachment and secured to its bed with two cobalt-chromium wires passed through the fragment and through the medial cortex of the tibia. All the osteotomies healed, and the average flexion of these patients was almost 100 degrees.[62]

Table 80–1. ANATOMIC CONSIDERATIONS AND IMPLANT SELECTION IN REVISION TOTAL KNEE ARTHROPLASTY

Anatomic Problem				
Soft Tissue		**Bone Loss**		
PCL	Collaterals	Tibia	Femur	**Implant Selection**
Intact	Intact	Minimal	Minimal	PCL-retaining, -sacrificing, or -substituting condylar prosthesis
Intact	Intact	Moderate	Moderate	PCL-sacrificing or -substituting condylar prosthesis with intramedullary stems
Absent	Intact	Minimal	Minimal	PCL-sacrificing or -substituting condylar prosthesis
Absent	Intact	Moderate	Moderate	PCL-sacrificing or -substituting condylar prosthesis with intramedullary stems
Absent	Absent	Minimal or moderate	Minimal or moderate	Collateral ligament–substituting prosthesis with intramedullary stems

PCL, posterior collateral ligament.

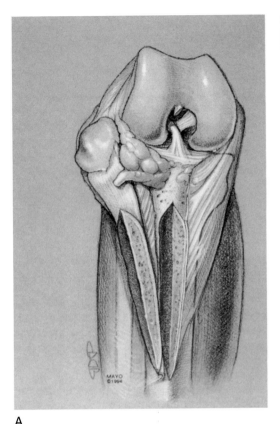
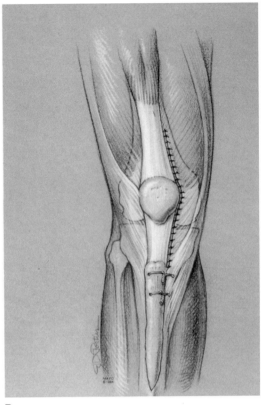

A   B

Figure 80–5. (**A**) A tibial tubercle osteotomy allows ready access to the knee with contracted extensor mechanisms (**B**). (Adapted from Whiteside L, Ohl MD: Tibial tubercle osteotomy for exposure of the difficult total knee arthroplasty. Clin Orthop 260:6, 1990.)

Implant Removal

Once the knee has been adequately exposed, tissue should be obtained for culture and pathologic evaluation. If the components are loose, the one in the femur is removed first, followed by the tibial and patellar components. If the implants are not loose, a high-speed cutting instrument such as the Midas Rex with an AM-10 tip is used for dissections at the implant-cement, not the bone-cement, interface (Fig. 80–6). Alternatives for freeing the cement-prosthesis interface include an oscillating saw with a thin, flexible blade or the Gigli saw, which is particularly useful for the anterior flange of the femoral component. The prosthesis must be freed completely before removal is attempted or severe bone loss from the distal femur or tibia may occur. Once the

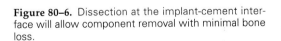

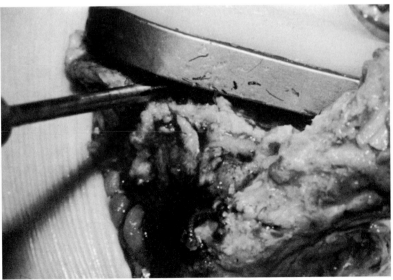

Figure 80–6. Dissection at the implant-cement interface will allow component removal with minimal bone loss.

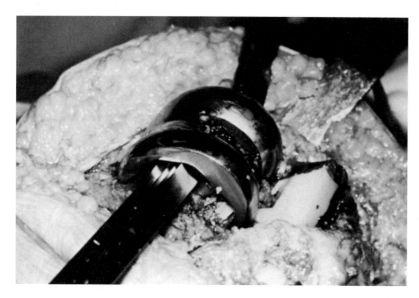

Figure 80–7. Use of multiple osteotomes as wedges to loosen the prothesis.

dissection is complete, a series of osteotomes are utilized as wedges to gradually free the component (Fig. 80–7). Alternatively, the femur can be disimpacted with care using a slap-hammer extractor or square-tip punch and mallet.

If the tibia is all-polyethylene, the plateau may be freed with the Midas Rex or saw similar to the femoral component. If the stem is securely fixed, the polyethylene is transected and the plateau is removed. The exposed stem now can be freed in a similar manner and extracted. A metal-backed tibial component is a more difficult problem. The tibial plateau portion should be freed by using the Midas Rex or saw. If the stem remains fixed, an impactor is positioned beneath the tray and and successive blows are directed proximally to free the stem. If the stem remains securely fixed, access to the stem must be obtained.

A diamond-tip cutting wheel or bit is utilized to transect the tibial tray at the junction with the stem (Fig. 80–8). It is helpful to cover the entire field, except for the tibial tray, with a sterile drape to minimize metallic debris in the wound. Continuous irrigation will minimize heat from friction and aid in debris removal. Once the stem of the implant is accessible, the stem is mobilized and the implant is removed.

Care must be exercised in removal of the patellar implant, or severe bone loss or fracture may occur. Use of a Midas Rex with a B-1 tip will allow dissection at the implant-cement interface. Once the implant is free except for the stem, osteotomes used as wedges will free the implant. Well-fixed metal-backed patellas can be removed with a diamond-tip cutting wheel that severs the fixation pegs.

Preparation for Reimplantation

Once the implant has been removed, all loose cement and any underlying fibrous membrane must be removed. Cultures of the membrane should be obtained to rule out infection. A meticulous débridement should

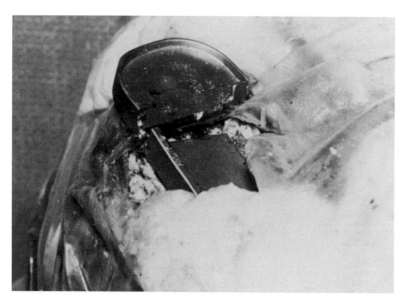

Figure 80–8. Transection of the tibial component tray to expose the stem for implant removal.

be performed. High-speed pulsed lavage will aid in the identification of remaining fibrous tissue and cement. Once all foreign material has been removed, the soft tissue scar should be addressed.

A thickened joint capsule invariably is present, especially posteriorly. If the thick posterior capsule is not thinned, it can impair joint motion and cause the knee to hinge open in flexion. One must be able to reduce the tibia under the femur at 90 degrees of flexion to ensure that the knee does not hinge open in flexion. Care must be taken to avoid injury to the neurovascular structures that lie in the layer of fat immediately behind the thick capsule. The collateral ligaments should be preserved. All hypertrophic synovium should be excised. Once the scarred tissues have been removed, soft tissue balance in flexion and extension may be assessed. Soft tissue balance should be obtained by using the same techniques as in primary arthroplasty.

Bone deficiencies are assessed, and the remaining bone surfaces are oriented. The proximal tibial and distal femoral cuts should be evaluated. The proximal tibial cut should be perpendicular to the mechanical axis of the tibia in the coronal and sagittal planes. Many total knee arthroplasty instrumentation systems have a jig that lies on the cut tibial surface with a rod that extends over the anterior tibial surface to assess this cut. If a long-stemmed tibial implant will be utilized, an intramedullary alignment cutting jig should be employed. A trial implant with an extended stem can be utilized similar to a T-square to check the accuracy of the cut and ensure seating of the tibia tray on the cut tibial bone surface. In the assessment of the tibial cut, the peripheral cortical rim should be utilized. Minimal resection of high portions of the rim should be performed to produce a level surface. Bone deficiencies in the central portion of the tibia may be ignored in the assessment of the tibial cut.

The accuracy of the distal femoral cut should be assessed next. A 5- to 7-degree valgus cut on the distal femur typically will result in a correct mechan-

ical axis of the limb. The peripheral bone should be utilized to assess this cut. Combined intramedullary and extramedullary guides from many primary instrumentation systems can be utilized. An alternative method is to place the distal femur against the tibial surface and assess the mechanical axis of the limb.

So-called rod-and-sleeve instruments for revision arthroplasty have been devised and improved on greatly in recent years. With the advent of offset stems for both the femoral and tibial sides, intramedullary instrumentation is now quite helpful in the revision setting. Nonetheless, trial fitting of the components is still the best method to assess fit and stability. An intraoperative radiograph with the trial components in place is often an excellent investment of time and effort.

To select the prosthesis for trial reduction, the status of the posterior cruciate and collateral ligaments as well as the extent of bone loss must be considered. Prosthesis selection has been discussed in preoperative planning. Usually, the collateral ligaments are intact and the posterior cruciate ligament is deficient. Therefore, a prosthesis that has a posterior-stabilized design will be selected. The location and extent of bone loss will influence the specific implant choice. The femoral implant selected should have an interior dimension that fits the remaining femoral bone stock. The exterior dimension of the femoral component should create equal flexion and extension spaces. The femoral component may require augmentation of its distal and/or posterior aspects to achieve these goals. An attempt should be made to restore the joint line to its correct position, approximately 2.5 cm distal to the femoral epicondyles.

Rotational alignment of the femoral component is important to ensure correct patellar tracking. Because the posterior femoral condyles are absent, rotational alignment must be set parallel to the femoral epicondyles where the collateral ligaments are attached. The lateral epicondyle should lie slightly posterior to the medial femoral epicondyle (Fig. 80–9). Careful removal of the overlying synovial tissue allows good

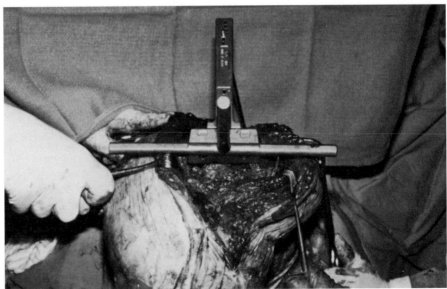

Figure 80–9. Assessment of rotational alignment by use of the femoral epicondyles.

visualization of the medial and lateral epicondyles. Confirmation of the attachment sites can be done by placing a nerve hook deep to each collateral ligament and palpating proximally.

Bone Loss

In revision surgery, bone loss may be considered in three degrees of severity. Type I bone deficiency is limited bone loss with an intact peripheral rim of bone and adjacent metaphyseal bone. Type I bone loss is encountered in the revision of a failed unicompartmental arthroplasty.[4,32,35] Bone loss of this type can be managed by bone grafting or cement filling. In type II bone loss, there is an intact peripheral rim of bone but deficient metaphyseal bone (Fig. 80–10). Type II bone loss occurs in revision of a failed condylar arthroplasty. Bone loss of this magnitude will require a long-stemmed implant to achieve fixation in intact bone and bone grafting of the metaphysis.[5] Type III bone loss is deficient peripheral and metaphyseal bone (Fig. 80–11).[39] Bone loss of this magnitude is encountered with longstanding loose condylar prostheses or failed hinged designs. Management of type III bone loss requires long-stemmed prostheses with metaphyseal augmentation and extensive bone grafting.

Bone loss from the tibia is located centrally and may extend to the periphery of one area of the tibial plateau. If more than 50 percent of the tibial bone surface is deficient

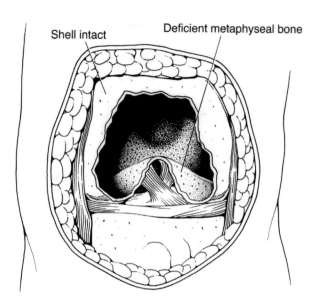

Figure 80–10. Type II bone loss with intact peripheral shell but deficient metaphyseal bone.

or if the bone deficiency extends to the periphery of the joint, a long-stemmed tibial component should be considered. The long stem will transfer the stress past the deficient bone area. On the femoral side, bone loss occurs distally and posteriorly. Bone loss usually is symmetric but may be asymmetric. If a standard resurfacing implant

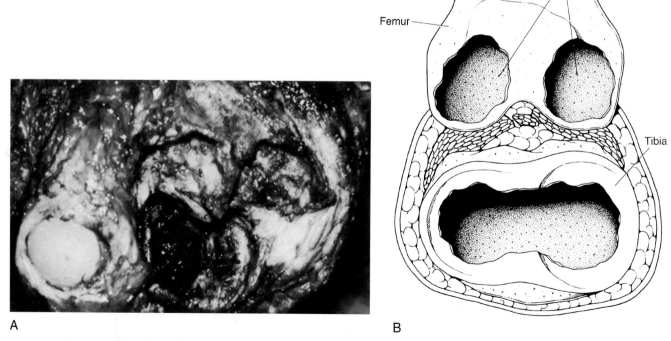

A

B

Figure 80–11. Type III bone loss with deficient peripheral and metaphyseal bone. (**A** from Rand JA: Revision total knee arthroplasty. *In* Evarts CM [ed]: Surgery of the Musculoskeletal System, 2nd ed, vol 4. New York, Churchill Livingstone, 1990, p 3645, with permission.)

is placed on the femur combined with a thicker tibial polyethylene component, stability may be achieved. However, the joint line will be displaced proximally (elevated) and an iatrogenic patella infra will be created. The result of the proximal joint line will be abnormal knee kinematics and patellar impingement against the tibial component. Therefore, bone lost from both the distal and posterior femur must be replaced. If only one aspect of the femoral bone loss is addressed, the knee will be unstable in either flexion or extension.

Bone loss at revision surgery can be managed by cement filling, bone grafting, or augmented components. Cement filling with or without screws or wire mesh will not provide optimal loading, and stress must be relieved by a stemmed implant. Cement is useful for small defects in older patients. Chen and Krackow have shown that it is advantageous biomechanically to convert defects into a step-shaped configuration when cement is used (Fig. 80–12).[10] Autogenous local bone or allograft can be used to fill bone deficiencies. Bone graft is particularly attractive for the younger patient in whom it is desirable to preserve bone stock for the future. To achieve bone graft healing, the recipient host bone bed must be prepared with a bur to expose bleeding bone. Large contained defects can be filled well with impacted morselized cancellous bone. Noncontained defects may require a bulk structural graft. Structural grafts should be configured into geometric shapes to obtain stability with the host bone and then supplementally fixed to the host bone. Cement must not be allowed to intrude into the interface between the bone graft and host bone. Large structural bone grafts cannot be expected to carry large loads alone and must be relieved of stress by a stemmed implant.

Augmented components can be of three types: (1) custom components (Fig. 80–13), (2) commercially augmented designs, or (3) modular wedges fitted to the standard implant in the operating room. Augmented components have the advantage of replacing lost bone with metal.[38] The augmented implant avoids the problems of weak cement filling of defects and the biologic uncertainty of bone graft incorporation. Custom components have distinct disadvantages: They are expensive, require prolonged time for manufacture, and do not always fit as anticipated.

Augmented components are available such as those with the original porous-coated anatomic (PCA) revision system (Fig. 80–14). Unfortunately, the PCA system does not address asymmetric bone loss on the femur or provide for management of peripheral bone deficiency on the tibia. Modern, modular total knee systems address those problems with the ability to selectively augment the distal or posterior femur as well as the proximal tibial bone defects (Fig. 80–15). These modular systems have proved useful in addressing many of the difficult bone loss problems. One other approach is the use of so-called metaphyseal cones to fill large defects.[26] These augments are attached to the intramedullary stem of an implant and are successively broached until rotational stability is obtained in the metaphyseal-diaphyseal junction. The augmentation cones are porous coated for

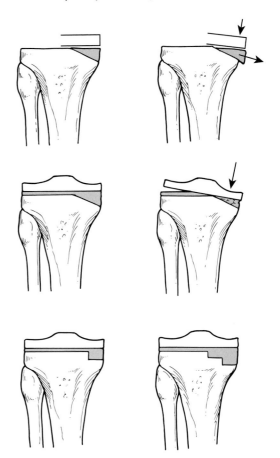

Figure 80–12. Wedge-shaped defects that are to be filled with cement are best converted to step-like defects because cement performs well under compression but relatively poorly under shear loads. (From Chen F, Krackow KA: Management of tibial defects in total knee arthroplasty: a biomechanical study. Clin Orthop 305:249–257, 1994.)

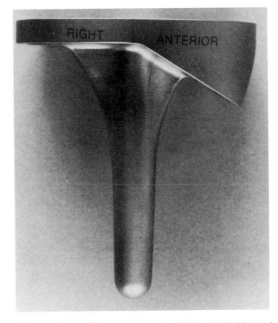

Figure 80–13. Custom tibial component for large medial bone defect.

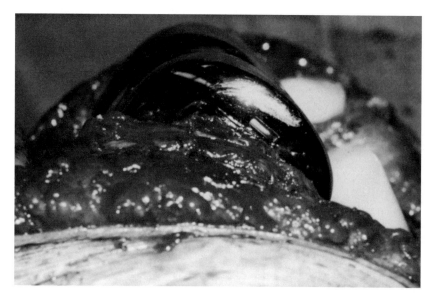

Figure 80–14. Augmented femoral component of the PCA revision type.

ingrowth, while the condylar portion of the implant can be inserted with cement (Fig. 80–16).

Fixation

Once a component system has been selected and a satisfactory trial reduction has been accomplished with correct limb alignment and stability, fixation must be considered. Cement fixation of the condylar portion of the implant remains the accepted technique. Whether a press-fit or a cemented intramedullary stem should be utilized is controversial.[20,34,52] With early revision implant designs, the intramedullary stems were too small to achieve a predictable press fit. Newer designs with modular stems are available that allow the option of a press-fit stem.[22]

If cement fixation of the stem is selected, the technique is similar to preparation of the femur for a cemented total hip arthroplasty. Plugging of the intramedullary canal is utilized, as is pulsatile lavage. A cement gun is used to introduce cement into the femoral and tibial medullary canals. Bone grafts must be sealed with Gelfoam at their interface with the tibia or femur to prevent cement interposition at the interface (Fig. 80–17).

The tibial component should be cemented first and the trial femoral component placed. The cement is allowed to harden with the knee in extension to allow assessment of rotational alignment with the tibial tuberosity and congruity between the femoral and tibial components.

The femur should be prepared with pulsatile lavage and cemented in a similar manner. Once the components are secure, motion, stability, and patellar tracking should be assessed.

The Patella

The patella has been neglected too often in discussions of total knee arthroplasty revision. The patella usually

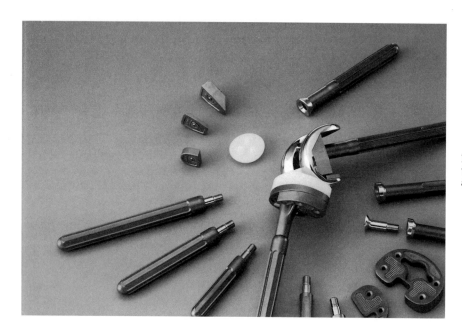

Figure 80–15. Modular revision total knee system with femoral and tibial augments, wedges, and stems.

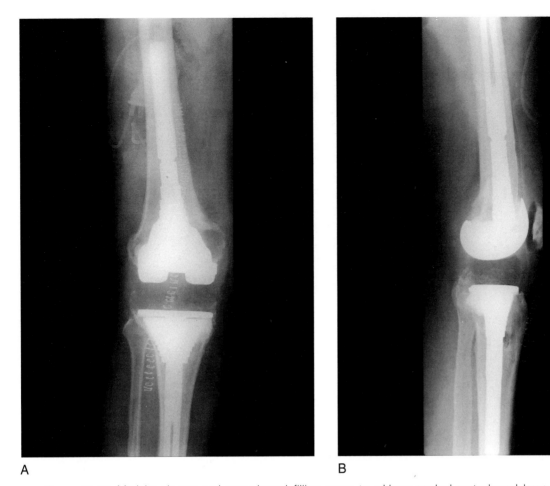

Figure 80–16. Modular sleeves and metaphyseal filling cones to address marked metaphyseal bone deficiency. Anteroposterior (**A**) and lateral (**B**) view.

has a concave bone deficiency in its center from the old fixation lug (Fig. 80–18). The patella should be measured with a caliper to determine its thickness and the symmetry of the bone resection. If the remaining bone is 10 mm or less, a new patellar implant may not have adequate bone for fixation. The alternatives then are either patelloplasty or patellar bone grafting.[21,37] Patellectomy is used rarely now if ever.

If adequate bone stock remains on the patella, patellar resurfacing may be considered. The patellar bone should be symmetric in thickness to within 2 mm on medial, lateral, proximal, and distal measurements with the caliper. The concave deficiency provides poor fixation for a central patellar fixation lug. The alternatives to a central fixation lug design are either a component with peripheral fixation pegs or a biconvex design (Fig. 80–19). The peripheral fixation lugs must be able to be placed in adequate-quality bone. The biconvex design is inset into a peripheral rim of bone created in the patella (Fig. 80–20). The peripheral rim of bone provides support for the implant, and the biconvex patellar implant fills the central bone defect.

Once the patella has been treated in the appropriate manner, tracking of the extensor mechanism and patellar tilt should be assessed. Lateral retinacular release and vastus medialis advancement or a proximal realign-

ment procedure should be performed as necessary to ensure correct patellar tracking.

Closure

Typically closure includes leaving the lateral retinacular release open if this has been performed, and the medial retinaculum and deep structures are closed with multiple interrupted sutures. A deep drain is typically placed and a compressive dressing applied.

RESULTS OF REVISION

Revision total knee arthroplasty results are difficult to compare because of differences in the criteria of success and differences in the implants used. The early results of revision total knee arthroplasty were not encouraging. Satisfactory results were achieved in 37 to 64 percent of knees when early implant designs were used.[1,2,8,9,13,14,41] In the initial experience at the Mayo Clinic with 427 revision total knee arthroplasties between 1970 and 1980, 357 (84 percent) had one revision, 60 (14 percent) had two revisions, and 10 (2 percent) had three revisions.[6,41,48] In the majority of these patients, the failures were of early resurfacing designs such as the geometric and polycentric prostheses.

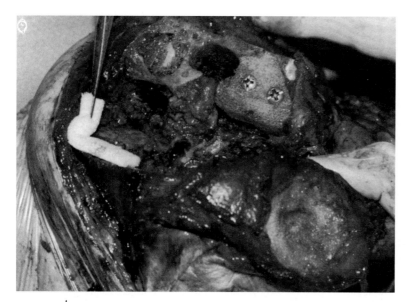

Figure 80–17. Sealing of the interface between bone graft and host bone prior to introduction of cement. (From Rand JA: Revision total knee arthroplasty. *In* Evarts CM [ed]: Surgery of the Musculoskeletal System, 2nd ed, vol 4. New York, Churchill Livingstone, 1990, p 3645.)

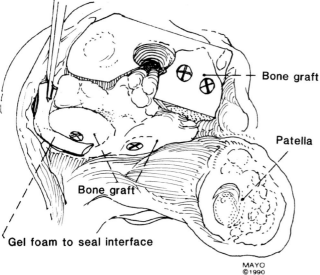

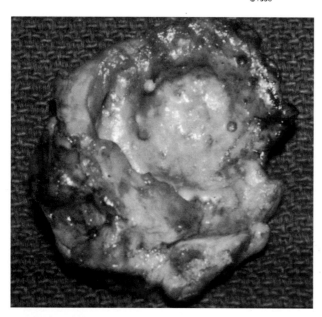

Figure 80–18. Patellar bone deficiency after a prosthesis failed.

Using earlier revision designs, actuarial survival analysis was utilized to estimate the duration of prosthetic function after revision. Patients with rheumatoid arthritis had a 90-percent probability of continued function at 5 years after revision compared with 65 percent for those with osteoarthritis (Fig. 80–21). Patients who were at their ideal body weight had a slightly better implant survival than those who were overweight (Fig. 80–22). Implant

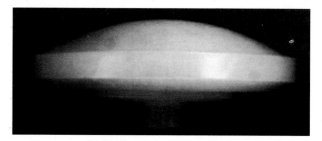

Figure 80–19. Biconvex patellar implant of the Genesis design for revision patellar arthroplasty.

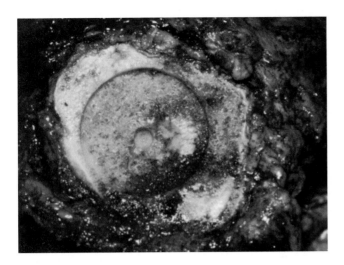

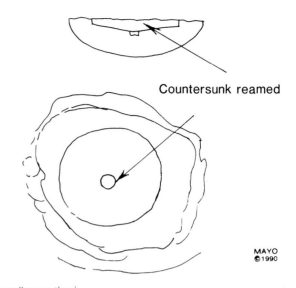

Countersunk reamed

MAYO
©1990

Figure 80–20. Patella prepared to accept the biconvex patellar prosthesis.

survival was better when condylar implants were used for revision than when older resurfacing designs were used (Fig. 80–23). Implant survival was better with the newer resurfacing implants such as a condylar prosthesis than with the more constrained rotating hinge or Total Condylar III implants ($P < 0.04$) (Fig. 80–24).

In view of the best results being observed with a condylar implant, a second study of 50 revision arthroplasties with condylar implants in 1980 and 1981 was performed.[43] These revision procedures used a posterior cruciate–sparing Total Condylar implant, a Kinematic condylar implant, or a Total Condylar implant. The patients were observed for 5 years. Seventy-six percent of the knees achieved a good or excellent knee score at final examination.

Dupont et al.[14] found 65 percent satisfactory results in 103 knees. With a Stanmore hinge, only 23 percent of 52 knees had good results at 3.5 years.[27] In rheumatoid patients, 60 percent of 48 revisions, with various

implants, were satisfactory at 5 years.[50] Cameron and Hunter[8] obtained only 37 percent satisfactory results in 73 knees. Kim and Finerman[30] reported pain relief in 81 percent of cases, and Thornhill et al.[58] reported a 40-point improvement in knee scores in 156 of 170 knee revisions. Good to excellent results in 68 percent of 28 knees was reported with the PCA system.[25]

Revision of various failed resurfacing implants to posterior-stabilized or hinge prostheses provided 46 percent good to excellent results in 65 knees at 5 years.[18] Revision of 14 failed prostheses to a Total Condylar III device provided a mean improvement in knee score from 58 to 81 at 4 years.[31] In a review of 36 revisions using the Total Condylar III prosthesis followed for 45 months, good or excellent results were achieved in 25 knees (76 percent).[51] Radiolucent lines were present in 60 percent, of which 16 percent were progressive. In the Mayo Clinic experience, the Total Condylar III prosthesis provided good or excellent results in 50 percent of 21

Figure 80–21. Prosthesis survival probabilities for rheumatoid knees and for osteoarthritic knees after revision of failed arthroplasty ($P < 0.001$). (From Rand JA, Peterson LFA, Bryan RS, Ilstrup DM: Revision total knee arthroplasty. Instr Course Lect 35:305, 1986.)

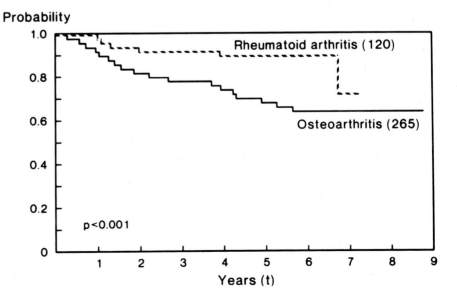

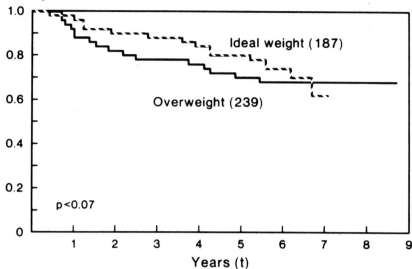

Figure 80–22. Prosthesis survival probabilities according to body weight. "Overweight" is 20 percent above ideal weight. (From Rand JA, Peterson LFA, Bryan RS, Ilstrup DM: Revision total knee arthroplasty. Instr Course Lect 35:305, 1986.)

knees at 4 years after revision.[40] A subsequent 15 year follow-up study showed that the Total Condylar III prosthesis remained durable and reliable.[59] The results were not affected if the prior implant was a resurfacing or constrained type or by the number of revisions. Insall and Dethmers[23] reported 89 percent good to excellent knee scores in 72 knees at 2 years with primarily posterior-stabilized designs.

Of 53 knees treated at the Mayo Clinic by revision with a Kinematic stabilizer prosthesis, results were good to excellent in 81 percent at 3 years.[21] These results were less satisfactory than those in 26 primary arthroplasties with the same implant, which gave 92 percent good to excellent results ($P < 0.05$).[21] With a Kinematic rotating-hinge prosthesis, 76 percent of the revision and 66 percent of the primary arthroplasties had good to excellent knee scores at 4 years.[45] A subsequent study of 77 Kinematic rotating-hinge prostheses used for complex primary and revision total knee arthroplasty was done with an average 6-year follow-up. Complications were numerous and required reoperation in 20 knees. Knee Society scores improved from 29 points preoperatively to 76 points at last follow-up. The average range of motion postoperatively was from 1 to 94 degrees.[20]

Seventy-six revision total knee replacements done at the Hospital for Special Surgery with modular components and stems inserted without cement were followed for an average of 3.6 years. Excellent or good results were obtained in 84 percent of patients. Eight percent had been re-revised at last follow-up.[19]

Sixteen knees with complex reconstructive problems were revised using a second-generation modular rotating-hinge design and were followed for an average of 4.2 years. Clinical and radiographic results were comparable to those of a group of 87 patients revised with a standard condylar design.[3]

The results of revision of 40 total knees in the presence of a bone defect of at least 1 cm and comprising 50 percent of either the femur or tibia were reviewed at 41 months after revision.[15] Good or excellent results were achieved in 75 percent, but with a complication rate of 30 percent and a failure rate of 10 percent. The authors concluded that an intramedullary stem should be used for fixation in the presence of bone loss. Using survivorship analysis with an endpoint of removal of the prosthesis, 97-percent survivorship was predicted at 6 years in 37 revision total knees.[49] In a survivorship analysis of 9200 total knees from the Mayo Clinic using an endpoint of implant removal, a survivorship of 72 percent at 10 years was predicted for the 1131 revision knees.[47]

COMPLICATIONS

Complications after revision surgery are of the same type as those after primary arthroplasty. Complications are influenced by the extent of previous surgery, host immunocompetence, and the adequacy of surgical technique in performing the reconstruction. Infection after revision may be related to the prolonged duration of the operation, problems in wound healing, and unrecognized sepsis as the cause of failure of the initial arthroplasty. The incidence of deep infection in the 427 revision arthroplasties performed at the Mayo Clinic was similar to the incidence of infection in 5643 primary total knee arthroplasties performed in the same time interval, 2.1 and 1.9 percent, respectively.[48] There was little correlation between a positive intraoperative culture and subsequent clinical infection. In our condylar revision experience, there was only one superficial and no deep infections in 54 knees.[43] In two previously infected knees, the Kinematic stabilizer prosthesis was used for revision and reinfection developed in both.[21] With the Kinematic rotating hinge for revision, there was a deep infection rate of 19 percent.[45]

Other complications include postoperative hematomas, delayed wound healing, bone or prosthesis fractures,

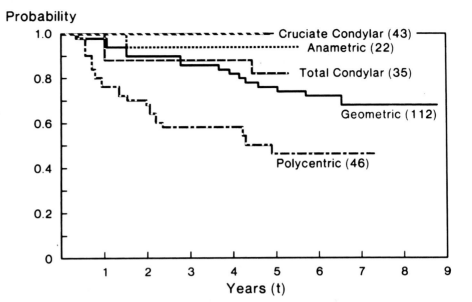

Figure 80–23. Prosthesis survival probabilities for semiconstrained implants from first to second revision, by actuarial technique. The number of implants is indicated for each survival curve. (From Rand JA, Peterson LFA, Bryan RS, Ilstrup DM: Revision total knee arthroplasty. Instr Course Lect 35:305, 1986.)

patellar instability, peroneal palsy, patellar tendon rupture, thromboembolism, and loosening of the revision implant. The frequency of these complications is lowest with condylar revision and highest when a rotating hinge is required.[45,48,56]

Radiolucent lines are common after revision arthroplasty because cement cannot penetrate sclerotic bone well. The exact thickness of a radiolucent line that suggests possible loosening is poorly defined. A circumferential radiolucency of 2 mm or greater raises concern. Radiolucent lines were evaluated in 81 knees with a condylar, posterior-stabilized, or rotating-hinge design at a mean of 3 years after revision. Radiolucent lines were present in 86 percent of the knees.[48] A complete radiolucency 1 to 2 mm wide was seen adjacent to 7 percent of the femoral components and 3 percent of the tibial components. Radiolucency greater than 2 mm wide was seen adjacent to 5 percent of the femoral and 1 percent of the tibial components. In the condylar revision

knees, radiolucent lines 1 mm or greater in width were seen adjacent to 14 percent of the tibial (5 percent were complete) and 7 percent of the femoral components.[43] Radiolucent lines were present adjacent to 29 percent of the Kinematic stabilizer implants.[21] With the Kinematic rotating hinge, lucent lines 1 mm or greater were present adjacent to about 29 percent of the femoral and 48 percent of the tibial components.[45] Therefore, radiolucent lines are frequently present and are more prevalent about large constrained implants.

AUTHORS' PREFERENCE

Our preference for revision total knee arthroplasty is to achieve a reconstructed joint line, soft tissue balance, range of motion of at least 90 degrees, and stability. Modular implants are utilized to accomplish these goals. The implant selected should be augmented on the

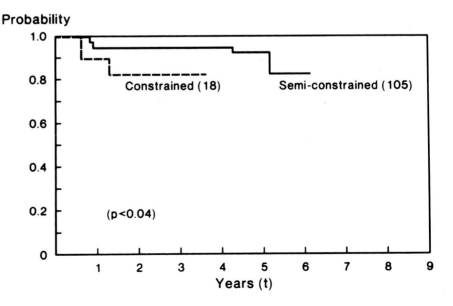

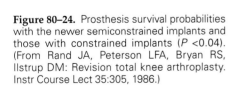

Figure 80–24. Prosthesis survival probabilities with the newer semiconstrained implants and those with constrained implants (P <0.04). (From Rand JA, Peterson LFA, Bryan RS, Ilstrup DM: Revision total knee arthroplasty. Instr Course Lect 35:305, 1986.)

femoral side distally and posteriorly to restore the joint line 2.5 cm distal to the femoral epicondyles. The interior dimension of the implant should match the remaining femoral bone while the exterior dimension of the implant results in equal flexion and extension spaces. The extent of distal augmentation affects the extension gap, and the extent of posterior augmentation on the femoral side affects the flexion gap. The thickness of the tibial component will affect both the flexion and extension gap. Therefore, the femoral implant is selected that will create even flexion-extension gaps. This may necessitate independent augmentation of variable amounts distally and posteriorly, as well as medially or laterally.

In revision surgery, a stemmed implant is generally utilized. It has been our preference to press fit intramedullary stems on the femur and tibia when feasible. One must not be a slave to the stem, however, and, if a press-fit intramedullary stem dictates malposition of a component, then the surgeon must switch to a shorter cemented stem. In most revision circumstances, a posterior-stabilized prosthesis is appropriate because it is difficult to retain and balance the posterior cruciate ligament. A collateral ligament–substituting (constrained condylar) prosthesis would only be utilized if soft tissue balance could not be obtained or if a collateral ligament were markedly deficient.

References

1. Ahlberg A, Lund A: Secondary operations after knee joint replacement. Clin Orthop 156:170, 1981.
2. Bargar WL, Cracchiolo A III, Amstutz HC: Results with the constrained total knee prosthesis in treating severely disabled patients and patients with failed total knee replacements. J Bone Joint Surg Am 62:504, 1980.
3. Barrack RL, Lyons TR, Ingraham RQ, Johnson JC: The use of a modular rotating hinge component in salvage revision total knee arthroplasty. J Arthroplasty 15:858, 2000.
4. Barrett WP, Scott RD: Revision of failed unicondylar unicompartmental knee arthroplasty. J Bone Joint Surg Am 69:1328, 1987.
5. Bertin KC, Freeman MAR, Samuelson KM, et al: Stemmed revision arthroplasty for aseptic loosening of total knee replacement. J Bone Joint Surg Br 67:242, 1985.
6. Bryan RS, Rand JA: Revision total knee arthroplasty. Clin Orthop 170:116, 1982.
7. Bryan RS, Rand JA: Indications, results, and complications of revision of total knee arthroplasty for mechanical failure. In Ranawat CS (ed): Total-Condylar Knee Arthroplasty: Technique, Results, and Complications. New York, Springer-Verlag, 1985, p 249.
8. Cameron HU, Hunter GA: Failure in total knee arthroplasty: mechanisms, revisions, and results. Clin Orthop 170:141, 1982.
9. Cameron HU, Hunter GA, Welsh RP, Bailey WH: Revision of total knee replacement. Can J Surg 24:418, 1982.
10. Chen F, Krackow KA: Management of tibial defects in total knee arthroplasty: a biomechanical study. Clin Orthop 305:249–257, 1994.
11. Dolin MG: Osteotomy of the tibial tubercle in total knee replacement: a technical note. J Bone Joint Surg Am 65:704, 1983.
12. Dorr LD, Conaty JP, Schreiber R, et al: Technical factors that influence mechanical loosening of total knee arthroplasty. In Dorr LD (ed): The Knee: Papers of the First Scientific Meeting of the Knee Society. Baltimore, University Park Press, 1985, p 121.
13. Ducheyne P, Kagan A II, Lacey JA: Failure of total knee arthroplasty due to loosening and deformation of the tibial component. J Bone Joint Surg Am 60:384, 1978.
14. Dupont JA, Campbell ED Jr, Lumsden RM II: Total knee arthroplasty revisions [abstract]. Orthop Trans 4:321, 1980.
15. Elia EA, Lotke PA: Results of revision total knee arthroplasty associated with significant bone loss. Clin Orthop 271:114, 1991.
16. Ewald FC, Jacobs MA, Miegel RE, et al: Kinematic total knee replacement. J Bone Joint Surg Am 66:1032, 1984.
17. Figgie HE III, Goldberg VM, Heiple KG, et al: The influence of tibial-patellofemoral location on function of the knee in patients with the posterior stabilized condylar knee prosthesis. J Bone Joint Surg Am 68:1035, 1986.
18. Goldberg VM, Figgie MP, Figgie HE III, Sobel M: The results of revision total knee arthroplasty. Clin Orthop 226:86, 1988.
19. Haas SB, Insall JN, Montgomery W, Windsor RE: Revision total knee arthroplasty with use of modular components with stems inserted without cement. J Bone Joint Surg Am 77:1700, 1995.
20. Hanssen AD: Hinges: the Mayo experience. Presented at the Knee Society Specialty Day Scientific Program, San Francisco, March 3, 2001.
21. Hanssen AD, Rand JA: A comparison of primary and revision total knee arthroplasty using the kinematic stabilizer prosthesis. J Bone Joint Surg Am 70:491, 1988.
22. Insall JN: Revision of total knee replacement. Instr Course Lect 35:290, 1986.
23. Insall JN, Dethmers DA: Revision of total knee arthroplasty. Clin Orthop 170:123, 1982.
24. Insall JN, Kelly M: The total condylar prosthesis. Clin Orthop 205:43, 1986.
25. Jacobs MA, Hungerford DS, Krackow KA, Lennox DW: Revision total knee arthroplasty for aseptic failure. Clin Orthop 226:78, 1988.
26. Jones RE: Management of complex revision problems with a modular total knee system. Orthopedics 19:802, 1996.
27. Karpinski MRK, Grimer RJ: Hinged knee replacement in revision arthroplasty. Clin Orthop 220:185, 1987.
28. Kaufer H, Matthews LS: Spherocentric arthroplasty of the knee: clinical experience with an average four-year follow-up. J Bone Joint Surg Am 63:545, 1981.
29. Kaufer H, Matthews LS: Revision total knee arthroplasty: indications and contraindications. Instr Course Lect 35:297, 1986.
30. Kim L, Finerman G: Results of revisions for aseptic failed knee arthroplasties [abstract]. Orthop Trans 7:535, 1983.
31. Kim Y-H: Salvage of failed hinge knee arthroplasty with a Total Condylar III prosthesis. Clin Orthop 221:272, 1987.
32. Lai CM, Rand JA: Revision of failed unicompartmental total knee arthroplasty. Clin Orthop 287:193, 1993.
33. Lotke PA, Windsor R, Ecker ML, Cella J: Long term results after total condylar knee replacement: significance of radiolucent lines [abstract]. Orthop Trans 8:398, 1984.
34. Murray PB, Rand JA, Hanssen AD: Cemented long-stem revision total knee arthroplasty. Clin Orthop 309:116, 1994.
35. Padgett DF, Stern SH, Insall JN: Revision total knee arthroplasty for failed unicompartmental replacement. J Bone Joint Surg Am 73:186, 1991.
36. Pagnano MW, Hanssen AD, Lewallen DG, Stuart MJ: Flexion instability after primary posterior cruciate retaining total knee arthroplasty. Clin Orthop 356:79, 1998.
37. Pagnano MW, Scuderi GR, Insall JN: Patellar component resection in revision and reimplantation total knee arthroplasty. Clin Orthop 356:134, 1998.
38. Pagnano MW, Trousdale RT, Rand JA: Tibial wedge augmentation for bone deficiency in total knee arthroplasty: a follow-up study. Clin Orthop 321:151, 1995.
39. Rand JA: Revision total knee arthroplasty. In Evarts CM (ed): Surgery of the Musculoskeletal System, 2nd ed, vol 4. New York, Churchill Livingstone, 1990, p 3645.
40. Rand JA: Revision total knee arthroplasty using Total Condylar III prosthesis. J Arthroplasty 6:1, 1991.
41. Rand JA, Bryan RS: Revision after total knee arthroplasty. Orthop Clin North Am 13:201, 1982.
42. Rand JA, Bryan RS: Alignment in porous coated anatomic total knee arthroplasty. In Dorr LD (ed): The Knee: Papers of the First Scientific Meeting of the Knee Society. Baltimore, University Park Press, 1985, p 111.
43. Rand JA, Bryan RS: Results of revision total knee arthroplasties using condylar prostheses: a review of fifty knees. J Bone Joint Surg Am 70:738, 1988.
44. Rand JA, Bryan RS, Chao EYS, Ilstrup DM: A comparison of cemented versus cementless porous-coated anatomic total knee

arthroplasty. *In* Rand JA, Dorr LD (eds): Total Arthroplasty of the Knee: Proceedings of the Knee Society, 1985–1986. Rockville, MD, Aspen Publishers, 1987, p 195.

45. Rand JA, Chao EYS, Stauffer RN: Kinematic rotating-hinge total knee arthroplasty. J Bone Joint Surg Am 69:489, 1987.
46. Rand JA, Coventry MB: Ten-year evaluation of geometric total knee arthroplasty. Clin Orthop 232:168, 1988.
47. Rand JA, Ilstrup DM: Survivorship analysis of total knee arthroplasty. J Bone Joint Surg Am 73:397, 1991.
48. Rand JA, Peterson LFA, Bryan RS, Ilstrup DM: Revision total knee arthroplasty. Instr Course Lect 35:305, 1986.
49. Ritter MA, Eizenber LE, Fechtman RW, et al: Revision total knee arthroplasty, a survival analysis. J Arthroplasty 6:351, 1991.
50. Rööser B, Boegård T, Knutson K, et al: Revision knee arthroplasty in rheumatoid arthritis. Clin Orthop 219:169, 1987.
51. Rosenberg AG, Verner JJ, Galante JO: Clinical results of total knee revision using the Total Condylar III prosthesis. Clin Orthop 273:83, 1991.
52. Samuelson KM: Bone grafting and noncemented revision arthroplasty of the knee. Clin Orthop 226:93, 1988.
53. Scott RD: Revision total knee arthroplasty. Clin Orthop 226:65, 1988.
54. Scott RD, Siliski JM: The use of a modified V-Y quadricepsplasty during total knee replacement to gain exposure and improve flexion in the ankylosed knee. Orthopedics 8:45, 1985.
55. Sculco TP: Technique of revision of total knee arthroplasty. *In* Ranawat CS (ed): Total-Condylar Knee Arthroplasty: Technique, Results, and Complications. New York, Springer-Verlag, 1985, p 238.
56. Stuart MJ, Larsen JE, Morrey BF: Reoperation after condylar revision total knee arthroplasty. Clin Orthop 286:168, 1993.
57. Thornhill TS, Dalziel RW, Sledge CB: Alternatives to arthrodesis for the failed total knee arthroplasty. Clin Orthop 170:131, 1982.
58. Thornhill TS, Hood RW, Dalziel RE, et al: Knee revision in failed non-infected total knee arthroplasty—the Robert B. Brigham Hospital and Hospital for Special Surgery experience [abstract]. Orthop Trans 6:368, 1982.
59. Trousdale RT, Beckenbaugh JP, Pagnano MW: 15 year results of the total condylar III implant in revision total knee arthroplasty (Paper #117). Presented at the 68th annual meeting of the American Academy of Orthopaedic Surgeons, San Francisco, February 28–March 4, 2001.
60. Trousdale RT, Hanssen AD, Rand JA, Cahalan TD: V-Y quadricepsplasty in total knee arthroplasty. Clin Orthop 286:48, 1993.
61. Whiteside LA: Cementless revision total knee arthroplasty. Clin Orthop 286:160, 1993.
62. Whiteside L, Ohl MD: Tibial tubercle osteotomy for exposure of the difficult total knee arthroplasty. Clin Orthop 260:6, 1990.
63. Wolff A, Hungerford D, Krackow K, Jacobs M: Osteotomy of the tibial tubercle during total knee replacement. J Bone Joint Surg Am 71:848, 1989.

81

Management of the Infected Total Knee Arthroplasty

• ARLEN D. HANSSEN, JAMES A. RAND, and DOUGLAS R. OSMON

Deep infection remains one of the most common reasons for failure of a total knee arthroplasty and occurs in approximately 1 to 2 percent of patients.[6] Diligence with recognized prevention measures to reduce bacterial contamination, augment the host response, and optimize the wound environment in the preoperative, perioperative, and postoperative time periods are necessary to reduce the incidence of deep infection (see Chapter 10). Although management methods and surgical techniques have improved significantly, rapid diagnosis and diagnosis and expeditious use of established treatment principles are essential to a successful outcome.

DIAGNOSIS

Infection may be diagnosed in four different clinical settings (Table 81–1). These are characterized by positive culture(s) discovered after a revision procedure (type 1), an acute infection diagnosed within the first 30 days after arthroplasty (type 2), chronic or late indolent infections (type 3), and acute hematogenous infections in an otherwise well-functioning prosthesis (type 4).[94] The basic fundamentals of diagnosis in any of these clinical settings include a high index of suspicion combined with a thorough history, physical examination, plain radiographs, arthrocentesis, and several simple hematologic studies. Radionuclide studies and evaluation of surgical tissue specimens occasionally may be helpful. This classification system is also a useful guide to select between the various treatment options for the infected knee arthroplasty.

Pain is the most common presenting symptom in the patient with an infected knee arthroplasty and typically occurs while at rest. Persistent pain or progressive stiffness since the time of arthroplasty should also alert one toward the possibility of deep infection. Persistent wound drainage is strongly suggestive of infection and should probably be treated with arthrotomy, débridement, and irrigation within the first several weeks after surgery.[104] Cultures of serous wound drainage are difficult to interpret and potentially misleading, and the use

of these cultures is discouraged. Empiric use of antibiotics for persistent wound drainage should be avoided because this practice only suppresses the clinical symptoms and delays diagnosis. If diagnosis is established early, it is possible to treat the infection without removal of the prosthesis.[14,91,97]

Early Postoperative Period

Diagnosis of infection in the early postoperative setting is best established by joint arthrocentesis because the erythrocyte sedimentation rate (ESR) and C-reactive protein (CRP) levels are nonspecific in the early postoperative period. The response of CRP following knee arthroplasty is greater than that following hip arthroplasty; however, rising levels after the third postoperative day may be indicative of deep periprosthetic infection.[105] In the early postoperative period, assertive management of delayed wound healing or marginal skin necrosis by débridement of necrotic skin and primary wound closure is preferable to empiric antibiotic treatment, prolonged observation, and eventual development of deep infection.[61] Although soft tissue reconstruction is occasionally invaluable in the prevention of deep periprosthetic infection for an exposed knee prosthesis, these procedures alone cannot be expected to cure an infection involving a total knee arthroplasty and must be considered only as adjunctive treatment methods.[1,16,35,42,65]

Delayed

An acute hematogenous infection typically presents with sudden onset of clinical symptoms in a previously well-functioning arthroplasty.[7] Specific risk factors, such as a remote source of infection or a recent invasive procedure causing a significant bacteremia, which may be associated with the possibility of hematogenous infection, should be ascertained.[63] The severity of symptoms, with pain, effusion, and restricted range of knee motion, in this setting facilitates rapid diagnosis. Although the

Table 81–1. CLASSIFICATION OF DEEP PERIPROSTHETIC INFECTION

	Type 1	Type 2	Type 3	Type 4
Timing		Early postoperative infection	Acute hematogenous infection	Late (chronic) infection
Definition	Positive intraoperative culture	Infection occurs within the first	Hematogenous seeding of	Chronic indolent clinical course;
	2 or more positive cultures	mo after surgery	previously well-functioning arthroplasty	infection present for more than 1 mo
	at surgery			
Treatment	Appropriate antibiotics	Attempt at débridement with	Attempt at débridement with prosthesis	Prosthesis removal
		prosthesis salvage	salvage or prosthesis removal	

ESR and CRP are typically elevated in these patients, the cornerstone of diagnosis is arthrocentesis and culture for aerobic and anaerobic bacteria.

The vast majority of patients with an infected total knee arthroplasty are diagnosed in the subacute or chronic setting. Historical factors such as persistent pain since the arthroplasty, prolonged postoperative wound drainage, antibiotic treatment for difficulties with primary wound healing, and knee stiffness despite extensive rehabilitation efforts may be associated with deep infection. Sequential comparison of plain radiographs may reveal progressive radiolucencies, focal osteopenia or osteolysis of subchondral bone, and periosteal new bone formation.[72]

Arthrocentesis is considered an essential element of the investigative process for several reasons.[5,28,60] Patients should be off antibiotics for several weeks prior to aspiration; failure to stop antibiotics often accounts for the inability to isolate organisms. In one series of 69 knees, the preoperative aspiration had a sensitivity of 55 percent, specificity of 96 percent, and accuracy of 84 percent.[5] However, 12 of the patients with infected knees were on antibiotics at the time of aspiration and 7 (58 percent) of these knee cultures had no growth. After antibiotics were discontinued, four knees were reaspirated, all had a positive culture, and the overall sensitivity improved to 75 percent, specificity to 96 percent, and accuracy to 90 percent.[5] These authors recommended routine aspiration prior to any revision knee arthroplasty.[5]

The use of molecular genetic diagnostic methods, such as the polymerase chain reaction technique, with joint aspirates is potentially promising, but these remain experimental modalities for diagnosis of the infected joint arthroplasty.[64] Currently, this technique is complex and the equipment for this technology is expensive.

The use of radioisotope scans to facilitate diagnosis of the chronically infected knee prosthesis is occasionally useful.[90] We currently use these imaging studies only for enigmatic painful prostheses. A screening technetium-99 study may be helpful when the study demonstrates the absence of significant tracer uptake because this rules out the possibility of deep infection. Indium-111–labeled leukocyte scanning alone appears to be more accurate (78 percent) than technetium-99 diphosphonate bone scanning alone (74 percent); however, the accuracy of indium-111–labeled leukocyte scanning combined with technetium-99 sulfur colloid marrow scintigraphy provides an improvement in accuracy to 95 percent.[79] The sensitivity of indium-111 scanning appears to be dependent on the activity of the infection, with reduced sensitivity in chronic and indolent infections.[36] False-positive results indium-111 scans have been observed in association with rheumatoid arthritis and massive osteolysis.[85] Technitium-99– or indium-111–labeled immunoglobulin imaging techniques have shown some promise but still require additional evaluation.[24,76]

Ultimately, intraoperative evaluation of surgical tissue specimens may be necessary to confirm the diagnosis in difficult cases. We have abandoned the use of Gram stain testing because it is notoriously unreliable, with a high percentage of false-negative results and an extremely low sensitivity.[3,23] The accuracy of frozen section testing to detect infection is inconsistently reported.[22,31,62,77] The positive predictive value of frozen sections is significantly better ($P < 0.05$) when the index was increased from 5 to 10 polymorphonuclear leukocytes per high-power field.[62] We believe that this test is a reasonable and reliable method when an accomplished pathologist evaluates appropriate tissue samples.

Although it is difficult to perform quantitatively, the surgeon's intraoperative assessment during the course of aseptic revision surgery is also very helpful. If there is any reason to suspect deep periprosthetic infection, several carefully selected tissue specimens are taken and final results awaited. Our current definition of prosthetic infection includes a combination of clinical signs and symptoms, histologic analysis of tissue, and results of cultures. The diagnosis of definite infection is made if evaluation of the knee establishes at least one of the following criteria: (1) two or more cultures obtained by aspiration or deep tissue specimens obtained at surgery yield the same organism, (2) histopathologic evaluation of intra-articular tissue reveals changes of acute inflammation, (3) gross purulence is observed at the time of surgery, or (4) an actively discharging sinus tract is found.[44]

Staphylococcus aureus is the most common microorganism (30 percent) recovered from an infected total knee arthroplasty, and coagulase-negative staphylococci (21 percent) are the second most common.[43] Prolonged antibiotic treatment prior to presentation accounts for 9 percent of infected total knee arthroplasties being culture negative.

TREATMENT

Once the diagnosis has been established, the variables that must be considered before initiating treatment include (1) the duration of time elapsed between the arthroplasty and diagnosis of infection, (2) identification of host factors that may adversely affect the treatment of the infection, (3) involvement of the soft tissue envelope surrounding the knee and specifically the integrity of the extensor mechanism, (4) consideration of the pathogen(s) responsible for the infection, (5) determination of whether the implant is loose or well fixed, (6) the physician's ability to provide the proper level of care required, and (7) careful assessment of the patient's expectations and functional requirements (Fig. 81–1).

Treatment goals for the infected total knee arthroplasty include eradication of infection, alleviation of pain, and maintenance of a functional extremity.

Careful patient assessment and counseling are extremely important aspects of the decision-making process. The patient or his or her family are often angry or afraid about the presence of infection, and the discussion is often emotional and prolonged. The probability for a successful outcome is most likely when the first treatment attempt has been appropriately selected and

Variables	Options	Goals
• *Depth of infection*	• *Antibiotic suppression*	• *Eradication of infection*
• *Time elapse since surgery*	• *Debridement*	• *Alleviation of pain*
• *Soft-tissues*	• *Resection arthroplasty*	• *Maintenance of function*
• *Prosthesis fixation*	• *Arthrodesis*	
• *Pathogens*	• *Amputation*	
• *Host factors*	• *Reimplantation*	
• *Physician capabilities*		
• *Patient expectations*		

Figure 81–1. Treatment of the infected total knee arthroplasty requires careful assessment of the treatment variables and selection of the proper treatment option to achieve the final treatment goals.

expertly performed. Secondary treatment attempts are often adversely affected by progressive scarring, devitalization of the soft tissue envelope, antibiotic-resistant organisms, and the continued bone loss associated with prior failures.

The six basic treatment options include (1) antibiotic suppression, (2) open débridement, (3) resection arthroplasty, (4) arthrodesis, (5) amputation, and (6) reimplantation of another prosthesis.

Antibiotic Suppression

Antibiotic treatment alone will not eliminate deep periprosthetic infection but can be used as suppressive treatment when the following criteria are met: (1) prosthesis removal is not feasible (usually because of a medical condition that precludes an operative procedure); (2) virulence of the microorganism is low; (3) the microorganism is susceptible to an oral antibiotic; (4) the selected antibiotic is without serious toxicity; and (5) the prosthesis is not loose.[98] The presence of other joint arthroplasties is a relatively strong contraindication to chronic antibiotic suppression. Despite the fact that most patients fail to meet all of the above-mentioned selection criteria, antibiotic suppression is commonly practiced, which unfortunately prolongs the presence of infection and often complicates subsequent treatment attempts. This method of treatment should be rarely initiated and only considered when all treatment criteria are met.

In a multicenter study, antibiotic suppression was successful in only 40 of 225 knees (18 percent).[8] Combining several series reveals that antibiotic suppression was successful in 62 (24 percent) of 261 knees.[8,40,55,98,109] Use of a combined regimen of rifampicin with a quinolone has been reported to be more successful than treatment with a single antibiotic.[26]

Débridement with Prosthesis Retention

Open débridement may be indicated for the occasional acute infection in the early postoperative period (type 2) or for acute hematogenous infection (type 3) of a securely fixed and functional prosthesis. Suggested criteria for this treatment technique include (1) short duration of symptoms (<2 weeks), (2) susceptible gram-positive organisms, (3) absence of prolonged postoperative drainage or development of a draining sinus tract, and (4) no prosthetic loosening or radiographic evidence of infection.[14] A relative contraindication for débridement and attempted salvage of the prosthesis is the presence other joint replacements.

Results of débridement are difficult to determine because of differences in microbiology and subsequent antibiotic management, variability in the time to treatment, quality of the soft tissue envelope, extent and completeness of débridement, status of implant fixation, and the criteria for success in each report. A multicenter study reported success with open débridement in 30 (19.5 percent) of 154 knees.[8] Combining multiple series describes success in a total of 140 (31.5 percent) of 445 knees.[8,10,12,18,33,40,46,53,55,71,88,94,97,104,109] Many of these débridement reports include patients with chronically infected prostheses.[81]

The importance of the timing of the débridement in relationship to the onset of symptoms or the period of time elapsed since the insertion of the prosthesis cannot be overemphasized.[14,70,91,94,96] When defining acute infection of less than 2 weeks' duration, débridement was successful in 3 of 5 acute infections (60 percent) compared with 3 of 16 (19 percent) chronic infections followed for an average of 3.5 years.[97] In one of the series that categorized the infection types, only 1 of 11 patients with a chronic infection were successfully treated with débridement.[94] It is quite clear that débridement with prosthesis retention should not be attempted in patients with chronic infections (type 3).[12,55,94]

Débridement must be performed urgently for early postoperative (type 2) and acute hematogenous (type 3) infections because delay of the débridement procedure while awaiting culture reports results in a significant decrease in the success of the débridement attempt. Expeditious treatment as soon as possible after the diagnosis has been established is the paramount concern. This is particularly true for *S. aureus*—delay beyond 48 hours after onset of symptoms resulted in a significant decrease in the success rate.[14] *Staphylococcus aureus* prosthetic joint infection is associated with the lowest success rate following débridement.[91,109]

The likelihood of success following débridement in the early postoperative period is much higher with cemented implants compared with uncemented implants, which may be due to more efficient sealing of the bone-cement interface of the cemented components in the early postoperative period. Unconstrained knees are more likely to have a successful outcome than hinged, constrained prostheses.[58,91] The ability to adequately débride the zone around loose components is compromised and therefore precludes the use of this treatment approach.

Although arthroscopy has been recommended as a method of débridement for the infected total knee arthroplasty, the ability to perform satisfactory débridement of proliferative synovitis and scar associated with deep periprosthetic infection is usually limited. Modular implants cannot be adequately débrided between the metal tibial tray and polyethylene tibial insert with the arthroscope. In a series of 16 infected total knee arthroplasties treated by arthroscopic débridement, there were 4 type 2 and 12 type 4 infections.[100] Only six (38 percent) of the knees were successfully treated, which was significantly worse than the 71 percent success rate obtained with open débridement performed by these authors.[71] We concur with the authors, who recommended open arthrotomy for débridement of the acutely infected knee arthroplasty.

We currently administer intravenous antibiotics for 4 weeks following débridement, based on the results of cultures, and then decide whether additional chronic

oral suppressive antibiotics are also desirable. The use of an implantable antibiotic pump to deliver antibiotics locally in combination with surgical débridement and salvage of an acutely infected prosthesis has been reported.[81] Duration of treatment averaged 18 weeks (range 10 to 32 weeks), with reported success in 10 (78 percent) of 12 knee replacements. This technique requires further evaluation before it becomes an accepted method of treatment for the infected total knee arthroplasty.

Resection Arthroplasty

Definitive resection arthroplasty is implant removal with no intention of subsequent knee reconstruction. The ideal candidate for definitive resection arthroplasty is a patient with polyarticular rheumatoid arthritis with limited ambulatory demands; resection arthroplasty allows the patient to sit more readily than is feasible with a knee arthrodesis. Patients with less disability are likely to be less satisfied with a resection arthroplasty.[30] The primary disadvantage of resection arthroplasty is the frequent occurrence of knee instability associated with pain during transfer or ambulation (Fig. 81–2).

Of 28 knees treated in 26 patients in one study, only 11 patients had rheumatoid arthritis, and 89 percent were free of infection at an average of 5 years following their resection arthroplasty.[30] Functional results were

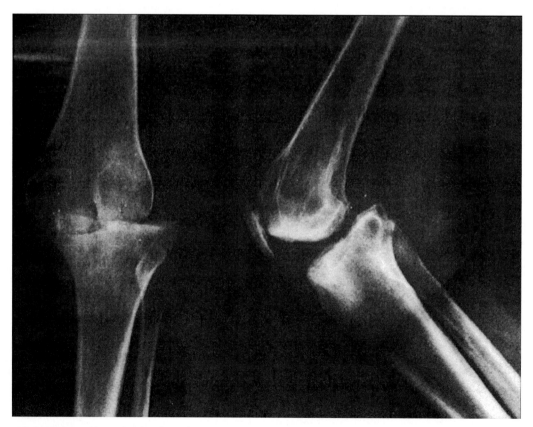

Figure 81–2. Patient with a painful and unstable resection arthroplasty after the treatment of an infected total knee arthroplasty.

suboptimal: 15 patients had been independent walkers but all now used walking aids, only 5 had sufficient knee stability for walking without external support, 8 required a knee-ankle-foot orthosis, and 2 used a splint. In 15 knees (15 patients) with infected constrained total knee arthroplasties treated by resection arthroplasty, infection was eradicated in all knees at 4 years' follow-up.[58] Fourteen patients needed walking aids, and persistent pain occurred in three patients. Although resection arthroplasty usually achieves satisfactory resolution of infection, most patients experience some pain, have knee instability, and have limited ambulatory capacity. Definitive resection arthroplasty is rarely utilized unless the patient has severe polyarticular involvement and limited ambulatory demands.

The three basic fundamentals of the operative technique include (1) initial débridement and removal of all infected tissue and foreign material, (2) temporary fixation with pins or sutures to maintain alignment and apposition of the tibia and femur, and (3) cast immobilization, permitting weight bearing, for at least 6 months.

Arthrodesis

Arthrodesis has traditionally been considered the gold standard treatment option for the infected total knee arthroplasty because of the excellent potential of resolving infection, alleviating pain, and providing stable knee function. Indications for knee arthrodesis with the failed total knee arthroplasty include (1) individuals with high functional demand, (2) single-joint disease, (3) young age, (4) extensor mechanism disruption, (5) a poor soft tissue envelope requiring extensive soft tissue reconstruction, (6) systemic immunocompromise, and (7) microorganisms requiring highly toxic antibiotic therapy or resistant to conventional antibiotics. Relative contraindications include (1) bilateral knee disease, (2) ipsilateral ankle or hip disease, (3) severe segmental bone loss, and (4) contralateral extremity amputation.[84]

In addition to excision of all necrotic, infected, and foreign material, resection of surrounding scar tissue permits healthy soft tissue to assist vascularization of bone at the arthrodesis site. The number of débridements required before wound closure usually depends on the surgeon's philosophy and ability to remove all infected material. One thorough débridement may be adequate; however, additional débridements should probably be performed in the presence of extensive tissue necrosis to allow a secondary evaluation of tissue viability. Inherent difficulties encountered in accomplishing a knee arthrodesis for an infected total knee arthroplasty are bone loss and extremity shortening. Adequate apposition of vascularized cancellous bone is the most important factor influencing the success of arthrodesis.

Usually, resection of several millimeters of bone from the distal femur and the proximal tibia exposes vascular bone in the knee with a resurfacing design. Hinged designs and implants with intramedullary stems often induce additional bone loss and are associated with a lower rate of successful arthrodesis.[57] Likewise, the knee

with multiple revisions usually has severe bone loss, and interdigitation of bone ends or insetting of the tibia inside the distal femur improves bone apposition and stability. Because the intramedullary bone circulation has often been compromised by the implant, bone deficiency should be augmented with cancellous bone graft placed peripherally around the arthrodesis site to allow revascularization from the surrounding soft tissues. Arthrodesis in patients with severe segmental bone loss can be addressed by the use of intercalary bone grafts or with adjunctive distraction histiogenesis to correct leg length inequality.

The optimum position for a knee arthrodesis is 10 to 20 degrees of flexion, which allows foot clearance without hip circumduction during the swing phase of gait. Knee flexion should not exceed 20 degrees, and, in the presence of bone loss, knee position near full extension maintains maximal extremity length and still allows foot clearance. Several fixation techniques may be used.

External Fixation

Use of an external fixation device has the advantage of leaving no residual foreign implants. Furthermore, this allows the potential for adjustment of fixator position and access to the soft tissues. Disadvantages include nonrigid fixation, potential for neurovascular injury during pin insertion, pin site complications, and the requirement of a second procedure for fixator removal.

The prior operative incision should be used, efforts are made to preserve bone vascularity, and a healthy surrounding soft tissue envelope should be achieved. Instrumentation can be used to facilitate accurate bone cuts, apposition, and alignment. Once proper limb alignment and rotation with optimal bone apposition have been attained, the bone ends are provisionally fixed with large crossed Steinmann pins, which markedly simplify and shorten the time required to apply the external fixator.

If a biplanar device is used, three centrally threaded 5-mm transfixing pins are placed in the distal part of the femur from medial to lateral to avoid the femoral vessels and three proximal tibial pins are placed from lateral to medial to avoid the peroneal nerve and anterior tibial vessels.[87] Two anterior half-pins are placed in the distal femur and proximal tibia as far as possible from the arthrodesis site to improve stability. We have also used small-wire external fixation devices for knee arthrodesis and have been favorably impressed with this external fixation technique (Fig. 81–3). Bone grafting is performed in knees with less than 50 percent surface bone contact between the tibia and femur. Morselized cancellous bone prepared with a bone mill or acetabular reamer provides excellent graft material. Posterior bone graft should be placed before the external fixator is tightened.

External fixation is maintained until clinical and radiographic union of the arthrodesis site is achieved (Fig. 81–4). Minimal bone loss usually requires external fixation of 10 to 12 weeks, but the presence of bone

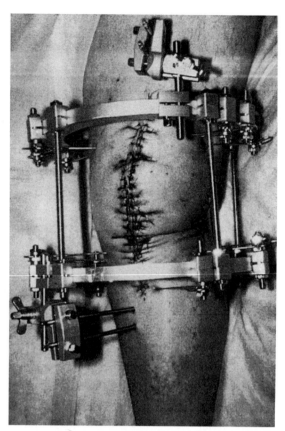

A

Figure 81–3. A, Clinical photograph of a small-wire fixation device used for knee arthrodesis. **B**, Anteroposterior and lateral radiographs of a patient with small-wire fixation device.

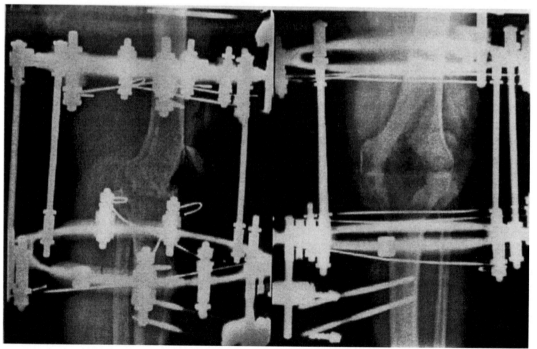

B

deficiency or need for bone graft usually necessitates a frame time of 16 weeks or longer. After the external fixator is removed, a cylinder or long-leg cast is applied for 6 to 12 weeks or until arthrodesis is achieved. Premature fixator removal must be avoided to achieve a successful arthrodesis.

Intramedullary Nailing

Arthrodesis with an intramedullary nail is not recommended in the presence of active infection because of the potential for extension of infection into the femoral or tibial medullary canals.[25,29] The technique is associ-

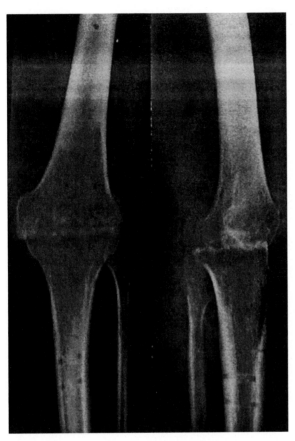

Figure 81–4. Anteroposterior and lateral radiographs of patient with solid knee arthrodesis treated with an external fixation device.

ated with prolonged operative times, averaging 6 hours, and an average blood replacement of 3000 ml.[29] Radiographic markers to define radiographic magnification are used on full-length anteroposterior radiographs and lateral radiographs of the femur and tibia to assist preoperative planning. Modular intramedullary nails have been developed to reduce the incidence of nonunion and complications, and to simplify the surgical procedure.[2,101]

After the knee is exposed, a tibiofemoral angle of 0 degrees is accomplished to allow passage of the nail. The tibia is initially prepared until the intramedullary reamers establish firm cortical contact in the isthmus of the medullary canal, followed by a trial fitting to make sure that the nail will not incarcerate during insertion. The femur is then reamed antegrade to accommodate the diameter of the femoral portion of the nail. Posterior bone graft is positioned just before the intramedullary nail is inserted into the tibia, and then the arthrodesis site is reduced. A long-leg cast may be used postoperatively to provide additional stability and to allow progressive weight bearing.

Plate Fixation

Arthrodesis with plate fixation typically employs two staggered dynamic-compression 12-hole plates.[75] A long-leg cast is used postoperatively until radiographic union

is present. Occasionally, in the face of severe bone loss, it may be necessary to augment intramedullary fixation with unilateral plate fixation.[95] Although plates provide excellent mechanical fixation, soft tissue coverage over dual plates can be difficult, and plate contouring can be arduous and requires considerable soft tissue dissection. Plate fixation can be considered to salvage pseudarthroses occurring after the use of external fixation (Fig. 81–5).

Results of Arthrodesis

The type of the prior knee implant, extent of bone deficiency, and arthrodesis technique affect success of knee arthrodesis following total knee arthroplasty. Time to union ranges from 2.5 months for a prior resurfacing implant up to 22 months for a hinged implant.[15,25] The success rate ranges from 71 to 81 percent following resurfacing implants and is 56 percent following hinged implants.[84] A multicenter study of 91 cases revealed that union was obtained in 86 percent of cases with a prior unicompartmental arthroplasty, 53 percent with a prior resurfacing procedure, and 51 percent with a prior hinged prosthesis.[57] Union occurred in 62 percent of knees where infection was controlled compared with 19 percent of knees with persistent infection.[57] Arthrodesis with a biplanar external fixator accomplished union in 66 percent of cases, whereas uniplanar fixation achieved union in only 33 percent. In our experience, use of biplanar external fixation provided a success rate of 71 percent in 28 knees.[87] Intramedullary nailing appears to a more reliable technique for achieving union when compared with external fixation techniques.[2,15,29,83,84,101,108]

Complications

Inherent complications of arthrodesis following total knee arthroplasty include nonunion, recurrent infection, and ipsilateral limb fracture, with the most frequent being nonunion. The etiology of nonunion includes bone deficiency, persistent infection, poor bone apposition, malalignment, and inadequate immobilization.[15,87] Specific complications associated with the external fixation technique include neurovascular injury during pin insertion, pin site infection, and fractures through pin sites, and complications have been reported in 20 to 65 percent of patients.[84] Complications inherent with intramedullary nailing include nail breakage and nail migration, and complications associated with intramedullary nailing for arthrodesis have been reported in 40 to 56 percent of cases.[84]

Amputation

Amputation is rarely indicated except for life-threatening systemic sepsis or persistent local infection associated with massive bone loss. The frequency of amputation is estimated to be less than 5 percent in patients who are treated for an infected total knee arthroplasty.[8,10,18,33,40,55,59,72,88,89,94,109,110] The most common factors leading to amputation include multiple revision

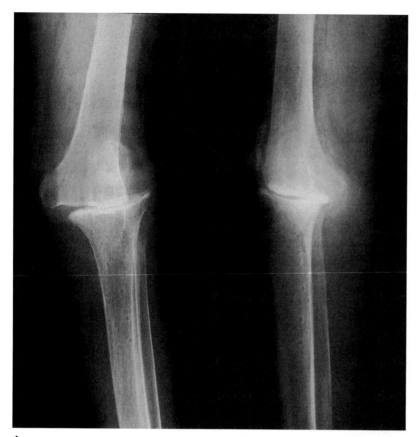

A

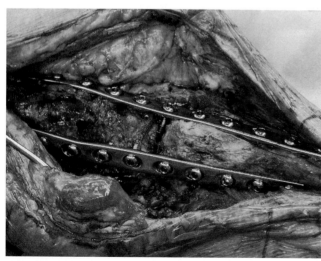

B

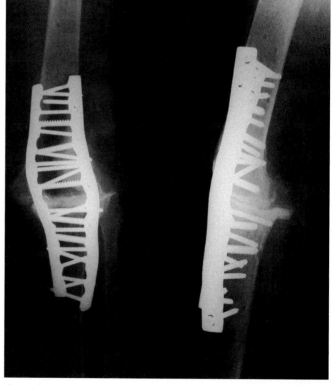

C

Figure 81–5. A, Anteroposterior and lateral radiographs of an established nonunion after an attempted arthrodesis with an external fixation device. **B**, Intraoperative photograph of double plates used for arthrodesis. **C**, Anteroposterior and lateral radiographs of double-plate fixation used for knee arthrodesis.

attempts for chronic infection, severe bone loss, and intractable pain.[52] Following amputation, many elderly patients remain limited ambulators or are nonambulatory because of the increased energy expenditure required for walking. Of 23 patients treated with above-the-knee amputation for a failed total knee arthroplasty, only 7 could ambulate regularly, 20 of the 23 used a wheelchair part of the day, and 12 (55 percent) were confined to the wheelchair.[82]

Insertion of Another Prosthesis (Reimplantation)

Reimplantation of another prosthesis after thorough débridement and administration of appropriate antimicrobial therapy has become an accepted method of treatment for most, but selected patients with an infected total knee arthroplasty.[8,39,44,51,86,110] Generally accepted contraindications for insertion of another prosthesis include (1) persistent or recalcitrant infection, (2) medical conditions that prevent multiple reconstructive procedures, (3) extensor mechanism disruption, and (4) a poor soft tissue envelope about the knee joint.

Controversies and questions regarding the reimplantation of another prosthesis include (1) the proper duration of antibiotic therapy, (2) the proper time delay from removal of the infected prosthesis to insertion of another prosthesis, and (3) the role of local antibiotic delivery systems, such as antibiotic-impregnated bone cement spacers or antibiotic-loaded prostheses.[56]

Antibiotics

The optimal duration and route of antibiotic delivery for treatment of the infected knee arthroplasty has not been clearly determined. A 6-week course of intravenous antibiotic administration prior to reimplantation has provided excellent success rates and represents the most commonly accepted clinical standard.[39,51,110] Most of these 6-week intravenous regimen studies did not routinely use adjunctive methods such as antibiotic-impregnated cement spacers or antibiotic-impregnated cement for prosthesis fixation.[51,110] There are no published trials that directly compare different durations of antibiotic treatment.

Excellent success with a shorter duration of intravenous antibiotics has been reported using 3 or 4 weeks of intravenous antibiotic therapy.[12,107] Antibiotic-impregnated cement was used at the time of reimplantation in both of these reports. In a retrospective analysis of 89 infected knee arthroplasties, there were no differences between the patient groups treated with 4 weeks or 6 weeks of intravenous antibiotics.[44] Most of these patients also received antibiotic-impregnated cement at the reimplantation.

In truth, the duration of antibiotic therapy likely needs to be individualized for each patient based on the virulence of the microorganism, the patient's comorbidities, and whether antibiotic-impregnated spacers or beads are also being used to deliver adjunctive antibi-

otics. The duration of antibiotic therapy should be longer rather than shorter for direct-exchange techniques as compared with a two-stage reimplantation approach.[17] The efficacy of oral antibiotics compared with intravenous antibiotics has not been formally evaluated.

Timing of Reimplantation

Reimplantation can be performed as a direct-exchange technique or by delayed reinsertion of the new prosthesis after antibiotic therapy. Success with direct exchange appears to be dependent on the presence of gram-positive infection, use of antibiotic-loaded cement for fixation of the new prosthesis, and prolonged use of antibiotics after the revision surgery. It would appear that the use of antibiotic-loaded bone cement is particularly important because direct-exchange procedures performed without the use of antibiotic-loaded cement were successful in only 11 (58 percent) of 19 knees.[40,44,86,97] When multiple series are combined, the success rate for a one-stage exchange technique using antibiotic-impregnated bone cement is 131 (74 percent) of 176 knees.[8,12,17,33,37,44,55,92,99]

Although there has been some increased interest in direct exchange, it is clear that delayed reconstruction provides the better chance for cure (Fig. 81–6). The chances for success are most probable with an appropriately selected and properly performed first treatment attempt. Secondary treatment attempts are often affected adversely by progressive scarring, soft tissue devitalization, and continued bone loss.[58] Delayed reconstruction is the most commoly accepted approach both in the United States and worldwide.[27,102]

The delayed reimplantation protocol includes soft tissue débridement and removal of the infected prosthesis and cement, followed by 6 weeks of intravenous antibiotics, maintaining a minimum bacteriocidal titer of 1:8, and subsequent reimplantation.[51] The success of this protocol was confirmed in a follow-up report of 64

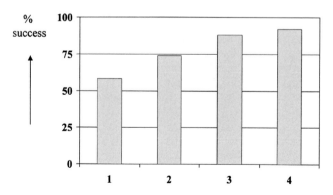

Figure 81–6. Graph demonstrating the independent beneficial effects of delayed reconstruction and the use of antibiotic-loaded bone cement for prosthesis fixation at the time of reimplantation 1, direct exchange without antibiotic-loaded bone cement (58 percent success); 2, direct exchange with antibiotic-loaded bone cement (74 percent success); 3, delayed reimplantation without antibiotic-loaded bone cement (87 percent success); and 4, delayed reimplantation with antibiotic-loaded bone cement (92 percent success).

infected knee replacements with a success rate of 97 percent for treatment of the original microorganism.[37] When patients who developed reinfection with a different organism were also considered, the ultimate cure rate free of infection was 90.6 percent at an average 7.5 years of follow-up. These early reports thus established the commonly accepted time delay of 6 weeks before reimplantation, but it is important to note that antibiotic impregnated-cement was not used in either study.

Most subsequent reports have used antibiotic-loaded cement spacers or beads in the interval between removal of the infected prosthesis and eventual reimplantation, and many also used antibiotic-loaded cement for prosthesis fixation at reimplantation.[11,13,34,44,50,54,66,94,107] The use of adjunctive antibiotic delivery has gradually led to decreased antibiotic duration and shorter time delays prior to reimplantation. Some investigators have shortened this time frame to several weeks.[19] In our practice, the majority of patients are treated with a 4-week course of antibiotics followed by reimplantation within the next week or so. Patients with systemic immunocompromise or infections caused by antibiotic-resistant microorganisms are treated with the traditional 6-week protocol of antibiotics and time delay before reimplantation. Large prospective trials will eventually be required to provide the scientific data to direct treatment decisions.

Antibiotic-Loaded Bone Cement

Local antibiotic delivery can be from beads or spacer blocks used prior to reimplantation and may also be from antibiotic-loaded bone cement used for prosthesis fixation at reimplantation. Theoretically, local antibiotic delivery supplements parenteral antibiotics; however, studies using these beads or spacers have not conclusively demonstrated superior efficacy.[48,74] When reimplanting, most reports have used antibiotic ratios of 1 g antibiotic per 40-g batch of bone cement.[43,44,109] Much higher dosage ratios, such as 4 to 6 g of antibiotics per 40-g batch of bone cement, are used with the spacers and beads.[41,80] The efficacy of these high antibiotic ratios has not yet been determined.

The use of antibiotic-impregnated cement for prosthesis fixation has been reported to exert a beneficial effect at the time of reimplantation.[44] Of 89 infected knee arthroplasties treated by reimplantation, antibiotic-impregnated bone cement for prosthesis fixation was a significant treatment variable because 7 (28 percent) of the 25 knees without the use of antibiotic-impregnated cement developed reinfection compared with only 3 (4.7 percent) of 64 knees with antibiotic-impregnated cement for prosthesis fixation.[44] This difference was statistically significant irrespective of the duration of intravenous antibiotics ($P = 0.0025$).

Several interesting trends are apparent when analyzing the benefits obtained from antibiotic-loaded cement and time delay before the insertion of a new prosthesis (see Fig. 81–6). Early reimplantation in less than 3 weeks without antibiotic-loaded cement provided success in only 58 percent of cases,[40,44,86,97] whereas the direct-exchange techniques with antibiotic-loaded cement for prosthesis fixation were successful in 74 percent of cases.[8,12,17,33,37,44,55,92,99] In the reports detailing delayed reimplantation, reimplantation without any antibiotic-loaded cement was successful in 65 (87 percent) of 74 knees,[7,39,44,53,54,97,109] whereas the use of antibiotic-loaded bone cement resulted in success in 254 (92 percent) of 277 knees.[10–13,34,41,44,50,54,89,92,94,107,108] This would suggest that a time delay, even in the absence of antibiotic-loaded cement, yields higher success rates than direct-exchange techniques when using antibiotic-loaded bone cement and that the best chance for cure is both with antibiotic-loaded bone cement and a two-stage reconstruction.

Spacer Blocks

Block spacers were introduced in the 1980s as a method to treat the infected knee arthroplasty between the time of infected prosthesis removal and eventual reinsertion of another prosthesis.[11] Over the past decade, the use of these block spacers has evolved to facilitate the ease of reimplantation for both the surgeon and patient. The primary functions of block spacers are delivery of local antimicrobial agents and maintenance of collateral ligament length.[11] Potential disadvantages of block spacers include the presence of a foreign body and bone loss incurred while awaiting reimplantation.

Essentially, the different types of block spacers include a simple tibiofemoral block, the molded arthrodesis block, articulating mobile spacers, and medullary dowels. The simple tibiofemoral block was the original spacer block and was preformed and then inserted into the tibiofemoral space after the cement had polymerized. These blocks were shaped as either simple "hockey pucks" or L-shaped spacers inserted into the tibiofemoral space (Fig. 81–7). Additional antibiotic beads or thin disks were often placed into the suprapatellar pouch or lateral gutters. Difficulties with this type of block spacer included the inability to match the surfaces of the block with the irregular surfaces of the distal femur and proximal tibia, subluxation of the bony surfaces off of the spacer surface, instances of extensor mechanism necrosis, wound breakdown, and progressive bone loss.[20]

The molded arthrodesis block method avoids some of the difficulties encountered with preformed spacer blocks. These spacers are fabricated so that the cement is placed within the knee in a doughy state and polymerized within the knee so that it can conform to the irregular contour of the femur and tibia (Fig. 81–8). This macrointerdigitation of the cement into bone defects and the intercondylar notch, with extension into the medullary canals and suprapatellar pouch, creates stability of the knee joint. This stability is helpful for patient comfort and prevents the difficulties of spacer migration and progressive bone erosion. Removal of these spacers requires fragmentation of the spacer into several large pieces with an osteotome at the time of reimplantation.

The mobile articulating spacer technique allows the patient to place the knee though a range of motion

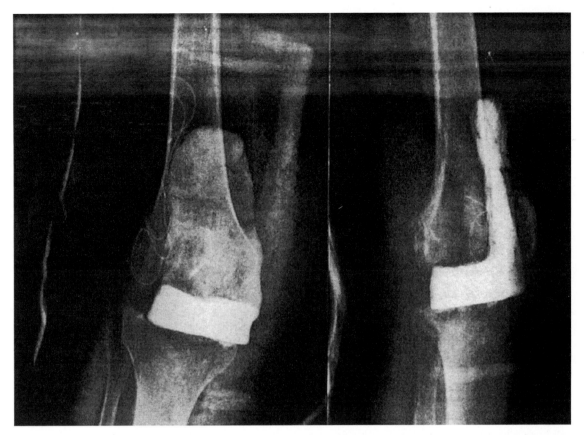

Figure 81–7. Anteroposterior and lateral radiographs of patient with an antibiotic-loaded cement spacer fabricated to fill the tibiofemoral and suprapatellar spaces.

Figure 81–8. A, Anteroposterior and lateral radiographs of a patient with a chronic infection of his total knee arthroplasty caused by *Enterococcus* species.

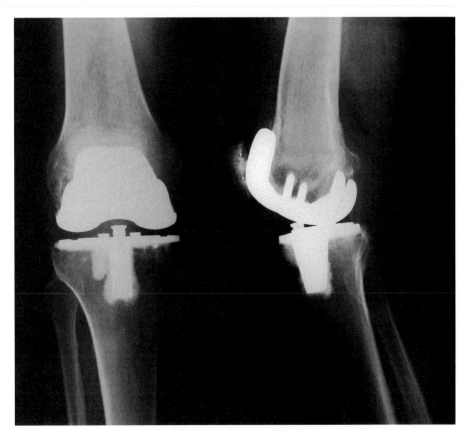

A

Illustration continued on following page

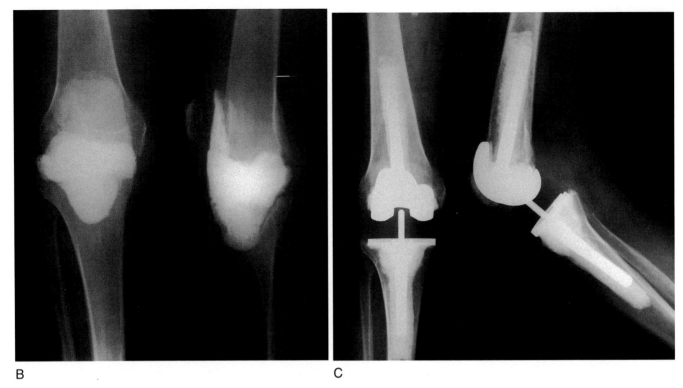

B

C

Figure 81–8. *Continued.* **B**, Anteroposterior and lateral radiographs of the molded arthrodesis spacer, which is composed of three 40-g batches of polymethylmethacrylate, 6 g of vancomycin powder, and 7.2 g of tobramycin. Note the interdigitation of the spacer into the tibial and femoral defects. **C**, Reimplantation total knee arthroplasty on the 42nd day after removal of infected prosthesis and completion of 42 days of intravenous antibiotics. The prosthesis is posterior stabilized and has vancomycin and tobramycin–loaded bone cement for prosthesis fixation.

during the time period between prosthesis removal and insertion of the new prosthesis.[41,50] These spacers, originally antibiotic-impregnated cement shaped into facsimiles of femoral and tibial components, allowed knee motion through articulation of the acrylic cement surfaces.[41] Eventually, a system of molds was introduced to develop low friction and more functional articulation by incorporating small metal runners and polyethylene tibial trays. This prevented the cement surfaces from articulating against each other.[41] One alternative has been to sterilize the prosthesis just removed and then incorporate the femoral component and tibial tray into the antibiotic loaded spacer.[50]

The theoretical advantages of mobile articulating spacers include the potential for improved functional outcomes and better range of motion. To date these benefits have not been documented. In a series of 55 patients, 25 with solid spacers and 30 with mobile articulating spacers, there was no difference between the two groups with respect to knee scores or final range of motion.[32] Articulating spacers do simplify the surgical exposure at reimplantation and are particularly helpful for patients requiring simultaneous removal of bilateral infected knee replacements.

Because extension of the infectious process into the medullary canals occurs in roughly one third of infected knee replacements without stems,[68] insertion of antibiotic-impregnated medullary dowels instead of beads

facilitates removal at reimplantation. A tapered cement dowel fashioned from the nozzle of a cement gun provides an excellent size and shape to be inserted into the medullary canal and facilitates easy removal at reimplantation (Fig. 81–9).

Combining two antibiotics in bone cement will improve elution of both antibiotics, and the two most commonly used antibiotics in clinical practice are vancomycin and tobramycin.[43] The use of at least 3.6 g of tobramycin and 1 g of vancomycin per package of bone cement is recommended by some.[66,80] However, the significant difference in cost between tobramycin and vancomycin may also be considered when determining the specific regimen for a given patient and organism. Several technical tips are helpful when mixing high-dose antibiotic-loaded cement. Mixing the monomer and powder together to form liquid cement before adding the antibiotic powder avoids mixing difficulties. Vancomycin powder is crystalline in nature, and, by leaving the large crystals intact, the volume of antibiotic elution from the final spacer is enhanced. In contrast, when mixing vancomycin into cement being used for prosthesis fixation, complete pulverization of all crystals is recommended because defects significantly weaken the cement. Creating surface patterns in the cement to produce an increased surface area facilitates antibiotic elution.[67] Creating micromotion of the cement spacer during curing creates macrointerdigitation into the irregular bony

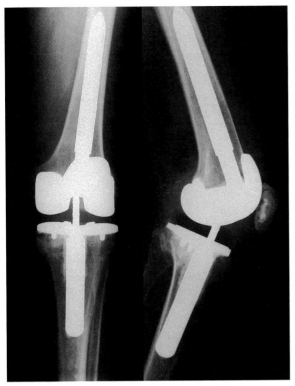

A

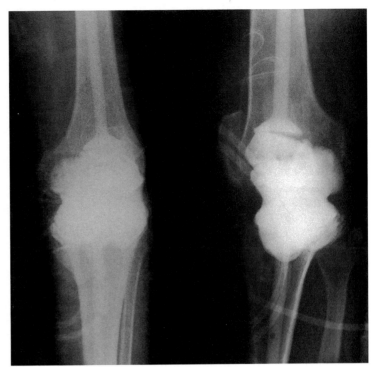

B

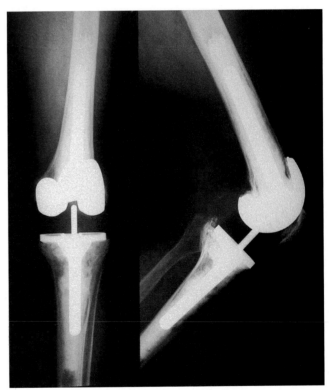

C

Figure 81–9. A, Anteroposterior and lateral radiographs of a patient with a chronic infection of his stemmed revision total knee arthroplasty caused by *Streptococcus viridans*. **B,** Anteroposterior and lateral radiographs of the molded arthrodesis spacer and dowel spacers fabricated with vancomycin and tobramycin antibiotic-loaded bone cement. **C,** Reimplantation total knee arthroplasty on the 35th day after removal of infected prosthesis and completion of 28 days of intravenous antibiotics. The prosthesis is posterior stabilized and has vancomycin and tobramycin–loaded bone cement for prosthesis fixation. The proximal tibial bone defects were filled with antibiotic-soaked cancellous bone graft.

contours but prevents integration of the cement into the cancellous bone. Overdistraction of the tibiofemoral space with these cement spacers may render flexion and extension gap balance difficult at reimplantation.

Interval Resection Arthroplasty

The effect of time delay between resection arthroplasty and reimplantation on optimal functional outcome has not been clearly established. Scarring and joint stiffness worsen with extended time delays, and spacers, which maintain the collateral ligament and extensor mechanism length, appear to facilitate reimplantation. Additional potential benefits of block spacers include local patient comfort and mobility during the time interval between resection arthroplasty and reimplantation, and this seems particularly true of mobile articulating spacers. There have been no significant differences between the knee scores, functional scores, or range of motion arc when the knees were analyzed according to the length of delay, type of knee prosthesis used at reimplantation, or use of a block cement spacer.[44] The final functional result appears to be more dependent on the patient's overall medical and musculoskeletal functional status.[103]

Despite the lack of evidence for improved functional outcomes with the use of spacers, the advantages of mechanical stability for the patient and reduction of difficulty with surgical exposure at reimplantation have led to their common acceptance. Block spacers should be supplemented by external immobilization, such as a brace or cast. In our opinion, casting is preferable because patients can be partially weight bearing and the wound, which is protected, heals more efficiently. Patients with mobile articulating spacers are encouraged to participate in range-of-motion exercises and are allowed up to 50 percent partial weight bearing.[41] The motion permitted by mobile articulating spacers particularly helps patients undergoing removal of bilateral infected knees.

Patients undergoing delayed reimplantation are typically anemic, and 88 percent require allogeneic blood transfusions.[78] The presence of infection precludes traditional alternatives such as reinfusion or autologous blood donation. Alternative solutions are reflected by a study of 39 consecutive two-stage reimplantations using recombinant human erythropoietin.[21] Compared with a control group of 81 cases, the transfusion requirement was significantly lowered ($P < 0.001$), and 52 percent of those treated avoided transfusion for the entire time period encompassing both stages of treatment.

One of the most important issues for both patient and surgeon is the determination of when it is safe and appropriate to proceed with reimplantation.[43] Unlike the ESR, the CRP levels typically normalize by the 21st day after surgery, so, if the levels remain elevated, this may suggest a persistent infection.[43,105] Aspiration has been suggested before proceeding with reimplantation.[71] This has not been totally satisfactory in our practice, and we prefer an intraoperative decision process

based on the appearance of the knee joint and analysis of frozen sections. However, this method requires considerable experience on the part of the surgeon and the pathologist, and the use of spacers or beads may alter the appearance of the tissues at reimplantation. In our study, analysis of frozen sections at reimplantation had a sensitivity of 25 percent, a specificity of 98 percent, a positive predictive value of 50 percent, a negative predictive value of 95 percent, and an accuracy of 94 percent.[22] If there is concern about the presence of persistent infection, it is prudent to perform another débridement, insert new spacers, close the wound, and await culture and sensitivity testing.

Reimplantation Procedure

The surgical approach is typically more difficult if the time delay is more than 6 to 8 weeks. Patients who have performed range-of-motion exercises with an articulating spacer are generally easier to expose when compared with patients who have had the knee immobilized. The patellar tendon attachment is at greatest risk because the infection and treatment often cause considerable scarring and loss of tissue compliance. Associated bone deficiencies and attendant ligamentous insufficiency may require more constrained prosthetic designs to achieve knee stability.[9] Currently, the majority of implants used for reimplantation at our institution are posterior-stabilized prostheses fixed with antibiotic-loaded cement (see Fig. 81–9).

Stemmed prosthetic components are typically used to augment prosthetic fixation, and, although the use of stemmed-cemented implants provides excellent fixation, the extraction of these prostheses is more difficult should reinfection occur.[45] When possible, cementation of the distal femur and proximal tibia with fluted press-fit stems can be done, and, if reinfection should occur, these implants are easier to remove. The use of hinged constrained prostheses is avoided if at all possible but is occasionally required.[9,52] Although the use of bone graft has been reported for reimplantation, there are no comparative studies of the effect of bone graft on the incidence of reinfection. Soaking of bone graft with antibiotic solution is an alternative mechanism of providing local antibiotic delivery, particularly when using uncemented implants. In a series of 33 patients treated with interval antibiotic-loaded beads, 6 weeks of intravenous antibiotics, and use of an uncemented prosthesis augmented with antibiotic-soaked bone graft, there was only one reinfection for an infection cure rate of 97 percent.[106] Unless one chooses to use an uncemented implant, bone graft is rarely required for the reimplantation arthroplasty. This avoidance of bone graft is accomplished by utilizing other alternatives such as modular wedges or filling of bone defects with antibiotic-loaded bone cement.

Occasionally after insertion of the new prosthesis, it is difficult to close the soft tissue envelope. Not reimplanting a patellar device facilitates capsular closure. Simultaneous use of a gastrocnemius rotational flap during the reimplantation procedure to achieve wound closure has been reported.[68] Another alternative for patients with multiple skin incisions or a tightly scarred soft tissue envelope is gradual soft tissue expansion prior to the reimplantation.[38,73] This procedure has allowed successful wound closure and avoids the use of soft tissue muscle transfer.

Reinfection After Reimplantation

Failure is more likely when treating an infected revision than an infected primary total knee arthroplasty.[49] These patients also have more bone loss and compromise of the soft tissue envelope. Patients with severe medical comorbidities and soft tissue compromise are also more likely to develop reinfection.[69] Although reimplantation has become a commonly accepted treatment modality for the infected knee prosthesis, the poor outcome of patients who develop reinfection after reimplantation has not been fully appreciated.

Among 24 knees treated for reinfection after reimplantation, 10 cases had successful arthrodesis, 5 were being maintained on suppressive oral antibiotics, 4 had knee amputations, and 3 had persistent pseudarthroses.[45] Three of the four amputations were for failed hinged knee prostheses. A successful arthrodesis was more predictable for prostheses without stems (75 percent) than with stemmed prostheses (40 percent).

A more recent report of 12 patients is more optimistic.[4] Nine knees underwent another salvage attempt, and, at an average of 31 months' follow-up, the average Knee Society knee score was 79 and the average functional score was 73, with no instance of recurrent infection. Nonetheless, the difficulties encountered in obtaining a healed wound, attaining a successful knee arthrodesis, and successful eradication of infection with nonprosthetic salvage procedures after a failed reimplantation are considerable. The morbidity and increased likelihood of amputation associated with reinfection must be carefully considered and presented to the patient before proceeding with reimplantation for treatment of the infected total knee arthroplasty.

COST ISSUES

It has been documented that the treatment of an infected knee replacement incurs an estimated net loss of approximately $15,000, and this loss is doubled for the Medicare patient.[47,93] These procedures have increased operative times, hospital stays, number of hospitalizations, number of surgical procedures, and blood loss when compared with aseptic revision knee surgery. These issues should be, but to date are not, considered in health care reimbursement schemes. Recognition of the numerous variables that are discretionary versus those based on data, as well as treatment by experienced and interested surgeons, does help minimize the cost of providing the best treatment for these patients. This is particularly true if the first treatment attempt of an infected knee arthroplasty is successful.

AUTHORS' PREFERRED METHOD

Treatment Options

The patient with an acute deep infection in the first few postoperative weeks or acute onset of deep infection in a previously well-functioning and well-fixed prosthesis is aggressively managed with open débridement and postoperative intravenous antibiotics for 4 weeks. Additional chronic oral antibiotics are considered on an individual basis and are generally administered if the patient would subsequently be considered a candidate for chronic suppression based on advanced age or poor medical condition. Occasionally, elderly patients with a well-fixed prosthesis, absence of drainage, and minimal to moderate pain are treated with aspiration and chronic oral antibiotic suppression if the offending microorganism is sensitive to a nontoxic antibiotic that can be tolerated by the patient. In the chronic setting, the treatment method chosen depends on the patient's functional requirements, the status of the soft tissue envelope about the knee joint, the extent of bone loss, and the integrity of the extensor mechanism. Definitive resection arthroplasty or above-the-knee amputation is rarely required. Disruption of the extensor mechanism or a poor soft tissue envelope (requiring soft tissue reconstruction or severe periarticular scarring) usually mandates knee arthrodesis. If there will be adequate bone apposition (more than 50 percent), an external fixation technique is preferred. For those patients with more severe bone deficiency, a two-stage intramedullary nailing is performed.

Arthrodesis

When there are no absolute contraindications to arthrodesis or reimplantation of another prosthesis, the benefits of arthrodesis being a definitive procedure with a better chance of eradicating infection are carefully presented to the patient. Additionally, the patient must be aware that reimplantation of another prosthesis does "burn some bridges." If there should be a reinfection, the nonprosthetic salvage options are less successful and the potential for amputation is increased. If the decision is made to proceed with reimplantation, we prefer a delayed two-stage approach. After removal of the infected prosthesis, the knee is closed over antibiotic-impregnated beads or spacers using an antibiotic that will be effective for the offending organism. The most common antibiotic used is vancomycin, followed by tobramycin or a combination of both antibiotics. The ratio of antibiotic powder per 40-g batch of bone cement is 3 or 4 g of vancomycin or 3.6 g of tobramycin. The capsule is closed with a running absorbable monofilament suture, braided subcutaneous sutures are avoided, and the skin is closed with a nonabsorbable monofilament suture. Postoperatively, the patient is placed in a knee immobilizer or a long-leg cast. Most patients are treated with a 4-week course of intravenous antibiotics under the supervision of our orthopedic infectious disease specialists. Most patients receive erythropoietin-α to improve their hemoglobin level between the time of the resection arthroplasty and the reimplantation.

Reimplantation

Reinsertion of another prosthesis is performed as soon as is convenient after the conclusion of the intravenous antibiotics. If there is concern about persistent deep infection, aspiration or débridement and tissue culture delays implantation until culture results are available. Most patients are empirically reimplanted based on the appearance of tissues at revision surgery and histologic analysis of fresh frozen tissue samples. Tissue for culture is obtained at the reimplantation. We prefer the use of antibiotic-impregnated bone cement for prosthesis fixation and choose the antibiotic based on sensitivity tests from the original offending organism(s). Vancomycin and tobramycin are most commonly used in a ratio of 1 to 2 g per batch of bone cement because higher dosages weaken the mechanical strength of the cement.

Implant Selection and Antibiotic Treatment

Currently, most prostheses used for reimplantation are posterior-stabilized or constrained condylar designs. Bone graft is avoided if possible, and the patella with severely compromised bone stock is often left unresurfaced. Postoperatively, the patient is continued on antibiotics until the results from the intraoperative cultures are available. If these cultures are negative, all antibiotics are discontinued. If these cultures are positive and the organism is the same as the original offending organism, a 4-week course of intravenous antibiotics is administered and then additional chronic oral antibiotics are considered. If the culture results are considered to be a laboratory contaminant, additional antibiotics are not recommended. Patients are then evaluated with a clinical examination, ESR, CRP level, and plain radiographs at 3 months postoperatively and annually thereafter. A global summary of this approach is shown in a treatment algorithm in Figure 81–10.

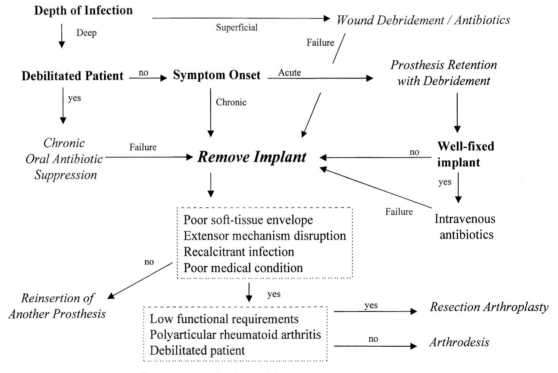

Figure 81–10. Treatment algorithm for the infected total knee arthroplasty.

References

1. Adam RF, Watson SB, Jarratt JW, et al: Outcome after flap cover for exposed total knee arthroplasties: a report of 25 cases. J Bone Joint Surg Br 76:750–753, 1994.
2. Arroyo JS, Garvin KL, Neff JR: Arthrodesis of the knee with a modular titanium intramedullary nail. J Bone Joint Surg Am 79:26–35, 1997.
3. Atkins BL, Athanasou N, Deeks JJ, et al: Prospective evaluation of criteria for microbiological diagnosis of prosthetic-joint infection at revision arthroplasty. The OSIRIS Collaborative Study Group. J Clin Microbiol 36:2932–2939, 1998.
4. Backe HA Jr, Wolff DA, Windsor RE: Total knee replacement infection after 2-stage reimplantation: results of subsequent 2-stage reimplantation. Clin Orthop 331:125–131, 1996.
5. Barrack RL, Jennings RW, Wolfe MW, Bertot AJ: The Coventry Award: The value of preoperative aspiration before total knee revision. Clin Orthop 345:8–16, 1997.
6. Bengtson S: Prosthetic osteomyelitis with special reference to the knee: risks, treatment and costs. Ann Med 25:523–529, 1993.
7. Bengtson S, Blomgren G, Knutson K, et al: Hematogenous infection after knee arthroplasty. Acta Orthop Scand 58:529–534, 1987.
8. Bengtson S, Knutson K: The infected knee arthroplasty: a 6-year follow-up of 357 cases. Acta Orthop Scand 62:301–311, 1991.
9. Berman AT, O'Brien JT, Israelite C: Use of the rotating hinge for salvage of the infected total knee arthroplasty. Orthopedics 19:73–76, 1996.
10. Bliss DG, McBride GG: Infected total knee arthroplasties. Clin Orthop 199:207–214, 1985.
11. Booth RE Jr, Lotke PA: The results of spacer block technique in revision of infected total knee arthroplasty. Clin Orthop 248:57–60, 1989.
12. Borden LS, Gearen PF: Infected total knee arthroplasty: a protocol for management. J Arthroplasty 2:27–36, 1987.
13. Bose WJ, Gearen PF, Randall JC, Petty W: Long-term outcome of 42 knees with chronic infection after total knee arthroplasty. Clin Orthop 319:285–296, 1995.
14. Brandt CM, Sistrunk WW, Duffy MC, et al: Staphylococcus aureus prosthetic joint infection treated with debridement and prosthesis retention. Clin Infect Dis 24:914–919, 1997.
15. Brodersen MP, Fitzgerald RH, Peterson LFA, et al: Arthrodesis of the knee following failed total knee arthroplasty. J Bone Joint Surg Am 61:181–185, 1979.
16. Browne EZ Jr, Stulberg BN, Sood R: The use of muscle flaps for salvage of failed total knee arthroplasty. Br J Plast Surg 47:42–45, 1994.
17. Buechel FF: Primary exchange revision arthroplasty using antibiotic-impregnated cement for infected total knee replacement. Orthop Rev 19:83, 1990.
18. Burger RR, Basch T, Hopson CN: Implant salvage in infected total knee arthroplasty. Clin Orthop 273:105–112, 1991.
19. Cadambi A, Jones RE, Maale GE: A protocol for staged revison of infected total hip and knee arthroplasties: the use of antibiotic-cement-implant composites. Orthop Int 3:133–145, 1995.
20. Calton TF, Fehring TK, Griffin WL: Bone loss associated with the use of spacer blocks in infected total knee arthroplasty. Clin Orthop 345:148–154, 1997.
21. Cushner FD, Barrack RL, Hanssen AD, et al: The use of EPO in two stage exchange TKA for infection. Presented at the Interim Meeting of the Knee Society, Boston, September 14–16, 2000.
22. Della Valle CJ, Bogner E, Desai P, et al: Analysis of frozen sections of intraoperative specimens obtained at the time of reoperation after hip or knee resection arthroplasty for the treatment of infection. J Bone Joint Surg Am 81:684–689, 1999.
23. Della Valle CJ, Scher DM, Kim YH, et al: The role of intraoperative Gram stain in revision total joint arthroplasty. J Arthroplasty 14:500–504, 1999.
24. Demirkol MO, Adalet I, Unal SN, et al: 99Tc(m)-polyclonal IgG scintigraphy in the detection of infected hip and knee prostheses. Nucl Med Commun 18:543–548, 1997.
25. Donley BG, Matthews LS, Kaufer H: Arthrodesis of the knee with an intramedullary nail. J Bone Joint Surg Am 73:907–913, 1991.
26. Drancourt M, Stein A, Argenson JN, et al: Oral treatment of Staphylococcus spp. infected orthopaedic implants with fusidic acid or ofloxacin in combination with rifampicin. J Antimicrob Chemother 39:235–240, 1997.
27. Drobny TK, Munzinger UK, Chomiak J: 2-stage exchange in the treatment of infected knee prosthesis. Orthopade 24:360–366, 1995.
28. Duff GP, Lachiewicz PF, Kelley SS: Aspiration of the knee joint before revision arthroplasty. Clin Orthop 331:132–139, 1996.
29. Ellingsen DE, Rand JA: Intramedullary arthrodesis of the knee after failed total knee arthroplasty. J Bone Joint Surg Am 76:870–877, 1994.
30. Falahee MH, Matthews LS, Kaufer H: Resection arthroplasty as a salvage procedure for a knee with infection after a total arthroplasty. J Bone Joint Surg Am 69:1013–1021, 1987.
31. Fehring TK, McAlister JA Jr: Frozen histologic section as a guide to sepsis in revision joint arthroplasty. Clin Orthop 304:229–237, 1994.
32. Fehring TK, Odum S, Calton TF, Mason JB: Articulating versus static spacers in revision total knee arthroplasty for sepsis. Clin Orthop 380:9–16, 2000.
33. Freeman MA, Sudlow RA, Casewell MW, Radcliff SS: The management of infected total knee replacements. J Bone Joint Surg Br 67:764–768, 1985.
34. Gacon G, Laurencon M, Van de Velde D, Giudicelli DP: Two stages reimplantation for infection after knee arthroplasty: Apropos of a series of 29 cases. Rev Chir Orthop Reparatrice Appar Mot 83:313–323, 1997.
35. Gerwin M, Rothaus KO, Windsor RE, et al: Gastrocnemius muscle flap coverage of exposed or infected knee prostheses. Clin Orthop 286:64–70, 1993.
36. Glithero PR, Grigoris P, Harding LK, et al: White cell scans and infected joint replacements: failure to detect chronic infection. J Bone Joint Surg Br 75:371–374, 1993.
37. Goksan SB, Freeman MA: One-stage reimplantation for infected total knee arthroplasty. J Bone Joint Surg Br 74:78–82, 1992.
38. Gold DA, Scott SC, Scott WN: Soft tissue expansion prior to arthroplasty in the multiply-operated knee. J Arthroplasty 11:512–521, 1996.
39. Goldman RT, Scuderi GR, Insall JN: 2-stage reimplantation for infected total knee replacement. Clin Orthop 331:118–124, 1996.
40. Grogan TJ, Dorey F, Rollins J, Amstutz HC: Deep sepsis following total knee arthroplasty: ten-year experience at the University of California at Los Angeles Medical Center. J Bone Joint Surg Am 68:226–234, 1986.
41. Haddad FS, Masri BA, Campbell D, et al: The PROSTALAC functional spacer in two-stage revision for infected knee replacements: prosthesis of antibiotic-loaded acrylic cement. J Bone Joint Surg Br 82:807–812, 2000.
42. Hallock GG: Salvage of total knee arthroplasty with local fasciocutaneous flaps. J Bone Joint Surg Am 72:1236–1239, 1990.
43. Hanssen AD, Rand JA: Evaluation and treatment of infection at the site of a total hip or knee arthroplasty. J Bone Joint Surg Am 80:910–922, 1998.
44. Hanssen AD, Rand JA, Osmon DR: Treatment of the infected total knee arthroplasty with insertion of another prosthesis: the effect of antibiotic-impregnated bone cement. Clin Orthop 309:44–55, 1994.
45. Hanssen AD, Trousdale RT, Osmon DR: Patient outcome with reinfection following reimplantation for the infected total knee arthroplasty. Clin Orthop 321:55–67, 1995.
46. Hartman MB, Fehring TK, Jordan L, Norton HJ: Periprosthetic knee sepsis: the role of irrigation and debridement. Clin Orthop 273:113–118, 1991.
47. Hebert CK, Williams RE, Levy RS, Barrack RL: Cost of treating an infected total knee replacement. Clin Orthop 331:140–145, 1996.
48. Heck D, Rosenberg A, Schink-Ascani M, et al: Use of antibiotic-impregnated cement during hip and knee arthroplasty in the United States. J Arthroplasty 10:470–475, 1995.
49. Hirakawa K, Stulberg BN, Wilde AH, et al: Results of 2-stage reimplantation for infected total knee arthroplasty. J Arthroplasty 13:22–28, 1998.
50. Hofmann AA, Kane KR, Tkach TK, et al: Treatment of infected total knee arthroplasty using an articulating spacer. Clin Orthop 321:45–54, 1995.

51. Insall JN, Thompson FM, Brause BD: Two-stage reimplantation for the salvage of infected total knee arthroplasty. J Bone Joint Surg Am 65:1087–1098, 1983.

52. Isiklar ZU, Landon GC, Tullos HS: Amputation after failed total knee arthroplasty. Clin Orthop 299:173–178, 1994.

53. Ivey FM, Hicks CA, Calhoun JH, Mader JT: Treatment options for infected knee arthroplasties. Rev Infect Dis 12:468–478, 1990.

54. Jacobs MA, Hungerford DS, Krackow KA, Lennox DW: Revision of septic total knee arthroplasty. Clin Orthop 238:159–166, 1989.

55. Johnson DP, Bannister GC: The outcome of infected arthroplasty of the knee. J Bone Joint Surg Br 68:289–291, 1986.

56. Kendall RW, Duncan CP, Smith JA, Ngui-Yen JH: Persistence of bacteria on antibiotic loaded acrylic depots: a reason for caution. Clin Orthop 329:273–280, 1996.

57. Knutson K, Hovelius L, Lindstrand A, Lidgren L: Arthrodesis after failed knee arthroplasty: a nationwide multicenter investigation of 91 cases. Clin Orthop 191:202–211, 1984.

58. Kramhoft M, Bodtker S, Carlsen A: Outcome of infected total knee arthroplasty. J Arthroplasty 9:617–621, 1994.

59. Lettin AW, Neil MJ, Citron ND, August A: Excision arthroplasty for infected constrained total knee replacements. J Bone Joint Surg Br 72:220–224, 1990.

60. Levitsky KA, Hozack WJ, Balderston RA, et al: Evaluation of the painful prosthetic joint: Relative value of bone scan, sedimentation rate, and joint aspiration. J Arthroplasty 6:237–244, 1991.

61. Lian G, Cracchiolo A III, Lesavoy MA: Treatment of major wound necrosis following total knee arthroplasty. J Arthroplasty 4(Suppl):S23–S32, 1989.

62. Lonner JH, Desai P, Dicesare PE, et al: The reliability of analysis of intraoperative frozen sections for identifying active infection during revision hip or knee arthroplasty. J Bone Joint Surg Am 78:1553–1558, 1996.

63. Maniloff G, Greenwald R, Laskin R, Singer C: Delayed postbacteremic prosthetic joint infection. Clin Orthop 223:194–197, 1987.

64. Mariani BD, Martin DS, Levine MJ, et al: The Coventry Award: Polymerase chain reaction detection of bacterial infection in total knee arthroplasty. Clin Orthop 331:11–22, 1996.

65. Markovich GD, Dorr LD, Klein NE, et al: Muscle flaps in total knee arthroplasty. Clin Orthop 321:122–130, 1995.

66. Masri BA, Duncan CP, Beauchamp CP: Long-term elution of antibiotics from bone-cement: an in vivo study using the prosthesis of antibiotic-loaded acrylic cement (PROSTALAC) system. J Arthroplasty 13:331–338, 1998.

67. Masri BA, Duncan CP, Beauchamp CP, et al: Effect of varying surface patterns on antibiotic elution from antibiotic-loaded bone cement. J Arthroplasty 10:453–459, 1995.

68. McPherson EJ, Patzakis MJ, Gross JE, et al: Infected total knee arthroplasty: two-stage reimplantation with a gastrocnemius rotational flap. Clin Orthop 341:73–81, 1997.

69. McPherson EJ, Tontz W Jr, Patzakis M, et al: Outcome of infected total knee utilizing a staging system for prosthetic joint infection. Am J Orthop 28:161–165, 1999.

70. Mont MA, Waldman B, Banerjee C, et al: Multiple irrigation, debridement, and retention of components in infected total knee arthroplasty. J Arthroplasty 12:426–433, 1997.

71. Mont MA, Waldman BJ, Hungerford DS: Evaluation of preoperative cultures before second-stage reimplantation of a total knee prosthesis complicated by infection: a comparison-group study. J Bone Joint Surg Am 82:1552–1557, 2000.

72. Morrey BF, Westholm F, Schoifet S, et al: Long-term results of various treatment options for infected total knee arthroplasty. Clin Orthop 248:120–128, 1989.

73. Namba RS, Diao E: Tissue expansion for staged reimplantation of infected total knee arthroplasty. J Arthroplasty 12:471–474, 1997.

74. Nelson CL, Evans RP, Blaha JD, et al: A comparison of gentamicin-impregnated polymethylmethacrylate bead implantation to conventional parenteral antibiotic therapy in infected total hip and knee arthroplasty. Clin Orthop 295:96–101, 1993.

75. Nichols SJ, Landon GC, Tullos HS: Arthrodesis with dual plates after failed total knee arthroplasty. J Bone Joint Surg Am 73:1020–1024, 1991.

76. Nijhof MW, Oyen WJ, van Kampen A, et al: Hip and knee arthroplasty infection: In-111-IgG scintigraphy in 102 cases. Acta Orthop Scand 68:332–336, 1997.

77. Pace TB, Jeray KJ, Latham JT Jr: Synovial tissue examination by frozen section as an indicator of infection in hip and knee arthroplasty in community hospitals. J Arthroplasty 12:64–69, 1997.

78. Pagnano M, Cushner FD, Hanssen A, et al: Blood management in two-stage revision knee arthroplasty for deep prosthetic infection. Clin Orthop 367:238–242, 1999.

79. Palestro CJ, Swyer AJ, Kim CK, Goldsmith SJ: Infected knee prosthesis: diagnosis with In-111 leukocyte, Tc-99m sulfur colloid, and Tc-99m MDP imaging. Radiology 79:645–648, 1991.

80. Penner MJ, Masri BA, Duncan CP: Elution characteristics of vancomycin and tobramycin combined in acrylic bone-cement. J Arthroplasty 11:939–944, 1996.

81. Perry CR, Hulsey RE, Mann FA, et al: Treatment of acutely infected arthroplasies with incision, drainage, and local antibiotics delivered via an implantable pump. Clin Orthop 281:216–223, 1992.

82. Pring DJ, Marks L, Angel JC: Mobility after amputation for failed knee replacement. J Bone Joint Surg Br 70:770–771, 1988.

83. Puranen J, Kortelainen P, Jalovaara P: Arthrodesis of the knee with intramedullary fixation. J Bone Joint Surg Am 72:433–442, 1990.

84. Rand JA: Alternatives to reimplantation for salvage of the total knee arthroplasty complicated by infection. Instr Course Lect 42:341–347, 1993.

85. Rand JA, Brown ML: The value of indium 111 leukocyte scanning in the evaluation of painful or infected total knee arthroplasties. Clin Orthop 259:179–182, 1990.

86. Rand JA, Bryan RS: Reimplantation for the salvage of an infected total knee arthroplasty. J Bone Joint Surg Am 65:1081–1086, 1983.

87. Rand JA, Bryan RS, Chao EYS: Failed total knee arthroplasty treated by arthrodesis of the knee using the Ace-Fischer apparatus. J Bone Joint Surg Am 69:39–45, 1987.

88. Rasul AT Jr, Tsukayama D, Gustilo RB: Effect of time of onset and depth of infection on the outcome of total knee arthroplasty infections. Clin Orthop 273:98–104, 1991.

89. Rosenberg AG, Haas B, Barden R, et al: Salvage of infected total knee arthroplasty. Clin Orthop 226:29–33, 1988.

90. Scher DM, Pak K, Lonner JH, et al: The predictive value of indium-111 leukocyte scans in the diagnosis of infected total hip, knee, or resection arthroplasties. J Arthroplasty 15:295–300, 2000.

91. Schoifet SD, Morrey BF: Treatment of infection after total knee arthroplasty by debridement with retention of the components. J Bone Joint Surg Am 72:1383–1390, 1990.

92. Scott IR, Stockley I, Getty CJ: Exchange arthroplasty for infected knee replacements: a new two-stage method. J Bone Joint Surg Br 75:28–31, 1993.

93. Sculco TP: The economic impact of infected total joint arthroplasty. Instr Course Lect 42:349–351, 1993.

94. Segawa H, Tsukayama DT, Kyle RF, et al: Infection after total knee arthroplasty: a retrospective study of the treatment of eighty-one infections. J Bone Joint Surg Am 81:1434–1445, 1999.

95. Stiehl JB, Hanel DP: Knee arthrodesis using combined intramedullary rod and plate fixation. Clin Orthop 294:238–241, 1993.

96. Tattevin P, Cremieux AC, Pottier P, et al: Prosthetic joint infection: when can prosthesis salvage be considered? Clin Infect Dis 29:292–295, 1999.

97. Teeny SM, Dorr LD: Treatment of the infected knee arthroplasty: irrigation and debridement versus two-stage reimplantation. J Arthroplasty 5:35–39, 1990.

98. Tsukayama DT, Wicklund B, Gustilo RB: Suppressive antibiotic therapy in chronic prosthetic joint infections. Orthopedics 14:841–844, 1991.

99. von Foerster G, Kluber D, Kabler U: Mid- to long-term results after treatment of 118 cases of periprosthetic infections after knee joint replacement using one-stage exchange surgery. Orthopade 20:244–252, 1991.

100. Waldman BJ, Hostin E, Mont MA, Hungerford DS: Infected total knee arthroplasty treated by arthroscopic irrigation and debridement. J Arthroplasty 15:430–436, 2000.

101. Waldman BJ, Mont MA, Payman KR, et al: Infected total knee arthroplasty treated with arthrodesis using a modular nail. Clin Orthop 367:230–237, 1999.

102. Wang CJ: Management of infected total knee arthroplasty. Chang Keng I Hsueh 20:1–10, 1997.

103. Wasielewski RC, Barden RM, Rosenberg AG: Results of different surgical procedures on total knee arthroplasty infections. J Arthroplasty 11:931–938, 1996.

104. Weiss AP, Krackow KA: Persistent wound drainage after primary knee arthroplasty. J Arthroplasty 8:285–289, 1993.

105. White J, Kelly M, Dunsmuir R: C-reactive protein level after total hip and total knee replacement. J Bone Joint Surg Br 80:909–911, 1998.

106. Whiteside LA: Treatment of infected total knee arthroplasty. Clin Orthop 299:169–172, 1994.

107. Wilde AH, Ruth JT: Two-stage reimplantation in infected total knee arthroplasty. Clin Orthop 236:23–35, 1988.

108. Wilde AH, Stearns KL: Intramedullary fixation for arthrodesis of the knee after infected total knee arthroplasty. Clin Orthop 248:87–92, 1989.

109. Wilson MG, Kelley K, Thornhill TS: Infection as a complication of total knee-replacement arthroplasty: risk factors and treatment in sixty-seven cases. J Bone Joint Surg Am 72:878–883, 1990.

110. Windsor RE, Insall JN, Urs WK, et al: Two-stage reimplantation for the salvage of total knee arthroplasty complicated by infection: further follow-up and refinement of indications. J Bone Joint Surg Am 72:272–278, 1990.

VII
The Foot and Ankle

HAROLD B. KITAOKA • SECTION EDITOR

82

Anatomy and Surgical Approaches

• GORDON G. WELLER, TODD A. KILE, and MARTIN G. ELLMAN

The most common complications in reconstructive procedures of the foot and ankle are many times directly related to poor wound healing. These complications can be devastating, particularly when most of the commonly exposed structures are superficial and even subcutaneous.[17,18] A keen understanding of the surgical anatomy and pitfalls associated with the various surgical approaches is needed and may help to avoid wound healing difficulties. This chapter reviews the pertinent foot and ankle anatomy, as well as several operative exposures utilized in adult reconstructive surgery.

Preoperative evaluation of the patient's sensation and circulation may prevent disaster. The presence of ischemia or neuropathy may preclude a satisfactory result. When they occur together, as in diabetes, elective surgery may need to be deferred until the distal neuro-circulatory status has been optimized.

Attention to technique is particularly important when undertaking surgery about the foot and ankle. Well-placed incisions with full-thickness flaps are created and care is taken to avoid forceful, blunt retraction. With an understanding of the regional anatomy, solutions to difficult problems can be achieved, particularly when dictated by previous trauma or incisions.

ANATOMY

Osseous

The foot is composed of 26 bones and two sesamoids, and can be categorized into three regions: the forepart, the midpart, and the hindpart (Figs. 82–1 and 82–2). The forepart of the foot contains five metatarsals, 14 phalanges, and usually two sesamoids. Each toe has three phalanges, except the great toe or hallux, which has two. The midportion of the foot contains the three cuneiform, the cuboid, and the navicular bones. The hindpart of the foot consists of the talus and the calcaneus.

The astragalus or talus is made up of the body, neck, and head. It is the only bone in the foot without any muscle attachments.[20] The body contains the convex dome, which articulates superiorly with the distal tibia at the talocrural joint. It also articulates with the medial malleolus of the tibia and the lateral malleolus of the fibula. Together this is known as the ankle mortise.

Because the dome of the talus is wider anteriorly, the malleoli must move, relative to one another, to allow for full plantar and dorsiflexion. This uniaxial configuration, coupled with the greater width anteriorly, provides maximum stability in dorsiflexion.[16] The neck of the talus projects forward, separating the body from the head, which articulates with the navicular. Inferiorly, the talus articulates with the calcaneus.

The sulcus tali is located on the inferior surface of the talus between the posterior and middle articular facets of the calcaneus. This sulcus tali combines with the opposing sulcus calcanei of the calcaneus to form the tarsal canal. The anterolateral expansion of the tarsal canal is termed the sinus tarsi.

The calcaneus articulates superiorly with the talus by way of the anterior, middle, and posterior facets. The middle facet is located on the upper surface of the sustentaculum tali, which is a medial projection from the calcaneus. A groove for the flexor hallucis longus tendon is located under the sustentaculum tali.

The cuboid articulates with the calcaneus proximally and with the bases of the fourth and fifth metatarsals distally. The inferior surface of the cuboid contains a sulcus for the peroneus longus tendon.

The navicular articulates proximally with the talus and distally with the three cuneiforms. The tuberosity of the navicular is located medially and inferiorly, and is one of the major attachments of the tibialis posterior tendon.

The transverse tarsal joint, commonly referred to as Chopart's joint, is formed by the talonavicular and calcaneocuboid articulations. The three cuneiform bones are wedge shaped, with the apex directed plantarward on the intermediate and lateral cuneiforms, and dorsally on the medial cuneiform. They are located between the navicular proximally and the first, second, and third metatarsals distally.

The tarsometatarsal (Lisfranc's) joints are the articulations between the five metatarsals distally and the three cuneiforms and cuboid proximally. The metatarsals help to form the transverse arch proximally and a relatively flat horizontal plane distally.

The first metatarsal is the largest of the five and bears approximately one third of the body's weight through the forepart of the foot. There are two grooves on the plantar surface of the first metatarsal head for the sesamoid articulations. The base of the first metatarsal is defined by its

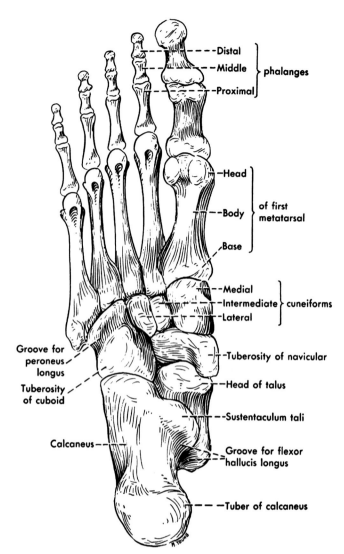

Figure 82–1. Dorsal and plantar views of the osseous anatomy of the foot. (From Hollinshead WH, Rosse C: Textbook of Anatomy, 4th ed. New York, Harper & Row, 1985, p 451, by permission of the Mayo Foundation.)

plantar tuberosity, while the plantar lateral enlargement at the base of the fifth metatarsal is its characteristic feature.

Soft Tissue

Muscular

The muscles of the foot and ankle are divided into extrinsic and intrinsic systems (Table 82–1). The extrinsic muscles originate proximally in the leg and send tendons to insert into the foot. There are many anatomic variations that may occur in the foot.[3,4,8,14,15] Extrinsic muscles located within the anterior compartment of the leg include the tibialis anterior, extensor hallucis longus (EHL), and extensor digitorum longus (EDL) (Fig. 82–3). These act as the dorsiflexors of the foot and ankle. The peroneus tertius assists with dorsiflexion and eversion of the foot. The lateral compartment of the leg contains the peroneus longus and brevis extrinsic muscles, which

assist with eversion of the foot and plantar flexion (Fig. 82–4). The three superficial posterior compartment extrinsic muscles are the gastrocnemius, the soleus, and the plantaris, which act as powerful plantar flexors to the foot and ankle. The deep posterior compartment contains the tibialis posterior, flexor digitorum longus, and flexor hallucis longus muscles (Fig. 82–5). The tibialis posterior tendon provides support to the longitudinal arch of the foot. The long toe flexors help to maintain balance and assist in push-off during gait.

The intrinsic muscles are arranged in four layers within the plantar surface of the foot[12] (Fig. 82–6). The first and most superficial layer includes the abductor hallucis, flexor digitorum brevis, and abductor digiti minimi (Fig. 82–7). The second layer contains the quadratus plantae, the lumbrical muscles, and the tendons of the flexor digitorum longus and flexor hallucis longus (Fig. 82–8). The third layer consists of three intrinsic muscles: the flexor digiti minimi brevis, adductor hallucis, and flexor hallucis brevis (Fig. 82–9). The fourth layer is made up of the seven interossei, divided into four dorsal and three plantar (Fig. 82–10).

The only intrinsic muscle on the dorsum of the foot is the extensor digitorum brevis. It is quite useful for reconstructive purposes as an island flap or as a muscle transfer distally to cover defects.[13] The most medial portion is known as the extensor hallucis brevis.

Vascular

The anterior tibial artery is accompanied by the deep peroneal nerve as it descends the leg. In the ankle region, the anterior tibial artery gives rise to the medial and lateral malleolar arteries. Once the anterior tibial artery enters the foot, it is called the dorsalis pedis artery. The lateral tarsal artery branches from the dorsalis pedis, as does the arcuate artery more distally. The dorsal metatarsal arteries arise from the arcuate artery. As the dorsal metatarsal arteries continue distally, they divide into the dorsal digital arteries.

The posterior tibial artery is accompanied by the tibial nerve into the distal leg. The posterior tibial artery passes deep to the flexor retinaculum and then divides as it reaches the plantar aspect of the foot, into the medial and lateral plantar arteries. The lateral plantar artery continues with the lateral plantar nerve and then courses medially to become the plantar arch. The plantar metatarsal arteries originate from the plantar arch and branch into plantar digital arteries. The medial plantar artery is accompanied by the medial plantar nerve.

The plantar digital veins continue into the plantar metatarsal veins, which then flow into the plantar venous arch. Likewise, the dorsal digital veins continue into the dorsal metatarsal veins that drain into the dorsal venous arch. The medial venous arch system becomes the great saphenous vein. The lateral venous arch becomes the small saphenous vein.

Neural

Innervation of the foot is supplied primarily by the sciatic nerve and the saphenous nerve.[28] The saphenous

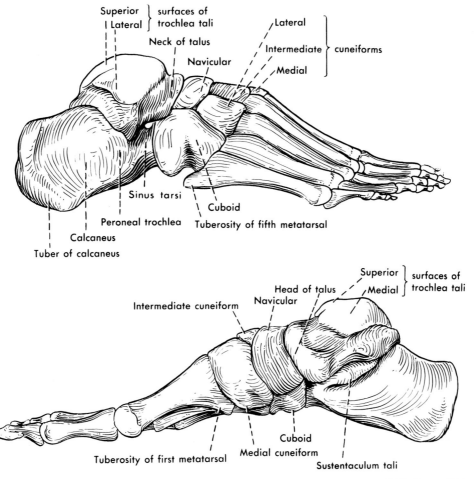

Figure 82–2. Lateral and medial views of the osseous anatomy of the foot. (From Hollinshead WH, Rosse C: Textbook of Anatomy, 4th ed. New York, Harper & Row, 1985, p 451, by permission of the Mayo Foundation.)

nerve, which is a branch of the femoral nerve, descends down the leg with the great saphenous vein. It travels anterior to the medial malleolus and then continues along the medial aspect of the foot to supply sensation to the area of the first metatarsophalangeal joint.

The sural nerve, a sensory nerve, descends down the leg near the small saphenous vein. It passes posterior and distal to the lateral malleolus and courses forward to the dorsolateral aspect of the foot to become the lateral dorsal cutaneous nerve. This nerve usually continues out to the lateral aspect of the fifth toe.

The superficial peroneal nerve descends down the anterolateral lower leg, where it divides and continues on the dorsum of the foot as both the medial and the intermediate dorsal cutaneous nerves. The medial dorsal cutaneous nerve divides and supplies sensation to the medial side of the great toe and adjacent sides of the second and third toes. The intermediate dorsal cutaneous nerve divides and supplies sensation to adjacent sides of the third and fourth and the fourth and fifth toes.

The deep peroneal nerve is located lateral to the anterior tibial artery in the distal leg. As the deep peroneal nerve descends in the ankle area, it divides into medial and lateral branches. The lateral branch crosses the tarsal area for motor innervation to the extensor digitorum brevis and interosseous muscles. The medial branch continues forward on the foot just lateral to the dorsalis pedis artery and branches in the first intermetatarsal space to supply sensation to adjacent sides of the great and second toes.

In the distal leg, the tibial nerve is in close proximity to the posterior tibial artery. The tibial nerve travels to the medial ankle level and provides medial calcaneal branches to the skin of the heel. The tibial nerve continues behind the medial malleolus and becomes the medial and lateral plantar nerves. These nerves provide terminal motor branches to the plantar intrinsic muscles, as well as sensation to the medial and lateral plantar aspects of the foot.

Sensation to the ankle joint is provided by branches from the deep peroneal and tibial nerves.[9]

Joints of the Ankle and Foot

Ankle Joint and Ligaments

The ankle (talocrural) joint consists of the proximal articulating surfaces of the talus and the distal ends of the tibia and fibula. This uniaxial joint is wider anteriorly,

Table 82–1. MUSCLES OF THE FOOT AND ANKLE

Muscle	Origin	Insertion	Function	Arterial Supply	Nerve Supply
Tibialis anterior	Lateral tibia, interosseous membrane	Medial cuneiform, base of 1st metatarsal	Dorsiflexor of foot, invertor of foot	Anterior tibial	Deep peroneal
Extensor hallucis longus	Fibula, interosseous membrane	Base of distal phalanx of great toe	Great toe extensor, dorsiflexor of foot	Anterior tibial	Deep peroneal
Extensor digitorum longus	Tibia, fibula, interosseous membrane	Middle and distal phalanges of lateral 4 toes	Extensor lateral 4 toes, dorsiflexor of foot	Anterior tibial	Deep peroneal
Peroneus terius	Fibula, intermuscular septum	Base of 5th metatarsal	Dorsiflexor and evertor of foot	Anterior tibial	Deep peroneal
Peroneus longus	Tibia, fibula	Medial cuneiform, base of 1st metatarsal	Plantar flexor of foot, evertor of foot	Anterior tibial and peroneal	Superficial peroneal
Peroneus brevis	Fibula	Base of 5th metatarsal	Plantar flexor of foot, evertor of foot	Peroneal	Superficial peroneal
Gastrocnemius	Femoral condyles	Posterior aspect of calcaneus	Plantar flexor of foot, flexor of knee	Posterior tibial	Tibial
Soleus	Tibia, fibula	Posterior aspect of calcaneus	Plantar flexor of foot	Posterior tibial and peroneal	Tibial
Plantaris	Lateral femoral condyle; knee joint capsule	Medial side of posterior calcaneus, tendocalcaneus	Plantar flexor of foot, flexor of leg	Posterior tibial	Tibial
Tibialis posterior	Interosseous membrane, tibia, fibula	Navicular, all cuneiform bones, 2–4 metatarsals, cuboid, sustentaculum tali	Plantar flexor of foot, invertor of foot	Peroneal	Tibial
Flexor digitorum longus	Posterior surface of tibia	Distal phalanges of lateral 4 toes	Flexor of lateral 4 toes, plantar flexor of foot	Posterior tibial	Tibial
Flexor hallucis longus	Fibula	Base of distal phalanx of great toe	Flexor of great toe, plantar flexor of foot	Peroneal	Tibial
Abductor hallucis	Medial tubercle of calcaneus, flexor retinaculum, plantar aponeurosis	Medial base of proximal phalanx of great toe	Abductor of great toe	Medial plantar	Medial plantar
Flexor digitorum brevis	Medial tubercle of calcaneus, plantar aponeurosis	Middle phalanx of lateral 4 toes	Flexor of lateral 4 toes	Medial plantar	Medial plantar
Abductor digiti minimi	Medial and lateral tubercles of calcaneus, plantar aponeurosis	Lateral side of base of proximal phalanx of little toe	Abductor and flexor of little toe	Lateral plantar	Lateral plantar
Quadratus plantae	Calcaneus, long plantar ligament	Tendons of flexor digitorum longus	Flexor of terminal phalanges lateral 4 toes	Lateral plantar	Lateral plantar
Lumbricales	Tendons of flexor digitorum longus	Bases of terminal phalanges of 4 lateral toes	Flexor of toes at MTP joints and extensor at interphalangeal joints	Plantar metatarsal	Medial plantar, lateral plantar
Flexor digiti minimi brevis	Base of 5th metatarsal bone, sheath of peroneus longus	Lateral side of base proximal phalanx of little toe	Flexor of little toe	Lateral plantar	Lateral plantar
Adductor hallucis	Sheath of peroneus longus, 2–4 metatarsal bases, 3–5 MTP joint capsules, transverse ligament	Lateral side of base of proximal phalanx of great toe	Adductor and flexor of great toe	First plantar metatarsal	Lateral plantar
Flexor hallucis brevis	Cuboid, cuneiform	Base of proximal phalanx of great toe	Flexor great toe	First plantar metatarsal	Medial plantar
Dorsal interossei	Metatarsal bones	2–4 proximal phalanges	Abductors 2–4 toes	Dorsal metatarsal	Lateral plantar
Plantar interossei	Metatarsal bones	3–5 proximal phalanges	Adductors 3–5 toes	Plantar metatarsal	Lateral plantar
Extensor digitorum brevis	Calcaneus, inferior extensor retinaculum	Medial 4 toes	Extensor of joints medial 4 toes	Dorsalis pedis	Deep peroneal

MTP, metatarsophalangeal.

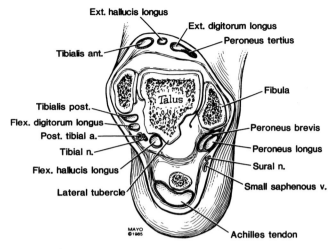

Figure 82–3. Diagrammatic view of the ankle region.

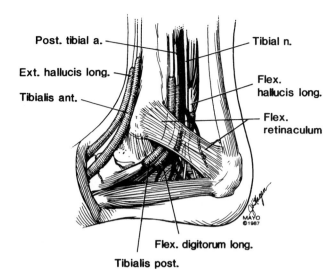

Figure 82–5. Soft tissue structures of the medial aspect of the foot and ankle.

causing it to be more stable in dorsiflexion. The lateral malleolus of the fibula extends more distally than does the medial malleolus, suggesting to Inman that this osseous arrangement is necessary to accommodate the axis of ankle motion and to allow minimal tension on the ligaments.[19] The superior articulating surface of the talus is convex from anterior to posterior. There is a smooth ridge on each side of this surface to continue the articular surface on the medial and lateral malleolar facets that articulate with the tibia and fibula.

The capsule of the ankle joint is thin anteriorly and posteriorly.[6] The medial and lateral aspects of the capsule are thickened by the strong collateral ligaments, thus providing reinforcement to the bony support. The medial collateral ligament (deltoid ligament) is quite strong, and fracture through the medial malleolus usually occurs before disruption of the deltoid ligament.[1] It also resists talar tilt.[11] The deltoid ligament is composed of superficial and deep layers. The superficial portion consists of the tibionavicular, tibiocalcaneal, and posterior tibiotalar

ligaments, which provide medial stability to the ankle joint. The two anterior components (tibionavicular and tibiocalcaneal) also help to stabilize the subtalar joint (Fig. 82–11). The deep portion of the deltoid is the anterior tibiotalar ligament, which stabilizes the mortise by maintaining the talus close to the medial malleolus.

The lateral collateral ligament of the ankle is composed of the anterior talofibular ligament, the calcaneofibular ligament, and the posterior talofibular ligament (Fig. 82–12). The most common ankle injury, the ankle sprain, usually involves tearing one or more of these ligaments. Lateral ankle stability is also provided by the anterior tibiofibular (syndesmotic) ligament as well as by the posterior inferior tibiofibular ligament (Fig. 82–13).

Subtalar Joint and Ligaments

The subtalar (talocalcaneal) joint is composed of facets on the plantar surface of the talus and their corresponding calcaneal articulations. The posterior facet of the talus is a large, concave surface and represents the majority of the articular surface area. A thin capsule surrounds the joint, separating it from other tarsal joints. Four ligaments provide stability to the subtalar joint complex. They include the medial, lateral, and interosseous talocalcaneal ligaments and the cervical ligament. The lateral entrance to the sinus tarsi is covered by the cervical ligament, which serves to prevent excess inversion. Excess eversion is limited by the interosseous talocalcaneal ligament.

Talonavicular Joint and Ligaments

The talonavicular, or talocalcaneonavicular, joint is a complex multiaxial joint created by the dome-shaped head of the talus and the articulations with the concave navicular, the middle and anterior facets of the calcaneus, and the dorsal surface of the plantar calcaneonavicular (spring) ligament. The dorsal surface of the neck of the talus and the navicular are covered by the thin,

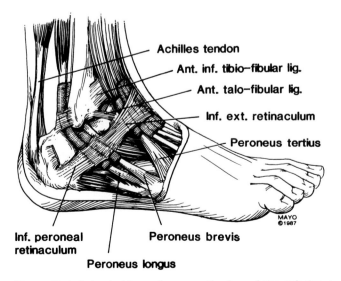

Figure 82–4. Lateral oblique diagrammatic view of the soft tissue structures of the foot and ankle.

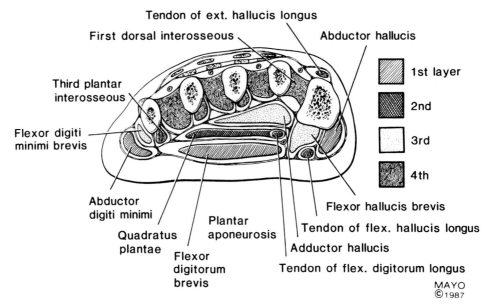

Figure 82–6. Diagrammatic cross-sectional view at the diaphyseal level of the metatarsals.

flat talonavicular ligament. The spring ligament is a stout structure joining the sustentaculum tali to the navicular, supporting the talonavicular joint. Lateral support comes from the calcaneonavicular portion of the bifurcate ligament. This joint forms the medial portion of the midtarsal (Chopart's) joint.

Calcaneocuboid Joint and Ligaments

The calcaneocuboid joint is saddle shaped and forms the remaining portion of the midtarsal joint of Chopart. The capsule thickens dorsally and forms the dorsal calcaneocuboid ligament. Plantarward, the long plantar ligament attaches to the cuboid and continues distally to

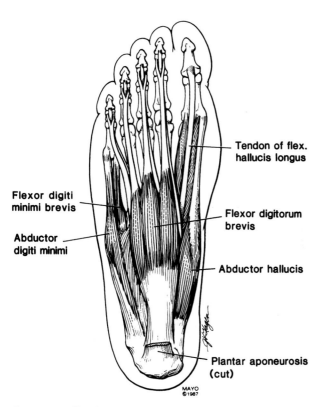

Figure 82–7. First layer, plantar muscles.

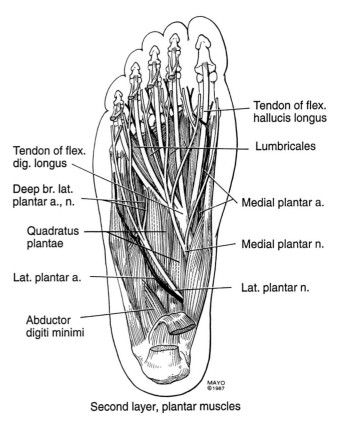

Second layer, plantar muscles

Figure 82–8. Second layer, plantar muscles.

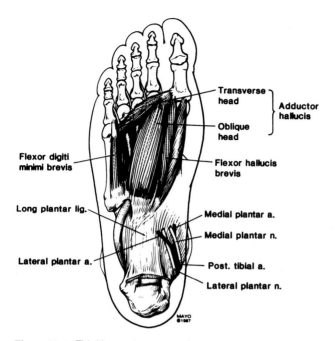

Figure 82–9. Third layer, plantar muscles.

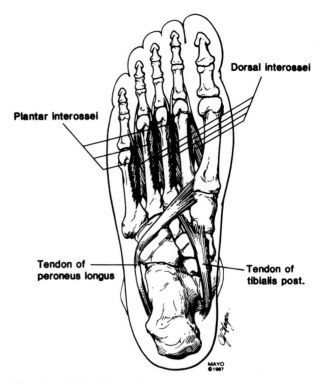

Figure 82–10. Fourth layer, plantar muscles.

insert on the plantar surfaces of the bases of the third, fourth, and sometimes fifth metatarsals. The fibers of the short plantar ligament lie deeper and do not continue beyond the cuboid bone. Both plantar ligaments provide support to the longitudinal arch, with a number of varying configurations of these ligaments.[39] Dorsolaterally, the bifurcate ligament is made up of the calcaneonavicular and the calcaneocuboid components and has classically been considered the principal support of the midtarsal joint of Chopart.

Tarsometatarsal Joints and Ligaments

There are five tarsometatarsal joints and, except for the first, they are contiguous with each other and the intercuneiform and cuneonavicular joints. They are synovial

joints and are known collectively as Lisfranc's joint. The base of the second metatarsal projects more proximally, about 3 mm, and its articulation with the intermediate cuneiform bone forms the keystone to the midportion of the foot and the transverse arch. The tarsometatarsal joints are stabilized by dorsal and plantar ligaments, as well as interosseous cuneometatarsal ligaments. Insertions, number, and course of the ligamentous structures can vary.[10] The lesser tarsometatarsal joints have small excursions, while the first ray can exhibit significant degrees of dorsiflexion and plantar flexion as well as rotation. The bases of the lateral four metatarsals are tightly bound by dorsal,

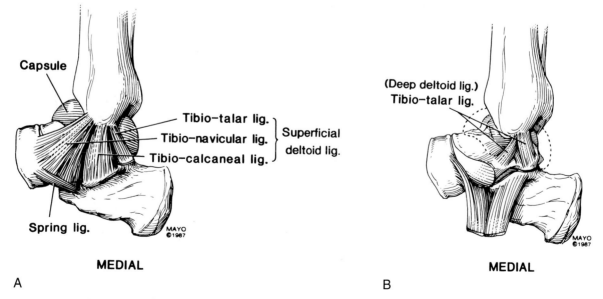

Figure 82–11. A, Diagrammatic view of superficial deltoid ligament. B, Deep deltoid ligament.

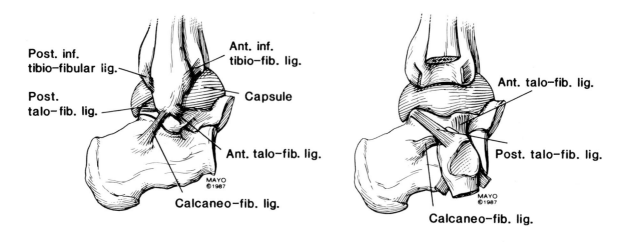

Figure 82–12. A, Diagrammatic view of superficial lateral ankle ligaments. **B,** Deeper view with fibula transected and reflected inferiorly.

plantar, and interosseous ligaments. The bases of the first and second metatarsals are not connected to one another; however, they are attached distally.

First Metatarsophalangeal Joint

The first metatarsophalangeal joint is considerably more complex than the lesser metatarsophalangeal joints and is described separately.

The first metatarsophalangeal joint is formed by the convex head of the first metatarsal and the concave articulating base of the proximal phalanx. The entire joint is referred to as the sesamoid complex, containing seven muscles, eight ligaments, and two sesamoid bones.[2] The two sesamoids are plantar to the first metatarsal head and articulate through two corresponding grooves located on the plantar aspect of the first

metatarsal head. These grooves are separated by a ridge known as the crista.

The medial and lateral collateral ligaments attach to their respective sides of the first metatarsal head and run obliquely forward and plantarward to attach on the base of the proximal phalanx. The medial and lateral sesamoidal ligaments also attach to the first metatarsal head and insert into the sesamoids and plantar pad. The tibial and fibular sesamoids are joined by the intersesamoid ligament. The first metatarsophalangeal joint is surrounded by a separate joint capsule.

Stability and function of the first metatarsophalangeal joint are further enhanced by seven muscle-tendon units. The EHL traverses the dorsal aspect of the joint longitudinally and inserts into the dorsal base of the distal phalanx of the great toe. This tendon forms an expansion over the first metatarsophalangeal joint capsule. An

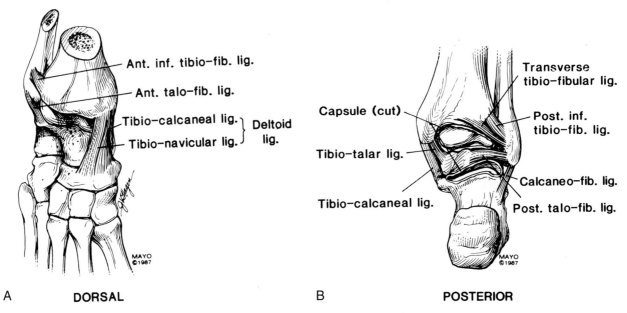

Figure 82–13. A, Diagrammatic view of anterior tibiofibular ligament. The anterior deltoid and lateral ligaments are also seen. **B,** The posterior tibiofibular ligament and other posterior stabilizers are also seen.

accessory tendon from the EHL, the extensor hallucis capsularis, attaches to the medial dorsal joint capsule. The extensor hallucis brevis approaches the hallux lateral to the longus tendon to insert into the dorsal base of the proximal phalanx of the hallux. Plantarward, the flexor hallucis brevis divides into two heads to encompass the tibial and fibular sesamoids and then inserts into the base of the proximal phalanx. The flexor hallucis longus passes through the groove between the two sesamoids and inserts on the plantar aspect of the base of the distal phalanx. The oblique and transverse heads of the adductor hallucis unite and insert into the lateral sesamoid complex with the lateral head of the flexor hallucis brevis. The abductor hallucis attaches to the medial sesamoid complex with the medial head of the flexor hallucis brevis.

Lesser Metatarsophalangeal Joints

The lesser metatarsophalangeal joints lie 2 to 3 cm proximal to the natural webs of the toes. They are formed by the rounded heads of the metatarsal bones fitting into the shallow concave facets of the proximal phalanges. Stability is provided by two collateral ligaments that are obliquely oriented, attaching proximally to the metatarsal head and distally to the base of the proximal phalanx and plantar joint capsule. The plantar aspect of the joint is further reinforced by the fibrous plantar ligament or plantar plate. Although the dorsal aspect of the joint capsule is relatively thin, it is reinforced by the extensor aponeurosis.

The plantar ligaments of the metatarsophalangeal joints are joined by the deep transverse metatarsal ligament. This ligament resists medial and lateral separation of the metatarsal heads under normal conditions.[5] The interosseous muscle tendons are located dorsal to the deep transverse metatarsal ligament, while the lumbrical tendons are positioned plantar to the ligament.

Motion of the lesser metatarsophalangeal joints includes flexion, extension, abduction, adduction, and rotation. Extension is usually greater than flexion and, during normal gait, can reach as much as 90 degrees at toe-off.[26]

EXPOSURES

Ankle and Hindpart of the Foot

Anterior Approach to the Ankle

The anterior approach provides excellent exposure to the ankle joint and as a result has been utilized for total joint arthroplasty, ankle arthrodesis, débridement of loose bodies or infections, and open reduction and internal fixation of intra-articular distal tibial fractures.[24,29–34] Wound healing problems can be minimized through the use of longer incisions, properly oriented with respect to the skin cleavage lines and relaxed skin tension lines, and postoperative compression with immobilization.[1,7,25,27,35]

A 10- to 15-cm longitudinal incision is made over the anterior aspect of the ankle joint, centered between the two malleoli (Fig. 82–14). This placement helps to avoid

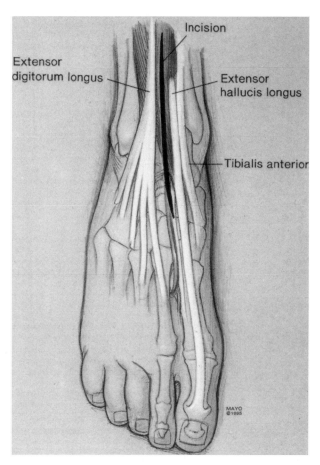

Figure 82–14. Diagrammatic anterior incisional approach to the ankle joint.

the medial branch of the superficial peroneal nerve, although care is taken to cut only the skin (Fig. 82–15).[18] As the incision is deepened, the fascia and extensor retinaculum are opened, exposing the long extensors and the anterior neurovascular bundle. The interval between the EHL and EDL tendons reveals the anterior tibial artery and deep peroneal nerve. With careful mobilization and gentle retraction, the anterior joint capsule can be exposed and incised for entry into the ankle joint. An alternate interval between the tibialis anterior and EHL tendons provides wide exposure without disturbing the neurovascular structures.[21] Alternatively, a lazy-S skin incision can be utilized as an anterior approach to the ankle.[37]

Pitfalls include injury to the medial dorsal cutaneous nerve, branching from the superficial peroneal nerve, which lies just beneath the skin. Above the ankle, the deep peroneal nerve and anterior tibial artery lie between the tibialis anterior and EHL muscles. At about the level of the ankle joint itself, the EHL tendon crosses to the medial side of the neurovascular bundle, such that the bundle is then located between the EHL and EDL tendons as they course onto the dorsum of the foot.

Approach to the Medial Malleolus

A direct approach to the medial malleolus can provide excellent visualization for medial malleolar fractures,

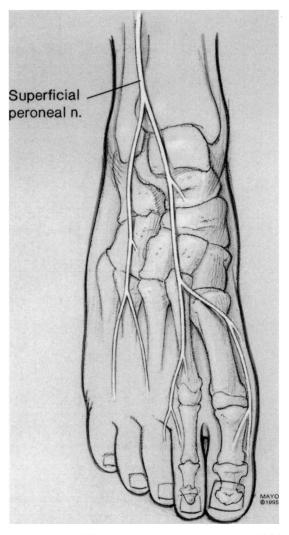

Figure 82–15. Dorsal diagrammatic representation of superficial peroneal nerve distribution.

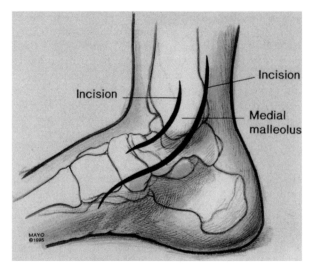

Figure 82–16. Medial approach to the ankle. The anterior or more posterior route may be chosen, depending on the lesion.

osteotomies, or talar dome lesions. A slightly anterior incision also allows inspection of the anteromedial joint surfaces of the tibia and talar dome. A posteriorly directed incision facilitates exposure of posteromedial talar dome lesions and the posterior margin of the tibia.

A 10-cm curvilinear incision is made, centered over the medial aspect of the ankle and curving forward toward the midportion of the foot (Fig. 82–16). Depending on the approach, its midpoint can be anterior or posterior to the tip of the medial malleolus. The anterior incision is deepened, preserving the long saphenous vein and branches of the saphenous nerve. The deep incision through the deltoid ligament and joint capsule provides access to the anterior articular surfaces. The posterior incision is carried down through the flexor retinaculum behind the malleolus, taking care not to injure the posterior tibial tendon (Fig. 82–17). Retracting the posterior structures allows visualization of the posterior aspect of the medial malleolus.

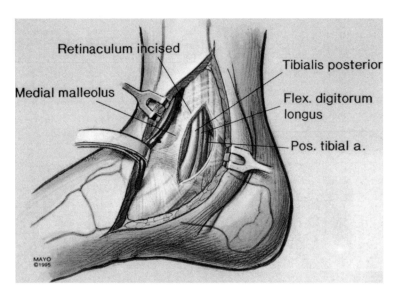

Figure 82–17. The deeper structures are depicted through the more posterior incision.

Pitfalls include damage to the long saphenous vein and nerves running anterior to the medial malleolus, resulting in subsequent neuroma formation. This can be minimized by preserving them as a unit. Posteriorly, the tibialis posterior tendon is most vulnerable, although the neurovascular bundle is not far from potential harm.

Approach to the Lateral Malleolus

The lateral approach to the distal fibula is most commonly used for open reduction and internal fixation of displaced lateral malleolar fractures. It can also provide access to the posterolateral tibia. When combined with fibular osteotomy or ostectomy, it affords excellent visualization of the tibiotalar joint for arthrodesis procedures.

A 10- to 15-cm longitudinal incision is made along the posterior margin of the fibula and is curved anteriorly at its distal end (Fig. 82–18). Full-thickness flaps are created down to periosteum, taking care not to damage the sural nerve and the short saphenous vein, both of which travel posterior to the lateral malleolus. The periosteum is incised to expose the fracture, stripping only enough to provide accurate reduction (Fig. 82–19). At the distal end of the fibula, the lateral ligaments can be visualized.

Pitfalls include injury to the sural nerve, which may lead to painful neuroma formation and dysesthesias along the lateral aspect of the foot. The perforating branches of the peroneal artery lie just deep to the medial aspect of the distal fibula. The peroneal tendons are also vulnerable to injury, particularly if they have subluxed anteriorly.

Lateral Approach to the Hindpart of the Foot

The lateral approach, also known as the Ollier approach, provides excellent exposure to the talocalcaneal (subtalar) joint and can easily be modified to include the calcaneocuboid joint.[23] It is particularly useful when performing arthrodeses of these joints.

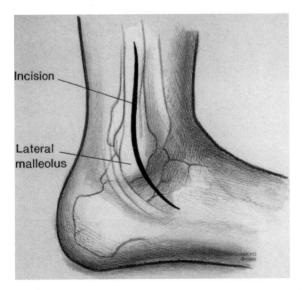

Figure 82–18. The lateral approach to the ankle is usually through this incision.

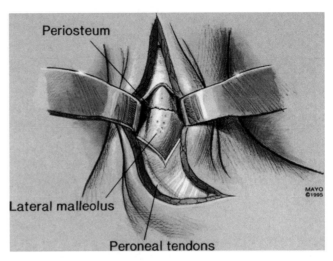

Figure 82–19. The periosteum is incised, revealing the fracture site.

An 8- to 10-cm incision is made obliquely over the sinus tarsi region. It extends from the lateral margin of the extensor digitorum brevis muscle back to the peroneal tendons (Fig. 82–20). The sural nerve, which is 1 to 2 cm beneath the tip of the distal fibula, is avoided. Sharp dissection is continued posteriorly and inferiorly until the peroneal sheath is encountered. The inferolateral margin of the extensor brevis is carefully elevated superiorly and distally. This allows identification of the calcaneocuboid joint anteriorly and the talocalcaneal joint posteriorly.

Pitfalls include forceful, blunt retraction causing skin necrosis. Careful positioning of the incision and full-thickness flaps may help to avoid this complication. The peroneal tendons are vulnerable as the incision is deepened.

Posterior Approach to the Ankle and Subtalar Joints

A posterior approach to the ankle has previously been described for placement of prostheses.[38,40] The ankle and subtalar joints can be exposed simultaneously, and this approach is particularly useful in salvage situations.[22] Failed total ankle arthroplasties, pseudarthroses from attempted ankle arthrodeses, and post-traumatic avascular necrosis of the talus all pose significant reconstructive challenges. This approach provides maximum exposure and allows for correction of significant deformities. Previous incisions or traumatic scars can be avoided.

In the prone position, a 20-cm curvilinear incision is made with the convexity toward the medial aspect of the leg. The apex of the curve should lie just medial to the Achilles tendon (Fig. 82–21). Full-thickness flaps are created with special attention to gentle handling of the skin and subcutaneous tissues. The tendo Achillis is transected in the coronal plane at its distal third (Fig. 82–22). The cut is completed anteriorly at the distal end and posteriorly at the proximal extent of the coronal split. The deep fascia is opened in the

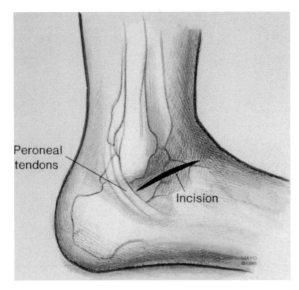

Figure 82–20. The incision for the lateral approach to the subtalar joint.

midline, exposing the flexor hallucis longus muscle belly. The origin of the flexor hallucis longus is elevated from the fibula and interosseous membrane and is retracted medially, protecting the tibial nerve and artery. The posterior capsules of the two joints of the hindpart of the foot are elevated subperiosteally from the posterior aspects of the tibia, the talus, and the calcaneus (Fig. 82–23). With care, the medial and lateral malleoli can also be exposed for resection when needed.

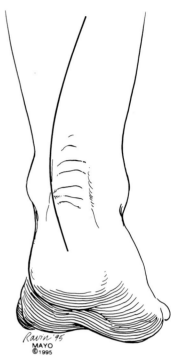

Figure 82–21. The curvilinear incision for the posterior approach to the ankle and subtalar joints.

Pitfalls include injury to the sural nerve as the skin incision crosses the midline proximally. Deep to the tendo Achillis, the midline is considered safe, although, with severe deformities, the neurovascular structures

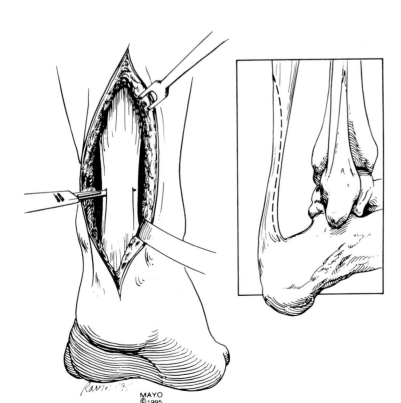

Figure 82–22. The Achilles tendon is split obliquely in the coronal plane. The cut ends are reflected to expose the deep fascia and the flexor hallucis longus muscle.

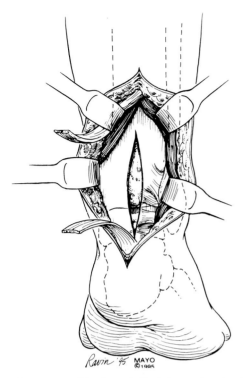

Figure 82–23. The flexor hallucis longus is retracted medially to protect the neurovascular bundle. The capsule and periosteum are incised in the midline, and the joints are exposed.

may be displaced. The tendon of the flexor hallucis longus is also prone to damage as the dissection proceeds deeper and medially. Once down to bone, the approach remains relatively safe.

Midportion of the Foot

Dorsal Approach to the Midportion of the Foot

The midpart of the foot can be approached dorsally for procedures involving Chopart's and Lisfranc's joints. Also, the medial intertarsal (naviculocuneiform and intercuneiform) joints can be accessed from this route.

A longitudinal incision is made directly over the area to be exposed. Should more than one incision be necessary, a 5- to 7-cm bridge of skin between the incisions will help to ensure a viable flap. Remaining medial to the EHL tendon avoids damage to the deep peroneal nerve and the dorsalis pedis artery (Fig. 82–24**A**). When a more lateral incision is needed, palpating the pulse and marking its course on the skin prior to exsanguinating the limb will also help to prevent injury to these structures (Fig. 82–24**B**). The neurovascular bundle can be found just deep to the tendons of the extensor digitorum brevis. Full-thickness flaps and minimal blunt retraction are necessary to prevent skin necrosis. The incision is carried directly down to the structures that are to be exposed, taking care to avoid any cutaneous nerves that can be identified.

Pitfalls include injury to the dorsalis pedis artery or the deep peroneal nerve. More laterally, branches of the superficial peroneal nerve are vulnerable.

Forepart of the Foot

Dorsomedial Approach to the Great Metatarsophalangeal Joint

The dorsomedial incision is most often utilized for procedures designed to treat symptomatic bunions or degenerative arthritis, or both. Bony excisions, soft tissue realignments, and arthrodeses can all be accomplished through this approach.

A 6-cm longitudinal incision is made over the dorsomedial aspect of the great toe metatarsophalangeal joint (Fig. 82–25). Beginning along the medial shaft of the distal metatarsal, the incision is gently curved over the dorsomedial aspect of the joint, remaining medial to the EHL tendon and the dorsal digital nerve, and may continue distally to the medial aspect of the great toe

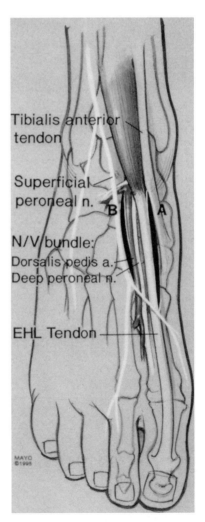

Figure 82–24. Diagrammatic view of dorsal approach to the midportion of the foot. Incision **A** is relatively safe, just medial to the EHL tendon. Incision **B** is used when a more lateral exposure is needed.

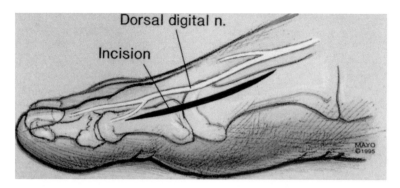

Figure 82–25. Dorsomedial incision to the great metatarsophalangeal joint. The dorsal digital nerve is also seen.

interphalangeal joint. The incision is carried through the fascia, and the dorsal digital branch of the medial cutaneous nerve is gently retracted. The capsule may then be incised longitudinally or a flap created to expose the joint, and subperiosteal dissection performed as needed (Fig. 82–26).

Pitfalls include painful neuroma formation within the dorsal digital nerve as a result of its proximity to the skin incision. The tendon of the flexor hallucis longus

muscle is vulnerable during subperiosteal stripping at the base of the proximal phalanx.

Dorsal Approach to the Great Metatarsophalangeal Joint

The dorsal approach to the great toe metatarsophalangeal joint is widely utilized for excision of metatarsal bony exostoses and dorsal wedge osteotomies of

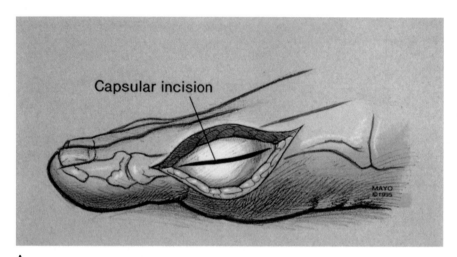

A

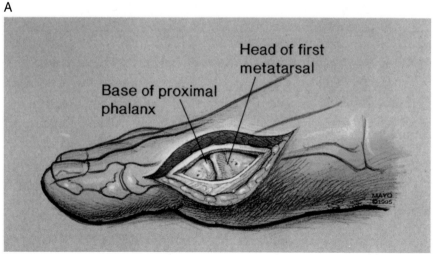

B

Figure 82–26. A, A longitudinal capsular incision is shown, although a flap is also commonly utilized. **B,** The base of the proximal phalanx and metatarsal head.

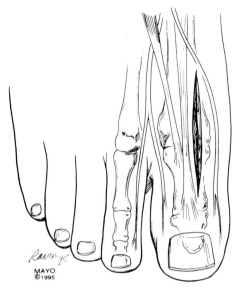

Figure 82–27. Dorsal approach to the great metatarsophalangeal joint, with the incision just medial to the EHL tendon.

the proximal phalanx in cases of hallux rigidus. Arthrodesis of the metatarsophalangeal joint can be stabilized with a dorsal plate and screws through this approach.

A dorsal longitudinal incision is made just medial to the tendon of the EHL, 2 to 3 cm proximal to the joint, and can be carried distally to the interphalangeal joint (Fig. 82–27). The fascia is divided, leaving a cuff of tissue with the tendon, and the EHL tendon is retracted laterally. The capsule is then incised and the joint exposed subperiosteally.

Pitfalls include scarring and postoperative adhesions in the EHL tendon, which may be avoided by leaving a

cuff of tissue medially as the incision is carried through the fascia. The dorsal cutaneous sensory branches are also vulnerable and should be preserved where possible.

Dorsal Approach to the Lesser Metatarsophalangeal Joints

A common approach to a single lesser metatarsophalangeal joint is through a 2- to 3-cm longitudinal incision over the dorsal or dorsolateral aspect of the joint (Fig. 82–28). The incision may be placed parallel and lateral to the EDL tendon, preserving the dorsal digital nerves. The joint capsule may then be incised and the joint exposed. When multiple joints require exposure, two dorsal incisions are placed, one each in the second and fourth web spaces.

Dorsal Web Space Approach

This approach is useful in salvage situations for deformity and instability at the lesser metatarsophalangeal joints.[36] Resection arthroplasty of the bases of the proximal phalanges or resection of the metatarsal heads can be performed through this incision. When combined with extensor tenotomies and subtotal webbing, this approach provides excellent exposure with minimal soft tissue trauma.

A Y-shaped incision is made in the second or fourth web spaces, or both. It begins dorsally, just proximal to the level of the metatarsal heads, and is carried distally to the inner aspects of both adjacent toes (Fig. 82–29). Sharp dissection down to bone is performed, and the metatarsophalangeal joints are exposed. The incision may be extended proximally for improved visualization or distally to allow for more bony resection.

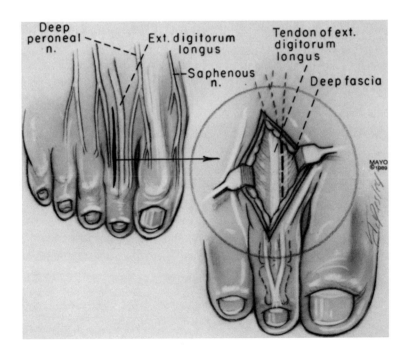

Figure 82–28. Diagrammatic view of the dorsal incisional approach to the second metatarsophalangeal joint.

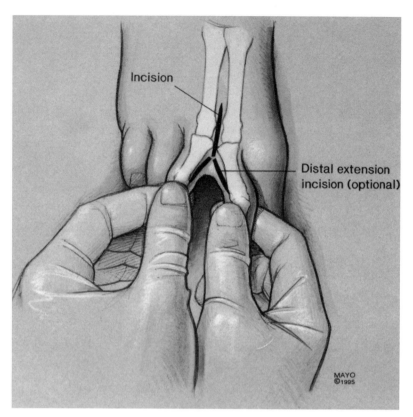

Figure 82–29. The dorsal approach to the second web space is depicted, with the Y-shaped incision centered over the lesser metatarsophalangeal joints.

Pitfalls include malposition of the toes relative to one another if the incision is placed too dorsal or plantar to the midline. The proper digital nerves are vulnerable if the dissection strays from the midline.

References

1. Acton R: Surgical principles based on anatomy of the foot: preoperative planning. Foot Ankle 2:200, 1982.
2. Alvarez R, Haddad RJ, Gould N, Trevino S: The simple bunion: anatomy at the metatarsophalangeal joint of the great toe. Foot Ankle 4:229, 1984.
3. Bareither DJ, Schuberth JM, Evoy PJ, Thomas GJ: Peroneus digiti minimi. Anat Anz 155:11, 1984.
4. Bejjani FJ, Jahss MH: Le Double's study of muscle variations of the human body. II. Muscle variations of the foot. Foot Ankle 6:157, 1986.
5. Bojsen-Moller F: Anatomy of the forefoot, normal and pathologic. Clin Orthop 142:16, 1979.
6. Clemente CE (ed): Gray's Anatomy, 30th Am ed. Philadelphia, Lea & Febiger, 1985, p 410.
7. Cox HT: The cleavage lines of the skin. Br J Surg 29:234, 1941.
8. Cralley JC, Schuberth JM, Fitch KL: The deep band of the plantar aponeurosis of the human foot. Anat Anz 152:189, 1982.
9. Cunningham DJ: Textbook of Anatomy, 12th ed. Oxford, England, Oxford University Press, 1981, p 255.
10. De Palma L, Santucci A, Sabetta S, Rapali S: Anatomy of the Lisfranc joint complex. Foot Ankle Int 18:6, 1997.
11. Harper MC: Deltoid ligament: an anatomical evaluation of function. Foot Ankle 8:19, 1987.
12. Henry AK: Extensile Exposure. London, Churchill Livingstone, 1973, p 300.
13. Hing DN, Buncke HJ, Alpert BS: Applications of the extensor digitorum brevis muscle for soft tissue coverage. Ann Plast Surg 19:530, 1987.
14. Hiramoto Y: Variation of the long plantar ligament [in Japanese]. Okajimas Folia Anat Jpn 60:401, 1984.
15. Hirsch BE, Vekkos LE: Anomalous contrahentes muscles in human feet. Anat Anz 155:123, 1984.
16. Hollinshead WH, Rosse C: Textbook of Anatomy, 4th ed. New York, Harper & Row, 1985, p 451.
17. Holmes GB: Surgical Approaches to the Foot and Ankle. New York, McGraw-Hill, 1994.
18. Hoppenfeld S, deBoer P: Surgical Exposures in Orthopedics: The Anatomic Approach, 2nd ed. Philadelphia, JB Lippincott, 1994, p 514.
19. Inman VT: The Joints of the Ankle. Baltimore, Williams & Wilkins, 1976, p 30.
20. Jahss M: Disorders of the Foot and Ankle: Medical and Surgical Management, 2nd ed. Philadelphia, WB Saunders, 1991, p 12.
21. Johnson KA: Surgery of the Foot and Ankle. New York, Raven Press, 1989, p 274.
22. Johnson KA: Tibiocalcaneal arthrodesis. In Johnson KA (ed): Master Techniques in Orthopaedic Surgery: The Foot and Ankle. New York, Raven Press, 1994, ch 36.
23. Jordan C, Mirzabeigi E: Atlas of Orthopedic Surgical Exposures. New York, Thieme, 2000, p 176.
24. Kirkup J: Richard Smith ankle arthroplasty. J R Soc Med 78:301, 1985.
25. Mahan KT: Plastic surgery and skin grafting. In McGlamry ED (ed): Comprehensive Textbook of Foot Surgery, vol. 2. Baltimore, Williams & Wilkins, 1987, ch 22.
26. Mann RA, Hagy JL: The function of the toes in walking, jogging, and running. Clin Orthop 142:24, 1979.
27. Miller WE: Operative incisions involving the foot. Orthop Clin North Am 7:785, 1976.
28. Myerson M: Foot and Ankle Disorders. Philadelphia, WB Saunders, 2000, p 29.
29. Newton St E III: An artificial ankle joint. Clin Orthop Rel Res 142:141, 1979.
30. Samuelson KM, Freeman MAR, Tuke MA: Development and evolution of the ICLH ankle replacement. Foot Ankle 3:32, 1982.

31. Scholz KC: Total ankle arthroplasty using biological fixation components compared to ankle arthrodesis. Total Ankle Arthroplasty 10:125, 1987.

32. Stauffer RN: Total joint arthroplasty: the ankle. Mayo Clin Proc 54:570, 1979.

33. Stauffer RN: Salvage of painful total ankle arthroplasty. Clin Orthop 170:184, 1982.

34. Stauffer RN, Segal NM: Total ankle arthroplasty: four years' experience. Clin Orthop 160:217, 1981.

35. Swiontkowski M, Post P: Surgical approaches to the lower extremity. *In* Chapman M (ed): Operative Orthopaedics. Philadelphia, JB Lippincott, 1988, p 47.

36. Teasdall RD: Resection arthroplasty of the second and third toes. *In* Johnson KA (ed): Master Techniques in Orthopaedic Surgery: The Foot and Ankle. New York, Raven Press, 1994, ch 12.

37. Tubiana R, Masquelet AC, McCullough CJ: Atlas of the Surgical Exposures of the Upper and Lower Extremities. London, Martin Dunitz, 2000, p 302.

38. Unger AS, Inglis AE, Mow CS, Figgie HE III: Total ankle arthroplasty in rheumatoid arthritis: a long-term follow-up study. Foot Ankle 8:173, 1988.

39. Ward KA, Soames RW: Morphology of the plantar calcaneocuboid ligaments. Foot Ankle Int 18:10, 1997.

40. Waugh TR, Evanski PM, McMaster WC: Irvine ankle arthroplasty. Clin Orthop Rel Res 114:180, 1976.

83

Biomechanics

• HAROLD B. KITAOKA and THOMAS R. JENKYN

Multiple attempts have been directed toward producing suitable replacement arthroplasties for the ankle, subtalar, and metatarsophalangeal (MTP) joints. The failure rates of these implants have limited their use in the past. Questions have been raised regarding whether implant arthroplasty offers superior clinical results over more conventional nonimplant alternatives. Design of a successful replacement arthroplasty for the ankle, subtalar and first MTP joint depends on a clear understanding of the geometry and constraints of each of these mechanically complex joints. Because these joints fulfill antigravity and locomotive roles, design success also depends on quantifying the kinematics and resulting forces of these joints during activities of daily living.

ANKLE AND SUBTALAR JOINTS

Design of a single ankle replacement arthroplasty suitable for all individuals is confounded for a number of reasons: the complexity of ankle joint mechanics, the obligatory consideration of functional status of the subtalar joint, and the great variability in geometry, axis of rotation, and normal range of motion of the ankle joint. One of the reasons for the limited success of ankle implants to date, as a consequence, is poor reproduction of normal mechanics. Failure may result from the surgeon's inability to retain critical ligamentous stabilizers; shortcomings in the implant design, which may not adequately deal with component fixation; and incomplete understanding of physiologic loading in the joint. The expectedly high magnitude of vertical and shear forces within the ankle are well recognized to contribute to implant failure.[7,13,18,21]

Geometry

The ankle joint (talocrural joint) is formed by the articulations between the tibial plafond and the talar trochlear surface and between the medial and lateral malleolar surfaces of the tibia-fibula and talus. The two malleoli form a fork within which the talus is tightly held. The plafond surface is concave and the trochlea convex, so the talus tends to rotate about an axis that runs primarily medial-lateral. The axis of the ankle joint has been located in various cadaver studies performed on fresh and unfixed specimens.[6,12,16] The shape of the articulation of the talus with the tibial plafond is that of a frustum of a cone, with a mean conical angle of 24 ± 6 degrees[6] (Fig. 83–1). The axis of this laterally diverging cone is downward in the frontal (coronal) plane and posteriorly in the transverse plane, passing slightly below the tips of the malleoli. Inman showed that the axis of rotation of the ankle joint runs distal to the tip of the medial malleolus at 5 ± 3 mm below and just lateral and anterior to the tip of the lateral malleolus, at 3 ± 2 mm below and 8 ± 5 mm to the anterior. The axis is therefore oriented distally and laterally in the frontal plane and posterolaterally in the transverse plane. This orientation of the axis is plotted in Figure 83–2.

The alignment of the ankle axis to the knee and foot markedly varies from individual to individual, but mean external tibial torsion is 23 degrees (with variation of ± 30 degrees) and mean transverse plane offset of the foot relative to the talar axis is approximately 6 degrees. The congruity of the ankle joint, and in particular the fit of the wedge-shaped talus in the mortise, has stimulated considerable investigation and discussion. The mean difference in anterior and posterior talar width (measured parallel) is 2.4 ± 1.3 mm (range 0 to 6 mm). The mean capacity for malleolar separation through the syndesmosis is 1 mm on average, with a maximal separation in any specimen of 2 mm. Thus, it is difficult to understand how the talus would have a tight fit in the mortise in full dorsiflexion and in full plantar flexion.

The answer to this enigma came with measurement of the articular diameters along lines that converge to the apex of the cone representing the shape of the talar body. Measured in this manner, differences in anterior and posterior width of the talus were negligible and were always less than 2 mm, explaining the excellent congruence of the ankle throughout its range.[6] The medial convergence of the frustum of the cone representing the talar body also produces obligatory discrepancies in the medial and lateral articular facets of the trochlea. Both the radius of the curvature of the talus and the arc described by the articular facet are greater on the lateral side. In addition, the lateral malleolus extends more distally than the medial malleolus to allow skeletal attachment of the lateral ligaments close

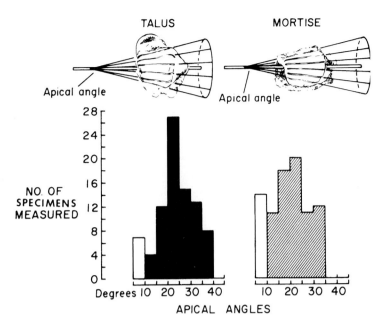

Figure 83–1. The talus as a frustum of a cone with a variable apical angle. (From Inman VT: The Joints of the Ankle. Baltimore, Williams & Wilkins, 1976.)

to the axis of rotation of the joint. This maintains ligament isometry throughout normal ankle range of motion and therefore limits change in ligament tension.

Finally, of geometric importance, in addition to the high degree of ankle joint congruity, the articular contact area of the tibiotalar articulation is large. This contact area, 11 to 13 cm², means that forces acting externally on the ankle result in lower local pressure on the articular surfaces within the ankle relative to those in the hip and the knee.[7,21] Minimal talar shift[14] and distal tibial malalignment[23] significantly decrease contact area and so increase local stresses. Investigations have also demonstrated talar shift with axial loading of intact normal ankles.[8] Lateral transition of the talus of up to 2 mm

was observed. These phenomena in normal joints would be magnified in a replacement arthroplasty that is either malaligned or unstable in the transverse plane.

Intimately involved with the function of the ankle joint is the subtalar joint (talocalcaneonavicular joint). The subtalar joint is composed of two separate joints that function together as a single mechanism inferior to the talus. These two subjoints are the articulations (1) between the posterior and middle talocalcaneal surfaces and (2) between the talar head and navicular socket. The axis of rotation is oriented generally posterior to anterior, moving superomedially as it travels anteriorly. Cadaver studies by Inman[6] demonstrated the variability in the orientation of the axis in normal populations (Fig. 83–3).

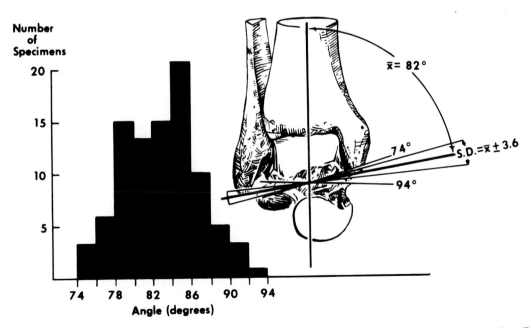

Figure 83–2. Variability between individuals of the orientation of the ankle joint rotational axis in the normal population. (From Inman VT: The Joints of the Ankle. Baltimore, Williams & Wilkins, 1976.)

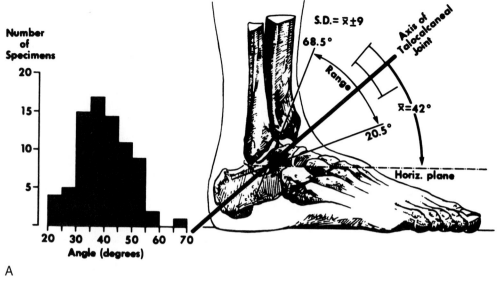

A

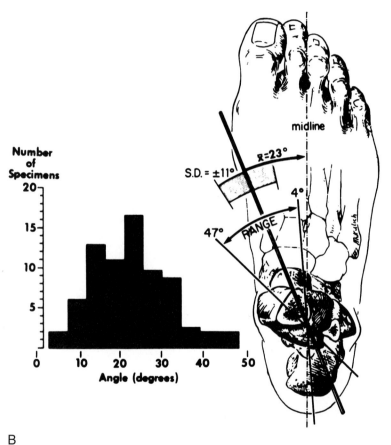

B

Figure 83–3. Variability between individuals of the orientation of the subtalar joint rotational axis in the normal population. (From Inman VT: The Joints of the Ankle. Baltimore, Williams & Wilkins, 1976.)

The angle of the rotation axis from horizontal in the sagittal plane was on average 42 degrees, with a range of 20.5 to 68.5 degrees. The angle of the axis with respect to the midline of the foot in the transverse plane was an average 23 degrees, with a range of 4 to 47 degrees. Because of the dependence of subtalar joint function on the clinical state of the ankle joint, degeneration of this joint can results from malaligned or unstable arthroplasty of the ankle joint. Maintenance of the congruency and geometry of the subtalar joint is of great relevance for successful outcome of replacement arthroplasty of the ankle joint.

Kinematics

The major motion allowed by the ankle joint is dorsiflexion and plantar flexion of the foot. However, because the rotational axis is not horizontal and transverse, there are small amounts of foot abduction and adduction coupled to dorsiflexion and plantar flexion. The motion and instantaneous centers of rotation of the ankle have been studied extensively. An important distinction in these studies is between functional ankle motion and maximal ankle motion. Maximal weight-bearing total ankle range of motion averages 43 degrees (range 24 to 75 degrees), with mean dorsiflexion and plantar flexion being 21 and 23 degrees, respectively.[16] Radiographic analysis reveals a migrating instantaneous center of rotation for the ankle joint with joint distraction associated with initiation of motion and articular jamming in the termination of movement.[16] Surface velocities indicate that sliding motion predominates, even in the majority of loaded ankles.[16] The mean normal total functional ankle range of motion is 24.4 degrees (range 20 to 31 degrees), with a mean of 10.2 degrees (range 6 to 16 degrees) of dorsiflexion and 14.2 degrees (range 13 to 17 degrees) of plantar flexion.[21]

The instantaneous rotational axis migrates as the ankle joint moves through its range of motion.[7] When dorsiflexed, the axis is oriented downward laterally. As the foot moves into neutral, the axis migrates into a more horizontal position, and in full plantar flexion the axis is oriented upward laterally in the frontal plane. The reason for this migration is anatomic. The radius of curvature of the lateral border of the talar trochlear surface in the sagittal plane is larger than that of the medial border. The surface of the lateral border is almost circular through all of its arch in the sagittal plane. However, the curvature of the medial border of the surface is not circular. The radius of curvature of the anterior portion of the medial border is smaller than the posterior portion. The radius of curvature of the medial border goes from being smaller than the lateral in its anterior portion to being almost equal in its posterior portion. Therefore, as the talus moves through its range of motion and the radius of curvature of the portion of surface in contact with the mortise changes, the axis of rotation migrates.

The subtalar joint motions are primarily inversion and eversion. Unlike the ankle joint rotational axis, the axis of the subtalar joint does not seem to migrate as the joint moves through its range of motion. The geometry of the socket of the navicular is not congruent with the talar head surface. Therefore, as the subtalar joint moves through its range of motion, the midfoot bones, the navicular and cuboid, rotate with respect to the calcaneus and talus to avoid dislocation of the socket-head articulation[5] (Fig. 83–4). This subtle motion between the hindfoot and midfoot can be considered as a part of the overall motion of the subtalar joint.

Consideration of ankle kinematics requires a broader view that includes the normal kinematics of the entire lower extremity because motions of the leg (specifically, the tibia), talus, and calcaneus are highly interdependent in stance phase.[12] Mean transverse plane rotatory motion of the tibia in stance phase amounts to 15 degrees.[11] Physiologic loading of the normal foot during stance causes plantar flexion of the talus relative to the tibia[5] that is proportional to the magnitude of the loading. Although the frontal plane obliquity of the ankle axis and the transverse plane offset of the foot and ankle axis produce some pronatory and supinatory displacements with dorsiflexion and plantar flexion, the ankle is not designed to accommodate the rotatory stresses imposed by the leg on the planted foot.[6] The subtalar joint, with an axis oriented upward 42 degrees (mean) in the sagittal plane and 23 degrees (mean) medially in the transverse plane, is ideally suited to absorb the rotational stress imposed. In a theoretical model, a 45-degree sagittal plane axis would produce 1 degree of accommodative subtalar eversion for each degree of tibial internal rotation. Similarly, 1 degree of subtalar inversion would result for each degree of tibial external rotation. Limited or absent subtalar motion can produce rotatory stresses in the ankle joint, which prosthetic designs with greater inherent stability and 1 degree of freedom of motion could not withstand.

Constraints

Both the articular geometry and the ligamentous supports contribute significantly to ankle stability. Of primary interest has been stability of the joint in rotation in the transverse plane and with inversion in the frontal plane. The contribution of bony geometry to stability depends on whether the ankle is loaded or unloaded. Stormont et al. found that, in the loaded state, articular geometry accounted for 30 percent of transverse plane rotational stability and 100 percent of inversion stability in the frontal plane.[22] In the unloaded state, the primary restraints were the anterior talofibular ligament to internal rotation and the calcaneofibular ligament to external rotation. The calcaneofibular ligament was also the primary restraint to inversion and the deltoid to eversion. Fraser and Ahmed found that torsional stability of the ankle was largely dependent on the degree of compression load applied to the ankle as well as the position of the ankle when the torsional load was applied.[4] A dorsiflexed ankle was more resistant to internal rotation than external rotation; in the plantar-flexed ankle, the opposite was found.

Rotatory stresses on the ankle joint are dissipated through motion at the subtalar joint and the joints of the foot more distally. Integrity of the subtalar joint, as with the ankle joint, is maintained with the articular geometry and the ligamentous structures. Distraction of the joint is stopped by the combined effort of the cervical and interosseus ligaments, which connect the inferior talus to the superior calcaneus in the volume of the sinus and canalis tarsi. With distraction of the joint not permitted, the significant convexity-concavity of the

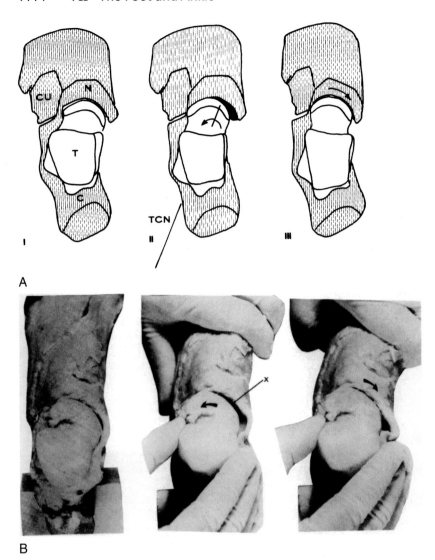

A

B

Figure 83–4. A, Movement of the navicular with respect to the talar head as the foot moves from eversion (**I**) into inversion (**III**). **B,** Dislocation of talus-navicular articulation resulting from this movement is not allowed. (From Huson A: Een Ontleedkundig-Functioneel Onderzoek van de Voetworte {An Anatomical and Functional Study of the Tarsal Joints}. Leiden, Drukkerij, 1961, pp 133–142.)

posterior talocalcaneal surface and the confinement of the talar head in the navicular socket withstand any dorsiflexion–plantar flexion stresses imposed on the joint through compression.[17] Medial-lateral and anterior-posterior translations of the joint are also opposed by the articular geometry.

The rotational and shear stresses of the ankle joint, which are likely to be major factors in ankle component loosening, can be decreased considerably by meniscal design replacement arthroplasty utilizing a polyethylene spacer with one flat surface. Lacking the geometric constraints of the normal ankle contour, which have been incorporated into most prosthetic ankles, the meniscal ankle is highly dependent on intact and correctly tensioned ligamentous constraints. The suitability of this arthroplasty design for the ankle has been questioned. In vitro, using an experimental prosthesis inserted under controlled conditions with the tightest possible meniscal fit, Bruge and Evans found excellent version and rotational stability with the ankle neutral but a twofold increase in anteroposterior laxity.[2]

Internal Joint Forces

The most important piece of biomechanical information for the surgeon is the magnitudes and timing of the internal loading of the ankle and subtalar joints. Without an understanding of these stresses, the successful design of replacement devices is confounded by uncertainty. If a device is to be able to withstand physiologic loading, this loading must be determined prior to design of the device and fully accounted for in the design. Unfortunately, direct measurement of the internal loading of these joints in vivo is technically very difficult, if not impossible. Therefore, the internal loading must be indirectly calculated.

Internal loading calculations begin with force and torque measurements of the external loading on the joints due to contact with the ground (ground reaction force [GRF]). This can be measured using motion data and force plate data collected in gait analysis laboratories. Using three-dimensional free-body analysis and the GRF, external joint torques are calculated along with the compression and shear forces on the joints.

Although it can be a counterintuitive idea, the internal loading of the joint arises mostly from the action of the muscles, and is usually much larger than the externally measured loading. The difficulty with calculating internal joint loading (i.e., the tension in the ligaments and the forces on the articular surfaces) is that the muscle tensions cannot be measured directly, or calculated with certainty. This is because several combinations of muscle tensions can produce the same external movement of the joints. The difference between the combinations is the amount of co-contraction of different muscle groups.

Assuming no co-contraction (or antagonism) between muscle groups, Stauffer and co-workers calculated that the aft shear force reaches a maximum of 70 percent of body weight at foot flat, and fore shear force reaches a maximum of 30 percent of body weight at push-off[21] (Fig. 83–5A). Compressive forces in the ankle plateau are 3 times body weight during foot flat and peak at 4.5 times body weight at heel-off (Fig. 83–5B). Although the majority of this compressive force is taken by the tibia, the fibula is a significant contributor, transmitting approximately one sixth of the load.[10]

In a more complex calculation of the entire lower extremity, Seireg and Arvikar predicted some antago-

nism between the plantar flexors and the dorsiflexors during stance phase. The joint loading of the ankle joint compression therefore climbed as high as 5.6 times body weight in late stance phase, and the shear force rose to 2 times body weight[18] (Fig. 83–6). In another model of internal loading that included both the ankle and subtalar joints and all the articular, ligamentous, and musculotendinous structures, the loading was found to be even greater during fast walking and quick turning.[1] In these conditions, the joint force was calculated as high as eight times body weight (Fig. 83–7). This high loading was due to the great amount of antagonism measured between the dorsiflexors, the peroneal muscles, and the plantar flexors during the awkward gait of fast walking. The joint loading during running has been calculated as anywhere between 9 and 13.3 times body weight.[3] Clearly the magnitude of the internal loading of the ankle is a hurdle in the design of a successful replacement device.

Design Considerations

After reviewing the geometry, the kinematics, and the internal loading environment of the ankle and subtalar

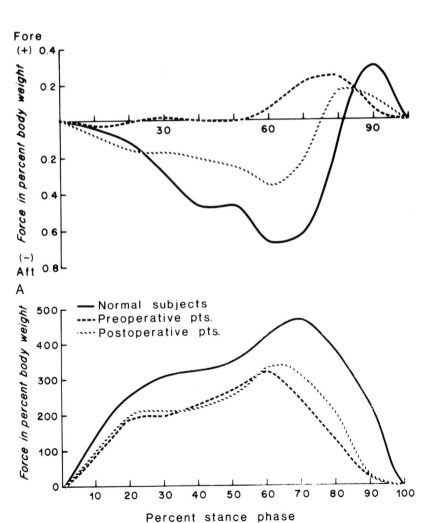

Figure 83–5. Mean patterns of ankle force. **A**, Tangential. **B**, Compressive. (From Stauffer RN, Chao EYS, Brewster RC: Force and motion analysis of the normal, diseased, and prosthetic ankle joint. Clin Orthop 127:189, 1977.)

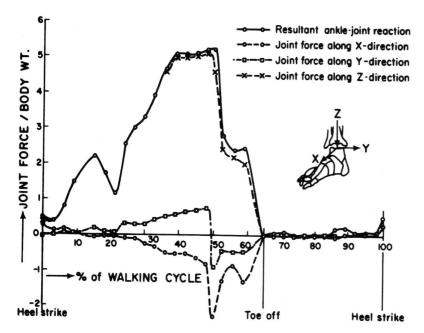

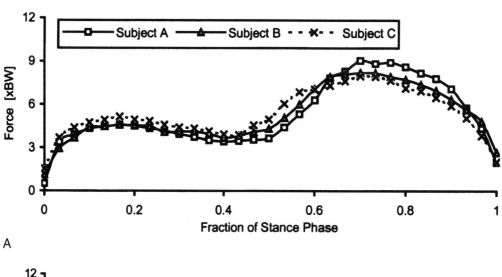

Figure 83–6. Joint compressive loading at the hip (*top*), knee (*middle*), and ankle (*bottom*) as calculated by the Seireg model. (From Seireg A, Arvikar RJ: A mathematical model for evaluation of forces in lower extremities of the musculoskeletal system. J Biomech 6:313–326, 1973.)

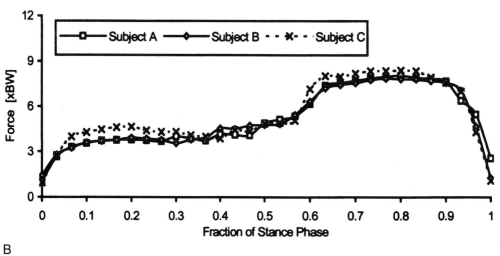

Figure 83–7. Joint force resultants for the ankle (**A**) and subtalar (**B**) joints during fast walking.

joints, it is clear that a successful replacement arthroplasty device must fulfill a number of requirements. First, because the loading in the ankle joint during common activities of daily living can be many times body weight, the device must be able to withstand these compressive and shearing loads without aseptic loosening, component failure, or nonphysiologic loading of the soft tissue.

Second, a replacement device must preserve the natural range of motion of the ankle and subtalar joints so as not to disrupt the walking gait pattern. Such a disruption inevitably leads to nonphysiologic loading of the knee and hip joints as a result of compensatory mechanisms and can hasten the development of joint degeneration in these areas.

Third, the anatomic geometry of the ankle and subtalar joints should be reflected in the device geometry, and the ligamentous structures should be left as intact as possible. This is because, while under such large internal loading, these joints maintain stability through ligament tension and joint surface compression. Joint stability is necessary to minimize the already large physiologic loading and maintain normal joint kinematics.

Design of replacement arthroplasty devices for the ankle is perhaps the most difficult of all the joints for a number of reasons. The forces to be withstood by the replacement are the highest in the body. Also, the range of motion of the ankle and subtalar joints is relatively large. Finally, fixation is confounded by the lack of bone stock within which the device can be implanted in the talus and by the minimal vascularization. Each of these factors has perhaps held progress in successful ankle replacement back while hip and knee replacement have become reliable and commonplace.

FIRST METATARSOPHALANGEAL JOINT

Geometry

The unique articular contour of the first metatarsal head plays an important role in stabilizing the first MTP joint, and a knowledge of its shape is essential to appreciate the forces across and the kinematics of the articulation. The articular geometry also is critical in the design of prosthetic replacements, particularly of unipolar and resurfacing types.

The first MTP joint is composed of three distinct, yet smoothly interrelated, articular surfaces: the phalangeal surface and the tibial and fibular sesamoidal articular surfaces. The sesamoidal grooves on the inferior aspect of the metatarsal head are separated by the longitudinally oriented intersesamoid ridge. The shape of the sagittal curvature of the first metatarsal head depends on the level of section of the head because of the depressions of the sesamoidal trochlea.

Sagittal sections in the plane of the intersesamoid ridge produce an articular rim that is virtually round, with a mean arc of 161 degrees and a mean radius of 11.4 mm.[25] Frontal or coronal plane sections show that, dis-

tally, the deep sesamoidal grooves on the inferior aspect of the head become less distinct and ultimately mold into the smooth phalangeal surface of the metatarsal head. At maximal depth, the trochlea for the tibial sesamoid is 1.5 to 2 mm deeper than the fibular groove.[25] Matching this, the tibial sesamoid is larger, longer, and closer to the base of the proximal phalanx than the fibular sesamoid.[17,25] The functional importance of the tibial sesamoid is also stressed by the orientation of the metatarsal head to the floor. The mean 13-degree medial rotation of the dorsal plantar axis of the normal first metatarsal head to the floor places the transverse axis of the tibial sesamoid and its trochlea parallel to the floor[17,25] (Fig. 83–8). As a result, the majority of the static vertical forces on the first metatarsal head are transmitted by the tibial sesamoid.

Sesamoid stability in the frontal (coronal) plane depends on the intersesamoid ridge. With MTP extension of greater than approximately 30 degrees, the restraint provided by the midline ridge progressively decreases, making the sesamoids potentially unstable in the frontal plane and prone to lateral subluxation.[25]

Kinematics

In normal circumstances, the first MTP joint has two degrees of freedom of motion: in the sagittal and in the transverse planes. Active and passive sagittal plane ranges of motion of the first MTP joint were found to be mean active flexion of 23 degrees, mean active extension of 51 degrees, and combined active and passive extension of 74 degrees.[8] The findings in a cadaver study were similar: the mean dorsiflexion was 76 degrees and plantar flexion 34 degrees, and the mean total angular displacement of the sesamoid relative to the first metatarsal head in the sagittal plane was 49 degrees.[19]

Instant centers of motion of the great toe phalanx on the metatarsal head were studied by Sammarco[15] and by Shereff et al.[19] Their findings were identical. In the sagittal plane, instant centers of rotation fell within the metatarsal head in normal joints, but their positions varied considerably (Fig. 83–9). Instant surface velocity vectors indicated tangential sliding motion through the range except that, at maximal extension, there was com-

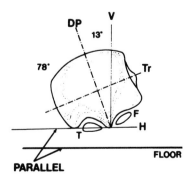

Figure 83–8. Orientation of the tibial sesamoid and its trochlea. (From Yoshioka Y, Siu DW, Cooke TDV, et al: Geometry of the first metatarsophalangeal joint. J Orthop Res 6:878, 1988.)

pression and jamming of the articular surfaces. Shereff et al. found that, with hallux valgus and hallux rigidus, sagittal plane centers of rotation were widely dispersed and fell outside the metatarsal head.[19] Surface velocity vectors of these specimens did not remain tangential to the joint surface as seen in normal subjects, indicating articular distraction and jamming.[19]

Transverse plane motion during flexion and extension of the first MTP joint ranged from 14 to 20 degrees in normal subjects (mean 15.4 degrees).[19] This motion was significantly decreased in hallux rigidus (mean 8.3 degrees) and minimally affected by hallux valgus (mean 14.6 degrees).

Constraints

Frontal and transverse plane motions at the first MTP joint are restricted by the bony contours of the metatarsal head—in particular, the anatomic relationship of the sesamoids to the plantar aspect of the head—and by ligamentous supports. The laterally directed force on the hallux produced by the toe box of shoes places continuous stress on these constraints. Snijders et al. produced the biomechanical model of transverse plane mechanics of the first MTP joint.[20] Two moments are demonstrated in the transverse plane (Fig. 83–10). One is the moment of the flexor hallucis longus on the hallux, producing valgus deviation of the great toe. The other is the medially directed first MTP joint reaction force, which causes progressive varus angulation of the first metatarsal. The laterally directed force of the shoe on the hallux increases the lateral deviation of the hallux, which accentuates the intrinsic deviating forces.

The stabilizing effect of the sesamoids, which restrict lateral migration of the long flexor tendon, is critical in maintaining long flexor alignment. Lateral subluxation of the sesamoids increases the laterally directed moment of the long flexor. The medial soft tissue restraints to valgus angulation of the hallux gradually attenuate in the face of persistent laterally directed extrinsic and intrinsic forces. Dorsal migration of the lateral sesamoid, which is associated with lateral subluxation, produces

frontal plane rotation of the hallux, a motion that appears to occur only in this abnormal circumstance.

In planning prosthetic replacement of the first MTP joint, there is a definite need to consider transverse and frontal plane mechanics and to retain stability in these planes that is normally provided by the sesamoids.

Reaction Forces

Reaction forces in the first MTP joint have been derived indirectly through free-body analysis using forces exerted by the hallux on force plates. Wyss et al. used a LOCAM camera synchronized with a force platform to obtain a record of sagittal plane kinematics at 50 Hz and combined this with foot radiographs with radiopaque markers to create a biomechanical model for the first MTP joint.[24] For each cine frame (sampled at 50 Hz), the GRF recorded by the force platform was used to determine the pulling force of the flexor hallucis longus and, in turn, the forces acting between the sesamoid and the first metatarsal head and between the phalangeal base and the first metatarsal head. These two forces were combined to determine the magnitude and vector of the resultant joint reaction forces.

There was considerable variation in the maximal joint reaction force, from 0.99 N/kg of body weight to 7.44 N/kg (mean 3.7 N/kg) in barefoot individuals. Maximal forces were slightly changed when shoes were worn (mean 3.59 N/kg), with a disproportionate increase in sesamoid loads. The mean angle between the vector of maximal joint reaction force and the axis of the first metatarsal (defined by the dorsal ridge of the first metatarsal shaft) was 4.8 degrees in barefoot individuals and 3.5 degrees in those wearing shoes, indicating that loading of the first metatarsal head was primarily axial. Histologic evaluation of the trabecular patterns of the metatarsal head by the same investigators showed maximal trabecular density in the region of maximal joint reaction force as determined by vector analysis, supporting the data.

The angle of the metatarsal shaft to the plane of the floor at maximal joint load averaged 66.8 degrees barefoot and 70.4 degrees in comfortable shoes.[24] Because of the loss of sesamoid stability with increasing extension, it is apparent that high-heeled shoes may contribute significantly to the development of hallux valgus by generating maximal loads in the first MTP joint in a position where the sesamoids are most susceptible to lateral subluxation. The implications also are clear for replacement arthroplasty, which also needs to ensure rotational stability of the prosthetic joint.

CONCLUSIONS

Successful replacement of the ankle and first MTP joint will ultimately be achieved, but not without an understanding of and respect for the normal mechanics of these articulations.

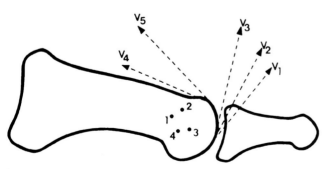

Figure 83–9. Instant centers of motion of the first metatarsophalangeal joint. (From Shereff MJ, Bejjani FJ, Kummer FJ: Kinematics of the first metatarsophalangeal joint. J Bone Joint Surg Am 68:392, 1986.)

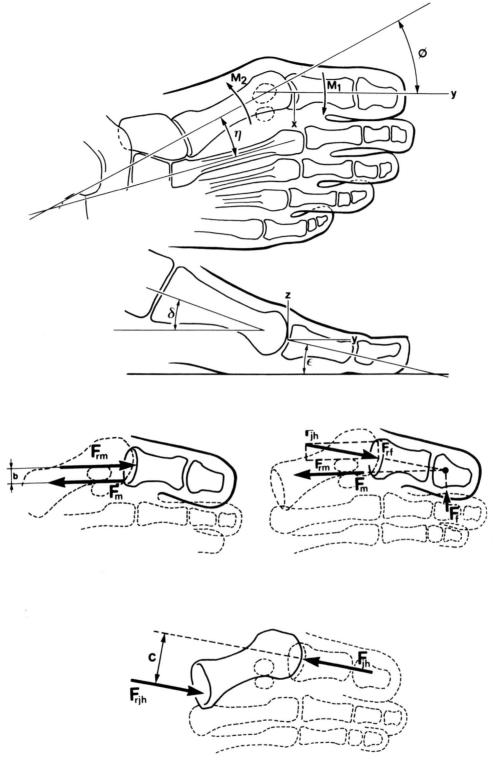

Figure 83–10. Transverse plane moments and forces in the first ray of the foot. (From Snijders CJ, Snijder JGN, Philippens MMGM: Biomechanics of hallux valgus and spread foot. Foot Ankle 7:26, 1986.)

References

1. Barnett CH, Napier JR: The axis of rotation at the ankle joint in man: its influence upon the form of the talus and mobility of the fibula. Anatomy 86:156, 1952.
2. Bruge P, Evans M: Effect of surface replacement arthroplasty on stability of the ankle. Foot Ankle 7:10, 1986.
3. Burdett RG: Forces predicted at the ankle during running. Med Sci Sports Exerc 14:308–316, 1982.
4. Fraser GA, Ahmed AM: Passive rotational stability of the weight-bearing talocrural joint—an *in-vitro* biomechanical study [abstract]. Orthop Trans 7:248, 1983.
5. Huson A: Een Ontleedkundig-Functioneel Onderzoek van de Voetwortle {An Anatomical and Functional Study of the Tarsal Joints}. Leiden, Drukkerij, 1961, pp 133–142.
6. Inman VT: The Joints of the Ankle. Baltimore, Williams & Wilkins, 1976.
7. Jenkyn T: Biomechanics of the Ankle Joint Complex using a Muscle Model Assisted Optimisation Model. PhD Thesis, University of Strathclyde, Glasgow, Scotland, UK, 1999.
8. Joseph J: Range of movement of the great toe in men. J Bone Joint Surg Br 36:450, 1954.
9. Kitaoka HB, Lundberg A, Luo ZP, An K-N: Kinematics of the normal arch of the foot and ankle under physiologic loading. Foot Ankle 16:492–499, 1995.
10. Lambert KL: The weight-bearing function of the fibula: a strain gauge study. J Bone Joint Surg Am 53:507, 1971.
11. Levens AS, Berkeley CE, Inman VT, Blosser JA: Transverse rotation of the segments of the lower extremity in locomotion. J Bone Joint Surg Am 30:859, 1948.
12. Michelson JD, Clarke HJ, Jinnah RH: The effect of loading on tibiotalar alignment in cadaver ankle. Foot Ankle 10:280, 1990.
13. Procter P, Paul JP: Ankle joint biomechanics. J Biomech 15:627–634, 1983.
14. Ramsey PL, Hamilton W: Changes in tibiotalar area of contact caused by lateral talar shift. J Bone Joint Surg Am 58:356, 1976.
15. Sammarco GJ: Biomechanics of the foot. *In* Frankel VH, Nordin M (eds): Basic Biomechanics of the Skeletal System. Philadelphia, Lea & Febiger, 1980, p 193.
16. Sammarco GJ, Burstein AH, Frankel VH: Biomechanics of the ankle: a kinematic study. Orthop Clin North Am 4:75, 1973.
17. Sarrafian SK: Anatomy of the Foot and Ankle: Descriptive, Topographic, Functional. Philadelphia, JB Lippincott, 1993.
18. Seireg A, Arvikar RJ: A mathematical model for evaluation of forces in lower extremities of the musculoskeletal system. J Biomech 6:313–326, 1973.
19. Shereff MJ, Bejjani FJ, Kummer FJ: Kinematics of the first metatarsophalangeal joint. J Bone Joint Surg Am 68:392, 1986.
20. Snijders CJ, Snijder JGN, Philippens MMGM: Biomechanics of hallux valgus and spread foot. Foot Ankle 7:26, 1986.
21. Stauffer RN, Chao EYS, Brewster RC: Force and motion analysis of the normal, diseased, and prosthetic ankle joint. Clin Orthop 127:189, 1977.
22. Stormont DM, Morrey BF, An K-N, Cass JR: Stability of the loaded ankle: relation between articular restraint and primary and secondary static restraints. Am J Sports Med 13:295, 1985.
23. Wagner KS, Tarr RR, Resnick C, Sarmiento A: The effect of simulated tibial deformities on the ankle joint during the gait cycle. Foot Ankle 5:131, 1984.
24. Wyss U, McBride I, Murphy L, et al: Joint reaction forces at the first MTP joint in a normal elderly population [abstract]. J Biomech 21:863, 1988.
25. Yoshioka Y, Siu DW, Cooke TDV, et al: Geometry of the first metatarsophalangeal joint. J Orthop Res 6:878, 1988.

84

Prosthetic Intervention of the Great Toe

• NORMAN S. TURNER III and DONALD C. CAMPBELL II

Through a process of both gradual and rapid redesign, the art and science of joint replacement have evolved. Some joints lend themselves to replacement more readily than others. This may be due to differences in anatomic configuration, joint forces, functional demands, and the level of scientific understanding of the joint in question. In addition, when there are alternatives to replacement that give functional, if not ideal, results, then joint replacement will have to perform at a very high level to be a reliable alternative.

These issues are certainly prominent when considering the metatarsophalangeal joints. Most of the effort directed at these joints has involved the first metatarsophalangeal joint, but the lesser joints have not been ignored.

It should be emphasized at the outset that many complaints offered by patients with forefoot pain are a result of overuse, inappropriate or ill-fitting shoes, or dissatisfaction with the appearance of the foot. Although disorders of other joints may share these features, the foot is in a class of its own in this regard. Recognizing these factors, the surgeon must first exhaust all reasonable nonsurgical methods of treatment; this should include patient education, as well as the willingness to refuse surgery to a patient with unreasonable expectations. K. A. Johnson put it this way: "A disgruntled patient without a surgical scar is much better off than a disgruntled patient with a surgical scar."[19]

HISTORICAL PERSPECTIVE

In 1952, A. B. Swanson, serving as an army surgeon, developed a cobalt-chromium metal hemispherical cap with an intramedullary stem to replace the metatarsal head in cases of gunshot wounds to the foot.[46] The results were not satisfactory because of the rigidity of the material, shear stresses at the joint, and poor soft tissue tolerance.

In 1965, Swanson introduced a single-stemmed silicone hemi-replacement for the metatarsal head, but, because it was considered preferable to replace the "non–weight bearing side of the joint," a single-stemmed device to replace the base of the proximal phalanx was developed in 1967 (Fig. 84–1). This was intended to supplement the popular Keller resection arthroplasty.

In 1969, silicone finger joint implants became available, and some surgeons began using these for arthroplasty of the first metatarsophalangeal joint.[49] Breakage of these devices was a problem.

In 1974, high-performance silicone elastomer was introduced, with a 400-percent greater tear propagation resistance than the earlier material. At that time, a double-stemmed flexible hinge implant was designed to be used at the first metatarsophalangeal joint (Fig. 84–2). These devices have had problems with breakage, and Swanson et al. introduced metal collars (press-fit titanium grommets) to protect the silicone implant from the bone edges.[44] In addition, they introduced another hemi-arthroplasty implant with a medullary stem for the base of the proximal phalanx, constructed of titanium.

Kampner[21] reported on the use of another design of a silicone flexible-hinge implant with a Dacron sleeve. This sleeve improved fixation to the bone; however, silicone breakage was a problem. The stem was then redesigned with ribs to provide better fixation (Fig. 84–3). Sebold and Cracchiolo reported on a double-stemmed silicone implant with titanium grommets.[41] With intermediate follow-up, it was thought that these grommets would protect the silicone stems. There are other designs of silicone devices available, such as the silicone "ball spacers," which are a ball-shaped implant with stems to fit into the canals.[3,15]

In 1981, Johnson and Buck[20] reported the Mayo Clinic experience with a total joint replacement for the first metatarsophalangeal joint. This was an unconstrained, stemmed, cemented stainless steel and polyethylene device (Fig. 84–4). Because of difficulties with loosening and a greater than 50-percent incidence of radiolucent lines at the bone-cement interface, its use has been discontinued. Merkle and Sculco,[32] using a semiconstrained total joint implant, reported 63 percent unsatisfactory results with 54 percent loosening, and have likewise discontinued its use.

Blair and Brown,[1] in 1993, presented a new implant design with a nonconstraint, two-component total joint replacement. The implant is constructed of titanium, cobalt-chrome, and ultra-high-molecular-weight polyethylene. Currently, there are no clinical studies on this device.

In addition to the devices listed above, there have been scattered reports of various ingenious but largely

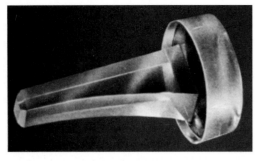

Figure 84–1. Silicone elastomer implant for the base of proximal phalanx of the hallux.

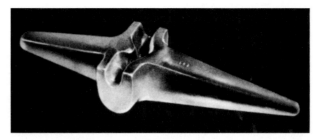

Figure 84–2. Silicone elastomer double-stemmed flexible hinged implant for the first metatarsophalangeal joint.

unproven caps and plugs that have been used for the metatarsophalangeal joints. Regnaud, in his 1986 textbook, refers to concave metal disks that are inserted into the joints as an interposition arthroplasty, then removed after 1 or 2 years.[38]

INDICATIONS

Considerable controversy surrounds the practice of replacement of the metatarsophalangeal joints. Some surgeons specializing in foot surgery use them rarely, if

at all. Others use them widely for a variety of indications. The literature offers occasional glimpses of a number of devices, but the most widely used and studied devices are the silicone elastomer implants. There is no unanimity of opinion regarding the usefulness or safety of these implants, as evidenced by the current literature. The manufacturer of the Swanson Silastic implants (Dow Corning Wright, Arlington, TN) distributes a booklet[46] outlining the characteristics and indications for that line of implants, citing a list of 126 references of which 124 are authored by Swanson. Each surgeon who proposes to treat patients with these devices should conduct a personal review of the literature to satisfy the

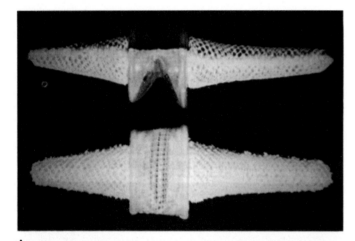

A

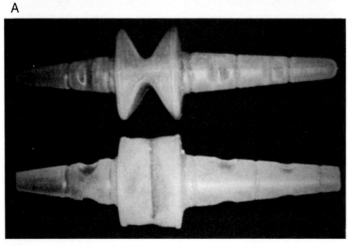

B

Figure 84–3. A, Silicone flexible hinge implant with Dacron sleeves. **B,** Silicone flexible hinged implant without Dacron sleeves.

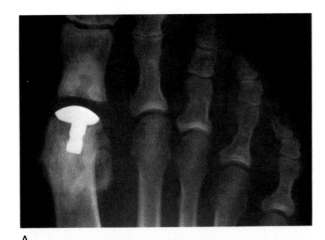

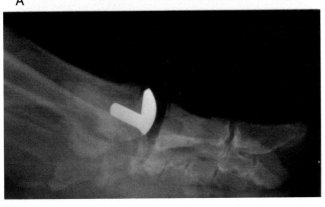

Figure 84–4. Anteroposterior (**A**) and lateral (**B**) radiographs of cemented unconstrained stainless steel and polyethylene total joint replacement designed by K. A. Johnson.

necessity of having a clear understanding of the indications, techniques, and potential problems.

Although various devices have been used in the lesser metatarsophalangeal joints, they have been even less well studied.[10] Cracchiolo et al.[8] reported experience with silicone implant arthroplasty of the second metatarsophalangeal joint in which a variety of other procedures were done concomitantly. In rheumatoid arthritis, double-stemmed hinged silicone implants have been used in the lesser metatarsophalangeal joints, but there are no comparative studies to demonstrate an advantage over other methods. Satisfaction remains high in patients treated without implants. The value of silicone implants in the second as well as the other metatarsophalangeal joints is not established. For this reason, only the first metatarsophalangeal joint is addressed in the remainder of this chapter.

Hemi-Arthroplasty

Because of the high rate of failure with these devices, the indications are limited. Consideration could be given to a patient with arthritis of the metatarsophalangeal joint with preservation of the contour of the metatarsal head, if that patient is elderly and relatively inactive. In such

circumstances, the alternatives to the use of an implant are usually more attractive.

Double-Stemmed Hinged Implant Arthroplasty

Indications include osteoarthritis of the first metatarsophalangeal joint, with or without hallux valgus, or failure of other procedures resulting in damage to the joint and perhaps bone loss as well. The patient must have expectations that can reasonably be met and be aware of the possible long-term problems. The patient must be cooperative, not only in the immediate postoperative period but for the long term as well. Finally, the performance of the operation must be within the surgeon's ability.

PHYSICAL EXAMINATION

Examination of the foot is essential to the development of a successful surgical plan. Palpating the pulses of the foot and ankle each time a patient's foot is handled is an excellent habit to cultivate. At the same time, one can acquire an opinion as to temperature and skin quality, noting the presence of hair or of scars that might indicate previous problems with wound healing. In addition, this technique allows the physician to reassure an anxious patient that the examination will be thorough and gentle. Once an overall assessment is made, attention may be directed to the deformity in question or to the area of patient complaint.

The flexibility of all joints should be assessed, not only the symptomatic ones. In the case of the metatarsophalangeal joints, the range of motion, the stability of the joints, and the ease with which any deformity may be passively corrected are noted. Osteophytes should be noted, recognizing that they may be a block to normal motion.

One should be especially alert to the presence of infection. This may be obvious, as in the case of a draining wound, or subtle, as in the situation of a mild ingrown nail with purulence that is seen only with elevation of the nail edge.

Finally, the physician must be aware of other musculoskeletal abnormalities that may have an impact on the results of foot surgery. Spinal deformities, hip joint disorders, genu varum or valgum, leg length inequalities, calf muscle tightness or contracture, ankle instability, pes planus or cavus, or deformities related to malunited fractures all should be noted. These problems may cause significant alteration in the manner in which forces are applied to the metatarsophalangeal joints.

RADIOGRAPHIC EXAMINATION

Standing anteroposterior and lateral radiographs as well as an oblique projection will allow adequate assessment of the angular deformities and the status of the joint. Overall bone quality should be noted. Abnormalities in joints other than the first metatarsophalangeal should be noted; this may have an important bearing on the overall treatment plan.

SURGICAL TECHNIQUE: DOUBLE-STEMMED HINGED IMPLANT

A thigh or calf tourniquet is applied. The first metatarsophalangeal joint is exposed through a straight medial incision (Fig. 84–5).[7] By keeping tension on the skin, the incision may be easily made through the skin without jeopardizing the cutaneous sensory nerves. Careful dissection will allow visualization of the capsule, which is incised longitudinally. It is important not to detach too much capsule from the metatarsal or from the proximal phalanx. An appropriate size of trial implant will assist in judging where to cut the metatarsal head. Cracchiolo[6] advises caution in making this cut in order to preserve the portion of metatarsal head that articulates with the sesamoids when the toe is in neutral position.

A broach or bur is then used to enter and enlarge the medullary canal of the metatarsal and proximal phalanx. The bone should be contoured to match the shape of the implant. Metal grommets are available for some devices to protect the implant from abrasion by the cut bone edges.[44]

Trial reduction will allow the surgeon to decide whether the alignment and tension are adequate. Release of the lateral capsule and common adductor tendon may be needed. In cases of severe hallux valgus with metatarsus primus varus, osteotomy at the base of the metatarsal may be required to properly align the metatarsophalangeal joint.

In order to avoid damage to the implant, it must be handled carefully, using blunt instruments. Careful closure is critical in order to maintain capsular integrity and the corrected alignment, and also to minimize wound complications. The abductor hallucis tendon may be advanced and incorporated into the capsular repair if needed. A drain should be left in the wound. Forceps should not be used on the skin edges, and care must be exercised to avoid injuring a cutaneous nerve during the skin closure. A gentle compression bandage should be applied in such a way that it helps to maintain and protect the corrected alignment.

Aftercare

Strict elevation of the foot should be maintained during the first 24 hours, at which time the drain is removed. The dressing may be changed then or in 3 or 4 days. In general, weight bearing may be permitted after the first day but should be minimized during the first 2 weeks. Some surgeons[15,37] recommend a splint, which maintains the corrected hallux valgus but allows flexion and extension. This is to be used for about 1 month, in combination with a wooden-soled postoperative shoe. Patients who have had an osteotomy for the first metatarsal must be cautioned against full weight bearing in the early period and may require a cast for 4 to 8 weeks.

RESULTS

In a 1979 report, Swanson et al.[45] reviewed 165 feet treated with the single-stemmed implant and 105 feet treated with the double-stemmed flexible hinged implant. In the single-stemmed group, indications were hallux rigidus, hallux valgus with osteoarthritis, rheumatoid arthritis, and failed previous surgery, such as McBride, Keller, or arthrodesis procedures. The hallux rigidus patients "were uniformly free of pain and satisfied with the cosmetic and functional results." The hallux valgus patients "stated they were free of pain and very pleased with the result." The nature of patient satisfaction is not reported, but recurrent hallux valgus was a problem, causing the author to advise use of the double-stemmed implant in this group. Only one patient, in the group with hallux valgus with osteoarthritis, experienced an inflammatory reaction to the implant, and this resolved over a 4-week period. In the double-stemmed group, all patients were reportedly free of pain postoperatively, although one patient had the implant removed because of infection.

Kampner,[21] using a silicone double-stemmed device of slightly different design from that of Swanson, reported a series of 130 implants in the first metatarsophalangeal joint in 98 patients, with 12 months' minimum follow-up. Excellent or good relief of pain was noted in 81.5 percent of patients, while 73 percent were satisfied with the cosmetic result. There were 11 implant fractures, all but one occurring in devices with Dacron sleeves. The author considered rheumatoid arthritis to be a relative contraindication because these patients had poorer results. This was largely attributed to the loss of the "buttressing or stabilizing effect that the lesser toes have" on the hallux following metatarsophalangeal joint resection. As a result, the hallux tends to drift into valgus, causing increased tensile stresses in the hinge of the implant. Seven of the 11 implant fractures were in such patients.

Swanson et al.[44] reported satisfactory results using a grommet bone liner for flexible hinged implant arthroplasty of 90 first metatarsophalangeal joints, with "favorable bone response" around the implant stems and at the bone-grommet interface. Most of the patients were pain free, with excellent functional results. There were no complications caused by particulate reactivity, implant fracture, or grommet fracture.

Hetherington et al.[16] reported results with 19 first metatarsophalangeal implants. Within an average time of follow-up of 5.9 years, complications were noted radiographically as implant deformation, bony erosions, and bony encroachment. Postoperative clinical evaluation revealed that several of the patients complained of pain and stiffness. Despite the clinical objective findings, patient satisfaction was very favorable.

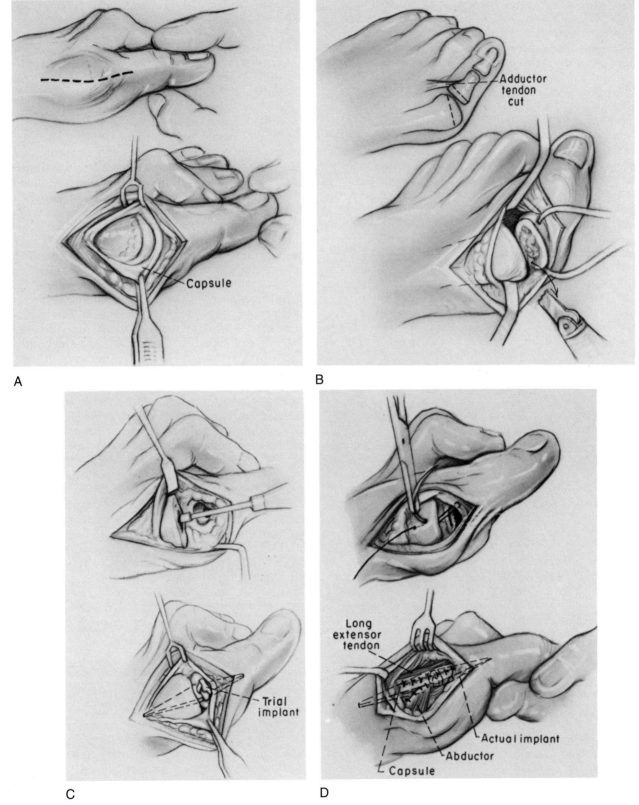

Figure 84–5. A, A standard medial surgical approach is made to the first metatarsophalangeal joint. **B**, In the case of hallux valgus, the adductor tendon is divided. The base of the proximal phalanx and the distal part of the metatarsal head is resected with a small surgical saw. **C**, The medullary canals of the metatarsal and proximal phalanx are prepared to receive the trial implant. **D**, Care is taken with the capsular closure. The joint must be balanced. The abductor hallucis tendon may be useful in achieving this goal. (Modified from Cracchiolo A III: Prosthetic arthroplasty of the hallux. In Evarts CM [ed]: Surgery of the Musculoskeletal System, 2nd ed. New York, Churchill Livingstone, 1990, p 4113.)

Moeckel et al.[34] reported their results in 67 feet of 45 patients who had rheumatoid arthritis and were followed for an average of 6 years (range 4 to 10 years). The forefoot operation included resection of the metatarsophalangeal heads or joints and the insertion of a double-stemmed silicone rubber implant in the first metatarsophalangeal joint. There were 42 women and 3 men, and the average age at the time of the operation was 56 years (range 36 to 79 years). Resection of the metatarsophalangeal heads or joints was performed through a plantar approach in 41 feet and a dorsal approach in 26 feet. A double-stemmed silicone rubber implant was placed in the first metatarsophalangeal joint in all feet. A good or excellent result was obtained in 58 feet (87 percent). Complications were infrequent. In three feet there was delayed healing of the wound, three implants were removed because of dislocation and infection, and four feet had revision to correct deformities of the lesser toes.

Cracchiolo et al.[9] reported detailed results in 66 patients who had a total of 86 double-stemmed silicone implants in the first metatarsophalangeal joint and were followed prospectively for an average of 5.8 years (range 2 to 15 years). There were two groups of patients: 34 patients (37 implants) who had degenerative joint disease and 32 patients (49 implants) who had rheumatoid arthritis. The implants were used only if the patient was a candidate for an excisional arthroplasty or an arthrodesis; they were not used in patients who wished to maintain or adopt very active use of the foot or to wear very high heels. Twenty-eight (82 percent) of the 34 patients in the first group were completely satisfied and 3 (9 percent) were somewhat satisfied. However, three patients (9 percent), all of whom had had a failed bunionectomy before the implant surgery, were dissatisfied; the ages of these three patients were less than the average age of all patients in the first group. Radiographs showed a fracture in three implants, but the patients had a good clinical result and an additional operation was not warranted. Twenty-seven (84 percent) of the 32 patients in the second group were completely satisfied, 4 (13 percent) were somewhat satisfied, and 1 (3 percent) was dissatisfied. Radiographs showed a fracture in five implants. Four of the fractures caused no symptoms and the result was good; the fifth one was fragmented and was removed because of symptoms. Radiographs showed radiolucent areas around the implant and hypertrophic changes in many patients. There was no evidence of synovitis, such as that caused by silicone, either clinically or radiographically. The authors found the double-stemmed silicone implant to be effective in reconstructing the first metatarsophalangeal joint but emphasized that it should be used only in carefully selected patients.

Granberry et al.[13] reported a series of 90 consecutive total joint replacements of the first metatarsophalangeal joint with a flexible hinged prosthesis within an average duration of follow-up of 3 years. Although subjectively the results were satisfactory in most of the patients, and pain, the most common preoperative symptom, was reduced, mechanical failure of the implant was common as determined radiographically. The range of motion of the metatarsophalangeal joint was decreased from nor-mal. Dorsiflexion averaged 26 degrees and plantar flexion 18 degrees. Callosities under at least one metatarsophalangeal joint were noted in 50 (69 percent) of the feet that had a physical examination. Pedobarographic analysis of the distribution of plantar pressure revealed that none of the patients exerted weight-bearing pressures on the affected great toe. However, the subjective results were not significantly associated with radiographic evidence of failure of the implant. Despite its success in relieving the symptoms of patients, the authors did not recommend this procedure because of the high and increasing rate of failure of the implant, as demonstrated radiographically.

In 1995, Shankar reported a series of 36 patients with 40 Silastic single-stemmed implants for hallux rigidus.[42] The average age of the patients was 54 years, with 110-month follow-up. "The majority of the patients were satisfied with the results in the short term." However, at the time of review, 36 percent were not satisfied with the results. Twenty-five feet had complete pain relief. The average range of motion was 20 degrees of dorsiflexion and 12 degrees of plantar flexion. On radiographic follow-up, 42.5 percent of the implants had evidence of fragmentation. Six implants were removed. The conclusion was that "the results in the long term are not acceptable and other options should be considered."

In rheumatoid arthritic patients, Clayton et al. compared silicone double-hinged implants without grommets in the great toe and resection of the metatarsal heads and pinning to resection arthroplasty with a medial capsular arthroplasty in the great toe and plantar plate arthroplasty of the lesser toes.[4] Thirty feet were treated in the nonimplant group and 49 feet in the implant group. The average follow-up was 75.8 months in the implant group versus 44.7 months in the nonimplant group. Patient satisfaction for appearance was 88 percent in the nonimplant group and 78 percent in the implant group. Functional results were comparable between the two groups. Mild to no pain was reported in 67 percent of the implant group and 88 percent of the nonimplant group. The overall results were good and comparable for the two groups and equal to the published results of arthrodesis combined with rheumatoid forefoot procedure.

COMPLICATIONS

The complications include infection, breakage of implant (Fig. 84–6), implant fragmentation and medullary lysis, cortical osteophytic proliferation, recurrence of hallux valgus, and synovitis, which can be associated with lymphadenopathy.[11] Also, implant wear with osteolysis that results in great toe shortening has been reported.[48]

Another complication is a stress fracture of the lateral metatarsals, possibly caused by an overloading of the lateral metatarsals secondary to some shortening of the hallux metatarsal or to re-establishing motion to the hallux metatarsophalangeal joint. Kitaoka and Cracchiolo[23] reported a 3-percent incidence of lateral metatarsal

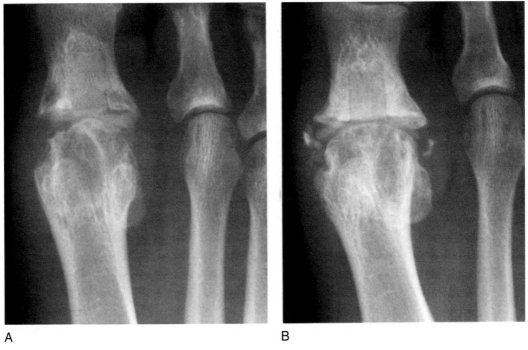

A   B

Figure 84–6. (**A** and **B**) Typical wear and breakage pattern with silicone elastomer hemi-arthroplasty in a patient with bilateral implants.

stress fracture during the first year following use of a double-stemmed silicone implant.

BIOCOMPATIBILITY

In Swanson and colleagues 1987 report[47] of 103 cases, reactive synovitis was noted in 4, 3 of which were revised. In two of the cases the implant had fractured. In the other there was bony overgrowth and the midsection of the implant was abraded. Numerous authors have reported experience with silicone implants without worrisome reaction to the material.[6,8,12,21,35]

There are several reports of problems related to silicone implants, especially the hemi-arthroplasties. Shereff and Jahss[43] presented a series of seven cases, five of which failed. Three of these were Swanson single-stemmed implants that, at revision, showed bone resorption at the bone-implant interface. Lemon et al.[26] described seven cases of inflammation following hemi-arthroplasty in six patients in whom the implants were removed and synovial biopsies were performed. Histologic examination revealed foreign body giant cell reaction with phagocytosis of silicone elastomer debris. The implants all revealed erosion of the articular surface (Fig. 84–7). Jasim and Weerasinghe[17] described four patients in a series of 215 implants who developed silicone lymphadenopathy, synovitis, and osteitis. Worsing et al.[50] made similar observations and demonstrated in an animal model that it is the particulate silicone material that provokes the response. Sammarco and Tabatowski[40] reported a case of ipsilateral femoral lymphadenopathy 3 years after replacement of a first metatarsophalangeal joint with silicone prosthesis in a

tennis player. The implant was noted to have failed. Fine-needle aspiration of the lymph node revealed a foreign body giant cell reaction to particulates morphologically compatible with silicone elastomer.

Mayo Clinic Experience

The results of the first metatarsophalangeal implant arthroplasty operations performed at Mayo Clinic between 1971 and 1986 have been reported.[36] Overall, 93 primary first metatarsophalangeal implant arthroplasty

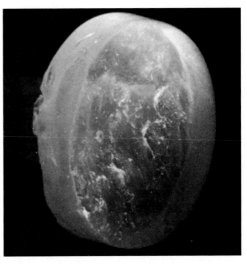

Figure 84–7. Close-up view of silicone elastomer hemi-joint implant showing eroded articular surface.

operations were performed in 79 patients (12 male and 67 female) with a mean age of 56 years (range 19 to 75 years). Fourteen were bilateral. The preoperative underlying diagnosis was hallux valgus in 22, hallux rigidus in 38, inflammatory arthritis in 32, and avascular necrosis of the metatarsal head in 1 foot. Twenty-four feet (26 percent) had previous operations of the first metatarsophalangeal joint, such as hallux valgus operation (13 feet), cheilectomy (4 feet), and resection arthroplasty (7 feet). Four types of implants were used: a single-stemmed silicone prosthesis (Dow Corning Wright) in 36 feet; a double-stemmed hinged silicone prosthesis (Dow Corning Wright) in 27 feet; a cemented stainless steel and polyethylene Johnson prosthesis (DePuy Orthopaedics) in 27 feet; and the cemented stainless steel and polyethylene Richards prosthesis in 3 feet.

At the last follow-up, 13 feet (14 percent) underwent reoperation and were considered failures. Clinical examination or interview was available for 75 feet in patients who were alive and without reoperation. Follow-up averaged 12 years (range 2 to 17 years). The overall probability that an implant would not have been removed 10 years after the arthroplasty was 86 percent, and at 15 years after arthroplasty was 82 percent (Fig. 84–8). No effect has been shown on implant survival of preoperative diagnosis, gender, relative weight, previous operation, and type of implant. Younger age was significantly related to poorer implant survival ($P < 0.03$). Patients 58 years or younger had a lower implant survival at 10 years (82 percent) compared to patients who were older than 58 years (90 percent).

Postoperatively, pain was present in 26 feet (35 percent). Including the 13 failed procedures, this makes 39 feet with pain (44 percent). Fifty feet (66.6 percent) had no functional restriction. Acceptable alignment was present in 35 feet (47 percent). Overall, the patients considered their response to surgery as worse in 3 feet (4 percent), the same in 13 feet (17 percent), improved in 30 feet (40 percent), and much improved in 29 feet (39 percent). Including the 13 failures, only 67 percent of feet were improved by surgery.

Objective Measurements

There was no significant difference in the total range of motion of the first metatarsophalangeal joint before surgery (24 degrees) and at the last follow-up (31 degrees).[36] The lateral metatarsophalangeal angle before surgery was 17 degrees and postoperatively was 29 degrees, which was a significant difference ($P < 0.0001$, paired t-test) and indicated the tendency for hallux extensus deformity to develop. The ratio of the first ray to second metatarsal length changed from 1.23 in the immediate postoperative radiographs to an average of 1.14 in the radiographs obtained at the last follow-up, indicating the significant degree of shortening that occurred after arthroplasty.

Bone resorption was present around the silicone implant, at the phalangeal and/or metatarsal level, in 13 feet. There was evidence of cyst formation in three feet. In eight feet (25 percent), there was evidence of severe silicone implant wear or deformation, with fracture of the implant in one case (Fig. 84–9). Definite loosening of the phalangeal and/or metatarsal cemented component was present in 57 percent. Definite migration of the phalangeal cemented component was present in 31 percent and definite migration of the metatarsal component in 31 percent (Fig. 84–10). A complete radiolucent zone was recognized at the bone-cement interface in 40 percent of feet at the phalangeal side and 10 percent of feet at the metatarsal side. Superficial infection occurred in four feet and deep infection in one foot (5 percent) (see Fig. 84–9). Plantar forefoot pain attributed to transfer metatarsalgia occurred in 10 feet. A lesser metatarsal stress fracture occurred in two feet. Implant dislocation occurred in six feet (6 percent).

Fifteen feet underwent reoperation: implant removal and synovectomy in nine feet, implant removal and

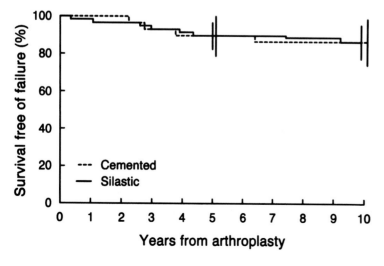

Figure 84–8. Survivorship analysis of first metatarsophalangeal joint arthroplasty with 95 percent confidence interval, according to type of implant. (From Papagelopoulos PJ, Kitaoka HB, Ilstrup DM: Survivorship analysis of implant arthroplasty for the first metatarsophalangeal joint. Clin Orthop 302:164, 1994.)

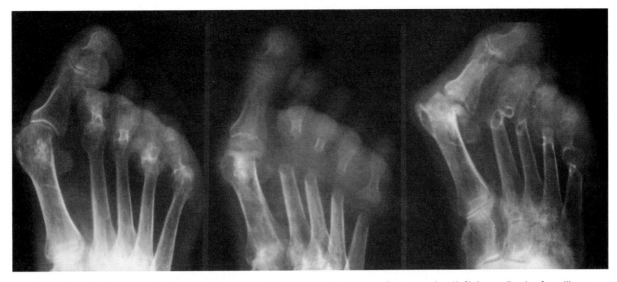

Figure 84–9. Radiographs of a 64-year-old woman with rheumatoid arthritis before operation (*left*), immediately after silicone implant arthroplasty with a hinged prosthesis (*middle*), and 5 years postoperatively (*right*). Note the implant deformation and fracture of the proximal stem of the implant with recurrence of the hallux valgus. Patient experienced a late deep infection and underwent component removal and arthrodesis. (From Papagelopoulos PJ, Kitaoka HB, Ilstrup DM: Survivorship analysis of implant arthroplasty for the first metatarsophalangeal joint. Clin Orthop 302:164, 1994.)

arthrodesis in two feet, and revision implant arthroplasty in two feet. One patient with a superficial infection was treated with débridement and another had a capsular release; in both cases the implants remained in situ and were not considered failures.[36]

REVISION PROCEDURES

In the event of failure of implant arthroplasty of the first metatarsophalangeal joint, there are a limited number of salvage options available. Usually removal of the device

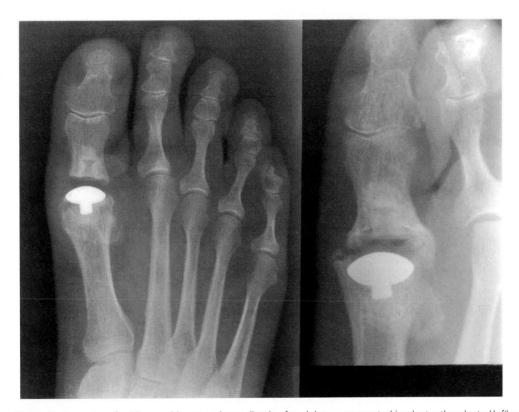

Figure 84–10. Radiographs of a 57-year-old woman immediately after Johnson cemented implant arthroplasty (*left*) and 15 years postoperatively (*right*). Patient was satisfied with the results. Note the subsidence of the metatarsal component with bony impingement medially and laterally. (From Papagelopoulos PJ, Kitaoka HB, Ilstrup DM: Survivorship analysis of implant arthroplasty for the first metatarsophalangeal joint. Clin Orthop 302:164, 1994.)

results in a resection arthroplasty, which may give a satisfactory result without other surgery.

Implant removal and synovectomy were used to treat the failure of 14 first metatarsophalangeal joint implant arthroplasties an average of 3.1 years after arthroplasty.[24] Follow-up of 5 years in 10 patients revealed excellent outcomes in 7 patients, good in 1 patient, fair in 1 patient, and poor in 1 patient. No significant changes in alignment occurred, although a trend toward toe extension was noted. Dynamic force plate studies in these patients demonstrated less pressure under the first metatarsal head and greater loading under the lateral forefoot. The great toe had less contact time during gait in the involved feet than in the control feet.

Koenig[25] presented a 3-year study of 10 cases of revision arthroplasty utilizing the Biomet Total Toe System. The procedure is performed to eliminate pain and restore function in cases of metatarsophalangeal joint silicone elastomer implant failure.

Arthrodesis remains a possibility, although it will be more difficult to accomplish because the medullary bone has been removed and bone has been resected from the joint. Therefore, arthrodesis may be slow to unite, and the result will be significant shortening of the toe. An alternative approach is interpositional bone grafting, in which a large corticocancellous graft is shaped to fit the space previously occupied by the implant. Fixation is very important. Coughlin and Mann[5] recommended double heavy-threaded Steinmann pins, placed axially through the hallux into the metatarsal head. Plate-and-screw fixation can be effective (Fig. 84–11). Hecht et al. reported 15 feet with a symptomatic silicone implant that underwent arthrodesis.[14] Bone graft (10 tricortical bone graft) was used in all patients, and fixation included Steinmann pins and plate-and-screw fixation. Thirteen of the feet went on to radiographic fusion. Patients noted improvement in pain, function, and appearance. There were no infections, and one patient developed a painful neuroma. This was considered to be a better alternative to resection arthroplasty in the active patient. Brodsky et al. presented 12 feet that were salvaged with first metatarsophalangeal arthrodesis with tricortical iliac crest graft with a 22-month follow-up.[2] Eight of these feet were the result of failed implants. Clinical arthrodesis was obtained in 11 feet in an average of 12 weeks. All but one patient had minimal or occasional activity pain. No patient had complete pain relief. There were three major complications. Two patients required skin flap for infection and skin necrosis. One patient developed a painless nonunion.

Finally, if revision is being performed because of implant breakage, it may be possible to simply remove the broken implant and insert a new one.

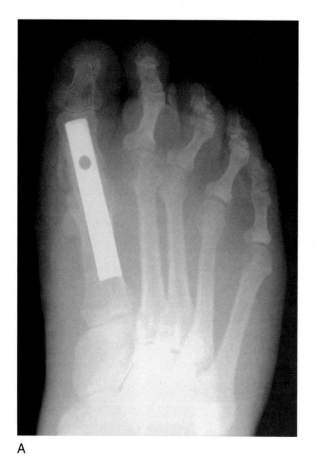

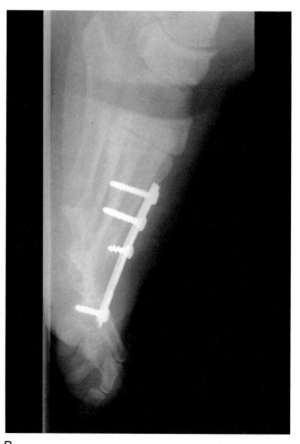

A   B

Figure 84–11. First metatarsophalangeal joint arthrodesis with interpositional iliac bone graft utilizing plate-and-screw fixation.

SUMMARY

Reports of implant arthroplasty of the metatarsophalangeal joints show a wide range of results, especially if hemi-arthroplasties are included. Excluding these, the results compare favorably with resection arthroplasty or arthrodesis. Raunio et al.[37] compared similar groups of patients with resection arthroplasty and arthrodesis of the first metatarsophalangeal joint. Roughly 80 percent of patients in both groups were satisfied. In the arthrodesis group, if one excludes the patients fused in more than 35 degrees or less than 20 degrees of extension from the floor plane, the satisfaction rate would be clearly higher. In the lesser metatarsophalangeal joints, implants may be an alternative, but their value in this role remains unclear. The patient's activity level may be a very important factor, but little has been reported regarding the *intensity* of activity following implant arthroplasty. The surgeon must question the patient regarding expectations, especially for strenuous occupational, vocational, or athletic activities. Finally, evidence of silicone lymphadenopathy in patients with these devices must signal caution in their use.

AUTHORS' PREFERENCE

Implant arthroplasty of the forefoot is a subject that generates strong opinions, attitudes, and feelings. Some practitioners have developed reputations for applying very liberal indications for the use of implants. For an orthopedist practicing in a referral center, the abuses and problems may be seen in a disproportionate number. Nevertheless, there is an obvious message. First, conservative, nonsurgical treatment must be stressed initially. Second, the surgeon must be certain that the patient's expectations are reasonable, and can likely be met by the proposed surgery. Third, the decision to implant a device must be based on scientific knowledge and sound, well-documented, clinical experience. The manufacturer and its representative cannot always be expected to provide unbiased information or recommendations.

At present at the Mayo Clinic, metatarsophalangeal implants are much more commonly removed than inserted.[24] Most of the joints removed have been hemi-arthroplasties, all of which either have shown severe abrasion or have been actually fragmented. Reports of silicone lymphadenopathy in such patients are worrisome, especially in view of our ignorance of the long-term consequences of this phenomenon. These devices should no longer be used, their manufacture should be stopped, and existing devices should be recalled. Double-stemmed devices appear to have more to offer, particularly in the patient who will make only mild demands on the foot.

Until independent clinical studies support the use of an implantable device, great caution should be exercised in its application. Improving our skills in the performance of established treatment methods will yield better results for most of our patients, without the problems currently inherent in implant techniques. Currently there is not a reliable implant on the market; therefore, reconstructive options without prosthetic devices are recommended.

References

1. Blair MP, Brown LA: Hallux limitus/rigidus deformity: a new great toe implant. J Foot Ankle Surg 32:257–262, 1993.
2. Brodsky JW, Ptaszek AM, Morris SG: Salvage first MTP arthrodesis utilizing ICBG: clinical evaluation and outcome. Foot Ankle Int 21:290–296, 2000.
3. Broughton NS, Doran A, Meggitt BF: Silastic ball spacer arthroplasty in the management of hallux valgus and hallux rigidus. Foot Ankle 10:61, 1989.
4. Clayton ML, Leidholt JD, Clark W: Arthroplasty of rheumatoid metatarsophalangeal joints. Clin Orthop 340:48–57, 1997.
5. Coughlin MJ, Mann RA: Arthrodesis of the first metatarsophalangeal joint as salvage for the failed Keller procedure. J Bone Joint Surg Am 69:68, 1987.
6. Cracchiolo A III: Management of the arthritic forefoot. Foot Ankle 3:17, 1982.
7. Cracchiolo A III: Prosthetic arthroplasty of the hallux. In Evarts CM (ed): Surgery of the Musculoskeletal System, 2nd ed. New York, Churchill Livingstone, 1990, p 4113.
8. Cracchiolo A III, Kitaoka HB, Leventen EO: Silicone implant arthroplasty for second metatarsophalangeal joint disorders with and without hallux valgus deformities. Foot Ankle 9:10, 1989.
9. Cracchiolo A III, Weltmer JB Jr, Lian G, Dorey F: Arthroplasty of the first metatarsophalangeal joint with a double-stem silicone implant: results in patients who have degenerative joint disease, failure of previous operations, or rheumatoid arthritis. J Bone Joint Surg Am 74:552, 1992.
10. Fox IM, Pro AL: Lesser metatarsophalangeal joint implants. J Foot Surg 26:159, 1987.
11. Freed JB: The increasing recognition of medullary lysis, cortical osteophytic proliferation, and fragmentation of implanted silicone polymer implants. J Foot Ankle Surg 32:171, 1993.
12. Gould N: Surgery of the forepart of the foot in rheumatoid arthritis. Foot Ankle 3:173, 1982.
13. Granberry WM, Noble PC, Bishop JO, Tullos HS: Use of a hinged silicone prosthesis for replacement arthroplasty of the first metatarsophalangeal joint. J Bone Joint Surg Am 73:1453, 1991.
14. Hecht PJ, Gibbons MJ, Wapner KL, et al: Arthrodesis of the first metatarsophalangeal joint to salvage failed silicone implant arthroplasty. Foot Ankle Int 18:383–390, 1997.
15. Helal B, Gibb P: Freiberg's disease: a suggested pattern of management. Foot Ankle 8:94, 1987.
16. Hetherington VJ, Mercado C, Karloc L, Grillo J: Silicone implant arthroplasty: a retrospective analysis. J Foot Ankle Surg 32:430, 1993.
17. Jasim KA, Weerasinghe BD: Silicone lymphadenopathy, synovitis and osteitis complicating big toe Silastic prostheses. J R Coll Surg Edinb 32:29, 1987.
18. Johansson JE, Barrington TW: Cone arthrodesis of the first metatarsophalangeal joint. Foot Ankle 4:245, 1984.
19. Johnson KA: Surgery of the Foot and Ankle. New York, Raven Press, 1989, p 35.
20. Johnson KA, Buck PG: Total replacement arthroplasty of the first metatarsophalangeal joint. Foot Ankle 1:307, 1981.
21. Kampner SL: Long-term experience with total joint prosthetic replacement for the arthritic great toe. Bull Hosp Joint Dis 47:153, 1987.
22. Keller WL: The surgical treatment of bunions and hallux valgus. N Y Med J 80:741, 1904.
23. Kitaoka HB, Cracchiolo A III: Stress fracture of the lateral metatarsals following double-stem silicone implant arthroplasty of the hallux metatarsophalangeal joint. Clin Orthop Rel Res 239:211, 1989.
24. Kitaoka HB, Holiday AD Jr, Chao EY, Cahalan TD: Salvage of failed first metatarsophalangeal joint implant arthroplasty by

implant removal and synovectomy: clinical and biomechanical evaluation. Foot Ankle 13:243, 1992.

25. Koenig RD: Revision arthroplasty utilizing the Biomet Total Toe System for failed silicone elastomer implants. J Foot Ankle Surg 33:222, 1994.

26. Lemon RA, Engber WD, McBeath AA: A complication of Silastic hemiarthroplasty in bunion surgery. Foot Ankle 4:262, 1984.

27. Mann RA, Clanton TO: Hallux rigidus: treatment by cheilectomy. J Bone Joint Surg Am 70:400, 1988.

28. Mann RA, Coughlin MJ: Hallux valgus and complications of hallux valgus. *In* Mann RA (ed): Surgery of the Foot, 5th ed. St. Louis: CV Mosby, 1986, p 65.

29. Mann RA, Thompson FM: Arthrodesis of the first metatarsophalangeal joint for hallux valgus in rheumatoid arthritis. J Bone Joint Surg Am 66:687, 1984.

30. McGarvey SR, Johnson KA: Keller arthroplasty in combination with resection arthroplasty of the lesser metatarsophalangeal joints in rheumatoid arthritis. Foot Ankle 9:75, 1988.

31. McKeever DC: Arthrodesis of the first metatarsophalangeal joint for hallux valgus, hallux rigidus, and metatarsus primus varus. J Bone Joint Surg Am 34:129, 1952.

32. Merkle PF, Sculco TP: Prosthetic replacement of the first metatarsophalangeal joint. Foot Ankle 9:267, 1989.

33. Moberg E: A simple operation for hallux rigidus. Clin Orthop 142:55, 1979.

34. Moeckel BH, Sculco TP, Alexiades MM, et al: The double-stemmed silicone-rubber implant for rheumatoid arthritis of the first metatarsophalangeal joint: long-term results. J Bone Joint Surg Am 74:564, 1992.

35. Molster OA, Lunde OD, Rait M: Hallux rigidus treated with the Swanson Silastic hemi-joint prosthesis. Acta Orthop Scand 51:853, 1980.

36. Papagelopoulos PJ, Kitaoka HB, Ilstrup DM: Survivorship analysis of implant arthroplasty for the first metatarsophalangeal joint. Clin Orthop 302:164, 1994.

37. Raunio P, Lehtimäki M, Eerola M, et al: Resection arthroplasty versus arthrodesis of the first metatarsophalangeal joint for hallux valgus in rheumatoid arthritis. Rheumatology 11:173, 1987.

38. Regnaud B: The Foot. Berlin, Springer-Verlag, 1986.

39. Riggs S, Johnson E: McKeever arthrodesis for the painful hallux. Foot Ankle 3:248, 1983.

40. Sammarco GJ, Tabatowski K: Silicone lymphadenopathy associated with failed prosthesis of the hallux: a case report and literature review. Foot Ankle 13:273, 1992.

41. Sebold EJ, Cracchiolo A: Use of titanium grommets in silicone implant arthroplasty of the hallux metatarsophalangeal joint. Foot Ankle Int 17:145–151, 1996.

42. Shankar NS: Silastic single-stem implants in the treatment of hallux rigidus. Foot Ankle Int 16:487–491, 1995.

43. Shereff MJ, Jahss MH: Complications of Silastic implant arthroplasty in the hallux. Foot Ankle 1:95, 1980.

44. Swanson AB, de Groot Swanson G, Maupin BK: The use of a grommet bone liner for flexible hinge implant arthroplasty of the great toe. Foot Ankle 12:149, 1991.

45. Swanson AB, Lumsden RM, Swanson DG: Silicone implant arthroplasty of the great toe. Clin Orthop Rel Res 142:30, 1979.

46. Swanson AB, Swanson DG: Treatment Considerations and Resource Materials for Flexible (Silicone) Implant Arthroplasty. Arlington, TN, Dow Corning Wright, 1987.

47. Swanson AB, Swanson DG, Mayhew DE, Khan AN: Flexible hinge results in implant arthroplasty of the great toe. Rheumatology 11:136, 1987.

48. Verhaar J, Bulstra S, Walenkamp G: Silicone arthroplasty for hallux rigidus: implant wear and osteolysis. Acta Orthop Scand 60:30–33, 1989.

49. Wenger RJJ, Whalley RC: Total replacement of the first metatarsophalangeal joint. J Bone Joint Surg Br 60:88, 1978.

50. Worsing RA Jr, Engber WD, Lange TA: Reactive synovitis from particulate Silastic. J Bone Joint Surg Am 64:581, 1982.

85

Ankle Replacement Arthroplasty

• HAROLD B. KITAOKA and RICHARD J. CLARIDGE

Following the outstanding success of hip replacement surgery in the 1970s, implant arthroplasty of the ankle was developed to offer the advantages of replacement arthroplasty to patients with end-stage ankle disease. Joint débridement offered limited benefits in established ankle arthritis. With techniques popular at that time, ankle arthrodesis could be difficult to achieve, with nonunion in up to 40 percent of cases[1,15,24,34,37,45] and overall complication rates between 34 and 60 percent.[36] The stage was set for an alternative to ankle arthrodesis. Replacement arthroplasty of the ankle seemed to fill this need.

Ankle replacement is most applicable in elderly patients with more sedentary lifestyles. It has the potential of providing pain relief while preserving joint motion. The implant must withstand unusually large compressive, shear, and rotatory forces across a relatively small area at the ankle level. Although a spectrum of designs have been used, most utilize metal alloy and high-density polyethylene components.

HISTORY OF ANKLE REPLACEMENT

Early Ankle Implant Designs

Early designs varied with respect to their ability to resist torsion and displacement forces, with relatively unconstrained or multiaxial types such as the Smith, Newton, and Waugh devices (Fig. 85–1) and more constrained types such as the ICLH, Mayo, Oregon, St. George-Buchholz, Conoidal, Conaxial, and TPR devices (Figs. 85–2 and 85–3).[6,7,11,33,35,44] There are advantages to each design type. Unconstrained devices allow for motion in multiple axes (flexion and extension, inversion and eversion, and rotation). Stress distribution may be better than in the more constrained devices. The unconstrained types, however, tend to be less stable and may therefore lead to problems such as impingement medially and laterally against the malleoli. Constrained devices are less prone to subluxate and may provide better protection against malleolar fractures or ligament rupture resulting from torsional stresses, but problems with implant failure and loosening occur because greater torque is transferred to the bone-cement-prosthesis interfaces with cyclic torsional loads.[47,49]

Efforts to address the recognized problems of impingement include resurfacing of the malleoli (e.g., Oregon ankle), resection arthroplasty of the medial and lateral malleolar surfaces, and distraction of these malleolar surfaces by the implant.[38] Many implants consist of two components, a metal tibial and a polyethylene talar component, although in others these are reversed. A third component, such as a polyethylene bearing, may be interposed between two metal components.[5] Efforts to address the problem of component loosening and subsidence have included adjustment of implant constraint, addition of porous ingrowth surfaces, and construction of a bony synostosis between the tibia and fibula.

Numerous investigators have played a role in the development of total ankle joint replacement for more than 20 years. Buchholz[4] was credited in one text[2] as a pioneer in ankle replacement, both as a designer and as a patient. Clinical results using implants such as the Buchholz design were reported.[9,10,16,20,32,50] Helal developed an implant in 1968 featuring a polyethylene convex articular surface fitting into a metal concave surface.[2] Lord and Marotte[31] reported ankle and subtalar replacement with a metal ball on a stem cemented into the tibia and a polyethylene cup cemented into the calcaneus.

In 1972, Freeman began using the ICLH prosthesis, in which the horizontal surfaces of the tibiotalar joint were replaced with a highly constrained prosthesis and resection arthroplasty of the malleoli was performed to reduce impingement.[14] This was further modified by the addition of medial and lateral articular surfaces.[3] Long-term results were reported in 1985, and both a high complication rate and poor clinical results were realized, with 13 of 41 considered satisfactory.[3] Other investigators have reported their experiences with total ankle replacement using this implant type.[16,19,20,43]

The New Jersey cylindrical replacement reported in 1976 by Pappas et al.[39] was not successful because of the degree of constraint with lack of axial rotation capability. Subsidence of the talar component and adequate tibial fixation were also recognized as problems. The Irvine ankle arthroplasty featured a toroidal design that was believed to add to implant stability.[51] Results using this implant were reported by Evanski and Waugh[13] and Demottaz et al.[10]

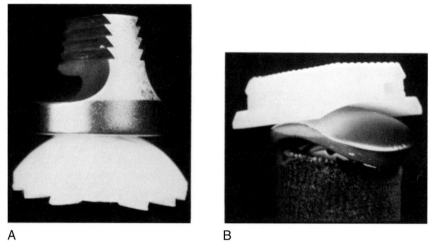

Figure 85–1. Unconstrained total ankle replacement design types. **A**, Smith. **B**, Newton.

The Mayo implant (Figs. 85–2**A** and 85–3) was highly constrained, and complications were reported by Stauffer,[47,49] particularly in younger patients with osteoarthritis. Overall the success rate was 76 percent, and results were better in patients with rheumatoid arthritis (88 percent). This implant type was successful in all 15 rheumatoid arthritis cases reported by Lachiewicz et al.,[30] although many had signs of component migration with radiolucent lines at the bone-cement interface.

The Smith prosthesis is dome shaped and therefore unconstrained (Fig. 85–1**A**). This is a ball-and-socket or

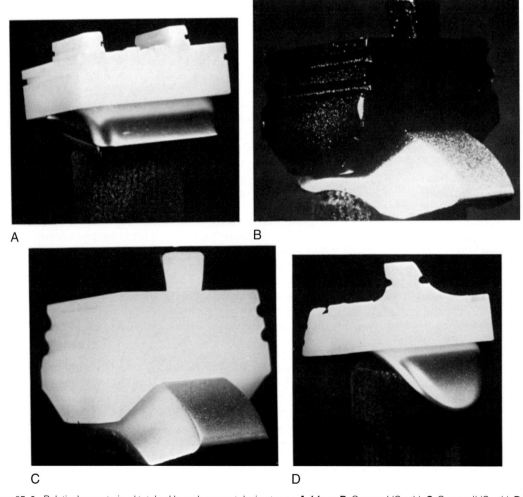

Figure 85–2. Relatively constrained total ankle replacement design types. **A**, Mayo. **B**, Oregon I (Groth). **C**, Oregon II (Groth). **D**, TPR.

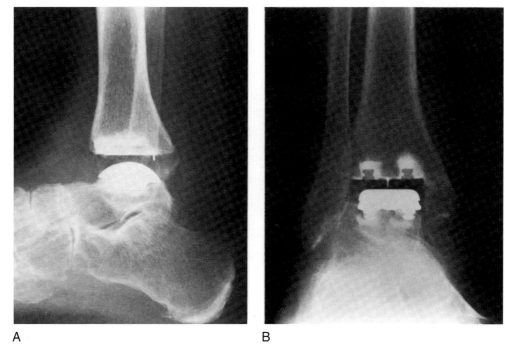

Figure 85–3. **A**, Lateral view of a well-positioned Mayo total ankle arthroplasty. **B**, Anteroposterior view with a good interface between the methacrylate and bone.

spherocentric design. Results of clinical trials were reported by a number of investigators.[9,10,12,13,21,52] Kirkup[21] described results of 24 cases and no longer recommends its use.

In 1972, Groth[17,18] began use of the Oregon ankle, which included not only resurfacing at the superior tibiotalar level but also medial and lateral articular surfaces. Results published in 1977 of 44 implants available for follow-up were considered good in 15 of 30 patients with degenerative arthritis and 9 of 10 with rheumatoid arthritis. He suggested application in rheumatoid arthritis and selected, older, debilitated, degenerative arthritic patients. Carbon-reinforced polyethylene was used in the tibial component (Fig. 85–2**B**, **C**). The TPR implant (Fig. 85–2**D**) is a single-axis design, and results using this type were reported by several investigators.[9,10,20]

Newton[38] reported his results with a relatively unconstrained design in 50 cases (Fig. 85–1**B**). His results were better in osteoarthritic patients compared with those with rheumatoid arthritis, particularly in those receiving long-term corticosteroids or with erosive changes.

In 1987, Scholz described the Scholz-PCA design, which is a semiconstrained ankle replacement with porous coating. Detailed results have not yet been published. Buechel and colleagues,[5] in 1988, reported their experience with a cementless, unconstrained low-contact-stress total ankle replacement, which they first used in 1981. This featured a polyethylene bearing between the two metallic implants. This evolved from an earlier experience with the New Jersey cylindrical ankle replacement and modifications. Eighty-seven percent of patients had mild or no pain.

Results

An interesting variety of implant types have been developed, and it is difficult to compare clinical results. One study by Demottaz et al.[10] reported results of 21 implants of multiple types, such as single axis (Mayo, TPR, Buccholz, Oregon) and multiple axis (Waugh et al.,[51] Smith[46]). There did not appear to be a correlation between the type of prosthesis and the incidence of mechanical complications, but the types of mechanical complications did seem to be related to the prosthesis design. Only 2 of the 21 designs were considered to provide good results, and problems of residual pain and signs of loosening were present in many.

There are additional concerns regarding the results of implant arthroplasty with time. Unger et al.,[50] in 1988, reported the results of 22 Mayo implants and one Buccholz design with a minimum of 2 years of follow-up. Eighty-three percent of the outcomes were considered satisfactory, but deterioration of clinical results with time was noted, with migration of the talar component in 14 of 15 cases and a radiolucent line at the bone-cement junction in 14 of 15 cases.

As long-term results of early ankle designs emerged, failures and complications such as loosening, instability, impingement, fractures, heterotopic bone, inadequate motion, wound healing problems, infection, and peroneal tendonitis led to a re-evaluation of the indications for ankle replacement. Salvage was often a difficult task because of the large soft tissue and bone defects. In a review of the London Hospital experience, Bolton-Maggs and co-workers concluded "In view of our results, and of the early results reported by others, . . . the overall results and long-term outlook of ankle arthroplasty is so poor as to warrant offering only ankle arthrodesis as the surgical treatment of the disabling arthritic ankle."[3] After reviewing 160 Mayo ankle implants, Kitaoka et al.[25] concluded that the Mayo implant was not recommended for osteoarthritis or rheumatoid arthritis of the ankle. Newton concluded that "Ankle fusion remains the procedure of choice for most painful ankle conditions . . . ."[38] By the 1980s, the reputation of ankle arthroplasty was severely tarnished, leaving ankle arthrodesis as the standard treatment for arthritic disorders of the ankle through most of the 1980s and 1990s.

Modern Ankle Designs

Several investigators persisted with ankle replacement, in spite of the initially discouraging results. Advances included the use of porous surfaces, incorporating a syndesmosis fusion, resurfacing the medial and lateral recesses, and the use of a three-component mobile-bearing design. Designs that incorporate bone ingrowth for prosthetic fixation eliminate the need for cement, allowing less bone resection. A syndesmosis fusion creates a larger surface area for tibial component fixation. A

mobile bearing provides another interface for motion, theoretically reducing stresses to the prosthesis-bone interface. The Buechel-Pappas, STAR, and Agility ankle designs have incorporated some of these concepts.

Buechel-Pappas Design

The original cylindrical New Jersey ankle developed by Buechel and Pappas had limited success because of its high degree of constraint and lack of axial rotation. A new, less constrained design incorporates a polyethylene meniscal bearing that allows flexion-extension at the polyethylene talar surface and rotation at the tibial polyethylene surface. A porous coating allowing bone ingrowth eliminates the need for bone cement. Early results of the first 23 ankles were encouraging, with only two patients dissatisfied.[5] Stability of the meniscal bearing was an occasional problem. The implant has been redesigned with an additional talar fixation fin and a deeper talar sulcus to contain the meniscal bearing and is available as a Food and Drug Administration (FDA) Class III device. Results on 30 ankles were excellent in 13 patients, good in 6, fair in 6, and poor in 5.[42] Three patients with avascular necrosis had poor results. An example is shown in Figure 85–4.

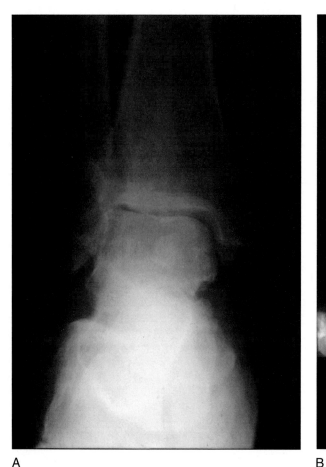
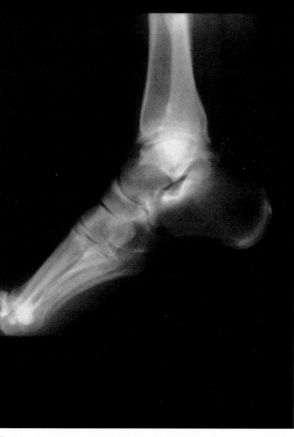

A   B

Figure 85–4. Radiograph of a patient with post-traumatic ankle arthritis in anteroposterior (AP) (**A**), lateral (**B**), and mortise (**C**) views. **D** and **E**, Radiographs taken immediately following Buechel-Pappas (New Jersey Low Contact Stress) total ankle arthroplasty (TAA) in AP (**D**) and lateral (**E**) views.

Illustration continued on opposite page

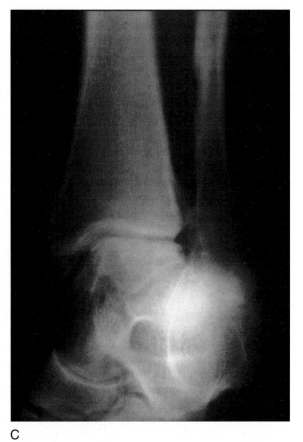

C

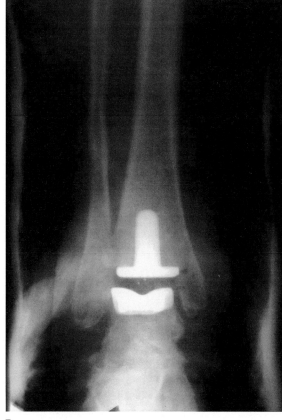

D

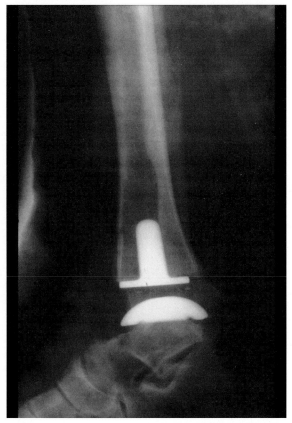

E

Figure 85–4. *Continued.*
Illustration continued on following page

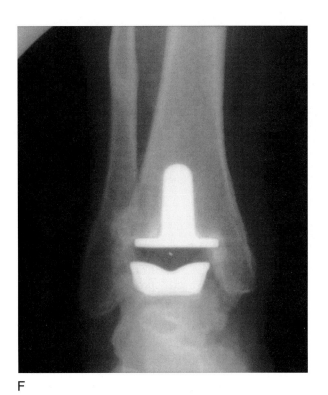

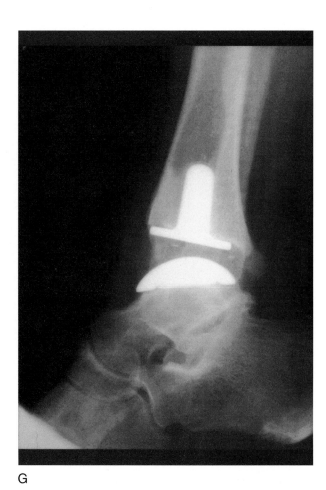

F   G

Figure 85–4. *Continued.* Anteroposterior (**F**) and lateral (**G**) radiographs taken 2 years following TAA showing that the patient had a successful result. (Courtesy of Dr. Sheldon Lin.)

STAR Design

Hakon Kofed reported on the Scandinavian Total Ankle Replacement (STAR) in 1995.[27] The initial design was a cemented two-component cylindrical design. The talar component consisted of a stainless steel cap that covers the talus with a central ridge to capture the tibial component. Estimated survival rate was 70 percent at 12 years in the first 28 ankles. Four patients required revision to arthrodesis. In a subsequent publication,[29] a three-component design was introduced that incorporates a polyethylene meniscal bearing with a flat tibial component (Fig. 85–5). Results using cement were similar for patients with rheumatoid arthritis and osteoarthritis. Survivorship analysis for the two groups was similar, with 72.7 percent survival for patients with osteoarthritis and 75.5 percent for those with rheumatoid arthritis at 14 years.

In its current form, as an FDA Class III device, a hydroxyapatite coating is used for component fixation.[53] In a series of 100 prospective cases that included the early cylindrical design as well as cemented and uncemented versions of the three-component design,[28] no difference was noted between patients older or younger than 50 years of age. Survivorship analysis revealed 75 percent survival at a median 6.8 years for those younger than 50 and 80.6 percent at 6 years for those older than 50. Twelve patients required revision, seven to fusion and five with component exchange.

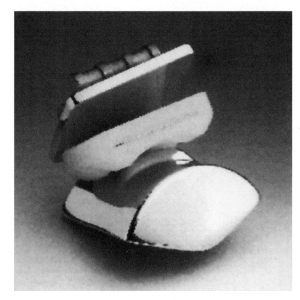

Figure 85–5. STAR three-component ankle arthroplasty.

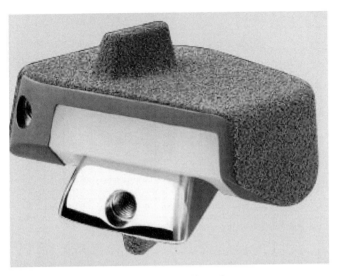

Figure 85–6. Two-component Agility ankle replacement.

Agility Design

Dr. Frank Alvine developed a semiconstrained, two-component ankle replacement (Fig. 85–6). The two components were initially made of titanium, but problems with talar wear led to a cobalt-chromium talar component. Design characteristics include a beaded porous coating on the nonarticulating surfaces of a large tibial and a smaller talar component and a tibiofibular syndesmosis to maximize tibial component fixation. The medial and lateral malleolar recesses are resurfaced. External rotation of the tibial component mimics the natural transmalleolar axis. An external fixator is used to align and distract the ankle prior to sizing and site preparation. Initially available in three sizes, right and left, six sizes are now available. Other design improvements include a larger and thicker tibial component and a thicker polyethylene insert for revisions.

The first consecutive 100 patients were reviewed independently.[40] Twelve patients with 14 ankles had died prior to review, leaving 83 patients with 86 ankle implants. Five patients required revision, four with implant revision and one with arthrodesis. Overall, 79 percent of patients were extremely satisfied and 13 percent satisfied. Ninety-five percent of patients would have the surgery again.

EVALUATION

Examination of the patient under consideration for total ankle replacement should parallel that of a patient who is considered for total hip or knee arthroplasty. In addition to a general medical evaluation, an examination of the lower extremities for skin integrity, neurovascular status, range of motion, and ligamentous stability is done. Limb length discrepancies, fixed deformities, and

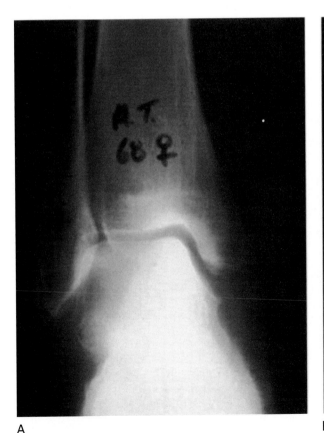

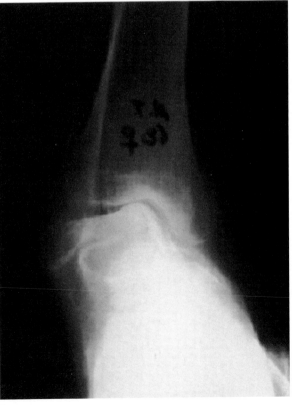

A   B

Figure 85–7. A, Non–weight-bearing anteroposterior (AP) view of a 68-year-old woman with ankle pain. Note the sclerosis of the medial tibial plafond. **B,** Radiograph taken 2 weeks later, showing the same patient on a weight-bearing AP view.

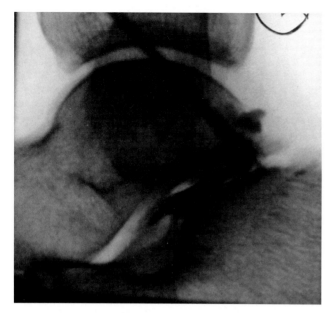

Figure 85–8. Diagnostic block of the subtalar joint relieves most of this patient's pain. Note needle placed in subtalar joint.

prior surgical procedures are considered. Nonoperative measures such as analgesics, anti-inflammatory medications, orthotics, splints, and lifestyle modifications may be appropriate.

Standing anteroposterior, lateral, and mortise view radiographs of the ankle are obtained. Figure 85–7 demonstrates the importance of weight-bearing radiographs. Stress views can be obtained when deemed necessary to help demonstrate instability. Radiographs of other joints of the lower extremity are often helpful in assessing associated degenerative changes. Not infrequently, ankle and subtalar degeneration develop coincidentally. Given that hindfoot function is better if one of these joints can be preserved, diagnostic injections, performed under fluoroscopy, can help determine if one of these joints can be preserved (Fig. 85–8).

Table 85–1. RELATIVE CONTRAINDICATIONS TO TOTAL ANKLE ARTHROPLASTY

Patient
Youth (60 yr)
Osteoarthritis (primary or post-traumatic)
Peripheral neuropathy
Corticosteroid use
Vascular insufficiency
Ankle
Hindfoot malalignment
Avascular necrosis of talus
Painful arthrodesis
Pseudoarthrosis
Distorted anatomy
Sepsis
Poor bone stock
Instability
Neuropathic arthropathy

INDICATIONS

Selection of patients for total ankle arthroplasty is still controversial, but certain guidelines can be provided. Elderly patients with end-stage ankle disease with minimal deformity and adequate bone stock are the most appropriate candidates.[8] With a relatively sedentary lifestyle, limited physical demands, and stiffness in adjacent joints, patients with rheumatoid arthritis are often ideal candidates provided they have adequate bone stock. Caution should be exercised, however, when considering patients with prior infection, compromised vascular status, avascular necrosis of the talus, or pseudarthrosis following attempted arthrodesis, or those who are under steroid treatment (Table 85–1). Ankles with significant instability, fixed varus or valgus deformities of the ankle and/or subtalar joint, or dynamic muscle imbalance are probably not appropriate for arthroplasty. Patients with multiple scars, poor soft tissue envelope from prior trauma, or vascular disease are poor candidates. Absolute contraindications include active infection and neuropathic arthropathy.

SURGICAL TECHNIQUE

The anterior approach has been the most widely used exposure for total ankle replacement. This technique allows fair exposure and provides anatomic landmarks that permit reasonable orientation of the components. Not uncommonly, an equinus contracture is part of the overall deformity and must be addressed with lengthening of the tendo Achillis complex. The approach is between the tibialis anterior and extensor hallucis longus tendons, reflecting the neurovascular bundle laterally (Fig. 85–9). By keeping slightly lateral to the tibialis anterior, it is possible to preserve its retinacular restraints, facilitating closure. The anterior ankle capsule is excised and the joint débrided. Although modifications may be necessary based on the specific prosthesis design, the basic procedure for bone resection and device implantation is somewhat standard. Particular care is taken to locate the anterior margin of the tibia after cheilectomy. The inner margin of the medial malleolus is located and used as the medial buttress of the tibial component.

With the ankle in neutral position, traction is applied to the foot to allow determination of appropriate lines of resection for the tibia and talus. A wafer is cut from the distal tibia with an oscillating saw, taking care not to deviate posteriorly and laterally into the fibula. Removal of the talar dome is accomplished so that ligament length will ultimately be re-established and subfibular impingement avoided. Distraction with an external fixator can facilitate bone resection. Troughs or fixation holes are fashioned appropriately in the tibia and talus. If methyl methacrylate is to be used, posterior cortical margins are retained to restrict posterior extravasation with compression of the prosthesis. The medial and lateral margins should be inspected for adequate clearance from the malleoli. Proper

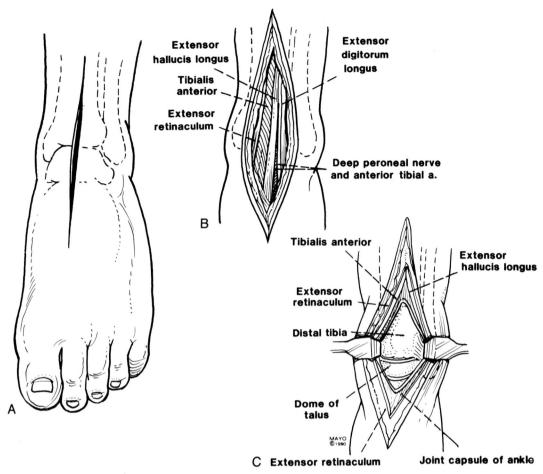

Figure 85–9. A, Skin incision for anterior exposure for total ankle arthroplasty. **B**, Deep dissection interval between tibial and extensor hallucis longus tendons. **C**, Excellent exposure of anterior joint.

component position is essential to preserve adequate flexion and extension (Fig. 85–10). Meticulous soft tissue technique is essential to minimize wound complications. The extensor retinaculum must be carefully repaired to prevent bowstringing of the tibialis anterior tendon, or wound necrosis can result.

The technique for the Agility ankle implant differs from the standard technique in that an external fixator is temporarily applied to distract and realign the diseased joint. Applied medially, it is used to obtain proper alignment and to facilitate the tibial and talar cuts (Fig. 85–11A, B). An alignment jig is applied after the exposure is complete (Fig. 85–11C, D). The appropriate-sized cutting jig is attached, and, with the use of an image intensifier, the cutting jig is aligned and the cuts begun (Fig. 85–11E, F). The guides are removed and the cuts completed. Prior to insertion of the trial components, a slot is cut in the talus for the talar fin, in 20 degrees of external rotation with respect to the axis of the tibial component (Fig. 85–11G). The final components are inserted and alignment is checked radiographically (Fig. 85–11H). A tibiofibular syndesmosis is created by débriding the space between the distal tibia and fibula, packing morselized bone graft into the space, and fixing the syndesmosis with two screws. An example of a suc-

cessful result following agility TAA is shown in Figure 85–12.

Insertion of the STAR prosthesis uses a tibial alignment system (Fig. 85–13A) but not an external fixator. After the tibial cut is made, the guide is removed and the talus fashioned to accept the talar component (Fig. 85–13B, C). The tibial guide is then replaced and the holes for tibial component fixation barrels are made (Fig. 85–13D), using a spacing block to simulate the polyethylene spacer. Insertion of the tibial component is completed and the final spacer inserted (Fig. 85–13E, F). Figure 85–14A and B shows a 78-year-old woman who developed post-traumatic arthritis following an ankle fracture. One year following her STAR ankle replacement, she is pain free (Fig. 85–14C, D).

Although the postoperative regimen may vary, bulky compressive dressings, elevation, and antibiotics are often employed for the first 24 hours. To achieve a syndesmosis fusion, at least 6 weeks of immobilization is required. Active range-of-motion exercises followed by partial early weight bearing is delayed until wound healing is achieved. Full weight bearing is begun once wound healing and syndesmosis fusion, if required, are attained.

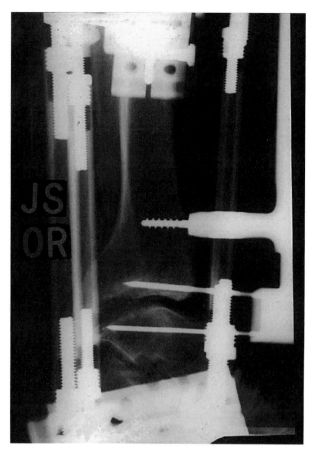

Figure 85–10. Correct orientation of the tibial and talar osteotomies is crucial for component orientation, as seen in this lateral view.

RESULTS

When the insertion is done properly, the result can be gratifying. Series that report long-term results of total ankle arthroplasty are difficult to compare. The variability in diagnosis, age, and follow-up and the absence of a uniform scoring system are contributing factors. Several early studies are noteworthy when considering the experience with ankle replacement. Enthusiasm was initially very high with the successes of joint replacement in the hip and knee. As a result of this unbridled enthusiasm, ankle prostheses were inserted in patients with traumatic degenerative arthritis of a younger age group, with avascular necrosis of the talus, with painful pseudoarthroses, and with malunited or painful arthrodeses. Many of these groups have subsequently been shown to be inappropriate for ankle replacement. The problem, then, is not so much with the specific prosthesis but in the selection of the proper patient.

Stauffer and Segal,[49] reviewing 102 ankle arthroplasties at the Mayo Clinic, found that the best results were obtained in patients with rheumatoid arthritis and those with post-traumatic or degenerative arthritis who were at least 60 years of age. Kitaoka et al. reported survivorship analysis of the Mayo total ankle arthroplasty.[25] From 1974 until the end of 1988, 204 primary Mayo total ankle arthroplasties were performed at the Mayo Clinic.

By means of actuarial analysis, we determined the cumulative rates of survival, with failure (defined as removal of the implant) as the endpoint. The average duration of follow-up was 9 years (range 2 to 17 years). By applying the Cox proportional-hazards general linear model, we identified two independent variables that were associated with a significantly higher risk of failure: a previous operative procedure on the ipsilateral foot or ankle and an age of 57 years or less. The overall cumulative rates of survival at 5, 10, and 15 years were 79, 65, and 61 percent, respectively (Fig. 85–15). The cumulative rate of survival was lower in patients 57 years old or less (Fig. 85–16). The probability of an implant being in situ at 10 years was 42 percent for patients who were 57 years old or less and who had had previous operative treatment of the ipsilateral ankle or foot and 73 percent for those who were more than 57 years old and who had had no such previous operative treatment (Fig. 85–17).

Modern ankle designs have proven more reliable. Kofed and Sorensen[29] reported survival rates of 72.7 percent for osteoarthritis and 75.5 percent for rheumatoid arthritis patients at 14 years for 52 cemented arthroplasties, 25 for osteoarthritis and 27 for rheumatoid arthritis.

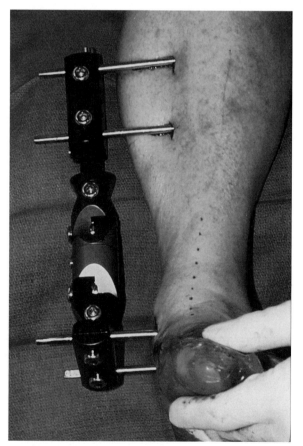

A

Figure 85–11. Agility total ankle replacement. **A,** A medial external fixator is applied. Correction of any fixed equinus deformity is required before this step. **B,** Diagram showing pin placement. **C,** The anterior ankle exposure is completed. **D,** Traction is applied at this time to correct any deformity and restore ligamentous balance.

Illustration continued on opposite page

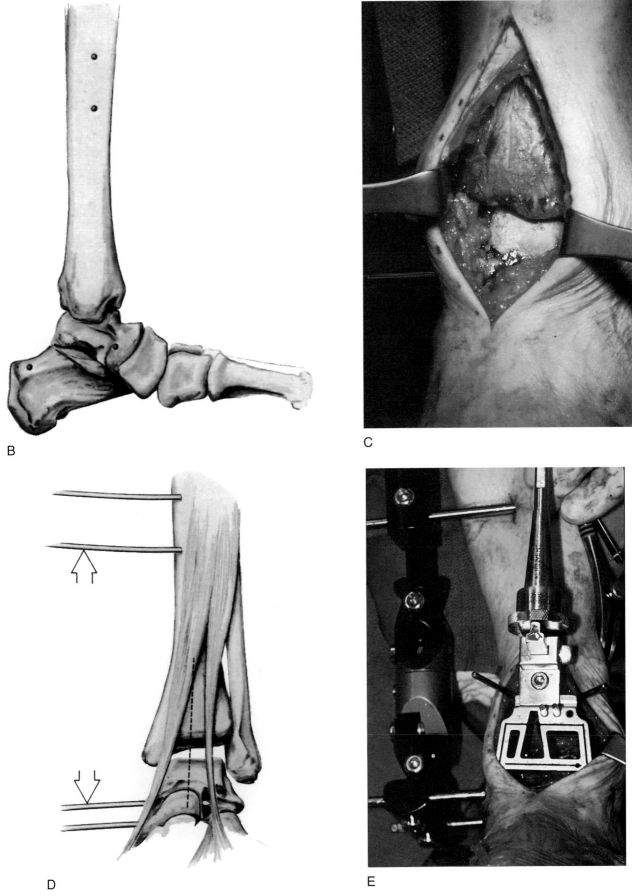

B

C

D

E

Figure 85–11. *Continued.*

Illustration continued on following page

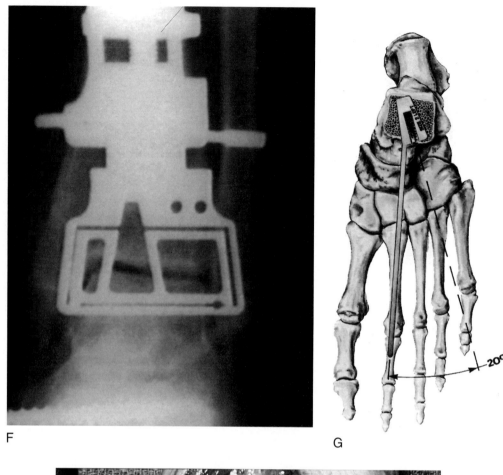

F

G

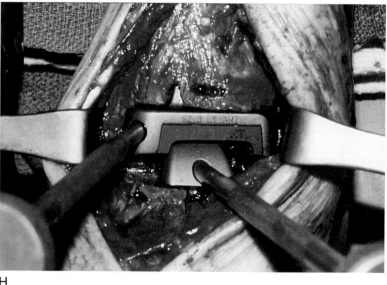

H

Figure 85–11. *Continued.* **E** and **F**, An alignment jig is applied and the position checked with the image intensifier. **G**, The keel for the talar component is cut in 20 degrees of external rotation. **H**, Position of the trial components is checked, followed by insertion of the final components.

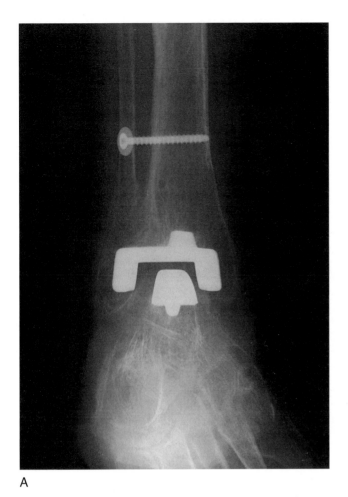

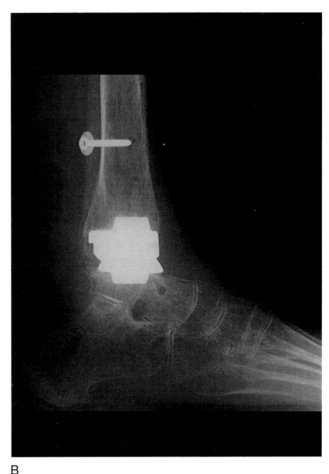

A   B

Figure 85–12. Mortise (**A**) and lateral (**B**) views of Agility total ankle replacement with a good alignment and ingrowth at 2 years.

Eleven ankles required revision or arthrodesis. In a consecutive series of 100 patients mixing two-component and three-component implants, with and without cement, the results were similar for patients older and younger than 50 years.[28] Seven ankles required an arthrodesis and five were revised. The remaining patients had good or excellent scores.

Buechel and Pappas reported their first 23 patients using a cementless implant in 1988.[5] Since then, the implant has been modified and results in the 30 of 38 ankles followed for an average of 4.5 years were reported by Saltzman.[42] Thirteen patients had results rated as excellent, six good, six fair, and five poor. Three patients had osteonecrosis, all with poor results. Six patients used a cane.

The Agility ankle was reviewed independently by Pyevich et al. in 1998.[40] Of 100 consecutive replacements in 95 patients, 12 patients with 14 ankle replacements had died and 1 was revised to an arthrodesis, leaving 85 ankles in 82 patients for review. Four ankles were revised. Forty-seven ankles were pain free, 24 had mild pain, and 14 had moderate pain. Seventy-nine percent of patients were extremely satisfied, 13 percent satisfied, 4 percent indifferent, and 4 percent

dissatisfied with the result. Nonunion of the syndesmosis fusion was associated with migration of the tibial component, but this did not appear to affect the clinical outcome.

AUTHORS' PREFERENCE

The proper selection of patients as well as design characteristics and surgical technique for total ankle arthroplasty are still evolving. At present, an elderly patient with limited activity demands is the best candidate. Patients with rheumatoid arthritis with adequate bone stock are ideal candidates. The ideal implant incorporates bone ingrowth for fixation, a semiconstrained design, minimal bone resection, replacement of worn components, and easy revision to arthrodesis.[22,23,26,41,48] The anterior surgical approach offers the best exposure, but care must be taken to carefully repair the retinaculum to minimize wound complications. Improvements in design and surgical technique may allow the orthopedic surgeon eventually to increase the application of replacement arthroplasty for degenerative arthritis of the ankle.

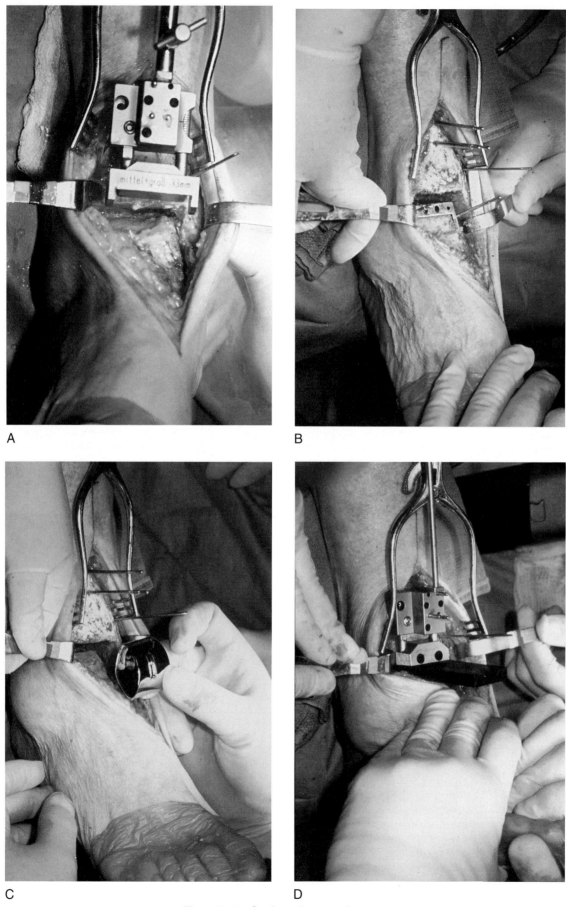

A

B

C

D

Figure 85–13. *See legend on opposite page*

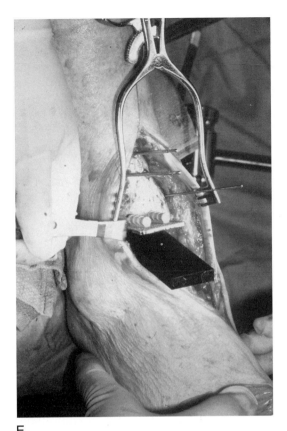

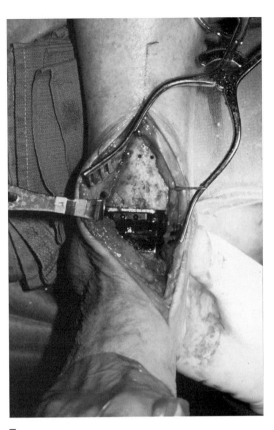

E   F

Figure 85–13. STAR total ankle replacement. **A,** The tibial alignment guide has been applied in preparation for the tibial cut. **B** and **C,** The guide is removed and the talus fashioned to accept the talar component. **D,** The holes for tibial component fixation are made. **E** and **F,** The tibial component is inserted with the final spacer.

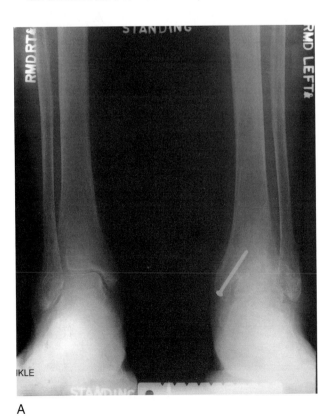

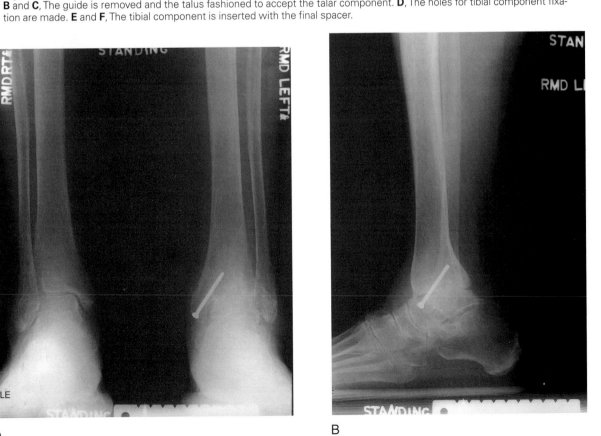

A   B

Figure 85–14. A and **B,** A 78-year-old woman with post-traumatic arthritis.

Illustration continued on following page

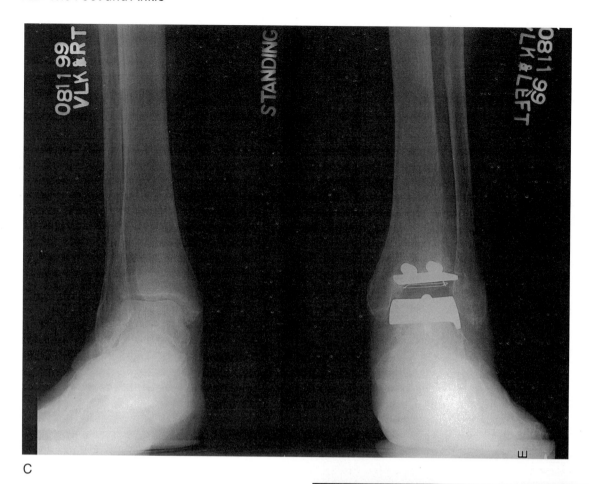

C

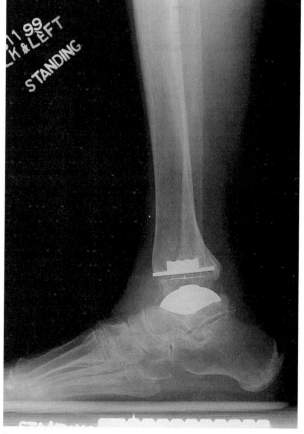

D

Figure 85–14. *Continued.* **C** and **D**, One year after surgery, she is doing well with no pain following STAR total ankle arthroplasty.

Figure 85–15. Graph of the cumulative rates of survival for 204 primary arthroplasties, with 95 percent confidence intervals (vertical bars). The endpoint was defined as removal of the implant. The rates of survival at 5, 10, and 15 years were 79, 65, and 61 percent, respectively. TAA, total ankle arthroplasty. The number below the curve indicates the number of patients remaining at the last time interval. (From Kitaoka HB, Patzer GL, Ilstrup DM, Wallrichs SL: Survivorship analysis of the Mayo total ankle arthroplasty. J Bone Joint Surg Am 76:974, 1994.)

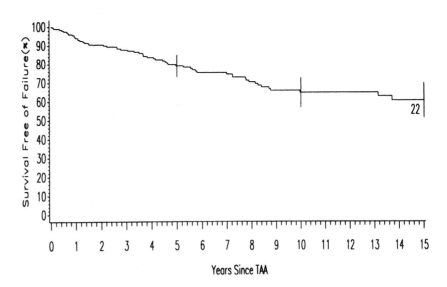

Figure 85–16. Graph of the cumulative rates of survival for 204 primary arthroplasties, with 95 percent confidence intervals (vertical bars), according to the age of the patient. At 10 years, the rate was 59 percent for the 104 ankles of the 89 patients who were 57 years old or less and 74 percent for the 100 ankles of the 85 patients who were more than 57 years old ($P < 0.02$). TAA, total ankle arthroplasty. The number below the curve indicates the number of patients remaining at the last time interval. (From Kitaoka HB, Patzer GL, Ilstrup DM, Wallrichs SL: Survivorship analysis of the Mayo total ankle arthroplasty. J Bone Joint Surg Am 76:974, 1994.)

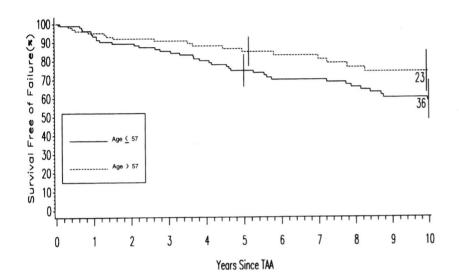

Figure 85–17. Graph of the cumulative rates of survival for 204 primary arthroplasties, with 95 percent confidence intervals (vertical bars), according to previous operative treatment of the ipsilateral foot or ankle. The rate was 84 percent at 5 years and 70 percent at 10 years for the 162 ankles (134 patients) that had not been operated on previously and 61 percent at 5 years and 47 percent at 10 years ($P < 0.001$) for the 42 ankles (42 patients) that had been operated on previously. TAA, total ankle arthroplasty. The number below the curve indicates the number of patients remaining at the last time interval. (From Kitaoka HB, Patzer GL, Ilstrup DM, Wallrichs SL: Survivorship analysis of the Mayo total ankle arthroplasty. J Bone Joint Surg Am 76:974, 1994.)

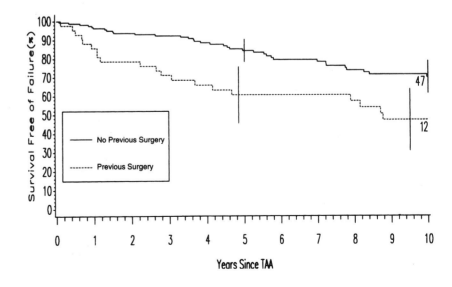

ACKNOWLEDGMENTS

The authors gratefully acknowledge the contributions of selected figures from Sheldon Lin, M.D., and James DeOrio, M.D.

References

1. Alexakis P, Smith RC, Wellish M: Indications for ankle fusion versus total ankle replacement versus pantalar fusion. Orthop Trans 1:87, 1977.
2. Benjamin A, Helal B: Surgical Repair and Reconstruction in Rheumatoid Disease. New York, John Wiley & Sons, 1980, p 206.
3. Bolton-Maggs BG, Sudlow RA, Freeman MAR: Total ankle arthroplasty: a long-term review of the London Hospital Experience. J Bone Joint Surg Br 67:785, 1985.
4. Buchholz H, Engelbrecht E, Siegel M: Total ankle endoprosthesis "St. Georg" model. Chirurg 44:241, 1973.
5. Buechel FF, Pappas MV, Cloris LJ: New Jersey low contact stress total ankle replacement, biomechanical rationale and review of 23 cementless cases. Foot Ankle 8:279, 1988.
6. Burge P, Evans M: Effect of surface replacement arthroplasty on stability of the ankle. Foot Ankle 7:10, 1986.
7. Calderale PM, Garro A, Barbiero R, et al: Biomechanical design of the total ankle prosthesis. Eng Med 12:69, 1983.
8. Claridge RJ, Hart MB, Jones RA, Johnson KA: Replacement arthroplasties of the ankle and foot. In Jahss MH (ed): Disorders of the Foot and Ankle. Philadelphia, WB Saunders, 1991, p 2647.
9. DeBastiani G, Vecchini L: Arthro-prosthesis of the ankle joint. Ital J Traumatol 7:31, 1981.
10. Demottaz JD, Mazur JM, Thomas WH, et al: Clinical study of total ankle replacement with gait analysis. J Bone Joint Surg Am 61:976, 1979.
11. Demottaz JD, Mazur JM, Thomas WH, et al: Clinical study of total ankle replacement. Clin Orthop 146:228, 1980.
12. Dini AA, Bussett FH: Evaluation of the early results of Smith total ankle replacement. Clin Orthop 146:228, 1980.
13. Evanski PE, Waugh TR: Management of arthritis of the ankle: an alternative to arthrodesis. Clin Orthop 122:110, 1977.
14. Freeman MAR, Kempson GE, Tuke MA, Samuelson KM: Total ankle replacement with the ICLH prosthesis. Int Orthop 2:327, 1979.
15. Frey C, Halikus NM, Vu-Rose T, Ebramzadeh E: A review of ankle arthrodesis: predisposing factors to nonunion. Foot Ankle 15:581, 1994.
16. Goldie IF, Herverts P: Prosthetic replacement of the ankle joint. Reconstr Surg Traumatol 18:205, 1981.
17. Groth HE: The Oregon ankle: a total ankle designed to replace all three articular surfaces. Orthop Trans 1:86, 1977.
18. Groth HE: Total ankle replacement with the Oregon ankle: evaluation of 44 patients followed two to seven years. Orthop Trans 7:488, 1983.
19. Herberts P, Goldie IF, Kornsi L, et al: Endoprosthetic arthroplasty of the ankle joint. Acta Orthop Scand 53:687, 1982.
20. Kaukenen JP, Raunio P: Total ankle replacement in rheumatoid arthritis: a preliminary review of 28 arthroplasties in 24 patients. Ann Chir Gynaecol 72:196, 1983.
21. Kirkup J: Richard Smith ankle arthroplasty. J Soc Med 78:301, 1985.
22. Kitaoka HB: Salvage of nonunion following ankle arthrodesis for failed total ankle arthroplasty. Clin Orthop 268:37, 1991.
23. Kitaoka HB: Fusion techniques for failed ankle arthroplasty. Semin Arthroscopy 3:51, 1992.
24. Kitaoka HB, Anderson PJ, Morrey BF: Revision of ankle arthrodesis with external fixation for non-union. J Bone Surgery Am 74:1191, 1992.
25. Kitaoka HB, Patzer GL, Ilstrup DM, Wallrichs SL: Survivorship analysis of the Mayo total ankle arthroplasty. J Bone Joint Surg Am 76:974, 1994.
26. Kitaoka HB, Romness DW: Arthrodesis for failed ankle arthroplasty. J Arthroplasty 7:277, 1992.
27. Kofoed H: Cylindrical cemented ankle arthroplasty: a prospective series with long-term follow-up. Foot Ankle 16:474, 1995.
28. Kofoed H, Lundberg-Jensen A: Ankle arthroplasty in patients younger and older than years: a prospective series with long-term follow-up. Foot Ankle 20:501, 1999.
29. Kofoed H, Sorensen TS: Ankle arthroplasty for rheumatoid arthritis and osteoarthritis. J Bone Joint Surg Br 80:328, 1998.
30. Lachiewicz PF, Inglis AE, Ranawat CS: Total ankle replacement in rheumatoid arthritis. J Bone Joint Surg Am 66:340, 1984.
31. Lord G, Marrotte JH: L'Arthroplastie totale de Cheville: experience sur 10 ans, à propos de 25 observations personelles. Rev Chir Orthop 66:527, 1980.
32. Manes HR, Alvarez E, Leving LS: Preliminary report of total ankle arthroplasty with osteonecrosis of the talus. Clin Orthop 127:200, 1977.
33. Matejczyk MB, Greenwald AS, Black JD: Ankle implant systems: laboratory evaluation and clinical correlation. Orthop Trans 3:199, 1979.
34. McGuire MR, Kyle RF, Gustilo RB: Total ankle arthroplasty and arthrodesis: a retrospective evaluation of a series of patients in Minneapolis and St. Paul. Orthop Trans 6:376, 1972.
35. McMaster WC: Total ankle arthroplasty. Adv Orthop Surg 9:264, 1985.
36. Mears DC, Gordon RG, Kann SE, Kann BA: Ankle arthrodesis with an anterior tension plate. Clin Orthop Rel Res 238:70, 1991.
37. Moran CG, Pinder IM, Smith SR: Ankle arthrodesis in rheumatoid arthritis. Acta Orthop Scand 62:538, 1991.
38. Newton SE: Total ankle arthroplasty. J Bone Joint Surg Am 64:104, 1982.
39. Pappas J, Buechel F, DePalma A: Cylindrical total ankle joint replacement. Clin Orthop 118:82, 1976.
40. Pyevich MT, Saltzman CL, Callaghan JJ, Alvine FG: Total ankle arthroplasty: a unique design. J Bone Joint Surg Am 80:1410, 1998.
41. Russotti G, Johnson K, Cass JR: Tibiotalocalcaneal arthrodesis for arthritis and deformity of the hind part of the foot. J Bone Joint Surg Am 70:1304, 1988.
42. Saltzman CL: Total ankle arthroplasty: state of the art. ICLS 48:263, 1999.
43. Samuelson KM, Freeman MAR, Tuke MA: Development and evaluation of the ICLH ankle replacement. Foot Ankle 3:32, 1982.
44. Scholz KC: Total ankle replacement arthroplasty. In Bateman JE (ed): Foot Science. Philadelphia, WB Saunders, 1976, p 106.
45. Scholz KC: Total ankle arthroplasty using biological fixation components compared to ankle arthrodesis. Orthopedics 10:125, 1987.
46. Smith FD: STA operation for pronated foot in children. Clin Podiatr 1:155, 1984.
47. Stauffer RN: Total ankle joint replacement. Arch Surg 112:1105, 1977.
48. Stauffer RN: Salvage of painful total ankle arthroplasty. Clin Orthop 170:184, 1982.
49. Stauffer RN, Segal NM: Total ankle arthroplasty: four years experience. Clin Orthop 160:217, 1981.
50. Unger AS, Cluglis AE, Mow CS, Figgie HE: Total ankle arthroplasty in rheumatoid arthritis: a long-term follow-up study. Foot Ankle 8:173, 1988.
51. Waugh RT, Evanski PM, McMaster WC: Irvine ankle arthroplasty: prosthetic design and surgical technique. Clin Orthop 114:180, 1976.
52. Wiedel JD: Total ankle arthroplasty with Smith prosthesis. Orthop Trans 1:154, 1977.
53. Zerahn B, Kofoed H, Borgwardt A: Increased bone mineral density adjacent to hydroxyapatite-coated ankle arthroplasty. Foot Ankle 21:285, 2000.

86

Complications of Replacement Arthroplasty of the Ankle

• HAROLD B. KITAOKA

In recent years, there has been increasing interest in replacement arthroplasty of the ankle. It is recognized that the complication and failure rates of total ankle arthroplasty (TAA) are considerably higher than for total hip or total knee arthroplasty. With new, innovative designs, recently reported clinical results have been very encouraging. Regardless of one's philosophy about the role of current ankle replacements, a rational approach to the assessment and treatment of the patient with painful TAA is needed.

TOTAL ANKLE ARTHROPLASTY COMPLICATIONS

Stiffness

The potential value of replacement arthroplasty of the ankle is the preservation of joint function and motion. It is discouraging for patients to undergo a major reconstruction operation and recognize a range of motion similar to that prior to surgery. There are at least five longer term studies that demonstrated no appreciable improvement in range of motion in the sagittal plane after TAA.

Stiffness may be related to multiple causes, such as ineffective rehabilitation after surgery. Most patients are able to perform ankle rehabilitation exercises independently, but others desire a more structured course of physical therapy. Another reason for stiffness is a poor soft tissue envelope about the ankle as a result of factors such as the severity of the initial injury (in post-traumatic arthritis), multiple previous operations of the ankle, and previous infection. Prolonged immobilization following the initial injury or subsequent multiple operations can contribute to the development of stiffness. Patients who suffer from ankle pain for years tend to avoid loading the affected extremity aggressively and limit their activities in order to minimize symptoms, thus encouraging the development of stiffness. Technical problems during ankle replacement, such as suboptimal component placement, or selection of an oversized implant may also play a role. In the past, with cemented prostheses, a mechanical block to full motion occasionally resulted from excessive polymethylmethacrylate. Heterotopic bone formation may occasionally lead to joint stiffness (Fig. 86–1). Because the motion that occurs in the sagittal plane is due to combined ankle and midfoot mobility, patients who have advanced midfoot arthritis or ankylosis are more cognizant of any decrease in ankle movement.

The stiff ankle may be treated with various physical modalities, such as physical therapy. Treatment such as manipulation under anesthesia, removal of excessive cement, removal of heterotopic bone, and exchange of one or more TAA components are options, but are rarely utilized. Fortunately, ankle stiffness is not always associated with pain and impaired function.

Delayed Wound Healing

In conventional surgical approaches, wound healing problems may occur in as many as 40 percent of patients who undergo TAA.[1] This complication may be a particular problem in patients with limited subcutaneous tissues and thin, fragile skin, such as those with rheumatoid arthritis who are dependent on corticosteroids, methotrexate, and other medications. Patients with post-traumatic arthritis often have sustained significant soft tissue injury or even a crush injury and have previous skin loss, healed free tissue transfer operations, healed skin grafts, healed lacerations, history of open fractures, previous deep infection, and adhesions in the region of the typical TAA incision. These concerns may not preclude ankle replacement surgery, but patients need to be informed of the potential for wound complications.

It is advisable to carefully plan the placement of surgical incisions and to exercise caution when handling soft tissues intraoperatively. It may be helpful to extend longitudinal incisions proximally and distally in order reduce the tension on the skin margins caused by retraction. When delayed wound healing occurs, it often affects the central portion of the incision and is superficial. This is usually managed by oral antibiotics, limiting

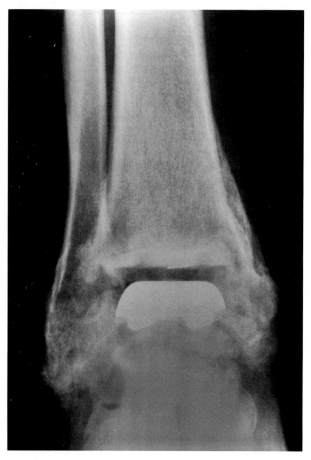

Figure 86–1. Heterotopic bone formation. (From Kitaoka HB, Patzer GL: Clinical results of Mayo total ankle arthroplasty. J Bone Joint Surg Am 78:1658–1664, 1996.)

activities, immobilization, and occasionally débridement. In many instances, the final results of surgery will not be affected if the problem is identified early and treatment initiated. When wound dehiscence is observed affecting a large section of the incision and involves full-thickness skin loss, urgent débridement procedures, antibiotics, and sometimes soft tissue coverage operations are required.

Infection

Deep infection is a serious complication of any joint replacement procedure. Following TAA, the rate of deep infection is about 3 to 5 percent.[1,23] In spite of the relatively low rate of occurrence, the consequences may be devastating. Prophylactic antibiotics are recommended in the perioperative period. It is necessary to be aware of the potential of a low-grade infection in patients who present with persistent pain following TAA. Infection is probable in patients with intermittent drainage from an incision that is almost, but not completely, healed. Symptoms and signs may overlap among various conditions such as superficial infection, deep infection, and sympathetically maintained pain. Because this distinction may not be clear, it may be necessary to obtain special investigative studies, such as an indium bone scan or arthrocentesis for culture, Gram stain, and cell count in patients with suspected infection.

The management of a superficial infection involves activity restrictions, antibiotics, and close observation, with or without immobilization. Occasionally, a superficial infection may progress to a deep infection and require urgent débridement and antibiotics. If there

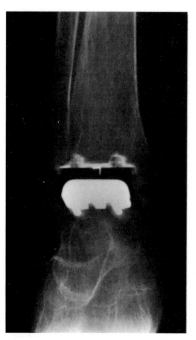
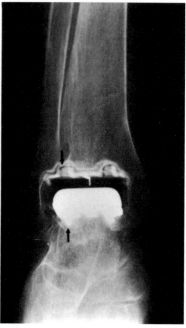

A   B

Figure 86–2. Septic loosening. **A**, Early postoperative anteroposterior (AP) radiographs show absence of a halo at the methacrylate-bone interface. **B**, Fifty-three months later, an increasing radiolucency is evident (*arrows*) at the interface secondary to deep infection.

is septic loosening (Fig. 86–2), the components are removed, the wound is débrided, an antibiotic-impregnated polymethylmethacrylate spacer is placed, the wound is closed, and the patient is immobilized in a cast or brace. Parenteral antibiotics are administered. If antibiotic treatment is completed (e.g., 6 weeks postoperatively), the patient is observed for an additional 2 weeks or so off of antibiotics. If there are no overt signs of residual infection, the definitive arthrodesis is performed in a delayed fashion at about 8 weeks postoperatively. During the delayed reconstruction, if the surgical pathology specimens demonstrate no evidence of acute inflammation, arthrodesis is performed. If there are still signs of infection based on the appearance of the wound or intraoperative pathology demonstrating acute inflammation, the process of débridement, antibiotic spacer placement, antibiotics, and immobilization is repeated. Rarely, for a TAA patient with a severe deep infection that cannot be eradicated via conventional means, amputation is an option.[17,22]

Loosening

Loosening of one or both of the components is a common the cause of pain and impairment after TAA. Loosening rates of between 6 and 25 percent after 3 to 5 years have been reported, with the talar component most often involved.[9] These rates are highly dependent on how loosening is defined. Radiolucent zones at least 2 mm in width at the methylmethacrylate-bone interface were noted by Demottaz et al.[7] in up to 88 percent of prostheses at 1 year follow-up. In another series, at an average 6-year follow-up, talar subsidence occurred in 14 of 15 cases, while 12 of 15 tibial components had tilted.[24] The implications for possible increased loosening rates with longer follow-up are evident.

The implant design can be related to the incidence of loosening. A TAA type that is relatively constrained is more likely to develop problems with loosening, as in joint replacement arthroplasty in other areas.[8] These types include the Mayo, ICLH, conoidal, and con-axial prostheses. This concern was recognized, and more recently developed implants have limited constraint. Larger implants that require resection of a significant portion of the talar body may be more prone to loosening. An osteopenic talar body may not support even a properly sized and well-positioned talar component when subjected to forces of 3 to 5 times body weight during normal level walking and exceeding 10 times body weight during running.

The lack of a standard definition for loosening may account for variation in incidence among different reports. Present methods of determining loosening, such as plain film radiography, underestimate the rate of occurrence. A modification of the femoral component loosening definition has been applied to the ankle replacement.[11,14] This is a more critical method of defining loosening based on radiolucency about the components and component migration (Table 86–1).

Table 86–1. DEFINITION OF TAA COMPONENT LOOSENING

Definite	Obvious migration of one prosthetic component or both*
Probable	Continuous radiolucent line surrounding the entire cement-bone interface but no evidence of migration
Possible	Radiolucent line extending along at least one half but less than the entire cement-bone interface

*Migration is defined as any discernable change in the position of the component.
From Kitaoka HB, Patzer GL: Clinical results of Mayo total ankle arthroplasty. J Bone Joint Surg Am 78:1658–1664, 1996.

The observation of probable or definite loosening may not demand operative treatment. In a long-term study of a relatively constrained prosthesis, patients who met the criteria for loosening did not always have disabling symptoms.[14] It is not unusual for the loose components to migrate to the extent that the malleoli come in contact and the joint becomes progressively stiff, even painful. In fact, complete bony ankylosis around the prosthesis has been observed following TAA, similar to that which has been observed after implant arthroplasty of the first metatarsophalangeal joint. Patients may also be debilitated from joints other than the ankle, and their more sedentary lifestyle, with limited demands on the ankle, may limit the symptoms. Parttime use of a polypropylene ankle-foot orthosis may suffice.

In patients with painful, loose prostheses, implant exchange has been attempted, but the standard operative treatment is implant removal and arthrodesis. Resection arthroplasty is not a viable option.

Hindfoot Arthritis

Arthritis of the adjacent joints is not unusual in association with TAA. The subtalar joint is frequently affected. The incidence is dependent on how arthritis is defined. In a study of a relatively constrained TAA device, many of the patients had moderate or severe subtalar arthritis or ankylosis of the subtalar joint.[14]

The etiology of hindfoot arthritis is multifactorial. The hindfoot joints may have sustained occult injury from the original trauma in the case of post-traumatic arthritis. Hindfoot arthritis may result from migration of the talar component of the prosthesis through the body of the talus and into the subtalar joint (Fig. 86–3). Patients with systemic rheumatic diseases may have evidence of hindfoot arthritis well before ankle replacement surgery. Subtalar stiffness may be accentuated by inadvertent placement of fixation into the joint or by application of compression across the intact joint for weeks with an external fixation device. If possible, it is advisable to place transfixion pins into the talar body, rather than in the calcaneus, when using an external fixator for tibiotalar arthrodesis.

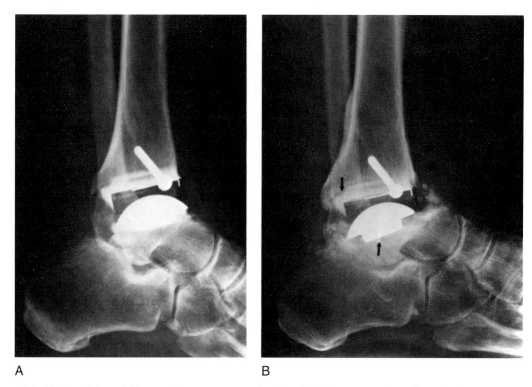

A   B

Figure 86–3. Hindfoot joint arthritis caused by component migration. **A,** Early postoperative radiograph shows poor positioning of the talar component in an angulated configuration. **B,** Forty-two months later, subsidence of the component into the cancellous bone of the talus body is seen.

Hindfoot arthritis may be adequately relieved with nonoperative management, such as anti-inflammatories, corticosteroid injections, and a hindfoot orthosis designed to limit hindfoot motion and permit ankle mobility. Occasionally, operative treatment is indicated. Because there are no proven subtalar joint prostheses available, standard surgical treatment is arthrodesis. In the case of subtalar arthritis associated with a failed ankle replacement, a single-stage tibiotalocalcaneal arthrodesis is indicated.

Malleolar Impingement

Impingement of the talar component beneath the lateral or medial malleolus is another possible cause of pain. Excessive tibial resection and inadequate resection of the talus beneath the lateral malleolar articulation are likely causes. Patients who initially experience satisfactory results following TAA and later develop pain and stiffness usually have component loosening with migration. The malleoli then become apposed, and symptoms of impingement occur.

The implant design can be directly related to the incidence of impingement. A TAA type that is relatively unconstrained is more likely to develop problems with malleolar impingement. These include older designs such as the Newton, Smith, and TPR.

The symptoms of malleolar impingement are said to improve with the use of a medial or lateral heel wedge, depending on the side of the impingement. Frequently, there is impingement of both malleoli. Decompression of malleolar impingement may be performed, but it has not been consistently successful. One reason for the inconsistent results is that the impingement may be secondary to prosthesis migration, a process that often progresses even after decompression surgery. Arthrodesis may be indicated.

Malleolar Fracture

Acute malleolar fracture may occur intraoperatively. It was observed in multiple reports, perhaps related to the specific prosthesis design and/or selection of a larger sized implant. In published reports, it occurred more commonly in the medial than the lateral malleolus. Technical problems sometimes play a role as well, such as removal of an excessive amount of bone medially or laterally.

Malleolar fractures may also occur postoperatively with progressive tibial component migration. Some prostheses, such as the Johnson TAA, had a tibial component designed similar to a wedge or cone (Fig. 86–4), which eventually migrated sufficiently to lead to a medial malleolar fracture. When recognized intraoperatively, the fracture may be fixed with two screws.

Total Ankle Arthroplasty Malalignment

Malalignment following TAA may be due to several factors, such as malposition of one or more components, subluxation or dislocation of the components from ligament instability, or a hindfoot disorder such as a concomitant flatfoot deformity. Care should be taken to select the correct implant size and properly align the components. Ligament stability should be restored and tested following component placement, and ligament tension adjusted as needed. A hindfoot deformity should be recognized prior to TAA because it may contribute to early failure of the TAA. Some surgeons recommend reconstructing the hindfoot with calcaneal osteotomy or an arthrodesis operation prior to or at the same time as the TAA.

Total Ankle Arthroplasty Instability

An important part of the TAA operation is achieving the proper soft tissue tension of the ankle ligaments. Excessive tension leads to a stiff joint. Ligament laxity is more a common problem, leading to prosthesis subluxation. There is evidence that patients with significant ligament instability before TAA will tend to have an unstable ankle afterward. Patients with severe instability may not be suitable candidates for ankle replacement. The stability of the soft tissue constraints should be tested intraoperatively and, if necessary, ligament repair/reconstruction performed.

EVALUATION OF PATIENT WITH PAINFUL ANKLE REPLACEMENT

Evaluation of the patient with a painful total ankle replacement should parallel that of a patient with pain following other arthroplasty types. Prior surgical procedures are considered. The specific complaints are carefully considered. For example, a skin abrasion or ulceration with footwear from a localized bony prominence is more easily addressed than deep pain from loosening. In addition to a general medical evaluation, an examination of the lower extremities to document skin integrity, neurovascular status, range of motion, painful motion, antalgic gait, alignment, tenderness, swelling, fluctuance, and stability is performed. In the instance where pulses are difficult to palpate and there is a question of the integrity of the vascular supply to the foot, noninvasive vascular studies are useful. Limb length discrepancy is measured.

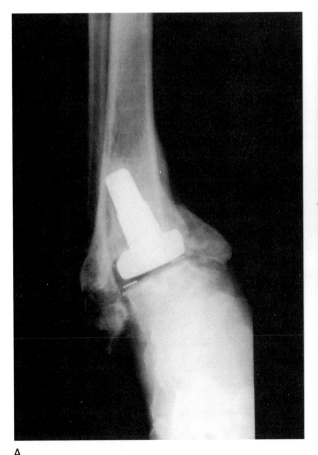

A

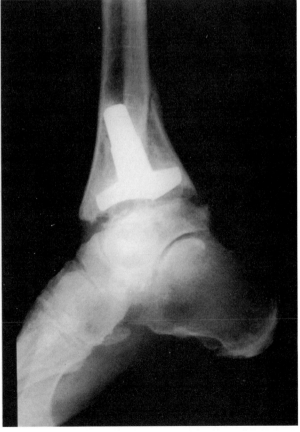

B

Figure 86–4. Failed TAA. **A,** Anteroposterior radiograph reveals acute malleolar fracture and varus deformity. **B,** Lateral view shows malposition of the tibial component. The subtalar joint does not appear to be compromised.

Standing anteroposterior, lateral, and mortise view radiographs of the ankle are obtained. Serial plain film radiographs should be carefully compared to determine changes in component position or alignment, development of radiolucencies about the implant, and condition of the hindfoot joints. Radiographs of other joints of the lower extremity are often helpful in assessing associated degenerative changes. Stress views can be obtained when necessary to document instability. Special studies are useful when there is a question of associated pathology such as deep infection. These include indium and technetium bone scans, arthrocentesis for cultures, and blood tests such as a complete blood count, sedimentation rate, and C-reactive protein.

Nonoperative measures such as anti-inflammatory medications, immobilization in an ankle-foot orthosis, and lifestyle modifications are offered.

SURGICAL TECHNIQUE: IMPLANT REMOVAL AND ARTHRODESIS

The failed TAA is often best salvaged by arthrodesis.[6,12,13,16,17,22] This is particularly true in cases of infection. For loosening alone, some have advocated revision of the components for selected ideal patients with adequate bone stock. Arthrodesis after failed TAA has generally been successful.[6] For septic loosening, débridement, antibiotic-impregnated cement spacer placement, immobilization, and then late arthrodesis with external fixation is preferred.

There are several options available for TAA removal and arthrodesis, such as malleolar (joint) resection arthrodesis, modified Campbell arthrodesis, posterior tibiotalocalcaneal arthrodesis, and modified Chuinard arthrodesis (Fig. 86–5).

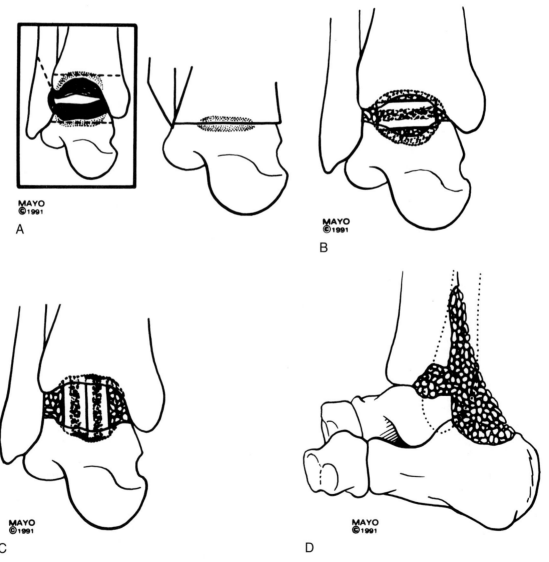

Figure 86–5. Arthrodesis techniques for failed TAA. **A,** Malleolar resection. **B,** Modified Chuinard arthrodesis. **C,** Modified Campbell arthrodesis. **D,** Posterior tibiotalocalcaneal arthrodesis. (From Kitaoka HB, Romness DW: Arthrodesis for failed ankle arthroplasty. J Arthroplasty 7:277–284, 1992.)

Malleolar Resection Arthrodesis

Perhaps the simplest technique of ankle arthrodesis with failed TAA involves implant and cement removal followed by resection of the margins of the tibia, fibula, and talus in order to achieve satisfactory bony apposition.[18] There is a direct bone-to-bone contact with this technique rather than the use of an intercalated bone graft, and therefore the arthrodesis readily unites. Supplemental morselized corticocancellous bone graft may be added. Following preparation of the bone surfaces, rigid external or internal fixation is applied.

This method has the advantages of simplicity and greater bony apposition of the tibia and fibula to the talus. It is applicable in the treatment of the infected TAA after the acute infection is addressed; this is an instance where supplemental bone graft may be less desirable. It does have the distinct disadvantage of accentuating the degree of shortening of the extremity, which may require a heel and sole lift on the shoe postoperatively. There may be an adverse effect on tendon function because of the degree of shortening. Tendon subluxation may occur from the malleolar resection.

Modified Campbell Arthrodesis

Campbell et al.[3] reported an ankle arthrodesis technique featuring vertically oriented struts of tricortical iliac crest bone graft inserted into a rectangular-shaped mortise. The mortise created by osteotomes in the original report is not unlike the bone defect caused by implant removal in the case of failed TAA. The operation can be modified by packing morselized bone graft around the vertical struts and applying an external fixation device. This operation has the advantage of preserving some of the height of the ankle in patients with large bone deficiencies. It requires a separate incision for harvesting the bone graft. This technique has been occasionally applied in patients with failed TAA, but there has not been any published series utilizing this technique for failed ankle replacement.

Posterior Tibiotalocalcaneal Arthrodesis

Another alternative is implant removal and posterior tibiotalocalcaneal arthrodesis[19] with bone grafting. This allows prosthesis removal and realignment, and may be applicable if the subtalar joint is also diseased.

Russotti et al.[20] reported an operation for arthrodesis of the ankle and subtalar levels in patients who had arthritis and deformity of the ankle and hindfoot. The operation is applicable in patients who have subsidence of the talar component into the subtalar joint, severe talar bone loss, and painful arthritis affecting the subtalar joint. As opposed to the previously described operations, this procedure is performed in the prone position and a posterolateral incision is made at the lateral margin of the Achilles tendon. The tendon is transected obliquely, and the ankle and subtalar joints are exposed posteriorly through the interval between the flexor hallucis longus medially and the peroneus brevis tendon laterally. The implant and cement are removed, and a trough is created in the posterior tibia, talus, and calcaneus. An iliac crest bone graft is morselized with a bone mill and packed into the trough, followed by application of an internal fixator. One of the potential advantages of this approach is that it utilizes a posterolateral incision in which the soft tissue envelope is usually not disturbed from previous operations. It does require exposure of the iliac crest to harvest the bone graft. The procedure has been applied for patients with failed ankle replacement with success.

Modified Chuinard Arthrodesis

The late Richard Stauffer, a pioneer in TAA design and salvage treatment,[21,22] modified an ankle arthrodesis technique of Chuinard and Peterson, using compression and a spacer of iliac crest bone graft designed to preserve length after prosthesis removal. Others[17] advocated compression and stabilization via external fixation and used a bone graft spacer if greater than 0.75-inch shortening is anticipated.

When the operation was originally described by Chuinard and Peterson,[5] the block of iliac crest bone graft was interposed between the resected tibial and talar bone surfaces with no fixation. It was thought that fixation was not required because the soft tissues around the distracted ankle provided adequate compression. Unlike the more conventional arthrodesis techniques, with resection of the joint surfaces this operation was associated with less shortening. The authors believed that it was applicable in growing children because of the limited disturbance to the physis.

Stauffer modified the operation by adding an external fixation device and used the procedure for patients with large bony deficiencies from failed TAA. After removal of the TAA components and cement, a tricortical block of iliac crest is placed horizontally in the defect to act as a spacer. Alignment of the ankle is adjusted and then maintained by a percutaneous longitudinal Steinmann pin passed through the heel. Additional morselized corticocancellous graft obtained from the iliac crest is packed around the tricortical structural graft and an external fixation is applied with pins in the talus and in the tibia. External fixation such as the Calandrucio triangular external fixation device, a unilateral fixator, or an Ace-Fisher fixator may be used (Fig. 86–6). Internal fixation such as compression screws may also be applicable. The selection of the specific fixation technique is dependent on a number of factors, such as whether it is a tibiotalar or tibiotalocalcaneal arthrodesis, degree of

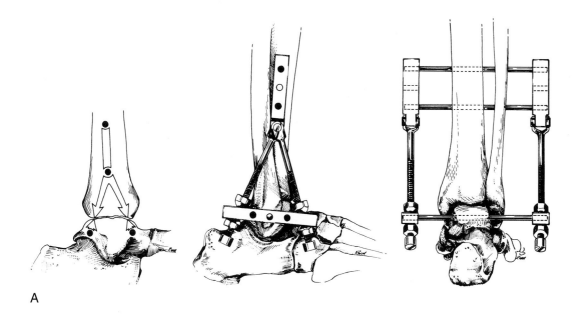

A

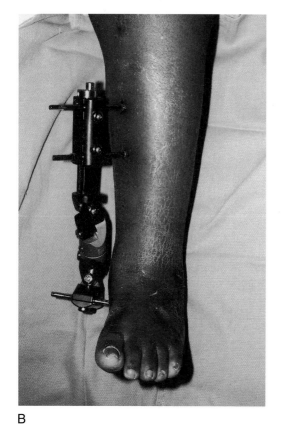

B

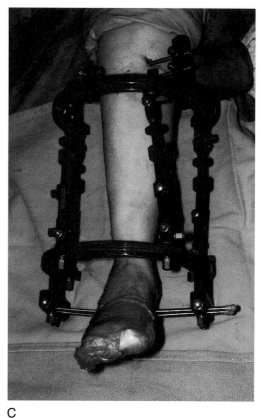

C

Figure 86–6. Fixation methods. **A**, Calandruccio triangular compression device. **B**, Unilateral external fixator (Orthofix). **C**, Ace-Fisher external fixator.

Illustration continued on opposite page

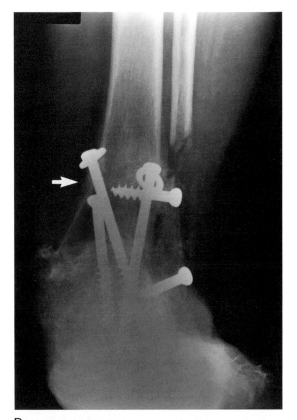

D

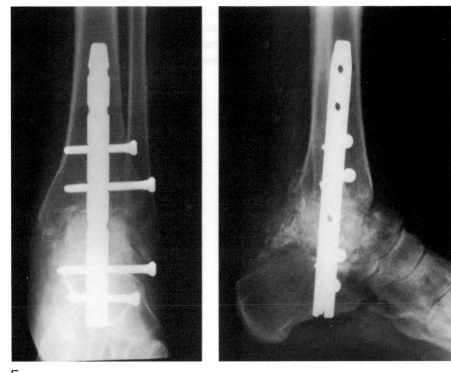

E

Figure 86–6. *Continued.* **D**, Screw fixation, lateral malleolar onlay graft. **E**, Intramedullary nail fixation. (From Kitaoka HB, Romress DW: Arthrodesis for failed ankle arthroplasty. Arthroplasty 7:27–284, 1992.)

bone loss, degree of osteopenia, recent infection, and preference and experience of the surgeon.

The advantages of this method compared to malleolar resection are good preservation of ankle height, high rate of union, good appearance, and lower potential for tendon problems about the ankle. The modified Chuinard arthrodesis requires a separate iliac crest incision.

POSTOPERATIVE MANAGEMENT

Following one-level or two-level arthrodesis operations for failed ankle replacement, patients are immobilized in a Robert-Jones compressive dressing for approximately 2 days. The dressing is changed, and, when the swelling is acceptable, a short-leg cast may be applied in patients who have internal compression arthrodesis. Those with external fixation devices are instructed on care of the pin sites and dressing changes. All patients will remain non–weight bearing for 8 weeks and even as long as 12 weeks postopera-

tively depending on the type of arthrodesis performed and the stability of fixation.

In general, the external fixation device is removed at approximately 8 to 12 weeks after surgery and a short-leg walking cast is then applied. The total length of immobilization is variable, again depending on the type of arthrodesis performed and the appearance of postoperative radiographs. The majority of patients are united by 4 or 5 months after surgery. Patients will require an extended period of rehabilitation. Following final cast removal, some patients will prefer the use of a walking shoe or athletic shoe, although the option of footwear modification with a Sach heel and rocker-bottom sole is offered.

RESULTS

The results of TAA removal and arthrodesis have been favorable, in spite of the complexity of the reconstruction (Figs. 86–7 through 86–10).[15] Kitaoka and Romness[16] reported results of 38 ankles in 36 patients

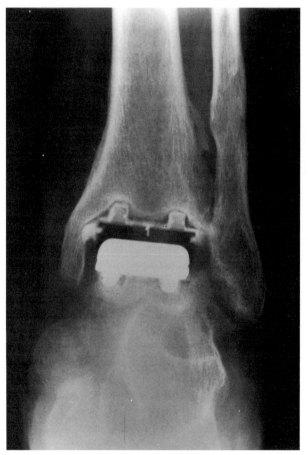

A

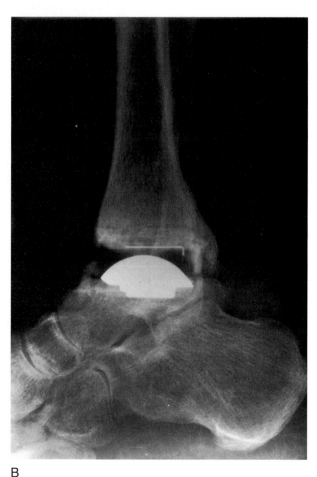

B

Figure 86–7. One-level modified Chuinard arthrodesis with good result. **A** and **B**, Radiographs of a 41-year-old man with a painful ankle after TAA. **A**, Anteroposterior view showing loosening, subsidence, and malleolar impingement. **B**, Lateral radiograph.

Illustration continued on opposite page

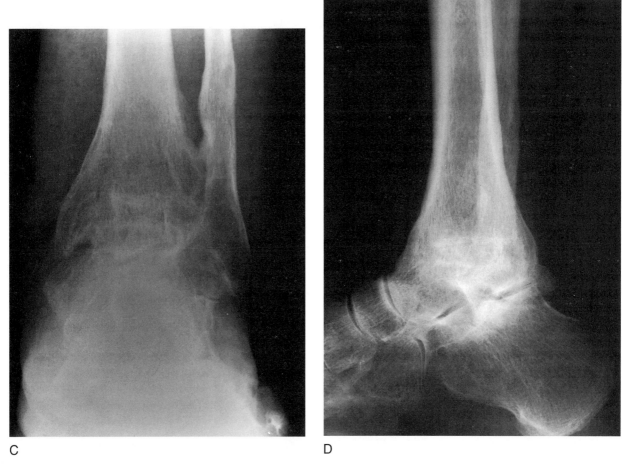

C   D

Figure 86–7. *Continued.* Anteroposterior (**C**) and lateral (**D**) views 14.5 years after successful modified Chuinard operation with external fixation. Note the preservation of ankle height. (From Kitaoka HB, Romness DW: Arthrodesis for failed ankle arthroplasty. J Arthroplasty 7:277–284, 1992.)

who underwent ankle arthrodesis for failed TAA between 1975 and 1988. Patients who had had previous fusion attempts before the TAA and patients who underwent multiple TAA attempts were excluded. All 36 patients were studied to determine union rate and also the occurrence and significance of perioperative complications. Five patients died and two could not be located, which left 31 ankles in 29 patients for follow-up study.

The average duration of follow-up was 8.3 years (range 2 to 14 years).[16] Twenty-two patients were women and 14 were men, and their mean age was 57 years (range 27 to 87 years). Eighteen patients were considered obese on the basis of abnormal body mass index. The primary diagnosis was post-traumatic arthritis in 23 ankles, degenerative arthritis in 5, and inflammatory arthritis in 10. Avascular necrosis was present in one ankle. Six ankles had the following associated neurologic disorders: neuropathic arthropathy in one, poliomyelitis in one, peripheral neuropathy in three, and Parkinson's disease in one. Three patients

had diabetes mellitus, 17 used tobacco, 27 had a hindfoot disorder, and 6 had malalignment. Before arthrodesis, patients underwent an average of two ankle operations (range one to five operations), such as débridement, open reduction–internal fixation, and soft tissue coverage. Infection occurred in nine ankles: infected arthroplasty in six, superficial wound infection in two, and remote infection after open fracture in one. The previous arthroplasty was a Mayo type of constrained device in 30 ankles and other types of implant in 8. Typically, patients did well immediately after the ankle arthroplasty but developed recurrent ankle pain that was resistant to nonoperative efforts such as anti-inflammatory medication, footwear modifications, corticosteroid injections, and decompression of the malleolar impingement. Usually patients with acutely infected arthroplasties had débridement operations before arthrodesis.

The cause of arthroplasty failure was infection in six ankles, avascular necrosis in one, neuropathic arthropathy in one, major ankle trauma in one, and

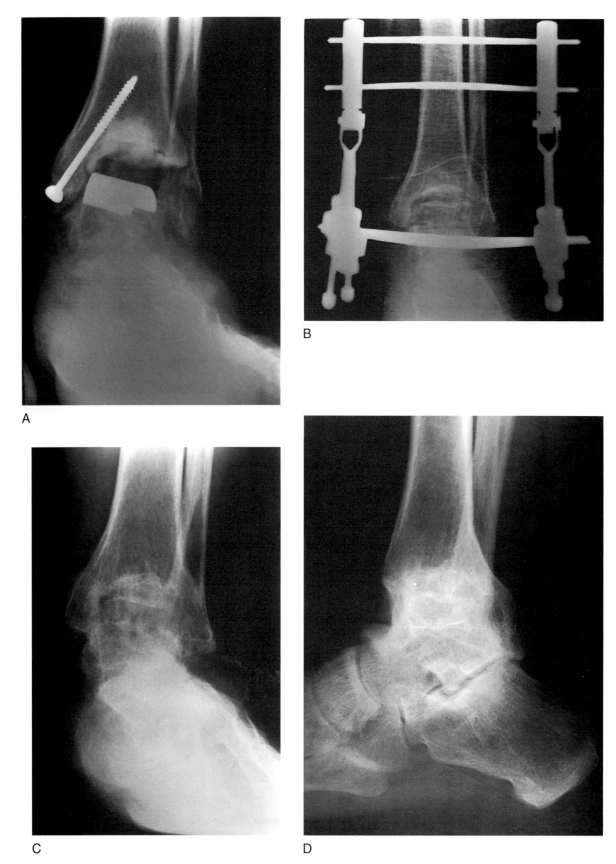

Figure 86–8. One-level modified Chuinard arthrodesis with good result in a 57-year-old male carpenter who had a painful TAA. **A**, Intraoperative radiograph before revision operation. **B**, Immediately after implant removal and modified Chuinard operation with Calandruccio external fixator. **C**, Three years later, the patient had no significant pain, returned to work without functional restrictions, and was satisfied. **D**, Lateral radiograph shows good alignment and preservation of ankle height. (From Kitaoka HB: Fusion techniques for failed ankle arthroplasty. Semin Arthroscopy 3:51–57, 1992.)

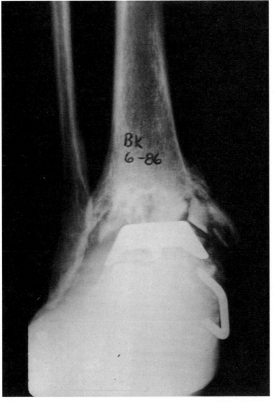

A

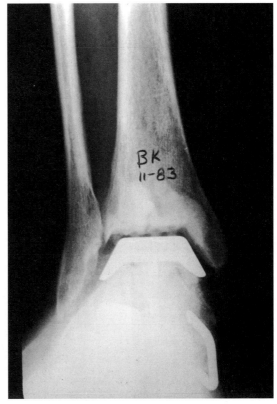

B

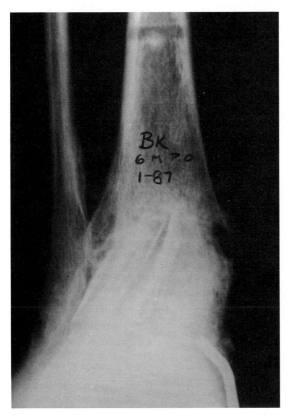

C

Figure 86–9. One-level modified Campbell arthrodesis with good result in a female patient who had rheumatoid arthritis. **A,** Radiograph after successful TAA. **B,** Four years later, the patient presented with a painful TAA. Note subsidence of implant. **C,** After successful modified Campbell operation with external fixation. (From Kitaoka HB: Fusion techniques for failed ankle arthroplasty. Semin Arthroscopy 3:51–57, 1992.)

undetermined in the remainder.[16] The salvage operations were performed at an average of 3.5 years after their previous total ankle arthroplasty. Appropriate laboratory studies were performed to evaluate the possibility of infection. The usual surgical approach was through the previous incision site, which was anterior in most cases. The implant components and cement were removed and intraoperative specimens for cultures were obtained. Four arthrodesis techniques were used. Malleolar resection to obtain adequate bony apposition was performed in 13 ankles and fixation was then applied. A modified Chuinard operation was used in 18 ankles, and a modified Campbell operation was used in 2. Posterior tibiotalocalcaneal arthrodesis was performed in 5 ankles. Fusion was attempted at the ankle level in 30 ankles and at the ankle and subtalar levels in 8 ankles. Supplemental bone graft was used in 32 ankles. External fixation was used in 36 ankles for an average of 9 weeks (range 7 to 17 weeks) and internal fixation with compression screws was used in 2 ankles. Cast immobilization was discontinued at an average of 18 weeks (range 11 to 3 weeks).

One patient died two months after surgery, before the arthrodesis had united.[16] Union was achieved in 33 of the remaining 37 ankles (87 percent). Four ankles

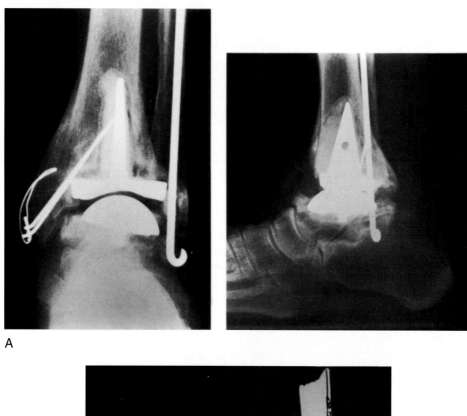

A

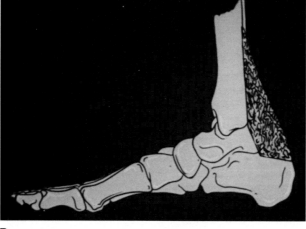

B

Figure 86–10. Posterior tibiotalocalcaneal arthrodesis. **A,** Anteroposterior (*left*) and lateral (*right*) radiographs show a loosened TAA that has subsided into the subtalar joint. **B,** Diagrammatic representation of arthrodesis from tibia to calcaneus.

Illustration continued on opposite page

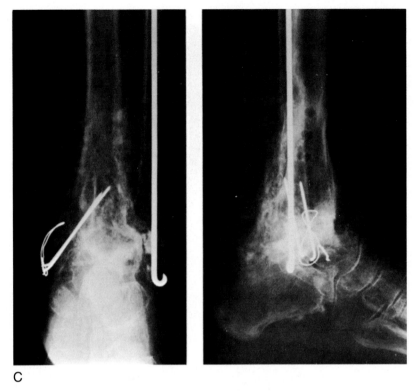

Figure 86–10. *Continued.* **C**, Anteroposterior (*left*) and lateral (*right*) views of postoperative tibia-to-calcaneus arthrodesis following removal of the ankle arthroplasty components.

failed to unite. One patient had neuropathic arthropathy and underwent arthroplasty elsewhere. The salvage procedure used was malleolar resection arthrodesis with external fixation. A second patient with severe talar bone loss and talar component subsidence into the subtalar joint had a modified Campbell fusion with a graft placed between the tibial, talar, and posterior facet of the calcaneus. The tibiotalar level united but the subtalar level did not. A third patient with Parkinson's disease and diabetes mellitus had malleolar resection and fusion with external fixation. The alignment was adjusted twice in the first 2 weeks after surgery. The fourth patient had rheumatoid arthritis with spontaneous ankylosis in most of the hindfoot and midfoot joints; this patient had modified Campbell arthrodesis, which was further revised 9 months after surgery.

Union correlated with patient satisfaction.[16] Clinical results were available in 29 patients (31 ankles). One patient had reoperation for nonunion. Patients were satisfied with the results in 24 ankles, satisfied with reservations in 4, and dissatisfied in 3. Nonunion was the reason for dissatisfaction in two patients. The third patient was dissatisfied because of limitation in footwear and the occurrence of postoperative complications (avulsion fracture of the anterior superior iliac spine). Of the 30 ankles that did not undergo revision arthrodesis, 20 (67 percent) had no pain, 5 (13 percent) had mild pain, 5 (17 percent) had moderate pain, and 1 (3 percent) had severe pain. Patients had no activity restrictions in 17 ankles (57 percent), and seven patients (23 percent) had restricted recreational but not daily activities. Three patients (10 percent) had severely restricted recreational and daily activities. Eight of the 38 ankles underwent reoperation: one patient had revision fusion 9 months after surgery (union), one had multiple débridement and soft tissue coverage operations, one had multiple débridements and partial wound closure, two had exostectomy, one had a soft tissue coverage procedure, one had pin tract exploration, and one had adjustment of the external fixator.

Carlsson et al. reported results of 21 patients who underwent arthrodesis 6 months to 15 years after ankle replacement.[4] Arthrodesis fixation was usually with a Hoffman external fixator. Thirteen of 21 ankles fused with the first attempt (62 percent).

COMPLICATIONS

Nonunion following ankle arthrodesis for failed ankle replacement is a concern (Fig. 86–11). Efforts should be directed toward identifying reasons for failure of the arthrodesis. Patients with upper extremity impairment such as shoulder, elbow, wrist, or hand pathology may have difficulty negotiating the use of crutches or a walker. If this is a significant factor, then revision

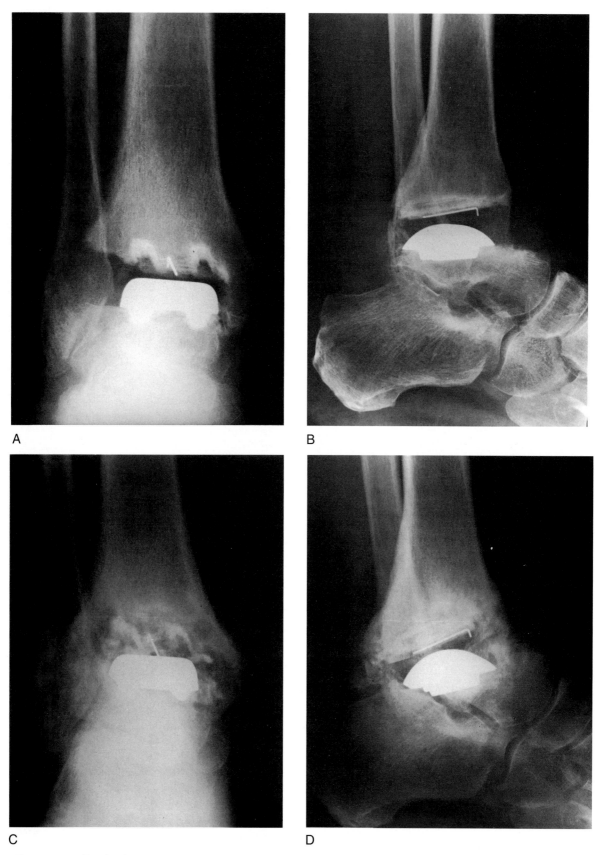

A

B

C

D

Figure 86–11. Two-level arthrodesis with nonunion at subtalar level in a 54-year-old man who had a TAA for degenerative arthritis. Anteroposterior (**A**) and lateral (**B**) views 2 months after TAA. **C**, Anteroposterior view 8 years after arthroplasty. **D**, Lateral view at 8 years postarthroplasty showing subsidence of the talar component into the subtalar joint. (From Kitaoka HB, Romness DW: Arthrodesis for failed ankle arthroplasty. J Arthroplasty 7:277–284, 1992.)

arthrodesis will likely fail. Patient compliance plays a role as well. Those who failed to comply with postoperative management are likely to behave similarly following revision arthrodesis. The relationship between tobacco use and nonunion has been previously reported. Smoking cessation is recommended, advice that is inconsistently followed.

Treatment of the arthrodesis nonunion involves determining whether it is an infected nonunion, and, if so, addressing the infection first.[6] Some patients have a painless nonunion following ankle arthrodesis, but this is rare. Ankle-foot orthosis treatment is recommended. Further operative treatment for nonunion can be challenging (Figs. 86–12 and 86–13). Patients usually are osteopenic, which affects fixation stability. Revision arthrodesis may entail the application of an external fixator, which is less appealing. Bone graft may be required. Patients often have hindfoot pathology, which may require a two-level (i.e., tibiotalocalcaneal arthrodesis) fusion. Patients often are emotionally exhausted and the prospect of further surgery is discouraging.

The published results of revision arthrodesis for nonunion following failed TAA are good. In a report of revision operations for nonunion following TAA, 10 patients underwent revision surgery at an average of 2 years after the prior arthrodesis attempts.[12] The revision procedures utilized included external fixation in seven, internal fixation in one, percutaneous fixation in one, and cast immobilization only in one. Supplemental bone graft was used in seven, union was achieved in 78 percent of the ankles, and the one complication was an infection in a patient with prior sepsis. The overall results were considered excellent in three, good in one, fair in three, and poor in two of the nine patients with adequate follow-up evaluation at an average of 7 years after revision surgery. Despite success of the arthrodesis in terms of union, it was common for patients to have residual symptoms because of other factors such as hindfoot degenerative arthritis and malalignment.[2] These patients, however, preferred the revision procedure to the alternatives, which were accepting the pain and impairment or even amputation surgery.

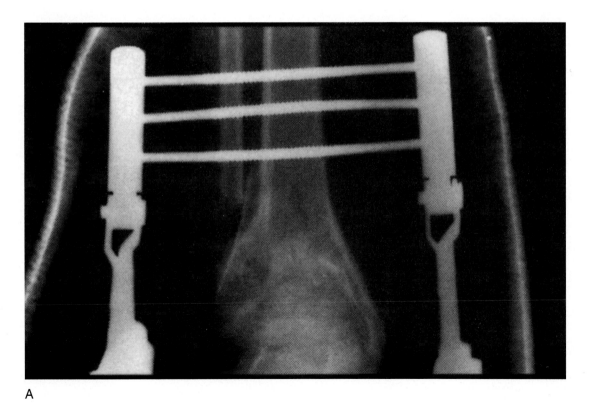

A

Figure 86–12. Revision tibiotalocalcaneal (TTC) arthrodesis with pin fixation, for nonunion after posterior TTC arthrodesis showing good result. A 45-year-old woman sustained multiple trauma, including major lower extremity vascular injury with painful ankle, stiff hindfoot, malalignment, and chronic edema, following two total ankle replacement operations elsewhere.

Illustration continued on following page

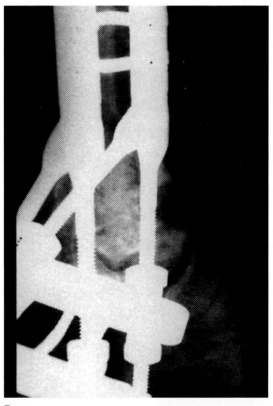

B

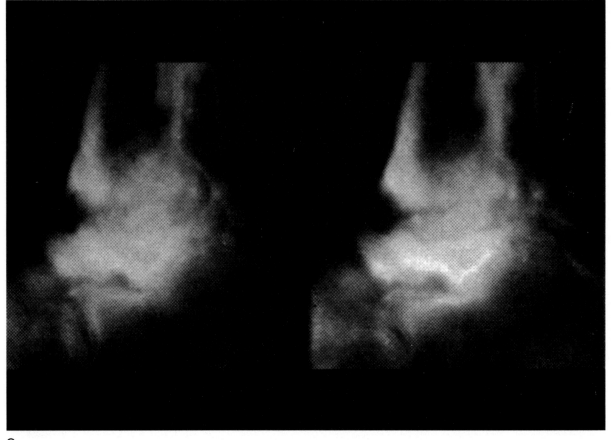

C

Figure 86–12. *Continued.* Anteroposterior (AP) (**A**) and lateral (**B**) radiographs immediately after posterior tibiocalcaneal arthrodesis with external fixation and iliac crest bone graft. **C**, Lateral radiographs 1.4 years later demonstrate nonunion and significant bony deficit. *Illustration continued on opposite page*

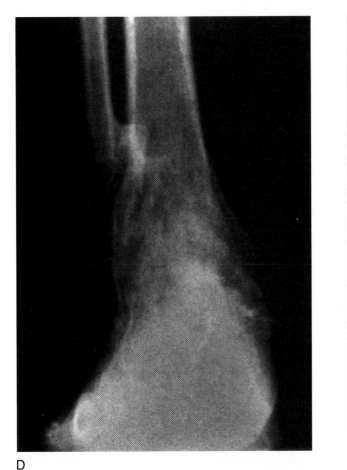

D

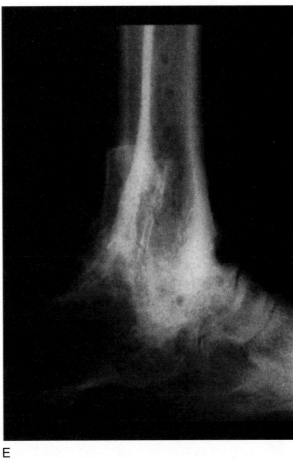

E

Figure 86–12. *Continued.* AP (**D**) and lateral (**E**) radiographs 3.4 years after revision demonstrate arthrodesis union and good alignment. (From Kitaoka HB: Salvage of nonunion following ankle arthrodesis for failed total ankle arthroplasty. Clin Orthop 268:37, 1991.)

Figure 86–13. Revision ankle arthrodesis with external fixation for nonunion after arthrodesis for failed TAA, showing union but hindfoot degenerative arthritis. A 54-year-old woman had salvage of nonunion following ankle arthrodesis for failed total ankle replacement. **A**, Immediate postoperative anteroposterior (AP) radiographs following revision ankle arthrodesis with external fixation without bone graft.

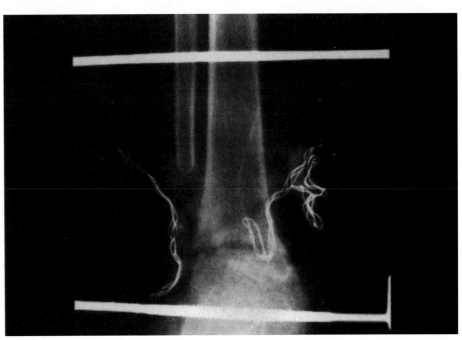

A

Illustration continued on following page

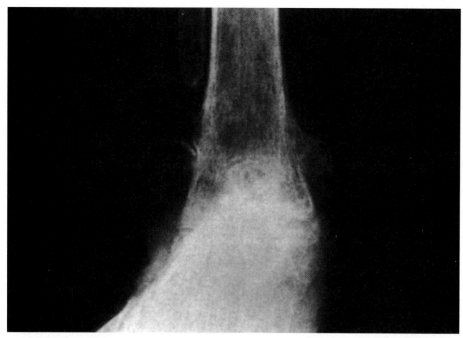

B

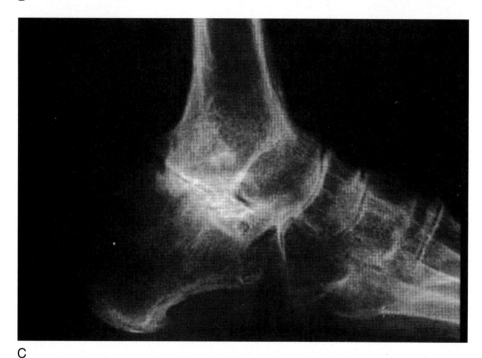

C

Figure 86–13. *Continued*. AP (**B**) and lateral (**C**) radiographs taken 10.6 years later. In spite of successful union and good alignment, the patient had symptoms because of the level of hindfoot degenerative arthritis. (From Kitaoka HB: Salvage of nonunion following ankle arthrodesis for failed total ankle arthroplasty. Clin Orthop 268:37, 1991.)

References

1. Bolton-Maggs BG, Sudlow RA, Freeman MAR: Total ankle arthroplasty: a long-term review of the London Hospital Experience. J Bone Joint Surg Br 67:785, 1985.
2. Buck P, Morrey BF, Chao EYS: The optimum position of arthrodesis of the ankle: a gait analysis study of the knee and ankle. J Bone Joint Surg Am 69:1052, 1987.
3. Campbell CJ, Rinehart WT, Kalenak A: Arthrodesis of the ankle: deep autogenous inlay grafts with maximum cancellous-bone apposition. J Bone Joint Surg Am 56:63, 1974.
4. Carlsson AS, Montgomery F, Besjakov J: Arthrodesis of the ankle secondary to replacement. Foot Ankle Int 19:240–245, 1998.
5. Chuinard EG, Peterson RE: Distraction-compression bone-graft arthrodesis of the ankle: a method especially applicable in children. J Bone Joint Surg Am 45:481, 1963.
6. Cierny G III, Cook WG, Mader JT: Ankle arthrodesis in the presence of ongoing sepsis: indications, methods, and results. Orthop Clin North Am 20:709, 1989.
7. Demottaz JD, Mazur JM, Thomas WH, et al: Clinical study of total ankle replacement with gait analysis. J Bone Joint Surg Am 61:976, 1979.

8. Groth HE: The Oregon ankle: a total ankle designed to replace all three articular surfaces. Orthop Trans 1:86, 1977.

9. Groth HE: Total ankle replacement with the Oregon ankle: evaluation of 44 patients followed two to seven years. Orthop Trans 7:488, 1983.

10. Groth HE, Fitch HF: Salvage procedures for complications of total ankle arthroplasty. Clin Orthop 224:244, 1987.

11. Harris WH, McCarthy JC Jr, O'Neill DA: Femoral component loosening using contemporary techniques of femoral cement fixation. J Bone Joint Surg Am 64:1063–1067, 1982.

12. Kitaoka HB: Salvage of nonunion following ankle arthrodesis for failed total ankle arthroplasty. Clin Orthop 268:37, 1991.

13. Kitaoka HB: Fusion techniques for failed ankle arthroplasty. Semin Arthroscopy 3:51, 1992.

14. Kitaoka HB, Patzer GL: Clinical results of Mayo total ankle arthroplasty. J Bone Joint Surg Am 78:1658–1664, 1996.

15. Kitaoka HB, Patzer GL, Ilstrup DM, Wallrichs SL: Survivorship analysis of the Mayo total ankle arthroplasty. J Bone Joint Surg Am 76:974, 1994.

16. Kitaoka HB, Romness DW: Arthrodesis for failed ankle arthroplasty. J Arthroplasty 7:277–284, 1992.

17. McMaster WC: Total ankle arthroplasty. Adv Orthop Surg 9:264, 1985.

18. Newton SE III: Total ankle arthroplasty: clinical study of fifty cases. J Bone Joint Surg Am 64:104, 1982.

19. Pappas J, Buechel F, DePalma A: Cylindrical total ankle joint replacement. Clin Orthop 118:82, 1976.

20. Russotti GM, Johnson KA, Cass JR: Tibiotalocalcaneal arthrodesis for arthritis and deformity of the hind part of the foot. J Bone Joint Surg Am 70:1304, 1988.

21. Stauffer RN: Total ankle joint replacement. Arch Surg 112:1105, 1977.

22. Stauffer RN: Salvage of painful total ankle arthroplasty. Clin Orthop 170:184, 1982.

23. Stauffer RN, Segal NM: Total ankle arthroplasty: four years experience. Clin Orthop 160:217, 1981.

Index

Note: Page numbers followed by f refer to figures; page numbers followed by t refer to tables.